BROCKLEHURST'S TEXTBOOK OF GERIATRIC MEDICINE AND GERONTOLOGY

BROCKLEHURST'S TEXTBOOK OF GERIATRIC MEDICINE AND GERONTOLOGY

SEVENTH EDITION

Howard M. Fillit MD
Clinical Professor of Geriatrics and Medicine
The Mount Sinai Medical Center
Executive Director
The Alzheimer's Drug Discovery Foundation and the Institute for the Study of Aging
New York, New York

Kenneth Rockwood MD MPA FRCPC FCAHS FRCP
Professor of Medicine
Division of Geriatric Medicine
Dalhousie University
Geriatrician
Queen Elizabeth II Health Sciences Centre
Halifax, Nova Scotia
Canada

Kenneth Woodhouse MD FRCP FHEA
Pro Vice-Chancellor
Professor of Geriatric Medicine
Cardiff University
Cardiff, Wales
United Kingdom

SAUNDERS
ELSEVIER

SAUNDERS
ELSEVIER

1600 John F. Kennedy Blvd.
Ste 1800
Philadelphia, PA 19103-2899

BROCKLEHURST'S TEXTBOOK OF GERIATRIC MEDICINE AND GERONTOLOGY ISBN: 978-1-4160-6231-8

Notice

Knowledge and best practice in this field are constantly changing. As new research and experience broaden our knowledge, changes in practice, treatment and drug therapy may become necessary or appropriate. Readers are advised to check the most current information provided (i) on procedures featured or (ii) by the manufacturer of each product to be administered, to verify the recommended dose or formula, the method and duration of administration, and contraindications. It is the responsibility of the practitioner, relying on his or her own experience and knowledge of the patient, to make diagnoses, to determine dosages and the best treatment for each individual patient, and to take all appropriate safety precautions. To the fullest extent of the law, neither the Publisher nor the Editors assume any liability for any injury and/or damage to persons or property arising out of or related to any use of the material contained in this book.

The Publisher

Library of Congress Cataloging-in-Publication Data

Brocklehurst's textbook of geriatric medicine and gerontology / [edited by] Howard M. Fillit, Kenneth Rockwood, Kenneth Woodhouse. -- 7th ed.
p. ; cm.
Includes bibliographical references and index.
ISBN 978-1-4160-6231-8 1. Geriatrics. 2. Gerontology. I. Fillit, Howard. II. Rockwood, Kenneth. III. Woodhouse, K. W. IV. Brocklehurst, J. C. (John Charles) V. Title: Textbook of geriatric medicine and gerontology. VI. Title: Geriatric medicine and gerontology.
[DNLM: 1. Geriatrics. 2. Aging. WT 100 B8641 2009]
RC952.B75 2009
618.97--dc22
2009008517

Acquisitions Editor: Druanne Martin
Developmental Editor: Anne Snyder
Editorial Assistant: Taylor Ball
Publishing Services Manager: Hemamalini Rajendrababu
Project Manager: Sukanthi Sukumar
Design Direction: Steven Stave
Marketing Manager: Helena Mutak

Printed in the United States of America
Last digit is the print number: 9 8 7 6 5 4 3 2 1

Contributors

MUHANNED ABU-HIJLEH MD FCCP
Assistant Professor of Medicine
Director of Interventional Pulmonology and Clinical Pulmonary Services
Department of Medicine
Rhode Island Hospital – The Alpert Medical School of Brown University
Providence, Rhode Island

ENRIQUE AGUILAR MD
Assistant Professor of Medicine
Department of Medicine
University of Miami, Miller School of Medicine;
Associate Chief of Staff, Geriatrics and Extended Care Service
Assistant Professor
Department of Geriatrics Research, Education, and Clinical Center
Miami Veterans Affairs Healthcare System
Miami, Florida

SONIA ANCOLI-ISRAEL PhD
Professor
Department of Psychiatry
University of California;
Director of Education
Sleep Medicine Center
University of California
San Diego, California

MELISSA K ANDREW MD MSc (PH) FRCPC
Assistant Professor
Department of Geriatric Medicine
Dalhousie University;
Assistant Professor
Internal Medicine and Geriatric Medicine
Capital District Health Authority
Halifax, Nova Scotia, Canada

WILBERT S ARONOW MD FACC FAHA FCCP AGSF
Clinical Professor of Medicine
New York Medical College;
Attending Physician
Divisions of Cardiology, Geriatrics, and Pulmonary/Critical Care and Chief, Cardiology Clinic
Westchester Medical Center/New York Medical College;
Senior Associate Program Director and Research Mentor for Residents and Fellows
Department of Medicine, Westchester Medical Center/ New York Medical College,
Divisions of Cardiology, Geriatrics, and Pulmonary/Critical Care
New York Medical College
Valhalla, New York

LODOVICO BALDUCCI MD
Chief, Senior Adult Oncology Program
H. Lee Moffitt Cancer Center and Research Institute
Tampa, Florida

MARIO BARBAGALLO MD PhD
Professor of Geriatric Medicine
Department of Internal Medicine and Emergent Pathologies
University of Palermo
Palermo, Italy

ANTONY BAYER MB BCh FRCP
Senior Lecturer in Geriatric Medicine
Department of Medicine
Cardiff University;
Director, Cardiff Memory Team
Rehabilitation Directorate
Cardiff and Vale University Local Health Board
Cardiff, Wales, United Kingdom

CERI BEATON BM BS BMedSci MRCS
Department of Surgery
Royal Gwent Hospital
Newport, South Wales, United Kingdom

PAUL E BELCHETZ MA MD MSc FRCP
Senior Clinical Lecturer
Faculty of Medicine
University of Leeds;
Consultant Physician/Endocrinologist
Leeds Nuffield Hospital;
Consultant Physician/Endocrinologist
Spire Leeds Hospital
Leeds, United Kingdom

STEVEN L BERK MD
Dean, School of Medicine
Health Sciences Center
Texas Tech University
Lubbock, Texas

RAVI S BHAT MBBS DPM MD FRANZCP
Associate Professor of Psychiatry
School of Rural Health
The University of Melbourne;
Consultant Old Age Psychiatrist and Director of Psychiatry
Goulburn Valley Area Mental Health Service
Goulburn Valley Health
Shepparton, Victoria, Australia

ARNAB BHOWMICK MBChB FRCS (Gen Surg)
Department of Surgery
Lancashire Teaching Hospitals NHS Trust
Lancashire, United Kingdom

ITALO BIAGGIONI MD
Professor of Medicine and Pharmacology
Vanderbilt University
Nashville, Tennessee

SIMON G BIGGS BSc PhD AFBPsS
Professor of Gerontology
Director, Institute of Gerontology
King's College London
London, United Kingdom

DAVID A. BLACK MA MBA FRCP
Dean and Director
Kent, Surrey and Sussex Postgraduate Medical and Dental Deanery;
Consultant Physician
South London Healthcare Trust
London, United Kingdom

HARRISON G BLOOM MD
Associate Clinical Professor
Brookdale Department of Geriatrics and Palliative Medicine
Mount Sinai School of Medicine;
Senior Associate and Director, Clinical Education and Consultation Service
International Longevity Center
New York, New York

CHARLOTTE E BOLTON MD MRCP
Associate Professor in Respiratory Medicine
Nottingham Respiratory Biomedical Research Unit
University of Nottingham;
Honorary Consultant in Respiratory Medicine
Nottingham City Hospital
Nottingham, United Kingdom

JULIE BLASKEWICZ BORON MS PhD
Assistant Professor
Department of Psychology
Youngstown State University
Youngstown, Ohio

CLIVE BOWMAN FRCP FFPH
Medical Director
BUPA Care Services
Leeds, United Kingdom

SIDNEY S BRAMAN MD FCCP
Professor of Medicine
Director, Division of Pulmonary and Critical Care Medicine
Department of Medicine
Rhode Island Hospital, The Alpert Medical School of Brown University
Providence, Rhode Island

LAWRENCE J BRANDT MD MACG FACP FAAPP
Professor of Medicine and Surgery
Albert Einstein College of Medicine;
Chief of Gastroenterology
Montefiore Medical Center
Bronx, New York

ROBERTA DIAZ BRINTON PhD
Professor
Department of Pharmacology and Pharmaceutical Sciences
School of Pharmacy, Pharmaceutical Sciences Center and Program in Neuroscience
University of Southern California
Los Angeles, California

SCOTT E BRODIE MD PhD
Associate Professor
Department of Ophthalmology
Mount Sinai Medical Center
New York, New York

GINA BROWNE RN PhD
Professor
School of Nursing, Clinical Epidemiology and Biostatistics and Ontario Training Centre in Health Services and Policy Research
McMaster University
Hamilton, Ontario, Canada

PATRICIA BRUCKENTHAL PhD APRN
Clinical Associate Professor
School of Nursing
Stony Brook University
Stony Brook;
Nurse Practitioner
Pain and Headache Treatment Center, Department of Neurology
North Shore University Hospital
Manhasset, New York

ANDREW K BURROUGHS MBChB (Hons) FEBG FRCP
Professor of Hepatology
Centre for Liver Studies
University College London;
Professor and Consultant Physician
The Royal Free Sheila Sherlock Liver Centre
Royal Free Hospital
Hampstead, London, United Kingdom

ROBERT N BUTLER MD
President and CEO
International Longevity Center—USA
New York, New York

RICHARD CAMICIOLI MSc MD FRCP(C)
Professor of Medicine (Neurology)
University of Alberta
Edmonton, Alberta, Canada

IAN A CAMPBELL FRCP
Consultant Physician
Chest Department
Llandough Hospital
Cardiff, Wales, United Kingdom

ROBERT VICTOR CANTU MD
Assistant Professor of Orthopaedic Surgery
Dartmouth-Hitchcock Medical Center
Lebanon, New Hampshire

MARGRED CAPEL
Consultant in Palliative Medicine
George Thomas Hospice Care
Cardiff, Wales, United Kingdom

HARVINDER S CHAHAL BMedSci MBBS MRCP
Specialist Registrar in Endocrinology
Department of Endocrinology
St Bartholomew's Hospital
London, United Kingdom

HERMAN S CHEUNG PhD
James L. Knight Professor
Department of Biomedical Engineering and Medicine
University of Miami;
Senior VA Career Scientist
Geriatric Research, Education, and Clinical Center
Bruce W. Carter VA Medical Center
Miami, Florida

SEAN D CHRISTIE MD FRCSC
Associate Professor
Department of Surgery (Neurosurgery)
Dalhousie University
Queen Elizabeth II Health Sciences Centre
Halifax, Nova Scotia, Canada

DAVID E C COLE BSc FRCPC MD PhD
Senior Scientist
Division of Genomic Medicine
Toronto General Research Institute
Toronto, Ontario, Canada

CLAUDIA COOPER BM MRCPsych MSc PhD
Senior Lecturer
Psychiatry of Older People
Research Department of Mental Health Sciences
University College of London
London, United Kingdom

TARA K COOPER MBBCh MRCOG
Department of Medicine and Veterinary Medicine
University of Edinburgh
Edinburgh;
Department of Obstetrics and Gynaecology
St Johns Hospital
Livingston, United Kingdom

RICHARD A COWIE BSc(Hons) MBChB FRCSE(SN)
Consultant Neurosurgeon
Greater Manchester Neuroscience Centre
Salford Royal Hospital
Salford, United Kingdom

PETER CROME MD PhD DSc FRCP (Lond, Edin and Glasg) FFPM
Professor of Geriatric Medicine
School of Medicine
Keele University
Newcastle-under-Lyme
Staffordshire, United Kingdom

SIMON C M CROXSON MD FRCP
Consultant Physician
Department of the Elderly
Bristol General Hospital
Bristol, United Kingdom

STUTI DANG MD MPH
Assistant Professor of Medicine
Department of Medicine
Geriatrics Institute, University of Miami Miller School of Medicine;
Researcher, Physician, and Director, T-Care and TLC
Geriatric Research, Education, and Clinical Center
Bruce W. Carter VA Medical Center;
Stein Gerontological Institute
Miami Jewish Home Health Systems
Miami, Florida

GWYNETH A DAVIES MRCP MD
Senior Clinical Lecturer
School of Medicine
Swansea University;
Honorary Consultant
Department of Respiratory Medicine
Singleton Hospital, ABMU Health Board
Swansea, Wales, United Kingdom

TIMOTHY J DOHERTY MD PhD FRCP(C)
Associate Professor
Department of Clinical Neurological Sciences
The University of Western Ontario
London, Ontario, Canada

LIGIA J DOMINGUEZ MD
Assistant Professor of Geriatric Medicine
Department of Internal Medicine and Emergent Pathologies
University of Palermo
Palermo, Italy

WILLIAM M DRAKE DM FRCP
Consultant Endocrinologist
Department of Endocrinology
St Bartholomew's Hospital
London, United Kingdom

EAMONN EELES MBBS MRCP MSc
Assistant Professor
Department of Geriatrics and Internal Medicine
Dalhousie University
Halifax, Nova Scotia, Canada;
Consultant Physician
Department of Geriatrics and General Medicine
Llandough Hospital
Cardiff, Wales, United Kingdom

WILLIAM B ERSHLER MD
Senior Investigator
Clinical Research Branch
National Institute on Aging
National Institutes of Health
Baltimore, Maryland

WILLIAM J EVANS PhD
Adjunct Professor
Department of Medicine, Division of Geriatrics
Duke University
Durham;
Vice President and Head
Muscle Metabolism Discovery Performance Unit
GlaxoSmithKline
Research Triangle Park, North Carolina

MARTIN R FARLOW MD
Professor and Vice Chair of Neurology
Indiana University School of Medicine;
Neurologist
University Clinical Neurologists
Indianapolis, Indiana

RICHARD C FELDSTEIN MD MSc
Department of Gastroenterology
New York University School of Medicine;
Attending Faculty
Department of Gastroenterology
Woodhull Medical and Mental Health Center
Brooklyn, New York

HOWARD M FILLIT MD
Clinical Professor of Geriatrics and Medicine
The Mount Sinai Medical Center
Executive Director
The Alzheimer's Drug Discovery Foundation and the Institute for the Study of Aging
New York, New York

ANDREW Y FINLAY MBBS FRCP (Lond and Glas)
Professor of Dermatology
Department of Dermatology
Cardiff University School of Medicine
Cardiff, Wales, United Kingdom

ILORA FINLAY MBBS FRCP FRCGP
Professor of Palliative Medicine
Cardiff University;
Consultant in Palliative Medicine
Velindre Hospital
Cardiff, Wales, United Kingdom

ROGER M FRANCIS MB ChB FRCP
Professor of Geriatric Medicine
University of Newcastle upon Tyne;
Consultant Physician Bone Clinic
Musculoskeletal Unit
Freeman Hospital
Newcastle upon Tyne, United Kingdom

ANTHONY J FREEMONT MD FRCP FRCPath
Professor of Osteoarticular Pathology
School of Clinical and Laboratory Sciences
University of Manchester;
Honorary Consultant in Osteoarticular Pathology
Department of Histopathology
Central Manchester NHS Foundation Trust
Great Manchester, United Kingdom

JAMES E GALVIN MD MPH
Associate Professor
Department of Neurology
Washington University School of Medicine
St Louis, Missouri

NICHOLAS J R GEORGE MD FRCS FEBU
Senior Lecturer and Consultant in Urology
Department of Urology
University Hospital South Manchester
Manchester, United Kingdom

NEIL D GILLESPIE BSc(Hons) MBChB MD
Senior Lecturer in Medicine (Ageing and Health)
Ninewells Hospital and Medical School
University of Dundee
Dundee, United Kingdom

ROBERT GLICKMAN DMD
Professor and Chair
Department of Oral and Maxillofacial Surgery
New York University College of Dentistry;
Director
NYU Medical Center/Bellevue Hospital Center
New York, New York

ADAM G GOLDEN MD MBA
Assistant Professor of Medicine
Department of Medicine
Geriatrics Institute, University of Miami Miller School of Medicine;
Researcher and Physician
Geriatric Research, Education, and Clinical Center
Bruce W. Carter VA Medical Center
Miami, Florida

LESLIE B GORDON MD PhD
Associate Professor of Pediatrics Research
Department of Pediatrics
Warren Alpert Medical School of Brown University
Hasbro Children's Hospital
Providence, Rhode Island;
Medical Director
The Progeria Research Foundation Peabody, Massachusetts

MICHELLE GORENSTEIN PsychD
Psychology Intern
Department of Psychiatry
The Mount Sinai Medical Center
New York, New York

MARGOT A GOSNEY MD FRCP
Director
Department of Clinical Health Sciences
University of Reading;
Professor of Elderly Care Medicine
Department of Elderly Care
Royal Berkshire NHS Foundation Trust
Reading, United Kingdom

JOHN TREVOR GREEN MB Bch MD FRCP
Clinical Senior Lecturer
Department of Medical Education
Cardiff University;
Consultant Physician
Department of Gastroenterology
University Hospital Llandough
Cardiff, Wales, United Kingdom

DAVID A GREENWALD MD FACG FASGE AGA-F
Associate Professor of Clinical Medicine
Albert Einstein College of Medicine;
Gastroenterology Fellowship Director
Montefiore Medical Center
Bronx, New York

CELIA L GREGSON BMedSci(Hons) MRCP(UK) MSc
Wellcome Clinical Research Fellow
Academic Rheumatology
University of Bristol
Bristol, United Kingdom

MICHAEL L GRUBER MD
Clinical Professor of Neurology and Neurosurgery
New York University School of Medicine;
Attending
Department of Neurology and Neurosurgery
NYU Langone Medical Center
New York, New York;
Director, Brain Tumor Center of New Jersey
Department of Neurology
Overlook Hospital
Summit, New Jersey

DAVID R P GUAY PharmD
Professor
College of Pharmacy
University of Minnesota
Department of Geriatrics
HealthPartners Inc.
Minneapolis, Minnesota

RENATO MAIA GUIMARÃES MD MSc
Director
Geriatric Medical Center
Hospital Universitario de Brasilia
Brasilia, Brazil

KHALID HAMANDI MB BS BSC MRCP PhD
Consultant Neurologist
Welsh Epilepsy Unit
Department of Neurology
University Hospital of Wales and University Hospital Llandough
Cardiff, Wales, United Kingdom

PETER HAMMOND BM BCh MA MD FRCP
Consultant Physician
Department of Diabetes and Endocrinology
Harrogate District Hospital
Harrogate – North Yorkshire, United Kingdom

STEVEN M HANDLER MD MS
Division of Geriatric Medicine
Department of Medicine
Department of Biomedical Informatics
School of Medicine
University of Pittsburgh
Geriatric Research Education and Clinical Center
Veterans Affairs Pittsburgh Healthcare System
Pittsburgh, Pennsylvania

JOSEPH T HANLON PharmD MS
Division of Geriatric Medicine, Department of Medicine, School of Medicine, and Department of Pharmacy and Therapeutics, School of Pharmacy, University of Pittsburgh
Geriatric Research Education and Clinical Center and Center for Health Equity Research and Promotion
Veterans Affairs Pittsburgh Healthcare System
Pittsburgh, Pennsylvania

MALENE HANSEN PhD
Assistant Professor
Center for Neuroscience, Aging, and Stem Cell Research
Burnham Institute for Medical Research
La Jolla, California

DANIELLE HARARI MB BS FRCP
Honorary Senior Lecturer
Division of Health and Social Care Research
Kings College London;
Consultant Physician in Geriatric Medicine
Department of Ageing and Health
Guy's and St Thomas' NHS Foundation Trust
London, United Kingdom

MUJTABA HASAN MD MSc FRCP
Senior Lecturer
Department of Geriatric Medicine
Cardiff University
Cardiff;
Consultant Physician
Department of Geriatric Medicine
Aneurin Bevan Health Board
Caerphilly, Wales, United Kingdom

GEORGE A HECKMAN MD MSc FRCPC
Department of Medicine, Divisions of Geriatric Medicine and Cardiology
McMaster University
Hamilton Health Science, General Division
Hamilton, Ontario, Canada

PAUL HIGGS BSc PhD
Professor of the Sociology of Ageing
Division of Research Strategy
University College London
London, United Kingdom

DAVID B HOGAN MD FACP FRCPC
Professor and Brenda Strafford Foundation Chair in Geriatric Medicine
Department of Medicine
University of Calgary;
Medical Director, Cognitive Assessment Clinic
Department of Clinical Neurosciences and Medicine
Alberta Health Services – Calgary;
Medical Director, Calgary Falls Prevention Clinic
Department of Medicine
Alberta Health Services – Calgary
Calgary, Alberta, Canada

SØREN HOLM BA MA MD
Professor of Bioethics
School of Law
The University of Manchester
Manchester, United Kingtom;
Professor of Medical Ethics
Section for Medical Ethics
University of Oslo
Oslo, Norway

BEN HOPE-GILL MD FRCP
Consultant Respiratory Physician
Department of Respiratory Medicine
Cardiff and Vale NHS Trust
Cardiff, Wales, United Kingdom

SUSAN E HOWLETT BSc (Hons) MSc PhD
Professor of Pharmacology and Medicine
Division of Geriatric Medicine
Dalhousie University
Halifax, Nova Scotia, Canada

RUTH E HUBBARD MSc MD MRCP
Consultant Geriatrician
Department of Geriatric Medicine
Cardiff and Vale NHS Trust
Cardiff, Wales, United Kingdom

JOANNA HURLEY MB BCh MRCP (UK)
Specialist Registrar in Gastroenterology
Department of Gastroenterology
University Hospital Llandough
Penarth, Wales, United Kingdom

C SHANTHI JOHNSON PhD RD FACSM FDC
Professor and Associate Dean (Research and Graduate Studies)
Faculty of Kinesiology and Health Studies
University of Regina
Regina, Saskatchewan, Canada

LARRY E JOHNSON MD PhD
Associate Professor
Department of Geriatrics and Family and Preventive Medicine
University of Arkansas for Medical Sciences;
Medical Director
Community Living Center Central Arkansas veterans Healthcare System
Little Rock, Arkansas

BINDU KANAPURU MD
Clinical Research Fellow
Clinical Research Branch
National Institute on Aging, National Institutes of Health
Baltimore, Maryland

ROSALIE A KANE PhD
Professor of Public Health
Health Policy and Management
School of Public Health
University of Minnesota
Minneapolis, Minnesota

CORNELIUS KATONA MD FRCPsych
Professor
University of Kent
Wingham Barton Manor
Westmarsh, Canterbury, Kent, United Kingdom

SEYMOUR KATZ MD FACP MACG
Clinical Professor of Medicine
Department of Medicine
Albert Einstein College of Medicine
Bronx;
Attending Physician
Department of Medicine
North Shore University Hospital/Long Island Jewish Health System
Manhasset;
Attending Physician
Department of Medicine
St. Francis Hospital
Roslyn, New York

HORACIO KAUFMANN MD FAAN
Professor of Neurology and Medicine
Department of Neurology
New York University School of Medicine
New York, New York

NICHOLAS A KEFALIDES MD PhD
Professor of Medicine-Emeritus
Department of Medicine
University of Pennsylvania
Philadelphia, Pennsylvania

HEATHER H KELLER RD PhD FDC
Professor
Department of Family Relations and Applied Nutrition
University of Guelph
Guelph, Ontario, Canada

ROSE ANNE KENNY MD FRCPI FRCP
Chair of Geriatric Medicine
Department of Medical Gerontology
Trinity College Dublin;
Consultant Physician in Geriatric Medicine
Department of Medicine for the Elderly
St. James's Hospital
Dublin, Ireland

THOMAS B L KIRKWOOD MA MSc PhD
Director, Institute for Ageing and Health
Newcastle University
Newcastle upon Tyne, United Kingdom

BRANDON KORETZ MD
Assistant Clinical Professor
UCLA Medical Center
UCLA Santa Monica Orthopedic Hospital
Department of Medicine
University of California, Los Angeles
Los Angeles, California

MARK A KOSINSKI DPM
Professor
Department of Medical Sciences
New York College of Podiatric Medicine
New York, New York

KENNETH J KOVAL MD
Professor of Orthopaedic Surgery
Dartmouth-Hitchcock Medical Center
Lebanon, New Hampshire

GEORGE A KUCHEL MD FRCP
Professor of Medicine Citicorp Chair in Geriatrics and Gerontology
University of Connecticut Center on Aging
University of Connecticut Health Center
Farmington, Connecticut

CHAO-QIANG LAI PhD
Research Molecular Biologist
Department of Nutrition and Genomics Laboratory
Jean Mayer USDA Human Nutrition Research Center on Aging at Tufts University
Boston, Massachusetts

W CLARK LAMBERT MD PhD
Professor and Associate Head, Dermatology
Professor of Pathology
Chief, Dermatopathology
Department of Dermatology
New Jersey Medical School
Newark, New Jersey

ALEXANDER LAPIN MD Dr Phil (Chem) Dr Theol
Associate Professor
Clinical Institute of Medical and Chemical Diagnostics;
Head of the Laboratory Department
Laboratory Medicine
Sozialmedizinisches Zentrum Sophienspital
Vienna, Austria

MYRNA I LEWIS PhD†
Assistant Professor
Mount Sinai School of Medicine
New York, New York

STUART A LIPTON MD PhD
Professor (Adjunct)
Department of Neurology
University of California, San Diego;
Neurologist
Department of Neurology
UCSD Medical Center
La Jolla, California

GILL LIVINGSTON MBChB FRCPsych MD
Professor
Department of Mental Health Sciences
University College of London;
Consultant Psychiatrist
Mental Health Care of Older People
Camden and Islington Foundation Trust
London, United Kingdom

JORGE H LOPEZ MD
Professor of Internal Medicine and Geriatrics
Department of Internal Medicine
Universidad Nacional de Colombia;
President
Asociacion Colombiana de Gerontologia Y Geriatria
Bogota, Colombia

MARY V MACNEIL MD FRCPC
Assistant Professor
Department of Medicine
Dalhousie University;
Medical Oncologist
Department of Medicine
Division of Medical Oncology
Queen Elizabeth II Health Sciences Centre and Nova Scotia Cancer Centre
Halifax, Nova Scotia, Canada

†Deceased

ROBERT L MAHER PharmD BCPS CGP
Assistant Professor of Pharmacy Practice
Mylan School of Pharmacy
Duquesne University
Pittsburgh, Pennsylvania

JILL MANTHORPE MA
Professor of Social Work
Director, Social Care Workforce Research Unit
King's College London
London, United Kingdom

KENNETH G MANTON PhD
Research Professor
Office of Dean of Arts and Sciences
Duke University
Durham, North Carolina

BRYAN MARKINSON DPM
Assistant Professor of Orthopaedics and Pathology
Center for Advanced Medicine
Mount Sinai School of Medicine
New York, New York

MAUREEN F MARKLE-REID RN MScN PhD
Associate Professor
School of Nursing
McMaster University;
Career Scientist
Ontario Ministry of Health and Long-Term Care
Hamilton, Ontario, Canada

JANE MARTIN PhD
Assistant Clinical Professor
Co-Director
Neuropsychological Testing and Evaluation Center
Department of Psychiatry
Mount Sinai Medical Center
New York, New York

EDWARD J MASORO PhD
Emeritus Professor
University of Texas Health Science Center
San Antonio, Texas

CHARLES N McCOLLUM MB ChB FRCS MD
Professor of Surgery
University Hospital of South Manchester
Manchester, United Kingdom

MICHAEL A McDEVITT MD PhD
Assistant Professor
Department of Medicine and Oncology
Johns Hopkins School of Medicine and Sidney Kimmel Comprehensive Cancer Center at Johns Hopkins
Baltimore, Maryland

BRUCE S McEWEN PhD
Professor and Head
Laboratory of Neuroendocrinology
The Rockefeller University
New York, New York

JOLYON MEARA MD FRCP
Senior Lecturer in Geriatric Medicine
University of Wales
College of Medicine
Rhyl, North Wales, United Kingdom

MYRON MILLER MD
Professor
Department of Medicine
Johns Hopkins University School of Medicine;
Director
Division of Geriatric Medicine
Department of Medicine
Sinai Hospital of Baltimore
Baltimore, Maryland

ARNOLD MITNITSKI PhD
Associate Professor
Department of Medicine
Dalhousie University
Halifax, Nova Scotia, Canada

PAIGE A MOORHOUSE MD MPH FRCPC
Assistant Professor
Department of Medicine
Division of Geriatric Medicine
Dalhousie University;
Clinical Researcher
Division of Geriatric Medicine
Capital District Health Authority
Halifax, Nova Scotia, Canada

JOHN E MORLEY MB BCh
Professor of Gerontology
Director
Division of Geriatric Medicine;
Director
Geriatric Research, Education and Clinical Center
St Louis, Missouri

LATANA A MUNANG MBChB MRCP (UK)
Specialist Registrar in Geriatric Medicine and General Internal Medicine
Department of Geriatric Medicine
Western General Hospital
Edinburgh, United Kingdom

JAMES W MYERS MD
Professor, Infectious Diseases
Department of Internal Medicine
Quillen College of Medicine
East Tennessee State University
Johnson City, Tennessee

TOMOHIRO NAKAMURA PhD
Research Assistant Professor
Center for Neuroscience, Aging, and Stem Cell Research
Burnham Institute for Medical Research
La Jolla, California

JAMES NAZROO MBBS BSc MSc PhD
Professor of Sociology
Department of Sociology
School of Social Sciences
University of Manchester
Manchester, United Kingdom

MICHAEL W NICOLLE MD FRCPC DPhil
Associate Professor
Department of Clinical Neurological Sciences
University of Western Ontario
London, Ontario, Canada

SEAN M OLDHAM PhD
Assistant Professor
Cancer Center and Center for Neuroscience, Aging and Stem Cell Research
Burnham Institute for Medical Research
La Jolla, California

JOSE M ORDOVAS PhD
Professor
Friedman School of Nutrition Science and Policy
Tufts University;
Director
Nutrition and Genomics Laboratory
Jean Mayer USDA Human Nutrition Research Center on Aging at Tufts University
Boston, Massachusetts

JOSEPH G OUSLANDER MD
Professor of Clinical Biomedical Science
Associate Dean for Geriatric Programs
Charles E. Schmidt College of Biomedical Science;
Professor (Courtesy)
Christine E. Lynn College of Nursing
Florida Atlantic University
Boca Raton;
Professor of Medicine (Voluntary)
Associate Director
Division of Gerontology and Geriatric Medicine
University of Miami Miller School of Medicine
Miami, Florida

JAMES T PACALA MD MS
Associate Professor and Distinguished Teaching Professor
Family Medicine and Community Health
University of Minnesota Medical School
Minneapolis, Minnesota

LAURENCE D PARNELL PhD
Computational Biologist
Nutrition and Genomics Laboratory
Jean Mayer USDA Human Nutrition Research Center on Aging at Tufts University
Boston, Massachusetts

GOPAL A PATEL MD
Department of Dermatology
New Jersey Medical School
Newark, New Jersey;
Department of Medicine
Memorial Sloan Kettering Cancer Center
New York, New York

THOMAS T PERLS MD MPH FACP
Associate Professor of Medicine;
Director
The New England Centenarian Study
Boston University School of Medicine
Boston University Medical Center
Boston, Massachusetts

THANH G PHAN MBBS
Assistant Professor
Department of Medicine
Monash University;
Assistant Professor
Department of Neurosciences
Monash Medical Centre
Clayton, Australia

KATIE PINK MBBCH (Hons) MRCP
Specialist Registrar
Department of Respiratory Medicine
Llandough Hospital
Cardiff, Wales, United Kingdom

VALERIE M POMEROY PhD FCSP BA Grad Dip Phys
Professor of Rehabilitation for Older People
Section of Geriatric Medicine
Division of Clinical Developmental Sciences
St George's University of London
London, United Kingdom

JOHN F POTTER BM BS DM FRCP
Professor of Ageing and Stroke Medicine
School of Medicine
University of East Anglia
Norwich, United Kingdom

MALCOLM C A PUNTIS MB Bach PhD FRCS
Senior Lecturer
Department of Surgery
Cardiff University;
Consultant Surgeon
University Hospital of Wales
Cardiff, Wales, United Kingdom

GANGARAM RAGI MD
Director
Advanced Laser and Skin Cancer Center
Teaneck, New Jersey

HOLLY J RAMSAWH PhD
Assistant Project Scientist
Department of Psychiatry
University of California San Diego
San Diego, California

M SHAWKAT RAZZAQUE MD PhD
Department of Oral Medicine, Infection and Immunity
Harvard School of Dental Medicine
Boston, Massachusetts;
Department of Pathology
Nagasaki University School of Medicine
Nagasaki, Japan

DAVID B REUBEN MD
Professor of Medicine
Department of Medicine
UCLA Medical Center
UCLA Santa Monica
Orthopedic Hospital
University of California, Los Angeles
Los Angeles, California

KENNETH ROCKWOOD MD MPA FRCPC FCAHS FRCP
Professor of Medicine
Division of Geriatric Medicine
Dalhousie University;
Geriatrician
Queen Elizabeth II Health Sciences Centre
Halifax, Nova Scotia, Canada

CHRISTOPHER A RODRIGUES PhD FRCP
Consultant Gastroenterologist
Department of Gastroenterology
Kingston Hospital
Kingston-upon-Thames, Surrey, United Kingdom

YVES ROLLAND
Service de Médecine Interne et de Gérontologie Clinique
Hôpital La Grave-Casselardit
Toulouse, France

BERNARD A ROOS MD
Professor and Director
Geriatrics Institute
Department of Medicine, Neurology, and Exercise and Sport Sciences
University of Miami Miller School of Medicine;
Director
Geriatric Research, Education, and Clinical Center
Bruce W. Carter VA Medical Center;
Director
Stein Gerontological Institute
Miami Jewish Home Health Systems
Miami, Florida

SONJA ROSEN MD
Assistant Clinical Professor
UCLA Medical Center
UCLA Santa Monica Orthopedic Hospital
Division of Geriatric Medicine
Department of Medicine
David Geffen School of Medicine at University of California Los Angeles
Los Angeles, California

DAVID H ROSENBAUM MD
Associate Clinical Professor of Neurology
Mount Sinai Medical Center
New York, New York

PHILIP A ROUTLEDGE OBE MD FRCP FRCPE FBTS
Professor of Clinical Pharmacology
Section of Pharmacology, Therapeutics and Toxicology
Cardiff University;
Department of Clinical Pharmacology
University Hospital Llandough
Cardiff and Vale University Health Board
Cardiff, Wales, United Kingdom

LAURENCE Z RUBENSTEIN MD MPH
Professor of Geriatric Medicine
University of California Los Angeles School of Medicine
Los Angeles;
Geriatric Research Education and Clinical Center
Greater Los Angeles VA Medical Center
Sepulveda, California

LISA V RUBENSTEIN MD MSPH
Professor of Medicine and Public Health
University of California Los Angeles School of Medicine
Los Angeles;
Department of Medicine
Greater Los Angeles VA Medical Center
Sepulveda, California

GORDON SACKS PharmD
Clinical Associate Professor
School of Pharmacy
University of Wisconsin
Madison, Wisconsin

GERRY J F SALDANHA MA (Oxon) FRCP
Consultant Neurologist
Department of Neurology
Maidstone and Tunbridge Wells NHS Trust
Tunbridge Wells, Kent;
Consultant Neurologist
Department of Neurology
King's College Hospital NHS Foundation Trust
London, United Kingdom

LUIS F SAMOS MD
Assistant Professor of Medicine
Department of Medicine
University of Miami Miller School of Medicine;
Medical Director
Nursing Home Care Unit
Geriatrics and Extended Care Service
Miami Veterans Affairs Healthcare System
Miami, Florida

MARY SANO PhD
Professor of Psychiatry
Director of the Alzheimer's Disease Research
Mount Sinai School of Medicine
Director of Research and Development
Bronx Veterans Administration Hospital
Bronx, New York

ROBERT SANTER BSc PhD DSc
School of Biosciences
Cardiff University
Cardiff, Wales, United Kingdom

K WARNER SCHAIE PhD ScD(Hon) DrPhil (Hon)
Affiliate Professor
Department of Psychiatry and Behavioral Sciences
University of Washington
Seattle, Washington

KENNETH E SCHMADER MD
Department of Medicine (Division of Geriatrics), and Center for the Study of Aging and Human Development
Duke University Medical Center
Geriatric Research, Education and Clinical Center
Veterans Affairs Medical Center
Durham, North Carolina

ANDREA SCHREIBER DMD
Clinical Professor
Department of Oral and Maxillofacial Surgery
New York University College of Dentistry;
Associate Attending
Department of Oral and Maxillofacial Surgery
Bellevue Hospital Center;
Director
New York University Medical Center/Bellevue Hospital Center
New York, New York

ROBERT A SCHWARTZ MD MPH
Professor and Head
Department of Dermatology
Professor of Medicine
Professor of Preventive Medicine and Community Health
Professor of Pathology
New Jersey Medical School
Newark, New Jersey

DAVID L SCOTT BSc MD FRCP
Professor of Clinical Rheumatology
Kings College London;
Honorary Consultant Rheumatologist
Kings College Hospital
London, United Kingdom

MARGARET C SEWELL PhD
Assistant Clinical Professor of Psychiatry
Mount Sinai School of Medicine
Director, Education Core
Alzheimer's Disease Research Center
New York, New York

D GWYN SEYMOUR BSc MD FRCP
Emeritus Professor of Medicine (Care of the Elderly)
University of Aberdeen
Aberdeen, United Kingdom

KRUPA SHAH MD MPH
Instructor in Medicine
Division of Geriatrics and Ageing
University of Rochester, School of Medicine
Rochester, New York

HAMSARAJ G M SHETTY BSc MBBS FRCP (London)
Honorary Senior Lecturer
Department of Integrated Medicine
Cardiff University Medical School;
Consultant Physician
Department of Integrated Medicine
University Hospital of Wales
Cardiff, Wales, United Kingdom

FELIPE SIERRA PhD
Director
Division of Aging Biology
National Institute on Aging
Bethesda, Maryland

ALAN J SINCLAIR MSc MD FRCP
Director
Institute of Diabetes for Older People
University of Bedfordshire
Luton, Bedfordshire, United Kingdom

KRISTEL SLEEGERS MD PhD
Assistant Professor
Department of Molecular Genetics
VIB and University of Antwerp;
Laboratory of Neurogenetics
Institute Born-Bunge
Antwerp, Belgium

OLIVER MILLING SMITH MBChB BSc MD MRCOG
Department of Medicine and Veterinary Medicine
University of Edinburgh;
Department of Obstetrics and Gynaecology
Royal Infirmary Edinburgh
Scotland, United Kingdom

PHILLIP P SMITH MD
Department of Surgery
University of Connecticut Health Center
Farmington, Connecticut

VELANDAI K SRIKANTH
Assistant Professor
Department of Medicine
Southern Clinical School
Monash University;
Assistant Professor
Department of Neurosciences
Monash Medical Centre
Clayton, Australia;
Honorary Member
Department of Epidemiology
Menzies Research Institute
Hobart, Australia

JOHN M STARR FRCPEd
Professor of Health and Ageing
Geriatric Medicine Unit
University of Edinburgh
Scotland, United Kingdom

RICHARD G STEFANACCI DO MGH MBA AGSF CMD
Director
Institute for Geriatric Studies
Director
Center for Medicare Medication Management
University of the Sciences in Philadelphia;
Medical Director
Department of LIFE
NewCourtland Elder Services
Philadelphia, Pennsylvania

PAUL STOLEE PhD
Associate Professor
Department of Health Studies and Gerontology
University of Waterloo
Waterloo, Ontario, Canada

MICHAEL STONE BA MBBS DM FRCP
Professor
Bone Research Unit
Department of Geriatrics
Cardiff University
Cardiff, Wales;
Geriatric Medicine
University Hospital of Llandough
Penarth, Wales, United Kingdom

BRYAN D STRUCK MD
Associate Professor
DW Reynolds Department of Geriatric Medicine
University of Oklahoma Health Sciences Center–College of Medicine;
Medical Director
Palliative Care Unit
Department of Geriatrics and Extended Care
Oklahoma City Veterans Administration Medical Center
Oklahoma City, Oklahoma

ALLAN D STRUTHERS BSc MD FRCP FESC
Professor of Cardiovascular Medicine
Division of Medical Sciences
University of Dundee;
Consultant Physician
Department of Medicine
Ninewells Hospital
Dundee, United Kingdom

STEPHANIE A STUDENSKI MD MPH
Professor
Department of Internal Medicine
University of Pittsburgh;
Staff Physician
Geriatric Research Education and Clinical Center
Pittsburgh Veterans Affairs Health System
Pittsburgh, Pennsylvania

DENNIS H SULLIVAN MD
Professor of Geriatrics and Internal Medicine
Executive Vice Chairman
Donald W. Reynolds Department of Geriatrics
University of Arkansas for Medical Sciences;
Director
Geriatric Research Education and Clinical Center
Central Arkansas Veterans Healthcare System
Little Rock, Arkansas

RAWAN TARAWNEH MD
Fellow
Department of Neurology
Washington University School of Medicine
Alzheimer's Disease Research Center
St Louis, Missouri

DENNIS D TAUB PhD
Senior Investigator
Clinical Immunology Section
Laboratory of Immunology
Gerontology Research Center
National Institute on Aging/National Institute of Health
Baltimore, Maryland

ROBERT E TEPPER MD FACP FACG
Associate Attending Physician
Department of Medicine
North Shore University Hospital
Manhasset;
Attending Physician
Department of Medicine
St Francis Hospital
Roslyn, New York

LaDORA V THOMPSON PhD BS PT
Professor
Program in Physical Therapy
University of Minnesota
Minneapolis, Minnesota

AMANDA G THRIFT BSc (Hons) PhD PGDipBiostat
Adjunct Associate Professor
Department of Epidemiology and Preventive Medicine
Monash University;
Head of Unit
Department of Stroke Epidemiology
Baker IDI Heart and Diabetes Institute
Melbourne, Victoria, Australia

ANTHEA TINKER CBE PhD FKC AcSS
Professor of Social Gerontology
Institute of Gerontology
King's College London
London, United Kingdom

MOHAN K TUMMALA MD MRCP
Department of Hematology and Oncology
Marshfield Clinic
Minocqua, Wisconsin

JANE TURTON MD
Medicine and Geriatric Medicine
Cardiff University
Cardiff, Wales, United Kingdom

CHRISTINE VAN BROECKHOVEN PhD DSc
Professor and Department Director
Department of Molecular Genetics
VIB and University of Antwerp;
Research Director
Laboratory of Neurogenetics
Institute Born-Bunge
Antwerp, Belgium

BRUNO VELLAS MD PhD
Centre de Gériatrie
Toulouse, France

NORMAN VETTER FFPH MD
Department of Primary Care and Public Health
Cardiff University;
National Public Health Service
Temple of Peace
Cardiff, Wales, United Kingdom

EMMA C VEYSEY MBChB MRCP
Dermatology Department
Singleton Hospital
Swansea, United Kingdom

ANDREW VIGARIO BA
Research Coordinator
Alzheimer's Disease Research Center
Mount Sinai Medical Center
New York, New York

DENNIS T VILLAREAL MD
Professor of Medicine
Department of Medicine
University of New Mexico School of Medicine;
Chief, Geriatrics Section
Department of Medicine
New Mexico VA Health Care System
Albuquerque, New Mexico

OLEG VOLKOV PhD
Senior Research Associate
International Longevity Center
New York, New York

ADRIAN WAGG MB FRCP FHEA
Consultant and Senior Lecturer in Geriatric Medicine
Department of Geriatric Medicine
University College London;
Consultant and Senior Lecturer in Geriatric Medicine
Department of Geriatric Medicine
University College London and St Pancras Hospitals
London, United Kingdom

ARNOLD WALD MD
Professor of Medicine
Section of Gastroenterology and Hepatology
University of Wisconsin School of Medicine and Public Health
Madison, Wisconsin

MARION F WALKER PhD MPhil Dip COT
Professor in Stroke Rehabilitation
School of Community Health Sciences
Institute of Neuroscience
The University of Nottingham
Nottingham, United Kingdom

KATHERINE WARD DPM DABPS
Palisades Podiatry Associates
Pomona, New York

HUBER R WARNER PhD
Associate Dean for Research
College of Biological Sciences
University of Minnesota
Minneapolis, Minnesota

BARBARA E WEINSTEIN PhD
Professor and Executive Officer
Health Sciences Doctoral Programs–Audiology, Nursing Sciences, Physical Therapy, Public Health
Graduate Center
The City University of New York
New York, New York

SHERRY L WILLIS PhD
Research Professor
Department of Psychiatry and Behavioral Sciences
University of Washington
Seattle, Washington

MILES D WITHAM BM BCh PhD
Clinical Lecturer in Ageing and Health
University of Dundee
Dundee, United Kingdom

JEAN WOO MD
Professor
Department of Medicine and Therapeutics
The Chinese University of Hong Kong
Hong Kong, China

KENNETH WOODHOUSE MD FRCP FHEA
Vice-Chancellor
Professor of Geriatric Medicine
Cardiff University
Cardiff, Wales, United Kingdom

ELIAS XIROUCHAKIS MD
Research Fellow
The Sheila Sherlock Hepatobiliary Pancreatic and Liver Transplantation Unit
Royal Free and UCL Medical School
London, United Kingdom;
Consultant Gastroenterologist and Hepatologist
Department of Gastroenterology and Hepatology
Athens Medical, P. Falirou Hospital
Athens, Greece

JOHN YOUNG MB(Hons) MSc MBA FRCP
Professor of Elderly Care Medicine
Leeds Institute of Health Sciences
Leeds University
Consultant Geriatrician
Bradford Teaching Hospitals NHS Trust
Leeds, United Kingdom

ZAHRA ZIAIE BS
Laboratory Manager
Science Center Port at University City Science Center
Philadelphia, Pennsylvania

Acknowledgments

Dr. Fillit wishes to thank his wife Janet and children, Marielle and Michael, for their support, patience, and encouragement. He also expresses his appreciation to Leonard Lauder and Ronald Lauder, founders and chairmen of the Institute for the Study of Aging, for their vision and dedication to aging research. He also thanks Filomena Machleder, whose tireless and excellent assistance made this book possible.

Howard M. Fillit

Professor Rockwood would like to thank many organizations that supported research on aging, including the Canadian Institutes of Health Research, the Dalhousie Medical Research Fund, and the Fountain Innovation Fund of the Queen Elizabeth II Health Sciences Foundation. He expresses special thanks for the support from his wife, Susan Howlett, and their sons, Michael and James.

Kenneth Rockwood

Professor Woodhouse would like to thank his wife, Judith, and his children for their unwavering support and encouragement. The support of his colleagues is very much appreciated and acknowledged. He would also like to thank his assistant, Shirley Green, whose knowledge of journal and book production procedures has proved invaluable in assisting him to fulfill his editorial commitment to the book.

Kenneth Woodhouse

All three editors wish to pay special tribute to the outstanding editorial support from Anne Snyder and Druanne Martin at Elsevier.

BROCKLEHURST'S TEXTBOOK OF GERIATRIC MEDICINE AND GERONTOLOGY

Contents

Section I: Gerontology
Introduction to Gerontology

1 Introduction: Aging, Frailty, and Geriatric Medicine 1
Howard M. Fillit, Kenneth Rockwood, and Kenneth Woodhouse

2 The Epidemiology of Aging 3
Norman Vetter

3 The Future of Old Age 11
Kenneth G. Manton

Biological Gerontology

4 Evolution Theory and the Mechanisms of Aging 18
Thomas B. L. Kirkwood

5 Methodological Problems of Research in Older People 23
Antony Bayer

6 Biology of Aging 30
Huber R. Warner, Felipe Sierra, and LaDora V. Thompson

7 Genetic Mechanisms of Aging 38
Chao-Qiang Lai, Laurence D. Parnell, and Jose M. Ordovas

8 Cellular Mechanisms of Aging 42
Robert Santer

9 Physiology of Aging 51
Edward J. Masoro

10 A Clinico-Mathematical Model of Aging 59
Kenneth Rockwood and Arnold Mitnitski

11 The Premature Aging Syndrome Hutchinson-Gilford Progeria: Insights Into Normal Aging 66
Leslie B. Gordon

Medical Gerontology

12 Connective Tissues and Aging 73
Nicholas A. Kefalides and Zahra Ziaie

13 Clinical Immunology: Immune Senescence and the Acquired Immune Deficiency of Aging 82
Mohan K. Tummala, Dennis D. Taub, and William B. Ershler

14 Effects of Aging on the Cardiovascular System 91
Susan E. Howlett

15 Age-Related Changes in the Respiratory System 97
Gwyneth A. Davies and Charlotte E. Bolton

16 Neurologic Signs in the Elderly 101
Rawan Tarawneh and James E. Galvin

17 Geriatric Gastroenterology: Overview 106
Richard C. Feldstein, Robert E. Tepper, and Seymour Katz

18 Aging of the Urinary Tract 111
Phillip P. Smith and George A. Kuchel

19 Bone and Joint Aging 117
Celia L. Gregson

20 Aging and the Endocrine System 123
Harvinder S. Chahal and William M. Drake

21 Aging and the Blood 127
Michael A. McDevitt

22 Aging and the Skin 133
Emma C.Veysey and Andrew Y. Finlay

23 The Pharmacology of Aging 138
David R. P. Guay

24 Antiaging Medicine 145
John E. Morley, Ligia J. Dominguez, and Mario Barbagallo

Neurogerontology

25 The Neurobiology of Aging: Free Radical Stress and Metabolic Pathways 150
Tomohiro Nakamura, Malene Hansen, Sean M. Oldham, and Stuart A. Lipton

26 Allostasis and Allostatic Overload in the Context of Aging 158
Bruce S. McEwen

27 Neuroendocrinology of Aging 163
Roberta Diaz Brinton

28 Normal Cognitive Aging 170
Jane Martin and Michelle Gorenstein

29 The Aging Personality and Self: Diversity and Health Issues 178
Julie Blaskewicz Boron, K. Warner Schaie, and Sherry L. Willis

Social Gerontology

30 Successful Aging: The Centenarians 184
Thomas T. Perls

31 Social Gerontology 187
Paul Higgs and James Nazroo

32 Productive Aging 193
Robert N. Butler

33 Social Vulnerability in Old Age 198
Melissa K. Andrew

Section II: Geriatric Medicine
Evaluation of the Geriatric Patient

34 Presentation of Disease in Old Age 205
Sonja Rosen, Brandon Koretz, and David B. Reuben

35 Multidimensional Geriatric Assessment 211
Laurence Z. Rubenstein and Lisa V. Rubenstein

36 Laboratory Medicine in Geriatrics 218
Alexander Lapin

37 Social Assessment of Geriatric Patients 223
Rosalie A. Kane

38 Surgery and Anesthesia in Old Age 230
D. Gwyn Seymour

39 Measuring Outcomes of Multidimensional Interventions 245
Paul Stolee

Cardiovascular System

40 Chronic Cardiac Failure 272
Neil D. Gillespie, Miles D. Witham, and Allan D. Struthers

41 Diagnosis and Management of Coronary Artery Disease 286
Wilbert S. Aronow

42 The Frail Elderly Patient with Heart Disease 295
George A. Heckman and Kenneth Rockwood

43 Hypertension 300
John F. Potter

44 Valvular Heart Disease 312
Wilbert S. Aronow

45 Cardiac Arrhythmias 327
Wilbert S. Aronow

46 Syncope 338
Rose Anne Kenny

47 Vascular Surgery 348
Arnab Bhowmick and Charles N. McCollum

48 Venous Thromboembolism in the Elderly 356
Hamsaraj G. M. Shetty, Ian A. Campbell, and Philip A. Routledge

The Respiratory System

49 Asthma and Chronic Obstructive Pulmonary Disease 362
Sidney S. Braman and Muhanned Abu-Hijleh

50 Nonobstructive Lung Disease and Thoracic Tumors 376
Katie Pink and Ben Hope-Gill

The Nervous System

51 Dementia Diagnosis 385
Richard Camicioli and Kenneth Rockwood

52 Presentation and Clinical Management of Dementia 392
Antony Bayer

53 Neuropsychology in the Diagnosis and Treatment of Dementia 402
Margaret C. Sewell, Andrew Vigario, and Mary Sano

54 Alzheimer's Disease 411
Martin R. Farlow

55 Vascular Cognitive Impairment 421
Paige A. Moorhouse and Kenneth Rockwood

56 Frontotemporal Dementia 428
Kristel Sleegers and Christine Van Broeckhoven

57 Functional Psychiatric Illness in Old Age 433
Cornelius Katona, Gill Livingston, and Claudia Cooper

58 The Older Adult with Intellectual Disability 445
John M. Starr

59 Epilepsy 453
Khalid Hamandi

60 Headache and Facial Pain 466
Gerry J. F. Saldanha

61 Stroke: Epidemiology and Pathology 478
Amanda G. Thrift and Velandai K. Srikanth

62 Stroke: Clinical Presentation, Management and Organization of Services 484
Velandai K. Srikanth and Thanh G. Phan

63 Disorders of the Autonomic Nervous System 498
Horacio Kaufmann and Italo Biaggioni

64 Parkinsonism and Other Movement Disorders 511
Jolyon Meara

65 Neuromuscular Disorders 520
Timothy J. Doherty and Michael W. Nicolle

66 Intracranial Tumors 533
David H. Rosenbaum, Michael L. Gruber, and Mary V. MacNeil

67 Disorders of the Spinal Cord and Nerve Roots 539
Sean D. Christie and Richard A. Cowie

68 Infections of the Central Nervous System 546
Steven L. Berk and James W. Myers

Musculoskeletal System

69 Metabolic Bone Disease 553
Roger M. Francis

70 Arthritis in the Elderly 566
David L. Scott

71 Connective Tissue Diseases 577
Anthony J. Freemont

72 Orthopedic Geriatrics 583
Robert Victor Cantu and Kenneth J. Koval

73 Sarcopenia 587
Yves Rolland and Bruno Vellas

74 Podiatry 594
Katherine Ward, Mark A. Kosinski, and Bryan Markinson

Gastroenterology

75 Geriatric Dentistry: Maintaining Oral Health in the Geriatric Population 599
Andrea Schreiber and Robert Glickman

76 The Upper Gastrointestinal Tract 608
David A. Greenwald and Lawrence J. Brandt

77 The Pancreas 626
Ceri Beaton and Malcolm C. A. Puntis

78 The Liver 635
Joanna Hurley and John Trevor Green

79 Biliary Tract Diseases 645
Elias Xirouchakis and Andrew K. Burroughs

80 The Small Bowel 652
Christopher A. Rodrigues

81 The Large Bowel 661
Arnold Wald

82 Nutrition in Aging 678
C. Shanthi Johnson and Gordon Sacks

83 Obesity 685
Krupa Shah and Dennis T. Villareal

The Urinary Tract

84 Diseases of the Aging Kidney 690
Latana A. Munang and John M. Starr

85 Disorders of Water, Electrolyte, and Mineral Ion Metabolism 697
M. Shawkat Razzaque

86 The Prostate 701
Nicholas J. R. George

Women's Health

87 Gynecologic Disorders in the Elderly 716
Tara K. Cooper and Oliver Milling Smith

88 Cancer of the Breast in the Elderly 726
Lodovico Balducci

Endocrinology

89 Adrenal and Pituitary Disorders 730
Paul E. Belchetz and Peter Hammond

90 Disorders of the Thyroid 737
Myron Miller

91 Disorders of the Parathyroid Glands 755
Jane Turton, Michael Stone, and David E. C. Cole

92 Diabetes Mellitus 760
Alan J. Sinclair and Simon C. M. Croxson

Hematology and Oncology

93 Blood Disorders in the Elderly 775
Bindu Kanapuru and William B. Ershler

94 Geriatric Oncology 791
Margot A. Gosney

Skin and Special Senses

95 Skin Disease and Old Age 801
Gopal A. Patel, Gangaram Ragi, W. Clark Lambert, and Robert A. Schwartz

96 Aging and Disorders of the Eye 810
Scott E. Brodie

97 Disorders of Hearing 822
Barbara E. Weinstein

Section III: Problem-Based Geriatric Medicine
Prevention and Health Promotion

98 Health Promotion for the Community-Living Older Adult 835
Maureen F. Markle-Reid, Heather H. Keller, and Gina Browne

99 Preventive and Anticipatory Care 848
James T. Pacala

100 Sexuality in Old Age 854
Robert N. Butler and Myrna I. Lewis

101 Exercise for Successful Aging 859
William J. Evans

102 Injury in Older People 865
Mujtaba Hasan

103 Rehabilitation: Therapy Techniques 870
Valerie M. Pomeroy and Marion F. Walker

103B Rehabilitation: General Principles
Available online only at www.expertconsult.com
John Young

Geriatric Syndromes

104 Geriatric Pharmacotherapy and Polypharmacy 880
Joseph T. Hanlon, Steven M. Handler, Robert L. Maher, and Kenneth E. Schmader

105 Impaired Mobility 886
Ruth E. Hubbard, Eamonn Eeles, and Kenneth Rockwood

106 Falls 894
Stephanie A. Studenski

107 Delirium 903
Eamonn Eeles and Ravi S. Bhat

108 Constipation and Fecal Incontinence in Old Age 909
Danielle Harari

109 Urinary Incontinence 926
Adrian Wagg

110 Pressure Sores 939
Bryan D. Struck

111 Sleep, Aging, and Late-Life Insomnia 943
Holly J. Ramsawh, Harrison G. Bloom, and Sonia Ancoli-Israel

112 Malnutrition in Older Adults 949
Larry E. Johnson and Dennis H. Sullivan

113 The Mistreatment and Neglect of Older People 959
Anthea Tinker, Simon G. Biggs and Jill Manthorpe

114 Pain in the Older Adult 965
Patricia Bruckenthal

115 Palliative Medicine for the Elderly Patient 973
Ilora Finlay and Margred Capel

116 Ethical Issues in Geriatric Medicine 983
Søren Holm

Section IV: Health Systems and Geriatric Medicine

117 The Elderly in Society: An International Perspective 988
Robert N. Butler and Oleg Volkov

118 Geriatrics in Europe 997
Peter Crome

119 Geriatrics in North America 1005
David B. Hogan

120 Geriatrics in the Rest of the World 1010
Jean Woo

121 Geriatrics in Latin America 1016
Jorge H. Lopez and Renato Maia Guimarães

122 Long-Term Care in the United Kingdom 1021
Clive Bowman

123 Institutional Long-Term Care in the United States 1026
Luis F. Samos, Enrique Aguilar, and Joseph G. Ouslander

124 Education in Geriatric Medicine 1032
Ruth E. Hubbard

125 Improving Quality of Care in the United Kingdom 1038
David A. Black

126 Preserving Medicare Through a "Quality" Focus 1046
Richard G. Stefanacci

127 Managed Care for Older Americans 1057
Richard G. Stefanacci

128 Telemedicine Applications in Geriatrics 1064
Stuti Dang, Adam G. Golden, Herman S. Cheung, and Bernard A. Roos

Index 1071

BROCKLEHURST'S TEXTBOOK OF GERIATRIC MEDICINE AND GERONTOLOGY

Color Plates

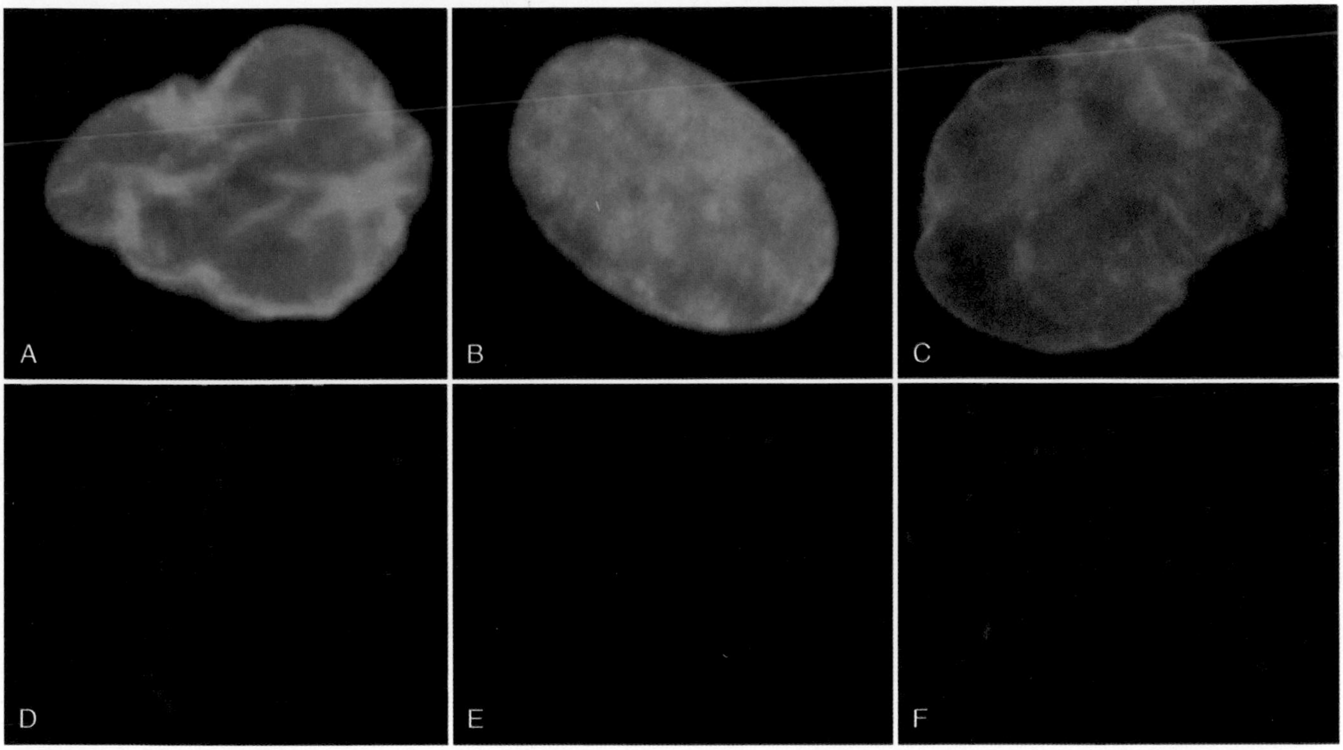

Plate 11-3. Nuclear blebbing and presence of progerin in HGPS and aging. Fibroblast nuclei stained with antilamin antibody **(A)** passage 4 HGPS, **(B)** passage 10 normal, **(C)** passage 40 normal; skin biopsies stained with antiprogerin antibody and shown here at 40× for **(D)** HGPS donor age 10 years old; **(E)** normal newborn, **(F)** normal, donor age 90 years old.

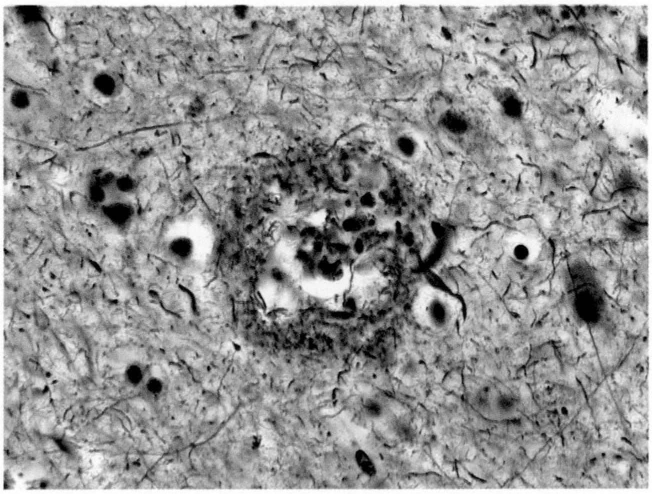

Plate 54-1. Neuritic plaques revealed by silver stain from cortex of patient with Alzheimer's disease.

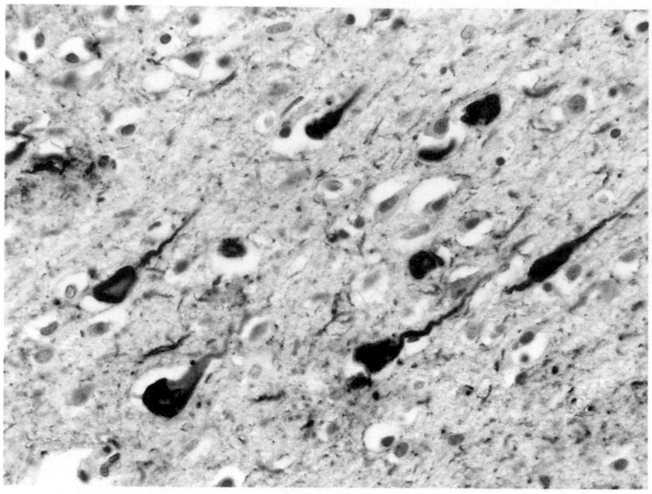

Plate 54-2. Neurofibrillary tangles in cortical section of brain from patient with Alzheimer's disease.

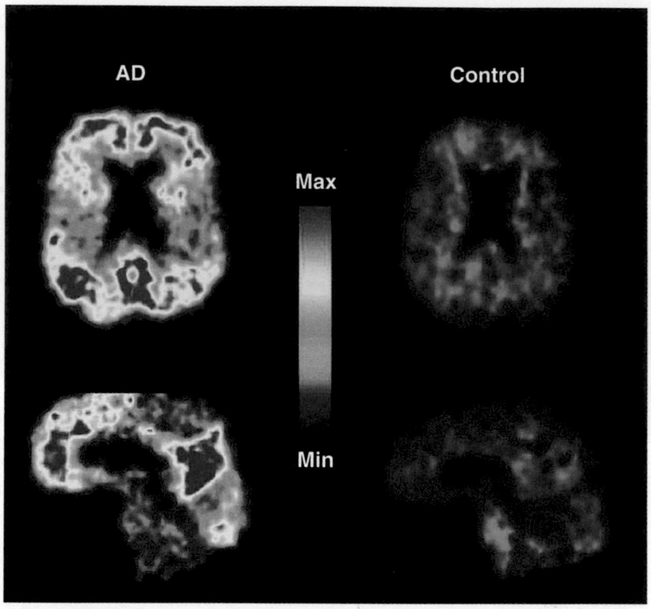

Plate 54-6. Agent labeling amyloid, PIB illustrating significant uptake in frontal and parietal regions.

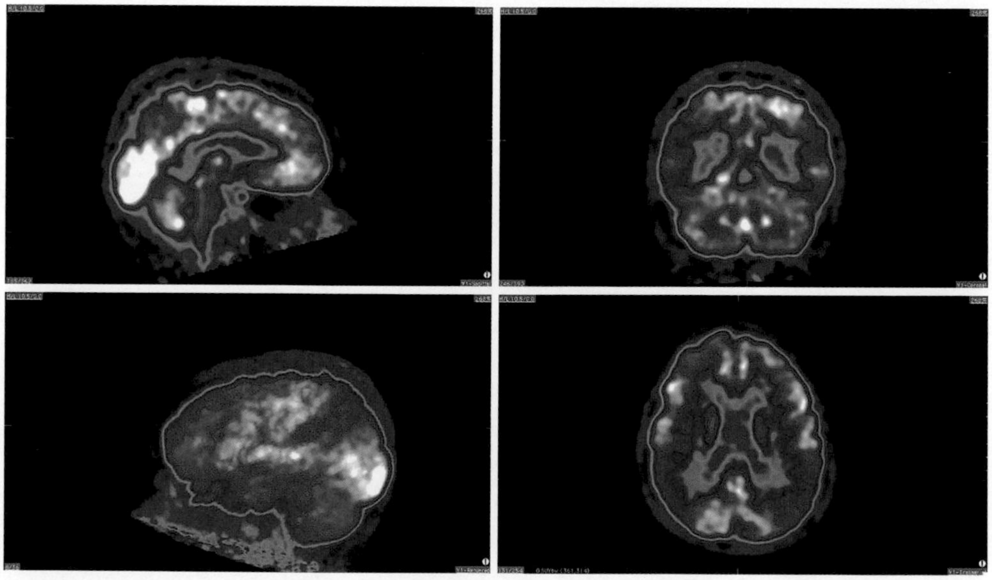

Plate 54-5. Views from PET study using 18-fluorodeoxyglucose obtained in a patient with Alzheimer's disease. The image demonstrates decreased signal or metabolism in the posterior parietal regions as may characteristically be seen with this illness.

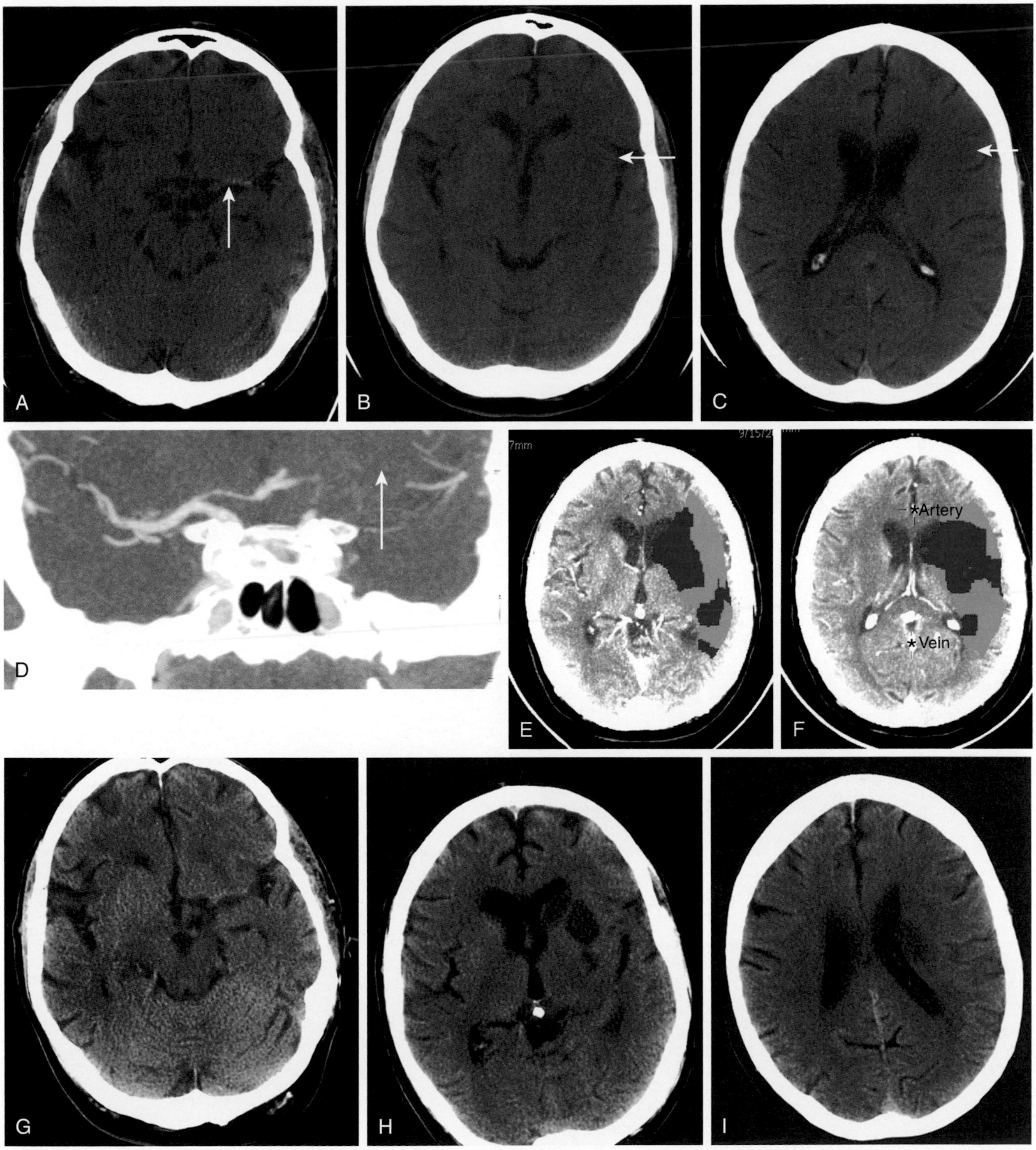

Plate 62-2. CT imaging revealing salvageable tissue in acute ischemic stroke. An 84-year-old man had acute left MCA occlusion resulting in aphasia and dense right hemiparesis while playing golf. This man was known to have AF and not on warfarin. The acute CT scan (**A**) showed the hyperdense MCA sign, which corresponded with CT angiography (**D**) evidence of left MCA occlusion. There is obscuration of the lentiform nucleus and edema in the left frontal cortex (**B** and **C**). The CT perfusion pictures (**E** and **F**) showed that the striatocapsular region (in red) was likely to be infarcted, whereas the surrounding area in green was at risk of infarction. He was treated with tissue plasminogen activator and the CT scans performed (**G–I**) 2 days later showed infarction of **only** the left striatocapsular region.

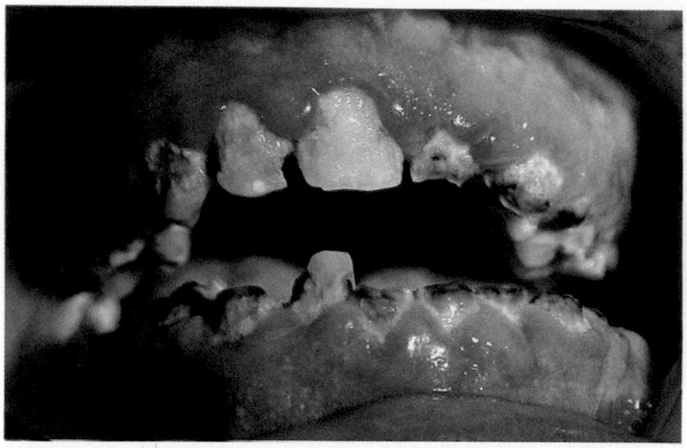

Plate 75-1. Rampant dental caries. *(Reprinted with the permission of Mirriam Robbins, DDS, New York University College of Dentistry.)*

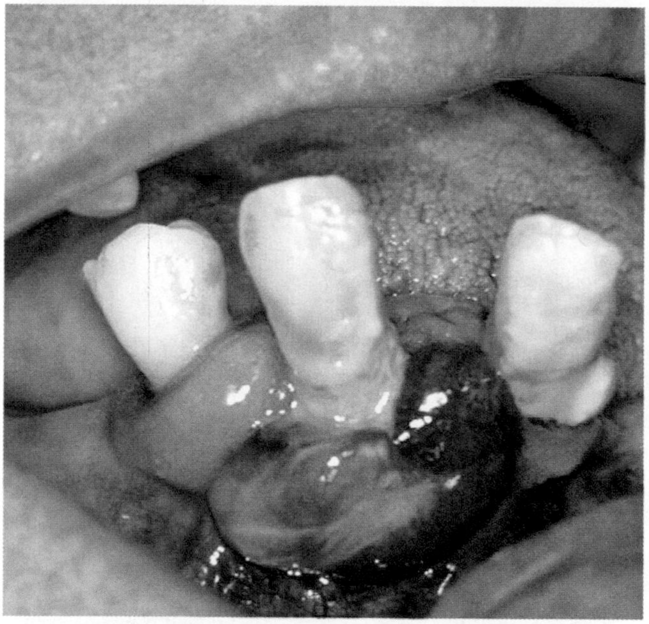

Plate 75-2. Periodontal abscess: associated with bone loss around root of tooth. *(Reprinted with the permission of Mirriam Robbins, DDS, New York University College of Dentistry.)*

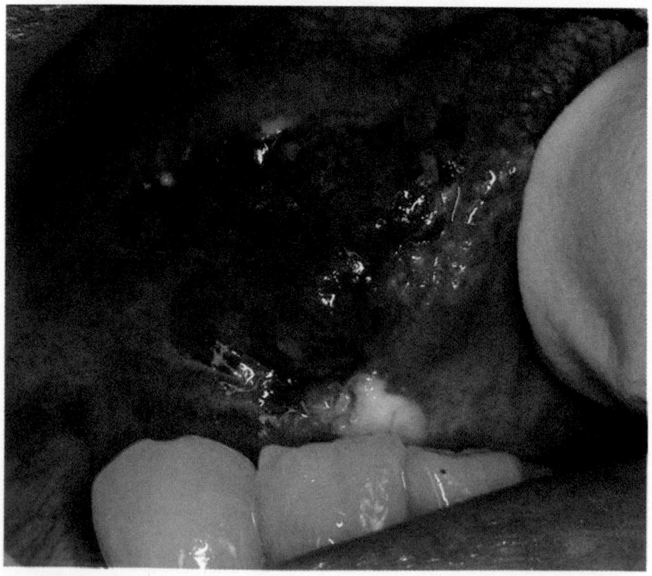

Plate 75-3. Oral dysplasias: right lateral border of tongue. *(Reprinted with the permission of Mirriam Robbins, DDS, New York University College of Dentistry.)*

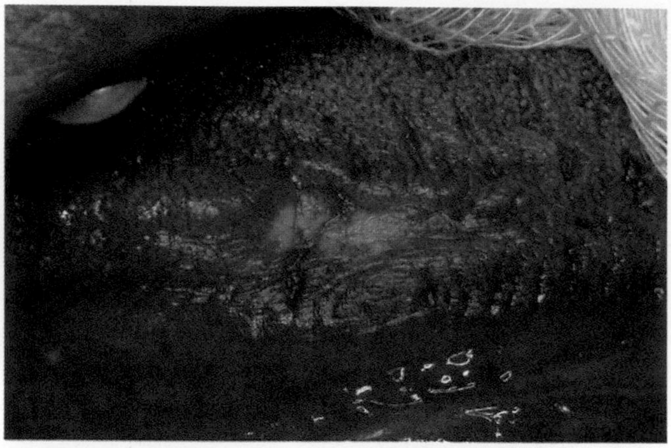

Plate 75-4. Leukoplakia or white lesion: left lateral border of tongue. *(Reprinted with the permission of Mirriam Robbins, DDS, New York University College of Dentistry.)*

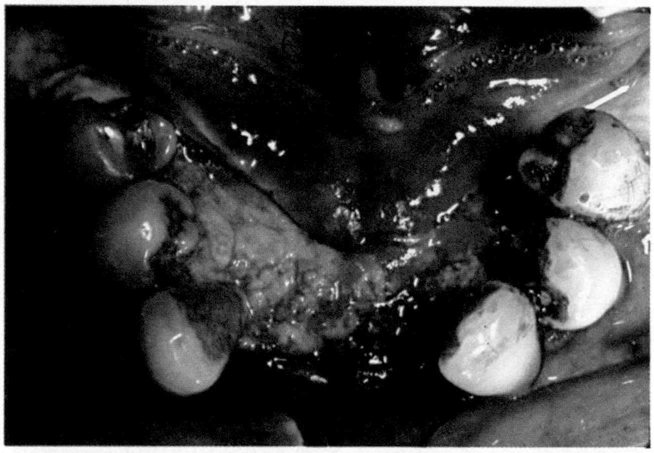

Plate 75-5. Squamous cell carcinoma: floor of mouth. *(Reprinted with the permission of Mirriam Robbins, DDS, New York University College of Dentistry.)*

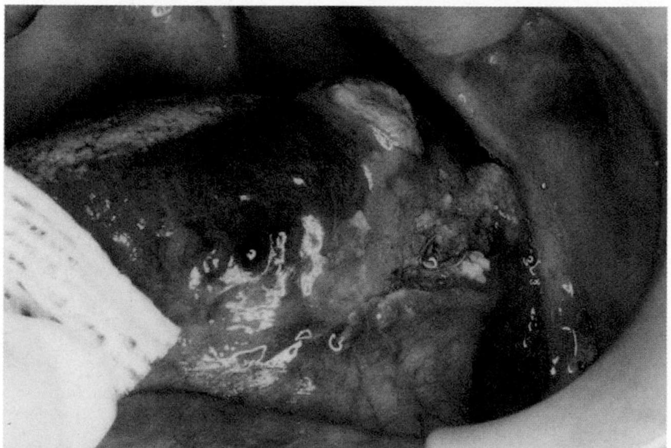

Plate 75-6. Squamous cell carcinoma: left lateral border of tongue. *(Reprinted with the permission of Mirriam Robbins, DDS, New York University College of Dentistry.)*

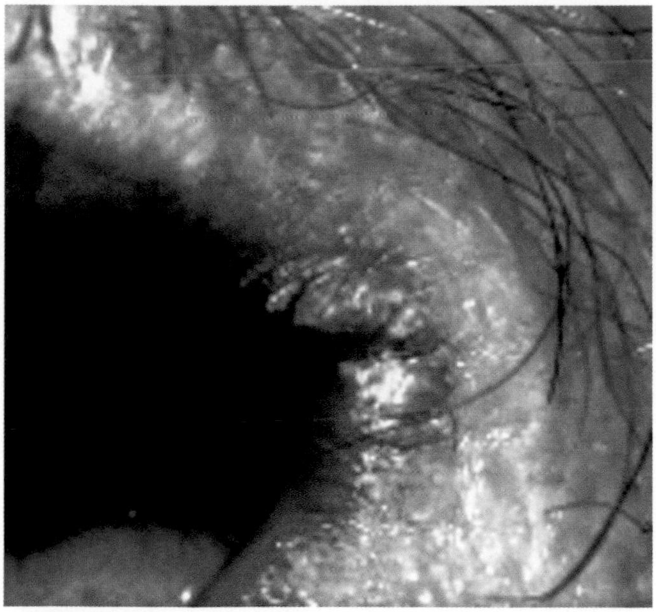

Plate 75-7. Angular cheilitis caused by loss of dentition, poor diet, and candidiasis. *(Reprinted with the permission of Mirriam Robbins, DDS, New York University College of Dentistry.)*

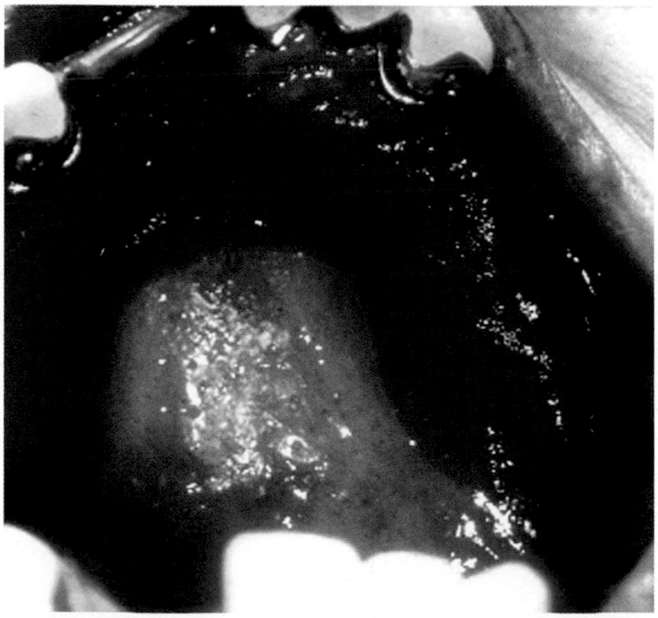

Plate 75-8. Denture stomatitis: ill-fitting denture and candidiasis. *(Reprinted with the permission of Mirriam Robbins, DDS, New York University College of Dentistry.)*

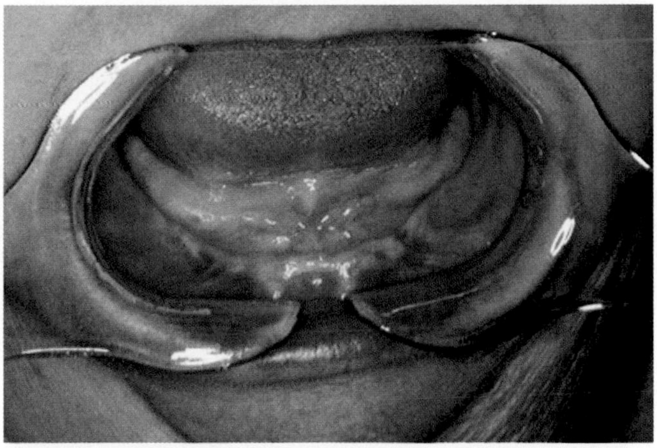

Plate 75-9. Atrophic mandible: early loss of dentition and long-term denture wear. *(Reprinted with the permission of Kenneth Fleisher, DDS, New York University College of Dentistry.)*

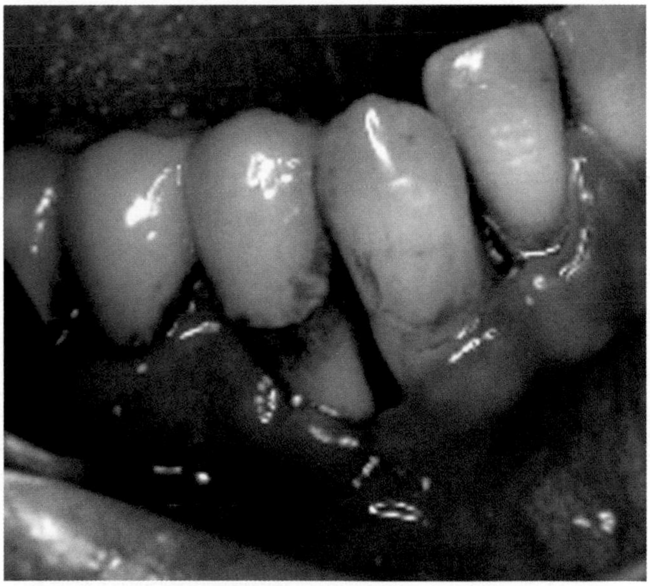

Plate 75-10. Severe periodontal bone loss. *(Reprinted with the permission of Mirriam Robbins, DDS, New York University College of Dentistry.)*

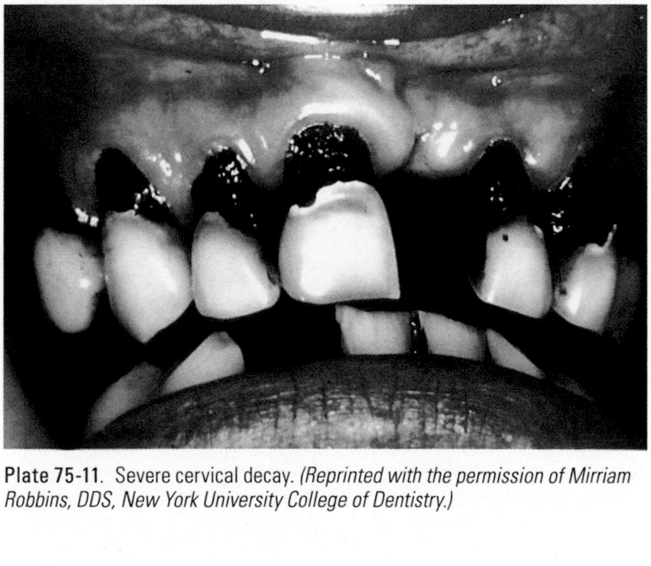

Plate 75-11. Severe cervical decay. *(Reprinted with the permission of Mirriam Robbins, DDS, New York University College of Dentistry.)*

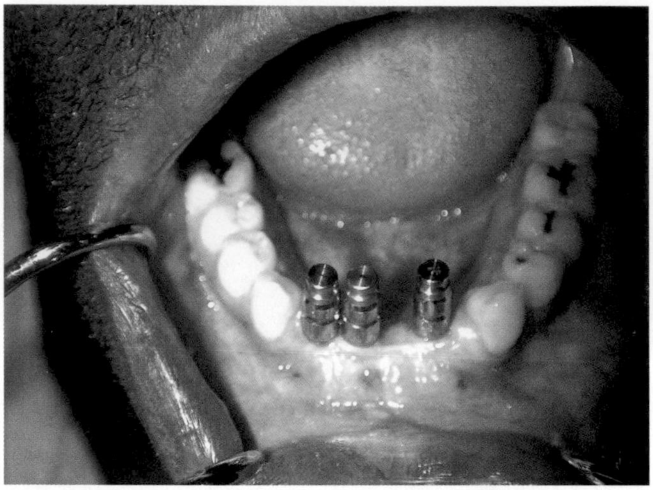

Plate 75-12. Dental implants: before fabrication of prosthesis/bridge. *(Reprinted with the permission of Mirriam Robbins, DDS, New York University College of Dentistry.)*

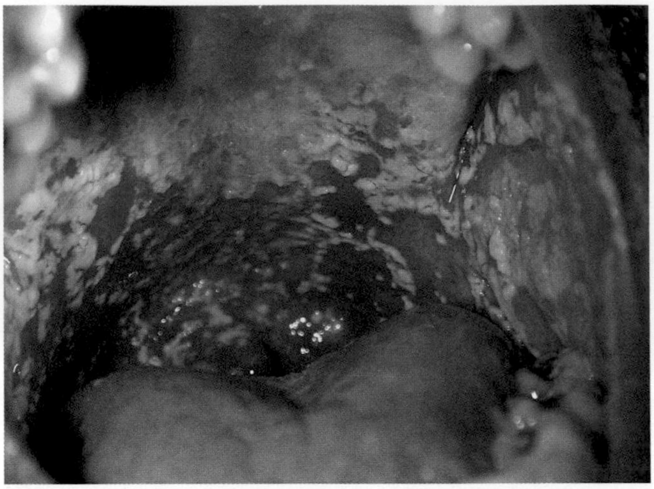

Plate 75-13. Oral candidiasis: note striae throughout indicative of fungal infection. *(Reprinted with the permission of Mirriam Robbins, DDS, New York University College of Dentistry.)*

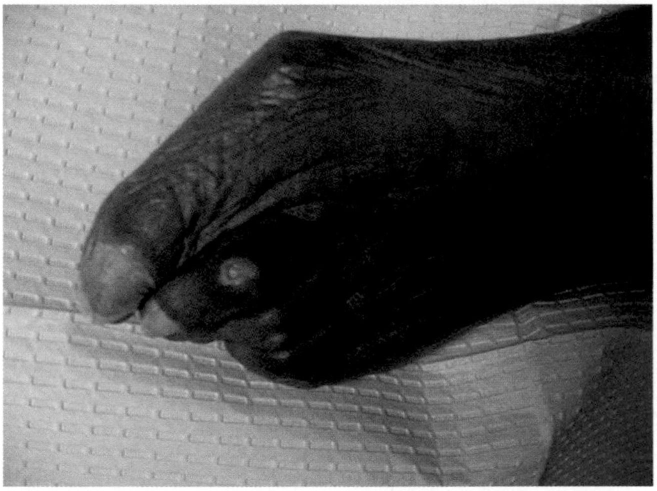

Plate 74-1. A bunion deformity with hammer toe of the second digit. Note preulcerative lesion over proximal phalangeal joint of second toe secondary to shoe pressure.

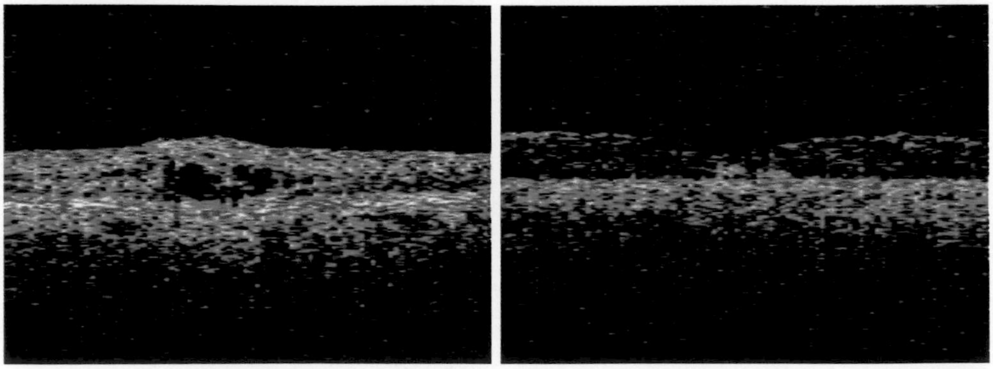

Plate 96-12. Treatment of wet age-related macular degeneration in a 90 year-old woman with intravitreal ranibizumab. Baseline images *(left)* show macular edema in fluorescein angiogram *(top – note patch of white fluorescence at temporal edge of fovea)* and in retinal cross-section as seen in OCT scan image *(bottom – extracellular fluid appears as dark clefts within retinal layers)*. After three injections of ranibizumab, edema has resolved *(right, top and bottom.* Note absence of white fluorescence in angiogram, and resolution of intraretinal clefts in OCT image, with restoration of normal foveal contour). Visual acuity improved from 20/100 (6/30) to 20/40 (6/12).

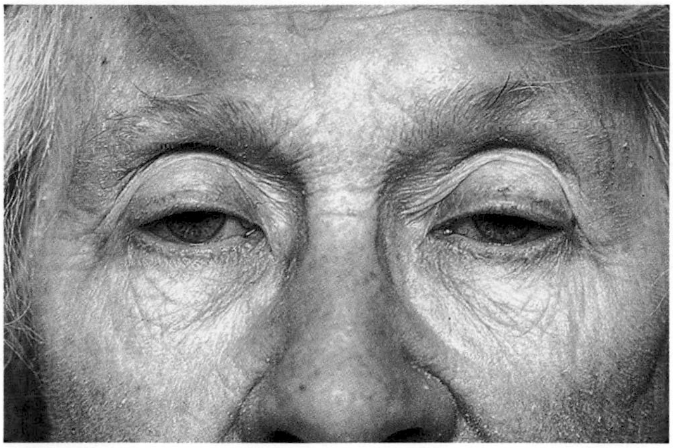

Plate 96-1. Senile ptosis. Note the low lid level and the loss of the normal lid folds. *(Courtesy of Murray Meltzer, MD.)*

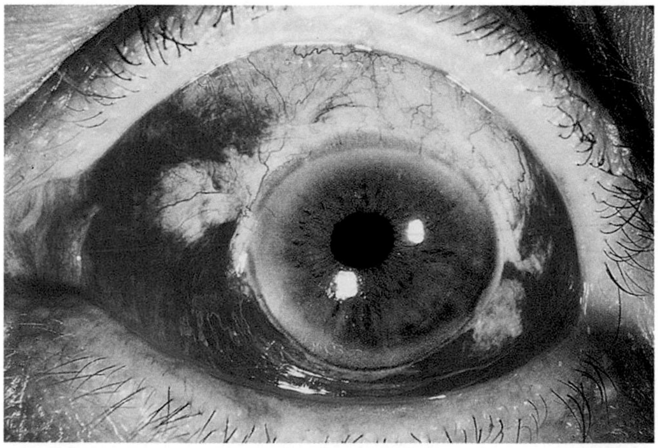

Plate 96-2. Subconjunctival hemorrhage. This small hematoma, seen through the transparent conjunctiva, is benign unless recurrent.

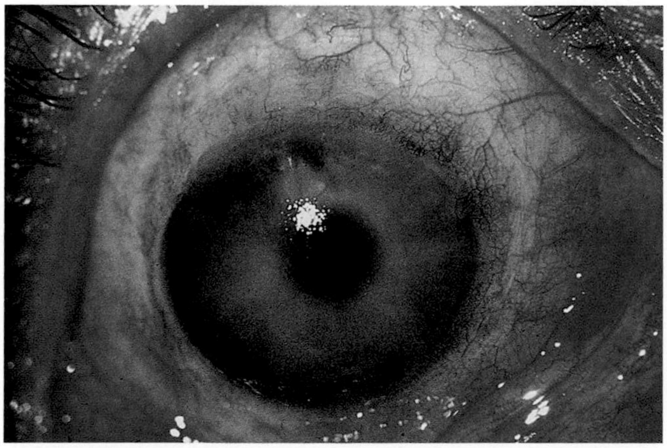

Plate 96-3. Corneal edema. The cornea is thickened and cloudy because of failure of the corneal endothelium to adequately dehydrate the tissue. *(Courtesy of Calvin Roberts, MD.)*

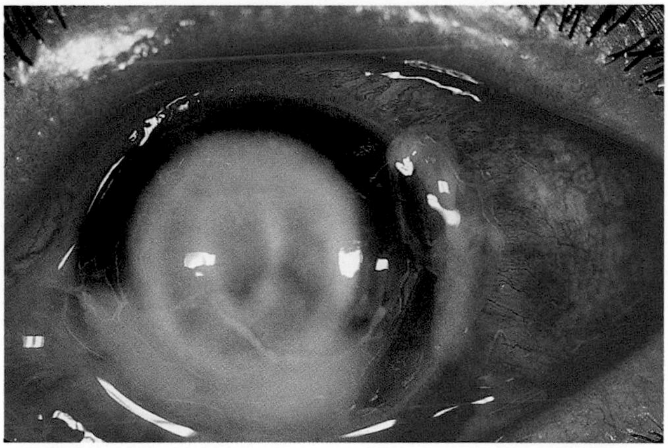

Plate 96-4. Corneal ulcer. A localized infection causes an epithelial defect and attracts an infiltrate of white blood cells. *(Courtesy of Michael Newton, MD.)*

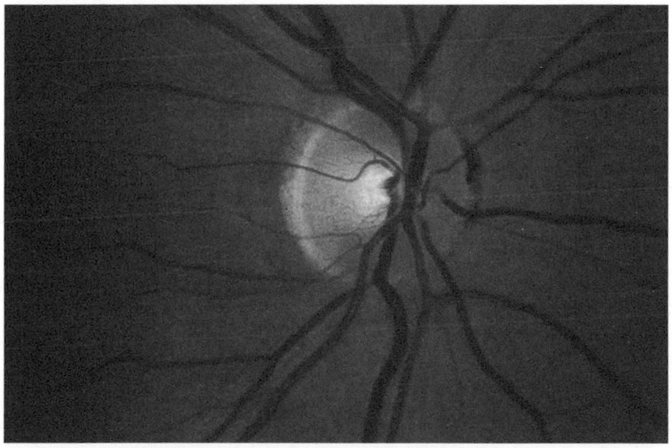

Plate 96-5. Normal optic nerve head. Cup-to-disc ratio is about 0.3.

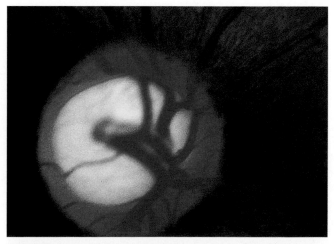

Plate 96-6. Glaucomatous optic nerve head cupping. Loss of neural tissue is seen as narrowing of the neural rim of the optic disc and enlargement of the central cup. (Compare with Figure 96-8.)

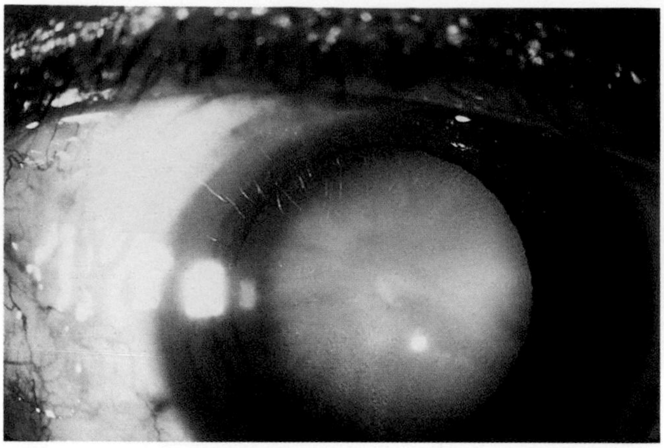

Plate 96-7. Cataract. Loss of transparency of the crystalline lens impairs visual acuity. *(Courtesy of Calvin Roberts, MD.)*

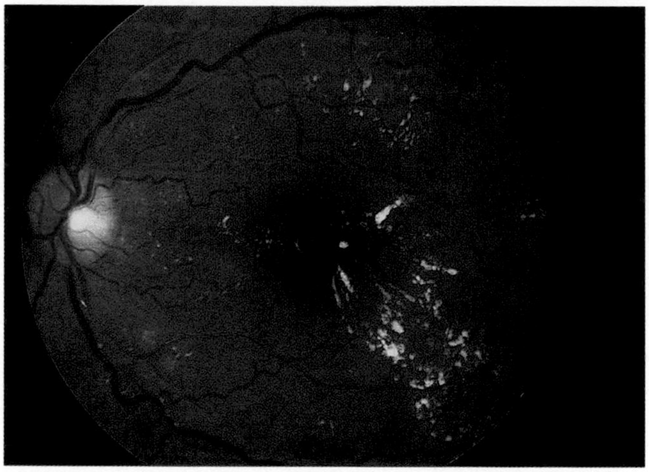

Plate 96-8. Background diabetic retinopathy. Microaneurysms ("dot hemorrhages"), intraretinal hemorrhages ("blot hemorrhages"), and "hard" exudates indicate deterioration of the retinal microcirculation.

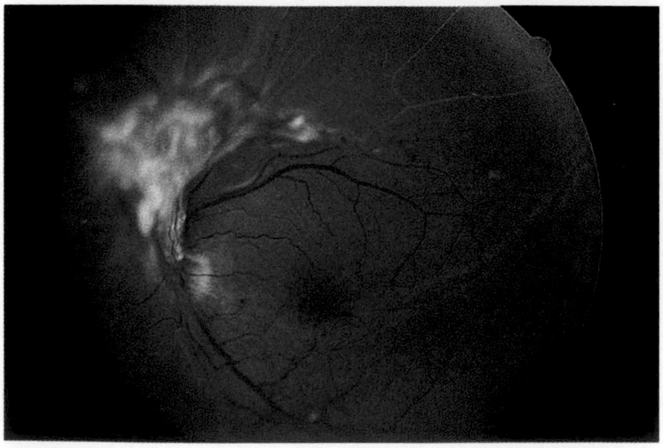

Plate 96-9. Proliferative diabetic retinopathy. A membrane of fibrovascular tissue has sprouted from the optic disc in response to prolonged retinal ischemia.

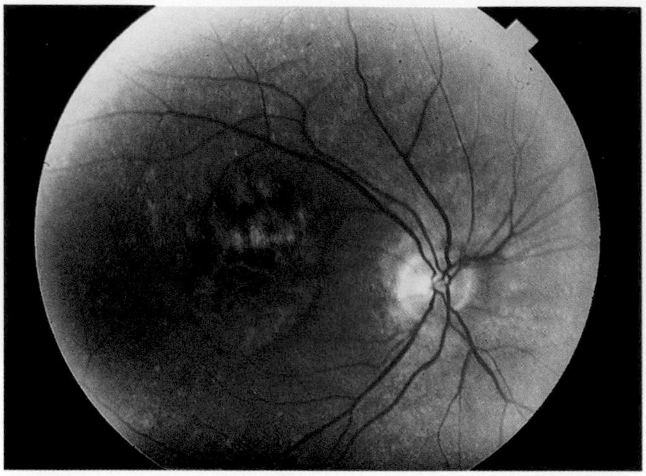

Plate 96-10. Atrophic ("dry") age-related macular degeneration. Geographic atrophy of the retinal pigment epithelium causes loss of central vision.

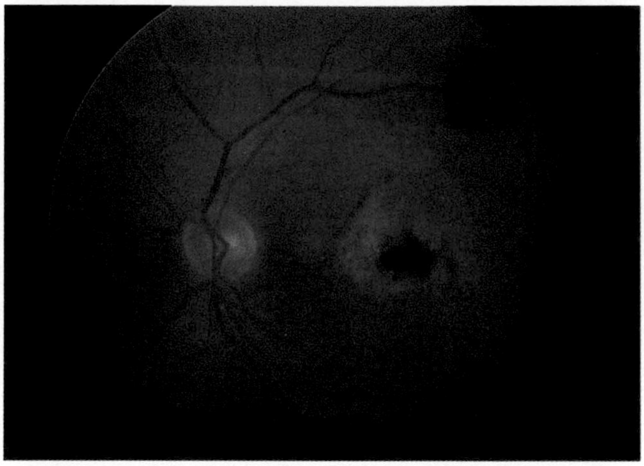

Plate 96-11. Exudative ("wet") age-related macular degeneration. Leakage and scarring from a subretinal neovascular membrane destroys central retinal function.

CHAPTER 1

Introduction: Aging, Frailty, and Geriatric Medicine

Howard M. Fillit
Kenneth Rockwood
Kenneth Woodhouse

There are many landmarks in the history of care for older adults. In ancient times, Hippocrates and Cicero wrote on aging and health. The first medical textbook on aging was published by Charcot in 1881 (Clinical lecture on senile and chronic diseases, London, New Sydenham Society). The term *geriatrics* was coined by Ignatz Nascher in 1909:

> *"Geriatrics, from geras, old age, and iatrikos, relating to the physician, is a term I would suggest as an addition to our vocabulary, to cover the same field that is covered in old age that is covered by the term pediatrics in childhood, to emphasize the necessity of considering senility and its disease apart from maturity and to assign it a separate place in medicine"* (New York Medical Journal 1909; 90:358–359).

Nascher, who was later recognized as the father of geriatrics, published the first American textbook of geriatric medicine in 1914 (Geriatrics: The diseases of old age and their treatment, Philadelphia, P. Blakiston's Son & Co). The book had three major sections: physiologic old age, pathologic old age, and hygiene and medicolegal relations. Geriatrics was first embedded as a component of a modern health system and became a specialty in 1948 within the National Health Service in the United Kingdom. As a result, the first "modern" textbook of geriatrics was published in 1973, edited by John Brocklehurst. We are proud, then, to present the heir of this lineage, the Seventh Edition of *Brocklehurst's Textbook of Geriatric Medicine and Clinical Gerontology*.

The first edition of *Brocklehurst* contained 39 chapters written by 44 authors. The current edition contains 128 chapters and 205 authors. This growth reflects our increasing knowledge, based on research, about gerontology and geriatric medicine. There has also been a significant advance in our understanding, in our perspective, and in our health systems, which also contribute to the evolution of our knowledge. Nevertheless, we have remained true to the original concept.

In the seventh edition, we have attempted to make the book more useful and valuable to the gerontologist, be they a biologic, social, psychological, or medical gerontologist. Indeed, the study of aging as an interdisciplinary field of research has expanded exponentially since the first edition. Consequently, the content on gerontology has been significantly reorganized and expanded. Although the effort to effectively combine gerontology and geriatric medicine in one comprehensive book is ambitious, we believe it is necessary since the clinician clearly requires knowledge of the gerontologic basis of geriatric practice, whereas the gerontologist needs the clinical perspective for his or her work to be relevant. Whether for the gerontologist, the geriatrician, the primary care physician, the specialist, or the care managers and other providers, we hope the book has value as a resource to improve the care of elderly persons, to create better systems of care, and to advance knowledge and research in gerontology.

Fundamentally, geriatric medicine encompasses three essential "bodies of knowledge." The first is gerontology, essential to the practice of geriatrics. One cannot effectively practice geriatrics without understanding the basic fundamentals of aging itself, much as a pediatrician cannot practice pediatrics without understanding child development. Indeed, geriatricians often refer to "adult development," not aging, as key to the practice of geriatric medicine. For example, evaluating the cognition of an aged person requires a working knowledge of the degree and nature of "normal" changes in cognition at that age. Gerontology, the study of aging, is also a fundamentally interesting scientific field relevant to geriatric medicine in that it encompasses the demography of aging, the biology of aging, the neuropsychology of aging, and medical gerontology.

The second component of the body of knowledge in geriatrics is disease specific. That is, geriatrics requires knowledge of the diseases that are more common in the aged than in the middle-aged (such as Alzheimer's disease), and knowledge of how common diseases such as pneumonia, hypertension, diabetes, or hypothyroidism differ in their presentation in old age.

The third component of geriatric medicine knowledge may be called complexity. Complexity, a focus on function, and an emphasis on multidisciplinary coordinated care management are each critical to geriatric medicine. Complexity refers to the fact that many older patients (in contrast to most middle-aged "internal medicine" patients with single illnesses) often have many comorbid illnesses, are on multiple medications, and suffer problems in the multiple spheres of physical, functional, psychological, and social health.

Complexity is further reflected in the "geriatric syndromes"—falls, polypharmacy, delirium, sleep disorders, and others—that are presented in the section on "geriatric syndromes." The focus on function is important in the evaluation of complexity in the frail elderly patient and key to the practice of geriatric medicine.

Because of the preponderance of chronic illness, complexity, and the resulting frailty (a state of increased vulnerability that arises from multiple, interacting medical and social problems), geriatric patients require effective health systems of chronic care, a multidisciplinary team approach, comprehensive yet efficient means of evaluation (such as geriatric assessment), and the increasing use of technology, such as electronic medical records and telemedicine. In particular, physicians and other care providers need to know how to participate in and to lead and manage health systems critical to the provision of quality and efficient geriatric care, which is presented in the section on health systems.

In the twenty-first century, with the emergence of billions of persons into a newly globalized world, we have expanded our international perspective. Aging is clearly now a global challenge, with all societies needing new and effective ways to provide quality, cost-effective care to the elderly with a focus on quality of life and continuing productivity.

This edition also aims for easier ways for readers to provide feedback for future editions, through the "contact us" button on the book's Web site (www.expertconsult.com). The introduction of a Web site for the book also reflects our aim to move from an exhaustive referencing style of textbook. We have given thought to why anyone might read—much less write—a textbook when so much information is readily available, and so quickly, on the web. The immediacy and proliferation of information is both the triumph and the challenge of the Internet, a "place" where the quality of information can be questionable. Since information is not knowledge, we are persuaded that there remains a role for a textbook that provides practitioners and scientists, in one text, a compendium of useful and validated information. We hope that as you read the chapters, you will get the sense that they were written by experts who care about their field and care about what you should know about it.

With the seventh edition, we aim to build on what has been achieved in geriatric medicine and gerontology, and to renew our commitment to provide gerontologists, geriatricians, and other academics and practitioners with updated, useful information to aid them in their special mission of providing care for older persons. To do this, we have recruited new editors: Professors Kenneth Rockwood (from Canada) and Kenneth Woodhouse (from the United Kingdom). Each has undertaken major research in the field and each brings a wealth of clinical, scholarly, and health systems experience and perspective to this important endeavor.

Thus, when colleagues or patients question "what is geriatrics?," we often reach for our "body of knowledge," here, a textbook weighing several pounds with more than 1350 pages of "small print."

In the twenty-first century, there can be no more important subject in medicine than gerontology and geriatrics. We believe this textbook represents the knowledge base for that effort.

CHAPTER 2

The Epidemiology of Aging

Norman Vetter

It must be obvious that, senescence apart, old animals have the advantage of young. For one thing, they are wiser. The Eldest Oyster, we remember, lived where his juniors perished.

SIR PETER MEDAWAR[1]

INTRODUCTION

Epidemiology is about measuring and understanding the distribution of the characteristics of populations. The origin of epidemiologic methods relates to the study of epidemics, initially set up by the rich to know when it was time to leave the area when a new epidemic spread among the poor. Epidemiologists are still concerned about the distribution of disease, but apart from being perhaps less likely to head for the hills when infection is rife, they have also added noninfectious diseases and the determinants of disease to their interests. Some have strayed into areas which are not disease-related, but are characteristics of the population itself; one such area is the epidemiology of aging.

The body of knowledge of the epidemiology of aging has evolved into concentrating on three main areas: the causes and results of the aging of populations, the natural history of diseases of old age, and the evaluation of services set up to assist older people. This chapter will concentrate on the first of these; the other two will be covered elsewhere in the textbook.

The causes and results of the aging of populations

The early twenty-first century is unique in a number of aspects, but in relation to the people of the world it is most remarkable as a time when humans live appreciably longer than ever before. Perhaps even more remarkably this rate of prolongation of average life expectancy shows little sign of abating. This extraordinary piece of good luck for those of us who live at this time is tempered a little by the knowledge that life insurers and those calculating pensions have been betting our money on our not living so long, as a result of which we may be poorer than we had hoped.

Longevity

The increase in human life expectancy over the past 10 years has taken both scientists and the population generally by surprise.[2] Until recently, demographers were confidently predicting that once the gains made by reducing mortality in early and middle life had reached completion, growth in longevity would stop and we would see the fixed reality of the aging process. This has not happened. Mortality experts who have repeatedly asserted that life expectancy is close to an ultimate ceiling have repeatedly been proven wrong. The apparent leveling off of life expectancy in individual countries has been an artifact of laggards catching up and leaders falling behind. In the developed world, average prolongation of life continues at 4 to 5 hours a day. Late-life mortality, which people theorized was likely to remain stable, has steadily increased (Figure 2-1).

The probable causes for the linear quality of this increase in life expectancy are twofold. Before 1950, most of the gain in life expectancy was due to reductions in death rates at younger ages. In the second half of the twentieth century, improvements in survival after age 65 caused the increase in the length of people's lives. Most forecasts of the maximum possible life expectancy in recent years have been broken within five years of the forecast.[3] World life expectancy has more than doubled over the past 200 years. So where will this lead? Life expectancy has increased by 2.5 years per decade for a century and a half; a reasonable suggestion would be that this trend will continue in coming decades. If so, average life expectancy will reach 100 in about 60 years.

Why do we age?

There now appears to be a reasonably clear consensus that the aging process is caused by an accumulation over time of molecular damage. The rate of aging in an individual is therefore a complex interaction between damage, maintenance, and repair. These interactions are, of course, influenced by both genetic and environmental factors. It has been said that whoever created humans, whether nature or a creator, did a poor job, but being aware of it, put in a lot of back-up systems. On the other hand it may be a universal law that hyperefficiency is less effective in the long run than flexibility. This may be a useful lesson beyond the realms of longevity in a world more fussed about efficiency than effectiveness.

It is assumed that genetic changes are unlikely to alter appreciably, under evolutionary pressure, over the short period, during which longevity has dramatically increased. The reason for the increasing longevity is therefore said to be caused by the interplay of advances in income, nutrition, education, sanitation, and medicine, with the mix varying over age, period, cohort, place, and disease. It seems likely then that these changes are largely a result of a wide range of environmental factors.

That being said, the birth cohorts of people born around the early 1900s experienced huge changes in socioeconomic conditions, hygiene, lifestyle, and medical care, leading to dramatic falls in infant mortality and infectious and respiratory diseases. The main effects were socioeconomic, leading to smaller families, better housing, and nutrition, though later in the century vaccination must have played some part. In later years it seems to have been the survival of older people that has led to the extension of life expectancy. The reason for this survival is not fully understood. The best we can do is to guess that it may be the availability of specific treatments for diseases of old age.[6]

However, it may be that we were working to the wrong theory of maximum human lifespan all along. Studies of large populations of humans, wasps, fruitflies, nematodes, and yeast have revealed a leveling off, and in some species even a decline, in mortality late in life instead of a continuously increasing rate. The possible reason that this has been

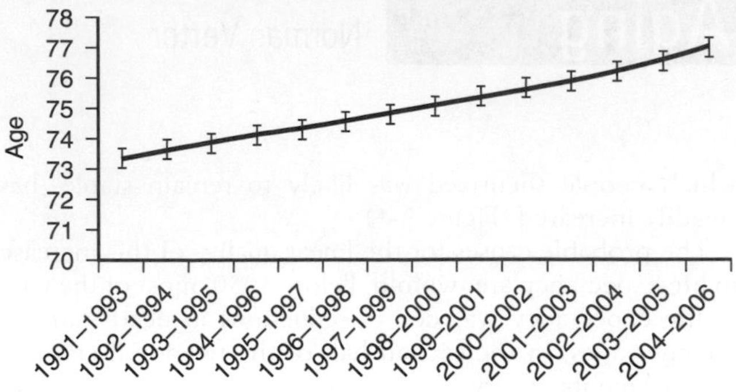

Figure 2-1. Life expectancy by time (United Kingdom ± 95% confidence intervals).

missed until now in humans may be that the deceleration in age-specific death rates does not seem to begin in humans until after 80 years of age, the plateau is not seen until after 110 years of age, and it requires the observation of large populations.[4]

In addition, genetics and environment are known to be intimately entwined. The length of telomeres has been said to be a measure of aging. Telomeres are the ends of chromosomes that help to protect the DNA from wearing down during the replication process that replenishes cells. Telomeres shorten over an individual's lifetime and are thought be a marker for aging. For instance it is known from matched twin studies that telomeres in a physically active group of people (who performed more than 3 hours and 20 minutes of exercise a week) were 200 nucleotides longer than those in a less active group (who performed less than 16 minutes exercise a week). Smokers and obese people are known to have shorter telomeres than their healthier counterparts.[5]

QUALITY OF LIFE AND DISABILITY

The measurement of quality of life on older people is self-evidently a vital outcome measure for deciding upon, for instance, the comparative effectiveness of different treatments. Many approaches have been made to this. For an overview for large populations, questionnaire methods are most commonly used, including the Bartel index, the SF-12, and more recently the WHOQOL-OLD, a generic health-related QOL measure developed for the World Health Organization.[7] A number of good reviews of measuring quality of life have been written by Bowling[8] and Haywood.[9]

The latter explored 122 articles relating to 15 measuring instruments. The most extensive evidence was found for the SF-36, COOP Charts, EQ-5D, Nottingham Health Profile (NHP), and Sickness Impact Profile (SIP). Four instruments had evidence of both internal consistency and test-retest reliability: the NHP, SF-12, SF-20, and SF-36. Four instruments lacked evidence of reliability: the HSQ-12, IHQL, QWB, and SQL. Most instruments were assessed for validity through comparisons with other instruments, global judgments of health, or clinical and sociodemographic variables. The author concluded that there was good evidence for reliability, validity, and responsiveness for the SF-36, EQ-5D, and NHP. There is more limited evidence for the COOP, SF-12, and SIP. The SF-36 was recommended where a detailed and broad-ranging assessment of health is required, particularly in community-dwelling older people with limited morbidity. The EQ-5D was recommended where a more succinct assessment is required, particularly where a substantial change in health is expected.

Another study of more than 16,000 in the health survey for England provided evidence that the SF-6D is an empirically valid and efficient alternative multiattribute utility measure to the EQ-5D, and is capable of discriminating between external indicators of health status.[10]

Figure 2-2 shows data from the above study for EQ-5D data by age. EQ-5D is an especially useful measure, where valid, because it can be used directly to measure utilities in cost-effectiveness studies when using the measure to build up quality-adjusted life-years (QALYs). QALY maximization as a means of, for instance, comparing two treatments, is sometimes criticized for being ageist, because other things being equal, the elderly with a shorter life expectancy will be given lower priority.

It is not the place of this chapter to go into detail on this argument, but some people believe that everyone, when faced with a sudden illness or accident at least, should be regarded as equal no matter what their state of health or likely longevity. This seems untenable at one extreme, say elderly patients with severe dementia. In that case it would seem that "not striving to keep alive" makes sense. However, a fit 90-year-old is usually able to benefit from high

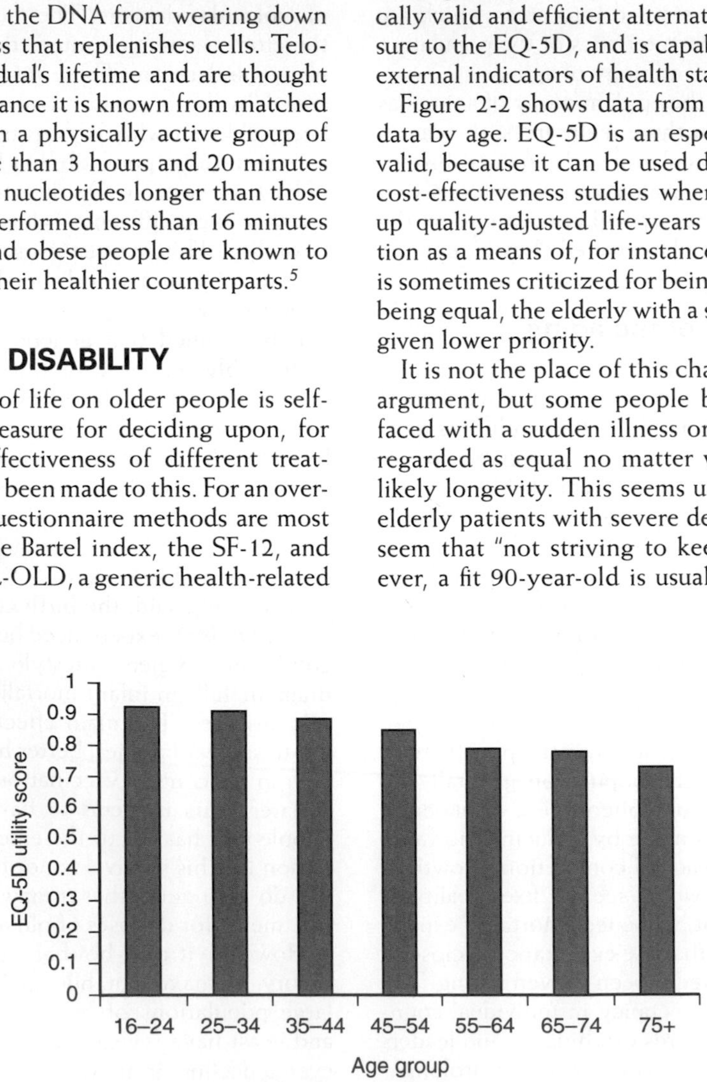

Figure 2-2. EQ-5D utility data by age.

technology solutions to his or her disease process as anyone else.

In contrast some people believe that QALYs are not ageist enough (e.g., the QALY-based view would give the same weight to treating a 10-year-old with a quality-adjusted life-expectancy of 10 years as to an 80-year-old with the same life expectancy). This does not account for the greater benefits that the old person has already received so that some people think that younger people should have priority over older people, regardless of life expectancy.[11]

Changes with time

It is a truism to say that older people nowadays are fitter than they were in the past. Measuring this between successive generations of the same age has been attempted. At the level of overall quality of life, it has been reported that people in their late 70s in the 1990s were less functionally impaired than was a similar group in the 1980s.[12] Since then various other longitudinal studies conducted in the United States, Europe, and in other developed countries have examined this. Although the findings are not consistent, several consensus publications and a meta-analysis that stratified results based upon the adequacy of measurement concluded that there appeared to have been a significant reduction in the rate of functional decline over the last 3 decades and that this finding was robust with respect to measurement approach, methodology, and to some extent by country.[13] This was difficult to pinpoint in the face of an approximately 1% reduction in mortality in older people, but most researchers conclude that there has been at least a 2% reduction in disability over the last several decades.

Turning to more specific problems that are common in older people, it is thought that, for example, average blood pressure measurements in successive cohorts of older people appear to be declining. Thus in the Gothenburg study, it was found that successive cohorts of 70-year-olds had lower arterial blood pressure with time.[14] Others have agreed that although the prevalence of disability and need for help increases with advancing age, within an age group these improve over time from one birth cohort to another.[15,16] The exception to this, until recently, has been fractures in older people where age-adjusted fracture incidence seemed to be rising steadily during the 1990s. However, since then, in Finland where the best data have been collected over time, the rate is changing rapidly, rising for some fractures[17] and falling for others.[18,19]

The exact reasons for the secular change in the risk of hip fracture are unknown. A cohort effect toward healthier elderly populations in the developed countries cannot be ruled out: in earlier birth cohorts, the early-life risk factors for fracture, such as perinatal nutrition, may have had stronger impact on the late-life fracture risk than in the others. A second reason could be the rising average body weight and body mass index (BMI). In all adult age groups in developed countries, the prevalence of obesity has increased since the 1980s. A low BMI is a strong risk factor for hip fracture, and it has been estimated that a one unit increase in the BMI of a population could result in an 7% decrease in the fracture incidence—the effect being greatest with weight gain among the thinnest older adults.

Measuring differences: predicting future quality of life

Data from the English longitudinal study of aging have been used to investigate whether longstanding illnesses, social context, and current socioeconomic circumstances predict quality of life.[20] This was a nationally representative sample of noninstitutionalized adults living in England using a standardized quality of life scale. The quality of life of the group was found, where adversely affected, in rank order to be reduced by depression, a poor financial situation, limitations in mobility, difficulties with everyday activities, and limiting longstanding illness. Quality of life was improved, again in rank order, by trusting relationships with the family, friends, and frequent contacts with friends; living in a good neighborhood; and having two cars. The regression models explained 48% of the variation in quality of life scores.

The authors concluded that efforts to improve quality of life in early old age need to address financial hardships, functionally limiting disease, lack of at least one trusting relationship, and inability to move out of a disfavored neighborhood. They did not mention the possible provision of extra cars.

This importance of the perceptions of older people about their neighborhood was also underlined by a further study of over-65-year-olds in the community.[21] In this study, perceptions of problems in the area (noise, crime, air quality, rubbish/litter, traffic, and graffiti) were predictive of poorer health. The good news about these findings is that many of these factors are modifiable and could have an important impact on the quality of life of older people.

A 65-year-old person with severe disability will have differences in need for support when compared with an 85-year-old person. The severe disability is likely to be complicated by multiple problems, especially social and mental problems, so that their health needs are likely to be greatly complicated by housing and financial needs and by isolation and loneliness.

Measuring differences: cross-sectional versus longitudinal data

Much of the research done on the aging process has been performed on cross-sectional data. This is not particularly surprising because such studies are easier and much less complicated to perform than longitudinal studies. Generally speaking, cross-sectional data indicate that aging has a more marked deleterious effect on the study group than longitudinal. The process of aging for us all is demonstrably longitudinal, so that wherever possible we should be guided by such data.

A number of examples of the differences between cross-sectional and longitudinal studies exist. A classic longitudinal study showed that cognitive decline appeared to be much more closely related to age in cross-sectional studies than in longitudinal.[22] Other cross-sectional studies that originally were thought to show that smoking had a protective effect on Alzheimer's disease were shown by longitudinal studies to be the opposite of the true effect, probably because smokers died before they had a chance to suffer from Alzheimer's.[23] In addition, marked effects have been seen in different cohorts born more recently. Age cohorts born only 5 years apart show notable differences in their height, weight, and other measures associated with changes in activity level.[24] It is therefore important to distinguish between the sorts of data that are available when making judgments about populations of older people. Generally, cross-sectional data paint a bleaker picture of the impact of aging than do longitudinal data.

Measuring differences: age

The age distribution of older men and women is very different, especially in the oldest age groups. For example, 3.8% of older women compared with 1.7% of older men are aged 90 and above. This situation is expected to persist for some time, but gender differences according to age will become less notable in the future.

When describing age groups there is a particular problem for the oldest group and sometimes for those below that. The groups 65 to 69, 70 to 74, 75 to 79, 80 to 84, and 85+ are commonly used in the literature and in research findings. This is a means of summarizing the data when looking at trends and other differences. However, closer examination of these groups compared with single year of age data may show that, although the first four of these represent 5-year age groups, the 85+ group can, depending on the population studied, only go up to 90 years of age or may continue beyond 100. In other words the 85+ group is not strictly comparable with the other two. By grouping the data, one is making the assumption that the group represents a midpoint. This, together with the likelihood of small numbers in the oldest age group, can account for anomalous findings in that group.

Table 2-1 shows data for a population based in a large general practice in South Wales by year of age and divided into age groups. It can be clearly seen that the 85+ age group is heavily skewed with the frequency midpoint of the group between 86 and 87 years, nowhere near the 5 years which is the midpoint of the others.

Figure 2-3 shows a typical example of how the top age group is out of line with previous groups. It shows the prevalence of breathlessness in the group shown in Table 2-1. The difference in value in the oldest age group may reflect a true difference or it may be due to assuming that the oldest group is at the midpoint, as explained above.

Measuring differences: sex

The average life expectancy at birth of females born in the United Kingdom is 80 years compared with 76 years for males. Women are more likely than men to be living with high blood pressure, arthritis, back pain, mental illness, asthma, and respiratory disease. Men are more likely than women to be living with heart disease. Older men are much more likely than older women to drive. Among people aged 75 and over, 58% of men and 33% of women have access to private transport. Among people aged under 75, women are more likely than men to be providing unpaid

Table 2-1. Year of Age by Age Groups

	AGE GROUPS					
Age	**65 to 69**	**70 to 74**	**75 to 79**	**80 to 84**	**>85**	**Total**
65	145	0	0	0	0	145
66	106	0	0	0	0	106
67	100	0	0	0	0	100
68	81	0	0	0	0	81
69	90	0	0	0	0	90
70	0	83	0	0	0	83
71	0	84	0	0	0	84
72	0	74	0	0	0	74
73	0	75	0	0	0	75
74	0	68	0	0	0	68
75	0	0	72	0	0	72
76	0	0	52	0	0	52
77	0	0	45	0	0	45
78	0	0	56	0	0	56
79	0	0	62	0	0	62
80	0	0	0	37	0	37
81	0	0	0	26	0	26
82	0	0	0	46	0	46
83	0	0	0	37	0	37
84	0	0	0	42	0	42
85	0	0	0	0	22	22
86	0	0	0	0	25	25
87	0	0	0	0	21	21
88	0	0	0	0	11	11
89	0	0	0	0	6	6
90	0	0	0	0	12	12
91	0	0	0	0	5	5
92	0	0	0	0	6	6
93	0	0	0	0	2	2
94	0	0	0	0	1	1
95	0	0	0	0	1	1
96	0	0	0	0	1	1
99	0	0	0	0	1	1
Total	522	384	287	188	114	1495

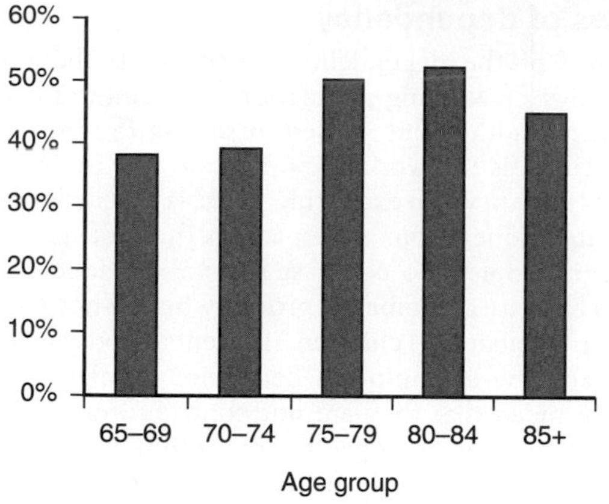

Figure 2-3. Breathlessness by age group.

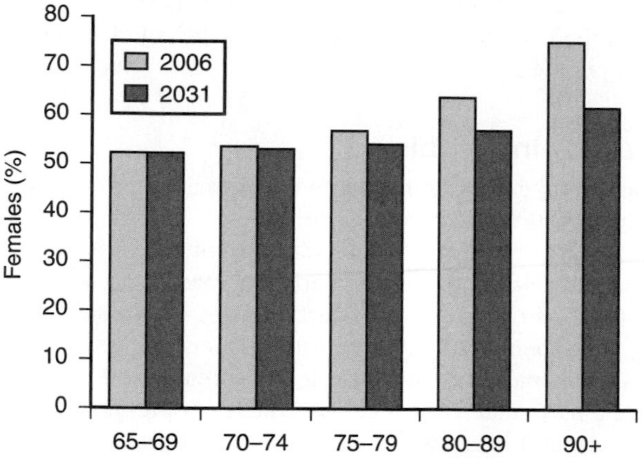

Figure 2-4. Projected percentage of older women by age in the United Kingdom.

care to relatives, neighbors, or friends; but among people aged 85 and over, men are more likely than women to be providing unpaid care. This is because of different average lifespans—older women are more likely to live alone, whereas older men are more likely to be married. Figure 2-4 shows the projected percentage of older women by age group.

Population aging is particularly rapid among women because of lower mortality rates among women. In older age groups, the proportion of women is therefore higher than men; increasingly so with advancing age. Therefore, when studying older people, it is essential to study gender as a basis of differentiation. For example, it has been suggested that older women's much higher level of functional impairment coexists with a lack of gender differences in self-assessed health. Some studies have reported no gender differences in self-reported health status among elderly people, whereas higher levels of more objectively measured disability existed among women. It has been shown that gender differences in health depend on the indicator and the age stratum analyzed. It could very well be that among older adults the impacts of different measures of socioeconomic position differ by health indicator and that disability-related indicators may be more sensitive to gender inequalities than

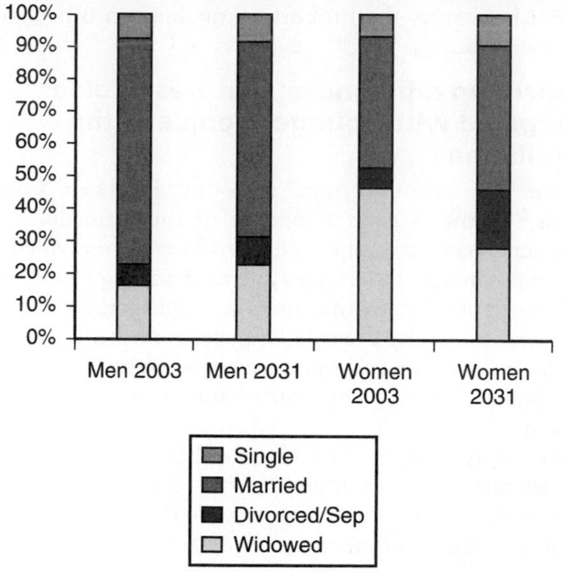

Figure 2-5. Projected percentage of older people by sex and marital status (England and Wales).

broad indicators of general health such as self-perceived health status.[25]

Among some older married couples, the man controls household finances, meaning that his partner may be left in a difficult position if suddenly she has to take over money management. Women's pension entitlement is often lower than men's and their risk of poverty in later life significantly greater.

Although the gender differences in the structure by age of the older population is expected to persist in the future, things will slowly change. As a result of the faster increase in life expectancy of men, gender differences in the composition of the older age groups will most likely shrink over time. Thus it is estimated that between 2006 and 2031, women will remain in the majority, but their share is due to decrease. For example, the percentage of women aged 80 to 89 is expected to decrease from 63.2% in 2006 to 56.3% in 2031.

Measuring differences: marriage

Older men and women are very different with respect to their marital status: 61% of men are married compared with 36.7% of women, whereas 16.5% of men are widowed compared with 46.1% of women. This gender imbalance varies by age, becoming more marked with time or among older cohorts. In the future these differences are expected to decrease dramatically. Figure 2-5 shows these changes.

There is predicted to be a dramatic increase in the share of divorced and separated individuals in the younger age groups of the older population between 2003 and 2031. Among the 65–74 year olds, one in five women will belong to this group, whereas now the percentage stands at just below 9%. The increase in the proportion of divorced and separated men will not be as great because men have a higher propensity to remarry, but the proportion of single men will reach more than 16%. In short, for both genders, but particularly so for men aged 65–74, the proportion married will diminish whereas the proportion of those in other groups will increase.

Measuring differences: features of older compared with younger people in the population

Figure 2-6, adapted from work by Professor Grimley Evans,[26] shows a general outline of the main differences between young and older people. These are divided into two main groups, differences due to the aging process itself and those not due to that process. Aging may be primary and intrinsic, set by the cellular makeup of the individual or it may be extrinsic and due to environmental challenges—the day-to-day wear and tear of the environment on that person.

Secondary aging is said to be either individual, such as the adaptations in an older person's gait because of poor proprioception or a tendency to write down things to overcome problems with memory. They are not themselves due to aging but are a response to some aspect of the aging process. Some aspects of old age give an advantage to the species. Thus humans with their odd need to stand on their swhich have to go through those pelvises at birth, have as a result very immature offspring who take many years to become independent beings. It appears that, in evolutionary terms, additional help in child care in the shape of grandmothers provided an advantage. Thus the menopause gave a major advantage to humankind and was adopted generally.

Then there are three main categories of difference which are not due to the aging process per se: selective survival, the fact that people who take more risks, whether by smoking or by dangerous sports, are less likely to be found in the older age group so that that group is lacking in such individuals. The second, a cohort effect, which I have mentioned elsewhere in the chapter and the third differential challenges for older people compared with those for the young, which I will now describe more fully. In many countries older people live in low quality housing as a consequence of social policy as well as poverty. More pervasive is the poorer quality of medical care provided for older people, largely as a result of discrimination against those who are older.

Indices of dependency

The ratio of the dependent population to the economically active or working population is sometimes called the dependency ratio. This is used in setting taxation policies, in particular, as the working population pay income tax. In fact the taxman, when extracting taxes, is much cleverer than just taking money from wage packets these days; so that all groups of people who purchase pay value-added and other taxes. There are a number of groups who are not part of the working population: children, students, housewives, husbands, and the unemployed. Being not formally employed does not mean that they are not contributing to the economy. In particular grandparents contribute hugely in terms of child care for working people and retired people, especially women, and are one of the biggest groups caring for elderly disabled relatives, most often a spouse.

Another indicator of the age structure is the aging index, defined as the number of people aged 65 and over divided by the number under age 15. By 2030 it is thought that all developed countries will have more people aged 65 and over than people under 15.

Is aging inevitable?

The old joke says "aging is inevitable, maturing is optional." However, lifestyle factors seem able to have an impact on aging. The best-known and obvious of these is smoking, which is related to a wide range of problems, some well known, as in lung disease, heart disease, and cancers, resulting in its being the most important predictor for mortality in a combination of six large longitudinal studies.[27] Others have a particular resonance with older people, notably bone strength and hearing ability.[28] These changes are so ubiquitous that there is a suggestion that smoking may accelerate the aging process itself.

On the positive side, there are also a number of studies that show the importance of continuing to perform exercise[29,30] and others that have shown that muscular strength in old age can, with training, be increased proportionately to a similar extent to that found in younger people[31] and that training appears to have some effect on the prevention of falls.[32]

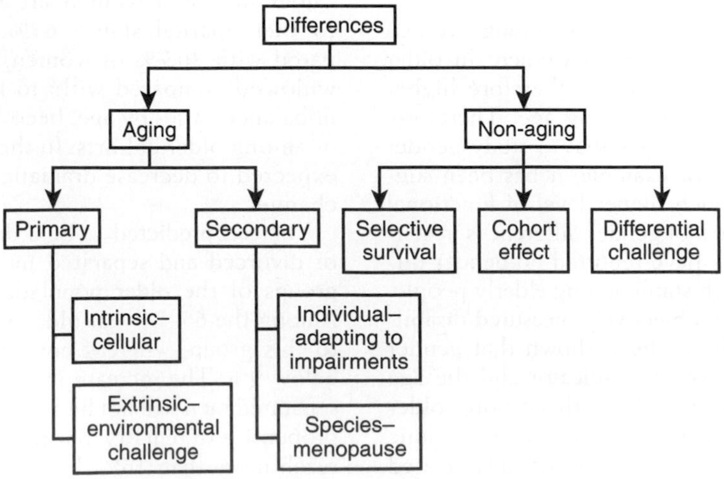

Figure 2-6. Differences between young and older individuals.

Living alone

The vast majority of those who live alone are widowed, although this percentage is much higher for women than men. The distribution of those who live with a partner (the vast bulk of older people) is similar between men and women and consists mainly of married or remarried individuals. By contrast, the category "living with others" is quite heterogeneous. Men are more likely to be married, perhaps living with a younger wife, whereas women in this group are for the most part widowed (Figure 2-7).

Living alone is likely to be increasingly common as the millennium advances. It is likely that a quarter of people born in the 1960s will be lone householders by age 60 and that close to a half of the 1960s Baby Boomers will be living solo by age 75.[33] Living alone is not directly related to loneliness, but the cause of living alone, especially widowhood, is closely related, so they are often associated.

Ethnicity, emigration, and immigration (internal and external)

Because of the youthfulness of immigrants, immigration is often seen as a solution to the "problem" of population aging in countries with low fertility. Presently the lack of people to take jobs in developed countries draws young people from developing countries, lowering the average age of the population. The overall large numbers and proportions emigrating again among the overseas-born population suggest that this U.K. subpopulation ages more slowly than does the U.K.-born subpopulation. This implies that the currently observed processes of immigration and emigration among U.K.s overseas-born immigrants will lower the U.K.s old-age dependency ratio in the long run as well as in the short run.

Table 2-2 shows the proportion of older people in the 2001 census by ethnic origin. There are a great preponderance of white people in the United Kingdom, with only very minor differences in the proportion between males and females.

Inequalities

Older people have tended to be neglected in research on health inequalities compared with people in other stages of life. Similarly, there has been a lack of research on how class interacts with gender in later life. One of the central reasons for this has been the difficulty of assigning people to social groupings after retirement because the approach has traditionally been based on occupational status and this is difficult to attribute when older people are mainly retired.

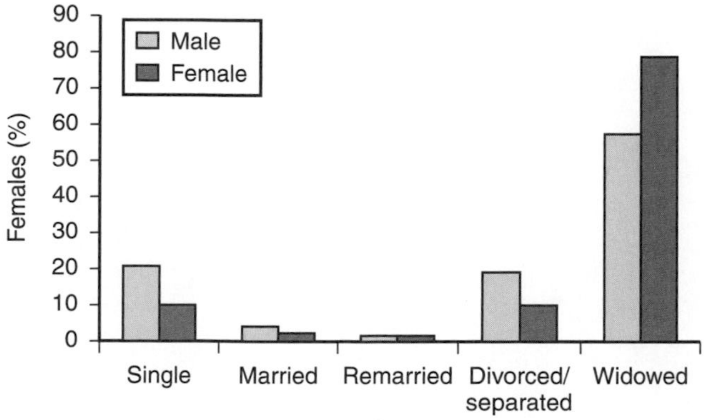

Figure 2-7. Marital status of older people living alone. *(Data from United Kingdom 2001 census.)*

Table 2-2. Older People by Sex and Ethnicity – United Kingdom

Ethnicity	Male	Female	Total
White	96.9	97.7	97.4
Asian	1.8	1.3	1.5
Black	1.0	0.7	0.8
Other	0.3	0.3	0.3
Total	100.0	100.0	100.0

Data from Census (2001) Office of National Statistics, United Kingdom.

There is evidence that increasing inequalities will occur between future cohorts of elderly people. Inequalities will persist between those who will have experienced full work histories, have acquired pension rights and housing wealth, and those who have not. The 1960s baby boomers, in particular, faced high unemployment levels when they first entered the labor market. Some of them have never had a full-time job, whereas others benefited from the Thatcher era, giving rise to the 1980s "yuppies." Inheritance of housing wealth primarily goes to individuals who are already owner-occupiers, further increasing the trend toward increased inequality and Richard Titmuss' notion of "two nations in old age."[34]

Inequalities by socioeconomic group continue even up to the end of life. During the last year of life, older people were still reluctant to take up their entitled benefits.[35] Primary health care professionals saw nearly all of the people who died during their last year. They could play an important role in ensuring that the elderly and the less well-off are aware of the services and benefits available to them.

CONCLUSIONS

Epidemiology is about measuring and understanding the distribution of the characteristics of populations. In relation to aging, the early twenty-first century is unique in the span of human existence for the longevity of the race. The aging of the population is a global phenomenon that requires international coordination nationally and locally.

The United Nations and other international organizations have developed a number of recommendations intended to reduce adverse effects of population aging. These include reorganization of social security systems, changes in labor, immigration, and family policies, promoting active and healthy life-styles, and more cooperation between governments in resolving socioeconomic and political problems

KEY POINTS
The Epidemiology of Aging

- The world population is older than it has ever been.
- Measuring the effect of an aging population is not straightforward; longitudinal approaches more accurately describe people's experience than do cross-sectional studies.
- Older people at a given age are fitter than they used to be in nearly all objective parameters measured.
- Inequalities between different social groups of older people, both for health and income, appear to be increasing in the U.K.

related to population aging. A country with an aging population may be helped by immigration of young workers to enlarge the working population, potentially with benefit to both countries as long as it is carefully monitored.

On the positive side, the health status of older people of a given age is improving over time because recent generations are fitter and have had less diseases. As a result, older vigorous and active people live to a much later age than previously, and given the opportunities, they can contribute economically. We have already extended the healthy and productive period of human life and this shows little sign of abating.

For a complete list of references, please visit online only at www.expertconsult.com

CHAPTER 3

The Future of Old Age

Kenneth G. Manton

The future of old age in the twenty-first century in the United States and other economically developed countries will be dynamic and will generate historically unprecedented demographic, social, economic, and medical conditions. This is due to quantitative and qualitative population, social, economic, and health factors. Some quantitative demographic factors are well known, although details of their operation are still not fully appreciated.

First, in the United States, there were rapid declines in mortality at young ages from at least 1900 because of reductions in infectious disease risks and infant and maternal mortality. Responsible for these declines were improved nutrition, new antibiotic therapies, immunization and vaccination programs for childhood diseases, and improved public hygiene (e.g., improved sanitation, drinking water, and, recently, air quality). The likelihood of surviving to 65 for United States' males in 1900 was 37.3%; for females 41.0%.[1] By 1950, this had increased to 61.8% for males and 74.3% for females. By 2005 this increased to 78.8% for males and 87.0% for females. From 1954 to 1968, United States mortality was viewed as static—male mortality rates increased 0.2% per year; although female mortality rates, in contrast, declined 0.8% per year. Federal agencies began to plan, and operate, as if the upper limit to population life expectancy had been reached.[2] Projections of the Social Security beneficiary population in the mid-1970s assumed that mortality would decline no further.[3] This view was also expressed by many epidemiologists who suggested that the third phase of the epidemiologic transition involved increases in the prevalence of chronic degenerative diseases[4] caused by adverse social[5] and public health conditions intrinsic to industrial society.[6] Additionally, some authors suggested there were few medical innovations successfully reducing chronic disease progression in the elderly.[7]

Second, the size of birth cohorts increased. Post–World War II baby boom cohorts reached a maximum in 1963 in the United States. The first of those cohorts reaches age 65 in 2012, and age 85 in 2032. The largest cohorts reach age 65 in 2029 and 85 in 2049. The larger size of recent cohorts, and improved mortality up to age 65, will produce large future increases in the elderly population in the United States. Similar population dynamics operate in other developed, and some major developing (e.g., China, India) countries. This will produce severe strains on economic and medical programs for elderly populations.

Third, after being static from 1954 to 1968, mortality in the United States above age 65 began to decline, in part because of the start of national research programs on chronic diseases. The National Heart Institute was created in 1949. The Framingham Heart Study began in 1950. Actually, although reductions in chronic disease mortality were identified as starting in 1968, a more comprehensive examination suggests that mortality declines for select chronic diseases began earlier. Declines in stroke mortality can be traced back to at least 1925.[8] Declines in male heart disease prevalence became evident after examining data on U.S. Civil War veterans age 65 and over who were assessed for pensions in 1910. A comparison of heart disease prevalence in Civil War veterans in 1910 with World War II veterans aged 65 and over in 1985 showed a decline of 66% in the intervening 75 years.[9] From 1950 to 1998, age-standardized heart disease mortality rates declined 58.8%; stroke mortality declined 71.7%.

Reductions in chronic disease mortality raised concern about society's "carrying" capacity for a growing elderly population because it suggested that the number of years individuals live after age 65 would be significantly extended. Although Social Security finances benefit from an increasing number of persons living through their labor force years to age 65, living beyond 65 increases the financial burden on Social Security, Medicare, and Medicaid programs. Recognition of the declines after 1968 in chronic disease mortality, and life expectancy increases above age 65, raised concerns about the long-term fiscal stability of the U.S. Social Security system. In 1982, in addition to payroll tax increases, increases in the Social Security normal retirement age from 65 to 67 were scheduled to occur from 2003 to 2017. Increases in the retirement age to age 70, or even 74, are currently being debated in Britain and Japan. A Japanese study suggested that future economic growth could be compromised by population aging. That study anticipated that one quarter of Japan's population will be over 65 by 2025 using estimates of life expectancy limits that were exceeded by 3 years by Japanese females in 1992.[10,11] Japanese life expectancy continues to be the world's highest, with 85.6 years for females in 2005.

Policy and social responses to population aging depends upon a fourth dynamic—changes in the average health of the elderly. Was the health of a person age 70 in 2005 better on average than the health of a 70-year-old in 1970; will the health of an 80-year-old in 2040 be better than the health of an 80-year-old in 2005? U.S. data suggest that the answers to these questions are yes. Significant declines in the prevalence of chronic disability and morbidity in the elderly population were observed from 1982 to 2004–2005, and appear likely to continue to 2006 and beyond.[12–17]

Even recent concerns over an obesitty epidemic in the United States seem to be overstated. Although obesity (measured by BMI >30.0) prevalence did increase in the United States from 1980 to 2000, its adverse health effects seem to have been muted by improvements from 1960 to 2006 in the ability to manage the circulatory disease risk factors that link obesity to diabetes and circulatory disease and death. Indeed, even the linkage of obesity to chronic disability seems to have been modulated.[18] Thus the obesity epidemic will not aggravate U.S. Medicare spending to the degree suggested by some U.S. economists.[19]

Such health changes have profound effects on the social and economic institutions of a country and on its health care delivery and financing system.[20] There are already popular responses in the perceived lower limit to "old age" in the United States. A recent survey suggested that persons age 50 thought a person has to reach age 80 before being "elderly." This was due to changing social perceptions and economic realities due to the growing proportion of the total U.S. population over age 65, and the effects on housing, insurance, and other private markets along with physical changes in younger old persons. Fundamental research issues involve determining parameters of the population health dynamics underlying changing social perceptions and economics. Whether or not improvements in health and functioning continue at late ages, and can be accelerated by judicious public health and medical innovations and investments, will affect how the United States' and other developed countries' social and economic institutions respond in the future to a growing elderly population.

A difficulty in anticipating future improvements in health at, for example, ages 85 and 95, is that changes depend in part upon both historical and future conditions. Historical factors are important because the individuals who will be the elderly and oldest-old cohorts in the next 65 years are already alive and have accumulated significant early exposures that partly determine the age trajectories of health parameters. Historical factors determine both the number of elderly persons (by reducing early mortality), and the mix of health problems they present (i.e., parameters of individual's health change with age and vary due to differences in the prior risk factor experiences of birth cohorts). That is, depending both upon the cohort an elderly person is in and the individual's life experiences, the principal health manifestations of aging may vary considerably. For example, very elderly cohorts may have little early smoking experience, and hence, little chronic pulmonary disease. Recent cohorts of postmenopausal females, because of the early use of exogenous estrogens, may have reduced osteoporosis and coronary heart disease (CHD) risks. An analysis of future conditions is necessary because we are in a historically unique period where many biomedical technologies and their clinical application are maturing so that many conditions once palliatively managed are now subject to disease-modifying treatments (e.g., rheumatoid arthritis[21] and, recently, osteoarthritis using orthobiologics[22]). Next, we briefly review historical and future inputs to the health dynamics of the elderly population, and then forecast what "old age" will signify in the future.

HISTORICAL DETERMINANTS OF THE FUTURE HEALTH OF THE ELDERLY

The realized human life span is increasing. The first well-documented case of a centenarian was reported in 1800.[23] The first well-documented achievement of the age of 110 years was in 1932. The first well-documented achievement of the age of 120 years (Jean Marie Calment; who lived over 122 years) was in 1995. There are partly documented reports of ages of 125 years being achieved for a Brazilian female; and 127 years for a U.S. Hispanic female. Thus the maximum documented human life span increased 10 years from 1800 to 1932, and over 12 years from 1932 to 1997 (i.e., at over twice the earlier rate). The number of centenarians in the United States increased 7% per year from 1960 to 1987. That growth continued with 54,000 centenarians estimated to be alive in 1995 and 82,000 centenarians estimated to be alive in 2007 (a 51% increase).[24] Similar annual rates of increase in the number of centenarians are found in other developed countries.[25] Thus centenarians are no longer a rarity, although population studies of their current and past health characteristics are.[26] One U.S. population study, the National Long Term Care Survey (NLTCS), oversampled persons 95 and above in 1994, 1999, and 2004. The age range of new elderly and extreme elderly cohorts is now broad enough (e.g., 65 to 115 years of age) that the parameters of the health consequences of aging can differ significantly across the cohorts.[27]

Evidence suggests that the health of the extreme elderly is improving and that interventions can be successful at late ages. Indeed, one recent study showed active life expectancy increased relatively faster at age 85 than at age 65.[17] One factor in health improvements is the effect of early mortality on the health of very elderly populations; "high" early mortality in a cohort "selects out" its genetically less fit members between ages 50 to 85. In a Swedish study, the relative risk of CHD mortality in monozygotic twin pairs was roughly 15 to 1 in middle age. Above age 85, the relative risk was 1.0.[28] Selection caused thyroid autoantibodies in Italian centenarians to be only as prevalent as they were at 50, even though their prevalence increased from ages 50 to 85.[29] Genetically determined lung cancer (because of defects in the cytochrome P-450 enzyme system) peaks at 70% at age 50; by age 70 the genetic form of the disease is 20% of cases.[30] ApoE4 (apolipoprotein E4), associated with heart disease and dementia risk, declines with age from a prevalence of more than 20% at age 80 to about 5% at age 100.[31] The null allele *C4B*Qo* is associated with heart attack risk in middle-aged males, with such risks (and selection against the genotype) occurring at later ages for females.[32,33]

If mortality selection were the only factor determining the health of extreme elderly cohorts, average health would decline as the proportion surviving from birth to late ages increased. Indeed, in recent analyses, younger cohorts had higher active life expectancies than older cohorts (M837). Thus factors other than selection must affect the health of the extreme elderly including medical innovations.

A study of surgery performed on patients aged 90 to 103 showed that intraoperative mortality declined from 29% in the 1960s to 8% by 1985.[34] The study was performed because surgery rates over age 90 increased fivefold from 1979 to 1989. The 5-year survival of this surgical group (mean age 93.5 years) was better than the general population (i.e., a 5-year survival of 21% versus 16% in regional life tables). A factor in the success of surgical interventions was the small number of "ever smokers" in the cohort and the low prevalence of chronic pulmonary disease.

Nutritional factors were thought to cause the reductions in chronic morbidity in Fogel's[9] study of Civil War veterans. One theory suggests that prenatal nutrition affects the risk of chronic disease at late ages[35–37] because the prenatal development of major organ systems is affected by maternal nutrition. In U.S. Civil War veterans born 1825 to 1844, the high prevalence of chronic disease was thought to be a result of poor maternal and early nutrition differentially affecting the development of major organ systems. Improvements from 1910 to 1985 in physiologic status at late ages was argued to be a result of improved early nutrition between the experience of the 1825 to 1844 and 1900 to 1920 cohorts. Fogel traced this to temporal increases in stature and body mass index (BMI) on Waaler surfaces.[38] Similar improvements were found in functional and strength measures between Civil War recruits and military personnel post–World War II in the Gould samples.[39]

Another theory suggests that improved food hygiene reduced exposures to viral and other chronic "slow" infections (e.g., cytomegalovirus [CMV], herpesvirus, and *Chlamydia pneumoniae*[40,41]) in animal food sources causing later reductions in atherosclerosis in adults.[42] They suggest that thermal food processing and tighter regulations on livestock production reduced the risk of chronic circulatory diseases and certain cancers[43] by reducing the risk of chronic viral and other infections.[42,44] That is, recent declines in heart disease mortality were traced to the ingestion of atherogenic viruses in pre–World War II and postwar declines in infection rates as food hygiene improved. A number of events shaped these trends; vesicular exanthema, a viral disease of swine, was discovered in 1932. Controls for this and other livestock infections began in California in 1945 to 1949, a state showing early (1950) declines in heart disease. An outbreak of vesicular exanthema in 1952 mandated national regulations requiring thermal processing of livestock feed. Hog cholera eradication programs began in 1962. The Swine Health Protection Act was passed in 1980 to prevent another virus from entering the food chain. Thermal processing of prepared foods, although existing as a technology at the turn of the century, expanded rapidly after World War II. Some early models of atherosclerosis[45,46] suggested that infectious agents were involved in addition to inflammatory processes, homeostatic factors, and blood lipids.[47] However, the technical ability (e.g., polymerase chain reaction [PCR] or fluorescence in situ hybridization [FISH]) to detect the presence of agents, their genetic effects, or persistent immunologic responses is relatively recent.[48]

Another model suggests that chronic circulatory disease change was in part due to changes in the dietary levels of micronutrients, such as vitamins A, B, C, E, and D. Vitamins A, C, and E are antioxidants and may reduce the rate of oxidation of low-density lipoprotein (LDL) cholesterol in macrophages (producing "foam cells")—a factor in atherogenesis.[47] Vitamins A and E are cellular redifferentiating agents possibly reducing the risk of some cancers.[49] The dietary levels of vitamins A (and other retinoids) and C depend upon the availability of fresh fruits and vegetables—foodstuffs difficult to preserve before refrigeration and transportation technologies allowed persons in northern temperate climates to continue to consume such foodstuffs through the winter. This also could affect hypertension and stroke risk in that refrigeration reduced the use of salt as a food preservative. Increased consumption of fruits may also have increased potassium intake and lowered hypertension.

Vitamin D has long been a supplement. Moon et al[50] noted that the curative effects of cod liver oil on rickets were documented in 1917. By 1923, the United States imported half a million gallons of fish liver oil; nearly 3 million gallons in 1930. Ultraviolet radiation of milk began in the United States in 1924. Production of vitamin D rose from 35 lb in 1948 to 14,000 lb in 1972. Supplementation became problematic in that vitamin D is a potent hormonal agent with a narrow therapeutic trough. Reductions in supplementation were mandated by the Food and Drug Administration (FDA) in 1972.

Vitamin D metabolism is complex, including effects on cellular calcium metabolism and parathyroid hormone production, possibly leading to hypertension.[51] Vitamin D interferes with the uptake of magnesium. Concomitant with increased vitamin D supplementation were declines in magnesium in the United States diet because of the use of nitrogen-based fertilizers. Vitamin D also increases the absorption of iron, so oversupplementation could affect heart disease by reducing magnesium (which could increase production of aldosterone[52]) and by increasing iron absorption—increasing LDL oxidation (also by causing increases in serum calcium and calcification of plaque), stroke (by affecting hypertension), and osteoporosis (by direct effects on osteoclasts and bone resorption). It is relatively recent that the standards for vitamin D supplementation, especially in the elderly, are now argued to be too low with increases of vitamin D intake in the elderly suggested.

A fourth model involves elevated homocysteine because of increased meat consumption and genetic or dietary deficiencies of vitamin B_6 and B_{12}. Decreasing renal function with age may adversely affect physiologic vitamin B levels, as may age changes in liver metabolism through the eighth decade of life. The homocysteine model suggests that atherosclerosis is partially a disease of protein toxicity whereby failure to detoxify certain sulfur-based amino acid products of protein metabolism leads to damage in arterial endothelium.[53] The homocysteine model may not only explain initiating events in circulatory disease,[54] but also possibly osteoarthritic and rheumatoid arthritic changes (by affecting cartilage matrix formation) and increases in dementia.[55] Vitamin B_6 also has a wide range of physiologic effects (e.g., DNA binding and nuclear localization) on a super family of ligand activated transcription factors that exert biologic effects by regulating target gene expression.[56,57] Recently, however, folic acid supplementation mandated in Canada and the United States was associated with considerable reduction in stroke risk as compared to Britain, where such supplementation did not occur.[58]

CURRENT AND FUTURE BIOMEDICAL INPUTS TO AGING

The factors described above determined health parameters of persons now entering advanced age ranges. To respond to this heterogeneity of aging parameters, and recent changes in the physiologic manifestation of aging changes, are treatment modalities made possible by recent biomedical research. Research focused on aging began in the United States with the creation of the National Institute on Aging (NIA) in 1974. In the 1960s, biologic senescence was often viewed as a genetically determined cellular process operating universally in all tissue types, with chronic diseases believed to be manifestations of its effects. Hayflick[59] suggested such a model after observing that human fibroblasts could reproduce only 50 to 60 times. An experiment[60] challenging this view examined the number of cell replications remaining for fibroblasts drawn from persons aged 30 to 80 years. Cells lost one replication for every 5 years of life. Cristofalo et al[61] found similar results. Thus, if this is the basic mechanism of senescence, it would not limit life spans near current levels. It has been suggested that defects in mitochondrial DNA may be a more likely biologic limitation to the maximum human life span, suggesting a limit of 129 years.

In the 1970s it became clear that many aging studies had design flaws (i.e., the rate of loss of physiologic function was tracked in "representative" elderly populations). This confounded the intrinsic physiologic rate of aging with the age-dependent prevalence of chronic disease determined by the history of environmental exposures. Studies of populations screened for existing chronic diseases lowered estimates of the age rate of loss of physiologic functions (e.g., the age rate of loss of cardiac function in an active elderly population was one half that in earlier studies).[62] Age-related disease processes were found to be physiologically more complex, with much wider variation in expression than previously thought.[63,64]

In the 1980s, medical science began to demonstrate significant potential for modifying chronic disease processes. Atherosclerosis was once thought to be a product of an aging circulatory system. Now it appears to be reversible by nutritional modification (e.g., cholesterol reduction) and other interventions,[65,66] with functional responses evident before anatomic changes[67,68] and facilitated by antioxidant therapy.[69] Left ventricular hypertrophy (LVH) was thought to be because of age-related remodeling of cardiomyocytes. However, angiotensin-converting enzyme (ACE)-II inhibitors and controlling hypertension can also cause regression of LVH,[70] possibly by blocking the effects of aldosterone in remodeling myocytes as fibrotic tissue.[71] Many classic signs of senescence, or old age, are now well-defined pathologic processes (e.g., frailty and osteoporosis, cognitive impairment, and Alzheimer's disease). With the pathologic mechanisms identified, it is possible to develop disease-modifying interventions, especially at the molecular level, and thus to remold the aging process.

Some early chronic disease and aging interventions were initiated serendipitously. Exogenous estrogens were used by 3 million U.S. women in 1985 for post menopausal symptoms. By 1994 this had grown to 10 million women. It appears that exogenous estrogens reduce the risk of osteoporosis and CHD[72] in postmenopausal women.[73] Research[74] suggested that estrogen supplementation could reduce the risk of dementia by 50%. A recent major clinical trial, however, calls those benefits into question, although reanalysis of those data suggested female Hormone Replacement Therapy has to be initiated shortly after menopause to have positive effects. Negative effects of HRT seemed most manifest in very elderly women where HRT was initiated 15 to 20 years postmenopause. Further analysis is needed to clarify the dynamics of treatment and response. Evidence suggests that testosterone supplementation may have benefits for males in terms of reduced dementia risk. Data from the 1999 NLTCS suggested there have been large declines in dementia risk from 1982 to 1999.[15]

Aspirin has long been used as an analgesic and to control fever. Recently, its potential in secondary prevention of stroke and heart attack by affecting platelet adhesion has been realized.[75] An association of aspirin consumption with reduced risk of colorectal cancer was found, as has a speculative association with reductions in Alzheimer's disease risks.[76] Nonsteroidal anti-inflammatory drugs (NSAIDs), by blocking inflammatory tissue responses, may affect other cancers by affecting the ability of tumor cells to metastasize and clonally organize.

Modeling senescence as the genetic control of the number of cell replications was given impetus by investigations of the end-segment of the human chromosome, the telomere, and an enzyme, telomerase, that induces its lengthening.[77] The evidence for the telomere controlling senescence is mixed. The telomere does decrease in length as the cell replicates but may correlate more strongly with oxidative stress. However, even when a given length is reached, although the cell ceases to divide, it may exhibit stable metabolism and function. Bone marrow and blood cells express low levels of telomerase, with that activity distributed across different cell types. Furthermore, its production may be controlled hormonally and by growth factors in damaged (e.g., the lung) tissues. Thus there may not be an absolute shutoff of telomerase in somatic cells but continuing production at low levels and with continuing genetic potential for production. This is consistent with templates of telomerase ribonucleic acid (RNA) existing in somatic cells and the ability of tumor cells to express telomerase after a crisis phase.[78]

Evidence of the role of telomerase in neoplastic growth is clear. Normally, cells stop replicating while the telomere is still long. It may be that the p53 mediated pathway to apoptosis[79] is activated when the telomere drops below a functionally suboptimal length. Then the cell enters a crisis phase that leads either to cell death or a reactivation of telomerase, a stabilized telomere length, and an immortal cell line.[80] Confirmation was found in that telomerase activity was present in 68% of stage I, and 95% of advanced stage breast tumors, but not in normal tissue. Telomerase was expressed in 45% of fibroadenomas, benign breast lesions.[81]

The search for mechanisms of senescence is difficult.[82] Many physiologic mechanisms associated with aging and cell growth have proved to be more mutable by environmental factors, even at the genetic and molecular level, than once thought.[47,83,84] Some authors[85] argued that human life expectancy is limited to 85 years unless medical science develops interventions at the molecular level to modify parameters of aging. The problem with these arguments is in defining molecular interventions; many existing interventions operate at a molecular level. Nutritional factors (e.g., vitamins A, B) may affect receptor structure in the cell membrane, the message to DNA, and the transcription of genetic code to specific proteins. Some interventions have been used for a long time, even though their mechanisms were initially not understood. Doxorubicin, an anthracycline, is a potent chemotherapeutic agent that disrupts cell replication by affecting nuclear proteins: Topoisomerase II α and β.[83] Early chemotherapeutic techniques were based on relatively simple principles where cell death was a function of drug concentration. The ways (e.g., interactions of c-*myc*, *bcl*-2, and *p53* genes[48]) in which apoptosis is induced, and interventions in ancillary processes such as angiogenesis, growth factor dependency, metastatic invasion, and cellular redifferentiation, are therapeutic avenues being investigated at the molecular level.

To illustrate, an agent in use a long time, for which the mechanisms of molecular action are still being elaborated, is the antiestrogen, tamoxifen. This compound was given to older women with advanced estrogen receptor positive breast cancer to control its growth.[86] At first, growth inhibition was attributed to competitive binding with estrogen in a tumor cell's estrogen receptors. This initially raised concern that tamoxifen would exacerbate osteoporosis and heart disease. However, tamoxifen's interaction with the receptor was more complex—sometimes being an agonist (i.e., it was protective against bone loss and circulatory disease). It appears that tamoxifen affects the ability to induce transcriptional activity in the carboxy-terminal ligand binding domain.[87] Of further interest was that tamoxifen affected estrogen receptor–negative tumor cells, and in interaction with chemotherapeutic agents (e.g., cisplatin),[88] by synergistically interacting in inducing apoptosis with other agents (e.g., vitamin D)[89]—possibly by increasing the expression of estrogen receptors or by blocking the action of drug-resistant genes by affecting the calcium channel membrane transport of the drug.[90,91] The effects on estrogen receptor–negative breast cancer cells may be due to the induction of apoptosis by overexpression of c-*myc*, mRNA, and protein.[92] These effects may be enhanced by retinoic acid and vitamin D_3 analogs.[93,94] Interventions into the transcriptional expression of genotypes by known agents is interesting, given growing insights into the relation of carcinogenesis and senescence.[80,95,96]

THE FUTURE OF AGING

The above suggest that (1) the physiologic expression of aging changes will vary in the future because of major changes in nutrition, infectious disease risks, and hygiene, some exposures inducing stable genetic aberrations,[48,84] and (2) that we already have many agents and therapies affecting the molecular transcriptional expression of genotype, although our knowledge of the details of those mechanisms, and how to intervene, are not complete. It can be argued, however, that we have only recently developed the scientific tools (e.g., PCR, restriction fragment length polymorphism [RFLP]; chromosome painting[48,84]) to accelerate our understanding of these mechanisms, and the techniques and agents for intervening (e.g., rational drug design; nonimmunosuppressive cyclosporin, PSC833).[97]

Techniques intervening at a molecular level are not restricted to cancer treatments but also apply to many other disorders.[98] A promising area is the improved regulation of the aging immune system.[99] A promising recent development was the observation that interleukin-10 (IL-10) suppressed tumor growth and inhibited spontaneous metastasis.[100,101] This was a surprise because IL-10 suppressed macrophage and helper T-cell function, and delayed hypersensitivity reactions. In suppressing macrophage activity, IL-10 suppressed release of proinflammatory cytokines, nitric oxide, and reactive oxygen intermediaries. It, however, stimulated natural killer (NK) cells and chemoattraction of CD8+ cells and neutrophils. Inhibition of macrophage activity may have a tumor suppressive effect by reducing the local production of multiple growth or angiogenesis factors. Alterations of immune function (e.g., by vitamin A, C, or E supplementation[102,103]), and inflammatory responses and angiogenesis may be important in autoimmune disorders[104] and in certain stages of atherogenesis.[105,106] As in other cases, nutritional factors hold promise for modifying abnormal immunoresponse (e.g., the role of fish oil supplementation on MHC-II molecules and the membranes of human white blood cells affecting auto-immune disorders).[107] Omega 3 fatty acids may protect against chronic obstructive lung disease in ever smokers.[108]

Thus there is a matrix of interrelations of physiologic processes that underlie the major chronic diseases expressed in old age. For example, the expression of Lp(a), a factor in circulatory disease risks, also has a strong association with breast cancer risk and its ability to metastasize.[109] The role of inflammatory response, and of the local production of growth factors, is likely crucial to both tumor growth and the development of atherosclerotic plaque.[101,105,106] There are likely associations of osteoporosis and atherosclerosis due to altered calcium metabolism.[110] Osteoporosis may be linked to hypertension and renal function by vitamin D metabolism.[98,111]

Because of this rapidly increasing understanding of disease process and therapeutic intervention at the molecular level, it is reasonable to anticipate future and accelerating changes in disease, function, and mortality risks at late ages. One of the crucial factors is to develop therapeutics with positive effect profiles. This is possible because of the above-mentioned matrix of physiologic functions that interrelate many age-dependent pathologies at the molecular level. For example, ACE-II inhibitors have positive effects on lipid and glucose metabolism, reduce LVH, possibly increase β-receptor density, and control hypertension.[112–114] Certain β-blockers may improve β-receptor activity in the myocardium by downregulating both the response to norepinephrine and to activity as an antioxidant.[115] The reason that IL-10 is promising is because it does not produce the serious side effects found with many other cytokines.[116]

An area of molecular medicine that is likely to strongly affect the health and functioning of the U.S. elderly population is in the management of osteoarthritis. Osteoarthritis is currently viewed as a medically untreatable condition in the United States (less so in Europe where glucosamine supplementation is more accepted), with current clinical responses involving surgical joint replacement (especially of the knee and hip). Although reasonably effective, alternative surgeries (e.g., hip resurfacing approved for use in the United States only last year by the FDA) and orthobiologic approaches to cartilage regeneration (using growth factors, stem cells for chondrocytes, and new materials for cartilage growth matrices) are finishing phase II trials and may represent improved approaches to deal with the 50% to 60% of elderly with some degree of osteoarthritis.[22] This, combined with new immunomodulatory drugs for rheumatoid arthritis, could greatly enhance the functionality of the U.S. elderly population.

One argument may be that this increased understanding of disease mechanisms may produce medical interventions too expensive to provide en masse to a rapidly growing elderly population (e.g., the prescription of human growth hormone). This may, however, be due to a misunderstanding of the economics of biomedical innovation in that while the initial development of new technologies is expensive the evolution of subsidiary production technologies reduces unit costs and more of the population is treated (i.e., research and development costs are amortized over larger numbers of patients and the full benefits for the population are realized).[117] For example, ACE-II inhibitors reduce the number of days of hospitalization required for congestive heart failure (CHF).[118] As a result, the cost benefit ratio of ACE-II inhibitors, appropriately applied, can be quite high.[70] *Helicobacter pylori* was characterized in 1984. The role of *H. pylori* in the mechanism for most ulcers and gastric cancers[119] identified new treatment modalities that are very cost-effective.

Antibiotic treatment for *H. pylori* costs about $200 compared with about $100 per month for the use of histamine blockers, which do not cure the disease. Given that there may be 4.5 million ulcer cases in the United States, the savings would be significant. Other technologies have proven cost-effective, such as day surgery and plastic lens implants for cataracts[120]; pacemakers more appropriate for cardiac functional decline at late ages with dual chambers which respond to the increasing importance of arterial pulse in regulating cardiac output with age.[121] Thus the correct understanding of a disease mechanism and linkages may produce synergistic interventions that eventually prove economic, especially if disease control is also accompanied by functional increases at late ages.[122] Estimates of the savings to Medicare of reductions in functional disability prevalence from 1982 to 1995 could be more than 7% of costs; or $180 billion to $200 billion (in 1995 dollars[12]).

Even more important is the failure of economic evaluations of medical costs to compare costs to the benefits of improved health (i.e., the return on investment). For example, the U.S. labor force rate of growth is projected to slow from 1.2% in 1996 to 0.8% in 2006, and 0.3% in 2016 with the consequence of slowing economic growth. Improving health at later ages, at the rates achieved from 1982 to 2004, could prove to be a strong stimulus to economic growth by enhancing the size and quality of the human capital pool at later ages.[123] In addition, economically, the share of GDP expended on health services could usefully grow as other consumer goods (e.g., electronics) markets saturate and disposable income grows.[124]

If costs are not such an important limiting factor to advancement of health at late ages when improved health is properly economically evaluated, what might aging in the mid-twenty-first century look like? Projections for the United States suggest that control of major circulatory disease risk factors, over a long enough time for their regulation to affect existing disease, could significantly increase the mean age at which CHD and stroke deaths occur.[125] The predominant forms of CHD would involve interactions of hypertension, atherosclerotic change, and age-related declines in cardiac function (e.g., age-related loss of β-receptor binding efficiency) that would become further dominated by the age-related changes in cardiac function. Cancer mortality has begun to show significant declines (e.g., 16% drop from 1990 to 2006) because of a variety of factors, with many new treatments now in clinical trials. Evidence suggests that significant breast cancer mortality reductions have occurred because of the use of tamoxifen in estrogen receptor–positive disease and adjuvant therapy in early node–negative disease.[126,127] Greenspan[128] suggests current chemotherapy, rigorously applied, could reduce the number of U.S. breast cancer deaths by one third. The aging of the population could promote this trend, as recent studies indicate that very young women with breast cancer may respond less favorably than older women to chemotherapy.[129,130] This is due to the generally less aggressive nature of disease in older women and probably to better management of the adverse effects of more aggressive treatments at later ages (e.g., use of granulocyte-colony stimulating factor [G-CSF]). However, progress is evident even for the more aggressive forms of breast cancer because of the development of monoclonal antibodies against specific growth factors, such as Herceptin.

The mix of cancers affecting an older population will change significantly. This will be related to the nature of the host tissue in which the tumor arises. For example, cancer related to infectious processes (liver cancer, gastric cancer) or food spoilage may decline. Other neoplasia related to biologic aging processes (e.g., prostate cancer, multiple myeloma, certain types of lymphoma, late-onset breast cancer) will increase in importance, although the mean age of death from those cancers will also increase. The effects of viral diseases on cancer risks and possibly on atherogenesis and general immunologic dysfunction (e.g., plasma cell dyscrasias of unknown significance, which often progress to multiple myeloma)[99] will become more treatable as antiviral agents improve and as our understanding of the chronic effects of viruses on the immune system advances. Thus there are a number of areas where therapeutic advances could occur, affecting multiple stages of very lengthy chronic disease processes. In addition, therapeutic advances could be supported by behavioral and lifestyle changes among middle-aged and elderly persons. This can be anticipated in that (1) the proportion of elderly cohorts who are better educated is increasing (i.e., better educated populations tend to be more amenable to public health messages)[131] and (2) physical activity has been shown to have benefits to extreme ages.[132–134]

These changes could increase life expectancy in the next 50 to 60 years (i.e., by 2050 to 2060) to 95 to 100 years.[135,136] This compares with U.S. Census Bureau high life expectancy projections for 2050 of 86.4 years for males and 92.3 years for females.[24] Census Bureau life expectancy estimates are based on extrapolations of mortality trends. Our higher estimates are based on using multiple risk factor data, their dynamics, and assumptions about the ability to jointly control those factors.[135,136] For example, in Kravchanko et al,[137] comparison of stringent risk factor control versus programs for progenitor cell replacement to reduce the arterial damage caused by atherosclerosis shows the potential benefits of such stem cell therapies.

These projections do not assume that heart disease, stroke, and cancer are eliminated. They do assume that the mean age at death for each is increased because of preventive and disease-modifying interventions on risk factor profiles. Those changes will also affect the proportion of deaths because of specific causes. Male cancer mortality could increase from about 20% to 40% of deaths at all ages. The largest changes would come from increased proportions of cancer deaths above age 85. For females, cancer mortality would increase relatively more (to about 60% of all deaths) because the adverse effects of menopausal changes in multiple cardiovascular disease (CVD) risk factors are assumed controlled in the projections. CVD risks would decline moderately (from 65% to 50%) for males as a proportion of all deaths, but those deaths would occur at later ages. For females, the projected declines in CVD deaths are much larger.

Such projections imply different things for U.S. society's carrying capacity for the elderly. In census projections, the high life expectancy series projects a U.S. population of 416 million by 2050. In this projection, 1% would be over age 100 (4.1 million), 7.2% would be over age 85 (30 million), and 23.3% would be over age 65 (97 million). The proportion of the population above a given age in the census projections is strongly affected by fertility assumptions. For example, Social Security Administration (SSA) cohort life tables for persons born in 1950 (which use less favorable mortality assumptions) imply that 5.6% of females and 1.5% of males live to age 100. Assuming a 3 to 1 survival advantage for females to age 100, this suggests that 4.6% of the 1950 cohort survives to age 100. For the 1990 cohort, survival to age 100 is 10.2% for females and 3.3% for males, or 8.4% combined. Thus in a stable population, a large proportion of persons reach age 100 even in less optimistic SSA 1990 life tables. In risk factor–based projections, the U.S. population is projected to be 456 million persons in 2050, with 14% over age 85, and 33% over age 65. Although these proportions are larger than in the census projections, they are not grossly different from the 25% of the Japanese population expected to be over age 65 in 2025. If fertility and immigration is lower than assumed in Japanese census projections, then the proportion of the population over age 65 and over 85 would be higher. Even the extreme projections made from risk factor data do not take into account recent studies suggesting that human mortality never exceeds 40% at any age (i.e., 40% is the maximum mortality rate)—an assumption built into the Society of Actuaries 1994 group annuity tables.[138] Such estimates are consistent with estimates from multiple studies showing that the annual increase in mortality rates slows to very low values (2% to 3%) about age 100.[26] These slow increases in mortality are apparently because of the high mortality rates of very elderly persons with high levels of disability. Thus the average level of disability about age 95 tends to stabilize because of the equilibrium with mortality rates at those ages.[125] Recent analysis even suggests prospects for mortality risk decline at advanced (i.e., 105+) ages.[139]

The question emerges of how a society and economy must change to deal with a population with such a high proportion of elderly, and quite possibly healthy and functional, persons. This is primarily a problem only if the commensurate change in the age-specific health status of the population does not occur. The health-mortality factors discussed above suggest that the natural dynamics of mortality, disability, and mortality (i.e., their dynamic equilibrium[140]) enforce this in part. There is also evidence of such changes in current health expenditures. Lubitz et al[141] found that the average Medicare expenditure for those who died at age 70 was $35,511, compared with $65,633 for those who survived to age 101. Thus the average Medicare expense per year for centenarians from ages 65 to 101 was $1,823 compared with $7,100 per year for those who died at age 70. Thus the pattern of a declining rate of Medicare expenditures with age contrasts to the accumulated liability of increased life expectancy for Social Security.

If disability declines, as observed from 1982 to 2004–2005, health costs may decrease even more rapidly at later ages.[17,123] This pattern also seems consistent with the different patterns of medical problems that may be faced at late ages in the future. Disability will not only be prevented but, in the future, functional loss will be increasingly reversed by "regenerative medicine" (e.g., orthobiologic management of osteoarthritis). Thus the primary response to the social costs of such large elderly populations might be increases in the normal retirement age for Social Security. Each year of increase in the normal retirement age for Social Security has a large fiscal impact. Thus, if the normal retirement age could be increased to age 70 (or 74), because the average physiologic status at those ages is now equivalent to the physiologic status at age 65 in, say, 1982—then a large portion of the fiscal burden of population aging could be addressed. Indeed, given restrictions on the ultimate size of human populations, improvements in health at advanced ages may be an economic necessity in the United States and other developed nations with rapidly changing population age structures.

KEY POINTS

The Future of Old Age

- Population aging
- Morbid conditions prevalent at advanced ages
- Centenarians and growth of extreme elderly
- Barker's hypothesis
- Nutritional supplementation and exercise as modifiers of aging
- Biologic inputs to aging and drug therapies
- Regenerative medicine: hormonal modulation
- Epidemiologic transition
- Disability prevalence declines
- Mortality declined in the second half of the twentieth century

For a complete list of references, please visit online only at www.expertconsult.com

CHAPTER 4

Evolution Theory and the Mechanisms of Aging

Thomas B. L. Kirkwood

The question "Why does aging occur?" calls for answers both at the level of proximate, physiological mechanisms and also at the level of ultimate, evolutionary origins. This chapter provides an understanding of why aging has evolved and examines what evolution theory can tell us about the kinds of mechanisms we might regard as prime candidates to explain senescence.

Evolution theory is well recognized as a powerful tool with which to inquire about the genetic basis of the aging process.[1–4] Although human aging has its roots long ago in our past, the study of its evolution can throw important light on key present-day challenges. For example, a range of population-based studies, including one based on genealogical analysis of the entire population of Iceland, has shown consistent evidence for a generic contribution to human longevity.[5] There is growing interest in knowing how many and what kinds of genes are likely to be involved in this heritability.[6,7] There is also interest in human genetic disorders such as Werner's syndrome and Hutchinson-Gilford progeria that are characterized by acceleration of many aspects of the senescent phenotype (see Chapter 11).

Before addressing questions about the evolutionary origin of aging it is important to be precise about how the term "aging" is to be understood. In this chapter, aging is defined as "a progressive, generalized impairment of function, resulting in a loss of adaptive response to stress and in a growing risk of age-related disease." The overall effect of these changes is summed up in the increase in the probability of dying, or age-specific death rate, in the population.

This definition of aging—in terms of a mortality pattern showing progressive increase in age-specific mortality—allows comparisons to be made even among species where the detailed features of the aging process may differ markedly. In phylogenetic terms, aging is widespread but by no means universal.[9–12] The fact that not all species show an increase in age-specific mortality indicates that aging is not an inevitable consequence of wear-and-tear. On the other hand, the fact that very many species do show such an increase is evidence that the evolution of aging has occurred under rather general circumstances.

EVOLUTION OF AGING

Theories on the evolution of aging seek to explain why aging occurs through the action of natural selection. The decline in survivorship, which is often also accompanied by a decline in fertility, means that there is an age-associated loss of Darwinian fitness that is clearly deleterious to the organism in which it occurs. Natural selection acts to increase fitness, so it is at once clear that selection should be expected, other things being equal, to oppose aging. The challenge to evolution theory is thus to explain why aging occurs in spite of its drawbacks.

Programmed or "adaptive" aging

It is sometimes suggested that despite its disadvantages to the individual, aging is beneficial and even necessary at the species level, for example, to prevent overcrowding.[13,14] In this case, genes that actively cause aging might have evolved specifically to program the end of life, in the same way as genes program development.

The difficulty with this view is that there is little evidence that intrinsic aging serves as a significant contributor to mortality in natural populations,[15] which means that it apparently does not play the adaptive role suggested for it. The theory also embodies the questionable supposition that selection for advantage at the species level will be more effective than selection among individuals for the advantages of a longer life. Aging is clearly a disadvantage to the individual, so any mutation that inactivated the hypothetical adaptive aging genes would confer a fitness advantage, and therefore, the nonaging mutation should spread through the population unless countered by selection at the species or group level. Conditions under which "group selection" can work successfully are highly restrictive,[16] especially when there is selection in the opposite direction acting at the level of the individual. Briefly, it is necessary that the population be divided among fairly isolated groups, and that the introduction of a nonaging genotype into a group should rapidly lead to the group's extinction. The latter condition is necessary to provide the selection between groups that might, in principle, counter the tendency for selection at the level of individuals to favor the spread of nonaging mutants. Although theoretical special cases have been constructed that might permit the selection of genes to cause aging, it appears unlikely that the necessary conditions will be met with sufficient generality to explain the evolution of aging.

Selection weakens with age

An observation of central importance to the evolution of aging is that the force of natural selection—that is, its ability to discriminate between alternative genotypes—weakens with age.[15,17–20] Because natural selection operates through the differential effects of genes on fitness, its discriminatory power must decline with age in proportion to the decline in the remaining fraction of the organism's lifetime expectation of reproduction. This is true whether or not the species exhibits aging.

The attenuation in the force of natural selection with age means inevitably that there is only loose genetic control over the later portions of the life span. For this reason it has been suggested that aging might be due to an accumulation in the germ line of mutations, which potentially are deleterious but are not expressed, or which produce no phenotypic effect until late in life.[15]

The idea is that if deleterious mutations are expressed so late that most individuals will already have died from some other cause, such as predation, even though the genes involved have the potential to cause harm they will be subject to very little selection against them. Over the generations, a large number of such genes might accumulate. These would cause aging and death only when an individual is removed to a protected environment, away from the hazards of the wild, and so lives long enough to experience their negative effects.

A stronger version of this theory was proposed by Williams,[18] who suggested that because of the declining force of natural selection with age, any gene that conferred an advantage early in life would be favored by selection even if the same gene had deleterious effects at older ages. Such "pleiotropic" genes could explain aging. The decline in the force of natural selection with age would ensure that even quite modest early benefits would outweigh severe harmful side effects, provided the latter occurred late enough.

Disposable soma theory

The disposable soma theory[1,4,21–23] explains aging through asking how best an organism should allocate its metabolic resources, primarily energy—between, on the one hand, keeping itself going from one day to the next, and on the other hand producing progeny to secure the continuance of its genes when it has itself died. No species is immune to hazards such as predation, starvation, and disease. All that is necessary by way of maintenance is that the body remains in sound condition until an age after which most individuals will have died from accidental causes. In fact, a greater investment in maintenance is a disadvantage because it eats into resources that, in terms of natural selection, are better used for reproduction. The theory concludes that the optimum course is to invest fewer resources in the maintenance of somatic tissues than are necessary for indefinite survival (Figure 4-1). The result is that aging occurs through the gradual accumulation of unrepaired somatic defects, but the level of maintenance will be set so that the deleterious effects do not become apparent until an age when survivorship in the wild environment would be extremely unlikely.

Comparison of the evolutionary theories

The adaptive program theory is in a category of its own and support for this theory is weak; it will not be considered further in this chapter. The disposable soma and pleiotropic genes theories are adaptive in the sense that aging is the result of positive selection for aspects of the organism's life history, but the essential difference is that aging itself is not adaptive but is a negative trait that arises only as a by-product or tradeoff of some other benefit. The late-acting deleterious mutations theory assumes an essentially neutral evolutionary process, the accumulation of mutations reflecting the inability of natural selection to maintain tight control over the later portions of the life span.

Among the nonadaptive theories there is a common strand, namely that old organisms count less. This is not due to any implicit assumption of frailty or obsolescence (this would render the theories circular), but to the simple mathematics of mortality. Even if old organisms retain exactly the same vigor as young ones, to the extent that old and young are physiologically indistinguishable, the fact that each cohort becomes numerically attenuated with age means that the selection force weakens. The nonadaptive theories are not mutually exclusive. Therefore, aging might in principle be due to a combination of any of them.

As regards the nature of gene action, the disposable soma theory is the most specific of the evolutionary theories, for it suggests not only why aging occurs but also predicts that the genetic basis of aging is to be found in the genes that regulate levels of somatic maintenance functions. Neither the pleiotropic genes theory nor the late-acting deleterious mutations theory is specific about the nature of the genes involved.

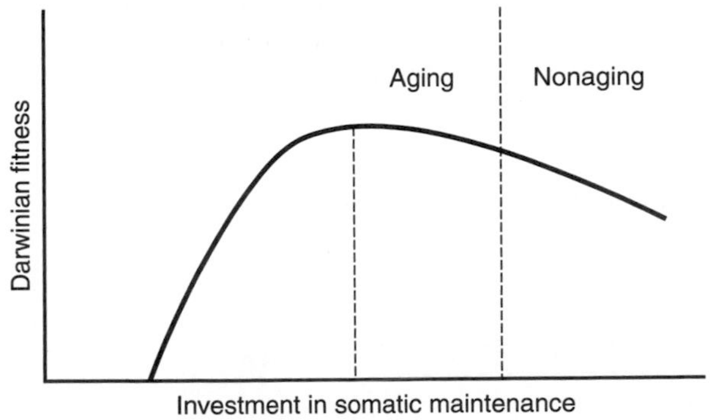

Figure 4-1. Relation between Darwinian fitness and investment in somatic maintenance predicted by the disposable soma theory of aging. Fitness is maximized at a level that is less than that which would be required for indefinite longevity (nonaging).

GENETICS OF LIFE SPAN

This section looks at the genetics of life span, first from the point of view of interspecies comparisons. That is, it will ask the question Why do species have the life spans they do? It will then look at intraspecies variation and heritability of life span. Finally, there is a brief discussion of human progeroid syndrome, such as Werner's and Hutchinson-Gilford progeria, as models of genetically accelerated senescence.

Species differences in longevity

In addition to explaining why aging occurs, evolution theory also must account for differences in species life spans. This raises basic questions about the genetic control of aging: specifically, how many genes are involved and how are these modified by selection to produce changes in life span?

For each of the nonadaptive theories, the generality of the selection forces that are involved suggests that multiple genes will be implicated. If there is a very large number of independent genes causing aging, however, the life span may be slow to change, because modifying a single gene may have little effect by itself and the probability of simultaneous independent modifications will be low. This suggests that either a reasonably small number of primary genes are responsible for aging, or that there exists some mechanism for coordinate regulation.

The evolution of increased life span is most readily explained if it is assumed that an adaptation occurs that results in a general lowering of the accidental (age-independent) death rate. In the late-acting deleterious mutations theory, this may result in new pressure to eliminate or postpone the deleterious gene effects. In the pleiotropic genes theory, the balance between early benefit and late cost may be shifted in favor of reducing the harmful effects on late survival. In the disposable soma theory, there may be selection to tune the optimum investment in maintenance to a higher level.

Variation within species

The variability in life span observed within a species or population clearly owes much to chance, but there is a significant heritable component as well.[5] Martin et al[3] have applied the terms "public" and "private" to denote genetic factors related to aging that may either be specific to individuals or shared across a population (perhaps even across species). Late-acting deleterious mutations are strong candidates for private genes because the fate of such alleles is determined largely by random genetic drift. Public genes are more likely to be those that arise through tradeoffs. In particular, the genes involved in regulating mechanisms of somatic maintenance are likely to be public genes of considerable importance. Although these genes are "public" in the sense that all individuals have them, there may nevertheless be variations within a population in the precise levels at which these functions are set. These variations in setting may in turn be the cause of genetic variation in life expectancy.

As predicted by the disposable soma theory, the level of individual somatic maintenance systems should be set high enough so that the organism remains in sound condition through its natural expectation of life in the wild environment, but not much higher than this, or resources will be wasted. Numerous maintenance systems operate in parallel to preserve viability (Figure 4-2). Depending on the levels at which they are set, each maintenance system can be thought of as "assuring" a given span of life (see also Cutler[24] and Sacher[25] for earlier discussion of the concept of "longevity assurance"). When any one of these critical mechanisms has exhausted its potential for assuring longevity, which happens because the accumulated defects threaten survival, the organism is liable to die.

If we now recall the shape of the fitness curve in Figure 4-1, we see that its peak—the point towards which natural selection is expected to exert evolutionary pressure—is rounded instead of sharp, and so we can expect a fair amount of intrapopulation variance in the precise settings of maintenance processes. Selection is expected to direct these settings toward the peak, but once within the region of the peak, the fitness differences on which selection can operate become quite small.

Putting these ideas together generates the prediction summarized in Figure 4-2. On the average, we expect the longevity assured by individual maintenance systems to be similar. This is because if the setting of any one mechanism is so low that it consistently fails before any of the others, then selection will tend to increase the level at which it is set. Conversely, if any mechanism tends always to fail after the others, then to the extent that this mechanism involves a metabolic cost, there will be selection to tune down the level at which it is set. In individuals, however, the genetic variance within the population is expected to result in variation in the extent to which the organism is predisposed to age from specific causes. For example, some individuals are likely to be less well protected against oxygen radicals than others, and these individuals will therefore experience greater oxidative damage.

Instances of extreme longevity, such as human centenarians, are of special interest for they are likely to be endowed with unusually high levels of each of the important ingredients of the cellular defense network.[6] Such individuals may also be distinguished by their freedom from alleles that predispose toward diseases that otherwise might shorten life expectancy. Schächter et al[27] performed the first genetic study comparing centenarians with younger adult controls, which validated the general potential of this approach. Since then a number of further studies have been conducted to examine the genetics of human longevity.[7]

It is anticipated that the next few years will see the publication of results from several large investigations looking either at individuals of extreme longevity (e.g., centenarians) or at families where there is reason to expect that family members share a genetic endowment predisposing to above-average longevity. Examples of the latter design include studies that are recruiting nonagenarian siblings (i.e., instances where two or more members of the same family are still alive past age 90). The technological advances that are presently being made in the capacity to assess DNA samples for possession of very large numbers of genetic markers at very high speed mean that the focus is now increasingly on genome-wide association studies and the linkage analyses that can be made using family groups. Herein lies both the strength of modern human genetics and a potential difficulty when studying a trait like longevity, which is likely to prove highly polygenic. If large numbers of genetic loci contribute to the longevity phenotype, but these individually make only small contributions, the difficulty of extracting the signals from the statistical noise will be formidable.

Human progeroid syndromes

A number of inherited human diseases have been characterized as showing a phenotype of accelerated aging. The best studied of these conditions is Werner's syndrome, a rare autosomal recessive disorder affecting around 10 in 1 million people, who prematurely develop a variety of major age-related diseases, including arteriosclerosis, ocular cataracts, osteoporosis, malignant neoplasms, and type II diabetes. Cells grown from Werner-syndrome patients show reduced

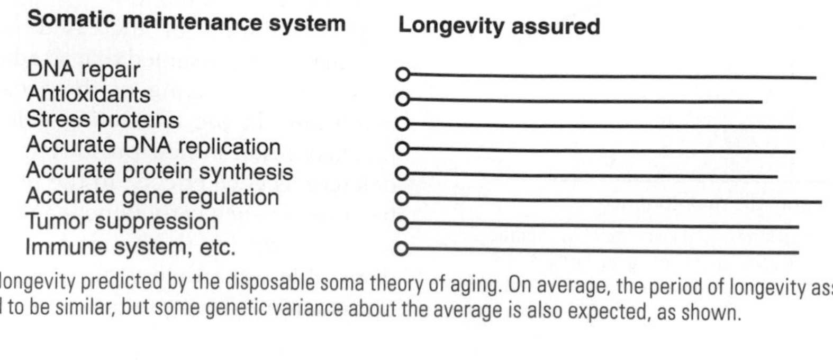

Figure 4-2. Polygenic control of longevity predicted by the disposable soma theory of aging. On average, the period of longevity assured by individual somatic maintenance systems is predicted to be similar, but some genetic variance about the average is also expected, as shown.

division potential and increased chromosomal instability compared with age-matched controls, and there is evidence that the pathology associated with Werner's syndrome may be related rather generally to impaired cell proliferation.

Yu et al[8] identified the gene responsible for Werner's syndrome as a DNA helicase, an enzyme responsible for unwinding DNA for purposes of replication, repair, and expression of the genetic material. This discovery strongly supports the concept that accumulation of somatic defects is important in aging, and it well illustrates the predicted involvement of longevity-assurance genes in determining the rate of aging. A defective helicase increases the rate of accumulation of DNA defects in actively dividing cell populations. A defect in this gene leads to accelerated aging, particularly in tissues in which cell division continues throughout life. In terms of the scheme shown in Figure 4-2, the mutation responsible for Werner's syndrome can be considered equivalent to shortening the line for longevity assurance through DNA repair. However, as Figure 4-2 illustrates, DNA repair is but part of the network of longevity assurance mechanisms that determine the overall rate of aging. It is striking that Werner's syndrome is not associated with accelerated aging in postmitotic tissues, such as brain and muscle, which is consistent with the fact that these tissues, by virtue of having little or no cell division during adult life, are relatively unaffected by having a defective DNA helicase.

Another striking example is Hutchinson-Gilford progeria. In this condition features of aging develop even faster than in Werner's syndrome. The discovery that Hutchinson-Gilford syndrome is associated with mutation in the lamin A gene, which affects the integrity of the cell's nuclear membrane, has again confirmed the association between rapid aging and accelerated accumulation of molecular and cellular damage.[28]

TESTS OF THE EVOLUTIONARY THEORIES

A key prediction of the evolutionary theories is that altering the rate of decline in the force of natural selection will lead to the evolution of a concomitantly altered rate of aging. This has been tested by applying artificial selection on life history variables or by making comparisons within and between species on the effects of different levels of extrinsic mortality. For practical reasons, most studies have focused on short-lived species, in particular the fruit fly *Drosophila melanogaster* and the nematode worm *Caenorhabditis elegans*.

Evidence for tradeoffs between early and late fitness components, as predicted by both the disposable soma and pleiotropic genes theories, comes from the success of artificial selection for increased longevity in *Drosophila*.[29–34] A general correlate of delayed senescence has been reduced fecundity in the long-lived flies. A similar tradeoff has also been reported for a human population, based on analysis of birth-and-death records of British aristocrats.[35]

The nematode *Caenorhabditis elegans* has yielded a growing number of long-lived mutants in which increased longevity has been consistently associated with increased resistance to biochemical and other stresses. Many of the affected genes are linked to pathways that control a switch between the normal developmental process of the worm and an alternative long-lived form called the *dauer* larva, which is invoked during times of food shortage. The emerging picture points to a fundamental link between metabolic control, growth and reproduction, and somatic maintenance.[36–38] These findings are directly consistent with the disposable soma theory, which predicts that at the heart of the evolutionary explanation of aging is the principle that organisms have been acted upon by natural selection to optimize the use of metabolic resources (energy) between competing physiologic demands, such as growth, maintenance, and reproduction. Consistent with this prediction it is striking that insulin signaling pathways appear to have effects on aging that may be strongly conserved across the species range. Insulin signaling regulates responses to varying nutrient levels. Allied to the role of insulin signaling pathways is the recent discovery that a class of proteins called sirtuins appears to be centrally involved in fine-tuning metabolic resources in response to variations in food supply.[39] It has long been known in laboratory rodents that restricted intake of calories simultaneously suppresses reproduction and upregulates a range of maintenance mechanisms, resulting in an extension of life span and the simultaneous postponement of age-related diseases. What is not at all clear, however, is whether the large effects on life span of modulating these pathways in very short-lived animals, such as nematodes and fruit flies, will be found to operate in longer-lived species. On evolutionary grounds it seems likely that there will have been greater evolutionary pressure to evolve a capacity to produce large responses to extreme environmental variation in small, short-lived animals. Therefore the scope for such modulation in humans, including through dietary restriction, is expected to be much less. Nevertheless it will be surprising if there are no metabolic consequences of varying food supply.

From the comparative perspective, the evolutionary theories predict that in safe environments (those with low extrinsic mortality) aging will evolve to be retarded. Adaptations that reduce extrinsic mortality (wings, protective shells, large brains) are generally linked with increased longevity (bats, birds, turtles, humans). Field observations comparing a mainland population of opossums subject to significant predation by mammals, with an island population not subject to mammalian predation, found the predicted slower aging in the island population.[40]

At the molecular and cellular levels, the disposable soma theory predicts that the effort devoted to cellular maintenance and repair processes will vary directly with longevity. Numerous studies support this idea. A direct relation between species longevity and rate of mitochondrial ROS production in captive mammals has been found[41,42] as has a similar relationship between mammals and similar-sized but much longer-lived birds.[43] DNA repair capacity has been shown to correlate with mammalian life span in numerous comparative studies,[44] as has the level of poly(ADP-ribose) polymerase,[45] an enzyme that plays an important role in the maintenance of genomic integrity. The quality of maintenance and repair mechanisms may be revealed by the capacity to cope with external stress. Comparisons of the functional capacity of cultured cells to withstand a variety of imposed stressors have shown that cells taken from long-lived species have superior stress resistance to that of cells from shorter-lived species.[46,47]

Tests of the evolutionary theories support the idea that it is the evolved capacity of somatic cells to carry out effective maintenance and repair that mainly governs the time taken for damage to accumulate to levels where it interferes with the organism's viability, and hence regulates longevity.

CONCLUSIONS

Our answers to the question "Why does aging occur?" have broad implications for how we perceive the likely genetic basis of aging. Firstly, evolution theory can illuminate a long-running debate about whether programmed or stochastic events, such as DNA damage, drive the aging process. The weakness of evolutionary support for the adaptive aging genes hypothesis calls the program theory into question. Any notion of an aging "clock" needs to be qualified by recognition of this fact. The existence of temporal controls in development and in cyclic processes such as diurnal and reproductive cycles does not provide a sufficient basis to suggest the existence of a clock that regulates aging. Nor does the broad reproducibility of many features of aging provide any real evidence for an underlying active program. This is not to say, however, that the nature and rate of aging are not genetically determined. The issue that distinguishes programmed from stochastic theories of aging is not whether the factors that determine longevity are specified within the genome, but rather, how this is arranged.[48]

Secondly, evolution theory clearly indicates a polygenic basis for aging. Different mechanisms and even different kinds of genes may operate together. This presents a major challenge, and progress is likely to require a combination of approaches, including (1) transgenic animal models in which candidate genetic factors are altered by genetic manipulation, (2) comparative studies to identify factors that correlate positively or negatively with species' life spans, (3) studies of the extremely long-lived (e.g., human centenarians) to identify factors associated with above-average expectation of life, and (4) selection experiments to investigate the response of life span to artificial selection pressures.

KEY POINTS
Aging

- We are not programmed to die.
- Aging occurs because, in our evolutionary past, when life expectancy was much shorter, natural selection placed limited priority on long-term maintenance of the body.
- Aging is caused by gradual accumulation of cell and tissue damage. Much of the damage arises as a side effect of essential biochemical processes, such as the use of oxygen to generate chemical energy through oxidative phosphorylation.
- Accumulation of damage begins early and continues progressively throughout life, resulting after several decades in the overt frailty, disability, and disease associated with aging.
- Multiple processes cause the damage that contributes to aging, and multiple genes regulate the efficacy of "longevity-assurance" processes, such as DNA repair, that together influence the rate of aging.
- Nongenetic factors, such as nutrition and exercise, can have important effects in modulating the rate of buildup of damage within the body.

For a complete list of references, please visit online only at www.expertconsult.com

CHAPTER 5

Methodological Problems of Research in Older People

Antony Bayer

INTRODUCTION

The relentless aging of society, the accompanying growth in age-related diseases, and the disproportionate use of health and social care resources by older people might be expected to be a powerful incentive to prioritize research into aging and geriatric medicine. However, ageist attitudes and beliefs persist among many funding agencies and researchers and some older people themselves. These, together with the many practical and methodological challenges that must be overcome to deliver high-quality studies in older people continue to act as barriers to effective delivery of research in this heterogeneous and often vulnerable population.

The difficulty of undertaking research involving older people tends to be exaggerated. It is wrongly assumed that too many will have significant comorbidity leading to a poor signal-to-noise ratio, an unacceptably high risk of adverse events, inability to complete necessary assessments, poor compliance, and high rate of drop-out. This can translate into arbitrary, unscientific, and unnecessary upper age limits. Yet many of the changes commonly attributed to aging are typically because of reasons other than chronologic age, notably physical and cognitive comorbidities leading to frailty, and psychosocial factors, such as relative lack of education and cigarette smoking. Furthermore it is often the old who have the greatest morbidity and mortality associated with the condition under study and who therefore will have the greatest absolute benefit from any effective intervention.

Ethical concerns about experimenting on elderly populations, who are considered "vulnerable" on the basis only of chronologic age, may be cited as justification for their exclusion, demonstrating misguided paternalism of younger research workers and ignoring the older person's right to autonomous decision making. The majority of even the oldest old will have no significant cognitive impairment and will generally have the capacity to make an informed decision about participation. The consequences of excluding older people from therapeutic research, where they are left to either receive treatments in the absence of evidence-based trials, or are denied drugs because they have been untried in their age group, might be considered especially unethical[1] and imply that clinicians have a duty to actively promote their inclusion in clinical trials.[2] All researchers should be careful that ageist attitudes do not influence their research design, and funding bodies and research ethics committees should challenge unnecessarily restrictive entry criteria, including inappropriate upper age limits.[3]

Ill-informed beliefs about the supposed high risk of developing mental incapacity and perceived low life expectancy after age 65 are sometimes used to exclude older people from longitudinal studies because it is wrongly assumed that few will stay the course. In reality, the annual incidence of dementia in those over 65 is about 1% and healthy life expectancy at age 65 in England is about 12 to 14 years.

Study Designs

The optimum choice of design to study aging and age-related conditions and to understand the mechanisms underlying change and their consequences will depend on the research question to be answered.[4] Qualitative studies; ecologic studies using available data; and quantitative studies using cross-sectional, case-control, and cohort designs will help to generate hypotheses. These can then be tested in experimental studies, using randomized controlled trial designs. Each design presents its own challenges and limitations.

Qualitative Methodologies

Qualitative research has its roots in anthropology and sociology and is an umbrella term for a heterogeneous group of methodologies with different theoretical underpinnings.[5] They aim to gain an in-depth understanding of peoples' behavior by exploring their knowledge, values, attitudes, beliefs, and fears. This allows subjects to give "richer" answers to questions and the researcher to explore the full complexity of human behaviors, thereby providing detailed insights that might be missed by other methods. For example, it may illuminate the reasons behind patients', carers', and clinicians' decisions about management[6,7] or explore important issues such as dignity that may be difficult to quantify.[8]

Qualitative studies are hypothesis-generating rather than hypothesis-testing, but results can identify specific issues that need to be tested using quantitative methods or can help to explain outcomes of experimental studies. Thus the two methods can usefully complement each other and increasing numbers of studies are using "mixed" methodologies (for example, a study trying to understand the attitudes of the elderly towards enrollment into cancer clinical trials).[9]

Samples in qualitative research tend to be small and labor-intensive, with data collected usually by direct observation or active participation in the setting of interest, or by in-depth individual interviews (unstructured or semistructured), focus groups (guided group discussions), or examination of documents or other artifacts. Other methods used in qualitative research studies include diary methods, role play and simulation, narrative analysis, or in-depth case study. Although potential areas of interest may be identified beforehand, there is no predetermined set of questions, and subjects are encouraged to express their views and ideas at length. Rather than formal sample size calculations, numbers of participants may be decided by analyzing interviews alongside data collection, which is stopped when no new themes are emerging (so-called "saturation"). Sampling tends to be purposive rather than comprehensive or random, deliberately aiming to reflect a specific range of experience and attitudes judged to be of likely relevance to the research question. The results are analyzed by exploring the content and identifying patterns or themes, often through an iterative process allowing meaning to emerge from the data, rather than by the deductive statistical approach of quantitative methods.

Critics of qualitative analysis are concerned that it is too influenced by the views and attitudes of the researchers when they are collecting and analyzing data, so it introduces unacceptable bias and problems with generalization and reproducibility of findings. Qualitative research can be challenging with older people, but because it can be less intrusive than more structured quantitative methodologies, it may be especially suited to those who are frail. They may be unable or unwilling to take part in lengthy interviews because of communication deficits or fatigue and several shorter interviews may be more practical. Focus groups may work best with just four or five elderly participants and need a skilled facilitator to ensure a high level of participant interaction. Extra effort is needed to ensure representative samples and to support those who are less confident, easily fatigued, or have cognitive or physical deficits. Participant or nonparticipant observation may be especially useful in institutional settings, but time must be given to establish trust with the researcher if residents and staff are not to feel threatened. Assurances of confidentiality and commitment from management are essential. However, once trust has been established, attrition rates tend to be low as participation tends not to be burdensome.[10]

ECOLOGIC STUDIES

Ecologic studies use available data to characterize samples and to generate hypotheses, although evidence for causality is generally weak. Data may be aggregated, such as census data and records of disease incidence by hospital, or individual, such as hospital discharge summaries or death certificates. As the data are already available, there are advantages of speed and economy, and impact of factors operating at population level (e.g., improved access to education, banning smoking in public places) may be difficult to measure at an individual level. However, measures may not be comparable over time or place, quality is always outside the researcher's control, and the available data may be selective. Many official statistics that are broken down by age will lump all the over-65s together or will only report information on adults of working age. When older people are included, they often exclude those not living in the community and those with cognitive impairment. Nevertheless, temporal data such as the effect of daily variations in air pollution or temperature on mortality of elderly people—where individual confounding factors remain constant over time—can provide robust evidence suggesting a causal effect, and ecologic data are also of value in studying the effects of early life factors on later health or disease in "life course epidemiology."[11]

CROSS-SECTIONAL STUDIES

Cross-sectional studies record information over a short period of time and are suited to report prevalence and the relationship between variables and age or dependency. They are relatively fast and simple to conduct as each subject is examined only once and several outcomes or diseases can be studied simultaneously. For example, recent data from the Health and Retirement Study of 11,000 adults aged 65 years or older (representing the 34.5 million older Americans) highlighted the important finding that common geriatric conditions (cognitive impairment, falls, incontinence, etc.) were similar in prevalence to common chronic diseases, such as heart disease and diabetes in older adults, and strongly and independently associated with dependency in activities of daily living.[12] However, cross-sectional studies give no information about incidence or causality and are of limited value when studying rare conditions or acute illness.

Data can be presented as the mean value for each age group, or age can be used as a continuous independent variable in a regression analysis, with the outcome of interest as the dependent variable. Associations can be confounded when the variable of interest affects the survival of subjects, with selective mortality leading to a survival bias.

Misinterpretation can also arise from birth cohort effects, with associations and differences not arising due to age differences, but due to the era in which people were born and brought up. Sometimes such differences from one generation to the next are of particular interest and a time series design may then be appropriate, sequential samples of a particular age group being studied every few years. For example, comparison of comparable datasets from the Health and Retirement Study in 1993 and 2002 suggests a falling prevalence of dementia in the United States.[13] Selection of subjects needs to ensure that they are well matched at each time point and methodologies need to be identical to ensure that differences are solely due to temporal changes and not to selection bias.

CASE CONTROL STUDIES

Case control studies choose groups with (cases) and without (controls) the outcome of interest and look back at what different exposures they may have had to identify possible risk factors. Case control studies have been widely used in genetic studies to identify susceptibility genes and are the best design to study rare conditions, as they are efficient in use of time and money, collecting a lot of relevant information on targeted individuals. Case control studies may be "nested" within cohort studies.

Bias can be introduced when cases and controls differ in ways other than just the outcome of interest (selection bias) or when cases are not "typical" (representativeness bias). Given the increasing heterogeneity characteristic of aging, bias can be a significant problem and care needs to be taken to well match cases and controls. Recall bias may arise because subjects are able to remember events better because of their significance, or unintentionally they may be prompted to remember by investigators, who should therefore be blinded to whether the person is a case or control when assessing exposures. People who have died do not make it into case control studies and their representatives are likely to be less reliable than the person themselves at remembering exposures, introducing a potential survival bias. Although case control studies can play a pivotal role in suggesting important associations, as in the original studies linking cigarette smoking and lung cancer,[14] confounding can also lead to highly misleading conclusions, as in the observational studies of combined hormone replacement therapy and cardiovascular disease in postmenopausal women.[15]

COHORT STUDIES

In a cohort or longitudinal study, a group of subjects are followed over time as they age to determine who develops a particular outcome or the rate at which a variable changes. Prominent cohort studies relevant to old people include the Baltimore Longitudinal Study of Aging,[16] the Rotterdam study,[17] and the Caerphilly cohort study.[18] Along with risk, the number of people who actually develop the outcome of interest can be calculated (incidence). Inevitably such studies take a long time and often require a large sample size (the rarer the outcome, the larger the sample needs to be) and so are expensive. The frequency of testing needs to be decided, based on the rate of change, the precision of the measures being used, available resources, and the stamina of both researcher and research subjects. Analysis of longitudinal data by slope analysis or other techniques is likely to require specialist knowledge.

Recall bias is avoided as subjects are enrolled before the outcome(s) and the sequence of events can be more clearly established, although the possibility of reverse causality must always be considered. Cohort effects are minimal because all the subjects are generally from a single birth cohort. Ideally, longitudinal aging studies would follow subjects from birth to the grave, but this is unlikely, as they would then outlive the research team. When age range in a longitudinal study is wide, cohort effects can be identified by plotting rates of change within age groups and seeing if the plots join up smoothly (a true age effect), or are a disjointed group of line segments similar to that often seen in repeated cross-sectional studies.

Potential bias may arise when outcomes are not measured or not recorded in a consistent fashion over time, with small changes in methodology such as new equipment, a change in assay technique, or differences in study personnel appearing to suggest age-related changes (detection bias). Ensuring a common period of training for all involved in the research, with periodic refresher courses and measures of interrater and intrarater reliability, can minimize problems, but researchers must stay alert to possible methodological error throughout data collection and analysis.

Important outcomes may be missed if follow-up is too short or too long, so that subjects die before they are reassessed. Inevitably, some subjects will drop out or be lost to follow-up (excursion bias), and there are various approaches to dealing with missing data by imputing values based on available records.

CLINICAL TRIALS

A clinical trial is the methodology of choice to examine causality, with the randomized controlled trial (RCT) acknowledged as the gold standard experimental design.[19] In a RCT, the researcher controls exposure to a single variable, the risk or treatment, by randomly assigning subjects to one group (intervention) or another (control, often involving a placebo intervention) and all subjects are then followed up to determine the outcome. When an effective intervention exists already, a placebo control is unethical and the new experimental intervention is then compared against an active control (the current standard of care). In rare cases, when the size of the treatment effect relative to the expected prognosis is dramatic, randomization may not be necessary or ethical, and historical controls (apparently similar, past patients) may be used.[20]

Parallel group RCT designs are generally preferred, intervention and control groups being treated simultaneously. Thus half the subjects receive treatment A (intervention) and the other half receives treatment B (control). In a crossover design, subjects swap groups half way through the study (half the subjects receiving treatment A followed by treatment B, with the other half receiving treatment B then A) and so each subject can act as their own control, assuming that there are no carry-over or seasonal effects. In a factorial design, two (and occasionally more) interventions, each with their own control, are evaluated simultaneously in the one study. For example one group tests treatment A, another tests treatment B, a third group tests A and B combined, and the control group tests neither A nor B. Such designs are used already extensively in cancer and cardiovascular studies and are likely to be needed increasingly in other conditions with multiple therapeutic options. Although they are an efficient method to test therapies in combination, achieving two comparisons for little more than the price of one, interactions between the interventions can complicate analysis of the outcomes and their interpretation.

Bias in clinical trials is reduced by the use of random allocation and blinding. Randomization increases the likelihood (but does not assure) that the groups will be well matched except for the intervention, distributing potential confounders both known and unknown between the intervention and control groups. Stratified randomization can be used to ensure particular groups (for example, the very old) are evenly distributed. Cluster randomization designs randomize groups of individuals (e.g., all those in a ward or nursing home) rather than individuals themselves and are increasingly common in health services research. Blinding means that the subject or investigator ("single-blind"), or both ("double-blind"), do not know to which group the subject is assigned. This prevents people from being treated differently in any way other than the intervention itself and helps to ensure that outcome assessments are unbiased.

National regulatory authorities, such as the U.S. Food and Drug Administration (FDA) and European Medicines Agency (EMEA), require positive outcomes from RCTs before a drug or medical device is given marketing approval for patient use. They will have been preceded by extensive preclinical in vitro (laboratory) and in vivo (animal) testing that, when appropriate, may include studies with nonhuman primate models of aging or transgenic animal models of disease. Clinical trials then progress through an orderly series of steps, commonly classified into Phases I to IV. Recently the concept of preliminary Phase 0 trials has also been introduced to describe exploratory, first-in human studies using single subtherapeutic (micro-doses) of study drug or agent, designed to confirm that the drug broadly behaves in man as predicted from preclinical testing.

In Phase I trials, the study drug or agent is tested in a small group of subjects (20 to 80) in single ascending dose (SAD) and multiple ascending dose (MAD) studies to assess a safe dosage range, the best method of administration and tolerance and safety (pharmacovigilance). The changes in the pharmacokinetics and pharmacodynamics of many drugs in older people, especially the frail, may significantly impact on the choice of dose and dosing frequency for clinical use. A Phase I trial usually recruits healthy young adults and so care must be taken with extrapolating results to elderly patients. When the study indication is common in older people, Phase I trials may recruit elderly healthy volunteers or patients with the relevant condition (e.g., as happened in initial studies of immunotherapy for Alzheimer's disease).

In Phase II trials, the study drug or agent is given to a larger group of subjects (100 to 300), generally patients with the study indication, to further assess safety and dosing requirements (Phase IIA) and to undertake preliminary studies of efficacy (Phase IIB). Usually these "proof of concept" studies recruit a homogeneous group of younger subjects to maximize the chances of success and minimize adverse events related to altered pharmacokinetics and pharmacodynamics, comorbid conditions, and drug interactions more characteristic of older patients. However, there have been recent calls for regulatory authorities to require performance of Phase II studies of new agents in individuals aged 70 and older.[21]

In Phase III trials, the efficacy and safety of the study drug or agent is evaluated in RCTs, usually two positive trials being required to gain approval from regulatory authorities. These require the recruitment of up to several thousand patients from multiple centers and generally last for 6 months to several years depending on the study indication. It is at this phase that arbitrary exclusion criteria based on chronologic age is especially difficult to justify. Randomization, stratified by age, and predetermined subgroup analysis will allow any issues specific to the elderly patients to become apparent. Phase IV (postmarketing) trials are designed to provide additional information about benefits and risks of treatment in long-term use in clinical practice. Serious adverse effects identified at this late stage in elderly patients have resulted in withdrawal or restricted use of several prominent drugs.

The carefully controlled nature of RCTs may themselves mean that they have limited generalizability as subjects are often a very well-defined, highly selected group. Extensive lists of inclusion and exclusion criteria may exclude those with other comorbidities or those taking other medications and the resulting trial population can end up bearing little resemblance to patients normally presenting in the clinic. This can result in unintended harm to future patients.[22,23] Certainly perceived gains from narrow eligibility criteria are often outweighed by the loss in generalizability and clinical applicability of the results and less opportunity to test preplanned subgroup hypotheses (including any effect of age).[24] Pragmatic clinical trials tend to take all comers and best reflect the effectiveness rather than merely the efficacy of an intervention.

Exclusion of older people from research

Elderly people, especially the frail and the very old, are too often excluded from RCTs, usually inappropriately and without justification.[25,26] A review of eligibility criteria of RCTs published in high-impact medical journals from 1994 to 2006 found that, after inability to consent, age was the second commonest exclusion criterion, with 38% of trials excluding the over-65s.[27] Similarly, an analysis of research papers published in four major medical journals in 1996 and 1967 found that one third of studies excluded subjects over 65 without providing justification,[28] although when the analysis was repeated in 2004 the proportion had fallen to 15%, with 5% of trials specific to older people.[29] The age bias can be present in clinical trials in most common conditions of older people, including cancer,[30,31] cardiovascular disease,[32,33] Parkinson's disease,[34] and urinary incontinence.[35] A search for RCTs specifically involving very elderly subjects identified only 84 trials published between 1990 and 2002, but concluded that their methodological quality did not differ from comparable trials in the general population.[36]

Reasons given for excluding elderly subjects from research include concerns about gaining consent, protocol eligibility criteria with restrictions on comorbidities and concomitant medications, worries about poor compliance, and high attrition and fears of an unacceptable level of adverse events. However, many of these concerns are unfounded or can be easily overcome.[37,38] A systematic review[39] examining participation of elderly patients in Phase III publicly funded RCTs in cancer between 1955 and 2000 found that in those trials with sufficient numbers of elderly enrollees, survival, event-free-survival, and treatment-related mortality outcomes were similar to outcomes reported in the remainder of the studies, with the authors concluding that the similarity in these two groups showing that the enrollment of elderly in experimental RCTs is not associated with increased harm. A review[40] of patients with various solid tumors entering Phase II cancer trials in Europe concluded that, compared with younger patients, the old did not have an increased risk of more severe or frequent adverse effects and there was no difference in response rate. However, doses did need more frequent adjustment in elderly patients and treatment discontinuation increased with age because of greater loss to follow-up and treatment refusal.

Informed consent

Seeking truly informed and freely given consent is fundamental to all research involving human subjects. The research participant must be able to retain and understand the relevant facts explained to them, be allowed sufficient time to weigh the benefits and risks to make a choice (without coercion), and then be able to communicate their decision to the researcher.[41] Consent is more than getting a signature in triplicate on a consent form and should be regarded as a continuous process involving ongoing open dialogue between researchers and participants.

Elderly patients may have more difficulty comprehending consent information (mainly because of education differences rather than age itself), and particular attention should be given to compensating for communication and sensory deficits, improving readability of information sheets and consent forms, and considering the use of innovative consent procedures. However, most older people are cognitively intact and, in empirical studies of competency to consent to medical treatment, elderly control individuals were nearly all judged fully capable using various legal standards.[42,43] Gaining informed consent may require more time because of characteristics of the older person and his or her wish to involve family members in the decision.

Those with cognitive impairment and the institutionalized are especially vulnerable to exploitation and require special consideration and management, although even then, lack of capacity should not be assumed.[44–46] The MacArthur Competence Assessment Tool for Clinical Research (MacCAT-CR)[47] is a semistructured assessment of a potential research subject's decision-making capacity to choose, understand, appreciate, and reason through information needed to make an informed decision and can be a useful aid, although it is time-consuming to administer and requires specialist training. Simple cognitive screens, such as the Mini Mental State Examination (MMSE),[48] are very imprecise guides to judging capacity.[49] If a prospective research participant is considered incapable of giving consent, the relevant legal framework must be followed.[50,51] Generally, research is allowed to go ahead with the subject's permission, an appropriate surrogate decision maker (usually the patient's next of kin) providing proxy consent, ethics committee approval, and if the study has the potential to benefit the subject (so called "therapeutic research") or when the research entails minimal risk and burden and cannot be undertaken with individuals able to consent ("nontherapeutic research"). Research advance directives or advance decisions clearly document an individual's views on research participation, but have not been widely adopted.[52]

Recruitment and retention

Research is dependent on recruiting and retaining sufficient numbers of suitable study subjects. There is no consistent evidence that chronologic age influences recruitment rate into trials.[53,54] Rather, the problem is that elderly patients are not given sufficient encouragement to take part. Thus a study of breast cancer trials found that older age remained predictive of not being invited to take part after adjustment for comorbidity, cancer stage, functional status, and race, yet a similar proportion of younger and older patients were recruited when they were asked.[55] As well as ageism, clinician apathy and inexperience of research may also contribute to the exclusion of older patients. A survey of French geriatricians found that nearly all considered that RCTs including very elderly subjects were scientifically necessary, but less than half of the elderly participated actively in such studies and many were never approached to do so.[56] Researchers have the greatest motivation and are therefore the most efficient recruiters. Elderly patients themselves do not appear to actively seek clinical trials, possibly because of a lack of knowledge, and are dependent on others to inform them of what is available.[9] Inclusion of people living in nursing homes is especially challenging given the particular issues around consent, loss of autonomy and negative staff attitudes, confidentiality, and resident rights.[46] Involving older people themselves as active partners in research design and conduct has become a policy requirement in the United Kingdom and may be helpful, although little is known about how involvement changes the research process.[57,58]

Although curiosity may prompt the initial interest of patients in research, anticipated personal benefits, such as health screening and regular monitoring and the possibility to help others, are the most important motivators for subsequent enrollment and for continued participation.[54,59] The main reasons for refusing enrollment are inconvenience and not wanting to be experimented upon or a self-perception of not being a suitable research candidate. Older research participants are more motivated than the young by feelings of altruism and "paying back" those who treat them and are less concerned about financial compensation for volunteering.[60] Studies in which all patients receive the active treatment, as part of a crossover design or open label extension after a placebo control phase, seem to be preferred.

A systematic review of factors that limit the quality, number, and progress of RCTs (in all age groups) identified many clinician- and patient-based barriers to participation (Table 5-1) but no effective strategies to improve recruitment,[61] a finding similar to that of a recent Cochrane Review.[62] An earlier literature review specific to older people had identified a number of factors open to modification to increase their participation in research studies. These included positive attitudes of staff toward research, acknowledgement of altruistic motives, gaining approval of family members, protocols designed for patient rather than staff convenience, and having a physician rather than a nurse approach the patient.[63] In a study of recruitment of frail older adults living at home into a RCT of geriatric assessment, yield (defined as the percentage of individuals contacted who later enrolled) was highest from community physician solicitations and presentations to religious or ethnic groups and lowest from media and mailing (and often problematic because of frequent misunderstandings).[53]

Table 5-1. Barriers to Participation in a Randomized Controlled Trial[61]

Clinician Based
- Time constraints
- Lack of staff and training
- Worry about the impact on doctor-patient relationship
- Concern for patients
- Loss of professional autonomy
- Difficulty with the consent procedure
- Lack of rewards and recognition

Patient Based
- Additional procedures and appointments for patient
- Additional travel problems and cost for patient
- Patient preferences for a particular treatment 9 or no treatment 0
- Worry about uncertainty of treatment or trials
- Patients' concerns about information and consent
- Protocol causing problem with recruitment
- Clinician concerns about information provided to patients

Once entered into a study, maintaining good communications—primarily by regular face-to-face or telephone contacts with the researchers, but also using regular newsletters about study progress and lunchtime meetings to meet staff involved and other participants—will aid subject retention.[59] Token gifts—such as study-related calendars, fridge magnets, and pens and pads—can also be given, but can be counterproductive if they appear too costly. Test sessions should aim to last no longer than 1 to 2 hours to prevent fatigue, and spacing data collection over multiple visits should be considered. Time must be allowed for social interaction and refreshments to stop contacts from becoming too impersonal. It should be remembered that most older people (and their accompanying caregivers) have other commitments and timing of research sessions should fit around these.

Transport provision is critically important. Mobility and cognitive problems may make travel more difficult and distance from home to the research center influences recruitment of older persons more than the young.[64,65] A prepaid taxi to and from the research center has many advantages. When research participants make their own travel arrangements, they should be reimbursed and convenient car parking ensured. Consideration should be given to easy access to the research office, which should be wheelchair-friendly and with suitable areas for accompanying relatives and caregivers to wait. Assessments that can be reliably performed by telephone or at the subjects' homes may be preferable to visits to the research center and are more likely to ensure that the subject is at ease. However, it is more difficult for researchers to set the agenda when they are guests in the subject's home, and ensuring that well-meaning relatives and pets do not interrupt testing sessions can be challenging. Regular delivery of study medication by mail may reduce the number of necessary visits. A formal "thank you" when the study ends and feedback of the final outcome is appreciated and expected.

Outcomes

Along with the standard outcome measures of morbidity and mortality, research in older people commonly needs to consider broader issues that impact quality of life, especially functional, cognitive, and social outcomes. Chosen measurement instruments must be valid (recording the attribute that it purports to measure), reliable (recording consistent results under varying conditions of measurement), and responsive (able to detect change). Other factors to be considered when selecting an instrument are whether it is self-administered or researcher-administered, whether it measures capability (what can be done relevant to experimental designs) or performance (what is done, relevant in pragmatic studies), and, perhaps most importantly, how long it takes to complete. Attention should also be given to the readability and style of self-completed questionnaires (Table 5-2).

The lack of validation of measurement instruments for use in elderly populations is a problem. Scales must be able to encompass the heterogeneity that is characteristic of elderly populations, avoiding floor and ceiling effects, and they must be acceptable to the study subjects. Even an apparently simple measure such as height becomes an issue when the person cannot stand. Use of validated alternatives such as knee-floor height then need to be considered, perhaps even in those who can stand, to ensure consistency across the whole study population.

Table 5-2. Checklist When Choosing Outcome Measures

- Is the measure proven to be valid and reliable in the study population?
- Is the measure responsive to clinically significant change?
- Is it acceptable to research subject and user? Could presentation be improved?
- Who is administering? Training need? Can a proxy respondent complete reliably?
- How long does it take to administer? Is the environment appropriate?
- Is scoring simple and are results presented ready for analysis?
- Has the measure been piloted in the study population?

Table 5-3. The 25-Item GMDS

A. General Parameters
- I. Full medical record including all past and present diseases, organ impairments, fractures, and surgical interventions.
- II. Full drug history, including number and type of generic medications and adverse effects reported.
- III. Charlson index
- IV. Vision and hearing evaluation
- V. EuroQol

B. Cardiovascular Risk Factors
- I. Assessment of diabetes and hypertension
- II. Assessment of alcohol and smoking habits (pack years)
- III. Blood pressure (BP) and heart rate (HR) in both sitting and standing positions measured at minutes 1 and 3

C. Functional Status
- I. Katz index (B-ADL)
- II. Lawton's instrumental activities of daily living (I-ADL)
- III. Timed Up and Go
- IV. Falls: 3 months recall record of the number, frequency, time of the day, and mechanisms of falling, assistive devices, pain, and fear of walking
- V. Frailty index

D. Cognitive and Psychological Status
- I. Years of schooling and educational level
- II. MMSE
- III. NPI
- IV. 15-item Geriatric Depression Score

E. Nutritional Status
- I. MNA-SF followed by MNA if at risk
- II. BMI
- III. Weight loss measured as 4% in 1 year or 5 kg in 6 months

F. Biologic Parameters
- I. Electrolytes (sodium, potassium creatinine, glucose), hepatic function (GGT, ASAT, ALAT), lipids (T-Chol, HDL-Chol, LDL-Chol), thyroid function, vitamin B_{12} and folic acid, albumin, and total protein levels, Hb A_{1c}, CRP, hemoglobin level, red and white blood cell count, and platelets
- II. Creatinine clearance by Cockcroft formula

G. Social Status
- I. Housing status
- II. Caregivers: number and type of formal/informal caregivers
- III. Time spent on formal care giving measured as hours per week

From Abellan van Kan G, Sinclair A, Anreieu S, et al. The geriatric minimum data set for clinical trials (GMDS). J Nutr Health Aging 2008;12:197–200.

KEY POINTS
Methodological Problems of Research in Older People

- Elderly people are too often excluded from research because of concerns about gaining consent, unnecessarily strict protocol restrictions on comorbidities and concomitant medications, worries about poor compliance and high attrition, problems with assessments and fears of an unacceptable level of adverse events. Many of these concerns are unfounded or may be easily overcome.
- Optimum choice of design to study aging and age-related conditions depends on the research question to be answered. Qualitative studies, ecologic studies using available data and quantitative studies using cross-sectional, case-control, and cohort designs, will help to generate hypotheses. These can then be tested in experimental studies, ideally using randomized controlled trial designs.
- Curiosity, anticipated personal health benefits, and the possibility to help others are the most important motivators for enrollment and for continued participation in research. The main reasons for refusing are inconvenience and not wanting to be experimented upon or a self-perception of being unsuitable. Older research participants are more motivated than the young by feelings of altruism and "paying back" those who treat them and are less concerned about financial compensation.
- Cognitively intact older people may have more difficulty comprehending consent information and special attention should be given to compensating for communication and sensory deficits, improving readability of information sheets and allowing sufficient time for the consent process. People with cognitive impairment and those in institutions may require alternative consent procedures.
- Once entered into a study, retention is promoted by maintaining good communications, good transport provision, and test sessions that are no longer than necessary and arranged at times to suit the participant. Outcome measures must be acceptable, valid, reliable, and responsive and focus on quality of life, especially functional, cognitive, and social outcomes, along with morbidity and mortality.

Experience with measures in younger, fit subjects cannot reliably be extrapolated to older patients with their higher prevalence of mobility, sensory, and communication deficits. When norms for the over-65s are available, they may be derived from small numbers of atypical, healthy, young-elderly subjects and of little relevance to the frail octogenarian in a nursing home. Ideally, reliability should be established in each population sample where the measure is to be used. Certainly all raters need to be trained to ensure consistency (interrater and intrarater reliability) and to help minimize bias. Piloting of all outcome measures in the population to be studied will ensure that the final choice is feasible and reduce the number of subsequent subject dropouts.

There are a growing number of measurement instruments that have established validity and reliability in elderly and frail subjects, with some approaching the status of gold standard. Examples are the Mini Mental State Examination (MMSE) for cognition,[48] the Geriatric Depression Scale (GDS),[67] the Barthel index,[67] and Katz index[68] for basic activities of daily living, the Lawton and Brody index for instrumental activities of daily living,[69] the frailty index,[70] the Mini Nutritional Assessment (MNA),[71] the timed up-and-go test (TUG) for falls risk,[72] and the Zarit Burden scale for caregiver burden.[73] Clinical trials in dementia have their own extensive battery of assessment measures.[74]

Recently, expert groups on both sides of the Atlantic have considered suitable functional outcome measures for clinical trials in frail older people.[75–77] The GerontoNet collaboration of leading European geriatric research centers has developed and piloted a 25-item geriatric minimum data set (GMDS).[77] This aims to achieve a uniform nomenclature and standardization of the assessment tools that will act as the minimum set of information to be included in future clinical studies involving older people. It claims to be straightforward, rapid to complete, easily accessible on the Internet, inexpensive, valid in a wide spectrum of research areas, and has been translated into the common European languages (Table 5-3).

For a complete list of references, please visit online only at www.expertconsult.com

CHAPTER 6

Biology of Aging

Huber R. Warner
Felipe Sierra
LaDora V. Thompson

INTRODUCTION

For this discussion about the biology of aging, we begin with a definition of what is meant by aging and the aging process. There are many definitions proposed, but the one provided by Richard Miller of the University of Michigan seems particularly useful for this chapter in a textbook on geriatric medicine.[1] He defines aging as the "process that progressively converts physiologically and cognitively fit healthy adults into less fit individuals with increasing vulnerability to injury, illness, and death." Thus the two most important general problems to overcome during human aging are (1) the increasing loss of physical and cognitive function with increasing age, and (2) the increasing susceptibility to a variety of morbid conditions.

The study of the biology of aging began with discovery research, which mostly focused on describing and cataloging aging changes. To understand how these age-related changes relate to Miller's definition, the challenge is then to distinguish among:

- Pathologically neutral age-related changes, such as the graying of hair
- Changes such as the accumulation of oxidatively damaged molecules or senescent cells that are believed to contribute to the development of one or more adverse age-related conditions
- Changes that cause overt pathology, such as the development of plaque and tangles in the brain of Alzheimer's disease patients
- Changes that are the result of such pathology

Three very important milestones occurring during the early discovery phase of aging research include the observations that: (1) restricting caloric intake increases longevity and delays the onset of age-related disease in rodents[2]; (2) oxygen radicals are produced in vivo and continuously damage cellular macromolecular components[3]; and (3) when human fibroblasts are grown in culture they have a finite life span.[4] Although these three concepts still provide much of the basis for biogerontologic research, so much progress has been made in fleshing out the details that *Cell* devoted its entire February 25, 2005, issue to reviews of basic aging research. Even so, in its July 1, 2005, issue, *Science* included the question "How much can human life span be extended?" as one of the 125 major scientific puzzles driving basic research today.[5]

Over the years a large number of theories of aging have been proposed to explain how age-related changes promote aging,[6] but the complexity of the process diminishes the possibility that any one theory will completely explain aging. The concept that aging is due to both genetic and environmental/stochastic factors is now generally accepted, but it remains difficult to distinguish between the process of aging itself, and the effects due to age-related diseases.

The chapter will first focus on cellular pathways now known to regulate longevity in a variety of animal model organisms. This knowledge resulted from the ability to isolate long-lived mutants of short-lived species such as nematodes, fruit flies and mice, which in turn has been greatly facilitated by success in sequencing the human genome and the genomes of these popular model organisms. We then discuss age-related changes related to cell proliferation and age-related changes due to damage to important cellular macromolecules, such as DNA, proteins, and lipids. These include, but are not limited to, free radical damage to DNA, proteins, and lipids[3]; DNA repair[7]; nonenzymatic glycation[8]; protein cross-linking and protein turnover. Such stochastic changes can become important risk factors in the development of the many degenerative age-related processes and diseases that must be dealt with by geriatricians. Beckman and Ames have written an excellent review of the free radical theory of aging,[9] which includes a discussion of many aspects of these overlapping phenomena, but a recent review of oxidative stress in transgenically altered mouse models by Han et al[10] argues that the level of damage and its relationship to late-life pathology, such as cancer, is still poorly understood. However, the chapter then includes one example of an age-related condition, sarcopenia, which may be at least partly due to oxidative damage to skeletal muscle proteins. The chapter concludes with a brief discussion of the general value of research on the basic mechanisms of aging.

THE INSULIN-SIGNALING PATHWAY AND LONGEVITY REGULATION

Our understanding of the molecular and genetic basis of aging has witnessed a significant advance in the last decade. The prevailing view until the mid-1980s[11] was that aging was stochastic and genetics probably played little direct role in a process that occurred after the reproductive period, and therefore beyond the power of genetic selection. However, hundreds of genes with effects on longevity have been uncovered in a variety of organisms. This was done partially as a result of the Longevity Assurance Genes Initiative of the National Institute on Aging. Genetically tractable species such as nematodes (*Caenorhabditis elegans*), fruit flies (*Drosophila melanogaster*), and yeast have been used extensively to interrogate the genetics of the aging process. Although phylogenetically far away from humans, these models have been chosen primarily because of their ease of manipulation, powerful genetics, and short life span. The earliest gene that was found to control the rate of aging in any organism was the *age-1* gene in *C. elegans*,[12] and subsequent work by several laboratories identified *daf-2* and *daf-16* as additional genes controlling life span in nematodes.[13–15] As it turned out, these genes all cluster within the insulin-signaling pathway: daf-2 is the nematode homolog of the insulin/IGF-like receptor, age-1 codes for the catalytic subunit of PI3K, and daf-16 codes for a forkhead transcription factor whose nuclear translocation is under the control of the insulin receptor/PI3K axis (Figure 6-1). In nematodes, binding of the Daf-2 receptor by any or some of the 38 known ILPs (insulin-like peptides) activates a signal transduction cascade that negatively regulates the activity of Daf-16. Under basal conditions, Daf-16 is phosphorylated and sequestered in the cytoplasm, and decreased activity of the Daf-2 pathway results in its dephosphorylation and subsequent translocation to the nucleus where it acts as a transcription factor, and activates a series of genes primarily involved in stress resistance, metabolism, and development. This pathway is inhibited by another gene involved in longevity regulation, *daf-18*, which is the nematode homolog of PTEN.

After this seminal work in *C. elegans*, the insulin/IGF pathway has been confirmed to play a role in regulating life span in other organisms, including *Drosophila* and mice. *Drosophila* has 7 different Dilps (*Drosophila* ILPs), and mutation of the insulin receptor substrate (IRS) chico leads to increased longevity. Mice (and humans) have a family of insulin-like receptors, including the insulin receptor (InsR) and the insulin-like growth factor receptors I and II (IGFR). Because neither *Drosophila* nor *C. elegans* has an "IGF receptor," it becomes relevant to establish which of the two pathways, insulin or IGF, is relevant to aging in mammals.

Several mouse models with increased longevity due to changes in the Ins/IGF pathway have been described. Most studied are the Ames[16] and the Snell[17] dwarf mice. These have mutations in the *Prop-1* and *Pit-1* genes, respectively, both of which are required for pituitary development, thus leading to a disruption of the somatotropic axis, which through the action of growth hormone (GH) regulates IGF-I levels. Furthermore, it has been observed that GH receptor knockouts[18] and IGF-1 receptor heterozygotes[19] are also long-lived. Many of these models have compensatory changes in both the insulin and IGF pathways, so the results are still not fully clear about the relative role of each of these pathways in longevity regulation. Interestingly, a recent report suggests that disruption of insulin signal in the brain through heterozygote deletion of one of the two IRS species, IRS2, leads to an extension of life span (18%) comparable to that observed by systemic IRS2 deletion.[20] These observations suggest a central control of insulin/IGF action that affects animal longevity, but the results have been contested by another group.[21] Further details are provided by the work of Conover and Bale,[22] which has shown that reduction of bioavailable IGF-1 (by deletion of PAPP-A, a protease that cleaves an IGF binding protein) also leads to an extension of life span. Certainly, many details still remain to be elucidated, but the available data support the hypothesis that the longevity extension observed in nematodes through manipulation of the Daf-2/Daf-16 pathway holds true in mice as well. Humans display an age-related decrease in GH release and IGF-1 synthesis, and the data from animal models leave open the possibility that this decrease in the activity of this axis might in fact be a protective mechanism. Indeed, supplementation of normal aged individuals with recombinant GH has resulted in significant adverse effects, with no clear benefits.[23] On the other hand, recent studies suggest that centenarian Ashkenazi Jews have a mutation in the IGF-I receptor, which in vitro correlates with a decrease in IGF signaling.[24]

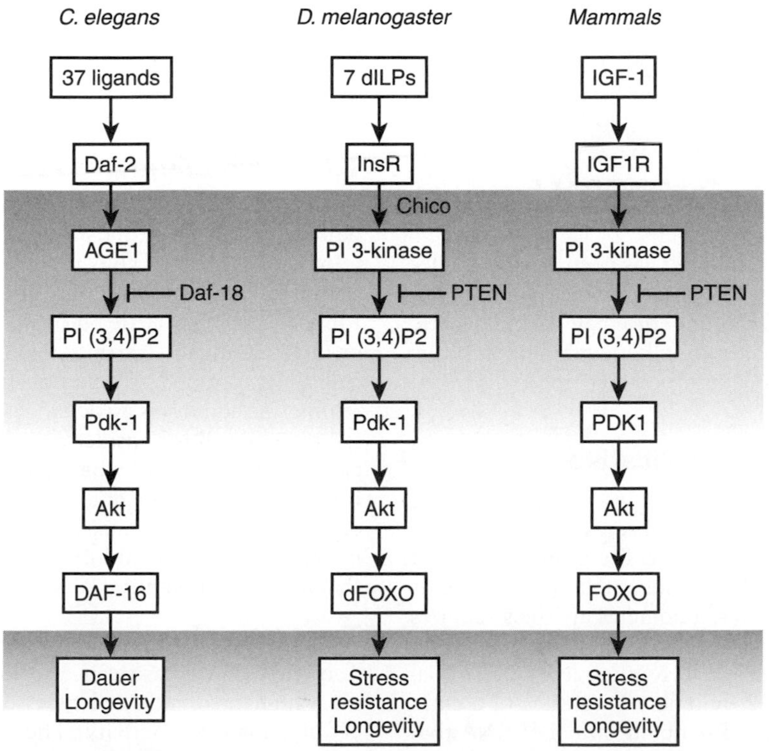

Figure 6-1. The insulin/IGF pathway is evolutionarily conserved, and has been shown to regulate longevity in several species, including *C. elegans, D. melanogaster,* and mammals. The figure depicts the similarities among the pathways in these three species. Of note, in both *C. elegans* and *D. melanogaster* there is only one pathway, whereas in mammals this has evolved into two separate ones, the insulin pathway and the IGF pathway. Although there is some debate, much of the evidence favors the IGF pathway as being relevant to longevity, and it is depicted here. There are also differences in the effectors that activate the pathways: in mammals there is only insulin and two IGFs, but in the lower species there are several ligands. The relative relevance of each of these ligands on aging has not yet been elucidated.

How does the insulin/IGF pathway regulate longevity? As mentioned above, the final result of the signal transduction cascade initiated at the receptor affects the translocation of Daf-16 to the nucleus. Daf-16 is the nematode homolog of mammalian FOXO (see Figure 6-1), and translocation of FOXO has been shown to be affected by several additional pathways involved in longevity.[25] Thus in addition to phosphorylation via the InsR/Akt pathway, FOXO phosphorylation is inhibited by a lipophilic signal sent from the gonads, and it is phosphorylated by activated AMP kinase in response to low energy, a pathway that could link FOXO to the mechanism of caloric restriction. FOXO is also modified in response to oxidative damage, both by phosphorylation through the JNK pathway and deacetylation by SirT1.[25] Thus it appears that FOXO lies at a nodal point that regulates organismal longevity in response to a variety of cues, both internal and external.[26] After translocation to the nucleus, FOXO acts as a transcription factor, upregulating the expression of a variety of genes involved in regulating the stress response, energy metabolism, cell proliferation, inflammation, and others.[27,28] It should be noted that nuclear translocation does not seem to be a sine qua non for FOXO's role in longevity. An increase in nuclear Daf-16 is not observed in *age-1* mutants, and constitutive nuclear localization of the transcription factor does not result in increased life span.[29]

It is important to keep in mind that although these genetic studies are aimed at unraveling the molecular mechanisms underlying the aging process, genetic manipulation of humans with the goal of extending life expectancy poses considerable ethical issues and is not the goal of aging research. Nevertheless, an understanding of the genetic basis of aging can provide valuable targets for therapeutic intervention and a solid theoretical foundation for age-delaying strategies (see later discussion under Why invest in basic aging research—the longevity dividend).

CELL PROLIFERATION, TELOMERASE, AND TELOMERE FUNCTION

The early work of Leonard Hayflick[4] has been interpreted by some to mean that aging itself is programmed. Although the number of doublings a cell can undergo may have a genetic basis, the number of doublings a cell actually undergoes is subject to stochastic events. This aspect of aging is discussed below.

Telomere structure and replicative senescence

The mechanistic basis of Hayflick's observation that human cells grown in culture have a limited life span remained a mystery until Harley et al[30] demonstrated that telomeres shorten each time a cell divides. Telomeres are the structures at the ends of chromosomes containing long noncoding repetitive sequences, and they are synthesized by a special enzyme called telomerase.[31] Telomerase consists of a catalytic protein complexed with a template strand of RNA that determines the repeating sequence of the telomeric DNA. Because most somatic cells do not express telomerase, as these cells continue to divide, the length of the telomeric DNA gradually shortens until a lower limit is reached (called the Hayflick limit), at which point proliferation ceases. This nonproliferative state is referred to as cell or replicative senescence. The idea that telomere length is critical to the proliferative potential of cells was strengthened by the observation that increasing cellular telomerase activity transgenically also increases the number of doublings a cell can undergo before reaching the senescent state.[32]

Telomeres consist of more than the long noncoding repetitive sequence at the 5′ end of each DNA strand. The telomeric DNA binds a large number of proteins that are important in the multiple functions of telomeres.[33] These proteins are not only involved in DNA replication, but they also protect the coding sequences near the ends of chromosomes, and prevent the recombination of chromosome ends with each other or with the double-stranded DNA ends transiently produced during the normal metabolism of DNA.

Telomere length and telomerase activity can impact human health in at least three general ways. One is through the altered phenotype of senescent cells, but negative effects can also be observed if there is either too much or too little telomerase activity present in the cell.

Altered phenotype and cancer

Phenotypical changes due to replicative senescence are best understood in the human fibroblast. Whereas fibroblasts normally facilitate the synthesis of the basement membrane that helps to repress the proliferation of the cells attached to it, senescent fibroblasts secrete enzymes that degrade this matrix material.[34] This degradation destroys the regulatory properties of the membrane, and Krtolica et al[35] have directly demonstrated that the presence of senescent cells promotes carcinogenesis of nearby preneoplastic cells. Thus replicative senescence is an example of antagonistic pleiotropy by preventing uncontrolled proliferation of cells in young animals,[36,37] but promoting cancer in their vicinity, a process of potential relevance as senescent cells accumulate with increasing age.[38]

Too much telomerase activity and cancer

Telomeres progressively shorten with time in proliferating human cells because most human cells contain little if any telomerase activity. Thus every time a cell proliferates, the telomeres get shorter because the cell replicative machinery cannot replace the little bit of DNA lost during the initiation of DNA synthesis. Exceptions include germ cells and stem cells,[39] lymphocytes,[40] and transformed cells.[41,42] Thus high telomerase activity is associated with the proliferative potential of cells and is considered to be a possible biomarker for cancer. The details of what actually causes telomerase activity to reappear in cancer cells, thus maintaining uncontrolled cancerous growth, remain to be worked out, but developing cancer drugs that inhibit telomerase is still a sought-after therapeutic intervention.

Too little telomerase activity and aging

Too little telomerase can also be a problem even though most human somatic cell types do not have significant levels of telomerase activity. The ability to replace damaged cells well into late life depends upon having robust stem cell pools, as the stem cells in these pools divide asymmetrically to produce the needed replacement cells. Telomerase activity is required to maintain the telomere length of the original mother cell. Individuals born with a mutation in either the telomerase catalytic protein or the associated template

RNA are defective in telomerase activity, and develop a condition known as dyskeratosis congenita (DC) because of their abnormal skin pigmentation. These patients may also present with nail dystrophy, premature hair graying, anemia, and/or bone marrow failure.[43,44] Bone marrow is a good source of hematopoietic and mesenchymal stem cells, so it is perhaps not surprising that defective telomere maintenance in stem cells might be associated with bone marrow failure. If failure to maintain tissue homeostasis contributes to the development of aging phenotypes, then decreased telomerase activity in stem cells is likely to accelerate aging indirectly because of decreased regenerative capacity of the pools.[45]

Rudolph et al[46] generated mice deficient in the RNA component of telomerase, and therefore lacking telomerase activity. Because mice have much longer telomeres than humans, the first three generations of these mice were fairly normal. However, by the sixth generation the mice were infertile, and their life span was reduced to 75% of normal. The sixth generation mice also had a reduced capacity to respond to stress or to repair wounds; they exhibited premature hair graying and had a higher spontaneous cancer incidence. Although increased telomerase activity is associated with cancer in humans, the loss of telomerase activity can also lead to genetic instability and cancer, indicating the complex and poorly understood relationships among telomere structure, cancer, and aging.

At least one other protein found in these telomeric complexes is related to a premature aging syndrome. Patients with Werner's syndrome (WS) lack a DNA helicase activity that results in growth retardation and early development of age-related pathologies beginning in the late teenage years.[47] Neither the role this DNA helicase plays in telomere structure and function, nor why its absence leads to premature aging, is known, but patients with WS typically develop cancer and osteoporosis prematurely, and die in their early fifties.

Telomere length as a biomarker of physiologic age

A surprising number of studies have reported an association between telomere length in lymphocyte DNA and some independent measure of human health and well-being. These include mortality,[48] Alzheimer's disease status,[49] exposure to psychologic stress,[50] cardiovascular disease,[51] and parental life span.[52] In every case these studies report a positive correlation between telomere length and healthy aging.[53] Neither the mechanistic basis for these associations, nor why these phenotypes correlate with telomere length in lymphocyte DNA, is well understood. However, they do support the concept that environmental factors also have an impact on aging.

CELL DEATH AND CELL REPLACEMENT — A CRITICAL ROLE FOR STEM CELLS?

Oxidative damage to cell components is random, although it may be concentrated in certain organelles such as the mitochondria, where most oxygen free radicals are generated. If the damage is severe enough, subsequent repair may be inadequate and apoptotic death may result, particularly mediated through the action of the $p66^{shc}$ and ATR proteins.[54,55] Cells lost through apoptosis must be replaced either through division of a nearby somatic cell, by a progenitor cell resident in the tissue where the cell has been lost, or by recruitment of a stem cell from an appropriate niche. Progenitor cells have long been known to be present in skeletal muscle in the form of satellite cells, but it has become clear that progenitor cells reside even in brain tissue.[56] Sharpless and DePinho[45] have recently proposed that "... ageing—once thought to be degenerative—might reflect a decline in regenerative capacity of resident stem cells across many tissues." Such an idea is certainly consistent with the time dependence of appearance of the many age-related pathologies that humans experience: osteoporosis, diabetes, sarcopenia, neurodegenerative diseases, end-stage renal disease, etc. It is not known why mesenchymal-derived tissues seem to be particularly vulnerable during aging.

An important question is whether the stem cell deficiency is quantitative (number of stem cells) or qualitative (function of stem cells). Available data suggest it may be either or both, depending on the tissue, the niche, and other signals and variables. For example, hematopoietic stem cell (HSC) number may be maintained, while HSC function declines.[57] Similarly, Conboy et al[58] showed that mouse satellite cells from old donors are rejuvenated in young recipients. These results suggest that stem cell function may decline during normal human aging. Such a decline could reflect either an altered ability to differentiate normally[59] or simply the decreased ability to replicate at all.[60] Recent evidence suggests that such declining stem cell functionality can be caused by DNA damage leading to excessive apoptosis,[61] and genetic mouse models also link this to premature aging phenotypes.[62,63] Excessive apoptosis forcing increased proliferation of stem cells to maintain tissue homeostasis, even in the absence of external DNA-damaging agents, can thus have adverse effects on stem cell niches resulting in accelerated aging.[33,45,55] In contrast, the presence of an overactive p53 protein[64,65] appears to cause premature aging by attenuating stem cell proliferation, leading to development of aging-related phenotypes, presumably due to inadequate cell replacement from stem cell niches.

In humans, telomerase activity is normally found only in the germline, stem cell niches, and activated lymphocytes. It would be of interest to know whether decreasing telomerase function is a factor in stem cell aging. Telomerase deficiency does lead to the development of age-related phenotypes in mice, but not until telomeres have been shortened by serial breeding of telomerase-deficient mice,[46] and replicative life span of hematopoietic stem cells is decreased by telomerase deficiency.[33,66]

PROGEROID SYNDROMES AND NORMAL AGING

Much progress in understanding human disease has been made by studying mouse models of the disease. Similar arguments can be made to support studies of aging of short-lived animal models such as yeast, nematodes, fruit flies, and mice. What is less accepted is whether there are appropriate accelerated human aging syndromes that may be informative about normal aging, in particular Werner's syndrome and Hutchinson-Gilford progeria syndrome (HGPS). Despite obvious differences with normal aging, these and other progeroid syndromes may provide uniquely informative opportunities to formulate and test hypotheses regarding the biology of aging and age-related diseases.[47,67] The phenotypes of these syndromes emerge at well-defined ages and include progressively degenerative changes similar to those observed during normal aging. The most common feature of both human and mouse mutations that accelerate the appearance of progeroid features is dysfunctional DNA metabolism, including replication, transcription, repair, and recombination. It remains to be determined whether such DNA dysfunction, and the cell death it may subsequently trigger, explains the time dependence of the appearance of progeroid phenotypes, and whether similar mechanisms are afoot although at a slower pace during normal aging. Such models may also provide clues about why mesenchymal stem cells might be particularly vulnerable in HGPS, as suggested by Halaschek-Wiener and Brooks-Wilson.[68]

PROTEIN DAMAGE AND SARCOPENIA—DOES PROTEIN OXIDATIVE DAMAGE PLAY A CAUSAL ROLE?

Aging is associated with a progressive decline of muscle mass, strength, and quality, a condition described as sarcopenia. The prevalence of sarcopenia in older adults is about 25% under the age of 70 years, and increases to 40% in adults 80 years or older.[69] Sarcopenia is a risk factor for frailty, loss of independence, and physical disability.[70] Sarcopenia and its detrimental correlates have an immense economical impact.[71] Thus understanding the mechanisms leading to muscle dysfunction (e.g., weakness) at advanced age represents a high public health priority.

The *free radical theory* of aging, formulated 50 years ago, proposes that aging can be attributed to deleterious effects of reactive oxygen species.[3] This hypothesis has been extensively investigated and debated, and although oxidative damage may not be the only cause of adverse age-related changes, it clearly has been linked to a number of them.[9] Overall, the *oxidative stress theory* states that a chronic state of oxidative stress exists in cells even under normal physiologic conditions because of an imbalance between prooxidants and antioxidants. This imbalance results in a net accumulation of oxidative damage in a variety of cellular macromolecules. Such oxidative damage increases during aging, which results in a progressive loss in the functional efficiency of various cellular processes.[72] Three tenets of this theory include: (1) there are many oxygen-derived metabolites and reactive nitrogen species produced during normal metabolism; (2) these metabolites damage the phospholipids, proteins, and DNA of the mitochondria and other critical cellular components; and (3) oxidative stress influences signaling, transcriptional control, and other normal processes within cells.

Skeletal muscle is particularly vulnerable to oxidative stress, due in part to the rapid and coordinated changes in energy supply and oxygen flux that occur during contraction, resulting in increased electron flux and leakage from the mitochondrial electron transport chain. Skeletal muscle also contains a high concentration of myoglobin, a heme-containing protein known to confer greater sensitivity to free radical-induced damage to surrounding macromolecules by converting hydrogen peroxide to other more highly reactive oxygen species.[73] Fundamental differences in skeletal muscle fiber type metabolism (slow-twitch aerobic fibers and fast-twitch glycolytic fibers) may confer differing degrees of susceptibility to oxidative stress and may be mechanistically related to the aging phenotype. The extent and time course of the deterioration of muscle function depend on many factors, such as the fiber type composition of the specific muscle studied and the selected age group. There is significant muscle atrophy, reductions in the force-generating capacity, slowing of contraction, and alterations in protein structure in fast-twitch fibers with normal aging.[74,75] In contrast, the age-associated atrophy and significant functional declines of the slow-twitch fibers occur later (well into senescence).[76]

The hypothesis that age-related deterioration of muscle function involves oxidative damage of muscle proteins by reactive oxygen and nitrogen (ROS and NOS) species[77] was suggested by a series of in vitro studies showing that ROS and NOS—such as peroxynitrite, hydroxyl radicals, H_2O_2, and nitric oxide—inhibit force production and induce changes in the regulation of calcium metabolism in skeletal muscle.[78–84] Studies on in vivo oxidative modifications of specific muscle proteins such as sarcoplasmic Ca^{2+}-ATPase (SERCA), actin, and myosin focused on a few selected markers, such as nitration of tyrosine (3-NT), formation of HNE (4-hydroxy-2-nonenal) adducts, oxidation of cysteine side chains, and glycation.[85–88]

The SERCA protein is probably the most extensively investigated muscle protein. These investigations focus on what sites are vulnerable to oxidative stress, and how the modification or damage alters protein function with increasing age. Normal aging of skeletal muscle is associated with increased nitration; in particular, specific nitration of the SERCA2a isoform in slow-twitch muscle.[85,89] Nitration can alter protein function and is associated with acute and chronic disease states.[90] 3-NT is formed when tyrosine is nitrated by peroxynitrite, a highly reactive molecule generated by the reaction of nitric oxide with superoxide. Muscle fibers are exposed to periodic fluxes of nitric oxide and superoxide, thus providing favorable conditions for the formation of peroxynitrite. Tyrosine nitration has the potential to inhibit protein function by altering protein conformation, imposing steric restrictions to the catalytic site, and preventing tyrosine phosphorylation.[91] Moreover, the functional significance of tyrosine nitration depends on both the site of modification and the extent of the protein population containing functionally significant modifications. Tyrosine nitration increases by at least threefold in skeletal muscle during normal aging, and correlates with a 40% loss in Ca^{2+}-ATPase activity during normal aging. Mass spectrometry analysis reveals an age-dependent accumulation of 3-NT at positions 294 and 295 of the SERCA2 protein, suggesting that these tyrosines play a critical role in muscle function. In vitro studies also demonstrate that SERCA2a is inherently sensitive to tyrosine nitration with concomitant functional deficits.[85,89] Because the physiologic role of the Ca-ATPase is to mediate muscle relaxation, the consequence of nitration-induced inhibition of SERCA2a most likely explains the slower contraction and relaxation times observed in skeletal muscle with normal aging.

Aging also leads to a partial loss of SERCA1 isoform activity, and a molecular rationale for this phenomenon may be the age-dependent oxidation of specific cysteine residues. Mapping of the specific cysteine residues reveals nine cysteine residues targeted by age-dependent oxidation in vivo, and six cysteine residues partially lost upon oxidant treatment in vitro.[92] Interestingly, the residues affected in vivo do not completely match those targeted in vitro, suggesting that modification of some residues do not contribute significantly to the loss of SERCA function with age. Taken together, these studies provide some insights about the molecular mechanisms responsible for age-related alterations in calcium regulation in skeletal muscle.

Myosin and actin are two key contractile proteins responsible for force generation and contraction speed. Age-related oxidative damage of myosin and actin are probably increased by decreased muscle protein turnover.[93] In the presence of reactive oxygen and nitrogen species, force is inhibited and contraction speed is altered.[78,79,94] Studies of in vivo oxidative modifications of myosin and actin have focused on selective markers of oxidative damage, such as nitration, formation of HNE adducts, and oxidation of cysteines.[86,88] During normal aging, myosin and actin do not significantly accumulate 3-NT or HNE-adducts. In contrast, an age-related decrease in cysteine content is detected in myosin, but not in actin with increasing age. Because the physiologic role of myosin and actin is to produce force and speed, the lack of accumulation of these oxidative stress markers is unlikely the explanation for age-related inhibitory changes in muscle contractility.

Another possible explanation of age-related inhibitory effects in muscle proteins is glycation. Accumulation of advanced glycation end products (AGEPs) resulting from the Maillard reaction alters the structural properties of proteins and reduces their susceptibility to degradation.[95] Decreased susceptibility of glycated proteins to degradation by the proteasome, the function of which is also compromised during aging,[96,97] might also contribute to the buildup of damaged proteins. Generally, muscle shows the least glycation of biologic tissues, with a basal level of glycation in muscle protein of 0.2 mmol/mol lysine,[98] but normal aging of skeletal muscle is associated with a tenfold increase in the percentage of fibers containing glycated proteins.[87] Subsequent mass spectrometry analysis identified the glycated proteins as creatine kinase, carbonic anhydrase III, β-enolase, actin, and voltage-dependent anion channel 1, with β-enolase showing an accumulation of CML with age in muscle. β-enolase may be a scavenger of AGE because lysines are at the exposed surface of the protein. This scavenging process may spare other proteins from AGE-modification and consequent functional impairment. β-enolase is a good candidate for this role because glycation of this protein has only a limited impact on cell physiology. Indeed, although glycation leads to a decrease in β-enolase activity, no changes were detected in glycolytic flux.[99] The significance of glycation of other skeletal muscle protein on muscle function is unknown, yet in vitro studies show that glycation decreases myosin and actin interactions.[100]

Taken together, these studies provide some insights about potential molecular mechanisms responsible for age-related alterations in contractility. An important limitation in the characterization of damaged proteins from muscle tissue is the fact that the data provide only a snapshot of a dynamic process because proteins are constantly being synthesized and degraded in most tissues. Furthermore, current knowledge about posttranslational modification due to oxidative stress, and the techniques available to measure them, may not permit the quantitative analysis of all potential modifications of a given protein of interest and its functional characterization. It is likely that the future will see a significant increase in the number of specific modifications of proteins known, and an increase in our ability to associate them with specific aging phenotypes.

In summary, reduced muscle function and its attendant decrease in physical performance with age is a significant public health problem. Sarcopenia affects more than half of Americans older than age 50,[101] at an estimated annual cost of $18.5 billion.[71] The cumulative effect of the reductions in skeletal muscle mass and function with age is a decrease in the capacity for physical work. This manifests as an inability to perform simple tasks of everyday life[101–105] and has been shown to contribute to disability,[69,101,106,107] greater risk for falls and fractures,[69] increases in all-cause mortality,[108] and, in general, a poor quality of life. People 85 and older are the fastest growing segment of the U.S. population, and estimates indicate that by 2030 almost 1 in 5 Americans, or 72 million people, will be 65 years or older (U.S. Census Bureau, 2005). Thus the incidence and prevalence of age-related decrements in muscle performance will increase, necessitating greater health care expenditures for supportive services and long-term care. Oxidative damage to key skeletal muscle proteins may be a contributing factor in sarcopenia. However, conclusive results require a more complete determination of the extent and location of oxidized sites, with parallel assessment of functional interactions of the proteins. Thus future research in the field of sarcopenia will attempt to identify and quantify all of the posttranslational modifications that a specific muscle protein accrues in vivo, and determine their functional implications.

WHY INVEST IN BASIC AGING RESEARCH?—THE LONGEVITY DIVIDEND

Much of current research into the biologic mechanisms of aging use death (life span) as an end point. Most biogerontologists agree that this is not the ideal end point, but it is used because we currently do not have any good biomarkers of the process, and ascertaining biologic age, as opposed to chronologic age, in laboratory animals is not an easy task. As a corollary to that choice, some believe that the purpose of basic aging research should be to increase human life span. Not only is that perception incorrect, but it is also dangerous. Indeed, it has been a long-held view that increasing the life span of humans will lead to a dramatic increase in the incidence of disease and disability.[109] If modern medicine succeeds in increasing life span without a concomitant increase in health span, the result could be a society of sick and infirm individuals, with poor quality of life, who will exert an enormous pressure on the economy by increasing the investment required for pensions, retirement, and health care costs.

Unfortunately, that is what appears to have happened during the last century, when median life span in the United States increased from 47 to 77.8 years, and at the same time, there has been a dramatic increase in the number of people with chronic disabilities and disease. As an example, Alzheimer's disease was not even described until 1907, and currently more than 4 million Americans have been diagnosed with the disease. So the prevalent view is that increasing the human life span any further will only lead to an ever more crippled society.

Most of the efforts of modern medicine are focused on addressing (and hopefully defeating) each of the major diseases burdening our population. For the aged, major fatal chronic diseases include cardiovascular diseases, cancer, dementias, and diabetes, but the quality of life is also impoverished by nonfatal diseases and conditions, such as osteoporosis, arthritis, sarcopenia, and others.[110] Enormous progress has been made in understanding and treating several (but not all) of these disorders. Although such treatments and cures "benefit" a few individuals (those afflicted), it has been calculated that curing any of the major fatal diseases will only have a marginal impact on median life span, usually in the order of 3 to 6 years.[111] Furthermore, the benefit to those cured may be only relative because usually the elderly suffer from multiple disease conditions in parallel (comorbidities), so that curing any one of them will still leave them exposed to the ravages of the others. As an example, let us imagine that suddenly all cardiovascular diseases are conquered, and no one will ever again die of this. Many people who currently have semiclogged arteries would be elated by the news, and many of them would indeed go on to live useful lives for a few extra years. But the preponderant majority of individuals currently affected by cardiovascular disease are in a general state of diminished health and comorbidities, and the extra years of life are more than likely to be spent in an ever more frail state, as other age-related diseases (diabetes, Alzheimer's) take hold. Thus the increase in life span observed in the last century has led to an increase in the incidence of these other diseases. We have indeed conquered a major previous killer, infectious disease, and that led to the increased incidence of previously uncommon illnesses, such as cancer, diabetes, Alzheimer's.

What is then to be done? Aging is the major risk factor for most, if not all, age-related diseases.[112] For example, a high cholesterol diet will have only a minor immediate impact on the health of a young individual, but could be fatal for an older one (or for the same young individual, once he or she ages). If we accept that age is a major risk factor for these diseases, then as a corollary, slowing the rate of aging should be expected to result in a delay in the appearance of all or most age-related diseases, conditions, and ailments.[113,114] If instead of addressing one disease at a time, as if their causes were independent, we recognize that age-related biologic changes are the main cause behind most age-related illnesses, then addressing the biologic changes that drive the process of aging is much more likely to have beneficial effects for humanity.[115] In effect, it has been calculated that a small decrement in the slope of the aging rate curve could result in a significant increase in the proportion of our life span spent in a healthy, disease-free state. A delay of just 7 years in the appearance of major age-related illnesses could result in a net increase in health span of 50% based on the fact that age-related decline rises exponentially with age, with a doubling time of approximately 7 years.[116]

At this time, such a goal seems within reach based on results obtained in animal models. Although much longevity research is performed in *C. elegans*, with few exceptions[117] there is a clear scarcity of reports dealing with physiologic data in these animals, so we cannot ascertain for sure whether or not extension in life span in this model occurred in a healthy or diseased state. On the contrary, a more modest but generally reproducible increase in both median and maximal life span has been observed in rodents subjected to caloric restriction by 40%.[2] It is not clear whether a similar increase can be obtained in humans, but the observations in a variety of mammals indicate that the increase in life span afforded by caloric restriction is accompanied by a general delay in the aging process, such that restricted animals show a delay in the appearance of most age-related declines and diseases measured, both at the physiologic and pathologic level. Independently of whether caloric restriction (or a mimetic thereof) will work in humans, the data show that the rate of aging can be externally manipulated. Thus by delaying the onset of age-related decline, it is possible to postpone the entire range of age-related ailments, leading to a significant extension of the period of healthy living. This concomitant effect at a host of different levels has been termed *The Longevity Dividend*.[5,6]

Interestingly, the longevity dividend concept extends well beyond health and well-being. A significant concern in many societies is the potential economic impact of the oncoming onslaught of age-related disease and disability, which threatens to break our pension and health care systems. The longevity dividend concept predicts that by addressing the basic mechanisms of aging, humans could live longer productive lives. This would translate into tangible economic benefits because people would be able to stay in the workforce longer (thus allowing for further wealth production and savings), and would withdraw less funds from pensions and the health care system. The economic implications of the longevity dividend have been explored in further detail elsewhere.[113]

KEY POINTS
Biology of Aging

- Decreasing the activity of the insulin-signaling pathway at any one of many steps, in a variety of animal models (fruit flies, nematodes, mice), shifts the focus of the organism from growth and reproduction to stress response and survival, thereby increasing its longevity.
- Damage to critical proteins changes their structure and compromises their function, and unless repaired or replaced, ultimately may decrease tissue function.
- Damage to DNA sufficient to block one of its critical functions (replication, transcription, repair, or recombination) may lead to cell death, and the need to replace that cell from a relevant progenitor cell pool.
- Excessive cell death can ultimately lead to exhaustion of the relevant progenitor cell pools responsible for maintaining tissue homeostasis in the presence of stress.
- Elucidating the biologic causes of aging is inherently important because aging is a major risk factor for development of most age-related pathology.

If we do manage to postpone aging, are there new diseases that will appear? Yes, that is a distinct possibility and a caveat to what has been exposed above. Even though so far we have been unable to increase maximal life span in humans,[111] modifying the aging process in animal models (e.g., by caloric restriction) does achieve that goal. If this is extrapolated to humans, it is indeed possible that currently rare or even new ailments will make their mark, just as defeating infectious diseases and many causes of childhood deaths did lead to an increase in the incidence of what we now call age-related diseases and conditions. Similarly, significantly extending median and maximal life span might lead to an increase in the prevalence of now rare diseases, such as liver amyloidosis. In this context, it is relevant to note that in studies conducted to date, it has been observed that most centenarians and super centenarians die of the same array of causes as younger individuals (with maybe a slightly lower incidence of cancer).[118] Nevertheless, if half of the human population reaches 100 years, and then are afflicted by these diseases, we still would have achieved an important goal: keep them healthy until their 90s. That could be one goal of modern medicine.

For a complete list of references, please visit online only at www.expertconsult.com

CHAPTER 7

Genetic Mechanisms of Aging

Chao-Qiang Lai
Laurence D. Parnell
Jose M. Ordovas

INTRODUCTION

Our society is experiencing unprecedented demographic changes where improvements in health care and living conditions together with decreased fertility rates have contributed to the aging of the population and a severe demographic redistribution.[1] Over the last 50 years, the ratio of people aged 60 years and over to children younger than 15 increased by about half, from 24 per hundred in 1950 to 33 per hundred in 2000. Worldwide by the year 2050, there will be 101 people 60 years and older for every 100 children 0 to 14 years old,[2] and many people over age 60 suffer from chronic illnesses or disabilities.[3] Therefore, to better understand the mechanisms of aging and the genetic and environmental factors that modulate the rate of aging, it is essential to cope with the impact of these demographic changes.[4] Aging can be defined as "a progressive, generalized impairment of function, resulting in an increased vulnerability to environmental challenge and a growing risk of disease and death."[5] It is generally assumed that accumulated damage to a variety of cellular systems is the underlying cause of aging.[5] To date, a large proportion of aging research has focused on individual age-related disorders compromising adult life expectancy and healthy aging, including cardiovascular disease (heart disease, hypertension), cerebrovascular diseases (stroke), cancer, chronic respiratory disease, diabetes, mental disorders, oral disease, and osteoarthritis and other bone/joint disorders. Environmental factors, such as diet, physical activity, smoking, and sunlight exposure, exert a direct impact on these disorders, whereas significant genetic components make separate contributions. Although individual genetic factors could be small differences in DNA sequences—single nucleotide polymorphisms or small insertions/deletions—in both the nuclear and mitochondrial genomes, the overall genetic contribution to aging processes is polygenic and complex.

The complexity of aging is reflected in that numerous models have been proposed to explain why and how organisms age and yet they address the problem only to a limited extent. The models that are more widely accepted include: (1) the oxidative stress theory implicating declines in mitochondrial function[6]; (2) the insulin/IGF-1 signaling (IIS) hypothesis suggesting that extended life span is associated with reduced IIS signaling[7]; (3) the somatic mutation/repair mechanisms focusing on the cellular capacity to respond to damage to cellular components, including DNA, proteins, and organelles[8]; (4) the immune system plays a central role in the process of aging[9]; (5) the telomere hypothesis of cell senescence, involving the loss of telomeric DNA and ultimately chromosomal instability[10]; and (6) inherited mutations associated with risk for common chronic and degenerative disorders.[11,12] In this work we will elaborate on the genetic component of each of these six hypotheses and the need for a more integrative approach to aging research.

MITOCHONDRIAL GENETICS, OXIDATIVE STRESS, AND AGING

The central role of mitochondria in aging, initially outlined by Harman,[13] proposed that aging, and associated chronic degenerative diseases, could be attributed to the deleterious effects of reactive oxygen species (ROS) on cell components. As the major site of ROS production, the mitochondrion is itself a prime target for oxidative damage. Moreover, this is the only organelle in animal cells with its own genome, (mtDNA), which is mostly unprotected, closely localized to the respiratory chain, and subject to irreversible damage by ROS. Specifically, accumulation of mtDNA somatic mutations, shown to occur with age,[14] often map within genes encoding 13 protein subunits of the electron transport chain (ETC) or 24 RNA components vital to mitochondrial protein synthesis. Not surprisingly, this mtDNA damage has been associated with deleterious functional alterations in the activity of ETC complexes. These mutations, whether single point mutations or deletions, have been shown in many studies to be associated with aging and with multiple chronic and degenerative disorders.[15] An early report examining the integrity of mtDNA found accumulated mtDNA damage more pronounced in senescent rats compared with young animals.[16] Other reports followed, including age-associated decreases in the respiratory chain capacity in various human tissues.[17] Hypotheses put forward stated that acquired mutations in mtDNA increase with time and segregate in mitotic tissues, eventually causing decline of respiratory chain function leading to age-associated degenerative disease and aging.[17] Furthermore, mtDNA haplotypes are associated with longevity in humans.[18,19] In sum, this mitochondrial genome–ROS production theory of aging is mechanistically sound and appealing.[20]

Deletions are the most commonly reported mtDNA mutations accumulating in aging tissues, and evidence for their role in aging is considered supporting.[21] In order to solidify the importance of mtDNA damage in aging, Trifunovic et al[22] developed a mouse model that indicated a causative link between mtDNA mutations and aging phenotypes in mammals. This "mtDNA mutator" mouse model was engineered with a defect in the proofreading function of mitochondrial DNA polymerase (Polg), leading to the progressive, random accumulation of mtDNA mutations during mitochondrial biogenesis. As mtDNA proofreading in these mice is efficiently curtailed, a phenotype develops with a threefold to fivefold increase in the levels of point mutations.[22] However, the abnormally higher rate of mutation took place during early embryonic stages, and mtDNA mutations continued to accumulate at a lower, near normal rate during subsequent life stages.[23] Although these mice display a completely normal phenotype at birth and in early adolescence, they subsequently acquire many features of premature aging, such as weight loss, reduced subcutaneous fat, alopecia, kyphosis, osteoporosis, anemia, reduced fertility, heart disease, sarcopenia, progressive hearing loss, and decreased spontaneous activity.[22] Such results confirm that mtDNA point mutations can cause aging phenotypes if present at high enough levels, but alone do not prove that the lower levels measured in normal aging are sufficient to cause aging phenotypes. Hence, attention turned to the focal distribution of mtDNA mutations rather than the overall amount as key in disrupting the efficiency of the respiratory chain and thus driving the observed aging phenotypes. To prove this hypothesis, Müller-Höcker examined hearts from individuals of different ages and reported focal respiratory chain deficiencies in a subset of cardiomyocytes in an age-dependent manner.[24] This was subsequently supported by evidence from a number of other cell types.[25–27] In sum, intracellular mosaicism, resulting from uneven distribution of acquired mtDNA mutations, can cause respiratory chain deficiency and lead to tissue dysfunction in the presence of low overall levels of mtDNA mutations.

The mitochondrial hypothesis of aging is conceptually straightforward, but in reality is much more complex[28] because a minimal threshold level of a pathogenic mtDNA mutation must be present in a cell to cause respiratory chain deficiency, and this threshold may vary between experimental models.[29] With 100 to 10,000 mtDNA copies per cell, mtDNAs that are mutated and normal at a given position coexist within a cell, tissue, or organ—a condition termed heteroplasmy. Different types of heteroplasmic mtDNA mutations have different thresholds for induction of respiratory chain dysfunction.[17] Moreover, subjects carrying heteroplasmic mtDNA mutations often display varying levels of mutated mtDNA in different organs and even in different cells of a single organ.[17] Furthermore, the intracellular distribution of mitochondria could play a role in the manifestation of the effects of mtDNA mutations.[30]

Although significant advances in our understanding of the role of mitochondria in aging have been made, it is likely that current theories will be revised as the link between mtDNA mutations and ROS production is more deeply probed.[31] Moreover, as the role of mitochondria in the response to caloric restriction is gaining relevance, available data are contradictory and not easily reconciled.[32] Thus research efforts will continue to describe the role of the mitochondrion in influencing the mechanisms of aging, but several boundaries should be heeded: (1) the difference in complexity between humans and model organisms at genetic, cellular, and organ levels; (2) the particular life span of each species, especially as medicine has allowed humans to live beyond a "normal" age of death; (3) the genetics of inbred animals often used in experiments contradicts humans who are highly outbred; and (4) the environmental conditions in which animals (highly standardized) and humans (quite different for anthropologic and cultural reasons) live.[33]

CHROMOSOMAL GENE MUTATIONS AND AGING

Genetic factors associated with human longevity and healthy aging remain largely unknown. Heritability estimates of longevity derived from twin registries and large population-based samples suggest a significant but modest genetic contribution to human life span of about 15% to 30%.[34] However, genetic influences on life span may be greater as an individual ages.[35] Moreover, the reported magnitude of the genetic contribution to other important aspects of aging such as healthy physical aging (wellness), physical performance, cognitive function, and bone aging are much larger.[34] Both exceptional longevity and a healthy aging phenotype have been linked to the same region on chromosome 4,[36,37] suggesting that although longevity per se and healthy aging are different phenotypes, they may share some common genetic pathways.

A number of potential candidate genes in a variety of biologic pathways have been associated with longevity in model organisms. Most of these genes have human orthologs and thus have potential to yield insights into human longevity.[38]

First, the most prominent hypothesis of aging states that mutants with decreased signaling through the insulin/IGF-1 signaling (IIS) pathway have extended life span. This pathway is evolutionarily conserved from nematodes to humans.[39] Thus genes of this pathway are promising candidate genes for influencing human longevity and healthy aging. Several studies have reported the association between genetic variants at *IGF1R* and *PI3KCB* and reduction of insulin-IGF-1activation and longevity.[40,41] The finding that a nonsynonymous mutation in *IGF1R* was found to be overrepresented in centenarians of shorter stature when compared with controls[42] supports a role for the IIS pathway in life-span extension in humans, thus extending observations in model organisms.

Second, macromolecule repair mechanisms regulate the process of aging.[6] Dysfunctional systems for damage repair to cellular constituents, such as DNA, proteins, and organelles, could curtail life span. These repair mechanisms are evolutionarily conserved across species.[43] Many studies support the detrimental effects of defective repair on reduced life span. Examples are human premature aging patients with mutations in a RecQ helicase, a crucial enzyme responsible for DNA strand break repair.[44] Variation at this gene has shown association with cardiovascular diseases.[45] However, few studies have demonstrated that an enhanced repair ability increases life span.[46] In addition, the altered protein/waste accumulation in the process of aging could aggravate cellular damage.[10] Thus dysfunction in clearance of cellular waste, which is also called autophagy, would accelerate aging. Downregulation of autophagy gene expression, such as *Atg7* and *Atg12*, has shortened the life span of both wild type and *daf-2* mutant *C. elegans*.[47]

Third, the immune system plays a central role in the process of aging.[9] Although inflammation is an essential defense of immune systems, chronic inflammation often leads to premature aging and mortality.[48] One key player of inflammation is the cytokine interleukin 6 (*IL6*). *IL6* overexpression has been linked to many age-related that such as rheumatoid arthritis, osteoporosis, Alzheimer disease, cardiovascular diseases, and type 2 diabetes.[49,50] Human studies have also demonstrated that *IL6* genetic variation is associated with longevity.[51,52]

Finally, cardiovascular disease is the major cause of morbidity and mortality in industrialized countries and thus a major obstacle to healthy aging and longevity. Much attention has been placed on genes encoding proteins functioning in lipid metabolism. Plasma lipid levels are highly dependent on age, gender, nutritional status, and other behavioral factors. It is therefore difficult, at least in cross-sectional studies, to determine to what extent a particular lipoprotein phenotype is causally associated with aging. One way to circumvent this issue is to rely on long-term prospective studies or to perform family-based studies.[11] Well-designed case-control genetic studies may also be advantageous because identification of particular variants associated with longevity may provide some hints to the biologic pathways leading to exceptional longevity. To that end, a large number of allelic variants in genes encoding apolipoproteins (*APOE, APOB, APOC1, APOC2, APOC3, APOA1, and APOA5*), transfer proteins (microsomal transfer protein [MTP], cholesteryl ester transfer protein [CETP]), proteins associated with HDL particles (PON1), and transcription factors involved in lipid metabolism (peroxisome proliferator-activated receptor gamma [PPARG]) have been examined in elderly populations. Similar to many other aspects of lipoprotein metabolism and cardiovascular disease risk, the most explored locus in terms of associations with longevity has been that of the *apolipoprotein E* (*APOE*) gene. Since the initial observation by Davignon et al,[53] reports from different parts of the world have observed a higher frequency of the *APOE4* allele in middle-aged subjects compared with older subjects (octogenarians, nonagenarians, and centenarians), concluding that the presence of the *APOE4* allele was associated with decreased life span.[54]

To summarize, data accumulated so far illustrate that a variety of genes are involved in several mechanisms of aging, age-related diseases, and to a certain extent with longevity. Although thus far tenuous, there are a number of clues indicating that there is crosstalk between genes involved in longevity and those involved in age-related diseases that could be involved in longevity beyond effects on healthy aging.

Genetics is a valuable tool to expand our understanding of the molecular basis of aging. However, most studies published so far have been limited by design (i.e., cross-sectional study, small sample size, limited SNP coverage of a small number of candidate genes, interethnic differences) and so results have been inconsistent.[55] Most recently, genomewide association studies (GWAS) offer a more comprehensive and untargeted approach to detect genes with modest phenotypic effects that underlie common complex conditions.[56] Some notable findings are emerging from GWAS with a focus on aging-related phenotypes.[34,57,58] However, to benefit fully from the contribution of genetics, large prospective studies need to be undertaken and fully supported by extensive genotyping and analytical capacities to collect adequate phenotype data. Even more important is the urgent need for a reliable intermediate phenotype for aging, both for genetic studies and for therapeutic interventions.[57]

Telomeres and aging

Telomeres are repetitive DNA sequences that are wrapped in specific protein complexes and located at the ends of linear chromosomes. Telomeres distinguish natural chromosome ends from DNA double-stranded breaks and thus promote genome stability.[59] Although traditionally considered as silent structural genomic regions, recent data suggest that telomeres are transcribed into RNA molecules, which remain associated with telomeric chromatin, suggesting RNA-mediated mechanisms in organizing telomere architecture.[60]

Telomere length has been proposed as a potentially reliable marker of biologic age, shorter telomeres reflecting more advanced age. Thus telomeres fit within mechanisms explaining the Hayflick limit[61] because they shorten progressively with each cell division. When a critical telomere length is reached, cells undergo senescence and subsequent apoptosis. Initial telomere length is mainly determined by genetic factors.[62,63] Although telomere shortening may be a normal biologic occurrence with each cell division, exposure to harmful environmental factors may affect its rate, accelerating telomere shortening.[64] To counter telomere shortening, telomerase, a cellular reverse transcriptase, promotes maintenance of telomere ends in human stem cells, reproductive cells, and cancer cells by adding TTAGGG repeats onto the telomeres. Moreover, recent studies suggest the existence of chromosome-specific mechanisms of telomere length regulation determining a telomere length profile, which is inherited and upheld throughout life.[65] Telomerases also may be involved in several essential cell signaling pathways without apparent involvement of well-established functions in telomere maintenance.[66] However, most normal human cells do not express telomerase and thus each time a cell divides some telomeric sequences are lost. When telomeres in a subset of cells become short (unprotected), cells enter an irreversible growth arrest state called replicative senescence.[67] The crucial role of telomeres in cell turnover and aging is highlighted by patients with 50% of normal telomerase levels resulting from a mutation in one of the telomerase genes. Short telomeres in such patients are implicated in a variety of disorders, including dyskeratosis congenita, aplastic anemia, pulmonary fibrosis, and cancer.[68] In addition to this manifestation in rare genetic disorders, short telomeres have been reported in the general population for several common chronic diseases, such as cardiovascular diseases[69,70] hypertension,[71] diabetes,[72] and dementia.[73] With respect to cancer[74] dysfunctional telomeres activate the oncoprotein p53 (TP53) to initiate cellular senescence or apoptosis to suppress tumorigenesis. However, in the absence of p53, telomere dysfunction is an important mechanism to generate chromosomal instability commonly found in human carcinomas.[75] Telomerase is expressed in the majority of human cancers, making it an attractive therapeutic target. Emerging antitelomerase therapies, currently in clinical trials, might prove useful against some human cancers.[76]

Based on current evidence, telomere shortening clearly accompanies human aging, and premature aging syndromes often are associated with short telomeres. These two observations are central to the hypothesis that telomere length directly influences longevity. If true, genetically determined mechanisms of telomere length homeostasis should significantly contribute to variations of longevity in the human population. Unraveling cause versus consequence of telomere shortening observed in the course of many aging-associated disorders is not an easy task. In addition, it remains unclear whether the biomarker value in a particular disease depends on shorter telomere length at birth or rather if it is merely a reflection of an accelerated telomere attrition during lifetime, or a combination of both. Although the importance of telomere attrition is supported by cross-sectional evidence associating shorter telomeres with oxidative stress and inflammation, longitudinal studies are required to accurately assess telomere attrition and its presumed link with accelerated aging.[77]

Epigenetics and aging

There is wide recognition that the fetal environment may strongly influence the risk of cardiovascular diseases and diabetes, both age-related disorders, as supported by epidemiologic data in humans and experimental animal models. It has been widely assumed that these long-lasting consequences of early-life exposures depend on the same mechanisms as those underlying "cellular memory" (i.e., epigenetic inheritance systems). There is a growing body of evidence that environmentally induced perturbations in epigenetic processes (such as DNA methylation and histone modification) can determine different aspects of aging, and the etiology and pathogenesis of age-related diseases.[78] Moreover, epigenetic alterations, such as global hypomethylation and CpG island hypermethylation, are progressively accumulated during aging and contribute to cell transformation, a hallmark of cancer.[79] Epigenetic tagging of genes controls expression of the genome and maintains cellular memory after many cellular divisions. Thus there is great importance in studying the epigenome to better comprehend genome health and the genetic mechanisms of aging. Moreover, tagging can be modulated by the environment, implying that environmentally induced changes in the epigenome could decrease or accelerate the process of unhealthy aging.[80]

An integrative approach to aging mechanisms

Caloric or dietary restriction (CR or DR)[81] is considered a universal mechanism that prolongs the life span of many organisms.[82] Although there is no unified explanation, multiple mechanisms and networks are thought to be involved. First, CR can extend life span through shifting energy metabolism. Although yeast under CR display enhanced respiration and decreased fermentation,[83] CR-mammals shift energy expenditure toward metabolizing fat and glycogen over glucose. One molecular mechanism potentially linking caloric restriction with longevity involves the PPARG pathway, possibly via lipid metabolism.[84] Picard et al[84] have shown that Sirt1 (sirtuin 1), the mammalian SIR2 ortholog, promotes fat mobilization in white adipocytes by repressing the effects of PPARG. Second, CR can extend life span by reducing ROS-mediated damage. Upon CR, SIRT1 also activates peroxisome proliferator-activated receptor gamma-coativator-1α (PPARGC1A), which regulates a series of nuclear receptors and controls mitochondrial function, oxidative phosphorylation, and cellular energy metabolism.[85] Upregulation of PPARGC1A reduces ROS production,[86] thus limiting mtDNA damage. PPARGC1A variants are associated with type 2 diabetes, CVD, DNA damage, and high blood pressure in humans.[87,88] Third, CR-animals are resistant to stress and inflammation through Foxo1 and Sirt1 inhibition of NF-κB signaling.[89] The most likely mechanism of CR-extension of life span adopts the hormesis hypothesis, a positive response of the organism to a low-intensity stressor.[90] CR is an evolutionarily conserved stress response using stress-responsive survival pathways that evolved long ago to provide for increased likelihood of survival in diverse environments.[82] Therefore, it is important to recognize the complexity of mechanisms involved in aging and the need to integrate several pathways and cellular mechanisms in understanding healthy aging. The term *network theory of aging* has been proposed[91] to overcome the reduction nature of individual models and to allow for interactions between individual contributing mechanisms. A proof of concept example is to consider interactions between two individual mechanisms that contribute to aging: DNA damage response and telomere maintenance. The key framework for considering these interactions is the integrative model, which predicts that telomere maintenance is an integral part of DNA damage response machinery. The integrative model predicts the dual phenotype, namely dysfunctional DNA damage response and dysfunctional telomere maintenance, where one of these mechanisms is the cause of aging. In line with this prediction, between 87% and 90% of mouse models and human examples of premature aging show this dual phenotype. Hence the integrative model is consistent with the network theory of aging. Others have provided evidence suggesting the connection between DNA damage in telomeres and mitochondria during cellular senescence.[92] Accordingly, improvement of mitochondrial function results in less telomeric damage and slower telomere shortening, whereas telomere-dependent growth arrest is associated with increased mitochondrial dysfunction. Moreover, telomerase, the enzyme complex known to re-elongate shortened telomeres, also appears to function independently of telomeres to protect against oxidative stress. Together, these data suggest a self-amplifying cycle between the genetics of the mitochondrion and the telomere: DNA damage during cellular senescence promotes aging and age-related disorders.

ACKNOWLEDGMENTS

Supported by the National Institutes of Health, National Institute on Aging, Grant 5R03AG023914 and NIH/NHLBI Grant HL54776 and NIH/NIDDK DK075030 and contracts 53-K06-5-10 and 58-1950-9-001 from the U.S. Department of Agriculture Research Service.

KEY POINTS

Genetic Mechanisms of Aging

- Important links between ROS production, mtDNA mutations, and aging, while strong, require further research.
- The mitochondrial role in the response to caloric restriction is coming to light.
- A number of nuclear encoded genes and their genetic variants affect any of several mechanisms of aging and longevity
- Genomewide association studies hold promise to identify genetic variants pertinent to aging, but intermediate biomarkers of aging are critically needed.
- Shorter telomeres accompany human aging, and premature aging syndromes often associate with telomere shortening but deciphering the causal role of telomere length in aging remains.
- The environment affects epigenetic processes and can influence the progression of aging and age-related diseases.
- The network theory of aging serves to link the genetic aspects of mtDNA damage, telomere maintenance with aging and age-related disorders.

For a complete list of references, please visit online only at www.expertconsult.com

CHAPTER 8

Cellular Mechanisms of Aging

Robert Santer

This chapter is an account of the subcellular mechanisms that are currently believed to have a major role in age-associated changes in cells that will ultimately result in cell death. Research into aging at a cellular level has burgeoned in recent years and is currently gathering pace as more and more is revealed about the causes and consequences of aging at this level. It is now generally accepted that age-associated cellular damage principally affects membrane lipids, proteins involved in metabolic and structural roles, nuclear and mitochondrial DNA, and intracellular signaling processes. There is also a reduction in aging of cellular maintenance and repair as a result of which cells are unlikely to recover from age-associated damage. It is also becoming clear that many cellular mechanisms of aging are closely tied to and interface with cellular mechanisms of diseases such as cancer and of certain degenerative diseases.

DESTRUCTIVE AGENTS IN CELLULAR AGING

Environmental agents

Ultraviolet (UV) solar radiation, the amount of which reaching the surface of the earth is increasing, causes damage to DNA; proteins, and lipids in the skin; and in the cornea, lens, and retina of the eye. DNA bases absorb UV light, resulting in structural changes that can be mutagenic such that a base becomes noncoding or miscoding.[1] Furthermore other abundant UV-induced mutagenic or lethal base lesions are cyclobutane-pyrimidine dimers and 6-4 photoproducts, which are potentially lethal because they can inhibit DNA polymerases from successful transcription.[1] An early cellular response to UV-induced DNA damage is by UV-damaged, DNA-binding proteins, which bind selectively to UV-irradiated DNA to switch on the cell's response to radiation damage.[2] UV-induced protein damage results in the accumulation of high molecular weight aggregates and reduced protein synthesis. Plasma membrane lipid damage by UV is mainly photo-oxidation of thiol groups and peroxidation of lipids themselves. UV-induced molecular mutations are greatly enhanced by the presence of oxygen. Thus, although oxygen is essential to life, it is the source of potentially damaging reactive oxygen species (ROS) that are found in the environment. Many sources of ROS are present in the environment ranging from exposure to additional ionizing radiation (from industry, nuclear radiation, and medicinal X-irradiation), ozone and nitrous oxide (primarily from automobile emissions), heavy metals (mainly cadmium, mercury, and lead), cigarette smoke (from both active and passive exposure), unsaturated fats, and many other chemicals intentionally or unintentionally present in foodstuffs.

Reactive oxygen species

The generation of reactive oxygen species (ROS) is a continuous process and a normal part of metabolism, especially the oxidative phosphorylation that takes place in mitochondria for the production of ATP. Thus the moment a new cell comes into existence following cell division, it will become a source of ROS production. ROS (originally called free radicals) were suggested to be a fundamental source of subcellular damage leading to cellular aging by Harman[3] more than 50 years ago and have come to be accepted as major, proven agents of such age-associated damage. ROS are ubiquitous and are extremely reactive clusters of atoms on account of the fact that they have an unpaired electron in the outermost shell of electrons. This is an extremely unstable configuration and they search for stability by rapidly extracting an electron from another molecule to achieve the stable configuration of four pairs of electrons in the outermost shell; thus they are very short-lived species. ROS, as indicated above, are formed by the interaction of many environmental factors with biologic molecules or as an unavoidable byproduct of cellular respiration. Four main sites of ROS generation are generally cited in the literature (the mitochondrial electron transport chain, cytochrome P-450 reactions, peroxidation of fatty acids, and phagocytic cells), but to this list must now be added skeletal muscle contraction,[4,5] which causes a widespread increase in ROS levels. The major source of ROS is mitochondria, where oxygen is partially reduced in the electron transport system at the NADH dehydrogenase stage and at the ubiquinone/cytochrome b intersection. However, mitochondrial electron transport does not work perfectly and a single electron reduction of oxygen to the superoxide anion $O_2^{-\cdot}$ takes place. Enzymatic dismutation of the $O_2^{-\cdot}$ by Mn-superoxide dismutase (SOD) in mitochondria and Cu-Zn-SOD in the cytoplasm leads to the formation of hydrogen peroxide (H_2O_2). Thus the generation of $O_2^{-\cdot}$ and H_2O_2 is a major byproduct of oxidation reduction reactions. It is also possible to remove H_2O_2 from tissues by catalases or by glutathione peroxidase. Unlike the $O_2^{-\cdot}$ anion, H_2O_2 easily crosses plasma membranes. If it is not removed and free Fe^{2+} ions are locally present in the cytoplasm, H_2O_2 can generate the hydroxyl radical (.OH), which can be regarded as the most damaging and reactive member of the ROS family compared with hydrogen and superoxide. The hydroxyl radical has a very short half-life, and does much damage to proteins, lipids, and DNA close to its site of production, but it can penetrate deep within cells unlike $O_2^{-\cdot}$, which is more likely to damage plasma membranes. The reaction that forms .OH is a two-stage process called the iron-catalyzed Haber-Weiss or Fenton reaction, which can be summarized:

$$H_2O_2 + O_2^- - Fe^{2+}/Fe^{3+} \rightarrow OH + OH^- + O_2$$

Another highly reactive ROS is peroxynitrite ($ONOO^-$), which is derived from the reaction of nitric oxide (NO) (produced by inducible, constitutive, or neuronal nitric oxide synthase) and $O_2^{-\cdot}$. The reaction is extremely fast, exceeding the ability of SOD to break $ONOO^-$ down. Again, $ONOO^-$ is a strong oxidant and the .OH radical formed when it breaks down is highly reactive.

An example of the damaging effects of ROS, at a molecular level, is that of an .OH radical removing a hydrogen atom from one of the carbon atoms in a side chain of a fatty acid forming a molecule of water. The carbon atom is left with an unpaired electron, which is very likely to react with a molecule of oxygen to form a peroxyl radical. The peroxyl radical can steal a hydrogen atom from a nearby side chain, thus making it into a radical. Thus, in interacting with other molecules to attain stability, ROS turn their target molecules into a radical. This initiates a chain reaction that will continue until two radicals encounter one another and each contributes its unpaired electron to form a covalent bond to link the two.

ROS derived from the mitochondrial electron transport chain at complex I (NADH dehydrogenase) and at complex III (ubiquinone-cytochrome *c* reductase), the process that consumes about 90% of a cell's oxygen intake, takes place on the inner membrane of the mitochondria and is at a very high level even in a state of low cellular activity. It has been estimated that about 1% to 2% of the oxygen intake is converted into ROS in mitochondria,[6] but this is a constant, unremitting source of ROS production. In addition, increased ROS production can result from disorders of the respiratory chain and cause an increase in the expression of Mn^{2+}-superoxide dismutase (MnSOD) leading to the production of H_2O_2. Although mitochondria are the prime site of ROS production, they possess antioxidant defense mechanisms such as MnSOD and glutathione peroxidase (GSH). The increase of oxidation of GSH that occurs in aging and in certain diseases of the liver and skeletal muscle[7] results in an increase of oxidation of mitochondrial DNA. Evidence such as this contributes to the concept that mitochondria are a prime source of ROS in aging.[8]

Among other subcellular sources of ROS are (1) cytochrome *P*-450 enzymes, which use a wide variety of endogenous and exogenous compounds as their substrates in many metabolic processes throughout the body. They are also involved in the oxidative metabolism of many drugs that in turn may increase or decrease their activity. Cytochrome P-450 enzymes are located in mitochondria and on the endoplasmic reticulum. Their most common reaction is a monooxygenase reaction, but they can reduce O_2 to $O_2^{-\cdot}$, possibly leading to oxidative stress. (2) Peroxisomes are organelles present in all cell types and whose role is to metabolize fatty acids. Peroxisomes contain high concentrations of oxidative enzymes whose activity generates H_2O_2 as a byproduct, which can leak out into the cytoplasm. However, they contain catalase, which can theoretically restrict the potential for damage by H_2O_2. Catalase levels, however, have rarely been shown to decrease in aging; in elderly humans higher plasma catalyze activity has been reported,[9] suggesting that compensatory antioxidant mechanisms may be present. (3) Phagocytic activity, induced by whatever pathologic reason, employs a combination of ROS and oxidants in large amounts and this activity generally increases with age. (4) ROS production as a result of the contraction of skeletal muscle has been shown to increase with age[4,5] and its release into the extracellular space suggests the potential for inflicting more distant tissue damage. (5) In the brain the metabolism of dopamine by monoamine oxidase produces H_2O_2, which has been implicated in the dopaminergic cell loss that is characteristic of Parkinson's disease. Indeed mesencephalic dopamine cells are particularly sensitive to H_2O_2-induced cell death.[10]

Molecular targets of ROS production and activity are principally proteins, lipids, and DNA and it is now well documented that such ROS-inflicted damage and its functional consequences increases with age. Peroxidative chain reactions of lipids eventually yield unsaturated aldehydes, which are highly reactive, inactivating enzymes, damaging DNA, and reacting with proteins to form cross-links. Evidence that lipid peroxidation increases with age is provided by the increase in the amount of lipofuscin (age pigment) in aged cells, representing a visible biomarker of aging. The most important consequence of lipid peroxidation is to decrease plasma membrane fluidity, thereby altering membrane properties and affecting membrane bound proteins. This will tend to have deleterious effects on the proper functioning of ion pumps and channels, receptors and/or their subunits and transmembrane molecules, such as integrins and other adhesion proteins by which cells interact with the extracellular environment. It may be significant that there is a correlation between the higher content of oxidation-resistant phospholipids in the plasma[11] and mitochondrial[12] membranes with greatly increased longevity in certain rodent species. A more widespread consequence of the oxidation of low-density lipoproteins at a cellular level is the formation and buildup of atherosclerotic plaque in the arterial system. ROS damage proteins by oxidizing individual amino acids, resulting in the induction of protein-protein cross-links and changing the conformation of proteins such that their function is impaired. Conformational changes of proteins with aging include those of structural proteins affecting cell shape or functions (such as axoplasmic transport in neurons), specific activities, and efficiencies of enzymes and membrane-bounded receptors. Proteins—such as myosin, creatine kinase, and ATPases, which are high in -SH groups—are particularly susceptible to oxidation by ROS as is the conversion of histidine residues to asparagine on account of the proximity of histidine residues to metal-binding sites of proteins. It should not be forgotten that age-associated damage as a result of ROS also causes cross-linking in extracellular proteins such as collagen. Nucleic acids are particularly vulnerable to damage by ROS, in particular by the superoxide radical, which can attack individual bases and sugars and cause several variants of DNA strand breaks and alterations that have mutagenic potential (see later discussion). Estimations of the amount of ROS-induced DNA damage can be made by assaying levels of the DNA oxidation product 8-hydroxydeoxyguanosine (8-OHdG), which has been shown to increase with aging. In relation to this, levels of DNA repair glycosylases such as those specific for 8-OHdG are positively correlated with longevity. DNA, however, possesses a wealth of repair mechanisms (see later discussion) that constantly attempt to repair ROS-induced damage.

In summary, the constant generation of ROS leads to molecular damage, which will cause damage to subcellular organelles leading to dysfunction at the cellular level and eventually to cell death. Together with ROS-induced damage to extracellular molecules, tissue and organ damage will eventually occur. As ROS generation commences with the formation of a zygote, it could be argued that cellular aging begins at conception! It is important to note that ROS can induce apoptosis in cells or activate nuclear transcription factors leading to the upregulation of death proteins or inhibition of survival proteins as part of the turnover of cells during the course of life. ROS-induced cell damage or death is implicated in a wide spectrum of age-related disorders, particularly of the nervous and musculoskeletal systems. The effects of ROS-induced damage on the life span has been demonstrated in wild-type and short-lived mutants of the nematode *Caenorhabditis elegans*, which can be extended by less than 50% after treatment with a synthetic antioxidant ROS scavenger.[13]

The damaging effects of ROS can be counteracted by antioxidants, which either occur endogenously or can be supplied exogenously. Antioxidants act by combining with ROS, thereby inactivating them and breaking ROS chain reactions. The cellular antioxidant capacity is, however, not 100% efficient. Naturally occurring, endogenous antioxidants vary in their concentrations from one cell type to another, between species and with age. Their concentrations do not necessarily decline with age because age-associated elevations of some antioxidants occur in organs such as the brain. The main endogenous antioxidants are enzymes such as (1) superoxide dismutase (SOD), which occurs in two forms—a mitochrondrial form containing Mn^{2+} (MnSOD) and a cytoplasmic form containing Cu^{2+} and Zn^{2+} (CuZnSOD), which converts superoxide anions into H_2O_2; (2) catalase, which converts H_2O_2 to molecular oxygen and water; and (3) GSH, which is a selenium (Se)-containing glycoprotein occurring in both the cytoplasm and in mitochondria (where it is imported from the cytoplasm) that also breaks down H_2O_2. The antioxidant defense provided by GSH is most important for mitochondria and for other cytoplasmic components.

Certain micronutrients, such as vitamins C, E, and ß-carotene, have long been regarded as potent antioxidants. Consequently, health promotion advice is constantly given for individuals to eat plenty of prunes, blueberries, spinach, strawberries, and hazelnuts to boost vitamin E intake because it is the most abundant fat soluble antioxidant. Similarly intake of fruits with high vitamin C levels is highly recommended. More recently α-lipoic acid, which inactivates hydroxyl and superoxide radicals and is claimed to protect both lipoproteins and membranes, unlike other antioxidants.[14] α-Lipoic acid is involved in carbohydrate metabolism. It is easily reduced to dihydrolipoic acid, which stabilizes peroxyl and peroxynitrite radicals. Both α-lipoic acid and dihydrolipoic acid regenerate by redox cycling other antioxidants, such as vitamins C and E, and increase intracellular glutathione levels, making it theoretically the perfect antioxidant. However, as endogenous levels are low, dietary supplementation is required and this has proved an effective antioxidant strategy.[15,16] The list of antioxidants is constantly increasing: β-carotene and lycopene, reddish plant pigments present in red fruit and vegetables, are also potent antioxidants; estrogens are antioxidants that have protective effects on the nervous system; curcumin oil, which is extracted from turmeric, induces the enzyme hemoxygenase (HO-1), which is a potent antioxidant.

When there is a shortfall in the levels of the naturally occurring antioxidants or an increase in the production of ROS, a state of "oxidative stress" can occur in which permanent damage to proteins, lipids, and DNA results. Aged cells, particularly those exposed to UV light, show increased ROS generation and an increased tendency toward oxidative stress as judged by increased amounts of protein, lipid, and DNA damage.[17] The cellular response to a state of oxidative stress can be summarized as: (1) an increase in the expression of antioxidant enzymes; (2) increased expression of genes encoding chaperones (heat shock proteins); (3) expression of immediate early genes (such as cFOS); (4) increased expression of genes encoding DNA repair enzymes; and (5) increased expression of genes encoding apoptosis-related proteins. Aged cells are less able to respond in these ways and consequently have a reduced potential for antioxidant capabilities and therefore in their ability to repair ROS-induced damage. Thus the effects that ROS production on a wide range of genes whose expression is vital for normal cell function and survival is now considered to be an important factor in determining longevity.[18]

Intracellular calcium homeostasis

The intracellular concentration of free calcium (Ca^{2+}) is instrumental in many processes of normal cellular activity and can be responsible for dysfunctional changes in cell function. The regulation of the passage of Ca^{2+} into a cell and throughout the cytoplasm has to be strictly regulated for normal cellular activity to continue. In aging cells, Ca^{2+} homeostasis involves many different mechanisms including calcium channels, pumps, transporters, and intracellular buffers and binding proteins; one or more of these mechanisms may be disrupted with potentially fatal consequences.[19,20,21] Ca^{2+} homeostasis has been extensively studied in mammalian neurons where it is intimately involved in neuron-specific activities such as the synaptic release of neurotransmitters and the regulation of genes encoding cytoskeletal elements essential for the elaborate morphology of neurons and the conduction of action potentials.

Extracellular Ca^{2+} levels are approximately 2 mM, whereas intracellular Ca^{2+} levels are 100 nM. Voltage operated Ca^{2+} channels (VOCCs) and nonspecific cationic channels are the key types of channels involved in the influx of extracellular Ca^{2+}. Of the six known VOCCs, the L-type VOCC is the main channel involved in events associated with aging and neurodegeneration. The very low intracellular Ca^{2+} levels are maintained by uptake into smooth endoplasmic reticulum (SER) involving Ca^{2+} ATPase activity, into mitochondria through the activity of Ca^{2+} uniporters and by Ca^{2+} binding proteins and Ca^{2+} ATPases in the plasma membrane. Additionally the endoplasmic reticulum is involved in the release of Ca^{2+} via the inositol 1,4,5-triphosphate pathway or through ryanodine receptors. If intracellular Ca^{2+} is elevated it can cause cytotoxic cell death, particularly if the cell is hypoxic. This is a common feature of all cell types but neurons are more vulnerable to this as many CNS neurons have nonspecific cationic channels, such as NMDA (*N*-methyl D aspartate) and AMPA ligand-gated glutamate receptors in their plasma membranes, which promote the influx of Ca^{2+} into the neuronal cytoplasm. Age-associated ROS damage to plasma membranes, ion pumps, and channels, coupled with altered gene expression for receptor and channel subunits, will all contribute to the challenge of maintaining low intracellular Ca^{2+} levels.

Increased intracellular Ca^{2+} leads to increased ROS generation and to the activation of the calmodulin-dependent enzyme nitric oxide synthase (NOS). NO interacts with the superoxide radical to produce peroxynitrite. Peroxynitrite levels therefore increase intracellularly and it diffuses rapidly to other neurons and causes cell damage by oxidizing lipids, proteins, and DNA (i.e., it is highly and rapidly cytotoxic). In astrocytes, age-associated depletion of glutathione in mitochondria greatly increases the sensitivity of astrocytes to peroxynitrite. It is critical for a cell to maintain and control a submicromolar Ca^{2+} level since the level of Ca^{2+} has important roles in many physiologic processes, controlling for example hormone secretion, ion channel activity, enzyme activity, assembly of the cytoskeleton, and also in the expression of many of the genes involved in these processes.[22] The regulation and/or restoration of Ca^{2+} levels is energetically demanding for a neuron because it is a highly ATP-dependent process. ROS damage to mitochondria results in a disruption of oxidative phosphorylation and in consequence reduced ATP production, which is likely to be the underlying source of perturbed Ca^{2+} regulation. With increased age there is a decrease in the mitochondrial membrane potential, which results in Ca^{2+} leaking out into the cytoplasm. Recently it has been confirmed in peripheral neurons that, with increasing age, the ability of the SER to take up Ca^{2+} decreases.[23] This can be demonstrated by depleting Ca^{2+} stores with caffeine and then measuring the reuptake by the SER. Ca^{2+} flow in and out of the SER is mediated by ryanodine receptors and, with age, the expression and numbers of these receptors is reduced.[23]

Decreases in intracellular calcium binding proteins (CBP)—such as calbindin-D28k, calretinin, and parvalbumin, which regulate the amount of calcium free in the cytoplasm—may also contribute age-associated changes in intracelluar Ca^{2+} concentrations in neurons. There is much variation in the age-associated changes in CBPs in differing parts of the CNS: their levels are unchanged in the cerebellum but reduced in the hippocampus, retina, and in lower motor neurons. Changes such as these have been implicated in motor neuron disease where neuron death has been linked to disruption of intraneuronal Ca^{2+} buffering. In the peripheral nervous system, there are striking differences in the effects of age on CBPs in postganglionic neurons. Many, but not all, sympathetic but not parasympathetic ganglionic neurons contain calbindin-D28k and the number of neurons containing calbindin falls by 50% in aged rats. On the other hand, all neurons of the rat major pelvic ganglion contain neurocalcin and there is an equal decrease in neurocalcin-positive neurons in both the sympathetic and parasympathetic neuron populations of this ganglion in old age.[24]

CELL SENESCENCE

Cultured cells normally only divide a limited number of times after which they enter a growth-arrested state called replicative senescence.[25] They do not produce any new DNA by replication but they do not die, remaining metabolically active in vitro for several months. Human diploid fibroblasts taken from a 40-year-old and cultured in vitro cease dividing after about 40 mitotic divisions, but those taken from an 80-year-old can only manage about 30 mitoses. The phenomenon of adult cells undergoing fewer mitotic divisions than cells from younger donors, originally described by Leonard Hayflick,[26] has given rise to the concept of the Hayflick limit and has been reported in human cells taken from a wide variety of tissues.[27] It is also well documented that cultured cells from short-lived species enter replicative senescence after fewer mitotic divisions than cells from longer-lived species, suggesting that replicative senescence is an indicator of longevity. But how may replicative senescence contribute to human aging? There are two possibilities: either on account of a cell's exhaustion of the capacity to divide or altered cell biology. Many organs, such as skin, the intestinal lining, the liver, the immune system, and hair follicles, rely on cell division for day-to-day functioning to replace naturally occurring cell loss. In such instances a decrease in cell division will have a serious impact on the proper functioning of the organ in question. Also, some tissues retain the ability for cell division in response to damage or cell loss (a burst of cell division is a major feature of wound healing); however, lower rates of wound healing is a feature of elderly humans. The effects of replicative senescence on cell biology may be manifested by differing patterns of postmitotic gene expression, which is often represented by an overexpression of proteins (e.g., aged human dermal fibroblasts increase their production of collagenase, which leads to the breakdown of the extracellular matrix [ECM] which damages the skin contributing to formation of the wrinkles seen with increasing age).

In vitro experiments have proven very productive in aging research but in vivo experiments present a greater challenge in detecting and evaluating age-associated cellular changes, particularly in a very long-lived species such as man. In consequence a significant proportion of aging research is conducted on short-lived species such as the fruit fly *Drosophila melanogaster* and the nematode *Caenorhabditis elegans*. However, there is a marker for human senescent fibroblasts—an abnormal form of the enzyme galactosidase—that is expressed late in a cell's life called senescence-associated β-galactosidase (SA-β-gal), which is a lysosomal enzyme.[28] Detecting SA-β-gal by histochemistry[29] has demonstrated that there are almost no senescent skin cells in people in their thirties but those in their 70s have clusters of SA-β-gal–positive cells in the dermis and epidermis. Senescent cells are, in addition, characterized by the production of high levels of ROS and consequent DNA damage,[30] increased levels of p53 tumor suppressor protein in response to DNA damage and high content of lipofuscin (age pigment). Senescent cells are generally harmful to an organism: senescent skin cells produce increased amounts of collagenase (metalloproteinase) as mentioned above and less TIMPS (tissue inhibitors of metalloproteinases) and other ECM degrading proteases, and senescent endothelial cells produce the cytokine interleukin-1α, which causes inflammation. Perhaps the most significant factor associated with dysfunctional senescent cells is that they increase in number with aging, possibly contributing to the greater incidence of tumors in the elderly.

What is the cellular mechanism that stops cells from dividing so that they enter the nondividing state of replicative senescence? A possible solution is the existence of one or more mutated genes that prevent mitosis from taking place and interrupting the cell cycle, perhaps by suppressing genes responsible for the synthesis of certain growth factors. Alternatively or additionally, ROS-induced metabolic changes that influence the synthesis or adversely affect critical signaling molecules and the inability of aged cells to activate antioxidant defense mechanisms may well be contributory factors. Most interest has, however, focused on telomeres, the repeat sequence DNA terminal regions of chromosomes that gradually shorten with successive mitotic divisions.

Telomeres and telomerase

Telomeres are nucleoprotein complexes that contain hexanucleotide repeat sequences of DNA at each end of a chromosome. They are required for successful replication of chromosomes during mitosis because they maintain chromosome length and protect chromosomes against damage. Telomeres are made up of tandem repeats of the bases TTAGGG whose nucleotides are complexed with specific telomere repeat-binding factors and another enzyme called tankyrase to form a cap at the end of the chromosome. The hexanucleotide repeats are added to the ends of the chromosomes by an enzyme called telomerase, which uses an RNA template and a reverse transcriptase (TERT) in contrast to the normal DNA polymerase. Thus telomeres are not replicated in the same way as the rest of the chromosomal DNA. Telomere replication is not as accurate as true DNA replication and the number of repeats in the telomeric DNA will decrease over time. Telomere length is also aided by a repair (recombination) protein called RAD51D (normally associated with the repair of double strand breaks in DNA) but this mechanism acts independently of telomerase. Cell senescence is associated with the gradual reduction in the number of TTAGGG repeats as cells continue to divide and the telomeres become so shortened and worn that eventually the chromosomes lose their ability to replicate and the DNA is thus at risk of being damaged by not being replicated. However, the gene which codes for the synthesis of telomerase at the same time helps to prevent the telomeres from shortening. In most cell types in man, this gene is rarely switched on to produce the enzyme. Therefore the cells become deficient in telomerase and gradually lose their ability to divide (i.e., they enter the state of replicative senescence). It was first demonstrated by Harley[31] that the telomeres in human cultured fibroblasts become shorter as a function of age, and from this arose the idea that measurement of shortening telomeres represented a "biologic clock" ticking away on a cell's journey toward replicative senescence. Oxidative stress has been shown to speed up telomere shortening as telomeric DNA is less well repaired than the remainder of the nuclear DNA.[32] The part of the telomerase enzyme that actually synthesizes the TTAGGG repeats is called TERT. Is it possible to insert the TERT telomerase gene by gene therapy so that the telomeres do not shorten and cells never enter the senescent state? This cellular immortalization has been attempted on cultures of skin fibroblasts from Werner's syndrome (progeroid) patients and on adult smooth muscle cells with success. Moreover, such immortalized cells have not shown any changes indicating that they have developed a cancer cell phenotype. Telomere shortening is not a characteristic of all cell types. In germ cells, cell division continues for decades and the telomeres never shrink because the telomerase gene is always active and the telomeres are constantly being replaced/synthesized. Germ cells can therefore be regarded as having been immortalized. Also the immune system relies on the constant and rapid production of T and B cells for which maintenance of telomeres is absolutely vital. It is thought that T-cell aging, combined with telomere shortening, may lead to increases in autoimmune responses and explain the increased susceptibility to inflammatory diseases in the elderly. In certain very active tumor cells, the telomerase gene is switched on and consequently the cells' ability to divide is maintained and tumors continue to grow. Cells with artificially lengthened telomeres live longer in culture and there are DNA-like molecules that make cancer cells grow much longer telomeres, thereby doubling their life span and potentially slowing down the rate of growth of tumors.

The contribution of telomere shortening to the other factors previously mentioned as leading cells into the state of replicative senescence clearly indicates that this is a very complex cellular process in aged cells. In view of the increased numbers of senescent cells with increasing age, Von Zglinicki[32] suggested that "telomeres act as cellular 'sentinels' for genomic damage and remove 'dangerous' cells from further proliferation." Whether this anthropomorphic idea is correct or not, there is no doubt that the genome is at great risk on account of telomere shortening and that it will have a profound effect on the proper functioning of the aging cell.

Genomic instability

DNA MUTATIONS

The declining force of natural selection in postreproductive life applies to senescent cells (i.e., as there are no further meiotic cell divisions, the opportunity for beneficial gene mutations for passing on to successive generations to occur has passed). On the other hand senescent cells may generate deleterious DNA mutations that, unlike DNA damage, are irreversible and may cause cellular or metabolic damage likely to decrease longevity. Using the mouse lacZ reporter gene, it has been possible to quantify point and rearrangement DNA mutations[33] in the heart and liver of young and aged mice where approximately threefold increases in mutation frequency occurred with age. The increase in the mutation frequency in the aged small intestine was even higher.

GENE REPRESSION

Gene repression is the switching off of individual genes whose products are needed to maintain the function of the cell such as the production of vital enzymes or cofactors. This is especially important if the products of such genes are not long-lived and deteriorate, or are metabolized. Unless these products can be supplied in the diet, the decrease in concentration will inhibit functioning dependent on a particular gene product. In senescent human fibroblasts, there is a range of genes that are repressed or underexpressed. The genes include, among others, those involved in signaling pathways, transcription factors, heat shock proteins, TIMPS, cytokines, and DNA polymerases. Gene repression is distinct from gene silencing where regions of chromosomal DNA become transcriptionally inactive on account of the tight wrapping of the histone proteins that prevent access to DNA polymerases, which would normally align the nucleotides into a new nucleic acid chain. In yeasts, aging may be regulated by DNA silencing[34] that is undertaken by several "silent information regulator" (Sir) proteins or sirtuins—the evolutionarily conserved lysine deacetylase Sir2 together with its partner proteins Sir3 and Sir4. In mammals the number of sirtuins increases to seven, indicating a more complex process of DNA silencing.

GENE OVEREXPRESSION

Gene overexpression is the switching on of genes in aging cells. Most of these have been demonstrated in senescent human fibroblasts and are functionally associated with the degradation of the ECM and the production of cytokines (i.e., these are deleterious functions that will lead to tissue damage). Gene dysregulation, where regions of chromosomes are activated inappropriately leading to the dysfunctional expression of certain genes, may be a contributory factor in age-associated gene overexpression. The use of high-density oligonucleotide microarrays provides a powerful method to visualize gene-expression profiles in tissues. This methodology has been used to investigate age-associated changes of thousands of genes simultaneously. Among many tissues examined, the gene-expression profile in aged mouse skeletal muscle was generally indicative of a lower expression of metabolic and biosynthetic genes.[35] In the neocortex and cerebellum of aged mice, the gene-expression profile indicated inflammatory responses, oxidative stress, and a reduction of neurotrophic support,[36] very similar to that seen in neurodegenerative diseases of the human brain. In a large study on the human frontal cortex in brains from individuals ranging in age from 26 to 106 years,[37] transcriptional profiling indicated downregulation of genes involved in synaptic transmission, Ca^{2+} homeostasis, signaling pathways, and mitochondrial function among others. Among the genes that are upregulated in this study were those involved with stress responses, antioxidant defenses, and DNA repair. These results raise the following questions: why is it that certain genes are selectively vulnerable to aging, what controls this vulnerability, and to what extent can the compensatory upregulation of defensive/repair gene activity be effective?

The effects of dietary (caloric) restriction on aging cells is normally associated with reduced metabolic rate and a decrease in the amount of ROS produced. However, dietary restriction has been shown to have distinct effects on gene expression that are beneficial to mice. Lee et al[36] and Weindruch et al[35] demonstrated that more than 100 genes were switched on as mice aged—many being genes that are activated when cells are damaged but in mice that had been fed a low calorie (but vitamin and protein supplemented) diet, less than a third of these genes were switched on, supporting the theory that dietary restriction is beneficial at the level of the genome.

GENOMIC DNA DAMAGE

Genomic or nuclear DNA is a highly complex and inherently unstable molecule and is susceptible to damaging agents, such as UV, ROS, and environmental chemicals. As the basis for the genome, it is a prerequisite that DNA is absolutely stable and perfectly aligned to ensure accurate replication, transcription, and minimalization of mutations. DNA strand breaks, which may occur spontaneously, are very prone to recombination and fusion with other chromosomes, thereby disrupting part of the genome. Thus DNA requires constant maintenance to repair the damage that occurs spontaneously and frequently. DNA is the only molecule in cells that is actively scanned to detect errors in synthesis and for DNA damage for which a multiplicity of repair mechanisms exists. If the repair mechanisms fail, then a mutation is more likely to occur and because of that potential threat, it is clear that the stability of the genome depends on DNA repair. Some of the changes in DNA structure that can be induced by ROS UV radiation (mainly hydroxyl radicals) can be listed as follows:

1. Point mutations (base deletion or substitution). The most common is the oxidation of guanine to 8-oxoguanine, which pairs with adenine rather than cytosine.
2. Translocation or transposition of a segment of DNA from one chromosome to another
3. Inversions — removal of a DNA segment and its reinsertion in reverse order
4. Double-stranded DNA breaks resulting in fragmented chromosomes
5. Insertion of nonchromosomal (usually viral) DNA
6. Deletion of whole genes
7. Single-stranded DNA breaks will interfere with gene transcription during replication

Among the DNA protective mechanisms, GSH is present in the nucleus and is important in protecting not only DNA from ROS attack but also the nuclear membrane itself. Specific repair of oxidative damage of DNA by enzymes is now evident. In the human genome, there are 130 DNA repair genes which are classified as follows:

1. Base excision repair genes which encode for enzymes that excise and replace damaged DNA purines and pyrimidines. Specific enzymes such as glycosylases recognize damaged or deficient C, G, T, and A bases and remove them. DNA repair polymerases and DNA ligases, normally involved in DNA replication, resynthesize a new strand using the undamaged one as a template. This is similar to DNA "proofreading," which is a very energy-demanding process that slows down replication but one that has evolved over time; nevertheless it is not a 100% perfect mechanism. One of the unsolved mysteries of this process is how the glycosylases detect damaged bases that are located deep within the DNA helix.
2. Nucleotide excision repair genes express enzymes that excise a series of adjacent nucleotides of a particular sequence.
3. Mismatch repair genes can rectify errors of DNA replication and recombination. Some enzymes are specialized for distinct types of mismatch.
4. Double-stranded breaks can be repaired by genes that encode proteins that are involved in strand pairing during recombination such as RAD51D, which is also involved in protecting telomeres.
5. Translesional DNA repair deals with damaged bases that impede the progression of a replicating DNA polymerase.

With regard to DNA repair in the aging cell, there is good evidence (by 8-OHdG measurement) that DNA damage is increased, that long-lived species have more efficient DNA repair mechanisms than short-lived ones, and that aged cells are less efficient at DNA repair. In general the machinery for selective gene expression, determined by chromosomal DNA, leading to the normal phenotype, changes little during life thanks to DNA repair.

MITOCHONDRIAL DNA

Mitochondrial DNA (mtDNA), attached to the inner mitochondrial membrane, codes for 13 of the 60 polypeptides of the mitochondrial respiratory complexes and is therefore an integral part of mitochondrial function. It is much more easily damaged than nuclear DNA due to its proximity to ROS production from oxidative phosphorylation and the fact that it is naked, lacking the protection of histone proteins. It is likely that the components of the electron transport chain most susceptible to ROS are Complex I (NADH ubiquinone reductase) and Complex IV (cytochrome oxidase). However, a beneficial effect of this location is that confining oxidative phosphorylation to mitochondria may reduce mitochondria-derived ROS from gaining access to the cytoplasm, entering the nucleus, and damaging nuclear DNA. Unlike nuclear DNA, mtDNA lacks repair mechanisms but mitochondria have their own antioxidant defenses, including GSH and MnSOD, both of which decrease in content in aging[6] as does total mtDNA content in a variety of tissues.[38,39] Consequently, 10 to 20 times more mtDNA bases are modified or deleted by ROS in aging compared with nuclear DNA, resulting in a reduction of mitochondrial transcripts and proteins derived from mtDNA. Levels of 8-OHdG are higher in mtDNA than in nuclear DNA. Because 8-OHdG is mutagenic, mtDNA mutations increase with age, and it is likely that this may be a factor contributing to the determination of life span[40] and rate of aging.[41] The rates of mitochondrial ROS production and accumulation of mtDNA mutations are higher in short-lived as opposed to long-lived mammals.

PROTEIN SYNTHESIS AND DEGRADATION

Cellular proteins are in a constant state of turnover involving synthesis and degradation, with individual proteins having half-lives that vary from a few minutes to several days. Overall there is a general reduction in protein synthesis and content in aging, but this masks the fact that synthesis of some proteins decreases, for others it remains static, and for other proteins, levels of synthesis increase with age. Also levels of protein synthesis vary with aging from one tissue to another and between species. Age-associated levels of proteins may not only relate to levels of synthesis but to malfunctioning of the mechanisms for protein breakdown. Proteins are integral to all aspects of cell function as they interact with all other macromolecules and are required for every aspect of cellular maintenance and repair. The integrity of the cytoskeleton, vital for giving a cell its shape and for processes such as axoplasmic transport, is also dependent on proper protein turnover. Many proteins that are not turned over rapidly undergo posttranslational modifications, such as phosphorylation, oxidation, glycation, or methylation; such altered proteins, which tend to accumulate in the cytoplasm with age, are implicated as the cellular basis of a range of pathologic conditions.

Although there is only one process for protein synthesis, there are multiple subcellular processes for the degradation of proteins. Protein degradation is a highly complex and tightly regulated process that plays major roles in a variety of basic cellular processes during the life and death of cells, and hence in both health and disease. The two main pathways are the lysosomal pathway and the ubiquitin-proteasomal pathway. A third proteolytic mechanism, however, exists involving the calpains (calcium dependent neutral proteases). The lysosomal pathway is mainly an indiscriminate cellular pathway for proteolysis that contributes to the general maintenance of a cell, resulting eventually in the formation of lipofuscin (age pigment), which tends to accumulate in cells with age. Lipofuscin is formed by ROS-induced oxidation of macromolecules derived from subcellular organelles. Some cell types are particularly prone to lipofuscin accumulation with aging, of which cardiac myocytes are a prime example in which almost a fifth of the cell volume may become occupied by lipofuscin in old age. Although regarded as being chemically inert, the disruptive effect on efficient contraction of the myofibrils may well contribute to myocardial dysfunction in old age. The accumulation of lipofuscin with age can be reduced by the antioxidant vitamin E, thus implicating ROS in lipofuscin formation. The efficiency of the lysosomal pathway declines with age as the binding of macromolecular targets to the lysosmal membranes and their transport into the lysosome becomes less effective[42,43] and there is leakage of certain lysosmal enzymes into the cytoplasm.[44]

In the ubiquitin-proteasome pathway, proteins are first covalently tagged by ubiquitins, which are small (76 amino-acid) proteins that control the system responsible for degradation of proteins. The ubiquinated protein can then be recognized by a 26S proteosome complex (of a 20S proteasome and a 19S cap). These are barrel-shaped, widely distributed cytosolic organelles that act effectively as a protease complex into which tagged proteins pass. The proteins have to unfold themselves as far as possible to enter the pore of the proteasome after which the ubiquitins are recycled. Proteasomes are large complexes of proteolytic enzymes that have three main types of proteolytic activity: chymotrypsin-like, trypsin-like, and caspase-like activity. The degraded proteins (i.e., amino acids or small peptides) can then be recycled. During aging, proteasomal function becomes impaired, with chymotrypsin-like activity in particular decreasing, but that of catalase-like activity not declining.

The third proteolytic pathway—the calpains (calcium dependent neutral proteases), which are ATP- and Ca^{2+}-dependent—have specific substrates in both the cytoplasm and the nucleus. In the event of oxidative stress-induced elevations of intracellular Ca^{2+} concentrations, the amount of DNA damage and repair, as indicated by reduced levels of 8-OHdG, implicates calpain-mediated degradation.[45] Given the trend toward increased oxidative stress and consequent perturbations of intracellular Ca^{2+} homeostasis in aging, the proteolytic involvement of calpains, which are very widespread, is also likely to be revealed as a major contributor. That there is an overall decrease with age in proteolytic activity is not disputed but the exact contribution made by the different pathways for protein degradation has yet to be resolved. Nevertheless the age-associated (and pathologic) aggregation of and cytoplasmic accumulation of oxidized or otherwise transformed proteins is not in doubt.

The tertiary structure of large protein molecules is achieved not by "self-assembly" because linkages between certain surfaces or polypeptide chains are necessary to attain the correct molecular configuration. Assistance in the noncovalent folding of polypeptide chains is supplied by molecular chaperones. Heat shock proteins (HSPs) are a group of such proteins that bind to such surfaces during assembly of large molecules and prevent the occurrence of incorrect union/interactions between parts/surfaces of the molecules. Many molecular chaperones are also HSPs, in that they are proteins expressed in response to raised temperatures or other cellular stressors,[46] but are not expressed when cells are performing their normal biologic functions. A major function of chaperones is to prevent newly assembled polypeptide chains from aggregating into nonfunctional structures such as protein aggregates that characterize some neurodegenerative diseases.[47] Chaperones also help in restoring correct conformation if a large protein becomes distorted during a biosynthetic process such as protein synthesis or during passage through a narrow membrane channel or pore. Chaperones are also involved in the constant removal and replacement of damaged proteins that occurs during the continual remodeling of cell structure by protein turnover. As proteins are turned over rapidly, the continued expression of chaperones is vital for normal cellular functioning. Chaperone expression is induced by stress such as a decrease in temperature, which reveals the need for chaperone production to cope with intracellular damage. When not required, chaperone expression decreases.

In aging cells ROS-induced DNA damages genes encoded to produce chaperones. Reduced levels of HSP expression occur in aged cells such as fibroblasts, which have lower expression of Hsp70—a collagen-specific chaperone—and also of Hsp90, which is required for the assembly and functioning of telomeres.[48] Chaperone-mediated autophagy (CMA) is a selective pathway for the degradation of damaged proteins in lysosomes. The processes whereby the proteins are targeted by the lysosome and cross the lysosomal membrane are aided by chaperones, can be induced by oxidative stress, and are adversely affected by aging.[49,50] The importance of molecular chaperones in cellular aging is indicated by the extension of life span that has been demonstrated in mice, *C. elegans,* and in *Drosophila* by the overexpression of chaperones or by the reduction in life span following inhibition of HSP translation and expression.[48]

SIGNALING PATHWAYS

Cells interact with their environment and respond to changing environmental conditions. Most stimuli are chemical ligands that bind to receptors in the plasma membrane but a much smaller number of stimuli, such as gases and steroid hormones, cross the plasma membrane and interact with intracellular receptors. Activation of a receptor by the bound ligand transduces the stimulus into an intracellular chemical signal, which can act as a messenger. The messenger molecule usually amplifies the signal and in turn activates some form of effector system for the cell to make the appropriate response to the initial stimulus. This process is known as a signaling pathway or signal transduction pathway. As most of the molecules involved in signaling pathways are proteins and the biology of proteins is adversely affected by many factors associated with cellular and molecular aging, such as ROS, DNA damage, gene expression, mRNA translation, and Ca^{2+} levels, it is to be expected that signaling pathways will also be affected in aging. Two of the most significant signaling pathways that have been shown to be involved in aging are the:

1. Insulin/IGF-1 pathway. This pathway is involved in the regulation of life span and is evolutionarily conserved.[51] Reduced receptor and PI3 kinase function impair insulin/IGF-1 signaling, resulting in a dramatically extended life span.[52]
2. Target of rapamycin (TOR) pathway. The TOR nutrient sensing pathway is an important regulator of cell growth, development, and aging, which interacts with processes such as transcription, mRNA translation protein turnover, and cytoskeletal organization.[53] TOR signaling generally conserves cellular energy, which can be diverted to cellular maintenance and repair mechanisms that will be beneficial to aging cells.

EXTRACELLULAR MATRIX

The interaction between cells and their immediate environment can be vital for their survival. Integrins, for example, are transmembrane molecules that are attached directly to the ECM and crucial to the cell's survival. Other molecules of the ECM are involved in relaying signals from cytokines or growth factors to receptors in the plasma membrane. There is some evidence for alterations in membrane properties and in the number and type of receptors with age. The process of glycation is a factor that causes changes in large proteins, such as collagen, with increasing age and in certain progressive diseases of aging—such as atherosclerosis, joint stiffness, arthritis, urinary incontinence, and congestive heart failure. Essentially, blood sugars chemically bond to proteins and DNA. Over time they become chemically modified to form advanced glycation end products (AGEs). AGEs interfere with the proper functioning of proteins and some form covalent cross-links with adjacent protein strands in the case of collagen and elastin. The mechanical result is that formerly flexible or elastic tissues become stiff. Also the chemical changes due to glycation and cross-linking can initiate harmful inflammatory and autoimmune responses. In addition, one of the effects of mechanical stress or inflammation on chondrocytes is to induce the production of ROS and as chondrocytes are isolated from one another in cartilage, they cannot be replaced and cartilage will degenerate.

KEY POINTS

Cellular aging is characterized by:

- The generation of reactive oxygen species (ROS)
- Damage to molecules and organelles by ROS
- Variably effective cellular antioxidant defense mechanisms
- Dysregulation of intracellular calcium homeostasis
- Alterations in telomere structure and telomerase expression
- Genomic DNA damage affecting gene expression
- Mitochondrial DNA damage affecting ATP production
- Alterations in protein synthesis and degradation
- Alterations in molecular chaperone activity
- Alterations in signaling pathways
- Alterations in cellular relations with the extracellular matrix

CONCLUSION

The cellular mechanisms of aging described above may provide a convincing account of the cellular processes that determine the length of survival and fate of a cell as individuals grow older. Accumulated molecular and cellular damage by UV, ROS, Ca^{2+}, and changes in genomic function can be demonstrated in aging cells. However, some of the scientific literature of the twenty-first century questions whether theories of aging such as accumulated oxidative damage are universally applicable across the animal kingdom.[54] Clearly these complex theories of aging at a cellular level are far from being completely understood. Another emerging realization is the close connection between perceived cellular mechanisms of aging with those underlying the development of cancer, for which increasing age is the largest risk factor.[55] This realization should, ideally, focus the minds of investigators in both fields in their quest for complete understanding of the mechanisms underlying these two critically important cellular processes.

For a complete list of references, please visit online only at www.expertconsult.com

CHAPTER 9

Physiology of Aging

Edward J. Masoro

When broadly defined, aging refers to all time-associated events that occur during the life span of an organism. During this time, many changes occur in the physiologic processes. These changes may be beneficial, neutral, or deteriorative. During the developmental period of life, most changes are due to the maturation of the physiologic processes and tend to be beneficial. However, during the postmaturational period of life, most changes are detrimental, although some may be neutral, such as the graying of the hair. Indeed, the term "senescence" is used to specifically denote this postmaturational deterioration. Senescence is defined as the deteriorative changes with time during postmaturational life that underlie an increasing vulnerability to challenges, thereby decreasing the ability of the organism to survive. Although senescence is a subset of aging, in common usage, aging is often used to only mean senescence. Unfortunately, this specialized meaning is usually not explicitly stated. In this chapter, aging and senescence will be used as synonyms, a usage particularly appropriate in a textbook of geriatric medicine.

This brief chapter can cover only concepts and provide a limited number of examples. Section 11 of the *Handbook of Physiology* series published by the American Physiological Society is dedicated to the physiology of aging.[1] That volume provides in-depth coverage of most age changes in the physiologic systems and should be consulted by readers who desire further information in a particular subject area.

PHYSIOLOGIC DETERIORATION AND THE AGING PHENOTYPE

A major characteristic of the aging phenotype is the deterioration of the physiologic processes exemplified by comparing elderly people with young adults. Indeed, physiologic deterioration plays an important role in the age-associated increase in the age-specific mortality rate. Thus, knowledge of the age changes in the physiologic systems is invaluable for both the geriatric physician tending elderly patients and the biologic gerontologist in the quest for an understanding of the biologic nature of aging.

Causes of age-associated physiologic deterioration

The progressive deterioration with age of the physiologic systems that starts during young adulthood is caused by the many damaging processes and agents that organisms encounter during life. Apparently, repair systems during postmaturational life are not able to fully eliminate the damage. The result is a progressive functional inadequacy of the physiologic systems due to the accumulation of damage. The extent of this functional inadequacy and its rate of occurrence vary among species and among individuals within a species, and among the physiologic systems of an individual. It is convenient to classify the damaging processes responsible for the age-associated physiologic deterioration in the following three categories: (1) damage resulting from intrinsic living processes, (2) damage caused by extrinsic factors, and (3) damage resulting from age-associated diseases.

DAMAGE RESULTING FROM INTRINSIC LIVING PROCESSES

Many of the processes essential to life also have damaging aspects. For example, aerobic metabolism, which enables organisms to readily generate metabolic energy from ingested nutrients, has the negative aspect of the generation of highly reactive compounds, such as superoxide radicals, hydroxyl radicals, and hydrogen peroxide because of the univalent reduction of oxygen. These oxygen-containing compounds are potentially highly damaging. Protection from, and repair of, damage due to these substances has evolved, but is not totally effective. Therefore, an accumulation of oxidative damage with increasing age occurs.[2] The extent of protection and the ability to repair damage varies among species. Thus, it is not surprising that there is interspecies variation in the rate of accumulation of oxidatively damaged macromolecules. Another example involves glucose, a most important fuel for most organisms. However, in addition to serving as an energy source, glucose also participates in the glycation and glycoxidation of proteins and nucleic acids and, in this way, alters their biologic functions.[3] Again, there are protective mechanisms and processes that eliminate the damaged macromolecules, which vary in efficacy among species. Probably there is no intrinsic living process that does not also have the ability to cause damage.

DAMAGE CAUSED BY EXTRINSIC FACTORS

There is general agreement that extrinsic factors contribute to the aging phenotype. Despite this, many do not subscribe to the view that these extrinsic factors are part of the aging process. This view is based on long-held criteria for aging processes enumerated by Strehler[4] in 1977. One of the criteria is "intrinsicality," the view that aging is entirely an intrinsic phenomenon. Busse[5] recognized the conceptual difficulty that this criterion caused and tried to resolve the problem by proposing the concept of primary and secondary aging. Primary aging was defined as universal changes occurring with age within a species or population, changes not caused by environment. Secondary aging was defined as changes as a result of the interactions of primary aging with disease processes and environmental factors. This concept may be faulty for two reasons. First, if aging results from progressive accumulation of unrepaired damage, it is irrelevant whether that damage originates from intrinsic processes or is caused by extrinsic agents. Second, extrinsic agents cause damage only because of interactions with biologic structures and processes. For example, it has been shown that the effect of genes on the life span and aging of *Drosophila melanogaster* is dependent on environmental interactions.[6]

In a sense, all damage is intrinsic whether it originates as a result of basic living processes or from reactions to extrinsic factors. However, this view downplays the importance of environmental factors that are not desirable because such factors can be modified and thus should be the focus of research on aging interventions.

Indeed, the notable effect that environmental factors can have on the aging process is particularly well illustrated by the

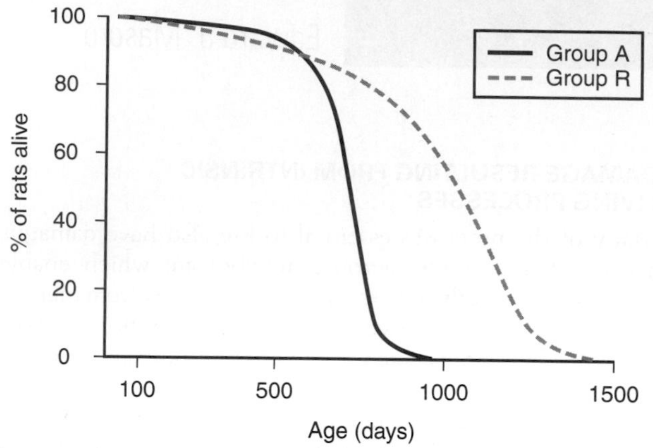

Figure 9-1. Survival curves for ad libitum–fed male F344 rats (group A, n = 115) and rats restricted to 60% of the mean ad libitum intake (group R, n = 115). *(Reprinted with permission Yu BP, Masoro EJ, Murata I, et al. Life span study of SPF Fischer 334 male rats fed ad libitum or restricted diets: longevity, growth, lean body mass and disease. J Gerontol 1982;37:130–141, Fig 6.)*

effects of long-term restriction of food intake by laboratory mice and rats.[7] Restricting the food intake by 30% to 50% of that eaten by ad libitum–fed animals markedly increases longevity (see Figure 9-1 for its typical effect on population survival characteristics[8]), prevents or delays age-associated disease, and maintains a broad array of physiologic processes in a youthful state until very advanced ages. Examples of the scope of these beneficial effects include: immune function,[9] cardiac function,[10] female reproductive function,[11] and gene expression.[12] Indeed, reduction of food intake retards most, but not all, age-associated changes in physiologic processes of rats and mice that have been studied. It has been established that the reduction in energy (calorie) intake is the dietary factor responsible for this retardation of age changes in the physiologic systems.[7] Thus, this phenomenon is often referred to as caloric restriction (CR). Although there is no evidence that CR during the adult life of humans would globally retard age-associated physiologic deterioration, it has been shown to influence the physiologic systems of nonhuman primates in a fashion similar to its effects on mice and rats.[13] Moreover, there is evidence that CR influences the occurrence and progression of age-associated human disease processes,[14] such as atherosclerosis,[15] hypertension,[15] and insulin resistance and impaired glucose tolerance.[16]

The lifestyle factor that has received the most attention relates to the fact that with increasing age many people become increasingly sedentary.[17] Studies on the effect of exercise training in old human subjects indicate that some of the decline in physiologic function with advancing age in sedentary people is due to the effects of exercise deficiency and probably can, at least in part, be reversed by physical activity even at advanced ages.[18] Skeletal muscle mass and strength decrease with increasing age,[19] and both the mass and the strength can be increased by resistance training even at very advanced ages.[20] It is likely that the frequently occurring increase in body weight in people between the ages of 20 and 70 years is primarily the result of a sedentary lifestyle.[21] Exercise has also been found to attenuate the age-associated increase in body fat content.[22] Most importantly, exercise improves the distribution pattern of body fat in elderly men and women.[23] There is also evidence that exercise increases insulin sensitivity and thereby alleviates insulin resistance and impaired glucose tolerance that commonly occur with advancing age.[24] There is little doubt that the increasingly sedentary lifestyle with advancing age contributes greatly to the deterioration of physiologic functions observed in old people.

There is no clear demarcation between lifestyle factors and personal habits. For example, exposure to the sun results in changes in skin structure and function,[25] referred to as photoaging by dermatologists and commonly viewed as a marker of aging by laypersons. Excessive sun exposure may be an inevitable consequence of the occupation of a person or of the climatic conditions of the geographic region in which the individual resides. If so, the effect of excessive skin sun exposure probably should be in the lifestyle category. However, recreational choice leading to excessive skin sun exposure such as sunbathing can be viewed either as lifestyle or as personal habit. A personal habit that has received much attention in regard to aging is cigarette smoking. It is established that aging of the skin is promoted by smoking.[26] Also, age-associated diseases that cause notable physiologic deterioration are promoted by smoking. Examples are chronic obstructive lung disease[27] and atherosclerosis.[28]

Psychosocial factors such as engaging in social activities have been shown to significantly lower the age-specific mortality rate of people in the retirement age range.[29] Since this type of engagement has also been found to enhance the execution of activities of daily living (ADL), it is likely that it retards or reverses age-associated deterioration of the physiologic system. Indeed, there is clear evidence that social support retards age-associated decline in cognitive function.[30] Although these psychosocial findings are intriguing, remarkably little is known regarding the underlying biologic mechanisms. Indeed, our understanding of this intriguing subject has progressed little since the last edition of this book.

DAMAGE RESULTING FROM AGE-ASSOCIATED DISEASES

Age-associated diseases are generally viewed as the cause of much of the physiologic deterioration that occurs with advancing age.[31] These diseases usually cause morbidity and mortality at advanced ages and are chronic or when acute are the result of long-term processes, such as bone loss or atherogenesis. It is also recognized that the occurrence and progression of age-associated diseases are strongly influenced by age-associated physiologic deterioration. However, there is disagreement regarding two fundamental questions. Are age-associated diseases an integral part of the aging process? Is there a fundamental difference between the aging of physiologic processes and the progression of what are called pathophysiologic processes?

In addressing these questions, the concept of "normal aging" has emerged[31] and is widely used by those conducting physiologic studies on aging humans. It is defined as senescence in the absence of disease; probably more appropriately, it should be called "atypical aging" rather than "normal aging." Most elderly people have one or more age-associated diseases. Moreover, Scully[32] points out that any definition of disease is problematic because what is called a disease is influenced by medical advances and societal culture. For example, Lakatta and Levy[33] view hypertension as a disease and point out that a systolic blood pressure of 140 to 160 mmHg is now considered to be hypertension, whereas in 1990 it was considered to be in the normal range. Indeed, it is to be expected that the fraction of the elderly free of age-associated disease will become vanishingly small as advances in medicine increasingly uncover occult disease. Moreover, to study what many investigators call "normal aging," great effort is made to exclude from the population to be studied subjects with age-associated disease. Although such studies are invaluable by providing a reductionist approach to the study of aging, a powerful tool in dissecting the details of the aging processes, they provide little assessment of what is occurring as the general population ages.

Furthermore, the view that normal aging does not involve the occurrence of age-associated disease is not conceptually sound in terms of basic biology. Evolutionary biologists propose that aging (senescence) occurs because of the decline in the force of natural selection with advancing age.[34] Thus, biologic processes that result in detrimental effects expressed late in life cannot be selected against. It is for this reason that physiologic deterioration increases with increasing age, and it is for the same reason that age-associated disease increasingly expresses with advancing age. It is true that some people (a very small subset) may age without evidence of discernible age-associated disease, but this may relate more to the fact that the distinction between age-associated disease and age-associated physiologic deterioration is arbitrary. For example, loss of bone mass is a well-recognized age-associated physiologic deterioration and osteoporosis is a major age-associated disease; the boundary in this case of when to label a physiologic change as a disease is arbitrary.

For all of the above reasons, in this chapter, deterioration of physiologic systems secondary to age-associated disease will be considered to be an integral part of aging. Of course, it is always important to know the specific reason for the altered physiology, and when age-associated disease is the major immediate cause, it should be identified.

INTERSPECIES AND INTRASPECIES VARIATION IN AGE-ASSOCIATED PHYSIOLOGIC DETERIORATION

In general terms, mammalian species are remarkably similar in that a progressive, but usually not linear, deterioration in the physiologic systems occurs with advancing postmaturational age.[35] However, there is considerable interspecies variation in the details of these physiologic changes.

There is also great intraspecies heterogeneity in age changes in the physiologic systems, a phenomenon that has been well characterized in humans. Rowe and Kahn[36] have developed the concept of "usual aging" and "successful aging" for considering the differences among individuals in age changes in physiologic functions. "Usual aging" refers to elderly who are functioning well but are at risk for disease, disability, and premature death. They may exhibit modest increases in systolic blood pressure and abdominal fat, and deterioration of one or more physiologic systems. "Successful" aging refers to a small group of disease-free elderly people who exhibit the following characteristics:

- Low risk of disease or disability
- High level of mental and physiologic function
- Active engagement in life

Rowe and Kahn focus on environment and lifestyle as the major determinants for achieving "successful aging" and point to adequate physical exercise, good diet, good personal habits (not smoking or abusing drugs and using alcohol in moderation), and good psychosocial environment as being particularly important. Surprisingly, they barely mention the role of genetics in achieving "successful aging."

Although the concept of "successful aging" is provocative, there are questions regarding its value and usefulness. One question is how common is "successful aging" now or is it likely to become if most people were to live in a good environment and adhere to an appropriate lifestyle. As of now, only a small fraction of those in the eighth decade of life would meet the criterion of being free of chronic disease (i.e., almost all suffer from one or more of the following diseases: osteoarthritis, coronary heart disease, cerebrovascular disease, congestive heart failure, dementia, type II diabetes, Parkinson's disease, cancer, benign prostate hyperplasia, and cataracts).[31] And this does not fully cover the list of such diseases.

A related question is what fraction of those who meet the criteria of "successful aging" in the eighth decade of life will continue to when in the ninth and tenth decades of life or when they are centenarians. If most of them undergo notable physiologic deterioration before death, what does the concept of "successful aging" provide in addition to the well-known fact that individuals age at different rates? The concept of biologic age as distinct from chronologic age was proposed long ago.[37] Thus the question arises as to whether the concept of "successful aging" is useful or misleading. It is likely that most centenarians were in the "successful aging" category when in the eighth decade of their lives. However, they exhibit notable physiologic deterioration, which must have occurred progressively during the ninth and tenth decades of life culminating after becoming centenarians.[31] It seems more appropriate to say that these centenarians undergo a slow rate of aging rather than "successful aging." This is not merely an academic issue but also one with societal implications because "successful aging" implies that physiologic deterioration due to aging can be prevented rather than merely delayed. Such a view may misguide public policy based on the view that an appropriate lifestyle and environment will enable people to reach very old age without the disabilities that are so costly in the use of societal resources. Unfortunately, it is possible that the environment and lifestyle advocated for "successful aging" may have just the opposite effect. Indeed, centenarians have greatly increased in numbers during the twentieth century[38] and may become commonplace during the twenty-first century. Furthermore, since the environment and lifestyle advocated for the achievement of "successful aging" is likely to increase the number of centenarians, it may result in an increase in the fraction of the population that consume societal resources because of notable physiologic deterioration.

AGE CHANGES IN THE PHYSIOLOGY OF SPECIFIC ORGANS AND ORGAN SYSTEMS

All organs and organ systems exhibit age-associated physiologic deterioration, if not in all individuals, at least in a significant fraction of the population. This subject area is so vast that it cannot begin to be covered in this brief chapter. The volume on aging[1] of the *Handbook of Physiology* series of the American Physiological Society provides a systematic and extensive coverage for those needing in-depth information about a particular organ or organ system. Also many other chapters in this textbook provide a substantial discussion of age changes in the physiology of specific organs and organ systems relevant to the subject matter of the chapter. In this chapter a few specific examples have been selected for discussion solely for the purpose of illustrating general concepts.

Before starting this discussion, it is important to point out that most of the studies on age changes in the physiology of organs and organ systems have used the cross-sectional study design. The interpretation of cross-sectional studies is often confounded by factors not related to aging.[39] What are called "cohort effects" is a major confounder.[40] For example, during the twentieth century, the number of years of education progressively increased in the developed nations.[41] Therefore, when comparing cognitive abilities of 30-year-olds and 80-year-olds in a cross-sectional study, the difference in educational levels confounds any conclusions about the effects of aging. What is referred to as "selective mortality" is the other major type of confounder of cross-sectional studies.[42] The older the age group being studied, the smaller is the fraction of its birth cohort still alive. Members of the birth cohort with risk factors for fatal diseases tend to die at younger ages than others in the birth cohort. Thus, for example, a difference in the blood level of HDL-cholesterol between those in the age range of 80 to 90 years compared with those in the age range of 50 to 60 years may relate more to "selective mortality" than to aging.

Aging broadly affects the cardiovascular system, ranging from structural and functional alterations of the heart and vasculature to changes in the neural reflexes regulating cardiovascular functioning.[43] Left ventricular hypertrophy commonly occurs with advancing age and its extent varies among individuals.[44] Notable left ventricular hypertrophy is associated with heart failure, coronary heart disease, and stroke. Left ventricular compliance commonly decreases with advancing human age and may be a contributor to heart failure.[45] The ability to increase heart rate in response to exercise-induced peak oxygen consumption declines with increasing human age.[46] Also, there is a decrease with advancing age in the ability of β-adrenergic agonists to increase heart rate.[33] There is an age-associated decrease in left ventricular contractility during maximal exercise and this is also a manifestation of reduced β-adrenergic responsiveness.[47] With increasing age, the large arteries dilate, stiffen, and the intima thickens.[48] Systolic blood pressure and pulse pressure commonly increase with increasing age, a phenomenon primarily due to age-associated arterial structural changes.[49] The extent of the increase in pulse pressure is a strong predictor of risk of cardiovascular disease.

Many of these age-associated changes in cardiovascular physiology may underlie the occurrence of cardiovascular disease, while cardiovascular disease may play an important role in many of the age changes in cardiovascular function. Moreover, lifestyle and other environmental factors undoubtedly are major players in the physiologic deterioration of the cardiovascular system and in the progression of cardiovascular disease. Of course, some of the deterioration may be due to intrinsic aging processes and thus inevitable. However, it is difficult to identify such processes with certainty because one cannot be sure that they do not arise from yet-to-be-recognized extrinsic factor or disease. Moreover, it is important to emphasize that those age changes in cardiac function that are secondary to lifestyle and other environmental factors are not inevitable and may be modifiable even at advanced ages, at least to some extent. Lakatta[50] points out that the cardiovascular age-changes are being studied at the molecular level in rodent and nonhuman primate models and that the findings of these studies hold promise for developing interventions for even the intrinsic aging processes underlying cardiovascular disease.

Cross-sectional studies of apparently healthy human populations report a decrease in kidney function after age 40, with the glomerular filtration rate decreasing about 1% per year of age increase.[61] However, a longitudinal study[52] conducted on subjects of the Baltimore Longitudinal Study of Aging has revealed that not all people exhibit an age-associated decline in glomerular filtration rate (Figure 9-2). The mean decrease in creatinine clearance in 446 male subjects followed over a 23-year period was 0.87 mL per minute per year. However, one third of the subjects showed no decline in creatinine clearance. Others in this study exhibited a small but statistically significant decline and still others had a notable decline in creatinine clearance. It is interesting to note that the mean decline in creatinine

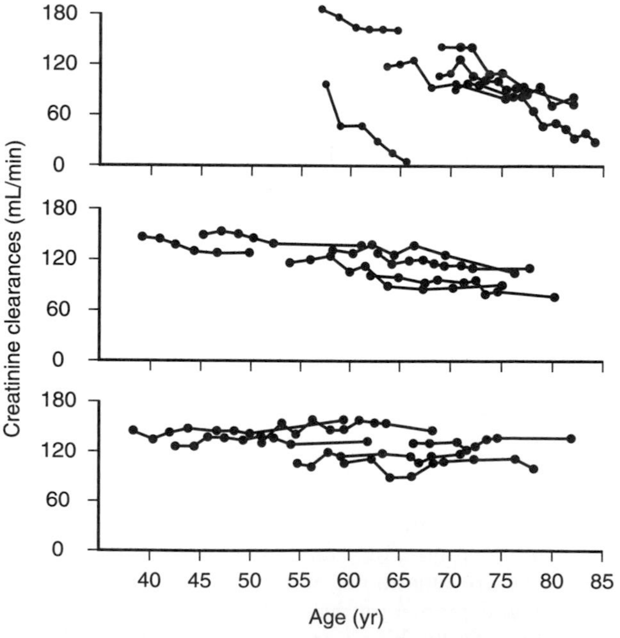

Figure 9-2. Age changes in creatinine clearance of male subjects studied serially in the Baltimore Longitudinal Study of Aging. The top panel presents the findings of six subjects from the group who exhibited notable decreases in creatinine clearance with increasing age; the middle panel presents the findings of six subjects from the group who exhibited a small but significant decrease in creatinine clearance with increasing age; the bottom panel presents the findings of six subjects from the group who exhibited no decrease in creatinine clearance with increasing age. *(From Lindeman et al[52] with permission of Blackwell Science Inc.)*

clearance of the subjects in this study group was similar to what has been observed in many cross-sectional studies. The reasons for the differences among people in changes with age in kidney function have not been established. Lindeman[51] has suggested that the decline in renal function noted in cross-sectional studies may be due to the fact that many in the populations studied suffered from undetected pathologic processes and that a decrease in glomerular filtration rate is not an inevitable involutional process. Indeed, it has been shown that elevated blood pressure accelerates the age-associated decline in renal function.[53] It is also possible that lifetime dietary preferences play a role since excessive dietary protein is believed to promote renal functional deterioration. Indeed, if the deterioration of renal function with age is primarily due to disease and/or environmental factors, then it is potentially modifiable by public health measures.

The appearance of the skin is widely used as an indicator of the age of a person. The skin, indeed, undergoes many structural and functional age-associated changes.[54] The skin wrinkles, loses elasticity and is increasingly more fragile. The barrier function of the skin is compromised, as is its immune function. The loss of sebaceous glands leads to dry skin and the loss of melanocytes causes alterations in pigmentation. There is a decrease in subcutaneous fat, which adversely affects the ability to cope with cold environments. However, the magnitude of most of these changes does not result from intrinsic aging processes but is the result of cumulative sun damage since their extent is much reduced in skin areas protected from the sun.[25] Cigarette smoking is the other major factor that promotes skin aging.[26] Indeed, sun exposure and cigarette smoking appear to act synergistically to promote skin aging.[26] Thus, commonly used skin markers of aging have little relation to intrinsic processes but primarily relate to environmental factors and can be readily modified by altering lifestyle.

These three examples make clear that many age changes are not primarily because of intrinsic aging processes but, to varying degrees, are secondary to (or are at least promoted by) age-associated disease or extrinsic factors or both. To view them as not being part of the aging process removes from consideration major problems that confront aging individuals nor is there any biologic basis for such a view. It is true that deterioration due to disease or extrinsic factors may be preventable and, in some cases, reversible, but that hardly lessens their involvement in aging. Indeed, much of what we currently consider to be intrinsic may ultimately be found to be of extrinsic origin or at least influenced by extrinsic factors. And what is considered to be extrinsic has its actions by interacting with intrinsic processes. Indeed, what is considered to be lifestyle may have a strong intrinsic basis (e.g., the sedentary lifestyle adopted by many people as they age also occurs in laboratory rats,[55] which in the case of the rodent is probably better viewed to be intrinsic rather than a lifestyle choice). Moreover, as discussed earlier, there are strong reasons to believe that most age-associated diseases are part of the aging process, making their separation from other aspects of aging arbitrary.[31] Nevertheless, identification of age-associated diseases is obviously essential in the practice of geriatric medicine and is also invaluable in experimental biogerontology by providing the detailed information needed for interpretation of the findings of human and animal studies.

AGE CHANGES IN ORGANISMIC FUNCTION

Given the many deteriorative changes that occur in the physiology of organs and organ systems, it is to be expected that the functional competence of the organism is compromised with advancing age. Indeed, organismic functional deficits occur that can be classified in the following way: (1) decreased ability to cope with challenges, (2) reduced functional capacity, and (3) altered homeostasis. A few examples of these organismic functional deficits are presented next.

Ability to cope with challenges

The reduced ability to cope with challenges, or what are often called stressors, is a hallmark of the aging phenotype.[56] It is well known that secretion of glucocorticoids by the hypothalamic-hypophyseal-adrenocortical system and increase in the activity of the adrenal medullary-sympathetic nervous system are responses common to all stressors, and that they play an important role in enabling mammalian organisms to cope with all stressors.[57] Also, induction of the heat shock protein system is a common response, enabling organisms of almost all species to withstand many different cellular stressors.[56] Of course, in addition to these general responses, there are defenses that are specific for particular stressors or challenges. However, because the loss with advancing age in ability of organisms to cope appears to occur with all types of stressors, it might be expected that there is deterioration of one or more of the general mechanisms. The currently available evidence does not indicate that the ability of the hypothalamic-hypophyseal-adrenocortical system to respond to challenges by increasing the secretion of glucocorticoid hormone is compromised by aging.[58] Of course, that does not rule out the possibility of a reduced ability of the glucocorticoid target site to respond to the hormone, but studies designed to address this possibility have yet to be done. There is some indication that the response of the adrenal medullary-sympathetic nervous system to challenges may be attenuated with advancing age,[59] but these findings are hard to interpret because basal levels of catecholamines are elevated with increasing age. There is also evidence that there is a blunting with age of at least some adrenergic responses in target tissues (e.g., the heart as discussed previously). Nevertheless, based on current information, it does not seem that an inadequate response of the adrenal medullary-sympathetic nervous system plays a major role in the age-associated reduction in the ability of the organism to meet challenges. In contrast to these neuroendocrine responses, the evidence is clear that the ability to induce heat shock proteins in response to cellular stressors markedly decreases with the increasing age of mammals,[56] and this may play a major role in the loss in ability to cope with stressors. However, because the physiologic deterioration occurs with advancing age in most organs and organ systems, functional deficits in specific responses may underlie the reduced ability to deal with a broad scope of challenges. A case in point is the decrease in the ability of the immune system to protect the organism from damage due to infectious agents.[60] Thus, although it has long been known that successfully meeting challenges is compromised with advancing age, the basis of this deficit remains to be fully elucidated.

Aerobic exercise capacity

The capacity of the cardiopulmonary system to supply oxygen to exercising muscles along with the capacity of the muscles to use this oxygen in energy metabolism is referred to as the aerobic exercise capacity. It is a measure of the maximum ability to carry out exercise and is determined by measuring the maximum rate of oxygen consumption attainable when performing an exercise test of increasing intensity that requires a large proportion of the total muscle mass. Aerobic exercise capacity decreases in healthy sedentary men and women at the rate of about 10% per decade.[61] Since physical fitness markedly influences aerobic exercise capacity, some of this decrease may be a result of the fall in physical activity with advancing age. The loss of aerobic exercise capacity is associated with a decrease in forced expiratory volume per second (FEV_1) and maximum heart rate. Hollenberg et al[61] believe that these pulmonary and cardiovascular changes play the major role in the age-associated decrease in aerobic capacity. Thus it is not surprising that the decline in aerobic exercise capacity is much greater in elderly people suffering from chronic disease, particularly atherosclerotic disease. Well-trained endurance athletes at all ages have a higher aerobic exercise capacity than untrained people of the same age.[62] Katzel et al[62] carried out a longitudinal study on the changes in aerobic fitness in endurance athletes of advanced ages. They found that some exhibited a greater longitudinal decline in aerobic exercise capacity than what was observed in sedentary people of the same age. Other old endurance athletes exhibited a very small longitudinal decline in aerobic exercise capacity. The former group was found to have decreased the magnitude of their endurance training during the course of the study, whereas the latter group had not. Katzel et al concluded that the rate of decline in aerobic exercise capacity in older endurance athletes is highly dependent on the intensity of their training. The aerobic exercise capacity of elderly sedentary men and women can be increased by physical training.[63]

Acid-base homeostasis

It has long been held that healthy elderly people have no problem maintaining normal acid-base balance when living the usual relatively unchallenged existence.[64] However, a careful meta-analysis of published data has challenged this view.[65] It was found that that there is a progressive increase in blood hydrogen ion concentration and a progressive decrease in the blood concentration of bicarbonate ion and carbon dioxide from age 20 to 80 years. The apparent steady-state plasma concentration of hydrogen ion was found to increase by 6% to 7% and the bicarbonate ion to decrease by 12% to 16%. It is likely that an age-associated deterioration of kidney function is responsible for the increase in the blood hydrogen ion because, when challenged with an acid load, the ability of the kidneys to excrete the acid load decreases with advancing age.[51]

Fat-free mass (FFM)

Body mass is divided into two components: fat mass and FFM. The constituents of FFM are skeletal muscle mass, body cell mass, total body water, and bone mineral mass. In men, peak FFM is reached in the mid-30s and progressively declines thereafter; in women, it is stable in young adulthood until about age 50 when it begins to progressively decline with advancing age.[66] Clearly, the homeostatic system regulating FFM is deranged at advanced age. An important component in the age-associated decrease in FFM is the loss of skeletal muscle mass, an important factor in the decrease in muscle strength with age.[66] Although physical exercise with an emphasis on weight-training can decrease the loss of muscle mass in the elderly, even individuals who maintain their fitness have some age-associated loss of muscle.[67]

Fat mass

Body fat mass increases with age in both men and women through middle age; a slow decrease occurs after age 70.[66] Even in those people whose body weight does not increase with age, body fat increases as lean body mass decreases. The homeostatic regulation of fat mass becomes faulty with advancing age. Sedentary lifestyle plays a role in the age-associated increase in fat mass since exercise is associated with a decrease in fat mass in the elderly.[68] However, exercise attenuates but does not totally prevent the age-associated increase in body fat. There is also a redistribution of fat to the abdominal region with increasing age.[66] Exercise not only decreases the age-associated increase in body fat but, most importantly, it also preferentially attenuates the disproportionate increase in abdominal fat.[69] The great concern about abdominal fat is due to the extensive evidence indicating that it is a risk factor for several age-associated pathologic problems such as coronary heart disease and type 2 diabetes.[70] Indeed, abdominal fat mass is positively associated with mortality in the elderly.[71] Thus interventions aimed at preventing the abdominal accumulation of fat with advancing age are most important to develop.

Bone mass

Bone mineral density (BMD), which accounts for 70% of bone strength, declines in both men and women starting in midlife.[72] Osteoporosis refers to a disease condition in which the extent of the decrease in BMD makes the individual prone to bone fracture; the age-associated decrease in BMD is probably the major reason that about 75% of all hip, spine, and distal forearm fractures occur in persons older than 65. In many women there is an age-associated postmenopausal increased rate of bone loss that can last for years.[73] Since women also have a less massive skeleton than men, it is not surprising that elderly women are more prone to bone fracture than elderly men. Middle-aged and older blacks of both genders have greater bone mass than whites.[74] They also have a substantially lower fracture rate, which is only partly due to maintaining a higher BMD. Cross-sectional studies have shown a positive correlation between exercise and BMD.[75] Although in postmenopausal women, low dietary calcium intake increases the risk of osteoporosis, this effect is often countered by such women having an increased body mass index.[76] Cigarette smoking lowers the BMD.[77]

Hormone replacement therapy has been the primary method for retarding bone loss in postmenopausal women. Treatment with low-dose conjugated estrogens or low-dose estradiol increases BMD in postmenopausal women.[78] Recent concern about the nonskeletal risks associated with long-term use of estrogens (e.g., breast cancer and cardiovascular disease) has lessened the enthusiasm for hormone replacement.

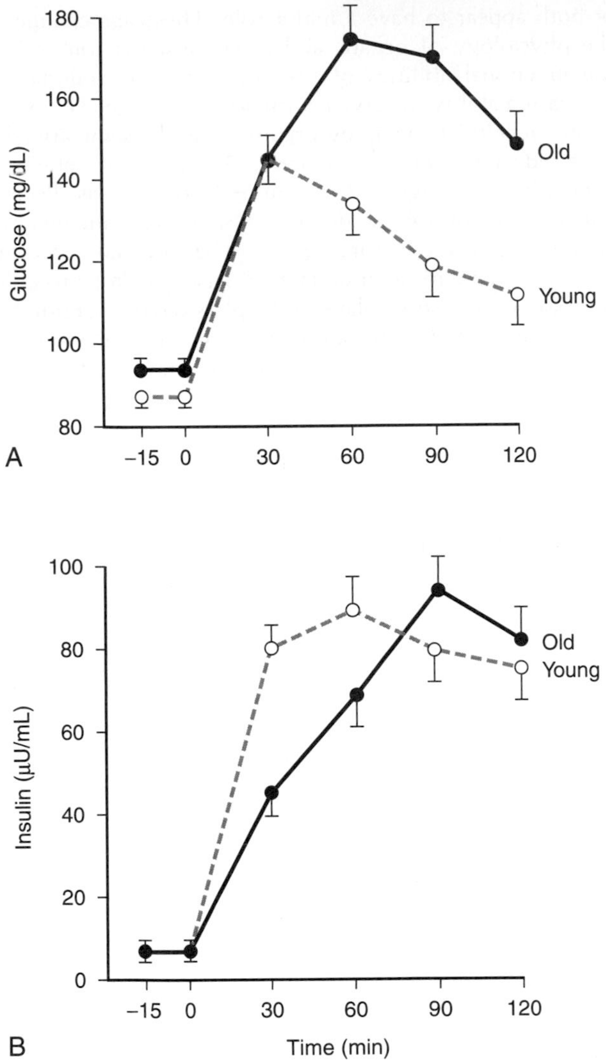

Figure 9-3. Influence of age on the response of plasma glucose and insulin concentration to an oral load of glucose. Young and old healthy human subjects were given 100 g of glucose orally. *(From Chen et al[86] with permission of Blackwell Science Inc.)*

Body temperature

The thermoregulatory system has the following components: thermal sensors (cutaneous and central); afferent neural pathways; central system integration; efferent neural pathways (somatic and autonomic); effectors (skeletal muscle shivering thermogenesis, brown adipose tissue nonshivering thermogenesis, cutaneous vasomotor activity, sweat gland activity). With increasing age, there are deficiencies at several levels of the thermoregulatory system.[79] Aging is associated with a progressive deficit in the ability to sense heat and cold, and also a reduced ability to generate heat (lower muscle mass for shivering thermogenesis) and dissipate heat (alterations in cardiovascular function and atrophy of sweat glands).[80] Also, there is impairment in nonshivering thermogenesis due to a decreased quantity of brown adipose tissue with advancing age.[81] The circadian rhythm of core temperature deteriorates at advanced ages.[82] Unlike in young men, body temperature in old men continues to increase following the cessation of a submaximal exercise.[83] Indeed, the deterioration of the thermoregulatory system makes old people extremely vulnerable to high and low environmental temperature.[84]

Glucose homeostasis

A diminished homeostatic regulation of plasma glucose concentration is a common characteristic of the aging phenotype.[85] When this regulatory ability declines sufficiently, a diagnosis of type II diabetes is made—a common age-associated disease. A major tool for examining glucose homeostasis has been the oral glucose tolerance test. Typical of the findings are those reported by Chen et al (Figure 9-3).[86] They administered orally 100 g of glucose to groups of healthy old and young subjects; plasma glucose rose to higher levels and remained elevated longer in the old than in the young, whereas the rise in plasma insulin level was delayed in the old, but with time reached that of the young. With increasing age, there is a reduced ability to secrete insulin[87]; however, it is not known how important a role it plays in the alteration in glucose homeostasis with age. In contrast, there is strong evidence that an increased resistance to insulin action is a major factor in the diminished homeostatic glucose regulation in old people.[88] As discussed previously, people become increasingly sedentary and have increased body fat, particularly in the abdominal region, with advancing age; these two factors are known to increase insulin resistance and to blunt the glucose homeostatic responses. Indeed, the effect of aging on glucose homeostasis can be ameliorated by increasing physical activity and in so doing decreasing adiposity, particularly in the abdominal region.[89] It is the increase in visceral fat that appears to be the major factor in increasing insulin resistance with advancing age.[90] Indeed, probably exercise increases insulin sensitivity[91] because it decreases abdominal fat.

KEY POINTS
Physiology of Aging

- Physiologic deterioration occurs during the adult life of most, if not all, mammalian species.
- The rate of age-associated physiologic deterioration and its character varies among species and among individuals within species.
- Age-associated physiologic deterioration results from the following three sources of damage: intrinsic living processes, environmental factors, and age-associated disease.
- Whether age-associated disease is an integral part of aging is a fundamental question that has yet to be resolved.
- Whether the concept of "normal aging," defined as aging in the absence of disease, is useful or misleading is an open question as is the related concept of "successful aging."
- The cross-sectional design has been used in most studies on the physiology of human aging; such studies can be confounded by factors other than aging, which makes it imperative that the possibility of confounders be carefully evaluated when interpreting the findings.
- The ability to cope with stressors is diminished with advancing adult age.
- The capacity to carry out activities (e.g., the aerobic exercise capacity), declines with advancing adult age.
- Homeostatic regulation deteriorates with advancing adult age.

SUMMARY AND CONCLUSIONS

Physiologic deterioration is a hallmark of the aging phenotype. This deterioration is caused by (1) damage resulting from intrinsic living processes; (2) damage due to extrinsic factors, such as diet, lifestyle, personal habits, and psychosocial factors; and (3) age-associated diseases. Although mammalian species are similar in that all show a progressive deterioration of physiologic processes with advancing age, the details of this deterioration vary among species. Thus the detailed characteristics of the deterioration probably have a strong genetic component. There is also a considerable intraspecies variation in the rate and character of physiologic deterioration with advancing age. Many of the differences among individuals of the same species appear to relate to extrinsic factors. Age-associated deterioration occurs in all organs and organ systems. The extent to which extrinsic factors and age-associated disease play a role varies among organ systems and among individuals but, in most cases, one or both appear to have a major role. These age changes in the physiology of organs and organ systems compromise the functional abilities of the organism and underlie the decreasing ability to survive with advancing age. The physiologic deficits of the aging organism can be summarized as (1) a reduced functional capacity, (2) a decreased ability to cope with challenges, (3) an altered homeostasis. Because much of the physiologic deterioration with advancing age is caused by extrinsic factors, aging can be modified by altering lifestyle and environmental factors. Also, the large role that age-associated disease plays in the physiologic deterioration can be modulated by presently available medical and public health measures and undoubtedly much more by those that will be developed in the future.

For a complete list of references, please visit online only at www.expertconsult.com

CHAPTER 10

A Clinico-Mathematical Model of Aging

Kenneth Rockwood
Arnold Mitnitski

INTRODUCTION

Overview of frailty

Geriatricians have an affinity for frail elderly people, or should. The complex care of elderly people who are frail is argued—including in the Foreword of this book—to be the very stuff of geriatric medicine.[1] This chapter, building on recent reviews,[2,3] addresses the issue of frailty in relation to complexity to argue that the formal assessment of complexity can usefully be employed to understand the scientific basis of the analyses of frailty, with insights for the practice of geriatric medicine.

Frail, elderly patients are at an increased risk—compared with others of the same chronologic age—as a consequence of having multiple, interacting, age-related physiologic impairments, some of which cross clinical thresholds to be recognized as diseases and others as disabilities. These impairments, diseases, and disabilities typically interact with various social vulnerability factors, which commonly travel with the frail to further increase the risk of adverse health outcomes.

The view of frailty as a multiple-determined at-risk state is reasonably noncontroversial.[4–8] By contrast, how best to operationalize frailty is more controversial. As outlined in various reviews, some of the proposed operational definitions receive more widespread support than others. In particular, the "phenotypic" definition of frailty used in the Cardiovascular Health Study (CHS)[9] has been endorsed at consensus conferences[6,7] and employed by several groups.[10–13] Indeed, it has even been claimed that the terms "frail" and "frailty" should be avoided except when used in the context of a CHS assessment.[14]

Overview of complexity

The idea of complexity is proving to be one of the most important conceptual advances in science.[15] Briefly, complexity arises from systems. Systems can be defined in many ways because there is an irreducible extent to which the definition of a system depends on the context in which it is considered. To start, it might work best to contrast a *system* with a *set of elements*. The elements of a set exist as members of the set because of some shared characteristic, but they do not become a system until there is interconnectedness between them. Interconnectedness exists when changes in one element result in changes in other elements, and these changes result in further changes, and so forth. It is the nature of the interrelated changes that defines complexity: complexity is the phenomenon of dynamic interactions in the elements of a system. The goal of complexity analyses is to quantify and summarize these changes.

The use of complexity analyses in aging has not been noncontroversial. For example, in 2002, an entire issue of *Neurobiology of Aging* was devoted to complexity. Some of the papers in the special issue gave examples in which complexity, as measured in one specific context, appeared to decrease with aging,[16] whereas others gave opposite examples.[17] Although some commentators despaired,[18] this result is typical when complex systems are first investigated. Commonly, with better specification of the context, (e.g., specification of intrinsic dynamics or of the time scale under consideration) apparent contradictions resolve. Such specification can lead to the implementation of new interventions that are based on a better appreciation of changes in dynamic complexity of biologic variability, such as the application of subsensory noise to the feet to improve postural stability in older adults.[19]

It is evident that aging humans constitute aging systems, both as individuals and as groups, and that within the human organism, there are different organ systems, although their specification—where does the vascular system end and the immunologic system begin?—often results in some arbitrariness. Such arbitrariness is best not ignored when considering a phenomenon as all-encompassing as the passage of time. How to specify the interconnectedness of the organs in the body as people age is not clear. It is clear, however, that there is (there must be, if it is a system) interconnectedness of health characteristics (interdependence of variables). One way to specify the interconnectedness of health characteristics is by the use of connectivity graphs (Figure 10-1). Such graphs are constructed to represent interconnectedness between variables, so that a line between variables is portrayed when some specified level of connectivity—say a correlation >0.2 exists. As the graph illustrates, some variables are more highly connected than others (i.e., some have more lines between them than others do.[20] (It is this high connectivity between some items more than others, that means that the items of the frailty index do not need to be weighted—an issue to which we will come.)

The connectivity graph illustrates two fundamental points about complex states, which are multiplicity and interconnectedness. Another way to think about interconnectedness is that a system is "more than a sum of its parts"; this is sometimes referred to as the system having "emergent properties." (The idea of emergent properties is controversial and need not be considered further here.) What will be evident is that an individual's state of health can be summarized by a single number—it is what we will refer to later as the frailty index—and that the properties or behavior of that number (for example, how the frailty index changes with age) can be considered as an area of investigation in and of itself. To continue that example, we have shown that the distribution of the frailty index with age has distinctive characteristics.[21] These characteristics can be studied using network models, which offer an apparatus for such analyses, based on stochastic dynamics.[22–28] One example is the idea that heterogeneity (here, of the distribution of the frailty index with age)[21,26] arises as a consequence of the stochastic dynamics of complex systems. This approach to studying heterogeneity is readily summarizable using a network approach, and has had wide applicability from cortical networks in Alzheimer's disease[29] to capital markets,[30] to gas furnace pressures.[31] Finally, the connectivity graph also shows that a complex system is summarizable. We will refer to this later, in terms of both the frailty index, and of the more general case of a clinical state variable. For now, we will simply note that a complex system can be summarized in ways that are not necessarily

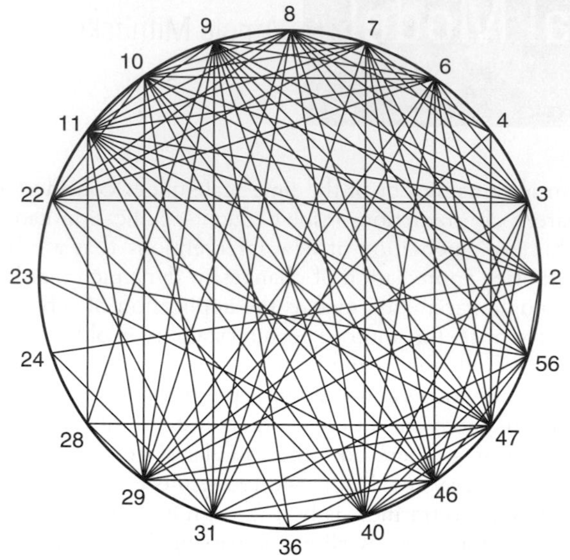

Figure 10-1. Connectivity graph. Nodes indicate the deficits (codes correspond to the deficits listed in reference 20) and edges indicate statistically significant relationships between deficits (i.e., when the conditional probability of one deficit, given another is statistically different ($p < 0.05$; *t*-test) from the unconditional probability of the first deficit. It is clear that not all elements are equally well connected. *(Copyright A Mitnitski et al, used with permission.)*

complicated. That is the goal of the bulk of initiatives in bringing the tools of complexity analysis to studying what happens as people age and become frail. As a start, the simplicity of the output of these analyses is a good measure by which the merit of the analyses might be judged.

THE PHENOTYPIC DEFINITION OF FRAILTY

A very popular approach to defining frailty is by means of a clinical phenotype. This operational definition, developed by a consensus and tested in the Cardiovascular Health Survey,[9] has been validated in several studies[12,13,32–39] and endorsed by several groups.[6–8] The phenotypic definition concentrates on five clinical characteristics: a self-report of exhaustion, self or observer report of a decline in activity level, demonstrated or reported weight loss, impaired strength (commonly operationalized as impaired grip strength using a dynamometer), and slow gait (e.g., defined as the slowest 20% of the population was defined at baseline, based on time to walk 15 feet, adjusting for gender and standing height).[9] People who have none of the five characteristics are said to be robust, and those with three or more are said to be frail. People who have only one or two problems are at an intermediate risk grade, referred to as being "prefrail." In several studies, the three groups have been shown to have ascending levels of risk of a number of adverse health outcomes, including worsening mobility, falls, disability, fracture, mortality, and institutionalization.[9,12,32–35,37]

A comprehensive series of studies have evaluated a wide range of markers that are seen in association with increasing grades of frailty. People who are frail have been found to have, among other impairments, higher levels of inflammatory markers,[40–42] worse glucose control[43] and lower antioxidant[13] and hemoglobin[44] levels.

The ready operationalization of the phenotypic definition, especially in epidemiologic studies, is a clear asset. So too has been the attempt to disentangle physical frailty from disability and comorbidity.[45] On the other hand, the phenotype has been criticized for an artificial distinction between physical and cognitive (including affective) states,[46] for requiring performance tests that can be impracticable in the clinical setting[47] and for problems of both sensitivity and specificity in relation to both mortality prediction[48] and to what many experienced clinicians would accept as frail.[46]

Frailty in relation to deficit accumulation

Our group has proposed that frailty can be understood in relation to deficit accumulation.[49] The fundamental idea to this approach is that the more deficits that people have (the more things people have wrong with them), the more likely they are to be frail. We have been encouraged to continue with this approach by the insights that can be gained from the study of the frailty index itself. Our group, and others[48,50] have described how the frailty index changes in characteristic ways. These changes are susceptible to precise analyses, which we will outline below, and which also appear to have useful clinical implications. In this way, we hope to move beyond cartoon models of frailty. For example, Figure 10-2 is one such cartoon model.[51] It represents frailty as a state that arises from a dynamic interplay between a variety of factors. When people are well, their assets outweigh their deficits. As they experience illness, the balance can shift, but as this is a dynamic state, it can shift back. The model also suggests that people with, for example, many social assets, will be harder to tip into frailty than those with fewer social assets.

Although cartoon models have many uses, and the advantage of readily illustrating complicated ideas, they cannot offer the precision of formal, quantitative models, as depicted in Figure 10-3.[52] It demonstrates changes in frailty states, from having n deficits at baseline, to k deficits at follow-up. The formal model shows that these probabilities can be modeled as a modified Poisson distribution. Here is what the formula says: the chance of having k deficits at follow-up is a function of the number of deficits n, at baseline. First, we must consider that to have k deficits at follow-up, the person must be alive, so the chance of moving from n to k must be adjusted for the chance of surviving. The term P_{nd} is the chance of dying during the interval between baseline and follow-up (or between any two consecutive assessments) so $1–P_{nd}$ is the chance of surviving. For any given n state (e.g., $n = 1$, $n = 2$, etc.), the chance of having any k deficit proceeds in a highly ordered way, with incremental change (this is what is implied by the Poisson distribution). For example, for most baseline states, the single most likely number of deficits that an individual will have at follow-up is one more than they had at baseline. (Formally, this can be summarized as saying that the mode of k is $n + 1$.) There is a slightly smaller chance of staying the same and about the same chance of having two things wrong more than at baseline, a smaller chance again of improving and so on. The probabilities of achieving any given k therefore arise as a function of n, and follow an ordered set of changes. On average, n increases, but for virtually any value of n, there is a chance of improvement (or stabilization or decline). Large jumps in n to k states are uncommon; when large changes in the value of n do occur, they usually go from a low n state (i.e., few deficits, good health) to a high k state.

Two other points are especially of note. One is that the chance of moving from any given n state to any k state

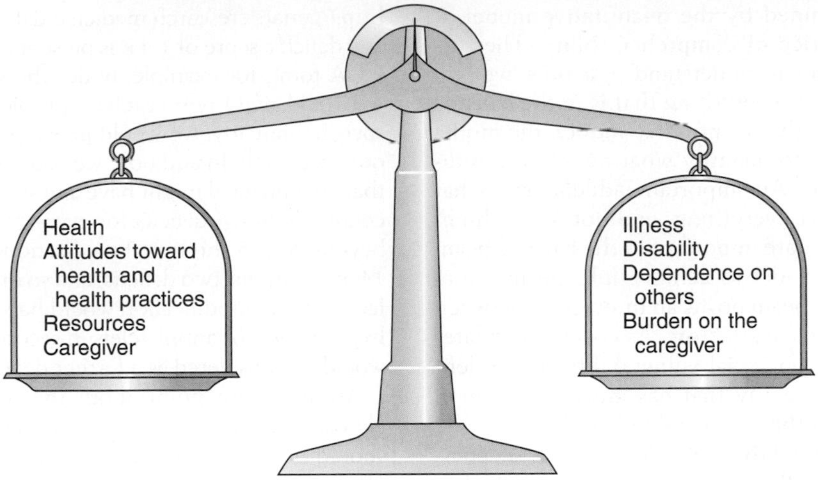

Figure 10-2. The balance beam model of changes in frailty states. The beam illustrates a multicomponent, dynamic state. *(Copyright CMAJ and used with permission.)*

$$P_{nk} = \frac{\rho_n^k}{k!}\exp(-\rho_n)(1 - P_{nd})$$

Figure 10-3. A formal mode of changes in frailty states, expressed as the probability of a person with *n* deficits at baseline surviving to have *k* deficits at follow-up. P_{nd} is the chance of dying; $P_{nd} = P_{0d}\, exp(b_2 n)$. Note that {I}$\rho_n = \rho_0 + b_1 n${/I}; {I}$\rho_0$ {/I} and P_{0d} are the characteristic risks associated with no deficits. The two parameters b_1 and b_2 describe, respectively (given the current number of deficits, *n*), the increments of their expected change, and the risk of death. Note that the model can be elaborated to include the effects of specific covariates, such as age, sex, or social vulnerability. In that case, the antilog of the ratio of the regression coefficients associated with each covariate is an estimate of the relative risk associated with that coefficient.

depends on both the present value of n, and the general (or ambient, or background) changes in that environment. This is captured in the formula by saying that {I}$\rho_n = \rho_0 + b_1 n${/I}, where {I}ρ_0 {/I} describes the chance of accumulating deficits for people who have nothing wrong at baseline (i.e., who at baseline are in the "zero [deficit] state.") The parameter b_1 describes, given the current nonzero number of deficits, the increments of their expected change.[25] Of course, the same obtains for the risk of death [i.e., $P_{nd} = P_{od}\, exp(b_2 n)$]; P_{od} is the chance of dying for people who have nothing wrong at baseline. Here, parameter b_2 describes, again given the current (nonzero) number of deficits, the associated risk of death.[25] In this way, it can be seen that the zero state appears to be informative about the environment in which a given population ages. Finally, we note that this is a simplified model, which can be adjusted to evaluate the impact of various covariates. For example, to understand the impact of high versus low level of education, we can evaluate its impact on {I}ρ_0 {/I} and P_{nd}.

The move from the operationalization of the concepts of deficits in dynamic balance in Figure 10-2 to the terms specified in Figure 10-3 took place over some years, but each agrees on the following essential points: Frailty is a multiply with agreement on determined state of risk that is complex (component parts which interact in ways that are not always summarizable at the level of the individual parts) and dynamic (the interactions produce further interactions, and change with time). In Figure 10-2, items that relate to health are envisaged as weights on the balance beam. For example, various health assets, such as a positive health attitude[53] or positive health practices such as exercise,[54] fit on the left hand side of the balance, giving positive weight to assets. Others, such as illness, and the particular illness which gives rise to disabilities, and the particular disabilities that result in dependence on others are seen to weigh on the negative side. As more health deficits mount up and a person becomes more frail, the assets and deficits come into a precarious balance. In this context, an acute illness can be an important deficit, and can even "tip the balance" between assets and deficits. As attractive as this model is—it is easy to understand, accommodates multiple factors, and is complex and dynamic—unless and until it can be quantified, it cannot rise beyond the status of a metaphor. (In its earliest operationalization, the deficits were quantified as grades of disability, cognitive impairment, and poor health attitude.)[55,56]

By contrast, Figure 10-3 proposes that changes in health status—changes in grades of frailty—occur as a function of the number of things that people have wrong with them. It says that the chance that people with that number of things wrong with them will change their health status in relation to a known distribution of the range of chances. These changes can be stability, worsening, or improvement. The distribution suggests that most people do not change their health status that much (i.e., a person with n things wrong with them is most likely, when followed up, to have $n+1$ things wrong, or to show a slight worsening) but also could stay at just n things wrong, or improve to $n-1$ things wrong. For most people, the chance of improvement to $n-1$ is about the same as the chance of worsening to $n+2$ things wrong. But those discrete states (slightly better, the same, or 1 or 2 more things wrong) consist of over half of the possible outcomes. The model assigns all possible outcome states (better, same, worse, or dead) typically with high precision based on just four parameters—a staggering degree of dimensionality reduction compared with most multivariable models. As the equation shows, each of the four parameters becomes an object of investigation, in and of itself. So the motivation to continue this line of inquiry is very strong.

Even so, most readers—especially most medical readers, for whom the mathematics is stereotypically not their strong suit—will worry that whatever apparent precision in these estimates might be obtained by the quantitative model, it comes at a very high price of comprehensibility. The balance beam is much easier to understand. For now, we will make the claim that almost everything that is in the balance beam can be included in the quantitative model: the model helps us understand how to quantify what our clinical intuition tells us is the case. An important addendum—what compels us to say "almost everything" and not "everything" is that some elements that are important in the balance beam need a more elaborate model to achieve full specification. For example, the balance beam posits an interaction between so-called "medical" and "social" factors. As covered in a later chapter of this textbook on social vulnerability, social deficits appear to operate in a way that has much in common with frailty, but at a level that is separable from it.[57]

A useful way to understand the dynamics of deficit accumulation is to consider what Benjamin Gompertz quantified in 1825[58]: the older people are, the more likely they are to die, as a precise function (+/– one or two error terms)[59,60] of the logarithm of their age (see Figure 10-3). But it is not as though people suddenly drop dead as they age. Instead, before death, they accumulate deficits, and they accumulate them exponentially with age.[61] In fact, it is the deficit count, more than chronologic age, which correlates most with the risk of death at any age.[48,49,61,62] The deficits that we can see accumulate clinically—the symptoms, signs, diseases, disabilities, and laboratory abnormalities that we typically count in frailty indices—presumably begin as subcellular impairments.[63] So the line of reasoning goes that barring sudden death or accidents, the more impairments people have, the more deficits they have; the more deficits they have, the more frail they are; and the more frail they are, the more likely they are to die.

DEVELOPMENT OF A FRAILTY INDEX BASED ON COMPREHENSIVE GERIATRIC ASSESSMENT

We began work on the frailty index by counting deficits in existing databases, chiefly epidemiologic ones. Over the years, we have collaborated with several groups to build a frailty index in their databases, usually epidemiologic, not clinical ones. This has justifiably caused concern in some quarters about the clinical usefulness of the approach,[64] especially as an optimal frailty index should contain no fewer than 30 to 40 items. (The lowest practical limit seems to be about 10, although at that point, selection of which items are to be counted becomes more important.)[65] Most recently, we have begun to build a frailty index prospectively from the standardized comprehensive geriatric assessment form that is used on all clinical geriatric medicine services at the Capital District Health Authority in Halifax, Nova Scotia. The CGA form (Figure 10-4) is the basis of our consultation assessment on the consultation services, and of care planning on each of our inpatient services (acute and rehabilitation services) and the day hospital. It is worth noting that the form readily can count up to 50 items (+10 items relating to social vulnerability) but can still fit on a single page.

The frailty index that is derived from the CGA form is built like any other, which is to say that it counts deficits. (We have built other frailty index measures based on CGA.)[66,67] In a recent open access journal publication, we have spelled out how to create a frailty index.[68] A video is also available at http://geriatricresearch.medicine.dal.ca. By convention, we give any deficit a score of 1 if it is present and 0 if it is absent. On the CGA form, for example, under the section "Communication" we would give 1 point each for problems of vision, hearing, and speech. Similarly, we would give a point for impaired mobility or a recent fall. In addition, we count each of the comorbidities that an individual might have and score one point for each. We count additional deficits for every five medications prescribed beyond five (5 through 9 medications, one deficit; 10 through 14 medications, two deficits, and so on). Any asymptomatic risk factor where modification would have a mortality benefit (e.g., hypertension or antiplatelets in secondary vascular prevention) would be considered as a further deficit if left untreated.

An important point about the frailty index-CGA is that almost all deficits can be measured in every patient, so there should be few missing data—typically less than 5% for any given item. This requirement has the effect of excluding many performance-based measures from frailty index variables, at least from survey data in which they typically have considerably more than 5% missing data.[47] If they are to be included, then it seems to be useful to assign missing data the score associated with worst performance status.[47]

Validation of the frailty index

The frailty index has been validated by our group and by others, typically using a three-part approach that considers content, construct, and criterion validity.[69] The content validity of a measure that counts what people have wrong with them, and assumes that the more they have wrong with them, the more likely they are to be frail, seems secure. In addition, it offers the idea of grades of frailty. On the other hand, many commentators have been concerned about the idea that the frailty index weights all items equally. A common specific objection is that it seems implausible that both "cancer" and "skin disease" should have the same weights (i.e., "0" if absent and "1" if present). The usual rejoinder is that although cancer more often is more lethal than skin disease, not all cancers are lethal, and not all skin diseases are benign. When skin disease is lethal (e.g., psoriasis with vasculitis and skin breakdown), it will have more deficits associated with it. The same would hold for a cancer that impacted the overall state of health. This detection of multiple deficits has the effect of weighting more serious illness higher, regardless of the cause of the illness.

Construct validity has been tested chiefly by convergent construct correlation (i.e., by correlating the frailty index with other frailty measures, and measures of disability, cognitive impairment, and comorbidity).[70] Correlations between the frailty index and other measures of frailty—including the phenotypic definition—typically run in the range of ~0.6 to 0.8. As reviewed elsewhere[2,3] slightly lower correlations (in the range of ~0.4 to 0.6) typically are seen with global measures of function, comorbidity, and cognition.

One aspect of construct validation that lends some insight into the nature of frailty is the relationship between the frailty index and age (Figure 10-5). Consistently in epidemiologic samples, we have found that the average value of the frailty index is highly associated with age (correlation coefficients >0.95).[2,3] Although the average value of the frailty index increases with age (typically about 3% per year on a log scale—see Figure 10-5, lower best fit line), individuals have variable numbers of deficits at any given age. People who have a large number of deficits (e.g., people with a frailty index score of more than 0.5,

Comprehensive Geriatric Assessment

Division of Geriatric Medicine, Dalhousie University

○ **Cognitive Status** ☐ WNL ☐ Dementia MMSE: ________ ☐ CIND/MCI ☐ Delirium FAST: ________ ☐ Chief lifelong occupation: ________ Education (years): ________

○ **Emotional** ☐ WNL ☐ ? Mood ☐ Depression ☐ Anxiety ☐ Fatigue ☐ Other

○ **Motivation** ☐ High ☐ Usual ☐ Low **Health Attitude** ☐ Excellent ☐ Good ☐ Fair ☐ Poor ☐ Couldn't say

○ **Communication** **Speech** ☐ WNL ☐ Impaired **Hearing** ☐ WNL ☐ Impaired **Vision** ☐ WNL ☐ Impaired

○ **Strength** ☐ WNL ☐ Weak Upper: PROXIMAL DISTAL Lower: PROXIMAL DISTAL

		BASELINE (two weeks ago)	CURRENT (today)	NOTES
○ **Mobility**	Transfer Walking AID	I A D I A D ________	I A D I A D ________	
○ **Balance**	Balance Falls	WNL IMPAIRED N Y Number ________	WNL IMPAIRED N Y Number ________	
○ **Elimination**	Bowel Bladder	CONT CONSTIP INCONT CONT CATHETER INCONT	CONSTIP CONT INCONT CATHETER CONT INCONT	
○ **Nutrition**	Weight Appetite	GOOD UNDER OVER OBESE WNL FAIR POOR	STABLE LOSS GAIN WNL FAIR POOR	
○ **ADLs**	Feeding Bathing Dressing Toileting	I A D I A D I A D I A D	I A D I A D I A D I A D	
○ **IADLs**	Cooking Cleaning Shopping Medications Driving Banking	I A D I A D I A D I A D I A D I A D	I A D I A D I A D I A D I A D I A D	

○ **Sleep** ☐ Normal ☐ Disrupted ☐ Daytime drowsiness **Socially Engaged** ☐ Freq. ☐ Occ. ☐ Not

○ **Social** ☐ Married ☐ Divorced ☐ Widowed ☐ Single

Lives ☐ Alone ☐ Spouse ☐ Other

Home ☐ House (levels___) ☐ Steps (number___) ☐ Apartment ☐ Assisted living ☐ Nursing home ☐ Other

Supports ☐ Informal ☐ HCNS ☐ Other ☐ None ○ **Req. more support**

Caregiver relationship ☐ Spouse ☐ Sibling ☐ Offspring ☐ Other

Caregiver stress ☐ None ☐ Low ☐ Moderate ☐ High

Caregiver occupation:(CG) ________

Patient contact: (Pt.)
☐ Inpatient
☐ Clinic
☐ GDH
☐ NH
☐ Outreach
☐ Home
☐ Assisted living
☐ ER
☐ Other

How many months since last well?

Current Frailty Score:

Score	Pt.	CG
1. Very fit		
2. Well		
3. Well c̄ Rx'd co-morbid disease		
4. Apparently vulnerable		
5. Mildly frail		
6. Moderately frail		
7. Severely frail		
8. Terminally ill		

ACTION REQUIRED (check appropriate circles)

Problems:	Med adjust req.	Associated medications: (*mark meds started in hospital with an asterisk)
1 RFR	○	
2	○	
3	○	
4	○	
5	○	
6	○	
7	○	
8	○	
9	○	
10	○	

Assessor/Physician: Date: ________ YYYY / MM / DD

Figure 10-4. A standard Comprehensive Geriatric Assessment (CGA) form used at the Centre for Health Care of the Elderly, Capital Health, Halifax, Nova Scotia. The individual items on it can be scored to derive a frailty index based on the CGA (FI-CGA). *(Copyright Geriatric Medicine Research Unit, Dalhousie University, Halifax, Nova Scotia, Canada. Used with permission.)*

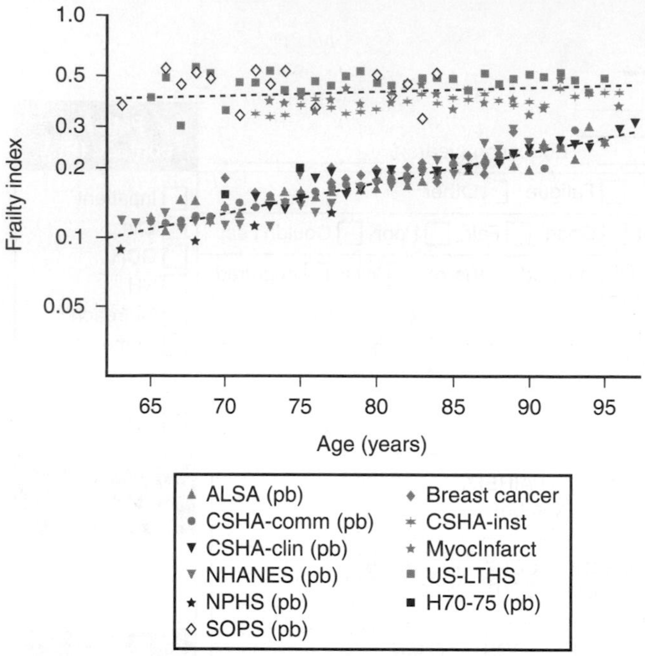

Figure 10-5. The relationship between the frailty index and age. Across several surveys, the frailty index accumulates in community dwelling older adults at a rate of about 3% per year, on a log scale (lower line). By contrast, in clinical samples and among institutionalized older adults, the values of the frailty index are much higher on average and show almost no accumulation with age.

and who had half or more of all deficits that were measured) typically show no mean accumulation with age; that is, they have, on average, about as many deficits as they can tolerate, so that if more deficits occur, they die. This is also typical of the mean value of people who come from clinical and institutional samples (see Figure 10-5, upper best fit line).[61,71]

Even though the average value of the frailty index increases with age, there is considerable individual variability, so that some people are well above and others well below the mean value. If the frailty index quantifies a risk state, then people with high frailty index values should have a higher risk of death than people with lower frailty index values. As noted, this is the case; it also holds for institutionalization,[65,72] health service use,[67] and worse health status.[52,73,74] In each case, the higher the frailty index count, the more likely the person is to experience an adverse outcome. The relationship between the frailty index and the risk of death, like the relationship between age and the risk of death, is also exponential.

The frailty index as a clinical state variable

If variation in grades of the frailty index reflects variation in the risk of adverse health outcomes, then it is reasonable to suppose that these grades in the frailty index represent different states of health. To this end, we have proposed that the frailty index can be considered as a clinical state variable.[2] A state variable is one that quantitatively summarizes the state of an entire system; a classic example is temperature, which can be measured has a single number on a graded scale. The number has a known meaning, as the average of the kinetic energies of the molecules which make up a given system. These individual kinetic energies are indeterminate. By contrast, temperature is more stable, and can behave in ways that can be known with precision. An important trait of a state variable is that it can be described using plain language descriptions. Temperature can be meaningfully communicated as, for example, hot, warm, cool, cold, or freezing. These descriptions can also be contextualized. In a biologic context, scalding would have a precise clinical meaning. These attributes appear to be particularly worthwhile in grading frailty and allow some precision to be brought to the question of what procedures might safely be entertained in a "frail" patient. This grading of risk in relation to the severity/load of the intervention and the responsiveness/frailty of the individual is an active area of inquiry. For now, the interim answer seems to be to translate the frailty index into terms used. One aspect of the frailty index as a clinical state variable that has yet to be fully explored is its translation into plain language: what is the analog to "hot" versus "tepid" with respect to frailty? Pending this answer being fully worked out, the high correlation between the frailty index and the Canadian Study of Health and Aging Clinical Global Frailty Scale[70] makes that measure seem to be a reasonable way to quickly grade degrees of fitness and frailty (Table 10-1).

Another consequence to flow from the idea that the frailty index defines discrete health states is that how these states change might be informative. As noted, this appears to be the case (see Figure 10-3). The probability for a given individual of a change in the number of deficits that they have depends on two factors. The first is the number of deficits that that individual has at baseline and the number of deficits that are accumulated, on average, by a person who has no deficits at baseline. Another notable feature of the reproducibility of the changes in health states represented by variable deficit counts/grades of frailty is that these estimates are very robust. The estimates noted above do not just come from different countries, but were developed using different versions of the frailty index, which typically has not been constructed in the same way in any two studies (see Figure 10-5). The examples quoted above employ iterations of the frailty index that use different types of variables (e.g., self-reported in the NPHS, clinically assessed [CSHA, H-70], or laboratory data H-70), and often different numbers of variables (from 39 in the NPHS to 70 in the CSHA to 100 in H-70).

The frailty index has often been referred to as a measure of biologic age.[20,50,75] If we consider that biologic age derives its rationale not as time since birth—that is already well handled by chronologic age—but as the time to death, then the high correlation between the frailty index and mortality can be usefully exploited to calculate biologic age. Here is how. Consider two people ("A" and "B") of the same chronologic age, say 80 years old (Figure 10-6). One has a frailty index score of 0.11, which by interpolation we can see is the mean value on average of the frailty index at age 65. We can this say that this person has a biologic age of 65 years. The second person has a frailty index value of 0.28, which corresponds to the mean value of the frailty index at age 95, meaning that this person has a biologic age of 95. In multivariable models, which include both chronologic age and the frailty index, each contributes independently, but with more information typically coming from the frailty index.[48,49] In addition, people who accumulate deficits more quickly have a higher mortality rate.

The frailty index-CGA is one instance of a clinical state variable, with a single number summarizing the overall clinical state of the individual. Other candidate clinical state variables can be considered. Recalling that a system is different from a set of elements by virtue of its interconnectedness,

Table 10-1. Clinical Frailty Scale

Grade	Plain Language Descriptor	Common Characteristics	Usual Frailty Index Values
1	Very fit	Robust, active, energetic, well motivated, and fit; these people commonly exercise regularly and are in the fittest group for their age. Commonly describe their health as "excellent."	0.09 (0.05)
2	Well	Without active/symptomatic disease, but less fit than people in category 1.	0.12 (0.05)
3	Well, with treated comorbid disease	Disease symptoms are well controlled compared with those in category 4.	0.16 (0.07)
4	Apparently vulnerable	Although not frankly dependent, these people commonly complain of being "slowed up" or have disease symptoms or self-rate health as "fair," at best. If cognitively impaired, do not meet dementia criteria.	0.22 (0.08)
5	Mildly frail	Shows limited dependence on others for instrumental activities of daily living.	0.27 (0.09)
6	Moderately frail	Help is needed with both instrumental and some personal activities of daily living. Walking commonly is restricted.	0.36 (0.09)
7	Severely frail	Completely dependent on others for personal activities of daily living.	0.43 (0.08)
8	Terminally ill	Terminally ill	

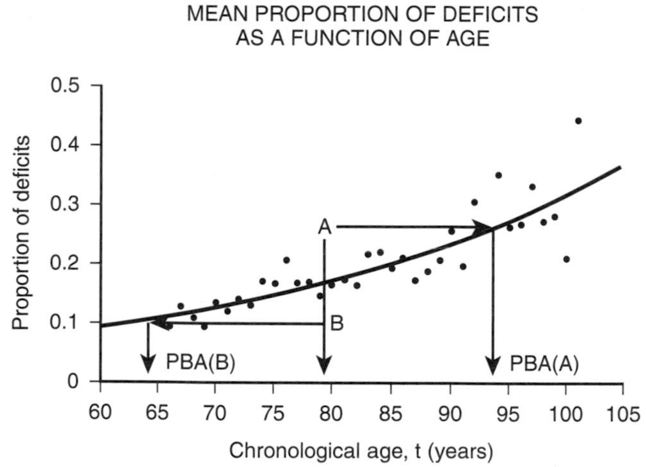

Figure 10-6. Personal biologic age. Because the mean value of the frailty index is so highly correlated with mortality (r^2 typically >0.95), it can be used to estimate personal biologic age, understood as a measure of the proximity to death. Consider two men, each with the same (chronologic) age of 78 years. Person A has a value of the frailty index that corresponds to the mean frailty index value for 93-year-olds. In that sense he has a personal biologic age of 93 years. By contrast, person B has a value of the frailty Index that is seen, on average, at age 63 years. That person would have a mortality risk that corresponds to that of 63-year-olds.

clinical state variables need to integrate information about connectedness of the component parts. In this way, decline in connectivity can be considered as a manifestation of frailty, a point that can be illustrated with connectivity graphs.[20] In this way too, it is evident that any clinical state variable should represent the functioning of a system, so from that standpoint must be high order. For humans, the evolutionary high order functions are upright bipedal ambulation, opposable thumbs, divided attention, and social interaction. In consequence, candidate clinical state variables logically can be sought in measures of mobility and balance, function, divided attention, and social withdrawal. Any geriatrician will recognize in this a short list of important "geriatric giants," those being impaired mobility ("taking to bed," "off legs"), falls, functional decline, and social withdrawal, or caregiver distress. This textbook has chapters on each topic and each is moving toward better quantification of the underlying phenomena. The valuation of mobility and balance appears to hold particular promise as a candidate for a clinical state variable that changes acutely.[76] Recently, too, a frailty index has been employed using data available in the emergency department record.[77]

Good geriatric medicine has always had an intuitive grasp of the nature of complexity as manifest in the frail elderly patients for whom geriatricians are privileged to care. The intent in making the analysis of complexity explicit is to build on this intuition, not substitute for it. As has been argued, providing a scientific basis for the specialty of geriatric medicine, rather than it existing as a set of utilitarian values (we do these things because they seem to work), is essential to advancing the care of frail elderly patients with complex needs.[78]

KEY POINTS

Models of Aging

- Frailty is an important issue for geriatricians; geriatric medicine chiefly consists in the complex care of elderly people who are frail.
- Frailty is a state of increased risk of adverse health outcomes.
- Operationalization of frailty is controversial, with three approaches to measurement: classification from preset descriptors; criteria based on the idea of common frailty phenotypes, and a count of deficits.
- An attractive feature of the deficit count approach is that it allows insights from formal analyses of complexity to be applied to clinical problems associated with frailty.
- One insight from complexity analyses is the notion of clinical state variables (i.e., single numbers that allow the overall clinical state to be summarized). The frailty index, a deficit count, is one example of the chronic health state. Mobility and balance, appropriately measured, appears to be another clinical state variable, more applicable for acute changes in health.
- Another idea that can be imported from complexity analyses is that instruments meant to convey information should be presented in ways that allow for easy pattern recognition.
- The formal analysis of complexity also makes clear why comprehensive geriatric assessment, and the evaluation of delirium, falls, and immobility are intrinsic to geriatric medicine. Each is a response to the analysis of complex systems at high risk for failure.

For a complete list of references, please visit online only at www.expertconsult.com

CHAPTER 11

The Premature Aging Syndrome Hutchinson-Gilford Progeria: Insights Into Normal Aging

Leslie B. Gordon

INTRODUCTION

Hutchinson-Gilford progeria syndrome (HGPS) is an extremely rare, uniformly fatal, segmental "premature aging" disease in which children exhibit phenotypes that may give us insights into the aging process at both the cellular and organismal levels. This chapter will compare HGPS with normal aging with respect to its genetics, biology, clinical phenotype, clinical care, and treatment. By looking carefully at one of the rarest diseases on earth, we gain novel and important insight into the most common conditions affecting quality and longevity of life—aging and cardiovascular disease.

HGPS: disease description

Hutchinson-Gilford progeria syndrome is, in most cases, a sporadic, autosomal dominant, "premature aging" disease in which children die of heart attacks or strokes at an average age of 13.[1,2] Children experience normal fetal and early postnatal development. Between several months and 1 year of age, abnormalities in growth and body composition are readily apparent (Figure 11-1). Severe failure to thrive ensues, heralding generalized lipoatrophy,[3,4] with apparent wasting of limbs, circumoral cyanosis, and prominent veins around the scalp, the neck, and trunk. Children reach a final height of approximately 1 m and weight of approximately 14 kg. Bone and cartilaginous changes include clavicular resorption, coxa valga, distal phalangeal resorption, facial disproportion (a small, slim nose and receding mandible), and short stature. Dentition is severely delayed.[5,6] Eruption may be delayed for many months, and primary teeth may persist for the duration of life. Secondary teeth are present, but may or may not erupt. Skin looks thin with sclerodermatous areas and almost complete hair loss.[7–9] Skin findings are variable in severity and include areas of discoloration, stippled pigmentation, tightened areas that can restrict movement, and areas of the dorsal trunk where small (1 to 2 cm) soft bulging skin is present. Joint contractures, due to ligamentous and skin tightening, limit range of motion. Intellectual development is normal in HGPS. Transient ischemic attacks and strokes may ensue as early as 4 years of age, but more often they occur in the later years. Death results from sequelae of widespread arteriosclerosis between the ages of 8 and 21 years, almost exclusively from myocardial infarction or stroke.[1,2,10]

Molecular genetics and cell biology

LAMIN A

HGPS is a member of the family of genetic diseases known as the laminopathies, whose causal mutations lie along the *LMNA* gene (located at 1q21.2).[11–13] The *LMNA* gene codes for at least four isoforms, of which only the lamin A isoform is associated with mammalian disease.[14,15] The lamin proteins are the principal proteins of the nuclear lamina; a structure located inside the inner nuclear membrane.[16] Lamin A, like all lamin molecules, contains an N-terminal head domain, a coiled-coil a-helical rod domain, and a carboxy terminal tail domain[17] (Figure 11-2). It is derived from a larger molecule, prelamin A, which undergoes multistep proteolytic processing, which includes the addition and then cleavage of a farnesyl group to become mature lamin A.[18–20] The loss of the farnesyl anchor presumably releases prelamin from the nuclear membrane, rendering it free to participate in the multiprotein nuclear scaffold complex just internal to the nuclear membrane, affecting nuclear structure and function.[19] The integrity of the lamina is crucial to many cellular functions, including mitosis, creating and maintaining structural integrity of the nuclear scaffold, DNA replication, RNA transcription, organization of the nucleus, nuclear pore assembly, chromatin function, cell cycling, and apoptosis.

MUTATIONS IN *LMNA* CAUSE HGPS

HGPS is almost always a sporadic autosomal dominant disease, with only one proven case of mosaicism.[21] Ninety percent of HGPS patients have a single C to T transition at nucleotide 1824, which activates a cryptic splice site[22–24] (Figure 11-2). Translation followed by posttranslational processing of this altered mRNA produces a shortened abnormal protein with a 50 amino acid deletion near its C-terminal end, henceforth called "progerin." The 50 amino acid deletion does not affect the ability of progerin to localize to the nucleus or to dimerize because the necessary components for these functions are not deleted.[19] Importantly, however, it does remove the recognition site that leads to proteolytic cleavage of the terminal 18 amino acids of prelamin A (see Figure 11-2), along with the phosphorylation site(s) involved in the dissociation and reassociation of the nuclear membrane at each cell division.[18,19]

The multisystem and primarily postnatal disease manifestation in HGPS is not surprising, since lamin A is normally expressed by most differentiated cells, preserving function in undifferentiated cells that dominate fetal development.[16] Lamin A expression is developmentally regulated and displays cell and tissue specificity, primarily in differentiated cells including fibroblasts, vascular smooth muscle cells, and vascular endothelial cells.[14,25,26] Although the alternate splicing in HGPS leads to decreased levels of lamin A, this does not seem to affect cell function at all. In fact, a mouse model entirely lacking lamin A shows no signs of disease.[27] HGPS is therefore a *dominant negative* disease; it is the action of progerin, not the diminution of lamin A, that causes the disease phenotype.

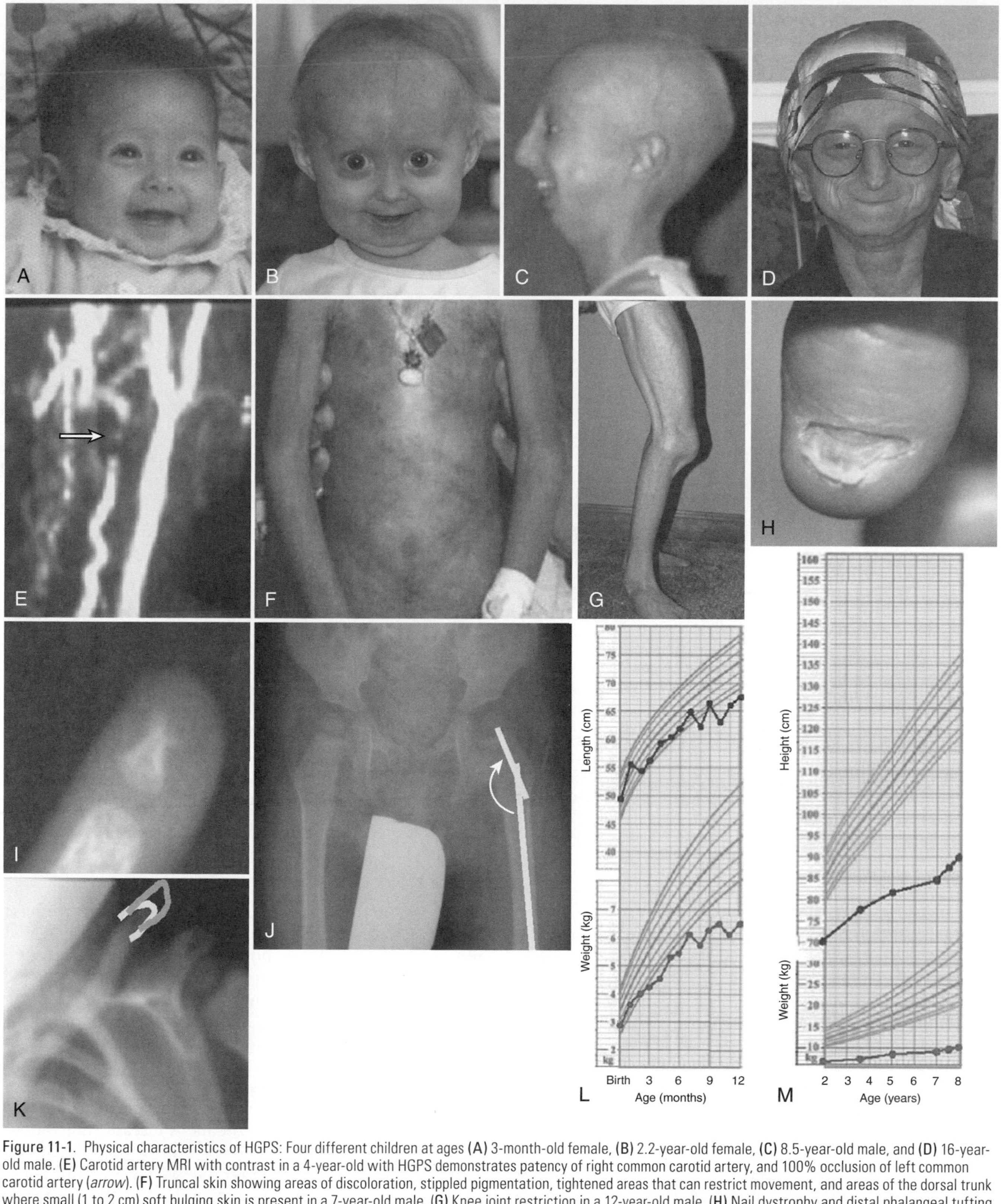

Figure 11-1. Physical characteristics of HGPS: Four different children at ages **(A)** 3-month-old female, **(B)** 2.2-year-old female, **(C)** 8.5-year-old male, and **(D)** 16-year-old male. **(E)** Carotid artery MRI with contrast in a 4-year-old with HGPS demonstrates patency of right common carotid artery, and 100% occlusion of left common carotid artery (*arrow*). **(F)** Truncal skin showing areas of discoloration, stippled pigmentation, tightened areas that can restrict movement, and areas of the dorsal trunk where small (1 to 2 cm) soft bulging skin is present in a 7-year-old male. **(G)** Knee joint restriction in a 12-year-old male. **(H)** Nail dystrophy and distal phalangeal tufting in a 10-year-old male. Typical x-ray findings: **(I)** acro-osteolysis of the distal phalange, **(J)** clavicular shortening, **(K)** coxa valga. Growth characteristics showing normal birth weight and length, followed by failure to thrive. Average length (blue) and weight (black) for age for 10 females during **(L)** birth to 12 months and **(M)** 2 to 8 years. Standard deviation less than 6% for each data point. Data for males is not significantly different from those of females ($p < 0.05$) (data not shown). *(Photos courtesy from The Progeria Research Foundation. Data courtesy from the PRF Medical and Research Database. Growth charts adapted from those developed by the National Center for Health Statistics in collaboration with the National Center for Chronic Disease and Health Promotion, published May 30, 2000,* www.cdc.gov/growthcharts.)

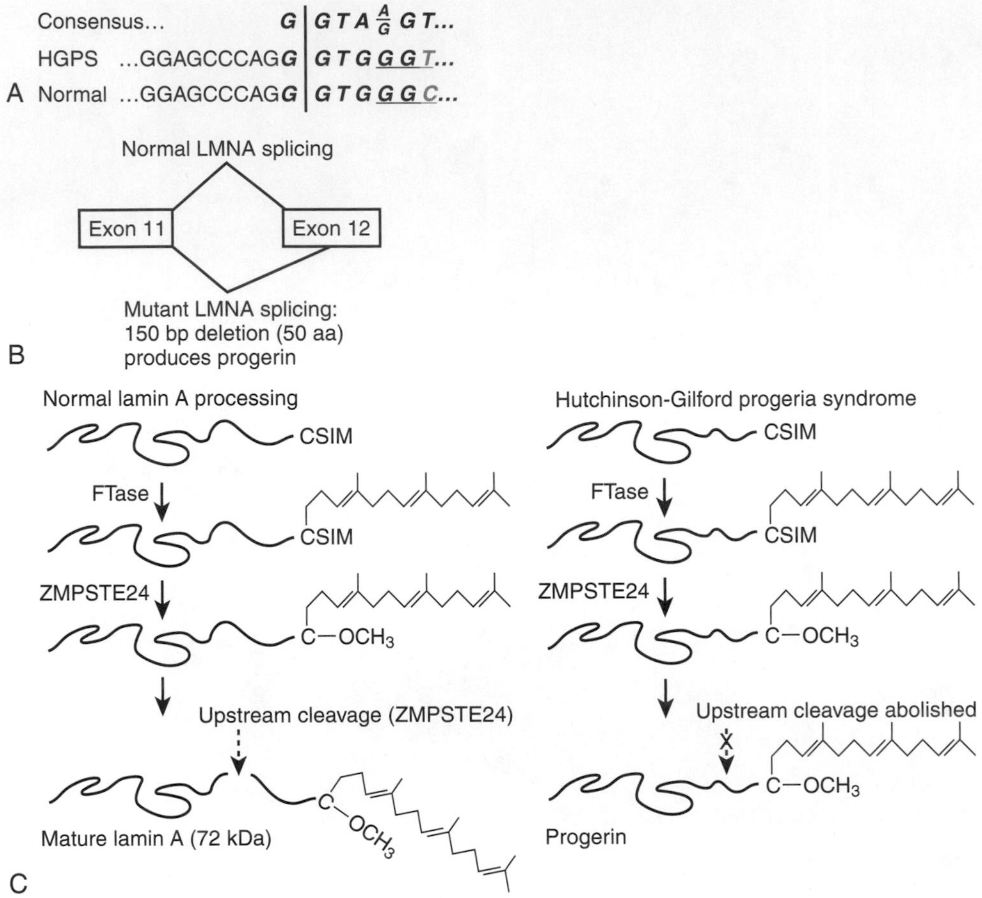

Figure 11-2. Abnormal splicing in HGPS and normal *LMNA*. (**A**) Sequences in bold and italics represent potential splice donor sequence. Partial DNA sequence for ideal consensus splice donor sequence (seven bases, *Top line*), which shares six of seven bases with HGPS (*Middle line*), and five of seven bases with normal *LMNA* (*Bottom line*). Codes for glycine are underlined. Mutant transition (C to T) in red. Vertical red line represents splice point used variably in HGPS, and in normal cells (less frequently). (**B**) Representation for mutant splicing that results in 50 amino acid deletion from lamin A, thus creating progerin. (**C**) Translation of the *LMNA* gene yields the prelamin A protein, which requires posttranslational processing for incorporation into the nuclear lamina. The prelamin A protein has the amino acids CSIM at the C terminus. This comprises a CAAX motif (where C is cysteine, A is an aliphatic amino acid, and X is any amino acid), which signals for isoprenylation (in this case, the addition of a farnesyl group to the cysteine by the enzyme farnesyltransferase [FTase]). After farnesylation, the terminal three amino acids (SIM) are cleaved by the ZMPSTE24 endoprotease, and the terminal farnesylated cysteine undergoes carboxymethylation. A second cleavage step by ZMPSTE24 then removes the terminal 15 amino acids, including the farnesyl group. This final cleavage step is blocked in Hutchinson-Gilford progeria syndrome. *(Copyright 2006. Nature Reviews Genetics.)*

FARNESYLATION AND HGPS

A key to disease in HGPS is the presumably persistent farnesylation of progerin,[24] which renders it permanently intercalated into the inner nuclear membrane, where it can accumulate and exert progressively more damage to cells as they age. That the failure to remove the farnesyl group is at least in part responsible for the phenotypes observed in HGPS is strongly supported by studies on both cell and mouse models, which have either been engineered to produce a nonfarnesylated progerin product, or treated with a drug that inhibits farnesylation, rendering a nonfarnesylated progerin product. Drugs tested include farnesyltransferase inhibitors, statins, and nitrogen-containing *bis*-phosphonates, all of which work at different points along the pathway leading to farnesylation of the abnormal lamin A proteins produced in progeria.[28] By preventing the initial attachment of the farnesyl group to newly synthesized preprogerin molecules, progerin is thought to be unable to effect its aberrant function at the inner nuclear membrane. In many in vitro and mouse model studies, some or all of the phenotypes of HGPS were reversed toward normal. This included reversing vascular disease in an HGPS mouse model that mimics progressive arteriosclerosis,[29] increased life span by 50%, fewer bone breaks, and increased size using farnesyltransferase inhibitor (FTI),[30] and increasing life span by 80%, improved growth, hair, and bone breakage in a ZMPSte24 –/– model.[31]

Aging and HGPS

HGPS is described as a "segmental" premature aging syndrome because it shares some phenotypes with normal aging, but not all. Cancer, Alzheimer's disease, and various other sequelae of aging are not present in HGPS. Clinical characteristics common to both, but accelerated in HGPS, include progressive vascular disease, bone loss (osteopenia or osteoporosis), loss of subcutaneous fat (lipoatrophy), and hair loss. A number of laminopathies have both progeroid and nonprogeroid phenotypes, but HGPS is the best studied for its commonalities with aging, senescence, and arteriosclerosis.[28]

HGPS and aging share a variety of cellular elements key to aging at the cellular level, including decreased resistance to oxidative stress, increased DNA damage, and decreased ability to repair that damage; abnormal nuclear shape (blebbing) (Figure 11-3; see also color plate 11-3); decreased resilience in response to mechanical strain; and a host of signaling pathways that change with senescence and age, including the Notch pathway.[32] Perhaps our most exciting new clue to the aging process is the presence of progerin protein at increasing concentrations as both HGPS and normal cells age.

Normal fibroblasts senesce, but HGPS fibroblasts senesce more rapidly (i.e., usually within 15 passages[33]). Oxidative stress, in the form of superoxide radicals and hydrogen peroxide, has been found to induce senescence and apoptosis and is implicated in the cause of atherosclerosis[34] and normal aging.[35,36] Antioxidants such as superoxide dismutase, catalase, and glutathione peroxidase help eliminate superoxide radicals and hydrogen peroxide. Yan et al[37] demonstrated significantly decreased glutathione peroxidase, magnesium superoxide dismutase, and catalase levels in HGPS fibroblast cultures compared with normal control cultures. Normal cellular senescence is also marked by increasing rates of DNA damage and a decline in the ability to repair this damage.[38] Progeria cells accumulate double stranded DNA (dsDNA) breaks and impaired DNA repair[39–41] Aberrant nuclear shape (called blebbing or lobulation) occurs in normal fibroblasts undergoing apoptosis as an antecedent to apoptosis and senescence[16] (see Figure 11-3; see also color plate 11-3). A consistent phenotype in HGPS cells is the same aberrant shape of their nuclei, which is readily detected following staining with antilamin antibodies.[16,24] The blebbing is a structural sign of cellular decline in both normal and HGPS cell cultures. Another structural weakening associated with aging cells, development of cardiovascular disease, and HGPS is the response to mechanotransduction (applied force).[42,43] When strain is applied to early passage wild-type fibroblast nuclei, they remain stiff.[44] Although progeria fibroblasts show normal rigidity at early passages (when progerin levels and nuclear blebbing are at a minimum), late passage nuclei show dramatically *increased* rigidity over wild-type fibroblasts. In addition, whereas wild-type cells enter S phase and G2 phase in response to mechanical stretch, HGPS cells do not proliferate in response to stretch. Microarray studies have revealed significant overlap between cell signaling in senescing cells and HGPS fibroblasts as compared with early passage normal cells.[45–47] The Notch regulatory pathway in particular stands out because Notch is important for maintenance of stem cells (including mesenchymal stem cells), differentiation pathways, and cell death. Significantly, both HGPS cells and non-progeria cells induced to produce progerin display up-regulation of three genes in the Notch pathway: Hes 3, Hes 4, Hey 1.

The discovery that progeria is caused by a mutation in lamin A, which had not previously been implicated in mechanisms of aging, brought in an entirely new question: Are defects in lamin A implicated in normal aging? The first positive evidence was reported by Scaffidi et al in 2006,[49] who showed that cell nuclei from normal individuals have acquired similar defects as progeria patients, including changes in histone modifications and increased DNA damage. Younger cells

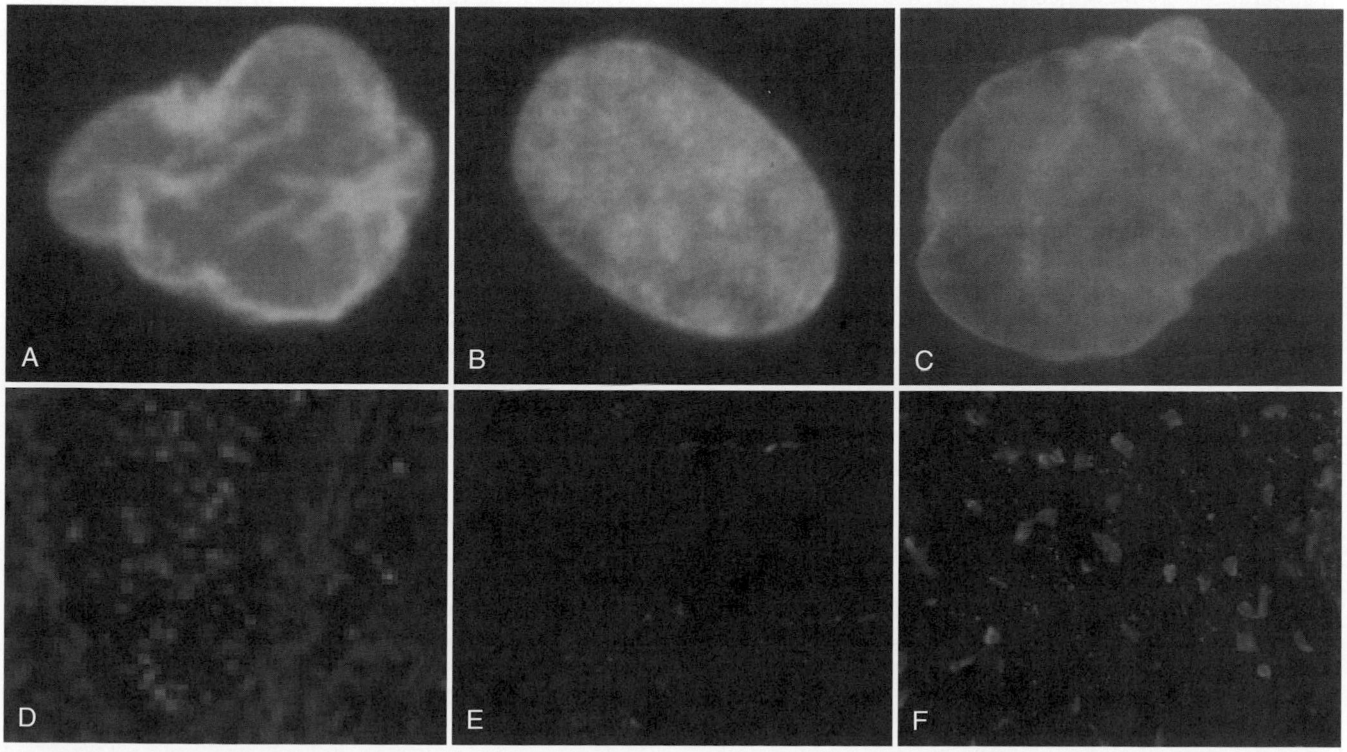

Figure 11-3. Nuclear blebbing and presence of progerin in HGPS and aging. Fibroblast nuclei stained with antilamin antibody (A) passage 4 HGPS, (B) passage 10 normal, (C) passage 40 normal; skin biopsies stained with antiprogerin antibody and shown here at 40× for (D) HGPS donor age 10 years old; (E) normal newborn, (F) normal, donor age 90 years old.

show considerably less of these defects. They further demonstrated that the age-related effects are the result of the production of low levels of preprogerin mRNA produced by activation of the same cryptic splice site that functions at much higher levels in progeria, and is reversed by inhibition of transcription at this splice site. Cao et al,[50] studying the same phenomenon, showed that among interphase cells in fibroblast cultures, only a small fraction of the cells contained progerin. The percentage of progerin-positive cells increased with passage number, suggesting a link to normal aging. Notably, McClintock et al found progerin in skin biopsies of older donors, while young donors had no detectable progerin. This is the first human in vivo demonstration of a buildup of progerin with normal aging[51] (see Figure 11-3; see also color plate 11-3). The newly discovered relationship between HGPS and lamin A has opened the doors of scientific exploration into how lamins play a role in heart disease and aging in the general population. Scaffidi et al[49] have shown that normal fibroblasts also produce some progerin by using this same splice site to a lesser degree than do HGPS fibroblasts.

A key element when considering treatment for HGPS, or for arteriosclerosis and normal aging, is progerin's dosage effect. In HGPS, the nonmutated *LMNA* gene splices normally produce full length lamin A, and only rarely uses the cryptic splice site to produce progerin. The other (mutated) *LMNA* gene produces both progerin in substantial amounts and a minor amount of lamin A. Reddel and Weiss showed that the mutant allele in cultured HGPS fibroblasts uses the cryptic splice site 84.5% of the time.[52] Different individuals may produce more or less progerin, and within an individual, different cell types may produce varying amounts of progerin versus normal lamin A. In normal fibroblast cells in culture, the cryptic splice site is used about fiftyfold less as compared with HGPS fibroblasts. However, because progerin protein accumulates with increasing age in skin biopsies[51] (see Figure 11-3; see also color plate 11-3) and in vitro with increasing passage number,[16] the influence of progerin on health in the general population probably also increases as we age. Clinical support for the dosage effect hypothesis is found in the study of a 45-year-old man with a progeroid laminopathy, whose mutation in T623S produced a cryptic splice site abnormality in *LMNA*, but the splice site was used 80% less frequently than in classic HGPS.[53] His phenotype mimicked HGPS, but to a milder degree. Therefore we can assume that decreasing the levels of progerin by a relatively modest percentage will significantly ameliorate disease. In addition, it is highly possible that one component of genetic predisposition to atherosclerosis lies in the amount of progerin that an individual accumulates in his or her lifetime.

OVERLAP BETWEEN HGPS AND ARTERIOSCLEROSIS OF AGING

Individuals with HGPS develop premature severe arteriosclerosis in childhood and frequently succumb to resulting heart attacks or strokes in the second decade of life.[1,54] Hypertension, angina, cardiomegaly, and congestive heart failure are common end-stage events.[55–58] The disease progression of progeria blood vessels does not fit the typical atherosclerotic description, which includes intima-media thickening, atherosclerotic plaque (rich lipid core) with ruptured cap and superimposed thrombosis, inflammation and endothelial destruction, and proliferating medial smooth muscle cells. In HGPS, intima-media thickness of the carotid artery is normal,[59] as are cholesterol, low-density lipoprotein (LDL), and high sensitivity C-reactive protein levels—all factors in chronic lipid-driven inflammation of atherosclerosis.[60]

Instead, the HGPS vascular phenotype resembles an arteriosclerosis, which is characterized by hardening of the vessels (decreased compliance) in medium and large vessels, and affects millions of aging individuals. Meredith et al, studying a cohort of 15 patients with HGPS, found that younger children displayed normal vascular compliance but that, with age, compliance decreased, and in a number of children this led to left atrial enlargement.[59] Blood pressure and heart rate were in the normal range in younger children, whereas the older children had increasing blood pressures and variable heart rates. Electrocardiograms were normal in most, although a few had long Q-T intervals suggesting fibrosis of the conduction system.

Gordon et al[60] found serum levels of cholesterol, triglyceride (TG), LDL, and C-reactive protein (a mediator of inflammation) within normal limits in 19 patients, but showed decreasing high-density (HDL) and adiponectin (a secretory product of adipose tissue) with increasing age in HGPS. In fact, adiponectin values exhibited a strong positive correlation with HDL values in progeria children. Declines in HDL and adiponectin have been implicated in other lipodystrophic syndromes and lipodystrophy associated with type 2 diabetes.[61–65] Adiponectin is emerging as an independent cardiovascular risk factor, which may directly regulate endothelial function[61–65] and which also correlates with HDL in type 2 diabetes.[66]

The fewer than 20 autopsies on children with HGPS have revealed focal plaque throughout large and small arteries, including all coronary artery branches.[1,57,58,67–70] The plaque is markedly calcified and contains cholesterol crystals and a nearly acellular hyaline fibrosis. Vessel cross-sections at autopsy of one 22-year-old woman with clinical features of HGPS revealed no indication of vasculature inflammation.[54] The vascular media no longer contained smooth muscle cells and the elastic structure was destroyed and replaced with extracellular matrix or fibrosis, with profound adventitial thickening and a depleted media. Presumably the primary loss of smooth muscle cells initiates vascular remodeling by secondary replacement with matrix in large and small vasculature.

Apoptosis occurs in vascular smooth muscle cells before the development of calcification,[71] and may even be required for calcification to occur. Since vascular calcification is a requisite event in plaque formation,[72] apoptosis may be a key element in the development of disease in HGPS and arteriosclerosis.[33,42,73]

HGPS is a disease involving abnormalities in the extracellular matrix, with increased collagen and elastin secretion, disorganized dermal collagen, decreased decorin, and increased aggrecan and ankyrin G compared with normal controls.[45,47,74–77] Extracellular matrix molecules have both structural and cell signaling functions in skin, bone, and the cardiovascular system,[78–84] all of which are severely affected in HGPS. In pathologic and clinical studies, mesoderm-derived tissues and their extracellular matrices are targets of principal defects. Gene expression studies of HGPS fibroblasts are consistent with these findings.[46,85] Aneurysms, noted in several cases of HGPS,[10,67,70] derive from medial necrosis, which could reflect either a connective tissue problem and concurrent death of smooth muscle cells.

In summary, the study of HGPS has provided a completely new molecule, progerin, which may play an integral role in general vascular biology and health. The progeria vasculature is characterized by global stiffness, tortuosity, and a loss of smooth muscle cells in the media with subsequent extracellular replacement. Biochemical abnormalities include progressively decreasing HDL and adiponectin. Smooth muscle cell dropout is unique to progeria, whereas global stiffness and tortuosity, decreased HDL, and adiponectin are observed in arteriosclerosis and type 2 diabetes in the normal aging population. Although progerin was found in arterioles of an HGPS patient,[25] future studies in this young field will need to assess for the presence of progerin in non-HGPS vasculature, and its potentially causal relationship to cardiovascular disease with aging.

Clinical care

DIAGNOSTICS AND GENETIC COUNSELING

Initial indications for HGPS include failure to thrive, skin signs, stiffened joints, delayed dentition, gradual hair loss, and subcutaneous loss of fat with normal developmental milestones. Average age at diagnosis is 2 years (see www.genetests.org). The Progeria Research Foundation (www.progeriaresearch.org) is the only patient advocate organization worldwide that is solely dedicated to discovering the cause, treatments, and cure for progeria. The organization provides services for families and children with progeria, such as patient education and communication with other progeria families. It serves as a resource for physicians and medical caretakers of these families via clinical care recommendations, a diagnostics facility, a clinical and research database, and funding for basic science and clinical research in progeria.

CARDIAC CARE AND LOW-DOSE ASPIRIN

Children with HGPS are at high risk for heart attacks and strokes at any age. The earliest published incidence of stroke is at the age of 4 years.[59] In one case, seizures were the presenting cerebrovascular event.[10] Importantly, stroke (cerebral infarction) may occur while the child exhibits a normal EKG and may be caused by occlusion of a small cerebral vessel in the absence of large-vessel intracranial blockages.[86]

Studies in adults have shown that the benefits of low-dose aspirin therapy increase with increasing cardiovascular risk.[87,88] Recommendations here are extrapolated from this evidence in adults. *Low-dose aspirin should be considered for all children with HGPS at any age*, regardless of whether the child has exhibited overt cardiovascular abnormalities or abnormal lipid profiles. Low-dose aspirin may help to prevent atherothrombotic events, including transient ischemic attacks (TIA), stroke, and heart attacks, by inhibiting platelet aggregation. Dosage is determined by patient weight, and should be 2 to 3 mg/kg given once daily or every other day. This dosage will inhibit platelet aggregation but will not inhibit prostacyclin activity.

Once a child begins to develop signs or symptoms of vascular decline, such as hypertension, TIA, strokes, seizures, angina, dyspnea on exertion, EKG changes, echocardiogram changes, or heart attacks, a higher level of intervention is warranted. Antihypertensive medication, anticoagulants, antiseizure and other medications usually administered to adults with similar medical issues have been given to children with HGPS. All medication should be dosed according to weight, and carefully adjusted according to accompanying toxicity and efficacy.

INTUBATION

Intubation is difficult in the child with progeria due to the small oral aperture with retrognathia, little flexion or extension in the cervical spine, relatively large epiglottis, and small glottic opening. Nasal fiberoptic may be difficult to place because of an unusual glottic angle. Intubation with direct visualization is recommended because glottic angle may make fiberoptic intubation difficult. For nonoral procedures, mask ventilation, or laryngeal mask airway is recommended over intubation.

PHYSICAL THERAPY (PT) AND OCCUPATIONAL THERAPY (OT)

Children with progeria need PT and OT as often as possible (optimally two to three times each per week) to ensure maximum range of motion and optimal daily functioning throughout their lives. The role of PT and OT is to maintain range of motion, strength, and functional status. Proactive PT and OT are important since all children with progeria develop restrictions in range of motion in a progressive manner (see Figure 11-1). Bony abnormalities are almost always evident in x-rays by the age of 2 years.[89–93] Range of motion may be restricted because of progressive joint contractures, primarily in the knees, ankles, and fingers as a result of tendinous abnormalities; hip abnormalities due primarily to progressive coxa valga; and shoulder restrictions due to clavicular resorption. Tightened skin can also restrict range of

KEY POINTS

The Premature Aging Syndrome Hutchinson-Gilford Progeria

- HGPS is a rare segmental premature aging syndrome in which children die of heart attacks or strokes between ages 7 and 20 years.
- HGPS is an autosomal dominant disease caused by a single base mutation in *LMNA*, leading to a silent mutation that creates a cryptic splice site.
- Lamin A is an inner nuclear membrane protein that is central to cellular structure and function, primarily in differentiated cells.
- The abnormal lamin A protein produced in HGPS, called progerin, is not only generated in HGPS, but is also generated to a lesser extent in the normal population.
- Cardiovascular disease in HGPS resembles arteriosclerosis of aging, with hypertension, vascular stiffening, vessel wall remodeling with abnormal extracellular matrix, plaque formation in the face of normal cholesterol levels, and finally stroke and heart attacks.
- Progerin accumulates with increased age and is likely associated with cellular aging and vascular disease in the general population.
- Preclinical studies show that preventing farnesylation of progerin improves disease phenotype both in cell culture and in mouse models, including reversal of vascular disease.

motion. Skin tightening can be almost absent in some children, or can be severe and restrict chest wall motion and gastric capacity in others.

Each regimen should be tailored to the child's individual needs, and tailored according to cardiac status in consultation with the child's physician. Any child who develops dyspnea (shortness of breath), angina (chest pain), or cyanosis (blue discoloration of lips and skin) during exertion should stop immediately. If symptoms do not rapidly resolve, the child should receive emergency medical care. If oxygen is available, it should be administered. Therapy personnel should be trained in cardiopulmonary resuscitation and have access to an automated external defibrillator with pediatric capability.

Common protocols for PT and OT include but are not limited to the following: Tracking progress through regular joint range of motion measurements is advised at least every 3 to 4 months. Due to the orthopedic conditions commonly seen in the hip and shoulder, range of motion in these joints should be closely monitored. Tightness is also seen in the heel cords, low back muscles, finger flexors, and triceps muscles. To maintain range of motion, a combination of myofascial release techniques followed by more traditional passive, active, and active-assisted stretching exercises are effective. Due to the possibility of weakened joint integrity due to coxa valga in the hips and clavicular resorption in the shoulders, it is advisable to avoid passive stretching in these joints and instead focus on active stretching. Weight-bearing activities in hands and knees are helpful for stretching finger flexors. To help maintain range of motion, traditional stretching can be followed by functional activities. Strengthening activities should target core strengthening for the hips and abdominals with activities such as sit-ups, bridges, and leg lifts. Due to orthopedic deformities, tendinous, and muscular and skin tightness, gait deviations often occur. It is advisable to focus on maintaining heel cord flexibility and hip internal rotation to minimize gait deviations.

ACKNOWLEDGMENT

I wish to gratefully acknowledge the children with progeria and their families, for participation in progeria research. Thank you to Frank Rothman, PhD, for review of the chapter and helpful suggestions.

For a complete list of references, please visit online only at www.expertconsult.com

CHAPTER 12

Connective Tissues and Aging

Nicholas A. Kefalides
Zahra Ziaie

Aging is a continuous process that constitutes a cycle studded with events that affect all systems in the body, including the connective tissues. The interrelationship between the aging process and connective tissues is complex, involving a variety of factors and interactions acting in a reciprocal fashion. One could inquire into the effects of aging on connective tissues and, conversely, one may ask how the components of connective tissue contribute to the aging process. To answer these questions, it is important to have some understanding of the structural biochemistry of connective tissues, some knowledge of the processes involved in their biosynthesis, modification, extracellular organization, and molecular genetics, and the factors affecting the properties of connective tissue cells and the extracellular matrix (ECM). In the period since the last edition, new data became available which highlight the progress made in the area of the mechanisms responsible for the alterations in connective tissue components in diseases associated with aging. Armed with this knowledge, it becomes apparent that there can be a huge number of events in the development of connective tissues that may be associated, directly or indirectly, with the processes or effects of aging. These have been and continue to be areas of intensive research.

This chapter presents an abbreviated discussion of the various components of the ECM, their structure, molecular organization, biosynthesis, modification, turnover, and molecular genetics. It discusses some concepts on the effects of aging on the ECM and the effects of aging on the properties of various connective tissues and the involvement of connective tissue physiology on diseases associated with aging.

THE PROPERTIES OF CONNECTIVE TISSUES

The properties of connective tissues are derived primarily from the properties of the components of the ECM surrounding, and secreted by, the cells of those tissues. Some connective tissues, such as cartilage or tendons, may be composed primarily of a single-cell type e.g., chondrocytes or fibroblasts), whose synthesis and secretion of ECM and other factors largely determine the properties of the tissue. Some tissues, such as bone, blood vessels, and skin, contain a number of different connective tissue cell types (e.g., osteoblasts and osteoclasts) in bone, endothelial, and smooth muscle cells in blood vessels, and fibroblasts and epithelial cells in skin, which contribute to both their structural and functional properties. Other tissues, such as cardiac muscle and kidney, may have properties dependent upon connective tissue components whose biologic roles are separate from the major physiologic function of the tissue and which may have influence over the properties of that tissue during the process of aging. Different cell types will exhibit different phenotypic patterns of ECM production, which in turn will influence the structural properties of a given connective tissue.

The major components of the ECM fall into three general classes of molecules: (1) the structural proteins, which include the collagens (of which there are now 28 types recognized) and elastin; (2) the proteoglycans, which contain several structurally distinct molecular classes, such as heparan sulfate and dermatan sulfate; and (3) the structural glycoproteins, exemplified by fibronectin (FN) and laminin (LM), whose contribution to the properties of connective tissues has been recognized only within the past 35 to 40 years. The interactions among these materials determine the development and properties of the connective tissues.

The collagens

STRUCTURE

The collagens are a family of connective tissue proteins having a triple-stranded organization and containing molecular domains within which the strands are coiled around one another in a triple helix. The reader is referred to two recent reviews on collagen biochemistry.[1,2]

The genes of at least 28 distinct collagen types have been characterized.[3] The interstitial collagens—types I, II, III, and V—exist as large, extended molecules that tend to organize into fibrils.[1] There may be more than one collagen type within these fibrils.[4] Type IV collagen, also known as *basement membrane (BM) collagen*, does not exist in fibrillar form, but rather in a complex network of collagen molecules linked by disulfide and other cross-linkages and associated with noncollagenous molecules, such as LM, entactin, and proteoglycans, to form an amorphous matrix.[5,6] Although at least 28 collagen types are recognized, the protein of only the first 11 collagens has been isolated from tissues.

There are 46 genes corresponding to the α chains of 28 collagen types.[3] Collagen type I is the most abundant collagen and the most abundant protein in the body. The basic unit of the type I collagen fibril is a triple helical heterotrimer, tropocollagen, consisting of two identical chains, termed α1(I), and a third chain, α2(I).[1] The other collagen types have been given similar designations; however, some of the types are homotrimers containing three identical chains and some contain three genetically distinct α chains.

The collagen α chain has a unique amino acid composition with glycine occupying every third position in the sequence. Thus the collagenous domains consist of a repeating peptide triplet, -Gly-X-Y-, in which X and Y are amino acids other than glycine. A large percentage of amino acids in the Y position is occupied by proline. In addition, collagen contains two unique amino acids derived from posttranslational modifications of the protein, 4- and 3-hydroxyproline and hydroxylysine. The presence of 4-hydroxyproline provides additional sites along the α chain capable of forming hydrogen bonds with adjacent α chains, which are important in stabilizing the triple helix so that it maintains its structure at body temperatures. If hydroxyproline formation is inhibited, the triple helix dissociates into its component α chains at 37° C.

The presence of glycine in every third position, along with the extensive hydrogen bonding, provides the triple helix with a compact protected structure resistant to the action of most proteases. The α chains of the collagen superfamily are encoded with information that specifies self-assembly into fibrils, microfibrils, and networks that have diverse functions in the ECM.[6] The structures of collagens can be stabilized further through the formation of covalent cross-linkages derived from modification and condensation of certain lysine and hydroxylysine residues on adjacent α chains.[2] Cross-linkage formation is important in stabilizing collagen fibrils and contributes to their high tensile strength.

BIOSYNTHESIS[7]

Type I collagen α chains are synthesized as a larger precursor, procollagen, containing noncollagenous sequences at their C and N termini. As each pro-α chain is synthesized, intracellular prolyl and lysyl hydroxylases act to form hydroxyproline and hydroxylysine. The triple helix is formed intracellularly and stabilized by the formation of interchain disulfide bonds near the carboxyl termini of the component pro-α chains. After secretion of the triple helical collagen, procollagen peptidases remove most of the noncollagenous portions at each end of the procollagen. Extracellular lysine and hydroxylysine oxidases oxidize the amino groups of lysine or hydroxylysine to form aldehyde derivatives, which can go on to form Schiff base adducts, the first cross-linkages. These can rearrange and become reduced to form the various other cross-linkages. Increased numbers of collagen cross-linkages have been reported in a pathologic state known as scleroderma.

DEGRADATION OF CONNECTIVE TISSUE COMPONENTS

The role played by matrix metalloproteinases (MMPs) in connective tissue turnover has gained prominence in the past 35 years as information on the mechanisms by which MMPs mediated synovial joint inflammation and ECM turnover in arthritides became available.[8] Extracellular degradation of collagen is accomplished by enzymes known as tissue collagenases. These enzymes cleave triple helical collagen at a site three quarters from the amino acid terminus, resulting in the formation of two triple helical fragments (225 nm plus 75 nm respectively), which denature at temperatures above 32° C to form nonhelical peptides that can be degraded by tissue proteinases. Cleavage by tissue collagenase is considered to be the rate-limiting step in collagenolysis of triple helical collagen. Collagenolysis is the subject of reviews by Kleiner and Stetler-Stevenson[9] and Tayebjee et al.[10]

Collagenolysis is an important physiologic process responsible to a large extent for the repair of wounds and processes of tissue remodeling in which undesired accumulations are removed as new connective tissue is laid down. However, in conditions such as rheumatoid arthritis, osteoporosis (OS), and aging, the production of collagenases may be stimulated, resulting in an elevated degradation of synovial tissue or bone.

Degradation of elastin by elastases—belonging to a family of serine—metalloproteinases, or cysteine proteinases, gives rise to the generation of elastin fragments, designated as elastokines.[11]

Tissue collagenases are secreted by connective tissue cells as a precursor, procollagenase, which must be activated to become enzymatically active. This can be achieved in vitro by the action of trypsin on the latent enzyme. Other proteinases, including lysosomal cathepsin B, plasmin, mast cell proteinase, and plasma kallikrein, also can activate latent collagenases. Thus inflammatory cells can secrete factors that lead to collagenase activation, accounting for the inflammatory sequelae of the arthritides. Collagenases are also under the influence of plasma inhibitors, of which α2 macroglobulin accounts for most of the inhibitory process. In addition, inhibitors of plasminogen activation can indirectly prevent the activation of procollagenases by plasmin. Fibroblasts and other connective tissue cells also secrete inhibitors of collagenases, suggesting a complex system of extracellular control of collagenolysis.[9,10]

Elastin

The biochemistry and molecular biology of elastin have been subjects of excellent reviews.[12,13] As in interstitial collagens, glycine makes up about one third of the amino acid content of elastin. Unlike collagen, however, glycine is not present in every third position. In addition, elastin is an exceedingly hydrophobic protein, with a large content of valine, leucine, and isoleucine.

Elastin is synthesized as a precursor molecule, tropoelastin, with a molecular weight of about 70 kDa. However, in tissues, elastin is found as an amorphous, macromolecular network. This is due to the condensation of tropoelastin molecules through the formation of covalent cross-linkages unique to elastin. These cross-linkages arise through the condensation of four lysine residues on different tropoelastin molecules to form the cross-linking amino acids, desmosine and isodesmosine, characteristic of tissue elastin. The reader is referred to reviews by Bailey et al[2] and Wagenseil and Mecham[13] for discussions of the details of collagen and elastin cross-linking.

The hydrophobicity, together with the formation of cross-linkages, endow elastin with its elastic properties and an extreme insolubility and amorphous structure. Elastin accounts for most of the elastic properties of skin, arteries, ligaments, and the lungs. The presence of elastin has been demonstrated in other organs, such as the eye and the kidney. In most tissues, elastin is found in association with microfibrils, which contain several glycoproteins, including fibrillin. Microfibrils have been identified in many tissues, and the importance of their assemblies as determinants of connective tissue architecture has been brought into focus by the identification of mutations in fibrillin in the heritable connective tissue disorder Marfan syndrome.[14]

An elegant review summarizes the current knowledge of the structure of the elastin gene, including consideration of the heterogeneity observed in immature mRNA as a result of alternative splicing in the primary transcript.[15] Analysis of the bovine and human elastin genes revealed the separation of those exons coding for distinct hydrophobic and cross-linking domains. Comparison of the cDNA, genomic sequences, and S1 analyses demonstrated that the primary transcript of both species is subject to considerable alternative splicing. It is likely that this accounts for the presence of multiple tropoelastins found in several species. It is suggested that the differences in alternative splicing may be correlated with aging.[15]

The proteoglycans

Proteoglycans are characterized by the presence of highly negatively charged, polymeric chains (glycosaminoglycans or "GAGs") of repeating disaccharide units covalently attached to a "core" protein. The disaccharide units comprise an *N*-conjugated amino sugar, either glucosamine or galactosamine, and a uronic acid, usually D-glucuronic acid or—in the instances of dermatan sulfate, heparan sulfate, and heparin—L-iduronic acid. In cartilage and in the cornea, another GAG, keratan sulfate, containing D-glucose instead of a uronic acid has been demonstrated. The amino group of the hexosamine component is usually acetylated and the GAGs are usually O-sulfated in hexosamine residues with some *N*-sulfation, instead of acetylation, in the instances of heparan sulfate and heparin. Depending on the source and type of proteoglycan, the number of GAGs attached to the core protein can vary from three or four all the way up into the twenties, with each GAG having a molecular size in the tens of thousands of daltons. In addition, as in the case of the cartilage proteoglycans, there may be more than one type of GAG attached to the core protein. In cartilage, several proteoglycan molecules may be associated with another very large GAG, hyaluronic acid, consisting of disaccharide units of glucuronyl *N*-acetylglucosamine. The compositional structure of the GAGs is summarized in Table 12-1.

The overall effect of these structures is the creation of huge, negatively charged highly hydrophobic complexes. The hydration and charge properties of these complexes cause them to become highly extended, occupying a hydrodynamic volume in the tissue much larger than would be predicted from their chemical composition. In the instance of synovial cartilage, it is suggested that the hydration endows the tissue with shock-absorbing properties in which applied pressure to the joint is counteracted by the extrusion of water from the complex, forcing a compression of the negative charges within the molecule. Upon the release of pressure, the electronegative repulsive forces drive the charges apart with a concomitant influx of water to restore the initial hydrated state. The metachromatic staining properties of connective tissues are due mainly to their proteoglycan content. Several excellent reviews of proteoglycan biochemistry have already been written.[16–18]

In recent years, several proteoglycans have been identified in the pericellular environment, either associated with cell surfaces or interacting with ECM components such as interstitial collagens, FN, and TGF-ß. Current reviews by Groffen et al[16] and Schaefer and Iozzo[17] describe the structures of the protein cores, their gene organization, their functional characteristics, and tissue distribution. Several of the proteoglycans described by Schaefer and Iozzo on the list constitute a group of small leucine-rich proteoglycans (SLRP). Notable among them are decorin[18] and perlecan.[19] They are multidomain assemblies of protein motifs with relatively elongated and highly glycosylated structures having several protein domains shared with other proteins. In their review, Groffen et al[16] discuss the role of perlecan as a crucial determinant of glomerular BM permselectivity and suggest that the additional presence of agrin, another heparan sulfate proteoglycan species, makes the latter an important contributor to glomerular function.

Lumican, one of the leucine-rich proteoglycans, is found in relative abundance in articular cartilage,[18] which, along with its size, varies with age. In adult cartilage extracts, it exhibited a molecular size in the range of 55 to 80 kDa. Extracts from juvenile cartilage had a more restricted size variation corresponding to the higher molecular size range present in the adult. In the newborn, the sizes were in the range of 70 to 80 kDa.

The biosynthesis of proteoglycans begins with the synthesis of the core protein. The sugars of the GAG chain then are sequentially added to, in most instances, serine residues of the protein, using uridine diphosphate conjugates of the component sugars, with sulfation following as the chain elongates. Most of the chain elongation and sulfation is associated with the Golgi apparatus. The degradation of proteoglycans is mediated through the action of lysosomal glycosidases and sulfatases specific for the hydrolysis of the various structural sites within the GAG chain. Genetic abnormalities in the production or synthesis of these enzymes have been shown to be the main causes of "mucopolysaccharidoses," whose victims may exhibit severe tissue abnormalities and a high incidence of mental retardation.

Table 12-1. Properties and Tissue Distribution of Glycosaminoglycans

GAGs	Composition	Tissue Distribution
Hyaluronic acid	*N*-acetylglucosamine D-Glucuronic acid	Blood vessels, heart, synovial fluid, umbilical cord, vitreous
Chondroitin sulfate	*N*-acetylgalactosamine D-Glucuronic acid 4- or 6-O-sulfate	Cartilage, cornea, tendon, heart valves, skin, etc.
Dermatan sulfate	*N*-acetygalactosamine L-Iduronic acid 4- or 6-O-sulfate	Skin, lungs, cartilage
Keratan sulfate	*N*-acetyglucosamine D-Galactose O-sulfate	Cornea, cartilage, nucleus pulposus
Heparan sulfate	*N*-acetylglucosamine	Blood vessels, basement membranes, lung, spleen, kidney
Heparin	*N*-sulfaminoglucos-amine D-Glucuronic acid L-Iduronic acid O-sulfates	Mast cells, lung, Glisson membranes

The structural glycoproteins

In addition to the collagen and elastin components of connective tissues, there are groups of glycoproteins, the structural glycoproteins, that have important roles in the physiology and structural properties of connective and other types of tissues. These proteins, which include FN, LM, entactin/nidogen, thrombospondin (TSP), and others, are involved during development, in cell attachment and spreading, and in tissue growth and turnover.

FIBRONECTIN

One of the best characterized of the structural glycoproteins is fibronectin (FN). It was originally isolated from serum where it was referred to as "cold-insoluble globulin" (CIG). As it became recognized that FN was an all important secretory product of fibroblasts and other types of cells, and was involved in cell adhesion, the term "FN" replaced CIG. Comprehensive reviews on the structure and function of FN have been published by Lafrenie and Yamada[20] and Mao and Schwarzbauer.[21]

FN exists as a disulfide-linked dimer with a molecular weight of about 450 kDa, each monomer having a molecular size of 250 kDa. FN exists in at least two forms, a tissue form and plasma FN. Plasma FN is somewhat smaller and is more soluble at physiologic pH than the cellular form. Spectrophotometric and ultracentrifugal studies indicate that both forms are elongated molecules composed of structured domains separated by flexible, extensible regions. Limited proteolytic digestion has revealed the presence of specific binding sites for a number of ligands, including collagen, fibrin, cell surfaces, heparin (heparan sulfate proteoglycan), factor XIIIa, and actin.

FN plays a role in blood clotting by becoming cross-linked to fibrin through the action of factor XIIIa transamidase, which catalyses the final step in the clotting cascade.[22] Fibroblasts and other cell types involved in the repair of injury adhere to the clot by interacting with the cell-binding domain of FN. FN also enables cells to migrate in developing embryos. FN contains a unique peptide sequence, arginylglycylaspartylserine (RGDS or RGD), that binds to specific cell surface proteins (integrins), which span the plasma membrane.[21] Purified RGD can inhibit FN from binding the cells and can even displace bound FN. The integrins have a complex molecular organization and appear to interact with certain intracellular proteins, thereby providing a mechanism for the control of a number of events by components of the extracellular environment.

FN is encoded by a single gene and its complete primary structure has been determined by the DNA sequencing of overlapping cDNA clones.[23] From such studies, it became recognized that there are peptide segments derived from alternative splicing of FN mRNA at three distinct regions, termed extra domain A (ED-A), ED-B, and connecting segment (III CS). A middle region of the polypeptide containing homologous repeating segments of about 90 amino acids, called type III homologies, has been identified.[24,25] Using immunologic techniques with monoclonal antibodies, it was shown that the ED-A exon is omitted during splicing of the FN mRNA precursor in arterial medial cells, while the expression of FN containing ED-A is characteristic of modulated smooth muscle cells, such as those in culture or those involved in intimal thickening and atherosclerotic lesions. It would appear that this process of alternative splicing is used during embryonic development or tissue repair as a mechanism to generate different forms of FN in the ECM by the inclusion or exclusion of specific segments. This could be the source of differences between the plasma and cellular forms of FN. This phenomenon of alternative splicing may also be involved in the synthesis of collagens and elastin, and may well be implicated in processes of aging.

LAMININ

Laminin (LM) is the major structural glycoprotein of BMs. In addition to its association with the molecular components of BMs (e.g., type IV collagen, entactin/nidogen, and heparan sulfate proteoglycan), it plays an important role in cell attachment and neurite growth.[26–28] LM is difficult to isolate from whole tissues or from BMs owing to its poor solubility, and so most of our knowledge of it is derived from extracts of tumor matrices.

LM is a very large complex composed of at least three protein chains associated by disulfide linkages. The largest of these, the α1, has a molecular weight of about 440 kDa, whereas the smaller units, β1 and γ1 chains, have molecular weights of about 200 to 250 kDa. Several LM isoforms have been described in recent years,[28] necessitating a new nomenclature of its component chains.[29] The authors describe 15 isoforms of LM. The first new chain α2 has been found in preparations from normal tissues but is absent from those from neoplastic tissues.[30,31] LM has been shown to have a twisted cruciform shape consisting of three short arms and a single long arm with globular domains at the extremities of each arm. In several of the newer isoforms of LM, the α1 chain has a smaller molecular size, lacking a portion of its amino terminus.

LM can influence processes of differentiation, cell growth, migration, morphology, adhesion, and agglutination. It plays a major role in the structural organization of BMs.[32] LM exhibits a preferential binding to type IV collagen compared with other collagen types. LM contains domains similar to those of FN that bind to different proteins, and cell surface components containing an RGD sequence on the α1 chain and a YIGSR sequence on the β1 chain, both of which bind to different integrins on the cell surface and are involved in cellular attachment and migratory behaviors.

ENTACTIN/NIDOGEN

Entactin/nidogen, a novel sulfated glycoprotein, is an intrinsic component of BMs. Entactin was first identified in the ECM synthesized by mouse endodermal cells in culture.[33] Subsequently, a degraded form, termed nidogen, was isolated from the Englebreth-Holm-Swarm sarcoma and mistakenly identified as a new BM component.[34] Both terms, entactin and nidogen, are used interchangeably in the modern literature. Entactin-1/nidogen-1 and entactin-2/nidogen-2 are differentially expressed in myogenic differentiation.[35]

Entactin/nidogen forms a tight stoichiometric complex with LM. Rotary shadowing electron microscopy has revealed its association with the γ1 chain of LM. Entactin/nidogen has been shown to promote cell attachment via an RGD sequence, and calcium ions have been implicated in its properties.[36] Its role along with LN in BM assembly and in epithelial morphogenesis has already been noted in the previous section. It has been shown that entactin-1/nidogen-1 regulates LM-1 dependent mammary specific gene expression.

THROMBOSPONDIN

Thrombospondins (TSPs) are a family of extracellular, adhesive proteins that are widely expressed in vertebrates. Five distinct gene products—designated TSP 1-4 and cartilage oligomeric matrix protein (COMP)—have been identified. TSP-1 and -2 have similar primary structures. The molecule (450 kDa) is composed of three identical disulfide-linked protein chains. It is one of the major peptide products secreted during platelet activation, and it is also secreted by a diversity of growing cells. TSP has 12 binding sites for calcium ion and depends upon it for its conformational stability. It binds to heparin and heparan sulfate proteoglycan and to cell surfaces, and appears to modulate a number of cell functions, including platelet aggregation, progression through the cell cycle, and cell adhesion and migration.[37,38] Recent genetic studies have shown associations of single nucleotide polymorphisms in 3 of the 5 TSPs with cardio vascular disease.[37] Both TSP 1 and 2 are best known for their antiangiogenic properties and their ability to modulate cell-matrix interactions.[38]

INTEGRINS AND CELL ATTACHMENT PROTEINS

As indicated above, cell surfaces contain groups of proteins, the integrins, that mediate cell-matrix interactions. The integrins behave as receptors for components of the ECM and interact with components of the cytoskeleton.[39] This provides a mechanism for the mediation of components of the ECM of intracellular processes, including control of cell shape and metabolic activity. The integrins exist as paired molecules containing α- and β-subunits. They appear to have a significant degree of specificity for ECM proteins, which apparently is conferred by combination of different α- and β-subunits.

In addition to the integrins, cell attachment proteins (CAMs) are present on the cell surface. These confer specific cell-cell recognition properties. For reviews on integrins and CAMs, see Albelda and Buck,[39] Danen and Yamada,[40] Takagi,[41] and Lock et al.[42]

AGING AND THE PROPERTIES OF CONNECTIVE TISSUES

From the foregoing discussion, it becomes apparent that there can be a multitude of possible loci in the development, structural organization, metabolism, and molecular biology of connective tissues for the introduction of alterations in the properties of these tissues. For a given tissue, changes in the composition of the ECM or changes in the factors that control the production of ECM can feed back through complex mechanisms to induce changes in the properties of the tissue. The process of aging may well involve some of these factors. It is probable that, during the aging process, the phenotypical expression of ECM (i.e., the patterns of ECM composition) will change. It is also probable that many of the components of the ECM may evolve with time as a function of their long biologic half-lives and the enzymatic and nonenzymatic modifications that take place. These can include processes of maintenance and repair, responses to inflammation, nonenzymatic glycosylation, cross-linkage formation, etc.

In a sense, it may be important to differentiate between those processes of senescence that are genetically programmed (i.e., innate senescence), and the contributions to aging induced by "environmental" factors. However, it becomes difficult to distinguish whether a given alteration is an effect or a cause of aging.

In this section an attempt is made to discuss some of the factors and conditions involving connective tissues that may be associated with the aging process. These include aspects of cellular senescence, inflammatory and growth factors, photoaging of the skin, diabetes mellitus, nonenzymatic glycosylation, the cause of OS, osteoarthritis (OA), atherosclerosis, Werner's syndrome (WS), and Alzheimer's disease (AD).

Cellular senescence

A large body of research has established conclusively that normal diploid cells have a limited replicative life span and that cells from older animals have shorter life spans than those from younger animals. Thus the process of aging could be attributed to cellular senescence. A number of observations suggest that connective tissue proteins may be affected during cellular senescence. In an extensive study on the properties of murine skin fibroblasts, van Gansen and van Lerberghe[43] concluded that among the main effects of cellular mitotic age were a depression of chromatin plasticity, changes in the organization of cytoplasmic filaments, and changes in the organization of the ECM. They implicated an involvement of collagen fibers in the intracellular events both in vivo and in vitro. Although senescent fibroblasts may not be dividing, they are biosynthetically active, showing an increased synthesis of FN and increased levels of FN mRNA. However, both senescent and progeroid cells demonstrated a decreased chemotactic response to FN and developed a much thicker extracellular FN network than did young fibroblasts.[44] There is some indication that, with increasing age, cells become less able to respond to mitogens, which may have a bearing on age-related differences in wound healing.[45] It was also shown that the presence of senescent chondrocytes increases the risk of articular cartilage degeneration that is associated with fibrillation of the articular surface and increased collagen cross-linking.[46] Thus it would appear that there is some correlation between cellular senescence and changes in the regulation of connective tissue metabolism and cellular interactions.

Inflammatory and growth factors

One of the active areas of contemporary connective tissue biology is the study of the influence of inflammatory and growth factors on the properties of connective tissues. It is well recognized that inflammatory cells accumulate in damaged and infected tissues as part of the inflammatory response. These cells secrete lymphokines, such as the interleukins, and other factors which may influence connective tissue metabolism. In addition, a number of growth factors, including epidermal growth factor (EGF), platelet-derived growth factor (PDGF), fibroblast growth factors (FGFs), and transforming growth factors (TGFs), can have extensive control over connective tissue metabolism. As indicated earlier, senescent cells may not respond to these factors as do young cells. In addition, it is possible that stimulation of cell replication by certain of these factors may accelerate the progression of cells toward senescence. To add to the complexity are the findings that many cells can synthesize certain of these factors including interleukin-1, PDGF, FGFs, and TGFs, endowing the cellular components of tissues with autocrine and paracrine properties.

In studies reported by Furuyama et al,[47] alveolar type II epithelial cells cultured on collagen fibrils in a medium supplemented with TGF-β-1 synthesized a thin continuous BM. Immunohistochemical studies revealed the presence of type IV collagen, LM, perlecan, and entactin/nidogen. Similar stimulatory effects of TGF-β-1 on BM protein synthesis in rat liver sinusoids were reported by Neubauer et al.[48] The role of a variety of growth factors and cytokines in the development of inflammatory synovitis accompanied by destruction of joint cartilage was demonstrated in studies by Gravallese.[49] Recent studies by Takehara[50] suggest that the growth of skin fibroblasts is regulated by a variety of cytokines and growth factors with a resultant increase in ECM protein production.

The extent of involvement of these interacting factors in the aging process is not clear, but it is probable that they contribute to the process.

Mechanisms of cutaneous aging

Cutaneous aging is a complex biologic activity consisting of two distinct components: (1) intrinsic, genetically determined degeneration, and (2) extrinsic aging due to exposure to the environment, also known as "photoaging." These two processes are superimposed in the sun-exposed areas of skin, with their profound effects on the biology of cellular and structural elements of the skin.[51,52] The symptoms of photoaging are different from those of intrinsic aging, and evidence suggests that these two processes have different mechanisms.

A variety of theories have been advanced to explain aging phenomena and some of them may be applicable to innate skin aging as well. It was postulated that diploid cells, such as dermal fibroblasts, have a finite life span in culture.[50] This observation, when extrapolated to the tissue level, could be expected to result in cellular senescence and degenerative changes in the dermis. Others have suggested that free radicals may damage collagen in the dermis,[53] and a third theory implicates nonenzymatic glycosylation of proteins, such as collagen, leading to increased cross-linking of collagen fibrils. It is postulated that this process is the major cause of dysfunction of collagenous tissues in old age.[54] Finally, cutaneous aging may be attributed to differential gene expression of ECM of connective tissue. It has been demonstrated that the rate of collagen biosynthesis is greatly reduced in the skin of elderly people.[55] Collectively, the observations on dermal connective tissue components in innate aging suggest an imbalance between biosynthesis and degradation, with less repair capacity in the presence of ongoing degradation.

Additional changes in the aged dermis concern the architecture of the collagen and elastin networks. The spaces between fibrous components are more compact owing to a loss of ground substance. Collagen bundles appear to unravel and there are signs of elastolysis. Scanning electron microscopic studies of the three-dimensional arrangement of rat skin from animals ranging in age from 2 weeks to 24 months showed that, during postnatal growth, there was a "dynamic rearrangement" of the collagen and elastic fibers, with an ordered arrangement of mature collagen bundles being attained by producing distortions of relatively straight elastic fibers. During adulthood, there is a tortuosity of these elastic fibers coupled with an incomplete restructuring of the elastic network that was deposited to interlock with the collagen bundles.

The effects of photodamage on dermal connective tissue are exemplified in the histopathologic pictures of photoaging. The hallmark of photoaging is the massive accumulation of the so-called "elastotic" material in the upper and middermis. This phenomenon, known as "solar elastosis," has been attributed to changes in elastin.[56] Solar elastotic material is composed of elastin; fibrillin; versican, a large proteoglycan; and hyaluronic acid. Even though the elastotic material contains the normal constituents of elastic fibers, the supramolecular organization of solar elastotic material and its functionality are severely perturbed. It was also known that elastin gene expression is notably activated in cells within the sun-damaged dermis. In addition, it has been shown that accumulation of elastotic material is accompanied by degeneration of the surrounding collagen meshwork. Parallel studies provide evidence implicating MMPs as mediators of collagen damage in photoaging.[55]

It would appear that the main culprit in photoaging appears to be the UV-B portion of the ultraviolet spectrum, although UV-A and infrared radiation also contribute to the damage. In UV-A irradiated hairless mice, there appears to be alteration in the ratio of type III to type I collagen in addition to the elastosis. It has been shown that UV irradiation of fibroblasts in culture enhances expression of MMPs.[55] There is also an increase in the levels of the components of the ground substance in photoaged skin (predominantly dermatan sulfate, heparan sulfate, and hyaluronic acid). In human aged skin, mast cells are numerous and appear to be degranulated. These cells are known to produce a variety of inflammatory mediators so that photoaged skin is chronically inflamed. In innate aging, the skin tends to be hypocellular. The microcirculation of the skin is also affected, becoming sparse, with the horizontal superficial plexus almost destroyed. Although atrophy may be presented in end-stage photoaging in the elderly population, ongoing photoaging is characterized by more, not less.

The effects of photoaging could be totally prevented by broad-spectrum sunscreens. Although severe photoaging in humans is considered to be irreversible, in hairless mice it was found that repair could take place after the cessation of irradiation, with the newly deposited collagen appearing totally normal. A similar repair was observed in biopsies of severely photo-damaged human skin after several years of avoidance of exposure to the sun.

Diabetes mellitus

Currently two types of diabetes mellitus are recognized clinically, type-1 diabetes (DM-1), which is insulin dependent and is caused by β-cell destruction, and type-2 (DM-2), formerly known as noninsulin dependent. Diabetics often show signs of accelerated aging, primarily as a result of the complications of vascular disease and impaired wound healing so common in this disease. It is well documented that diabetics will exhibit a thickening of vascular BMs.[5] The biologic basis for this thickening is as yet obscure, but could well be related to abnormalities in cell attachment, or the response to factors affecting BM formation to excessive nonenzymatic glycosylation of proteins, or to an abnormal turnover of BM components. Fibroblasts from diabetic individuals exhibit a premature senescence in culture.[57] The role of inhibitors of aldose reductase was investigated by Sibbitt et al.[58] They showed that, in normal human fibroblasts, the mean population doubling times, population doublings to senescence, saturation density at confluence, tritiated thymidine incorporation, and response to PDGF were inhibited with increasing glucose concentrations in the media. They found that inhibitors of aldose reductase, sorbinil and tolrestat, completely prevented these inhibitions. Myoinositol had similar effects; however, no data were presented to indicate that aldose reductase inhibitors would reverse the premature senescence in fibroblasts from diabetic individuals. Thus it is not clear whether prevention of the formation of reduced sugars can have a therapeutic effect, nor is it clear that all of the aging effects of diabetes are mediated by reduced sugars.

One of the less known complications of DM-1 and DM-2 is bone loss. This complication is receiving increased attention because DM-1 diabetics are living longer due to better therapeutic measures; however, they are faced with additional complications associated with aging, such as OS.[59] Both DM-1 and DM-2 diabetic patients are under high risk of cardiovascular disease. Uncontrolled hyperglycemia may give rise to nonenzymatic glycosylation of proteins, which may lead to the generation of reactive oxygen species, increased intermolecular and intramolecular cross-linking with subsequent vessel damage, and atherogenesis.[60,61]

Nonenzymatic glycosylation and collagen cross-linking

When enzymes attach sugars to proteins, they usually do so at sites on the protein molecule dictated by the specificity of the enzyme for the regional sequence to be glycosylated. On the other hand, nonenzymatic glycosylation, a process long known to cause food discoloration and toughness, proceeds nonspecifically at any site sterically available.[61] The longer a protein is in contact with a reducing sugar, the greater the chance for nonenzymatic glycosylation to occur. In uncontrolled diabetics, elevated circulating levels of glycosylated hemoglobin and albumin are found. Since erythrocytes turn over every 120 days, the levels of hemoglobin A_{1c} are an index of the degree of control of hyperglycemia over a 120-day period. The same is true for glycosylated albumin over a shorter period. Proteins such as collagen, which is extremely long-lived, have also been shown to undergo nonenzymatic glycosylation. Paul and Bailey[62] demonstrated that glycation of collagen forms the basis of its central role in complications of aging and diabetes mellitus.

The nonenzymatic reactions between glucose and proteins are collectively known as the Maillard or Browning reaction. The initial reaction is the formation of a Schiff base between glucose and an amino group of the protein. This is an unstable structure and can spontaneously undergo an Amadori rearrangement in which a new ketone group is generated on the adduct. This can condense with a similar product on another peptide sequence to produce a covalent crosslinkage.[60] Initially, glycation affects the interaction of collagen with cells and other matrix components, but the most damaging effects are caused by the formation of glucose-mediated intermolecular cross-linkages. These cross-linkages decrease the critical flexibility and permeability of the tissues and reduce turnover. Another fibrous protein that is similarly modified by glycation is elastin.[62] Verzijl et al[63] have shown that, during aging, nonenzymatic glycation results in the accumulation of the advanced glycation end-product pentosidine in articular cartilage aggrecan.

The arthritides—osteoarthritis

The development of rheumatoid diseases, particularly OA, is a common event in aging individuals. The cause of OA and OS is based on a variety of factors ranging from genetic susceptibility, to endocrine and metabolic status, to mechanical and traumatic injury events.[64] With aging, the bone loss in OA is lower compared with OS. The lower degree of bone loss with aging is explained by the lower bone turnover, as measured by bone resorption-formation parameters.[65] In the initial stages of OA, there is increased cell proliferation and synthesis of matrix proteins, proteinases, growth factors, and cytokines synthesized by adult articular chondrocytes. Other types of cells and tissues of the joint, including the synovium and subchondral bone, contribute to the pathogenesis.[66]

In inflammatory arthritis, degradative enzymes including tissue collagenases and metalloproteinases are present in the rheumatoid lesion, leading to degradation of both cartilage and bone. It is believed that inflammatory factors stimulate abnormal levels of these enzymes.[67] Studies by Iannone and Lapadula[68] demonstrated that interleukin-1 (IL-1) is produced by synovial cells. IL-1, TNF-β, and other cytokines are also mitogenic for synovial cells and can stimulate the production of collagenases, proteoglycanases, plasminogen activator, and prostaglandins. It is suggested that IL-1 plays an important role in the pathogenesis of rheumatoid arthritis.

Osteoporosis

OS is a systemic skeletal disease, comprising rarefaction of bone structure and loss of bone mass, leading to increased fracture risk. The frequency of this disorder increases with aging. Twin and family studies have demonstrated a genetic component of OS regarding parameters of bone properties, such as bone mineral density, with a heredity component of 60% to 80%.[69] OS affects most women above 80 years of age; at the age of 50, the lifetime risk of suffering an OS-related fracture approaches 50% in women and 20% in men. Studies indicate that genetic variations explain as much as 70% of the variance for bone mineral density in the population.[70] The National Organization of Osteoporosis recommends bone density testing for all women over 65 and earlier (around the time of menopause) for women who have risk factors.

Viguet-Carrin et al[71] demonstrated that different determinants of bone quality are interrelated, especially the mineral content and modifications in collagen. Different processes of maturation of collagen occur in bone, involving enzymatic and nonenzymatic reactions. The latter type of collagen modification is age related and may impair the mechanical properties of bone. In a study of human trabecular bone taken at autopsy, Oxlund et al[72] examined both collagen and reducible and nonreducible collagen cross-linkages in relation to age and OS. The extractability of collagen from vertebral bone of control individuals was increased with age. Bone collagen of OS individuals showed increased extractability and a marked decrease in the concentration of the divalent reducible collagen cross-linkages compared with sex- and age-matched controls. No alterations were observed in the concentration of trivalent pyridinium cross-linkages. These changes would be expected to reduce the strength of the bone trabeculae and could explain why the OS individuals had bone fractures although the collagen density did not differ from that of the sex- and age-matched controls.

Croucher et al[73] have quantitatively assessed cancellous structure in 35 patients with primary OS. Their data demonstrate that, for a given cancellous area, structural changes in primary OS are similar to those observed during age-related bone loss in normal subjects. These findings strongly implicate an abnormal increase in the activity(ies) of osteoclast-derived resorption enzymes, acting on the degradation of the ECM, in the cause of OS.

Arterial aging

In young healthy individuals, the cushioning function of elastic arteries—principally the aorta—results in optimal interaction with the heart, and optimal steady flow through peripheral resistance vessels. As the arteries age, changes in their composition and structure lead to an increase in the stiffness of their walls, resulting in increased pulse pressure, hypertension, and a greater risk of cardiovascular disease. Another effect of aortic stiffening is transmission of flow pulsations downstream into vasodilated organs, principally brain and kidney, where pulsatile energy is dissipated and fragile microvessels are damaged. This accounts for microinfarcts and microhemorrhages, with specialized cell damage, cognitive decline, and renal failure.[74]

The arterial media responsible for arterial stiffness and resilience is composed of elastin, collagen, vascular smooth muscle cells, and ground substance. Elastin comprises 90% of arterial elastic fibers. The generalized age-related stiffening (arteriosclerosis) is confined primarily to the media of arteries. Although the absolute amounts of both collagen and elastin in arteries fall with age, the ratio of collagen to elastin increases. In addition, with age, elastic lamellae undergo fragmentation and thinning, leading to ectasia and a gradual transfer of mechanical load to collagen, which is 100 to 1000 times stiffer than elastin. Possible causes of this fragmentation are mechanical (fatigue failure) or enzymatically driven by MMP activity.[75] MMPs navigate the behavior of vascular wall cells in different atherosclerosis stages, in adaptive remodeling, in normal aging, and in nonatherosclerotic vessel disease.[76] In arteries, accumulation of advanced glycation end products over time leads to cross-linking of collagen and consequent increases in its material stiffness. Furthermore, the remaining elastin itself becomes stiffer, owing to calcification and the formation of cross-links due to advanced glycation end products, a process that affects collagen even more strongly.[75] These changes are accelerated in the presence of disease such as hypertension, diabetes, and uremia. Most studies show that arterial stiffening occurs across all age groups in both DM-1 and DM-2. Arterial stiffening in DM-2 results partially from the clustering of hyperglycemia, dyslipidemia, and hypertension, all of which may promote insulin resistance, oxidative stress, endothelial dysfunction, and the formation of proinflammatory cytokines and advanced glycosylation end products.[77]

Although there is ample evidence for the link between arteriosclerosis and the degradation and remodeling of collagen and elastin, much remains unknown about the detailed mechanisms.

Werner's syndrome

WS is a rare autosomal recessive premature aging disease manifested by age-related phenotypes, such as atherosclerosis, cataracts, OS, soft tissue calcification, premature graying, and loss of hair, and a high incidence of some types of cancer.[78] The gene product, WRN, which is defective in WS, is a member of the RecQ family of DNA helicases.[79] Clinical and biologic manifestations in four major body systems—the nervous, immune, connective tissues, and endocrine systems—similar to normal aging, appear at an early stage of the patient's life. WS may cause abnormalities in the cardiovascular system manifested as restrictive cardiomyopathy.[80] Ostler et al[81] reported that WS fibroblasts show a mutator phenotype, abbreviated replicative life, and accelerated cellular senescence. They also demonstrated that T-cells derived from WS patients have the mutator phenotype. Increased collagen synthesis in fibroblasts from two WS patients has been reported. This was accompanied by a near doubling of the levels of procollagen mRNA over normal controls. Similarly, studies by Hatamochi et al[82] demonstrated that WS fibroblast-conditioned medium brought about activation of normal fibroblast proliferation but failed to alter the relative rates of collagen and noncollagenous protein synthesis by such fibroblasts.

Alzheimer's disease

AD is a disease of old age. The characteristic pathophysiologic changes at autopsy include neurofibrillary tangles, neuritis plaque, neuronal loss, and amyloid angiopathy. Mutations in chromosomes 1, 12, and 21 cause familial AD. Susceptibility genes do not cause the disease by themselves but in combination with other genes modulate the age of onset and increase the probability of AD.[83] Significant progress has been made in identifying the mutations in the Tau protein and dissecting the cross-talk between Tau and the second hallmark lesion of AD, the Aβ peptide-containing amyloid plaque.[84]

Recent studies with familial AD have demonstrated reduction or loss of smooth muscle actin in the media of cerebral arterioles. Intracerebral arterioles and numerous capillaries were laden with amyloid deposits. There was marked expression of collagen type III and BM collagen type IV. Fibers of both amyloid and collagen were found within the BM.[85]

Clinical and experimental studies have shown that cerebral perfusion is progressively decreased during increased aging, and this decrease in brain blood flow is significantly greater in AD. Studies by Carare et al[86] have shown that capillary and arteriole BMs act as "lymphatics" of the brain for drainage of fluid and solutes. Amyloid β (Aβ) is deposited in BM drainage pathways in cerebral amyloid angiopathy and may impede elimination of amyloid β and interstitial fluid from the brain in AD.

The localization of BM components, such as LM, entactin/nidogen, and collagen type IV, to the amyloid plaque has suggested that these components may play a role in the pathogenesis of AD.[87] The work of Kiuchi et al[88] has shown that entactin/nidogen, collagen type IV, and LM had the most pronounced effect on preformed Aβ 42 fibrils, causing disassembly of amyloid β-protein fibrils. Circular dichroism studies indicated that high concentrations of BM components induced structural transition in Aβ 42 β-sheet to random structures.

It has been suggested that the vascular BM may serve as a nidus for senile plaque, playing a role in the development of both amyloid and neuritic elements in AD.

SUMMARY

This chapter has reviewed some aspects of biochemistry and molecular biology, and the involvement of connective tissue in the process of aging. There is a complexity

KEY POINTS
Connective Tissues and Aging

- Changes in the structural integrity and production of connective tissue macromolecules are associated with the process of aging.
- Loss of tissue function in aging is associated with increased cross-linking of collagen and elastin fibrils and subsequent decrease in their turnover.
- Alternative splicing in the mRNA of the connective tissue macromolecules has been implicated in the process of aging.
- There is a correlation between cellular senescence and changes in the regulation of connective tissue metabolism.
- Nonenzymatic glycosylation of collagen and elastin is accelerated with aging and may be associated with changes in diabetes.
- In age-related osteoporosis, a decrease in divalent reducible collagen cross-linkages may lead to reduced bone strength and may explain increased bone fractures.
- In aging and in senile dementia of the Alzheimer type, there is colocalization of type IV collagen, laminin, heparan sulfate proteoglycan and amyloid plaque in the brain vasculature.

inherent in the control of connective tissue structure, metabolism, and molecular biology, and aging might contribute to alterations in these and vice versa. Among the phenomena that may prove central to the aging process are the processes of collagen cross-linking and nonenzymatic glycosylation, alternative gene splicing, effects of solar radiation, the interplay of cytokines and growth factors on the control of connective tissue phenotype, production and action of degradative enzymes, factors that affect cell replication, connective tissue diseases, and intracellular factors that control senescence. The causes and effects of aging are an active area of contemporary research in which the involvement of connective tissue is an important element.

For a complete list of references, please visit online only at www.expertconsult.com

CHAPTER 13

Clinical Immunology: Immune Senescence and the Acquired Immune Deficiency of Aging

Mohan K. Tummala
Dennis D. Taub
William B. Ershler

As a fundamental organ necessary for the maintenance of life, the immune system first appeared in primitive organisms about 480 million years ago.[1] The intricate relationship between acquired immunity and infection was apparent early in recorded history. Observing an epidemic of plague in 430 BC, Thucydides reported that anyone who had recovered from the disease was spared during future outbreaks. The era of modern immunology was launched with Jenner's report in 1798 of an effective vaccine employing cowpox pustules to prevent smallpox in humans. Improved understanding of immunity and infection continued throughout the nineteenth and twentieth centuries. For example, identification of bacterial organisms ultimately resulted in the discovery of antibodies that could neutralize these microbes and/or their toxins, eventually leading to endorsement of the concept of vaccination. The discovery of antibody structure during the 1960s finally began the era of modern immunochemistry. With regard to cellular immunity, despite the early work of Metchnikoff and his followers, the role of cells in acquired immunity was not truly appreciated until the 1950s. Although theories of "self-recognition" and "autoimmunity" appeared early in the twentieth century, autoimmune diseases remain incompletely understood.

As a concept, immunogerontology is a relatively recent focus of interest. In 1969, Walford proposed that declining immune function contributes to the biologic processes of aging.[2] He speculated that disorders in the immune system that occur with aging account for three major causes of disease in old age: (1) increased autoimmunity; (2) failing surveillance allowing the expression of cancers; and (3) the increased susceptibility to infectious diseases. Current evidence supports the notion that the decline in immune function with aging may be viewed as a form of acquired immunodeficiency of modest dimension. Complicating the assessment of aging on immune function, older people are more likely to have diseases, conditions, or exposures that contribute to declining immune function.[3]

CHANGES IN THE HUMAN IMMUNE SYSTEM WITH AGING

Nonspecific host defense

Primary (innate) immunity is the first line of defense against invading pathogens. It differs from secondary (acquired) immunity in that it does not require sensitization or prior exposure to offer protection. Primary immunity involves tissues (e.g., mucocutaneous barriers), cells (monocytes, neutrophils, natural killer [NK] cells) and soluble factors (cytokines, chemokines, complement) coordinated to mediate the nonspecific lysis of foreign cells.

A feature of innate immunity is the detection of pathogens using pattern recognition receptors such as Toll-like receptors (TLRs) that recognize specific molecular patterns present on the surface of pathogens triggering a variety of signaling pathways. After processing of antigen by the antigen presenting cells, the peptide fragments are presented along with major histocompatibility (MHC) class II molecules to $CD4^+$ T cells or with MHC class I molecules to $CD8^+$ T cells to generate efficient T-cell responses. The antigen presenting cells also provide additional co-stimulatory stimulus (e.g., ligation of B7.1 or CD80 on antigen-presenting cells with CD28 on T cells) to lower the threshold of T-cell activation and survival following the recognition of antigens. The ligation of TLRs on antigen presenting cells enhances the phagocytosis of the pathogen through the release of chemokines and other peptides, which then result in activation and recruitment of immune cells to the sites of infection.

Phagocytosis

Phagocytosis involves the engulfment and lysis and/or digestion of foreign substances. The capacity of neutrophils, macrophages, and monocytes for phagocytosis is determined by their number and ability to reach the relevant site, adhere to endothelial surfaces, respond to chemical signals (chemotaxis), and complete the process of phagocytosis.[4] The study of alterations in phagocytosis with age must then involve examinations of each of these steps, and are inherently more difficult in human populations than in disease-free inbred animals. Extrapolation of studies of senescent mice to humans suggests age itself does not attenuate response to bacterial capsular antigens in a well-vascularized area such as the lung.[5,6] Niwa et al reported a deterioration in neutrophil chemotaxis and increase in serum lipid peroxidase in the nonsurviving cohort of a 7-year longitudinal study, suggesting a preterminal but not necessarily "normal" aging alteration in these factors.[7] However, age-related effectiveness in chemotaxis may be reduced in less vascular tissues in vivo, such as in the skin, which also has a number of other changes that may impair the ability of cells in the vascular compartment to reach a site of infection.[8] Although elderly persons preserve the number and overall phagocytic capacity, in vitro neutrophil functions (including endothelial adherence, migration, granule secretory behavior such as superoxide production, nitric oxide, and apoptosis) appear to be reduced with age,[9–11] and significantly fewer neutrophils arrive at the skin abrasion sites studied in older people.[12] How this translates to immune response and immune-mediated repair in infected or otherwise physiologically stressed older people remains unknown. Although the expression of TLRs and GM-CSF receptors are not diminished, ligation of these receptors results in altered signal transduction. With aging, alterations in signal transduction of these receptors may be involved in the defective function of neutrophils with decreased response to stimuli such as infection with gram positive bacteria.[13,14] These changes in the elderly, unlike in the young, could be the result of changes in the recruitment of TLR4 into lipid rafts and no-raft fractions (the domains on plasma membrane that play an important role in cell signaling) with LPS stimulation.[15] And similarly, the activation through GM-CSF on the surface of these cells is also altered in the elderly because of an age-related presence of a phosphatase in the lipid raft blocking cell activation and contributing to decreased response to GM-CSF in neutrophils from older people.[16]

Macrophage activation also appears to change with age; this may be partially attributable to a reduced gamma interferon signal from T lymphocytes.[17,18] A decrease in the number of macrophage precursors and macrophages is observed in bone marrow.[19] Although it is not clear if there is an age-associated decrease of TLR on the surface of aged macrophages, defective production of cytokines has been observed after TLR stimulation, possibly due to altered signal transduction.[20,21] With aging, there is diminished expression of MHC class II molecules both in humans and in mice, resulting in diminished antigen recognition and processing by these antigen presenting cells.[19,22] In addition, activated macrophages from humans and mice produce higher levels of prostaglandin E2, which may negatively influence antigen presentation.[19] Fewer signals at the site of infection may be a consequence of reduced numbers of activated T cells locally due to reduced antigen processing capacity of macrophages. Fewer T cells and the defective expression of homing markers to attract T cells from peripheral blood into inflamed tissues[23] suggests that increased susceptibility of old mice to, for example, tuberculosis, reflects an impaired capacity to focus mediator cells and the additional cytokine they may express at sites of infection (see more on T-cell changes with age in later discussion). These observations may help explain why late-life tuberculosis or reactivation tuberculosis occurs and remains clinically important in geriatric populations. The change in function of antigen-presenting dendritic cells (DC) with aging is less well defined. A decrease in number and migration of Langerhans cells in skin has been described in elderly people,[24] but their function remains sufficient for antigen presentation.[25] In contrast, DCs from the elderly who are considered "frail" have been demonstrated to have reduced expression of costimulatory molecules, secrete less interleukin (IL)-12, and stimulate a less robust T-cell proliferative response when compared with those who are not "frail.[26]"

Cell lysis

Cell lysis is mediated through a variety of pathways, including the complement system, natural killer (NK), macrophage/monocyte, and neutrophil activity. Complement activity does not appear to decline significantly with age, and neutrophil function also appears intact. However, in longitudinal studies of nonhuman primates, NK activity does appear to be affected by age[27] and acute stressors such as illness.[28] The functioning status of NK cells is dependent on a balance of activating and inhibitory signals delivered to membrane receptors.[29] A well preserved NK cell activity is observed in healthy elderly individuals[30] explaining, in part, a lower incidence of respiratory tract infections and higher antibody titers after influenza vaccination.[31] However, elderly individuals with chronic diseases and frailty are characterized by lower NK cytotoxicity and a greater predisposition to infection and other medical disorders.[32,33]

Although little is known about any changes in expression of activating and inhibitory receptors in the elderly, NK activation and cytotoxic granule release remain intact.[30,34] Secretion of IFN-γ after stimulation of purified NK cells with IL-2 shows an early decrease, which can be overcome with prolonged incubation.[35] IL-12 or IL-2 can upregulate chemokine production, although to a lesser extent than that observed in young subjects.[36] These observations suggest that NK cells have an age-associated defect in their response to cytokines with subsequent detriment in their capacity both to kill target cells and to synthesize cytokines and chemokines.

Specific host defense

There are well-defined alterations in both cellular and humoral immunity with advancing age. In the cellular immune system, most studies show no significant changes with human aging in the total number of peripheral blood cells, including total lymphocytes, monocytes, NK cells, or polymorphonuclear leukocytes.[35,37–41] The appearance of lymphocytopenia is associated with mortality in elderly people, but is not an age-related finding.[42–44] Most studies show no changes in the percentages of B- and T-lymphocyte populations in the peripheral blood,[45,46] although chronically ill elderly people may particularly have a decline in total T-cell numbers. Equivocal changes in the ratio of helper cells to suppressor cells (T4/T8) occur in normal aging.[39,40,45,47,48] These findings are in contrast to human immunodeficiency virus (HIV)-induced acquired immunodeficiency syndrome (AIDS) associated with a decreased T4/T8 ratio. Finally, there is a specific age-related increase in memory cells, cells that express the CD45 surface marker.[49–52]

Qualitative changes in T-cell function

The function of lymphocytes is altered with aging. This may be a consequence of decreased thymic function, an important factor for age-related changes in thymic dependent immunity-adaptive T-cell immunity. Declines in serum thymic hormones precede the decline in thymic tissue. By the age of 60, few of the thymic peptides are measurable in human peripheral blood,[53] and the thymus undergoes progressive reduction in size associated with the loss of thymic epithelial cells and a decrease in thymopoiesis. Thymic hormone replacement may improve immune function in old age,[54,55] but there are no current clinical indications in this regard.

T cells may be considered either "naïve" or "memory" on the basis of prior antigen exposure, and with advancing age, there has been noted a relative expansion of the memory T-cell pool. The competency of adaptive immune function declines with age primarily because of a dramatic decline in production of naïve lymphocytes because of a decline in thymic output and an increase in inert memory lymphocytes (see later discussion). Naïve $CD4^+$ T cells isolated from aged humans and animals display a decreased in vitro responsiveness and altered profiles of cytokine secretion to mitogen stimulation and expand poorly and give rise to fewer effector cells when compared with naïve $CD4^+$ T cells isolated from younger hosts. Naïve $CD4^+$ T cells from aged animals produce about half the IL-2 as young cells on initial stimulation with antigen-antigen presenting cells. Also the helper function of naïve $CD4^+$ T cells for antibody production is also decreased.[56] But newly generated CD4+ cells in aged mice respond quite well to antigens and are able to expand with adequate IL-2 production with good cognate helper function. Thus these age-related defects in naïve CD4+ T cells appear to be a result of the chronologic age of naïve CD4+ T cells rather than the chronologic age of the individual. These aged naïve CD4+ T cells proliferate less and produce less IL-2 in response to antigenic stimulation than naïve CD4+ T cells that have not undergone homeostatic divisions in the peripheral blood. The mechanism underlying homeostasis associated dysfunction of naïve CD4 T cells is not known. But in contrast to naïve cells, memory CD4+ T cells are long lived, maintained by homeostatic cytokines, and are relatively competent with age. Isolated CD4+ T cells from healthy elderly human and old mice are normal in antigen proliferation in vitro.[57] Memory CD4+ T cells generated from young age respond well to antigens over time, whereas memory CD4+ T cells derived from older age respond poorly.[58] Memory T cells generated from aged naïve T cells, upon stimulation, survive and persist well, but they are markedly defective in proliferation and cytokine secretion during recall responses with impaired cognate help for humoral immunity. Healthy elderly are able to mount a CD4+ T-cell response comparable to that observed in younger individuals when vaccinated with influenza, but they exhibit an impaired long-term CD4+ T-cell immune response to the influenza vaccine.[59] Vaccination with influenza results in increased IL-2 secretion in response to viral antigen in vitro.[60,61] But the number of influenza-specific cytotoxic T cells declines with age, with no increase after vaccination.[62]

Alteration in cell surface receptor expression (e.g., the loss of costimulatory receptor CD28 on the surface of CD8+ T cells) is one of the most prominent changes that occur with aging. CD28−CD8+ T cells are absent in newborns but become the majority (80% to 90%) of circulating CD8+ T cells in the elderly. Functionally, these CD28−CD8+ T cells are relatively inert and have a reduced proliferative response to TCR cross-linking, but maintain their capacity for cytotoxicity and are resistant to apoptosis.[63] This loss of CD28 expression is associated with a gain of expression of stimulatory NK cell receptors in CD28−CD8+ memory T cells, enabling their effector function as a compensation for impaired proliferation.[64]

There is a reduction of naïve CD8+ T cells with some degree of oligoclonal expansion of CD8+ T cells with age observed in the healthy elderly.[65] This expansion may reflect a compensatory phenomenon to control a latent viral infection or to fill available T-cell space as a result of diminished output of naïve T cells from the thymus. When this clonal expansion reaches a critical level, the diversity of T-cell repertoire is reduced and its ability to protect against new infections is compromised as seen when elderly humans are exposed to new antigens. For example, the effect of host age was studied in the recent severe acute respiratory syndrome (SARS) outbreak, and it was discovered that the antigen recognition repertoire of T cells was approximately 10^8 in young adults but only 10^6 in the elderly.[66] Notably, most of the SARS mortality was observed in infected persons over the age of 50 years. Accumulation of CD28−CD8+ T cells are also found in viral infections, such as CMV, EBV, and hepatitis C, so CD28−CD8+ T cells may be derived from CD28−CD8+ T cells after repeated antigenic stimulation.[67] This clonal expansion of CD28−CD8+ T cells appears to be associated with increased infections and failed response to vaccines in the elderly. As a result of the combination of thymic involution, repeated antigenic exposure and alteration in susceptibility to apoptosis (increased for CD4 and decreased for CD8), the thymic and lymphoid tissue in the aged host becomes populated with anergic (nonresponsive) memory CD8+CD28− T cells resulting in impaired cell mediated immunity. The potential for far-reaching effects of the presence of senescent T cells is illustrated by the correlation between poor humoral response to vaccination in the elderly and an increase in the proportion of CD8 T cells that lack expression of CD28.[68,69]

There is also a decline in delayed-type skin hypersensitivity (DTH)[70–73] and the assessment of this has become a useful measure of cell-mediated immunity. Generally, a battery of skin test antigens (usually four to six antigens) is required to adequately assess DTH. The number of skin test positive reactions declines with age from more than 80% in young individuals to less than 20% in older individuals.[73] As with most functional measures in geriatric populations, there is remarkable heterogeneity. In one study,[72] 17.9% of subjects over age 66 years and living at home were anergic compared with 41% who were living in a nursing home but able to care for themselves and 60% who were functionally impaired and living in a nursing home. Although skin testing is a good indicator of cell-mediated immunologic health, it is heavily influenced by both acute and chronic illnesses and the component of anergy because of "aging" is difficult to discern. Furthermore, concomitant in vitro testing suggests that not all anergic patients have impaired in vitro responses,[37,74] suggesting that some of the observed skin test anergy may be either technical (i.e., due to difficulty in intradermal injection in the skin of elderly people) or because of a deficit in antigen presentation, as described above. Thus both in vivo cutaneous DTH assessment and in vitro lymphocyte testing may be necessary to more adequately identify individuals who are truly anergic and presumably immunodeficient. The relevance of this type of determination is apparent by the repeated demonstrations of an association between anergy and mortality.[43,72,73,75–77]

The issue of an age-associated decline in DTH has particular relevance for the testing of past or current tuberculosis exposure.[78–82] Acknowledging the high incidence of anergy in elderly patients, care must be given to assess response to control antigens, such as *Candida*, mumps, or streptokinase-streptodornase (SKSD) before concluding a negative tuberculin reaction indicates absence of TB exposure. Furthermore, for the healthy elderly, false positive skin tests may be observed in those who have had repeated testing ("booster" effect).[82]

Qualitative changes in B-cell function

In the humoral immune system, there are no consistent changes in the number of peripheral blood B cells with age. The decline in antibody production following vaccination in the elderly is the result of reduced antigen-specific B-cell expansion and differentiation, leading to production of low titres of antigen-specific IgG. Most studies indicate a mild to moderate increase in total serum immunoglobulin (Ig)G and IgA levels with no change in IgM levels.[83,84] Declines in antibody titers to specific foreign antigens have been noted, including naturally occurring antibodies to the isoagglutinins,[85] and titers of antibody to foreign antigens such as microbial antigens.[86–90] Both the primary[91] and secondary immune responses to vaccination are impaired. Elderly patients tend to have lower peak titers of antibody and more rapid declines in titers after immunization[92,93] and the peak titer occurring slightly later (2 to 6 weeks rather than 2 to 3 weeks postvaccination) than in younger people.[94] In contrast, serum autoantibodies may have organ specificity, such as antiparietal cell, antithyroglobulin, and antineuronal antibodies.[46,95–101] With aging, there is a decreased generation of early progenitor B cells resulting in low output of new naïve B cells with clonal expansion of antigen-experienced B cells. This results in limited repertoire in immunoglobulin generation (through class switch) in B cells as observed in elderly humans and old mice[102] with limited antigen-specific B-cell expansion and differentiation, leading to production of reduced titers of antigen-specific IgG. The antibodies produced by older B cells are commonly of low affinity due to reduced class switching and somatic recombination in the variable region of the immunoglobulin gene that is necessary for antibody production and diversity. The generation of memory B cells is highly dependent on germinal centers, the formation of which are known to decline with age. The formation of germinal centers is dependent to some extent on interactions of B cells with CD4+ T helper cells, and the age-related quantitative and qualitative changes in T and B cells may account, in large part, for the clinically observed diminished response to vaccines. For example, although 70% to 90% of individuals less than 65 years old are effectively protected after influenza vaccination, only 10% to 30% of frail elderly are protected.[105]

Organ-nonspecific autoantibodies, such as antibodies to DNA and rheumatoid factors, also increase with age. Circulating immune complexes may also increase with advancing age.[95,106] The reason why auto-antibodies increase with age is not known. Several explanations are possible, including alterations in immune regulation and an increase in stimulation of B-cell clones because of recurrent or chronic infections or increased tissue degradation.

Cytokine dysregulation and aging

There has been an increased awareness of alterations in the production and degradation of cytokines with age (Table 13-1). In vitro studies to assess functional aspects of lymphocytes after stimulation with mitogens show a decline in proliferative responses possibly as a result of decreased T-cell lymphokine production and regulation, particularly interleukin-2 (IL-2).[44,48,107,108] Decreases in the percentage of IL-2 receptor positive cells, IL-2 receptor density, and in the expression of IL-2 and IL-2 receptor specific mRNA in old humans have been reported.[48,109] IL-2 production in response to specific antigens also declines. There is a profound decline in the proliferative capacity of T lymphocytes to nonspecific mitogens.[46,48,73,110] In addition, antigen-specific declines in the proliferative potential of T cells have been demonstrated.[70,111] The number and affinity of mitogen receptors on T lymphocytes do not change with age.[112] However, the number of T lymphocytes capable of dividing in response to mitogen exposure is reduced, and the activated T cells do not undergo as many divisions.[80]

Table 13-1. Immunologic Markers of Aging

Decreased	Increased
Thymic output	Memory T and B cells
Naïve peripheral T cells	Oligoclonal expansion of memory lymphocytes
Diversity of T- and B-cell repertoire	
Co-stimulatory stimuli to T cells	CMV specific CD8+/CD4+ T cells
CD28+ T cells	CD45 RO+ T cells
CD45+ T cells	CD 28− T cells
IL-2, INF-γ, IL-12, IL-10, IL-13	IL-6, SCF*, LIF†
Proliferation with mitogens	
Delayed type hypersensitivity	Anergic T cells
Response to vaccination	

*Stem cell factor
†Leukemia inhibitory factor

Superimposed upon the accumulation of a relatively inert naïve T-cell fraction observed with advancing age, there appears also to be a shift in predominance of helper T-cell responses from type 1 (TH1) to type 2 (TH2). Cells of the TH1 type produce IL-2, interferon-γ, and TNF-α and predominantly mediate cell-mediated immune and inflammatory responses, whereas cells of the TH2 type produce IL-4, IL-5, IL-6, and IL-10, factors that enhance humoral immunity (Figure-13-1).[56] Whereas the decline in IL-2 and IL-12 may contribute to the observed decline in cellular immune function, the increase in proinflammatory cytokines (particularly IL-6) may contribute to the metabolic changes associated with frailty. It has been proposed that a chronic exposure to such proinflammatory signals contributes to the phenotype of frailty.[113] In fact, elevated IL-6 levels have been shown to correlate well with functional decline and mortality in a population of community-dwelling elderly people.[114] Thus the inflammation-related biomarkers are powerful predictors of frailty and mortality[115,116] in the elderly and this phenomenon is referred to as "inflamm-aging.[49]"

In the steady state (i.e., in the absence of stress, trauma, infection, or disease), IL-6 is tightly controlled and levels in the serum are typically measured in the very low picogram range. Among the regulators of IL-6 are sex steroids (estrogen and testosterone), and, at menopause, detectable IL-6 levels appear in the blood in apparently healthy individuals. This inappropriate presence of a circulating proinflammatory molecule has garnered great interest among biogerontologists because it provides a rational explanation for many of the phenotypic features of frailty and levels associated with a number of age-associated disorders, including atherosclerosis, diabetes, Alzheimer's disease,[117,118] and osteoporosis.[119,120]

CLINICAL CONSEQUENCES OF IMMUNE SENESCENCE

Autoimmunity

Waldorf[91] speculated that autoimmunity plays an important role in the aging process. Cohen and others have alternatively proposed that autoimmunity may play an important physiologic role in the regenerative and reparative process that is ongoing during aging.[121] Certain autoimmune diseases have

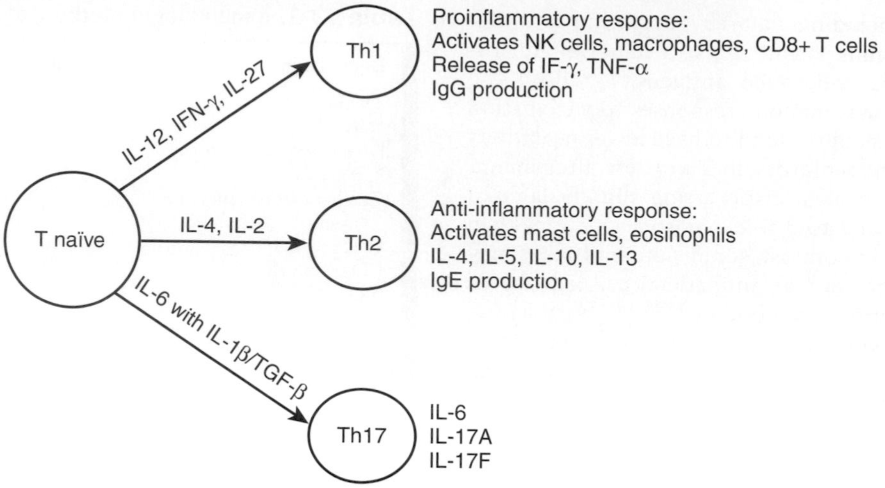

Figure 13-1. Differentiation of naïve TH cell into effector T cells. The differentiation of naïve T cells into various effector T-cell subsets occurs in response to stimulation by distinct antigen-presenting cells and cytokine exposure. These functional subsets include TH1, TH2, TH17, and Treg cells. These subsets play distinct roles in the genesis and control of cell-mediated immunity and inflammation. Traditionally, the TH1 responses have been implicated in many autoimmune and inflammatory disease states and cytokines produced by these cells, primarily IL-2, IFN-γ, and TNF-α induce both mononuclear and polymorphonuclear cell infiltration and activation in the target tissues. In this fashion, deregulated expression of proinflammatory cytokines is thought to play a central role in the development of autoimmune diseases and chronic inflammatory responses. In contrast, TH2 cells secrete IL-4 and IL-10 that promote humoral immunity and inhibit TH1 responses and have been implicated in amelioration and remission of autoimmune and inflammatory diseases. A third TH subset, named TH17, has recently been described that depends on IL-23 for survival and expansion, and has been identified as a major mediator of pathogenic inflammatory responses associated with autoimmunity, allergy, organ transplantation, and tumor development. Over the last few years, regulatory T (Treg) cells of several types have been identified and shown to play an active role to suppress autoreactive T cells; however, these cells are also capable of suppressing the host's ability to mount an optimal cell-mediated immune response to antigens and tumor cells if their numbers and activity are not controlled.

their highest incidence in old age, such as pernicious anemia, thyroiditis, bullous pemphigoid, rheumatoid arthritis, and temporal arteritis, suggesting that the age-related increase in autoantibodies may have clinical relevance,[122–127] although this latter point remains unproven.

Autoimmunity may also play a role in vascular disease in old age.[128] Giant T-cell arteritis is a common disease in old age[124,129] and is associated with degenerative vascular disease. Indeed, immune mechanisms may result in atherosclerosis, a final common pathway of pathology secondary to a variety of vascular insults.[130] A number of antivascular antibodies have been described in man[131–134] that are associated with diseases of the vasculature. Antiphospholipid antibodies are associated with a variety of pathologic states of the vasculature, including stroke and vascular dementia,[135,136] temporal arteritis, and ischemic heart disease.[137,138] However, the exact mechanism by which antiphospholipid antibodies cause vascular injury remains unknown.[139] The increased occurrence of antiphospholipid antibodies with age[140–142] and the association of these autoantibodies with vascular disease may represent a predisposing immunologic factor for immune-mediated vascular disease in elderly people. Autoantibodies to vascular heparan sulfate proteoglycans (vHSPG) may also be important in vascular injury in old age,[133] since vHSPG plays an important role in normal anticoagulation and cholesterol metabolism.[143]

Immune senescence and cancer

Age is the single greatest risk for cancer.[144] It has long been postulated that immune mechanisms play an important role in recognizing and destroying tumor cells, and thus an age-associated decline in immune function might be invoked to explain the increased rate of cancer in old age. The problem with this hypothesis is that, as rational as it sounds, it has been very difficult to prove (see later discussion). Furthermore, there are other explanations for the observed increased malignant disease in the elderly, not the least of which is the estimated prolonged time (measured in decades for many epithelial tumors) it takes to sustain the multiple genetic and epigenetic events required for malignant transformation and tumor growth to the point of clinical detection. An alternative explanation suggests that the host and host factors change over time, favoring progression and expression in later life. These two hypotheses to explain the increase in late-life malignancy have aptly been described as "seed vs. soil."[145]

From an immunologic and "soil" standpoint, there are two principal observations that relate to malignancies and age: (1) deregulation of proliferation of cells directly controlled by the immune system and (2) evidence of increased malignancies in late life that could be hypothetically restrained by nonsenescent immunity. These will be discussed sequentially.

Proliferative disorders of the lymphocyte are common in old age. Although bimodal in incidence, the peak in late-life lymphoma includes a disproportionate incidence of nodular B-cell types.[146] Both old humans and mice have commonly exhibited a monoclonal gammopathy (paraprotein) in the last quartile of the life span.[47–150] Monoclonal gammopathies increase with age and may occur in 79% of sera from subjects over the age of 95 years.[151–153] Radl[151] has defined four categories of age-associated monoclonal gammopathy: (1) myeloma or related disorders; (2) benign B-cell neoplasia; (3) immune deficiency, with T cell greater than B-cell loss; and (4) chronic antigenic stimulation. He speculates that the third category is by far the most common, and that this is what occurs with immune senescence. It is possible that age-associated immune dysfunction is initially associated with markers of aberrant immune regulation, such as increased levels of paraproteinemia and/or autoantibody, which may later contribute to the pathogenesis of lymphoma. Monoclonal gammopathies may cause morbidity, particularly renal disease in the absence of overt multiple myeloma.[154] In a minority of cases of monoclonal gammopathies, a malignant evolution may occur.[154–156] Multiple myeloma also demonstrates an age-related increase in incidence.[157] Although treatment is not generally indicated for monoclonal gammopathies,[152] treatment of myeloma is often useful. Another common malignant transformation of the lymphocyte in old age is chronic lymphocytic leukemia.[158] Non-Hodgkin's lymphoma also increases in incidence with age, whereas Hodgkin's lymphoma has a bimodal distribution.[159]

Finally, a discussion of cancer development and aging would not be complete without considering the importance of the decline in immunity and associated failure of "immune surveillance."[160–163] It has long been proposed that the decline in immune function contributes to the increased incidence of malignancy. However, despite the appeal of such a hypothesis, scientific support has been limited and the topic remains controversial.[164] Proponents of an immune explanation point to experiments in which outbred strains of mice with heterogeneous immune functions were followed for their life span.[165,166] Those that demonstrated better functions early in life (as determined by a limited panel of assays available at the time on a small sample of blood) were found to have fewer spontaneous malignancies and a longer life than those estimated to be less immunologically competent. Furthermore, it is difficult to deny that profoundly immunodeficient animals or humans are subject to a more frequent occurrence of malignant disease. Thus it would stand to reason that others with less severe immunodeficiency would also be subject to malignancy, perhaps less dramatically so. However, the malignancies associated with profound immunodeficiency (e.g., with AIDS or after organ transplantation) are usually lymphomas, Kaposi's sarcoma, or leukemia and not the more common malignancies of geriatric populations (lung, breast, colon, and prostate cancers). Accordingly, it is fair to say that the question of the influence of age-acquired immunodeficiency on the incidence of cancer in elderly people is unresolved. There is much greater consensus on the importance of immune senescence in the clinical management of cancer, including the problems associated with infection and disease progression.

Immune senescence and infections in old age

An aging immune system is less capable of mounting an effective immune response after infectious challenge and thus infection in elderly people is associated with greater morbidity and mortality.[167,168] Most notable in this regard are infections with influenza virus, pneumococcal pneumonia, and various urinary tract pathogens. However, older individuals are also more susceptible to skin infections, gastroenteritis (including *Clostridium difficile*), tuberculosis, and herpes zoster (shingles). There is also an increase in hospital- and nursing home–acquired infections in elderly people. These susceptibilities to infection are due to both immune senescence and other changes more common among older individuals, such as a reduced ciliary escalator efficiency and cough reflex predisposing to aspiration pneumonia; urinary and fecal incontinence predisposing to urinary tract and perineal skin infections; and immobility predisposing to pressure sores and wound infections.

Infections in older people frequently present atypically.[74,144,169] Old individuals may not have typical "hard" signs of infection, such as spiking fever, leukocytosis, prominent inflammatory infiltrates on chest x-rays, or rebound tenderness for those with an acute abdomen. Thus a change in mental status or mild malaise might be the only clinical indication of urinary tract infection or even pneumonia. Lower baseline temperatures may require the need for monitoring the change in temperature, rather than the absolute temperature. This is particularly true in the frail elderly, for whom infections caused by unusual organisms, recurrent infections with the same pathogen, or reactivation of quiescent diseases such as tuberculosis or herpes zoster virus can be counted on to present atypically and also to be resistant to standard therapy.

Influenza

Most of the significant morbidity and excess mortality during influenza epidemics occurs in older adults.[170] Age itself, in addition to and separate from the many comorbid conditions of older people, is a significant risk factor for severe complications of influenza.[171] It is widely held that much of the increased susceptibility of elderly people to influenza and its complications are attributable to immunologic factors, including reduced antibody responsiveness and influenza-specific cell-mediated immunity as discussed above. The role of humoral immunity, especially in the form of neutralizing antibodies, is perhaps most important for preventing and limiting the initial infection[172] rather than promoting recovery. T-cell-mediated responses appear to be more important and primarily involved in postinfection viral clearance and recovery; influenza-specific cytotoxic T lymphocyte (CTL) activity correlates with rapid clearance of virus in infected human volunteers, even in the absence of detectable serum antibody.[173] This has been experimentally confirmed in several studies through the adoptive transfer of influenza-specific CTLs in mouse models.[174,175] No doubt influenza-specific antibody declines with age, whether because of natural infection or vaccination,[176–178] and this presumably translates to an increased risk of influenza infection. However, and perhaps equally important, CTL,[62,179] human leukocyte antigen (HLA) restriction by influenza-specific T-cell clones, and lymphocyte proliferative responses also decline with age. T cell-mediated cytokine responses, most notably IL-2, also decrease with age, although this has not been as clearly established for healthy elderly people[61] as it has been for frail elderly people.[60] Together these observations account for much of the age-related increase in influenza susceptibility and morbidity. Furthermore, although influenza in otherwise healthy unvaccinated elderly people leads to an illness that lasts nearly twice as long as their younger counterparts, influenza illness duration in those elderly people previously vaccinated (i.e., vaccine failures) is comparable to the illness duration in vaccinated healthy young adults. This observation remains true when the vaccine-to-circulating strain match is poor, negating poor vaccine match as a reason not to vaccinate seniors annually. In the long-term care setting, influenza vaccination was found to be effective in reducing influenza-like illness and preventing pneumonia, hospitalization, and deaths (both infectious and "all cause" mortality). Among the elderly residing in the community setting, the benefits of annual vaccination have been demonstrably modest in some studies,[180] and more effective in others.[81,182] Among many efforts to increase the immune response and hence protection from influenza vaccination in the elderly, component hemagglutinin dose within the vaccine and higher doses were found to be more immunogenic.[183] It is important to note that, despite all of the changes occurring with age and comorbid conditions of age, influenza vaccine still is highly cost-effective in reducing influenza-related infections and complications, especially in the high-risk elderly population.[171,182,184]

Pneumococcal disease

Reduced immune competence, whether due to age, disease, or drug therapy, introduces risk for complications from pneumococcal disease. For example, one study found the incidence of pneumococcal disease to be 70 cases per 100,000 in individuals over the age of 70 compared with 5 cases per 100,000 in younger adults.[185] *Streptococcus pneumoniae* is a gram-positive lancet-shaped diplococcus that normally colonizes the nasopharynx and was present in up to 70% of individuals in the preantibiotic era. The pathogenic form is encapsulated, and antigenic variants of the polysaccharide capsule are sufficiently immunogenic to be useful as vaccine targets. The rising prevalence of penicillin-resistant *Pneumococcus*[186] renders infection treatment more difficult and reinforces the need for prevention as a primary management strategy for pneumococcal disease.

Pneumonia is the most prevalent expression of infection with *S. pneumoniae* but other sites of infection are also clinically important. These include otitis media, sinusitis, meningitis, septic arthritis, pericarditis, endocarditis, peritonitis, cellulitis, glomerulonephritis, and sepsis (especially postsplenectomy). Chronic obstructive pulmonary disease is an independent risk factor for occurrence of and complications from pneumococcal infection, and this might relate to the altered mechanics of clearing secretions and altered immunity within the lung itself. Risk factors for pneumococcal infections also include conditions that predispose an individual to aspiration of pneumococci, such as swallowing disorders, a feature not uncommon in stroke survivors.

Prevention is the best form of defense, and the polysaccharide antigens of the pneumococcal vaccine have been used to generate T-cell independent responses, a theoretical advantage for older adults because immune senescence is thought to primarily perturb T-cell more so than B-cell responses (see previous discussion). Yet, studies on pneumococcal vaccine efficacy in disease prevention often have been disappointing or inconclusive,[178,187] with more recent studies suggesting efficacy and cost-effectiveness.[188–191] Consequently, underuse of pneumococcal vaccine has been held accountable for the development of outbreaks in nursing facilities in which vaccination rates were low.[192,193] Currently, revaccination is recommended for persons aged 65 and older if they received vaccine 5 or more years prior and were less than 65 years of age at the time of vaccination. Meanwhile, new vaccine designs aim to better stimulate the immune response in older adults by recruiting T-cell help through polysaccharide conjugation with a peptide combined with cytokine[194] or by using a peptide target.[195] Whether these approaches are superior for an immune senescent patient remains to be defined.

Varicella-zoster virus

Herpes zoster (shingles) is caused by varicella zoster virus (VZV) and is increasingly prevalent with advancing age, as are its severity and complications.[196–200] The majority of cases occur after the age of 60 years[201] and by 80 years, the annual attack rate is 0.8%. Two major complications of herpes zoster, postherpetic neuralgia and cranial nerve zoster (often of the ophthalmic nerve, and not infrequently resulting in lower motor neuron paresis), are the most disabling. Postherpetic neuralgia occurs in more than 25% of patients 60 years and older and is strongly associated with sleep disturbance and depression.[202–206] Bell's palsy[207] and Ménière's[208] disease, both conditions associated with advanced age, have also been linked to herpes zoster. VZV-specific cell-mediated immunity correlates closely with susceptibility to herpes zoster in large populations, such as patients with lymphomas, bone marrow transplant recipients, and immunocompetent elderly persons.[209–216] Whereas a decline in VZV-specific cell-mediated immunity is a major precipitant for VZV reactivation,[217] demonstrable VZV immunity limits the viral replication and spread.[218] In a randomized clinical trial with a live attenuated VZV vaccine among adults aged 60 years and over, vaccination reduced the incidence of herpes zoster, and postherpetic neuralgia compared with those who received a placebo.[219] The magnitude of benefit with reduction in postherpetic neuralgia was more pronounced in those aged 70 years or more. This study led to approval of vaccine among the elderly greater than 60 years of age in the United States, and also in Europe and Australia.

SECONDARY CAUSES OF ACQUIRED IMMUNODEFICIENCY IN OLD AGE

In contrast to the normative changes that may result in a mild idiopathic-acquired immunodeficiency with aging, a variety of secondary causes of acquired immunodeficiency occur in elderly people that may be severe, yet reversible. The distinction between secondary causes of immune deficiency from "normal" age-related changes is an important clinical distinction. The clinician needs a high index of suspicion for acquired immunodeficiency in old age, since many causes are reversible and can be the primary reason for infection risk, altered presentation of infection, or inadequate response to usual therapy.

Malnutrition

The effects of malnutrition on the immune system may be profound, and clearly increase the risk of infection in elderly people.[220,221] Immune deficits in undernourished ambulatory elderly people may be reversed by nutritional supplementation. Malnutrition affects up to 50% of hospitalized elderly people and is highly associated with poor acute care outcomes, including death.[222–224] Severe protein, calorie, vitamin, and micronutrient deficiencies may cause immune impairment resulting in poor outcomes in response to infection.[225,226] An absolute lymphocyte count below 1500 cells/mm^3 often indicates some degree of malnutrition, and a count below 900 cells/mm^3 is a frequent correlate of both severe malnutrition and immunodeficiency.

Comorbidity

Chronic illnesses such as congestive heart failure[230] and Alzheimer's disease may be associated with progressive cachexia despite adequate food intake, and may be mediated by tumor necrosis factor or other inflammatory mediators.[94,102] In patients with dementia, despite adequate food intake, malnutrition is common and is associated with a fourfold increase in infection.[102] Diabetes mellitus, common in geriatric populations, is frequently associated with diminished immune function.

Polypharmacy

Since elderly people frequently consume a number of prescription or over-the-counter medications, drug-induced acquired immunodeficiency is probably far more common than is generally appreciated. Numerous commonly prescribed drugs cause neutropenia and lymphocytopenia. Analgesics, nonsteroidal antiinflammatory agents, steroids, antithyroids, antibiotics, antiarthritic drugs, antipsychotics, antidepressants, hypnotics/sedatives, anticonvulsants, antihypertensives, diuretics, histamine type-2 (H2) blockers, and hypoglycemics are among a long list of commonly prescribed medications that may suppress inflammatory and/or immune responses.[227–229] T lymphocytes also have calcium channels along with cholinergic, histaminic, and adrenergic receptors, and drugs that work on these targets may have unappreciated effects on immune function.[230] Hypogammaglobulinemia may also be induced by medications.[231] Recent studies have also demonstrated that medications may also be associated with an impaired or enhanced response to vaccination.[232,233]

HIV and other infections

HIV infection may be a cause of acquired immunodeficiency in elderly people and should always be considered part of the differential diagnosis of acquired immunodeficiency in elderly patients with lymphopenia and appropriate risk factors.[234–238] The most common source of AIDS in the elderly was until recently transfusion, but now it is acquired through sexual activity.[239–241] Dementia is often a common presenting feature of AIDS,[242] and AIDS should be considered part of the differential diagnosis of dementia in aged patients with appropriate risk factors. The possibility that many cases of AIDS will go undetected in the elderly has considerable implications for geriatric-health care workers. In the United States, approximately 11% of patients with AIDS are over 50 years of age—a recognized health issue in geriatric population—and age could be an independent risk factor in rapid progression of the disease.[240,243]

Stress

Psychosocial isolation, depression, and stress are probable causes of immune dysfunction in old age.[244,245] There is an increased incidence of cancer during periods of psychosocial stress and depression related to bereavement.[246,247] Social isolation and marital discord may impair immune function.[248] Chronic stress in the form of care giving for a demented spouse also reduces influenza vaccine response.[249] Interventions to enhance social contact demonstrably improve immune function as measured by a variety of laboratory measures.[250] Immobility may also cause immune dysfunction, and exercise may maintain function in old age in both animals and humans.[251] These aspects of psychoneuroimmunology obviously have particular relevance in the interdisciplinary practice of geriatrics, given the high prevalence of psychosocial problems in elderly people.

Immune function assessment

The tests necessary to perform an immunologic evaluation to establish the diagnosis of acquired immunodeficiency in old age are readily available to the clinician.[252] The humoral immune system is readily tested by measuring total serum protein and quantitative immunoglobulin (IgG, IgA, and IgM) levels. Serum protein electrophoresis, and immunoelectrophoresis are useful to rule out monoclonal gammopathy, myeloma, and some forms of lymphoma, and may also provide clues to chronic inflammatory disease (polyclonal gammopathy, reduced albumin). Specific antibody titers such as isoagglutinins also provide additional information regarding B-cell function. The integrity of the cellular immune system is tested by blood leukocyte counts (including absolute lymphocyte counts), delayed skin test hypersensitivity employing a panel of at least six antigens, and in vitro testing such as measurements of lymphocyte subsets, the proliferative capacity of lymphocytes in response to mitogen or specific antigens, and cytokine production. The latter tests are often performed in a standard clinical immunology laboratory. Other more sophisticated immune tests are also available from the clinical immunology consultant and research laboratory.

Specific potentially reversible causes of acquired immunodeficiency, such as malnutrition or medications, should be sought in aged patients with recurrent or unusual infections, particularly those with lymphocytopenia and/or anergy. At a minimum, a medication review and a nutritional assessment should be performed, with monitoring of neutrophil or lymphocyte counts during nutritional supplementation or medication withdrawal. HIV infections should always be considered in high-risk patients, including the very old, particularly because the risks for spread of HIV among health care workers and family members caring for frail elderly persons.

Immune enhancement and other clinical strategies

Numerous interventions have been employed in an attempt to enhance immune function in old age. The use of thymic and other hormones, mediations, and cytokines have been proposed as immunoenhancing agents, but none of these has gained clinical acceptance.[253] In animals, calorie restriction without undernutrition clearly prolongs life and is associated with immune competence into late life; however, the benefits of calorie restriction in man remain unknown.[254] Supplemental zinc and other trace metals may also have benefit in some older patients in restoring lymphocyte proliferation in vitro, and in enhancing delayed-type skin hypersensitivity reactions, but their effects in preventing or reducing the morbidity of infections or other problems potentially related to immunodeficiency in old age have not been demonstrated.[255–258] Vitamin C and other antioxidants may also have beneficial effects on immune function.[259,260] Megadose dietary supplementation does not significantly improve immune function in the normal-aged animal.[261]

Vaccinations are critically important in maintaining the health of elderly people in the face of declining immunity and are effective in preventing pneumococcal pneumonia, influenza, and tetanus and in reducing mortality from these illnesses.[251,262–264] Although elderly people achieve lower peak titers and more rapid declines of serum antibody levels, the majority of healthy elderly people achieve titers that are generally presumed protective.[89,92,265,266] However, chronically ill, frail elderly people, particularly institutionalized, malnourished individuals, may not achieve adequate protective peak antibody titers against pneumococcal pneumonia or influenza when immunized with a single dose of vaccine, and supplemental doses are recommended by some experts.[267–269] Older persons may require revaccination with tetanus toxoid more frequently than every 10 years (as currently recommended) to maintain protective levels of antibodies in the serum.[88,270] The use of new protein conjugate and immunoconjugate vaccines may improve the response in older people.[271–273]

CONCLUSIONS

There are mild to moderate changes within the immune system with normal aging, and these render an individual susceptible to certain infections and may also affect clinical presentation. A more profound deficit in immune function is commonly observed in geriatric populations, but when this occurs, the clinician should be highly suspicious that secondary (i.e., causes other than just "aging") are involved. Reversible causes of acquired immunodeficiency in this age group include comorbid diseases, malnutrition, medications, stress, and possibly infections, including HIV. Newer therapeutic approaches may ultimately be useful in the treatment of acquired immunodeficiency in elderly people, particularly in high-risk individuals who are substantially impaired by the effects of aging and diseases of old age on the immune system.

KEY POINTS

Clinical Immunology of Aging

- The immune system changes with age, primarily affecting T-cell and B-cell functions
- Changes in the immune system are relevant to the changing clinical presentation and expression of disease.
- Immune senescence affects vaccine effectiveness.

For a complete list of references, please visit online only at www.expertconsult.com

CHAPTER 14

Effects of Aging on the Cardiovascular System

Susan E. Howlett

Advanced age is a major risk factor for the development of cardiovascular disease. Why age increases the risk of cardiovascular disease is debatable. The increased risk might arise simply because there is more time to be exposed to risk factors such as hypertension, smoking, and dyslipidemia. In other words, the aging process itself has little impact on the cardiovascular system. However, an emerging view is that the accumulation of cellular and subcellular deficits in the aging heart and blood vessels renders the cardiovascular system susceptible to the effects of cardiovascular diseases. Although increased exposure to risk factors likely contributes to the development of cardiovascular disease in aging, there is considerable evidence that the structure and function of the human heart and vasculature change importantly as a function of the normal aging process. These changes occur in the absence of risk factors other than age, and in the absence of overt clinical signs of cardiovascular disease.

AGING-ASSOCIATED CHANGES IN VASCULAR STRUCTURE

Studies in blood vessels from apparently healthy humans have shown that the vasculature changes with age. The large elastic arteries dilate, something that is evident to the naked eye, and that is well seen in arterial radiographic studies. These readily visible changes arise from microscopic changes in the wall structure of the centrally located, large elastic arteries.[1,2] The arterial wall is composed of three different layers, which are known as tunics. The outermost layer, or tunica adventitia, is composed of collagen fibers and elastic tissue. The middle layer, known as the tunica media, is a relatively thick layer composed of connective tissue, smooth muscle cells, and elastic tissue. The contractile properties of the arterial wall are determined primarily by variations in the composition of the media. The innermost layer of the arterial wall, or tunica intima, consists of a connective tissue layer and an inner layer of endothelial cells. Endothelial cells are squamous epithelial cells that play an important role in regulation of normal vascular function, and endothelial dysfunction contributes to vascular disease.[3] Age-associated changes in these different layers have a profound effect on the structure and function of the vasculature in older adults.

The process by which the structure of the arterial wall is modified by the aging process is known as remodeling. Structural changes due to remodeling are apparent even in early adulthood and increase with age.[2] Aging-related arterial remodeling is thought to provide an ideal setting in which vascular diseases can thrive. Indeed, structural changes that occur in the arteries of normotensive aging humans are observed in hypertensive patients at much younger ages.[2]

One of the most prominent age-related changes in the structure of the vasculature in humans is dilation of large elastic arteries, which leads to an increase in lumen size.[4] In addition, the walls of large elastic arteries thicken with age. Studies of carotid wall intima plus media (IM) thickness in adult human arteries have shown that IM thickness increases between twofold and threefold by 90 years of age.[1] Increased IM thickness is an important risk factor for atherosclerosis independent of age.[2] Thickening of the arterial wall in aging is due mainly to an increase in the thickness of the intima.[1] Whether thickening of the media occurs in aging is controversial. However, studies have shown that the number of vascular smooth muscle cells in the media declines with age, while the remaining cells increase in size.[5] Whether these hypertrophied smooth muscle cells are fully functional or whether this is one way in which aging is deleterious to vascular function is not yet clear. The major structural changes in the vasculature with age are summarized in Figure 14-1.

Age-associated thickening of the intima is due, in part, to changes in connective tissues in aging arteries. The collagen content of the intima and collagen cross-linking increase markedly with age in human arteries.[1,3,6] However, the elastin content of the intima declines, and elastin fraying and fragmentation have been reported.[1,6] It has been proposed that repeated cycles of distention followed by elastic recoil may promote the loss of elastin and the deposition of collagen in aging arteries.[1] These changes in collagen and elastin content are believed to have important effects on the distensibility or stiffness of aging arteries, as discussed in more detail in the "Arterial Stiffness in Aging Arteries" section.

In addition to alterations in intimal connective tissues in aging, studies in human arteries have shown that the aging process modifies the structure of the endothelial cells themselves. Endothelial cells increase in size with age or hypertrophy. In addition, endothelial cell shape becomes irregular.[7] The permeability of endothelial cells increases with age and vascular smooth muscle cells may infiltrate the subendothelial space in aging arteries.[1,7] There also is considerable evidence that many of the substances released by the endothelium are altered in aging arteries.[8] The impact of these changes on vascular function is discussed in more detail in the next section.

ENDOTHELIAL FUNCTION IN AGING

Once regarded as an almost inert lining of the blood vessels, the vascular endothelium is now recognized to be metabolically active tissue involved in the many changes needed to maintain and regulate blood flow. The structure and function of the endothelium changes notably with age.[3,8,9] In younger adults, the vascular endothelium synthesizes and releases a variety of regulatory substances in response to both chemical and mechanical stimuli. For example, endothelial cells release substances, such as nitric oxide, prostacyclin, endothelins, interleukins, endothelial growth factors, adhesion molecules, plasminogen inhibitors, and von Willebrand factor.[10] These substances are involved in the regulation of vascular tone, angiogenesis, thrombosis, thrombolysis, and many other functions. There is evidence that the aging

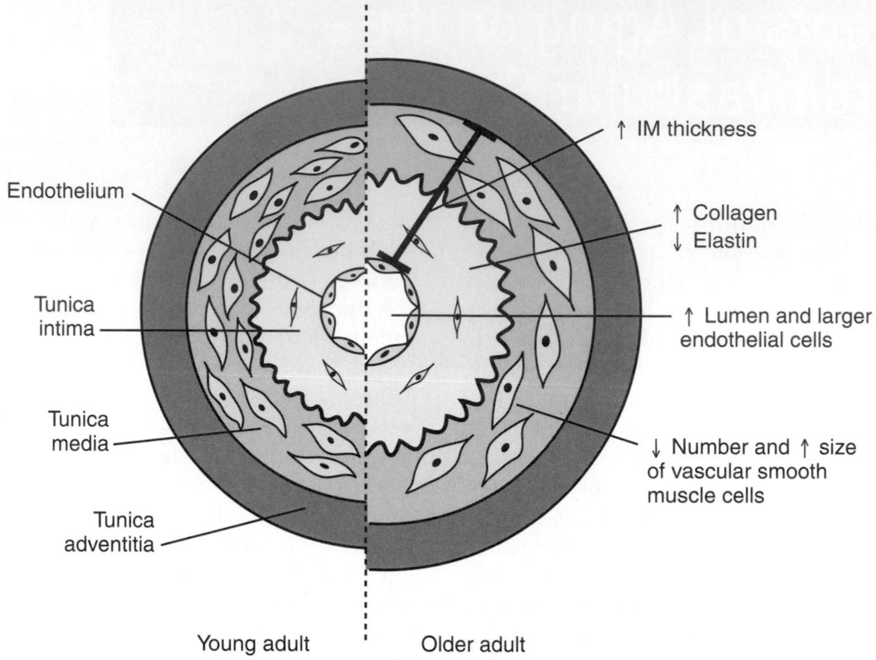

Figure 14-1. Remodeling of the central elastic arteries with age. The layers of the arterial wall are labeled as indicated. There are marked changes in central elastic arteries as a consequence of the aging process. The diameter of the lumen increases with age. Intima plus media (IM) thickness also increases, primarily as a consequence of an increase in the thickness of the tunica intima. An increase in collagen deposition and a decrease in elastin are responsible for intimal remodeling in aging arteries. The number of vascular smooth muscle cells in the tunica media decreases, whereas the remaining cells hypertrophy. Endothelial cell hypertrophy also occurs in aging arteries.

process may disrupt many of these normal functions of the vascular endothelium.

Endothelial dysfunction is most often measured as a disruption in endothelium-dependent relaxation. Endothelium-dependent relaxation is mediated by nitric oxide, which is released from the endothelium by mechanical stimuli, such as increased blood flow (shear stress), and by chemical stimuli (i.e., acetylcholine, serotonin, bradykinin, or thrombin).[10] When nitric oxide is released from the endothelium, it causes vascular smooth muscle relaxation by increasing intracellular levels of cGMP. The increased cGMP prevents the interaction of the contractile filaments actin and myosin.[11] Thus blood vessel relaxation is impaired with age. The age-related increase in vascular stiffness is, in part, related to the reduced ability of the vascular endothelium to produce nitric oxide as people age.[12] The decrease in nitric oxide release with age appears to be mediated by less effective acetylcholine activity.[13]

The mechanism by which nitric oxide activity is reduced in aging remains controversial. Nitric oxide is synthesized in endothelial cells by a constitutive enzyme called endothelial nitric oxide synthase (eNOS or NOS III).[14] There is some evidence that the levels of eNOS are reduced in aging, which could account for the decrease in nitric oxide activity in aging vasculature.[15] However, other studies suggest that factors such as the production of oxygen free radicals in aging endothelial cells may impair nitric oxide production in aging.[13] Further studies will be needed to fully understand the mechanism or mechanisms responsible for endothelial dysfunction in aging vasculature.

There is good evidence that endothelial dysfunction is an important cause of cardiovascular disease, independent of age.[3,8,9] Therefore age-related endothelial dysfunction is likely to make a major contribution to the increased risk of vascular disease in older adults.

ARTERIAL STIFFNESS IN AGING ARTERIES

Aging-related remodeling of the large, central elastic arteries has a major impact on the function of the cardiovascular system. One of the best-characterized functional changes in aging arteries is a decrease in the compliance or distensibility of aging arteries.[2] This resistance of aging arteries to deflection by blood flow is known as an increase in arterial stiffness.[16] This increase in arterial stiffness impairs the ability of the aorta, and its major branches, to expand and contract with changes in blood pressure. This lack of deflection of the blood flow increases the velocity at which the pulse wave travels within large arteries in older adults.[16] An increase in pulse wave velocity is related to hypertension, but pulse wave velocity can be measured separately from blood pressure. An increase in pulse wave velocity in aging is an important risk factor for future adverse cardiovascular events.[17]

The structural changes in the arterial wall described above are implicated in the increase in arterial stiffness observed in central elastic arteries in the aging heart. The increased collagen content and increased collagen cross-linking that occur in aging arteries are believed to increase arterial stiffness in aging.[1,3] Other factors such as reduced elastin content, elastin fragmentation, and increased elastase activity also are thought to increase stiffness in aging arteries.[3] Changes in the endothelial regulation of vascular smooth muscle tone and changes in other aspects of the arterial wall and vascular function also may contribute to the age-associated increase in arterial stiffness.[1,3]

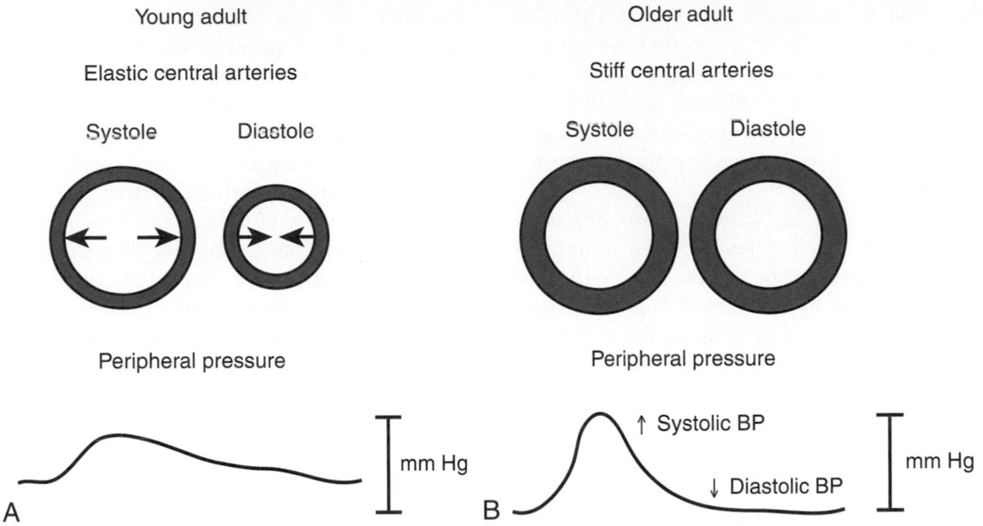

Figure 14-2. The age-associated increase in central artery stiffness has important effects on peripheral pressure. **A,** In young adults, the elastic central arteries expand with each cardiac contraction, so that a part of the stroke volume is transmitted peripherally in systole and the remainder is transmitted in diastole. **B,** In older adults, stiff central arteries do not expand with each contraction, so stroke volume is transmitted in systole. This leads to an increase in systolic blood pressure and a decrease in diastolic blood pressure in older adults. *(Modified from Izzo JL Jr: Arterial stiffness and the systolic hypertension syndrome. Curr Opin Cardiol 2004;19: 341–352.)*

Arterial stiffness is thought to be responsible for some of the changes in blood pressure that are reported in older adults.[18] In younger adults, recoil in the elastic central arteries transmits a portion of each stroke volume in systole and a portion of each stroke volume in diastole, as illustrated in Figure 14-2, *A*. However, in aging arteries, the increase in stiffness of large arterial walls is thought to contribute to the increased systolic arterial pressure and the decreased diastolic pressure that are characteristically observed in aging.[18] In this way, stiff central arteries can lead to an increase in pulse pressure in aging.[18] These changes occur because increased stiffness abolishes elastic recoil in central elastic arteries. This means that blood flow is transmitted during systole, which leads to a high systolic pressure.[18] As blood flow is transmitted in systole, the elastic recoil does not dissipate in diastole and diastolic pressure declines with age, as shown diagrammatically in Figure 14-2, *B*. This increase in systolic pressure with no change or a decrease in diastolic pressure leads to isolated systolic hypertension, which is the most common form of hypertension in older adults.[19] Studies have shown that isolated systolic hypertension increases the risk of cardiovascular disease.[20] Therefore aging-related changes in stiffness of large elastic arteries can explain many of the changes in blood pressure observed in aging and may contribute to the increased risk of cardiovascular disease in older adults. In addition, this increase in central artery stiffness is thought to play a role in some of the age-associated changes in the heart, both by increasing the work of the heart and decreasing coronary artery flow, as discussed in the next section.

Age-related changes in blood vessels may vary between different vascular beds. The structural changes that lead to increased arterial stiffness are much more pronounced in large, elastic arteries, such as the carotid artery, than in smaller, muscular arteries such as the brachial artery.[1,4] However, there are age-related changes in vascular reactivity in vessels other than the central elastic arteries. For example, the responsiveness of arterioles to drugs that stimulate α_1-adrenergic receptors declines with aging.[21] Vascular responsiveness to either endothelin or angiotensin receptor agonists also may decline with age, although this has not been extensively investigated and there is no evidence for such changes in humans.[21] Few studies have investigated the impact of age on vascular responsiveness in veins, but most studies report that age has little impact on the responsiveness of veins to a variety of pharmacologic agents.[21] Investigation of age-dependent alterations in vascular reactivity is an important area of inquiry; such changes would affect the responsiveness of the aging vasculature to drugs that target blood vessels in humans. Table 14-1 summarizes the major age-associated changes in the vasculature, along with the clinical consequences of these alterations.

Table 14-1. Age-Related Changes in the Vasculature

Age-Associated Changes in Vasculature	Clinical Consequences
↑ Intimal thickness	Promotes atherosclerosis
↑ Collagen, reduced elastin, ↑ vascular stiffness	Systolic hypertension
Endothelial cell dysfunction	↑ Risk of vascular disease

EFFECT OF THE AGING PROCESS ON THE STRUCTURE OF THE HEART

The aging process has obvious effects on the structure of the heart at both the macroscopic and microscopic levels. At the macroscopic level, there is a noted increase in the deposition of fat on the outer, epicardial surface of the aging heart.[22,23] Calcium deposition in specific regions of the heart, known as calcification, is commonly observed in the aging heart.[23] There also are changes in the gross morphologic structure of individual heart chambers with age. There is an age-associated increase in the size of the atria. Furthermore, the atria dilate and their volume increases with age.[24] Although some studies have reported that the mass of the left ventricle increases with age, others have concluded that ventricular mass does not increase with age if subjects with underlying heart disease are excluded.[25] However, there is general agreement that left ventricular wall thickness increases progressively with age.[7,24]

Age-related changes in cardiac structure are apparent not just macroscopically, but at the level of the individual heart cell. Briefly, there are fewer more active heart cells and more fibroblasts. Beginning at age 60, there is a noticeable decline in the number of pacemaker cells in the sinoatrial node, which is the normal pacemaker of the heart.[26] The total number of muscle cells in the heart, which are known as cardiac myocytes, also declines with age and this decrease is greater in males than in females.[22] Indeed, the population of cardiac myocytes in the heart declines by approximately 35% between the ages of 30 and 70 years old.[27] This cell loss is thought to occur through both apoptotic and necrotic cell death.[28] The loss of cardiac myocytes in the aging heart leads to an increase in size (hypertrophy) of the remaining myocytes, something that is more pronounced in cells from men than in cells from women.[22] This cellular hypertrophy may compensate, at least in part, for the loss of contractile cells in the aging heart. However, unlike cellular cardiac hypertrophy that occurs as a result of exercise, hypertrophy of cells in the aging heart results from the age-related loss of myocytes, which may increase the mechanical burden on the remaining cells.[28]

In addition to the cardiac myocytes, the heart contains large numbers of fibroblasts, which are the cells that produce connective tissues such as collagen and elastin. Collagen is a fibrous protein that holds heart cells together, whereas elastin is a connective tissue protein that is responsible for the elasticity of body tissues. As the number of myocytes progressively declines with age, there is a relative increase in the number of fibroblasts.[23] The amount of collagen increases with age, and there is thought to be an increase in collagen cross-linking between adjacent fibers with aging.[7,24,29] Increased collagen in the aging heart leads to interstitial fibrosis.[30] There also are structural changes in elastin in the aging heart and these changes may reduce elastic recoil in the aging heart.[23] Together with changes in the myocytes with aging, these structural changes in connective tissues increase myocardial stiffness, decrease ventricular compliance, and thereby impair passive left ventricular filling.[30] The impact of these changes on myocardial function is considered in more detail next.

MYOCARDIAL FUNCTION IN THE AGING HEART AT REST

There are significant age-associated abnormalities in cardiac function in older adults, especially diastolic function and especially with exercise. These changes are most apparent during exercise, although some changes are evident even at rest. When individuals are reclining at rest, the heart rate is similar in younger and older subjects. However, when older individuals move from the supine to the seated position, the heart rate increases less in older adults than in younger adults.[24] This decreased ability to augment heart rate in response to positional change may be linked to the age-related impairment in responsiveness to the sympathetic nervous system discussed in the "Response of the Aging Heart to Exercise" section. In contrast, left ventricular systolic function, which is a measure of the ability of the heart to contract, is well preserved at rest in older adults.[7,24,25] Other measures of cardiac contractile function at rest also are unchanged with age. The volume of blood ejected from the ventricle per beat (stroke volume) is generally comparable or slightly elevated in older adults when compared with their younger counterparts.[7,24] Similarly, the left ventricular ejection fraction, which is the ratio of the stroke volume to the volume of blood left in the ventricle at the end of diastole, is unchanged in aging.[7,24] Thus systolic function is relatively well preserved in healthy older adults at rest.

Unlike systolic function, diastolic function is profoundly altered in the hearts of older adults at rest. The rate of left ventricular filling in early diastole has been shown to decrease by up to 50% between 20 and 80 years of age.[24] Several mechanisms have been implicated in the reduction of left ventricular filling rate in the aging heart. It has been proposed that age-associated structural changes in the left ventricle impair early diastolic filling. The aging heart is characterized by increased collagen deposition and structural changes in elastin, both of which combine to increase left ventricular stiffness in the aging heart.[23] This increased ventricular stiffness reduces the compliance of the ventricle and impairs passive filling of the left ventricle.[30] An additional mechanism that has been implicated in the decrease in ventricular filling rate in aging is changes at the level of the cardiac myocytes. Uptake of intracellular calcium into internal stores is disrupted in myocytes from the aging heart.[24,30] As a result, residual calcium from the previous systole may cause persistent activation of contractile filaments and delay relaxation of cardiac myocytes in the aging heart.[30] It also has been suggested that diastolic dysfunction reflects, at least in part, an adaptation to the age-related changes in the vasculature. Increased vascular stiffness leads to increased mechanical load and subsequent prolongation of contraction time.[30] The age-associated increase in stiffness of the aorta increases the load the heart must work against (afterload), which is thought to promote the increase in left ventricular wall thickness observed in the aging heart.[25] These adaptive changes may serve to preserve systolic function at the expense of diastolic function in the aging heart.

In the hearts of young adults, left ventricular filling occurs early and very rapidly, due primarily to ventricular relaxation. Only a small amount of filling occurs as a result of atrial contraction later in diastole in the young adult heart.[24] In contrast, early left ventricular filling is disrupted in the aging heart. This increased diastolic filling pressure results in left atrial dilation and atrial hypertrophy in the aging heart.[29] The more forceful atrial contraction observed in the aging heart promotes late diastolic filling and compensates for the reduced filling in early diastole.[24] Because the atria make an important contribution to ventricular filling in older adults, loss of this atrial contraction due to conditions such as atrial fibrillation can lead to a marked reduction in diastolic volume and can predispose the aging heart to diastolic heart failure.[30] Atrial dilatation also can promote the development of atrial fibrillation and other arrhythmias in the aging heart.[24] Despite this evidence for diastolic dysfunction in the aging heart, left ventricular end diastolic pressure does not decline with age in older healthy adults at rest. Indeed, aging is actually associated with a small increase in left ventricular end diastolic pressure, in particular in older males.[24] Thus although the filling pattern in diastole is altered in aging, this does not lead to notable changes in end diastolic pressure in older hearts at rest.

RESPONSE OF THE AGING HEART TO EXERCISE

Although many aspects of cardiovascular performance are well preserved at rest in older adults, aging has important effects on cardiovascular performance during exercise. The decline in aerobic capacity with age in individuals with no evidence of cardiovascular disease is attributable in part to peripheral factors, such as increased body fat, reduced muscle mass, and a decline in O_2 extraction with age.[29,31,32] However, there is strong evidence that age-associated changes in the cardiovascular system also contribute to the decrease in exercise capacity in older individuals. Studies have shown that the VO_{2max}, which is the maximum amount of oxygen that a person can use during exercise, declines progressively with age starting in early adulthood.[31,32] Age-related changes in maximum heart rate, cardiac output, and stroke volume described below compromise delivery of blood to the muscles during exercise and contribute to this decline in VO_{2max} in aging.

The maximum heart rate attained during exercise decreases gradually with age in humans, a fact well known by widely distributed posters commonly seen in exercise facilities.[33] Interestingly, this decrease is not affected by physical conditioning because it is present in both sedentary and fit individuals.[25] Several mechanisms have been implicated in the reduction in maximum heart rate during exercise in aging. One mechanism involves a decrease in the sensitivity of the aging myocardium to sympathetic stimulation. Normally, the sympathetic nervous system becomes activated during exercise, and releases catecholamines (noradrenaline and adrenaline) to act on β-adrenergic receptors in the heart. This β-adrenergic stimulation leads to an increase in heart rate and augments the force of contraction of the heart. However, it is well established that the responsiveness of the heart to β-adrenergic stimulation declines with age.[24] This is thought to be due to high circulating levels of noradrenaline that are present in older adults.[34] These high levels of catecholamines in older adults arise from a decrease in plasma clearance of noradrenaline and an increase in the spillover of catecholamines from various organ systems into the circulation in older adults.[34] Chronic exposure to high levels of catecholamines may desensitize elements of the β-adrenergic receptor signaling cascade in the aging heart and limit the rise in heart rate during exercise.[24] An additional mechanism that is thought to limit the maximum heart rate in exercise is the decrease in the total population of sinoatrial nodal pacemaker cells in the aging heart.[31] This decrease in the number of pacemaker cells may impair the response of the heart to sympathetic stimulation during exercise.

The decrease in maximal heart rate during exercise has a major impact on the response of the aging cardiovascular system to exercise. Both heart rate and stroke volume are important determinants of cardiac output. Therefore a decrease in maximum heart rate during exercise would be expected to have an impact on cardiac output during exercise in older adults. Although this has not been extensively investigated, there is evidence that cardiac output during exercise is lower in older adults compared with their younger counterparts.[7,25] This decrease in cardiac output during exercise is not attributable to age-associated alterations in stroke volume.[7,29] However, the reduced responsiveness to β-adrenergic receptor stimulation in the heart may limit the increase in myocardial contractility in response to exercise in older adults.[7,25,29] These changes in cardiovascular function in aging are thought to be mitigated by an increase in left ventricular end-diastolic volume during exercise in older adults.[33] This increases the amount of blood in the ventricle at the end of diastole, and increases the stretch on the heart. It is well established that an increase in the amount of blood in the ventricle at the end of diastole results in an increase in the strength of contraction of the heart, a property known as the Frank Starling mechanism. Thus an increase in the reliance on the Frank Starling mechanism may at least partially compensate for the decrease in heart rate and contractility during exercise in aging.[7,25,33]

Although a decrease in cardiovascular performance and an increased susceptibility to cardiovascular diseases are inevitable consequences of the aging process,[35] there is evidence that regular exercise has numerous beneficial effects on the aging cardiovascular system. Endurance exercise blunts the decline in VO_{2max} that occurs as a consequence of the aging process.[31] Additionally, the age-associated decline in cardiac output can be partially overcome by regular aerobic training.[31] However, endurance training does not modify the age-related decline in maximal heart rate during exercise.[25,31] This might occur because exercise increases the levels of circulating catecholamines, which have been implicated in the decline in maximal heart rate in older adults as discussed earlier.[31] Regular endurance exercise also attenuates the increased arterial stiffness that is observed in central elastic arteries from sedentary older adults.[36] Finally, habitual aerobic exercise can protect the aging heart from detrimental

KEY POINTS

Effects of Aging on the Cardiovascular System

- The structure and function of the human heart and vasculature change as a function of the normal aging process.
- The age-associated increase in stiffness of central elastic arteries promotes systolic hypertension in older adults.
- Diastolic dysfunction in the aging heart arises from impaired left ventricular filling, increased afterload, and prolonged availability of intracellular calcium.
- Decreased responsiveness to β-adrenergic receptor stimulation limits the increase in heart rate and contractility in response to exercise in older adults.
- Despite limits on the ability of the aging cardiovascular system to respond to exercise, regular exercise attenuates the adverse effects of aging on the heart and vasculature and protects against the development of cardiovascular disease in older adults.

Table 14-2. Age-Related Changes in the Heart

Age-Associated Changes in the Heart	Clinical Consequences
↑ Collagen, changes in elastin, ↑ left ventricular wall thickness	Impairs passive left ventricle filling
Prolonged availability of intracellular calcium	Diastolic dysfunction
Left atrial hypertrophy↑	
Susceptibility to atrial arrhythmias	
↓ Number of pacemaker cells in sinoatrial node	↓ Ability to elevate heart rate in response to exercise
↓ Sensitivity to β-adrenergic receptor stimulation	Impaired ability to ↑ heart rate and contractility in exercise

effects of cardiovascular diseases such as myocardial ischemia.[37] Therefore there is good evidence that exercise can mitigate at least some of the detrimental effects of age on the cardiovascular system. The major age-related changes in the heart and the clinical consequences of these changes are summarized in Table 14-2.

SUMMARY

There are prominent changes in the structure and function of the vasculature and the myocardium in older adults when compared to younger adults. These changes are apparent even in the absence of risk factors other than age and in the absence of overt cardiovascular disease. However, these age-related alterations in the vasculature and the heart may render the cardiovascular system more susceptible to the detrimental effects of cardiovascular disease.

For a complete list of references, please visit online only at www.expertconsult.com

CHAPTER 15

Age-Related Changes in the Respiratory System

Gwyneth A. Davies
Charlotte E. Bolton

RESPIRATORY FUNCTION TESTS

The commonly used respiratory function tests are presented in this chapter. In addition, patterns of lung function abnormality seen in some of the common types of condition are also presented.

The breathing parameters are:

- Forced expiratory volume in 1 second (liters): FEV_1. This is the volume of air expired during the first second of a forced expiratory maneuver from vital capacity (maximal inspiration). Measured by spirometry.
- Forced vital capacity (liters): FVC. This is the total volume of air expired during forced expiration from the end of maximum inspiration. A slow vital capacity (SVC) is the volume of air expired, but this time through an unforced maneuver. In the young these are similar but in emphysema, where there is loss of elastic recoil, FVC may fall disproportionately more than SVC. These are also measured by spirometry.
- Peak expiratory flow rate (liters/minute): PEFR. This is the maximal expiratory flow rate measured using a peak flow meter, a more portable method; therefore serial home measurements may be requested in patients.

The following measurements require more detailed lung function testing:

- Total lung capacity (liters): TLC. The volume of air contained in the lung at the end of maximal inspiration. Measured by helium dilution or body plethysmography together with the next two tests.
- Functional residual capacity (liters): FRC. This is the amount of air left in the lungs after a tidal breath out and indicates the amount of air that stays in the lungs during normal breathing.
- Residual volume (liters): RV. The amount of air left in the lungs after a maximal exhalation. Not all the air within the lungs can ever be expired.
- Transfer factor (mmol/minute): TL_{CO}. This is a measure of the ability of the lung to oxygenate hemoglobin. It is usually measured with a single breath hold technique using low concentration carbon monoxide.
- Transfer coefficient (mmol/minute/k/Pa/L_{BTPS}): K_{CO}. This is the TL_{CO} corrected for the lung volume.

In addition, blood gas measurements are often performed to assess both acid-base balance and oxygenation. The most important measures for respiratory disease are the partial pressure of oxygen (PaO_2), partial pressure of carbon dioxide ($PaCO_2$), and the pH. A low PaO_2 (hypoxemia) with a normal $PaCO_2$ indicates type I respiratory failure. An increased $PaCO_2$ with hypoxemia indicates type II respiratory failure. A rapidly rising $PaCO_2$ will result in a fall in the pH, for example, seen in an acute exacerbation of chronic obstructive pulmonary disease (COPD). Renal compensation occurs in response to chronically high $PaCO_2$ with correction of the pH to normal/near-normal levels; but this renal compensation takes several days to occur. Hyperventilation, associated with excess expiration of CO_2, as seen in anxiety attacks but also in altered respiratory control such as Cheyne-Stokes respiration, will result in an increase in pH as a result of a drop in $PaCO_2$. Pure anxiety-related hyperventilation will not cause hypoxemia but other causes for this altered respiratory control may cause hypoxemia.

There are two main characteristic patterns of respiratory disease based on spirometric evaluation. These are the obstructive and the restrictive patterns. The obstructive pattern, as seen in patients with asthma and COPD, is characterized by:

- Reduced FEV_1 and PEFR
- Normal or reduced FVC. (If FVC reduced, disproportionately less reduced than FEV_1)
- Reduced FEV_1/FVC ratio to less than 0.7

The restrictive pattern is characterized by:

- Reduced FEV_1
- Reduced FVC
- Normal or high FEV_1/FVC ratio

Conditions relating to both these spirometric patterns with more detail on lung function patterns and utility of other lung function parameters to characterize and diagnose conditions will be discussed in further chapters.

AGE-RELATED CHANGES IN THE RESPIRATORY SYSTEM

Lungs age over a lifetime but there is in addition an accumulation of environmental insults that an individual has been exposed to, given that the lungs have direct contact with the atmosphere. The key exposure is smoking in the form of direct smoke but also second-hand passive smoking, the impact of which is being increasingly recognized.[1,2] A quantitative evaluation of a person's smoking habit is usually classed as pack years (20 cigarettes a day (1 pack/day) for 10 years equates to 10 pack years).

Oxidative stress is an important mechanism of lung function decline, oxidants stemming both from cigarette fumes and from other causes of airway inflammation.[3,4] Oxidants and the subsequent release of reactive oxygen species (ROS) lead to reduction and inactivation of proteinase inhibitors, epithelial permeability, and enhanced nuclear factor κB (NF-κB), which promotes cytokine production, and in a cyclical fashion is capable of recruiting more neutrophils. There is also plasma leakage, bronchoconstriction through elevated isoprostanes, and increased mucus secretion. The lung has its own defense enzymatic antioxidants such as superoxide dismutase (SOD), which degrades superoxide anion and catalase, and glutathione (GSH), which inactivates hydrogen peroxide and hydroperoxidases. Both are found intracellularly and extracellularly. In addition there are nonenzymatic factors that act as antioxidants, such as vitamin C and E, β-carotene, uric acid, bilirubin, and flavonoids.[5]

Recently, there has been a renewed interest in the effect of critical early life periods determining peak lung function and the subsequent "knock-on" effect on lung function in later life and the effect on the adult and the elderly lungs. If peak lung function reserve is not attained, then the "natural" trajectory of decline may lead to symptomatic lung impairment in mid or later life. Such factors in early life would include premature birth, asthma, environmental exposure, nutrition, and respiratory infection.[6,7] In addition, the effect of environmental pollution, nutrition, respiratory infections, and physical activity on lung function decline are reported.[8,9] The mechanisms affecting respiratory function are likely to be multiple and cumulative. Interestingly, in the Inuit community, where lifestyle has gradually become more westernized—with a reduction in the fishing and hunting activities and the community developing a more sedentary lifestyle—there has been acceleration in age-related lung function decline.[10]

In the aging lung, there are structural and functional changes within the respiratory system and, in addition, immune mediated and extrapulmonary alterations. These are discussed in detail in this chapter.

Structural changes

There are three main structural changes in the aging lung. These include the (1) lung parenchyma and subsequent loss of elastic recoil; (2) stiffening of the lung (i.e., reduced chest wall compliance); and (3) the respiratory muscles.

The main change is the loss in the alveolar surface area as alveoli and alveolar ducts enlarge. There is little alteration to the bronchi. The small airways suffer qualitative changes far more than quantitative changes in the supporting elastin and collagen, with disruption to fibers and loss of elasticity leading to the subsequent dilatation of alveolar ducts and airspaces known as "senile emphysema." Alveolar surface area may drop by as much as 20%. This leads to an increased tendency for small airways to collapse during expiration because of the loss of the surface tension forces.[11] In a healthy elderly individual, this is probably of little or no significance but reduction in their reserve may unearth difficulties at the time of an infection or superadded respiratory complication. Amyloid deposition in the lung vasculature and alveolar septae occurs in the elderly, although its relevance is unclear. Within the large airways, with aging, there is a reduction in the number of glandular epithelial cells, resulting in a reduced production of mucus and thus impairing the respiratory defense against infection.

Chest wall compliance is decreased in the elderly. Contributing to this increasing stiffness of the lungs are loss of intervertebral disc space, ossification of the costal cartilages, and calcification of the rib articulatory surfaces, which combine with muscle changes to produce impaired mobility of the thoracic cage. In addition to these, additional insults from osteoporosis leading to vertebral collapse have been shown to result in a 10% reduction in FVC,[12] probably through developing kyphosis and increased anterior-posterior diameter—the barrel chest. Such vertebral collapse is frequently found in the elderly, increasing with age, if sought through appropriate imaging. These structural alterations lead to suboptimal force mechanics of the diaphragm and increasing chest wall stiffness. Rib fractures, again common in the elderly, may further limit respiratory movements.

The predominant respiratory muscle is the diaphragm, making up about 85% of respiratory muscle activity; with the intercostals, the anterior abdominal muscles and the accessory muscles also contributing. The accessory muscles are used by splinting of the arms, a feature commonly associated with the emphysematous COPD patient. Inspiration leading to chest expansion is brought about by these muscles contracting, whereas expiration is a passive phenomenon. The accessory muscles are used where there is increased ventilatory demand, such as in the COPD patient. The respiratory muscles are made up of type I (slow), type IIa (fast-fatigue resistant), and type IIx (fast-fatigable) fibers. The difference in the muscle fibers is based upon the aerobic capacity and ATP activity of the myofibrils and confers differing physiologic properties. The major age-related change in the respiratory muscles is a reduction in the proportion of type IIa fibers, which thus impairs both strength and endurance.[13] An increasing reliance on the diaphragm due to loss of intercostal muscle strength and the less advantageous diaphragmatic position to generate force add to breathlessness. Globally, there is reduced muscle myosin production and this is likely to confer disadvantage to the respiratory muscles also. Comorbid conditions, such as COPD and congestive heart failure, are associated with altered muscle structure and function as is poor nutrition.[14–16] Physical deconditioning and sarcopenia, hormone imbalance, and vitamin D deficiency will exacerbate the age-related lung structural changes—the body becomes less adaptive to the respiratory limitations. Medications, especially oral corticosteroids, may cause problems particularly with regard to respiratory and peripheral muscle strength. Acute infection puts added demand on the respiratory system and may expose the limited respiratory reserve.

Age-related functional changes

FEV_1 and FVC fall with age. Flow within the airways also falls. The ratio of FEV_1 to FVC falls by approximately 0.2% per year as a result of a greater reduction in the FEV_1 parameter relative to FVC with time, with changes more rapid in women.[17]

The total lung capacity (TLC) does not change significantly with age as the loss of elastic recoil and increased elastic load of the chest wall counteract. The RV and FRC increase due to reduced elastic recoil, causing the premature closure of the airways and stiffness of the chest wall. The elderly person thus breathes at higher lung volumes, placing additional burden on the respiratory muscles and has higher energy expenditure of up to 120% that of a young adult. The closing volume is the lung volume at which the dependent airways begin to close during expiration. This is increased in the elderly because of a lack of support and tethering of the terminal airways by collagen and elastin, and may lead to closure during normal tidal breathing,[18] leading to ventilation perfusion (V/Q) mismatch that may be responsible for lower resting arterial oxygen tensions.[17] Although arterial oxygen tensions tend to be lower in the elderly, unless there is coexistent respiratory disease, the PaO_2 is sufficient for adequate hemoglobin saturation. There is reduced gas transfer (TL_{CO})

because of the aforementioned structural changes and the V/Q mismatch. There is, in addition, reduction in pulmonary capillary blood volume and density of the capillaries.

The previously mentioned impaired respiratory muscle strength and endurance may be of little or no functional significance in the healthy elderly person, but may lead to impaired reserve to combat respiratory challenges consequent upon acute respiratory disease. Measures of respiratory muscle strength, such as the maximal inspiratory pressure (MIP), maximal expiratory pressure (MEP), and sniff nasal inspiratory pressure (SNIP), fall with age.[14]

In the elderly there are alterations in the regulation and control of breathing. The elderly breathe with similar minute ventilation to younger subjects but at smaller tidal volumes and a higher respiratory frequency. A blunted response to both hypoxia and hypercapnia has been reported,[19–21] with Poulin[22] demonstrating impaired response to hypoxia during sustained hypercapnia. Elderly people show an increased ventilatory response to exercise,[20] which may be more pronounced in males.[23] Maximal oxygen uptake (VO_{2max}) declines with age with a parallel decline in exercise capacity, having reached a peak as a young adult. This is due to a combination of both cardiovascular (such as reduced cardiac output) and respiratory causes, including ventilation perfusion mismatch. The decline in maximal oxygen uptake with age can be attenuated to some degree by maintaining regular exercise.[24,25]

Elderly people are less able to objectively perceive acute bronchoconstriction.[26,27] Moreover, airway β_2-adrenoceptor responsiveness is reduced in old age, as evidenced by impaired responses to β-agonists in healthy elderly subjects.[28] Altered chemoreceptor sensitivity to hypoxia, reduced ability to perceive elastic loads on inspiration or expiration, impaired perception of tactile sensation and joint movement, or age-associated central processing abnormalities may all be contributing factors.[29,30] Subsequently, this is likely to mask deteriorating respiratory symptoms and may delay presentation to health care services.

Sleep disordered breathing is more common in the healthy elderly,[31] yet older subjects appear less likely to seek medical review or have the sleep disorder diagnosed due to a high prevalence of tiredness, fatigue, and snoring in this age group generally along with concurrent other medical illness and sedating medication including benzodiazepines. Cerebrovascular disease is associated with sleep disordered breathing,[32] and in fact obstructive sleep apnea in stroke patients is a predictor of death.[33] There is increased upper airway resistance in the elderly with a reduced respiratory effort to try and overcome this obstruction. There is a high prevalence of sleep disordered breathing in patients with congestive heart failure,[34] and it is said to be greater in patients with Alzheimer disease,[35] both of which are increasingly prevalent in the elderly. In addition and conversely, sleep disordered breathing can contribute to both cardiovascular disease and impaired cognitive function.[36,37]

Effects of aging on pulmonary host defense and immune response

The immune system is described as comprising two separate but interacting components. Innate immunity is the rapid, nonspecific system which functions as the first line of defense against invading microorganisms. Adaptive (or acquired) immunity, mediated by B and T lymphocytes, is antigen-specific and involves the development of memory cells allowing a future antigen-specific response. There is impaired immune function in the elderly, both of the innate and adaptive components.

Aging leads to breakdown of the mucosal barrier of the lung and reduced mucociliary clearance enabling invasion by pathogenic organisms. In the aged lung, the innate immune system is increasingly challenged by greater contact with pathogens and cumulative exposure to environmental insults such as smoking. There is impaired chemotaxis and phagocytosis, reduced superoxide generation, and reduced bactericidal activity of neutrophils.[38] Dendritic cells are less efficient at antigen presentation. In addition, although the number of natural killer (NK) cells increases with advanced age, there is a reduction in NK cytotoxicity.[39] In vitro evidence suggests that macrophage function is impaired with age, with a reduced capacity to generate reactive oxygen species and proinflammatory cytokines, and reduced expression of certain pattern-recognition receptors, such as Toll-like receptors.[40,41]

Healthy elderly subjects have been shown to demonstrate a hyperinflammatory state, so-called "inflamm-aging."[42] This is associated with increased circulating proinflammatory cytokines, such as IL-6, TNF, IL-1β, prostaglandin E_2, and antiinflammatory mediators, including soluble TNF receptor, IL-1 receptor antagonist and acute phase proteins (C-reactive protein, serum amyloid A). This background proinflammatory state may contribute to a poorer outcome when host defenses are challenged in the aged lung.

Alterations in cell-mediated adaptive immunity include atrophy of the thymus together with aging within the T-cell pool, including altered memory T-cell function and a shift from a TH1 to TH2 profile.[41] There is a reduction in naïve T-lymphocyte production and absolute numbers of $CD3^+$, $CD4^+$, and $CD8^+$ T cells. Other changes include a smaller T-cell receptor repertoire and reduced proliferative responses to antigens. A decrease in B-cell numbers, impaired production of memory B cells, and reduced antibody responses affect humoral immunity in the elderly.

Immunosenescence explains a large part of the increased susceptibility to lower respiratory tract infection in the elderly.

KEY POINTS
Age-Related Changes in the Respiratory System

- There are both age-related changes and true aging changes in the respiratory system.
- Most of the available information comes from cross-sectional studies rather than longitudinal studies.
- There are structural and functional changes to the lung in the elderly. In addition, there are alterations to respiratory control and immunologic alterations that can all contribute to age-related changes of the respiratory system. Such alterations may be synergistic.
- Exercise exerts additional demands on the respiratory system that may reveal respiratory limitation. In addition, although alterations in the respiratory system may not be apparent in the healthy elderly person, acute illness may unearth the diminished respiratory reserve.
- Elderly people are less able to perceive bronchoconstriction and other symptoms. In parallel, there is thus relative underreporting of symptoms.

However, causes which contribute to pneumonia risk in this population are multifactorial. Bacterial colonization of the upper respiratory tract is not uncommon in the elderly.[43] This may be associated with colonization of the stomach, which itself is commoner in old age and may be preceded by antacids or H_2 blockers.[44,45] The elderly person with swallowing difficulties, particularly in association with cerebrovascular disease and other neurologic diseases where there is associated cognitive impairment, is more prone to aspiration. Similarly, tracheal intubation or the presence of nasogastric tubes increases aspiration risk. Malnutrition and the presence of chronic disease such as diabetes or renal failure will also contribute to pneumonia susceptibility. An age-related decline in immune function leads to a reduced response to vaccination including the influenza vaccination and increased susceptibility to respiratory infection and pneumonia.

In conclusion, there are both structural and functional changes in the lungs together with alterations in the control of breathing and more general immunologic alterations in the elderly. The changes are not just a direct consequence of age but are also affected by environmental exposure and coexistent comorbidities.

For a complete list of references, please visit online only at www.expertconsult.com

CHAPTER 16

Neurologic Signs in the Elderly

Rawan Tarawneh
James E. Galvin

Neurologic disorders are a common cause of morbidity and institutionalization in the elderly population.[1] Not only does advancing age increase the frequency and severity of neurologic disease, but it may also play an important role in modifying disease presentation. The geriatric neurologic examination can be challenging even for the experienced physician. Normal aging may be associated with the loss of normal neurologic signs or the exaggeration of others. It may be associated with the appearance of findings considered abnormal in younger patients or the reappearance of physical signs usually seen in infancy and early stages of development.

The geriatric neurologic examination is also influenced by involvement of other systems (e.g., rheumatologic disease), the frequent cooccurrence of multiple conditions in a single patient, and the presentation of nonneurologic disorders (e.g., myocardial infarction, urinary tract infection, fecal impaction) as neurologic signs (e.g., gait difficulty and confusion). Therefore, it is important for physicians to appreciate the multitude of age-related changes in both the central and peripheral nervous system (Table 16-1).

MENTAL STATUS

Because the frequency of cognitive disorders increases dramatically with advancing age, examination of mental status is one of the most important components of the neurologic examination. Unfortunately, it is often also one of the most difficult parts of the neurologic examination to interpret. In general, fund of knowledge continues to expand throughout life and learning ability does not appreciably decline with age. Cognitive changes associated with normal aging include a decrease in processing speed, cognitive flexibility, visuospatial perception (often in conjunction with decreased visual acuity), working memory, and sustained attention.[2] Other cognitive abilities such as access to remotely learned information and retention of new encoded information appear to be spared in aging, thus allowing their use as sensitive indicators for disease processes.[3]

Crystallized intelligence characterized by practical problem solving, knowledge gained from experience, and vocabulary[4] tends to be cumulative and does not generally decline with aging.[5] On the other hand, fluid intelligence characterized by the ability to acquire and use new information as measured by solutions to abstract problems and speeded performance (e.g., performance on the Raven's progressive matrices and Wechsler Adult Intelligence Scale digit symbol task) has been shown to decline gradually with aging.[6]

Longitudinal studies of memory and aging demonstrate considerable variability among cognitive abilities between different individuals (interindividual variability) and among different cognitive domains within the same individual (intraindividual variability).[3] At least part of this variability may be attributed to different study designs; however, it is very important to take the intraindividual and interindividual variability into consideration when defining neuropsychological norms for the elderly.[7] Some authors have suggested that age-weighted rather than age-corrected norms for cognition should be used,[8] whereas other investigators have stressed the influence of other factors such as culture, experience, educational background, and motor speed on cognitive performance.[7] For example, although older adults generally perform less well on both the verbal and performance subtests of the Wechsler Adult Intelligence Scale compared with young adults, these differences are minimized when corrected for motor slowing and educational level. Other situational factors that may affect individual performance on cognitive tasks include fatigue, emotional status, medications, and stress. Moreover, it may be very difficult to attribute impaired cognition to aging in the presence of underlying conditions such as depression, dementia, and delirium—all of which are common, and often unrecognized, in the elderly population.

The elements of a comprehensive mental status examination include assessment of cognitive, functional, and behavioral domains. The initial contact with the patient affords the opportunity to assess whether a cognitive, attention, affective, or language disorder is present. If available, questioning of an informant may bring to light changes in cognition, function, and behavior that the patient either is not aware of or denies.

Screening for cognitive disorders in the older adult may include both performance and informant measures. Examples of brief tests of mental status include the Mini Mental State Exam,[9] the Mini-Cog,[10] and the Montreal Cognitive Assessment.[11] These tests compare decrements in cognitive ability to published norms, often adjusted for age and education. Decrements in cognitive ability are compared with published norms, often adjusted for age and education. Examples of other brief informant assessments include the AD8,[12] and the Informant Questionnaire on Cognitive Decline in the Elderly.[13] These scales detect intraindividual decline by comparing current performance on cognitive and functional tasks to prior levels of performance. Combining performance and informant measures may increase the likelihood of detecting cognitive disorders.[14]

CRANIAL NERVE FUNCTION

Smell and taste

Normal aging is associated with decrements in olfaction at both threshold and suprathreshold concentrations. Elderly people also have reduced capacity to discriminate the degree of differences between odors of different qualities and have impaired performance on tasks that require odor identification.[15] Impaired olfaction with aging may be due to structural and functional changes in the upper airway, olfactory epithelium, olfactory bulb, or olfactory nerves.[15] It is important to recognize that while impaired smell can be associated with aging, it can also be the result of medications, viral infections, and head trauma. Moreover, there appears to be early involvement of olfactory pathways in neurodegenerative diseases such as Alzheimer disease (neurofibrillary tangles)[16] and Parkinson disease (Lewy bodies).[17] Taste, which in turn is greatly dependent on olfaction, also decreases with advanced age, with a reduced sensitivity for a broad range of

Table 16-1. Neurologic Changes Associated With Normal Aging

Psychomotor slowing
Decreased visual acuity
Smaller pupil size
Decreased ability to look upward
Decreased auditory acuity, especially for spoken language
Decreased muscle bulk
Mild motor slowing
Decreased vibratory sensation
Mild swaying on Romberg test
Mild lordosis and restriction of movement in neck and back
Depression of Achilles tendon reflex

tastes compared to young adults.[18,19] Although the number of taste buds does not seem to be significantly decreased in the elderly, some studies have suggested decreased responses in electrophysiologic recordings from taste buds.[20] Multiple other factors such as medications, smoking, alcohol, and dentures may contribute to decreased taste.

Vision

Age-related changes have been documented in visual acuity, visual fields, depth perception, contrast sensitivity, motion perception, and perception of self-motion in relation to external space (optical flow).[7] Anatomic and physiologic studies have demonstrated a gradual decline in photoreceptors after the age of 20, resulting in decreased visual acuity in elderly.[21] This is especially apparent in conditions with low contrast and luminance.[22] There is also a decline in visual field sensitivity with aging.[23] The mechanisms responsible for this are not well understood. There is also an age-related impairment in accommodation that leads to farsightedness (presbyopia) and a decrease in accommodation because of rigidity of the lens.[7] Relaxation and accommodation times increase progressively and peak around the age of 50. Therefore, many elderly are forced to use glasses for reading. Moreover, ophthalmologic conditions, such as cataracts, glaucoma, and macular degeneration occur commonly with age and contribute significantly to decreased visual acuity seen with aging.

Pupillary abnormalities have also been described with normal aging. These include smaller pupils (senile miosis), which may be due to decreased preganglionic sympathetic tone,[24] sluggish reaction to light, and decrease or even loss of the near or "accommodation" response.[25,26] Some authors have reported loss of pupillary reaction in 5%–19% of normal elderly in the absence of neurologic disease.[27]

Age-associated changes in extraocular motility include decreased velocity of saccades, prolonged latency, decreased accuracy, and prolonged duration and reaction time. There is also an age-related limitation of upgaze,[28] but not downgaze, slowing of smooth pursuits, and impaired visual tracking.[27,29–32] Vertical gaze changes begin in middle age and decline in the upward plane from 40 degrees between the ages of 5 and14 years, to 16 degrees between the ages of 75 and 84.[33,34] Vertical gaze palsy is an important consideration in the evaluation of driving abilities in older adults (street signs, traffic lights). Other changes of eye movements with aging include loss of Bell's phenomenon (upward and outward deviation of the eyes in response to attempted forced closure of the eyelids).

Hearing and vestibular function

Gradual loss of cochlear hair cells, atrophy of the stria vascularis, and thickening of the basement membrane may account for the impaired hearing that is commonly seen with aging. This is often referred to as "presbycusis" and predominantly affects higher frequencies.[2] Other changes include impaired speech discrimination, increase in pure tone threshold averages (approximately 2 dB/yr), and decreased discrimination scores.[35]

Vestibular function may also be affected with aging. There is a decrease in vestibulospinal reflexes, and in the ability to detect head position and motion in space. These may be secondary to loss of hair cells and nerve fibers along with neuronal loss in the medial, lateral, and inferior vestibular nucleus in the brainstem.[7]

MOTOR SIGNS

There is a progressive decline in muscle bulk associated with aging, sometimes referred to as sarcopenia. This is most obvious in the intrinsic muscles in the hands and feet, particularly the dorsal interossei and thenar muscles as well as around the shoulder cap (deltoid and rotator cuff muscles). Atrophy of the thenar muscles, without weakness or fasciculations, may be present in more than 50% of elderly patients.[36] Results of different longitudinal studies have been inconsistent regarding the predominant fiber type affected by aging, with reports of loss of type IIb fibers or "fast twitch" fibers[37]), reduction in the percentage of type 1 fibers with no change in type I or II mean fiber area, a decrease in the capillary to fiber ratio,[38] and an increase in the percentage of type I fibers.[39] The decrease in muscle mass is associated with electrophysiologic evidence of denervation and muscle fiber atrophy.[40] However, fasciculations are not a normal sign of aging, and if present, should warrant search for pathologic causes (e.g., motor neuron disease, compressive cervical myelopathy, multifocal motor neuropathy).[7]

Decrease in muscle strength often accompanies the decrease in muscle bulk.[41] One study reported up to 50% decrease in maximum voluntary contraction force and twitch tension in the quadriceps in elderly patients compared with younger ones.[42] Hand grip strength decreases significantly after the age of 50, but strength in the arms and shoulders does not change until after the age of 60. Weakening of abdominal muscles may accentuate lumbar lordosis and contribute to low back pain. Other studies have suggested that changes in muscle strength are not frequent[25] or significant in the absence of underlying disease states.[27] Differences in the results of these studies can be attributed to different evaluation techniques and the examination of different muscle groups.

In addition to motor bulk and strength, there also appears to be loss of speed and coordination of movement with aging. Speed of hand and foot tapping was found to be reduced by 20% to 23% in one study.[41] A mild terminal tremor and hesitation in finger nose testing,[25] mild bradykinesia,[43] rigidity, and mild dysmetria on finger-nose and heel-shin testing have also been described in isolation in 1.8% to 44% of elderly.[2,27,29] In one study of 467 patients, the prevalence of parkinsonian signs defined as the presence of signs of two or more categories (ridigity, bradykinesia, tremor, gait disturbance) increased gradually from 14.9% for people aged 65 to 74 to

52.4% for those 85 and older.[43] These may interfere with activities of daily living, such as dressing, eating, and getting out of a chair and may be an important source of disability. Another finding of that study was that the presence of parkinsonism was associated with a twofold increase in mortality mostly as a result of gait instability.

Paratonia

Paratonia (Gegenhalten) represents increased motor tone with rapid passive movements of the limbs (i.e., flexion and extension), often suggestive of deliberate resistance. Unlike the rigidity of Parkinson, it is not constant and tends to disappear with slow movements of the limbs. Paratonia can be detected when the patient's arms, suspended 15 cm above the lap, remain elevated after being released despite instructions to the patient to relax.[2]

The prevalence of paratonia increases with advancing age with a prevalence 4% to 21%.[31] It is considered by some to be a postural reflex or a cortical release sign. Similar to other primitive release signs, its prevalence is higher in patients with advanced Alzheimer's and correlates with the severity of cognitive impairment. Other investigators consider paratonia as a sign of age-related changes in the basal ganglia.[32]

Tremor and other abnormal movements

Physiologic tremor may occur at any age. There are different types of physiologic tremor: rest tremor with a frequency of 8 to 12 Hz, postural tremor when the patient holds out the arms during isometric contractions of the muscles against gravity (with a frequency of 8 to 12 Hz), and action or volitional tremor during isotonic contraction (with a frequency of 7 to 12 Hz).[44]

The prevalence of physiologic tremor in healthy elderly is controversial.[44] Postural tremor is more likely secondary to other causes, such as medications, alcohol, disease states such as hyperthyroidism, hyperadrenergic states, or dystonia. When no obvious secondary factors are evident, essential tremor should be considered in the diagnosis. Its prevalence has been reported to range from 1.7% to 23% of healthy elderly aged 65 years or older in different studies.[45] In the absence of secondary causes for tremor, and when the tremor does not fit the criteria for essential tremor, it is often referred to as senile tremor. Senile tremor is very common, affecting 98% of elderly patients in one community-based case control study. It is often a mild asymptomatic tremor and frequently does not require treatment. It is unclear if it represents an exaggerated physiologic tremor or a mild form of essential tremor.[2] A rhythmic, usually asymmetric rest tremor is often indicative of Parkinson disease.[5]

Senile chorea is a rare condition with late onset of generalized chorea in the absence of dementia and absence of a family history of a similar condition. It is probably better considered a prodromal syndrome rather than a separate disease entity as many patients diagnosed with senile chorea later develop other neurologic disorders such as Huntington's disease. Some pathologic reports have demonstrated its association with abnormalities in the putamen, globus pallidum, and cerebellar nuclei.[2]

The frequency of idiopathic lingual-facial-buccal dyskinesia is elevated in patients over the age of 60 with a prevalence of 1.5% and can be as high as 38% in hospital-based populations. Tardive dyskinesia associated with neuroleptic medications should be considered in the differential diagnosis.[2]

CHANGES IN GAIT AND STATION

There is a tendency to develop flexed posture with advanced age. This may be due to decreased neuromuscular power, increased tone (paratonia), and degenerative joint disease. Increased postural sway is a normal phenomenon in the elderly and is seen in two different frequencies. Fast oscillations are dependent on proprioceptive input from the lower extremities and slow oscillations are dependent, at least partially, on vestibular input. Looking at the feet exaggerates this normal sway by interfering with visual compensation. Postural righting reflexes may be slowed and with reduced amplitude in the elderly. Control of stance, as judged by the amplitude of sway, is poor in childhood, peaks in adulthood, and decreases with age. In one study, almost one third of patients above the age of 60 were unable to minimize their sway with visual endeavors and therefore had a significant risk for falls.[44]

Examination of gait in the elderly is an essential part of the neurologic examination, given the high risk of falls in the population. Gait is composed of equilibrium (maintaining an upright posture) and locomotion (gait ignition and steppage); both of which appear to be decreased in aging.[7] Healthy elderly people have difficulty maintaining balance on one foot with eyes closed. Quantitative studies have also shown that older people have greater body sway[46] and exhibit significant reduction in the velocity of gait and length of stride.[47] Therefore, the elderly may have difficulty with tandem gait or heel to toe walking for extended periods of time.

The term idiopathic senile gait[48] is sometimes used to describe the clinical picture of stooped posture, posteriorly rotated immobile pelvis, excessive flexion at the hips and knees, a reduced toe-floor clearance, a slightly broad base, and reduced arm swing.[49] However, this term remains poorly defined and does not include all forms of gait disorders that can be seen with aging. There is also substantial overlap with the gait associated with many pathologic conditions, such as normal pressure hydrocephalus, parkinsonism, and lacunar state.[50]

Other factors that contribute to impaired gait in the elderly include decreased muscle strength, weakening of abdominal muscles, arthritis and degenerative joint disease, diminished vibration and position sense, impaired visual and vestibular systems, and impaired motor speed and coordination. Despite these multiple factors, some authors suggest that age alone does not generally affect postural righting reflexes or cause recurrent falls. If present, these should be investigated to rule out underlying disorders such as Parkinson's disease.

DEEP TENDON REFLEXES

The ability to detect reflexes can be limited by conditions such as apprehension or joint disease in the elderly. Hyporeflexia or areflexia of the ankle jerks has been reported in elderly people.[51] Asymmetry of reflexes was reported in 3% of the elderly in one study. Electrophysiologic studies report both afferent and efferent limbs of the reflex to be decreased with age.[7] The ankle jerk is usually the first reflex to decrease or disappear with aging although, there have been reports of loss of patella tendon reflexes as well.[44]

Superficial reflexes (abdominal, cremasteric, and plantar response) may become sluggish or disappear with advanced age. Corticospinal lesions above T6 may lead to loss of all superficial abdominal reflexes, whereas all are spared in lesions below T12. Lesions between T10 and T12 may lead to selective loss of the lower reflexes only with a positive Beevor's sign (upward movement of the umbilicus in a supine patient attempting to flex the head).[7]

Extension or dorsiflexion of the big toe with fanning of the toes induced by stroking the lateral aspect of the sole is called the Babinski sign. It is considered to be a primitive reflex that, when present beyond the first 2 years of life, is a reliable sign of upper motor neuron pathology. No consistent changes have been documented with normal aging, and there is often some degree of interobserver variability in eliciting this reflex.[7]

SENSORY SIGNS

The most common and evident abnormality in sensory examination associated with aging is decreased vibration and to a lesser extent proprioception. Both of these sensory modalities are carried by the dorsal column; their impairment with age may be due to proliferation of connective tissue, arteriosclerotic changes in the arterioles, degeneration in the nerve fibers,[52] or loss of axons in the dorsal column.[53]

Vibration sense is impaired in 12% to 68% of elderly between the ages of 65 to 85 years old and becomes more impaired with advanced age.[27] The loss of vibration affects both upper and lower extremities and often begins distally.[2] This can be demonstrated with a 128 tuning fork at the metatarsals or medial malleolus of the ankle. One study reported that vibration sense might be absent in the soft tissues of the abdomen, thighs, and legs and the plantar surfaces of the toes even when it is present over bony prominences.[44] Using quantitative measurements, it has been shown that the sensitivity of vibration decreases with age in the high frequency range but does not change in the low frequency range (25 to 40 Hz).

Proprioception is also affected to a lesser extent with a prevalence ranging from 2% to 44% in different studies.[27,31] This often manifests as a mild sway on the Romberg test. There is paucity of data regarding the involvement of tactile sensation in the elderly. Some reports suggest that age is associated with increased thresholds for light touch.[55] However, these changes are often not significant enough to be detected clinically. Other studies found no change in quantitative measures of touch or two-point discrimination.[41] The results of different studies regarding changes in thermal sensitivity have been conflicting.[2]

Despite an increased pain threshold in the elderly, subjective sensory symptoms such as paresthesias, formications, postherpetic neuralgia, and tic douloureux are commonly encountered in the elderly population.[44]

PRIMITIVE REFLEXES

Primitive reflexes, or so called "archaic" or developmental reflexes represent loss of cortical inhibition on reflex associations present at early stages of development and later suppressed with brain maturation. Their reappearance in adult life has been associated with atrophic changes predominantly involving the frontal lobes (e.g., dementia syndromes, demyelinating disease, or cerebrovascular disease) and are sometimes referred to as "cortical release signs." However, these reflexes are sometimes seen in otherwise healthy elderly and some (such as the palmomental reflex) can be elicited at all ages. The exact pathophysiologic mechanisms underlying these reflexes are not completely understood. In isolation, they are neither sensitive nor specific for any neurologic disease. Although some can be seen in normal aging, their occurrence in combination should necessitate investigation for underlying disease (neurodegenerative disease and dementia) and should not be attributed to normal aging alone.[2]

Palmomental reflex

Contraction of the mentalis muscle in the lower jaw is elicited by stroking the ipsilateral thenar eminence. It is a polysynaptic and nociceptive reflex with the afferent arm traveling through the median and ulnar nerves and the efferent arm in the facial nerve. The threshold for eliciting the palmomental reflex varies greatly between individuals.[56] The palmomental reflex is seen in up to 27% of individuals before age 50 and in more than 35% of individuals over age 85.[31] The appearance of the palmomental reflex may reflect frontal lobe dysfunction.[2]

Snout or pout reflex

This is elicited by pressing or gently tapping over the philtrum of the upper lip in the midline, which results in pouting or pursing of the lips. It is a nociceptive reflex of the perioral muscles carried by the trigeminal and facial nerves for the afferent and efferent limbs. Unlike the palmomental reflex, it is generally not seen before the age of 40 to 50 according to different reports.[57] However, the incidence increases with age, with a prevalence of 73% by age 85.[27] The occurrence of this reflex correlates well with impaired performance on psychometric testing[58] and corresponds to loss of large pyramidal neurons in the anterior cingulate gyrus.[2]

Suck reflex

This is elicited by stroking the lips with the index finger or a reflex hammer. The response could be incomplete with the lips closing around the finger or object, or could be complete— resulting in sucking movements in the lips, tongue, and jaw.[44] If the stimulus is applied to the lateral margins of the lips, the head turns towards the side of the stimulus. Although it can be seen in 6% of normal elderly,[59] it is more common in the presence of dementia[58] and correlates with the severity of cognitive impairment.[60] The snout and suck reflex appear to be more common with prolonged use of phenothiazines.[44]

Grasp reflex

There are three different types of grasp reflex that reflect three different levels of severity of cortical disinhibition.[2] The first called tactile grasp is elicited by applying firm pressure across the palm from the ulnar to the radial side while distracting the patient (e.g., asking the patient to count backwards from 20). It is considered positive if the patient grasps the examiner's fingers or flexes the fingers with adduction of the thumb in response to stroking the palm. Traction grasp is described as the patient counter pulling when the examiner attempts to pull away from the patient's grip. Magnetic grasp is when the patient follows or reaches for the examiner's hand to grasp it. It is generally considered a pathologic sign, and often occurs as a result of contralateral or bilateral damage to medial frontal or basal ganglia structures. However, some have reported its presence in 3% to 67% of normal elderly[27,31] and generally increases with advanced age. It is also more frequent in Alzheimer's disease[61] and correlates with the degree of cognitive impairment.[60] Analogous to the grasp reflex in the hand is flexion and adduction of the toes with inversion and incurving of the foot in response to tactile stimulation or pressure on the sole. This reflex is seen invariably in neonates and may reappear in the elderly and contribute to gait difficulty.

Glabellar tap reflex

Other names for this reflex include glabella tap sign, orbicularis oculi sign, blinking reflex, and Myerson's sign. It is elicited by tapping between the eyebrows with the finger, at a rate of 2 per second and avoiding a visual threat response. A normal response consists of blinking in response to the first 3 to 9 taps, followed by cessation of the response with further tapping. It is considered positive or abnormal if blinking continues with further tapping. An abnormal glabellar tap was first described in Parkinson's disease patients and was considered to be diagnostic for that disease. However, it can occur with normal aging and other neurodegenerative disorders. It is found in more than 50% of normal older adults and it is debatable whether it becomes more prevalent with older age.[31,32] It is different from the other primitive reflexes in that it mainly results from lesions of basal ganglia, rather than cortical disinhibition.[2]

CONCLUDING COMMENTS

A variety of neurologic disorders (e.g., stroke, Parkinson's disease, Alzheimer's disease) preferentially affect older adults. To document normal findings and detect abnormal signs, a comprehensive mental status and neurologic examination should be performed in every older adult.

Altered cognitive function in the setting of a clear sensorium is consistent with dementia secondary to a neurodegenerative process (Alzheimer's disease, Parkinson's disease, Pick's disease) or medical illness (cerebrovascular disease, vitamin B_{12} deficiency, hypothyroidism). Delirium on the other hand causes alteration in sensorium and level of consciousness and may be due to medications, infection, head injury, or metabolic derangements. Associated features include disruption of sleep-wake cycle, intermittent drowsiness and agitation, restlessness, emotional lability, and frank psychosis (hallucination, illusions, delusions). Predisposing factors include advanced age, dementia, impaired physical or mental health, sensory deprivation (poor vision or hearing), and placement in intensive care units.

A functional decline in some aspects of cranial nerve function (e.g., vision, hearing, vestibular function, taste, and smell) can be readily detected on examination. In the absence of other findings, this may be considered part of the normal aging process. However, a constellation of abnormalities usually represent a pathologic condition afflicting the nervous system. Similarly, older individuals experience decreased mobility, coordination, sensation, and strength as they age. However, more profound changes that significantly alter mobility or present as focal neurologic signs should alert the clinician to a neuropathologic disorder and warrants diagnostic testing.

In conclusion, neurologic findings of normal aging include subtle declines in cognitive function, mildly impaired motor function, and altered sensory perceptions. However, exaggerated impairments in cognitive, behavioral, motor, and sensory function suggest the onset of neurologic diseases that commonly afflict the older adult. A comprehensive mental status and neurologic examination in addition to a detailed general physical examination is the foundation for identifying neuropathologic conditions that necessitate further investigation.

ACKNOWLEDGMENTS

This chapter was supported by a grants from the National Institute on Aging (P50 AG005681, P01 AG03991, P01 AG026276), the Alzheimer Association, and a generous gift from the Alan A. and Edith L. Wolff Charitable Trust.

KEY POINTS

Neurologic Signs in the Elderly

- Neurologic disorders are a common cause of morbidity, mortality, and institutionalization in elderly populations, not only increasing in severity of neurologic disease but modifying disease presentation.
- Because the frequency of cognitive disorders increases dramatically with advancing age, examination of mental status is one of the most important components of the neurologic examination. The elements of a comprehensive mental status examination include assessment of cognitive, functional, and behavioral domains.
- Neurologic findings of normal aging include subtle declines in cognitive function, mildly impaired motor function, and altered sensory perceptions. However, exaggerated impairments in cognitive, behavioral, motor, and sensory function suggest the onset of neurologic disease.
- A functional decline in sensory cranial nerve function (e.g., vision, hearing, vestibular function, taste, and smell), in the absence of other findings, may be considered part of the normal aging process.
- Primitive or "pathologic" reflexes (glabellar, grasp, snout, palmomental) occurring in isolation may be seen in normal aging. However, their occurrence in combination or with other neurologic signs may represent processes affecting frontal lobe function (e.g., dementia syndromes, demyelinating disease, or stroke).

For a complete list of references, please visit online only at www.expertconsult.com

CHAPTER 17

Geriatric Gastroenterology: Overview

Richard C. Feldstein
Robert E. Tepper
Seymour Katz

More than 20% of our population is expected to exceed 65 years of age by 2030,[1] with the most rapidly growing segment over 85 years of age.[2] Of necessity, gastroenterologists will be increasingly confronted with digestive diseases in elderly patients. Gastrointestinal disease is the second most common indication for hospital admission of elderly patients,[3] who account for four times as many hospitalizations as do younger patients.[1] In the outpatient setting, patients 75 and older visit internists six times more frequently than do younger adults.[3]

NORMAL PHYSIOLOGY OF AGING

With a few notable exceptions, the digestive system maintains normal functioning in elderly people. To distinguish between the expected age-related alterations of the gut and symptoms attributable to pathologic conditions, the clinician must have an understanding of the normal physiology of aging. One must also appreciate the interactions between the gastrointestinal (GI) tract and longstanding exposures to environmental agents (e.g., medications, tobacco, and alcohol) and chronic non-GI disease states (e.g., congestive heart failure, diabetes mellitus, chronic obstructive pulmonary disease, dementia, depression).[4] With this knowledge, it will become apparent that most new GI complaints in otherwise healthy older people are due to disease rather than to aging alone and therefore merit appropriate investigation and treatment.

Aging is not associated with a difference in either the desire to eat or the hunger response before meal intake, but postprandial hunger and the desire to eat are reduced.[5,6] One explanation may be that fasting and intraduodenal lipid-stimulated plasma concentrations of cholecystokinin (CCK), a physiologic satiety factor, and leptin, a hormone that functions mainly as a signal of adiposity eliciting long-term satiety, have been found to be higher in older than in younger men.[7–10] However, anorexia in older individuals should not be attributed to advanced age alone. This symptom warrants evaluation to exclude a medical or psychological cause or a medication-induced adverse effect.[5]

Up to 40% of healthy elderly people subjectively complain of dry mouth. Although baseline salivary flow probably decreases with aging, stimulated salivation is unchanged in both healthy and edentulous geriatric patients.[11–15] Chewing power is diminished, probably because of the decreased bulk of the muscles of mastication,[16,17] although perhaps attributable in part to preclinical manifestations of neurologic disease rather than to the normal aging process.[15] Although many older patients are edentulous to some degree, better dental care has enabled more of them to have intact teeth now than in the past.[5,18,19]

Gustatory and olfactory sensation tend to decrease with aging.[10,20] The ability to detect and discriminate between sweet, sour, salty, and bitter tastes deteriorates as one gets older.[5,10,21,20] Thresholds for salt and bitter taste show age-related elevations, whereas that for sweet taste appears stable.[5,22] By the ninth decade, the olfactory threshold increases by about 50%, contributing to poor smell recognition.[5,10,23]

Despite early data to the contrary, the physiologic function of the esophagus in otherwise healthy individuals is well preserved with increasing age, with the exception of very old patients.[24,25] Studies from the early 1960s introduced the concept of the "presbyesophagus" based on cineradiographic and manometric data,[26,27] but the term has been abandoned.[28] A more recent study that excluded patients with diabetes or neuropathy found no increase in dysmotility in elderly men.[29] Investigators have also found that minor alterations may occur in some octogenarians, including decreased pressure and delayed relaxation of the upper esophageal sphincter and reduction in the amplitude of esophageal contraction.[30,31] Furthermore, a recent study has shown age-related changes of increased stiffness and reduced primary and secondary peristalsis in the human esophagus that is associated with a deterioration of esophageal function beginning after the age of 40.[27] In addition, in a study comparing esophageal manometry and scintigraphic examinations of gastroesophageal reflux in groups of healthy volunteers ranging from 20 to 80 years of age, it was determined that while the number of reflux episodes per volunteer was similar in the various age groups, the duration of reflux episodes was longer in older volunteers. The older participants had impaired clearance of refluxed materials due to a high incidence of defective esophageal peristalsis.[33] Similarly, in another study, age was shown to correlate inversely with LES pressure and length, UES pressure and length, and peristaltic wave amplitude and velocity suggesting that normal esophageal motility deteriorates with advancing age.[34] Together, the above findings may help explain the high prevalence of reflux symptoms in the elderly.

Most studies on gastric histology have found evidence of an increased prevalence of atrophic gastritis in people over 60.[35,36] Consequently, it has been suggested that aging results in an overall decline in gastric acid output.[24,37,38] However, more recent data have demonstrated that gastric atrophy and hypochlorhydria are not normal processes of aging. Rather, *Helicobacter pylori* infestation, which is common in the elderly, not advancing age itself, appears to be the more likely cause of these histologic and acid secretory changes.[35,39–43] The literature remains conflicted over the issue of whether aging alone, rather than factors such as increased *H. pylori* infestation and decreased smoking leads to altered pepsin secretion.[6,41,44–45] Intrinsic factor secretion is usually maintained into advanced age and is retained longer in the setting of gastric atrophy than is acid or pepsin secretion.[46,47] Gastric prostaglandin synthesis, bicarbonate, and nonparietal fluid secretion may diminish, making the elderly more prone to nonsteroidal anti-inflammatory drug (NSAID)-induced mucosal damage.[5,6,10] Finally, most (but not all) studies have shown that gastric emptying of solids remains intact in the elderly, although liquid emptying is prolonged.[48–53]

Small bowel histology[54–56] and transit time[10,52,57–59] do not appear to change with age in humans, although increased epithelial proliferation in response to cellular injury has been found in a rodent model.[60] Splanchnic blood flow is reduced in the elderly population.[6] Small bowel absorptive capacity for most nutrients remains intact, but there are some exceptions especially those due to effects of disease (e.g., chronic gastritis and bacterial overgrowth) and medications on micronutrient absorption.[10] No change with aging was found in duodenal brush border membrane enzyme activity of glucose transport.[61] D-xylose absorption testing remains normal after correction for renal impairment, except perhaps in octogenarians.[62,63] Jejunal lactase activity decreases with age, whereas that of other disaccharides remains relatively stable, declining only during the seventh decade.[64] Protein digestion and assimilation,[24,65] and fat absorption remain normal with aging, although the latter has a more limited adaptive reserve capacity.[67–70] Absorption of fat-soluble vitamin A is increased in the elderly population,[10,46,71] while vitamin D absorption may be impaired[46,66,72,73] and a reduction in vitamin D receptor concentration and responsiveness occurs.[5,18,66] Absorption of the water-soluble vitamins B_1 (thiamine),[74] B_{12} (cyanocobalamin),[67,69,75] and C (ascorbic acid) remains normal, whereas disparate data exist on folate absorption with aging.[77,78] Iron absorption is maintained in the healthy elderly who are not hypochlorhydric,[79,80] but absorption of zinc[46,81] and calcium[46,82–84] declines with age.

Several histologic changes have been demonstrated in the colon, including increased collagen deposition,[6] atrophy of the muscularis propria with an increase in the amount of fibrosis and elastin,[24,85] and an increase in proliferating cells especially at the superficial portions of the crypts.[60,86] Some studies have found that colonic transit time increases with aging to varying degrees,[70,87,89] perhaps due to the increase with age in the number of abnormally appearing myenteric ganglia in the human colon.[88] Other studies have not shown any change.[90,91] Current thinking holds that colonic motility and the colon's response to feeding are largely unaffected by healthy aging. Prolonged transit time in older people with constipation is due to factors associated with aging (e.g., comorbidity, immobilization, drugs) rather than aging per se.[92]

Anorectal physiologic changes have been well-documented. Aging is associated with decreased resting anal sphincter pressure in both sexes and decreased maximal sphincter pressure in women.[93,94,95] This may be due in part to age-related changes in muscle mass and contractility and in part to pudendal nerve damage associated with perineal descent in elderly women.[95,96] The closing pressure (i.e., the difference between the maximum resting anal pressure and the rectal pressure) also falls in elderly women.[97] Maximum squeeze pressure declines with age, particularly in postmenopausal women,[8] as does rectal wall elasticity.[98,99] An age-dependant increase in rectal pressure threshold producing an initial sensation of rectal filling has also been demonstrated.[100] Defecation dynamic studies in older women show a significant failure of rectal evacuation because of insufficient opening of the rectoanal angle and an increased degree of perineal descent compared with younger women.[92,101] Histologic[102] and endosonographic[103] studies on anorectal structure revealed that the internal anal sphincter develops fibro-fatty degeneration and increased thickness, respectively, with aging.

The pancreas undergoes minor histologic changes with aging.[24,104,105] There also appears to be a steady increase in the caliber of the main pancreatic duct, with other branches showing areas of focal dilatation or stenosis without any apparent disease or functional age-related changes.[104,106] In fact, 69% of patients older than 70 years of age without pancreatic pathology have a "dilated" duct when criteria developed for younger patients are applied.[107] High echogenicity of the pancreas is a normal finding on ultrasonography.[108] Aging reduces exocrine pancreatic flow rate and secretion of bicarbonate and enzymes, and the rate falls significantly with repeated stimulation.[8,104,105,109,110] However, other studies have shown a lack of reduced pancreatic secretions with age, independent of disease and the effect of drugs.[110]

Anatomical studies on the liver reveal an age-related decrease in weight, both absolute and relative to body weight, and in the number and size of hepatocytes.[111–112] Pseudocapillarization of the hepatic sinusoid (morphologic changes such as defenestration and thickening of the liver sinusoidal endothelial cell, increased numbers of fat engorged nonactivated stellate cells), lipofuscin accumulation, bile duct proliferation, fibrosis, and nonspecific reactive hepatitis are histologic changes more common in the elderly population.[112,113,114] The major functional changes in older patients are reduction in hepatic blood flow,[110,114] altered clearance of certain drugs, and delayed hepatic regeneration after injury.[113–117] The altered drug clearance is due to age-related reductions in phase I reactions (e.g., oxidation, hydrolysis, reduction), first pass hepatic metabolism, and serum albumin binding capacity. Phase II reactions (e.g., glucuronidation, sulfation), however, remain unaffected by aging.[111,112,115,116] There are no age-specific alterations in conventional liver blood tests.[117]

Although an early cholecystographic study found that gallbladder emptying remained stable with increasing age,[118,119] more recent data showed that gallbladder contraction in the elderly person may be less responsive to CCK.[119,120] Increases in the proportions of the phospholipid and cholesterol components of bile raise the lithogenicity index,[121,122] leading to increased occurrence of gallstones in the aged.[24] Choledocholithiasis is particularly common in elderly patients who have undergone an emergency cholecystectomy, the incidence of bile duct stones approached 50%.[123] Even in the absence of bile duct stones or other pathology, older patients generally have larger common bile duct diameters than do younger patients.[124]

ALTERED MANIFESTATION OF ADULT GASTROINTESTINAL DISEASES

Although there are certain disorders that occur almost exclusively in the elderly population, the majority of diseases afflicting older people are those that affect younger adults as well. However, these illnesses may have atypical features that must be recognized by clinicians and represent a formidable challenge. In elderly people with an "acute abdomen," the initial diagnostic impression has been found to be incorrect in up to two thirds of patients,[125] and the mortality in octogenarians is 70 times that in young adults.[126]

Acute abdominal pain appears to mute with age.[47,127] Theories explaining this phenomenon include increased endogenous opiate secretion, a decline in nerve conduction, and mental depression.[128] Pain localization is often atypical in elderly patients. For example, in a study on acute appendicitis, 21% of patients over 60 years of age have atypical pain distribution, while this occurred in only 3% of patients under 50 years of age.[129]

The causes of acute abdominal pain differ as well. Acute cholecystitis, rather than nonspecific abdominal pain or acute appendicitis, was found to be the most common cause in one large survey.[126,127] In this series, 10% of patients over 70 years of age were found to have a vascular cause for their pain, such as mesenteric ischemia, embolus, or infarction. Furthermore, retrospective studies have shown that in elderly patients with acute cholecystitis, more than 60% of elderly patients did not have the typical back or flank pain and 5% had no pain at all. In addition, 40% denied nausea, more than 50% were afebrile, and 41% had a normal white count. Overall, 13% of elderly patients had no fever, leukocytosis, or abnormal liver function tests.[127] A multicenter review found that 25% of emergency patients over the age of 70 had cancer (usually colorectal in Europe and North America, and hepatocellular in tropical regions)[126] as the cause of pain, whereas patients below age 50 had malignancy as the explanation in fewer than 1% of cases.[130]

Acute appendicitis may have few overt abdominal signs[127,131,129] and may therefore progress more frequently to gangrene and perforation.[132] Other intraabdominal inflammatory conditions, such as diverticulitis, may have rather nonspecific symptoms including anorexia, altered mental status, low-grade or absence of fever, relatively little tenderness, and late-stage complications (e.g., hepatic abscess). Even perforation of a viscus may lack the typical dramatic manifestations.[128,136] Possible explanations for the paucity of tenderness in some cases include altered sensory perception, use of psychotropic drugs, and absence of chemical peritonitis if the patient is hypochlorhydric.[47] The site of perforation also differs with age. Colonic perforation is more common than perforated peptic ulcer disease or appendicitis, the two most common causes for generalized peritonitis in younger patients.[126]

Studies vary regarding whether or not there is a higher prevalence of gastroesophageal reflux disease (GERD) in the elderly population,[134,137,139,140] but several studies suggest that the frequency of GERD complications is significantly higher in older people.[134,137,138] Severe esophagitis is much more common in patients beyond the age of 65 than in young people.[138,142] Esophageal sensitivity seems to decrease with age,[141] so very severe esophagitis may be associated with a relative paucity of symptoms. In fact one study showed that greater than 75% do not experience acid regurgitation as an initial symptom.[134] Therefore manifestations of GERD are more likely to be late-stage complications, such as bleeding from hemorrhagic esophagitis,[142] dysphagia from a peptic stricture, or adenocarcinoma in the setting of Barrett's esophagus. GERD-induced chest pain may mimic or occur concomitantly with cardiac disease; thus reflux must be excluded in any elderly patient with all but very typical angina.[25] Aspiration from occult GERD should be considered in elderly patients with recurrent pneumonia or exacerbations of underlying chronic obstructive pulmonary disease.[25] Early endoscopy is indicated in all elderly patients with GERD, regardless of symptom severity.[134,137] The medical and surgical treatment of GERD in the elderly follows the same principles as for young patients.[137] Proton pump inhibitors as a class are considered first-line treatment for GERD and erosive esophagitis in the elderly,[134,143] although the elderly may require a greater degree of acid suppression than young patients to heal their esophagitis.[140] And with the advent of newer proton pump inhibitors, studies have shown good tolerability even for long-term therapy due to minimal interactions with other drugs because of a lower affinity for cytochrome P450.[133]

Gastroduodenal ulcer disease has a several-fold greater incidence, hospitalization rate, and mortality in the elderly.[144–146] Up to 90% of ulcer-related mortality in the United States occurs in patients over 65.[146] This is due to an increase in injurious agents (e.g., *H. pylori* and nonsteroidal antiinflammatory drugs [NSAIDs], two factors which do not seem to act synergistically)[147,153] and to impaired defense mechanisms (e.g., lower levels of mucosal prostaglandins).[10,148] There may be a paucity or distortion of classic burning epigastric pain, temporal features related to food intake, and typical patterns of radiation.[47] Pain was absent in one third of elderly hospitalized patients with peptic ulcer disease.[149] As a result, elderly patients more frequently develop complications such as bleeding or perforation. Giant benign ulcers of the elderly can mimic malignancy by presenting with weight loss, anorexia, hypoalbuminemia, and anemia. Despite the increased morbidity and mortality of upper GI bleeding in the elderly, endoscopic and clinical criteria have been reported that would allow for successful outpatient management.[150–153]

The manifestations of celiac sprue differ considerably in the elderly since features are generally more subtle than in young patients.[47,157] Only one quarter of newly diagnosed elderly patients with celiac disease have primarily diarrhea and weight loss.[154] Vague symptoms, including dyspepsia or an isolated folate or iron deficiency, may be the patient's sole manifestation.[157,158] In one study, the mean delay to diagnosis in the elderly aged 65 years and older was 17 years.[159] Severe osteopenia and osteomalacia[157] and a bleeding diathesis due to hypoprothrombinemia are more common in the elderly than in the young.[47] Small bowel lymphoma may be particularly common when celiac disease occurs in the elderly person.[155,159] Therefore elderly patients with persistent symptoms including weight loss, pain, and bleeding—despite strict adherence to a gluten-free diet—require careful evaluation to exclude GI malignancy.[156]

Constipation is perceived by elderly patients to be straining during defecation rather than decreased bowel frequency,[160–162] and it may be manifested in unusual ways. Excessive defecatory straining in patients with underlying cerebrovascular disease or impaired baroreceptor reflexes can present as syncope or a transient ischemic attack. When unrelieved constipation progresses to fecal impaction, an overflow "paradoxical" diarrhea may occur, even in patients with relatively normal anal sphincter pressure. If the clinician does not recognize this and prescribes the standard antidiarrheal therapy, the underlying impaction will only worsen and potentially lead to other serious complications, such as stercoral ulcers and bleeding.[161,162]

Crohn's disease of new onset in elderly people has been commonly reported to be limited to the colon more often than it is in young patients.[164] The colitis is more often left-sided in the elderly, whereas proximal colonic involvement is more common in the young.[165,166] Older patients are less likely to have close relatives affected by Crohn's disease and to have abdominal pain as a presenting symptom.[167] Crohn's disease in the elderly group develops more rapidly and is characterized by a shorter time interval between onset of symptoms and first resection.[167] Elderly patients with Crohn's disease may suffer fewer relapses,[47] and their postoperative recurrence rate is lower than, or equal to, that of young people.[164] However, in older patients who do have postoperative recurrence, it occurs more rapidly than in younger patients.[167] Whereas those few young Crohn's disease patients who die do so of their disease, death in older patients is usually due to unrelated causes.[164] Older patients are more prone to steroid-induced osteoporosis;[156] bisphosphonates prevent and effectively treat bone loss in these patients[168] and their use must be strongly considered in this setting.

The manifestations of ulcerative colitis are generally the same in the young and the old, including extraintestinal manifestations.[166] In the elderly person, proctosigmoiditis is more common, whereas pancolitis and the need for surgery are less common.

Therapy for inflammatory bowel disease in the elderly can follow the same stepwise regimen as in the younger population. However, a clear distinction must be made between the "fit" elderly and the "frail" elderly. Studies have shown that the "fit" elderly can tolerate therapeutics similar to the younger generation, taking into account the natural decline in age-related drug metabolism with minimal additional risk or morbidity.[204]

The most common manifestations of gallstone disease in the elderly population are acute cholecystitis and cholangitis.[47] In fact, biliary tract disease is the most common indication for surgical intervention in patients having acute abdominal pain over the age of 55 years.[127] Cholecystitis in the elderly person may have nonspecific symptoms, including vague mental and physical disability.[127,169,170] Pain may be muted[127] or absent even in the presence of gallbladder empyema, leading to a delay in hospitalization.[171] Typical features of cholangitis may be absent. Therefore blood cultures are critical to exclude bacteremia as the sole evidence of an infected biliary tract, which can result in greater mortality in the elderly.[172,173] Elderly patients who require emergency cholecystectomy have a higher mortality rate than younger patients, but can do well with elective operations aside from longer operative times and postoperative hospital stays.[174] Thus surgery should not be denied to the healthy elderly patient with recurrent biliary colic based on age alone.[123,175] Minimally invasive procedures such as endoscopic retrograde cholangiopancreatography and laparoscopic cholecystectomy should be used whenever possible.[123]

The clinical course of liver disease in the elderly is usually similar to that in the young, although complications are tolerated less well.[47,176] Chronic hepatitis C, along with alcoholic liver disease, is emerging as the most common cause of chronic parenchymal liver disease in the elderly population.[117,178] Viral hepatitis more commonly has a prolonged and cholestatic picture in the elderly, although data are equivocal on whether older people are more or less likely to suffer severe or fulminant hepatitis.[112] Although the risk of death from fulminant liver failure from acute hepatitis A infection appears to increase with age,[178] acute hepatitis B in elderly patients is usually a mild, subclinical disease and the risk of fulminant disease is not increased.[177] However, a higher risk for progressing to chronic infection exists for those who acquire the disease after 65 years of age.[178] Advanced age at the onset of infection with hepatitis C is associated with an increased mortality rate.[177] This is related to a more rapid rate of fibrosis, the cause of which is unknown but presumed to be related to the decline in immune function with age.[178] When fulminant hepatic failure develops from any cause, advanced age is an adverse prognostic variable.[117] Certain conditions, including alcoholic liver disease, hemochromatosis, primary biliary cirrhosis, and hepatocellular carcinoma, are often seen in more advanced stages when they first present in older patients.[112]

Nonalcoholic fatty liver (NAFLD) is the most common liver disorder in the United States and worldwide[204] and is seen with increasing prevalence in the elderly.[205] However, recent studies have shown a lack of association with the metabolic syndrome, a clear distinction from the disease in adulthood.[205] In addition, the natural progression of NAFLD with associated liver complications is typically noted between the sixth and eighth decades of life.[206] Therefore the diagnosis of cryptogenic cirrhosis in the elderly may be directly related to the ever rising epidemic of fatty liver in adulthood.

GASTROINTESTINAL PROBLEMS UNIQUE TO THE ELDERLY POPULATION

Certain gastrointestinal symptoms and diseases occur primarily, or even exclusively, in the elderly population. In the esophagus, a posterior hypopharyngeal (Zenker's) diverticulum may form as a result of reduced muscle compliance of the upper esophageal sphincter.[179,180] The most common presentation is dysphagia; however, serious complications include aspiration and malnutrition. Neurologic disorders, particularly cerebrovascular insult (e.g., small basal ganglia infarcts)[10] and Parkinson's disease, account for 80% of cases of oropharyngeal dysphagia in elderly people.[181] Dysphagia aortica is a syndrome in which symptoms are caused by extrinsic compression of the esophagus by a large thoracic aneurysm or a rigid atherosclerotic aorta.[31] Although cervical osteophytes are common in the elderly population, they are thought to be a very rare cause of dysphagia.[31]

Stomach disorders generally confined to elderly people include atrophic gastritis, with or without pernicious anemia. As mentioned previously, prolonged *H. pylori* infection rather than aging alone may be responsible for this condition. A Dieulafoy's lesion, resulting from a nontapering ectatic submucosal artery, may be an obscure cause of upper GI bleeding in patients of all ages but is particularly frequent in the elderly population.[182,183]

The prevalence of small bowel diverticulosis increases greatly in older people.[185] The condition may be limited to a single large duodenal diverticulum or may be characterized by numerous diverticula throughout the jejunum. Although most cases are completely asymptomatic, some lead to perforation, hemorrhage, or bacterial overgrowth-induced malabsorption.[47,185,186]

Chronic mesenteric ischemia, manifested by intestinal angina, is a very rare form of mesenteric vascular disease seen in elderly patients with atherosclerosis.[187,188] In fact, mesenteric artery stenosis is found in 17.5% of elderly patients aged greater than 70 years.[187] Aortoenteric fistula, an uncommon cause of life-threatening GI hemorrhage, occurs in elderly patients with prior graft placement for an abdominal aortic aneurysm (AAA) or, rarely, with an untreated AAA. It can also occur in patients who have undergone aortoiliac bypass surgery (0.5%) and in patients with native anatomy and after enteral stent placement.[184]

NSAID-induced enteropathy, characterized by ulceration, leading to acute or occult bleeding, ileal stenosis, strictures, protein loss, or iron deficiency, has been increasingly recognized.[156]

Age is a strong risk factor for colon polyps and cancer. Guidelines that advise colorectal screening examinations beginning at age 50 in average-risk patients and at age 40 for certain high-risk patients do not provide upper age constraints for colorectal screening. Some experts have suggested an age cutoff at 80 years for screening[189] and 85 years for surveillance for patients who have had only small tubular adenomas.[190] Since these ages are somewhat arbitrary, colorectal screening and surveillance in the elderly group must be individualized based on comorbidity and life expectancy.[191,192] Colonoscopic polypectomy, rather than surgery, has been advocated for the treatment of large polyps in healthy elderly patients up to 90 years old in whom life expectancy is at least 5 years.[189]

Several other colonic disorders are seen far more commonly in older patients than in younger patients. These include colonic diverticulosis, a condition found on postmortem examination in more than 50% of people over the age of 70.[194] In fact, a recent study has estimated its prevalence to be 65% in elderly patients greater than 65 years of age.[193] Also common is segmental colitis associated with sigmoid diverticulosis;[195,196] sigmoid volvulus; vascular ectasia in the cecum;[197] stercoral ulcer in the setting of fecal impaction; fecal incontinence,[160,163,198,200] the second leading cause of institutionalization among the elderly;[96,200] and *Clostridium difficile* infection, a frequent cause of diarrhea in older people,[196,199] and the most common cause of nosocomial infectious diarrhea in the nursing home setting.[201]

The majority of elderly patients with jaundice have biliary tract obstruction as the cause, rather than hepatocellular disease. Malignancy is more common than choledocholithiasis as a cause of obstruction. Since an elderly person with malignant obstructive jaundice rarely survives more than 4 months, endoscopic rather than surgical biliary decompression is appropriate.[123] In this setting, endoscopic biliary stenting for palliation has been advocated to restore a sense of well-being, to avoid early liver failure and encephalopathy, and to improve the patient's nutritional and immunologic status.[123,202] However, with the advent of improved surgical techniques and postoperative mortality, surgery has expanded to a greater number of patients during the past decade and has found increased use in patients over 70 years old.[202] When acute hepatitis occurs, one third of cases are commonly[178] drug induced and not viral as in young people.[112] Pyogenic liver abscesses primarily affect elderly patients, and should be considered in the differential diagnosis of fever or bacteremia of unclear cause.[177]

SUMMARY

The gastrointestinal tract generally maintains normal physiologic functioning in the elderly population. Most new GI symptoms in otherwise healthy older patients are due to pathology rather than to the aging process alone. These patients merit attentive and expeditious evaluation and management since their ability to tolerate illness is lower than that of younger patients.

KEY POINTS
Evaluation and Treatment of GI Disorders

- Normal physiologic changes in the aged gastrointestinal tract are few, so clinicians must seek out and actively treat GI disorders (e.g., oropharyngeal dysphagia, malabsorption, abnormal liver enzymes) and not ascribe these signs and symptoms to the aging process.
- Elderly patients have diminished reserve capacity to accommodate illness and should be thoughtfully evaluated and treated early in the course of disease to prevent irreversible deterioration.
- Goals of treatment must be realistic and individualized, with an emphasis on returning the patient to a functional lifestyle.
- Comorbid conditions and concomitant medications have a dramatic effect on the presentation and prognosis of GI disease in elderly people.
- To improve compliance, clinicians must avoid prescribing medications that are expensive and/or are taken frequently throughout the day if alternatives are available because elderly patients may be on a fixed income, subject to "polypharmacy," or have memory impairment.
- Clinicians should avoid prescribing drugs more likely to cause adverse effects (e.g., isoniazid, corticosteroids, opiates, mineral oil, NSAIDs, anticholinergics) if reasonable alternatives are available, and avoid overprescribing tranquilizers and antidepressants for symptoms thought to be due to somatization.
- Although irritable bowel syndrome of new onset may occur in the elderly, 90% of cases first appear before the age of 50. Therefore this diagnosis should be rendered only after thorough evaluation to exclude other diseases, including malignancies or ischemia.
- Endoscopy and abdominal surgery can be performed safely in the elderly. Morbidity and mortality are related to the degree of concomitant disease and the emergent or elective nature of the procedure. An unnecessary delay in surgery is often lethal.
- Chronologic age need not be an absolute contraindication to aggressive therapeutic measures, such as chemotherapy or organ transplantation, as the tolerance of these interventions correlates more with the overall physiologic condition.

For a complete list of references, please visit online only at www.expertconsult.com

CHAPTER 18

Aging of the Urinary Tract

Phillip P. Smith
George A. Kuchel

INTRODUCTION

Although traditional classification considers the upper and lower urinary tracts as part of one system, each serves a distinct function. We are greatly indebted to Drs. Jassal and Oreopoulos, authors of this chapter (Aging of the Urinary Tract) in the previous edition, for their detailed discussion of renal aging. In this edition, both upper and lower urinary tract components will be considered, emphasizing the known effects of aging on each system. Nevertheless, a number of potentially pertinent topics will not be discussed in this chapter. For example, age-related changes in renal handling of water and electrolytes are addressed in Chapter 85, whereas diseases which commonly affect the aged kidney, prostate, and gynecologic structures are discussed in Chapters 84, 86, and 87, respectively. Of course, given the multifactorial systemic complexity inherent to aging and to common geriatric syndromes (Chapter 10),[1] the discussion will need to cross traditional organ-based boundaries. Therefore we will also discuss the ability of age-related declines in renal function to influence key geriatric measures, such as cognitive function and mobility performance. Conversely, given growing evidence that oxidative stress, inflammation, and nutrition can influence aging- and disease-related processes across many different tissues, the ability of these systemic factors to modify urinary tract aging will also be considered. Finally, the contribution of lower and upper urinary tract dysfunction to urinary incontinence, a major geriatric syndrome, is discussed in Chapter 109.

UPPER URINARY TRACT: KIDNEYS AND URETERS

Overview

Declines in renal function represent one of the best documented and most dramatic physiologic alterations in human aging. In spite of great progress, important issues remain. For example, it has been difficult to explain why renal aging can be so variable between seemingly "normal" individuals and to establish which of these changes may potentially be reversible. Nevertheless, recent developments and continuing research in this area offer unique opportunities for improving the lives of older adults.[2–5]

Glomerular filtration rate

Age-related declines in glomerular filtration rate (GFR) are well established; yet contrary to general belief, GFR does not inevitably decrease with age. Among Baltimore Longitudinal Study of Aging participants, mean GFR declined approximately 8.0 mL/min per 1.73 m^2/decade from the middle of the fourth decade of life.[6] However, these decrements were not universal, with approximately one third of these subjects showing no significant decrease in GFR over time.[6] This high degree of interindividual variability among relatively healthy older adults has raised the hope that age-related declines in GFR may not be inevitable and could ultimately be preventable even in the absence of an overt disease process. At the same time, clinicians wishing to prescribe renally excreted medications to healthy older adults clearly require reliable tools to accurately estimate GFR.

The decrease in GFR with age is generally not accompanied by elevations in serum creatinine[6] since age-related declines in muscle mass tend to parallel those observed for GFR, causing overall creatinine production to also fall with age. Thus serum creatinine levels generally overestimate GFR with age, and in women and underweight individuals serum creatinine is most insensitive to impaired kidney function.[7] Although many formulas have been devised for estimating creatinine clearance based on normative data,[8,9] their reliability in predicting individual renal function is poor.[10,11] In the frail and severely ill patients on multiple medications—where the need for accurate estimation is greatest—the reliability of such estimates may be the most questionable. In consequence, timed short duration urine collections for creatinine clearance measurement are generally recommended.[10,12] In contrast to the poor predictive ability of low creatinine, elevations in serum creatinine above 132 mmol/L (1.5 mg/dL) reflect declines in GFR greater than what would be typically expected with normal aging, indicating the presence of likely underlying pathology. Ultimately, even creatinine clearance has limitations and may underestimate GFR.[13] Cystatin C, a measure of kidney function that is independent of muscle mass, has been advocated as an improved marker of reduced GFR in the elderly with creatinine levels within the normal range.[14] Although FDA-approved kits for its measurement have been available since 2001 and in spite of its potential attraction in the management of frail older adults, the precise role of cystatin C measurements in clinical decision-making remains to be defined.

Renal blood flow

On average, aging is associated with a progressive decrease in renal plasma flow.[15,16] Losses of 10% per decade have been described, with typical values declining from 600 mL/min in a young adult to 300 mL/min at 80 years of age.[15,16] Perfusion of the renal medulla is maintained in the face of lower blood flow to the cortex, which can be observed as patchy cortical defects on renal scans obtained in healthy older adults. Regional renal flow and GFR are determined by a balance between the vascular tone involving afferent and efferent renal blood supply. Generally, renal vasoconstriction increases in old age, whereas the capacity of the vascular bed to dilate is decreased. Responsiveness to vasodilators (e.g., nitric oxide, prostacyclin) appears to be attenuated, whereas responsiveness to vasoconstrictors (e.g., angiotensin II) is enhanced.[5] Basal renin and angiotensin II are significantly lower in older adults, whereas the ability of various different stimuli to activate the renin-angiotensin system is blunted.

Tubular function

The ability of the tubules to excrete and reabsorb specific solutes plays a crucial role in maintaining normal fluid and electrolyte balance. The impact of aging and specific disease processes on the ability of tubules to handle specific solutes is discussed in another chapter (Chapter 85). Nevertheless, some overarching principles are worthy of note. First, overall tubular function appears to decline with aging. Second, the ability to handle water, sodium, potassium, and other electrolytes is generally impaired with aging. Third, such physiologic declines do not generally affect the ability of older adults to maintain normal fluid and electrolyte balance under basal conditions. Fourth, older adults are less able to maintain normal homeostasis when exposed to specific fluid and electrolyte challenges.[2,5,17]

For example, ability to both conserve and excrete sodium is impaired, with reduced salt resorption in the ascending loop of Henle, reduced serum aldosterone secretion, and a relative resistance to both aldosterone and angiotensin II.[2,5] As a result, older adults take longer to reduce their sodium excretion in response to a salt-restricted diet.[2,5] Conversely, older adults take longer to excrete a sodium load.[2,5] Qualitatively similar changes have been described as regards tubular capacity to adjust to changes in water.

Structural changes

As with other organs, there are both differences between individuals—some have more evident aging changes than others—and within individual kidneys (i.e., different parts of the kidney are affected differently by aging). In general, the aged kidney is granular in appearance, with modest declines in parenchymal mass.[2,5] The most impressive changes involve a reduction in both the number and size of nephrons in the renal cortex, with a relative sparing of the medullary regions.[2,5] Loss of parenchymal mass leads to a widening of interstitial spaces between the tubules and an increase in interstitial connective tissue. Numbers of visible glomeruli in aged kidneys decline in parallel with change in weight, with the percentage of glomeruli that are sclerotic increasing.[2,5] Sclerosis is associated with lost lobulation of the glomerular tuft, increased mesangial cells, and decreased epithelial cells, resulting in a smaller effective filtering surface. In response, remaining nonsclerotic glomeruli compensate by enlarging and hyperfiltering.

Even in the absence of hypertension and other relevant diseases, important changes of the intrarenal vasculature can be observed in old age.[2,5] Larger renal vessels may show sclerotic changes, whereas smaller vessels generally are spared. Nevertheless, arteriolar-glomerular units demonstrate distinctive changes in old age.[2,5,18] Cortical changes are more profound, with hyalinization and collapse of glomerular tufts, luminal obliteration within preglomerular arterioles and decreased blood flow. Structural changes within the medulla are less pronounced, whereas juxtamedullary regions demonstrate evidence of anatomic continuity and functional shunting between afferent and efferent arterioles.

Mechanistic considerations

The hyperfiltration theory suggests that a loss of glomeruli results in increased capillary blood flow through the remaining glomeruli and a correspondingly high intracapillary pressure.[2,5] Such age-related increases in intracapillary pressure (or shear stress) can also result in local endothelial cell damage and resultant glomerular injury, contributing to a progressive glomerulosclerosis.[2,5,19] Cytokines and other vasoactive humoral factors have been implicated in this type of pressure-mediated renal damage.[2,5,20] Also in support of the hyperfiltration theory, both restricted protein intake[21] and those antihypertensives that reduce single nephron GFR (e.g., ACE inhibitors and angiotensin II blockers)[21] reduce glomerular capillary pressure, attenuate glomerular injury, and prevent measurable declines in renal function.

Other factors and mechanisms contribute to age-related declines in renal function. For example, individuals born with a reduced nephron mass could be more vulnerable to all categories of renal injury, including that associated with aging. In fact, a growing body of research has linked renal aging to the damaging effects of normal metabolism through the accumulation of toxins, such as reactive oxygen species (ROS), advanced glycosylation end products (AGE), and advanced lipoxidation end products (ALE).[2,3,5,22,23] This "toxin-mediated" theory has many attractions. First, these toxins accumulate with aging and can induce structural and functional changes. Second, they provide vital linkages between efforts to understand aging at the level of a single organ to traditional gerontologic research into longevity (Chapter 4). Third, nutritional and eventual pharmacologic interventions may allow individuals to decrease exposure to such toxins and to ultimately prevent or delay renal aging. Fourth, such research has permitted the development of a pathophysiologic framework within which multiple different risk factors including underlying genetic predisposition, renal progenitor cell behavior,[24] gonadal hormone levels,[25] diet,[22] smoking,[26] and multiple subclinical processes can all influence how renal aging manifests in individuals.[2,5,23]

A system-based perspective

Renal aging cannot be viewed in isolation from aging at the systemic level. Not only are most individuals with chronic kidney disease (CKD) elderly, but these patients are frail and at high risk of being disabled.[4] Individuals with advanced CKD have an especially high risk of developing cardiovascular disease,[27] cognitive declines,[27–30] sarcopenia,[31–33] and poor physical performance.[27,34] It remains to be seen to what extent milder declines in renal function, more consistent with normal aging, may contribute to altered body composition and physiologic performance seen in generally healthy older adults. As discussed, creatinine-based estimates of GFR depend on skeletal muscle mass and tend to overestimate GFR in older adults. Thus it is interesting that even mild declines in GFR as measured using cystatin C were associated with poorer physical function, whereas creatinine-based GFR estimates demonstrated a relationship only when less than 60 mL/min/1.73 m^2.[35] Ultimately the development of an approach that places renal aging in a systems-based context where key functional issues are also considered may offer some of the most exciting opportunities for developing interventions that will help maintain function and independence in late life.

LOWER URINARY TRACT: BLADDER AND OUTLET

Overview

The function of the lower urinary tract (LUT) is to isolate the kidneys from the exterior environment, thus allowing urine storage and periodic evacuation. The anatomic arrangement of the non-refluxing ureterovesical junction, the fluid-tight urethral sphincteric mechanism, and the interposed chamber (the bladder) create an effective barrier to the retrograde passage of infectious agents into the kidneys and thence into the bloodstream. Presumably, as the result of evolutionary pressures, the bladder and its outlet normally function as a urine storage structure sufficiently capacious to accept several hours' volume of renal output, whereas an efficient evacuation mechanism under voluntary permissive control can be quickly and voluntarily activated and then returned to storage status.

The requirements for proper function of this system include normal sensory transduction of normal physiologic bladder filling; central transmission and subconscious processing; appropriate conscious recognition and processing; coordination of sphincteric relaxation and bladder pressurization via detrusor contraction; normal biomechanical function of the bladder and its outflow, and intact urethral/bladder guarding and voiding reflexes. In addition to the multiplicity of potential age-associated pathologies, which may disturb this complex process, biomechanical and functional changes as a result of the aging process per se also alter the storage and evacuation function of the LUT (Table 18-1). This section will discuss common LUT symptoms and how these may relate to changes due to "normal" aging versus pathologic aging.

Lower urinary tract symptoms are broadly categorized into irritability (overactive bladder; frequency/urgency/nocturia), obstructive/retentive (hesitancy, abnormal stream, incomplete emptying), and incontinence. The prevalence of all such symptoms increases with age and is population-dependent. The NOBLE study reported data on 5204 randomly selected participants. Overactive bladder symptoms were experienced by 5% to 10% of people under age 35, increasing to 30% to 35% over age 75, with no gender differences.[36] Overactive bladder symptoms including incontinence were experienced more commonly and earlier in life in women than in men, with 19% of women and 8% to 10% of men over age 65 reporting some degree of urinary incontinence. Similarly, in 550 symptomatic patients, lower urinary tract symptoms increased with age in both women and men.[37] The prevalence of moderate to severe symptoms roughly doubled between age 40 and 49 and over 80.[37] A urodynamic study of continent elderly people found that 63% were symptom-free, 52% were both symptom-free and free of any potential confounding disease or drug, and 18% were also free of any urodynamic abnormality.[38] Detrusor overactivity unrelated to identifiable disease was observed in 53%, with no correlation with either gender or age.[38] Bladder contractility decreased with age, as defined by postvoid residual volume after a strain-free void.[38] Finally, a urodynamic study of incontinent institutionalized elderly patients reported a prevalence of detrusor overactivity of 61%,[39] with a similar proportion (59%) showing detrusor underactivity.[39] In the same study, 92% of the nondemented individuals, but only 65% of the demented subjects, reported warning sensations.[39]

Table 18-1. Potential and Common Influences on LUT Function in the Elderly

"Normal" Aging
- Afferent/thresholding changes
- Diminished neuromuscular detrusor function
- Altered outflow tract characteristics
- Increased nocturnal urine production

Pathologic Internal Dysfunctions
- Afferent dysfunction: neural tissue damage (i.e., childbearing, biomechanical changes [injury, disease], surgery, chronic obstruction, diabetes)
- Efferent dysfunction: chronic obstruction, tissue damage (neurologic, myopathy), etc.
- Control/reflex dysfunction: disc or cord disease, CNS disease
- Defects of volition due to dementia, CVA, etc.

External Factors
- Fecal impaction and sensorimotor reflex suppression secondary to colorectal distention
- Medications: decreased urethral resistance (α-blockers, neuroleptics, benzodiazepines), increased bladder pressure (bethanechol, cisapride), increased urine production (diuretics), efferent/motor impairment (anticholinergics, antiparkinsonism agents, β-blockers, disopyramide); indirect effects (cough—ACE inhibitors, mental status changes—psychotropics).
- Environmental inadequacies

Physiologic assessment

Impaired detrusor and sphincteric function are common in old age, consistent with lower urinary tract symptoms being more common in older adults. However, the relative contributions of aging have yet to be disentangled from those of the menopause, pelvic organ prolapse, bladder outlet obstruction, and comorbidities (obesity, cardiovascular insufficiency, dementia, diabetic and other neuropathies).

The impact of prostatic hypertrophy (BPH) in men on lower urinary tract function is discussed elsewhere (Chapter 86). In women, pelvic organ prolapse may bear both direct and indirect relationships to lower urinary tract dysfunction.[40] About 40% of women with LUT symptoms have vaginal prolapse, and vice versa. Lower urinary tract symptoms correlate moderately well with the severity of vaginal prolapse.[41] Anterior and posterior vaginal prolapse to levels above the introitus may be associated with irritative and incontinence symptoms, and anterior and apical vaginal prolapse beyond the introitus may produce bladder outlet obstruction. Significantly, sphincteric incompetence may be masked by significant anterior prolapse; we await reliable methods to assess sphincteric competence in such patients.

The impact of estrogen loss with menopause and aging on lower urinary tract function is not well characterized. In mature rodents, oophorectomy results in decreases in detrusor smooth muscle, axonal degeneration, and EM findings of sarcolemmal dense band patterns with diminished caveolar numbers, suggesting impaired contractile properties as a result of de-estrogenization.[42,43] In a study of symptomatic premenopausal and postmenopausal women, a lower mean maximum detrusor pressure was observed during voiding in postmenopausal women, suggesting that menopause may influence LUT function either by impaired detrusor function or reduced outlet resistance.[44] The clinical impact of estrogen replacement on symptoms of bladder overactivity and incontinence are contradictory and incomplete.

Recent physiologic studies have associated aging with an increased volume at first desire to void, diminished capacity, decreased voiding volumes and flow rates, impaired detrusor contractility, increasing prevalence of detrusor overactivity, and impaired sphincteric function.[38,45–50] Even so, methodological problems prevent firm conclusions. Studies typically use selected populations, most are studies of symptomatic patients and such important physiologic factors as estrogenization status and pelvic floor support and function status, and bladder outlet patency assessments are not reported. Furthermore, cystometric interdependencies are inconsistently considered; for example, flow rates are dependent upon voided volumes. If voided volumes are diminished, flow rates can be expected to be lower. In the absence of bladder outlet obstruction, volume-corrected flow rates do not deteriorate with age.[50–52]

Bladder function and structure

Distinct morphologic changes of the detrusor relating to aging have been described. A decrease in detrusor muscle to collagen ratio[53] and nerve density in the detrusor[54] accompanies aging, although quantitative assessment in a rat model demonstrated no diminution in nerve density at the bladder neck in aged versus mature rats.[55] Classic associations of electron microscopy with urodynamic findings in an aged population were reported by Elbadawi et al.[56–59] Aging with normal urodynamic performance is associated with the so-called "dense band" pattern, in which the sarcolemma is dominated by dense bands with depleted caveolae and slight widening between muscle cells.[57] Impaired detrusor contractility is associated with widespread degeneration of muscle cells and axons, with sarcoplasmic vacuolation, sequestration/blebbing, cell shriveling and fragmentation, and presence of cellular debris in the intercellular spaces.[57,60,61]

Specific changes in the neuropharmacology of detrusor function have also been attributed to aging. The detrusor normally contracts in response to M3 muscarinic receptor activation via pelvic nerve efferent release of acetylcholine (M2 receptors are also present, but their precise role is not known).[61] M3 receptor numbers decrease with age[62] and M3-stimulated activity is diminished, although the clinical importance of decreased contractile sensitivity is unclear.[63] Against the decline in M3 responsiveness, other factors appear to become more important, including purinergic transmission,[64–66,67] nonneuronal urothelial acetylcholine release[64] and an increased contractile response to norepinephrine.[68] These findings suggest that receptor-mediated sensory and motor responses in addition to inherent muscular changes are important in the alterations of detrusor function with aging.[64,69]

Demonstrable detrusor motor dysfunction is associated with aging. The bladder may not contract well enough to ensure adequate emptying, or it may contract inappropriately. In both cases, irritative and obstructive symptoms can result, with varying degrees of urinary incontinence. Detrusor underactivity and overactivity can coexist; patients with both problems tend to be older than those with only detrusor overactivity or impaired contractility, suggesting these may reflect distinct, but related processes.

The ability of the bladder to create expulsive pressure against a relaxed outlet over a time sufficient to empty the bladder requires normal detrusor muscular function, conceptualized as detrusor contractility. Detrusor underactivity (i.e., the inability to generate sufficient bladder pressure over time to ensure normal emptying) is a common problem in elderly patients with LUTS such as urinary retention, poor urinary stream, and/or incontinence.[39,61] Neither detrusor contractility nor detrusor underactivity has an accepted cystometric definition; detrusor underactivity probably represents the clinical result of the physiologic entity of impaired detrusor muscle contractility. Although several studies have concluded detrusor contractility diminishes with age, their assessment of "contractility" is confounded by lack of pressure/flow assessment and population selection.[45,70] Furthermore, the use of "stop-test" to assess isovolumetric detrusor contractility has been inconclusive,[51,52] possibly due to the variable effects of methodologic perturbations of bladder outlet function. Total detrusor effort does not change with age; however, aging is associated with failure of contraction initiation and slowed contraction velocities.[71] Maximum detrusor pressure and detrusor pressure at maximum flow are not a function of age in symptomatic unobstructed, unoperated men and women over age 40, although unadjusted flow rates decrease and PVR volumes increase with age.[47] Maximum detrusor pressures associated with detrusor overactivity decrease with age,[72] suggesting larger absolute but decreased functional bladder capacity and diminished voiding efficiency. Maximal detrusor pressure responses occur at greater bladder volumes in aged animals than in mature animals.[73] The finding of greater contractility (by stop-test) in aged patients with detrusor overactivity at lower bladder volumes as compared with patients without detrusor overactivity[52] suggests that maximal contractility is preserved, and that functional deficits (evidenced as detrusor underactivity) are due to an inability to maintain a contractile state.

Animal studies provide evidence that age-related decrements in voiding efficiency are not a result of maximal pressure generating capabilities but rather the ability to maintain adequate pressurization. The maximal contractile response to acetylcholine increases with age in ex vivo rat bladder studies.[74] In a cystometric study of young, adult, and aged female rats, bladder compliance decreased with age, and the threshold bladder pressure for voiding contractions increased, suggesting altered afferent function affecting the micturition reflex. However, maximal voiding bladder pressures, bladder capacity, and voiding efficiency did not differ among groups. This study also reported more nonvoiding contractions, impaired compliance, increased bladder capacity, and diminished voiding efficiency in obstructed animals relative to their unobstructed counterparts. Of interest is that only the young animals were able to compensate for outlet obstruction with an increased voiding bladder pressure.[75] Similarly, other animal models have demonstrated an impaired ability of the aged detrusor to accommodate obstructive, ischemic, and fatigue stresses.[76–78] Thus, contractile deficiencies in the aged may include failure to accommodate altered bladder outlet, vascular, and sensory changes associated with aging, rather than only an inherent contractile failure of the muscle.

No changes in flow rates were observed over 27 months in asymptomatic postmenopausal women in a longitudinal study.[50] If impaired contractility is associated with aging, it develops over a relatively long period. Of interest is that in this same study, postmenopausal women with detrusor overactivity had impaired voiding function, which deteriorated over the same time period, suggesting that LUT dysfunction associated with aging is multidimensional and more rapidly progressive once initiated. This may be interpreted as age-related deterioration of multiple overlapping functions, with an eventual systemic decompensation at some threshold level.

Overactive bladder (irritative) symptoms such as urinary frequency, nocturia, urgency, and urge incontinence are more prevalent with age, and may be the result of abnormal sensory and/or motor activity. Detrusor overactivity (DO) is the undesired contraction of the detrusor, with or without urine loss. As a description of a urodynamic finding, the term replaces older and less accurate terms such as detrusor hyperreflexia and detrusor instability.[79] At very low levels it may be asymptomatic; no urodynamic standard for clinical significance exists, and studies reporting the incidence of DO have used differing urodynamic definitions. Detrusor overactivity is found in about one-half of elderly patients with irritative symptoms.[80] Most, if not all, elderly patients with urge incontinence have detectable detrusor overactivity.[52,80] A particularly vexing problem is the combination of DO with impaired contractility, historically referred to as DHIC (detrusor hyperreflexia with impaired contractility). Although the concept of an inefficient detrusor coupled with motor overactivity analogous to a fibrillatory heart is not difficult, the problems of defining DO and impaired contractility complicate a precise physiologic definition of DHIC. It is associated with more complex symptomatology, and is estimated to be the underlying problem in one third of incontinent institutionalized elderly.[45] In community-dwelling symptomatic elderly patients using conservative urodynamic definitions, detrusor underactivity was found in 48% of men and 12% of women. Among people with detrusor underactivity, two thirds of men and one half of women also had detrusor overactivity.[81] Coexisting neurologic disease is common in DHIC patients; 28% were found to have ALS, parkinsonian syndrome in 18%, MSA in 18%, and Alzheimer dementia in 13%.[82]

Several lines of research have suggested age-related changes in the afferent limb of the micturition reflex play important roles in the clinical changes observed with aging LUT function. Aged animals void less often, but with higher volumes, and demonstrate a greater pressure threshold for voiding, but no difference in maximal pressure,[83] suggesting a primary impact of aging on LUT sensory activity. Animal and human studies suggest that the decreased afferent signal results in larger bladder volumes. These diminished sensations can result in delayed sensations of bladder filling, diminished "warning time" between the first urge to urinate and urgency with leakage,[84] and impaired bladder emptying. The resultant decreased functional capacity may then aggravate symptoms of urinary frequency/urgency/urge incontinence by perpetuation of bladder volumes in the narrow functional zone between first urge to urinary and leakage.

Outlet function and structure

The urinary sphincter is under semivoluntary control. The concept of an internal and external sphincter is not anatomically precise. Rather, the sphincteric mechanism is more accurately divided into factors intrinsic and extrinsic to the urethra itself.[85] Intrinsic factors result in resting closure of the lumen, and include mucosal adherence and biomechanical properties relating to flow of fluid through a compliant tube. In addition to the inherent physical properties of urethral dimensions and connective tissue performance, urethral dynamics are actively modified by urethral smooth muscle, under autonomic influence. The extrinsic mechanisms are primarily responsible for the ability to voluntarily and/or reflexively increase urethral resistance to flow in response to sudden increases in bladder pressure, generated by coughing, laughing, etc. (so-called stress incontinence) or detrusor contraction as a result of detrusor contraction or overfilling. The extrinsic mechanisms are composed of the paraurethral connective tissues and their direct and indirect connections via striated muscle to the bony pelvis.

Age-related sarcopenia and changes in connective tissue composition result directly in changes in sphincteric efficiency and probably impact urine storage and voiding efficiency. Smooth and striated muscle thickness and fiber density in the bladder neck and urethra have been found to be diminished in older women relative to young women.[86-88] Striated muscle changes are circumferentially uniform, although the decrease in smooth muscle is most pronounced on the dorsal/vaginal aspect of the urethra.[88] These changes presumably result in alterations of urethra sphincter function, as suggested by the finding of lower detrusor pressures at the opening and closing of the urethra in older women.[55,89] Although the validity of urethral closure pressure (UCP) as a measure of sphincteric competency is debatable, it negatively correlates with age.[72] Although a decrease in urethral resistance may impair sphincteric efficiency, it may ameliorate potential obstructive/retentive problems resulting from impaired contractility; ex vivo animal studies have demonstrated that aged bladders are unable to maintain effective detrusor contractions against an increased outlet resistance.[90]

KEY POINTS
Aging of the Urinary Tract

- Average declines in renal function hide considerable variability, including an impressive proportion of people in whom age appears to have only a small influence on renal function.
- Although elderly people with chronic kidney disease are more likely to be frail, whether frailty itself is specifically associated with incident renal impairment is not clear. Aspects of the frailty state (e.g., sarcopenia) are associated with aspects of age-related urinary tract dysfunction (e.g., detrusor hypoactivity).
- In the upper urinary tract, several changes are seen with age that reduce glomerular filtration; serum creatinine is a poor estimate of actual GFR with age and with frailty.
- In the lower urinary tract, symptoms alone are generally inadequate to establish a diagnosis. Bladder irritative symptoms (frequency, nocturia, urgency) can result from detrusor overactivity (inappropriate contraction), underactivity (poor emptying performance), or sensory dysfunction. Incontinence and obstructive symptoms may result from detrusor and/or outlet dysfunctions.
- A challenge for rational therapy is that both detrusor underactivity and overactivity can exist in the same patient.
- In general, changes in bladder sensorimotor capabilities result in altered storage and voiding functions. Bladder volumes may increase in combination with less efficient sensation, resulting in less warning before an overwhelming urge to void.

As explained earlier, diminished urethral afferent activity related to aging may have a role in impaired voiding function. Conversely, urethral afferent activity may also impair successful urine storage and thus be an important contributor to age-related overactive bladder symptoms, including frank detrusor overactivity and urge incontinence. Urethral closure pressures negatively correlate with age, and are positively associated with detrusor overactivity in humans,[72] suggesting a role for inappropriate activation of prevoiding urethral-detrusor reflexes because of impaired sphincteric function in the age-related prevalence of detrusor overactivity.

A system-based perspective

Aging is associated with an increased prevalence of bothersome lower urinary tract symptoms and demonstrable alterations of function. Changes in tissue properties and sensorimotor function demonstrate complex interactions, producing functional changes which do not correlate well with symptoms. These alterations are complicated by other age-related physiologic changes and comorbidities. The determinants of urine storage and voiding functions include renal output, lower urinary tract biomechanical and sensorimotor function, central processing abilities, and mobility. Degradation of the ability to normally store and appropriately evacuate urine thus has many contributors, both external and inherent to the lower urinary tract.

For a complete list of references, please visit online only at www.expertconsult.com

CHAPTER 19

Bone and Joint Aging

Celia L. Gregson

The musculoskeletal system serves three primary functions: (1) it enables an efficient means of limb movement; (2) it acts as an endoskeleton, providing overall mechanical support and protection to soft tissues; and (3) it serves as a reservoir of mineral for calcium homeostasis. In the elderly population, the first two of these functions frequently become compromised; musculoskeletal problems are the major cause of pain and physical disability in people over the age of 65 years[1] and fracture incidence rises steeply with age[2] (Fig. 19-1). Several factors contribute to the age-related decline in musculoskeletal function:

1. Aging effects on components of the musculoskeletal system (i.e., articular cartilage, the skeleton, and soft tissues), contribute toward the increasing incidence of osteoporosis and osteoarthritis (OA), the reduced range of joint movement, and the stiffness and difficulty in initiating movement.
2. There is the age-related rise in the prevalence of common musculoskeletal disorders that begin in young adulthood or in middle age, and cause increasing pain and disability without shortening life span (e.g., seronegative spondylarthritides, musculoskeletal trauma).
3. There is a high incidence of certain musculoskeletal disorders in the elderly, such as polymyalgia rheumatica, Paget's disease of bone and crystal-related arthropathies.

A number of interrelated hypotheses have been advanced to explain the high prevalence of bone, muscle, and joint-problems in older humans[3–6]:

1. The long life span results in increasing accumulation of mechanical damage to the musculoskeletal system.
2. There is a lack of genetic investment in the repair of age-related tissue damage that develops in the post-reproductive phase of life.
3. The musculoskeletal system in humans has not adapted fully to the upright posture and prehensile grip because of lack of evolutionary pressure to do so, with the result that many of our bones and joints are inappropriately shaped and "underdesigned" to be able to cope with the stresses applied.
4. By virtue of their sedentary lifestyle, modern humans tend to be exposed to less mechanical stress than their ancestors. Because musculoskeletal strength is governed by the mechanical inputs to which that individual is exposed, this may result in a weaker musculoskeletal system, which is not well adapted for episodes of sudden major stress.

Several different mechanisms are involved in musculoskeletal tissue aging,[7] including:

- Reduced synthetic capacity of differentiated cells such as osteoblasts and chondrocytes, with a consequent loss of ability to maintain matrix integrity
- A decline in the mesenchymal stem cell populations
- Posttranslational modification of structural proteins, such as collagen and elastin
- The accumulation of degraded molecules, such as proteoglycan fragments, in musculoskeletal tissue matrices
- Decreased circulating and local levels of trophic hormones, growth factors, and cytokines, such as insulin-like growth factor-1 (IGF-1), involved in maintaining tissue integrity; or an altered ability of the cells to respond to them
- A decreased capacity for wound healing and tissue repair, which may be the result of some or all of the mechanisms described above
- Alterations in the loading patterns of tissue, or the tissue's response to loading

The major tissues that have received the most attention and which are pivotal to the integrity of the system are articular cartilage, the skeleton, and soft tissues. Age-related changes in these structures are now described in more detail.

ARTICULAR CARTILAGE

The structure of a mammalian synovial joint is summarized in Figure 19-2. Much of its function derives from the properties of articular cartilage, which cushions the subchondral bone and provides a low-friction surface necessary for free movement. Articular cartilage contains very few cells, is aneural and avascular, and yet its integrity is maintained throughout a lifetime of biomechanical stress. With increasing age, the cartilage surface often starts to break down, leading to OA. This is associated with changes in other tissues of the joint (Fig. 19-3). However, OA is not an inevitable consequence of aging; instead, aging adds to the risk of OA. With age, articular cartilage thins and changes color from a glistening white to a dull yellow. In addition, the mechanical features of the tissue change. There is a decrease in tensile stiffness, fatigue resistance, and strength, but no significant change in the compressive properties. These changes are partly caused by the decrease in water content that accompanies aging. The morphology and function of the cells (chondrocytes) and nature of the two main matrix components, aggrecan (aggregating proteoglycans) and type II collagen, also change with age. The density of cells in the tissue changes little, but their morphology alters with an increase in intracytoplasmic filaments and they change their secretion of matrix components, producing more variable proteoglycans. Aging is also associated with alterations in the response by chondrocytes to anabolic and catabolic stimuli, such as IGF-1 and interleukin-1. For example, immature cartilage degrades more readily when stimulated with interleukin-1. Generally with age, repeated cell divisions lead to progressive telomere shortening and replicative senescence. However, connective tissue cells and their stem cells may be less susceptible given their relatively slow turnover rates.[8] Stress-induced premature senescence (SIPS) has been proposed as

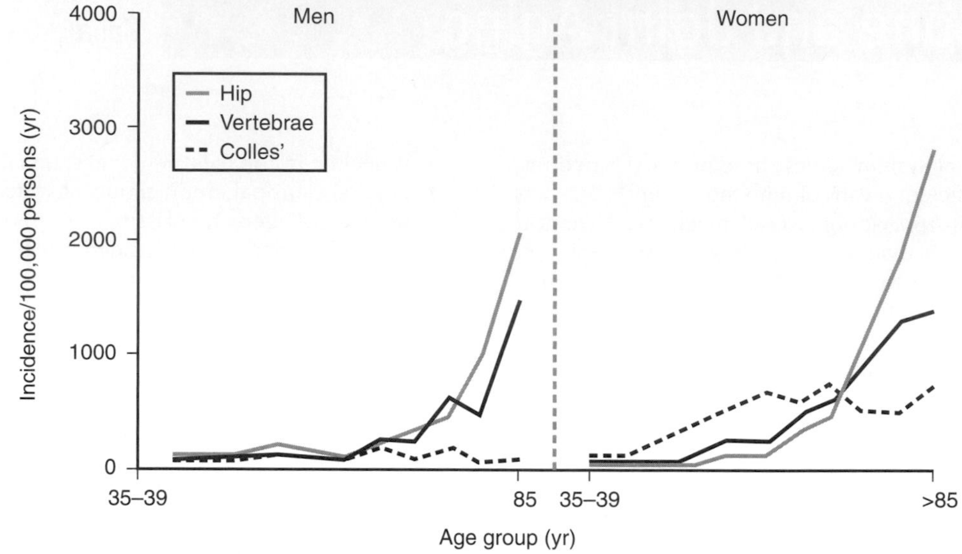

Figure 19-1. Age-specific incidence rates for hip, vertebral, and distal forearm (Colles') fracture in Rochester, Minn., men and women. *(Adapted from Cooper C, Melton LJ. Epidemiology of osteoporosis. Trends Endocrinol Metab 1992;3:224–9).*

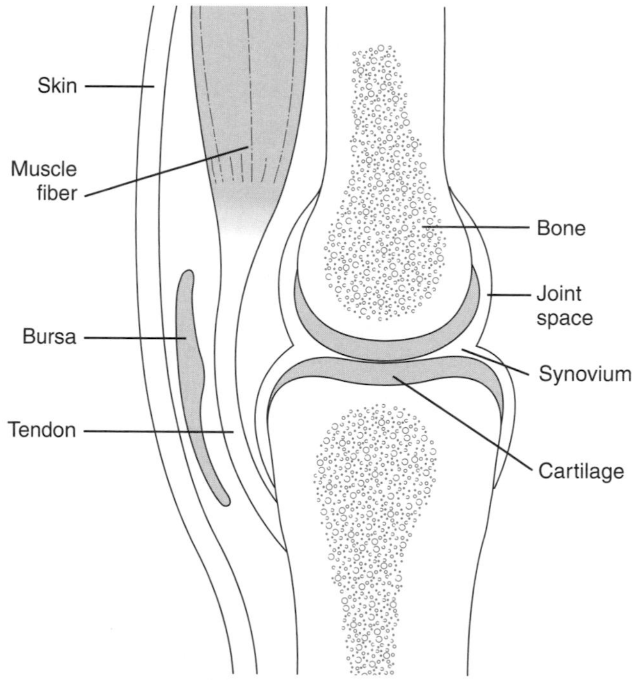

Figure 19-2. The synovial joint. The histologic appearances of the main tissues are highlighted. *(Courtesy Drs J. H. Klippel and P. A. Dieppe.)*

an alternative explanation to replicative senescence; insults such as mechanical loading, interleukin-1, and caveolin-1 lead to increasing expression of senescence biomarkers.[9,10]

Depletion of cartilage proteoglycan is one of the earliest signs of articular cartilage loss in OA. Proteoglycans consist of a protein core and two major glycosaminoglycan (GAG) side chains: chondroitin sulfate (CS) and keratan sulfate (KS). The CS is the predominant GAG chain in human articular cartilage. It is made up of oligosaccharide (sugar) chains containing a basic disaccharide repeat of two sugar molecules (*N*-acetylgalactosamine and glucuronic acid). These sugar molecules carry a sulfate group on either the sixth (C6) or fourth (C4) carbon atom of the sugar ring. Such sulfation patterns are often called C6 and C4 sulfation and show marked changes with aging and in OA.[11,12] More than 90% of the CS in adult human articular cartilage is C6, which is thought to interact with collagen and other extracellular matrix macromolecules and help maintain the integrity of the cartilage.[11] C4 accounts for less than 10% of the adult cartilage and is thought to be a characteristic of immature cartilage. In OA cartilage, there is an increase in C4 and decrease in C6. Changes in the C6:C4 ratio of the articular cartilage with aging and in OA may make the cartilage more susceptible to cytokine-mediated damage.[12]

The main proteoglycan, aggrecan, binds with hyaluronan to form massive, hydrophilic aggregates that expand the collagen framework of the tissue to provide it with its compressive and tensile strength. With age there is reduced proteoglycan aggregation, with smaller proteoglycans being synthesized with an increase in KS and reduced CS content, and increased aggrecanase production leading to aggrecan degradation. Synthesis of KS requires less oxygen than CS, thus the KS-CS balance has recently prompted research interest into changing oxygen tension patterns within connective tissues as a result of ischemia.[13,14]

Collagen also changes, with some increase in fiber diameter and an increase in cross-linking. This fiber cross-linking may be enzymic or nonenzymic, involving lysyl hydroxylase or not, respectively. In young growing skeletons, collagen turnover is high and enzymic divalent and trivalent cross-links stabilize the collagen fibers, with almost complete hydroxylation of telopeptide lysines. With age lysyl hydroxylase activity wanes, causing incomplete hydroxylation of telopeptide lysines, that is, until maturation is complete, after which enzymatic cross-linking remains constant. However, collagen fiber cross-linking does increase with age because of nonenzymatic reactions between glucose and lysine, forming glucosyl lysine and related molecules. Subsequent oxidative and nonoxidative reactions produce stable end products

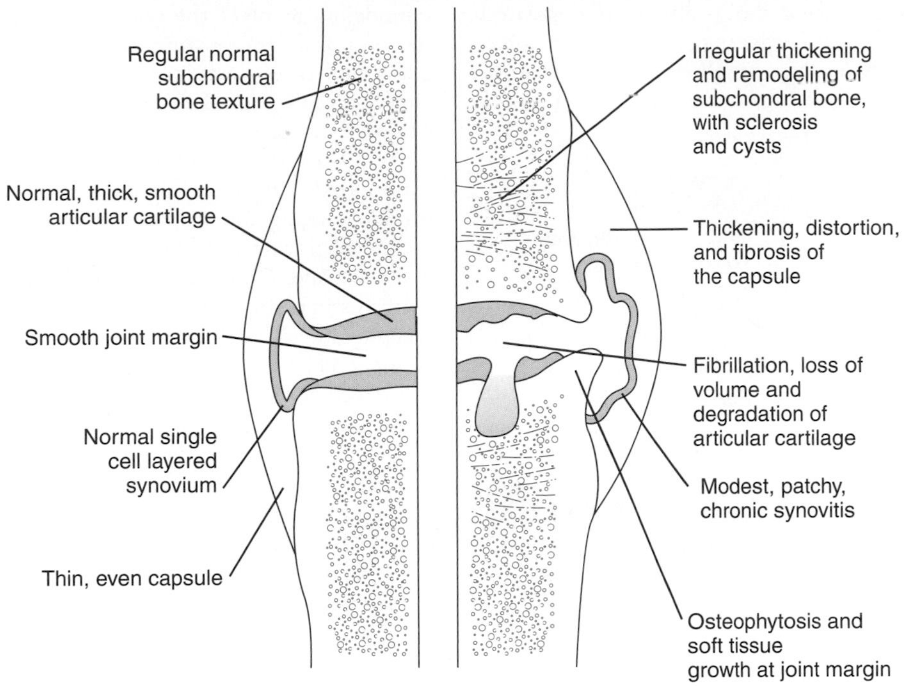

Figure 19-3. Normal versus osteoarthritic synovial joint. *(Courtesy Drs J. H. Klippel and P. A. Dieppe.)*

known as advanced glycation end products (AGEs), some of which can act as collagen cross-links producing fibers too stiff for optimal function.[15,16] Hyperglycemia and oxidative stress increase AGE production and dietary AGE intake may also be important.[17,18] Elastin, which conveys extensibility and elastic recoil in some ligaments, is also stabilized by cross-linking, and AGE production can also prompt age-related stiffening.[19]

Changes in calcified cartilage, the layer separating articular cartilage from subchondral bone, are felt to be important in the pathogenesis of OA; however, the underlying mechanisms remain unclear.[20] Estrogen receptors have been identified in articular chondrocytes with estrogens influencing cellular homeostasis.[21] The chondroprotective properties of estrogen are lost following menopause. A history of hormone replacement therapy has been associated with a reduced prevalence of OA.[22] In men, testosterone levels have been positively associated with cartilage volume.[23]

Cell death in cartilage

There has been much research interest into apoptosis, a normal physiologic process involved in the removal of potential carcinogenic and damaged cells. The process is also involved in development; for example, during endochondral ossification of the hyaline cartilage, cells (chondrocytes) die by apoptosis.[24] An age-related decrease in articular cartilage cellularity has been associated with cartilage fibrillation, thinning, and an increased prevalence of OA in elderly people.[25,26] Now chondrocyte apoptosis appears to be a crucial event in cartilage aging and the pathogenesis of OA. Cartilage matrix degradation by apoptotic bodies, abnormal loading, changes in nitric oxide synthesis, altered cytokine regulation, impaired mitochondrial functioning, and downregulation of the *Bcl*-2 gene have all been implicated in the control of chondrocyte apoptosis in animals.[27] How these all relate to human aging remains an area of interest.

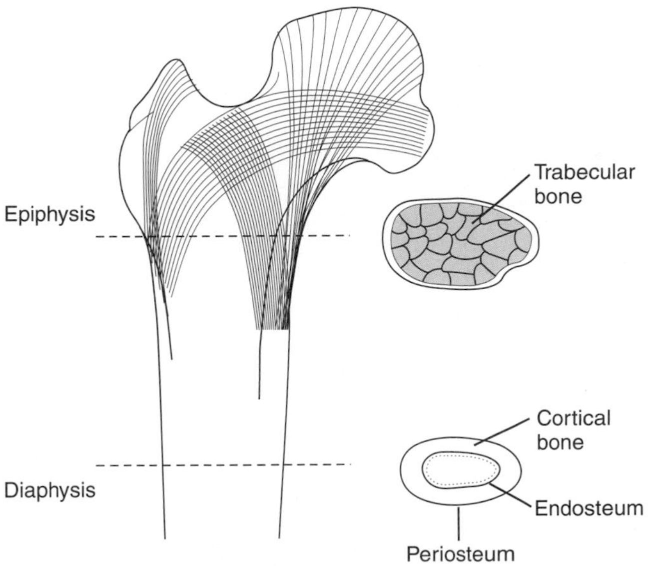

Figure 19-4. The macroscopic organization of bone. *(Courtesy Drs J. H. Klippel and P. A. Dieppe.)*

THE SKELETON

Weight-bearing bones consist of an outer shell of cortical bone; an arrangement designed for maximum strength. In addition, certain sites, such as vertebrae and metaphyses, contain an inner meshwork of trabecular bone to act as an internal scaffold (Figure 19-4). Microscopically, the skeleton is made up of interconnecting fibrils of type I collagen, which provide tensile strength. Hydroxyapatite crystals, which are made up of calcium and phosphate, are deposited in holes within the collagen fibrils, giving bone its rigidity. Adult bone continuously undergoes self-renewal. This process, known as bone remodeling, occurs at discrete sites throughout the skeleton called bone remodeling units. Bone remodeling involves the coordinated activity of those cells responsible for bone formation and resorption (i.e., osteoblasts and osteoclasts, respectively) in a continuous cycle aimed at replacing microdamage and at adapting bone density and shape to the patterns of forces it endures (Figure 19-5). Osteoclasts differentiate from hematopoietic precursors shared with macrophages, whereas osteoblasts, which produce osteoid and promote mineralization, arise from mesenchymal precursors that also give rise to fibroblasts, stromal cells, and adipocytes. Osteoblasts produce macrophage colony stimulating factor (M-CSF) and membrane-bound receptor activator of nuclear factor-kappa B ligand (RANKL), factors crucial for osteoclastogenesis.[28] RANKL, by binding to the osteoclast's RANK receptor, stimulates osteoclast differentiation, averting cell death. This process is regulated by osteoblasts that produce osteoprotegerin, a decoy receptor.[29] Multiple factors influence the RANK-RANKL interaction; PTH, vitamin D, cytokines, interleukins, prostaglandins estrogen, mechanical forces, transforming growth factor β and thiazolidinedione PPARg ligands commonly used in the treatment of type 2 diabetes mellitus, to name but a few, and work is underway to better understand these processes.

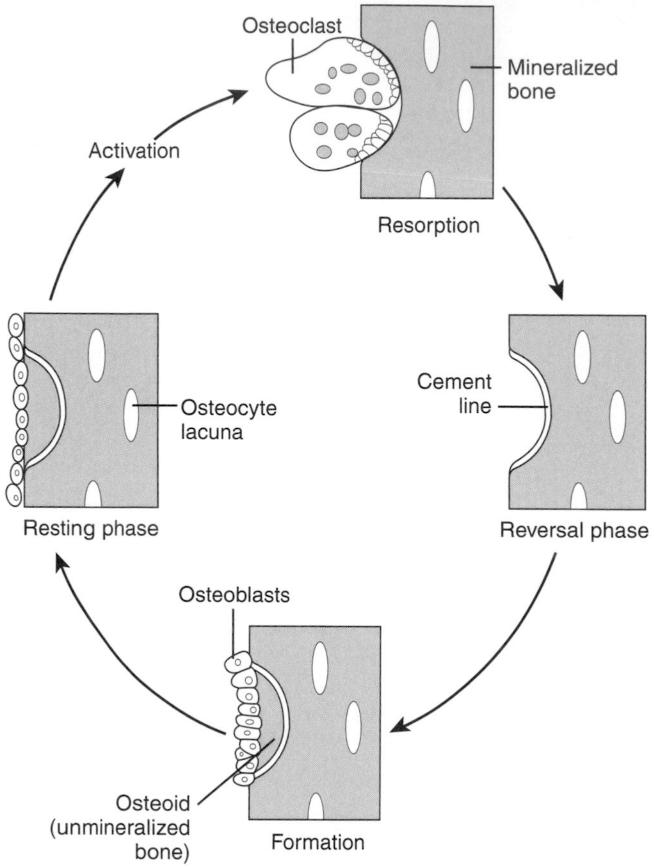

Figure 19-5. The bone remodeling sequence. This commences with osteoclastic bone resorption, following which a cement line is laid down (reversal phase). Osteoblasts then fill up the resorption cavity with osteoid, which subsequently mineralizes—the bone surface finally being covered by lining cells and a thin layer of osteoid.

Structural changes in the skeleton

Once middle age is reached, the total amount of calcium in the skeleton (i.e., bone mass) starts to decline—a process that is accelerated during the first few years following menopause in women.[30] This is associated with changes in skeletal structure by which the skeleton becomes weaker and more prone to sustaining fractures. Where these alterations affect trabecular bone, individual trabeculae undergo thinning followed by perforation and ultimately removal, leading to disruption of the trabecular network (Fig. 19-6). The bony cortex also becomes considerably weaker during aging, through a combination of thinning as a result of expansion of the inner medullary cavity and an increase in size, number, and clustering of Haversian canals. Along with deterioration in skeletal architecture, the material strength of bone may also decline significantly with age; microfractures are thought to accumulate within bone tissue with increasing

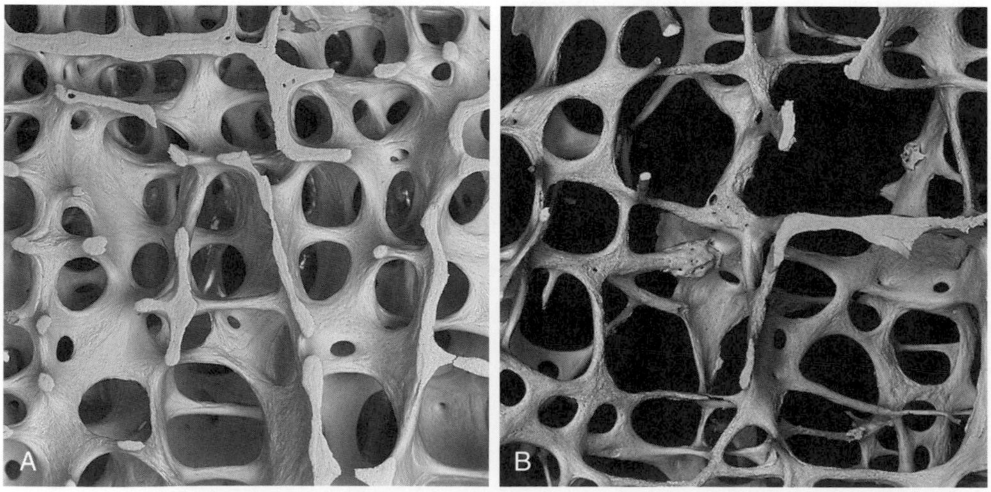

Figure 19-6. Changes in trabecular structure associated with osteoporosis. Scanning electron micrographs of lumbar vertebrae (magnification × 20) obtained from: (A) a 31-year-old male; (B) an 89-year-old female. Note the loss of bone tissue associated with thinning and removal of trabecular plates. *(Kindly supplied by Professor A. Boyde, Department of Anatomy and Developmental Biology, University College, London.)*

age, representing the accumulation of fatigue damage.[31] In addition, adverse biochemical changes may occur, such as a decline in cross-linking efficiency, required for stabilizing collagen fibrils.[32]

Changes in skeletal metabolism

Bone loss in the elderly population is largely a result of excess osteoclast activity,[33] which causes both an expansion in the total number of remodeling sites and an increase in the amount of bone resorbed per individual site, resulting in a bone remodeling imbalance. The rise in osteoclast activity in older women partly reflects the decline in ovarian hormone production following menopause because estrogens exert an important restraining influence on bone resorption by limiting RANKL production and promoting osteoclast apoptosis while also exerting antiapoptotic effects on osteoblasts.[34] The age-related decline in bone density had been felt to be due to falling estrogen levels in women and testosterone levels in men. However, more recently estrogens have emerged as the dominant sex steroid, regulating male bone loss later in life, and, in combination with testosterone, acquisition of peak bone mass early in life.[35] Strong positive correlations between serum estradiol, particularly bioavailable estradiol, levels and bone mineral density (BMD) have been observed, whereas correlations between testosterone and BMD have been weak or lacking.[36,37]

In addition, osteoclast activity may be elevated in the elderly population as a consequence of vitamin D deficiency, which is widespread among elderly people.[38] Dietary vitamin D insufficiency combined with reduced sunlight exposure and a reduced capacity to synthesize vitamin D in aging skin, lead to mild secondary hyperparathyroidism.[39–41] These effects of vitamin D insufficiency on bone metabolism are aggravated by an age-related decline in efficiency of gastrointestinal calcium absorption and an age-related decline in efficiency of renal 1α hydroxylation of vitamin D. Low vitamin D levels influence mesenchymal stem cell differentiation toward greater adipogenesis at the expense of osteoblastogenesis.[42] Despite subclinical evidence of osteomalacia, many of these patients present in the same way as osteoporosis, for example, with fractures of the femoral neck. Furthermore, an increased tendency toward bone marrow adipogenesis, to the detriment of osteoblast production, with consequent accumulation of bone marrow fat rather than trabecular bone, has been observed independent of estrogens.[42,43] Furthermore the peroxisome proliferator-activated receptor (PPAR) induced in humans treated for diabetes mellitus with thiazolidines, has through its effects on adipogenesis been implicated in the development of osteoporosis.[44] PPAR, together with the Wnt signaling pathway, are currently of interest as potential therapeutic targets for osteoporosis.

An age-related reduction in the bioavailability of other important regulatory factors such as IGF-1 have also been described. Aging leads to a gradual decline in circulating growth hormone (GH) and IGF-1, with consequent declines in bone density, lean body mass, and skin thickness; the so-called "somatopause."[45] Reductions in these trophic factors encourage local expression of molecules (e.g., TNF-α and interleukins), which increase osteoclast and decrease osteoblast activity and downgrade the differentiation potential of bone marrow stem cells.[28] Therapeutic GH has been shown to increase bone mineral density in GH-deficient osteoporotic patients.[46] Immobilization is recognized to cause bone loss whereas physical activity can help attenuate rates of age-related bone loss. Reductions in physical activity often accompany aging, thereby reducing the quality and quantity of mechanical inputs to the skeleton, which are important in maintaining osteoblast activity. Use of whole-body vibration exercise has been shown to increase femoral neck BMD and balance.[47] Cellular sensing of normal and abnormal mechanical loads and the consequent alterations in cell biology is known as mechanotransduction, a mechanism designed to maintain normal tissue homeostasis[48] and poorly understood in elderly human tissue.

SOFT TISSUES

Age-related changes occur in other bone- and joint-related tissues, largely as a result of reduced synthesis and posttranslational modification of collagen, which leads to reduced ligament elasticity. For example, the tensile strength of tendons and ligament-bone complexes declines with age and integrity of joint capsules may be lost. This may result in disorders such as dysfunction of the rotator cuff of the shoulder, which may be associated with communications between the shoulder joint and subacromial bursa. In addition, there is a gradual loss of connective tissue resistance to calcium crystal formation in the elderly population, leading to an increase in the incidence of crystal-related arthropathies. Functional impairment in soft tissues may also adversely affect biomechanics of the joint, which may be an important initiating factor in the development of OA. For example, age-related changes have been described in the metabolism and composition of the extracellular matrix in the meniscus,[49] which may contribute to the development of knee OA.

Back and neck pain and stiffness are common complaints in the elderly population, which are likely to reflect age-related changes in intervertebral discs. The latter consist of an outer fibrous ring called annlus fibrosus and an internal gelatinous (semifluid) structure called nucleus pulposus. As people get older, the diameter of the nucleus pulposus and the hydrostatic pressure within this region decreases, resulting in increased compressive stress within the annlus.[50] Thus with age the intervertebral disc becomes more compressed, causing a decrease in the intervertebral space and therefore an overall decrease in height of the individual. The extracellular matrix of the disc contains a network of collagen fibers (both type I and type II) that are responsible for the tensile strength, and aggregating proteoglycans that help the disc to resist compressive forces. Age-related changes in the distribution and concentrations of these macromolecules can also significantly alter the mechanical properties of the disc. In many ways, extracellular matrix metabolism is rather similar to articular cartilage; for example, with age there is increased degradation and reduced synthesis of type II collagen, and the glycosaminoglycan and collagen contents are decreased.[51]

Sarcopenia is the slow and progressive age-related loss of skeletal muscle, resulting in reduced muscle power and function. The consequences of increased falls and hence increased fracture risk with associated loss of independence can be devastating. Sarcopenia is predominantly due to a decline in muscle fiber number, although atrophy of fibers, especially type II fibers, also occurs. Sarcopenia has been associated with declining levels of anabolic factors: estrogen and vitamin D levels in women, testosterone and physical performance in men, in addition to waning GH and IGF-1 levels. Furthermore, increased levels of catabolic cytokines have also been implicated—interleukin-6, particularly in older women, and TNF-α, particularly affecting muscle mass in men.[52–54] Denervation resulting in motor unit reduction may also be important.

CONSEQUENCES OF BONE AND JOINT AGING

Musculoskeletal problems cause a huge burden of pain and physical disability in older people. The most important functional impairments include the marked loss of muscle strength, reduced range of movements of the spine and peripheral joints, and loss of joint proprioception contributing to problems of balance. In addition, spinal osteoporosis causes progressive kyphotic deformity and height loss, which in some individuals may be relatively asymptomatic. The key symptoms include pain and stiffness. Although pain thresholds may increase, there is also a very high prevalence of musculoskeletal pain. For example, some 25% of those individuals over the age of 55 years complain of current knee pain. Stiffness and difficulty in initiating movement are almost universal in those over the age of 70 years.

Changes in the bone and soft tissues make the whole system more susceptible to trauma. Periarticular pain syndromes and spinal disorders related to minor trauma are common, but by far the most important consequence is the high incidence of fractures. These partly reflect the age-related increase in skeletal fragility that characterizes osteoporosis, and partly the age-related increase in falls, which is multifactorial (see Chapter ***). Osteoporosis predisposes to an increased risk of fracture at all skeletal sites other than flat bones such as the skull, although fractures of the vertebrae, distal radius, and hip are by far the most common (see Fig. 19-1). The relative increase in hip fractures in the very elderly may also be related to changes in the pattern of falling since older subjects, with slower motor function, may be less likely to fall onto an outstretched arm.

The extent of the disability related to musculoskeletal changes is well described in community-based epidemiologic studies. Problems with reaching and with locomotion are particularly frequent, the latter contributing extensively to the isolation of elderly people. In addition, it is well recognized that in those who sustain a hip fracture the majority fail to regain their previous level of functioning, and there is also an appreciable excess mortality; 10% dying in hospital within the first month, with overall around a third dying within a year.[55]

THE FUTURE

An aging population, with a rising age-specific incidence of fracture, has serious implications for our projected fracture rates. Fragility fractures are expensive, both in terms of direct medical costs, but also through the costs of their social sequelae. Furthermore, globally the prevalence of obesity is rising at an alarming rate. The cumulative physical consequences of a life of repetitive excessive skeletal loading is likely to manifest in substantially greater morbidity in the elderly in the years to come. Although present treatments for osteoporosis mostly focus on suppressing bone resorption, future treatments are likely to be anabolic, following on from the identification and understanding of the genes and the gene products responsible for the regulation of bone mass.

KEY POINTS

Bone and Joint Aging

- Musculoskeletal problems cause a huge burden in elderly people through a combination of pain and functional impairment.
- These problems result partly from the increased incidence of common musculoskeletal disorders in the elderly, such as rheumatoid arthritis and polymyalgia rheumatica.
- The high burden of musculoskeletal disease in elderly people also reflects the impact of the aging process on tissues which make up the musculoskeletal system, such as articular cartilage and bone.
- There have been considerable advances in recent years in the understanding of the cellular and molecular mechanisms that underlie these age-related changes.

For a complete list of references, please visit online only at www.expertconsult.com

CHAPTER 20

Aging and the Endocrine System

Harvinder S. Chahal
William M. Drake

INTRODUCTION

As individuals age, complex endocrine changes occur, resulting in a decline of endocrine function involving the responsiveness of tissues and reduced hormone secretion from peripheral glands. This is associated with modifications in the central mechanisms controlling the temporal organization of hormonal release with a dampening of circadian hormonal and nonhormonal rhythms. The effects of aging can occur in any endocrine gland and many endocrine functions are so intertwined that reductions in function can adversely affect other glands. Changes in many endocrine systems occur with healthy aging, including the growth hormone/insulin-like growth factor-1 axis (somatopause), estrogen (menopause), testosterone (andropause), dehydroepiandrosterone and its sulfate (adrenopause), the hypothalamic-pituitary-cortisol axis and the hypothalamic-pituitary-thyroid axis. This chapter will delineate some aspects of the interplay between the aging process and endocrine function regulation and explores the age-related changes in hormone metabolism and production, with their associated clinical consequences. However, in evaluating the changes that occur in endocrine glands it is important to distinguish between the real aging effects on endocrine mechanisms from any confounding factors due to the higher prevalence of age-related illness.

Growth hormone/insulin-like growth factor-1 axis

Growth hormone (GH) has both an anabolic and lipolytic effect and its action on peripheral tissues is partly mediated by circulating (hepatic generated) or paracrine insulin-like growth factor-1 (IGF-1).[1] Throughout life the secretion of GH undergoes marked changes. Before puberty, GH secretion is relatively low; but during sexual maturation and adolescence, GH output increases, resulting in accelerated somatic growth.[2] However, with aging there is reduced GH secretion with a decline in both serum GH and IGF-1 levels.[1] There is a greater than 50% reduction in healthy older adults' GH production and IGF-1 concentrations[3] and this progressive decline has been termed *somatopause*. This decrease in GH secretion is known to cause a reduction of protein synthesis, a decrease in lean body mass and bone mass, and a decline of immune function.[1]

The exact neuroendocrine mechanism of somatopause remains unclear. Early studies suggested the occurrence of senescent changes in the pituitary,[4,5] but this has not been supported by several observations showing that there is no decrease in pituitary somatotroph cell numbers[6] or that neither exogenous growth hormone-releasing hormone (GHRH)[7,8] nor GH-releasing peptide analogues[9] can rejuvenate GH output and plasma IGF-1 levels in older subjects. Consequently, research has focused on the hypothalamic regulation of GH secretion whereby an age-dependent decrease in hypothalamic GHRH output contributes to the GH decline with aging.[10] Low physical fitness and higher adiposity seen in older individuals also contribute to decreased GH secretion,[11] although the underlying mechanism is uncertain. The low IGF-1 levels seen with aging are not due to hepatic responsiveness to the hormone because serum IGF-1 levels increase in both young and old men after exogenous administration of either GH or GHRH.[1]

The suggestion that older individuals have genuine GH deficiency that would benefit from GH treatment has arisen from the observation that nonelderly GH-deficient adults have changes in body composition similar to the aging phenotype, which are improved by long-term recombinant human GH therapy.[12] There is much uncertainty regarding the overall balance of benefits versus risks of GH replacement in older individuals.[13] In 1990, a study showed 6 months of treatment with recombinant GH in 12 healthy 61- to 81-year-old men with serum IGF-1 concentrations below those of healthy younger men resulted in a 9% increase in lean body mass and a 15% decrease in adipose tissue mass.[14] However, the weekly dose of GH was approximately twice as high as the dose used in nonelderly GH-deficient adults, the study was not double-blinded, and no assessment was made regarding muscle strength, exercise endurance, or quality of life.[15] A double-blind placebo-controlled study in healthy women (n = 57) and men (n = 74) aged 65 to 88 years found that GH with or without sex steroids increased lean body mass and decreased fat mass.[16] However, no change in muscle strength or maximal oxygen uptake during exercise was observed. These findings mirrored a previous randomized, controlled, double-blind trial in 1998 in which 6 months of physiologic GH doses administered to 52 healthy men aged older than 69 years with low baseline IGF-1 levels resulted in body composition improvement, but no functional ability change.[17] A further study was performed on 18 healthy men aged 65 to 82 years who initially underwent progressive weight training for 14 weeks to invoke a trained state and then were randomized to receive GH or placebo while continuing a further 10 weeks of strength training.[18] This study suggested that in older men GH supplementation does not augment the response to strength training.

The age-related testosterone decline in men may also contribute to the observed reduction in GH secretion. Nonpharmacologic doses of combined GH and testosterone in older men result in improvement in selected aspects of physical performance and increased muscle IGF-1 gene expression without measurably changing body composition or muscle strength.[19] In two more recent studies, coadministration of low dose GH with testosterone resulted in beneficial changes in midthigh muscle, aerobic capacity,[20] and whole-body protein turnover and synthesis.[21]

The original enthusiasm for the use of GH replacement in aging individuals has been severely dampened by the known adverse side effects, including arthralgia, carpal tunnel syndrome, edema, and hyperglycemia. There is also concern regarding the association of cancer and the GH–IGF-1 axis in the normal population.[15,16] GH replacement studies in aging individuals have been for a maximum of 12 months, so long-term safety data have not been published. In a recent systematic review of the GH trials, it was concluded that the increased rates of side effects of GH replacement outweighed the small beneficial effects on body composition in healthy older individuals.[22] Long-term studies are needed to determine the efficacy and safety of GH treatment in older adults who are not GH deficient. The beneficial effects of GH secretagogues in the elderly also need to be investigated.

Menopause

From the age of 40 ovulation frequency decreases and in most women reproductive ovarian function ceases within the next 15 years, resulting in menopause.[23] Ovarian follicles function less well during this period, with serum estradiol concentrations being lower and follicle-stimulating hormone (FSH) concentrations higher than in younger women, whereas luteinizing hormone (LH) is unchanged.[24] Follicular activity eventually ceases, estrogen concentrations fall to postmenopausal values, and both FSH and LH levels rise above premenopausal concentrations.[23] The changes in the hypothalamic-pituitary-gonadal axis result in an increased risk of cardiovascular events, rapid loss of skeletal mass, vasomotor instability, psychological symptoms, and atrophy of estrogen responsive tissue.

During the postmenopausal period, serum concentrations of atherogenic lipids deteriorate, with an increase in low-density lipoprotein and total cholesterol and a reduction in high-density lipoprotein, leading to a greater risk of cardiovascular disease.[25] These biochemical markers are favorably altered by hormone replacement therapy, but there is no improvement in cardiovascular disease outcome.[26,27]

There is rapid bone loss at the time of menopause as a result of estrogen withdrawal, which takes place on the background of age-related bone loss that begins from the fourth decade of life. A modest rise in serum ionized calcium occurs without any change in parathyroid hormone (PTH) levels, suggesting a possible change in the PTH set-point. There is also a decline in the estrogen-dependent components of intestinal calcium absorption and renal tubular calcium reabsorption. The associated high bone resorption with normal PTH also suggests an increased sensitivity of bone to PTH. There is no change in serum 1,25-vitamin D.[28] Estrogen replacement maintains bone mass and reduces fracture risk during the immediate menopausal period, when the rate of bone loss is greatest.[29] In postmenopausal women bone mass has also been maintained with bisphosphonates, which act by inhibiting bone resorption more than formation,[30] and raloxifene treatment, which is a selective estrogen receptor modulator acting selectively on bone and lipid profiles.[31]

Vasomotor symptoms originate in the hypothalamus with a resetting of the thermoregulatory system[23] and the hot flush is preceded by an LH surge.[25] Decreased estrogen levels reduce serotonin levels, resulting in hypothalamic 5-HT2A receptor upregulation, which leads to a change in the set-point temperature resulting in hot flushes.[32] However, the full mechanism is incompletely understood. These episodes are reduced with hormone replacement, but not entirely eliminated.[33] Cognitive disturbances are reported during menopause, which appear to be related to changes in estrogen levels; however, studies have shown inconsistent results regarding the effect of estrogen replacement on cognitive function in postmenopausal women.[34] The decline in estrogen levels in postmenopausal women results in vaginal mucosa atrophy, dysuria, urinary frequency, and incontinence. Local or systemic estrogen replacement therapy may improve these symptoms.[35] Loss of libido in postmenopausal women occurs partly due to a decline in both estrogen and testosterone levels because ovarian function ceases.[36]

The Women's Health Initiative (WHI) study has caused considerable debate regarding the risk benefit of hormone replacement therapy. The combined estrogen and progestin arm of the study was terminated early because women on combined hormonal therapy had an excess risk of breast cancer.[26] At the time the trial was stopped, the estrogen plus progestin group had significantly increased risks of coronary heart disease, stroke, and pulmonary embolism, whereas the risks of colorectal cancer and hip fracture were decreased and mortality risk was not significantly different.[37] In the postintervention follow-up period of 2.4 years, the increased risk of cardiovascular events and decreased fracture risk both disappeared. The group of patients that were initially randomized to combined hormonal therapy were more likely to develop breast cancer, and had a significantly greater risk of all malignancies.

The unopposed estrogen arm of the WHI study showed similar results to the combined treatment arm with regards to heart disease, stroke, and thromboembolic events. There was a trend toward a decrease in breast cancer incidence.[38] Further analysis from WHI showed that estrogen therapy alone or in combination with progestin treatment, increased the risk of both mild cognitive impairment and dementia.[39] Another trial of estrogen plus progestin in postmenopausal women with established coronary disease did not demonstrate beneficial effects of hormone replacement therapy for the secondary prevention of heart disease.[27] Careful explanation is needed for patients to understand that hormone replacement therapy may carry a modestly increased risk of ischemic stroke, coronary events, venous thrombosis, and possibly breast cancer. In order to minimize these hazards, hormone replacement therapy should be considered only for severe menopausal symptoms and for the shortest possible time in women who are fully informed of these risks.[40] For a more comprehensive review regarding the management and treatment of menopause, the reader is directed to a recent review article by Nelson.[41]

Andropause

For many years there was much debate regarding whether serum total testosterone levels were truly lower in healthy older men, or whether this decline was a result of confounding effects from chronic illness and medications. However, cross-sectional and longitudinal studies have shown a gradual, but progressive age-dependent decline in testosterone levels in healthy men, which has been termed *andropause*.[42,43] This is more noted for free testosterone than for total testosterone because there is an age-associated increase of sex hormone binding globulin levels.[44] Unlike the sharp decline in estrogen production at menopause, the age-related decline in testosterone level is more variable, with unclear clinical consequences.[45]

In elderly men the reduction in serum testosterone levels is mainly due to decreased production rates,[46] which occur at all levels of the hypothalamic-pituitary-testicular axis.[47] Both serum LH and FSH levels show an age-related increase in longitudinal studies, but the age-related decline in testosterone levels is not often reciprocated with changes in serum LH concentrations.[48] This is most likely due to the age-related impairment of gonadotrophin-releasing hormone secretion and alterations in gonadal steroid feedback mechanisms.[49] Aging decreases the testosterone response to LH and human chorionic gonadotrophin,[50] and the circadian rhythm of plasma testosterone secretion—with higher levels in the morning than in the evening—is generally blunted in older men.[51]

The typical phenotype associated with declining testosterone levels in aging men includes increased fat mass, loss of muscle and bone mass, fatigue, depression, anemia, poor libido, erectile deficiency,[42] insulin resistance,[52] and higher cardiovascular risk.[53] These clinical features are similar to changes associated with testosterone deficiency in young men, so the syndrome of androgen deficiency of the aging male (ADAM) has been described. However, this phenotype may also occur in older men with normal androgen levels and so the ADAM syndrome has not been universally accepted.[54]

Several clinical studies have been performed to determine whether testosterone supplementation may benefit aging individuals. Despite several trials examining various parameters, including body composition, muscle strength, bone density, metabolism, and lipid profile, there is still no consensus as to whether androgen treatment may be beneficial in older men.[55] Data from large clinical trials in elderly males is lacking and the short-term and long-term benefits of testosterone replacement therapy need to be critically evaluated.[56]

Dehydroepiandrosterone

Even though dehydroepiandrosterone (DHEA) and its sulfate-bound form (DHEAS) are the most abundant steroid hormones, their full physiologic functions are still unknown. DHEA(S) is an abundant circulating adrenal androgen, but may have cardioprotective, antidiabetic, antiobesity, and immunoenhancing properties.[57] Much debate has focused on the antiaging effects of DHEA and its potential use as the "hormone of youth.[58]" The major age-related change in the human adrenal cortex is a striking decrease in the biosynthesis of DHEA(S).[59–61] Serum DHEA levels decline rapidly and markedly after the age of 25,[60] with 80-year-old patients having DHEA levels 10% to 20% of those of younger counterparts.[62] However, the physiologic consequence of this decline is incompletely understood. Many speculate that administration of DHEA may reverse the aging effects, and there is widespread commercial availability of DHEA outside the regular pharmaceutical networks, without adequate scientific evidence.[63] Cross-sectional studies describe an association between the decline in DHEAS levels and cardiovascular disease, breast cancer, low bone mineral density, depressed mood, type 2 diabetes, and Alzheimer's disease, but this may be due to the actual aging process rather than being causally related.[64]

There is a noted sexual dimorphism in adrenal hormone regulation with healthy aging. In older women lower DHEA(S) and higher cortisol levels are seen compared with older men. This is in contrast to cortisol levels in men and women, which show a progressive, parallel increase with aging. The consequence of sexual dimorphism in adrenal hormones may have implications for age-related changes in cardiovascular disease, brain function, and bone metabolism.[65]

The largest study to date assessing the effect of oral DHEA in otherwise healthy older individuals was a double-blind randomized parallel study of 140 men and 140 women aged 60 to 79 years, who were given daily 50 mg doses of DHEA or a placebo.[66] No improvement in well-being or cognition was found. Other trials have failed to demonstrate any benefit of DHEA on well-being, mood, cognition, or activities of daily living,[67–69] suggesting that the decline in serum DHEA levels with aging does not have deleterious effects on well-being, cognition, and sexuality.[63]

In summary, there is no clear clinical consequence of the age-related decrease in serum concentration of DHEA and there are no clear benefits of DHEA replacement in older individuals.[63,70]

Hypothalmo-pituitary-adrenal axis

The hypothalamo-pituitary-adrenal (HPA) axis has an important role in the life-sustaining homeostatic and allostatic adjustments to internal and external stressors. This stress adaptive axis is a dynamic feedback network with circadian rhythmicity and pulsatile neurohormone secretion.[71] However, how this axis changes with aging is incompletely understood. There are variable age-related changes in the effects of ACTH on cortisol secretion or cortisol on ACTH secretion,[72] with no deficiency of adrenal production of corticosteroids.[73] Healthy aging disrupts the neuroendocrine mechanisms coordinating within axis pulsatility and 24-hour rhythmic cortisol release and alters the interaxis mechanisms that link LH and cortisol release. Serum cortisol secretion may vary more within a 24-hour period in older subjects, as compared with younger subjects.[71] There is a 20% to 50% increase in 24-hour mean cortisol levels between 20 and 80 years of age,[59] the evening nadir in serum cortisol concentrations may be higher and earlier in older subjects,[59,74] and there is no age-related change in corticosteroid binding globulin levels.[65] The inhibition of ACTH and cortisol secretion with dexamethasone is similar to that seen in younger individuals,[72] but may be slower in onset.[75] In older women, serum cortisol concentrations increase more with exogenous ACTH.[72] Older men have similar rises in serum concentrations as younger men and the cortisol response to stress is prolonged in older individuals.[71] There are gender-specific, age-related alterations of the HPA axis. With healthy aging there is an increase in the cortisol response to CRH challenge and diminished hypothalamic-pituitary sensitivity to glucocorticoid feedback inhibition, which is more profound in older women than older men.[65]

These age-related changes of the HPA axis could be of physiologic importance with chronic cortisol excess being implicated in hippocampal atrophy and cognitive impairments during aging. Cortisol circadian amplitude and phase changes may be relevant in the cause of sleep disorders in the elderly.[59] Additionally in older females, increasing levels of HPA-axis activity, as measured by urinary free cortisol excretion, are associated with declines in memory performance.[76] In healthy older men, cortisol levels are inversely related to both bone mineral density and the rate of bone loss, suggesting that bone density and the rate of involutional bone loss in healthy individuals might also be regulated by the HPA axis.[77] Furthermore in both men and women, cortisol levels are strongly associated with the risk of clinical fractures.[78] Lastly there is an association between 24-hour cortisol production rate and increased body fat in older men. Thus the increase in HPA-axis activity may play a role in the alterations in body composition and central fat distribution that are seen in aging.[79]

Hypothalamo-pituitary-thyroid axis

With aging there are a significant number of complex physiologic alterations. However, it is important to note that these direct age-related changes need to be distinguished from indirect alterations caused by simultaneous thyroidal or nonthyroidal illness, or other physiologic or pathophysiologic states whose incidence increases with age. Thyroid function tests in the elderly are difficult to interpret because several changes formerly believed to be a direct result of the aging process have subsequently been shown to be due to the increased prevalence of subclinical thyroid disease and/or the result of nonthyroidal illness.[80] With age, thyroid hormone clearance decreases, but there is also a decline in thyroid hormone secretion, resulting in unchanged total and free serum thyroxine (T_4) concentrations.[81] In contrast serum total and free triiodothyronine (T_3) concentrations are decreased with aging, most likely due to reduced peripheral conversion of T_4 to T_3 as a direct effect either of nonthyroidal illness or of aging itself.[80]

Apparently older euthyroid patients may have reduced serum thyroid-stimulating hormone (TSH) concentrations,[82,83] but this is usually a pathologic finding indicating either exogenous or endogenous thyrotoxicosis.[84] However, in elderly patients without clinical or subclinical hyperthyroidism, slightly decreased serum TSH may be seen.[83,85] An age-dependent reduction of daily TSH secretion rate has been reported,[86] the cause of which is unknown. It may be due to supersensitivity of thyrotrophs to the negative feedback from T_4, but other theories such as reduced hypothalamic thyroid-releasing hormone secretion have not been excluded.[80] The amplitude of the nocturnal pulses of TSH secretion, which results in the majority of 24-hour TSH secretion, is lower in older subjects,[87] leading to decreased T_4 secretion in response to the decrease in T_4 clearance.[81]

Thyroidal disease prevalence increases with age, with all types of thyroid disease being found, but the clinical manifestations are different from those in younger patients. In older individuals there is a higher prevalence of autoimmune hypothyroidism. Hyperthyroidism is mainly characterized by cardiovascular symptoms and is frequently due to toxic nodular goiters; differentiated thyroid carcinoma is more aggressive.[88] Aging is also associated with the appearance of thyroid autoantibodies, but the biologic and clinical significance of this finding is unknown. Thyroid autoantibodies are rare in healthy centenarians and in other highly selected aged populations, although they are observed in unselected or hospitalized elderly patients, suggesting that the appearance of these autoantibodies is due to age-associated disease rather than a consequence of the aging process itself.[89] However, even though physiologic changes are seen in the hypothalamo-pituitary-thyroid axis, their contribution to the pathogenesis of age-associated diseases, such as atherosclerosis, coronary heart disease, and neurologic disorders, still needs to be determined.[80]

CONCLUSION

Each endocrine system undergoes complex changes with aging, many of which occur independently from confounding factors because of the higher prevalence of age-related illnesses. These changes ultimately cause a decline in the peripheral levels of estrogen and testosterone, with an increase in luteinizing hormone, follicle-stimulating hormone, and sex hormone binding globulin. There is additionally a decline in serum concentrations of growth hormone, insulin-like growth factor-1, and dehydroepiandrosterone and its sulfate-bound form. The endocrine functions that are essential to life, such as adrenal and thyroid functions, show an overall minimal change in basal levels with aging even though there are complex changes that do occur within the hypothalamo-pituitary-adrenal/thyroid axis. The clinical significance of these deficiencies is variable and is still being evaluated. Menopause causes a series of changes in bone metabolism, lipid metabolism, vasomotor symptoms, and possibly cognition. Similarly, gonadal function decline in men is associated with loss of muscle and bone mass, increased fat mass, insulin resistance, higher cardiovascular disease risk, poor libido, erectile dysfunction, fatigue, depression, and anemia. Declines in the GH–IGF-1 axis result in reduced protein synthesis, decreased lean body and bone mass, and a decline of immune functions. The clinical significance of adrenal hormone changes is variable.

There have been many studies trying to reverse the endocrine effects seen in aging by restoring the serum hormonal levels of older individuals back into younger ranges. However, whether these therapies have true clinical benefit is still unclear. The "magic pill" to reverse the process of aging has still not been discovered and the quest for a "hormone of youth" continues.

For a complete list of references, please visit online only at www.expertconsult.com

CHAPTER 21

Aging and the Blood

Michael A. McDevitt

HEMATOPOIESIS

The production of blood

Normal blood cell development is reviewed with emphasis on recent developments and controversies related to blood cell development, function, and aging. In that blood and bone marrow have always been among the most accessible tissues for experimental study, any review of aging and the blood will contain historical insights into underlying mechanisms of cellular, immunologic, and genetic changes associated with aging. With recent advances, we can now add additional epigenetic, stem cell, molecular, and cellular insights.

SITES OF BLOOD CELL DEVELOPMENT, BONE MARROW, AND STROMA

Healthy individuals produce billions of red and white blood cells every hour of every day under normal conditions. With infection, bleeding, or other stresses, production is increased in response to complex physiologic mechanisms. The entire process of hematopoiesis begins with a limited number of hematopoietic stem cells (HSCs),[1] which serve as the reservoir for the progenitors that fuel mature blood cell production, while maintaining the stem cell compartment. The sites of hematopoiesis change with mammalian development.[2] During the first 6 to 8 weeks of human embryonic life, the yolk sac is the site of hematopoiesis, followed by a fetal liver stage. With further organismal development, the bone marrow becomes and remains the major site of hematopoiesis, outside of pathologic disorders such as thalassemia and myeloproliferative disorders (MPD), in which extramedullary hematopoiesis in spleen, liver, and elsewhere may occur. Elegant studies in mice have tracked the developmental migration of HSCs through these various tissues and identified the earliest site of origin of definitive HSC in the embryo proper as the aorta gonad mesonephros (AGM) region.[3]

The bone marrow is a specialized microenvironment. At birth the bone marrow is a fully hematopoietically active tissue, but with aging there is replacement of active hematopoietic tissue with inactive adipose tissue. An approximately 1% per year involution is a rough standard used to assess clinical bone marrow biopsy cellularity in different age individuals.[4] Bone marrow stroma includes a diverse cellular mix of fibroblasts, macrophages, mast cells, reticular cells, endothelial cells, osteoid, and adipocytes. Conventional histologic and immunohistologic analysis has identified a generally orderly arrangement of developing cells in the bone marrow, including the presence of early granulocytic cells along the bony trabecular margins, and erythroid islands, megakaryocytes, and occasional lymphoid nodules positioned in the intertrabecular spaces. Examples of special cellular relationships include erythroid islands with a central macrophage that facilitates red cell enucleation,[5] and megakaryocyte localization near draining venules to facilitate platelet release into the bloodstream.[6] Age-related histologic findings include marrow necrosis and fibrosis, loss of bone substance, increase in bone marrow iron stores, expansion of adipose tissue, and accumulation of benign lymphoid aggregates.[7] Although analysis of individual cytokines, cellular compositions, and supportive stromal functions can be measured to decrease with aging, the underlying mechanisms responsible for these changes are poorly understood.

Recent technological advances have helped to identify a specialized component of the bone marrow microenvironment, the "niche." This three-dimensional functional hematopoietic unit has specialized anatomic relationships between bone, blood vessels, and differentiating hematopoietic cells. As such, the HSC niche functions as an anatomically confined regulatory environment governing HSC numbers and fate.[8] An example of a molecular interaction facilitating specialized function in the niche is the tyrosine kinase containing receptor (Tie2) on HSCs, and the interacting ligand (Ang-1) produced by surrounding stroma to enhance the ability of HSCs to become quiescent and increase local adhesion to bone.[9] This interaction is thought to protect HSCs from stresses that suppress hematopoiesis.

Niche anatomic relationships include vascular endothelium and perivascular cells, sympathetic nervous system components, and osteoclasts. Osteoblasts and CXC chemokine ligand 12 expressing reticular cells have been identified as important regulatory components. Wnt family members, Ang-1/Tie-2, calcium-sensing receptor signaling, osteopontin, and other extracellular matrix components have also been implicated.[8] Two spacially and likely functionally distinct bone marrow microenvironment/niches have been proposed.[10,11] The endosteal HSC niche contains osteoblasts as the main supportive cell type. The vascular niche has HSCs associated with the sinusoidal endothelium in the bone marrow and spleen.[12] These environments serve as sites for local cytokine production. Factors implicated in HSC function include the Notch ligands—Delta and Jagged—involved in the generation, antidifferentiation, and expansion of HSCs.[13] Wnt signaling is involved in HSC generation and expansion and maintenance of HSCs in a quiescent state.[14] Bone morphogenic proteins (BMP) and transforming growth factor-β regulate HSC activity,[15] and BMP appears to regulate the size of the endosteal niche.[16] Many other soluble factors are also currently under investigation, including fibroblast growth factors, angiopoietin-like proteins, insulin-like growth factor 2, and others.[17]

In addition to maintenance of normal steady-state hematopoiesis, the microenvironmental niche appears to be involved in disease pathogenesis. Perturbations of the niche as a cause of hematologic disease are supported by the observation of Walkley et al, where mice null for the retinoic acid γ-receptor (RAR-γ−/−) develop a MPD dependent not on the HSCs of the null mice, but rather on the microenvironment.[18] Similarly, inactivation of the retinoblastoma gene in a murine model resulted in a profound myeloproliferative disorder as a consequence of impaired RB-dependent interaction between myeloid-derived cells and the microenvironment.[19] The human MPD primary myelofibrosis, long known as a disorder of abnormal marrow fibrosis leading to "wandering stem cells"[20] has been proposed to be a clonal disorder of stem cell niche deregulation and abnormal stroma.[21] Donor cell leukemia (DCL), a rare complication of bone marrow transplantation, has been potentially linked to niche damage from inflammation triggered by the primary underlying malignancy, or active chemotherapeutic and radiation conditioning, or transplant-related immune modulatory treatments—all leading to extrinsic leukemic influences on donor HSCs.[22]

Besides serving as a primary site of hematopoiesis, recent studies have identified the bone marrow as a potential source of cells for nonhematopoietic wound healing or regeneration. The precise nature of the source of the donor cells from the bone marrow remains controversial and the subject of much investigation. Examples of possible bone marrow-derived tissue contributors include mesenchymal stem or stromal cells,[23,24] and fibrocytes.[25] The heart,[26] cornea,[27] and liver[28] are among many tissues that are being examined as potential target organs for bone marrow–derived regenerating tissue grafts.

HEMATOPOIETIC STEM CELLS

The stem cell model of hematopoiesis starts with the totipotent HSC that has the capacity for self-renewal to prevent exhaustion of the HSC compartment, and the asymmetric proliferation and differentiation to produce large numbers of lineage-restricted hematopoietic cells daily, and the ability to reconstitute hematopoiesis in a lethally irradiated host.[1] Although intrinsic and extrinsic control of the early developmental steps from self-renewing HSC and cells committed to differentiation are poorly understood, these represent an excellent general model system to define basic mechanisms of mammalian cell development and differentiation. The ability of transferred HSCs to reconstitute hematopoiesis provides the clinical basis for bone marrow transplantation. The earliest description of HSCs was based on studies showing murine bone marrow transplanted into lethally irradiated mice, rescuing the recipient by reconstituting donor hematopoiesis.[29] Remarkably, intravenous injection is possible because the HSCs are able to home to the bone marrow, and identify and interact with the niche. The biology and physiology of the HSC is enormously complex and is the subject of many reviews[1,2,30] that include descriptions of the characterization and developmental origins of HSCs, enumeration and cellular sources, regulation of cell fate decisions, and clinical implications for bone marrow transplantation. Several areas of stem cell biology particularly relevant to aging stem cells are discussed later in this chapter.

TELOMERES AND SENESCENCE

Normal somatic cells appear to have a finite number of cell divisions available to them. In 1961 Hayflick and Moorhead described experiments that established this concept.[31] After completing this limiting number of cell divisions, a resting phase or senescence is entered. These postmitotic cells do not immediately die, but may survive for several years with normal function but with biochemical changes. Cellular senescence has long been used as a cellular model for understanding mechanisms underlying the aging process. Compelling evidence obtained in recent years demonstrates that DNA damage is a common mediator for both replicative senescence, which is triggered by telomere shortening, and premature cellular senescence induced by various stressors, such as oncogenic stress and oxidative stress.[32] Extensive observations suggest that DNA damage accumulates with age and that this may be due to an increase in production of reactive oxygen species (ROS) and a decline in DNA repair capacity with age. Mutation or disrupted expression of genes that increase DNA damage often results in premature aging. In contrast, interventions that enhance resistance to oxidative stress and attenuate DNA damage contribute toward longevity. There is significant evidence that deregulated accumulation of ROS in HSCs leads to abnormal hematopoiesis.[33,34] The precise levels of contribution of ROS production, oxidative damage, DNA repair machinery abnormalities, genomic instability, and other triggers of senescence to the aging process and age-related HSC dysfunction remain to be determined.

Telomeres and telomerase have been specifically investigated as potential components of age-related bone marrow failure and hematopoietic cell function. Human diseases characterized by mutation in the telomerase apparatus and associated with telomerase dysfunction have provided unique insights into tissue aging.[35] There are at least three human diseases that are associated with germ-line mutations of the genes encoding the two essential components of telomerase, TERT and TERC. Heterozygous mutations of these genes have been described for patients with dyskeratosis congenita, bone marrow failure, and idiopathic pulmonary fibrosis. The spectrum of mutations in TERT and TERC varies for these diseases and appears at least in part to explain the clinical differences observed. Environmental insults and genetic modifiers that accelerate telomere shortening and increase cell turnover may exaggerate the effects of telomerase haploinsufficiency, contributing to the variability of age of onset and tissue-specific organ pathology.

Warren et al, 2008, reviewed the general lack of direct evidence for progressive depletion of the HSC pool based on telomere shortening, however.[36] Serial bone marrow transplantation experiments in mice suggest that although the replicative potential of HSCs is finite, there is little evidence that replicative senescence causes depletion of the stem cell pool during the normal life span of either mouse or man. In fact extensive evidence suggests that HSC numbers substantially increase with advancing age in mice.[37] The expansion of the HSC pool is a cell-autonomous property as HSCs from aged donors exhibit a greater capacity than young controls upon transplantation into young recipients.[38] Although there is an increase in the number of HSCs with age, they have functional deficiencies, including altered homing and mobilization properties[39,40] and decreased competitive repopulation abilities.[37] Remarkably, a skewing of lineage potential from lymphopoiesis to myelopoiesis has been observed with age.[30] There are reduced lymphoid progenitors in old mice and maintained to increased myeloid progenitors. These HSC findings may explain some of the features of age-related immune cell senescence and an increase in the myelogenous hematological malignancy incidence noted with aging.

EPIGENETICS

Epigenetic marks represent DNA modifications of genomic DNA or associated proteins, other than the DNA sequence itself, that are heritable through cell division. These include

DNA methylation, a covalent modification of cytosine; histone modifications affecting the nucleosomes around which the DNA is coiled; and alterations in nucleosomal packing or higher-order folding of chromatin. Acquired epigenetic changes are common in human malignancy.[41] Epigenetic changes have been associated with the loss of responsiveness to stress that accompanies aging.[42] The intersection of cancer risk, which increases with age and is associated with epigenetic changes, with the normal aging process is an open question. A recent direct examination of longitudinal changes in global DNA methylation in the same individuals over time has provided insight into this problem.[43] Methylation was serially tested in two separate cohorts of individuals 11 or 16 years apart on average. Significant methylation change over time was identified. Also, familial clustering of methylation change was observed, suggesting that methylation maintenance may be under genetic control. There is growing evidence for significant epigenetic regulation of HSC function and behavior.

HSCs are defined by their self-renewal capacity and undifferentiated state. The mechanisms that control these are poorly understood. In vivo, in vitro, and gene expression profiling studies have revealed extensive heterogeneity in the phenotypes and properties of HSCs. Analysis of single HSC in long-term transplantation assays and genetic differences in HSC behavior in different strains of inbred mice demonstrate that many HSC behaviors are fixed intrinsically through genetic or epigenetic mechanisms.[30,44] A striking example of epigenetically fixed heterogeneity among HSCs is found in myeloid-biased HSCs. These HSCs make typical levels of myeloid cells but generate too few lymphocytes. The diminished lymphoid progeny have impaired response to IL-7.[45] Using highly purified HSCs from young and aged mice, Chambers et al also identified functional deficits but also an increase in stem cell number with advancing age.[46] Gene expression analysis identified approximately 1500 of more than 14,000 genes that were age-induced and 1600 that were age-repressed. Genes associated with the stress response, inflammation, and protein aggregation dominated the upregulated expression profile, whereas the downregulated profile was marked by genes involved in the chromatin remodeling and the preservation of genomic integrity. Many chromosomal regions showed coordinate loss of transcriptional regulation; an overall increase in transcriptional activity with age and inappropriate expression of genes normally regulated by epigenetic mechanisms was observed.

Application of chromatin-modifying/epigenetic drugs to normal HSC cultures with cytokines results in the preservation of marrow-repopulating activity and activation of several genes and their products implicated in HSC self-renewal compared with cells exposed to cytokines alone, which lost their marrow-repopulating activity.[47] Previous attempts to expand HSCs resulted in HSC differentiation and stem cell exhaustion or, at best, asymmetric cell divisions and maintenance of the same numbers of HSCs. These observations suggest chromatin modifying agents may allow symmetric division of HSCs and expansion of potential therapeutic grafts, with preservation of stem cell function. The demethylating agents 5-aza-2'deoxycytidine (decitabine, DAC) and 5-azacytidine (AZA) at low doses induce hematologic and cytogenetic remission in a subset of patients with myelodysplastic syndrome (MDS). The effects on platelet counts can be remarkable and response is correlated with increased survival.[48] Molecular analysis of patients with an informative clonal marker and a neutrophil response indicates that restoration of normal nonclonal hematopoiesis may be the predominant effect of DAC.[49] Further evaluation of the mechanisms that chromatin modifying agents alter normal and malignant hematopoiesis will be necessary to fully exploit these early observations.

PROGENITOR COMPARTMENT

Lineage-restricted progenitor cells derived from HSCs allow amplification of numbers and differentiation into separate lineage effector cells. Ultimately, more than 10 different mature cell types are derived from the HSC through these progenitors. Within a pathway, there are early and late progenitors, which differ in the number of potential proliferative cell divisions. Identification and study of progenitors has been greatly facilitated through the development of culture systems, including the identification of growth factors necessary to prevent apoptosis, an important default regulatory pathway in many if not all hematopoietic lineages. The regulation of hematopoietic cell lineage commitment remains controversial. As intrinsic determinants of cellular phenotype, transcription factors represent major components of the underlying process.[2,50]

The successful isolation of the common lymphoid progenitor (CLP), which can generate all lymphoid types but not any myeloid cells, and its counterpart—the common myeloid progenitor (CMP), which can be the source of all myeloid-cell types—provides important insights into developmental cellular pathways, suggesting that the myeloid and lymphoid developmental programs operate independently downstream of HSCs. Recent studies suggest that even these pathways, however, are much more complicated.[51,52] Key concepts related to underlying basic mechanisms responsible for progenitor cell development include the roles of qualitative and quantitative variations of transcription factor abundance, including transcription factor complexes, and even order of expression.[53] Some factors are dominant for specific lineages. Graded reduction of C/EBPα transcription factor in granulocyte monocyte progenitors (GMPs) results in a mast-cell production frequency inversely proportional to the abundance of the C/EBPα transcription factor.[53] Taking advantage of a PU.1-null mouse model, DeKoter and Singh[54] showed that high-level PU.1 expression is associated with macrophage differentiation, whereas low-level expression promotes B-cell formation. Lineage diversification also involves interplay of antagonistic competing lineage determining transcriptional programs. Continuing the PU.1 macrophage example, further investigation of PU.1 regulation of macrophage differentiation from upstream macrophage/granulocyte progenitors led to the discovery of a circuit of counter antagonistic repressors, Egr-1/2/Nab-2 and Gfi1.55 Previous work had revealed the antagonism of PU.1 and GATA-1 in erythroid vs. myeloid lineage determination.[56,57]

Based on the importance of transcriptional control mechanisms on hematopoietic regulation, it has been proposed that cumulative somatic mutations in transcription factors might contribute to the aging process by disrupting the transcriptional networks that regulate cell structure and function. This hypothesis was termed "transcriptional instability"; but experimental investigation has not supported this hypothesis to date.[58] Using a more evolutionarily distant model system, Budovskaya et al[59] did find an association between global aging in the nematode *Caenorhabditis elegans* and expression differences in three GATA transcription factors: ELT-3, ELT-5, and ELT-6. In old age, ELT-5 and ELT-6 expression increases and ELT-3 decreases, resulting in changes in a multitude of genes with GATA regulatory sites. These results suggest that aging in worms is caused by a drift in a GATA transcriptional regulatory network rather than accumulation of cellular damage. Interestingly, mammalian GATA binding transcription factors, particularly GATA-1, GATA-2, and GATA-3, have many critical roles in hematopoiesis from HSC, T cell, and myeloid effector cell biology.[2]

CIRCULATING BLOOD CELLS

Circulating blood cells represent the third class of hematopoietic cells in Metcalf's original classification of hematopoiesis.[60] The cellular components of circulating blood cells includes granulocytes, monocytes, eosinophils, basophils, erythroid cells, and lymphocytes. As critical physiologic cellular effectors, age-related changes in number and/or function have been proposed to contribute to the frailty that develops in some aging individuals.

GRANULOCYTES

Granulocytes, including neutrophils, eosinophils, and basophils, are components of the innate immune response to bacterial, fungal, and protozoal infections. It is well known that the immune response decreases during aging, leading to a higher susceptibility to infections, cancers, and autoimmune disorders. One of the most important cellular components of the innate immune response is neutrophils. Polymorphonuclear neutrophils (PMNs) are the first cells to be recruited to the site of inflammation. They have a short life span and die by apoptosis. However, their life span and functional activities can be extended in vitro by a number of proinflammatory cytokines, including the granulocyte-macrophage colony stimulating factor (GM-CSF). It has been shown that the functions and the rescue from apoptosis of PMNs tends to diminish with aging. With aging there is an alteration of other receptor-driven functions of human neutrophils as well, such as superoxide anion production and chemotaxis. Observations of molecular defects in neutrophil receptor mediated signaling[61-63] taken together describe an acquired defect in innate immunity with aging that at least in part might partially explain the higher incidence of sepsis-related deaths in the elderly population and may impact on frailty. Clinical studies investigating whether hematopoietic growth factors at pharmacologic doses (including GCSF and GM-CSF) improve outcome in older adults with cancer have demonstrated some success.[64]

EOSINOPHILS, BASOPHILS, AND MAST CELLS

Eosinophils function in host defense, allergic reactions, and other inflammatory responses, tissue injury, and fibrosis. Age-related changes in eosinophil function have been identified by Mathur et al.[65] The role of abnormal peripheral blood eosinophil "effector" functions in the pathophysiology of clinical entities such as asthma in the elderly remains to be determined. Basophils are the least common of the human granulocytes and are implicated in immediate hypersensitivity reactions, such as asthma, urticaria, allergic rhinitis, and anaphylaxis. Basophils and mast cells are effectors of immediate allergic reaction via their high-affinity receptors for IgE. Mast cells are derived from bone marrow hematopoietic progenitors in the bone marrow, although they only transiently circulate in blood enroute to tissue sites. Like other hematopoietic lineages, transcriptional networks responsible for mast cell lineage commitment and differentiation are areas of active investigation.[66] Nguyen et al[67] have identified age-induced reprogramming of mast cell degranulation and Sparrow et al identified inflammatory airway mechanisms involving basophils in older men, which may participate in inflammatory responses including asthma in the elderly patient.[68]

MONOCYTES AND MACROPHAGES

Monocytes and macrophages are closely related developmentally to neutrophils. Circulating monocytes give rise to a variety of tissue-resident macrophages throughout the body and specialized cells, such as osteoclasts and dendritic cells (DCs). Monocytes originate in the bone marrow from a common myeloid progenitor that is shared with neutrophils and are released into the peripheral blood where they circulate for several days before entering the tissues and replenishing tissue macrophage populations.[69] Circulating monocytes represent approximately 5% to 10% of human peripheral blood leukocytes in nonpathologic situations. Significant heterogeneity exists in the monocyte/macrophage phenotype, which has been investigated functionally, morphologically, through cell surface markers, and more recently through genetically altered mouse models.[70,71] For example, KLF4–/– mice were identified as having a lack of inflammatory monocytes,[72] producing fewer monocytic cells, and having increased granulocytic cells in clonogenic assays.[73] The many functional roles of monocyte, macrophage, dendritic, and osteoclast cells in maintenance of tissue homeostasis through clearance of senescent cells; remodeling and repair of tissues after inflammation; antigen presentation; and other immune function through production of inflammatory cytokines are only partially understood. Some tumors even recruit infiltrating monocytes for nefarious purposes such as enhancing tumor angiogenesis.[74] Similar to age-related changes in neutrophil signaling pathways impeding the immune response described earlier, monocyte macrophage signaling including Toll-like receptors has also been reported to be altered.[75]

RED CELLS

Erythrocytes transport hemoglobin, the major oxygen carrying pigment, and thus provide tissue gas exchange. Hormones that change with age, hypoxia, sex, and other poorly understood factors influence red cell numbers in mammals. The erythroid lineage was among the first of the hematopoietic lineages where tissue specific hematopoietic transcription factors were first cloned and then ablated in mice to identify their roles in hematopoiesis.[2] Recent discoveries place the erythroid and megakaryocyte lineages again at the forefronts of new developmental pathways. MicroRNAs (miRNAs) are a novel class of small, regulatory RNA molecules that play evolutionarily conserved roles in cellular function and development, and mediate target gene repression through 3′ untranslated region (UTR) interactions.[76] First implicated and confirmed to regulate lymphopoiesis in hematopoietic cells,[77] specific miRNAs have also been implicated as necessary for normal erythroid and megakaryocyte development.[78,79] The precise target genes and mechanisms remain under intense evaluation. Abnormal miRNA expression has been implicated in leukemia and lymphomas and mechanistic studies support a role for miRNAs in the pathogenesis of these disorders.[80]

Age-related changes in red cell numbers is unfortunately not an infrequent finding in aging adults. Anemia for all adult age ranges is one of the most frequent diagnoses on the medicine wards. Mechanisms explored to explain the anemia in the older adult include the identification of excessive circulating inflammatory cytokines such as IL-6, which may negatively impact on hematopoiesis through multiple mechanisms, including antagonizing function or impairing erythropoietin production.[81] Epidemiologic studies report that a third of the cases of anemia in older persons are unexplained, however. The diagnosis and treatment of anemia in older adults is more comprehensively reviewed in other chapters.

LYMPHOID DEVELOPMENT

Like myelopoiesis, lymphoid development has intrinsic and extrinsic controls and requires specific environmental interactions.[82,83] Understanding these developmental stages is critical to understanding normal and abnormal immunity and lymphogenesis. The peripheral immune system develops from stem cells originating in the bone marrow. Lymphoid progenitors migrate from the bone marrow (including B and T cells) to specialized peripheral sites, including the thymus, spleen, Peyer's patches, Waldeyer's ring, and lymph nodes to undergo further maturation, differentiation, and acquire self/non-self "training." Upon identification of a danger signal or foreign invader, innate immune cells respond by destroying infected cells (NK cells) and releasing cytokines and chemokines to recruit additional immune cells to fight the invader or infection and alter the host environment (inflammation). This innate immune response is often followed by an adaptive (antigen-specific) immune response with the recruitment of effector B and T lymphocytes. Following effective clearance of the invading pathogen, the host immune response must return to the quiescent state to prevent damage from an excessive immune response. A specialized subset of T cells recently described, called regulatory T cells (Treg), participate in this process.[84]

AGING AND T CELLS

T cells become specialized in the thymus to provide adaptive cellular immunity via CD8 cytotoxic T cells, and play important roles in B cell–mediated humoral immunity through helper functions. T cells have been identified as highly susceptible to age-related changes. A number of factors have been linked to the decline in T-cell function with age; however, it appears that age-induced thymic atrophy and decreased output of naïve T cells is a critical factor.[85] Changes in the composition of the bone marrow stroma with age and decreased nurturing of hematopoietic precursors contribute to decreased T-cell production with aging. Secretion of IL-7, an essential T-lineage survival cytokine, is decreased in aged bone marrow.[86] The precise nature and identity of the bone marrow–derived, earliest committed T cells remains controversial, which complicates quantitation with age. Early T-lineage progenitors (ETPs), which give rise to T cells, are generated in the bone marrow. Thymocyte progenitor cells then enter the thymus and begin their differentiation and education process with changes in surface marker expression, rearrangement of their T-cell receptor, and positive and negative cellular selection. The overall process of T-cell maturation and education is modulated by cytokines, hormones, epithelial cells, macrophages, dendritic cells, and fibroblasts in the thymic stroma. Increasing understanding of the thymic epithelial-hematopoietic cell interactions includes identification of Notch pathway receptors and ligands required for T-cell development.[87] As an individual ages, the thymus involutes and the output of T cells falls significantly.[88–89] By 70 years of age, the thymic epithelial space shrinks to less than 10%

KEY POINTS
Aging and the Blood

- Considerable progress is being achieved in identifying gene regulatory networks that direct hematopoietic cell fate. Harnessing this information may lead to more effective hematopoietic cell therapies.
- We are only beginning to appreciate the impact of regulatory RNAs including microRNAs (miRNAs) on normal and malignant hematopoietic development and function. Current examples include regulation of hematopoietic stem cell (HSC) and progenitor cell function, immune cell differentiation, response to infection, and development of immunologic disease and malignancy.
- Studies of the aging HSC are providing increased understanding and molecular insights into cellular senescence, aging, and the age-associated increase in malignancy and patterns of leukemia susceptibility.
- With increased understanding of the HSC niche we can anticipate improved approaches to HSC therapy, age-related disorders of lymphopoiesis and hematopoiesis, and the development of treatments for niche-derived diseases.
- Further characterization of leukemic stem cells will lead to more effective therapies for these typically poor prognosis disorders in adults, including novel therapies directed against the leukemic stem cell, not the bulk tumor.
- Identification and characterization of regulatory T cells (Tregs) are providing new insights into autoimmune and malignant immune disorders and may provide a cellular target for new therapies for these conditions.
- Continued study of acquired abnormalities in signaling and other underlying mechanisms of effector cell dysfunction with aging may provide insight and new effective therapies associated with hematopoietic contributions to frailty.
- The bone marrow continues to be evaluated as a source of alternative cellular regenerative therapies. Better understanding of stem cell biology and lineage plasticity are required to advance this burgeoning field.

of the total tissue. New techniques to monitor newly produced (naïve) recent thymic emigrants (RTEs) have provided powerful molecular tools to evaluate the attenuation of thymopoiesis with aging.[90] CD4:CD8 recent thymic emigrant numbers diminish with age, and RTE maturation and activation is suboptimal in aged mice. These and other observations[91] provide promise that therapeutic regeneration of functional thymic epithelial space in aging individuals could potentially reverse some of the age-related T-cell deficits.

With aging, the decrease in naïve T cells is accompanied by an increase in memory T cells in the periphery. Impaired T-cell contributions to humoral immunity are numerous including decreased IL-2 production,[92,93] germinal center defects,[94] reduced activation, differentiation, and cytokine production.[92,93] Impaired CD8 cytotoxic effector T-cell function is also diminished when influenza responses in murine models or humans are assayed.[95] These and other studies[96,97] provide some of the mechanisms that might explain disease-related immune system senescence effects associated with aging. Much recent work on the regulation of the immune system has focused on regulatory T cells (Tregs), $CD4^+/CD25^+/Foxp3^+$ regulatory T cells that play a key role in controlling the host immune response to prevent excessive immune response and damage.[84,98,99] Quantitation and functional evaluation of these cells in disease and aging is under active investigation.[100]

AGING AND B CELLS

B-lymphocyte development begins in the fetal liver and bone marrow in defined stages characterized by the status of immunoglobulin gene rearrangement in cells expressing combinations of specific cell surface antigens.[83] The production of B lymphocytes begins to decline steadily in adult life and is severely compromised in the elderly.[101,102]

In addition to reduced production of B-lineage cells in aged mice and man, studies have shown that the numbers of all B-cell progenitors, including ELP, CLP, pre-pro-B, and pro-B cells, are reduced in old bone marrow.[103] The decline in B-cell production is not restricted to very old mice.[104] Gene profiling of young and old HSC[30] suggests that age-related defects in the hematopoietic system appear to be different between lymphoid and myeloid lineages. The expression of lymphoid-specific gene sets was significantly reduced in old HSCs, whereas genes directing myeloid development were upregulated. Numerous biochemical and differentiation defects have also been identified in later developmental stages of B-cell production. Compromised CLP to pre-pro-B, and Pro-B to pre-B cell differentiation and proliferation and impaired responses to lymphopoietic cytokines IL-7 and TSLP all represent defects that may contribute to the reduced numbers of B-cell progenitors in the bone marrow of older mice.[103] Murine transplant studies that showed rescue of aged B-lineage progenitors transplanted into young but not old environments[105] are additional evidence for stromal contributions to B-cell, age-related senescence.

The translational impact of these elegant murine studies remains to be integrated with other immune defects identified in aging individuals and correlated with clinical outcomes and potential interventions. One recent approach to autoimmune diseases refractory to conventional treatments includes "rebooting the immune system." High-dose cyclophosphamide (HiCy) chemotherapy has been administered to patients with systemic lupus erythematosus, autoimmune hemolytic anemia, myasthenia gravis, multiple sclerosis, and other autoimmune disorders with the goal of largely eliminating the mature immune system while leaving the hematopoietic precursors intact.[106–108] These HiCy treatments have been effective, even in highly refractory patients, but are not always durable, indicating that continued immunosuppression or additional approaches (rebooting and retraining) may be necessary for cure.[109]

For a complete list of references, please visit online only at www.expertconsult.com

CHAPTER 22

Aging and the Skin

Emma C. Veysey
Andrew Y. Finlay

INTRODUCTION

The skin performs many vital functions including homeostatic regulation; prevention of percutaneous loss of fluid, electrolytes, and proteins; thermoregulation; sensory perception; and immune surveillance. In addition, skin forms the most visible indicator of age, the features of which are now widely considered cosmetically unacceptable. Through the effects of aging, skin becomes dry and itchy,[1] and more susceptible to infection,[2] immunologic disorders,[3] vascular complications and increased risk of cutaneous malignancy. In fact most people over the age of 65 have at least one skin disorder, and many have two or more.[4] The skin is subject to intrinsic (chronologic) aging, which is under genetic and hormonal influence, and to extrinsic aging, which is caused by environmental factors, principally UV radiation (UVR) and also smoking. UVR-induced aging is known as photoaging. The skin is particularly vulnerable to the effects of external insults and the appearance of the skin differs greatly between covered (e.g., buttocks) and sun-exposed (e.g., face, forearm) sites. There are distinct morphologic and histologic features differentiating intrinsic and extrinsic aging of the skin; however, there is also evidence that these two processes have some overlapping biologic, biochemical, and molecular mechanisms.[5] The overall result is loss of elasticity and tensile strength with wrinkle formation, increased fragility, and impaired wound healing. The skin is equipped with multiple inherent mechanisms that protect against the harmful processes that induce aging; however, the efficacy of these mechanisms decreases significantly over time.

INTRINSIC AGING

Intrinsic aging, although genetically predetermined, varies between populations and different sites on the same individual. The process of intrinsic aging falls into two categories: one that is engendered within the tissue itself and one which is caused by the influence of aging in other organs, for example, age-related hormonal changes. The former is largely controlled by progressive telomere shortening, compounded by low-grade oxidative damage to telomeres and other cellular constituents.[6] A study looking at normal human epidermis established that progressive telomere shortening associated with aging is characterized by tissue-specific loss rates.[7] Clinically, intrinsically aged skin is dry, lax, and finely wrinkled.[8]

EXTRINSIC AGING

Photoaging

Exposed sites, in particular the face, anterior chest, and extensor surfaces of the arms, display the hallmarks of extrinsically aged skin resulting from the cumulative effects of life-long UVR. It has been stated that photodamage accounts for up to 90% of age-associated cosmetic problems[9] and it is mostly preventable. Ultraviolet B (UVB, 280 to 320 nm) only penetrates as far as the epidermis and is responsible for sunburn, tanning, and photocarcinogenesis.[10] UVB is the major cause for direct DNA damage and induces inflammation and immunosuppression.[11] The effects of ultraviolet A (UVA, 320 to 400 nm), although less well understood, are thought to play a larger role than that of UVB in photoaging given UVA's far greater abundance in sunlight, far greater day-long and year-round average irradiance, and greater average depth of penetration into the dermis.[11] In pale-skinned individuals, the first signs of extrinsic aging on exposed sites are apparent by the age of 15 years,[12] whereas on nonexposed sites they are not apparent until age 30.[13] The pursuit of a tan remains a high priority in Western culture, resulting in ever-rising rates of skin cancer and prematurely aged skin. Clinically, photo-aged skin is characterized by deep wrinkles, laxity, roughness, a sallow or yellow color, increased fragility, purpura formation, pigmentary changes, telangiectasia, impaired wound healing, and benign and malignant growths. The mechanisms through which UVR induces accelerated aging are discussed later in the chapter.

Smoking

Smoking is an independent risk factor for premature facial wrinkling after controlling for sun exposure, age, sex, and skin pigmentation.[14] The relative risk of moderate-to-severe wrinkling for current smokers was found to be 2.3 for men and 3.1 for women.[15] There is a clear dose-response relationship, with facial wrinkling increasing in individuals who smoke for longer and also with increasing numbers of cigarettes per day.[14] Some studies have reported that women are more susceptible to the wrinkling effects of smoking.[15] When smoking and excessive sun exposure combine, the effect on wrinkling multiplies. The risk of developing wrinkles increases to 11.4 times that in a normal age-controlled population.[16] The exact mechanism for the aging effects of smoking is poorly understood. The effects may be topical due to the drying or irritating effect of cigarette smoke on the skin, or systemic with induction of matrixmetalloproteinase-1 (MMP-1),[17] or through affecting cutaneous microvasculature, which is constricted by acute and long-term smoking.[18]

Skin type

Pigmentation of the skin is protective against the cumulative effects of photoaging; those with skin type VI (black) showing little difference between exposed and unexposed sites.[19] In addition, the difference in skin cancer rates between Whites and African Americans indicates that pigmentation provides a 500-fold level of protection from UV radiation.[20] The appearance of photodamaged skin differs for those with skin types I and II (red hair/freckles/burns easily) and those with skin types III and IV (darker skin, tans easily). The former tend to show atrophic skin changes, with fewer wrinkles and sometimes focal depigmentation (guttate hypomelanosis) and dysplastic changes, such as actinic keratoses and epidermal malignancies. In contrast, those with III/IV skin develop hypertrophic responses, such as deep wrinkling, coarseness, a leather-like appearance, and lentigines.[11] Basal cell carcinoma and squamous cell carcinoma occur almost exclusively on sun-exposed skin of light-skinned people.

Wrinkling in Asian skin has been documented to occur later and with less severity than in Whites.[13]

EPIDERMIS

The epidermis is composed of an outer nonviable layer called the stratum corneum, and the bulk of epidermis consists primarily of keratinocytes, with smaller populations of Langerhans cells and melanocytes.

The stratum corneum is the body's principal barrier to the environment and also plays a major role in determining the level of cutaneous hydration. Its structure is often compared to the "bricks and mortar" model consisting of protein-rich corneocytes, which are embedded in a matrix of ceramides, cholesterol, and fatty acids.[21] These lipids form multilamellar sheets amid the intercellular spaces of the stratum corneum and are critical to its mechanical and cohesive properties, enabling it to function as an effective water barrier.[22] There is general agreement that the thickness of the stratum corneum does not change with age[23] and that barrier function does not alter significantly. However, certain features of aging skin do indicate an abnormal skin barrier, namely the extreme skin dryness (xerosis) and increased susceptibility to irritant dermatitis that accompanies old age. Furthermore there is evidence of altered permeability to chemical substances[24] and reduced transepidermal water flux in aged skin.[21] It seems that baseline skin barrier function is relatively unaffected by age.[23] However, if the skin is subjected to sequential tape stripping, the barrier function in aged skin (>80 years) is much more readily disrupted than in young skin (20 to 30 years).[23] In addition, the same study found that after tape stripping, barrier recovery was greatly disturbed in the older age group. The reason for this abnormality is not entirely understood; however, it appears that there is a global reduction in stratum corneum lipids, which affects the "mortar" that binds the corneocytes. More recently studies have confirmed that in moderately aged (50 to 80 years) individuals, abnormal stratum corneum acidification results in delayed lipid processing, delayed permeability barrier recovery, and abnormal stratum corneum integrity.[25] Not only does the rise in stratum corneum pH interfere with lipid production, it also accelerates the degradation of intercorneocyte connections, the corneodesmosomes.[26] The abnormal acidification is linked to decreased membrane Na^+/H^+ transport protein.[25] In addition, with age, stratum corneum turnover time lengthens with protracted replacement.[27]

Studies of epidermal thickness disagree, and no conclusion can yet be drawn on any change with age.[20] It appears that the epidermis thins with age at some body sites, such as the upper inner arm[28,29] and back of the upper arm,[30] but remains constant at others, such as the buttock, dorsal forearm, and shoulder.[31] This variation is clearly not accounted for by sun or environmental exposure alone.[20] Differences in study method, population, and body site likely account for these greatly different results. One author suggests that although epidermal thickness remains constant with advancing age, variability in epidermal thickness and keratinocyte size increases.[8]

The most consistent change found in aged skin is flattening of the dermoepidermal junction at sites that were highly corrugated in youth.[32] The flattening creates a thinner looking epidermis primarily because of retraction of the rete ridges.[20] With this reduced interdigitation between layers, there is less resistance to shearing forces.[13] There is also a reduced surface area over which the epidermis communicates with the dermis, accompanied by a reduced supply of nutrients and oxygen.[33]

There is general agreement that epidermal cell turnover halves between the third and seventh decades of life.[34,35] This is consistent with the observation that wound healing capacity deteriorates in old age.[36]

Keratinocytes

With age there is increasing atypia of the basal layer keratinocytes.[29] Involucrin, a differentiation marker normally expressed by irreversibly differentiated keratinocytes in the stratum corneum, has been found to have increased expression in sun-damaged skin.[37] This is consistent with the fact that keratinocyte differentiation is impaired by UVR. In addition, in basal epidermal cells there is downregulation of certain β_1-integrins,[37] which are markers of keratinocyte differentiation and adhesion to the extracellular matrix, suggesting that proliferation and adhesion of keratinocytes in photodamaged aged skin are significantly abnormal.

Melanocytes

With age there is a reduction in the number of melanocytes of between 8% and 20% per decade. This is manifest as a reduction in melanocytic nevi in older patients.[38] There is an associated loss of melanin in the skin, which means less protection against the harmful effects of UV radiation. Consequently, the elderly are more susceptible to skin cancers and sun protection remains very important for this group, despite the fact that the majority of an individual's harmful sun exposure occurs in the first 2 decades of life.[39]

DERMIS

The dermis consists predominantly of connective tissue, and contains blood vessels, nerves, and the adnexal structures including sweat glands and sebaceous glands. Its main role is to provide a tough and flexible layer that supports the epidermis and binds to the subcutis, the fatty layer deep to the dermis. Dermal connective tissue contains collagen and elastin. Collagen fibers comprise the biggest volume of the skin and give the skin its tensile strength, whereas elastin fibers contribute to elasticity and resilience.[33]

As with the epidermis, studies reveal conflicting results, with some showing thinning with age and others no change.[20] It has been suggested that the initial effect of photodamage in young is skin is thickening through solar elastosis; in contrast in the elderly more severe damage results in notable thinning.[40] However, despite extensive data, it is extremely difficult to define the effects of aging on skin thickness, partly because of individual and regional variations between different studies.[20]

It is generally accepted that changes in the dermis are responsible for wrinkling; however, the mechanism is not entirely understood.[32] There is general atrophy of the extracellular matrix, accompanied by a decrease in cellularity, especially of the fibroblasts, which also have reduced synthetic abilty.[41,42] There are more abnormalities of collagen and elastic fibers in sun-exposed sites.[43,44]

Collagen

Collagen is the most abundant protein found in humans, and as the primary structural component of the dermis is responsible for conferring strength and support to human skin. Alterations in collagen play an integral role in the aging process.[39]

In the dermis of young adults, collagen bundles are well organized; they are arranged in such a way that allows for extension, with return to their resting state facilitated by the interwoven elastic fibers.[32] In aging there is an increase in density of collagen bundles[45] and they lose their extensible configuration, becoming fragmented, disorganized, and less soluble.[46,47]

Both UVR and the intrinsic aging process, mainly through the production of reactive oxygen species (ROS), result in upregulation of the collagen degrading enzymes matrix metalloproteinases.[48] In addition, there is a decrease in collagen synthesis[49] and thus a shift in the balance between synthesis and degradation occurs.[8] Different collagens in the skin have different functions and they are all affected differently by the aging process. In young skin collagen I comprises 80% of dermal collagen and type III makes up 15%; however, with age there is a decrease in collagen I with a resultant increase in the ratio of type III to type I collagen.[47,50] There are also changes to levels of collagen IV and VII. Collagen IV, an integral part of the dermoepidermal junction, provides a structural framework for other molecules and plays a key role in maintaining mechanical stability[39] and collagen VII is critical for basement membrane binding to the underlying papillary dermis.[39] There are significantly lower levels of both collagen IV and collagen VII at the base of wrinkles and it is speculated that loss of these collagens contributes to wrinkle formation.[51]

Elastin

Elastin exhibits numerous age-related changes, including slow degradation[52,53] and accumulation of damage in existing elastin with intrinsic aging,[52] increased synthesis of apparently abnormal elastin in photo-exposed areas,[54] and abnormal localization of elastin in the upper dermis of photodamaged skin.[21]

Histologically, one of the most striking features of photodamaged skin is the change in elastotic material. On hematoxylin and eosin staining, there is an area of amorphous blue staining in the superficial to mid-dermis, and is referred to as "solar elastosis." This represents a tangled mass of degraded elastic fibers accompanied by amorphous material composed of disorganized tropoelastin and fibrillin in the upper dermis.[11] Even in sun-protected sites, most elastin fibers appear abnormal after the age of 70 years.[44,55] This abnormal elastotic material provides neither elasticity nor resilience to the skin.

Glycosaminoglycans and water content

Glycosaminoglycans (GAGs) along with collagen and elastin are major constituents of the skin, and include hyaluronic acid, dermatan sulfate, and chondroitin sulfate.[39] The key role of these molecules is to bind water, and their presence enables the skin to remain plump, soft, and hydrated.[39] In photoaged skin the level of GAGs increases[56,57]; however, these molecules are unable to exert their hydrating effect as they are deposited on elastotic material rather than scattered diffusely in the dermis, as in young or photoprotected skin.[57]

Young skin is well hydrated as most of the water is bound to proteins.[58] Water molecules that are not bound to proteins bind to each other and form what is known as tetrahedron or bulk water.[58] In intrinsically aged skin, water structure and binding does not appear to be altered significantly.[56] In photoaged skin there is an increase in total water content[56]; however, as proteins are more hydrophobic[59] and folded[56,58] than those in sun-protected skin, and GAGs are deposited on elastotic material, water binds to itself rather than to these molecules, and so is present mostly in the tetrahedron form.[56] In addition, tetrahedron water does not offer the same level of hydration and turgor as the bound form of water, thus contributing to the dry xerotic appearance of photoaged skin.[21]

Dermal vasculature

Although not all studies are in agreement, it appears that increased age may be associated with decreased cutaneous perfusion, especially in photo-exposed areas.[20] One study has demonstrated a 35% reduction in venous cross-sectional area in aged skin as opposed to young skin.[60] This reduction in vascularity is particularly noticeable in the papillary dermis (superficial dermis), where there is loss of the vertical capillary loops. Reduced vascularity results in skin pallor, depleted nutrient exchange, and disturbed thermoregulation.[39] There is some evidence that the vasoconstrictive or vasodilatatory responses to cold and heat, respectively, are delayed in the elderly, further diminishing thermoregulatory reponses.[20] In addition, dermal vasculature in mildly photodamaged skin displays venule wall thickening. However, in severely photodamaged skin the walls are thinned and become dilated, manifesting clinically as telangiectasia.[11]

SWEAT GLANDS

Eccrine sweat glands

There is a reduction in the number of eccrine sweat glands[61] and output per gland[62] with increasing age, which also impacts on thermoregulation. There is an equally reduced response to the effects of epinephrine in men and women in old age; however, there is a far greater decrease in response to acetylcholine in men than in women in old age. This suggests that the effects of cholinergic sweating are indirectly affected by hormones.[62] Further evidence for this is provided by the observation that the maximum rate of cholinergic sweating is far greater in adult males than in adult females or juveniles, and is probably therefore androgen-dependent.[63]

Apocrine sweat glands

Apocrine gland activity is diminished, probably as a consequence of declining testosterone levels, leading to a reduction in both pheromone secretion and consequent body odor.[64]

SEBACEOUS GLANDS

Age does not alter the number of sebaceous glands, although they become hyperplastic and larger,[65] particularly in photoaged skin and may present as giant comedones. Despite this increase in size, there is a 50% reduction in sebum production,[66] which contributes to xerosis of aged skin. Some investigators believe that this is due to decreased levels of testosterone,[67] although this does not explain the hyperplasia. In addition, the constituency of aged sebum is altered, in that it contains less free cholesterol and more squalene.[68]

Nails

Nail growth increases until about the age of 25 years, thereafter it starts to decrease.[32] Until the age of 70, nail growth is greater in men than women, after which the situation appears to be reversed.[69] Nails become more brittle in the elderly and develop beaded ridging. This brittleness may be caused by a reduction in lipophilic sterols and free fatty acids.[70]

Hair

Changes in hair color and density are very visible indicators of age and are the target of endless manipulation to maintain a youthful appearance. It is estimated that by the age of 50, approximately 50% of people are 50% gray, irrespective of hair color and sex.[71] Hair graying appears to be a consequence of an overall and specific depletion of hair bulb and outer root sheath melanocytes, as melanocytes are still detected in sebaceous glands and the surrounding interfollicular epidermis.[72] The mechanism for this steady depletion remains uncertain.

With age there are changes in hair follicle density, hair shaft diameter, and rate of hair growth. These changes are brought about through a variety of mechanisms and vary greatly according to site. Chest, axillary, and pubic hair all decrease in density with age; however, in men there is often increased hair growth in the eyebrows, around the external auditory meati, and in nostrils.[32] In elderly women there is conversion of vellus to terminal hairs on the chin and moustache.

Aside from intrinsic aging, a principal influence on hair with age is androgenetic alopecia. This is a genetically predetermined condition that results in patterned scalp hair loss and arises due to increased sensitivity of hair follicles to the effects of dihydrotestosterone, produced by breakdown of free testosterone by the enzyme 5a-reductase.[73] It affects at least 50% of men by the age of 50 years and 50% of women by the age of 60 years.[74] Hairs in the affected area become finer and less pigmented until they resemble vellus hairs.[74]

Immune function

The density of Langerhans cells in the skin decreases greatly in the elderly even in sun-protected sites.[75,76] Not only is there a reduction in the number of Langerhans cells, but they have reduced ability to migrate from the epidermis in response to tumor necrosis factor-α.[77] Similarly, T cells are reduced in number and become less responsive to specific antigens.[27,78] Aging skin also appears to have a reduced ability to produce certain cytokines such as interleukin-2,[79] whereas there is an increase in other cytokines such as interleukin-4.[79] The consequence of these changes is a reduced intensity to delayed hypersensitivity reactions[3] and increased susceptibility to photocarcinogenesis and chronic skin infections.[34]

Nerves and sensation

There is a decrease in sensory perception and an increase in pain threshold with age.[80] It has been demonstrated that there is loss of Meissner's corpuscles in the little finger, from over 30/mm^2 in young adults to approximately 12/mm^2 by the age of 70 years.[81]

Subcutaneous tissue

There are age-dependent changes in subcutaneous fat distribution. There is loss of fat from the face, dorsal aspects of the hands and the shins, with gains in subcutaneous fat in other areas, particularly the waist in women and abdomen in men.[38]

Women

Reduced estrogen levels in postmenopausal women contributes to wrinkling, dryness, atrophy, laxity, poor wound healing, and vulvar atrophy.[82] Studies suggest that loss of collagen is more closely related to postmenopausal age than chronologic age, and thus reflects hormonal effects.[83,84] Estrogen therapy appears to prevent collagen loss in women with higher baseline levels of collagen, and stimulates synthesis of collagen in those that have lower initial collagen levels.[85,86] Studies have also supported a relationship between estrogen deprivation and degenerative changes of dermal elastic tissue.[87] However, it remains uncertain whether there are beneficial effects of estrogen therapy on skin elasticity.[88] There is some evidence that hormone replacement therapy (HRT) improves skin dryness[89] and wound healing,[90] and increases skin surface lipids.[91,92]

Mechanism

The production of reactive oxygen species (ROS) or free radicals, through UVR, smoking, pollution, and normal endogenous metabolic processes, is thought to contribute to the process of aging in the skin. ROS induces gene expression pathways that result in increased degradation of collagen and accumulation of elastin.[93] ROS not only directly destroys interstitial collagen, but also inactivates tissue inhibitors of matrix-metalloproteases and induces the synthesis and activation of matrix degrading metalloproteases.[93]

Hormones have also been shown to play a role. Postmenopausal hormone changes are responsible for a rapid worsening of skin structure and functions, which can be at least partially repaired by HRT or local estrogen treatment.[84,94]

Mitochondrial DNA (mtDNA), due to repeated constitutional oxidative stress, incurs regular DNA damage and in particular deletion of a specific length of DNA, which is known as the "common deletion." This deletion is 10 times more common in photodamaged than in sun-protected skin. It results in decreased mitochondrial function and further accumulation of ROS, with additional damage to the cell's ability to generate energy. The extent of mtDNA damage in photodamaged skin does not correlate with the chronologic age of the person, but rather with photodamage severity (reviewed by Yaar and Gilchrest[11]).

UVR can accelerate telomere shortening, which occurs ordinarily with every cell division. This results in the activation of DNA damage response proteins such as p53, the tumor suppressor protein, thereby inducing proliferative senescence or apoptosis, depending on the cell type.[6,95]

Treatment and prevention

Sun avoidance and sunscreen use is central to preventing age-related skin changes. Aside from this there are a number of products of proven and still controversial efficacy.

Topical retinoids can cause a significant improvement in skin surface roughness, fine and coarse wrinkling, mottled pigmentation, and sallowness.[96] Histologically, there is reduction and redistribution of epidermal melanin, increased papillary dermal collagen deposition, and increased vascularity of the papillary dermis. Tretinoin treatment not only improves photodamage, but also reverses histologic changes associated with intrinsic aging.[97,98] These effects are thought to be mediated via the nuclear retinoic acid receptors (RARs). Retinoids not only improve the cosmetic appearance of aging, but also help prevent skin cancer.[11]

There are also many novel therapies undergoing investigation. For instance, the delivery of enzymes that assist in DNA repair, antioxidants such as the polyphenols, flavinoids, alpha-hydroxy acids, and many others. Dietary lipids appear to play a role in skin aging. There is evidence that a low-fat diet provides some protection against the development of actinic keratoses[99]; however, certain dietary fats appear to be protective against UV-induced damage.[11] Future treatments include inducing cutaneous pigmentation, thus protecting the skin from UVR damage, and various approaches to this are in development.[11] Nonmedical therapies include laser treatment, injectable fillers, botulinum toxin, and of course surgery.

CONCLUSION

Skin is subject to a complex blend of intrinsic and extrinsic aging processes and is particularly vulnerable to environmental insults, namely UVR. Although there are numerous defense mechanisms to protect the skin from damage, the efficacy of these diminish over time, resulting in the clinical features associated with aging and the development of skin cancers. Sun protection is the key to prevention and novel therapies are also emerging.

KEY POINTS

Aging and the Skin

- Aging of the skin is affected by intrinsic and extrinsic factors.
- UV radiation is responsible for most of the visible signs of aging and is known as photoaging.
- Photoaging is seen on sun-exposed sites, such as the face and forearms.
- Photoaging results in increased degradation of collagen and increased deposition of abnormal elastin in the dermis.
- Intrinsic aging is associated with fine wrinkling, xerosis (dryness), and skin laxity. Extrinsic aging is associated with coarse wrinkles, xerosis, mottled dyspigmentation, skin laxity, roughness, and the development of malignant neoplasms.
- The mechanisms for aging skin include the actions of ROS, mtDNA mutations, and telomere shortening.
- Hormonal changes, particularly in women, are important for skin aging.
- The key to treatment is prevention through sun protection, but other novel therapies are emerging.

For a complete list of references, please visit online only at www.expertconsult.com

CHAPTER 23

The Pharmacology of Aging

David R. P. Guay

Each day worldwide, elderly people consume millions of doses of medications. This remarkable amount of medication use benefits many elderly people greatly by preventing and treating disease, preserving functional status, prolonging life, and improving or maintaining good quality of life. However, this level of medication exposure may also harm elderly people via adverse drug reactions and is associated with problems such as drug interactions. The harmful and beneficial responses of elderly individuals to drugs are partially dependent upon age-related physiologic changes that influence how the body handles a given drug (i.e., pharmacokinetics) and what a drug does to the body (i.e., pharmacodynamics). To obtain the desired therapeutic response and prevent drug-related problems, it is also useful to have an understanding of drug use patterns in the elderly. Therefore, this chapter first examines the epidemiology of drug use in elderly populations around the world, followed by age-related alterations in drug pharmacokinetics and pharmacodynamics, and finally drug interactions.

EPIDEMIOLOGY OF DRUG USE

In general, the number of medications (prescription and nonprescription) used by older individuals is greater than the number used by younger persons.[1] The number and type of medications used by elders are based in part on living situations and access to medications, as detailed later.

In the community

More than 75% of community-dwelling elderly people use one or more medications, with percentages varying by country: Sweden (93%), Netherlands (90%), United States (88%), Italy (93%), Canada (75%), and Ireland (75%).[2–7] The average number of medications being used at a given time is higher for U.S. elders compared with elders elsewhere. The U.S. average ranges between 3 and 8, whereas the average in Sweden is 4.2, the average in Taiwan is 4.7, and the average in Italy is 3.5.[2,4,5,8–10] The most common types of medications are cardiovascular, gastrointestinal, central nervous system, analgesic, and vitamin agents.[1,2,5,6,10–13] The most common factor associated with medication use is gender, with females using more medications than males.[1,5,12–16] Increasing age has also been associated with increased medication use in the United States, Canada, and the United Kingdom.[11,12,14,16] In the United States, race has been associated with differences in medication use, with African Americans and Hispanic Americans demonstrating less use than whites.[9,17]

In hospitals

Medication use by elderly people at the time of hospital discharge is slightly higher than that of community-dwelling elders; it ranges, on average, from about 3 whites medications in Germany to 5 in the United States, Australia, and the Netherlands.[18–21] There is a paucity of information with regard to the types of medications used by elders in this setting. However, in small studies conducted in the Netherlands, the United States, and Australia, the most common types of medications are cardiovascular, gastrointestinal, central nervous system, and analgesic agents, with noticeably frequent use of antimicrobials and laxatives.[18–20] There are conflicting studies regarding whether sex, increasing age, and the number of medical conditions are factors enhancing medication use in this setting.[1,7,18–21]

In long-term care facilities

The level of medication use by elderly people in long-term care facilities (LTCFs) is generally higher than that of elders living at home.[22] For example, more than 75% of U.S. LTCF residents receive four or more medications compared with 51% of Italian residents, 41% of Japanese residents, and 27% of Irish residents.[7,8,23] There is also disparity worldwide in the percentages of LTCF residents taking large numbers of medications. In the United States and Iceland, 33% of LTCF residents take 7 to 10 medications, whereas only 5% of residents exhibit this degree of use in Denmark, Italy, Japan, and Sweden.[23] The average number of routinely scheduled medications in most LTCF populations ranges from 4 to 5, except in the United States and Sweden where the average is 6 to 7.[2,7,8,22,24–26]

The most common types of medications used are cardiovascular, central nervous system, laxative, and analgesic agents.[7,8,27] Overuse of certain centrally active medications, namely psychotropics, can be a particular problem in the LTCF setting.[28] Factors that have been associated with increased psychotropic use include dementia or mental illness and lack of drug monitoring.[29] Before 1987, there was a higher rate of usage of these agents in U.S. LTCFs.[28] Federal legislation was then enacted that defined clear indications for appropriate prescribing of these agents and mandated close monitoring of them (Omnibus Budget Reconciliation Act or OBRA 1987), resulting in a dramatic reduction in use.[29] Psychotropic medication usage rates are much higher in LTCFs in countries where there is no such monitoring.[29]

Access to medications

Universal public health insurance programs for elderly people in Australia, Sweden, Canada, France, Germany, Japan, New Zealand, and the United Kingdom provide some level of drug benefit coverage, with the drug benefits differing in the amount of cost sharing, the maximum amount of coverage, and the specific pharmaceuticals covered.[30] The U.S. health insurance program for the elderly, Medicare, began coverage of outpatient drugs in 2006 via Medicare Part D. Although characterized by substantial copayments and an absence of coverage over a small but fixed drug cost range (the so-called "doughnut hole"), U.S. elders are now protected from catastrophic out-of-pocket costs for outpatient drugs. This in turn has improved adherence and reduced the need for elders to forgo necessities to purchase medications.[31–33] Additionally, in developing countries, the supply of medications may be inadequate or too expensive for elders to purchase.[34]

ALTERED PHARMACOKINETICS

Table 23-1 illustrates an overview of age-related changes in drug pharmacokinetics.[35,36] The text herein details these changes in drug absorption, distribution, metabolism, and elimination.

Absorption

Numerous changes occur in the physiology of the gastrointestinal tract as a function of advancing age that might be expected to affect the absorption of drugs administered orally.[37] Gastric pH rises owing to the development of atrophic gastritis (as well as the use of acid-suppressive medications to treat age-related GI disorders, such as peptic ulcer and gastroesophageal reflux). Gastric emptying is somewhat delayed and decreases are seen in intestinal blood flow (30% to 40% from age 20 to 70 years), intestinal motility, and number of functional absorptive cells.

Most drugs administered orally are absorbed via the process of passive diffusion, a process minimally affected by aging. A few agents require active transport for GI absorption and their bioavailability may be reduced as a function of aging (e.g., calcium in the setting of hypochlorhydria). Of more significance is the decrease in first-pass hepatic extraction that occurs with aging, resulting in an enhancement in systemic bioavailability for drugs such as propranolol, morphine, and meperidine after oral administration.[37] The bioavailability of drugs that are cytochrome P450 (CYP450) isoenzyme 3A4 and/or P-glycoprotein substrates (e.g., midazolam, verapamil) may be increased in older women but no dosage adjustment recommendations have as yet been made.[38]

The effect of aging on drug absorption from other sites of administration such as the rectum, muscle, and skin is poorly understood. For example, conflicting results have been published regarding the effect of aging on the pharmacokinetics of transdermal fentanyl.[39]

Distribution

A number of changes in physiology occur with aging that may impact drug distribution. Body fat as a proportion of body weight rises from 18% to 36% in males and from 33% to 45% in females from age 20 to 70 years, whereas lean body mass decreases by 19% in males and by 12% in females, and plasma volume decreases by 8% from age 20 to 80 years. Total body water decreases by 17% from age 20 to 80 years and extracellular fluid volume decreases by 40% from 20 to 65 years of age. In addition, cardiac output declines approximately 1% per year from age 30 years, and brain and cardiac vessel blood flow rates decline 0.35% to 0.5% and 0.5% per year, respectively, beyond age 25 years. Additionally, frailty and concurrent disease may result in substantial changes in the serum concentrations of the two major drug-binding plasma proteins (albumin, which binds acidic drugs, decreases, while α1 acid glycoprotein, which binds basic drugs, remains the same or rises).[40]

As a result of the above factors, the volume of distribution of water-soluble (hydrophilic) drugs is decreased and that of fat-soluble (lipophilic) drugs is increased. Moreover, changes in volume of distribution can directly affect the loading doses of medications. For many drugs, loading doses will be lower in older versus younger patients and lowest in older white and Asian females (thus use weight-based

Table 23-1. Age-Related Changes in Drug Pharmacokinetics

Pharmacokinetic Phase	Pharmacokinetic Parameters
Gastrointestinal absorption	Unchanged passive diffusion and no change in bioavailability for most drugs
	↓ active transport and ↓ bioavailability for some drugs
	↓ first-pass effect and ↑ bioavailability for some drugs
Distribution	↓ volume of distribution and ↑ plasma concentrations of water-soluble drugs
	↑ volume of distribution and ↑ terminal disposition half-life ($t_{1/2}$) for fat-soluble drugs
	↑ or ↓ free fraction of highly plasma protein-bound drugs
Hepatic metabolism	↓ clearance and ↑ $t_{1/2}$ for some oxidatively metabolized drugs
	↓ clearance and ↑ $t_{1/2}$ of drugs with high hepatic extraction ratio
Renal excretion	↓ clearance and ↑ $t_{1/2}$ of renally eliminated drugs

↑ = increased; ↓ = decreased.

regimens routinely).[38] Decreases in serum albumin concentration can lead to a reduction in the degree of plasma protein binding of acidic drugs, such as naproxen, phenytoin, tolbutamide, and warfarin, thus increasing the drug-free fraction. Increases in α1 acid glycoprotein because of inflammatory disease, burns, or cancer can lead to enhancement in the degree of plasma protein binding of basic drugs such as lidocaine, β-blockers, quinidine, and tricyclic antidepressants, thus reducing the drug-free fraction. Provided there is no compromise in excretory pathways, these potential changes are unlikely to be clinically significant. However, plasma protein binding changes can alter the relationship of unbound (free) and total (unbound + bound) plasma drug concentrations, making drug concentration interpretation more difficult. In these cases, the measurement of free plasma drug concentrations may be preferable to the usual use of total plasma drug concentrations.

Metabolism

Although drug metabolism can occur in numerous organs, most of the available data concern the effects of aging on the liver. Over the age of 30 years, there is an approximate 1% per year decline in liver blood flow and liver mass.[41]

Drugs are metabolized by two types of reactions: phase I (oxidative reactions) and phase II (conjugative/synthetic reactions wherein an acetyl group or a sugar is conjugated to the drug to enhance its polarity, water-solubility, and hence, excretion via the kidneys). Most phase I reactions are mediated by CYP450 monooxygenase enzymes. Table 23-2 illustrates five CYP450 isoenzymes of clinical importance and selected substrates. Age-related declines in drug oxidation (which are substrate-specific in their extent) are thought to more closely relate to reductions in liver volume (i.e., hepatocyte mass) than reductions in hepatic enzymatic activity.[42] Age-related decreased phase I metabolism, resulting in reduced total body clearance and increased terminal disposition half-life, has been reported for diazepam, chlordiazepoxide, piroxicam, theophylline, and quinidine (Table 23-3). The activities of CYP450 isoenzymes 1X and 3A4, and the drug transporters P-glycoprotein and MDR1, are

Table 23-2. Selected Cytochrome P450 Substrates by Isoenzyme

CYP1A2	CYP2C9	CYP2C19	CYP2D6	CYP3A4
Caffeine	Diclofenac	Diazepam	Codeine	Alprazolam
Clozapine	Phenytoin	S-mephenytoin	Desipramine	Astemizole
Olanzapine	Tolbutamine	Omeprazole	Dextromethorphan	Cyclosporine
Theophylline	S-warfarin	Phenytoin	Encainide	Midazolam
			Haloperidol	Nifedipine
			Metoprolol	Quetiapine
			Paroxetine	Terfenadine
			Risperidone	Triazolam
			Thioridazine	Verapamil

Table 23-3. Drugs Whose Hepatic Metabolism Is Impaired With Advancing Age

Amlodipine	Nifedipine
Chlordiazepoxide	Nortriptyline
Diazepam	Phenytoin
Enalapril	Piroxicam
Erythromycin	Propranolol
Fosinopril	Quinidine
Imipramine	Theophylline
Levodopa	Triazolam
Lidocaine	Verapamil
Morphine	

not affected by aging or differences between the sexes.[38] In contrast, the activities of CYP450 isoenzymes 2C9, 2C19, and 2D6 are reduced by 20% to 25% in older versus younger patients and by a further 10% to 20% in females versus males.[38] The effect of aging on polymorphic drug metabolism has not been well studied, although available data suggest that advancing age has no significant effect on acetylator phenotype or cytochrome P450 isoenzyme 2D6 polymorphism.[43,44] Differences in enantiomeric disposition as a function of age are substrate-specific. For example, age-dependent changes in enantiomeric disposition have been reported for hexobarbital, propranolol, mephobarbital, and warfarin.[45–47] Phase II reactions appear to be generally spared from any adverse effect of aging.

Age-associated reductions in hepatic blood flow can reduce the clearance of high hepatic extraction ratio drugs, such as tricyclic antidepressants, lidocaine, several opioids, and propranolol (Table 23-3).[41] Numerous confounders such as race, gender, frailty, smoking, diet, and drug interactions can significantly enhance or inhibit hepatic drug metabolism in the elderly.[48]

Elimination

Few data are available regarding the effect of aging on the biliary system. However, aging is associated with a significant reduction in renal mass and number and size of nephrons. In addition, glomerular filtration rate (GFR), tubular secretion, and renal blood flow decrease approximately 0.5%, 0.7%, and 1% per year, respectively, over the age of 20 years. At all ages, these three parameters are lower in women than in men.[38] However, elderly people are a heterogeneous group, with up to one third of healthy elders having no decrement in renal function as measured by creatinine clearance, a surrogate for glomerular filtration. In addition, tubular secretion and glomerular filtration may not decline in parallel.[49] The estimation of creatinine clearance (CrCl), using any of a number of equations, serves as a useful screen for renal impairment in lieu of the use of serum creatinine (SCr), which is an imperfect marker of renal function in the elderly because of the reduction of muscle mass with advancing age (i.e., a "normal" serum creatinine does not equate with "normal" renal function in the elderly).[50] One useful estimation equation is that of Cockcroft and Gault[51]:

$$\text{CrCl (males)} = \frac{(140 - \text{age in years}) \times (\text{total body weight in kg})}{72 \times \text{SCr in mg/dL}}$$

For females, multiply the result by 0.85.

A more accurate estimation equation for renal function is the Modification of Diet in Renal Disease Simplified Algorithm[38]:

$$\text{estimated GFR(eGFR)(mL/min/1.73 sq.m)} = 186.3^{*} \times (\text{SCr}^{\dagger})^{-1.154} \times (\text{age in years})^{-0.203}$$

*Use 175 if using a standardized SCr assay.
†For SCr in SI units (μmol/L), divide by 88.4.
For African Americans, multiply the result by 1.212
For females, multiply the result by 0.742
An online calculator is available at www.kidney.org.

This equation is superior to that of Cockroft and Gault in elders and the obese. Adjustment for body surface area is only needed in very small or very large individuals. It must be remembered that all current drug dosage regimen adjustments for impaired renal function are based on CrCl as estimated using the Cockroft and Gault (or similar) equations. The utility of the MDRD equation in this area awaits further study.

Numerous medications are primarily renally excreted and/or have renally excreted active metabolites. Evidence exists of age-related reductions in the total body clearances of drugs that are primarily renally cleared (Table 23-4). The risk of adverse clinical consequences is likely increased for those drugs with narrow therapeutic margins (e.g., digoxin, aminoglycosides, chemotherapeutics). Dosage adjustment for renal impairment is easily accomplished once CrCl has been estimated. In fact, there are even guidelines available for dosage adjustment of cancer chemotherapeutic agents in elders with cancer.[52]

Table 23-4. Drugs Whose Renal Elimination Is Impaired With Advancing Age

ACEI	Furosemide
Acetazolamide	Lithium
Amantadine	Metformin
Aminoglycosides	Procainamide/NAPA
Chlorpropamide	Ranitidine
Cimetidine	Vancomycin
Digoxin	

ACEI, angiotensin-converting enzyme inhibitor; *NAPA,* N-acetylprocainamide.

Table 23-5. Drugs Whose Sensitivity Is Altered With Advancing Age

β-Agonists (↓)	H_1-antihistamines (↑)
β-Blockers (↓)	Metoclopramide (↑)
Benzodiazepines (↑)	Neuroleptics (↑)
Calcium antagonists (↓↑)	Opioids (↑)
Dopaminergic agents (↑)	Warfarin (↑)
Furosemide (↓)	Vaccines (↓)

↑ = increased; ↓ = decreased.

ALTERED PHARMACODYNAMICS

In contrast to the relationship of aging to altered pharmacokinetics, fewer data are available investigating the effect of aging on pharmacodynamics (drug response). Theoretically, altered pharmacodynamics could be due to two mechanisms: (1) altered sensitivity owing to changes in receptor number or affinity or changes in postreceptor response, and (2) age-related impairment of physiologic and homeostatic mechanisms.[53] This section reviews altered responses of elderly people to medications mediated by these two mechanisms.

Altered sensitivity

Table 23-5 lists those medications for which there are reasonable data documenting altered drug sensitivity in elderly people. Firm evidence exists that elders are less responsive to β-blockers and β-agonists.[54,55] There is a diminished maximal response to furosemide.[53] Firm evidence also exists that elders are more sensitive to the effects of benzodiazepines. Using psychomotor testing, this has been established for nitrazepam, temazepam, midazolam, loprazolam, and diazepam.[53,56] Enhanced sensitivity has also been demonstrated for opioids, metoclopramide, dopamine agonists, levodopa, and traditional neuroleptics.[53] It is well established that elderly people have enhanced sensitivity to the effects of oral anticoagulants. The underlying mechanism of this effect is unknown.[57] There is evidence for both enhanced and reduced sensitivity to calcium-channel blockers in elders measured as blood pressure response or electrocardiographic (P-R interval) response.[53,56]

Alterations in physiologic and homeostatic mechanisms

Physiologic and homeostatic impairments in elderly people that may affect drug response include autonomic nervous system dysfunction (orthostasis, bowel/bladder dysfunction), impaired thermoregulation, reduced nutrient intake, reduced cognitive function reserve, impaired postural stability, glucose intolerance, and immunosenescence.[58–64] The loss of efficiency of homeostatic mechanisms puts elders at risk of symptomatic orthostasis/falls (with antihypertensives, traditional neuroleptics, tricyclic antidepressants), urinary retention and constipation (with drugs with anticholinergic properties), falls and delirium (with virtually every sedating drug), and accidental hypothermia or heatstroke (with neuroleptics).

DRUG INTERACTIONS

Drug-drug interactions can be defined as the effect that the administration of one drug has on another drug.[65] The two major types of drug-drug interactions include pharmacokinetic interactions, wherein drug absorption, distribution, metabolism, and excretion are affected and pharmacodynamic interactions, wherein pharmacologic effect is altered. Drugs may also interact with food, nutritional status, herbal products, alcohol, and preexisting diseases.[66–69]

Table 23-6. Selected Cytochrome P450 Inducers and Inhibitors by Isoenzyme

CYP1A2	CYP2C	CYP2D6	CYP3A4
Inducers	**Inducers**	**Inducers**	**Inducers**
Char-broiled beef	Rifampin	None known	Carbamazepine
Cruciferous vegetables			Phenytoin
Omeprazole			Rifampin
Smoking			St. John's wort
Inhibitors	**Inhibitors**	**Inhibitors**	**Inhibitors**
Cimetidine	Amiodarone	Fluoxetine	Erythromycin
Ciprofloxacin	Fluconazole	Paroxetine	Ketoconazole
Fluvoxamine	Fluvastatin	Quinidine	Nefazodone
		Ritonavir	

Pharmacokinetic interactions

Increased drug bioavailability may be seen with the concurrent ingestion of grapefruit juice owing to its inhibitory effect on CYP450 isoenzyme 3A4-mediated first-pass metabolism in the gut wall and liver. This may result in exaggerated pharmacologic effects.[70] Decreased bioavailability can be seen when phenytoin is administered with enteral feedings.[71] Multivalent cations (e.g., antacids, sucralfate, iron, calcium supplements) can reduce the bioavailability of tetracycline and quinolone antimicrobials.[72]

Drug interactions involving drug distribution are primarily related to altered plasma protein binding. Although a number of drugs may displace other drugs from plasma protein binding sites, especially acids such as salicylate, valproic acid, and phenytoin, this type of drug interaction is rarely clinically significant.

Drug interactions most likely to be clinically significant are those that involve the inhibition or induction of metabolism of narrow therapeutic margin drugs.[73] Table 23-6 illustrates selected CYP450 enzyme inducers and inhibitors. It does not appear that young and elderly individuals differ in the magnitude of hepatic enzyme inhibition after exposure to drugs such as cimetidine, macrolide antimicrobials (e.g., erythromycin, clarithromycin), quinidine, and ciprofloxacin.[72,74] However, there is controversy regarding the effect of hepatic enzyme inducers in young versus elderly individuals, with some studies demonstrating no difference between the age groups, whereas others suggest that elders do not

Table 23-7. Most Common Herbal-Drug Interactions[81]

Interacting Drug	Herbs (Vernacular Names)	Description of the Effect of Herbs on Drug Kinetics/Activity
Warfarin	St John's wort, ginseng	↓ INR
	Garlic, danshen, gingko, devil's claw, dong quai, papaya, glucosamine	↑ INR
	Garlic, ginseng, gingko, ginger, feverfew	↑ bleeding time
ASA, NSAIDs, dipyridamole, clopidogrel/ticlopidine	Gingko	↑ bleeding time
Amitriptyline	St. John's wort	↓ drug concentration
Warfarin		
Theophylline		
Simvastatin		
Alprazolam		
Verapamil		
Digoxin		
Iron		
Ethanol	Ginseng	
Phenytoin	Shank hapusphi	
Phenytoin	Gingko	
Valproate		
Iron	Feverfew	
	Camomile	
Metformin	Guar gum	
Glibenclamide		
Digoxin		
Lithium	Psyllium	
ASA	Tamarind	↑ drug concentration
Nifedipine	Gingko	
Sertraline	St. John's wort	Serotonin syndrome (mild)
Paroxetine		
Trazodone		
Nefazodone		
Chlorpropamide	Garlic	↓ glucose concentrations
Antidiabetic drugs	Fenugreek	
MAOIs	Ginseng	Manic-like symptoms, headache, tremors
Thiazides	Gingko	↓ drug effect
	Dandelion	
	Uva-ursi	
Thyroxine	Horseradish	
	Kelp	
Phenytoin	Shank hapusphi	
Warfarin	Gingko	↑ drug effect
ASA		
NSAIDs		
Dipyridamole		
Clopidogrel/ticlopidine		
Benzodiazepines	Kava	
Barbiturates		
Opioids		
Ethanol		
Barbiturates	Valerian	
Other CNS depressants		
Digoxin	Hawthorne	
Thiazides	Gossypol	
Levodopa	Gingko	↑ "off" periods in Parkinson disease
Anabolic steroids	Echinacea	↑ Hepatotoxicity risk
Amiodarone		
Methotrexate		
Ketoconazole		
Caffeine	Ma huang	Hypertension, insomnia, tachycardia, nervousness, tremor, headache, seizures, ↑ MI/stroke risk
Stimulants		
Decongestants		
Tricylic antidepressants	Yohimbine	Hypertension
Heparin	Fenugreek	↑ bleeding risk
Clopidogrel/ticlopidine		
Warfarin		

Abbreviations: ↓ = decreased; ↑ = increased; *INR*, international normalized ratio (of prothrombin time); *ASA*, aspirin; *NSAID*, nonsteroidal anti-inflammatory drug; *MAOI*, nonselective monoamine oxidase inhibitor; *CNS*, central nervous system; *MI*, myocardial infarction.

Table 23-8. Drug-Disease Interactions to Avoid in the Elderly as Defined by Explicit Criteria by Canadian and U.S. Consensus Panels[82,83]

Drug or Drug Class	Disease
α-Agonist decongestants	Benign prostatic hypertrophy, insomnia, hypertension
α-Blockers	Stress incontinence
Anticholinergic antihistamines	Benign prostatic hypertrophy, stress incontinence, cognitive impairment, constipation
Anticholinergic tricylic antidepressants	Benign prostatic hypertrophy, stress incontinence, cognitive impairment, constipation, syncope/falls, arrhythmias, heart block, postural hypotension, glaucoma
Aspirin (>325 mg/day)	Peptic ulcer, blood clotting disorders or while taking anticoagulants
Barbiturates	Cognitive impairment
Benzodiazepines, long half-life	Chronic obstructive pulmonary disease, stress incontinence, depression, falls
Benzodiazepines, short-intermediate half-life	Syncope/falls
Bupropion	Seizures
Calcium-channel blockers	Heart failure, constipation
Chlorpromazine	Postural hypotension, seizures
Clopidogrel	Blood clotting disorders or while taking anticoagulants
Clozapine	Seizures
CNS stimulants	Hypertension, anorexia, malnutrition, cognitive impairment, insomnia
Dipyridamole	Blood clotting disorders or while taking anticoagulants
Disopyramide	Heart failure
Gastrointestinal, genitourinary antispasmodics	Benign prostatic hypertrophy, stress incontinence, cognitive impairment, constipation
Methylphenidate	Insomnia
Metoclopramide	Parkinson's disease
Monoamine oxidase inhibitors	Insomnia
Neuroleptics, traditional	Parkinson's disease
Nonsteroidal anti-inflammatory drugs	Chronic renal failure, heart failure, hypertension, peptic ulcer*
Olanzapine	Obesity
Propranolol	Chronic obstructive pulmonary disease
Pseudoephedrine, phenylephrine	Hypertension, benign prostatic hypertrophy, insomnia
Skeletal muscle relaxants	Benign prostatic hypertrophy, cognitive impairment
Tacrine	Parkinson's disease
Theophylline	Insomnia
Thiazide diuretics	Gout
Thioridazine	Seizures
Thiothixene	Seizures
Ticlopidine	Blood clotting disorders or while taking anticoagulants
Tolterodine	Benign prostatic hypertrophy

*Except celecoxib (in absence of ASA).

respond as well to enzyme induction.[45,75–77] It may be that these effects are substrate- and/or inducer-specific.

Inhibition of renal clearance of one drug by another drug can also result in clinically significant effects.[78] Many of these drug-drug interactions involve competitive inhibition of tubular secretion of anionic or cationic drugs. Cationic agents include amiodarone, cimetidine, digoxin, procainamide, quinidine, ranitidine, trimethoprim, and verapamil. Anionic agents include cephalosporins, indomethacin, methotrexate, penicillins, probenecid, salicylates, and thiazides.

Drug interactions with herbal and over-the-counter (OTC) products are frequently overlooked. In one series, 52% of all moderate- or high-risk interactions occurred between prescription drugs and herbal and/or OTC products.[79] The interaction potential of herbal products is enhanced because of frequent contamination with heavy metals and adulteration with prescription drugs (e.g., NSAIDs, corticosteroids, psychotherapeutics, and phosphodiesterase-5 inhibitors such as sildenafil).[80] Table 23-7 illustrates the most common herbal-drug interactions.[80,81]

Pharmacodynamic interactions

Some drugs may alter the response of another drug and produce adverse effects. A good example of this is the synergistic effect of taking more than one anticholinergic agent concurrently, which can result in delirium, urinary retention, constipation, and other problems.[65] Other examples include additive bradycardia when β-blockers are administered concurrently with verapamil or diltiazem, additive hypotension when several antihypertensives are administered concurrently, and sedation/falls when several CNS depressants (e.g., benzodiazepines, sedative-hypnotics, antidepressants, neuroleptics) are administered concurrently.

Drug-disease interactions

Drug interactions can also be considered in a broader sense when they involve medications that can affect and can be affected by disease states. Elderly people are at higher risk for adverse outcomes with drug-disease state interactions owing to alterations in homeostatic mechanisms, diminished physiologic reserve, and multiple comorbidities. Recently, a national expert panel from Canada and another from the United States developed a list of potentially clinically important drug-disease state interactions (Table 23-8).[82,83] Unfortunately, explicit quality indicators (such as the Beers list[83]) cannot be easily transferred from one country to another, or even from one setting to another, without being modified and revalidated because of contextual differences.[84]

SUMMARY

Elderly people consume a disproportionate share of medications. Factors enhancing medication use include the concurrent presence of multiple diseases, female gender, increasing level of care, and increasing age. Other factors that probably influence drug use in elderly people include provider prescribing behaviors, cultural milieu, psychosocial issues (i.e., living alone, anxiety, depression), and direct-to-consumer advertising by the pharmaceutical industry.

The most common classes of medications in the elderly include cardiovascular, gastrointestinal, central nervous system, and analgesic agents. Many studies have documented that the aging process alters drug disposition and response. Changes in body composition with aging result in an altered volume of distribution for many drugs. Age-related changes in plasma protein binding may alter the relationship of unbound and total plasma drug concentrations.

Phase I hepatic metabolism is often reduced in older patients, resulting in reduced clearance and increased terminal disposition half-life for many commonly used drugs. Age-related decline in renal function decreases clearance and increases the terminal disposition half-life of renally eliminated drugs. Pharmacodynamic studies indicate that elderly individuals tend to be more sensitive to the effects of benzodiazepines, opioids, dopamine-receptor antagonists, and warfarin. Drug-drug and drug-disease interactions may also impact elders' well-being.

Knowledge of this information is important for achieving the maximal benefits of medications in the elderly while minimizing or preventing drug-related problems.

KEY POINTS

Pharmacology of Aging

- The elderly are avid consumers of medications.
- Age-related alterations in drug pharmacokinetics are most pronounced in terms of the decline in the hepatic metabolism and renal elimination of certain drugs.
- Age-related alterations in drug pharmacodynamics are understudied, but older adults appear to be more sensitive to the effects of benzodiazepines, opioids, dopamine-receptor antagonists, and warfarin.
- Drug-drug and drug-disease interactions are common in older adults and may have a negative impact on health-related quality of life.

For a complete list of references, please visit online only at www.expertconsult.com

CHAPTER 24

Antiaging Medicine

John E. Morley
Ligia J. Dominguez
Mario Barbagallo

Attempts to reverse the aging process stretch back to the time when Adam and Eve were expelled from the Garden of Eden. Since then, both wise sages and charlatans have made numerous pronouncements on what the populace should do to extend their lifespan. In most cases this has required those who wish to benefit to pay exorbitant sums of money to those who have developed the magical elixir of longevity. This has led to the concept that antiaging medicine is a scam.

On the other hand, we have seen a remarkable extension in longevity over the last century. In the United States, at the start of the twentieth century half of the population was dead by 50 years of age, whereas by the dawn of the twenty-first century half of females lived to over 80 years of age. These dramatic changes were brought about by public health measures such as improved sanitation, a greatly improved and available food supply, the introduction of antibiotics, vaccinations, improved care of pregnant women and the birthing process, enhanced surgical techniques, and to a lesser extent a variety of new medications introduced in the second half of the twentieth century. One needs also to give credit to the improved work environment and the decrease in excessive manual labor.

The secret to longevity appears often to be following a healthy lifestyle and avoiding excesses. In the thirteenth century, Friar Roger Bacon in England wrote a best-selling antiaging book.[1] His secrets to longevity were:

- A controlled diet
- Proper rest
- Exercise
- Moderation in lifestyle
- Good hygiene
- Inhaling the breath of a young virgin

Clearly the first five recommendations, although relatively boring, remain today a reasonable approach to prolonging life and improving its quality. However, it was "the breath of a young virgin" that made the book popular. Modern antiaging books tend to follow this same formula with a set of sensible advice mixed in with the modern "breath of a virgin." These similarly ridiculous suggestions range the gamut from growth hormone, through herbs and megavitamins, to infusions to remove calcium from arteries.

George Valiant, a Harvard psychiatrist, studies inner city persons and Harvard graduates from their mid-50s.[2] His studies suggest that aging successfully occurred in those individuals who:

- Got some exercise
- Did not smoke
- Managed crises well
- Did not abuse alcohol
- Enjoyed a stable marriage
- Were not obese (although this applied only to inner city folk)

Recently, the Norfolk-EPIC study found that persons who followed four simple lifestyle habits were physiologically 14 years younger than those who did none of them.[3] The four magical ingredients that produced this greatly improved outcome were:

- Not smoking
- Getting some exercise
- Eating five helpings of fruit and vegetables each day
- Drinking 1 to 14 glasses of alcohol per week

As long-lived populations tend to come from places such as Japan, Macau, and Hong Kong, where there is a high preponderance of fish in the diet, it is most probably reasonable to suggest that fatty fish intake, rich in eicosahexanoic and docosahexaenoic acid, should be included in a diet of a person who wishes to live for a long time.[4]

A BRIEF HISTORY OF ANTIAGING MEDICINE

In ancient Egypt the olive leaf was used to improve beauty and extend life.[5] This is paralleled in the twenty-first century by the recognition that the Mediterranean diet is associated with longer and healthier lives. Ayurvedic medicine in India developed specific diets, lifestyle practices, and herbs that would extend life.

The search for the Fountain of Youth was first made famous by Ponce de Leon, the Governor of Puerto Rico, who went searching for Bimini, where it was believed that there was a fountain of youth. Instead he discovered Florida, a modern day haven for retirees in the United States. In 1933, in a fictitious book called "Lost Horizon," James Hilton created a paradise where no one aged, called Shangri-la. So riveting was this concept for the public that a number of expeditions set out to try and find this paradise in the Himalayan Mountains. Nobel Prize winner Elie Metchnikoff mistakenly believed that Bulgarians lived extremely long lives and this was due to yogurt. This created an antiaging cult based on eating yogurt.

The modern quasi-scientific approach to antiaging medicine was expressed in the book *Life Extension* by Durk Pearson and Sandy Shaw, published in 1982.[6] In an 858-page volume they provided detailed accounts of animal experiments that increased longevity, claiming that their book was "for anyone, regardless of age, who seeks greater youthfulness—*starting right now*." This book opened the door to multiple others where snippets of animal science were fed to the public, suggesting that these findings should be used by humans who wished to live a long life.

The American Academy of Anti-Aging Medicine (A4M) was founded in 1992 by Drs Ronald Klatz and Robert Goldman. Its avowed purpose is to advance "technology to detect, prevent and treat aging related disease and promote research into methods to retard and optimize the human aging process." It provides a number of certifications for physicians in antiaging medicine. It claims to have more than 20,000 members from more than 100 countries (www.worldhealth.net;

accessed Sept. 28, 2008). It produces the *International Journal of Anti-Aging Medicine*.

The Life Extension Foundation is based in Florida and produces the monthly magazine, *Life Extension*. Its readership is thought to be in the neighborhood of 350,000. It was founded by Saul Kent in 1980. It also sells dietary supplements by mail order.

Two more mainstream physicians whose books have promoted antiaging philosophies are Andrew Weil and Deepak Chopra.

Aubrey De Grey, a Cambridge-educated scientist, has developed a theory called "Strategies for Engineered Negligible Senescence." He has been extraordinarily successful at promoting his theories to the lay public. He suggests that there are seven types of aging damage, which are readily open to treatment.

- Cancer mutations
- Mitochondrial mutations
- Intracellular junk
- Extracellular junk
- Cell loss
- Cell senescence
- Extracellular cross-links

The De Grey SENS proposal has been widely criticized by gerontologists: "Each one of the specific proposals that comprise the SENS agenda is, at our present stage of ignorance, exceptionally optimistic," and it "will take decades of hard work, if (these proposals) ever prove to be useful."[7] His approach is a classic example of the quasi-scientific methods that have been used to create antiaging literature.

The most extensive criticism of the modern antiaging medicine came in 2002 from Olshansky, Hayflick, and Carnes.[8] The article stated, "no currently marketed intervention has yet been proved to slow, stop or reverse human aging.... The entrepreneurs, physicians and other health care practitioners who make these claims are taking advantage of consumers who cannot easily distinguish between the hype and reality of interventions designed to influence the aging process and age-related diseases."

Caloric restriction

In 1934, Mary Crowell and Clive McKay at Cornell University published a series of experiments showing that limiting the food intake of laboratory rats (dietary restriction) resulted in prolongation of their lives.[9] Subsequently, studies in some, but not all species, have shown that caloric restriction results in a prolongation of lives. Recent studies have suggested that caloric restriction needs to be started in younger animals and it fails to prolong life in older animals.[10]

Studies in monkeys have suggested that dietary restriction improves the metabolic profile (glucose, cholesterol) in these animals[11] and may attenuate Alzheimer's-like amyloid changes in their brains.[12] However, these animals also show a loss of bone and an increased propensity to develop hip fractures.

Numerous theories exist as to why caloric restriction may enhance longevity. The hormesis theory of caloric restriction suggests that caloric restriction represents a low level of stress, which allows the animal to develop enhanced defenses that slow the aging process. It has also been suggested that caloric restriction reduces oxidative damage, enhances insulin sensitivity, and decreases tissue glycation. The "silent information regulator" (Sir) gene is upregulated by caloric restriction in yeast and in mammals. However, the role of Sir genes in longevity is controversial.

The Caloric Restriction Society was founded in 1984 by Ray and Lisa Walford and Brian Delaney. Members of this society practice caloric restriction to varying degrees. Studies of members of this society suggest that they have lower blood pressure, glucose, and cholesterol values.[13] The National Institutes of Health have funded a number of short-term studies to determine the utility of caloric restriction in middle-aged persons. The enthusiasm for caloric restriction in older persons has been tempered by multiple studies in persons over 60 years of age showing that weight loss is associated with increased institutionalization, increased mortality, and increased hip fracture.[14]

At present, there are a number of caloric-restriction diets that are advertised to the public as a method for life prolongation. The CRON-diet (Caloric Restriction with Optimal Nutrition) was developed by Roy Walford and Brian Delaney. It was based on the research conducted in the Biosphere. In general this diet recommends a 20% caloric restriction based on determining one's basal metabolic rate. The Okinawa diet is a low calorie, nutrient-rich diet based on the original diet of the people living on the Japanese island of Okinawa (Ryukyu Islands). Its popularity is based on the large number of centenarians who used to live in the Ojime Village on Okinawa. The diet is calorie restricted compared with the Japanese diet. It predominantly consists of vegetables (especially sweet potatoes), a half a serving of fish per day, legumes, and soy. It is low in meat, eggs, and dairy products. The New Longevity Diet by Henry Mallek represents a popularization of other longevity diets. It needs to be recognized that none of these diets has been proven to extend longevity. It is interesting to note that Roy Walford, a major proponent of dietary restriction, died at 79 years of age of amyotrophic lateral sclerosis. Animal studies have suggested that caloric restriction is especially bad for animals with amyotrophic lateral sclerosis.

Exercise

Exercise in moderation appears to be a cornerstone of longevity. Mice with an excess of phosphoenolpyruvate carboxykinase (PEPCK-C) in their skeletal muscle are more active than their controls and can run for 5 km at a speed of 20 m/min compared with 0.2 km for control mice.[15] These mice live longer than controls and females remain reproductively active until 35 months of age.

Observational studies in humans have strongly suggested that those who are physically active live longer. In a study of 70- to 80-year-olds, those with higher total energy expenditure lived longer than those with less energy expenditure.[16] A major factor in enhancing energy expenditure was stair climbing.

Fries found that older runners compared with sedentary older persons tended to become disabled 13 years later.[17] The LIFE Pilot study showed that a structured physical activity program significantly improved functional performance. Walking speed is associated with decreased disability. Physical activity is associated with decreased dysphoria. Persons aged 50 years of age who exercise regularly are less liable to develop Alzheimer's disease as they age.[19] Regular physical activity reduces the rate of deterioration in persons with dementia.[20]

THE HORMONAL FOUNTAIN OF YOUTH

Since the publication of Wilson's "Feminine Forever" in the 1950s, touting the role of estrogen to maintain youth, there has been increasing interest in the antiaging effects of hormones.[5] Previously, toward the end of the nineteenth century, Brown-Séquard had suggested a testicular extract produced remarkable antiaging effects. It is unlikely that his extract had any testosterone, demonstrating the powerful effect of the placebo. This led to a large number of rich men in Europe and the United States receiving monkey testicular implants, which were claimed to rejuvenate them. Brinkley in the United States pioneered a series of "goat gland" extracts, which were equally ineffective but made him a rich man. Subsequently, almost every hormone has been touted to produce antiaging effects. In general it can be said that the more enthusiasm that the lay public has expressed in these hormones, the less likely they are to be effective.

25(OH) vitamin D levels decline with aging.[21] Low levels of vitamin D have been associated with increased mortality.[22] In persons with 25(OH) vitamin D levels below 30 ng/mL, replacement has been demonstrated to enhance function, decrease falls, and decrease hip fracture.[23] Vitamin D replacement of more than 625 IU per day in a meta-analysis decreased mortality.[24] It is now generally accepted that older persons should either get regular skin exposure (15 to 30 min/day) without sun block or they should take 800 to 1000 IU/day. All persons over 70 years of age should have their 25(OH) vitamin D levels measured at least yearly (preferably in winter) because they may need higher doses of vitamin D to raise their level above 30 ng/ml.

Studies on men with low testosterone have shown conflicting results concerning whether or not low testosterone is associated with an increased mortality rate (Table 24-1).[25–29] Overall, testosterone should be considered a quality of life drug and not a life extension drug. The major effects of testosterone are to enhance libido and sexual function.[30] Testosterone also increases muscle and bone mass and muscle strength in hypogonadal males.[31] No studies have evaluated its effect on hip fracture. Testosterone also increases visuospatial cognition.[32] Recent studies have suggested that testosterone may be cardioprotective.[33] Despite multiple potential positive effects of testosterone, recommendations for its use in older males as set out by the International Society for the Study of the Aging Male are that it should only be given to males who have symptoms and are biochemically hypogonadal.[34] Either the Aging Male Survey or the Saint Louis University Androgen Deficiency in the Aging Male [ADAM] questionnaire[36] (Table 24-2) can be used to screen for symptoms.

Testosterone levels decline rapidly in females between 20 to 45 years of age.[37] The reason for this rapid decline is uncertain. Recent studies have suggested that testosterone replacement in females may improve libido to a small extent.[38]

The role of estrogen replacement in females following the menopause was muddied by the Women's Health Initiative.[39,40] It appears clear that in women over 60 years of age, estrogen replacement will increase cardiovascular disease and mortality. This is similar to the finding of the HERS study.[41] It remains unclear whether there is a place for estrogen at the time of menopause. In women with premature menopause, estrogen replacement appears to be reasonable until the age of 52 years. Women with menopause between the ages of 45 to 55 may benefit from estrogen replacement in low doses, both to treat symptoms and delay the loss of bone. Its effect at this time on cardiovascular disease is uncertain, but some authorities believe it may be cardioprotective at this time period ("the critical period hypothesis"). In women with normal menopause, estrogen should most probably not be used for more than 5 years. Similar caveats exist for the use of progesterone and, when necessary to use, one should consider a progestagen with aldosterone antagonistic properties.

Dan Rudman and his colleagues[42] created a craze for growth hormone replacement as a "fountain of youth" by their publication in the *New England Journal of Medicine*. Their paper citing the negative effects of growth hormone in older males was published later in *Clinical Endocrinology* and has been generally ignored by antiaging pundits.[43] A meta-analysis published in 2007 could find no positive effects of growth hormone in older persons.[44] Studies with ghrelin agonists in older persons have been equally disappointing. Ghrelin is a peptide hormone released from the fundus of the stomach that increases appetite, releases growth hormone, and enhances memory.[45] A Google search for "growth hormone and aging" resulted in 1,200,000 citations. These included a large number of sponsored links selling growth hormone or physicians who prescribe it. These advertisements included statements such as "Using growth hormone combats the ravages of aging," "Can aging be reversed," and "Growth Hormone Releaser: Fight the Aging Process Effectively" (Accessed Sept. 28, 2008).

Table 24-1. Does Low Testosterone Predict Death?

Author, Year	Population	Predicts Death
Morley et al, 1996[25]	14-yr follow-up of healthy men in New Mexico	No
Shores et al, 2006[26]	Veteran population, 8-yr follow-up	Yes
Arajo et al, 2007[27]	Massachusetts Male Aging Study	No
Khaw et al, 2007[29]	Europe	Yes
Laughlin et al, 2008[28]	Rancho Bernardo 11.8-yr follow-up	Yes

Table 24-2. The Androgen Deficiency in the Aging Male [ADAM] Questionnaire

A positive answer represents yes to 1 or 7 or any 3 other questions.

[Circle one]

Yes	No	1. *Do you have a decrease in libido (sex drive)?*
Yes	No	2. *Do you have a lack of energy?*
Yes	No	3. *Do you have a decrease in strength and/or endurance?*
Yes	No	4. *Have you lost height?*
Yes	No	5. *Have you noticed a decreased enjoyment of life?*
Yes	No	6. *Are you sad and/or grumpy?*
Yes	No	7. *Are your erections less strong?*
Yes	No	8. *Have you noticed a recent deterioration in your ability to play sports?*
Yes	No	9. *Are you falling asleep after dinner?*
Yes	No	10. *Has there been a recent deterioration in your work performance?*

Dehydroepiandrosterone (DHEA) and its sulfate levels fall dramatically with aging.[46] This has resulted in multiple claims that DHEA can rejuvenate older persons. However, large well-controlled studies have failed to show any effects of DHEA on aging.[47] The Google search for "DHEA and Aging" yielded 758,000 citations. A quotation from one of these sites says: "DHEA stands out as a multitalented star with amazing ways..."

On the web, pregnenolone has been called "the feel-good hormone" or "the mother hormone." Our studies in mice have shown that pregnenolone is a potent memory enhancer.[48] However, the ability to demonstrate similar effects in humans has been largely negative; at present there is no evidence that in humans pregnenolone is a memory enhancer or an antiaging hormone.[49]

Melatonin, a hormone that is produced by the pineal gland, also declines with aging. It has antioxidant properties and as such has been touted as an antiaging hormone and a soporific. Overall, it appears to have minimal effects.

Marcus Tullius Cicero said "Old age must be resisted and its deficiencies restored." With the exception of vitamin D, there is little evidence that hormone replacement should be used in an attempt to reverse the aging process. Despite this it would appear that unscrupulous charlatans will continue to prescribe and supply them inappropriately and the aging populace will hungrily devour them with the hope of staying young forever.

ANTIOXIDANTS AND AGING

Multiple animal studies have shown a role for oxidative stress in aging.[50] Oxidative damage has also been implicated in the pathogenesis of age-related diseases, such as atherosclerosis and Alzheimer's disease. It is clear that consumption of fruits and vegetables that are rich in antioxidants appear to prevent disease. However, there is no evidence that persons taking vitamin supplements have a longer life than those who do not take supplements. Studies with vitamin E and cardiovascular disease in humans have found that supplementation either has no effect or is harmful.[51] Similarly, effects of vitamin E on cancer have suggested mixed results. Vitamin E had minimal effects on people with Alzheimer's disease.

β-carotene in the ATBC trial resulted in an increase in lung, prostate, and stomach cancer.[52] The CARET study also resulted in an increase in lung cancer death in people previously exposed to asbestos.[53] No positive effects of β-carotene on cardiovascular disease have been found in a number of studies.[54]

Similarly, vitamin C has been shown to have minimal beneficial effects.

α-Lipoic acid is a powerful antioxidant. It has been shown to be useful in the treatment of diabetic neuropathy.[55] It has reversed memory disturbances in SAMP8 mice, a partial model of Alzheimer's disease.[56] However, our unpublished studies in mice have shown that it increased mortality rate.

Overall, human studies do not support the use of antioxidant vitamin supplementation. The one exception may be the use of high-dose multivitamins in age-related macular degeneration. Based on the available data, high-dose vitamin supplementation cannot be considered to be benign.

Table 24-3. Cosmetic Antiaging Products

Product	Action	Side Effects
Sunscreens with a sun protection factor [SPF] greater than 15	Decrease actinic keratosis and squamous cell carcinoma	Allergic reactions occur in 1 in 5 persons
α- and β-hydroxyl acids	Exfoliants that decrease roughness and some pigmentation	Irritation of skin
Retinoids (tretinoin and tazarotene)	Decrease pigmentation, wrinkling, and roughness	Irritation of skin
Fluorouracil cream	Actinic keratosis	Irritation of skin
Laser therapy	Wrinkles, pigmentation, telangiectasia	Scarring, hypopigmentation, bruising
Dermabrasion	Wrinkles, actinic keratoses	Scarring, pain, infection
Skin fillers (collagen and hyaluronic acid)	Wrinkles	Pain, allergic reactions
Botox	Wrinkles	Bruising, ptosis, headaches

Photoaging

Aging of skin occurs because of environmental damage, which interacts with chronologic aging.[57] Photoaging occurs as a result of ultraviolet light exposure. With the aging of the population there has been an explosion of medication, cosmetics, and dermatologic procedures that attempt to reverse the aging process (Table 24-3). These agents are used to remove or prevent wrinkles, rough skin, telangiectasia, actinic keratosis, brown spots, and benign neoplasia. In 2002 more than $13 billion was spent on 5 million cosmetic procedures and more than 1 million "plastic" surgery procedures. Among relatively common antiaging plastic surgery procedures are rhytidectomy ("face-lift"), blepharoplasty, abdominoplasty ("tummy tuck"), and lipectomy or liposuction. These procedures are costly and pander to the vanity of our new aging population.

CONCLUSION

Amazing breakthroughs in the understanding of the aging process are occurring almost daily in cellular and animal models. Gerontologists, like Tantalus, are consistently being tempted to instantly apply these findings in humans before appropriate controlled trials are carried out. As history has shown, this is a dangerous precedent. Treatments that are highly effective in animals can be highly toxic in humans. The geriatrician plays an important role in being able to educate older persons regarding the positives and negatives of antiaging medicines.

Two areas that have the potential to totally change the antiaging field are stem cells and computers. Studies with stem cells carrying muscle IGF-1 in rodents have shown that they can reverse muscle loss in old animals.[58] The potential for stem cells to rejuvenate a variety of tissues is enormous but its application to humans is in its infancy.

We are beginning to see computer-enhanced technology used to reverse age-related deficits. Examples are cochlear implants and retinal computer chips. As computer technology advances, Kurzweil has suggested that hippocampal computer chips could be used to treat Alzheimer's disease.

Today's science fiction may well represent tomorrow's antiaging technology. The rapid advances in robotic prosthesis and exoskeletons will further enhance the ability of older persons to function well in late life.

Antiaging medicine raises a number of ethical issues. For instance, in a society of limited resources, is extending the life of the older population appropriate? Is extending life without improved quality appropriate? What if life extension was associated with cognitive impairment? How long is it appropriate to extend life: for 5 years, 10 years, 20 years, 50 years, or 100 years? There are no simple answers to any of these questions and the answers depend not only on scientific and philosophical areas, but also on religious views and fiscal realities.

Every year changes in medical knowledge are leading to increased longevity and improved quality of life. It needs to be recognized that not all advances in mainstream medicine have positive effects, but overall medical advances are at present the strongest antiaging medicine. In contrast the aging public continues to spend billions of dollars on antiaging potions of little proven value. Geriatricians will continue to be at the forefront of educators on how to age successfully.

KEY POINTS
Antiaging Medicine

- The factors best demonstrated to delay aging are fruit and vegetables, exercise, not smoking, drinking one or two glasses of alcohol daily, and fish consumption.
- Vitamin D replacement, in persons with low 25[OH] vitamin D levels, decreases hip fractures, improves muscle strength, enhances function, and decreases mortality.
- Antiaging medicine has been hijacked by charlatans who promote unproven or dangerous remedies to a naïve aging public.
- Too often animal studies that produce longevity are directly applied to humans before appropriate clinical trials have been carried out.
- There is no evidence that hormones or megadoses of vitamins prolong life.
- Numerous products of varying quality are available to slow photoaging and remove skin blemishes.

For a complete list of references, please visit online only at www.expertconsult.com

CHAPTER 25

The Neurobiology of Aging: Free Radical Stress and Metabolic Pathways

Tomohiro Nakamura
Malene Hansen
Sean M. Oldham
Stuart A. Lipton

Environmental stressors and several genetic pathways play complex and crucial roles in the neurobiology and control of aging. This chapter will summarize current knowledge on these two specific research areas divided into two sections: one on free radical stressors and the other on genetic control of metabolic pathways.

SECTION I: NITROSATIVE AND OXIDATIVE STRESS IN THE NEUROBIOLOGY OF AGING

Aging represents a major risk factor for neurodegenerative diseases, such as Parkinson's disease (PD); Alzheimer's disease (AD); amyotrophic lateral sclerosis (ALS); and polyglutamine (polyQ) diseases, such as Huntington's disease, glaucoma, human immunodeficiency virus-associated dementia, multiple sclerosis, and ischemic brain injury, to name but a few.[1–5] Although many intracellular and extracellular molecules may participate in neuronal injury and loss, accumulation of nitrosative and oxidative stress, because of the excessive generation of nitric oxide (NO) and reactive oxygen species (ROS), appears to be a potential factor contributing to neuronal cell damage and death.[6,7] A well-established model for NO production entails a central role of the *N*-methyl-D-aspartate (NMDA)-type glutamate receptors in nervous system. Excessive activation of NMDA receptors drives Ca^{2+} influx, which in turn activates neuronal NO synthase (nNOS) and the generation of ROS[8,9] (Figure 25-1). Accumulating evidence suggests that NO can mediate both protective and neurotoxic effects by reacting with cysteine residues of target proteins to form S-nitrosothiols (SNOs), a process termed S-nitrosylation because of its effects on the chemical biology of protein function. Importantly, normal mitochondrial respiration may also generate free radicals, principally ROS, and one such molecule, superoxide anion ($O_2^{\cdot -}$), reacts rapidly with free radical NO to form the very toxic product peroxynitrite ($ONOO^-$)[10,11] (Figure 25-2).

An additional feature of most neurodegenerative diseases is accumulation of misfolded and/or aggregated proteins.[12–15] These protein aggregates can be cytosolic, nuclear, or extracellular. Importantly, protein aggregation can result from either (1) a mutation in the disease-related gene encoding the protein, or (2) posttranslational changes to the protein engendered by nitrosative/oxidative stress.[16] A key theme of this chapter, therefore, is the hypothesis that nitrosative or oxidative stress contributes to protein misfolding in the brains of neurodegenerative patients. In this chapter, we discuss specific examples showing that S-nitrosylation of (1) ubiquitin E3 ligases such as parkin or (2) endoplasmic reticulum chaperones such as protein-disulfide isomerase (PDI) is critical for the accumulation of misfolded proteins in neurodegenerative diseases such as PD and other conditions.[17–20]

PROTEIN MISFOLDING IN NEURODEGENERATIVE DISEASES

A shared histologic feature of many neurodegenerative diseases is the accumulation of misfolded proteins that adversely affect neuronal connectivity and plasticity, and trigger cell death signaling pathways.[12,15] For example, degenerating brain contains aberrant accumulations of misfolded, aggregated proteins, such as α-synuclein and synphilin-1 in PD, and amyloid-β (Aβ) and tau in AD. The inclusions observed in PD are called Lewy bodies and are mostly found in the cytoplasm. AD brains show intracellular neurofibrillary tangles, which contain tau, and extracellular plaque, which contains Aβ. Other disorders manifesting protein aggregation include Huntington's disease (polyQ), ALS, and prion disease.[14] The above-mentioned aggregates may consist of oligomeric complexes of nonnative secondary structures and demonstrate poor solubility in aqueous or detergent solvent.

In general, protein aggregates do not accumulate in unstressed, healthy neurons due in part to the existence of cellular "quality control machineries." For example, molecular chaperones are believed to provide a defense mechanism against the toxicity of misfolded proteins because chaperones can prevent inappropriate interactions within and between polypeptides, and can promote refolding of proteins that have been misfolded because of cell stress. In addition to the quality control of proteins provided by molecular chaperones, the ubiquitin-proteasome system (UPS) and autophagy/lysosomal degradation are involved in the clearance of abnormal or aberrant proteins. When chaperones cannot repair misfolded proteins, they may be tagged via addition of polyubiquitin chains for degradation by the proteasome. In neurodegenerative conditions, intracellular or extracellular protein aggregates are thought to accumulate in the brain as a result of a decrease in molecular chaperone or proteasome activities. In fact, several mutations that disturb the activity of molecular chaperones or UPS-associated enzymes can cause neurodegeneration.[15,21,22] Along these lines, postmortem samples from the substantia nigra of PD patients (vs. non-PD controls) manifest a significant reduction in proteasome activity.[23]

Historically, lesions that contain aggregated proteins were considered to be pathogenic. Recently, several lines of evidence have suggested that aggregates are formed through a complex multistep process by which misfolded proteins assemble into inclusion bodies; currently, soluble oligomers of these aberrant proteins are thought to be the most toxic forms via interference with normal cell activities, whereas

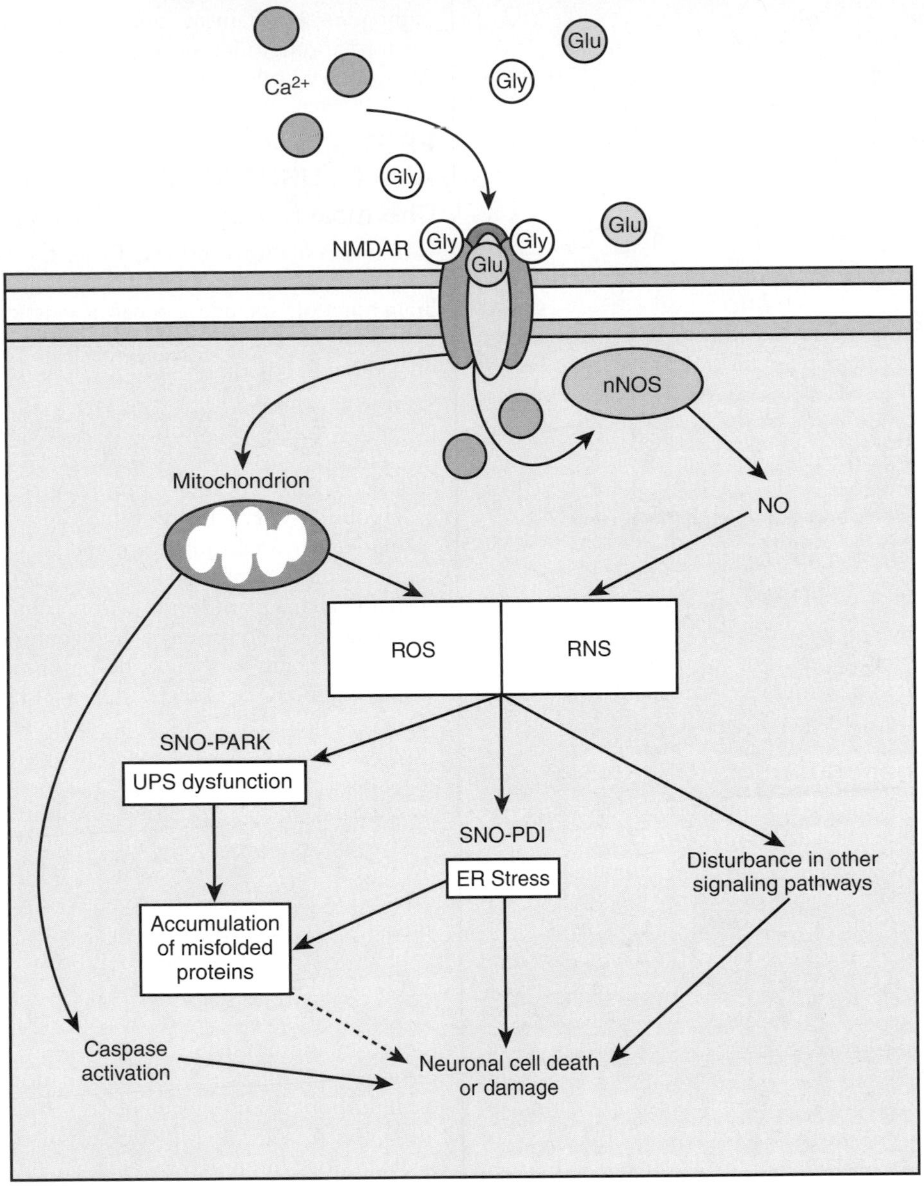

Figure 25-1. Activation of the NMDA receptor (NMDAR) by glutamate (Glu) and glycine (Gly) induces Ca^{2+} influx and consequent ROS/RNS production. NMDAR hyperactivation triggers generation of ROS/RNS and cytochrome C release from mitochondria associated with subsequent activation of caspases, causing neuronal cell death and damage. *SNO-PARK,* S-nitrosylated parkin; *SNO-PDI,* S-nitrosylated PDI.

frank aggregates may be an attempt by the cell to wall off potentially toxic material.[8,24]

GENERATION OF REACTIVE OXYGEN/ NITROGEN SPECIES (ROS/RNS)

NMDA receptor-mediated glutamatergic signaling pathways induce Ca^{2+} influx

It is well known that the amino acid glutamate is the major excitatory neurotransmitter in the brain. Glutamate is present in high concentrations in the adult central nervous system and is released for milliseconds from nerve terminals in a Ca^{2+}-dependent manner. After glutamate enters the synaptic cleft, it diffuses across the cleft to interact with its corresponding receptors on the postsynaptic face of an adjacent neuron. Excitatory neurotransmission is necessary for the normal development and plasticity of synapses, and for some forms of learning or memory; however, excessive activation of glutamate receptors is implicated in neuronal damage in many neurologic disorders ranging from acute hypoxic-ischemic brain injury to chronic neurodegenerative diseases. It is currently thought that overstimulation of extrasynaptic NMDA receptors mediate this neuronal damage, while in contrast synaptic activity may activate survival pathways.[25–27] Intense hyperstimulation of excitatory receptors leads to necrotic cell death, but more mild or chronic overstimulation can result in apoptotic or other forms of cell death.[28–30]

NMDA receptor-coupled channels are highly permeable to Ca^{2+}, thus permitting Ca^{2+} entry after ligand binding if the cell is depolarized to relieve block of the receptor-associated ion channel by Mg^{2+}.[31,32] Subsequent binding of Ca^{2+} to various intracellular molecules can lead to many significant consequences. In particular, excessive activation of

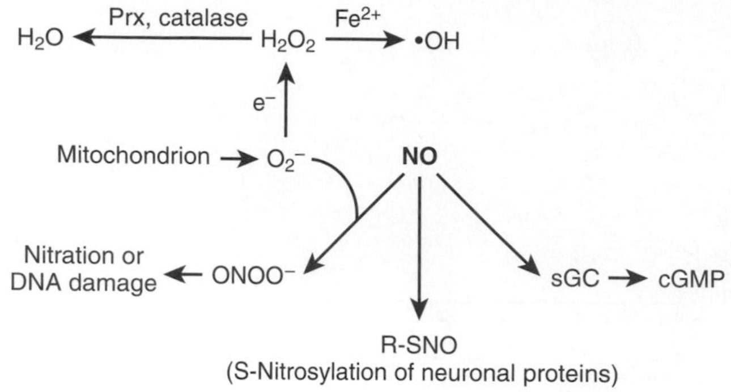

Figure 25-2. Pathways of ROS/RNS neurotoxicity. NO activates soluble guanylate cyclase (sGC) to produce cyclic guanosine monophosphate (cGMP), which in turn activates cGMP-dependent protein kinase. Excessive NMDA receptor activity, leading to the overproduction of NO, can be neurotoxic. For example, S-nitrosylation of parkin and PDI can contribute to neuronal cell damage and death, in part by triggering accumulation of misfolded proteins. Other neurotoxic effects of NO are mediated by peroxynitrite ($ONOO^-$), a reaction product of NO and superoxide anion (O_2^-). In contrast, S-nitrosylation can also mediate neuroprotective effects, for example, by inhibiting caspase activity and preventing overactivation of NMDA receptors.

NMDA receptors leads to the production of damaging free radicals (e.g., NO and ROS) and other enzymatic processes, contributing to cell death.[6,11,29,30,33,34]

Ca^{2+} influx and generation of ROS/RNS

Excessive activation of glutamate receptors is implicated in neuronal damage in many neurologic disorders. John Olney coined the term "excitotoxicity" to describe this phenomenon.[35,36] This form of toxicity is mediated at least in part by excessive activation of NMDA-type receptors,[6,7,37] resulting in excessive Ca^{2+} influx through a receptor's associated ion channel.

Increased levels of neuronal Ca^{2+}, in conjunction with the Ca^{2+}-binding protein Ca^{2+}/calmodulin (CaM), trigger the activation of nNOS and subsequent generation of NO from the amino acid L-arginine.[8,38] NO is a gaseous free radical (thus highly diffusible) and a key molecule that plays a vital role in normal signal transduction but in excess can lead to neuronal cell damage and death. The discrepancy of NO effects on neuronal survival can also be caused by the formation of different NO species or intermediates: NO radical (NO·), nitrosonium cation (NO^+), nitroxyl anion (NO^-, with high energy singlet and lower energy triplet forms).[11]

Recent studies further pointed out the potential connection between ROS/RNS and mitochondrial dysfunction in neurodegenerative diseases, especially in PD.[5,39] Pesticide and other environmental toxins that inhibit mitochondrial complex I result in oxidative and nitrosative stress, and consequent aberrant protein accumulation.[17,18,20,40,41] Administration to animal models of complex I inhibitors, such as MPTP, 6-hydroxydopamine, rotenone, and paraquat, which result in overproduction of ROS/RNS, reproduces many of the features of sporadic PD, such as dopaminergic neuron degeneration, upregulation and aggregation of α-synuclein, Lewy bodylike intraneuronal inclusions, and behavioral impairment.[5,39]

Increased nitrosative and oxidative stress are associated with chaperone and proteasomal dysfunction, resulting in accumulation of misfolded aggregates.[16,42] However, until recently little was known regarding the molecular and pathogenic mechanisms underlying contribution of NO to the formation of inclusion bodies, such as amyloid plaque in AD or Lewy bodies in PD.

PROTEIN S-NITROSYLATION AND NEURONAL CELL DEATH

Chemical biology of S-nitrosylation

Early investigations indicated that the NO group mediates cellular signaling pathways, which regulate broad aspects of brain function, including synaptic plasticity, normal development, and neuronal cell death.[33,43–45] In general, NO exerts physiologic and some pathophysiologic effects via stimulation of guanylate cyclase to form cyclic guanosine-3′,5′-monophosphate (cGMP) or through S-nitrosylation of regulatory protein thiol groups[9,11,42,46–48] (Figure 25-2). S-nitrosylation is the covalent addition of an NO group to a critical cysteine thiol/sulfhydryl (RSH or, more properly, thiolate anion, RS^-) to form an S-nitrosothiol derivative (R-SNO). Such modification modulates the function of a broad spectrum of mammalian, plant, and microbial proteins. In general, a consensus motif of amino acids comprised of nucleophilic residues (generally an acid and a base) surround a critical cysteine, which increases the cysteine sulfhydryl's susceptibility to S-nitrosylation.[49,50] Our group first identified the physiologic relevance of S-nitrosylation by showing that NO and related RNS exert paradoxical effects via redox-based mechanisms. NO is neuroprotective via S-nitrosylation of NMDA receptors (as well as other subsequently discovered targets, including caspases) and yet can also be neurodestructive by formation of peroxynitrite (or, as later discovered, reaction with additional molecules such as MMP-9 and GAPDH)[11,51–58] (Table 25-1). Over the past decade, accumulating evidence has suggested that S-nitrosylation can regulate the biologic activity of a great variety of proteins, in some ways akin to phosphorylation.* Chemically, NO is often a good "leaving group," facilitating further oxidation of critical thiol to disulfide bonds among neighboring (vicinal) cysteine residues or, via reaction with ROS, to sulfenic (–SOH), sulfinic ($–SO_2H$) or sulfonic ($–SO_3H$) acid derivatization of the protein.[18,20,57,66] Alternatively, S-nitrosylation may possibly produce a nitroxyl disulfide, in which the NO group is shared by close cysteine thiols.[67]

Analyses of mice deficient in either nNOS or iNOS confirmed that NO is an important mediator of cell injury and death after excitotoxic stimulation; NO generated from nNOS or iNOS is detrimental to neuronal survival.[68,69] In addition, inhibition of NOS activity ameliorates the progression of disease pathology in animal models of PD, AD, and ALS, suggesting that excess generation of NO plays a pivotal role in the pathogenesis of several neurodegenerative diseases.[70–73] Although the involvement of NO in neurodegeneration has been widely accepted, the chemical relationship between nitrosative stress and accumulation of misfolded proteins has remained obscure. Recent findings, however, have shed light on molecular events underlying this relationship. Specifically, we recently mounted physiologic and chemical evidence that S-nitrosylation modulates the (1) ubiquitin E3 ligase activity of parkin,[17–19] and (2)

*References 11,17,18,20,50,57–65

Table 25-1. Examples of S-Nitrosylated Proteins Confirmed in Neurons or Brains

SNO Targets	Effect of SNO	Reference No.
Caspases	• Decreased activity • Suppression of cell death	(54,52) (178,53)
Dexras1	• Activation of GTPase • Regulation of iron homeostasis	(179,180)
N-Ethylmaleimide sensitive factor	• Enhanced interaction with GluR2 • Regulation of exocytosis	(181,182)
GAPDH	• Enhanced interaction with Siah1 • Activation of p300/CBP • Augmentation of cell death	(58,183)
MAP1B	• Enhanced interaction with • Axon retraction	(184)
MMP-9	• Activation • Augmentation of cell death	(57)
NMDAR (NR1 and NR2A)	• Inhibition • Suppression of cell death	(11,56)
Parkin	• Decrease in E3 ligase activity • Augmentation of cell death	(17,18)
PDI	• Decreased activity • Accumulation of misfolded proteins • Augmentation of cell death	(20)
PrxII	• Decreased peroxidase activity • Augmentation of cell death	(185)

chaperone and isomerase activities of PDI,[20] contributing to protein misfolding and neurotoxicity in models of neurodegenerative disorders.

S-nitrosylation and parkin

Identification of errors in the genes encoding parkin (an ubiquitin E3 ligase) and UCH-L1 in rare familial forms of PD has implicated possible dysfunction of the UPS in the pathogenesis of sporadic PD as well. The UPS represents an important mechanism for proteolysis in mammalian cells. Formation of polyubiquitin chains constitutes the signal for proteasomal attack and degradation. An isopeptide bond covalently attaches the C-terminus of the first ubiquitin in a polyubiqutin chain to a lysine residue in the target protein. The cascade of activating (E1), conjugating (E2), and ubiquitin-ligating (E3) type of enzymes catalyzes the conjugation of the ubiquitin chain to proteins. In addition, individual E3 ubiquitin ligases play a key role in the recognition of specific substrates.[74]

PD is the second most prevalent neurodegenerative disease and is characterized by the progressive loss of dopamine neurons in the substantia nigra pars compacta. Appearance of Lewy bodies that contain misfolded and ubiquitinated proteins generally accompanies the loss of dopaminergic neurons in the PD brain. Such ubiquitinated inclusion bodies are the hallmark of many neurodegenerative disorders. Age-associated defects in intracellular proteolysis of misfolded or aberrant proteins might lead to accumulation and ultimately deposition of aggregates within neurons or glial cells. Although such aberrant protein accumulation had been observed in patients with genetically encoded mutant proteins, recent evidence from our laboratory suggests that nitrosative and oxidative stress are potential causal factors for protein accumulation in the much more common sporadic form of PD. As illustrated below, nitrosative/oxidative stress, commonly found during normal aging, can mimic rare genetic causes of disorders, such as PD, by promoting protein misfolding in the absence of a genetic mutation.[17–19] For example, S-nitrosylation and further oxidation of parkin result in dysfunction of this enzyme and thus of the UPS.[17,18,75–78] We and others recently discovered that nitrosative stress triggers S-nitrosylation of parkin (forming SNO-parkin) not only in rodent models of PD but also in the brains of human patients with PD and the related α-synucleinopathy, DLBD (diffuse Lewy body disease). SNO-parkin initially stimulates ubiquitin E3 ligase activity, resulting in enhanced ubiquitination as observed in Lewy bodies, followed by a decrease in enzyme activity, producing a futile cycle of dysfunctional UPS.[18,19,79] We also found that rotenone led to the generation of SNO-parkin and thus dysfunctional ubiquitin E3 ligase activity. Moreover, S-nitrosylation appears to compromise the neuroprotective effect of parkin.[17] Nitrosative and oxidative stress can also alter the solubility of parkin via posttranslational modification of cysteine residues, which may concomitantly compromise its protective function.[80–82] Additionally, it is likely that other ubiquitin E3 ligases with RING-finger thiol motifs are S-nitrosylated in a similar manner to parkin to affect their enzymatic function; hence, S-nitrosylation of E3 ligases may be involved in a number of degenerative conditions.

S-nitrosylation of PDI mediates protein misfolding and neurotoxicity in cell models of PD or AD

The ER normally participates in protein processing and folding but undergoes a stress response when immature or misfolded proteins accumulate.[83–86] ER stress stimulates two critical intracellular responses. The first represents expression of chaperones that prevent protein aggregation via the unfolded protein response (UPR), and is implicated in protein refolding, posttranslational assembly of protein complexes, and protein degradation. This response is believed to contribute to adaptation during altered environmental conditions, promoting maintenance of cellular homeostasis. The second ER stress response, termed ER-associated degradation (ERAD), specifically recognizes terminally misfolded proteins for retro-translocation across the ER membrane to the cystosol, where they can be degraded by the UPS. Additionally, although severe ER stress can induce apoptosis, the ER withstands relatively mild insults via expression of stress proteins such as glucose-regulated protein (GRP) and PDI. These proteins behave as molecular chaperones that assist in the maturation, transport, and folding of secretory proteins.

During protein folding in the ER, PDI can introduce disulfide bonds into proteins (oxidation), break disulfide bonds (reduction), and catalyze thiol/disulfide exchange (isomerization), thus facilitating disulfide bond formation, rearrangement reactions, and structural stability.[87] PDI has four domains that are homologous to thioredoxin (TRX) (termed a, b, b′, and a′). Only two of the four TRX-like domains (a and a′) contain a characteristic redox-active CXXC motif, and these two-thiol/disulfide centers function as independent active sites.[88–91] Several mammalian PDI homologues, such as ERp57 and PDIp, also localize to the ER and may manifest similar functions.[92,93] Increased expression of PDIp in neuronal cells under conditions mimicking PD suggest the possible contribution of PDIp to neuronal survival.[92]

In many neurodegenerative disorders and cerebral ischemia, the accumulation of immature and denatured proteins results in ER dysfunction,[92,94–96] but upregulation of PDI represents an adaptive response promoting protein refolding and may offer neuronal cell protection.[92,93,97,98] In addition, it is generally accepted that excessive generation of NO can contribute to activation of the ER stress pathway, at least in some cell types.[99,100] Molecular mechanisms by which NO induces protein misfolding and ER stress, however, have remained enigmatic until recently. The ER normally manifests a relatively positive redox potential in contrast to the highly reducing environment of the cytosol and mitochondria. This redox environment can influence the stability of protein S-nitrosylation and oxidation reactions.[101] Interestingly, we have recently reported that excessive NO can lead to S-nitrosylation of the active-site thiol groups of PDI, and this reaction inhibits both its isomerase and chaperone activities.[20] Mitochondrial complex I insult by rotenone can also result in S-nitrosylation of PDI in cell culture models. Moreover, we found that PDI is S-nitrosylated in the brains of virtually all cases examined of sporadic AD and PD. Under pathologic conditions, it is possible that both cysteine sulfhydryl groups in the TRX-like domains of PDI form S-nitrosothiols. Unlike formation of a single S-nitrosothiol, which is commonly seen after denitrosylation reactions catalyzed by PDI,[61] dual nitrosylation may be relatively more stable and prevent subsequent disulfide formation on PDI. Therefore we speculate that these pathologic S-nitrosylation reactions on PDI are more easily detected during neurodegenerative conditions. Additionally, it is possible that vicinal (nearby) cysteine thiols reacting with NO can form nitroxyl disulfide,[67] and such reaction may potentially occur in the catalytic side of PDI to inhibit enzymatic activity. To determine the consequences of S-nitrosylated PDI (SNO-PDI) formation in neurons, we exposed cultured cerebrocortical neurons to neurotoxic concentrations of NMDA, thus inducing excessive Ca^{2+} influx and consequent NO production from nNOS. Under these conditions, we found that PDI was S-nitrosylated in a NOS-dependent manner. SNO-PDI formation led to the accumulation of polyubiquitinated/misfolded proteins and activation of the UPR. Moreover, S-nitrosylation abrogated the inhibitory effect of PDI on aggregation of proteins observed in Lewy body inclusions.[20,102] S-nitrosylation of PDI also prevented its attenuation of neuronal cell death triggered by ER stress, misfolded proteins, or proteasome inhibition. Further evidence suggested that SNO-PDI may in effect transport NO to the extracellular space, where it could conceivably exert additional adverse effects.[61]

The UPS is apparently impaired in the aging brain. Additionally, inclusion bodies similar to those found in neurodegenerative disorders can appear in brains of normal aged individuals or those with subclinical manifestations of disease.[103] These findings suggest that the activity of the UPS and molecular chaperones may decline in an age-dependent manner.[104] Given that we have not found detectable quantities of SNO-parkin and SNO-PDI in normal aged brain,[17,18,20] we speculate that S-nitrosylation of these and similar proteins may represent a key event that contributes to susceptibility of the aging brain to neurodegenerative conditions.

SECTION II: METABOLIC-INSULIN SIGNALING IN THE CONTROL OF AGING AND NEURODEGENERATION

The insulin/IGF-1 signaling pathway and organismal aging

Experiments using model organisms have provided rapidly increasing evidence that reduced activity of the insulin and insulin-like growth factor (IGF) signaling (IIS) pathways extends lifespan. This discovery is particularly striking as impaired IIS function is also known to have detrimental effects, including death during embryogenesis and diabetes. In addition, alterations of IIS pathway activity can have profound effects on reproduction, stress resistance, and metabolism.[105] Recent research has started to unravel the underlying mechanism of IIS-mediated lifespan modulation. Furthermore, this research has also shown a mechanistic link between IIS and neurodegenerative diseases. In this section, we will provide an overview of the role IIS plays in organismal aging and highlight examples of how IIS, and other longevity genes with metabolic functions, regulate neurodegeneration.

Because of the complex regulatory systems that modulate lifespan, a successful approach to addressing this question has been the use of the simple invertebrate models: the nematode *Caenorhabtidis elegans*, and the fruitfly *Drosophila melanogaster*. Indeed, a short lifespan and genetic accessibility of *C. elegans* led to the discovery of the first long-lived IIS mutant (*age-1*) through a genetic screen for genes that alter lifespan.[106] This mutant encodes the worm phosphoinositide-3-kinase (PI3K),[107,108] which supported additional findings in *C. elegans* demonstrating that mutations in the insulin/IGF-1 receptor DAF-2 increased lifespan and that this effect depended on the FOXO transcription factor DAF-16.[106,109–111] With the discovery that mutations in the insulin receptor (InR) or its substrate CHICO could extend the lifespan of *Drosophila*,[112,113] these collective findings suggested that reduced IIS activity is an evolutionarily conserved mechanism to extend lifespan. This remarkable notion was further supported when rodents were shown to live longer if either the insulin or the IGF signaling pathways were disrupted,[114–117] indicating that the evolutionary conservation extends to mammals. This functional conservation may even extend to humans as alterations in the IGF signaling pathway has been observed in centenarians.[118] These findings also provided a possible explanation to the long lifespan observed in growth-hormone deficient Ames dwarf mice and growth hormone receptor knockout mice because growth hormone positively regulates the production of IGF-1.[119,120]

Figure 25-3 summarizes IIS interventions that have so far been shown to modulate lifespan in worms, flies, and mice.

IIS modulations that affect organismal lifespan

As IIS coordinates nutritional availability and growth, long-lived IIS mutants have effects on the metabolic reserves (altered fat content) and delayed development, decreased adult body size, reduced fecundity, and increased stress resistance.[105,121] Recent reports have shown that these processes

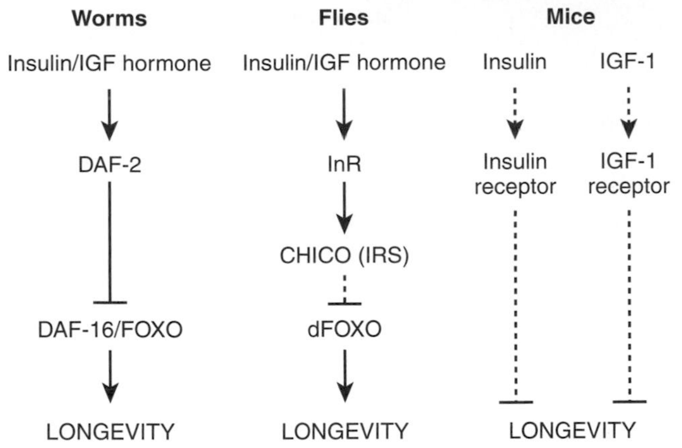

Figure 25-3. The insulin-IGF pathway regulates aging in multiple organisms. Molecular components of the insulin/IGF-1 signaling pathway that have been shown to influence the lifespan of worms, flies, and mice. *Dashed lines*, plausible regulatory relationships.

make individual contributions to the extended longevity phenotype because of reduced IIS pathway activity.[121] Another important feature of reduced IIS function is the promotion of a longer "healthspan" and longer lifespans in some instances. For instance, experiments have demonstrated protective effects of IIS mutants that extend lifespan in invertebrate models against specific aging-related diseases such as cancer,[122–124] cardiac failure,[125] and Alzheimer's disease[126,127] (see later discussion).

Recent research efforts have focused on understanding when and where IIS modulates lifespan. To address the temporal requirement for reduction of IIS in determining lifespan, IIS was decreased in *C. elegans* during adulthood by administration of bacteria engineered to express double-stranded RNA for *daf-2*, and this treatment was sufficient to extend lifespan.[128] Consistent with this, adult-only expression of dFOXO in the adipose tissue of flies was also demonstrated to be sufficient to extend lifespan.[129,130] Similarly, adult-specific overexpression of dPTEN[129] and ablation of the insulin-producing neurons in the last stage of preadult development is sufficient to enhance longevity.[131]

The tissue-specific requirements for IIS to modulate lifespan have also been investigated in some detail and have pointed towards important roles for neuronal and fat tissues. For instance, replacement of the insulin-IGF-1 receptor DAF-2 in neurons in *daf-2(−)* worms shortened lifespan back to that of wild-type.[132,133] This is in somewhat contrast to the downstream effector of the *daf-2* pathway, the FOXO transcription factor DAF-16, which has been found to primarily function in the intestine—the worms' adipose tissue—to regulate lifespan downstream of the *daf-2*/insulin/IGF-1 receptor.[134] Thus insulin signaling in neural tissues controls signals that act in the periphery to modulate lifespan. Consistent with specific roles in neuronal and fat tissues, as mentioned above, ablation of the insulin-producing neurons is sufficient to enhance longevity, whereas fat-specific overexpression of the pathway antagonists dPTEN or dFOXO can extend lifespan in flies via nonautonomous signaling to the insulin-producing neurons.[129,130] Finally, fat-specific knockout of the insulin receptor in mice can also extend lifespan.[115] Determining the nature of the signals and their cross-talk with the peripheral tissues remains a critical area of research. These results also highlight the potential autonomous and nonautonomous contributions, and acute versus chronic consequences of altering insulin-metabolic signaling in age-dependent diseases. How IIS orchestrates organ senescence, including neurodegenerative diseases, and longevity remains an important area of future studies. Thus these combined results indicate the existence of evolutionarily conserved, complex systemic responses regulated by IIS.

Mechanisms by which IIS affect organismal lifespan and neurodegenerative diseases

What is the basis of the beneficial lifespan effects that reduced IIS induce? Recent studies have used unbiased approaches, including gene-expression profiling to understand the FOXO transcriptome, in worms/flies to gain insight into the downstream effectors of IIS. Several studies have been reported using long-lived IIS mutants.[135–140] Importantly, genes required for metabolism, stress response, and detoxification of oxidative damage have been identified. Nonetheless, when the effect of altering expression of these genes individually has been investigated directly, their effect on longevity has been minor.[137] This has been taken to indicate that many FOXO-regulated genes are required to act additively to produce the profound lifespan effects seen in long-lived IIS mutants. In contrast, other genes might work in parallel to FOXO to extend lifespan by reducing IIS in *C. elegans*, for instance the heat-responsive transcription factor HSF-1[141,142] and genes involved in autophagy—a cellular process by which cytoplasmic components are degraded and recycled.[143,144] Clearly, these results point to a multimechanistic regulation of the aging process.

Importantly, the aging process has recently been directly linked to neurodegenerative diseases via the IIS pathway. Several studies performed in *C. elegans* and *Drosophila* proteotoxicity models indicate that IIS links directly to the onset of toxic protein aggregation, for example, of the Aβ peptide causing Alzheimer's disease and via PolyQ stretches as those found in Huntington's disease.[141,145–147] These studies have started to shed light on the mechanism by which IIS affects neurodegeneration and suggest that IIS can protect against misfolded aggregates in Alzheimer's disease by multiple mechanisms. The main mechanism involves disaggregation of toxic species to enable their degradation via small heat shock proteins (regulated by the HSF-1 transcription factor), whereas the secondary mechanism, regulated by DAF-16/FOXO, involves aggregation of proteins into high-molecular species that are less toxic to the cell.[145] Future research should address if the link between IIS and neurodegenerative diseases exists in mammalian systems.

Other metabolic longevity pathways and genes with links to neurodegeneration

Reduced food intake without malnutrition, referred to as dietary restriction (DR), also extends lifespan of a variety of species and has been extensively studied in model organisms.[148] In *C. elegans*, it was first conclusively addressed if DR regulates longevity via the IIS pathway. This is not likely to be the case because only IIS, but not DR, is completely dependent on the FOXO transcription factor DAF-16 in worms.[149] Similarly, *dFoxo* null mutant flies still show lifespan extensions following DR.[129,150] The effects of DR on IIS in mammals are less clear because long-lived Ames mice (mentioned previously) subjected to DR show further increase in lifespan,[151] whereas GHRKO mice subjected to DR failed to increase lifespan.[152] The complexity of mammalian Ins-IGF signaling suggests a more integrated interaction with DR because DR leads to increased insulin sensitivity. Importantly, dietary restriction protects against neurodegeneration in mouse models,[153] and dietary-restricted worms show reduced proteotoxicity mediated by the transcription factor HSF-1, similarly to IIS mutants.[154]

The sirtuins were the first reported genetic regulators of DR-induced longevity. These proteins encode NAD^+-dependent histone deacetylases.[155] There is some controversy about the level of conservation regarding the role in DR of these genes. Overexpression of Sir2 extends the lifespan of yeast, worms, and flies[155]; however, this appears to involve a DR-independent mechanism in *C. elegans*.[156–159] Sirtuins (which include 7 homologs in mammals, SIRT1-7, with SIRT1 being the mammalian ortholog of Sir2) also affect neurodegeneration in mammalian systems; yet, there is some controversy about this role. SIRT1 protects against neurodegeneration in mice,[160] and activation of SIRT2 in cell-based models for neurodegeneration leads to protection against neuronal cell death.[161] In contrast, however, loss of SIRT1 also provides protection against neuronal loss in mice.[162] One possibility is that sirtuin effects follow an "inverted U-curve" with benefit at high or low levels of activity. Taken together, these findings suggest that the mechanisms by which sirtuins regulate cellular protection and organismal longevity may be rather complex.

Another potential player in the regulation of lifespan by DR is the nutrient sensor TOR (target of rapamycin). TOR exists in two distinct complexes, termed TORC1 and TORC2.[163,164] Reduction of TOR function has been shown to increase lifespan in yeast, worms, and flies.[165–167] TOR regulates multiple processes, including metabolism, protein translation, and autophagy.[124,163,164] All of these processes have been linked to aging. Longer-lived TOR mutants have an altered metabolic profile.[165] Reduced protein translation extends lifespan in yeast, worms, and flies.[168] Autophagy is required for dietary-restricted animals to live long,[169] similar to IIS mutants (see previous discussion). In this way, it appears as autophagy is linked to longevity processes specifically involved in nutrient sensing. TOR interacts with the IIS pathway,[163] and this is also true in the context of aging. Inhibition of TOR and insulin/IGF-1 signaling does not further extend lifespan.[156,170] Furthermore, the TOR binding partner Raptor, called *daf-15* in worms, is a transcriptional target of DAF-16/FOXO.[166] However, mutants with reduced TOR pathway activity do not require the FOXO transcription factor DAF-16.[166,170] Indeed, the TOR binding partner Raptor is a transcriptional target of DAF-16/FOXO[166] and recent work in *Drosophila* has shown that TOR may function downstream of dFOXO.[165] TOR may also contribute to neuronal survival. Inappropriate activation of the cell cycle by misfolded proteins leads to cell death in postmitotic neurons. This response can be reversed by blocking the cell cycle via increasing cell cycle inhibitors and inhibiting the cell growth regulatory TOR protein.[127] How TOR regulates growth, metabolism, aging, and neurodegenerative diseases is a critical area of research.

The ATP sensor AMPK has also been suggested to play a key role in DR. Similar to TOR, AMPK plays a role in aging, stress resistance, and tumorigenesis.[171–173] AMPK also interacts with the IIS pathway because lifespan extension via reduced IIS is dependent on worm AMPK, *aak-2*, and overexpression of AAK-2 extends *C. elegans* lifespan.[173] Whether this effect is conserved in other organisms awaits confirmation. Additionally, AMPK may have a neuroprotective role because loss of AMPK causes a dramatic increase in neurodegeneration in flies.[174,175] AMPK may have additional roles in regulating neural function. The energy sensing factor AMPK may function downstream of actual chemosensory nutrient-sensing pathways, which allows the animal to detect and respond to changes in food availability. Interestingly, worms in which certain gustatory and olfactory neurons have been removed by laser ablation are long-lived.[176] These lifespan extensions are, however, dependent

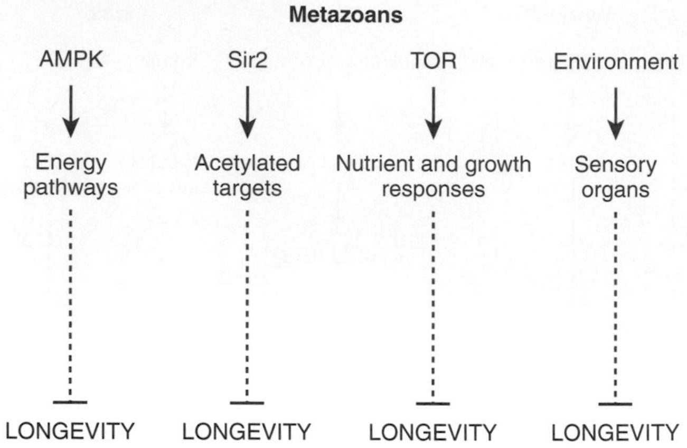

Figure 25-4. Signaling processes that regulate aging. Signaling by proteins and processes with metabolic functions that have been shown to modulate organismal aging in metazoans. *Dashed lines,* plausible regulatory relationships.

KEY POINTS

The Neurobiology of Aging: Free Radical Stress and Metabolic Pathways

- Excessive NMDA receptor activation and/or mitochondrial dysfunction trigger excessive nitrosative and oxidative stress that may result in malfunction of the UPS or molecular chaperones.
- Excessively produced ROS/RNS may contribute to abnormal protein accumulation and neuronal damage in sporadic forms of neurodegenerative diseases.
- S-nitrosylation of specific molecules such as parkin and PDI provides a mechanistic link between free radical production, abnormal protein accumulation, and neuronal cell injury in neurodegenerative disorders, such as PD and AD.
- Elucidation of these new pathways may lead to the development of additional new therapeutic approaches to prevent aberrant protein misfolding by targeted disruption or prevention of nitrosylation of specific proteins (e.g., parkin, PDI, and PrxII).
- Single gene mutations in the insulin and insulin-like growth factor signaling pathways can lengthen lifespan in worms, flies, and mice, implying evolutionary conservations of mechanisms.
- Such mutations can keep the animals healthy and disease-free for longer and can alleviate certain aging-related pathologies. Determining the tissue requirement, genetic interactions, and timing of these effects remain important areas for further research.

on DAF-16/FOXO, suggesting that nutrient sensing by these neurons is not involved in the longevity response to DR in *C. elegans*. On the other hand, flies exposed to the odor of abundant food no longer respond fully to the lifespan extending effects of DR treatments,[177] indicating that sensory perception indeed may play a role in DR-mediated longevity. Thus the environment can play an important role in determining lifespan. Future work will determine how IIS-metabolic pathways are linked to neurodegeneration, aging, and lifespan.

Figure 25-4 summarizes signaling by proteins and processes with metabolic functions that have been linked to organismal aging.

While this chapter was under review, too papers establishing longevity roles for TOR and S6 kinase in mammals were published.[186,187]

For a complete list of references, please visit online only at www.expertconsult.com

CHAPTER 26

Allostasis and Allostatic Overload in the Context of Aging

Bruce S. McEwen

INTRODUCTION

"Stress" is often identified as a factor in accelerated aging[1] and an important factor in disorders such as cardiovascular disease and depression, and a contributor to other disorders.[2] Being "stressed out" is a commonly used word that generally refers to experiences that cause feelings of anxiety, anger, and frustration because they push a person beyond his or her ability to successfully cope. Besides time pressures and daily hassles at work and home, there are stressors related to economic insecurity, poor health, and interpersonal conflict. More rarely, there are situations that are life-threatening—accidents, natural disasters, violence—and these evoke the classical "fight or flight" response. In contrast to daily hassles, these stressors are acute and yet they also can lead to depression, anxiety, posttraumatic stress disorder and other forms of chronic stress in the aftermath of the tragic event.

The most common stressors are, therefore, ones that operate chronically, often at a low level, and cause us to behave in certain ways. For example, being "stressed out" may promote anxiety or depressed mood, poor sleep, eating of comfort foods and overconsumption of calories, smoking, or drinking alcohol excessively. Being stressed out may reduce social interactions or regular physical activity. Not infrequently, anxiolytics and sleep promoting agents are used, but, with continuation of this state, the body may increase in weight, and develop metabolic dysregulation and atherosclerotic plaques.

The brain is the organ that decides what is stressful and determines the behavioral and physiologic responses, whether health promoting or health damaging. The brain is a biologic organ that changes under acute and chronic stress and directs many systems of the body—metabolic, cardiovascular, immune, renal—that are involved in the short and long-term consequences of being stressed out.

What does chronic stress do to the body and brain, particularly in relation to the aging process? This chapter summarizes some of the current information placing emphasis on how the stress hormones and related mediators can play both protective and damaging roles in brain and body, depending on how tightly their release is regulated, and it discusses some of the approaches for dealing with stress in a complex world.

DEFINITION OF STRESS, ALLOSTASIS, AND ALLOSTATIC LOAD

"Stress" is an ambiguous term and the actual stress response has protective and potentially damaging effects[3]: On the one hand, the body responds to almost any novel or challenging event by releasing catecholamines that increase heart rate and blood pressure and help adapt to the situation. Yet, chronically increased heart rate and blood pressure produce a chronic wear and tear on the cardiovascular system that can result, over time, in disorders such as atherosclerosis, strokes, and heart attacks. For this reason, the term "allostasis" was introduced by Sterling and Eyer[4] to refer to the active process by which the body responds to daily events and maintains homeostasis (*allostasis* literally means "achieving stability through change"). Because chronically increased allostasis can lead to disease, we introduced the term "allostatic load or overload" to refer to the wear and tear that results from either too much stress or from inefficient management of allostasis (e.g., not turning off the response when it is no longer needed). Other states that lead to allostatic overload are summarized in Figure 26-1 and involve not turning on an adequate response in the first place or not habituating to the recurrence of the same stressor, which then fails to dampen the allostatic response.[3]

PROTECTION AND DAMAGE AS THE TWO SIDES OF THE RESPONSE TO STRESSORS

Thus protection and damage are the two contrasting sides of the physiology that defend the body against the challenges of daily life, whether or not we call them "stressors." Besides adrenalin and noradrenalin, there are many mediators that participate in allostasis, and they are linked together in a network of regulation that is nonlinear (Figure 26-2), meaning that each mediator has the ability to regulate the activity of the other mediators, sometimes in a biphasic manner. Glucocorticoids are the other major "stress hormones." Proinflammatory and anti-inflammatory cytokines are produced by many cells in the body, and they regulate each other and are, in turn, regulated by glucocorticoids and catecholamines. Whereas catecholamines can increase proinflammatory cytokine production, glucocorticoids are known to inhibit this production.[5,6] The parasympathetic nervous system also plays an important regulatory role in this nonlinear network of allostasis since it generally opposes the sympathetic nervous system and, for example, slows the heart and also has anti-inflammatory effects.[7,8]

What this nonlinearity means is that when any one mediator is increased or decreased, there are compensatory changes in the other mediators that depend on time course and level of change of each of the mediators. Unfortunately, we cannot measure all components of this system simultaneously and must rely on measurements of only a few of them in any one study. Yet the nonlinearity must be kept in mind in interpreting the results.

MEASUREMENT OF ALLOSTATIC LOAD

Measurement of allostatic load and overload involves sampling of key mediators that may be elevated in what are called "allostatic states"[9] and markers of cumulative change such as abdominal fat. Allostatic states refer to the response profiles of the mediators themselves as shown in Figure 26-1. On the other hand, allostatic overload focuses on the tissues and organs and other end points that show the cumulative effects of overexposure to the mediators

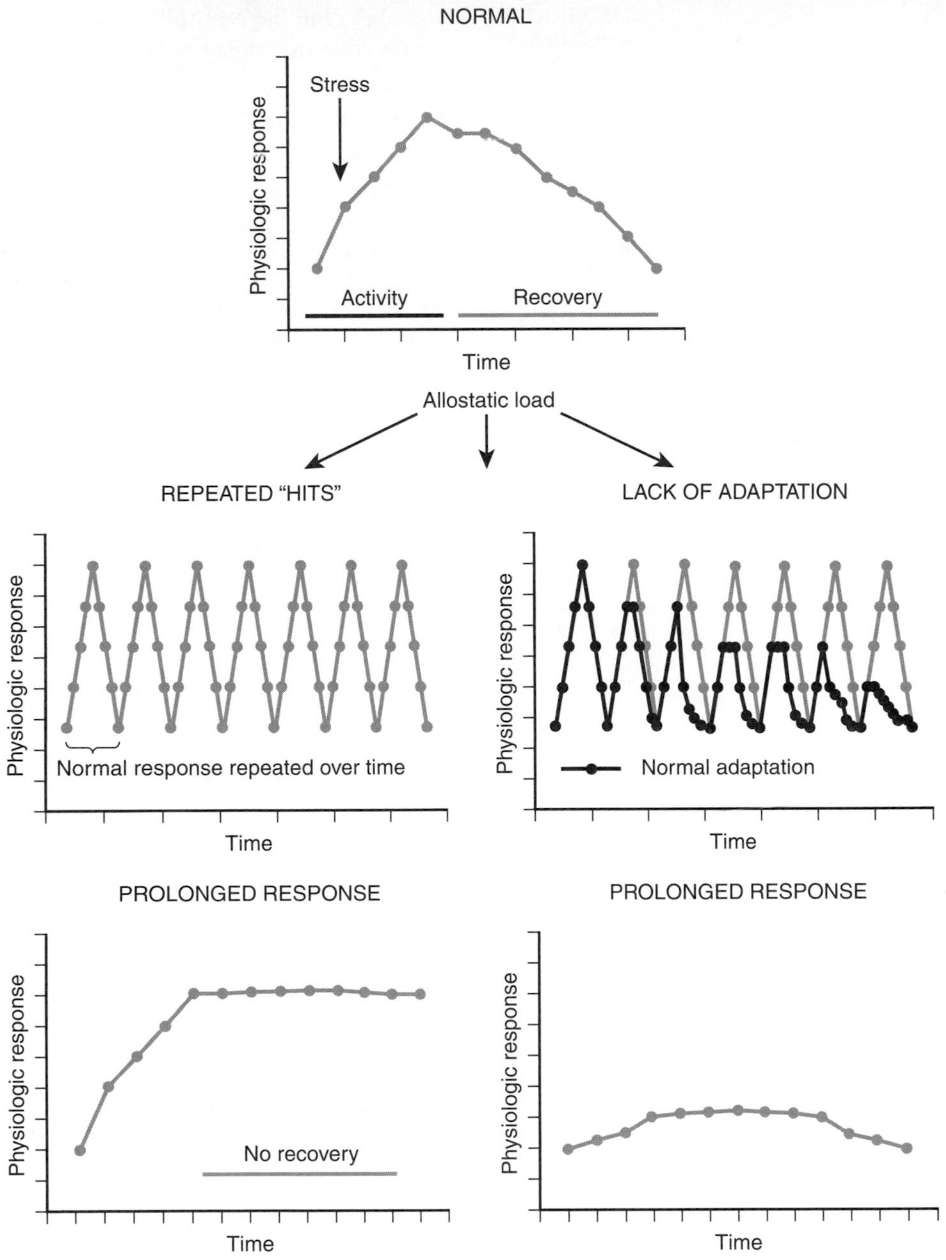

Figure 26-1. Four types of allostatic load. The top panel illustrates the normal allostatic response, in which a response is initiated by a stressor, sustained for an appropriate interval, and then turned off. The remaining panels illustrate four conditions that lead to allostatic load: *top, left* repeated "hits" from multiple stressors; *top, right* lack of adaptation; *bottom, left* prolonged response due to delayed shut down; and *bottom, right* inadequate response that leads to compensatory hyperactivity of other mediators (e.g., inadequate secretion of glucocorticoid, resulting in increased levels of cytokines that are normally counter-regulated by glucocorticoids). *(From McEwen BS. Protective and damaging effects of stress mediators. N Engl J Med 1998;338:171–9.)*

of allostasis. These are done by collecting samples from subjects in a minimally invasive and cost-effective manner. This limits the choice to the circulating mediators, such as glucocorticoids, DHEA, catecholamines, and certain cytokines. Salivary assays are particularly attractive, but then the question arises as to how to sample over time to get an adequate representation of a dynamic system since the levels of the mediators may fluctuate during the day and night. This is a topic unto itself and has been the subject of a number of methodological studies (see Web site for MacArthur SES and Health Research Network: www.macses.ucsf.edu/). Table 26-1 contains a list of some end points that can be used for cumulative assessment of allostatic overload in different systems of the body. These are currently in use in the Coronary Artery Risk Development In Young Adults (CARDIA) Study and have been shown to have predictive power for a number of health outcomes.[10–13]

BEING "STRESSED OUT," ESPECIALLY SLEEP DEPRIVATION AND ITS CONSEQUENCES

The common experience of being stressed out has as its core the elevation of some of the key systems that lead to allostatic load—cortisol, sympathetic activity, and proinflammatory

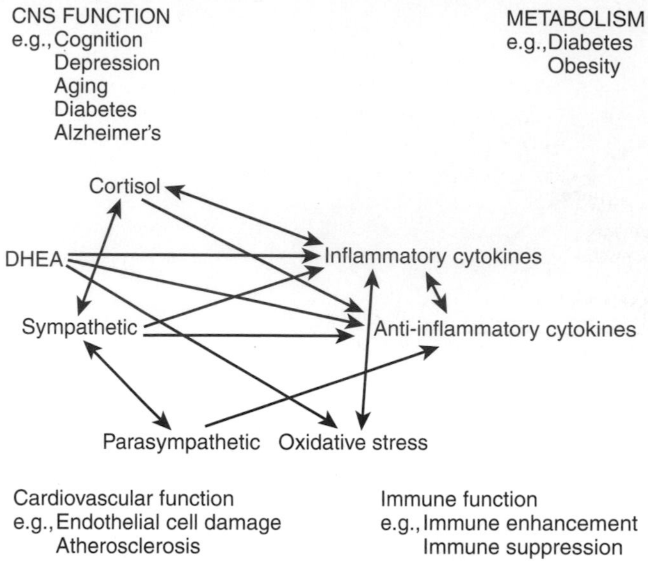

Figure 26-2. Nonlinear network of mediators of allostasis involved in the stress response. Arrows indicate that each system regulates the others in a reciprocal manner, creating a nonlinear network. Moreover, there are multiple pathways for regulation (e.g., inflammatory cytokine production is negatively regulated via anti-inflammatory cytokines, and via parasympathetic and glucocorticoid pathways, whereas sympathetic activity increases inflammatory cytokine production). Parasympathetic activity, in turn, contains sympathetic activity. *(From McEwen BS. Protective and damaging effects of stress mediators: central role of the brain. Dialogues Clin Neurosci 2006;8:367–81.)*

Table 26-1. Measurements of Allostatic States and Allostatic Overload in CARDIA Study[49–51]

Urine: 12 hr overnight
1. Urinary norepinephrine
2. Urinary epinephrine
3. Urinary free cortisol
Saliva: six saliva samples over 1 day assayed for cortisol
Blood
1. Total and HDL cholesterol
2. Glycosylated hemoglobin
3. IL-6
4. CRP
5. Fibrinogen
Other
1. Waist-hip ratio
2. Systolic and diastolic BP—seated/resting
3. Heart rate variability

cytokines, with a decline in parasympathetic activity. Nowhere is this better illustrated than for sleep deprivation, which is a frequent result of experiencing a lot of stress. Sleep deprivation produces an allostatic overload that can have deleterious consequences, which are particularly evident in aging: for example, poor sleep in aging women has been associated with elevated levels of IL-6.[14] Sleep restriction to 4 hours of sleep per night increases blood pressure, decreases parasympathetic tone, increases evening cortisol and insulin levels, and promotes increased appetite, possibly through increases in ghrelin and decreases in leptin.[15–17] Proinflammatory cytokine levels are increased, along with performance in tests of psychomotor vigilance, and this has been reported to result from a modest sleep restriction to 6 hours per night.[18] Moreover, reduced sleep duration has been reported to be associated with increased body mass and obesity in the NHANES study.[19] Sleep deprivation also causes cognitive impairment.[15]

KEY ROLE OF THE BRAIN IN RESPONSE TO STRESS

The brain is the master regulator of the neuroendocrine, autonomic, and immune systems, along with determining behaviors that contribute to unhealthy or healthy lifestyles, which, in turn, influence the physiologic processes of allostasis.[3] See Figure 26-3. Alterations in brain function by chronic stress can therefore have direct and indirect effects on the cumulative allostatic overload. Allostatic overload resulting from chronic stress in animal models causes atrophy of neurons in the hippocampus, prefrontal cortex, brain regions involved in memory, selective attention, and executive function, and hypertrophy of neurons in the amygdala, a brain region involved in fear, anxiety, and aggression.[15] Thus the ability to learn, remember, and make decisions may be compromised by chronic stress and may be accompanied by increased levels of anxiety and aggression. A recent study has shown increased reactivity of the amygdala to neutral facial expressions, indicating an increase in anxiety and reactivity, resulting from a few days of sleep deprivation.[20]

TRANSLATION TO THE HUMAN BRAIN

Much of the impetus for studying the effects of aging and stress on the structure of the human brain has come from the animal studies summarized elsewhere.[15] Age-related reductions in entorhinal and hippocampal volume have been associated with mild cognitive impairment and early stages of Alzheimer's disease, and a longitudinal study of aging Montreal residents revealed a smaller hippocampus and impaired hippocampal spatial and memory functions in those who showed rising cortisol levels during a yearly examination.[21] Although it is not possible to pinpoint causal factors in these age-related changes, stress and glucose regulation, along with depression and other mood and anxiety disorders, must be considered.

Regarding stress, although there is very little evidence regarding the effects of ordinary life stressors on brain structure, there are indications from functional imaging of individuals undergoing ordinary stressors (such as counting backwards) that there are changes in neural activity.[22] There are also long-term effects (e.g., chronic transcontinental air travel with short turnaround time, a type of chronic stress is associated with a smaller hippocampus,[23] and a 20-year history of high perceived stress has been associated with smaller hippocampal volumes).[24]

Stress causes depressive illness in individuals with certain genetic predispositions,[15,25] and the hippocampus, amygdala, and prefrontal cortex show altered patterns of activity in PET and fMRI and changes in volume: decreased volume of hippocampus and prefrontal cortex and amygdala, although amygdala volume has been reported to increase in the first episode of depression, whereas hippocampal volume is not decreased.[26]

There is hippocampal volume loss in Cushing's disease along with cognitive impairment and depressed mood that can be relieved by surgical correction of the hypercortisolemia.[27] Moreover, there are a variety of other anxiety-related disorders, such as posttraumatic stress disorder (PTSD) and

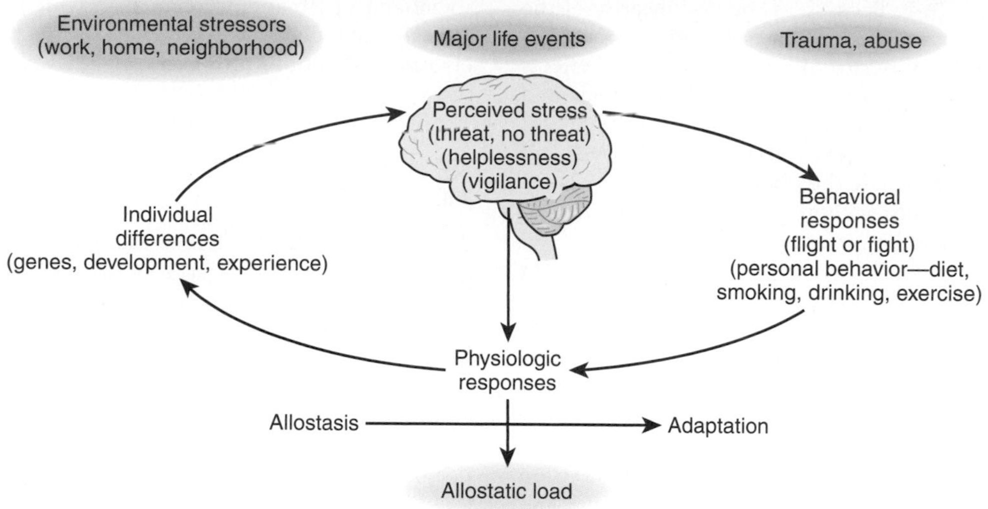

Figure 26-3. Central role of the brain in allostasis and the behavioral and physiologic response to stressors. *(From McEwen BS. Protective and damaging effects of stress mediators. N Engl J Med 1998;338:171–9.)*

borderline personality disorder, in which there is atrophy of the hippocampus.[15] Another important factor in hippocampal volume and function is glucose regulation. Poor glucose regulation is associated with smaller hippocampal volume and poorer memory function in individuals in their 60s and 70s who have "mild cognitive impairment" (MCI),[28] and in those with frank type 2 diabetes.[29]

POSITIVE AFFECT, SELF-ESTEEM, AND SOCIAL SUPPORT

Having a positive outlook on life and good self-esteem appear to have long-lasting health consequences,[30] and good social support is also a positive influence on the measures of allostatic load.[31] Positive affect, assessed by aggregating momentary experiences throughout a working or leisure day, was found to be associated with lower cortisol production and higher heart rate variability (showing higher parasympathetic activity), and a lower fibrinogen response to a mental stress test.[32]

On the other hand, poor self-esteem has been shown to cause recurrent increases in cortisol levels during a repetition of a public speaking challenge in which those individuals with good self-esteem are able to habituate (i.e., attenuate their cortisol response after the first speech).[33] Furthermore, poor self-esteem and low internal locus of control have been related to 12% to 13% smaller volume of the hippocampus in both younger and older subjects, and higher cortisol levels during a mental arithmetic stressor.[34]

Related to both positive affect and self-esteem is the role of friends and social interactions in maintaining a healthy outlook on life. Loneliness, often found in people with low self-esteem, has been associated with larger cortisol responses to wakening in the morning and higher fibrinogen and natural killer cell responses to a mental stress test, and sleep problems.[35] On the other hand, having three or more regular social contacts, as opposed to 0 to 2 such contacts, is associated with lower allostatic load scores.[31]

DELETERIOUS ROLE OF ADVERSE EARLY LIFE EXPERIENCE

The aging process begins at conception, and experiences early in life have a profound influence on the quality and length of life. Early life experiences perhaps carry an even greater weight in terms of how an individual reacts to new situations.[15] For example, adverse early life experiences involving physical and sexual abuse carry with it a life-long burden of behavioral and pathophysiologic problems, and cold and uncaring families produce long-lasting emotional problems in children. These adverse experiences impact upon brain structure and function and the risk for later depression and posttraumatic stress disorder.[36,37]

CONCLUSIONS

Because environmental factors and experiences play a large role in the aging process, understanding and manipulating those factors can reduce the accumulation of allostatic overload. There are a number of approaches to deal with stress and allostatic overload as they affect the life course and affect health later in life. For the individual, these include lifestyle, personal habits, and pharmaceutical agents. For society, there are policies of government and the private sector.

For the individual, life-long habits may be hard to change, and it is often necessary to turn to pharmacologic interventions: sleeping pills, anxiolytics, β-blockers, and antidepressants are all drugs that are used to counteract some of the problems associated with the accumulation of allostatic overload. Likewise, drugs that reduce oxidative stress or inflammation, block cholesterol synthesis or absorption and treat insulin resistance or chronic pain can help deal with the metabolic and neurologic consequences of being chronically stressed out. All of these agents have value, and yet each one has side effects and limitations that are based in part on the fact that all of the systems that are dysregulated in allostatic overload are also systems that interact with each other and perform normal functions when properly regulated, as described in Figure 26-2. Because of the nonlinearity of the systems of allostasis, the consequences of any pharmaceutical treatment may be either to inhibit the beneficial effects of the systems in question or to perturb other systems in a direction that promotes an unwanted side effect. Examples of the former include the problems with cox 2 inhibitors[38] and examples of the latter include the obesity-inducing effects of some of the atypical antipsychotics that are widely used to treat schizophrenia and bipolar disorder.[39]

The private sector has a powerful role, and businesses that encourage healthy lifestyle practices among their employees are likely to gain reduced health insurance costs and possibly a more loyal workforce.[40,41] Moreover, governmental policies are important, and the Acheson Report[42] from the United Kingdom in 1998 recognized that no public policy should be enacted without considering the implications for health of all citizens. Thus basic education, housing, taxation, setting of a minimum wage, and addressing occupational health and safety and environmental pollution regulations are all likely to affect health via a myriad of mechanisms. At the same time, providing higher quality food and making it affordable and accessible in poor and affluent neighborhoods, is necessary for people to eat better, providing they also learn what types of food to eat and can afford them. Likewise, making neighborhoods safer and more congenial and supportive[43] can improve opportunities for positive social interactions and increased recreational physical activity. For the elderly population, community centers and activities that promote social interactions and physical activity have been demonstrated to be beneficial.[44,45]

Finally, there are programs that combine some of the key elements just described, namely, education, physical activity, and social support, along with one other ingredient that is hard to quantify: namely, finding meaning and purpose in life. One example is the Executive Volunteer Corps and another is the Experience Corps, which takes elderly volunteers and trains them as teachers' assistants for younger children in the neighborhood schools.[46] Not only does this program improve the education of the children, it also benefits the elderly volunteers and improves their physical and mental health.[47] Thus finding ways of improving the social and physical environment in which people live their lives should reduce the need for more direct medical and psychiatric interventions for everyone, particularly the elderly.

KEY POINTS

Allostasis and Allostatic Overload in the Context of Aging

- Events of daily life can produce the feeling of being "stressed out" and elevate and sustain activities of physiologic systems and promote health damaging behaviors and poor sleep.
- Accumulated over time, this results in wear and tear on the body, which is called "allostatic load/overload." This accumulated wear and tear reflects not only the impact of experiences, but also genetic constitution, individual behaviors and lifestyle habits, and early life experiences that set life-long patterns of behavior and physiologic reactivity.
- Hormones and other mediators associated with stress and allostatic overload protect the body in the short run and promote adaptation by the process known as allostasis.
- The brain is the key organ of stress, allostasis, and allostatic overload because it determines what is threatening and therefore stressful, and also determines the physiologic and behavioral responses. Brain regions such as the hippocampus, amygdala, and prefrontal cortex respond to acute and chronic stress by undergoing structural remodeling, which alters behavioral and physiologic responses.
- Imaging studies of the human brain show smaller hippocampal volume in mild cognitive impairment in aging, Type 2 diabetes and prolonged major depressive illness, and in individuals with low self-esteem. Structural and functional alterations in amygdala and prefrontal cortex are also reported.
- Besides pharmaceutical agents, approaches to alleviate chronic stress and prevent diseases related to allostatic overload include changes in personal habits and lifestyle, and policies of government and business that would improve the ability of individuals to reduce their own chronic stress burden as they become older.

For a complete list of references, please visit online only at www.expertconsult.com

CHAPTER 27

Neuroendocrinology of Aging

Roberta Diaz Brinton

Neuroendocrine senescence is a multifactorial process with a high degree of interpersonal variability and subject to a host of beneficial or detrimental influences. As such, neuroendocrine aging is an illustrative example of both the aging process and of modifiers of aging[1] (also see Chapter 20). Neuroendocrine aging is inextricably linked with reproductive aging. In this regard, reproductive senescence and the stages therein provide a window into the dysregulation of endocrine systems that ultimately results in the aging profile. For both women and men reproductive aging results from the complex interplay of age-dependent endocrine changes and the hypothalamus-pituitary-gonadal axis.[2] Although reproductive senescence leads to a loss of function, the neuroendocrine profile is characterized by both gains and loss of function. This brief review focuses on reproductive aging in women and men as an illustrative case of neuroendocrine aging. Further reviewed is the impact of neuroendocrine changes of reproductive senescence on a hallmark of aging—decreased metabolism.

Reproductive Aging in Women

The female reproductive axis is composed of the hypothalamic-pituitary-ovarian-uterine axis and undergoes accelerated aging relative to other systems that are otherwise healthy. Reproductive senescence in women is defined by oocyte depletion, which begins at birth and proceeds as a continuum until menopause is achieved. A woman is endowed at birth with a finite number of oocytes that are arrested in prophase I of meiosis. Reproductive aging consists of a steady loss of oocytes through ovarian follicular atresia or ovulation, which does not necessarily occur at a constant rate.[3–5] The relatively wide age range (42 to 58 years) for menopause in normal women seems to indicate that women are either endowed with a highly variable number of oocytes or that the rate of oocyte loss varies greatly. Menopause occurs at an average age of 51.4 years with a Gaussian distribution from 40 to 58 years.[2] In the United States, approximately 1.5 million women reach menopause each year, and more than 45 million women will be over the age of 55 in 2020.[6]

Normal reproductive aging in women is characterized by three distinct phases that can span years: perimenopause (also known as the menopause transition), menopause, and postmenopause. According to the Stages of Reproductive Aging Workshop (STRAW),[6] reproductive senescence occurs over the span of years that can be subdivided into three distinct stages.[6] Variable cycle length, variable cycle intervals, and high FSH characterize the menopausal transition or perimenopause, subdivided into early and late transition states. A year of amenorrhea is considered the end to the perimenopause state. The end of the amenorrhic year constitutes the onset of the postmenopausal stage, which is also subdivided into early and late components. Early postmenopause is defined by 4 years since the last menstrual period. Subsequent to these 4 years, late stage postmenopause then ensues and lasts until the woman's death.

PERIMENOPAUSE TO MENOPAUSE

The menopause transition or perimenopause is characterized by menstrual and endocrine changes in the hypothalamic-pituitary-ovarian-uterine axis that lead inexorably to reproductive senescence.[7] During perimenopause, ovulation occurs irregularly as a result of fluctuations in the hypothalamic and pituitary hormones.[3,5,8] In late phase perimenopause, nearly half of cycles are anovulatory.[5] In the ovulatory cycles, FSH, LH, and E2 levels increase with progression of STRAW stage, and in the luteal phase, serum progesterone decreases. Early cycle (ovulatory and anovulatory) inhibin B decreases steadily across the STRAW stages and is largely undetectable during elongated ovulatory and anovulatory cycles during the transition. The decline of inhibin B during early perimenopause results in the rise in follicle-stimulating hormone (FSH), with no significant change in inhibin A or estradiol levels.[9] FSH levels may rise during some cycles but return to premenopausal levels in subsequent cycles.[9] Further complicating the determination of FSH concentration is the pulsatile pattern of secretion. The variability in hormone levels creates difficulties in interpreting a single laboratory test value[3] but an increase in FSH continues to be a clinical marker of ensuing menopause and postmenopause.[6]

In late stage perimenopause, concentrations of 17β-estradiol are highly variable.[5] Estrogen levels can be both persistently low, as might be expected, but can also be abnormally high. High 17β-estradiol concentration is associated with increased vulnerability to neurodegenerative insults and neuronal cell death.[10] A high level of 17β-estradiol does not reduce the persistently high FSH and LH levels.[4,5] Remarkably, the cyclicity of progesterone appears to remain generally intact, whereas the level of progesterone can vary between normal values, to high spikes of progesterone, to undetectable levels.[9]

Menopause is the final stage of perimenopause and is complete after 12 months of amenorrhea following the final menstrual cycle, which reflects a near complete but natural decrease in ovarian hormone secretion. Three to 11 months of amenorrhea or of irregular periods in women aged 45 to 55 years were most predictive of menopause within the following 3 years.[3]

Symptomatically, hot flashes (also referred to as flushes) are most likely to occur during late stage perimenopause and early stage postmenopause.[6] The prevalence of hot flashes in women is low but present in ~10% of women during the late stage of reproductive life.[11] Prevalence increases substantially in early perimenopause, reaches a maximum in late stage perimenopause, remains high into the early postmenopausal stage, and returns to a low but persistent prevalence in late stage postmenopausal women.[11] Prevalence for hot flashes can range from 30% to 80%.[12] Women aged 40 to 60 years who have had a hysterectomy and oophorectomy are at high risk for hot flashes.[11,12] In most women, hot flashes are transient. The condition improves within a few months in about 30% to 50% of women and resolves in 85% to 90% of women within 4 to 5 years. However,

10% to 15% of women continue to have hot flashes into late stage postmenopause. Although the mechanism leading to hot flashes remains unknown, the resemblance to heat-dissipation responses has led to the dysfunction of thermoregulation by the anterior hypothalamus hypothesis. The exact role of estrogen in the pathogenesis of hot flashes remains unresolved. While estrogen levels do not differ substantially between postmenopausal women who have hot flashes and those who do not, the withdrawal of estrogen can induce hot flashes in women with gonadal dysgenesis who received estrogen therapy that was subsequently discontinued, suggesting that estrogen withdrawal plays a role in the cause of hot flashes.[11] In the Study of Women's Health Across the Nation (SWAN), a large U.S. multicenter cohort study, higher levels of FSH were the only hormonal measure independently associated with flushing after adjustment for levels of estradiol and other hormones.[11] Women undergoing pharmacologic therapies to antagonize estrogen receptor activation by selective estrogen receptor modulators (SERMS) or to inhibit estrogen synthesis using 5α-reductase inhibitors for breast cancer experience a significant rise in the frequency of hot flashes.

POSTMENOPAUSE

Like the perimenopause, postmenopause is separated into an early and late stage. Early postmenopause is defined as 5 years since the final menstrual cycle.[6] Levels of FSH continue to be high during early menopause and remain elevated throughout the late stage of postmenopause.[6] During the early postmenopause phase there is a significant decline in ovarian hormones to a permanently low level, which is associated with accelerated bone loss.[13,14] Postmenopausal women undergo two phases of bone loss, whereas aging men undergo only one.[14] In women, the menopause initiates an accelerated phase of predominantly trabecular bone (also known as cancellous and spongy bone) loss that declines over 4 to 8 years, followed by a slow phase that disappears after 15 to 20 years when severe depletion of trabecular bone stimulates counter-regulatory forces that limit further loss.[14] The accelerated phase results from the loss of the direct repressive effects of estrogen on bone turnover, which is mediated by estrogen receptors in both osteoblasts and osteoclasts. During menopause, bone resorption increases by 90%, whereas bone formation markers increase by only 45%. In the ensuing slow phase, the rate of trabecular bone loss is reduced, but the rate of cortical bone loss can be increased.[14] Both serum-bioavailable estrogen and testosterone decline in aging men, and bioavailable estrogen is the major predictor of their bone loss. Thus both sex steroids are important for developing peak bone mass, but estrogen deficiency is the major determinant of age-related bone loss in both sexes.[14] Trabecular bone has low density and strength but very high surface area and fills the inner cavity of long bones. The external layer of trabecular bone contains red bone marrow, where hematopoiesis occurs and where most of the arteries and veins of bone organs are found. A wide range of pharmacologic agents are available to prevent and treat osteoporosis, including antiresorptive estrogen, selective estrogen receptor modulators (SERMS), bisphosphonates, calcitonin, or anabolic therapies including parathyroid hormone (PTH1-34 or PTH 1-84) and agents with yet undetermined mechanism of action such as strontium ranelate.[15,16] Corrections in general deficiencies in calcium, vitamin D, or both are a first line of therapeutic intervention.[15,16]

Therapeutic horizons

Multiple pharmacologic and nonpharmacologic interventions have been used to treat hot flashes, with the most common pharmacologic intervention being estrogen or hormone therapy.[11,17] Multiple types of estrogen, doses, and routes of administration have been developed. Each formulation targets cessation of hot flashes and prevention of osteoporosis with near equal efficacy depending on the dose.[11] A recent position statement from the North American Menopause Society (NAMS) supports initiation of estrogen or hormone therapy around the time of menopause to treat menopause-related symptoms.[18] Use of hormone therapy was supported to treat or reduce the risk of certain disorders, such as osteoporosis or fractures and hot flashes in select postmenopausal women.[19] Analysis of the benefit-risk ratio for menopausal hormone therapy indicated favorable benefit close to menopause but decreased benefit with aging and advanced time after menopause in previously untreated women.[18] The attendant risks and side effects of estrogen or hormone therapy are substantial,[20] which has led to behavioral and alternative therapies. However, there is no convincing evidence that acupuncture, yoga, Chinese herbs, dong quai, evening primrose oil, ginseng, kava, red clover extract, or vitamin E improve hot flashes.[11] Clinical trials of soy phytoestrogens have been inconsistent in showing benefit, with most randomized double-blind clinical trials indicating no significant benefit for treatment of hot flashes.[21]

The association between hormone therapy and increased risk of neoplasias in reproductive organs (see Chapter 89) has led to the development of selective estrogen receptor modulators in an attempt to selectively activate the beneficial effects of estrogen while reducing the risks of therapy. In recent years, an increasing number of estrogen receptor ligands and novel SERMs have been identified from nature, whereas others have been designed and synthesized de novo within academia and the pharmaceutical industry.[22] The FDA-approved indications for hormone therapy in women are for treatment of hot flashes and prevention of osteoporosis, whereas SERMs are approved for breast cancer prevention and treatment of osteoporosis. Thus pharmaceutical industry efforts focus on the FDA-approved indications along with antineoplastic action in the breast and uterus. Although these molecules are diverse, the unifying feature of these development efforts is that they do not specifically target estrogenic actions in the brain and they typically increase the occurrence and frequency of hot flashes.[22] The oldest and most studied SERM is tamoxifen (TMX), a triphenylethylene derivative, nonsteroidal first-generation SERM.[22] 4-hydroxytamoxifen (OHT) is a minor metabolite of TMX, with a shorter half-life but binds to ER with a binding affinity 20 to 30 times greater than TMX and equivalent to that of 17β-estradiol.[22] Tamoxifen functions as an ER antagonist in the breast, but can act as an ER agonist activity in bone, liver, and uterus.[22] Since 1971 TMX has been used to treat breast cancer in premenopausal and postmenopausal women and in 1999 TMX was recommended for use in breast cancer prevention.[22] Another nonsteroidal SERM for the treatment of osteoporosis is raloxifene (RAL), a benzothiophene derivative nonsteroidal second-generation SERM. Similar to TMX,

RAL has a mixed pharmacologic profile, acting as both an ER agonist and antagonist in a tissue-specific manner. In the breast and uterus, RAL acts as a classic antiestrogen to inhibit the growth of mammary or endometrial carcinoma, whereas in nonreproductive tissues, it acts as a partial estrogen agonist to prevent bone loss and lower serum cholesterol with a pharmacologic profile similar to that of 17β-estradiol in both ovariectomized rats and postmenopausal women.[22] In recent years, an increasing number of third and fourth generation novel SERMs has been identified and developed within both academia and the pharmaceutical industry.[22] With enhanced efficacy, specificity, and antineoplastic action in the breast and uterus, novel SERMs demonstrate more potential clinically therapeutic uses for prevention or treatment of menopause-related symptoms, such as hot flashes and osteoporosis. One such molecule is bazedoxifene, developed by Wyeth in collaboration with Ligand Pharmaceuticals. Available data for tolerability and efficacy suggest that bazedoxifene can significantly reduce bone loss, prevent fractures, and is expected to be an attractive choice for a wide range of postmenopausal women who are estimated to have osteoporosis or are at risk for developing the disease.[23] The combined use of bazedoxifene and conjugated estrogens is currently under clinical development for the prevention of postmenopausal osteoporosis and the treatment of vasomotor symptoms associated with menopause.[23] Eli Lilly, which originally developed RAL marketed under the trade name of Evista, is currently testing its next generation SERM arzoxifene in a phase III clinical trial for preventing or treating osteoporosis and breast cancer in postmenopausal women. Preclinical data have demonstrated that arzoxifene is a potent estrogen antagonist in mammary and uterine tissue while acting as an estrogen agonist to maintain bone density and lower serum cholesterol.[22,23] SERMs that target estrogen action in the brain are being developed as NeuroSERMs and PhytoSERMs and are in early stage preclinical development.[24,25]

Unresolved issues in reproductive senescence in women

To date, there is no pharmacogenomic strategy for identifying women appropriate for hormone therapy or which hormone therapy would be most efficacious. Genomic strategies to date have identified estrogen receptor polymorphisms associated with increased risk of cognitive impairment in aged women. However, several single nucleotide polymorphisms (SNPs) on *ERα* (*ESR1*) and *ERβ* (*ESR2*) genes have been associated with a range of hormone-sensitive diseases, such as breast cancer and osteoporosis. Estrogen receptor genetic variations may also influence cognitive aging and were investigated in a cohort of 1343 women (mean age 73.4 years) and 1184 men (mean age 73.7 years).[26] Among women, two of the *ERα* SNPs (rs8179176, rs9340799)[26,27] and two of the *ERβ* SNPs (rs1256065, rs1256030) were associated with the likelihood of developing cognitive impairment.[26] In men, one of the *ERα* SNPs (rs728524) and two of the *ERβ* (rs1255998, rs1256030) were associated with cognitive impairment. These findings suggest that estrogen receptor genetic variants may play a role in cognitive aging. Tailoring hormone therapy based on SNP profile remains uncharted territory.

Timing of hormone therapy intervention is of critical importance and several studies are underway to determine the impact of timing of hormone therapy. Emerging evidence supports a critical window of therapeutic opportunity[28] that is related to the healthy cell bias of estrogen action.[29,30] The healthy cell bias of estrogen action hypothesis predicts that estrogen therapy, if initiated at the time of perimenopause to menopause when neurologic health is not yet comprised, will be of benefit as manifested as reduced risk for age-associated neurodegenerative diseases, such as Alzheimer's and Parkinson's.[29,30]

The issue of whether oophorectomy before undergoing the menopause transition has implications for neuroendocrine and neurologic aging remains unresolved. However, increasing evidence indicates that the natural process of reproductive senescence is a systematic biologic strategy to transition from reproductive fertility to reproductive senescence. In contrast, women undergoing oophorectomy typically have not undergone this systematic transition that requires years to complete. Emerging evidence indicates that oophorectomy before menopause transition has profound consequences for subsequent risk of neurodegenerative disease. Women who underwent either unilateral oophorectomy or bilateral oophorectomy before the onset of menopause had significant increased risk of parkinsonism, cognitive impairment or dementia, and diagnosed depressive illness relative to referent women.[31–33] The increased risk for either parkinsonism or cognitive impairment was similar regardless of the indication for the oophorectomy, and for women who underwent unilateral or bilateral oophorectomy, they were considered separately.[31,32,34] The risk of parkinsonism and of cognitive impairment or dementia increased following oophorectomy with significant linear trends of increasing risk for either outcome with a younger age at oophorectomy.[34] In women who underwent bilateral oophorectomy at younger ages with depressive illness, treatment with estrogen to age 50 years did not modify the long-term risk of depressive and anxiety symptoms.[33] Further, mortality was significantly higher in women who had received a prophylactic bilateral oophorectomy before the age of 45 years relative to referent women (hazard ratio 1.67 [95% CI, 1.16–2.40], $p = 0.006$).[35] Increased mortality was observed principally in women who had not received estrogen therapy up to the age of 45 years.[35] Collectively, these emerging data indicate a significant and profound impact of prohibiting the menopause transition.

The long-lasting changes in the brain that underlie the transition are largely unexplored beyond the changes in hypothalamic hormones involved in the reproductive cycle. The early, unrelenting, and persistent elevated levels of FSH and the consequences at the cellular and systems level in the brain remain unknown. The rise in FSH is a remarkable example of a gain of function associated with aging.

Major challenges for optimal estrogen and hormone therapy remain. Beyond the timing issue,[28,29] the real and perceived risks of hormone therapy remain and are amplified by results of both the WHI and WHIMS trials.[36–38] It is clear that many, *but not all*, women could potentially benefit from estrogen or hormone therapy intervention. Biomarkers to identify women appropriate for treatment and the type of hormone regimen remains largely undeveloped beyond hot flashes. Hormone therapy interventions that selectively target the benefits of estrogen while avoiding untoward risk factors remain an unmet need in women's health. Estrogen alternatives that activate estrogen mechanisms in the brain but not in the breast or uterus, such as NeuroSERMs and PhytoSERMs, are promising strategies for sustaining the benefits of estrogen in the brain to prevent age-associated neurodegenerative disease.[30,39]

ANDROPAUSE

Like the female reproductive endocrine system, the male system reproductive axis is composed of the hypothalamic-pituitary-gonadal (HPG) axis, but unlike women the male reproductive system does not undergo accelerated aging, and fertility can be sustained throughout a man's lifespan.[40] Unlike women, for whom menopause leads to the irreversible end of reproductive life, an end of gonadal function and as a consequence low sex hormone levels in all postmenopausal women, fertility persists in men until very old age and the age-associated decrease in testosterone levels is slowly progressive.

Eventhough the age-associated decrease in testosterone levels is slowly progressive, a substantial proportion of men in their 80s still have bioavailable testosterone levels comparable to the normal range of young men. Therefore a significant decline in androgen levels is not a generalized feature of male aging, and as a rule androgen deficiency is only partial.[40] Moreover, the threshold level(s) of testosterone below which consequences of androgen deficiency become manifest, and which or how many clinical symptoms best establish the diagnosis of androgen deficiency, remains uncertain.[41] Thus the existence of andropause as a medically definable condition remains controversial.[42] Arguments in favor of clinical significance are the similarities between the symptomatology of aging and that of androgen deficiency in young hypogonadal men.[40] Opposing arguments cite the near ubiquitous decline of almost all physiologic systems and thus the decline in testosterone synthesis by the gonads is considered just one part of the complex mosaic of aging.[43] As such, the terms partial androgen deficiency of the aging male or late onset hypogonadism have been proposed as alternatives to andropause or male climacteric because of the connotation of a generalized phenomenon and of permanent infertility.

Consistent with a primary testicular cause of decreased testosterone production, mean serum luteinizing hormone (LH) levels in the male population tend to increase with age but this increase is of modest amplitude and is inconsistent.[40] For example, many elderly men with a serum testosterone concentration below that of young men do not have elevated LH levels. Moreover, the modest increases in basal serum LH in elderly men appear to result in part from a slower plasma clearance rather than from increased pituitary secretion.[40] Neuroendocrine aging in men is characterized by dysregulation of the pulsatile release pattern of LH secretion, whereas the regulation of FSH secretion is essentially maintained.[40] Therapeutically this is of significance as the testicular residual secretory capacity could allow many elderly men to substantially raise their serum testosterone levels, provided there was physiologically appropriate LH activation. The change in LH secretory pattern is due to changes in the feedback regulatory mechanisms within the hypothalamus as pituitary secretory capacity is preserved in the elderly.[40]

Testosterone is largely bound to plasma proteins, only 1% to 2% being free, with 40% to 50% loosely bound to albumin, and 50% to 60% specifically and strongly bound to steroid hormone binding globulin (SHBG).[40,44] Unbound testosterone diffuses passively through the cell membranes into the target cell, where it binds to the specific androgen receptor (AR).[40] Androgen concentration in target tissues depends on plasma concentration of bioavailable androgen, local androgen metabolism, and the presence of androgen receptor. As would be expected, total androgen (testosterone + dihydrotestosterone [DHT]) concentration is highest in the prostate and scrotal skin, and higher in pubic skin than in striated muscle. In prostate and scrotal skin, the concentration of DHT is 5 to 10 times higher than that of testosterone, whereas in muscle DHT levels are extremely low. In the prostate, almost all androgenic effects are exerted by DHT via conversion of testosterone by type 2 5α-reductase.[40] In many tissues DHT mediates most androgenic effects of testosterone. A notable exception is muscle, where testosterone is the active androgen.[40] Androgen deficiency is characterized by total testosterone levels of less than 300 ng/dL or bioavailable testosterone level of less than 5 ng/dL.[45]

Androgenic actions of testosterone and DHT are mediated via binding to the androgen receptor (AR). Although testosterone and DHT bind to the same receptor, the affinity of DHT for the AR is greater than that of testosterone. Expression of AR is increased by androgens and estrogens (especially in the prostate), and decreased in aging in different tissues. In addition to the well-characterized nuclear androgen receptor that activates gene transcription, testosterone can also exert rapid, nongenomic effects, in part via binding to a G protein-coupled membrane receptor. The SHBG-testosterone complex initiates a cAMP-mediated, transcription-independent signaling pathway affecting calcium channels.[40] AR is highly expressed in male accessory sex organs and in some areas of the brain, whereas a lower level of AR expression occurs in skeletal muscle, in the heart and vascular smooth muscle, and in bone.[40] Sensitivity of AR to androgens is modulated by polymorphisms of the AR. The AR gene contains a polymorphic trinucleotide CAG-repeat in exon 1, which encodes a functionally relevant polyglutamine tract of variable length. A CAG-repeat length exceeding the normal range of 15 to 31 results in diminished AR transactivation function. Clinical studies have indicated that AR polymorphisms are associated with a higher prevalence of several androgen-sensitive diseases, including prostate cancer.[40]

A subset of the physiologic actions of testosterone derives from its aromatization to 17β-estradiol, which binds to estrogen receptors (ERs).[40] Documented estrogen-mediated actions of testosterone in men include a role in the feedback regulation of LH, a role in the regulation of skeletal homeostasis, and a role in lipid metabolism and cardiovascular physiology; among other possible estrogen actions in men, there are indications for a role in the brain and in spermatogenesis.[40] It appears that similar to women, declining bioavailable estrogen levels can play a significant role in age-related bone loss and fracture risk in men.[46] Consistent with a role of estrogen in bone development and remodeling, males with a homozygous deletion of the *ERα* gene or aromatase deficiency have unfused epiphyses, elevated markers of bone remodeling, and low bone mass despite normal or elevated testosterone levels.[46] Moreover, aromatase-deficient males responded to estrogen therapy with marked increases in bone mass, consistent with an "anabolic" effect of estrogen, in contrast to its predominantly antiresorptive action in postmenopausal women.[46] As in women, aging in men is associated with continuous loss of bone and an exponential increase of the incidence of fractures of the hip and the spine.[46] Moreover, in older men the consequences of fractures in terms of morbidity and mortality appear to be more severe than in their female counterparts.[46] Acquired profound hypogonadism in men induces high bone turnover and accelerated bone loss, which parallels bone loss in elderly men.[46] Placebo-controlled clinical studies have shown that the benefits of testosterone to bone in older men are likely to depend largely, but not completely, on aromatization of the steroid to estradiol.[42] However, declining bioavailable testosterone levels may also contribute as testosterone is an antiresorptive agent and promote maintenance of bone formation along with being aromatized to estradiol.[46]

Therapeutic horizons

Androgen hormone therapy is available in multiple formulations that range from oral tablets to transdermal gels and patches to buccal adhesives to long-acting intramuscular injectables.[45] As with hormone therapy in women, testosterone therapy may be associated with increased risk of serious adverse effects in men. Metastatic prostate cancer and breast cancer are hormone-dependent cancers that may be stimulated to grow during testosterone treatment.[45] Consequently, the use of testosterone therapy, with its potential to increase risk and/or progression of prostate tumorigenesis, has been controversial and has led to the development of selective androgen receptor modulators (SARMs) that lack significant androgen action in the prostate but exert agonist effects in select androgen-responsive tissues of interest, including brain, muscle, and bone.[47] Several strategies of SARM design are being pursued.[48,49] The first strategy is to develop novel steroidal compounds that are not substrates for the enzyme 5α-reductase, which converts testosterone to DHT. As mentioned above, prostate growth is largely induced by DHT rather than testosterone as DHT exhibits ~tenfold greater potency for AR, which reflects both a higher binding affinity for AR and a slower dissociation rate from AR.[47] SARMs that are not 5α-reductase substrates and thus do not form DHT or DHT-like derivatives have relatively low androgen action in the prostate. There are several synthetic androgens in this class that are potentially promising candidates with varied affinity for AR and androgenic activity, including 7α-cyano-19-nortestosterone, 7α-acetylthio-19-nortestosterone, 19-Nor-4-androstene-3β,17β-diol 3β,19-nortestosterone, and 4-estren-3α17β-diol.[49] At this time, the most promising SARM in this category is 7a-methyl-19-nortestosterone, commonly referred to as MENT.[50–53] MENT, developed by the Population Council, is currently in clinical trials as an androgen therapy for hypogonadal men and exhibits low androgen activity in the prostate but is more potent than testosterone in other peripheral androgen-responsive tissues including bone.[49] Although not a substrate for 5α-reductase, MENT is a substrate for aromatase and thus, like testosterone, can be converted to estradiol. Because many cellular effects of testosterone result from aromatization to estradiol and subsequent activation of ER-dependent signaling, there is potentially strong benefit in a SARM that exhibits both androgen and estrogen functions. The effects of MENT on neural function are virtually unknown. The testosterone-based structure of MENT strongly suggests blood-brain barrier permeability. Another promising SARM in this class is 19-Nor-4-androstene-3β,17β-diol (also called estren-ß). Estren-ß has high affinity for both estrogen and androgen receptors, a property that has benefits and liabilities as a SARM.[49] A second SARM design strategy is the development of nonsteroidal synthetic AR ligands.[54] Of particular interest are compounds that bind AR but have altered interaction with AR binding pocket side chains that underlie tissue specificity.[49] An example of this class is BMS-564929, which is currently in clinical trials to improve musculoskeletal end points in hypogonadal men.

Unresolved issues in reproductive senescence in men

Many of the issues that are unresolved for reproductive senescence are applicable to men. The issue of hormone therapy for androgen deficiency remains controversial. Lowering of testosterone concentrations in adult men by surgical orchiectomy or by GnRH agonist or antagonist administration is associated with rapid and marked loss of bone mineral density, an increase in fat mass, and a loss of muscle mass and strength.[41,46] Lowering of testosterone concentrations also results in hot flashes and a decrease in overall sexual activity, thoughts, and fantasies.[45] Hot flashes are common among men treated with androgen deprivation therapy for prostate cancer.[11]

Testosterone therapy may be associated with increased risk of serious adverse effects in men. Metastatic prostate cancer and breast cancer are hormone-dependent cancers that may be stimulated to grow during testosterone treatment.[45] As prostate cancer is most typically a function of age, the long-term consequence of surgical or pharmacologic orchiectomy beyond the impact on bone and blood has not been established in men. Nor have biomarkers been developed to adequately identify men appropriate for androgen or SARM therapy.

Neuroendocrine aging and brain metabolism: implications for neurodegenerative disease

On average, the adult human brain represents approximately 2% of body weight but accounts for 20% of the oxygen and, hence, calories consumed by the body, which is 10 times that expected on the basis of its weight alone.[55] The high rate of metabolism is remarkably constant despite widely varying mental and motor activities.[55] Ongoing metabolic activity consists largely of the oxidation of glucose to carbon dioxide and water, resulting in the production of large amounts of energy in the form of ATP. Most of the energy used in the brain is required for the propagation of action potentials and for restoring postsynaptic ion fluxes after receptors have been stimulated by the neurotransmitter. Thus the greatest majority of the metabolic activity in the brain is devoted to synaptic processes.[55]

The significant portion of energy metabolism in the brain devoted to maintaining synaptic transmission and integrity suggests that decrements in energy production would first effect synaptic transmission and physiology. Consistent with this postulate, mounting evidence suggests that Alzheimer's disease (AD) begins with subtle alterations of hippocampal synaptic efficacy before frank neuronal degeneration.[56] Further, hypometabolism in the brain predicts cognitive decline years in advance of the clinical diagnosis of AD.[57] The association between mitochondrial dysfunction and neurodegenerative diseases, such as Alzheimer's and Parkinson's, is mounting along with evidence that hypometabolism and a concomitant reduction and dysfunction in mitochondrial gene expression in the brain are antecedents to the cognitive deficits of AD.[57–60] The association between hypometabolism and AD is based on multiple levels of analysis and experimental paradigms that range from genomic analyses in animal models and the postmortem autopsy human brain to in vitro cell model systems to brain imaging in humans. Overall, each of these levels of analyses indicate that dysfunction in glucose metabolism, bioenergetics, and mitochondrial function are consistent antecedents to development of Alzheimer pathology.[57,60–67] The decline in brain glucose metabolism and mitochondrial function can appear decades before diagnosis and thus may serve as a biomarker of AD risk and a therapeutic target.[57,63,67,68]

The circumstances that initiate hypometabolism remain to be fully determined but one clue is the shift in the brain from glucose as the primary energetic fuel to ketone bodies. Under metabolically challenging conditions (i.e., starvation, aging, and neurodegeneration), neurons can use acetyl-CoA generated from ketone body metabolism (ketolysis) produced by the liver or under conditions of starvation in neighboring glial cells.[30] In AD there is a generalized shift toward use of an alternative fuel, ketone bodies. This is evidenced by an observed 45% reduction in cerebral glucose use in AD patients,[69] which is paralleled by a decrease in the expression of glycolytic enzymes that are coupled to a decrease in the activity of the pyruvate dehydrogenase complex.[70] Further, although there is a 100:0 ratio of glucose to other substrates utilization in young controls, there is a 2:1 ratio in incipient AD patients compared with a ratio of 29:1 in healthy elderly controls.[71]

Basic science analyses indicate that the endogenous estrogen, 17β-estradiol, significantly increases glucose uptake, glucose metabolism, insulin growth factor signaling, and the energetic capacity of brain mitochondria by maximizing aerobic glycolysis (oxidative phosphorylation coupled to pyruvate metabolism).[30,39] The enhanced aerobic glycolysis in the aging brain would be predicted to prevent conversion of the brain to use alternative sources of fuel such as the ketone body pathway characteristic of AD.[30,39] The ability of estrogen to sustain glucose as the primary fuel source in the brain by enhancing glucose transport, uptake, and aerobic glycolysis (oxidative phosphorylation coupled to pyruvate metabolism) is likely linked to its ability to prevent age-associated metabolic decline in the brain and thus could be a key mechanism whereby estrogen reduces the risk of AD in postmenopausal women.[30,39]

A growing body of evidence indicates that postmenopausal women experience a decline in brain metabolism that is prevented by estrogen therapy. As part of a 9-year study in the Baltimore Longitudinal Study of Aging, Resnick et al conducted positron emission tomography (PET) to assess regional cerebral blood flow in a small cohort of women who were estrogen therapy (ET) users versus women who were not. Results of this analysis showed that ET users and nonusers showed significant differences in PET-regional cerebral blood flow–relative activation patterns during the memory tasks. ET users showed better performance on neuropsychological tests of figural and verbal memory and on some aspects of the PET activation tests.[72] In a follow-up longitudinal study of the same cohort of healthy menopausal women, Maki and Resnick[73] found that regional cerebral blood flow was increased in estrogen therapy users relative to nonusers in the hippocampus, parahippocampal gyrus, and temporal lobe, regions that form a memory circuit and that are sensitive to preclinical AD.[73] Further, these investigators found that the increase in regional cerebral blood flow was associated with higher scores on a battery of cognitive tests.[73] In a separate 2-year follow-up analysis, Rasgon et al detected a significant decrease in metabolism of the posterior cingulate cortex among postmenopausal women at 2-year follow-up who did not receive estrogen, whereas those women who were estrogen users did not exhibit significant metabolic change in the posterior cingulate.[74] These findings that estrogen use may preserve regional cerebral metabolism and protect against metabolic decline in postmenopausal women, especially in the posterior cingulate cortex, is particularly important given that metabolism in this region of the brain declines in the earliest stages of AD.[60,74]

As might be expected from reduced energy metabolism, postmenopausal women are at greater risk for developing metabolic syndrome. A longitudinal, 9-year study of 949 participants in the Study of Women's Health Across the Nation (SWAN) investigated the natural history of the menopausal transition in women of five ethnicities at seven geographic sites.[75] By the onset of menopause, 13.7% of the women had new-onset metabolic syndrome. Odds of developing the metabolic syndrome per year in perimenopause were 1.45 (95% confidence interval, 1.35–1.56); after menopause, 1.24 (95% confidence interval, 1.18–1.30). Surprisingly, an increase in bioavailable testosterone or a decrease in sex hormone-binding globulin levels increased the odds of developing metabolic syndrome. This longitudinal study of the largest cohort of middle-aged women undergoing the menopausal transition indicated that the prevalence of the metabolic syndrome increased significantly during the perimenopausal and early postmenopausal years, independent of aging and other known cardiovascular disease risk factors such as weight gain and smoking. Increased bioavailable testosterone emerged as an independent predictor, after controlling for aging and cardiovascular disease risk factors. These findings suggest that progression through menopause, with the associated decrease in estrogen level, results in a progressively androgen-dominated hormonal milieu, which then increases the risk of developing metabolic syndrome.[75]

In contrast to the positive association of testosterone and metabolic syndrome in women, in healthy men there is a negative correlation between serum testosterone and free testosterone with visceral fat.[40] In a cohort study of 571 men aged 30 to 79 years, low testosterone levels predicted central obesity in men 12 years later.[40] Increased adiposity is itself partially responsible for a decrease of testosterone levels. Moreover, decreased growth hormone levels, as observed in elderly males, may also play a role in the age-associated changes in body composition.[40] Genetic analyses, functional imaging, and animal models of differential aerobic capacity indicate a role of decreased mitochondrial function in inducing the metabolic disturbances characteristic of insulin-resistant states in men.[76] Dysfunctional mitochondria were evidenced by decreased maximal aerobic capacity and decreased expression of mitochondrial genes involved in oxidative phosphorylation in men of northern European descent with impaired glucose tolerance (IGT) and type 2 diabetes.[76] Hypogonadal men with low testosterone levels had a threefold higher prevalence of the metabolic syndrome relative to men with normal testosterone level.[76] Low serum testosterone levels were associated with an adverse metabolic profile to suggest that low testosterone levels and impaired mitochondrial function promote insulin resistance in men.[76]

Remarkably, cognitively normal children, both male and female of 50 to 80 years old, with a maternal but not paternal history of Alzheimer's disease showed a reduction in the cerebral metabolic rate of glucose use in the same regions as clinically affected AD patients, involving the posterior cingulate cortex/precuneus, parietotemporal and frontal cortices, and medial temporal lobes.[67] As mitochondrial DNA is maternally inherited, these findings strongly suggest a relationship between mitochondrial function and hypometabolism characteristic of AD.[67]

Collectively, these findings indicate that decrements in gonadal hormones are associated with hypometabolism in the brain, increased risk of metabolic syndrome, and decreased glucose metabolism in the brain characteristic of Alzheimer's disease. Further, early intervention with hormone therapy reversed the hypometabolism associated with hypogonadal hormone status.

ACKNOWLEDGMENTS

Research and preparation of this review were supported by grants from the National Institute on Aging (P01 AG026572), National Institute of Mental Health (1R01 MH67159), the Alzheimer's Drug Discovery Foundation, and the Kenneth T. and Eileen L. Norris Foundation to RDB.

KEY POINTS

Neuroendocrinology of Aging

- Neuroendocrine senescence is a multifactorial process with a high degree of interpersonal variability and subject to a host of beneficial or detrimental influences.
- Normal reproductive aging in women is characterized by three distinct phases that can span years: perimenopause (also known as the menopause transition), menopause which typically occurs between 49 and 51 years of age, and postmenopause.
- Increasing evidence indicates that an oophorectomy before the natural menopause transition has profound consequences for subsequent risk of neurodegenerative disease.
- In men, fertility persists until very old age and the age-associated decrease in testosterone levels is slowly progressive.
- Loss of gonadal hormones can be associated with dysfunction in glucose metabolism, bioenergetics, and mitochondrial function in the brain. Decreased brain metabolism precedes development of Alzheimer pathology, can be manifested decades before diagnosis, and may serve as a biomarker of Alzheimer disease risk and as a therapeutic target.

For a complete list of references, please visit online only at www.expertconsult.com

CHAPTER 28

Normal Cognitive Aging

Jane Martin
Michelle Gorenstein

This chapter provides an overview of the principal features of cognitive functioning in normal aging adults. The first part of this chapter considers intelligence and the importance of estimating premorbid intellectual ability to detect discrepancies in functioning, followed by the concept of cognitive reserve being protective as we age. The cognitive functions of attention and processing speed, memory, verbal abilities, and executive functions are discussed in turn before a final section regarding the lifestyle factors associated with cognitive functioning. "Normal" in the present context refers to older individuals with no discernible mental illness and whose physical health is typical of their age group.

Intelligence and Aging

The figure of 5 million Americans aged 85 and above in 2007 is expected to grow to more than 19 million by the year 2050 based on projections by the U.S. Bureau of the Census.[1] By 2050 it is estimated there will be approximately 600,000 Americans aged 100 and above. As a consequence, cognitive studies of this age group are a necessary area of research. There is a need to understand what is normal or typical aging in contrast to the development of a disease process and additionally to understand what factors contribute to improved cognitive status with increasing age.

Literature on cognitive aging is based on studies of performance on standardized intelligence and neuropsychological tests. "IQ" refers to a derived score used in many test batteries designed to measure a hypothesized general ability: intelligence. The accepted definition is that general intelligence is a measure of overall ability on all types of intellectual tasks. General intelligence can be more specifically divided into the concepts of *fluid intelligence* and *crystallized intelligence*.[2] Fluid intelligence is the primary factor of most intelligence tests, measuring the degree to which an individual can solve novel problems without any previous training. On the other hand, crystallized intelligence is the amount of knowledge and information from the world that one brings to the testing situation. It has been established that fluid intelligence declines in older adults and crystallized intelligence is well preserved. The general theory is that fluid intelligence increases throughout childhood into young adulthood, but then plateaus and eventually declines; crystallized intelligence increases from childhood into late adulthood.[2]

Since a multitude of cognitive functions are assessed in an intelligence battery and IQ scores represent a composite of performances on different kinds of items, the meaningfulness of IQ is often questioned.[3] The only widely agreed-upon value of IQ tests is that IQ scores are good predictors of educational achievement and consequently, occupational outcome. The argument about the usefulness of IQ scores is that a composite score does not highlight important information that is only obtainable by examining discrete scores and, for that reason, most widely used tests, such as the Wechsler's Adult Intelligence Scale (WAIS-III),[4] now include measures of more discrete factors and domains. Even with the limitations, IQ scores help to provide a baseline of overall intellectual functioning from which to assess performance on cognitive tests as we age.

PREMORBID ABILITY

Lezak, Howieson, and Loring caution that an estimate of premorbid ability should never be based on a single test score, but instead should take into account as much information about the individual as possible.[3] Thus a good premorbid estimation of intelligence in adults uses current performance on tasks thought to be fairly resistant to neurologic change and demographics, such as educational and occupational attainment. This approach uses test scores obtained in the formal testing session of "hold" tests (i.e., tests that tap the abilities that are considered resistant to the effects of cerebral insult).[5] Aspects of cognitive functioning that involve overlearned activities change very little in the course of aging, whereas functions that involve processing speed, processing unfamiliar information, complex problem-solving, and delayed recall of information typically decline with age.[6] On the WAIS-III,[4] tests such as vocabulary, information, and picture completion are considered relatively resistant to the effects of aging and thus are useful "hold" tests to help estimate overall premorbid levels of cognitive functioning. However, limitations exist that must be considered. For example, the information subtest reflects an individual's general fund of information and the score may be misleading because this test is strongly affected by level of education. Scores on word reading tests, such as the National Adult Reading Test (NART)[7] developed in Britain and the subsequent AMNART[8] for use in the United States, correlate highly with IQ and have been found to be relatively resistant to cerebral insult.[5] However, the AMNART is not useful for an aphasic individual or someone with visual or articulatory problems. Again, the practice of using many sources of information to estimate an individual's premorbid level of cognitive functioning is essential.

Premorbid estimation of overall intellectual functioning is important to establish to compare current performance against some standard measure. However, comparing an individual's performance to a general population average score is misleading because it is only useful if the individual matches the population in terms of demographic measures, such as IQ and education. For example, *average* performance may be considered functioning at a normal level for one individual and may represent a significant decline for another individual. Thus a more useful approach is to compare an individual's current performance against an individualized standard. Only in this way can deficits or a diagnosis be discerned. Since premorbid neuropsychological test data are rarely available, it becomes necessary to estimate an individual's premorbid level of intellectual functioning against which present test scores can be compared to determine a change in cognitive functioning. Assessing a deficit involves comparing an individual's present performance on cognitive tests to an estimate of the individual's original ability level (premorbid level) and evaluating the discrepancies.[3]

COGNITIVE RESERVE

The concept of cognitive reserve[9,10] proposes that there are differences in how individuals are able to compensate once pathology disrupts the brain networks that normally underlie performance. Thus variability exists across individuals in their ability to compensate for cognitive changes as they age. The cognitive reserve model evolved in response to the fact that often there is not a direct relationship between the degree of brain pathology that disrupts performance and the degree of disruption in actual performance across individuals. In other words, often individuals with a similar degree of brain pathology differ in their clinical presentation of functional ability. Reserve may represent naturally occurring individual differences in the ability to perform a task or deal with increases in task difficulty. These differences may be due to innate intellectual ability, such as IQ, and/or they may be altered by experiences of education, occupation, or leisure activities.[10] Stern et al[10] suggest that a higher neural reserve might mean that brain networks that are either more efficient or more flexible in the face of increased demand may be less susceptible to disruption. This model suggests that the brain actively attempts to compensate for the challenge represented by brain disease and hypothesizes that adults with higher initial cognitive ability are better able to compensate for the effects of aging and dementia.[9]

According to the cognitive reserve model, impairments in cognition become apparent only after a reserve is depleted. Individuals with less reserve are likely to exhibit clinical impairments because they have relatively fewer resources to maintain them in the course of normal aging and disease-related changes, whereas individuals with more initial reserve can function longer without obvious clinical impairments because their supply of resources is greater.[11] The initial level of cognitive reserve may be determined by numerous factors, such as innate intellectual ability and differences in cognitive activity as the brain matures throughout the lifespan. It has been found that early education and higher levels of intellectual ability and activity are associated with slower cognitive decline as individuals age.[11–14] Fritsch et al[11] found that IQ and education had direct effects on global cognitive functioning, episodic memory, and processing speed, but that other midlife factors, such as occupational demands, were not significant predictors of late-life cognition. Studies of the relationship between childhood intelligence and cognitive decline in later life have found that individuals with lower childhood mental ability experience greater cognitive decline than those with higher childhood mental ability, suggesting that higher premorbid cognitive ability is protective of decline in later life.[12] Kliegel, Zimprich, and Rott[13] found that both early education and life-long intellectual activities seem to be of importance to cognitive performance in old age; higher early education and the greater number of intellectual activities continued throughout life served as a buffer against becoming cognitively impaired. Cognitive reserve research suggests that an active, engaged lifestyle, emphasizing mental activity and educational pursuits in early life, has a positive impact on cognitive functioning in later life. Thus individuals whose baseline cognitive functioning is at higher levels and who have an engaged lifestyle that typically includes interpersonal relationships and productive activities, will likely show less cognitive decline with age.

Attention and Processing Speed

Attention relates to one's ability to focus and concentrate on a given stimuli for a sustained period of time. Attention is a complex process that allows one to filter stimuli from the environment, hold and manipulate information, and respond appropriately.[5] Models of attention typically divide attention into various processes, such as alertness/arousal, selective attention, divided attention, and sustained attention. There is a limited amount of information that the brain can process at a given time. Attention allows one to function effectively by selecting the specific information to be processed and filtering out the unnecessary information.

It is difficult to assess pure attention as many tests of attention overlap with tests of executive function, verbal and visual skills, motor speed, information processing speed, and memory. Traditional methods of assessing attention involve timed tasks and tests of working memory. The Wechsler subtest, Digit Span,[4] is a common method for assessing attention span for immediate verbal recall of numbers. Digit span involves the examiner reading progressively longer strings of digits for the individual to repeat both forwards and backwards. Thus both digits forward and backward require auditory attention and are dependent on short-term memory retention. Another commonly used test to assess attention is the Continuous Performance Test of Attention (CPTA).[15] The CPTA consists of the individual listening to a series of letters on an audiotape and tapping his or her finger each time the target letter is presented.

Attentional processes, like other cognitive functioning, change over the course of the lifespan, but attention is particularly vulnerable to the process of aging. However, the effects of aging on attention are related to the complexity of the task. Attention on simple tasks, such as digit span, is relatively well preserved into the 80s. On the other hand, on tasks that require divided attention, elderly individuals respond more slowly and make more errors. In normal aging there is typically a decline in sustained attention, selective attention, and an increase in distractibility.[16]

With regard to aging and cognition, attention is a prerequisite for healthy memory functioning. Attention is necessary in the process of encoding information for future retrieval from memory, and as we age, the complex processes of encoding and retrieving information require greater attentional resources. Intact attention is also required for the processing of information; processing speed is the rate at which one can process information. It is often difficult to assess pure processing speed because many tasks also reflect a visual and/or motor component. Timed tests can measure processing speed and also help the examiner to gain a better understanding of attentional deficits.[17] Slowed processing speed is demonstrated in slower reaction times and in a longer than average performance time.[5] One test frequently used to assess processing speed is the Trail Making Test, Part A.[5] The Trail Making Test, Part A is a timed sequencing test that requires individuals to draw a line from one number to the next in numerical order. Timed visual scanning tasks, requiring one to identify a target letter, number, or symbol, are also used to assess processing speed.

The processing-speed theory proposes that the decline seen in memory and other cognitive processes with normal aging is in part due to slow processing speed. It has been estimated that older adults' response time is approximately

1.5 times slower than younger adults.[18] It is hypothesized that slower processing speed impacts cognition in two ways: the limited time mechanism and the simultaneity mechanism.[19] The limited time mechanism occurs when relevant cognitive processes are performed too slowly and therefore, cannot be accomplished in the expected time. The simultaneity mechanism occurs when slower processing reduces the amount of information available for later processing to be completed. In other words, relevant information may not be accessible when it is needed because it was not encoded. However, slower processing speed associated with normal aging does not impact an individual's performance across all tasks. Processing speed has a stronger relationship with tasks of fluid intelligence than crystallized intelligence. Slower processing speed in the elderly accounts for the decline in fluid ability (e.g., memory and spatial ability) with aging, but not crystallized ability (e.g., verbal ability).[20]

Memory

Memory is commonly thought of as the ability to recall past events and learned information. However, aside from remembering information from the past, memory includes memory for future events (remembering an appointment), autobiographical information, and keeping track of information in the present (e.g., a conversation or reading prose). Memory can be discussed in terms of the complex processes by which the individual encodes, stores, and retrieves information. Memory can also be divided into the length of time the items have been mentally stored; thus the distinction between short-term memory and long-term memory. In addition, memory can be organized by the type of material being stored, such as visual or verbal or autobiographical information. Similar to other areas of cognitive functioning, different aspects of memory differ in how they change with aging.

WORKING MEMORY (SHORT-TERM MEMORY)

Working memory or short-term memory is seen as a limited-capacity store for retaining information over the short term (seconds to 1 to 2 minutes) and for performing mental operations on the contents.[5] Immediate memory, the first stage of short-term memory, temporarily holds information and may also be thought of as one's immediate attention span. The recognized limited capacity store of approximately seven bits of information[21] requires that information get transferred from short-term memory to a more permanent store for later recall. Baddeley and Hitch[22] proposed a model that divides short-term or working memory into two systems: one phonological, for processing language (verbal) information and one visual-spatial, for processing visual information.[22–24] This model holds that short-term memory is controlled by a limited-capacity attentional system and thus organized by a "central executive." The "central executive" assigns information to be remembered to either the visuospatial sketchpad (for memory of visual and spatial information) or the phonological loop (for verbal materials). The overall concept is that more specialized storage systems exist in the limited short-term store that distinguish between verbal and visual information to be stored. Through rehearsal in working memory (e.g., repetition), copies of the information are sent for long-term storage. Regardless of the particular memory model, the overall idea is that short-term memory is a temporary holding ground for information that can be processed or encoded into long-term memory.

Working memory is typically assessed by asking an individual to recall or repeat back words, letters, or numbers, often with sequences of varying length. Using this method, short-term memory span shows only a slight age effect.[3] However, short-term memory becomes vulnerable to aging when the task becomes more complex and requires mental manipulation. For example, on the Wechsler's subtest, Digit Span, individuals are presented with progressively longer strings of numbers verbally and are asked to immediately recall digits in a forward sequence and in reverse order. It is when the task requires more than attention span and individuals have to recall the numbers in reverse sequence, thus manipulating the material, that older adults perform disproportionately weaker than younger adults.[3]

The issue of how aging affects short-term or working memory is associated with the level of complexity of the particular task and the presence of a distracting task. Older adults have been found to have difficulty suppressing irrelevant information from the recent past.[25] Difficulties in processing due to changes in inhibitory control result in increased difficulty selecting relevant information on which to focus in working memory and difficulty in shifting focus while ignoring distracting information.[26] Although working memory capacity is an important facet in the process of learning new information, attention and processing speed are inextricably linked to one's ability to learn. In daily life, older adults perform cognitively best when they focus on one task at a time because attention and processing speed are not divided. Simple memory strategies, such as writing down information or rehearsing information aloud, can help to compensate for memory changes as we age. Such mental techniques aid older adults' ability to move information from short-term to long-term memory. It is important to note that short-term memory decline is part of normal aging and generally these age-related changes do not affect daily functioning in the disruptive way that the presence of dementia affects daily functioning.

LONG-TERM MEMORY

Long-term memory refers to the acquisition of new information that is available for access at a later point in time and involves the processes of encoding, storage, and retrieval of information. Although long-term memory typically means memory for information from the past, it also involves memory for future events or what is called *prospective memory*. An example of prospective memory is remembering a future doctor appointment or remembering to take medication and requires that a memory be maintained about what must be done before the action takes place. Despite numerous theories about the stages of memory or processing levels, the dual system conceptualization of two long-term memory systems (explicit and implicit) provides a useful model for clinical use to understand patterns of functioning and deficits.[3,5,24,27] *Explict memory* refers to the intentional recollection of previous experiences; an individual consciously attempts to recall information and events. To assess explicit memory, verbal or visual information (e.g., words or pictures) is presented and after a delay, the individual is asked to recall the material either through simple recall or a recognition task. *Implicit memory*, on the other hand, relates to knowledge that is observable in performance, but without the awareness that one holds this information. For example, the ability to ride a bicycle does not depend on the conscious awareness of the particular skills involved in the activity.

Explicit memory. Explicit memory, often referred to as declarative, can further be divided into episodic memory and semantic memory. Episodic memory refers to the ability to recollect everyday experiences.[28] More specifically, *episodic memory* is the conscious recollection of personal events along with the specific time and place (context) that they occurred. Episodic material includes autobiographical information, such as birth of a child or graduation from high school, and includes personal information, such as a meal from the previous day or a recent golf game; these are memories that relate to an individual's own, unique experience and include the details of "when and where" an event occurred. Most memory tests assess episodic memory and usually involve a free recall (retrieval), a cued recall, and a recognition trial, and rely on an individual's ability to recollect the material to which they were previously exposed.[5] Compared to younger adults, older adults typically perform better on recognition tasks as opposed to recall tasks. Recognition requires less cognitive effort since a target or cue is provided as a prompt to aid recall as opposed to a recall task, which requires an individual to recall the material to which they were previously exposed without any prompt. Overall, aged adults are most disadvantaged when tests use explicit memory, in particular episodic memory, compared with younger adults.[29,30]

Semantic memory is an individual's knowledge about the world and includes our memory of the meanings of words (vocabulary), facts, concepts, and contrary to episodic memory, is not context dependent. Knowledge is remembered regardless of when and where it was learned, such as word definitions or knowing the years that World War II occurred. Tests that assess semantic memory include vocabulary and word identification tests (AMNART),[8] category fluency tasks (e.g., Animal Naming Test),[31] and confrontational or object naming tests (e.g., Boston Naming Test).[32] When most aged adults report memory complaints, they are often referring to the difficulty remembering words and names of objects and people.[33]

Tests that require recall of semantically unrelated material, such as the Rey Auditory-Verbal Learning Test (RAVLT)[34] word lists, are seen as more difficult because they require more effortful strategies for encoding and retrieval than do story recall tests, such as Wechsler's Logical Memory (WMS-III Logical Memory)[35] or semantically related word lists, such as California Verbal Learning Test (CVLT).[36] When information is presented in a context or words on a list belong to a category and are semantically related, the material presented is already organized in a meaningful way, which aids the recall processes. Such aforementioned memory tests include both delayed recall and recognition trials to discern whether a deficit relates to the storage rather than to the retrieval of information.[3]

Implicit memory (procedural memory). Implicit memory, often referred to as nondeclarative, does not require the conscious or explicit recollection of past events or information and the individual is unaware that remembering has occurred. Implicit memory is usually thought of in terms of procedural memory, but also involves the process of priming. *Priming* is a type of cued recall in that an individual is exposed to material without his or her awareness and this prior exposure aids a future response. For example, having been shown the word *green*, individuals will be more likely to respond "green" when later asked to complete the word fragment g e_ _, even though *great* is a more common word.[37] Similarly, the prior brief presentation of a word increases the likelihood of identifying it correctly when presented with a choice of words at a later time.[38] Advertising is based on the concept of priming because the exposure to a product may lead to selecting that product for future purchase.

Procedural memory relates to skill learning and includes motor and cognitive skill learning, and perceptual or "how to" learning.[3] Riding a bicycle, driving a car, and playing tennis are examples of procedural memory. It is generally accepted that implicit memory processes are relatively unimpaired in older adults; on simple tasks there is little or no difference between older and younger adults although greater age deficits emerge when the implicit learning task is more complex.[29] A good example of how implicit (procedural) memory is preserved with aging is the observation of patients with amnesia who lack the ability to learn new information, but still remember how to walk, dress, and perform other skill-dependent activities.[39] Most research on implicit memory has focused on the finding that the repetition of information aids performance even when conscious memory of the prior experience is not needed.[38] The overall conclusion from research on implicit memory is that there is relatively little age-related change in this area compared with explicit memory tasks that involve active recall or recognition of information.

OVERALL AGE-RELATED CHANGES IN MEMORY

Retrieval of information is an important part of daily functioning. With normal aging, memory deficits are associated primarily with the storage of long-term episodic memories. Information that places little demand on attention, such as implicit memory tasks, results in very little age-related changes in performance. The advantage that older adults experience on recognition tasks indicates that their memory storage and retrieval may be much less efficient than that of younger adults. A processing speed perspective illustrates that normal aging is accompanied by a slowing in overall cognitive processing and it is accepted that older adults process information at a slower rate compared with younger adults. Salthouse[19] found that after statistically controlling for processing speed, age was only weakly related to memory. Memory functioning in normal aging is thus mediated by processing speed. The reduced attentional resources concept[18,40] suggests that a limited amount of cognitive resources are available for a given task and consequently, a more complex task requires more attentional capacity than a simpler task. It follows that because the amount of attentional resources is reduced with aging, the processes of encoding and retrieval of information use a larger proportion of available resources for older adults than for younger adults. In sum, research suggests that overall cognitive slowing and changes in attentional ability account for much of the change in memory functioning as we age.

Verbal Abilities

Most verbal abilities remain intact with normal aging.[41] Therefore vocabulary and verbal reasoning scores remain relatively constant in normal aging and may even show minor improvements. The two main areas of verbal abilities that are frequently discussed in terms of aging are verbal fluency (semantic and phonemic) and confrontation naming. Verbal fluency is the ability to retrieve words based on their meaning or their sounds. Confrontation naming describes the ability to identify an object by its name.

Two common tests used to assess verbal fluency are the Controlled Oral Word Association Test (COWAT)[42] and the semantic fluency test.[31] The COWAT is perhaps the most widely used test of phonemic fluency. The COWA task requires an individual to generate as many words that begin with a specific letter as quickly as they can. The semantic fluency task is a timed-test that requires the individual to generate examples in a specific category (e.g., animal naming test).

The Boston Naming Test[32] is a commonly used test to measure confrontation naming ability as individuals are required to name the object in the presented picture. Confrontation naming is composed of several different processes; an individual must perceive the object in the picture correctly, identify the semantic concept of the picture, and retrieve and express the appropriate name for the object.[43] Confrontation naming ability is associated with the tip-of-the-tongue (TOT) phenomenon. The TOT phenomenon occurs when an individual knows the name of a person or object and is able to retrieve the semantic information about the object, but cannot retrieve the name of the object.[44] Although an individual is unable to retrieve the target word, he or she will often try to describe the term using other words.[45] Throughout all of adulthood, proper nouns comprise the majority of TOT experiences. However, the increase in TOT phenomenon among older adults is due to their greater difficulty in retrieving proper nouns.[44] There is not a significant age difference in the frequency of TOT episodes for simple words. However, older adults have significantly more TOT experiences than younger adults for difficult words.[45] Thus, word-finding difficulty and TOT moments are the most common cognitive complaints of older adults.

The majority of cross-sectional studies have found that older adults have lower scores on the Boston Naming Test compared with younger individuals. It should be noted that while subjective complaints of word-finding difficulties increase with age, significantly lower performance on tasks of confrontation naming only emerges after age 70.[44] Zec et al[46] found that confrontation naming ability as measured by the Boston Naming Test improves when individuals are in their 50s, remain the same in their 60s, and decline in the 70s and 80s; it should be noted that the magnitude of these age-related changes is relatively small. It was found that there was an approximate one word improvement in the 50s age group and a 1.3 word decline in the 70s age group. There is some indication that there is an accelerated rate of decline in confrontation naming ability with age.[44]

Normal aging is associated with a decline in verbal fluency. It is important to note that the normal age-related decline seen in verbal fluency performance may be partially mediated by reduced psychomotor speed rather than true deficits in verbal ability. Slowed handwriting and reading speed in the elderly was predictive of poorer performance on verbal fluency tests.[47] Rodriguez-Aranda and Martinussen[48] found a decline in verbal fluency as measured by the COWAT after age 60. The ability to generate words beginning with a particular letter improves until the third decade of life and remains constant through the 40s. Subsequently, a significant decline occurs in phonemic naming ability and continues to worsen gradually until the late 60s. Phonemic verbal fluency ability continues to decline rapidly through the late 80s. Gender and education may impact one's phonemic verbal fluency across the lifespan. Women may slightly outperform men on tasks of phonemic verbal fluency. Individuals with higher levels of education (beyond high school) show greater verbal fluency ability as measured by the COWAT compared with individuals with lower levels of education (12 years or less).[49]

Executive Functions

Executive functions describe a wide range of abilities that relate to the capacity to respond to a novel situation.[16] Executive functions include abilities such as mental flexibility, response inhibition, planning, organization, abstraction, and decision-making.[50,51] Executive function can be thought of as having four distinct components: volition, planning, purposive action, and effective performance.[3] Volition is a complex process that refers to the ability to act intentionally. Planning is the process and the steps involved in achieving the goal. Purposive action refers to the productive activity required to execute a plan. Effective performance is the ability to self-correct and monitor one's behavior while working. All of the components of executive functioning are necessary for problem solving and appropriate social behavior.

Another term for executive functions is frontal lobe functions because these abilities are localized in the prefrontal cortex.[52] The frontal aging hypothesis refers to the idea that normal aging leads to deterioration of the frontal lobes. Deterioration is due to a loss of volume in the prefrontal cortex and is associated with cognitive deficits. Prefrontal deterioration plays a key role in many of the age-related changes in cognitive processes, such as memory, attention, and executive function.[53]

Like many cognitive processes, it is difficult to assess pure executive function as many of the measures used in its assessment rely on other cognitive processes such as working memory, processing speed, attention, and visual spatial abilities. The Wisconsin Card Sorting Test (WCST)[54] is a popular test used to measure executive function. The WCST requires an individual to sort a set of cards based on different categories. Individuals are not informed about how to sort the cards and must deduce the correct sorting strategies through the limited feedback that is provided. After a particular category is achieved (i.e., a set number of correct responses) based on a particular characteristic (e.g., color or shape), the sorting strategy changes and the individual must shift strategies accordingly. Once the test is completed, the examiner is provided with several measures related to executive function, for example, categories and perseverative errors. A category is achieved when a specific number of cards have been sorted correctly based on the particular criterion such as color. Perseverative errors occur when an individual continues to give the wrong response when provided the feedback that the strategy is not or is no longer correct, thus demonstrating a lack of cognitive flexibility.

On the WCST older adults achieve significantly fewer categories than younger adults.[52] The most significant decline in performance on this test is seen in adults age 75 and older. Individuals of this age group achieve significantly fewer categories and more perseverative errors compared with younger individuals. However, changes in executive functioning as measured by neuropsychological assessments, such as the WCST, can be seen in adults aged 53 to 64, but adults ages 53 to 64 do not show deficits on more real-world executive tasks.[55] Thus although individuals in midadulthood may show a decline in executive functioning on structured neuropsychological tests, their real-world executive skills remain intact.

Other measures used in the assessment of executive functioning included Trail Making Test, Part B[5] and the WAIS-III subtests,[4] Matrix Reasoning and Similarities. Trail Making, Part B, is a timed visual-spatial sequencing task requiring an individual to draw connecting lines alternating between numbers and letters in numerical and alphabetical order. Matrix Reasoning is an untimed task that measures one's nonverbal analytic thinking abilities. The Matrix Reasoning task requires an individual to identify the missing element of an abstract pattern from a variety of choices. Wechsler's Similarities subtest measures an individual's verbal abstract reasoning skills by asking an individual to describe how two different objects/concepts are alike.

Normal aging is generally associated with a decline in executive functioning.[56] When reasoning and problem-solving involve material that is novel, complex, or requires the ability to distinguish relevant from irrelevant information, the performance of older adults suffers because they tend to think in more concrete terms and the mental flexibility required to form new abstractions and concepts declines.[3] Compared with younger adults, older adults also show a decreased capacity to form conceptual links as mental flexibility diminishes.[3] Executive functions serve as the overseer of brain processing and are essential for purposeful, goal-directed behavior. Deficits in executive functioning can be seen in difficulties with planning and organizing, difficulties implementing strategies, and inappropriate social behavior or poor judgment.

Lifestyle Factors Associated with Cognitive Functioning

LEISURE ACTIVITIES

The mental exercise hypothesis refers to the notion that keeping mentally active will help maintain an individual's cognitive functioning and prevent cognitive decline. Many activities, such as playing bridge, doing crossword puzzles, studying a foreign language, and learning to play an instrument, have been suggested to help in preventing cognitive decline.[57] The research regarding the mental exercise hypothesis has been varied and there is currently not a definitive answer regarding the role of leisure activities in preventing cognitive decline.

It is suggested that engaging in leisure activities, especially ones that are cognitively demanding, maintains or improves cognitive functioning.[58] However, there is also evidence that individuals with high levels of intellectual functioning engage in more cognitively demanding activities, making it difficult to discern the exact role of mental activities in preventing cognitive decline. This line of research suggests that it is not the activity per se that is responsible for maintaining cognitive functioning, but rather specific lifestyles and living conditions.[58]

Although there is not conclusive evidence regarding the protective factors of leisure activities, several research studies[59,60] have shown that leisure activities reduce the risk of dementia in the elderly. Reading, playing board games, learning a musical instrument, visiting friends or relatives, going out (i.e., to movies or a restaurant), walking for pleasure, and dancing are associated with a reduced risk of dementia.[59,60] Such leisure activities have been shown to protect against memory decline even after controlling for age, sex, education, ethnicity, baseline cognitive-status, and medical illness. Participation in an activity for 1 day per week was found to reduce the risk of dementia by 7%.[59] Individuals who participated in many leisure activities (i.e., six or more activities a month) had a 38% less risk of developing dementia.[60]

It has been also hypothesized that leisure activities reduce the risk of cognitive decline by enhancing cognitive reserve. A decrease in activity results in reduced cognitive abilities.[61] Engaging in leisure activities may also provide structural changes in the brain that protect against cognitive decline given that certain areas of the adult brain are able to generate new neurons (i.e., plasticity). Stimulation, such as engaging in social, intellectual, and physical activities, is suggested to promote increased synaptic density. Enhanced neuronal activation has been proposed to hinder the development of disease processes, such as dementia.[60] However, research has also shown that changes in cognitive reserve are more likely to occur early in life; it is primarily the early experiences of education and intellectual activity that increases cognitive reserve the most.[11] Despite the varied findings,

> *"people should continue to engage in mentally stimulating activities because even if there is not yet evidence that it has beneficial effects in slowing the rate of age-related decline in cognitive functioning, there is no evidence that it has any harmful effects, the activities are often enjoyable and thus may contribute to a higher quality of life, and engagement in cognitively demanding activities serves as an existence proof—if you can still do it, then you know that you have not yet lost it."*[57]

PHYSICAL ACTIVITIES

It has been hypothesized that engaging in physical activities may enhance cognition and prevent decline in late life as physical activities enhance blood flow to the brain and oxygenation, processes which are known to slow biologic aging.[11] Physical activities reduce cardiovascular and cerebrovascular risk factors, which may reduce the risk of vascular dementia and Alzheimer disease.[62] There is also evidence that physical activity may directly affect the brain by preserving neurons and increasing synapses.[63]

Moderate and strenuous physical activity is associated with a decreased risk of cognitive decline. Moderate activity includes playing golf on a weekly basis, playing tennis twice a week, and walking 1.6 m/day. Research has found that long-term regular physical activity, such as walking, is associated with less cognitive decline in women.[64] The benefits of walking at least 1.5 hr/wk at a 21 to 30 min/mile pace are similar to being about 3 years younger and are associated with a 20% reduced risk of significant cognitive decline.

SOCIAL ACTIVITIES

Social support has also been suggested to serve as a protective factor in cognitive decline. Social support may serve as a buffer against stress and may lead to decreased cortisol production in the brain. Lower levels of cortisol result in better performance on tests of episodic memory.[65] Interacting with others may also prevent cognitive decline by providing an individual with increased mental stimulation[66] and may also protect an individual from depression, which has been shown to negatively impact cognition.[67] Depression and mood disorders are associated with an accelerated cognitive decline as people age.[68] Processing speed, attention, and consequently, memory may all be affected by depression. In addition, a lack of social interaction also impacts an older adult's well-being. It has been found that individuals who live alone or have no intimate relationships are at an increased risk of developing dementia; those individuals who are classified as having a poor social network are 60% more likely to develop dementia.[69] Individuals in their 70s who report having limited social support at baseline show greater cognitive decline at follow-up assessments.[67] On the other hand, individuals with greater emotional supports have better performance on cognitive tests.[67] Rowe and Kahn[70] proposed a model of successful aging as being composed of three main components: avoidance of disease-related disability, maintenance of physical and cognitive functioning, and active engagement in life. Active engagement with life involves maintaining interpersonal relationships and it has been found that social environment and emotional supports may be protective against cognitive decline and result in a slower decline in functional status.

HEALTH FACTORS

Several medical conditions are associated with cognitive decline. Hypertension is the most prevalent vascular risk factor in the elderly.[71] Chronic hypertension has been shown to result in deficits in brain structure including the reduction of white and gray matter in the prefrontal lobes, atrophy of the hippocampus, and increased white matter hypertensities.[72] Research has found that uncontrolled hypertension can lead to cognitive decline that is independent of normal aging,[71,73] aside from posing a risk for stroke. Older adults with hypertension have mild but specific cognitive deficits in the areas of executive function, processing speed, episodic memory, and working memory.[73]

Diabetes mellitus has also been associated with cognitive decline.[74,75] Lipids and other metabolic markers may play a role in the relationship between diabetes and cognition.[76] Diabetes may also impact cognition through confounding factors such as hypertension, heart disease, depression, and decreased physical activity.[76] Individuals with type 1 diabetes display a slower processing speed and a decline in mental flexibility.[75] Type 2 diabetes is also associated with cognitive decline; longer duration of type 2 diabetes results in greater cognitive decline.[77] Elderly women with type 2 diabetes have a 30% greater risk of cognitive decline compared with those without diabetes, with a 50% greater risk for individuals with a 15-year or greater history of diabetes.

Dietary factors and vitamin deficiencies have also been associated with cognitive decline in the elderly population. Individuals with cognitive decline associated with normal aging should be investigated for B_{12} deficiency. Research has demonstrated that vitamin B_{12} injections may improve executive and language functions in patients with cognitive decline, but will rarely reverse dementia.[78] Low vitamin B levels may be associated with impaired cognitive performance through several possible mechanisms including, multiple central nervous system functions, reactions involving DNA, and the overproduction of homocysteine that could potentially damage neurons and blood vessels.[79] Low levels of vitamin B_{12} and folic acid result in poorer performance on tasks of free recall, attention, processing speed, and verbal fluency.[80] Overall, research suggests that the effects of vitamin deficiency are most likely seen on complex cognitive tasks that demand greater executive functions.

Conclusion

Cognitive decline is a natural part of aging. However, the extent of decline varies across individuals and across the specific cognitive domain being assessed. The cognitive reserve perspective maintains that individual differences with regard to cognitive aging are related to an individual's reserve built upon early life factors (i.e., educational and intellectual experiences).[9]

Although cognitive reserve can be increased in later life, it is more amenable to change in early life. Although cognitive decline is inevitable, all areas of functioning do not change equally. It is well established that older adults process, store, and encode information less efficiently than younger adults. The cognitive functions related to fluid intelligence, such as the ability to solve novel or complex problems, tend to decline with aging, whereas cognitive functions related to crystallized intelligence, such as school-based knowledge, vocabulary, and reading, generally remain stable throughout life. Processing speed and attentional capacity are particularly vulnerable to aging, especially on more challenging tasks, and mediate multiple areas of cognitive functioning. For example, a memory problem is often, more accurately, a problem with poor attention and/or slowed speed of processing information.

KEY POINTS

Normal Cognitive Aging

- Variability exists across individuals in their ability to compensate for cognitive changes as they age.
- An active, engaged lifestyle, emphasizing mental activity and educational pursuits in early life, has a positive impact on cognitive functioning in later life.
- In normal aging there is typically a decline in sustained attention and selective attention and an increase in distractibility.
- Older adults' response time is approximately 1.5 times slower than younger adults.
- Most verbal abilities remain intact with normal aging.
- Normal aging is generally associated with a decline in executive functioning.
- Memory deficits associated with normal aging are primarily related to the storage of long-term episodic memories.
- Implicit memory tasks, results in very little age-related changes in performance.

Although research has found cognitive decline in the areas of attention, processing speed, episodic memory, and executive function, research has also shown that older adults have cognitive (or brain) plasticity and may benefit from cognitive training and other mental activities.[81] However, the results of cognitive training with normal aging adults has been varied; although improved performance on a specific task can be found, there is a lack of generalizability to daily functioning in the long term.[82] Nevertheless, maintaining an engaged and healthy lifestyle (social, physical, and intellectual) improves one's quality of life and may add to successful aging. One problem is the assumption that "successful aging" means that there is no discernable change in memory and overall cognitive functioning from one's previous level of functioning. Changes in cognition are a normal part of aging and not something that is necessarily a cause for concern or precursor to dementia. Older adults need to adjust their idea of normal aging to a more realistic standard.

ACKNOWLEDGMENT

Material in this chapter contains contributions from the previous edition, and we are grateful to the previous author for the work done.

For a complete list of references, please visit online only at www.expertconsult.com

CHAPTER 29

The Aging Personality and Self: Diversity and Health Issues

Julie Blaskewicz Boron
K. Warner Schaie
Sherry L. Willis

Personality may be defined as the pattern of thoughts, feelings, and behaviors that shape an individual's interface with the world, distinguish one person from another, and manifest across time and situation.[1–3] Personality is impacted by biologic, cognitive, and environmental determinants, including the impact of culture and cohort. Theoretical approaches to personality are as varied as the breadth of the construct they attempt to describe and explain. Yet each approach, to varying degrees, emphasizes stability and change within individuals across time and situations.

The impact of personality across the adult life span touches every domain: personal, professional, spiritual, and physical. Certainly, personality characteristics have direct and indirect influences on health status, health behaviors, and behavioral interactions with health care professionals. Although no single chapter can adequately condense such rich empirical and theoretical research, we will attempt to provide a concise overview of stage models, trait theory, and social-cognitive approaches to personality. As such, we will focus on aspects of personality development among cognitively intact older adults, not personality changes that may ensue as the result of dementia.

Each section of this chapter contains four subsections. For each of the three major approaches (stage, trait, social-cognitive), we first provide an overview of classic along with the most current research on stability and maturational and environmental change within adult personality. Our focus will be on findings from longitudinal data. Second, we include cross-cultural comparisons of adult personality where available. This focus provides a unique contribution to recent reviews of adult personality and aging.[4,5] Third, we examine the health correlates of adult personality, focusing on morbidity and mortality, well-being, life satisfaction, positive and negative affect, anxiety, and depression. Finally, we discuss measurement issues and provide examples of current assessment instruments.

PERSONALITY STAGES AND EGO DEVELOPMENT

Freudian theory

The psychoanalytic approach to adult personality development has its roots in the theories of Sigmund Freud. His theories encompassed four domains: level of consciousness, personality structure, defense mechanisms, and stages of psychosexual development.[6,7] Freudian theory postulates that adult personality is made up of three aspects: (1) the id, operating on the pleasure principle generally within the unconscious; (2) the ego, operating on the reality principle within the conscious realm; and (3) the superego, operating on the morality principle at all levels of consciousness. The interplay of these personality structures generates anxiety that must be reduced through various defense mechanisms. These mechanisms act to obscure the true, anxiety-laden reasons for one's behavior.

Although seminal in the expansion of our understanding of the human psyche, Freud's specific theories receive little attention in the scientific study of personality today.[6] His theories are not easily amenable to scientific inquiry in that they frequently lead to nonspecific hypotheses, wherein failure to find expected effects may simply be a result of unknown defense mechanisms. Additionally, having postulated that personality development associated with his stages of psychosexual development essentially ends in adolescence, Freud's theories have limited applicability to the fields of gerontology and geriatric medicine.

Post-Freudian theorists

In contrast, some post-Freudian theorists have conceptualized personality development as a continuing process focused on current interpersonal and/or family-of-origin issues as the source of individual distress and coping patterns. Carl Jung proposed that as individuals age, they achieve a balance between the expression of their masculine characteristics (animus) and feminine characteristics (anima).[8,9] Findings regarding increased balance of gender roles with age have emerged in different cultures, lending some support to Jung's hypothesis.[2]

Erik Erikson's stages of psychosocial development are perhaps the best known of the stage theories of adult personality. The sequence of Erikson's eight stages of development is based on the epigenetic principle, which means that personality moves through these stages in an ordered fashion at an appropriate rate.[3,10] Two of the eight stages describe personality change during the adult years. Although the identity crisis is placed in adolescence, deciding "who you are" is a continual process that is reflected throughout adulthood, even in old age.[11] In the midlife stage of *generativity versus stagnation*, individuals seek ways to give their talents and experiences to the next generation, moving beyond the self-concerns of identity and the interpersonal concerns of intimacy.[5] Successful resolution of this stage results in the development of a sense of trust and care for the next generation and the assurance that society will continue. Unsuccessful resolution of this stage results in self-absorption.

Ego integrity versus despair is Erikson's final stage of ego development, beginning around age 65 and continuing until death. In this stage, individuals become increasingly internally focused and more aware of the nearness of death. Successful resolution of this stage results in being able to look back on one's life and find meaning, developing a sense of wisdom before death. Alternatively, meaninglessness and despair can ensue if the process of life review results in focus on primarily negative outcomes.

Difficulties arising from attempts to empirically investigate Erikson's theory include the assertion that stages must be encountered in order and the lack of specification regarding how developmental crises are resolved so that an individual may move from one stage to the next. However, the environmental influences of culture and cohort on adult personality have been minimized. One 22-year investigation found significant age changes supportive of Erikson's theory.[12] Middle-aged adults expressed emotions and cognitions consistent with successful completion of more psychosocial developmental crises than younger adults. In addition, Ackerman et al found a stronger association between generativity in midlife compared with young adulthood.[13] Some theorists postulate that the ego integrity versus despair period initiates a process of life review.[14]

Life review

The concept of life review is the exception to this lack of empirical investigation regarding stage theories of adult personality.[14,15] *Life review* can be thought of as a systematic cognitive-emotional process occurring late in life in which an individual thinks back across his or her life experiences and integrates disparate events into general themes. The portion of life review focusing on recall of primarily positive life experiences is reminiscence. Reminiscence has been linked to successful aging[16] by contributing to sustained identity formation and self-continuity, a sense of mastery, meaning, and coherence in life, and acceptance and reconciliation of one's life.[17] Although this approach to adult personality development can be conceptualized as a cognitive process in which identity emerges from the story of one's life, we have chosen to include it with stage models because it is most frequently described as occurring near the completion of one's life. Nevertheless, it should be acknowledged that individuals likely undergo a process of life review periodically throughout the adult years including young adulthood[18] and midlife.[19,20]

Stage theories and diversity

Few studies investigating stage theories of personality have focused on diverse cultural or racial/ethnic groups. Most of the stage models, such as Freud's original theories, were based on highly select samples. Only a few investigations of life review have succeeded in recruiting participants reflecting the general population of interest.[21–23] In one study, cross-cultural evidence indicated life review programs have improved self-esteem and life satisfaction in Taiwanese elderly.[24] Data reflecting the broader diversity of the population is needed for examining the universality of life review and the generalizability of the basic assumptions.

Stage theories and health

There has been limited investigation of the relation between stage approaches to adult personality and health. Once again, the exception to this rule is the investigation of life review processes. Several intervention studies support the contention that life review, in comparison with nonspecific but supportive interventions, has a positive impact on health, life satisfaction, well-being, and depression.

A recent meta-analysis on reminiscence and well-being in older adulthood demonstrated that although reminiscence was moderately (effect size 0.54) associated with life-satisfaction and well-being in older adulthood, engaging in life review had a stronger effect.[17] This suggests that consideration of all major life events, both positive and negative, as is typical for life review, has a greater impact on well-being in older adulthood. Furthermore, another meta-analysis by Bohlmeijer et al investigated the effects of life review on late-life depression.[25] Results suggested that life review and reminiscence may be an effective treatment for depressive symptoms in older adults. Additional research has supported the utility of life review interventions to decrease depressive symptoms and improve life satisfaction in the elderly.[26–28] Finally, participants in life review programs have demonstrated wider psychological benefits, including increased autonomy, environmental mastery, personal growth, positive relations with others, purpose in life, and self-acceptance in comparison to control groups.[29]

Measurement issues

The primary methodological problem plaguing empirical research involving stage theory approaches to adult personality development is the lack of specification of change mechanisms and limitations in psychometrically reliable and valid measures. The most current stage approach to adult personality in our organizational scheme involves the concept of life review near the end of life. Bohlmeijer et al note the lack of standardized protocols to life review as a therapeutic technique in the delivery of interventions.[17]

A common methodological limitation in much of this research is the problem of making causal inferences of age-related personality change from cross-sectional studies. In these studies, age-related differences could be observed because of the impact of aging or due to cohort differences. Without cohort-sequential data, it is impossible to tease apart these influences. Thus, although stage theories of adult personality have intuitive appeal, their contribution is limited by vague delineation of constructs and methodology.

Personality traits

In contrast to stage approaches to adult personality development, empirical research regarding trait approaches has experienced a significant boom in recent years. The Big 5 Model of personality provides a broad framework for organizing the hundreds of traits, or individual differences, that characterize people.[30] These five core dimensions have been demonstrated at most life stages through extensive factor analyses of personality descriptors.[31,32] A description of the most commonly identified five factors can be found in Table 29-1.

Early studies suggested that maturational changes in personality occur in young adulthood until approximately age 30 with relative intraindividual stability in traits thereafter.[33–37] However, stability of personality across adulthood lacks consensus. The debate as to whether personality

Table 29-1. The Big 5 Personality Traits[30]

Emotional Stability vs. Neuroticism. Anxiety, depression, emotional instability, self-consciousness, hostility, and impulsiveness vs. relaxation, poise, and steadiness.

Extraversion or Surgency. Gregariousness, assertiveness, activity level, and positive emotions vs. silence, passivity, and reserve.

Culture/Intellect or Openness to Experience. Imagination, curiosity, and creativity vs. shallowness, imperceptiveness, and stupidity.

Agreeableness or Pleasantness. Attributes such as kindness, trust and warmth that are considered pleasant and attractive to others vs. hostility, selfishness, and distrust.

Conscientiousness or Dependability. Encompasses organization, responsibility, ambition, perseverance, and hard work vs. carelessness, negligence, and unreliability.

remains stable or changes in adulthood may be based upon different criteria for determining change. Roberts and Mroczek described various forms of change including mean-level change, rank-order consistency, structural consistency, and individual differences in change.[38] Most often, research supporting stability refers to rank-order consistency, whereas research emphasizing change focuses on individual differences in change. Consistent with cross-sectional results,[31] longitudinal assessments have shown small age-related declines in neuroticism, extraversion, and openness to experience, with age-related increases in agreeableness and conscientiousness in adults up to age 70 (declines in neuroticism persisted until age 80); however, this research is often cited as supporting stability of personality in adulthood. Although mean-level changes are shown, individuals maintain their rank-order on the personality domains.[39] Findings from other research teams contribute support for stability.[40–44]

Study of variability in individual rates of change has provided support for the notion that personality may change, even in adulthood.[45–48] Together these studies suggest that some individuals change more or less than other individuals in terms of personality traits. Thus recent research has attempted to investigate factors that may contribute to these varying rates of individual change. In a 12-year longitudinal study of middle-aged to older men, Mroczek and Spiro found cohort, incidence of marriage or remarriage, spousal death, and memory complaints to be associated with differential rates of change in personality.[47] Individual differences in life circumstances were also found to be associated with differential rates of change in personality in a sample of older women.[49] Social support, unmet needs, health, and psychosocial needs are examples of various life circumstances found to be significant predictors of differential rates of change in older women.[49] Thus specific life experiences may have an impact on personality. Consideration of the various definitions of change and the factors accounting for change is important when reviewing research on personality stability or change.

Trait theories and diversity

Cross-cultural studies have most frequently compared non-Hispanic whites in the United States with individuals living in other countries.[50–52] These studies seek to estimate the effects of environment on different age cohorts by comparing adults in cultures with different recent histories. Using the NEO Personality Inventor-R, McCrae et al studied parallels in adult personality traits across cultures in five countries: Germany, Italy, Portugal, Croatia, and South Korea.[51] Once again, different patterns of age changes would result if environmental factors play a major role in adult personality development. In contrast, intrinsic maturational perspectives would suggest that even widely different cultures should show similar age trends. Results showed that, across cultures, midlife adults scored higher on measures of agreeableness and conscientiousness and lower on neuroticism, extraversion, and openness than 18- to 21-year-olds. Congruence was strongest for openness and weakest for neuroticism, for which only two cultures (Germany and South Korea) replicated the American pattern.

Using the California Psychological Inventory (CPI), factor structures similar to the Big 5 were compared among adults in the United States and the People's Republic of China; comparisons revealed very similar patterns of age correlations.[50,52] In the Yang study, the Chinese sample was an average of 25 years younger than the U.S. sample, and age effects were smaller in the U.S. sample. Likewise, Labouvie-Vief et al found high congruence on all four personality factors derived from the CPI: extraversion, control/norm orientation, flexibility, and femininity/masculinity.[50] Older cohorts across cultures had lower scores on extraversion and flexibility and higher scores on control/norm orientation. Once again, age differences were more pronounced among Chinese than U.S. adults. Smaller cultural differences were found among the youngest age groups than among the oldest groups.

In general, the results of these cross-cultural studies are consistent with the hypothesis that there are universal intrinsic maturational changes in personality.[50–52] Yang et al reported, however, that across the span from 18 to 65 years, age never accounted for more than 20% of the variance in CPI scale scores.[52] Gender did not influence the pattern of results in these cross-cultural studies. The authors differed in their interpretation of the influence of environmental factors. In the Yang and McCrae studies, the authors maintained that the results offered little support for historical cohort effects being major determinants of cross-sectional age differences in adult personality traits. Although noting the high degree of similarity in personality traits across cultures, Labouvie-Vief et al also noted that cultural climate and cultural change do impact the relation between age and personality.

Trait theories and health

There is extensive literature on the relation of adult personality and health. Neuroticism is one of the traits most frequently studied in relation to health. Neuroticism has been associated with greater reactivity to stress,[53] whereas high levels of personal control or mastery serve as a protective factor in regards to the impact of stress on health.[54,55] Siegman et al found the dominance factor derived from the Minnesota Multiphasic Personality Inventory (2-MMPI) to be an independent risk factor for incidence of fatal coronary heart disease and nonfatal myocardial infarction among older men with an average age of 61.[56] Niaura et al found that among older men, greater hostility may be associated with a pattern of obesity, central adiposity, and insulin resistance, which can exert effects on blood pressure and serum lipids.[57] Finally, several studies have documented an association between personality and mortality, indicating that higher levels of neuroticism and lower levels of conscientiousness serve as risk factors of mortality.[58–61]

Measurement issues

There are multiple instruments of personality traits that measure the Big 5.[62–64] Regardless of the specific measurement instrument used, however, these measures demonstrate remarkable consistency in the derivation of five dimensions of personality via factor analysis.[30] However, multiple methodological issues remain. One major complication of stability estimates in adult personality research involves what kind of stability is under consideration. The impact of cohort and time of measurement on trait consistency within the longitudinal studies conducted to date has not been fully considered.[44] Studies of gender role differences have shown that age is not as good a predictor as the life experiences of different cohorts on personality traits of men and women across time.[65–67] Thus it may be that earlier-born cohorts developed more consistent personality traits earlier in life as the result of numerous social/historical and life span–related influences.

More extensive consideration of the relative impact of biologic and environmental variables on stability and change in adult personality is essential. Although the influence of genetic factors has been investigated in the development of personality among monozygotic and dizygotic twins over a 10-year period, no such investigations have addressed the contribution of genetics to the maintenance of personality across the adult age range. Regarding the impact of environmental influences, with time and age individuals may encounter fewer novel experiences.[44] Thus the stability of personality factors may be causally related to the decreasing novelty of the environment in which individuals live rather than genetic factors. Finally, prior research on traits has been primarily descriptive and would profit from a theory-driven approach.

SOCIAL-COGNITIVE APPROACHES TO PERSONALITY

The social-cognitive approach to the study of adult personality and the self focuses on the processes underlying stability and change in one's perception of the self, and emphasizes the impact of necessary, adaptive adjustments in one's personality. An individual's sense of self is proposed to develop through the interaction of internal and environmental factors, influencing maturational changes and cohort differences. Although the content of the developing self may change, this model proposes that the mechanisms by which changes are integrated into the concept of self are stable. Thus the development of the self as a dynamic construct reflects one's identity, perception of possible selves, need for affiliation, and perception of the remaining life span.

Identity and the self

Whitbourne describes a life span approach to one's core identity development. *Identity* is defined as an individual's developing sense of self, an organizing schema through which internal and external life experiences are interpreted.[68] Identity includes physical functioning, cognition, social relationships, and environmental experiences.[69] The identity process theory posits that changes in identity with age occur through assimilation, accommodation, and balance.[70] Successful aging consists of integrating information about the self and achieving equilibrium between assimilation and accommodation.

Whitbourne and Collins examined the self-reports of adults aged 40 to 95 years regarding the relation between identity and changes in physical functioning.[71] Forty-year-olds were sensitive to age-related changes. Individuals aged 65 and older reported paying particular attention to perceived changes in competence. These individuals were more likely to use identity assimilation (i.e., reinterpretation of experiences to coincide with the self) in the area of cognitive functioning than were other age groups. In a subsequent study, Sneed and Whitbourne found that identity assimilation and identity balance were associated with increased self-esteem, whereas accommodation resulted in decreased self-esteem.[72] Finally, in a study of identity and self- consciousness, identity accommodation was positively associated with self-reflection and public self-consciousness.[73]

Researchers interested in understanding the self from a life span perspective often use the theoretical framework provided by the "possible selves" model.[74] The construct of "possible selves" postulates that individuals are guided in their actions by aspects of the self that represent what the individual could become, would like to become, and is afraid of becoming. Possible selves serve as psychological resources that may motivate an individual and direct future behavior.

Ryff's research provides empirical support for the concept of possible selves.[75] Young, middle-aged, and older adults were asked to judge their past, present, future, and ideal selves on dimensions related to self acceptance, positive relations with others, autonomy, environmental mastery, purpose in life, and personal growth. Older people were more likely than younger adults to downwardly adjust their ideal self and to view their past more positively.[75] Over a 5-year period in old age, hoped and feared possible selves were found to remain stable.[76] Goal orientation shifted with age, specifically older adults focused on maintenance and loss prevention, and this orientation was associated with well-being.[77] A shift in goal orientation in regards to possible selves may contribute to perceived control and stability of possible selves. Perceived control over development is associated with subjective well-being across adulthood.[78]

Socioemotional selectivity theory

Carstensen's socioemotional selectivity theory (SST) focuses on the agentic choices made by adults in their social world for the purpose of regulating knowledge-oriented and emotion goals.[79–81] The purposeful selective reduction in social interaction begins in early adulthood, and emotional closeness remains stable or increases within selected relationships as one ages.[79–81] When time is perceived as open-ended, acquisition of knowledge is prioritized. When time is perceived as limited, however, emotional goals assume primacy. Older adults select social relationships in which they want to invest their resources and in which they expect reciprocity and positive affect, thereby optimizing their social networks. Thus older adult's social networks are reduced by choice, as individuals decrease contact with acquaintances but seek to maintain contact with relatives and friends as a function of increased saliency of emotional attachment to one's life goals.[79–81]

The perception of time left in life (future time perspective) is postulated to be fundamental to motivation, and age is correlated with time perspective.[82] Perceiving an ending plays an important role in identity processes, such that endings promote greater self-acceptance and less striving toward an abstract ideal.[75,83] Thus due to changes in the perceived time left to live, older adults have been shown to be more present-oriented than concerned about the past and less concerned than young adults about the future.[84] Rather than age being the causal factor in shifts in self-perception and social goals, it is the inverse association of chronologic age with number of years left to live that produces observed relations.

Social-cognitive theories and diversity

There have been few empirical investigations of cultural or racial/ethnic diversity in the study of social-cognitive approaches to adult personality development. Cross-cultural research on socioemotional selectivity theory mostly supports similarities in age differences across cultures, rather than cultural differences.

Waid and Frazier compared older Spanish-speaking natives and white non-Hispanic English-speaking natives.[85] Cultural differences in hoped and feared possible selves were present, primarily reflecting traditional differences in individualistic (English-speakers) and collectivist (Spanish-speakers) cultures. Common feared selves included physical concerns for English-speaking natives, and loss of loved ones for Spanish-speaking natives. Frequently cited hoped for selves included family-oriented domains for Spanish-speaking natives and advances in the abilities/education domain for English-speaking natives. Thus the cultural differences evident for possible selves and control revolve around differences attributed to individualistic and collectivist cultures.

Gross et al found consistent age differences in the subjective report of emotional experience and control across diverse cultures: Norwegians, Chinese-Americans, African Americans, European-Americans, and Catholic nuns.[86] Across all groups, older adults reported fewer negative emotional experiences and greater emotional control. Likewise, Fung et al found support for the notion that socioemotional selectivity is due to perceived limitations in time among adults in the United States and Hong Kong,[87] and among adults in Taiwan and Mainland China.[88]

An investigation exemplifying the importance of perceived time left to live was conducted following the terrorist attacks of September 11, 2001, in the United States, and the SARS epidemic in Hong Kong. By investigating social goals before and after these events, Fung and Carstensen found increased motivation to focus on emotional goals, regardless of age.[89]

Social-cognitive theories and health

In general, empirical research regarding identity and the self has explored relations with physical health outcomes, whereas research regarding socioemotional selectivity theory has focused on relations with emotional outcomes. As one advances in age, people define themselves increasingly in terms of health and physical functioning.[21] In a study of older adults aged 60 to 96 years, leisure was an important domain for the young-old, whereas health was the most important self-domain for the oldest-old.[90] It appears that adults cognitively manage their expectations and social comparison processes so that they are, in general, no less satisfied with their health status despite increasing physical limitations.

The content of possible selves and perceived control have been examined in relation to subjective well-being, health, and health behaviors. Hooker and Kaus found that having a possible self in the realm of health was more strongly related to reported health behaviors than was a global measure of health values.[91] Stability in perceived control provides a protective benefit to health. Older adults exhibiting variability in perceived control had poorer health, functional status, more physician visits and hospital admissions.[92,93]. Individuals with higher self-efficacy, the belief that one has the ability to exert control over themselves and their environments, interpret and manage stressors in ways that promote health.[94]

With regard to socioemotional selectivity theory, negative exchanges with one social network have a detrimental impact on daily mood, and if encountered frequently, can increase incidence of depression, whereas positive exchanges can serve to buffer the impact of negative exchanges.[95]

Measurement issues

Comparison of findings from studies focusing on possible selves compared with socioemotional selectivity are limited by the different measurement approaches used. The possible-selves construct is measured using a questionnaire inventory.[83] Socioemotional selectivity theory, in contrast, has relied on self-report, observation of marital interactions, and card sorting of potential social partners on the basis of similarity judgments, with the resulting categories submitted to multidimensional scaling analysis.[82]

A strength of social-cognitive approaches is the positing of explanatory processes for personality development; the identification of specific, testable processes such as identity assimilation, identity accommodation, possible selves, or socioemotional selectivity promotes theoretical advances via empirical hypotheses testing.

Social cognitive researchers interested in personality and self in later life investigate domains emphasizing growth and development in old age, and contribute to an individual's perception of possible selves, need for affiliation, and content of life review.

SYNTHESIS AND FUTURE DIRECTIONS

In this chapter, we have reviewed the psychological literature concerning personality development across the adult life span. We considered stage, trait, and social-cognitive approaches to the study of adult personality. Within each section, we reviewed literature on diversity and health outcomes where available. We also included a measurement section highlighting particular assessment instruments and providing an overview of methodological strengths and weaknesses for each approach.

This chapter has reviewed several issues central to the conceptualization of adult personality. The issue of stability versus maturational change or cohort differences in personality development is dependent on the theory and measurement approach used. For example, the relative stability found in the trait approaches (e.g., the Big 5) may be in part a result of the aggregation of multiple personality facets. Examination of stability at both the facet and aggregate level is needed to investigate whether personality may be dependent on genetic or biologic factors. In contrast, measurement of more precise traits (e.g., facets) may be more influenced by cognitive and environmental (i.e., cohort) influences. Thus specific individual traits would be expected to be less stable across time than the Big 5 personality aggregates. As stated in the section on trait theory, clarity in the definition of stability (i.e., intraindividual, mean-level, or ordinal) is critical to ensure that conclusions drawn from differing research methodologies are interpreted uniformly.

In the effort to tease apart the influence of environmental and biologic influences on stability and change, cross-cultural comparisons of adult personality have been particularly useful. Comparisons of adults of the same age who have experienced different environments across the life span provide evidence regarding the extent of environmental influence on personality. More research is needed, however, addressing personality development of very old individuals in diverse cultures. Additionally, investigation of health effects of adult personality in diverse cultures provides invaluable information for health service provision and the development of preventive interventions.

Finally, it would be useful to apply the wealth of accumulated information regarding personality across adulthood to the provision of services designed to enhance quality of life. Identification of personality processes that drive specific behaviors and choices (i.e., medical treatments) is needed. There is powerful evidence that personality characteristics can affect health status and health behaviors. For example, interventions such as life review have successfully enhanced quality of life. Using social-cognitive approaches to adult personality development and the processes of identity assimilation, identity accommodation, and socioemotional selectivity could inform interventions designed to improve the process of advance care planning for the implementation of life-sustaining or palliative treatments at the end of life.

Furthermore, applied intervention research will not only enhance service provision but also drive theoretical advances in the concept of the self in old age. For example, palliative care and/or hospice interventions designed to provide services targeting personal, physical, and spiritual needs can inform aspects of socioemotional selectivity theory involving present-time orientation and time remaining to live. Incorporating aspects of life review could also provide advances in theories driving therapeutic approaches for depression. Interventions for bereaved personal and professional caregivers and interventions for the terminally or chronically ill older adult are desperately needed. It is our contention that the time to apply our knowledge of adult personality across the life span is now, thereby deriving benefit from our accumulated knowledge and driving advances in theory.

ACKNOWLEDGMENT

Dr. K. Warner Schaie and Dr. Sherry L. Willis are now faculty at the University of Washington, Department of Psychiatry and Behavioral Sciences, Seattle Longitudinal Study, 180 Nickerson Street, Suite 206, Seattle, WA 98109.

KEY POINTS

The Aging Personality and Self

- Personality is the pattern of thoughts, feelings, and behaviors that shape an individual's interface with the world, distinguish one person from another, and manifest across time and situations. It is impacted by biologic, cognitive, and environmental determinants.
- Stage theorists include Freud, Jung, and Erikson. The psychoanalytic approach to adult personality encompasses four domains: level of consciousness, personality structure, defense mechanisms, and stages of psychosexual development. Erikson's eight stages of development are based on the idea that the growing personality moves through stages in an ordered fashion. Few studies investigating stage theories of personality have focused on diverse cultures, racial/ethnic groups, or health.
- Trait approaches are the standard method of personality assessment today with multiple instruments available. The Big 5 personality traits are: neuroticism. extraversion, openness to experience, agreeableness, and conscientiousness. In general, the results of cross-cultural studies are consistent with the hypothesis that there are universal intrinsic maturational changes in personality. Neuroticism in particular has been associated with several health outcomes including stress, chronic conditions, and mortality.
- The social-cognitive approach focuses on the individual's sense of self, developing through the interaction of internal and environmental factors. Social-cognitive theories have incorporated physical health and emotional outcomes.
- The socioemotional selectivity theory focuses on the agentic choices made by adults in their social world for the purpose of regulating knowledge-oriented emotion goals. In socioemotional selectivity theory, individuals alter their environmental interactions such that optimization of emotional experience is prioritized later in life. There are few empirical investigations incorporating diverse cultural or racial/ethnic groups in the study of social-cognitive approaches to adult personality development; existing evidence suggests similar age differences across cultures.

For a complete list of references, please visit online only at www.expertconsult.com

CHAPTER 30

Successful Aging: The Centenarians

Thomas T. Perls

Demography of centenarians

According to the United States Social Security Administration, in 2006 approximately 40,000 people age 100 years and older collected Social Security benefits. On the other hand, the U.S. census reported 50,000 centenarians for the year 2000.[1] Thus, in the United States, there can be substantial variation in the reported prevalence of centenarians. Suffice it to say that centenarians are relatively rare, somewhere in the range of 1 to 2 per 10,000 in the United States. Although the growth of centenarians has been noted to be the fastest of any age group, that growth appears to be slowing to about 4% in the United States.[2]

Other countries note similar findings. Scotland recently reported 680 centenarians for 2006, for a population of 5,116,900[3]; a rate of approximately 1 centenarian per 7500 people. The Scottish report also noted that the relative prevalence of male centenarians was rising, from 10% of centenarians in 2002, to 12.5% in 2006. In 2000, in the United States, male prevalence among centenarians was 14.1%.[2] In England plus Wales, centenarians have been noted to be the fastest growing age group since the 1950s. Since 2002, the annual growth rate is 5.8% according to a 2007 report.[4] In Canada, in 2006, there were 4635 people age 100 years and older or 1.5 centenarians per 10,000 in the population.[5] Statistics Canada states that the highest centenarian prevalence is in Japan, where there were 29,000 centenarians in 2006, a rate of about 2.3 centenarians per 10,000 people.[5]

Definitions of healthy aging

In the New England Centenarian Study (http://www.bumc.bu.edu/centenarian), we study centenarians and their family members primarily because of our long-held belief that these individuals are a model of successful aging. By determining exposure and genetic factors that are more or less common compared to other groups, we should be able to determine risk factors for premature versus healthy aging and to formulate strategies that enhance a person's ability to compress their disability toward the end of a longer life. An important question to ask, however, is: are centenarians and/or their family members in fact models of successful or healthy aging?

The answer depends upon the definition of successful or healthy aging, which geriatricians and gerontologists continue to grapple with. In a very helpful attempt at dealing with this issue, Depp and Jeste looked at various components of 29 different definitions of successful aging from 28 studies. For 26 of these definitions, the predominant feature was being disability-free.[6] Robine and Michel have also stressed the importance of quality of life and sense of well-being in considering a definition.[7]

Of factors important in successful aging, they stress the impact of genetics, environment, economics, and culture over the life span.[7] Crimmins notes the importance of allostatic load (the cost of compensating for and adapting to stressors) upon a person's ability to age well.[8,9] The ability to deal with stressors and more generally age-related diseases leads to the as-of-yet poorly defined notions of adaptive capacity, functional reserve, and resilience, which may be important distinguishing features in the ability to achieve exceptional old age.[10]

Based upon their ability to compress disability toward the end of their lives, we believe, at least retrospectively, that centenarians are a human model of healthy aging (based upon disability prevalence). Early on in our study of approximately 50 centenarians, we noted that approximately 90% of the centenarians in a population-based study were functionally independent at the average age of 92 years.[11] We subsequently also noted that a number of centenarians were compressing their disability well into their 90s while noting a long history of age-related disease(s). Christensen et al longitudinally studied Danish nonagenarians from the 1905 birth cohort from 1998 to 2005, quantifying at multiple time points their cognitive and physical function. Over this time period, the proportion of functionally independent individuals, beginning at 39% and ending at 32%, remained fairly stable.[12] Their results suggest that functional independence is an important marker of future survival at very old ages. From these and other studies, disease prevalence in some older individuals might not be a reliable marker of disability.

DISTINGUISHING BETWEEN COMPRESSION OF MORBIDITY AND COMPRESSION OF DISABILITY AND THE ROLE OF RESILIENCE (FUNCTIONAL RESERVE AND ADAPTIVE CAPACITY)

Many centenarians do not compress their illnesses (morbidity) toward the end of their lives. Approximately 45% have sustained some chronic age-related illness before age 80 years, 42% develop such a disease after the age of 80, and about 13% remain disease-free at age 100; we have termed these groups respectively, survivors, delayers, and escapers.[13] The Tokyo and Greek centenarian studies recently determined a similar prevalence of escapers in their study.[14,15]

Despite the fact that most centenarians do not compress their morbidity, we suspected from our previous work that most, nonetheless, compress their disability. We therefore hypothesized that compression of disability, perhaps more so than morbidity, is an important marker and determinant of exceptional longevity.[16] To investigate this hypothesis, Lara Terry led the analysis of disease and functional status history from 523 women and 216 men ages 97 years and older. Subjects were divided into those who developed age-related diseases (chronic obstructive pulmonary disease, dementia, diabetes, heart disease, hypertension, osteoporosis, Parkinson disease, and/or stroke) at or before the age of 85 years (termed "survivors") and those who developed any of these diseases after the age of 85 (termed "delayers"). We then also classified these individuals according to their last-assessed functional status (e.g., at age 97 years old or older).

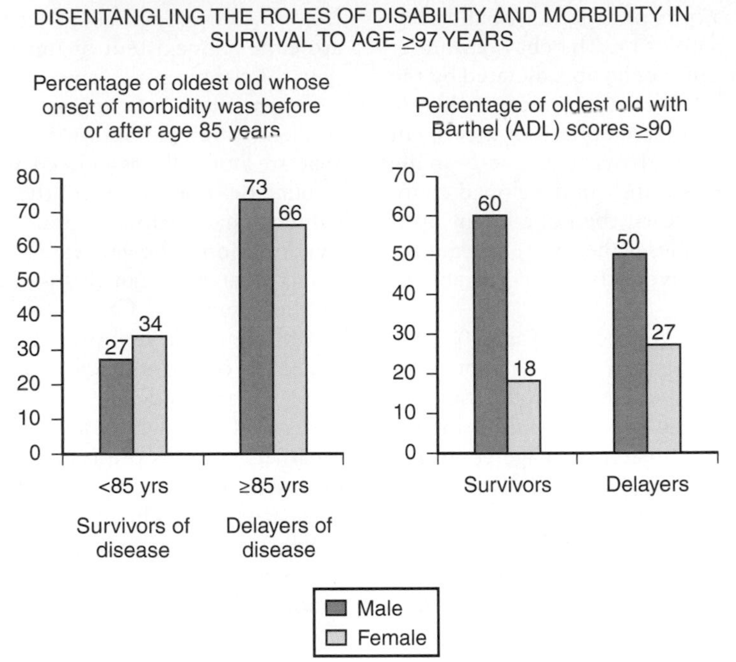

Figure 30-1. A group of 523 women and 216 men age greater than 97 years were studied retrospectively for age of onset for age-related diseases, and at the time of interview, their current level of function. Left panel: Frequency of men and women whose age of onset of age-related diseases was before age 85 years ("survivors" of disease) or at 85 years or older ("delayers" of disease). Right panel: Frequency of male and female survivors and delayers who at the time of interview (age >97 years) were independently functioning.

Overall, 32% of the subjects were survivors and 68% were delayers. Further results are depicted in Figure 30-1. As the first panel reveals, the majority of these very old subjects were delayers of disease (73% of males and 66% of females), and 27% of males and 34% of females were survivors of disease. In the second panel of Figure 30-1, we see that despite being survivors of disease, 60% of the males were independently functioning at age 97 years or older. On the other hand, just 18% of the female survivors were independently functioning. Among the disease delayers, 50% of the males and 27% of the females were independently functioning at age 97 years or older.

Therefore, it is remarkable that whereas many people have significant morbidity and mortality associated with numerous age-related diseases, the above centenarian survivors and delayers have a resilience (or functional reserve or adaptive capacity) that allows them to not only live to extreme old age, but to do so while compressing their disability until very old age. Quantifying and understanding the underlying determinants and mechanisms of this resilience should be an important priority in the study of healthy aging and exceptional survival.

The gender disparity

As seen in the second panel of Figure 30-1, male centenarians tend to have significantly better functional status than their female counterparts. The fact that male centenarians more frequently have better physical and cognitive function than their female counterparts has been noted in most centenarian studies, most notably the Italian Centenarian Study.[12] It might first seem paradoxical that male centenarians fare better than female centenarians, the females outnumber the males approximately 8:1. The female survival advantage begins at around age 50, when men generally begin to experience particularly vascular-related diseases such as myocardial infarction and stroke, whereas women delay the clinical expression of these diseases by 10 or so years, until their 60s to 70s. A plausible hypothesis for why male centenarians fare better is that only those who are functionally independent are able to achieve such extreme old age. Women on the other hand appear to be able to survive with age-related diseases more readily and thus experience the double-edged sword of being able to live longer while also more frequently living with age-related illnesses and disability. This hypothesis is supported by findings in the above- cited Danish study in which 38% of males at age 98 years were functionally independent but then this proportion rose to 53% among 100-year-olds.[12] The proportion of women who were independent, how ever, continued to fall, from 30% of 98-year-olds to 28% of 100-year-olds. The most obvious explanation for these trends would be a selection phenomenon among the men, where the frail die, leaving behind a cohort of exceptionally fit survivors. The other paradox I would mention here is that while the male centenarians might be exceptionally fit relative to the females, it would appear that they still have higher age-related disease associated mortality rates, so that once they do develop a disease, such as dementia or stroke, their mortality risk probably is much higher than it might be for women. Such hypotheses point to the possibility that women are much more resilient than men with regards to aging and age-related diseases.

Heritability and familiality of exceptional longevity

Twin studies demonstrate that only 20% to 30% of life expectancy is genetic, whereas 70% to 80% of the variation is due to environment, behavior, and luck.[18,19] Epidemiologic studies such as the Seventh Day Adventist Health

Study also suggest that the majority of variation around average life expectancy is due to people's health behaviors. Fraser and Shavlik found that the healthy behaviors dictated by the Seventh Day Adventist religion (e.g., no tobacco or alcohol use, regular exercise, vegetarian diet, emphasis of time spent with faith and family) can explain a 10-year advantage in life expectancy.[20] If average life expectancy in developed countries is approximately 78 to 80 years, then one might optimistically expect that most people, if they were to emulate the behaviors of Seventh Day Adventists, should be able to live to 88 to 90 years.

If optimal health behaviors can get people to age 90 years, then one must assume that genetics and luck come into play in achieving even older ages. A number of studies suggest that genetic variation might play an increasingly important role at the oldest ages (e.g., greater than age 90 years), which should be encouraging for the potential discovery of genetic determinants of exceptional longevity.[21–24] Such a genetic advantage likely takes the form of lacking variations that increase risk for premature mortality and more controversially, also variations that slow down the rate of aging and decrease the risk for age-related diseases.[25,26]

We have observed a marked predisposition of the siblings of centenarians to also achieve exceptional longevity.[27,28] The children of centenarians appear to be very much following in the footsteps of their parents with 50% to 60% reduced rates of cardiovascular disease, stroke, diabetes, hypertension, and cancer compared with the children of parents that belonged to the same birth cohort as the centenarians but who died at average life expectancy.[29,30] Furthermore, already in the septuagenarian years, the centenarian offspring experience 20% reduced mortality rates compared with the referent cohort.[31] Barzilai et al noted that both centenarians and their children, more frequently than their referent cohort (the spouses of the offspring), had large high- and low-density lipoprotein (HDL and LDL) particle size, which is associated with lower cardiovascular disease risk. This phenotype was associated with a higher frequency in both generations of a specific variation of the cholesteryl ester transfer protein (CETP) gene.[32]

Supercentenarians

Supercentenarians, who are people age 110 years and older, were virtually unheard of before 1960. Currently there are approximately 70 such individuals in the United States and approximately 300 worldwide. Over the past 10 years, we have enrolled enough supercentenarians to name a new study, The New England Supercentenarian Study (http://www.bumc.bu.edu/supercentenarian). The oldest supercentenarian whose age has been well validated was Jeanne Calment, who died at the age of 122 years in 1997. Even older claimed ages are immediately suspect and often come from less developed countries where such old vital records are either nonexistent or unreliable and there is secondary gain for claiming such ages.

Supercentenarians appear to be different in terms of their resilience and the ability to live with age-related diseases that are normally associated with increased mortality risk. In our case series review of the medical histories of 32 supercentenarians, we found cardiovascular disease, diabetes, and hypertension to be very rare (<3%).[33] Stroke was a bit more common at 10%, but this is still remarkable given the ages of these subjects. Cancer, though, was unexpectedly frequent, with 25% reporting a cancer history. We also found that 41% of the subjects required only minimal assistance or were independently functioning. Thus, the supercentenarians, 90% of whom are women, are similar to male centenarians in terms of probably lacking functional reserve to deal with an age-related disease and therefore once such a disease becomes clinically evident, the mortality risk is very high. The cancer history is interesting, particularly given the well-known interplay between mechanisms of aging and of cancer.[34] Anecdotally we have found extremely old individuals who present with unusually large tumors that have not metastasized. We suspect that cancers and their ability to spread behave quite differently in the extreme old compared with people of younger ages and this represents another important avenue of further research.

KEY POINTS
Successful Aging: The Centenarians

- Centenarians are among the fastest growing age groups in developed countries. Much of this growth is due to the few number of centenarians before 1960, major improvements in public health measures throughout the early to mid 1900s, and marked improvements in the health of people age 80 and older.
- Whereas the compression of both morbidity and disability are essential features of survival to old age for some centenarians, for others, the compression of disability alone may be the key prerequisite. Functional status and not necessarily the presence of disease, and certainly not age alone, are important factors to consider in assessing a person's prognosis.
- Although far fewer in number, male centenarians tend to have significantly better cognition and physical function than their female counterparts.
- Exceptional longevity runs strongly in families and the importance of genetic factors in achieving older age might increase at the most extreme ages.

For a complete list of references, please visit online only at www.expertconsult.com

CHAPTER 31

Social Gerontology

Paul Higgs
James Nazroo

INTRODUCTION

Social gerontology, as its name implies, is concerned with the study of the social aspects of old age. This remit is broad, encompassing a large range of topics, disciplines, and methods, and requiring a good understanding of the clinical and economic dimensions of aging. Factors studied cover: individual experiences of aging (age identities, social networks and supports, life events, coping and resilience, etc.); the social institutions that provide health and social care services to older people; how old age is socially constructed and the age-related inequalities that flow from this; the factors that drive social and health inequalities in older age, such as class, gender, and ethnicity/race; and the broad social impacts of our aging populations. But central to these studies has been a concern to understand the factors that promote or undermine the well-being, or quality of life, of older people.

The main conclusions from research on older people's quality of life, and their clinical implications, were well summarized in Hepburn's chapter in the previous edition of this volume, which focused on factors that contribute to "social functioning"—social status, social connections, occupations/activities, personal resources, and life events.[1] Here we take a broader view of the social context of aging, describing the development of approaches within social gerontology that seek to theorize and understand the aging experience. We illustrate how these ideas have developed in ways that reflect changes in the experience of aging and show how the drivers of these changes relate to social inequalities at older ages. We begin by describing the tendency within social gerontology to problematize the circumstances of later life, through accounts of adjustment, disengagement, dependency, and poverty and through a conceptualization of increasing life expectancy in terms of the potential difficulties that are brought about as populations age. We go on to argue that as later life becomes more of a potentially positive experience for greater numbers of people, such an approach is not the most useful way to view old age in today's world. We suggest that we are seeing dramatic changes in the experience of aging that need to be understood both in terms of changes to the health and wealth of older people and in terms of the cultural context of cohorts—such as the baby boomer generation—now entering retirement. These "new" older people challenge much of the thinking about old age and how it relates to gerontology. We conclude by returning to the theme of inequality, by exploring the heterogeneity of aging experiences and how these relate to class, gender and ethnicity/race.

THE "PROBLEM" OF OLD AGE

As Cole, Achenbaum, and Katz have observed, current academic concerns with aging have tended to focus on the "problem of old age."[2,3,4] Indeed, the perception of older people as a social problem has a long history in both social and health research, and this preoccupation with the problems of senescence characterizes the development of gerontology, including social gerontology. Katz[4] quotes the first article in the first issue of the newly established *Journal of Gerontology* in 1946, which stated that "Gerontology reflects the recognition of a new kind of problem that will increasingly command the interest and devotion of a variety of scientists, scholars, and professional workers.[5]" How this influenced the development of specifically social approaches to later life can be seen with the establishment of a Committee on Social Adjustment in Old Age by the Social Science Research Council in 1944 and a Research Unit into the Problems of Aging by the UK Nuffield Foundation in 1946. In this immediate postwar period, Sauvy (1947) suggested that Britain's economic difficulties were largely the result of an aging population. Furthermore he claimed that:

> *"The danger of a collapse of western civilization owing to a lack of replacement of its human stock cannot be questioned. Perhaps we ought to regard this organic disease, this lack of vitality of the cells, as a symptom of senility of the body politic itself and thus compare social biology with animal biology".[6], pg. 124*

This sense of foreboding had been a strong theme driving earlier developments in social policy. The introduction of old age pensions in Britain in 1908 was not only intended to eliminate extreme poverty in old age, but also to lower "poor law" expenditure on older people.[7] By the mid 1920s the effects of economic turbulence had moved the terms of debate in the direction of the capacity of retirement to alleviate unemployment. In this formulation removal from active participation in the workforce was the main motivation for retirement, which in time led to a lowering of the retirement age to 65.

In the United States there were similar concerns to take older workers out of the workforce, with the economic depression of the 1930s creating an impetus for change. However, several factors complicated matters, including the fact that the majority of older people in the United States were still in employment. In addition legislators had to deal with the federal structure of the government, the confusing pattern of Civil War pension entitlements that many were eligible for, and the wide array of pension schemes operating across companies and occupations.[8,9] In this context, the Townsendite movement of the 1930s (named after Dr. Francis E. Townsend) argued for a tax-funded state pension rather than one based on a contributory principle. Furthermore, in advocating the reflationary potential of creating a large number of state-funded consumers, the movement reconceptualized retirement with the slogan *"youth for work/age for leisure."*[9] However, the New Deal and its Social Security pension when it was established in 1935 was much more conventional in its conception, acting as both a poverty alleviation program and as a way of dealing with unemployment by using retirement to release jobs to younger workers.

The identification of the old as a problem that needed to be resolved continued along these lines for much of the second half of the twentieth century, although with different national emphases. In the United Kingdom the tradition that includes Rowntree's studies of poverty,[10,11] continued in the work of Townsend,[12] and has been a continuing theme of social gerontologists into the twenty-first century.[13] Conversely, in the United States, the successful selling of retirement after World War II led to research initiatives and programs on both successful and productive aging, concerned with investigating adaptation to the circumstances of retirement. Whatever the national differences, the collection of data to answer questions posed as the "problem of aging" has continued to the current day, although more recently within the context of population aging and the economic consequences that accompany it. Paradoxically, this has meant that research is now directed at the problems posed by "a rapidly growing population of rather healthy and self-sufficient persons whose collective dependence is now straining the economies of western nations".[4] We return to this theme shortly, but first describe the early theoretical perspectives that have underpinned social gerontology.

THEORETICAL APPROACHES: FROM FUNCTIONALISM TO STRUCTURED DEPENDENCY

Much of the reason for social gerontology's focus on the problems associated with later life lies in the emergence of retirement, in the 1940s in the United States,[9] and the 1960s in the United Kingdom,[14] as a distinct part of the life course. This led sociologists working within the functionalist tradition, such as Parsons and Burgess,[15,16] to worry about the "roleless role" of the retired person, a population defined by their permanent exit from the labor market rather than indigence. Obviously this referred mainly to men for whom social role and employment were seen as largely interchangeable, whereas a consistent domesticated role was assumed for women. Criticism of this view, and the corresponding assumption that retirement was therefore relatively nonproblematic for women, came from Beeson,[17] who pointed out that it was not based on any empirical evidence and ignored the existence of working women.

Some approached this "roleless" state through the prism of "disengagement" theory,[18] focusing on the social and psychological adjustment of the older person to postwork/postmarried life. Theorizing the wider processes that went alongside retirement, this hypothesized that older people in industrial societies disengaged themselves from the roles that they occupied so that younger generations would have opportunities to develop and take on their socially necessary roles. Consequently, disengagement was assumed to not only occur in relation to work roles, but also in relation to families, when retired generations became much less central to the lives of their children. Focusing on a psychological approach, disengagement theory saw itself as influenced by the work of Erikson and notions of life review.[19] A considerable amount of research was undertaken in the United States during the 1960s to provide evidence for this theory. A longitudinal study in Kansas City showed that older people did indeed "disengage", although women were observed to start this process at widowhood, whereas men began on retirement.[20] This approach, which for a long time was one of the dominant paradigms in social gerontology, saw the way in which old age occurred in modern societies as an inevitable and natural process. Questions about whether older people wanted to "disengage", or were forced to do so by society, were not asked. The emphasis on psychological adjustment also avoided looking at the very real social processes that structured old age.

Although disengagement theory centered on the perspective of the individual older person, the analysis put forward by the predominantly British "structured dependency" approach stressed the importance of social policy.[21] For writers in this school and those who described themselves as adopting the "political economy" approach to aging, the problem of old age was not one of individual social and psychological adjustment but of a dependency "structured" by the circumstances of retirement, something that was set by government social policy.[22,23,24] Townsend noted that retirement not only marks a withdrawal from the formal labor market, it also marks a shift from making a living through earning a wage to being dependent on a replacement income.[21] That this income was often funded by the state demonstrated the role of social policy in structuring the dependency that many older people experienced postretirement. In the United Kingdom, for example, the relatively low levels at which the state pension was paid out indicated the low priority older people had in decisions about state welfare. But as Walker,[22] and others, pointed out, the continuing impact of social class into later life was also indicated in the relative imbalance between the level of state retirement pensions, which funded the majority of working class retirees' old age, and the amounts paid out by the better funded occupational pensions enjoyed by the middle class. Those reliant on state retirement pensions, consequently, were seen as a residual category of the population drawing resources from public funds, a "problem" that led to considerable interest in researching poverty in later life.

It is also argued that structured dependency is not just limited to the economic sphere, but pervades social processes more generally. Townsend suggested that the association of age with infirmity and dependency not only "represents" the position of older people, but also justifies the inferior status of older people and their exclusion from various forms of social participation.[25] Ageism also emerges out of the cultural valorization of "youthfulness", which not only defines aging in negative terms, but also clears the way to make it acceptable to discriminate against older people. This can manifest itself in policies seeking to limit medical or health care resources to older people, in discriminatory employment practices, and in the treatment of physically frail or mentally confused older people.[25] For writers such as Townsend and Walker, with a focus on well-being and social inequality, the "disengaged" position of later life is not only a social construction, but also something that should be challenged by campaigns for the restoration of full citizenship rights to older people.[26]

INCREASING LIFE EXPECTANCY AND COMPRESSION OF MORBIDITY—A GOLDEN AGE

As described elsewhere in this volume, there are many who argue that the human life span is malleable, mortality only occurring as a result of an accumulation of damage in cells and tissues and limitations in investments in somatic maintenance.[27] And more controversially writers such as de Grey argue that longevity can be extended upwards once the basic biologic processes have been understood.[28] Although his views have been heavily criticized, at a population level there is now a widespread recognition that life expectancy is increasing rapidly, at an accelerating rate. For example, Rau et al show that for men aged 80 to 89 mortality rates dropped by 0.81% between the 1950s and 1960s, but by 1.88% between the 1980s and 1990s, whereas for women of the same age group the figures were 0.91% and 2.45%, and the rate of acceleration in decline in mortality rates is greatest for older people.[29] Given a focus on the problem of age, it is not surprising that concerns have been expressed that increased longevity might lead to higher rates of morbidity and/or disability; a "failure of success" where industrial societies have passed through an epidemiologic transition that has shifted the burden of disease onto chronic conditions in later life.[30] However, this conclusion has been challenged by evidence that suggests that increased life expectancy does not come at the cost of an "expansion of morbidity".[31] Writers such as James Fries have proposed a thesis built around a "compression of morbidity", where even under the conditions of increased life expectancy the proportion of life spent in ill health is concentrated into an ever shorter period before death.[32,33] Although this view challenged many of the assumptions made about the connection between aging and chronic illness, there has been considerable support for the claim that chronologic age in itself is not a factor in increasing levels of disability and chronic illness.[34] Although analysis based on subjective measures of health have suggested an increasing disease burden in later life,[35] more objective indicators of disability suggest a more positive view of healthy life expectancy.[36,37] Indeed, recent analyses of disability rates in the United States suggest that not only are disability rates falling, they are falling at an accelerating rate, much in the same way as mortality rates are falling at an accelerating rate. For example, in 1982–1984 rates were falling at a rate of 0.6% per annum, a figure that increased to almost four times that level (2.2%) by 1999–2004/2005, and rates decreased most rapidly for oldest people.[38]

However, to this must be added the emergence of an "obesity epidemic", which may reverse the decline in both mortality and disability and may lead to new patterns of chronic illness. Olshansky et al argue that current trends in obesity in the United States may result in a decline in life expectancy for future cohorts.[39] Based on current rates of death associated with obesity they predict that life expectancy will be reduced by between one third and three quarters of a year. So, the trends are complex. In Canada a study of health lifestyles among baby boomers identified a number of contradictory changes. A substantial fall in smoking rates, increase in levels of excessive drinking, and reductions in levels of exercise over the last quarter of the twentieth century were accompanied by a sharp increase in rates of obesity and diabetes.[40] Manton uses the notion of "dynamic equilibrium" to suggest that mortality in later life is affected by the rate of "natural aging" and the distribution of risk factors for specific diseases in the population.[41] Interventions aimed at risk factors will bring improvements in both mortality and reduce the severity of associated disabilities. Schoeni, Freedman, and Martin have noted how changes in smoking behavior, greater educational attainment, and declines in poverty have impacted on the decline in disability levels in the United States.[36] This, however, raises the issue of whether the achievement of a successful postretirement later life is the province of the disciplined individual, rather than the expectation of the ordinary person, and again raises questions as to the role, and contribution, of the healthy retired.

OPPORTUNITY AGE—SUCCESSFUL AGING AND THE THIRD AGE

The implicit concerns regarding the status of older people has also been a theme of what has come to be known as the "productive aging" approach.[42] This position has antecedents in Rowe and Kahn's notion of "successful aging",[43,44] which sought to separate this positive state, characterized by good health and social engagement, from what was termed "usual" aging. Productive aging adopts a broader approach than that of successful aging. It is concerned to make it possible for the increasing numbers of people who are living longer and healthier lives, under changes in the circumstances of retirement and in the nature of work, to make significant social or economic contributions, rather than simply retiring to a state of leisure. Again the focus is on social engagement, with productive aging going beyond conventional meanings of economic productivity to include volunteering and civic participation.[45,46] Older people acting in this way would therefore demonstrate that they were not just consumers of resources, but also made a valuable contribution to the societies in which they lived. The benefits of engaging in productive aging for the individual and society are argued to be considerable as they not only engaged individuals in society, but also used otherwise wasted capacities and capabilities.

Many of the criticisms of the productive aging approach have focused on the possibility that such laudable intentions could be easily interpreted as a simple invocation of the need to be productive in conventional economic terms.[47] Estes and Mahakian go further in their criticism by linking both successful and productive aging approaches with an extension of market principles into the process of aging itself, arguing that this acts to benefit what they call the "biomedically oriented medical-industrial complex" and ignores the social and economic disadvantages operating in both society and social policy.[48] As a result, while the advocates of the productive aging approach have moved the debate on aging away from a simple equation of age and dependency, a tendency to identify those aspects of later life that mesh with normative assumptions about desirable social and economic worth remains in this approach. So, the problematizing of old age has not occurred only around perceived role deficits and social exclusion, it has also focused on the responsibilities that older people should take on.

This is also reflected in discussions of the potential for older people to enjoy a fulfilling "third age" of relative good health and affluence. The idea of the third age is most associated with the work of Laslett, who argued that later life can no longer be viewed in a pessimistic fashion.[49] Not only is the portion of most people's lives spent in retirement increasing, the idea of a fixed retirement age is being challenged by the many individuals who have chosen to take retirement at ages other than that set by eligibility for the state retirement pension. For many, Laslett argued, retirement offers possibilities for undertaking the self-enriching activities denied earlier in life when the tasks of earning a living, or bringing up children, or both, got in the way.

> *"The life phase in which there is no longer employment and child raising to commandeer time, and before morbidity enters to limit activity and mortality brings everything to a close, has been called the third age. Those in this phase have passed through a first age of youth, when they are prepared for the activities of maturity, and a second age of maturity, when their lives were given to those activities, and have reached a third age in which they can, within fairly wide limits, live their lives as they please, before being overtaken by a fourth age of decline."*[49], pg. 3

In discussing a long positive third age underpinned by relatively good health and a short, but ultimately terminal, fourth age, Laslett demonstrated the opening up of the period of retirement away from a simple conflation with old age. However, in his focus on the third age, Laslett is wary that later life should not become self-indulgent. To this end he warns of the dangers of indolence and the importance of accepting the responsibilities of the third age. In particular, he identifies education as one of the key areas necessary for a successful third age, and to this end he was a proponent of the University of the Third Age. He also saw the duties of the third age as going much further than just using time well and explicitly called for older people to act as cultural trustees for society.[49] The challenge, as Laslett sees it, is to get those in the third age to accept their responsibilities rather than simply enjoy a leisure retirement.

However, this moral reading of the third age has become more difficult to maintain as the conflation between the third age and the baby boomer generation has become widely accepted, particularly in the United States.[50,51] For the baby boomer generation there is the real potential for retirement to be transformed into an arena of lifestyle and consumption, rather than education and responsibility. A blurring of the distinction between "middle" and "old" age is fostered by the increasing influence of lifestyle consumerism on significant numbers of older people, rather than just the younger age groups typically associated with these developments.[52] Here the third age can be seen as a space in which old age can be avoided and an ill-defined middle age can be extended further and further up the life course.[53] For example, the submergence of clear age-appropriate divisions in dress, along with the greater acceptability of leisure clothing, has meant that jeans and T-shirts can be worn by people of very different ages without social sanction.[54] The signs of old age become seen as a "mask" detracting from the person beneath.[52] This relates to the individualization, or destandardization, of the life course, where the idea of a linear life course, with clearly defined stages, has become less applicable.[55,56]

Gilleard and Higgs have argued that to better grasp the contemporary experiences of aging there is a need for an understanding of the implications of this increasing cultural engagement with lifestyle and consumerism by successive cohorts of retirees.[57] Such an approach suggests that we are witnessing the aging of generations whose adult life has been organized through the prism of a youth-oriented consumer culture. The postwar "baby boomer" cohorts who grew up in circumstances of expanding consumer choice and economic prosperity created a "generational schism" between themselves and those older than they, who had grown up in less prosperous times. This schism manifested itself in attitudes, music, and clothes, but most significantly in lifestyles, where there have been cumulative changes to the nature of families, relationships, and sexuality. And this has not been discarded as the teenagers of the sixties became the retirees of the twenty-first century.[51,58] It is this generationally located set of attitudes and behaviors that may lie behind many of the features of contemporary aging.

The identification of retirement in terms of its opportunities for leisure, rather than simply being a "roleless role," or a moment for life review, can be seen among those older workers who do not wait until the state retirement pension age, or forced redundancy, to retire. Retirement as choice is valorized by a consumer culture, whereas those who face redundancy or conventional retirement patterns are seen as less agentic and less able to deal with the new circumstances of later life. That contemporary retirement and later life is more structured by these contemporary cultural pressures than by concerns for the social worth of older generations can be seen in the concerns of governments and social commentators as they seek to reflect, and adapt, this image of later life to their more pressing objectives of deregulation and commodification of social policy. Indeed it is the emphasis on leisure retirement over civic participation, rather than inequality, that is most reflected in the writings of Laslett on the third age and those advocating productive aging. Whether the so called "greedy geezers" will take the resources without reciprocating is a question that motivates much of the research agenda.[59] Equally the opportunities of current retirees cannot be assumed to continue indefinitely as some of the unique factors associated with the "baby boomer" generation may disappear and the proretired stance of many welfare regimes may become the focus for reform.

INEQUALITIES IN LATER LIFE—CONTINUITIES AND IMPACT

The transformation of later life along the lines suggested in the preceding section depends on older people having the resources to be able to participate in the various cultural activities now open to them. The incomes and standard of living of the majority of retired people in the European Union and North America have improved greatly over the past few decades. For example, in 1979 in Britain 47% of pensioners were in the bottom fifth of the income distribution, but by 2005–2006 this had fallen to just under 25%.[60] So while the association of age with poverty has been a historic reality, the relationship is not deterministic and, as the figure of 25% in the bottom 20% of incomes indicates, is no longer the case. Indeed, as those writing from a structured dependency position have argued in a different context, income poverty is not driven by retirement *per se*. As the cohorts who were working in the latter part of the twentieth century, who were on average relatively more affluent than their predecessors, have retired, they have brought into retirement some of the benefits they had accrued during their working lives, allowing them to continue to pursue the lifestyles they had developed earlier in their lives. However, this affluence has not necessarily been equally shared among these cohorts. There is a diversity of locations within the older population, some of whom are not as well off as others. Levels of poverty are, of course, also influenced by state policies. For example, in England only 25% of those aged above the state pension age were in income poverty (defined as those receiving 60% or less of the median household income for all ages) in 2004–2005, and that this figure had fallen substantially from 31% over the short period since 2002–2003 as a result of changes in the tax benefit system.[61] But most relevant to changes in the average level of poverty among the postretirement population is the changing preretirement circumstances of successive cohorts moving into retirement.

These changed circumstances have not, however, led to reductions in the level of inequality among the older population (rather than between older and younger people). Analyses of the incomes of people aged 50 and older in England, for example, show the income distribution to be heavily skewed, with more than two thirds of individuals having household incomes below the mean level.[61] Single women are substantially more likely to be in income poverty than others, and women who are divorced, separated, or widowed face the highest risk of income poverty.[61] Not surprisingly, another key determinant of income poverty is education level, with higher levels of education negatively associated with income poverty.[61] Wealth is, perhaps, a more accurate reflection of economic well-being at older ages, reflecting as it does both the accumulation of advantage over the life course and resources to support consumption in postwork life. Data on the wealth distribution show similar levels of inequality. In England, those making up the top 10% of the wealth distribution of the 50 and older population have an average net total wealth (excluding pension wealth) of approximately £1,200,000, compared with the mean figure of approximately £300,000 and a median figure of approximately £205,000.[61] If housing wealth is excluded (on the basis that not all housing wealth can be realized to support nonhousing consumption), the figures are an average of £500,000 for the top 10% of the wealth distribution, compared with a mean of £110,000, a median of only £22,500, and approximately 20% of the population having no wealth.[61] The wealthiest tenth of the population aged 50 and older hold 40% of the total wealth and 63% of nonhousing wealth.[61]

Returning to the importance of preretirement circumstances, it is obvious to state that such inequalities among the older population reflect those occurring earlier in the life course. But there is a distinct possibility that they are aggravated by the retirement process. In England less than half of men and a third of women in the 5 years before state pension age are in paid employment, and a significant proportion of those in paid employment are part-time employment (a fifth of men and two thirds of women).[62] However, such early "retirement" is not unrelated to wealth, with those at the bottom of the wealth distribution being most likely to not be working followed by those at the top of the wealth distribution.[62] And route into retirement also varies by occupational grade and wealth, with those in the highest grades and with the highest wealth more likely to have taken some form of voluntary retirement, and those in the lowest grades and with the lowest wealth more likely to have left work because of poor health or redundancy.[63,64]

Such inequalities extend beyond the financial realm and extend to cultural activities, social and civic participation, and health. For example, in the 50 and older population in England, less than a quarter of those with managerial and professional occupational class backgrounds are not a member of an organization, compared with almost two fifths of those with an intermediate class background and almost half of those with a routine or manual class background.[65] Similarly, almost three quarters of those in the managerial and professional class group visit museums and art galleries, compared with close to three fifths of those in intermediate classes and just over a third of those in routine and manual classes.[65]

In terms of health, socioeconomic inequalities persist despite dramatic increases in life expectancy.[66] In terms of risk of mortality, in a 5-year follow-up of an English sample age 50 and over, 5% of men in the richest wealth quintile had died compared with 18% of men in the poorest wealth quintile, with equivalent figures of 3.3% and 15.6% for women.[67] Similar differences can be found in relation to morbidity, with measures of self-evaluated health, symptoms of disease, diagnoses of disease, limitations in physical and cognitive function, risky health behaviors, and biomarkers of disease all showing marked inequalities by occupational class, income, wealth, and education at older ages.[68–71]

Such inequalities in economic position, cultural activities, social participation, and health may be aggravated by the general move in developed countries toward individual responsibility for achieving a comfortable postretirement income. Those adopting the structured dependency approach see this increasingly individualized approach to social policy as perpetuating class, gender, and ethnic/race inequalities. Taking class inequality as their cue, the "political economy" strand has linked the position of older people to more neo-Marxist themes around the role of the older person within the capitalist economy.[22,23] Equally gender and ethnic/race inequality in relation to pensions and consequent postretirement economic inequalities have been explored.[72–75] And in more recent works the mixed fortunes of older people in the globalized economy have been a focus for theorizing.[76] All of this literature points to a need to consider the ways in which lives of older people are socially structured, but also how the nature of this might be changing (perhaps differentially across classes, genders, and ethnicities) with time and across generations.

CONCLUDING COMMENTS

Social gerontology's concern with the study of old age has meant that of necessity it has had to embrace the changes that have occurred to the nature of aging and old age over the past 60 years. Most significantly this has meant understanding the changing nature of retirement, a period that is an expected life stage for the vast majority of people in developed countries and a life stage that is no longer necessarily marked "by the shadow of the workhouse". Indeed, what it means to be retired, as well as the way in which age, health, and retirement interact, has undergone profound change. Many of the afflictions and disabilities of old age no longer define the whole period after working age, even if they are a constitutive part of old age. Such positive changes in retirement, postretirement life, and aging are distributed in unequal ways that reflect previously existing imbalances in resources, but this does not suggest that there has been no change, in the position of older people. The circumstances of older people reflect a diversity of experiences and a persistence of inequality, but older people can no longer be conceived in general terms as "roleless," disengaged, or forced into dependency. In a similar fashion, the circumstances of those living in the third age may merely seem to be precursors of the decline and disability of those living to older ages or those living with greater restrictions, but it would be a mistake to bracket both sets of experiences into one generic concept of old age. The distinctiveness of both the third and the fourth ages means that individuals experiencing them often have different needs and different capacities from one another. Subsuming them under one label runs the risk of failing to address the circumstances of either; suggesting less autonomy to one group and too much agency to another.

The role of social gerontology is to study how old age is lived and how it can be improved. There will be different ways of viewing the problems of "old age" in the future as there have been in the past, but such developments result from the fact that aging and old age are undergoing constant change and will throw up new challenges. It is in this context that the vulnerability of some sections of the older population can be addressed and moves toward the improvements in their lives more firmly situated in the more positive conceptualization of later life established by many of those in the third age.

KEY POINTS
Social Gerontology

- Social gerontology is the study of the social contexts of old age.
- There are a number of different approaches to understanding the social experience of old age.
- Some approaches in social gerontology problematize the situation of older people within society and present accounts that focus on individual adjustment, disengagement, or poverty.
- Other approaches see the emergence of new possibilities of aging as increased life expectancy is often accompanied by good health, especially at younger ages. These positions have been characterized as the "third age" and can be connected to ideas of productive aging.
- An important dimension of aging is the study of inequalities, either between older groups and younger ones or between older people themselves.
- The overall balance of health and illness in the older population, and unequal resourcing of old age, means that social gerontology needs to accept the heterogeneity of later life as a necessary starting point.

For a complete list of references, please visit online only at www.expertconsult.com

CHAPTER 32

Productive Aging

Robert N. Butler

INTRODUCTION

Productive aging is defined as the capacity of an individual or population to serve in the paid workforce and in volunteer activities, to assist in the family, and to maintain, to varying degrees, autonomy and independence for as long as possible. The concept was created primarily in response to stereotyped depictions of older persons as dependent and a burden to society. It served to draw attention to the fact that productivity does not stop when a person grows older, and that the older population is being underused by society. It reflected both the need for older persons to work longer in an older society, and the persistence and universality of prejudice against them in the workplace.[1] The concept of productive aging was also a reaction to the tendency of economists to omit the voluntary activities and informal contributions made by older adults when measuring a nation's gross domestic product (GDP).

The extent to which an older person can remain productive is determined by a variety of personal factors, including physical and emotional well-being, motivation, attitude, education, and experience, and by changing technologies and societal attitudes and structures. The interplay between personal issues and societal norms has an important influence on both paid and unpaid productive activities. Confirming the landmark study by the National Institute of Mental Health of healthy community-resident aged men conducted in the 1950s and 1960s, The MacArthur Study of Successful Aging in America found that engagement in meaningful activities contributes to good health, satisfaction with life, and longevity, along with providing a potentially effective means of reducing costs of physical and emotional illness in later life. Older persons who have goals and structure are more likely to live longer than people who lack motivation and purpose.

Paid work includes remunerative self-employment and work for others. For older employees, the central issue regarding participation in paid work is retirement. Many factors influence an individual's decision to retire, including health, economic status, the quality of the work environment, the structure of social security and private pension plans, the availability of part-time work and/or flexibility of work hours, and age discrimination. Other significant factors are education, marital status, and spouse's labor force participation. Race and gender may also influence a person's decision to retire.[2]

DEMOGRAPHY

Years are being added to both ends of the life course, and at the same time as the birth rate drops, there is also an unprecedented reduction in maternal, infant, childhood, and late life mortality and morbidity rates. Population projections from the Social Security Administration show a decline in the working age population (20 to 64) per capita after 2010.[3] In 1950, the ratio of Americans ages 20 to 64 to those 65 and above was 16.5:1. In 2001 it was 3.3:1. By 2030, it will decline further to 2:1.[4]

Viewed another way, the world's population is growing at an annual rate of 1.7% but the population over 65 increases by 2.5% per year. In the United States, workers aged 55 through 64 have become the fastest growing segment of the workforce.[5] Most developing countries as well are aging rapidly. In Latin America and most of Asia, the number of people over 60 will double by 2030 to 14% of the population. In China, that number will rise to 22%.

In Europe, projections indicate that by 2050 retirees will outnumber workers and some fear that nations will be unable to finance their public pension systems. There is concern that if older workers retire in large numbers, sometime after 2010 there will be fewer workers to support more retirees, with the consequent reduction of growth in material standards of living among many European nations. These fears stem in part from the inappropriate interpretation of the dependency ratio, which broadly applied compares the number of dependents in a population (children plus persons 65 and older) to the population of younger adults. However, given that not everyone between the ages of 18 and 64 is working, that fewer children are being born, and that many persons over 65 are economically independent, through continuing employment, savings, private pensions, and social security based on contributions they have made to society over the course of many years, a more accurate measure of dependency would compare the economically dependent population with the population that is economically active.[6] Moreover, the cost of raising a child to age 18 is estimated conservatively at $200,000 ($300,000 if the child goes to college).

Thanks to the technology revolution, productivity is a more important measure of a nation's economic well-being than the size of its workforce. For example, food is far more plentiful now than it was a century ago, even though 37% of Americans in 1900 were engaged in agriculture compared with 2% today. As productivity grows in a variety of industries there will be less need for workers of any age, and the continuing low birth rates in the industrialized world will not pose significant problems.

It has been suggested that if it were possible to maintain a constant number of years in retirement, rather than automatically leaving the workforce after completing a constant number of years in paid employment, labor force participation rates of older workers would increase. Thus the reduced growth in labor supply would not by itself cause living standards to be lower than they were in 1997.

RETIREMENT

Juanita M. Kreps[7] noted in 1977 that retirement was a relatively new life stage, and that it was quickly becoming a device for balancing the numbers of job seekers with the demand for workers. And in the 1950s, social gerontologists Eugene Friedmann and Robert Havighurst[8] wrote ". . . retirement is not a rich man's luxury or an ill man's misfortune. It is increasingly the common lot of all kinds of people. Some find it a blessing; others, a curse. But it comes anyway, whether blessing or curse, and it comes often in an arbitrary manner, at a set age, without direct reference to the productivity or the interest of the individual in his work."

Before the industrial revolution people worked until they died and retirement was virtually unknown. Following industrialization, in 1889, Germany's Chancellor Otto von Bismarck established the first national contributory pension program in the modern era. At the turn of the twentieth century, the rise of labor unions in industrialized countries created worker protection that included retirement benefits. During most of the twentieth century, early retirement was an important labor market tool, serving to balance the number of people looking for jobs with the demand for workers and in particular supporting the careers of younger workers. Between 1910 and 1998–99, there was a drop of 1.2 years per decade in the age at which men retired from paid employment, so that the average male retirement age fell from 74 years to 63. Since male life expectancy has increased about 0.8 year per decade in the same period of time as the retirement age fell, late twentieth century workers have spent an increasingly significant portion of their lives in retirement. It is estimated that for many, retirement will last longer than their lives from birth until their entrance into the workforce.[9] Having said that, it must be noted that a trend toward later retirement appears to be developing, with baby boomers indicating their intention to work beyond the age of 65.

In today's labor market demographic trends that include a longer life expectancy and fewer younger people entering the workforce are at odds with benefit programs inherited from an era that provided incentives for early retirement for older workers. Traditional defined benefit pensions still in force include provisions that often discourage people from working past a certain age. For example, pensions are denied some workers who wish to remain on their jobs in a part-time capacity after formal retirement and employers' concerns about legal or tax ramifications can also work against flexible work options. There is a shift away from defined benefit pensions to defined contributions, and therefore this problem is diminishing. This can favor staying on the job with less expense to the employer. It also permits workers to take pensions with them if they move from job to job, which contributes to continuing productive aging.

Retirement trends vary between nations due to differences in the overall job markets, and in countries with higher unemployment, financial disincentives are still used to discourage the continued employment of older workers. A 1998 study of 24 OPEC countries showed that in 1950 the average retirement age was 65 or higher, but by 1995 there was a drop to age 62 in many of these nations. The decrease in the average retirement age of women has been even faster.[10]

In the 1950s the United States placed in the middle of countries surveyed for retirement ages, but by 1995 it had one of the highest, with only Iceland, Japan, Norway, and Switzerland having a higher male retirement age, and Iceland, Japan, Norway, Sweden, and Turkey having a higher female retirement age. In Europe since the 1960s there has been a marked decline in labor force participation, especially by men ages 60 to 64. It is below 20% in Belgium; 35% in Italy, France, and the Netherlands; 50% in Germany; and 40% in Spain. There have also been declines in employment between ages 45 and 59. The rates of labor force participation between 55 and 64 are less than 50% for both men and women in Finland, France, and the Netherlands.[11]

In the United States, Social Security is the main source of cash income of households headed by an individual age 65 or older. It provides slightly more than 40% of the total cash income received by this population. Social Security replaces about 42% of the final wages earned by a fully employed single worker who earns the average wage and begins collecting at 65, and 63% of the final wages of a worker with a nonworking dependent spouse. Until recently, a retirement means test was used to prevent older workers who collected Social Security from continuing to earn more than a certain amount annually in paid employment. Workers between 65 and 69 lost $1 in benefits for every $3 they earned in excess of $17,000. In 2000 the United States passed the Senior Citizens' Freedom to Work Act, which eliminated earnings penalties of Social Security recipients aged 65 and older who were born before 1945, allowing potential retirees to receive full benefits regardless of other earnings. As a result, the number of older persons who rejoin the workforce on a part-time, seasonal, or full-time basis is expected to rise, adding an estimated $19.5 billion to the gross domestic product by 2008. Furthermore, for every $2 in annual earnings in excess of the designated limit ($10,800), a worker between 62 and 65 loses $1 in annual benefits.

Another step that might promote productive aging was passed by Congress in 1983, with implementation beginning in 2003. The age at which retirees can claim full Social Security benefits in the United States will gradually increase from 65, reaching 67 by 2027. Recommendations have been made to raise the retirement age to 70 by 2029 and as needed after that, in accordance with further increases in life expectancy. Many OECD nations are also gradually increasing the age at which workers become eligible for retirement benefits. Incentives are being considered to encourage people to delay retirement benefits or continue working while they receive benefits. For example, the United Kingdom has equalized retirement ages for men and women by raising the retirement age for women.

Increasing the average age of full pension entitlement and removing pension earnings rules and penalties for working past a certain age would allow healthy people to continue paid employment while increasing the length of time during which contributions are made to pension funds. However, it must be noted that at the same time as it extends years of salaried employment, it represents a cut in benefits to the beneficiary. Protection must also be made available to those unable to work for health reasons.

PAID EMPLOYMENT

Complete retirement is much less prevalent among older Americans than is commonly believed. At least 50% of all workers "partially retire" by taking part-time jobs toward the end of their working lives, and the chance that an individual will reenter the labor force after initial retirement is about one in four. Older workers employed in nontraditional paid work arrangements include independent contractors, on-call and temporary workers, and those engaged in home-based work, part-time work, and postcareer bridge jobs. In 2000, only about 13% of older Americans worked, but a recent survey conducted by the AARP (formerly the American Association for Retired Persons) found that about 80% of baby boomers plan to continue working after retirement, 35% at least part time.

With the drop in fertility in most industrialized nations, their future labor force will grow slowly, requiring them to invest in physical capital that will reduce labor needs, establish continuous education programs, liberalize immigration policies, train physicians to appropriately care for people as they grow older so they can continue to be productive, and encourage more women with children and older workers to remain in the workforce. Removing disincentives and creating positive incentives for older workers to stay employed can contribute to sustaining growth in industrialized nations. Policies that encourage phased retirement would include changing federal tax and pension laws to allow for the collection of partial benefits. Such laws would stimulate valued employees to remain on the job in flexible work situations, while eliminating some of the costs associated with their employment. Flexible employment options include job sharing, which allows two workers to split the responsibilities of one position, part-time work and temporary employment. Another option is work from home. Large companies report that between 1995 and at the turn of the twenty-first century, the percentage of employees who share jobs overall rose by 70%, and the number who work from home climbed 81%. A 1999 survey of more than 500 large corporations found that 16% are experimenting with flexible hours for older workers, and early quantitative data indicate a positive impact on productivity. Finally, long-time employees could serve as consultants or mentors.

A German flexible retirement proposal offers employees incentives higher than those already established by law. Unions and employers in Baden-Württemburg established a plan that allowed 55-year-old workers to work half time and receive 82% of their salary. If the employer did not wish to participate, at age 61 the worker could opt to work half time on 70% of full salary. Whatever the decision, the pension contribution would continue at 95% of the full time rate.

AGEISM IN THE WORKPLACE

Ageism is discrimination based on age, and it creates official and societal acceptance of limits on the employment of older persons, contributing to later-life displacement. Financial disincentives, workplace discrimination, and inadequate retraining are factors which must be considered when discussing the continued paid employment of older persons. National surveys conducted in the United States in the 1980s suggest that 80% of Americans in general and 61% of employers in particular believe that most employers discriminate against older people and make it difficult for them to find work.[12] Until 1967, when the Age Discrimination in Employment Act was passed in the United States, approximately one half of private sector job openings were advertised as closed to applicants over 55, and one quarter were barred to workers over 45. Age discrimination is the complaint most often lodged against employers, according to the Equal Employment Opportunity Commission, and a study in 1994 for the AARP showed that discrimination against older workers was about the same as that against African Americans and Hispanics of all ages.[13]

Although the relationship between age and job performance is exceedingly weak, misconceptions are common. They include the belief that most older workers are limited by health conditions, less flexible on the job, less educated, that they possess skills that are technologically obsolete, and are difficult to retrain. In a research study to determine whether worker performance declines with age, the literature showed that the only jobs for which performance appeared to decline with age were jobs that required manual labor. No correlation was found between age and work quality for supervisors and professionals, and job performance in sales was shown to improve with age.

British economist Richard Disney notes that although it is true that a younger workforce may be more adaptable and quicker to learn, it is also true that they have less training and experience. Although some individuals in an older workforce may experience a degree of depreciation in skills and difficulty in retraining during periods of rapid technological change, overall, they have greater experience and maturity, are more dependable, and embody high productivity and less absenteeism. Of course, continuing educational opportunities would further increase the value of continuing employment of older workers.

The proportion of chronically disabled older Americans has fallen steadily in the past decades, and fewer older people are unable to work because of disability. According to the National Long-Term Care Survey, the prevalence of chronic disability in Americans age 65 and older fell from 26.5% in 1982 to 19% in 2004–2005.[14] There can be some decline in mental and physical functioning, but in general, older workers remain productive in spite of these limitations, by finding ways to compensate for both functional conditions and chronic diseases. In fact, disabilities are more likely to involve hearing or eyesight problems than a complete inability to function. Employer accommodation can be relatively easy, for example, adjusting font sizes on computer monitors or being sensitive to an employee's need to take medications while at work.

Historically, a large number of the life-time contributions to scholarship, the arts and sciences were made by men and women in their later years. In fact, the period of life after age 50 accounts for the major portion of output in most scholarly and scientific fields. Ages 70 to 79 alone account for 20% of the output in the fields of scholarship and 15% in the sciences.[15] Today, employers report that their older workers are as creative as younger employees, more dependable, and far more experienced. According to a Harris Poll of 774 corporate human resource directors, 80% agree that older workers had less turnover, and 71% said they had as much ability as younger workers to acquire new skills.

Industrialized nations are just beginning to take action against persistent ageism. For example, Australia's Council on Ageing (COTA) has begun to urge employers, businesses, trade unions, academics, and workers themselves to look for solutions to age-based discrimination.

Effective laws are needed to ensure that older workers receive equal opportunities for training to keep up with changing technology and to encourage lifelong learning. Reforms must be passed to ensure that job opportunities are available for older workers, and that they are equipped with the necessary skills and level of competence. Restructuring the job environment to accommodate older workers and developing innovative ways to reorganize work for long-tenure employees can increase productivity and help skilled older employees remain competitive. For example, in Norway, the government has undertaken a major national lifelong learning initiative, which is known as Competence Reform. Employees who have been working at least 3 years and employed by the same employer for the last 2 years have the right to full-time or part-time study leave for up to 3 years. Its purpose is to raise the level of competence and provide the country with a highly skilled and flexible workforce, and one of its benefits will be to help older workers stay abreast of new technologies and remain competitive in the workplace.

It has become increasingly important that computer-related training, like training in general, be customized to physically accommodate older trainees (i.e., offering larger monitors, screen displays, and a keyboard and mouse that can accommodate a limited range of motion), in addition to research in new technology (i.e., perfecting a voice-activated computer that eliminates the need for keyboard and mouse). In a collaborative effort between the private and public sector, computer learning centers in the United States that accommodate older students, computer software companies and aging organizations have begun to work together to promote computer literacy among older adults.

UNPAID WORK

Free time was once the exclusive province of the well-to-do, especially women, but now millions of older persons have the time that younger persons lack. A 1999 survey[16] reports that nearly half of all Americans age 55 or older engage in some form of unpaid work.

Unpaid work includes volunteer work performed through formal organizations, such as hospitals, churches, and schools; informal help to relatives and friends, including caregiving and home maintenance; and unpaid help in a family business.[17] Formal volunteering in a community can be a substitute for paid labor, either producing services at a preexisting level, expanding the product of a community's public and private organizations, or creating a new service, such as volunteer service organizations. Examples include mentoring programs for inner city children, foster grandparent programs, and the recruitment of retired medical professionals in the development of free health clinics for the delivery of health care to the medically underserved.

Domestic activities include home maintenance and production of goods or services for home consumption. Older members add significantly to the nation's welfare in activities that include care of young, sick, or functionally limited family members and the transmission of values to younger generations.

Older people fill an important role as informal parent-surrogates to grandchildren. In 1998 this cohort was responsible for the care of nearly 4 million children, or 5.6% of all American children under the age of 18. Over 2.5 million maintained families with or without legal parents also in residence, and in more than 888,000 cases, they raised the children alone. Among families with preschoolers and employed mothers, 17% received primary child care from the child's grandparents. Family dynamics and financial constraints militate against adoption, and often lacking legal status as guardians, they can experience financial difficulties maintaining themselves and their grandchildren.

Unpaid labor by family members, which reduces labor costs of a family enterprise, is predominantly the purview of older persons. Beyond economic considerations, their participation may have the positive effect of enriching family relationships and enhancing the older person's sense of self-worth.

JAPAN

Japan's population is aging much faster than in any other industrialized country. It has one of the lowest birthrates of any developed nation and the longest-living population. Employment opportunities for older persons in Japan are limited, and **the unemployment rate has increased.** In the mid 1970s, twice as many workers entered the job market as were retiring and the legal minimum age at which employees could retire and receive a pension was 55. But, as the twenty-first century unfolds, two workers will retire for every worker entering the job market. Sooner or later, industries will find it impossible to recruit enough young workers to the labor market to replace workers who have left.

In 1998, the legal minimum age of retirement in Japan was raised to 60, and it will gradually be raised to age 65 by 2013 for men and by 2018 for women. Thirty-seven percent of Japanese men work after age 60, in contrast to 10% of American men. Japanese employers retain some of their older workers at lower wages, and transfer some others to subsidiaries or related firms. Workers also can find jobs with their old firm's suppliers or customers.

With a view to encouraging even further employment of older workers, the Japanese government is beginning to offer companies a variety of incentives to encourage their older workers to remain in the workforce. Incentives include subsidies to businesses whose total workforce has more than 10% older workers and to employers who have eliminated mandatory retirement. Other incentives include partial coverage of expenses for employers who have adapted facilities and equipment in the workplace to make them better suited for older workers.

DEVELOPING NATIONS

The United Nations estimates that by 2025, more than 75% of the over 60-population will live in developing nations, including 70% of the world's 604 million women over age 60. Forty percent of older people in developing nations will live in the countryside, but very few studies of this population have been undertaken.

Traditionally, old people who lived in rural poverty could depend upon their adult children to care for them as they aged. Today, modern industries and opportunities for advancement draw the young to the cities, leaving the elders in the community to cope as best they can with limited resources. Since rural economies depend predominantly upon heavy manual labor, frail older persons are often left without visible means of support. Women especially lack the resources, skills, and social independence to cope with the changing social conditions. International nonprofit organizations, such as the United Nations Subcommittee on Aging, the International Women's Movement, and Help

Age International, among others, are in the early stages of addressing the problems of impoverished older women in developing countries.

Small loan programs in developing nations limit credit availability to older persons; however, there are notable exceptions. Since 1976, a Bangladeshi nonprofit organization, Grameen Bank, has made small, unsecured loans available to people of all ages to begin small businesses, which are known as "microenterprises." Older women are particularly encouraged to participate in these entrepreneurial endeavors. Action for Welfare and Awakening in Rural Environment (AWARE), in Hyderabad, India, is one of several agencies that enable older workers to buy materials for individual work projects. In Colombia, Pro Vida, a nongovernmental agency, has developed programs to redirect or retrain the skills of older people (e.g., one town's innovative program gives impoverished older persons a monopoly on employment in a recycling program). In Ecuador, bakeries employ older people, and in the Philippines, they are trained in car repair and encouraged to open their own businesses. Laundries, home repair services, general merchandise shops, equipment rentals, industrial sewing, child care, and hand-made crafts are other types of enterprises that have provided work for older persons in developing nations.[18]

CONCLUSION

In the twenty-first century, declining mortality and disability rates in early old age measure the improved health of older people. In some ways, retirement has been a twentieth-century phenomenon. It was required when the majority of people labored in mines, factories, and foundries, and it continues to be humane and necessary for individuals who have reasons to stop working after a lifetime of toil. Analyses of a variety of occupations and their physical requirements show that a much smaller proportion of jobs require strenuous physical effort, and a large percentage require only moderate or light physical exertion. They suggest that the physical demands of work are easier to meet than they were in the past.[19]

A social norm that is appropriate to the new longevity and to a world trend toward human rights would be one in which all people are considered individually and collectively as a resource to meet their own and society's needs; one in which retirement remains a desired goal, as indeed it is, after a lifetime of work. At the same time, the new added life expectancy necessitates a commensurate increase in work expectancy, as long as there are jobs and people can work without age discrimination.

The responsibility for preserving one's human capital ultimately rests with the individual. If older individuals can continue to develop their productive potential, whether in paid employment, service to family and community, or by sharing artistic and avocational abilities, their lives will be enriched at the same time as they continue to benefit society. Late life productivity is multifaceted, encompassing altruism, citizenship, stewardship, creativity, and the search for faith. A study found that while older people think that older workers should not stand in the way of younger workers, they also believe that "life is not worth living if you cannot contribute to the well-being of others."[20]

KEY POINTS

Productive Aging

- Productive aging is the capacity of an individual or population to engage in paid work and in nonremunerative activities, such as volunteer service to the family and community. It is affected by both internal and external factors. Internal factors include physical and emotional health, motivation, attitude, and experience. External factors involve society's willingness and ability to accommodate the special needs of older persons.
- Factors that encourage paid employment in later years include worker demand, educational level, changing technologies that may require retraining, and societal attitudes and structures. The age at which a country mandates or encourages its workers to retire influences the productive aging of its citizens.
- Ageism is discrimination based on age, and it creates official and societal acceptance of limits on the employment of older persons. Financial disincentives, workplace discrimination, and inadequate retraining are factors that have an impact on their continued employment.
- Some benefit programs discourage workers from remaining on their jobs and provide incentives for early retirement. This is at odds with the projected demographics of greater life expectancy and fewer younger people entering the workforce. Removing disincentives to retirement and creating incentives for older workers to stay employed and employers to retain them can contribute to sustained growth in industrialized nations. Incentives include retraining older workers in new technologies, making accommodations for disabilities that do not impact on their ability to do the job, and developing options for job-sharing and part-time employment.
- Means tests penalize older workers who receive pension benefits if they earn more than a specified amount. For example, in 2000 the United States eliminated earnings penalties of Social Security recipients aged 65 and older. Many OECD nations are also gradually increasing the age at which workers become eligible for retirement benefits.
- Older persons contribute significantly to a nation's benefit in activities that contribute to the care of young, sick, or functionally limited family members and the transmission of values to younger generations. Unpaid labor by older family members can significantly reduce labor costs of a family enterprise.

For a complete list of references, please visit online only at www.expertconsult.com

CHAPTER 33

Social Vulnerability in Old Age

Melissa K. Andrew

People's lives are embedded in rich social contexts; many social factors impact on each of our lives every day. This is perhaps more noticeably so for older adults as declines in health and functional status may increase reliance on social supports and diminish opportunities for social engagement, even in the face of social circles dwindling due to declining health and function among peers.

This chapter will provide an overview of how social factors affect health in old age, through a discussion of the concept of *social vulnerability*. The association with health outcomes relevant to geriatric medicine (including function, mobility, cognition, mental health, self-assessed health, frailty, institutionalization, and death) will be the focus, with particular emphasis on the relationship between social vulnerability and frailty. Detailed discussion of social gerontology and of standardized instruments and measurement scales used in the social assessment of older people is beyond the scope of this chapter; interested readers are referred to the two chapters on these topics in this volume.

BACKGROUND AND DEFINITIONS

Many social factors influence health, including socioeconomic status, social support, social networks, social engagement, social capital, and social cohesion.[1–8] As such, the social context is key to a broad understanding of health and illness. Perhaps due in part to the numerous disciplines in which this line of inquiry has been investigated (including epidemiology, sociology, geography, political science, and international development, among others), terminology and methods of approach have differed. In some instances, the same terminology has been used to refer to different ideas, whereas in others, divergent terminology obscures underlying commonalities. There has also been debate surrounding the level, from individual to communal, at which some elements of the social context are relevant, and as such, how they can be measured.[1,9,10] In the following section, the various terms and concepts will be defined and discussed, and each will be placed in context on the continuum from individual to group influence (Figure 33-1).

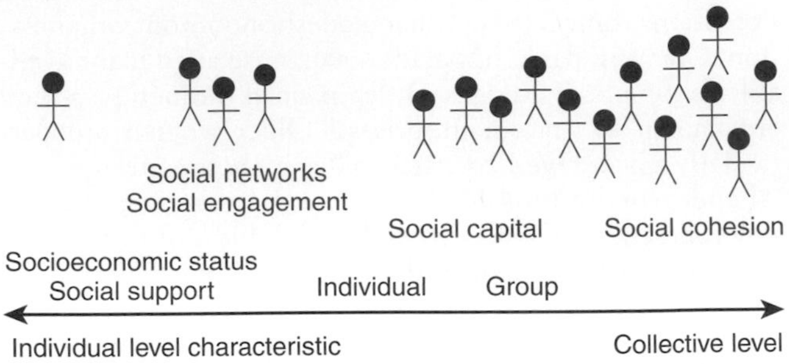

Figure 33-1. The continuum of social factors that influence health, acting from individual to group levels.

Socioeconomic status

Socioeconomic status (SES) is a broad concept that includes such factors as educational attainment, occupation, income, wealth, and deprivation. There are three broad theories of how socioeconomic status might relate to health.[11] The materialist theory states that gradients in *income and wealth* are associated with varying levels of deprivation, which in turn affects health status as those with fewer means have inferior access to health care and the necessities of life. Another view is that *education* influences health through lifestyle and health-related behaviors such as diet, substance use, and smoking. A third theory sees social status (often measured by *occupation*) and personal autonomy as key influences on health, particularly through the stresses that accompany low social status and low autonomy.[11] Measurement of each of these elements of SES may present difficulties in the older adult population. Older persons are likely to be retired and older women may never have worked outside the home, making occupational assessments problematic. Income is associated with employment status, and many income supplements and benefits are available to those with disability and poor health raising problems of reverse causation.[11] Educational opportunities available to older cohorts may have been limited, creating a "floor effect" in which it is difficult to differentiate among the majority whose educational attainment is low.[11] Additionally, information may be missing when a proxy respondent has been used, depending on how well the proxy knows the subject. Socioeconomic status is a property of individuals; however, aggregates of such measures can be used to describe the social context in which people live. For example, average income, employment rates, or educational attainment may be useful descriptors when applied to groups of people living in relevant geographic areas such as housing facilities or neighborhoods, and may allow for study of contextual effects on health.[12–18]

Social support

Social support refers to the various sources of help and resources obtained through social relationships with family, friends, and other care providers. Types of social support include emotional (including the presence of a close confidante), instrumental (help with activities of daily living, provided through labor or financial support), appraisal (help with decision making), and informational (provision of information or advice).[19] Various measures of social support have been studied, with some tending to be more "objective" (based on reports of actual use of services and tangible help received in the various domains) and others more "subjective," based on the individual's perception of the adequacy and richness of the supports to which they have access. Social support can also importantly be seen as a two-way transaction, with the older person receiving support in some areas while providing support in others. For example, within spousal relationships each spouse may have complementary strengths and weaknesses; between generations, older people may provide care for grandchildren and financial support for adult children, while receiving instrumental support.[20]

Social networks

Social networks are the ties that link individuals and groups in social relationships. Various characteristics can be measured, including size, density, relationship quality, and composition.[1] Both social networks and social support are generally seen as individual-level resources, and are measured at an individual level.[3,19,21] Through social networks, individuals can access social support, material resources, and various other forms of capital (cultural, economic, and social).[22]

Social engagement

Social engagement represents an individual's participation in social, occupational, or group activities, which may include formal organized activities such as religious meetings, service groups, and clubs of all sorts. More informal activities such as card groups, trips to the bingo hall, and cultural outings to see concerts or galleries can also be considered as social engagement. Volunteerism is often considered separately,[1] but can also be seen as an important measure of social engagement.

Social capital

Social capital is a broad term which has been used inconsistently in the literature, and there is ongoing debate about its nature and measurement. For example, Bourdieu defines social capital as "the aggregate of the actual or potential resources which are linked to possession of a durable network of more or less institutionalized relationships."[22] His definition is consistent with the idea that social capital is a resource that can be accessed and measured at an individual level, stating that "the volume of social capital possessed by a given agent thus depends on the size of the network of connections he can effectively mobilize and the volume of the capital ... possessed by each of those to whom he is connected."[22] However, his definition is also consistent with the view that social capital is a *property* of the relationships within the network—if there are no connections between individuals, there would be no social capital. Coleman makes a similar argument, stating, "Unlike other forms of capital, social capital inheres in the structure of relations between actors and among actors. It is not lodged either in the actors themselves or in the physical implements of production."[23] He also sees social capital as a resource accessible by individuals, writing, "social capital constitutes a particular kind of resource available to an actor."[23]

Putnam defines social capital as "the features in our community life that make us more productive—a high level of engagement, trust, and reciprocity"[24] and sees it as "simultaneously a 'private good' and a 'public good' "with both individual and collective aspects.[25] To access the "private good" benefits of social capital, an individual would need to be integrated into a network and have direct connections with other members. But the "public good" effects of social capital would accrue to everyone in the community, regardless of their personal connections to others. The "public good" concept of social capital is shared by others, including Kawachi et al, who see social capital as an ecologic level characteristic that can only properly be measured at a collective level, and state that "social capital inheres in the structure of social relationships; in other words it is an ecologic characteristic," which "should be properly considered a feature of the collective (neighborhood, community, society) to which an individual belongs."[3,14,21,26]

Measures of social capital are as varied as its definitions, and include both structural elements (such as social networks, relationships, and group participation) and cognitive ones (such as trust in others, voting behavior, newspaper subscription, feelings of obligation, reciprocity and cooperation, and perceptions of neighborhood security).[1,10,23]

Social cohesion

The concept of social cohesion implies collectivity of definition and measurement. Again, definitions vary, but generally relate to ideas of cooperation and ties that unite communities and societies. For example, Stansfeld defines social cohesion as "the existence of mutual trust and respect between different sections of society."[27] For Kawachi and Berkman, social cohesion relies on two key features of a society: absence of social conflict and presence of social bonds.[3]

Social isolation

Social isolation is another term that is encountered in the literature relating social circumstances and health. It is related to ideas of loneliness, reduced social and religious engagement, and reduced access to social supports. It may also incorporate properties of the older person's environment, such as difficulty with transportation. As with many other social factors, social isolation can be "subjective" (as perceived by the older person themselves, e.g., loneliness) or "objective" (based on outside measures or assessments by others).

Social vulnerability

The concept of social vulnerability addresses the understanding that the reason we are interested in the social environment is not merely as a descriptor, but to attempt to quantify an individual's relative vulnerability (or resilience/invulnerability) to perturbations in their environment, social circumstances, health, or functional status. Older people's social circumstances are complex, with multiple factors that may interact in potentially unforeseen ways. A global measure of social vulnerability would thus account for this complexity while providing descriptive and predictive value. A measure of social vulnerability should be broad enough to capture a rich description of the social deficits (or problems) that an individual has, be readily and practically measurable in population and clinical settings, be responsive to meaningful changes, and be predictive of important health outcomes.

HOW CAN WE STUDY SOCIAL INFLUENCES ON HEALTH?

Study of how social factors influence health requires careful consideration of analytic design in relation to the specific questions being asked (Table 33-1).

Possible approaches include traditional "one thing at a time" analyses in which a single social factor (for example, the social network) is related to the outcome of interest, ideally adjusting for possible confounders in a multivariable model. This approach has certain benefits, chief among them simplicity and clarity in execution and interpretation. For example, it allows for clear statements of important findings such as "An extensive social network seems to protect against dementia."[28] This approach can be done using single variables considered individually, a combination of variables relating to different aspects of the same theme (e.g., several

Table 33-1. Analytic Approaches for Studying Social Influences on Health

Analytic Approach	Benefits	Drawbacks
"One Thing at a Time"		
Single variables considered individually (*e.g., size of the social network*)	Simple and clear execution and interpretation	May result in overly simplistic understanding of associations
Combination of variables relating to the same theme (*e.g., several variables describing social network*)	Allows simultaneous investigation of several variables, adjusting for one another and for relevant confounders	• Validity considerations must be addressed • Models may become too complex with technical challenges (e.g., colinearity)
Validated measurement instrument (*e.g., Lubben Social Network Scale*)	Use of standardized and validated instruments enhances reliability and validity	• Lengthy administration time • Rigidity • Use may be limited with existing datasets if difficult to reconstruct faithfully
"Many Things at Once"		
Index approach: deficit accumulation (*e.g., social vulnerability index, frailty index*)	• Takes many aspects of social circumstances into account simultaneously • Does not rely on use of single variables, which may present measurement challenges in some older people • Related factors are not arbitrarily separated • Allows representation of gradations in exposure • Potential applicability to most datasets and clinical situations	• Represents risk relating to composite social circumstance rather than single identifiable factors in isolation • Complex modeling based on novel techniques
Options for Studying the Social Context		
"Horizontal" analyses (*e.g., multivariable regression modeling*)	Simple and clear execution and interpretation	• May not provide a full understanding of the social context • Technical problems for models: observations not really independent
"Vertical" analyses (*e.g., multilevel modeling, hierarchical linear modeling*)	• Yields more detailed understanding of contextual effects • Preserves independence of observations • Avoids loss of meaning due to data aggregation	• Not all datasets lend themselves to these models; need sufficient numbers in groups with shared characteristics • Complex models

variables that relate to the size and quality of the social network), or set instruments that have been previously validated to measure the social factor of interest (e.g., the Berkman-Syme Social Network Index and the Lubben's Social Network Scale).[29] The standardized psychometric properties of such scales add to the reliability and validity of studies that employ them, but their use does have drawbacks including relative rigidity and lengthier administration time. Their use may also be limited or impossible with existing datasets due to challenges encountered in their faithful reconstruction.

Deficit accumulation offers another potential approach to the study of social influences on health. Akin to the frailty index, which readers will find described elsewhere in this volume, a *social vulnerability index*, operationalized as a count of deficits relating to many social factors, offers a means of considering an individual's broad social circumstance and the potential vulnerability of their health and functional status. The index has a number of benefits, including: (1) the potential to include many different categories of social factors (for example SES, social support, social engagement, social capital), (2) the commonly encountered difficulty of embodying social and socioeconomic characteristics using single variables in studies of older adults is alleviated by including consideration of multiple different factors, (3) related factors are not arbitrarily separated into distinct categories for separate analysis, and (4) representation of gradations in social vulnerability is improved compared with consideration of one or a few binary or ordinal social variables. This last point is particularly important given that studies using the social vulnerability index in two cohorts of older adults have found that no one was completely free of social vulnerability (i.e., no individual had a "zero" score on the index).[30]

In addition to these analytic considerations of how the social factor(s) of interest is/are measured, incorporating the social context into the analyses can be done in different ways. More traditional "horizontal" approaches might add a summary variable that describes the individual's social context (e.g., mean neighborhood income or educational attainment) as a variable/confounder attached to the individual in the multivariable model.[16,17] This approach can yield useful findings and has the advantage of simplicity, but some might argue that it does not provide a full understanding of the importance of the contextual variable(s) and it presents statistical problems in terms of independence of observations (individuals are no longer truly independent if they share these important characteristics of the groups to which they belong). Multilevel (or "vertical") modeling (e.g., hierarchical linear modeling) is another option; here, the individual is nested within layers of group influence, with collective characteristics treated as attributes of the group rather than of the individual.[31] This approach offers the advantage of allowing for more detailed understanding of the contextual effects, preserving the independence of observations, and not losing information as happens when data are aggregated.[31]

The consideration of contextual or group-level variables such as neighborhood and community characteristics is particularly relevant to the study of how social factors affect health because many social factors are properties of the groups or communities in which individuals live and may be best measured on a group level. As we have seen, there is active debate about whether social capital is a property of individuals or of groups.[1,9] Most theories of social capital are consistent with the idea that it is a property of relationships between individuals and within societies rather than residing within individuals per se. The heart of the issue that continues to divide theorists is whether social capital is a resource that an individual can be said to draw upon, and thus, in practical research terms, whether or not it can legitimately be measured at an individual level. This debate has clear implications for the design and interpretation of research studies that aim to investigate how social factors influence health; valid and useful findings can rest only on sound theoretical foundations. In this regard, a second distinction may be helpful: the answer may depend on whether the question applies to *where social capital exists* (is it a property of individuals or of relationships?) or to *how it is measured and accessed*.[9] Practically speaking, measurement issues and data availability may strongly influence analytic design. The issue of how social factors should be studied in relation to older adults' health is therefore ideally guided by a balance of these theoretical considerations and analytic pragmatism.

SUCCESSFUL AGING

This concept has been the subject of numerous inquiries in both the academic literature and the popular press.[32] Interested readers are referred to the comprehensive chapter by T. A. Glass in the sixth edition of this text.[33] Definitions of successful aging vary, but generally fall into psychosocial and biomedical camps. Psychosocial conceptualizations emphasize compensation and contentedness, where biomedical definitions are based on absence of disease and disability.[33] The concept of successful aging recognizes that the aging process is variable, and that how older people adapt to later life changes associated with aging influences how "successfully" they will age. Ideally, research into this area would identify potentially modifiable factors at play that help some age "better/more successfully" than others.

There is a potential downside to the idea of successful aging: if successful aging is applied as a value judgment, it may be at the cost of blaming and further marginalizing the "unsuccessful agers," those who are not so fortunate as to have the good health and functional status that might allow them to be doing aerobics at 102 or volunteering with "the old people" at 99.[32] Such stereotypes, based on both rare aging successes and on the undercurrent of ageism that is common in our society, also influence portrayal of older people in the popular media. Both positive and negative stereotypes run the risk of perpetuating the marginalization of the most vulnerable older people, whether their "unsuccessful aging" is implied or emphasized.[32]

Another way to think about successful aging is those individuals who overcome their expected trajectory in the natural history of decline for a given level of frailty. Work with the frailty index has shown that trajectories of decline are established early, and that such declines are well-predicted using mathematical models.[34,35] However, there are some individuals who improve or transition to lower levels of frailty (who are able to "jump the curve" from their own predicted course and outcomes to attain the outcomes that would be expected for people with a lower baseline level of frailty); this might be a useful subgroup in which to study predictors and correlates of this "successful aging."

ASSOCIATIONS WITH HEALTH

The various social factors discussed here have been associated with health outcomes that are important for the older population. Readers interested in broad-based discussions of how social circumstances relate to health (and to other attributes of societies) are referred to the works of Putnam, Wilkinson, and Marmot, who have each made strong and comprehensive cases that weak social cohesion and declines in social capital contribute to poor health,[25] and may explain associations between poor health and income inequalities[36] and social status inequalities.[6] As in many areas of geriatric medicine, studies pertaining specifically to older adults are limited in number. These will be discussed here along with important findings from general population studies in relation to health outcomes that are important in geriatric medicine.

Survival

Numerous studies have found associations between social factors and survival. Perceived social support and social interaction were associated with lower 30-month mortality in a cohort of 331 community-dwelling adults aged 65 and older in Durham County, N.C.[37] In the Alameda County 1965 Human Population Laboratory study, those, including older adults, with a richer social network, more contact with friends and family, and church or other group membership (used to generate a social network index) had lower mortality over 9 years of follow-up.[38] Using 17-year follow-up data from the same study, social connectedness predicted better survival at all ages, including those aged 70 and older.[5] Older individuals with few social ties also had reduced survival in a cohort study conducted in Evans County, Ga.[2] In another study, increased social ties predicted 5-year survival in two of three community-based cohorts.[39] The Whitehall studies of men employed in the British civil service identified an impressive gradient in survival across levels in the occupational hierarchy: in middle age, office workers in the lowest ranking jobs had four times the mortality of those in the highest ranking "administers" category. This gradient persisted after retirement (though it diminished to twice the risk of mortality) in the oldest age group studied, age 70 to 89.[6,7] High social vulnerability, as measured using a social vulnerability index, increased the risk of mortality over 5 and 8 years follow-up in two separate longitudinal studies of older Canadians: the Canadian Study of Health and Aging (CSHA) and the National Population Health Survey.[30] Ecologic (collective-level) analyses using multilevel modeling have also linked high social capital, defined by high trust and membership in voluntary associations, with reduced mortality at state[18] and neighborhood[14] levels in the United States.

Cognitive decline and dementia

In a study of 2812 older adults living in New Haven, Conn., social disengagement was associated with 3-, 6-, and 12-year incident cognitive decline defined as a transition to a lower category of performance on the 10-item Short

Portable Mental Status Questionnaire.[40] Greater emotional social support predicted better cognitive function measured by a battery of tests assessing language, abstraction, spatial ability, and recall over 7.5 years in the MacArthur Studies of Successful Aging.[41] Among 2468 CSHA participants aged 70 and older, high social vulnerability was associated with a 35% increase in the odds of clinically meaningful cognitive decline (a decline of ≥ 5 points[42] on the Modified Mini Mental State Examination [3MS]) over 5 years.[43] In a cohort of 1203 older adults in Kungsholmen, Sweden, those with a limited social network (including consideration of marital status, living arrangement, and contacts with friends and relatives) had a 60% increased risk of dementia over an average of 3 years of follow-up, whereas the incidence of dementia decreased in a stepwise fashion with increasing social connectedness.[28] The association of strong social networks and participation in mental and physical leisure activities with reduced incidence of dementia was also supported by a systematic review.[44] An American study of 9704 older women found that a richer social network (defined as the top two tertiles on the Lubben Social Network Scale) was associated with maintenance of optimal cognitive function (i.e., not experiencing age-related declines in cognition) over 15 years of follow-up.[45] Loneliness has also been associated with lower levels of baseline cognition in older people, more rapid cognitive decline, and double the risk of pathologically diagnosed Alzheimer dementia.[46] Social interaction and engagement reduced the probability of declines in orientation and memory in a 4-year study of community-dwelling Spanish older adults[47] and greater social resources (networks and engagement) were similarly associated with reductions in cognitive decline in old age.[48]

Socioeconomic status has also been studied in relation to cognition and cognitive declines in late life. Low SES (as measured by education, income, and assets) was associated with cognitive decline (≥ 5 point decline in the 3MS over 4 years) independent of biomedical comorbidity in a cohort of 2574 older participants aged 70 to 79 in the Health, Aging, and Body Composition study.[49] In a study that measured performance on complex memory tasks and electroencephalography (EEG) recordings of event-related potentials, older women (aged 65 and older) of high socioeconomic status performed similarly to younger women in complex source memory tasks, and appeared to make use of neural compensation strategies not used by their lower SES counterparts and not required by the younger subjects.[50] In the Chicago Health and Aging project study of 6158 older people aged 65 and older, early life socioeconomic status (both of the individual's family and of their birth county) was associated with late life cognitive performance but not with subsequent rate of decline.[51] A report from the English Longitudinal Study of Ageing (ELSA) found that neighborhood-level SES was associated with cognitive function independent of individual SES.[16] Using hierarchical linear modeling, neighborhood-level educational attainment was associated with cognitive function of Americans aged 70 and older participating in the Study of Assets and Health Dynamics Among the Oldest Old (AHEAD). This was independent of individual factors including educational attainment and neighborhood measures of income, leading the authors to conclude that promoting educational attainment in the general population may help older residents to maintain cognitive function.[52]

Functional decline and dependence

Low levels of social engagement among older adults have been associated with increased disability (measured as impairment in activities of daily living, mobility, and upper and lower extremity function) over 9 years of follow-up.[4] Older adults (aged 72 and older) with dense social networks showed delayed onset of self-perceived disability over 8 years of follow-up in a panel study of 1000 residents of three retirement communities in Florida.[53] Social engagement through group participation, social support, and trust/reciprocity were each associated with reduced functional impairment in community-dwellers in a cross-sectional analysis of the Health Survey for England. The association between group participation and functional impairment was also statistically significant among residents of institutional care homes.[54]

Mobility

Various social factors have been associated with risk of falls and of subsequent injury. For example, one Australian population-based study found that older people with lower SES, those living alone, and those needing repairs to their home were more likely to have fallen.[55] Another study identified protective factors for fall-related hip fractures that included being currently married, living in the same place for more than 5 years, having private health insurance, and engaging in social activities.[56] Neighborhood-level deprivation has been associated with incident self-reported mobility difficulties and measured impairment in gait speed independent of individual SES and health status in the English Longitudinal study of Aging (ELSA).[17]

Institutionalization

As most studies in this field have been done using surveys or cohorts with community-based sampling frames, there has been a paucity of research including residents of long-term care facilities. However, severe lack of social support has been associated with higher odds of care home residence,[54] and is a risk factor for care home placement.[57,58] The issue of how social factors and social vulnerability affect the health of older residents of institutions requires further study. In a cross-sectional analysis of the Health Survey for England, where associations between social capital and health were found among care home residents, these associations were generally weaker than in the community setting, suggesting that the importance of social capital may vary according to living situation.[54]

Mental health

Low perceived neighborhood social capital and high social disorganization were associated with both psychiatric and physical morbidity in a study of British adults.[59] Mental health has also been found to be associated with the strength and nature of social ties, although protective effects do not appear to be uniform across all population groups.[60] For example, a study of 1714 older Cubans found that social networks (particularly those centered on children and extended family) were associated with reduced depressive symptoms in women, whereas being married and not living alone were more important for men.[61] Among community dwelling older adults, social support, group participation, and trust/reciprocity were each associated with better mental health as measured by the General Health Questionnaire, an instrument that has been validated to detect mild psychiatric morbidity. Social support was also associated with reduced psychiatric morbidity among older adults who resided in care homes.[54] Lower neighborhood SES and higher population density were associated with depression and anxiety among people aged 75 and older in Britain, but in this study the effect of neighborhood SES was explained by individual SES and health factors.[62]

Self-assessed health

Individual-level social capital, as defined by religious participation, trust, and having a helpful friend, was associated with better self-assessed health among Swedish-speaking adults in a bilingual region of Finland.[63] High community-level social trust and membership in voluntary associations were also associated with better self-assessed health among community-dwelling adults in multilevel analyses adjusting for individual-level influences on health in two large (N = 167,259 and 21,456) American studies.[13,15] Among 1677 community dwelling older adult participants in the Health Survey for England, higher levels of social support, group participation, and trust/reciprocity were associated with better self-assessed health.[54] At a neighborhood level, low SES (including poverty, unemployment, low education, and reliance on public assistance) was associated with poor self-assessed health of Americans aged 70 and older in the AHEAD study, independent of individual-level health and SES factors. This association with self-assessed health held even though the neighborhood-level attributes were not independently associated with cardiovascular disease and functional status.[64]

Frailty

In two cohorts of older Canadians, social vulnerability was moderately correlated with frailty, but was distinct from it. Both frailty and social vulnerability contributed independently to the risk of mortality.[30] Several social determinants of frailty were identified in an elderly Chinese population aged 70 and older; these included low SES (occupational category and inadequate income), having few or little contact with relatives and neighbors, low participation in community/religious activities, and reporting low social support.[65]

MECHANISMS

Various mechanisms have been proposed to explain how social factors might affect health. Broadly speaking, these can be broken down into four groups: biologic and physiologic, behavioral, material, and psychological. Study of neurophysiology and neuroanatomy may also contribute to understanding the relationship between social factors and health.

Physiological

Chronic and sustained stress responses exert powerful effects on health through complex hormonal regulatory systems, with myriad downstream effects on tissues and organs. Various animal studies have found effects on the hypothalamic-pituitary-adrenal axis. Chronically elevated levels of glucocorticoids in socially isolated rats accelerate aging processes including hippocampal cell loss and cognitive impairment.[19] Social support has also been linked to immune function in both humans and animals, with social isolation and loneliness compromising immunocompetence even among otherwise healthy medical students.[19]

Behavioral

Socioeconomic inequalities (including employment and educational opportunities) and the norms and influences exerted through social networks and communities may affect health-related behaviors such as diet, smoking, substance use, and exercise. This may partially explain social influences on health; however, many studies in which these behaviors are taken into account find that social circumstances exert additional independent effects on health.[13,19,37,38]

Material

Socioeconomic status and social support networks clearly affect access to goods and services. This access accrues in three broad ways: through financial resources (what you have), social status (who you are), and social contacts (who you know). Those with financial means and high social status can afford to make healthy lifestyle choices (e.g., balanced diet, opportunities for exercise, avoiding smoking, and substance abuse) and access health care services that may be difficult to obtain without such resources. There are also strong systemic and societal factors that serve to maintain the social exclusion of marginalized individuals and groups. Those with strong social support resources can access financial and instrumental assistance in time of need.

Psychological

Self-efficacy and adaptive coping strategies are important for health, and are some of the potential psychological mechanisms through which social factors may influence health.[19] Low self-efficacy (having low confidence in one's abilities) is associated with fear of falling, with important functional and mobility ramifications for older people.[66] Low self-efficacy has also been found to predict functional decline in older people with impaired physical performance.[4] Social supports and engagement may bolster feelings of self-efficacy and self-confidence.

Neurophysiology and neuroanatomy

Study of patients with neurologic conditions has historically been a rich source of insight into the function of the brain and nervous system. Whereas the potential mechanisms discussed in the last few paragraphs attempt to explain how social circumstances themselves might influence health, here we consider the reverse; by studying people with neurologic conditions including dementia we may be able to learn more about how the brain influences social factors like engagement, participation in social networks, and perceptions of others such as trust and reciprocity that are important to the idea of social capital. For example, some individuals with dementia become socially withdrawn and apathetic, suspicious and less trusting, or have other personality changes that influence their social function. Study of the localization and function (e.g., with functional imaging techniques and more traditional neuropathology) of such problems may add to the elucidation of the links between social function and social circumstances and health. This field is in its early stages, but as an example, "agreeableness" in frontotemporal dementia (which is often characterized by personality changes and problems with social function) has been shown to be positively correlated with the volume of the right orbitofrontal cortex and negatively correlated with left-sided orbitofrontal volume.[67] Animal studies may also contribute to this area of inquiry. For example, study of hyenas has shown that the four distinct species of hyenas can be placed on a continuum of increasing social complexity. Interestingly, the volume of the frontal cortex (as determined by internal measurements of their skulls) is directly proportional, with the hyenas that have the most complex social relationships having the greatest frontal lobe volumes.[68]

FRAILTY, EXCLUSION, AND "SILENCE BY PROXY"

Older adults who are frail and/or cognitively impaired present a unique challenge for research in this field for many reasons. These include exclusion from research, reliance on proxy informants, problematic assessment of social situation and socioeconomic status, and controversy regarding informed consent.

Many frail older adults may be excluded from population-based research if the sampling frame excludes nursing homes (as is commonly the case) or if persons unable to answer for themselves are not included in surveys. Even if efforts are made to include these groups by using proxy respondents, subjective reports and personal historical details may be missing or unreliable.[9,54]

This "silence by proxy" presents great challenges in research involving frail elderly people, as it is often hardest to gather information from those who are the most frail, particularly in institutions where family may be unavailable to fill in historical details. One might imagine that social support and social interactions could be more relevant to health in frail older people because they might be most reliant on family and friends for care and encouragement, and that benefits of social engagement could be greater in terms of mobility and optimizing function appropriate to their level of ability. As such, the associations found in studies from which they are excluded could be underestimated.

POLICY RAMIFICATIONS AND POTENTIAL FOR INTERVENTIONS

Although there are not many intervention studies in which social vulnerability is reduced and health outcomes studied, some studies do suggest hope in this regard. For example, there is evidence that participation in some types of voluntary groups may help to buffer the negative psychological effects of functional decline.[69] Intervention trials with so-called "befriending services," in which social support is offered by a volunteer visitor, have had mixed results, possibly due in part to limited uptake.[70] There is a large literature and clinical experience with structured peer support groups, for example, those provided through various disease-specific community organizations; discussion of these is beyond the scope of this chapter.

One area in which social interventions have the potential to improve health is in the design of seniors' housing. Given the mounting evidence that social engagement and interaction with neighbors improves health, these principles could be brought to bear as housing developments and facilities for older people are designed, built, and renovated. Cannuscio has described such senior housing strategies as a "promising mode of delivery of social capital to the aging population."[26] Long-term care facilities could be designed to encourage interaction among residents and with the wider community. Resident rooms spread out along long hallways, inaccessible to those with mobility impairment, might be replaced by rooms organized into pods around shared common areas.[27] "Planned care environments" in which a continuum of living arrangements from independent apartments to full nursing care exist within a single complex might foster neighborhood cohesion and reduce residential mobility, which has been shown to negatively impact the formation of social ties.[12,26] Community planning on a larger scale may also help to address many of the challenges to mobility and community interaction faced by older people. Sidewalks and crosswalks wide enough and in good enough repair to allow the use of mobility aids, traffic lights with cycles long enough to allow safe crossing, accessible public transportation, and availability of services in local residential neighborhoods are strategies that benefit the health of people of all ages. As an example of taking such policy considerations to national and international levels, these issues are at the core of the World Health Organization's Age-Friendly Cities project.[71]

CONCLUSIONS

Although further research is required to clarify and contextualize the relationships between social circumstances and health in older adults, it is becoming increasingly clear that social factors exert great influence. Here, the various social factors that have been studied in relation to health have been reviewed, along with their relationship to the concept of overall social vulnerability. Specific associations with health outcomes that are important in geriatric medicine, including frailty, have been discussed.

The social vulnerability index approach has numerous advantages, including theoretical grounding in an understanding of the continuum of social influences on health and in relation to work on frailty, consideration of numerous different domains of social factors at once, and great potential for clinical applicability. From the point of view of clinical services providing care in geriatric medicine, the issue is not only which deficits an individual has, but how they add up to contribute to that person's vulnerability in ways that might predispose them to adverse outcomes. As such, a composite measure of social vulnerability may be a useful and potentially clinically relevant starting point to conceptualize the social circumstance of older adults whom we encounter in the course of clinical care. This points to the need for clinical operationalization and testing of such measures of social circumstances.

For a complete list of references, please visit online only at www.expertconsult.com

CHAPTER 34

Presentation of Disease in Old Age

Sonja Rosen
Brandon Koretz
David B. Reuben

Not only are diseases more common in elderly people, they may be more difficult to diagnose accurately. Nonspecific symptoms, such as altered mental status, weight loss, fatigue, falls and dizziness may be the earliest or only manifestations in this age group. For example, many infections (e.g., pneumonia, urinary tract infection) may present with a change in mental status and fatigue, but few or no symptoms related to the source of the infection. Furthermore, classic presenting symptoms of common diseases may be absent. For example, older persons having myocardial infarction may not report having chest pain.

A number of possible explanations may account for such atypical presentations. Multiple comorbid conditions may alter the presentation of disease, and age-related physiologic changes may alter the perception of stimulus. For example, because of age-related changes in immunity, the febrile response may be absent in infected older persons.[1] Furthermore, cognitive impairment may prevent the patient from providing an accurate history. As a result, these atypical presentations may be more common than classic presentations. Moreover, an atypical presentation may predict a poor outcome for hospitalized elderly patients,[2] perhaps as a result of delays in diagnosis and initiation of appropriate therapy.

Because older patients may often have nonspecific symptoms and/or atypical symptoms for disease, we have chosen to present this material in two different formats. First, this chapter examines five nonspecific presentations of disease (altered mental status, weight loss, fatigue, dizziness, and falls and fever). Next, we review some common diseases, discussed by organ system, to explore the differences in disease presentation between younger and older patients.

NONSPECIFIC CLINICAL PRESENTATIONS OF DISEASE IN THE OLDER POPULATION

As noted in Table 34-1, six nonspecific presentations may be due to diverse disorders. We review the major diseases responsible for these presentations and provide approaches to determining the causes.

Altered mental status

Altered mental status (AMS) may often be the only indicator of a serious underlying disease.[3] Presenting symptoms can include disorientation, decreased or nonsensical verbalization, and somnolence or hyperactivity or a mixture of both. When altered mental status is of rapid onset accompanied by disturbed consciousness (especially decreased attention) and is due to a medical condition, it meets the criteria for delirium. Delirium can also be associated with sleep disturbances and hallucinations. Delirium is a common presentation of disease in the elderly, and is the most common complication associated with inpatient hospital admission for older people.[4] The symptoms of delirium may persist for months and are associated with adverse outcomes.[5]

The differential diagnosis of AMS in elderly patients is very broad, and encompasses many systems. The presence of a clinical history suggesting infection, low grade fever, or leukocytosis may suggest an infectious cause. As stated before, because of age-related changes in immunity, older persons may not necessarily mount a fever or leukocytosis.[1] The most common infectious causes of delirium include respiratory, urine, and skin infections. Another cause may be iatrogenic secondary to medications. Medications with a narrow therapeutic index and/or those that cross the blood-brain barrier are the most common culprits. These include anticholinergics and benzodiazepines. Alcohol intoxication or withdrawal should also be considered. Metabolic disorders include electrolyte imbalances, especially sodium disorders; dehydration; hypoglycemia; and hypoxia. Cardiovascular causes include heart failure and myocardial infarction.[6] Central nervous system causes such as infections (e.g., meningitis and encephalitis,[7] stroke, seizures, and subdural hematomas are less common. Finally, miscellaneous causes of altered mental status in the older population include urinary retention and fecal impaction.[8]

Altered mental status may also occur in the absence of delirium. For example, psychiatric causes, such as dementia with psychosis, psychotic depression, and bipolar disorder, may present with changes in mental status. Psychosis may be accompanied by delusions and hallucinations, and is one of the most common noncognitive symptoms associated with Alzheimer's dementia.[9] The second most common cause of psychosis in the elderly is depression.[10] Mania, though less commonly present in the elderly population, is characterized by hyperactivity, but patients should generally remain oriented.

When patients are too altered to give a reliable history, it is important to obtain a careful history and physical examination, which requires corroboration by family members, friends, caregivers, or health care workers, for patients who live in institutional settings. It is also important to review medications with a focus on recent changes and over-the-counter medications that may have anticholinergic properties (e.g., those containing diphenhydramine). For the most part, infection and other major medical causes can be identified with a set of simple laboratory studies, including a complete blood cell count with differential, comprehensive metabolic panel, urinalysis, chest x-ray, electrocardiogram, and, depending on patient's clinical status, cardiac enzymes.

Table 34-1. Nonspecific Clinical Presentations of Disease in the Older Population

Category	Disease Examples	Altered Mental Status	Weight Loss	Fatigue	Dizziness	Falls	Fever
Infection	Urosepsis	x	x	x	x	x	x
	Pneumonia	x		x		x	x
	Subacute endocarditis	x		x			x
	Cellulitis	x		x			x
	Meningoencephalitis	x					x
Metabolic disorders	Hypoxia	x	x	x	x	x	
	Dehydration	x		x	x	x	
	Hyponatremia	x		x	x	x	
	Hypoglycemia	x		x		x	
Cardiopulmonary	Heart failure		x	x			
	COPD		x	x			
Cancer			x	x			x
Psychiatric		x	x	x	x		
Cerebrovascular		x			x	x	
Rheumatologic	Pseudogout (CPPD)	x	x	x			x
	Rheumatoid arthritis	x		x			x
	Temporal arteritis	x		x			x
	Adult-onset Still disease			x			x
Endocrine	Hyperthyroidism	x	x	x			x
	Hypothyroidism	x		x			

If an infectious cause is suspected but no clear source can be found, a lumbar puncture may be warranted,[11] although a recent retrospective analysis of 232 hospitalized patients with fever and altered mental status demonstrated that lumbar punctures for suspected nosocomial meningitis in nonsurgical patients have a low yield.[12] Though altered mental status is unusual in meningitis, it may be a sign of other central nervous system infection, particularly meningoencephalitis. Furthermore, older patients may not mount the typical immune-response associated with these infections, such as fever or leukocytosis. Finally, brain imaging is of value in ruling out stroke or subdural hematoma if there is clinical suspicion of either diagnosis, or if the evaluation of AMS is otherwise unrevealing. Finally, EEG is helpful in diagnosing occult seizures.

Weight Loss

Undernutrition is indicated by unintentional weight loss of more than 5% within a year.[13] Unintentional weight loss occurs in up to 15% of community-dwelling older persons, between 20% to 65% of hospitalized patients, and 5% to 85% of institutionalized older persons.[14]

Unintentional weight loss is often a marker of severity of comorbidities or undiagnosed disease, and it may be divided into three causes: social, psychological, and medical.[14] Social reasons include poverty, functional impairment, social isolation, poor nutritional knowledge, and elder abuse. Most surveys have shown that poverty is the single most important social cause of weight loss.[15] Dependence in ADLs and IADLs, such as needing assistance with feeding, shopping, or food preparation, are also important factors. Psychological reasons include psychiatric problems such as depression, paranoia, and bereavement. Depression has been shown to be the major cause of weight loss in the outpatient setting.[16] Ninety percent of older adults with depression have weight loss, compared with 60% of younger adults.[17] It is also an important cause in institutionalized patients. Medical reasons include dementia; pulmonary and cardiac diseases; malignancy; medications; alcoholism; infectious diseases; poor dentition; endocrine abnormalities, especially hyperthyroidism and diabetes; malabsorption; and dysphagia.

The first step in determining the cause is to assess whether patients have adequate dietary intake.[18] If they have inadequate dietary intake, physiologic and psychosocial factors should be investigated. Physiologic factors include nausea, constipation, poor oral health, and functional dependence. Medication side effects also may contribute. For example, narcotics and anticholinergics may cause constipation, which in turn may cause bloating and poor appetite. Psychosocial factors including poverty, dementia, depression, and social isolation should be investigated. The use of geriatric screening instruments such as the Mini Mental State Examination[19] and the PHQ-9[20] can help elucidate the etiology.

On the other hand, if patients have adequate dietary intake, a search must be undertaken for underlying disease by careful history and physical examination, with special attention paid to symptoms that may suggest malignancy (such as cough, constipation, or gastrointestinal bleeding), cardiac, or pulmonary disease. The physical examination should evaluate for lymphadenopathy, palpable masses, and breast or thyroid abnormalities. Initial laboratory testing should include pre-albumin, complete blood cell count with differential, comprehensive metabolic panel, thyroid-stimulating hormone, urinalysis, erythrocyte sedimentalion rate (ESR), lactate dehydrogenase (LDH), and chest x-ray.[21] Depending on the patient's clinical findings and laboratory results, consideration should be given to abdominal ultrasound or CT.

Fatigue

Fatigue can be defined as tiredness or decreased energy, and excessive daytime fatigue is not a normal process of aging.[22] As the body protects its functional reserve, fatigue may be associated with generalized weakness that may occur if fatigue progresses.[23] Fatigue may be acute or chronic, the latter of which is the result of physical and/or psychological factors.

Physiologic causes of fatigue by body systems include hematologic/oncologic (e.g., anemia, cancer, and cancer-related therapy), cardiac (e.g., congestive heart failure), renal or liver disease, endocrine (thyroid disease, diabetes), and pulmonary (sleep-related breathing disorders, severe obstructive or restrictive lung diseases). Fatigue is one of the most common side effects of cancer treatment, with 70% of cancer patients receiving radiation and chemotherapy experiencing this symptom and may also persist for years after treatment.[24] Fatigue is also the most common symptom of congestive heart failure (CHF), and is the initial presenting complaint in 10% to 20% of new CHF diagnoses.[25] Obstructive sleep apnea (OSA) is common in patients over 60 years, with a reported prevalence of 37.5% to 62%; daytime sleepiness is a prominent symptom.[26] Other sleep disorders, such as insomnia or disturbances in sleep-wake cycles that may occur with dementia, can also lead to daytime fatigue. Some chronic infections, such as subacute endocarditis, may also present with fatigue as a chief complaint. Medications are also a common culprit of fatigue in the elderly, particularly antihistamines, anticholinergic medications, sedatives or nonsedating hypnotics, and antihypertensive medications (especially beta-blockers at high doses). Finally, psychiatric illnesses, most commonly depression, can cause excessive fatigue.

The evaluation of fatigue begins with history, with focus on any symptoms concerning for malignancy (e.g., weight loss) or other body system diseases that may suggest a cause (e.g., dyspnea suggesting anemia, congestive heart failure, ischemia, or pulmonary disease; recent bereavement suggesting depression). A cognitive assessment with the Mini Mental State Examination[19] should be performed to screen for cognitive impairment, and the PHQ-9[20] should be performed to screen for depression. Similarly, the physical examination should focus on any red flags (e.g., weight loss suggesting malignancy, edema suggesting congestive heart failure). A review of medications should focus on any potentially sedating medications, including over-the-counter medications such as antihistamines. The laboratory and diagnostic testing is then tailored toward identifying possible causes. In addition to basic labs (complete blood cell count, comprehensive metabolic panel, thyroid-stimulating hormone, urinalysis), additional diagnostic tests may be ordered based on history and physical findings (e.g., an electrocardiogram, echocardiogram, and BNP may be ordered in someone suspected of having CHF).

Dizziness

Dizziness occurs in more than 30% of the population over 60 years of age, and as many as 7% of elderly patients have this symptom.[27] Though common, dizziness is not a normal process of aging. It can be a vexing clinical problem, the cause of which is often difficult to both diagnose and treat. Most older patients who have dizziness have a benign cause, but dizziness may also be indicative of a more serious underlying medical condition. One study of patients older than 60 years of age having dizziness showed that 28% had a cardiovascular diagnosis and 14% had a central neurologic disorder. Of note, 22% had no attributable cause of symptoms identified.[28] Psychological disorders are rare as the primary cause of dizziness, but may be contributing or modulating factors in older persons with dizziness.[29] Furthermore, patients with dizziness may develop fear of falling, falls,[30] and subsequent disability in daily activities secondary to their symptoms.[31]

To determine the cause of dizziness, it is important to first determine the nature of the presenting symptoms. Dizziness can be classified into four symptom categories: vertigo, presyncope, dysequilibrium, and nonspecific dizziness.[32] *Vertigo* is defined as a feeling that one's surroundings are moving, and can be episodic or continuous. Causes of vertigo include benign paroxysmal positional vertigo, acute labyrinthitis, Meniere's disease, vertebrobasilar insufficiency, brain stem stroke, tumors, and cervical vertigo. *Presyncope* is defined as a lightheaded feeling or impending faint. Presyncope is commonly due to orthostatic hypotension, vasovagal attacks, and decreased cardiac output, such as significant valvular lesions or arrhythmias. *Dysequilibrium* is defined as a sense of unsteadiness or imbalance where one feels as if one is going to fall, and is usually constant and occurs primarily while standing. Dysequilibirum is usually the result of vestibular loss (e.g., acoustic neuroma), proprioceptive (e.g., cervical osteoarthritis) and somatosensory loss (e.g., peripheral neuropathy), cerebellar or motor lesions (e.g., subcortical or cerebellar infarct, tumors) or multiple neurosensory impairments, such as those occurring in Parkinson disease. Finally, some nonspecific dizziness symptoms do not fit into any of the above categories. These may be described as mild lightheadedness, but also may be difficult for patients to describe. Infections (e.g., urinary tract infections), anxiety, or hyperventilation are commonly responsible for nonspecific dizziness.

The evaluation of the differential diagnosis begins with a history and physical examination, with a focus on the nature of the patient's symptomatology. A dizziness simulation battery can be performed to further delineate which type of dizziness the patient suffers from.[33] For example, reproduction of symptoms with nystagmus in response to the Barany or Dix-Hallpike maneuver is diagnostic for vertigo. Further vestibular concerns can be evaluated with audiometry, brain MRI, and/or referral to an otolaryngologist. Presyncope should be evaluated with screening laboratory tests, including complete blood cell count, comprehensive metabolic panel, urinalysis and thyroid function, electrocardiogram, and possible further cardiac (e.g., event monitor, echocardiogram) or neurologic (carotid ultrasound, brain MRI) testing, depending on clinical presentation and history. In addition, dysequilibrium may require a neurology evaluation and further neurologic testing. Non-specific dizziness should also be evaluated with basic screening laboratory tests as indicated earlier.

Falls

Over one third of the community dwelling persons over 65 fall each year, and more than 50% of these patients have recurrent falls.[34] Falls are responsible for two thirds of accidental deaths, which are the fifth leading cause of death in older adults.[35] One in 10 falls results in serious injury, including hip fracture and subdural hematomas.[34] Falls are also independently associated with functional and mobility decline. All patients over 65 should be screened for a history of falling in the last year, as patients who have fallen in the last year are at higher risk for falling again.[36]

Though the cause of most falls is multifactorial in nature, it is useful to understand the separate entities that may be contributing factors or may independently cause falls. These include the following physiologic contributors: cardiac disease (e.g., orthostatic hypotension, arrhythmia, valvular lesions, ischemia); neurologic diseases (e.g., strokes, subdural hematomas in recurrent fallers, peripheral neuropathy; cognitive impairment); musculoskeletal (e.g., osteoarthritis, leg asymmetry, muscle weakness); sensory impairment (visual and hearing impairment); iatrogenic (medications; physical restraints in institutionalized settings); and primary gait and balance impairments. There are also several other nonphysiologic factors that may cause or contribute to falls, including: incorrect use of walking aids; environmental hazards (e.g., loose carpets), performing several activities simultaneously, inappropriate footwear, and hazardous behavior.[37]

If the physician learns that a patient has fallen in the last year, a multifactorial evaluation of the cause(s) should be undertaken. This begins with a history determining the circumstances surrounding the falls (e.g., loss of balance, tripping secondary to poor vision, or presyncopal symptoms). A review should be performed of both prescription and nonprescription medications that may be contributing to falls (e.g., sedatives, anticholinergics, nonsedating hypnotics). The physical examination should include orthostatic vital signs, visual acuity testing, and a gait and balance evaluation. The physician can most efficiently observe a patient's gait while the patient is entering and leaving the examination room. Simple tests of balance include observing the patient's ability to stand side-by-side, semitandem and full-tandem for 10 seconds; and stability during a 360-degree turn.[38] The neurologic examination should evaluate for any focal or generalized weakness, impaired cognition, signs of parkinsonism (e.g., rigidity, tremor) or poor proprioception. For patients who are found to have cognitive impairment or focal weakness, further evaluation may include brain imaging to assess for vascular disease. In addition, patients with focal weakness may require musculoskeletal imaging (e.g., to evaluate for osteoarthritis, spinal stenosis, mass lesions) and EMG studies to evaluate for possible peripheral neuropathy. The cardiovascular examination should include evaluation for valvular lesions, arrhythmias, or carotid lesions. An electrocardiogram should be performed with further cardiac testing if patients have presyncopal or syncopal symptoms (see Dizziness section). The musculoskeletal examination should focus on any muscle weakness or atrophy, joint abnormalities, foot deformities, or leg asymmetry. A complete blood count, basic metabolic panel, thyroid-stimulating hormone, and vitamin B_{12} level may identify a specific or contributing cause.

Fever

Fever is the prototypical sign of many infections (most commonly urinary tract, infections, pneumonias, skin, and intra-abdominal infections; less commonly endocarditis and osteomyelitis), and some malignancies (e.g., lymphoma, renal cell carcinoma, and hepatic cell carcinoma) and rheumatologic diseases (e.g., calcium pyrophosphate dihydrate deposition disease, rheumatoid arthritis, temporal arteritis, and adult onset Still's disease). Other less common causes include drug reactions, hematomas, and thyroid storm.

The presence of fever serves as a warning sign for potentially life-threatening diseases.[39] But, as already mentioned, the febrile response may be absent in infected older patients. While errors in measurement may account for some of this variability,[40] older patients, on average, have a lower basal temperature than younger persons.[41] To compensate for this, some have suggested that the use of change from basal temperature might be more sensitive for the presence of infection than absolute temperature.[40] In elderly individuals, an oral temperature of greater than 99° F should be considered elevated.[1] One study examined the importance of fever in 470 consecutive elderly patients who were seen in an emergency room with temperatures of 100.0° F or greater.[42] Three quarters of these patients were classified by the authors as seriously ill.

The fever workup should begin with a history focusing on evaluation for infection, malignancy, or rheumatologic disease. Physical examination should pay attention to cardiac (e.g., murmurs suspicious for endocarditis) and pulmonary examination (e.g., rhonchi indicating possible pneumonia), lymphadenopathy, skin findings, joint abnormalities, and gastrointestinal examination (e.g., pain, organomegaly or other masses). Laboratory evaluation should begin with complete blood cell count with differential, urinalysis, urine culture, and chest x-ray and ESR, the latter if there is clinical suspicion for osteomyelitis, endocarditis, temporal arteritis, or lymphoma. Further imaging may be warranted if there is clinical suspicion for occult disease, such as intraabdominal abscesses or neoplasm.

COMMON DISEASES AND THEIR ATYPICAL PRESENTATION IN THE OLDER POPULATION

As noted in Table 34-2, common diseases may often have atypical presentations in the older population. In this section, we review some of these common diseases and discuss the differences in disease presentation between younger and older patients.

Gastroesophageal reflux disease

Symptoms of gastroesophageal reflux disease (GERD) are common among elderly patients. The typical symptom in the older population is postprandial substernal burning exacerbated by reclining. Among older persons referred for endoscopy, almost 20% have erosive or complicated esophagitis.[43] People in this subgroup are more likely to complain of dysphagia, respiratory symptoms (chronic cough, hoarseness, or wheezing), and vomiting than patients without severe esophagitis.

Peptic ulcer disease

Among patients with endoscopically diagnosed ulcers, elderly people are less likely to have abdominal pain.[44] Conversely, they are more likely to have bleeding, a shorter duration of symptoms, and other symptoms not typically considered to be associated with peptic ulcer disease (nausea, vomiting, anorexia, or abdominal pain not relieved by eating or drinking).[45]

Appendicitis

Although appendicitis is more common in younger patients, its mortality is substantially higher among older persons.[46] The classic presentation is peri-umbilical pain that rapidly localizes to the right lower abdominal quadrant in association with peritoneal signs. Although this pattern may not be as common in elderly persons, most older patients will develop right lower quadrant pain at some time during the illness. Abdominal rigidity, decreased bowel sounds, and the presence of a mass appear to be more common in older

Table 34-2. Common Diseases and Their Atypical Presentations in the Older Population

Disease	Typical Presentation in Younger Persons	Atypical Presentation in Older Persons
GERD	Postprandial burning with reclining	Postprandial burning with reclining Dysphagia Chronic cough Hoarseness
PUD	Epigastric abdominal pain	Bleeding Nausea and vomiting Anorexia Abdominal pain not relieved by eating or drinking
Appendicitis	Peritoneal signs localizing to right lower quadrant Nausea/vomiting Leukocytosis	Abdominal rigidity Abdominal pain—generalized Decreased bowel sounds Nausea/vomiting Leukocytosis
Cholecystitis	Right upper quadrant pain Murphy sign Fever Nausea/vomiting Leukocytosis	Generalized abdominal pain Fever Nausea/vomiting
Myocardial infarction	Substernal chest pain radiating to left arm or jaw	Chest pain Dyspnea Vertigo Altered mental status Heart failure Weakness
Pneumonia	Fever Cough Chills Pleuritic chest pain	Tachypnea Altered mental status Decreased oral intake Fever Cough Chest pain
Gout	Male predominance Monoarticular	Indolent course Polyarticular
Rheumatoid arthritis	Indolent course	Acute onset Fever Weight loss Fatigue
Urinary tract infection	Dysuria Fever	Altered mental status Dizziness Nausea

patients.[47] Though variable, the frequency of nausea, vomiting, leukocytosis, and fever do not appear to be significantly different between older and younger patients.

Cholecystitis

The typical presentation of cholecystitis is right upper quadrant pain, fever, nausea, vomiting. Leukocytosis may not be present in elderly patients. In one retrospective cross-sectional study of 168 patients over the age of 65, 57% had nausea, 38% had vomiting, and 36% had back or flank pain radiation.[48] Surprisingly, 84% had neither epigastric or right upper quadrant pain, and 56% of patients were afebrile.

Myocardial infarction

Altered mental status, neurologic symptoms, weakness, and worsening heart failure are common presentations of an acute myocardial infarction in older persons.[49] Because pain perception decreases with aging, silent myocardial ischemia is more common. Even when older patients have the classic presentation of substernal discomfort, its intensity tends to be less severe.

Some studies have directly compared the presenting symptoms of MI in younger and older patients. In a Finnish study, typical presentations occurred more commonly in younger patients, whereas older patients more commonly had dyspnea, vertigo, and loss of consciousness.[50] A second study found that chest pain became less common as a presenting symptom of MI as patients aged; however, most patients of all ages had chest pain accompanying their MI.[51] The presence of syncope, stroke, and delirium as initial symptoms was also significantly associated with increased age.

Pneumonia

Pneumonia is the fifth leading cause of death among elderly people. Unlike the typical presentation of pneumonia consisting of fever, cough, chills, and pleuritic chest pain, atypical presentations occur more frequently in older persons.[52] These atypical presentations include decreased oral intake, falling, or confusion, or an abrupt worsening of an underlying chronic medical condition (e.g., hemiplegia from a prior stroke). Tachypnea is common; three quarters or more of elderly patients with pneumonia may present with respiratory rates greater than 20/min,[53,54] and may be one of the earliest signs of pneumonia, often occurring 24 to 48 hours before the clinical diagnosis.[55] Fever has been reported in 27% to 80% of older patients with pneumonia.[54,56,57,58] A cough has been noted in 54% to 82% of elderly patients admitted to the hospital with community-acquired pneumonia.[59,60] Chills or rigors are noted in about one quarter of patients and a similar percentage had falls.[48] Chest pain may be present in one third.[52] Delirium occurs in 15% to 47% of patients with pneumonia and seems to be more common among nursing-home patients (approximately 48%) than those who live independently.[54,56,57,60]

Gout

The presentation of gout in the older person may follow a more indolent course and be more likely to be polyarticular.[61] The male predominance noted in younger patients does not seem to be present among older persons.[62] There is a strong association with long-term diuretic use; renal excretion of uric acid is inhibited because of volume contraction.[63,64] For the same reason, tophaceous deposits are more likely to be present in elderly people.

Rheumatoid arthritis

Compared with younger persons, older patients who develop rheumatoid arthritis (RA) tend to have more constitutional symptoms (fever, weight loss, and fatigue), are more likely to have an acute onset of arthritis, have more shoulder involvement, and have a negative assay for rheumatoid factor.[65–68] However, there are some concerns about the methodological rigor of the studies on which these conclusions are based.[69]

Urinary tract infection and urosepsis

Bacteriuria becomes increasingly common with advancing age. In the absence of symptoms, its association with increased mortality is controversial.[70] It is clear, however, that the urinary tract is the most common source for bacteremia in elderly patients admitted to a hospital.[54] The typical symptoms associated with lower tract infections—dysuria, urgency, and suprapubic pain—are commonly absent in older patients with bacteriuria.[71] Similarly, the flank pain, fevers, and chills that typically accompany upper urinary tract infections may be absent. The clinical picture of urinary tract infections in older persons is variable. In one series of elderly patients with bacteremia from urinary sources, 30% had confusion, 29% had a cough, and 27% had dyspnea.[72] Other studies suggest that the febrile response to urinary tract infection remains intact, but also suggest that confusion is a common presenting sign.[73]

CONCLUSION

Many studies support the notion that common diseases present differently in the elderly population. What is less clear is whether it is appropriate to call these presentations atypical. In fact, when the atypical presentation is more common than the classic presentation described for younger persons, perhaps it should be termed the typical presentation in the older age group. Rather than using the 25-year-old as the reference standard for all age groups, practitioners should remain aware that diseases have different clinical features depending upon the age of the affected patient. Physicians should also be aware of common nonspecific presentations of illness, and their differential diagnosis and appropriate evaluation to help lead them to the right diagnosis.

KEY POINTS

Presentation of Disease

- Nonspecific presentations of disease may be the earliest or only manifestations of disease in older people.
- Six common nonspecific presentations of disease include altered mental status, weight loss, fatigue, falls, dizziness, and fever.
- Practitioners should remember that many common diseases may present differently in younger and older patients.

For a complete list of references, please visit online only at www.expertconsult.com

CHAPTER 35

Multidimensional Geriatric Assessment

Laurence Z. Rubenstein
Lisa V. Rubenstein

Geriatric assessment is a multidimensional, usually interdisciplinary, diagnostic process intended to determine a frail elderly person's medical, psychosocial, and functional capabilities and problems with the objective of developing an overall plan for treatment and long-term follow-up. It differs from the standard medical evaluation in its concentration on frail elderly people with their complex problems, its emphasis on functional status and quality of life, and its frequent use of interdisciplinary teams and quantitative assessment scales.

The process of geriatric assessment can range in intensity from a limited assessment by primary care physicians or community health workers focused on identifying an older person's functional problems and disabilities (screening assessment), to more thorough evaluation of these problems by a geriatrician or multidisciplinary team (comprehensive geriatric assessment), often coupled with initiation of a therapeutic plan. This chapter discusses both limited geriatric assessment, such as can be performed by a single practitioner in an office setting, and comprehensive geriatric assessment, usually requiring a specialized geriatric setting.

Because the ultimate goal of geriatric assessment is to improve quality of life for elderly people, readers may find Figure 35-1 helpful.[1] As diagrammed, quality of life includes health status and socioeconomic and environmental factors. Health status can be quantified both by measures of disease, such as signs, symptoms, and laboratory tests, and by measures of functional status. By functional status, we mean the individual's ability to participate fully in the physical, mental, and social activities of daily life. The ability to function fully in these arenas is strongly affected by an individual's physiologic health, and can often be used as a measure of the seriousness of a patient's multiple diseases. A comprehensive geriatric assessment should be able to evaluate and plan care for all these areas.

BRIEF HISTORY OF GERIATRIC ASSESSMENT

The basic concepts of geriatric assessment have evolved over the past 75 years by combining elements of the traditional medical history and physical examination, the social worker assessment, functional evaluation, and treatment methods derived from rehabilitation medicine, and psychometric methods derived from the social sciences. By incorporating the perspectives of many disciplines, geriatricians have created a practical means of viewing the "whole patient."

The first published reports of geriatric assessment programs came from the British geriatrician Marjory Warren, who initiated the concept of specialized geriatric assessment units during the late 1930s while in charge of a large London infirmary. This infirmary was filled primarily with chronically ill, bedfast, and largely neglected elderly patients who had not received proper medical diagnosis or rehabilitation and who were thought to be in need of lifelong institutionalization. Good nursing care kept the patients alive, but the lack of diagnostic assessment and rehabilitation kept them disabled. Through evaluation, mobilization, and rehabilitation, Warren was able to get most of the long bedfast patients out of bed and often discharged home. As a result of her experiences, Warren advocated that every elderly patient receive comprehensive assessment and an attempt at rehabilitation before being admitted to a long-term care hospital or nursing home.[2]

Since Warren's work, geriatric assessment has evolved. As geriatric care systems have been developed throughout the world, geriatric assessment programs have been assigned central roles, usually as focal points for entry into the care systems.[3] Geared to differing local needs and populations, geriatric assessment programs vary in intensity, structure, and function. They can be located in different settings, including acute hospital inpatient units and consultation teams, chronic and rehabilitation hospital units, outpatient and office-based programs, and home visit outreach programs. Despite diversity, they share many characteristics. Virtually all programs provide multidimensional assessment, using specific measurement instruments to quantify functional, psychological, and social parameters. Most use interdisciplinary teams to pool expertise and enthusiasm in working toward common goals. Additionally, most programs attempt to couple their assessments with an intervention, such as rehabilitation, counseling, or placement.

Today, geriatric assessment continues to evolve in response to increased pressures for cost containment, avoidance of institutional stays, and consumer demands for better care. Geriatric assessment can help achieve improved quality of care and plan cost-effective care. This has generally meant more emphasis on noninstitutional programs and shorter hospital stays. Geriatric assessment teams are well positioned to deliver effective care for elderly persons with limited resources. Geriatricians have long emphasized judicious use of technology, systematic preventive medicine activities, and less institutionalization and hospitalization.

STRUCTURE AND PROCESS OF GERIATRIC ASSESSMENT

Geriatric assessment begins with the identification of deteriorations in health status or the presence of risk factors for deterioration. These deteriorations include both worsening of disease and worsening of functional status. If disease alone has worsened, without affecting function, the patient should be able to be cared for in usual primary care settings. In addition, when functional status problems are mild and are not rapidly progressive, it is appropriate for a primary care practitioner to proceed with the assessment. However, because families and patients identify functional status problems early, and because internists and family practitioners often are unfamiliar with the concept of "treating" functional status impairment as a problem in its own right, patients often self-refer to geriatric care settings for these functional status problems when

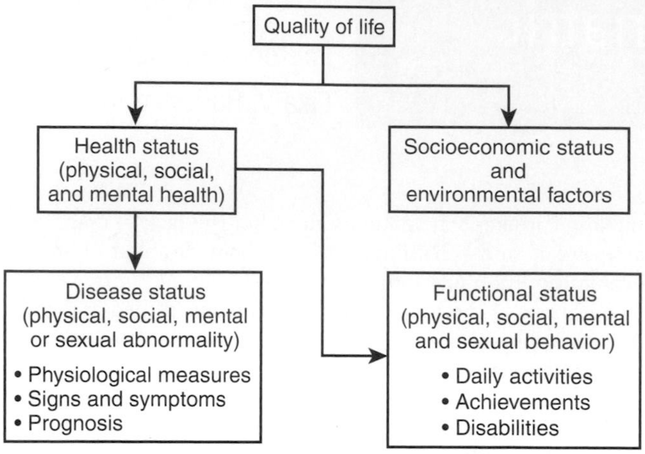

Figure 35-1. Conceptual components of quality of life—relationship to health and functional status. *(Adapted from Rubenstein LV, Calkins DR, Greenfield S et al. Health status assessment for elderly patients: reports of the Society of General Internal Medicine task force on health assessment. J Am Geriatr Soc 1989;37:562–9, with permission of Blackwell Science, Inc.)*

such settings are available. Patients who have new severe or progressive deficits should ideally receive comprehensive multidisciplinary geriatric assessment. Figure 35-2 outlines an approach for evaluating elderly outpatients with health status deterioration and deciding who should be referred to multidimensional geriatric assessment settings.

Using this approach, an elderly patient with a deteriorating health status of any kind, be it a markedly elevated blood glucose, a vertebral collapse, or a new inability to perform errands, should be evaluated briefly to determine the full extent of functional disabilities. Many experts believe that frail elderly people, defined generally as people over the age of 75, or over age 65 with chronic disease, should also be screened for functional disability or risk factors at regular intervals such as once a year, even when no known acute health insults have occurred.[1,4–7] When a new disability or high-risk state is detected through screening, such patients may also be appropriate for a full geriatric assessment.

A typical geriatric assessment begins with a functional status "review of systems" that inventories the major domains of functioning. The major elements of this review of systems are captured in two commonly used functional status measures—basic activities of daily living (ADL) and instrumental activities of daily living (IADL). Several reliable and valid versions of these measures have been developed,[8–12] perhaps the most widely used being those by Katz et al,[13] Lawton and Brody,[14] and Wade and Colin.[15] These scales are used by clinicians to detect whether the patient has problems performing activities that people must be able to accomplish to survive without help in the community. Basic ADL include self-care activities, such as eating, dressing, bathing, transferring, and toileting. Patients unable to perform these activities will generally require 12- to 24-hour support by caregivers. Instrumental activities of daily living include heavier housework, going on errands, managing finances, and telephoning—activities that are required if the individual is to remain independent in a house or apartment.

To interpret the results of impairments in ADL and IADL, physicians will usually need additional information about the patient's environment and social situation. For example, the amount and type of caregiver support available, the strength of the patient's social network, and the level of social activities in which the patient participates will all influence the clinical approach taken in managing deficits detected. This information could be obtained by an experienced nurse or social worker. A screen for mobility and fall risk is also extremely helpful in quantifying function and disability, and several observational scales are available.[16,17] An assessment of nutritional status and risk for undernutrition is also important in understanding the extent of impairment and for planning care.[18] Likewise, a screening assessment of vision and hearing will often detect crucial deficits that need to be treated or compensated for.

Two other key pieces of information must always be gathered in the face of functional disability in an elderly person. These are a screen for mental status (cognitive) impairment and a screen for depression. Of the several validated screening tests for cognitive function, the Folstein Mini Mental State Examination is one of the best because it efficiently tests the major aspects of cognitive functioning.[19] Of the various screening tests for geriatric depression, the Yesavage Geriatric Depression Scale[20] and the PHQ-9 (depression screen of the Patient Health Questionnaire)[21] are in wide use, and even shorter screening versions are available without significant loss of accuracy.[22]

The major measurable dimensions of geriatric assessment, together with examples of commonly used health status screening scales, are listed in Table 35-1.[7–36] The instruments listed are short, have been carefully tested for reliability and validity, and can be easily administered by virtually any staff person involved with the assessment process. Both observational instruments (e.g., physical examination) and self-report (completed by patient or proxy) are available. Components of them—such as watching a patient walk, turn around, and sit down—are routine parts of the geriatric physical examination. Many other kinds of assessment measures exist and can be useful in certain situations. For example, there are several disease-specific measures for stages and levels of dysfunction for patients with specific diseases such as arthritis,[30] dementia,[31] and parkinsonism.[32] There are also several brief global assessment instruments that attempt to quantify all dimensions of the assessment in a single form.[33–36] These latter instruments can be useful in community surveys and some research settings but are not detailed enough to be useful in most clinical settings. More comprehensive lists of available instruments can be found by consulting published reviews of health status assessment.[7–12,37]

A number of factors must be taken into account in deciding where an assessment should take place. These are outlined in Table 35-2. Mental and physical impairment make it difficult for patients to comply with recommendations and to navigate multiple appointments in multiple locations. Functionally impaired elders must depend on families and friends, who risk losing their jobs because of chronic and relentless demands on time and energy in their roles as caregivers, and who may be elderly themselves. Each separate medical appointment or intervention has a high time-cost to these caregivers. Patient fatigue during periods of increased illness may require the availability of a bed during the assessment process. Finally, enough physician time and expertise must be available to complete the assessment within the constraints of the setting.

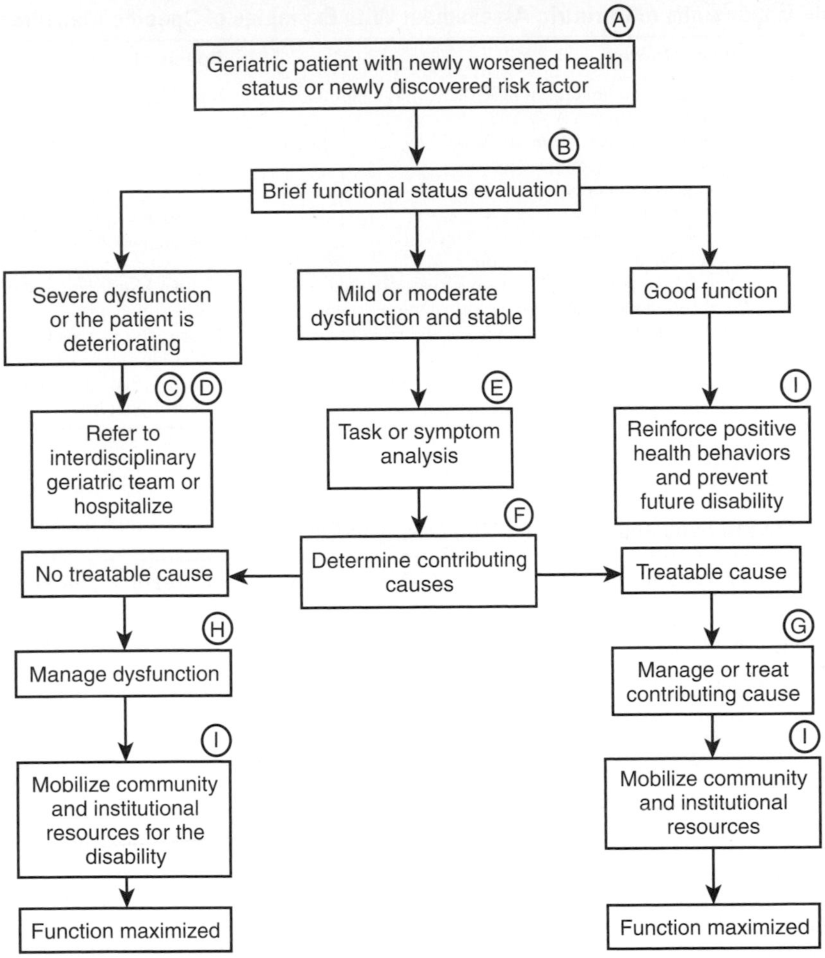

Figure 35-2. Evaluating and treating health status deterioration among geriatric outpatients.

A, Elderly patients with a new deterioration in health status or newly discovered risk factor(s) may need geriatric assessment. Examples of patients needing assessment include the following:

1. Frail elderly people with a new functional disability or risk factor for deterioration detected on routine screening
2. Elderly people with a new or worsened medical complaint or laboratory finding (e.g., "I fell last week" or the x-ray shows a new vertebral compression fracture)
3. Elderly people with a new or worsened functional disability complaint ("I can't go to church because of my health")

B, Brief functional status evaluation should include the following:

1. Activities of daily living (ADL)[13-15,23]
2. Instrumental activities of daily living (IADL)[14,23]
3. Mental status (e.g., Folstein Mini Mental State Examination)[19]
4. Affective status (e.g., Yesavage Geriatric Depression Scale)[20-22]

C, Full multidimensional geriatric assessment and/or hospitalization is necessary for elderly patients with new severe or progressive functional disability

D, Targeted assessment for patients in office practice is appropriate for the following:

1. Patients whose functional disabilities or medical problems are mild enough to make multiple appointment feasible
2. Patients whose disability is stable enough to permit assessment over weeks to months

E, To perform task or symptom analysis, select the patient's major symptom or disability or chief complaint (the one that bothers him/her the most, the disability upon which resolution of other health problems depends, or the one that is the most treatable). Then determine the exact maneuvers necessary to complete the task, or the exact components of the symptom (e.g., "difficulty getting dressed" due to difficulty putting on shoes because of inability to bend, or "difficulty with housework" because of failure to complete tasks despite adequate physical ability to perform them)

F, To determine contributing causes:

1. Perform a targeted history, guided by the functional disabilities detected and by the known common occult causes of disability in the elderly (see text)
2. Perform a targeted physical examination, always including postural blood pressure changes, vision and hearing screening, observations of gait (at least get up, walk 25 feet, turn around, sit down). Determine all specific physical disabilities, such as hip flexor weakness or poor hand mobility, that explain the observed functional disability.

G, Manage or treat contributing cause(s). Begin appropriate medical treatments and evaluations. Mobilize community and institutional resources as appropriate (low-vision resources for blindness; Alcoholics Anonymous for alcoholics, etc.). Identify key members of the multidisciplinary team and refer as needed (e.g., social worker for social isolation, physical therapist for gait disorder, or psychiatrist for depression).

H, When the disability cannot be reversed, maximize function using available services and behavioral or physical adaptation. For example, rearranging schedule to maximize activity, providing adaptive devices, or arranging for home support services might be indicated.

I, Always reinforce positive health behaviors.

Table 35-1. Measurable Dimensions of Geriatric Assessment With Examples of Specific Measures

Dimension	Basic Context	Specific Examples
Basic ADL[23]	Strengths and limitations in self-care, basic mobility, and incontinence	Katz (ADL)[13]; Lawton Personal Self-Maintenance Scale[14]; Barthel index[15]
IADL[23]	Strengths and limitations in shopping, cooking, house hold activities, and finances	Lawton (IADL)[14]; Older Americans Resources and Services, IADL Section[27]
Social activities and supports[24]	Strengths and limitations in social network and community activities	Lubben Social Network Scale[28]; Older Americans Resources and Services, Social Resources Section[27]
Mental health—affective[26]	The degree to which the person feels anxious, depressed, or generally happy	Yesavage Geriatric Depression Scale[20,22]; PHQ-921
Mental health—cognitive[27]	The degree to which the person is alert, oriented, and able to concentrate, and perform complex mental tasks	Folstein Mini-Mental State[19]; Kahn Mental Status Questionnaire[29]
Mobility—gait and balance[9,11]	Quantitative scale of gait, balance, and risk of falls	Tinetti Performance Oriented Mobility Assessment[16]; Get Up and Go Test[17]
Nutritional adequacy[18]	Current nutritional status and risk of malnutrition	Nutrition Screening Initiative Checklist[18]; Mini Nutritional Assessment[25]

Abbreviations: *ADL*, activities of daily living; *IADL*, instrumental activities of daily living.

Table 35-2. Determining the Intensity and Location of the Geriatric Assessment

	Office Setting	Outpatient/Homecare Team	Inpatient Unit/Team
Level of disability	Low	Intermediate	High
Cognitive dysfunction	Mild	Mild to severe	Moderate to severe
Family support	Good	Good to fair	Good to poor
Acuity of illness	Mild	Mild to moderate	Moderate to severe
Complexity	Low	Intermediate	High
Transportation access	Good	Good	Good to poor

Most geriatric assessments do not require the full range of technology nor the intense monitoring found in the acute-care inpatient setting. Yet hospitalization becomes unavoidable if no outpatient setting provides sufficient resources to accomplish the assessment fast enough. A specialized geriatric setting outside an acute hospital ward, such as a day hospital or subacute inpatient geriatric evaluation unit, will provide the easy availability of an interdisciplinary team with the time and expertise to provide needed services efficiently, an adequate level of monitoring, and beds for patients unable to sit or stand for prolonged periods. Inpatient and day-hospital assessment programs have the advantages of intensity, rapidity, and ability to care for particularly frail or acutely ill patients. Outpatient and in-home programs are generally cheaper and avoid the necessity of an inpatient stay.

Assessment in the office practice setting

A streamlined approach is usually necessary in the office setting. An important first step is setting priorities among problems for initial evaluation and treatment. The "best" problem to work on first might be the problem that most bothers a patient or, alternatively, the problem upon which resolution of other problems depends (alcoholism or depression often fall into this category).

The second step in performing a geriatric assessment is to understand the exact nature of the disability through performing a task or symptom analysis. In a nonspecialized setting, or when the disability is mild or clear-cut, this may involve only taking a careful history. When the disability is more severe, more detailed assessments by a multidisciplinary or interdisciplinary team may be necessary. For example, a patient may have difficulty dressing. There are multiple tasks associated with dressing, any one of which might be the stumbling block (e.g., buying clothes, choosing appropriate clothes to put on, remembering to complete the task, buttoning, stretching to put on shirts, or reaching downward to put on shoes). By identifying the exact areas of difficulty, further evaluation can be targeted toward solving the problem.

Once the history has revealed the nature of the disability, a systematic physical examination and ancillary laboratory tests are needed to clarify the cause of the problem. For example, difficulty dressing could be caused by mental status impairment, poor finger mobility, or dysfunction of shoulders, back, or hips. Evaluation by a physical or occupational therapist may be necessary to pinpoint the problem adequately, and evaluation by a social worker may be required to determine the extent of family dysfunction engendered by or contributing to the dependency. Radiologic and other laboratory testing may be necessary.

Each abnormality that could cause difficulty dressing suggests different treatments. By understanding the abnormalities that contribute most to the functional disability, the best treatment strategy can be undertaken. Often one disability leads to another. Impaired gait may lead to depression or decreased social functioning, and immobility of any cause, even after the cause has been removed, can lead to secondary impairments in performance of daily activities because of deconditioning and loss of musculoskeletal flexibility.

Almost any acute or chronic disease can reduce functioning. Common but easily overlooked causes of dysfunction in elderly people include impaired cognition, impaired special senses (vision, hearing, balance), unstable gait and mobility, poor health habits (alcohol, smoking, lack of exercise), poor nutrition, polypharmacy, incontinence, psychosocial stress, and depression. To identify contributing causes of the disability, the physician must look for worsening of the patient's chronic diseases, occurrence of a new acute disease, or appearance of one of the common occult diseases listed earlier. The physician does this through a refocused history guided by the functional disabilities detected and their differential diagnoses, and a focused physical examination. The physical examination always includes, in addition to usual evaluations of the heart, lungs, extremities, and neurologic function, postural blood pressure, vision and hearing screening, and careful observation of the patient's gait. The Mini Mental State Examination, already recommended as part of the initial functional status screen, may also determine what parts of the physical examination require particular attention as part of the evaluation of dementia or acute confusion. Finally, basic laboratory testing including a complete blood count, a blood chemistry panel, and tests indicated on the basis of specific findings from the history and physical examination, will generally be necessary.

Once the disability and its causes are understood, the best treatments or management strategies for it are often clear. When a reversible cause for the impairment is found, a simple treatment may eliminate or ameliorate the functional disability. When the disability is complex, the physician may need the support of a variety of community or hospital-based resources. In most cases, a strategy for long-term follow-up and often, formal case management should be developed to ensure that needs and services are appropriately matched up and followed through.

Comprehensive geriatric assessment

If referral to a specialized geriatric setting has been chosen, the process of assessment will probably be similar to that described above, except that the greater intensity of resources and the special training of all members of the interdisciplinary team in dealing with geriatric patients and their problems will facilitate carrying out the proposed assessment and plan more quickly, and in greater breadth and detail. In the usual geriatric assessment setting, key disciplines involved include, at a minimum, physicians, social workers, nurses, and physical and occupational therapists, and optimally may include other disciplines such as dieticians, pharmacists, ethicists, and home-care specialists. Special geriatric expertise among the interdisciplinary team members is crucial.

The interdisciplinary team conference, which takes place after most team members have completed their individual assessments, is critical. Most successful trials of geriatric assessment have included such a team conference. By bringing the perspectives of all disciplines together, the team conference generates new ideas, sets priorities, disseminates the full results of the assessment to all those involved in treating the patient, and avoids duplication or incongruity. Development of fully effective teams requires commitment, skill, and time as the interdisciplinary team evolves through the "forming, storming, and norming" phases to reach the fully developed "performing" stage.[38] Involvement of the patient (and caregiver, if appropriate) at some stage is important in maintaining the principle of choice.[38,39]

EFFECTIVENESS OF GERIATRIC ASSESSMENT PROGRAMS

A large and still growing literature supports the effectiveness of geriatric assessment programs (GAPs) in a variety of settings. Early descriptive studies indicated a number of benefits from GAPs, such as improved diagnostic accuracy, reduced discharges to nursing homes, increased functional status, and more appropriate medication prescribing. Because they were descriptive studies, without concurrent control patients, they were not able to distinguish the effects of the programs from simple improvement over time. Nor did these studies look at long-term, or many short-term, outcome benefits. Nonetheless, many of these early studies provided promising results.[40–44]

Improved diagnostic accuracy was the most widely described effect of geriatric assessment, most often indicated by substantial numbers of important problems uncovered. Frequencies of new diagnoses found ranged from almost one to more than four per patient. Factors contributing to the improvement of diagnosis in GAPs include the validity of the assessment itself (the capability of a structured search for "geriatric problems" to find them), the extra measure of time and care taken in the evaluation of the patient (independent of the formal elements of "the assessment"), and a probable lack of diagnostic attention on the part of referring professionals.

Improved living location on discharge from a healthcare setting was demonstrated in several early studies, beginning with T. F. Williams' classic descriptive pre-post study of an outpatient assessment program in New York.[45] Of patients referred for nursing home placement in the county, the assessment program found that only 38% actually needed skilled nursing care, while 23% could return home, and 39% were appropriate for board and care or retirement facilities. Numerous subsequent studies have shown similar improvements in living location.[46–59] Several studies that examined mental or physical functional status of patients before and after comprehensive geriatric assessment coupled with treatment and rehabilitation showed patient improvement on measures of function.[46–50,52,56]

Beginning in the 1980s, controlled studies appeared that corroborated some of the earlier studies and documented additional benefits such as improved survival, reduced hospital and nursing home use, and, in some cases, reduced costs.[46–67] These studies were by no means uniform in their results. Some showed a whole series of dramatic positive effects on function, survival, living location, and costs, whereas others showed relatively few if any benefits. However, the GAPs being studied were also very different from each other in terms of process of care offered and patient populations accepted. To this day, controlled trials of GAPs continue, and as results accumulate, we are able to understand which aspects contribute to their effectiveness and which do not.

One striking effect confirmed for many GAPs has been a positive impact on survival. Several controlled studies of different basic GAP models demonstrated significantly increased survival, reported in different ways and with varying periods of follow-up. Mortality was reduced for Sepulveda geriatric evaluation unit patients by 50% at 1 year, and the survival curves of the experimental and control groups still significantly favored the assessed group at 2 years.[46,60,61] Survival was improved by 21% at 1 year in a Scottish trial of geriatric rehabilitation consultation.[56] Two Canadian consultation trials demonstrated significantly improved 6-month survival.[52,53] Two Danish community-based trials of in-home geriatric assessment and follow-up demonstrated reduction in mortality,[47,58] and two Welsh studies of in-home GAPs had beneficial survival effects among patients assessed at home and followed for 2 years.[49,50] On the other hand, several other studies of geriatric assessment found no statistically significant survival benefits.[51,55,56]

Multiple studies followed patients longitudinally after the initial assessment and thus were able to examine the longer-term utilization and cost impacts of assessment and treatment. Some studies found an overall reduction in nursing home days.[46,56,62] Hospital use was examined in several reports. For hospital-based GAPs, the length of hospitalization was obviously affected by the length of the assessment itself. Thus some programs appear to prolong initial length of stay,[44,63,64] whereas others reduce initial stay.[58,65] However, studies following patients for at least 1 year have usually shown reduction in use of acute-care hospital services, even in those programs with initially prolonged hospital stays.[46,47,54]

Compensatory increases in use of community-based services or home-care agencies might be expected with declines in nursing home placements and use of other institutional services. These increases have been detected in several studies[47,49,52,66] but not in others.[46,54,59] Although increased use of formal community services may not always be indicated, it usually is a desirable goal. The fact that several studies did not detect increases in use of home and community services probably reflects the unavailability of community service or referral networks rather than that more of such services were not needed.

The effects of these programs on costs and utilization parameters have seldom been examined comprehensively, owing to methodological difficulties in gathering comprehensive utilization and cost data, and statistical limitations in comparing highly skewed distributions. The Sepulveda study found that total first-year direct health care costs had been reduced owing to overall reductions in nursing home and rehospitalization days, despite significantly longer initial hospital stays in the geriatric unit.[46] These savings continued through 3 years of follow-up.[60] Hendriksen's program[47] reduced the costs of medical care, apparently through successful early case-finding and referral for preventive intervention. Williams' outpatient GAP[54] detected reductions in medical care costs owing primarily to reductions in hospitalization. Although it would be reasonable to worry that prolonged survival of frail patients would lead to increased service use and charges—or, of perhaps greater concern, to worry about the quality of the prolonged life—these concerns may be without substance. Indeed, the Sepulveda study demonstrated that a GAP could improve not only survival but prolong high-function survival,[46,60] while at the same time reducing use of institutional services and costs.

A 1993 meta-analysis attempted to resolve some of the discrepancies between study results, and tried to identify whether particular program elements were associated with particular benefits.[68,69] This meta-analysis included published data from the 28 controlled trials completed as of that date involving nearly 10,000 patients, and was also able to include substantial amounts of unpublished data systematically retrieved from many of the studies. The meta-analysis identified five GAP types: hospital units (six studies), hospital consultation teams (eight studies), in-home assessment services (seven studies), outpatient assessment services (four studies), and "hospital- home assessment services" (three studies), the latter of which performed in-home assessments on patients recently discharged from hospitals. The meta-analysis confirmed many of the major reported benefits for many of the individual program types. These statistically and clinically significant benefits included reduced risk of mortality (by 22% for hospital-based programs at 12 months, and by 14% for all programs combined at 12 months), improved likelihood of living at home (by 47% for hospital-based programs and by 26% for all programs combined at 12 months), reduced risk of hospital (re)admissions (by 12% for all programs at study end), greater chance of cognitive improvement (by 47% for all programs at study end), and greater chance of physical function improvement for patients on hospital units (by 72% for hospital units).

Clearly not all studies showed equivalent effects, and the meta-analysis was able to indicate a number of variables at both the program and patient levels that tended to distinguish trials with large effects from those with more limited ones. When examined on the program level, hospital units and home-visit assessment teams produced the most dramatic benefits, whereas no major significant benefits in office-based programs could be confirmed. Programs that provided hands-on clinical care and/or long-term follow-up were generally able to produce greater positive effects than purely consultative programs or ones that lacked follow-up. Another factor associated with greater demonstrated benefits, at least in hospital-based programs, was patient targeting; programs that selected patients who were at high risk for deterioration yet still had "rehabilitation potential" generally had stronger results than less selective programs.

The meta-analysis confirmed the importance of targeting criteria in producing beneficial outcomes. In particular, when use of explicit targeting criteria for patient selection was included as a covariate, increases in some program benefits were often found. For example, among the hospital-based GAP studies, positive effects on physical function and likelihood of living at home at 12 months were associated with studies that excluded patients who were relatively "too healthy." A similar effect on physical function was seen in the institutional studies that excluded persons with relatively poor prognoses. The reason for this effect of targeting on effect size no doubt lies in the ability of careful targeting to concentrate the intervention on patients who can benefit, without diluting the effect with persons too ill or too well to show a measurable improvement.

Studies performed after the 1993 meta-analysis have been largely corroborative. A more recent meta-analysis confirmed that inpatient GAPs for elderly hospital patients may reduce mortality, increase the chances of living at home in 1 year, and improve physical and cognitive function.[70] However, with principles of geriatric medicine becoming more diffused into usual care, particularly at places where controlled trials are being undertaken, differences between GAPs and control groups seem to be narrowing.[71–76] For example, a 2002 study of inpatient and outpatient GAPs failed to demonstrate substantial benefits.[77] Other studies continue to reveal major benefits of inpatient programs.[78,79] Effects of outpatient GAPs have been less impressive, with a 2004 meta-analysis showing no favorable effects on mortality outcome.[80] For cost reasons, growth of inpatient units has been slow, despite their proven effectiveness, whereas outpatient programs have increased, despite their less impressive effect size in controlled trials. However, some newer trials of outpatient programs have shown significant benefits in areas not found in earlier outpatient studies, such as functional status, psychological parameters, and well-being, which may indicate improvement in the outpatient-care models being tested.[72 76,79]

A 2002 meta-analysis of preventive home visits revealed that home visitation programs are consistently effective if they are based on multidimensional geriatric assessments, employ multiple follow-up visits, and are offered to elderly persons with relatively good function at baseline.[81] The NNV (number needed to visit) to prevent one hospital admission in programs with frequent follow-up was shown to be about 40. An expanded 2008 meta-analysis of preventive home visits largely confirmed the earlier findings on the importance of multidimensional assessment and higher function, but not on multiple follow-up visits.[82] It has also been recently confirmed that a key component of successful programs is a systematic approach for teaching primary care professionals. These results have important policy implications. In countries with existing national programs of preventive home visits, the process and organization of these visits should be reconsidered on the basis of the criteria identified in this meta-analysis. In addition, there are a variety of chronic disease management programs specifically addressing the care needs of older adults.[83] Engrafting the key concepts of home-based preventive care programs into these programs should be feasible and cost-effective as they continue to evolve. Identifying risks and dealing with them as an essential component of the care of elderly persons is central to reducing the emerging burden of disability and improving the quality of life for older adults.

A continuing challenge has been obtaining adequate financing to support adding geriatric assessment services to existing medical care. Despite GAPs' many proven benefits, and their ability to reduce costs documented in controlled trials, health care financiers have been reluctant to fund geriatric assessment programs—presumably out of concern that the programs might be expanded too fast and that costs for extra diagnostic and therapeutic services might increase out of control. Many practitioners have found ways to "unbundle" the geriatric assessment process into component services and receive adequate support to fund the entire process. In this continuing time of fiscal restraint, geriatric practitioners must remain constantly creative to reach the goal of optimal patient care.

CONCLUSION

Published studies of multidimensional geriatric assessment have confirmed its efficacy in many settings. Although there is no single optimal blueprint for geriatric assessment, the participation of the interdisciplinary functional status and quality of life as major clinical goals are common to all settings. Although the greatest benefits have been found in programs targeted to the frail subgroup of elderly people, a strong case can be made for a continuum of GAP-screening assessments performed periodically for all older persons and comprehensive assessment targeted to frail and high-risk patients. Clinicians interested in developing these services will do well to heed the experiences of the programs reviewed here in adapting the principles of geriatric assessment to local resources. Future research is still needed to determine the most effective and efficient methods for performing geriatric assessment and on developing strategies for best matching needs with services.

KEY POINTS

Geriatric Assessment

- Geriatric assessment is a systematic multidimensional approach to improving diagnostic accuracy and planning care for frail elderly people.
- Controlled trials have documented many benefits from geriatric assessment, including improved functional status and survival and reduced hospital and nursing-home admissions.

For a complete list of references, please visit online only at www.expertconsult.com

CHAPTER 36

Laboratory Medicine in Geriatrics

Alexander Lapin

INTRODUCTION

The improvement of life style and health care, especially in industrialized countries created the phenomenon of the inverse demographic pyramid. As a result, the proportion of elderly within the general population is growing constantly. Many disciplines of geriatric medicine have become topics of growing interest. However, this is not the case in laboratory medicine where, besides an occasional stress on reference intervals for the elderly, a more fundamental discussion on consequences resulting from the actual demographic trend has not resulted until now. This chapter should provide some insights on this problem.

Objectivity as a basic principle of in vitro diagnosis

Since antiquity, in vitro diagnosis follows the same principle: A biologic sample (blood, urine) is drawn from the patient and subjected to analysis of its properties. The result is than interpreted in terms of clinical information concerning the health status of the patient. If such analysis is properly calibrated, the result can be expressed quantitatively (e.g., by numerals, not by words as is the case in other diagnostic disciplines, such as in pathology or radiology). Thereafter the result of a laboratory analysis is not an expertise, which results from the subjective experience of the operator, but is an objective measurement, which is always related to an à-priori postulated standard. Thus most of the results provided by laboratory investigations can be considered as data. In general, they are reproducible and comparable to each other and, as such, they represent a validated instrument of modern, evidence-based medicine.

To extend the principle of objectivity even on clinical interpretation, the laboratory report contains an indication of reference interval, which is stated aside from the numerical quotation of the result. It corresponds to the statistical distribution of the results that would be obtained when the analysis would be performed on a collective of healthy (not specifically diseased) individuals. Usually, such a reference group is taken as a demographic sample from the normal adult population while the term of normal is usually understood as a synonym for healthy.[1]

However, since the reference interval is determined statistically, on the basis of calculation of the 95th percentile of gaussian normal distribution, 5% of results obtained from healthy individuals will be always situated outside the reference range and this without any pathologic correlation. This means that performing an increasing amount of laboratory tests in the same healthy individual, the probability that one of the results would be outside of the reference interval increases constantly. Ironically the more one performs laboratory investigations, the probability that the individual will be found as not normal increases.[1]

This consideration illustrates the limits of the statistically based reference concept,[2] emphasizing the fact that a human being is first of all an unrepeatable personality, not just an anonymous element of a collective. And even this insight does not reveal the specificity of the problem of the geriatric laboratory medicine.

Geriatric individuality

From the sociologic point of view, the question of whether an older person is healthy or sick cannot be answered by productivity in his or her job, nor by fact that he or she brought a notification of illness to the employer, but actually by his or her subjective feeling, which is an aspect of his or her quality of life.

But there is another aspect which should be considered in geriatric laboratory medicine. It is a continuous decline of physiologic functions. Age-dependent impairment of renal and pulmonal function, progression of osteoporosis, decrease of various endocrine functions, and weakening of immunity at an older age are some such examples.[3–6] In view of this, and in an analogy to pediatrics, attempts have been made to establish—even for geriatrics—age-related reference intervals. Nevertheless, these intentions failed because of individuality and variability of the senescent process from both a clinical and a biologic point of view.

In pediatrics as in adult medicine, the majority of population is healthy and patients have usually one, but rarely several, causes for their illness. The primary aim of medicine here is to detect and to cure the disease as efficiently as possible to protect the future life chances of the individual and to return him or her as fast as possible back to normal (working) life. In geriatrics it is different. Here, since an old person has reached the last part of life, clinical history must be more complex then in previous phases of life. Passed crises, emergency situations, but also periods of prosperity and affluence, all had influence on the actual health state. Various diseases and trauma, which randomly occur in the course of life, have left more or less relevant aftereffects, which at the older age, contribute to the specificity of the clinical status of each aged person. Moreover, with advancing age, the probability of manifestation of a genetically or secondarily predisposed disease increases progressively. All together these inputs can be characterized by the term multimorbidity, which is a very important notion of clinical geriatrics. It characterizes the occurrence of several diseases or pathologic processes in one patient, which proceed often in an oligosymptomatic and atypical ways.

Of course, different involutive processes can be considered more or less as physiologic processes of older age, but they all can occur with individual accentuation and can be triggered by different random events at different moments of the life. In this context it becomes more and more difficult to define unequivocally the term of biologic age.[7] And finally, one has to accept that death itself is often a result of one or more diseases breaking out during the ultimate period of life (Figure 36-1).

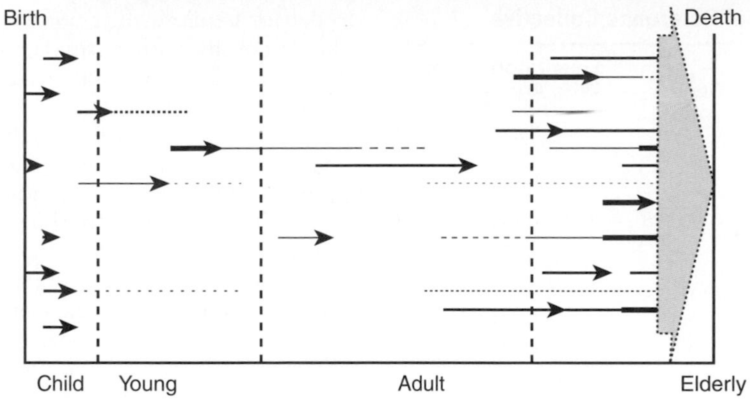

Figure 36-1. The course of life (horizontal axis) and randomly occurring diseases and traumas (→), and their aftereffects (—): At the end of life, they are contributing in an additive way to the final clinical status. *(From Lapin A, Böhmar F. Laboratory diagnosis and geriatrics: more than just reference intervals for elderly ... Wien Med Wochenschr 2005;155:1–2, :30–5.)*

In sum, when speaking about normality in geriatrics, one has to state that in age the perfectly healthy individual is a biologic rarity rather than the normal case.[8]

From screening to monitoring

The opinion that geriatric reference intervals can be estimated by large scale studies seems to be spurious even from a theoretical point of view. According to the publication of Harris,[9] the width of the reference interval is determined by three kinds of variation, which can be characterized by appropriated coefficients of variation C_V:

C_{VA} – **analytical variation** – which is due to the imprecision of an analytical method
C_{VB} – **biologic variation** – which concerns variations within one individual
C_{VC} – **interindividual variation** – which is due to differences between several individuals

The total variation (C_{VTOT}) results from the geometric sum of these three variations:

$$C_{VTOT} = \sqrt{C_{VA}^2 + C_{VB}^2 + C_{VC}^2}$$

In practice, it can be assumed that the analytical variation (C_{VA}) is almost negligible because of a high technical standard of the analytical method and that the total reference interval (C_{VTOT}) is determined by two other kinds of variation: the biologic (C_{VB}) and the interindividual (C_{VC}) one. Therefore two extreme constellations can be considered:

1. In the first case, the reference interval of the parameter is almost identical with the biologic variation (C_{VB}), which is nearly the same in all healthy individuals ($C_{VC} \rightarrow 0$) (this is, for example the case with glucose). Now, when in one particular individual a disease breaks out, the probability that the corresponding value will be shifted out of the reference range is increased. Thereafter, using such a test, the "pathology" would be detected early and the probability to obtain a result outside the reference interval will be increased by repeated measurement (Figure 36-2).
2. By contrast, another situation is given when the parameter shows narrow biologic variation ($C_{VB} \rightarrow 0$), but mean values (or medians) of this variation are different from individual to individual (this is, for example, the case with uric acid). In this case, the reference interval results preferentially from the distribution of mean values (medians) of such

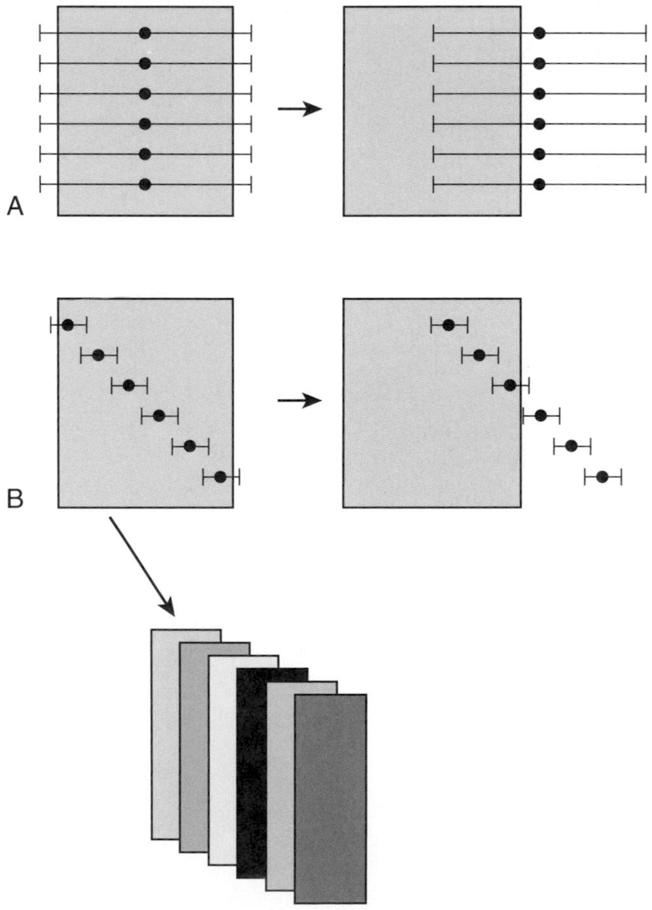

Figure 36-2. Influence of illness on two kinds of laboratory investigations (according to Harris EK 1974[9]). **A,** The width of the reference interval is determined by biologic factors (e.g., intraindividual variation [C_{VB}]). Due to an illness, all values are shifted out from the reference interval. **B,** The width of the reference interval is determined by intraindividual variation (C_{VC}), whereas intraindividual variation is negligible ($C_{VB} \rightarrow 0$). An illness would shift the values only in a segment of individuals of the considered collective. To improve the diagnostic relevance of this test, stratification (e.g., redefinition of the subreference intervals has to be performed.)

Table 36-1. Stratification of Reference Collective

Laboratory Parameter	Gender	Linear Correlation With Age
Creatinine	M	0.233
	W	0.041
Urea	M	0.196
	W	0.220
Chloride	M	0.168
	W	−0.050
AST	M	−0.088
	W	0.085
GGT	M	−0.004
	W	−0.007
Cholinesterase	M	−0.446
	W	−0.287
Albumin	M	−0.435
	W	−0.288
Iron	M	−0.243
	W	−0.178
RBC	M	−0.365
	W	−0.102
Hemoglobin	M	−0.363
	W	−0.122
Hematocrit	M	−0.323
	W	−0.126
MCV	M	0.164
	W	−0.047
CRP	M	0.160
	W	−0.050
Cholesterol	M	−0.446
	W	−0.090
Triglycerides	M	−0.191
	W	−0.070
Uric Acid	M	−0.104
	W	0.079
Glucose	M	0.087
	W	
TSH	M	−0.033
	W	0.019
FT4	M	0.101
	W	0.119
T3	M	−0.397
	W	−0.291

Abbreviations: *AST,* aspartate amino transferase; *CRP,* C-reactive protein; *FT4,* free thyroxin; *GGT,* gamma glutamyl transferase; *MCV,* mean cell volume of erythrocytes; *POCT,* point of case testing; *RBC,* red blood cell; T3, total triiodothyronine; *TSH,* thyroid stimulating hormone; *M,* men; *W,* women.

Modified from Lapin A, Böhmer F. What are "normal" laboratory parameters in elderly patients when examined on first admission to a geriatric hospital? A pilot study. Eur J Geriatr 2003;5(2):86–93.

individual variations (C_{VC}). Strictly speaking, such a test is less suitable for the diagnostic use, especially for early detection of a disease. A minor pathologic change, which occurs in one individual, would provide a shift merely out of his or her individual interval of biologic variation, but not necessarily outside the reference interval as determined for all considered individuals of the whole collective (C_{VTOT}). Evidently, such a pathologic change can remain undetected, even despite a repeated measurement.

To increase the diagnostic significance of such a test, it is necessary to perform stratification of the reference collective (e.g., to determine separately the reference intervals in different subpopulations, which in turn should be defined according to more specific criteria such as gender, age, other demographic parameters [Table 36-1]).

But for geriatrics it is not enough. The stratification also should consider other criteria, such as physical constitution, nutritional status, mobility, cognitive activity, predominant disease, and others.

By pushing stratification to the extreme, it becomes more and more difficult to find statistically relevant reference groups of individuals with the same characteristics. This is a major problem in establishing an age-dependent reference interval in geriatrics.[10,11]

On the other hand, the ultimate stratification may be when the actual result (measured value) is referred uniquely to the previous results of the same person. And here, parameters of narrow biologic variation but of wide interindividual differences are not useful for screening (e.g., to detect a new disease), but they are well suited for monitoring dynamic changes in the individual clinical status of a concrete patient. However, a basic condition for the realization of such "long-term monitoring" is the assessment of the long-time stability and quality of the applied laboratory tests. Unfortunately, especially in geriatrics, this can be sometimes put in question.

The monitoring in geriatrics

One of the actual trends of today's laboratory medicine is consolidation of laboratories, which is imposed by the improvement of economic efficiency of laboratory testing. Usually this means the concentration of medical laboratories in large semiindustrial diagnostic institutions.[12]

The outsourcing of laboratory medicine from clinical institutions entails a depersonalization of the communication between clinicians and laboratory specialists.[13,14] Consequently, certain aspects which have been theoretically known to affect the diagnostic significance of laboratory testing gain an unexpected actuality. One of these concerns the preanalytics.

Due to reduced physiologic reserves, many elderly patients who show larger biologic variation have to be considered for a number of laboratory parameters. Such preanalytical effects include orthostatic effects (especially in patients with edema), effects related to impaired mobility and/or nutritional status, and seasonal influences.[15] Moreover, poor venous status of some elderly patients can cause difficulties in the phlebotomy and blood collection, which is then responsible for hemolytic sera and inadequately small sample volume for an optimal analytical process.

The fact that the number of samples provided by geriatric practitioners is far inferior to those of an acute wards' can induce negligence and sloppiness resulting in the bad habit that geriatric samples are treated with less interest and without priority. Well known is the situation when, in a nursing home, the lab courier is missed and collected samples have to be left for the next day or for the later analysis batch. The increased turnaround time is always disadvantageous. For the stability of analytes*,[15] and for the actuality of diagnostic information that has be submitted to the clinician.

But the consolidation of laboratory medicine has induced another trend, which can be characterized as point-of-care testing (POCT). Using small testing devices mostly based on dry-chemistry principle, analyses can be performed close to the patient and therefore in a shorter and easier manner

*Analyte: substance, enzymatic activity, or other subject of chemical analysis.

Table 36-2. Examples of Possible Alteration of Clinical Significance of Some Laboratory Parameters When Used in Geriatrics

	Usual Significance in Adults	Possible Alternative Significance in Elderly
BUN	Renal insufficiency	Acute catabolism (often reversible)*
Albumin	Renal or hepatic insufficiency	Biologic age,† malnutrition, frailty
Cholesterol	Risk of atherosclerosis (high cholesterol)	Malnutrition,‡ marker of fatal prognosis§ (low cholesterol)
Gamma-GT	Alcoholism, cholestasis, hepatitis	Liver congestion (e.g., by heart insufficiency)
Amylase	Pancreatitis	Parotitis (often during summer season); macroamylase
LDH	Parenchymal damages, hemolysis	Phlebotomy problem
Total protein (normal)	Chronic inflammation	Exsiccation, myeloma
CRP	Inflammation, acute phase	Infection, necrosis (sometimes unique conclusive marker)
ESR	Chronic inflammation	Occult neoplasm
PTT	Heparin, hemophilia	Lupus inhibitor
Haemoglobin	Bleeding	Anemia of the elderly, myelodysplastic syndrome
MCV (normal)	Alcohol abuse	Vitamin B_{12} or folate deficiency

*For example, after an accidental episode of acute dehydration.
†Campion EW, deLabry LO, Glynn RJ. The effect of age on serum albumin in healthy males: report from the normative aging study. J Gerontol 1988;433:M18–M20.
‡Goichot B, Schlienger JL, Grunenberger F, et al. Low cholesterol concentrations in free-living elderly subjects: relations with dietary intake and nutritional status. Am J Clin Nutr 1995;62:547–53.
§Rudman D, Mattson DE, Nagraj HS, et al. Prognostic significance of serum cholesterol in nursing home men. JPEN 1998:12:155–8.

than by using a distant laboratory.[16] For geriatrics, the POCT is of particular interest, not the least because of the growing scope of available tests. Although the use of POCT has become a generally accepted procedure, some disadvantages such as calibration, documentation, and especially uncontrolled performance by untrained personnel represents a subject of many discussions in different meetings of the laboratory medicine.

Nevertheless, a serious problem can arise when laboratory data, provided by different sources (e.g., diagnostic institutions and by different POCT-devices), are clinically evaluated in the same patient's history.[17] Such a situation is quite frequent in geriatrics since aged patients can be treated within a short period by several medical providers: In a doctor's office, in a nursing home as a resident, and in a hospital as an emergency patient.

Medical significance of laboratory results in the aged

Finally there is the issue of medical significance of laboratory analyses in the context of clinical geriatrics. This can be different from adult medicine and not only in physiologic parameters, but also in demographic changes, life expectancy, and clinical consequences (Table 36-2).

An example for change in diagnostic significance in the course of life can be seen in the case of cholesterol (Figure 36-3). Usually the mean level of cholesterol in serum correlates with cardiovascular risk and increases with the age. However, from the sixth decade, this increase stops and the cholesterol level begins to decrease. This behavior is due to successive demographic change of the cohort. Individuals, which at their adult age revealed a high level of cholesterol, become now at the older age victims of their own increased risk being now continuously excluded from the higher-age cohort as a result of mortality.[18] At the same time, cholesterol also becomes a marker for nutritional status: its decrease correlates with malnutrition.[19] And finally, on the end of this age-dependent correlation, the sudden decrease of the cholesterol level can indicate a worsening life expectancy prognosis.[20]

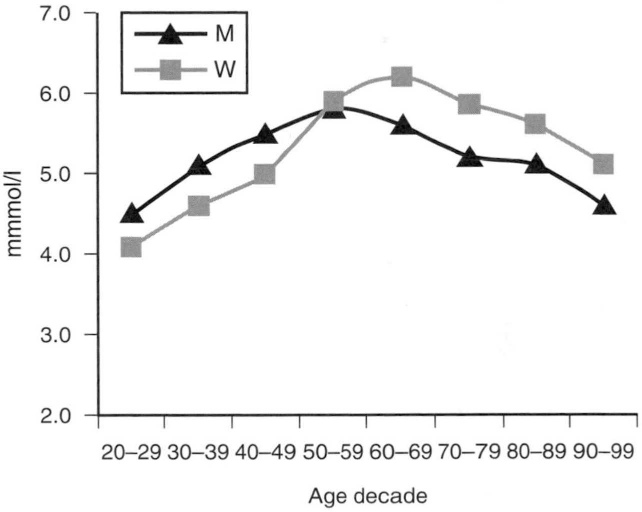

Figure 36-3. Age-dependent course of cholesterol (according to the author's data). *(From Lapin A, Böhmer F. Laboratory diagnosis and geriatrics: more than just reference intervals for elderly.... Wien Med Wochenschr 2005;155:1–2, 30–5.)*

Due to the symptomatic, supportive and palliative therapy, which is in geriatrics more important than in adult medicine, the geriatrician is sometimes forced to undergo therapeutic compromises; for example, using corticosteroids in patients with diabetes mellitus. In this situation, to optimize the individual therapeutic strategy, it is not enough to monitor the clinical status; more important can be the estimation of the still remaining functional capacity of different organs and systems. For example, it is useful to monitor renal function by measuring serum creatinine, but more conclusive can be to estimate the creatinine clearance to know which proportion of renal functional reserve remains intact. In other words, parameters, which enable the estimation of still remaining functional capacity and/or which provide prognostic information, are of particular importance for geriatrics. A good example of such parameters is natriuretic peptide (known as BNP), whose blood level provides quantitative information about the degree of cardiac insufficiency in sense of congestive heart failure.

Another important feature of geriatrics is the frequent presence of multimorbidity. In this context, Fairweather and Campbell demonstrate, that in the elderly, "failing to make diagnosis when the disease is present or making a diagnosis when a disease is not present is likely to occur twice as often as in younger patients."[20] In the same way, an actual autopsy study showed that the accuracy rate of the clinical diagnosis of the immediate cause of death is no higher than roughly 50%.[21]

In this sense it is meaningful to differentiate between multipathology and multietiology. Since multipathology can be seen as a complex of several impairments of the organism, the term of multietiology is a more complicated one. It characterizes several dynamic pathologic processes, often convoluted in each other. Often, pathologic conditions such as infections, cardiovascular diseases, acute abdomen, hyperthyroidism, and depression occur in the elderly in an atypical and nonspecific way and with correspondingly atypical symptoms, physical findings, and laboratory results.[22] But more difficult can be the adequate estimation of multiple etiological factors that are contributing to the current status of the patient. Often due to the propensity to think in terms of a single disease, it can be difficult for the clinician to decide which of the actual factors are important and will benefit the patient if treated. At the same time, the underestimation of multietiology together with the progressive decline of the cognitive and physical status of the patient can aggravate the problem of the degradation of the diagnostic information.[23] However, especially in view of the prognosis of the patient, there can be a growing discrepancy between the necessity of a diagnostic and therapeutic intervention and the need for conservation patient care into appropriate dignity. In this case, even laboratory medicine faces ethical limits.

CONCLUSION

With the growing of the elderly population in industrialized countries, the role of geriatric medicine will grow steadily. This in turn will create corresponding requirements for better efficiency in laboratory diagnoses. More than elsewhere in medicine, in geriatrics one has to deal with individuals rather than with collectives, and it can be expected that geriatric laboratory medicine will be subjected to a change of paradigms. Not only the statistically revealed evidence, as obtained from studies of a large number of individuals, but also the consideration of the individual patient, with his or her clinical individuality, status, predispositions, physiologic reserves, and prognosis, will need another, probably an alternative insight. It will not be sufficient to consider health solely from the deterministic point of view, observing differences between physiology and pathology of laboratory findings, but likewise it will be important to consider the clinical individuality as a relative risk in the dimension of time for the rest of the patient's life.[24]

From the practical point of view, it would be necessary to pay more attention to limits of the diagnostic significance of laboratory testing of the elderly. This should be considered especially for education programs of specialists in geriatric medicine. Research in geriatrics should be concentrated on new diagnostic parameters that would enable a better estimation of the clinical risk to the patients.

KEY POINTS

Laboratory Medicine in Geriatrics

- **Normality in geriatrics:** The perfectly healthy individual is a biologic rarity rather than the normal case. In geriatrics, it is a problem to postulate generally applicable references.[1]
- **Multimorbidity:** By approaching the end of life, the sum of aftereffects of previous diseases and the probability of manifestation of predisposed diseases increases. The individuality of a person increases by his or her life itinerary.
- **To keep the best possible quality of life** requires monitoring of individual clinical status, rather than screening for potentially occurring diseases, with the aim of a complete cure.
- **Laboratory parameters** that provide information about still available physiologic reserves are especially valuable. Clinical interpretation of some laboratory tests can be modified by life expectancy of the patient.
- **Laboratory medicine in geriatrics** should be performed with long-time quality assessment, professional logistics, and with special consideration of preanalytics.

[1]other terms used more or less correctly for the same purpose: reference range, normal values

For a complete list of references, please visit online only at www.expertconsult.com

CHAPTFR 37

Social Assessment of Geriatric Patients

Rosalie A. Kane

Social functioning is a broad concept, embracing all human relationships and activities. Social functioning therefore is multidimensional and cannot be measured meaningfully in a single scale. Physicians caring for older people will need routinely to assess at least some aspects of the social functioning of their patients. In some instances, physicians will also need to understand and use assessments done by the social worker on his or her own hospital teams, by local authority social workers (in the United Kingdom), or by case managers in community long-term care programs (in the United States). For these purposes, it is useful to consider the nature of available assessment technology, the particular aspects of social functioning that should be assessed, and the usefulness of the information derived for the actual planning of care.

SOCIAL ASSESSMENT AS PART OF COMPREHENSIVE ASSESSMENT

Particularly in the United States, but also in other developed countries, frail elderly persons often receive their first general, multidimensional assessment from a social worker or nurse who is defined as a case manager or care coordinator.[1–2] Such assessments are typically performed in the patient's own home, but they may also be performed in the hospital before the patient's discharge. The assessor uses a structured information-gathering schedule (often contained in a rather long booklet) to pose questions directly to the older person or (if the older person is incapable of participating) to a surrogate informant. Such assessments can take an hour or more to complete. They do not involve a physical examination or laboratory tests.

Multidimensional assessment used by case managers will typically include the following components:

- Factual information about the older person's marital status, household composition, housing situation, and income.
- Assessment of physical health based on some combination of the following checklist: symptoms; diseases the respondent believes he or she has; reports of overall use of hospitals, physicians, and other health care; reports of days sick; reports of medications used; summary of deficits in hearing, vision, speech, and dentition; and a self-reported estimate of the patient's health.
- Assessment of the ability to perform basic activities of daily living using a standardized scale. Such scales, at a minimum, measure independence in bathing, dressing, toileting, transferring out of bed or chair, and feeding, but may also include information about mobility, hand control, continence, and endurance.
- Ability to perform more complex social skills associated with independent living, sometimes called IADL (instrumental activities of daily living). Items that may or may not be scored on such a scale include cooking, cleaning, doing laundry, shopping, using transportation, communicating by telephone, managing money, and taking medications.
- Direct screening for cognitive impairment (to determine whether the respondent is reliable).
- Direct assessment of depressive affect and other possible psychological disturbances.
- Assessment of the social functioning of the older person in terms of the range of activities and relationships that the person pursues, the help available to or used by him or her, the presence of a confidante, and perhaps the subjective satisfaction of the older person with social interactions.
- Enumeration of the help the older person is receiving from family members and friends, from social programs, and from privately paid helpers directly employed by the older person and family.

Such batteries of questions are common in the United States, where they are in wide use in public programs. Many are derived from an assessment protocol developed at the Older Americans Research and Service (OARS) program at Duke University, commonly called the OARS methodology,[3] which has had extensive work done on its psychometric properties[4] and which has been extensively adapted. Another multidimensional tool that has had substantial work is the CARE (Comprehensive Assessment and Referral Evaluation) interview, developed by Gurland et al[5] for a collaborative study done in the United States and the United Kingdom and later refined by the development of scales.[5–9] But the protocols in actual use for case management programs vary enormously in the way they combine questions and scales.

Some general points can be made about these multidimensional assessment tools and their use by social workers and case managers with geriatric patients.

DESCRIPTIVE OVERVIEW

The batteries usually attempt a descriptive overview of physical and psychiatric functioning, but make no claims to diagnostic capability. Rather, in the context of an overall social assessment, the questions on physical and psychological health are designed to point out when fuller geriatric or psychogeriatric assessments should be sought. Thus the presence of questions about health status, health use, and medications are designed not to encroach on physicians' diagnostic prerogatives, but to identify persons needing medical attention and to take medical conditions into account in planning care.

SCORES

Scores may be derived for various subsections of the assessment, but the assessments seldom can generate an overall well-being score that has clinical significance.

COMPREHENSIVE ASSESSMENT PROTOCOLS

These vary in the extent to which the information is based on queries made directly to the older person versus judgments of the assessor on the enumerated items. Unless careful instruction and training accompanies the assessment instrument, it is likely that the resultant information will not distinguish well between the older person's responses and the assessor's judgments.

FUNCTIONAL ABILITIES

These are at the heart of the assessment, but are difficult to standardize and interpret. Although substantial agreement has been achieved on items for inclusion on ADL and IADL scales, variations occur in detail and approach to measurement. Sometimes, for example, the information about functioning is based on observation and sometimes on the older person's report. Sometimes the individuals are queried about what activities they are able to perform, and sometimes about activities they actually do perform. Sometimes the score is based on demonstration under test conditions, and sometimes professionals rate performance based on their observations. Widely varying time frames may be used (e.g., the last few weeks, the last few months, right now). There is also variation in the standard for adequate performance and the extent to which pain and discomfort of the older person, or elapsed time to complete a task, are taken into account. Recent work has been done to combine ADL and IADL items in a general scale. Rather than using the conventional but arbitrary system of according equal points for each item, Finch et al[10] did empirical work to develop a scale where items are weighted according to their overall importance in functional capacity.

SERVICE PROVISION

When used by case managers or social workers, the assessment protocol is meant to inform decisions about the services that should be arranged and the priority the particular older person's needs should get. However, there is seldom a clear set of rules to guide the assessor in translating the information from the assessment into guidelines for a service plan. Glass shows the intimate relationship between social factors and ADL functioning.[11] Taking advantage of a data set where respondents were asked about functioning in terms both of what they thought they could do and what they did do, he identified "underachievers" who failed to perform to their perceived capacity and, oddly enough, "overachievers" who claimed to do what they believed they were incapable of doing. Further inspection showed remarkable resourcefulness and creativity among the overachievers, and a variety of social and psychological factors (lack of wish to do the function, lack of transportation, lack of opportunity, lack of money, family factors) among the underachievers.[11]

ASPECTS OF SOCIAL FUNCTIONING

The multidimensional, comprehensive batteries described above are composed of constituent parts, designed to measure various aspects of functioning. The groundwork for measuring those dimensions is often laid in earlier research with the particular set of questions or scales. Let us now consider what aspects of social functioning should be measured.

All behavior of human beings might be termed social. But many aspects of social functioning hardly need be measured in detail for geriatric care. In a multivolume review of measures pertaining to old people, Mangen and Peterson[12] devote chapters to measurement of dimensions such as religiosity, interspousal relationships, and filial relationships. Relevant social dimensions for geriatric care constitute a shorter list, which has been summarized in a number of review works.[13,14] Suggested below is the information on social functioning that is needed, excluding health use and basic performance of ADL, which are important components but are covered elsewhere in this volume. Note, however, that ADL and IADL performance will be enhanced or impeded by social factors, and, conversely, social factors can influence the repercussions of ADL or IADL impairment. To deal with the latter, Allen and Mor[15] elaborated on functional measures by incorporating follow-up questions designed to assess any deleterious consequences of insufficient help (e.g., "Have there been times in the past month when you were not able to bathe as often as you would have liked because no one was available to help you?" or "Have there been times in the past month when you were unable to eat when you were hungry because no one was available to help you?"). They refer to these as indices of unmet need.

First, the ability to perform social roles, sometimes called social skills, is relevant. For younger people, such measures usually encompass their performance as employees, family members, and citizens.[16] For older people, perhaps shortsightedly, the measurement of role performance is usually limited to ability to perform the so-called instrumental ADL (cooking, cleaning, laundry), which are, in turn, related to household management and independent living.

Second, information about social relationships (their frequency, context, and quality), social activities (again their frequency, nature, and quality), social resources (including income, housing, and environmental conditions) is useful to geriatric providers. Third, social support is a salient concept to examine; it may include the help the patient is receiving and can expect to continue to receive from others in the environment, and the degree to which this help is perceived as supportive. Fourth, subjective social well-being can be measured more generally.

A fifth area of social function—family burden or family stress—has come into prominence in the last decade.[17] Although highly relevant to geriatric care, this measure pertains to family caregivers rather than to the older person receiving the care. The idea is that an understanding of the type and degree of burden that caregiving creates for the relative primarily responsible will help determine whether the arrangement is realistic, humane, and fair, and the extent to which relief for the family member is necessary.

A sixth emerging area concerns personal autonomy, values, and preferences. In recent years, there has been much interest in personal autonomy and values of older persons receiving long-term care.[18] This is fueled by growing social science literature that suggests that older people who perceive that they have lost control and choice over their lives experience adverse health outcomes, including depression, increased morbidity, and even increased mortality.[19–21] Some attempts have been made to estimate a measure of autonomy, although these measures are not ordinarily incorporated into everyday clinical practice. A related effort entails assessing the values and preferences that may be important to geriatric patients.[22]

Finally, substantial work has been done to seek a satisfactory approach to assessing the older person's satisfaction with the care and help received. Before briefly discussing each of these areas, some general comments about the problems of measuring social functioning are warranted.

Problems in assessing social functioning

First, social concepts such as social isolation, social support, or social well-being are value-laden abstract constructs, subject to interpretation. Thus several scales containing different items may purport to measure the same thing, whereas scales that seem to be similar in content carry different labels.[12] It is important not to be deceived by the name of the scale, but to examine its contents.

Second, most social variables have both an objective and a subjective component. For example, one can measure social support by quantifying the support network and its activities, or by asking whether the older people view themselves as supported in various ways. Similarly, one can examine the burden of caregivers by quantifying their objective tasks with the patient and their other obligations, or one can measure the extent to which they feel burdened. Both approaches may be important.

Third, adequate social functioning can be achieved through diverse patterns. One seldom finds clear norms for interpreting the results of social information. A person who states that he or she has 10 friends is not necessarily twice as well befriended as a person with five, nor can one say that a person who spends much time playing cards is better off than one who spends the same amount of time fishing. Growing out of this observation are two important points in interpreting social information: (1) a change in social functioning may be as important as the actual value on a scale; and (2) information about adequate thresholds of functioning is needed. Regarding the latter, the objective of social measurements for geriatric caregivers is not to achieve a perfectly scaled measure of a social property such as isolation or social support; rather, it is to determine whether these dimensions have fallen below some threshold that means that the patient is at risk.

Fourth, social role expectations for the elderly are unclear at best and vary according to ethnic groups and over time. Nobody seems to know what constitutes adequate role performance for a retiree, a grandparent, or an elderly widow or widower, and establishing these norms is more complicated because of their likely sensitivity to cultural differences.

Finally, much social functioning involves people in interaction with others. They fill social roles, cope with stress, receive help from family members, and so on. How well a particular older person functions socially is, in part, dependent on the behavior of others, which complicates the assessment process. Glass et al[23] have pioneered in expanding the range of social functioning examined in older people. In studies underway at Yale and later at Harvard, the team has attempted to develop better measures of social functioning related to productive aging in social and economic roles, incorporating housework, yard work, childcare, and other family roles, paid work, and volunteer work.

Social relationships, activities, and resources

The aggregated social relationships of a client, viewed descriptively, are sometimes called the social network. "Social network" refers to the web of social relationships and contacts that an individual may have. Although difficult because of the amount of data collection needed, objective properties of social networks can be described using terms such as size (how many people are in the network), density (the number of people who know each other in the network), homogeneity (similarity of network members on various characteristics), multiplexity (the number of different types of interactions exchanged), and reciprocity (the balance or imbalance between perception of giving and receiving support).[24] Researchers point out that "social network" is a static concept referring to relationships across the life span; the term "social convoy" has been suggested as a more dynamic concept.[25] Measures in this area have been extensively reviewed by Levin.[26]

Although social networks have properties—such as size, density, frequency, and intensity of contact, permeability, and directionality[24–29]—from the viewpoint of geriatric care, the large number of properties that can be elaborated upon for social research can be reduced to an interest in the frequency and nature of the patient's human contacts in the course of a day, week, or month. One approach, often incorporated into assessment, involves querying the patient about the frequency of contacts in person, by telephone, or by mail by categories of people (adult children, other relatives, friends, others), using a metric such as "frequently, occasionally, seldom, or never," or attempting more exact quantification (less than once a week, and so on). Such questions are sometimes followed up by asking the person whether he or she has contact with these people more than desired, about the right amount, or less than desired. The OARS methodology, a multidimensional assessment tool described earlier,[5] contains an often-used measure of social contacts.

Some efforts have been made to combine social contacts and social activities in brief social network scales, designed to predict the individual's well-being and need for service. The Berkman Social Network Scale,[30] developed in a general population, and the Lubben Social Network Scale,[31] developed for the elderly, are examples. Typically, marital status, membership in formal groups, and religious participation are included with other brief measures of social contact to form a short scale.

To assess social resources, well-planned, consistently asked questions are better than scales. Each assessment of social functioning does well to contain straightforward questions about household income and assets, and income and assets of the older person with the disability. It is also important to determine the composition of the household and the nature and adequacy of the housing. In some social contexts, access to a car and transportation is also an important social resource. Depending on the political context, information about insurance coverage, veteran status, and specific disability status may provide a key to resources that could be available for the person. Other information that is important in developing a plan and coming to know the individual includes information about the individual's occupation or former occupation, and interests; typically such items are overlooked.

Social support

A description of the social network does not automatically translate into an understanding of how well the patient's needs are met, nor does it permit a prediction of how well the needs may continue to be met in the future. Being enmeshed in a large network of family and friends may, depending on the network, be reassuring or stressful, helpful or harmful, informative or misleading. Social support is the positive tangible and intangible assistance drawn from the social network.[32] A social network or convoy has multiple functions, which also can be measured.[26,27] These include giving informational support, such as facts and advice; affective support, such as comfort, encouragement, and love; social support and stimulation, such as companionship; and tangible help, such as money or physical assistance. It is obvious that the geriatric team has an interest in knowing whether a given patient has a network that can or does provide such support. The social network is the potential vehicle for social support, but may be associated with negative and positive effects. Social scientists have studied the complex stress process that involves interaction of life events, chronic life strains, self-concepts, coping skills, and social supporters.[33]

If the geriatric patient already has tangible needs for physical help from others, one measure of social support is a straightforward tabulation of the kinds of help received and their frequency. Assessment tools usually attempt, however, to go beyond this simple count to an estimation of the likelihood that the help can continue into the future, and the prospects for a replacement, if the person giving most of the help cannot continue. Research suggests that often the patient's social support in terms of physical help depends on one person whose own health may be fragile, or who cannot continue indefinitely because of competing demands.[34] In such cases, planning can begin to broaden the base of social support. In other instances, additional relatives and friends are available to help, but the primary family caregiver assumes that nobody else is capable or willing. If the patient has not previously needed physical help, then an estimation of the likelihood of this help is needed. A few key questions can assist in making this prediction; for example: "If necessary, is there someone who could come and help you during the day?" or "Is there someone who could stay overnight with you if necessary?" Social support measures are also summarized in Levin's recent review.[26]

Subjective well-being

An overall measure of the patient's well-being is sometimes sought in a comprehensive assessment tool. Such measures are also often used to evaluate the worth of long-term care programs.[35,36] The two most frequently used measures in this regard are Lawton's Philadelphia Geriatric Center Morale Scale[37] and the Life Satisfaction Index (LSI-A) of Neugarten, Havighurst, and Tobin.[38,39] Both these scales are relatively brief and simple to administer, both have developed an extensive use history, and both measure elements of life satisfaction by asking clients to consider the extent to which their expectations in life were met. At the same time, both also measure aspects of existential well-being or happiness.

Although these two scales are often used for program evaluation, it is unclear how much these measures should change as a result of a worthwhile program. For example, a meal program may be performing an important and appreciated function, and yet the answer to the question "Overall, have I achieved most of my goals in life?" would remain the same. In general, it seems best to measure satisfaction with a program directly, through questions that specifically ask about satisfaction with various elements of the program itself.[13]

Caregiver burden

In both the United States and in Europe, social services authorities for the elderly recognize that their programs would be inadequate to meet the needs for care were it not for the volunteer efforts of family members. Indeed, unpaid family members give most of the personal care and housekeeping help that is received by community-dwelling older people. In the United States, almost 80% of in-home services for elderly people are given by family members. It has become a widespread program principle that social services should supplement and enhance family care, when appropriate, but should not replace it.

Given this situation, it becomes important to assess the well-being of family caregivers to estimate (1) how long such care may be expected to continue, and (2) legitimate needs for relief. Somewhat unfortunately because of its negative connotations, this area of measurement is often called measurement of "family burden." Many scales have been developed in the last decade to assess family caregiver burden.[40–45] These scales are often themselves multidimensional (including, for example, physical burden, emotional burden, social burden, and financial burden), and they may concentrate on subjective burden or objective burden, or both. Other scales designed especially to examine the stress-engendering aspects of family care for persons with dementia specifically measure the presence and frequency of a range of troublesome behavior. Pearlin et al[46] have contributed a careful conceptual model of the stress process related to family caregiving, complete with brief measures of the relevant aspects of the phenomenon (including problematic behavior, overload, relational deprivation, family conflict, job-caregiving conflict, economic strain, role captivity, loss of self, caregiving competence, personal gain, management of situation, management of meaning, and management of distress). This series of measures is designed for research rather than clinical practice, yet it reminds us that the concept of caregiver burden is by no means straightforward. In general, it has been well documented that objective needs of the older person and objectively defined tasks occasion varying degrees of burden. The Caregiving Hassles Scale[47] can be used to measure the extent to which care of an elderly relative causes small daily tribulations or, in the vernacular, "hassles." Some authorities believe that the daily hassles produce more stress than dramatic life crises. Less attention has been given to the positive aspects of caregiving, sometimes called "uplifts," though these, too, have been measured and studied.[48]

The stress or burden of family caregivers, balanced against positive aspects of the role, should be part of a comprehensive assessment of an older person. However, the social worker or case manager must then be prepared to interpret and use the information to decide when and how much relief should be offered to family members. It is important also to understand the information collected according to the relationship of the family caregiver to the patient (spouse, adult offspring, other relative) and the competing obligations of that family caregiver (which could include employment, care of younger children, care of another disabled or elderly relative, or even dealing with their own failing strength).

In addition to applying specific measures that generate scores, clinical teams can benefit by consulting a practical reference work by Lustbader and Hooyman,[49] which lists sets of assessment questions that are useful for specific caregiving situations. For example, when a spouse is a caregiver, they suggest that one ask about the length of the marriage before the illness; the health of the caregiving spouse; the predisability marital patterns; the timing of onset relative to the couple's retirement plans; the impact of the illness on the couple's financial resources; the impact on their sexual functioning; and the availability of backup help from other family and friends. If siblings are sharing caregiving, the assessment might include these questions: Is concern about a potential inheritance straining sibling relationships? Is there financial disparity among siblings? Is there a natural leader, a parental favorite? Is there a health care professional among them? Are there stepsiblings among them? What have been the adult siblings relationships to each other? And what obligations must each sibling meet in addition to parental care?

Personal autonomy, preferences, and values

In the last decade in the United States, there has been an attempt to record older people's preferences regarding life-sustaining medical treatment.[50–53] Such information is desired partly for legal reasons, to prevent liability, and partly to guide clinicians in giving good care. If taken seriously, however, assessment of such preferences is notoriously difficult. The validity of the data depends on whether accurate information has been adequately disclosed to the respondent and has been understood by the respondent. Some work has been undertaken to construct and study such measures, though in practice many assessment batteries merely contain a notation of the older person's preference for such services as cardiopulmonary resuscitation, artificial hydration, or respirators, and their preferences about who they want to act in their stead if they become temporarily or permanently unable to make decisions without any assurance that the questions were asked or comprehended in any consistent way.

Others have sought to assess values of geriatric patients directly, a pursuit that is fraught with conceptual and methodological difficulties.[54] Using a tool that is meant to be an exercise in self-discovery rather than precise measurement, Gibson, a philosopher, and her colleagues[55,56] developed a values history, which they recommend for distribution to clients to complete at their leisure and with discussion among families. At the other extreme, Doukas and McCullough[57] have developed an approach that uses a few true-false questions to tap into values about risk, life and death, and spirituality.

Work has been done to assess systematically the ordinary values and preferences of older people that might be related to their care. Although not amenable to generating an overall scale, it is feasible to incorporate a list of topics that the patient rates in terms of importance, providing descriptive detail. Using a stem that relates the topic to care that they might need now or in the future, the instrument developed asks the person to rate the importance of the following: performing everyday routines in a particular way; participating in certain activities at home or away from home; personal privacy; specific events or milestones being anticipated or projects being completed; freedom from pain; taking risks as opposed to being protected but less free; involving or not involving family in their care; qualities desired in a helper; and qualities desired in a place to live. Older clients were willing to respond to such questions, revealing differences in the importance these issues hold and in the content of what they deemed important. However, clinicians were often somewhat reluctant to enter into such discussions, partly because of the time involved (about 20 minutes) and partly because of a sense of being intrusive or being unable to act on the preferences expressed.[22,58]

Although considerable hubris is involved in attempting to assess values and preferences, and assessors doing so must guard against believing that they have encapsulated the essence of another human being in a few simple items, it seems equally improper to ignore this arena. In fact, systematic efforts to assess the patient's values and preferences are likely to restructure the encounter between social workers and geriatric patients in important ways. Moreover, insights into the values and preferences of the older persons served may be the best safeguard against inappropriate or paternalistic decision making about their lives.

Satisfaction

Although the technical quality of care procedures may be assessed by professionals using objective criteria, increasing emphasis has been given to seeking a reliable way to elicit the patient's perspective, particularly with reference to home help and personal assistance. It is argued that the intimacy of care and its close connections to daily life requires that professionals have a way of determining how patients view that care. Indeed, evidence suggests that older people are often reluctant to accept the help suggested, and speculation has been that this reaction is related to dislike of the way services are offered. Geron[59,60] conducted focus groups with older home care clientele from varying ethnic backgrounds to identify the elements of quality important to consumers. With great consistency across ethnicity, older people identified the following elements of good care: humaneness (helpers who were likable, pleasant, courteous, caring), competence, dependability, continuity (i.e., if the previous two criteria were met, consumers preferred consistency rather than change), adequacy in terms of amount of help, and choice in the type and timing of help received. They then developed and tested a satisfaction tool. It is noteworthy, however, that such tools are quite specific to the service context.

Satisfaction has come to be seen as a measure of experience mediated by expectations. As such, it is bedeviled by the propensity of people to adjust their expectations downwards or to hold low expectations in the first place. Measurement of satisfaction is also rendered technically difficult if those whose reports are sought are dependent on the services or, worse, feel intimidated—the latter being a possibility for those living in group residential settings. Nonetheless, substantial progress has been made in measuring satisfaction.[61]

Social functioning of people with dementia

A large number of scales have been developed for rating or assessing the social functioning of persons with dementia in terms of presence of appropriate behavior and absence of behaviors considered disruptive.[62,63] Initially these instruments relied on ratings by professional caregivers or family caregivers. More recently, observational and even physiologic tools have been used to measure social stress and social well-being on the part of those who cannot communicate.[64] In the late 1990s, several tools were developed and tested that depend on self-report from the person with dementia. Notably Brod et al[65] developed a short set of Likert type of quality of life ratings called the DqoL, and Logsdon et al[66] developed an even shorter set of 13 dichotomous questions for self-report of quality of life. Both these tools have reported good reliability. Teri and Logsdon[67] developed the Pleasant Events Schedule-AD, which is used either with the person with dementia or a proxy observer, to zero in on the existential experience of the person with dementia.

An emerging concern is the discordance found between the rating of the older person and that of a family or staff proxy when paired ratings are available. This has called proxy ratings into question without presenting any substitute to measure social well-being in those persons whose dementia is too advanced for self-report. It would seem prudent to use proxies most when highly objective information about social functioning is sought, and to provide clear definitions of the behavior being observed, an approach taken in the multidimensional observational scale for older adults (MOSES).[68]

Social assessment within congregate group settings

Assessments of social functioning and social well-being within the context of a nursing home or board-and-care home need to take into account the nature of the setting. Although elaborate approaches to examine how the individual fits into the community have been made for research purposes,[69] this area of assessment is in its infancy in terms of scale development to be applied to residents. Sometimes this work is lumped with satisfaction measures that are tailored to specific residential programs. A large ongoing project funded by the U.S. Department of Health and Human Services concentrates on measuring quality-of-life outcomes for nursing home residents and has developed short scales to tap 11 dimensions of quality of life: meaningful activity, individuality, dignity, privacy, enjoyment, relationships, comfort, functional competence, spiritual well-being, sense of security and order, and autonomy.[70] These measures largely deal with social as opposed to physical functioning, and choice or systematic attention, although elaborate measures of environmental climates have been made for research purposes.

EMERGING AREAS OF SOCIAL ASSESSMENT

Other areas of social assessment are amenable to measurement and may be important in specific situations, but measurement approaches are just evolving. Also some new themes are getting attention. The following are some examples:

- Measures of housing environments and housing satisfaction. This is an underdeveloped arena.[71] Some work has recently been done to separate factors related to assisted living environments (often called "housing with services"). One such study identified personal care services, general services, apartment, control/choice, and housekeeping/dining as separate constructs.[72]
- Assessment of formal support in the form of help from personnel from health care and social service organizations. Such a measure of assistance may or may not be thought of as part of the social assessment; but, however classified, it is necessary. It is often helpful to divide "formal care" into types of tasks: nursing tasks, such as help with medicines or procedures; personal care, such as help with bathing, toileting, eating, and transferring; housekeeping tasks, such as laundry, cooking, cleaning; help with transportation; help with business matters; and help with arranging for services, such as case management. Assessments usually develop indicators of frequency (days/visits per month, week, or day) and intensity (total hours of help of each type in a given period).
- Assessment of the specific tasks performed by family caregivers. Some assessment tools develop parallel questions to use in inquiring about the type of tasks and the frequency and intensity provided by both formal and informal sources. It is only by comparing formal and informal help received with needs for assistance that an estimation of unmet need is developed. Typically, care plans developed by social workers are designed to meet unmet needs.
- Assessing social well-being across cultures. Attention is now being given in general to the extent to which assessments of elderly people cross cultural lines. Cultural relativity would be particularly important for

KEY POINTS
Social Assessment

- Social functioning is a multidimensional construct that cannot be well measured in a single scale.
- Relevant domains of social functioning with available measures include: ability to perform social roles; social relationships; social support; family caregiver well-being; autonomy; values and preferences; and satisfaction.
- Measurement strategies for social functioning must take into account that most domains have an objective and subjective component; that normative social role definitions in old age are lacking; that there appear to be multiple ways to achieve satisfactory social functioning; and that research is needed to establish thresholds with clinical significance.
- Advances have been made in conceptualizing quality of life for persons with dementia and for eliciting reliable direct responses from those with substantial cognitive impairment. Observational approaches have been developed for those who cannot be interviewed.
- Measures of social well-being need to be modified or augmented for people who live in congregate group settings to receive care.
- Topics highlighted for developmental work include: housing environments and housing satisfaction; assessment of help from paid individuals and organizations; the type and intensity of care activities performed by family caregivers; and cross-cultural measures of social functioning.

making normative judgments about social well-being. This topic was flagged in an issue of the *Journal of Mental Health and Aging*, where both methodological and content considerations are reviewed.[72]

ASSEMBLING THE ASSESSMENT PROTOCOL

As this chapter has suggested, assessment of social functioning can be as detailed as the geriatric team desires, touching on many or few dimensions of social functioning. The assessment may also vary in its mix of scales, single items, clinical ratings, and reliance on open-ended, unstructured approaches. This chapter recommends a consistent and standardized approach to assessing aspects of social functioning. Commitment to consistency and routine approaches is probably more important than which particular instrument is selected. Initial parsimony is also suggested, followed by more detailed assessment as necessary. It is highly likely that there will be an inverse relationship between the amount of information collected and the reliability and validity of the assessment interview.

A social worker is highly accepted as a member of a geriatric team. However, the importance of social information—whether collected specifically by a social worker or collected by a generalist who is gathering information to be used by all professionals on the team—has been insufficiently appreciated.

For a complete list of references, please visit online only at www.expertconsult.com

CHAPTER 38

Surgery and Anesthesia in Old Age

D. Gwyn Seymour

This chapter provides a general overview of surgery and anesthesia in old age, but lays particular stress on those areas of the subject that are changing most rapidly and/or are attracting most clinical and research interest. After a brief introduction dealing with epidemiologic trends, the elderly surgical patient is evaluated from a predominantly medical viewpoint. It is not possible to go into details of anesthetic or surgical technique here, but these have been considered at length elsewhere.[1–4]

Rehabilitation of the elderly orthopedic patient, important though it is, is also not dealt with here because it is discussed elsewhere in this textbook.

TRENDS IN SURGERY AND ANESTHESIA IN OLD AGE

The surgical treatment of elderly patients is not a late twentieth century invention. Of 100 cases of strangulated hernia operated on by van Assen in Amsterdam between 1903 and 1906, 18 persons were between 50 and 70 years of age, 17 were between 70 and 80 years, and 3 were over 80.[5] Inhalational anesthesia was used in one third of the cases, with local anesthesia in the others. There were only two deaths, but one of those was a patient aged 81.

In the last 30 years, however, the increase in surgical activity in patients aged 65 and over has been much greater than would have been expected from demographic trends alone.[6] This increase has not just been in life-saving procedures, but has also been seen in procedures such as cataract surgery or total hip replacement, which are predominantly aimed at increasing the quality of life. Surgery for cataract and total hip replacement for osteoarthritis are two prime examples of high-technology approaches to a surgical problem that have had a major impact on the quality of life of elderly patients. They neatly refute the simplistic assumption that hightechology "cures" are for the young, and low-technology "care" is for the old—a policy which is ethically dubious, and often financially unsound, because of the high costs of long-term care.[7] As Grimley Evans puts it, in many circumstances, "curing is caring."[8] In recent years, some of the increased surgical activity in young and old alike has been because of technological advances such as minimally invasive surgery. These techniques have had a major impact in urology, gynecology, general surgery,[1,4,6,9] and even in cardiac surgery.[10,11,12]

Some of the changes in surgical activity in different age groups have followed naturally from changes in the incidence or prevalence of disease or the availability of effective nonsurgical therapy.[6] Thus surgery for peptic ulceration has become much less common in the last 30 years, but on the other hand there has been a marked increase in the number of hip fractures, partly due to demographic change but probably due to underlying changes in osteoporosis prevalence as well.[13] In an ideal world, we would first assess medical and surgical needs in the community and then provide the appropriate services to meet those needs. A number of reviews edited by Stephens and Raftery[14] are of interest in this respect, particularly those dealing with colorectal cancer, total hip replacement, total knee replacement, cataract surgery, hernia repair, varicose vein treatment, prostatectomy, peripheral vascular disease, and adult intensive care.

AGE, SURGERY, AND OUTCOME

The association between age, surgery, and postoperative outcome is a complicated one.

1. Many surgically treatable diseases become more common with age. For example, the incidence of colorectal cancer increases almost exponentially after the age of 40.[14]
2. Age may have an effect on surgical presentation; for instance, an acute abdomen in some older people may have less dramatic signs and symptoms.[15]
3. Agist attitudes may influence patients and professionals in decisions as to whether elective surgical referral is indicated. Whereas overall attitudes are changing, older patients in higher socioeconomic groups may have very different elective referral rates from older people who are socioeconomically deprived.[16]
4. The incidence of nonelective presentation of surgical disease tends to rise sharply with age[17] probably from a mixture of the above factors, and nonelective surgical procedures have much higher rates of morbidity and mortality than elective procedures.[17–19]
5. Elderly surgical patients often have one or more coexisting medical conditions.[20] When these involve major organs, such as the heart, lung, or kidney, then the risks of surgery and anesthesia tend to increase.[17,21]
6. Even in the absence of coexisting medical disease, gerontologic studies point to a diminution in homeostatic reserve with age, a condition that has been termed "homeostenosis."[22] Under conditions of extreme stress (such as severe burns or trauma), the fit elderly patient has less chance of survival than the fit young patient[23–25] but vigorous intensive therapy can improve survival rates at all ages.[25,26]
7. The increasingly common "league table" approach, by which the surgical mortality rates of individual institutions are widely publicized, may have a detrimental effect on the care of high-risk elderly surgical patients. There might be managerial pressures to avoid surgery because of the "detrimental" effect that a postoperative death would have on the league table. Case-mix stratification is a theoretical way around this problem, but is very difficult to achieve in practice.[27]

How can all these effects be disentangled? A fair summary of the available evidence is that it appears to be age-associated illness rather than the aging process itself that is the main reason for the increase in morbidity and mortality following surgery and anesthesia in old age.[28,29] Lines of evidence to support this assertion include:

- The APACHE III system, which looks at risk factors predicting mortality in intensive care unit patients, has indicated that almost 50% of the variability in mortality is a result of the intensity of the acute illness, whereas only 3% is because of chronologic age.[30]
- While univariate analyses in which age is the only predictor variable tend to show a strong relationship between old age and adverse outcome in general surgical patients, multivariable analyses relating several preoperative risk factors to postoperative outcome have usually shown age by itself to be less important as an independent predictor.[31–33]

Thus attempts to set upper age limits for certain operations are suspect not simply from an ethical point of view,[7] but are technically suspect because age by itself is such a poor predictor of adverse postoperative outcome in an individual elderly person. Even in groups of older people there are no distinct cut-off points.[30,34] Each person with a surgical problem—whatever his or her age—needs and deserves an individual assessment. In each case there is a need to estimate, on an individual basis, whether the potential benefits of a surgical operation outweigh the potential risks.[29,35]

ANESTHETIC FACTORS

For a more detailed account of anesthesia in old age, specialist texts should be consulted,[1–3] but the following section considers topics of general interest to the referring physician.

Morbidity and mortality following anesthesia

In some elderly individuals, factors such as the extent and type of surgical pathology and the presence of serious coexistent medical disease may suggest that the potential risks of surgical intervention outweigh the potential benefits. Under such circumstances, the nonanesthetist should resist the temptation to pronounce the patient "not fit for an anesthetic," as postoperative deaths occurring solely because of anesthesia are very rare at any age, and in any case, it should be the anesthetist who estimates anesthetic risk.[35] In Pedersen's[17] series of patients of all ages, nonfatal complications directly attributable to anesthesia occurred in 1 patient in 170, whereas the overall rate of postoperative cardiopulmonary complications was as high as 1 in 11. For complications directly attributable to anesthesia, there was no correlation with age. For problems not directly attributable to anesthesia, in-hospital mortality and cardiorespiratory complications were rare below the age of 50, but there was a steady increase in incidence of these postoperative problems for age groups 50 to 69, 70 to 79, and 80 and over. The total in-hospital postoperative mortality in Pedersen's series was 1.2%, but it was difficult to judge whether or not anesthesia contributed to individual deaths, many of which occurred in elderly patients having major surgery for malignant disease. Difficulties in attributing the relative contribution to postoperative mortality of multiple factors such as urgency of presentation, extent of medical and surgical pathology, type of surgical procedure, and anesthetic technique is a recurring problem in surgical audit.[38,39]

Anesthetic drugs in elderly patients

Dodds[40] has described anesthesia as "applied clinical pharmacology with enough pathophysiology to confuse the picture." The scope for confusion of the picture is greatly increased in old age, particularly if preexisting polypharmacy is present. The review of anesthetic drugs in the elderly population by Dodds,[40] and a shorter account in a recent handbook[41] are recommended as a concise guide to an enormous subject. However, nine key points from that review are highlighted here, with the permission of the author.

1. The minimum alveolar concentration (MAC) is that concentration of an anesthetic gas that suppresses movement in response to a surgical stimulus in 50% of subjects. MACs tend to fall with age; in one study, halothane had a MAC of 1.08% in children but 0.64% at age 81.
2. With increasing age, there is a tendency for increased shunting in the lungs and decreased cardiac output. These pathophysiologic changes have complex effects on the uptake of volatile gases, as a low cardiac output favors rapid uptake, whereas a decreased lung function produces the opposite effect.
3. Where there is preexisting ischemic heart disease, the patient may be vulnerable to the cardiac depressant effects of some anesthetics and there is also the theoretical risk that isoflurane, enflurane, sevoflurane, and desflurane might "steal" blood from ischemic myocardium through vasodilation of normal vessels.
4. Hepatic metabolism and/or clearance of drugs tends to be affected by age, but there is considerable variability. Insoluble anesthetic agents that require no hepatic metabolism should be safer than soluble agents. Some agents such as halothane also have potentially hepatoxic metabolites, and this agent may also produce a fall in protein synthesis.
5. Hepatic metabolism releases inorganic fluoride from some hydrocarbon anesthetics, and nephrotoxicity could theoretically occur.
6. Because of reduced neuronal density and a reduced metabolic rate, the elderly may be more sensitive to a given amount of anesthetic drug. Additionally, in patients with a delayed circulation time, there is a danger of overdosage when intravenous agents are given too fast because a delayed response may be mistaken for a lack of therapeutic effect. Smaller doses, slower rates of infusion, or repeated small boluses are recommended in elderly people.
7. Neuromuscular blocking agents can be classified into depolarizing and nondepolarizing types. The latter are usually favored in old age and atracurium has attractions because it is not dependent on renal and hepatic metabolism for its clearance.[42]
8. Elderly people appear to have an increased sensitivity to opiates.
9. Nonsteroidal anti-inflammatory agents (NSAIDs) are commonly used for analgesia in younger patients, but may present increased hazards in the elderly population because of nephrotoxicity, fluid retention, and tendency to gastric irritation.

Long-term medications

Although not exclusively an "anesthetic" topic, it is convenient at this point to mention that a number of long-term medications that the patient is taking may have important implications for anesthesia and surgery. The main preoperative role of the physician is to gather information about current prescribed and over-the-counter drugs and to inform the surgical/anesthetic team. Most cardiovascular drugs will need to be continued, and sudden withdrawal of β-blockers and statins may present particular problems.[43]

ACE inhibitors will usually be omitted on the day of surgery, but this needs to be discussed with the surgical/anesthetic team. Decisions on the continuation of warfarin will depend on the surgical procedure and the reason the drug is being given, but will usually be guided by local protocols. Of other antithrombotic drugs, clopidogrel may have persistent effects for 10 days after cessation and recent use of this drug should be drawn to the attention of surgeons and anesthetists. Local protocols for patients with diabetes are usually readily available. Patients with Parkinson's disease may present difficult anesthetic and perioperative problems and require special attention.[44] The physician should be aware that "nil-by-mouth" regimens may permit the administration of essential oral drugs, but details are best left to the anesthetic/surgical team.

Prophylactic preoperative β-blockade

On theoretical grounds, preoperative initiation of β-blockers might be expected to have a beneficial effect on postoperative cardiovascular complications. In 2007, an influential report, while acknowledging that the evidence base was incomplete, favored the use of β-blockers in patients undergoing vascular surgery if myocardial ischemia had been demonstrated on formal cardiac testing.[43] However, a recent editorial[45] advised caution in the use of both prophylactic β-blockers and statins, at least until the ongoing POISE and DECREASE IV trials had reported. The POISE results appeared in May 2008,[46] and came to the worrying conclusion that, in patients undergoing noncardiac surgery, extended-release metoprolol succinate significantly increased the rate of mortality and strokes postoperatively, even though the number of cardiac events was decreased. Thus while other studies raise the theoretical possibility that lower doses of long-acting β-blocker titrated 7 days in advance could be beneficial,[47] the administration of higher-dose β-blocker therapy in the perioperative period might well be associated with greater risk than benefit.

STRATEGIES OF PREOPERATIVE ASSESSMENT

What should be the preoperative role of the physician?

The anesthetist is the person best qualified to assess anesthetic risk, and is also the person responsible for deciding whether or not a patient is fit for anesthesia.[35] However, an authoritative document on perioperative care in older people[29] has concluded that preoperative cross-specialty advice involving anesthetists, surgeons, and physicians is beneficial in the preoperative assessment, particularly in patients aged 80 and over. Although some of the "physician advice" may be provided by organ specialists, such as cardiologists or respiratory physicians, a frail older person is likely to need a comprehensive geriatric assessment (CGA), which is the domain of specialists in old age medicine (i.e., geriatricians) and their associated multidisciplinary teams.

Although geriatricians and their teams have commonly been involved in the postoperative (and sometimes the preoperative) care of orthopedic patients,[48] formal structures leading to preoperative and postoperative involvement with older general surgical patients has been rare. The POPS (Proactive care of Older People undergoing Surgery) program is an interesting exception, and in the first POPS publication, Harari et al[49] describe how they targeted elective high-risk surgical patients aged 65 and over, hypothesizing that preoperative CGA and preoperative and postoperative monitoring and interventions would reduce postoperative complications and length of stay. The published results to date have not had randomized concomitant controls, and a formal randomized control trial is underway, but it appears that the POPS approach can have a favorable effect on postoperative morbidity (pain, pneumonia, delirium, wound infection, and pressure sores), speed of mobilization, mean lengths of stay, and rates of delayed discharge.[49] The current criteria for considering patients for a POPS assessment are shown in Table 38-1.

Another innovative system that incorporates elements of CGA with other assessments is PACE (Pre-operative Assessment of Cancer care in the Elderly).[50] Following an extensive survey of preoperative status and postoperative outcome, the PACE researchers have published details of the preoperative characteristics of their patient group, and a publication linking preoperative factors with postoperative outcome is awaited.[51]

General strategy of preoperative assessment

In their recent handbook, Dodds et al[2] list eight key points that need to be considered when assessing an older patient in whom major surgery is being planned. These are shown in Table 38-2. Focusing down, Dodds et al[2] propose a four-point approach to preassessment, along broadly traditional lines.

1. The **history**, to identify past and present medical and surgical problems, allergies, medication usage, and past anesthetic and surgical procedures.
2. A review of **organ systems**

Table 38-1. Referral Guidance for the POPS (Proactive care of Older People undergoing Surgery) Program, for Patients Aged 65 and Over Awaiting Surgery[49]

Cardiovascular: MI in past 2 years, or unstable angina, or treated heart failure, or untreated BP > 160/90
Poorly controlled DM
Previous stroke
On warfarin
Chronic lung disease (if thought to put patient at risk)
Poor nutrition (BMI <20, wt loss >5 kg in last 6 months)
Two or more falls from standing in past year
Memory problems, or history of confusion, or known dementia
ADL: Needing help with getting to toilet, bed to chair, standing, dressing, walking
Likely to need a complex discharge package

Table 38-2. Key Points for Preoperative Assessment and Preparation of Elderly Patients Undergoing Major Surgery

- Age as such is not a good predictor of surgical risk.
- Physiologic age-related changes increase the risks of surgery and anesthesia.
- Comorbidities increase with age.
- Anesthetic planning for surgery in elderly people is a challenge.
- Aim of assessment is to identify within the composite elderly patient what integrated responses are critically reduced, or have failed, and then to systematically review individual organ systems for functional reserve.
  - Incidence of ischemic heart disease and valve disease increases with age and is associated with increased morbidity and mortality.
  - Chest disease is common in the elderly, and pulmonary complications are more common in the postoperative period.
  - Presence of interval delirium or confusion indicates a very high risk of postoperative cognitive impairment and general anesthetic or sedation should be avoided.
  - Hepatic insufficiency usually results in a poor surgical outcome.
  - Renal insufficiency associated with uremia increases risk.
- Before emergency surgery, there may not be time for complete evaluation and correction of risk factors.
- Life-saving treatment can proceed without consent.
- Advance directives before surgery should be documented, and the name of the patient's surrogate should be recorded.

Reproduced from Dodds C, Chandra MK, Servin F. Anaesthesia for the Elderly Patient. Oxford, UK: Oxford University Press; 2007.

3. Estimates of **functional reserve** of various organs, especially the heart, lungs, and kidneys
4. **Investigations**, paying particular attention to symptoms and signs indicating a severe and/or evolving clinical problem

The implications of abnormalities in the major organ systems are considered later in this chapter, but the topics of functional reserve and "routine" preoperative testing will be considered at this point.

Estimating functional reserve

Numerous studies have demonstrated a mild decrease in *basal function* of many organ systems in apparently healthy older people, but have pointed to a much more marked decrease when *reserve capacity* systems are put under stress. For example, when the case of cardiac output, the differences between young and old subjects are much more notable on exercise than they are at rest.[52] When pathology is added to "normal" aging the loss of reserve capacity may be considerable, but the degree of deficit might become apparent only when the system is stressed by surgical disease, anesthesia, and/or a surgical procedure. It has been calculated[2] that major surgery and its associated systemic inflammatory response may see a rise of oxygen requirements from an average of 110 mL/min/m^2 to an average of 170 mL/min/m^2.

It is not practicable to carry out direct measurements of preoperative cardiorespiratory reserve in all older people undergoing moderate or major surgery, and the best indicator that further specialized investigation might be indicated is likely to be the history supplemented by observation of usual activities. An approximate quantification of cardiorespiratory reserve can be based on the number of Metabolic Equivalents (METS) a patient can achieve. One MET is broadly defined as the energy it takes to sit quietly, and is defined as 3.5 mL/kg/min based on the resting oxygen

Table 38-3. Classification of Functional Capacity[43,53]

Estimated energy requirements in metabolic equivalents (METs) of various activities:

1-4 METS:
- Can take care of self—eat, dress, use the toilet
- Can walk indoors around the house
- Can walk a block or two on level ground at 2-3 miles/hr
- Can do light housework, such as dusting or washing dishes

4-10 METS:
- Can climb a flight of stairs or walk up a hill
- Can walk on level ground at 4 miles/hr
- Can run a short distance
- Can do heavy housework (e.g., scrubbing floors/lifting furniture)
- Can play golf, go bowling, go dancing, play doubles tennis, throw a baseball

>10 METS:
- Can do strenuous sports (swimming, singles tennis, football, basketball, skiing)

requirement of a 70-kg male aged 40.[2] Typical METS for a number of standard activities are shown in Table 38-3. The basic research work on METS dates back 40 years or more, but the concept was brought to a wider audience by the 1996 ACC/AHA (American College of Cardiology and American Heart Association) guidelines of perioperative examination for noncardiac surgery, subsequently updated in 2002 and 2007.[43] The ACC/AHA guidelines regard the attainment of 7 METS as "excellent," 4 to 7 METS as "moderate," and less than 4 METS as "poor." An ability to climb two flights of stairs without stopping is equivalent to about 4 METS and is a criterion commonly employed by British anesthetists.[2]

According to the ACC/AHA guidelines, patients who require further cardiac testing (using criteria referred to later in this chapter) should undergo treadmill exercise ECG or pharmacologic stress testing. A possible alternative is to estimate the "anaerobic threshold" by means of a bicycle ergometer, as part of a general strategy of "hemodynamic optimization." This technique is now available in a number of U.K. hospitals.[54,55]

"Routine" preoperative testing

What tests (such as blood tests, electrocardiograms, and chest x-rays) are required "routinely" in asymptomatic patients who are about to undergo surgery? Over the years this has been a subject of a large amount of debate and a modest amount of research. Various guidelines have not always been concordant in their advice and much of their content has needed to be based on expert consensus opinion. The National Institute for Health and Clinical Excellence (NICE) guidelines on preoperative testing are pertinent to the present discussion because they give separate recommendations for adults aged 60 and over,[56] although NICE acknowledges that consensus among their expert advisers was hard to achieve.

In deciding to carry out a test preoperatively (or, for that matter, in any clinical situation) it is useful to reflect on the five possible functions of a test, as listed by Garcia-Miguel et al[57]:

1. To assess a preexisting health problem
2. To identify unexpected conditions

3. To predict preoperative or postoperative complications
4. To act as a baseline for later comparisons
5. To be an opportunistic screening for unconnected conditions

RESPIRATORY PROBLEMS IN THE OLDER SURGICAL PATIENT

Incidence of postoperative respiratory complications

Respiratory complications are common after surgery in elderly patients, and while the majority of such patients survive, deaths from respiratory causes still rank alongside cardiac and thromboembolic deaths as major potentially preventable causes of postoperative mortality. Sprung et al[58] estimate that 40% of perioperative deaths in people aged 65 and over have a respiratory cause.

The reported incidence of postoperative respiratory problems depends on the exact definitions used. In general surgical patients assessed prospectively in Cardiff (Wales), postoperative respiratory problems were found in 33% of those aged 65 to 74, and in 50% of those aged 75 and over; but these percentages became 20% and 24%, respectively, when uncomplicated atelectasis was disregarded.[59] The risk of postoperative respiratory complications in these patients was increased in the presence of preexisting lung disease, smoking, volume depletion, and incisions near the diaphragm.[60] Similarly, Brooks-Brunn[61] reported six risk factors to be independently associated with postoperative respiratory complications in adults aged 18 and over undergoing abdominal surgery. These were: age 60 or over; impaired preoperative cognitive function; smoking in the previous 8 weeks; body mass index 27 or more; history of cancer; and incision involving the upper abdomen (or upper and lower abdomen together). Pedersen et al[62] found that age, major abdominal surgery, emergency operation, preexisting chronic lung disease, prolonged anesthesia, and the presence of pancreatitis were all positively associated with an increased risk of postoperative respiratory problems. Much more recently, Qaseem et al[63] estimated that, relative to age less than 60, the odds ratios for postoperative respiratory complications were 2.09 for those aged 60 to 69 and 3.04 for those aged 70 to 79.

Pathophysiology of respiratory problems in elderly surgical patients

Lung abnormalities are common in older people even in the absence of smoking or known lung disease, although it is difficult to be sure how much of the abnormality is due to aging and how much to other factors such as recurrent respiratory infections or pollution. Pulford and Connolly[64] have pointed to an increased closing volume (i.e., the lung volume at which basal airways begin to collapse) as one of the most consistent abnormal respiratory findings in old age, and this appears to be important in the cause of many postoperative respiratory complications.[65] Because closing volumes tend to lie within the range of tidal ventilation when normal individuals aged 65 and over are sitting quietly, postoperative atelectasis is a constant threat in old age, especially in patients who are not mobilized promptly.[2] Sprung et al[58] recently focused on those age-related respiratory changes that were most likely to be adversely affected by anesthesia and surgery. These were reduced lung static recoil, increased chest wall stiffening, and reduced alveolar surface area, combining to cause a decrease in vital capacity and expiratory flow rates, and an increase in residual volume and ventilation-perfusion mismatch.

Simple atelectasis may produce only minor signs and a low-grade hypoxemia but becomes clinically important when the lungs are already compromised and/or where the atelectasis develops into frank pneumonia. It should be noted, however, that in the majority of postoperative patients, atelectasis is thought to be initiated not by retained secretions but by basal airways collapse.[21,65] In this situation, classic "expiratory" methods of percussion and encouragement of coughing may do more harm than good.[66]

Estimation of respiratory risk and possible preventive strategies

In thoracic surgery, there is a large amount of literature on the role of preoperative respiratory function testing as an aid to decision making.[67–69] A recent guideline from the American College of Physicians (ACP) is an important milestone in developing an evidence-based approach to respiratory assessment in adults undergoing nonthoracic surgery. The ACP guidelines deserve to be read in full,[63,70,71] but an abbreviated summary is given in Table 38-4. Drawing on the same material, Cartin-Ceba et al[73] have produced a strategy particularly aimed at older patients, which has separate schedules of recommendations for the preoperative, intraoperative, and postoperative period.

Late postoperative hypoxemia

In the early postoperative period, prompt detection of possible respiratory complications and/or hypoxemia has been greatly aided by the development of pulse oximetry (although the need for direct measurement of blood gases has not been removed entirely, as pulse oximeters indicate oxygen saturation rather than absolute oxygen tensions and give no indication as to carbon dioxide levels[74]). Pulse oximeters have also had a major role in identifying brief episodes of profound hypoxemia in some individuals 2, 3, 4, or even more days following surgery.[75] The basic underlying mechanisms for episodic hypoxemia are reasonably well understood, although the conventional explanation offered here is probably an oversimplification.[65] In some cases, a patient who has had little or no hypoxemia for the first 1 or 2 postoperative days starts to develop episodes of profound hypoxemia (perhaps going below 60% saturation of oxygen), during the second, third, or fourth postoperative night. These desaturations often coincide with the presence of rapid-eye-movement (REM) sleep, which causes a disturbance of the respiratory mechanism similar to obstructive sleep apnea. The stress of surgery and, in particular, the use of opiates at the time of operation appear to suppress REM sleep for 2 to 3 days after major surgery, and it is when the REM sleep reappears that the episodes of desaturation occur.[76] Initially, the suppression of REM sleep was blamed entirely on opiates, but the phenomenon also occurs in patients who have not been given opiates.

Table 38-4. Brief Summary of American College of Physicians Recommendations on "Risk Assessment for and Strategies to Reduce Perioperative Pulmonary Complications for Patients Undergoing Noncardiothoracic Surgery"[63,70–72]

A. In order to initiate appropriate preoperative and postoperative interventions:
  1. Evaluate preoperatively the following risk factors:
     - Chronic obstructive airways disease
     - Age over 60
     - Congestive cardiac failure
     - ASA class of II or more (i.e., the presence of even minimal impairment)
     - Impairment in activities of daily living
     - Smoking (but note that a smoking history shows only a modest correlation with increased postoperative chest complications once respiratory disease has been allowed for, and evidence suggests that smoking cessation probably needs to take place at least 2 months before surgery)
     - obesity and mild or moderate asthma are not proven risk factors for postoperative pulmonary complications.
  2. Recognize the following higher risk procedures, with concomitant risk factors:
     - Operations lasting >3 hr
     - Abdominal surgery
     - Thoracic surgery
     - Vascular surgery
     - Aortic aneurysm repair
     - Emergency surgery
     - General (as opposed to regional) anesthesia
  3. Note that a serum albumin of less than 35 g/L is a powerful marker for postoperative pulmonary complications

B. In those judged at higher risk, recommended procedures to reduce postoperative pulmonary complications are:
  1. Deep breathing exercises or incentive spirometry
  2. Selective use of nasogastric tube

C. Preoperative spirometry and chest radiography is not recommended routinely, but might be indicative for patients with previous diagnosis of chronic obstructive airways disease or asthma.

D. The following should not be used "solely for reducing postoperative pulmonary complication risk:"
  1. Right heart catheterization
  2. Total parenteral or enteral nutrition (for those who are malnourished or have low serum albumin levels).

Hypoxemia would be expected to cause arrhythmias and it is tempting to conclude that some unexplained postoperative deaths around the third postoperative day are because of the cardiac effects of unrecognized hypoxemia.[77–80] However, it has been difficult to demonstrate a one-to-one relationship between episodes of hypoxemia and cardiac disturbance,[81] and other factors such as carbon dioxide levels might be important as well. Hypoxemia would also be expected to have a detrimental effect on wound healing and cerebral function[82,83] but again, there is need for further research.

Episodes of late postoperative hypoxemia can be prevented almost entirely by giving continuous oxygen by nasal cannulae for several days after surgery.[84] Common regimens are "three days and five nights." However, there are practical difficulties in identifying the patients who will be at risk from hypoxemia, and there is a balance to be struck between trying to monitor large numbers of patients with pulse oximeters and the alternative strategy of giving oxygen to a high proportion of patients even though some may not need it.

CARDIAC PROBLEMS IN THE ELDERLY SURGICAL PATIENT

Incidence of postoperative cardiac complications

Clinical evidence of postoperative myocardial infarction has been reported in 1% to 4% of unselected general surgical patients aged 65 and over.[21] In patients aged 75 and over, and in populations of patients with known ischemic heart disease, the incidence is at least twice as high. The association between increasing age and postoperative myocardial infarction is likely to be due in part to a secondary association between age and preoperative ischemic heart disease. Additional risk factors repeatedly reported to increase the chance of postoperative myocardial infarction include myocardial infarction within the previous 6 months and active congestive cardiac failure.[85] Other risk factors for postoperative myocardial infarction and/or cardiac failure include age, angina, hypertension, diabetes, arrhythmias, peripheral vascular disease, valvular heart disease, smoking, and previous cardiac surgery.[85]

More extensive electrocardiographic monitoring in the perioperative period has revealed that many elderly patients have repeated episodes of subclinical myocardial ischemia that might be amenable to treatment. As mentioned above, some of these episodes might be precipitated by episodes of profound hypoxemia that are respiratory rather than cardiac in origin.

Diagnosis of myocardial infarction in the postoperative period is difficult because the symptoms may be masked by analgesia or anesthesia, and the expected cardiac enzyme changes (such as a rise in creatinine kinase) may be mimicked by surgical trauma to muscle. However, more specific enzyme tests such as troponin I and troponin C have allowed more precise diagnosis and enabled smaller infarcts to be detected.[86] Once clear clinical signs and symptoms of postoperative myocardial infarction are present, the death rate has been reported to be as high as 50%.[17,21] However, in the study by Badner et al,[87] which used troponin estimations as part of the diagnostic process, there were only three deaths out of the 18 patients with a postoperative myocardial infarction.

Cardiac assessment of the noncardiac surgical patient

It has been estimated that for every patient with heart disease undergoing cardiac surgery, there are about 10 patients with heart disease, recognized or unrecognized, undergoing noncardiac surgery.[85] Many such patients are elderly. A large amount of literature has therefore grown up on the "cardiac assessment of the noncardiac surgical patient."[88,89] Even though extensive use of high-technology screening of cardiac and respiratory function might in theory be able to predict many postoperative complications,[90,91] the large number of patients undergoing surgery every day would make such a policy impractical. Apart from the practical and economic implications, there are also scientific objections to high technology mass screening. Some of the cardiac tests are not without risk, and, in addition, widespread preoperative cardiac screening in relatively low-risk patients would inevitably throw up large numbers of false positive results, which could result in the unnecessary postponement of much-needed surgery.

Are there "low-technology" strategies based on simple clinical assessment that would increase our chances of predicting postoperative cardiac complications? The earliest studies looked at risk factors one at a time (univariate analysis).[85] Subsequently, Goldman et al[92] in 1977 produced the first multifactorial index of cardiac risk in general surgical patients aged 40 and over. The problem with any clinical risk index is that it tends to perform well on the dataset from which it was constructed (i.e., the training dataset) but usually performs less well on subsequent datasets (test datasets).[60] Attempts to validate the Goldman index in other datasets gave variable results, particularly in patients undergoing vascular surgery.[21] A modification of the Goldman index by Detsky in 1986[93] attempted to increase predictive power by taking into account the underlying surgical illness, but these early risk indices have now been largely superseded by other approaches, as is described later.

These newer approaches have employed a stepwise approach to risk prediction, with initial screening tests leading, where appropriate, to more complicated investigations.[88,89] The ACC/AHA guidelines, first published in 1996 and later updated in 2002 and 2007,[43] deserve close reading, but are briefly described in the section that follows. First, however, a more general point about risk prediction needs to be made, which has applications outside the field of cardiac assessment and also applies to medical and surgical situations. A major concept that is incorporated into the ACC/AHA guidelines is the principle that more complex evaluation of risk, by means of noninvasive or invasive investigations, is best applied in those patients whose risk has already been judged as being *neither very high nor very low*. The mathematical justification for this comes from Bayes' theorem and is related to the concept of prior probability. In essence this states that, because most medical tests are neither very good nor very bad but something in-between, they are most likely to influence decision making when the prior estimation of risk is neither very high nor very low.[88,89] Where the prior probability of disease is very low, then the available noninvasive tests do not usually have a sufficiently high sensitivity and specificity to "lift" the patient into the "moderate risk" group and so do not alter the clinical assessment. On the other hand, when the prior probability of heart disease is very high, say 90%, then even if the noninvasive tests are negative, this is not enough to "demote" the patient to a low-risk category, and so the tests again do not alter management.

The ACC/AHA guidelines[43]

The ACC/AHA guidelines of 1996, 2002, and 2007 have many features in common, with the latest guidelines being summarized in Table 38-5. With the exception of patients whose surgical problems are so urgent that they need to go for surgery straight away, the guidelines recommend one of four courses of action depending on patient circumstances:

1. Proceed to surgery without further investigations.
2. Perform noninvasive cardiovascular investigations to define risk with more precision (further management depending on the results of these investigations).
3. Do invasive cardiovascular testing straight away.
4. Delay or cancel surgery, or perform a lesser procedure, because the estimated cardiac risk is very high.

The broad basis of classifying patients is shown in Table 38-5. It can be seen that three types of risk factor are considered:

1. The nature and extent of the surgery being planned
2. Clinical predictors for increased perioperative cardiovascular risk
3. The functional capacity of the individual patient. (The method of estimating functional capacity has been described above and in Table 38-3. The ACC/AHA recommendation is that patients with a maximal functional capacity of 4 METS or less should be considered at high risk)

At the center of the ACC/AHA document is an algorithm which, on the basis of the three types of risk factor, recommends which of the four courses of action should be pursued. The original papers or Web site[43] should be

Table 38-5. ACC/AHA Guidelines[43] for Perioperative Cardiovascular Evaluation before Noncardiac Surgery

Consider three factors:

1. The nature and extent of the surgery being planned:
   - Vascular surgery (reported cardiac risk >5%) such as aortic and other major vascular surgery, and peripheral vascular surgery. (This category was referred to as "high surgical risk" in previous guidelines.)
   - Intermediate surgical risk (reported cardiac risk 1% to 5%), such as intraperitoneal and intrathoracic surgery, carotid endarterectomy, head and neck surgery, orthopedic surgery, and prostate surgery.
   - Low surgical risk (such as endoscopic procedures, superficial procedures, cataract surgery, breast surgery, ambulatory surgery)
2. Clinical predictors for increased perioperative cardiovascular risk:
   - "Active cardiac conditions" (referred to as "major risk" in earlier guidelines), such as unstable coronary syndromes (unstable or severe angina, acute [<7 days] or recent [<1 month] myocardial infarction), decompensated heart failure, significant arrhythmias, and severe valvular disease.
   - Clinical factors from the Revised Cardiac Risk Index (replacing the "intermediate" category referred to in earlier guidelines) including history of
     - o Heart disease (including previous myocardial infarction)
     - o Compensated or prior heart failure
     - o Cerebrovascular disease
     - o Diabetes mellitus
     - o Renal insufficiency
   - Minor, including
     - o Age over 70
     - o Uncontrolled hypertension
     - o Rhythm other than sinus
     - o ECG abnormalities (LV hypertrophy, left bundle branch block, ST-T abnormalities)
3. Functional capacity, based on MET levels of <4 or ≥ 4 (as described previously).

An algorithm incorporating information from these three elements (see reference 43) indicates who should:

1. Proceed to surgery without further investigations
2. Undergo further noninvasive cardiovascular investigations
3. Undergo invasive cardiovascular investigations
4. Be considered for a cancellation or delay of surgery, or performance of a lesser surgical procedure

From Fleisher LA, Beckman JA, Brown KA, et al. ACC/AHA 2007 guidelines on perioperative cardiovascular evaluation and care for noncardiac surgery: a report of the American College of Cardiology/American Heart Association Task force on practice guidelines (writing committee to revise the 2002 guidelines on perioperative cardiovascular evaluation for noncardiac surgery). J Am Coll Cardiol 2007;50(17):1707–32 (executive summary) and e159–e241 (full report).

consulted by those intending to use the algorithm in clinical practice.

While the ACC/AHA guidelines draw as far as possible on research evidence, many of their recommendations are not fully "evidence-based," with expert opinion being used to fill shortfalls in the published literature. It is therefore to be expected that refinements and alterations will be required as more research information becomes available. It should also be recognized that, as currently formulated, the ACC/AHA guidelines would lead to practical problems for many clinicians and health care administrators. For example, as peripheral vascular disease is classified as having a "high" surgical risk, the guidelines would indicate that all such patients should routinely undergo noninvasive cardiac testing before surgery. In most U.K. centers, this is not current common practice and would present considerable logistical problems.

A final point to make about all predictive systems is that they are only part of the process of risk reduction. While a broad stratification of preoperative risk is a reasonable aim (not least as a means of allowing the patient an informed choice as to whether he or she wants surgery), risk reduction also demands that a significant effort should be directed into the peri- and postoperative care of *all* patients. Such care requires careful monitoring at a level appropriate to the patient's condition, with adequate provision of high-dependency units and intensive-therapy units if clinically indicated. Within a U.K. setting, there is concern that existing facilities are not always sufficient to provide optimal levels of postoperative care, with the result that older, frailer patients who are being monitored extremely closely during the period of their operation may rapidly find themselves back on a general surgical ward soon afterwards.[37–39]

Cardiac surgery

Paradoxically, the prediction of risk in patients who are undergoing cardiac as opposed to noncardiac surgery is less of a problem, as most cardiac patients will have had sophisticated and invasive preoperative cardiac testing. Even more importantly, such patients are routinely monitored postoperatively, usually in an intensive therapy unit. A decade ago, in leading centers, the mortality rate following cardiac surgery in patients aged 70 and over was only of the order of 5%, compared with a rate of about 2.5% in patients under 69, and a quarter of all patients were over 70.[94,95] However, outside specialist teaching centers there has been concern that referral practices and cardiac surgical rates in older patients are suboptimal.[96–98] Research has shown that quality of life and functional improvement after successful cardiac surgery is at least as good after the age of 70 as it is for younger patients.[99–100] Such studies add weight to the argument that procedures such as angioplasty, and operations such as coronary artery bypass grafting and aortic valve replacement, should be more widely available in elderly people.

Another growth area of potential benefit to older surgical patients is "minimally invasive cardiac surgery." To those outside the field, minimally invasive cardiac surgery appears to be a contradiction in terms, but there is a growing interest in techniques such as "beating heart anastomoses," which can avoid the problems of cardiac bypass.[10,12,101] For anatomic reasons, minimally invasive techniques cannot replace all conventional coronary artery bypass procedures; but they could take their place alongside conventional surgery and percutaneous coronary angioplasty as one of a basket of techniques that could benefit elderly people.

UNDERNUTRITION

Poor nutrition has been reported to have adverse effects on immune response, wound healing, and gastrointestinal, cardiovascular, and respiratory function,[102] and undernutrition in adults with medical and surgical problems is at long last attracting significant clinical and research interest. Nutritional assessment should therefore be part of the routine evaluation of older patients who are being considered for surgical treatment, even if this policy requires extra training of doctors and health workers.[103]

Research interest in undernutrition in adult surgical patients in hospitals was prompted by studies such as that of Bistrian et al[104] in the 1970s. Although the accuracy of some of the early estimates of prevalence has been challenged,[105] such studies were important in drawing general attention to the existence of malnutrition in hospitals. One of the valid criticisms of the early studies was overreliance on the serum albumin as a purely nutritional marker, whereas in recent years, it has become clear that it is better to regard it as a general indicator of illness severity.[106,107] For instance, in a surgical patient with a low serum albumin and an intra-abdominal abscess, it is more likely that the inflammatory response is causing the low albumin than it is that malnutrition is causing the sepsis.

The review by Corish[102] indicated that the nutrition of older patients coming into surgical wards is often suboptimal and that this is clinically relevant to their management. Once within hospital, the older patient may not be nutritionally safe. Corish points to studies which indicate that elderly hospital inpatients who are "eating normally" have a dietary intake well below their estimated energy requirements, and observations of food wastage indicate that as little as 60% of the food that is served to older patients is actually consumed. A deterioration in nutritional status following admission is therefore quite common, and is compounded by "nil by mouth" episodes as the result of illness, investigations, or surgical procedures.

At a practical clinical level, how should we assess nutritional status in elderly patients on a busy surgical ward? Corish[102] discusses individual methods that could be used but points out that none has been developed specifically for the elderly surgical patient and comments that "all the traditional markers in nutrition lose their specificity in the sick adult." For a broad assessment of nutritional status, Corish highlights the American Society for Parenteral and Enteral Nutrition (ASPEN) guidelines. Risk factors for undernutrition and adverse outcomes listed by ASPEN include: involuntary loss or gain before hospital admission of more than 10% of usual body weight within 6 months (or 5% in 1 month); a weight of 20% over or under ideal body weight; the presence of chronic disease; increased metabolic requirements; alterations to the normal diet as a result of recent surgery, illness, or trauma; and an inadequate nutritional intake for greater than 7 days.

Along with the criteria listed above, different rules of thumb have been suggested for the detection of "clinically significant" weight loss in the elderly population. These include 4.5 kg over 2 years, 2 kg per year, 4% or 5% over 1 year and 7.5% over 6 months. Although there is a dispute about exact criteria, Corish points out that a loss of 20% of body weight is almost invariably associated with physiologic impairment, and that older people may well be less tolerant of weight loss than the young.

Additional nutritional indicators that have been used in some studies include anthropometry, various serum proteins, creatinine/height index, functional status, immunologic competence, and bioelectrical impedance.[102] Anthropometric methods of assessing nutrition may appear to be more "scientific" than other methods, but there are often practical problems in applying them to older people in general, and old surgical patients in particular. Anthropometric measurements that can potentially be used in routine clinical practice are weight, height, body mass index (BMI) (weight in kilograms divided by the square of the height in meters), triceps skinfold thickness, midarm circumference, midarm muscle circumference, hand-grip strength, and measured weight change. McWhirter and Pennington[108] remind us that the BMI by itself is not a sensitive indicator of protein-energy malnutrition in adults because it does not distinguish between depletion of fat or muscle. There are added problems in assessing BMI in older people, who may lose height as the result of osteoporosis. Some researchers substitute knee height or arm demispan for body height, but then, as for all the other anthropometric measurements, it is necessary to establish age- and sex-matched norms in a comparable general population.[108] Furthermore, in acutely ill surgical patients, even the measurement of body weight presents practical problems.

Multi-item nutrition risk indices reviewed by Corish include the Nutritional Risk Index, Nutritional Risk Score, Subjective Global Assessment, Mini Nutritional Assessment, Prognostic Nutritional Index, Likelihood of Malnutrition Index, and the Instant Nutritional Assessment.[102] All have strengths and weaknesses with the usual tradeoff between sensitivity and specificity and a varying requirement for specialized laboratory tests.

In an effort to improve nutritional assessment in all hospitalized patients, the British Society for Enteral and Parenteral Nutrition (BAPEN) has been promoting the use of "MUST" (Malnutrition Universal Screening Tool).[109] MUST-type information is designed to be easy to collect and includes height, weight (past, present, and including a % estimate of recent weight loss), and BMI (calculated using arm width span or knee height if there is severe kyphosis) and estimates of severity of illness and likely future intake of nutrition. It would seem to be good practice for the referring physician to include such information when referring patients for possible surgery and anesthesia. The recording of serum albumin would also be a reasonable routine strategy, provided that it is realized that it is primarily a marker of poor health. Routine recording of the BMI will also identify patients with a high BMI, who will present different anesthetic and surgical problems (see later discussion). MUST is intended to be a pragmatic tool for clinical use rather than a precise instrument for use by specialist researchers, but it incorporates two important principles from the early surgical work of Windsor and Hill, namely that recent weight loss may be more important than the absolute weight, and that patients who have a reduction in function alongside signs of undernutrition are much more at risk than those who do not.[106,110,111]

Nutritional supplementation

Although there is ample evidence that malnutrition is statistically associated with a range of problems in medical and surgical patients,[112] this does not necessarily prove that the relationship is one of cause and effect. Still less does it prove that nutritional enhancement will improve postoperative outcome. The only way to assess the benefits or otherwise of nutritional supplementation in undernourished elderly patients is to carry out randomized controlled trials.[102] Such trials are not easy to do, and two recent reviews of nutritional supplementation in the elderly population have commented on the poor quality of many of the trials.[113,114] The systematic review of Milne et al[113] looked at 49 randomized controlled trials of protein and energy supplementation involving a total of 4790 elderly people at risk of malnutrition. Twenty of the trials took place with hospital patients, of which eight involved hip fracture patients but only two involved general surgical patients. The overall conclusion, when all the studies were combined, was that nutritional supplementation produced demonstrable weight gain, and probably a reduction in mortality, although beneficial effects on complications and functional status could not be consistently demonstrated.

The systematic review of Avenell and Handoll[114] confined its attention to postoperative nutritional supplementation in elderly patients following hip fractures. Twenty-one randomized trials published before February 2006 were included, involving 1727 participants. Again, it was difficult to draw firm conclusions. The eight trials providing additional oral feeding (with a variety of feeds containing energy, protein, and some vitamins and minerals) were consistent with a beneficial effect provided that a combined endpoint of "mortality plus complications" was used in the statistical analyses. The four trials involving nasogastric feeding provided only limited data but did not show a convincing effect on mortality, and, moreover, tubes were poorly tolerated. Only five of the studies overall, and only two of the nasogastric tube studies specifically examined the effect of supplementation on malnourished patients. This might well have been an important omission because following nasogastric feeding in the classic early study by Bastow et al,[115] the hospital mortality in the "very thin" category of patients was reduced relative to the "thin" group (relative risk 0.37 vs. 1.12). However, the confidence intervals were very wide owing to small patient numbers, and so the results were not statistically significant. Similarly, when morbidity was the outcome measured by Bastow, it was the "very thin" group who appeared to benefit most. If the evidence that nutritional support is most likely to be of benefit when targeted on very malnourished patients is borne out by future research, this will be good news for both patients and health service managers. For instance, the study by McWhirter and Pennington[108] indicated that 27% of general surgical patients, 39% of orthopedic surgery patients, and 43% of medical elderly patients were "undernourished." However, when only severe malnutrition was considered, the figures became more manageable, being 1%, 6%, and 19%, respectively.

From a purely academic standpoint, we might conclude that the existing randomized controlled trials do not as

Table 38-6. ESPEN Guidelines on Enteral Nutrition for Surgery[116]

1. Enteral nutrition (by mouth, or if necessary, by tube) is indicated without delay, even in the absence of obvious undernutrition, if:
   - It is anticipated that the patient will be unable to eat for more than 7 days perioperatively, or
   - The patient cannot maintain oral intake above 60% of recommended intake for more than 10 days
2. Where patients are at "severe nutritional risk," a delay for preoperative enteral nutrition is recommended. Severe nutritional risk is defined by the presence of at least one of:
   - Weight loss >10%–15% within 6 months
   - BMI <18.5 kg/m²
   - Subjective Global Assessment Grade C
   - Serum albumin <30 g/L (with no evidence of hepatic or renal dysfunction).
3. Finally, it is important to start enteral nutrition therapy as soon as a nutritional risk becomes apparent, rather than waiting until severe undernutrition has developed.

yet permit the construction of authoritative guidelines. However, in the meantime, we need to offer the best nutritional advice that we can for our older surgical patients. Combining information from many sources, ESPEN (the European Society for Parenteral and Enteral Nutrition) has recently issued guidelines on enteral nutrition in surgery[116] that cover both the preoperative and postoperative period. The main preoperative recommendations are shown in Table 38-6.

OBESITY

The pathophysiology of obesity has been discussed by Bray,[117] who divides patients into five categories: individuals who are not obese (class 0) have BMIs of 20 to 25 kg/m², whereas the BMIs of individuals in class I (low risk from obesity), II (moderate risk), III (high risk), and IV (very high risk) are 25 to 30, 30 to 35, 35 to 40, and greater than 40 kg/m², respectively. In reviewing anesthetic risks, Wilson and Reilly[118] take 35 kg/m² or more as their definition of obesity, and discussed the physiologic and anatomic implications. However, even in patients with severe obesity it has been difficult to demonstrate an increase in postoperative mortality; the main excess risk appears to be postoperative wound infections, with some studies also reporting an increase in thromboembolic complications.[118]

Studies of postoperative outcome in mild or moderately obese patients are surprisingly uncommon in the literature.[118] Garrow et al[119] prospectively studied 469 patients undergoing abdominal surgery of whom 73 were classified as obese (defined as the top 15% of BMIs for men and women). The obese group had significantly more wound infections, but no differences were found in respect of deep venous thrombosis, pulmonary embolism, chest infections, urinary infections, and unexplained fever. Postoperative deaths (one in the obese group and six in the nonobese group) were too few for statistical analysis.

Garrow's series[119] was not confined to elderly people, but in a much earlier survey of general surgical patients aged 65 and over, patients above the 75th percentile of triceps thickness had twice the rate of postoperative wound infections, but no increase in postoperative chest infections or in-hospital mortality.[120] In a more recent study of elderly general surgical patients,[19] patients were classed as being underweight or overweight by simple visual inspection. It was the underweight group that had the worst in-hospital mortality[19] and 5-year mortality (Seymour et al, unpublished observations). This is of interest because there is evidence from population studies that, as a broad generalization, once a patient has achieved old age (often despite their obesity), it is being underweight rather than being overweight that tends to be associated with worse long-term survival.[121–123]

Looking at in-hospital events in more detail, a retrospective study of perioperative morbidity following primary knee and hip replacement defined obesity as 20% above ideal weight for height, based on life insurance tables.[124] On this criterion, 103 out of 154 patients were classified as obese (joint replacement patients with osteoarthritis tend to be overweight, in contrast to hip fracture patients who tend to be underweight). Although the obese patients had longer operative times, their stay in the hospital, number of days with a fever, number of transfusions, and analgesic use were no different from the nonobese.[124] In a retrospective study of coronary artery bypass graft patients aged between 60 and 86, obesity was significantly related to length of hospital stay, but was less important as a predictor than congestive cardiac failure, renal impairment, and being aged 75 years and over.[125] A detailed discussion of the technical problems that obesity presents to the anesthetist and intensivist is provided by Adams and Murphy.[126]

FLUID AND ELECTROLYTE IMBALANCE

Reports from NCEPOD (National Confidential Enquiry Into Perioperative Deaths)[37] have stressed the critical importance of fluid balance in elderly surgical patients. In the 1999 review,[38] which concentrated on patients aged 90 and over, examples of overadministration and underadministration of fluid were encountered. In regard to perioperative fluid management, the following six key points were made:

1. Fluid imbalance can contribute to serious postoperative morbidity and mortality.
2. Fluid imbalance is more likely in elderly people as they tend to have renal impairment or other comorbidity.
3. Accurate monitoring, early recognition, and appropriate treatment of fluid imbalance is essential.
4. Fluid balance should be accorded the same status as drug prescription.
5. Training in fluid management, for medical and nursing staff, is required to increase awareness and spread good practice.
6. There is a fundamental need for improved postoperative care facilities.

However, the assessment and treatment of fluid and electrolyte disturbance in surgical patients is difficult, particularly for emergency patients where the deficits are likely to be most severe. There is no simple "cookbook" approach that will guarantee perfect fluid balance every time, and the best strategy usually is to make an initial broad assessment, to start treatment on that basis, and to monitor progress constantly thereafter. If cookbook rules are difficult to formulate for young surgical patients, then they are even more difficult to draw up for older patients; here, the increased prevalence of preexisting renal disease and homeostatic impairment in the cardiovascular system and renal system[127] produces a need for tighter control, at the same time the signs and symptoms of salt and/or water depletion are more difficult to interpret.[21,128]

Assessment of fluid and electrolyte status

The standard surgical strategy when assessing perioperative fluid and electrolyte requirements in patients of any age is (1) to assess preexisting deficits, (2) to estimate maintenance needs, and (3) to allow for continuing losses.[21,129]

The assessment of preexisting fluid and electrolyte deficits is more difficult in elderly patients because many of the classic signs of water and salt depletion such as reduced skin turgor and postural hypotension are neither sensitive nor specific in old age. For example, postural hypotension or lax skin tone may exist in elderly patients who are not volume-depleted, whereas a compensatory tachycardia may fail to develop in elderly people who are.[21,128,130] There is a need not just to examine the patient but to look at the whole clinical context over the previous few days. For instance, a patient who has been vomiting for 2 days is likely to be depleted of both salt and water even if the clinical signs are equivocal.

Water depletion

Another basic principle of electrolyte/fluid balance is to try to estimate the type of fluid that has been lost and to identify the main body compartment that has been affected. It is helpful to remember that depletion of water alone has a very different effect from losses of salt plus water.[21,129,130] Pure water depletion primarily affects the intracellular compartment, and the initial symptoms and signs are nonspecific, being drowsiness, irritability, and perhaps low grade fever.[21,128] In healthy younger patients, thirst is a reliable indicator of water depletion, but this may not be true in a proportion of healthy older patients,[127,130] and the symptom may in any case be impossible to elicit in acutely ill surgical patients. The main fact to remember about water depletion is that hypernatremia tends to develop, and Lye[131] has estimated that 90% of cases of hypernatremia in geriatric clinical practice are a result of water depletion.

Salt and saline depletion

Loss of salt (or saline, as salt loss is usually associated with water loss as well) has its predominant effect on the extracellular compartment, which includes the vascular compartment.[21,129,130] Middle-aged patients with this type of depletion classically develop postural hypotension and tachycardia, but the presence or absence of these signs may be difficult to interpret in older patients where postural hypotension from other causes may occur in one quarter of patients, and where autonomic reflexes are often blunted.[130]

The patient with severe saline depletion will eventually develop circulatory collapse and poor peripheral circulation, but these are late signs. A low jugular venous pressure (obtained by lying the patient flat and observing the neck) is a test of volume depletion that is underused.[21] In severe cases, more invasive methods such as central venous pressure monitoring may be needed and noninvasive means of estimating intravascular volume are being developed[132,133] Whereas a high serum sodium can be used to diagnose water depletion, a low serum sodium is unfortunately not a good sign of salt depletion because hyponatremia can occur in a variety of clinical conditions, including congestive cardiac failure, where total body stores of sodium tend to be high, and where intravenous administration of saline might lead to clinical disaster.

In a younger patient with salt and water depletion, the appropriate kidney response is to produce a urine that is concentrated and low in salt. If a young patient develops oliguria, and the urine has these features, then a "prerenal" deficit can be presumed and fluid challenge can be given. In the elderly patient, where a degree of coincidental renal impairment is common, oliguria may develop as a result of prerenal causes, but the urine may be misleading because the preexisting renal damage does not allow for salt and water conservation. Again, there is the need to take into account the whole clinical situation and not one set of biochemical results. If the clinical signs and history point to a likely volume depletion, then the correct course of action is to treat cautiously and monitor closely.

Defining dehydration

Strictly the word *dehydration* should apply to water depletion on its own.[134] However, in general usage, dehydration is often taken to mean a deficit of water or salt or both, and the classic signs of dehydration under this usage are actually signs of salt depletion such as postural hypotension. An otherwise very useful review of salt and water depletion in elderly medical patients[130] appears to use the term dehydration in this more general sense. As the signs, symptoms, and treatment of saline depletion on the one hand, and water depletion on the other, are different, it is therefore unfortunate that the word dehydration is often used in a nonspecific sense to smudge both of these together. The best course of action is probably to avoid the word altogether and to try to specify the nature and amount of the fluid that has been lost, and which body compartment is primarily affected.

Practical aspects of fluid and electrolyte therapy

Some broad rules of thumb that have been suggested when treating fluid/electrolyte disturbance in elderly surgical patients are as follows:

1. A water loss of 2 kg or more is probably significant in an elderly patient.[131]
2. In younger adults, Shires and Canizaro[135] suggest that a saline loss of 4% of the body weight is "mild," 6% to 8% is "moderate," and 10% is "severe." Elderly patients are probably at more risk from a given percentage of saline depletion because of their more limited homeostatic reserve.
3. It has been estimated that, in the younger surgical patient, 4 L of saline are lost before signs of depletion appear, and 4 L of saline are gained before edema develops.[136] There appear to be no comparable estimates for older patients.

4. The recommended rate of fluid administration depends on the type of fluid that has been lost.

In cases of water depletion, rapid replacement may be hazardous, as cerebral edema can result. Van Zee and Lowry[129] recommended that only one half of the calculated water deficit should be administered over the first day, with the remainder being replaced over the next 1 to 2 days. Water repletion can be achieved by 5% dextrose infusions intravenously or subcutaneously. Water by the oral or nasogastric route is an alternative.

In cases of volume depletion, rapid replacement is usually desirable. In young patients with severe volume depletion, Shires and Canizaro[135] recommend an initial infusion rate of 2 L/hr, but state that this rate should be halved as soon as signs of improvement appear. Even then, when rates of infusion are above 1 L/hr, they recommend that a physician be in constant attendance. For older patients with severe volume depletion, Shires and Canizaro point out that the benefits of rapid repletion may be partly offset by the risks of fluid overload, and they state that monitoring by central venous line or a pulmonary artery catheter is desirable.

Wet, dry, or something else?

"Wet, dry or something else" is the title of a recent editorial by Bellamy,[137] which refers to the "great fluid debate" raging among anesthetists as to whether a patient should be given a liberal or a restricted fluid regimen over the perioperative period. This is of particular relevance to older patients because of their tendency to "homeostenosis," as described at the beginning of this chapter. Bellamy suggests that the wet and dry schools of thought can best be reconciled by individualizing the amount and timing of fluid administration depending on the measured cardiovascular status of the individual patient who is being treated. The key concept is circulatory "optimization," so that fluids are given to those who are depleted while being withheld from those who are fluid overloaded. With the increasing availability to the anesthetist of noninvasive or minimally invasive monitoring devices,[138] the concept of optimization has passed from a theoretical concept to a practical prospect, and although this is an area of more immediate interest to the anesthetist and intensivist than the referring physician, an awareness of such concepts will assist mutual understanding and has a general applicability outside the fields of surgery and intensive care. A related concept, which also merits a wider readership is that of ERAS (enhanced recovery after surgery). The central idea[139] of ERAS is to question the conventional approach to perioperative metabolic care, which accepts that a stress response to major surgery (with all its potential adverse effects in patients with homeostenosis) is inevitable. Fearon et al[139] describe how an ERAS group was set up in 2001 bringing together departments of surgery from Scotland, Sweden, Denmark, Norway, and the Netherlands, around the key concept that "a substantial element of the stress response can be avoided with the appropriate application of modern anesthetic, analgesic, and metabolic support techniques."[139] Early mobilization and a reduced postoperative stay in the hospital is also a key feature of ERAS, which has attractions for patients and hospital managers alike.

CENTRAL NERVOUS SYSTEM

Postoperative stroke

Postoperative stroke is a relatively rare complication following general surgery, although the incidence rises with age, being around 1% in those over 65 and 3% in the over 80 age group. Although age, cardiac disease, peripheral vascular disease, hypertension, smoking, and previous cerebrovascular events all appear to be risk factors, risk prediction in individual patients is difficult.[140] However, procedures on the carotid arteries, and coronary artery bypass procedures, carry a higher stroke risk than general surgical procedures. In the case of carotid endarterectomy for symptomatic stenosis, the balance of risks and benefits has been worked out in two controlled clinical trials, but the place of surgery in asymptomatic stenosis is still a matter for debate.[141–143]

The risk of stroke after open heart surgery appears to be falling but still remains higher than that for general surgery.[144] The improvement in outcome in cardiac bypass patients has usually been attributed to better techniques of extracorporeal circulation, but two studies of postoperative cardiac patients have claimed that the main risk of postoperative stroke is to be found in a small subset of patients with preexisting cerebrovascular or carotid disease.[145,146]

Postoperative delirium

Postoperative mental impairment following surgery has been a topic of interest for many years. A proportion of older patients will develop acute postoperative delirium. This has an incidence of 10% to 40% depending on the type of operation, on the exact definition of delirium employed, and on whether the study was prospective or retrospective.[59,147] Many of the precipitants of delirium in the postoperative situation are the same as those causing delirium in the medical patient;[148] they include acute illness (particularly infection), the effects of drugs, and withdrawal from alcohol or psychoactive drugs such as tranquilizers. However, delirium may also be due to premedication (especially with anticholinergics), anesthetic drugs, associated surgical complications, and episodes of late hypoxemia. Diagnosis of the cause of delirium may also be more difficult postoperatively. For instance, delirium tremens developing postoperatively in an emergency surgical patient who has been unwilling or unable to give a history of heavy alcohol intake before admission may be attributed to "surgical" causes.

A painstaking prospective study of the risk factors for postoperative delirium has been carried out.[149] Independent predictors of delirium were: an age of 70 or over; self-reported alcohol abuse; poor cognitive status; poor functional status; markedly abnormal preoperative sodium, potassium, or glucose; noncardiac thoracic surgery; and aortic aneurysm surgery. Although it is sometimes stated that delirium is less common after regional as opposed to general anesthesia, in a large randomized controlled study of patients undergoing elective total knee replacement, Williams-Russo et al[150] found no statistical difference between the incidence of postoperative delirium in patients following general anesthesia (12 of 128, or 9.4%) and that following epidural anesthesia (16 of 134, or 12%).

Although it is good practice to try to minimize risk factors that might cause delirium in elderly surgical patients, and minimal use of premedication in older surgical patients is one way of doing this, the main clinical requirement is probably to recognize delirium when it occurs and to treat the cause vigorously. However, as detailed in a number of recent reviews,[151–154] randomized trials of strategies aimed at reducing the incidence of delirium in older people in a variety of clinical situations are now being reported.[155] In a randomized controlled study of hip fracture patients, it was reported that daily visits from a geriatrician reduced the overall incidence of postoperative delirium.[156] Another recent study of hip fracture patients used a nurse-led intervention program, and although the incidence of delirium was not reduced, the duration of delirium episodes was shortened.[157]

Although there are still many unanswered questions, the preoperative cognitive status is an important piece of information for the referring physician to pass on to the surgical/anesthetic team, and anesthetists are becoming increasingly familiar with cognitive assessment scales such as the Abbreviated Mental Test or the Mini Mental State Examination.[2] Reasons for recording preoperative cognitive status include:

1. Considerations about whether the patient has the capacity to consent to a surgical procedure[158]
2. The fact that preexisting dementia is a major predisposing risk factor for delirium[151,152] and the need to identify patients who might benefit from intervention[152–154]
3. The practical consideration that postoperative delirium is easier to diagnose if there is a preoperative baseline

Postoperative dementia

The more difficult question in regard to postoperative mental status is whether dementia ever occurs as a primary event following uneventful surgery and anesthesia. There has been argument about this in the literature for 50 years following pioneering studies that attempted to identify patients who had "never been the same since their operation."[159,160] Many of the early studies in this area were uncontrolled and did not have a baseline mental assessment measurement.[161] Some were also associated with emergency surgical procedures where a number of factors such as hypotension or sepsis might have had a permanent effect on cerebral function that was not directly due to surgery or the anesthetic process.[161]

In recent years there have been attempts to carry out properly controlled trials, with detailed psychological testing before and after surgery.[161] An inevitable limitation of such trials is that the need to make precise preoperative psychological assessments tends to limit them to elective patients who are undergoing anesthesia under carefully controlled conditions and so the risk of postoperative complications of any type is likely to be small. Such formal trials have not demonstrated objectively that anesthesia, whether general or regional, has a permanent effect on cognitive functioning. For instance, in the study of Jones et al,[162] average scores on objective tests of cognitive function before surgery were not statistically significantly different from those obtained 3 months after surgery, although there was a group of 21 out of the 129 patients who reported some subjective changes. It is not clear whether these patients had real but subtle changes in cognitive function that could not be picked up by the standard tests, or whether they had other conditions such as depression or postoperative fatigue that were not primary dementing processes. A subsequent prospective randomized study of local versus general anesthesia for cataract surgery in patients aged 65 to 98 years found no cognitive decline at 3 months after surgery, and no difference between the two anesthetic groups.[163]

Subsequently, Williams-Russo et al found no long-term (6-month) difference in cognitive functioning between elderly patients undergoing elective orthopedic surgery under regional anesthesia and those undergoing general anesthesia.[150] However, the cognitive function of 12 out of the 231 patients (7 of 114 of those having an epidural anesthetic and 5 of 117 having a general anesthetic) was worse at 6 months than it had been preoperatively. In the absence of long-term follow-up information of nonoperative patients using the same cognitive assessment protocols, it is difficult to assess whether a decline of this amount would have occurred even in the absence of surgery.

Many of the earliest studies could be criticized because they had no controls and/or because preoperative psychological testing was limited or absent. However, the first ISPOCD (International Study of Post-Operative Cognitive Dysfunction) study was specifically designed with these criticisms in mind, and still came to the worrying conclusion that 25.8% of all patients had POCD (postoperative cognitive dysfunction) 7 days after surgery and that 9.9% of patients still had evidence of POCD on the repeat neuropsychological tests carried out at 3 months (with corresponding values for controls being 3.4% and 2.8%).[164] Contrary to expectations, no correlation was found between perioperative hypoxemia and/or hypotension and the subsequent development of early or late POCD. Indeed, despite analyses of the effects of more than 25 other clinical parameters, only age showed a statistically significant correlation with late POCD. Because the first ISPOCD study did not provide definitive guidance with regard to the prevention or treatment of POCD, ISPOCD2 was embarked upon,[165] but many of the key questions remain unanswered.[166]

So what should we advise an older patient who is concerned about the risk of cognitive impairment following an elective surgical procedure? This remains a difficult question, and in a recent review of central nervous system dysfunction after noncardiac surgery in old age, led by a senior ISPOCD researcher, no definitive answers were offered.[167] Rather, the following five points were made:

First, CNS dysfunction after anesthesia and surgery is predominantly a problem of old age. Second, postoperative delirium is an established clinical entity, although more research is required into the cause, prevention, and management. Third, POCD cannot yet be regarded as a single defined syndrome. Although there appear to be some older patients who show persistent cognitive dysfunction after an apparently uneventful surgery and anesthesia, the occurrence of cognitive problems in hospitalized nonsurgical patients makes it difficult to determine whether the link between surgery and/or anesthesia is causative. Fourth, more follow-up studies of patients with mild cognitive impairment are needed. Fifth, postoperative CNS dysfunction is a public health problem worthy of a large amount of future study.

ONLINE COMPUTERIZED RISK ASSESSMENT AND GUIDANCE

An interesting technical development in the last decade has been the growth and refinement of multivariable risk assessment tools that are intended to give estimates of surgical risk. Many of these tools are available online, raising the possibility that they might be used during or after a consultation with an older patient contemplating surgery, or perhaps directly by older people themselves. Although there are the usual technical problems in devising tools that can produce accurate predictions in groups of patients, let alone individuals, this is a development of great potential interest to patients, physicians, anesthetists, and surgeons. Two of the better known systems are the group of instruments bearing the POSSUM label, and the EUROSCORE system.

POSSUM stands for Physiological and Operative Severity Score for the enUmeration of Mortality and morbidity. The original POSSUM publication[168] established the principle of building a combined risk score from: (1) "physiologic" risk (based in more recent POSSUM versions on nonsurgical factors such as age, cardiac function, systolic blood pressure, pulse, urea and hemoglobin) and (2) "operative severity" (incorporating information about the procedure, urgency, stage of carcinoma if present, and degree of peritoneal soiling). Since then, a whole POSSUM family has arisen, including P-POSSUM (using updated coefficients from the initial POSSUM tool) O-POSSUM (esophageal procedures), AAA-POSSUM (abdominal aortic aneurysm) and CR-POSSUM (colorectal procedures). CR-POSSUM is of particular interest because colorectal cancer is a common surgical problem in old age with a good chance of surgical cure, but the operation is associated with significant morbidity and mortality. Tekkis and Smith have produced an excellent Web site[169] that not only provides updates of the latest POSSUM instruments (and other risk prediction instruments), but also carries out risk calculations on line. A new index for predicting postoperative mortality in patients aged 80 and over with colorectal cancer has also recently been proposed by Heriot et al.[170]

EUROSCORE is a multivariable risk prediction system with a focus on risk prediction after cardiac surgery. The calculations are based on (1) patient-related factors (including age), (2) cardiac-related factors, (3) operation-related factors, and, like POSSUM, the system is housed on an excellent Web site that allows individual patient details to be entered and estimated risks to be calculated.[171]

There are also a number of Web sites that give more general information about topics of relevance to the older surgical patient. Two such sites are those of the Age Anaesthesia Association (AAA)[172] based in the United Kingdom and the Society for the Advancement of Geriatric Anaesthesia (SAGA)[173] based in the United States.

SURGICAL AND ANESTHETIC AUDITS

Audit is a process that has been well established for many years among surgeons and anesthetists, and physicians have much to learn from their colleagues in these specialties. A major advance in Britain has been the establishment of a National Confidential Enquiry into Perioperative Deaths (NCEPOD) for the United Kingdom, excluding Scotland, and the corresponding Scottish Audit of Surgical Mortality (SASM).[37–39] Annual reports publish illustrative cases where deaths of individual surgical patients might have been avoided, and because about two thirds of all the deaths occurred in patients over the age of 70, they are particularly relevant to the present discussion. Recurrent themes over the years have been the necessity for nonelective patients to be treated in units with appropriate facilities and by staff with the appropriate levels of experience. In some of the individual case reports, potentially preventable factors have included a lack of medical stabilization of patients before surgery. It must be acknowledged, however, that this is a difficult judgment to make because excessive delay before surgery is also associated with increased complication rates in many conditions, including hip fractures. Audits such as NCEPOD and SASM have also stressed the importance of having appropriate organizational structures in place to deal with high-risk groups such as the elderly emergency surgical patient.[37–39]

KEY POINTS

Surgery and Anesthesia

- The association between age, surgery, and postoperative outcome is a complex one. However, there are scientific and ethical reasons to argue that age by itself should not be a barrier to surgery. Each patient, whatever his or her age, needs an individual assessment so that the potential benefits and risk of surgery and anesthesia can be identified.
- Respiratory problems are a common cause of postoperative morbidity, and an important cause of postoperative mortality. Research into the mechanism of postoperative respiratory complications has allowed a more logical approach to prevention and treatment and helpful guidelines are now emerging, but further research is required to define an optimal set of strategies. Pulse oximetry has made it easier to monitor and treat hypoxemia, but research is still going on into the underlying mechanisms.
- "Cardiac assessment of the noncardiac surgical patient" has been an area of research activity for many years. Guidelines issued by the American College of Cardiology and the American Heart Association (ACC/AHA) in 1996, 2002, and 2007 provide a coherent approach to the management of surgical patients who have coincidental cardiac disease. However, while there is a considerable evidence base supporting these guidelines, further research is needed.
- Undernutrition in middle-aged and elderly surgical patients has only recently attracted the research attention that it deserves. Broad guidelines for identifying older surgical patients at risk and for designing nutritional interventions are available, but the evidence base is still patchy.
- The ERAS (enhanced recovery after surgery) approach is an important development in perioperative care, which is based on the concept that a "substantial element of the stress response can be avoided with the appropriate application of modern anesthetic, analgesic, and metabolic support techniques." Developments in minimally invasive monitoring and therapeutic technologies are complementary to the ERAS approach.
- The causes of acute delirium in surgical patients are similar to the causes in elderly nonsurgical patients. A major and continuing concern over the years, however, has been whether permanent cognitive dysfunction can occur simply as a result of an uneventful anesthetic. The first International Study of Postoperative Cognitive Dysfunction (ISPOCD1) was designed to answer these questions once and for all, but doubts remain.

The establishment of audit, the general acceptance of well-designed guidelines for patient management, and evidence-based approach are examples of general measures that are likely to improve postoperative outcome of all elderly surgical patients. This approach is complementary to the more usually discussed method of risk reduction, which is to target high-risk patients before surgery and to put in maximum effort at this point. It is becoming clear, however, that perfect targeting of patients is unlikely ever to be achieved and that a combined approach involving selective targeting, perioperative and postoperative monitoring, and close attention to the general environment, structure, and interprofessional links of the surgical service is needed.[26,29] A wider look at the subject might also consider the process of referral in the first place, and would also examine the attitudes of society to high-technology treatment in old age.[7,8,16,174]

FUTURE TRENDS

Factors increasing the number of surgical procedures in old age

It is highly likely that the technical developments in surgery and anesthesia that have occurred in the recent past will continue in the future and will allow potentially beneficial surgery to be extended to ever older and frailer patients. Such developments are also likely to lead to more favorable attitudes to surgery in old age, so that more patients will be referred. Even if attitudes and techniques were not to change, demographic changes would lead to an increase in surgery in the old and the very old in the next two decades.

Factors decreasing surgical procedures in old age

It is to be hoped that preventive medicine or novel forms of medical therapy will reduce the need for surgical intervention in many conditions. This has already been seen in regard to modern medical therapy for peptic ulceration. An increase in minimally invasive techniques might also lead to a reduction in the number of major surgical operations being performed. For instance, gallbladder surgery is increasingly being performed by laparoscopic techniques rather than via a laparotomy.[9]

A reduction in surgical activity in some conditions because of better medical therapies or the substitution of less invasive procedures is obviously to be applauded. Much more sinister, however, is the tendency for politicians and health planners to contemplate that some forms of potentially beneficial surgery should be rationed on the basis of age, even though there is very poor evidence that age by itself has any significant effect on the ability of a patient to benefit from a given surgical procedure.

If elderly patients are denied surgery simply on the basis of their age, this is by definition agist and such practices need to be challenged vigorously.[16,34] However, more subtle forms of discrimination might occur because of reduced equity of access of older people to medical and surgical services, and a U.K. Medical Research Council review concluded that "research is needed to examine the extent of differences in access to the NHS according to age group."[175] Although detection of inequity of access is difficult for both medical and surgical conditions, the research is technically simpler in the surgical situation because interventions and endpoints tend to be more clearly defined. Preliminary investigations by Seymour and Garthwaite[16] suggested that inequity of access for surgical patients on the basis of age does exist, but that this interacts with inequity based on patient deprivation. Age-related inequity is probably decreasing with time, but inequity on the basis of deprivation might be more resistant to change.

For a complete list of references, please visit online only at www.expertconsult.com

CHAPTER 39

Measuring Outcomes of Multidimensional Interventions

Paul Stolee

Although frailty in older persons may be associated with an underlying loss of complexity in many physiologic systems,[1] the clinical conditions and geriatric syndromes[2] that are commonly present in frail older persons are often highly complex. This clinical complexity, including the multiple interacting medical and social concerns, is the challenge and also the joy[3,4] of geriatrics.

Geriatric services respond to this complexity with comprehensive approaches to assessment, multidisciplinary teams, and multidimensional interventions. Although there may be widespread agreement on the need for comprehensive, multidisciplinary, and multicomponent approaches, there is less agreement on the specific elements of these approaches. It is also not always clear which specific interventions or aspects of care (or combinations thereof) "make the difference" for an individual patient or for groups of patients—hence the references to the "black box" of geriatrics.[5,6] Clinical complexity and comorbidity have often meant that frail older persons are excluded from many clinical trials.[7] This is problematic both in terms of the interventions being tested—interventions targeting single diseases often have limited efficacy for the constituency of geriatric medicine patient[8]—and in terms of the results of these studies—which are not generalizable to many frail older patients.[8,9] Multicomponent interventions have been found to be more effective than single component interventions for frail older patients,[10] but these types of programs are much more difficult to evaluate in the context of clinical trials.[8] Allore and colleagues[11] make a distinction between statistical/analytical considerations and clinical considerations in the design of such trials. Statistical or analysis considerations would suggest one specific intervention should target a single outcome or risk factor (the basis on which power calculations are generally undertaken).[7] Clinically, however, it makes sense for interventions to target more than one outcome or risk factor, and many interventions are likely to have overlapping effects.[11] For studies of interventions for frail older patients, clinical and analytical considerations are particularly at odds.

Given the heterogeneity of the patient population, and the heterogeneity of clinical interventions, it is not surprising that evidence for the effectiveness of geriatric interventions has been hard to establish. Rubenstein and Rubenstein[12] have closely observed this literature over the years, and have pointed out a number of factors associated with an increased likelihood of demonstrating their effectiveness. These include appropriate targeting, more intensive interventions, control over longer-term management, and a usual care control group. To this list, it is suggested here that an additional consideration be added: the selection of meaningful and responsive outcome measures. The selection of appropriate outcome measures for geriatric interventions is not straightforward and has been identified as a priority for research.[13,14] In the early 1990s, a working group of the American Geriatrics Society achieved a consensus on measures appropriate for measuring outcomes of geriatric evaluation and management units.[15] The consensus statement recommended 12 physical outcomes, three psychological and social functioning outcomes, and 17 outcomes related to health care utilization and cost (reflecting concerns about future implementation and funding). The number and variety of these measures reflect the multidimensional nature of geriatric care and its potential system impact. While all of these measures may have relevance to specialized geriatric interventions, few, if any, of these measures would be relevant for all patients. The question therefore becomes how to achieve nonarbitrary dimensionality reduction from multidimensional interventions with multidimensional outcomes.

Some of the challenges associated with measuring outcomes of multidimensional geriatric interventions can be gauged by reviewing the outcome measures used in randomized controlled trials of these interventions. Relevant studies were identified from selected major systematic reviews and meta-analyses, beginning with the seminal meta-analysis of comprehensive geriatric assessment services published by Stuck and colleagues in 1993.[16] Other reviews included a review of studies specifically focused on outpatient geriatric assessment,[17] two reviews of studies focused on preventive home visits,[18,19] and one review that specifically targeted multi-component interventions.[11] Collectively, these reviews reported results from 56 randomized controlled trials (Appendix Table 1). Outcome measures were categorized into mortality; self-rated health; health care utilize; three assessment domains—physical function, cognitive function, and psychosocial outcomes; and an "other" category. In these 56 studies (Appendix Table 2),

- Physical function was measured in 54 studies, using 32 different measures, of which 23 were statistically significant.
- Cognitive function was measured in 33 studies, using 11 different measures, of which 6 were statistically significant.
- Psychosocial function was measured in 36 studies, using 29 different measures, of which 12 were statistically significant.
- Self-rated health was measured in 18 studies, using 8 different approaches, of which 4 were statistically significant.
- Health care use outcomes were measured in 45 studies, using 19 different measures, of which 24 were statistically significant.
- Other outcomes were measured in 32 studies, using 16 different measures, producing statistically significant results in 13 studies.

The collective data illustrate several points. Geriatric services were associated with statistically significant benefits in each category of outcome measure in at least some studies, but no category of outcome was significantly improved in all studies. None of the studies reported significant improvement in all of the outcomes measured. The review also highlights the range of outcomes considered meaningful, and plausible, for geriatric services. Death is a clear end point, and mortality is amenable to summation and comparison in meta-analyses but is not necessarily the most meaningful parameter for programs serving a frail clientele for whom life expectancy is limited.[7] Indicators related to health care use are of great relevance to the health system and while they may relate to an older person's quality of life (for example, for some older persons, quality of life may be higher in community settings than in a long-term care home), these are at best indirect measures of quality of life from a patient's perspective. Within each of the other domains, there is further evidence of heterogeneity—each domain has multiple aspects, and a large variety of instruments and approaches have been used to measure these. Even within the "other" category, an outcome such as "falls" is itself a multifactorial syndrome.[11]

Geriatric assessment outcomes and quality of life measures

The assessment domains commonly measured in geriatric intervention studies can be seen as major components of quality of life. If outcomes commonly targeted by multidimensional geriatric interventions can be considered collectively as a reflection of quality of life as the overarching domain of importance, then a sufficiently comprehensive quality of life measure could be a good choice as an outcome measure for common use in geriatric intervention studies. A candidate measure is the Medical Outcomes Study 36-Item Short Form General Health Survey (SF-36),[20] which has been very widely used as a health-related measure of quality of life.[21] Unfortunately, testing of its use with older persons has not been extensive,[7] and results of these studies suggest the utility of this measure in geriatrics may be limited.[22] The development of a measure that could achieve wide acceptance has been hindered by the lack of a common conceptual or theoretical understanding of the meaning of quality of life and by lack of agreement on its constituent elements.[23] Walter Spitzer has argued, however, that the development of a "gold standard" measure is possible even for a subjective construct such as quality of life: "We fail to have a Gold Standard…because no one has made it his or her primary objective to develop a Gold Standard either for measures of health status or for measures of quality of life…I believe Marilyn Bergner and her co-workers have a sufficiently long head start that they deserve support from all the rest of us."[24] Although Spitzer pointed to the work of Marilyn Bergner on the Sickness Impact Profile[25] as the best candidate for further development as a gold standard quality of life measure, Bergner turned out not to share this view: "The bitter truth is that there is no gold standard, there is unlikely ever to be one, and it is unlikely to be desirable to have one."[26]

Standardized assessment systems

Another approach that aims at providing a comprehensive assessment of health and social functioning is the use of a standardized assessment system, of which the interRAI Minimum Data Set (RAI/MDS) assessment systems are the most prominent. The interRAI instruments are a comprehensive assessment and problem identification system developed by an international consortium of researchers.[27] The original interRAI assessment was developed for long-term care homes (MDS 2.0) in response to U.S. government regulations (OBRA) aimed at improving nursing home quality.[28] The interRAI Home Care assessment instrument (RAI-HC, or MDS-HC),[29] has been developed for home care settings. Other versions have been developed for use in mental health,[30] acute care,[31] palliative care,[32] and other settings. RAI assessment items include personal items, referral information, cognition, communication and hearing, vision, mood, behavior, physical functioning, continence, disease diagnoses, preventive health measures, nutrition status, oral health, skin condition, environmental assessment, and formal and informal service use. Specific scales have been derived from RAI assessment items, including measures of activities of daily living (ADLs),[33] cognitive impairment,[34] depression,[35] and pain.[36] Application of the RAI system has been linked with reduced institutionalization and functional decline.[37] The approach to data collection is one of "best available information." This may be done by interview or observation of the older person, by interview of the caregiver (paid or unpaid), or through chart review. While this approach may suggest the possibility of inconsistent data collection, it should be noted that there is growing support for outcome measurement that incorporates a variety of perspectives, including self-report, proxy, and objective measures.[7,38]

An important advantage of the interRAI system is that it allows for consistency in data collection across sites and also across types of care settings—the various versions of the RAI instruments use similar questions and data collection approaches. This advantage is particularly strong when contrasted with the alternative practice of trying to achieve consensus on the "battery" of measures that should be used in clinical practice and outcome evaluation. Even if a particular group achieves consensus on a set of tools (e.g., Dickinson, 1993),[39] another group is likely to agree on a different set (e.g., Pepersack, 2008),[40] and it is unlikely that all members of either group will be consistent in their use of the prescribed measures.

A limitation of the interRAI assessment systems is the same as for other approaches aiming to achieve a comprehensive, multidimensional assessment: not all of the assessment areas will point to relevant clinical outcomes for all patients, and it would still be necessary to identify the specific outcomes of interest for a specific intervention or for a specific patient. In the interRAI system, this is addressed to some extent through the use of "triggers" that are used to identify issues warranting further investigation, referred to as resident assessment protocols (RAPs)[41] or clinical assessment protocols (CAPs).[42]

The inadequacies of outcome measures have often been suggested as a possible explanation for negative or ambiguous results of intervention trials. This is illustrated in the following comments from several studies:

"The fact that we observed no significant differences in the prevention of decline in activities of daily living or cognitive function in our study may be explained in several ways … (including) … insensitivity of our outcome measures to improvements that did occur."[43]

"There might, however, have been positive effects which we could not detect. Our measurements on the health state may not have been sensitive enough to show relevant effects."[44]

"The outcome variables may have been wrongly chosen to measure the effects of this kind of program."[45]

"Common measures of disability may be insensitive to change in the outpatient setting of the day hospital."[46]

"For most of the published programs, efficacy was tested on questionable indicators (e.g., mortality, health services use), on a crude proxy for functional decline (e.g., admission to a nursing home), or using a global unresponsive measure of functional autonomy."[47]

"It is possible that the measures we used to evaluate health related quality of life lacked sufficient sensitivity."[48]

A point made clear in the appendix is the lack of consensus and consistency in the selection of outcome measures for geriatric interventions. The heterogeneous and individualized nature of both geriatric programs and their patients makes such a consensus unlikely. Williams has argued strongly for the individualized nature of geriatric care:

"It is clear, first, that there are immense individual differences among older people, more than at any earlier age, in virtually all types of characteristics—physical, mental, health, and socioeconomic. Thus when we consider what quality of life means to an older person and what features of quality of care may contribute to that quality of life, we *must* arrive at highly individualized conclusions. This principle is of course recommended for all ages, but it may not be so essential in some aspects of earlier life as it is in the lives of older people."[49]

Individualized outcome assessment

One attempt to reflect the individualized nature of older persons in outcome measurement is the use of clinical judgment, with such measures as the Clinical Global Impression[50] or Clinician Interview-Based Impression.[51] These approaches allow a clinically experienced rater to reflect individual characteristics and health concerns in an overall assessment of improvement. These measures provide a role for informed clinical judgment in outcome assessment, but do not provide details on the specific aspects of a patient's health or quality of life that may have been improved as a result of an intervention.

The individualized nature of geriatric care can also be addressed through individualized outcome measures. Individualized outcome measures allow for specific measurement domains to be selected that are most relevant for individual patients. Individualized measures can be used to generate clinical insights into the nature of the effects of geriatric interventions, and particularly into understanding the effects of Alzheimer's disease treatment[52]:

"To the extent that standard measures do not record ways in which important improvements or deteriorations occur, they miss an opportunity to enhance our understanding of what Alzheimer's disease looks like when it gets better, and to provide clinical correlates of supposed pharmacologic changes. In this regard, I believe that the developments of individualized outcome measures may provide some useful insights into patterns of clinically important changes and heterogeneous disease conditions."[53]

A number of fully or semiindividualized measures have been developed for use in a variety of settings.[54] The most widely known of these is likely goal attainment scaling (GAS), which was proposed by Kiresuk and Sherman in the 1960s as a tool for evaluating human service and mental health programs.[55] GAS is an individualized goal-setting and measurement approach that enables users to individualize goals to the needs, concerns, and wishes of a specific patient, and also to individualize the scale on which attainment of these goals is measured. GAS accommodates multiple individualized goals, and also permits calculation of an overall score that enables comparisons between individuals or between groups of patients. GAS differs from other individualized measures in two important respects. First, GAS allows for the individualization of the scales on which goals are measured and the goals. Second, GAS requires a judgment to be made at the beginning of treatment on the level of goal attainment that will be considered to be a successful outcome (rather than, for example, subjectively rating achievement of outcome on 10-point scales, as in the Canadian Occupational Performance Measure).[56]

Individual goals are scaled on a five-point rating scale of expected outcomes, from −2: much less than expected; −1: somewhat less than expected; 0: expected level (program goal); +1: somewhat better than expected: +2 much better than expected. The steps to construct a GAS "follow-up guide" are detailed in Table 39-1. An example follow-up guide is provided in Table 39-2. Goals can be weighted in terms of their relative importance, although equally weighted goals are generally recommended.[57] A summary goal attainment score (T score) allows comparison of outcomes for different

Table 39-1. Developing a Goal Attainment Scaling (GAS) Follow-up Guide

1. Identify the issues that will be the focus of treatment.
   - Focus on problems that are important to the client and that the intervention is expected to change.
2. Translate the selected problems into goals—aim for at least three.
   - It must be possible to observe or elicit the client's level of attainment on these goals at the time of follow-up.
3. Choose a brief title for each goal.
4. Select an indicator for each goal.
   - The indicator is the behavior or state that clearly represents the goal, and can be used to indicate progress in meeting the goal.
5. Specify the expected level of outcome for the goal.
   - Predict the status of the client on the selected goal at the end of treatment or at a prespecified follow-up time.
6. Describe the client's current status in relation to the goal indicator.
   - Typically this is at the "somewhat less" or "much less" level. This is usually designated with a "checkmark" on the guide.
7. Specify the remaining "somewhat better" and "somewhat less" than expected levels of outcome for the goal.
   - These are more or less likely but still realistically attainable outcomes.
8. Specify the remaining "much better" and "much less" than expected levels of outcome.
   - Achievable, still realistic limits of the indicator.
   - Represent outcomes that might be expected 5%–10% of the time.
9. Repeat scaling steps for each of the goals.
   - Try not to skip any of the five levels for each goal.
10. Although GAS is an individualized approach, descriptors, items, or scores from standardized measures may be useful in scaling some GAS goals.
11. On follow-up, rate the level for each goal that best reflects the client's current state. This is usually designated with an asterisk on the guide.
12. Determine the GAS follow-up score.

patients or for groups of patients. GAS scores for a large group of patients are expected to have a mean of 50 and a standard deviation of 10. The GAS score can be calculated using a formula[55] or looked up in a table (e.g., Zaza, et al, 1999)[58] if goals are unweighted. A standardized menu approach has been proposed as a means to facilitate goal setting.[59]

The first published use of GAS in geriatrics was in 1992.[60] Since then, the measurement properties of GAS in geriatric settings have been tested in a number of studies.[61] GAS has been found to have good interrater reliability (intraclass correlation coefficients of 0.87 to 0.93)[60,62,63] and to correlate with standardized measures such as the Barthel Index and with global ratings.[63] Of particular significance for outcome

Table 39-2. Goal Attainment Scaling Follow-up Guide

Attainment Levels	Mobility	Activities of Daily Living (ADLs)	Future Care Arrangements
Much better than expected +2	*>200 yards with walker, or independent with cane*	*Independent in ADLs and instrumental ADLs*	*Home with no need for home support*
Somewhat better than expected +1	*independent with walker (100-200 yards)**	*Independent in ADLs and instrumental ADLs, except outside activities*	*Home with weekly home support*
Expected level (program goal) 0	*independent with walker, limited distance(<100 yards)*	*Independent with ADLs, needs help with meal preparation, housework, and transportation**	*Home with home support 2-3 times/week**
Somewhat less than expected −1	*Walker with assistance* ✓	*Dependent in ADLs, except dressing* ✓	*Discharged to nursing home*
Much less than expected −2	*Bedfast*	*Dependent in ADLs, including dressing*	*On rehabilitation unit >7 weeks* ✓
Comments			*Patient does not wish nursing home placement*

Appendix

Appendix Table 1. Randomized Controlled Trials of Geriatric Interventions and Associated Outcome Measures

OUTCOME MEASURES				
Study	**Setting**	**Study Description**	**Physical Function**	**Cognitive Function**
Allen et al, 1986[1]	IGCS USA	1 year N = 185 Evaluated whether a geriatric consultation service (GCS) can provide additional input into patient care and the strategies that improve compliance to this input	Katz Index of Independence in Activities of Daily Living (ADLs),[2] Older American's Resources and Services (OARS), Instrumental Activities of Daily Living Scale (IADLs)[3]	Pfeiffer Short Portable Mental Status Questionnaire[4]
Alessi et al, 1997[7]	HAS USA	3 years N = 202 Measured the process of comprehensive geriatric assessment (CGA) and determined (1) major findings in CGA, (2) emergence of annual clinical yield of CGA, and (3) factors that affect patient adherence with recommendations	Oral health assessment,[8] vision and hearing test,[9] gait and balance assessment,[10] functional status assessment,[11] hematocrit and glucose testing, urinalysis, fecal occult blood testing	Kahn-Goldfarb Mental Status Questionnaire[12]
Applegate et al, 1990[16]	GEMU USA	1 year N = 155 Evaluated whether care for older patients in an geriatric assessment unit would affect their function, rate of institutionalization, and mortality rate	Self-reported ability to perform physical activities,[17] performance on timed physical tests,[18] self-reported ADLs showed significant improvement in study group than control in first 6 months ($P < .05$)	Folstein Mini-Mental State examination (MMSE)[19]

measurement in geriatrics is that GAS has consistently been found to be very responsive to change. This has been demonstrated in before and after studies[3,62–65] and in the context of a randomized controlled trial.[66] GAS has been used as an outcome measure in randomized trials of a geriatric assessment team[67] and of an antidementia medication.[68,69] In both cases, GAS measured statistically significant benefits of the intervention. The clinical utility of GAS in geriatrics has been assessed using qualitative methods.[70]

GAS is a measure that seems to be a particularly strong fit for the measurement needs and constraints of geriatric interventions. It has potential both as a research measure and as a clinical tool. Although goal priorities may differ among patients, caregivers, and clinicians,[71,72] involving diverse perspectives can generate rich insights into the interventions that will most benefit older patients, and into the effects of these interventions.

CONCLUSION

Measuring the outcomes of multidimensional geriatric interventions presents significant challenges. These challenges have resulted in frail older patients often being excluded from studies of interventions from which they might benefit, and in potential benefits of geriatric interventions not being detected by the measures used. After a quarter century of controlled trials in geriatrics, it seems unlikely or perhaps even inappropriate that consensus will be achieved on a set of standardized measures that will have wide applicability. For consistency of data collection and to provide comprehensive assessment information, there is a strong rationale to move toward standardized health information systems such as the interRAI. In measuring outcomes, Goal Attainment Scaling is an effective and clinically useful approach to addressing the challenges of outcome measures for heterogeneous, frail older patients.

ACKNOWLEDGMENTS

The author is grateful to Sarah Meyer for assistance in reviewing background literature for the development of this paper.

Psychosocial	Self-Rated Health	Mortality	Health Care Utilization	Other
Center for Epidemiologic Studies Depression Scale (CES-D)[5]			Admitting service used, number of days in institution	Veterans Alcoholism Screening Test,[6] time of year of consultation, number of medical problems per patient, compliance rates of recommendation; direct discussion with house staff lead to increased compliance in intervention group ($P = .0030$)
Social assessment, Geriatric Depression Scale (GDS)[13]				Percentage of ideal body weight,[14] medication review,[15] environmental assessment, adherence to recommendations; subjects more likely to adhere to recommendations involving referral to a physician than to a nonphysician professional, for community service, or for recommendations involving self-care activities ($P < .001$)
CES-D[5]	Acute Physiology and Chronic Health Evaluation (APACHE) II score[20]	Control group patients who were at lower-risk of immediate nursing home placement had significantly higher mortality at 6 months (95% CI = 1.2 to 15.2; $P < .05$), there was no significance in the higher-risk stratum	After 6 weeks significantly less study patients were living in an institution ($P < .01$); no significance at 6 months; significantly less study patients institutionalized at 1 year ($P < .05$), risk of nursing home admission 3.3 times higher in control group (95% CI = 2.6 to 3.8; $P < .001$), study group spent more days in rehabilitation than control group ($P < .0001$)	

(Continued)

Appendix Table 1. Randomized Controlled Trials of Geriatric Interventions and Associated Outcome Measures—Cont'd

OUTCOME MEASURES

Study	Setting	Study Description	Physical Function	Cognitive Function
Beyth et al, 2000[21]	GEMU USA	6 months N = 325 Studied the effectiveness of a multicompontent management program of warfarin therapy and warfarin-related major bleeding in older patients	Recurrent venous thromboembolism, therapeutic control of anticoagulant therapy measured by the "patient-time" approach[22] and the international normalized ratio[23]; intervention group patients were within the therapeutic range at each time period significantly more often than controls ($P < .001$)	
Boult et al, 2001[25]	OAS USA	18 months N = 568 Studied the effectiveness and costs of geriatric evaluation management (GEM) in preventing disability	Bed disability days (BDDs), restricted activity days (RASs),[26] Sickness Impact Profile (SIP): Physical Functioning Dimension;[27] treatment group lost less function after 12 and 18 months (*aOR*=.67, 95% *CI* = .47–.99), they had fewer health related restrictions in ADLs (*aOR*=.60, 95% *CI* = .37–.96)	
Burns et al, 2000[30]	OAS USA	2 years N = 98 Aimed at comparing the effectiveness of long-term primary care management by an interdisciplinary geriatric team	Katz Index,[2] IADL deficits[31] significantly better in GEM group at 1 year ($P = .006$),[11] study subjects showed improvement in RAND general well-being inventory[32] ($P = .001$)	Study group showed increase in MMSE score[19] at 2 years ($P = .025$)
Carpenter et al, 1990[36]	HAS UK	3 years N = 539 Tested benefits of regular surveillance on elderly people living at home	Winchester Disability Rating Scale[36]	
Clarke et al, 1992[37]	HAS UK	3 years N = 523 Tested the effect of social intervention in terms of mortality and morbidity on elderly people living alone	ADLs[38]	Measure of cognitive impairment and a simple screening tool for dementia[39]
Cohen et al, 2002[43]	GEMU/ OAS USA	3 years N = 1388 Assessed the effects of inpatient units and outpatient clinics on survival and functional status	Survival and quality of life with Medical Outcomes Study 36-Item Short-Form General Health Survey (MOS SF-36),[44,45] Katz ADLs,[2,46] Physical Performance Test,[47] positive effects on bodily pain at 12 months in GEMU treatment group ($P = 0.01$)* * Variation in significance at other follow-up times	

Psychosocial	Self-Rated Health	Mortality	Health Care Utilization	Other
		No significant difference between groups		Bleeding Severity Index[24] showed significantly more incidence of bleeding in control group at 1, 3, and 6 months (P = .0498)
GDS[28]; treatment group was less depressed at 12 months (P < .01) and 18 months (P < .01)	Individual questions on general health.[29]	No significant difference	Costs, Medicare expenditure, individual questions on use of nursing home and home health services; treatment group used less home health services (aOR = .60, 95% CI = .37–.92)	
Study group showed improvement on perceived global social activity (GSA)[33–35] (P = .001), on the CES-D[5] (P = .003), and on the perceived global life satisfaction (GLS) scale[33–35] (P < .001) at 2 years	Study subjects showed improvement on Global health perception[33–35] (P = .001) at 2 years	No significant difference	Number of days in institution, study subjects had smaller increases in number of clinical visits (P = .019) at 2 years	
		No significant difference	Geriatric and psychogeriatric community support services, primary health care team contacts, use of community support services, control group spent 33% more days in an institution than study group (P = 0.03)	Falls
Wenger's Scale (measure of support networks),[40] the Philadelphia Geriatric Morale Scale,[41] social contact score[42]	Perceived health status significantly greater in treatment group* *No p-value given	No significant difference		
		No significant difference	Utilization of health services, costs, GEMU treatment group experienced more days in the hospital (P < .001)	

(Continued)

Appendix Table 1. Randomized Controlled Trials of Geriatric Interventions and Associated Outcome Measures—Cont'd

OUTCOME MEASURES

Study	Setting	Study Description	Physical Function	Cognitive Function
Counsell et al, 2000[48]	GEMU USA	3 years N = 1531 Tested whether a multicomponent intervention called Acute Care for Elders improved functional outcomes and the process of care in hospitalized elderly patients	Mobility index,[49] Physical Performance and Mobility Examination (PPME),[50] Charlson comorbidity score,[51] IADLs,[31] Katz Index[2] decline at 12 months favoured intervention group ($P = .037$); fewer intervention patients experienced the composite outcome of either ADL decline from baseline or nursing home placement at discharge ($P = .027$); persisted at 1 year follow-up ($P = .022$)	Pfeiffer Short Portable Mental Status Questionnaire[52]
Epstein et al, 1990[55]	HAS USA	1 year N = 600 Studied the effectiveness of consultative geriatric assessment and follow-up for ambulatory patients	Physical examination, new diagnoses, functional impact of patient diagnosis, Katz Index,[2] OARS (IADLs),[56] SIP[57]	MMSE[19] showed significantly better cognitive function at 3 months than controls ($P < .05$) and those over 80 years improved more than those who were younger ($P < .05$)
Fabacher et al, 1994[62]	HAS USA	1 year N = 254 Examined the effectiveness of preventive home visits in improving health and function in older adults	Physical examination, health behaviour inventory, gait and balance assessment,[63] Katz Index,[64] IADLs[31] were significantly higher in intervention group at 1 year ($P < .05$)	MMSE[19]
Fretwell et al, 1990[65]	IGCS USA	6 months N = 436 Assessed whether early interdisciplinary geriatric assessment could prevent mental, physical and emotional decline without increasing hospital stay or costs	Katz Index[66]	MMSE[67]
Gayton et al, 1987[69]	IGCS Canada	6 months N = 222 Evaluated the effects of a interdisciplinary geriatric consultation team in an acute care hospital	Barthel Index,[70] Level of Rehabilitation Scale (LORS)[71]	Pfeiffer Short Portable Mental Status Questionnaire[4]
Gilchrist et al, 1988[72]	GEMU UK	22 months N = 222 Tested the efficacy of an orthopaedic geriatric unit in managing elderly women with proximal femoral fractures	General medical assessment, hip and chest X-ray, more patients in study group were found to have new medical disorders than those in control (95% $CI = 3.4$ to 28.5, $P < .025$)	Mental function[73,74]
Gunner-Svensson et al, 1984[75]	ICGS Denmark	11 years N = 343 Assessed whether social medical intervention would help to avoid relocation in nursing homes	Unspecified questions on somatic symptoms, functions, activities	Unspecified questions on mental condition with emphasis on dementia

Psychosocial	Self-Rated Health	Mortality	Health Care Utilization	Other
CES-D (short form),[53] physicians more often recognized depression in intervention group than controls (P = .02), patient satisfaction with hospitalization[54] was higher in intervention group (P = .001), along with caregiver satisfaction (P < .05)	Overall health status, APACHE II[20]		Reason for hospitalization, time from admission to initiation of discharge planning, social work consultations, orders for bed rest, physical therapy consults, application of physical restraints, length of stay, costs, intervention, physicians significantly reported no difficulty getting treatment plans carried out (P = .010), and noted that they were often informed of useful information on discharge plans (P = .015), additionally, intervention nurses reported higher satisfaction with extent of care (P = .001) and extent to which issues were discussed (P = .001)	Medications
Social support, social activities,[58] coping style, emotional health adapted from RAND Health Insurance Study,[59] satisfaction[60] showed significant benefits for those that were in the lowest quintile of functional health at 1 year (P < .05)	Changes in health status, overall perceived health with adapted RAND[61]	No significant difference	Nursing home placement, incidence of hospitalization, costs, length of stay, office visits, use of diagnostic tests	Medications, nutrition, economic issues, environmental issues
GDS[28]			Intervention group had significantly increased likelihood of having a primary care physician at 1 year (P < .05)	Environmental hazards, falls, immunization rates significantly improved in intervention group at 1 year (P < .05), nonprescription drug use increased significantly for control group at 1 year (P < .05)
Zung Self-Rating Depression Scale (SDS),[68] treatment groups emotional function improved (P = .045) at 6 weeks		No significant difference	Costs, number of days in institution	
		No significant difference	Health care utilization, number of days in institution, place of residence at discharge	
		No significant difference	Placement of patients, length of hospital stay	
Unspecified questions on communication		No significant difference	Housing, medical contact, help in illness, relocations significantly differed in favour of the intervention group for women over 80 years old (P < .05)	Diet, demographic information (age, sex, and marital status)

(Continued)

Appendix Table 1. Randomized Controlled Trials of Geriatric Interventions and Associated Outcome Measures—Cont'd

OUTCOME MEASURES

Study	Setting	Study Description	Physical Function	Cognitive Function
Hall et al, 1992[76]	HAS Canada	3 years N = 167 Evaluated a local health program (long-term care program of the B.C. Ministry of Health) to assist frail elderly persons living at home	ADLs, chronic disease	
Hansen et al, 1992[82]	HHAS Denmark	1 year N = 344 Evaluated a nurse and physician led follow-up model of home visits to elderly patients after discharge from hospital	General medical data	
Harris et al, 1991[83]	GEMU Australia	1 year N = 267 Aimed at testing the differences in medical management and clinical outcome between a designated geriatric assessment unit and two general medical units.	ADLs,[84] radiology and pathology tests, discharge diagnosis	MMSE[19]
Hebert et al, 2001[85]	HAS Canada	1 year N = 503 Tested the efficacy of a multidimensional program aimed at functional decline of elderly people	Functional Autonomy Measurement System (SMAF),[86] hearing	
Hendrikson et al, 1984[90]	HAS Denmark	3 years N = 285 Measured the effects of preventative community measures for elderly people living at home		
Hjort Sorensen & Sivertsen, 1988[91]	HAS Denmark	3 years N = 585 Tested the effectiveness of a socio-medical intervention aimed at relieving unmet medical and social needs of elderly people	ADLs and IADLS[92]	
Hogan et al, 1990[93]	IGCS Canada	1 year N = 132 Conducted a trial of a GCS in an acute care setting	Improved Barthel Index[94] at 1 year in intervention group ($P < .01$)	Mental Status Scale[95]
Hogan et al, 1987[96]	IGCS Canada	1 year N = 113 Assessed the effectiveness of a GCS on outcomes related to hospital stay	Barthel Index[94].	Improvement in Metal Status Score[95] in intervention group ($P < .01$)
Inouye et al, 1999[97]	GEMU USA	2 years N = 852 Evaluated a multicomponent strategy for the prevention of delirium in hospitalized older patients	Katz Index,[2] Jaeger vision test, whisper test,[98] APACHE II[20]	Confusion Assessment Method,[99] MMSE,[19] Digit Span Test,[100] modified Blessed Dementia Rating Scale[101, 102] showed significantly less incidence of dementia ($P = .02$) and low total number days of delirium ($P = .02$) and total number of episodes ($P = .03$) in intervention group

Psychosocial	Self-Rated Health	Mortality	Health Care Utilization	Other
Memorial University Happiness Scale,[77] UCLA Loneliness Scale,[78] Social Readjustment Rating Scale,[79] social support	MacMillan Health Opinion Index,[80] Health Locus of Control (HLC)[81]	Significantly higher survival rates for those in the treatment group at 3 years (P = .054)	At 2 years, significantly more of the treatment group remained at home (P = .02), and at 3 years (P = .04)	Smoking, alcohol consumption, nutrition, number of prescription medications
Unspecified social data		No significant difference	Number of days in institutions, number of readmissions to the hospital, intervention patients were admitted to a nursing home significantly less than controls (P < .05) at 1 year follow-up	
		No significant difference	Accommodation prior to hospitalization, length of admission, accommodations at discharge	Procedures performed, medications on admission and discharge showed that patients in the geriatric assessment unit were discharged on fewer drugs (P < .04)
General Well-being Schedule,[87, 88] Social Provisions Scale[89]		No significant difference	Admissions, use of health services	Medications, risk of falls
		Significantly more deaths in control group than in intervention group (P < .05)	Contact with general practitioners, or primary care practitioners, significantly more medical calls registered to control group (P < .05), significant reduction in hospital admissions in intervention group (P < .05), admissions into nursing home significantly larger in control group (P < .05)	
Quality of life	Self-rated health	No significant difference	Practical help received, need for more help, number of institutionalizations	
		Intervention had improved 6 month survival (P < .05) at 4 months	Number of days in institution, living arrangements post discharge	
		Lower short-term death rates in intervention group (P < .05)	Costs, number of days in institution, number of referrals to community services at discharge higher in intervention group (P < .005)	Falls, treatment group received fewer medications at discharge (P = .05)
				Adherence to intervention

(Continued)

Appendix Table 1. Randomized Controlled Trials of Geriatric Interventions and Associated Outcome Measures—Cont'd

OUTCOME MEASURES

Study	Setting	Study Description	Physical Function	Cognitive Function
Jensen et al, 2003[103]	ICGS Sweden	34 weeks N = 362 Assessed the effectiveness of a multifactorial program for the prevention of falls and injury on elderly with high and low levels of cognition	Hearing and vision, Barthel ADL Index,[70, 104] Mobility Interaction Fall Chart,[105] DiffTUG (measures ability to walk and carry a glass of water)[106]	MMSE[19]
Kennie et al, 1988[108]	IGCS UK	18 months N = 144 Assessed whether prospective management could reduce various outcome measures in females with femoral fractures	Katz Index,[2] ADLs significantly better in treatment group ($P = .005$)	Pfeiffer Short Portable Mental State Questionnaire[4]
McEwen et al, 1990[109]	HAS UK	20 months N = 296 Tested the effectiveness of a nurse-run screening program	McMaster health index,[110] functional and problem evaluation interview[111]	
Melin et al, 1992[114]	HHAS Sweden	6 months N = 249 Assessed the impact of a primary home care intervention program on patient outcomes after discharge from a short-stay hospital	Katz Index,[17, 66, 115, 116] IADLs[117, 118] improved at follow-up in study group ($P = .04$), medical disorders declined in the study group at 6-month follow-up ($P < .001$)	MMSE[19, 119]
Newbury et al, 2001[120]	HAS Australia	2 years N = 100 Measured the effectiveness of a nurse-led health assessment of elderly people living independently at home	Hearing and vision, physical condition, Barthel Index,[70] mobility	MMSE[19]
Pathy et al, 1992[122]	HAS UK	3 years N = 725 Evaluation of a case finding and surveillance program of elderly patients at home	General health status, Townsend Score[123]	

Psychosocial	Self-Rated Health	Mortality	Health Care Utilization	Other
				Environmental hazards, medications, falls (number of residents suspected of falling, number of falls, and time to occurrence of first fall significantly longer in high MMSE intervention group ($P < .001$)), fall related injuries using Abbreviated Injury Scale[107] showed increased injuries in low MMSE control group ($P = .006$)
			Significantly fewer discharges of patients in treatment group to NHS or private nursing care ($P = .03$)	
Nottingham health profile,[112] Philadelphia Morale Scale,[113] significantly better in test group with respect to attitude in own ageing ($P < .01$) and loneliness ($P < .05$) at 20 month follow-up, emotional reaction ($P < .05$) and isolation ($P < .01$) perceived to be worse in control group at 20 month follow-up.		No significant difference	Contact with health and social services	Compliance with medication
Social function ratings on activities attended, contacts made during preceding week was significantly higher in study group ($P = .01$) at 6 month follow-up			Number of admissions to short term care and rehabilitative care hospitals, number of inpatient care days and outpatient care days showed that study group spent more days in home care than controls ($P < .001$) but fewer days in long-term hospital care than controls ($P < .001$)	Number of medications increased in control group at 6 month follow-up ($P = .02$)
Unspecified social factors, SF-36 Quality of Life Questionnaire[121] and GDS-15[13] showed significant improvement in intervention group at 1 year ($P = .032$ *and* $P = .05$, *respectively*)	Self-rated health	No significant difference	Housing, admission to institutions	Medication, compliance, vaccinations, alcohol and tobacco use, nutrition, number of problems in each group, number of participants with problems, number of self-reported falls showed significant improvement in intervention group ($P = .033$)
Nottingham health profile Life Satisfaction index[124]	Self-rated overall health significantly higher in intervention group ($P < .05$)	Significantly lower in intervention group ($P < .05$)	Use of services (domiciliary visits, contact with general practitioner, chiropody and attendance allowance), questions about Meals on Wheels and home help, hospital admissions did not differ but duration of stay was shorter in intervention group ($P < .01$)	

(Continued)

Appendix Table 1. Randomized Controlled Trials of Geriatric Interventions and Associated Outcome Measures—Cont'd

OUTCOME MEASURES

Study	Setting	Study Description	Physical Function	Cognitive Function
Powell & Montgomery, 1990[125]	GEMU Canada	3 months N = 203 Studied the effectiveness of an inpatient geriatric unit at a hospital	Functional activity	Cognitive function improved between discharge and home visit in intervention group* *No p-value given
Reuben et al, 1999[126]	OAS USA	15 months N = 363 Tested the effectiveness of outpatient CGA coupled with an adherence intervention	NIA lower extremity battery,[127] Functional Status Questionnaire,[128] MOS SF-36[129, 130] showed change scores for treatment group in physical functioning (P = .021), RAS and BDD[131] significantly lower in treatment group (P = .006), Physical Performance Test[47] showed treatment effect (P = .019)	MMSE,[19] mental health summaries showed significant treatment effect (P = .006)
Rubenstein et al, 1984[134]	GEMU USA	2 years N = 123 Assessed the effectiveness of a geriatric evaluation unit in improving patient outcomes	IADLs,[31] Personal self-maintenance scale[31] showed significant improvement in study patients (P < .01), almost 5 times as many new diagnoses were made in study group than controls (P < .001)	Kahn-Goldfarb Mental Status Questionnaire[12]
Rubin et al, 1992[135]	HHAS USA	1 year N = 200 Studied the effectiveness of a GEM program on health care charges and Medicare	Medical history, Katz Index,[66] IADLs	Sensory and communication abilities,[136] MMSE[56]
Rubin et al, 1993[137]	OAS USA	1 year N = 200 Assessed the effect of outpatient GEM on physical function, mental status and well-being	Katz Index,[66] IADLs[46] showed greater improvement and less decline in treatment group at 1 year (P = .038)	MMSE[52]
Shaw et al, 2003[139]	IGCS UK	1 year N = 274 Determined the effectiveness of multifactorial intervention after falls in older patients with cognitive impairments and dementia	General medical examination, mobility assessment,[140] assessment of walking aids, feet and footwear[141]	
Silverman et al, 1995[143]	OAS USA	1 year N = 442 Studied the process and outcome of outpatient CGA	ADLs,[3,144] Barthel Index,[94] urinary and bowel incontinence identified significantly more often in study group (P < .0001)	MMSE,[19] Clinical Dementia Rating Scale (CDR),[145] cognitive impairment identified significantly more often in study group (P < .0001)

Psychosocial	Self-Rated Health	Mortality	Health Care Utilization	Other
Depression, life satisfaction		Fewer patients died in intervention group* * No p-value given	Duration of stay longer in intervention group but overall admissions were lower* * No p-value given	
Patient Satisfaction Questionnaire,[132] Perceived Efficacy in Patient-Physician Interaction scale,[133] treatment group benefited on social functioning scale ($P = .01$), and emotional well being ($P = .016$) at 15 months	Treatment group reported less pain[129] than control group ($P = .043$)	No significant difference		Falls
Philadelphia Geriatric Morale Scale[113] showed significant improvement at 1 year follow-up for study patients ($P < .05$)		Mortality rate was significantly higher in control group at 1 year follow-up ($P < .005$)	Utilization costs, initial placement at discharge; significantly higher study patients were discharged to their home than controls ($P < .05$), more than twice as many controls were discharged to a nursing home ($P < .05$), study patients underwent more specialized screening examinations and consultations than controls ($P < .001$), at 1 year follow-up controls averaged more than twice as many nursing home days ($P < .05$)	Medications
Social history, affective and behavioural status[136]			Experimental group was significantly more likely to receive home health care than control group ($P < .01$), control group had significantly greater inpatient charges ($P < .03$) and Medicare reimbursement ($P < .005$)	Medications
Life Satisfaction Index-Z (LSI-Z)[138]	Self-perception of health status (OARS)[56] was significantly higher for the treatment group ($P = .006$); perceived less decline in health ($P = .007$) and fewer activity limitations ($P = .024$)	No significant difference	No significant differences between groups on long-term nursing placements	
		No significant difference	Fall related attendance at accident or emergency department, fall related hospital admissions	Number of falls, time to first fall, injury rates, medications, environmental hazards[142]
Measures of social support, patient satisfaction with care,[146] clinical depression and anxiety sections of Diagnostic Interview Schedule (DIS)[147, 148] showed significantly lessened anxiety in study group at 1 year ($P = .036$), depression identified significantly more often in study group ($P = .0004$)	Self-perceived health status		Nursing home institutionalizations	Changes in participant status, caregiver stress[149] was significantly less at 1 year in study group ($P = .002$)

(Continued)

Appendix Table 1. Randomized Controlled Trials of Geriatric Interventions and Associated Outcome Measures—Cont'd

OUTCOME MEASURES

Study	Setting	Study Description	Physical Function	Cognitive Function
Strandberg et al, 2001[150]	OAS Finland	5 years N = 400 Determined the effectiveness of a multifactorial prevention program for composite major cardiovascular events in the elderly with athero-sclerotic disease	General medical examination, cardio-vascular tests (blood pressure, heart rate and 12-lead resting electro-cardiogram), blood tests, physical function,[151] clinical events	Consortium to Establish a Registry for Alzheimer's Disease tool (CERAD)[152]
Stuck et al, 1995[155]	HAS USA	3 years N = 414 Evaluated the effect of in-home CGA and follow-up of elderly people	Geriatric Oral Health Assessment Index,[8] balance and gait,[156] vision and hearing,[9] treatment group required less assistance in basic ADLs[11] ($P = .02$) at 3 years	Kahn-Goldfarb Mental Status Questionnaire[12]
Stuck et al, 2000[159]	OAS Switzer-land	3 years N = 791 Examined the effects that preventive home visits with annual multidi-mensional assessments have on functional status and institutional-ization between high- and low-risk older persons	Gait and balance performance,[63] ADLs and IADLs[11]; intervention group at low baseline were less dependent in IADLs (95% *CI* = 0.3 to 1.0, $P = .04$)	MMSE[19]
Teasdale et al, 1983[161]	GEMU USA	1 year N = 124 Assessed whether a geriatric assess-ment unit using a multidisciplinary team approach impacted patient placement outcomes		
Thomas et al, 1993[162]	IGCS USA	1 year N = 120 Tested the effectiveness of a inpatient geriatric consultation team	Functional Assessment Inventory (FAI)[163]: physical and activities scales, Katz Index[2]	
Timonen et al, 2002[164]	OAS Finland	9 months N = 68 Studied the effects of a multi-component training program focused on strength training after hospitalization	Diseases, strength and physical performance tests, strength of knee extension significantly better after intervention in study group at 3 and 9 months ($P = .004$ *and* $P = .009$, *respectively*), isometric hip abduction strength significantly improved in intervention group at 3 months ($P = .004$), maximum walking speed improved significantly at 3 and 9 months in study group ($P = .004$ *and* $P = .022$, *respectively*), Berg Balance Scale[165] significantly better in study group at 3 and 9 months ($P = .004$ *and* $P = .001$, *respectively*)	
Tinetti et al, 1994[166]	HAS USA	1 year N = 301 Evaluated the effect of multiple-risk-factor reduction on incidence of falls	Presence of chronic disease, ADLs,[31] vision[167] and hearing,[168] Sickness Impact Profile (ambulation and mobility subscales),[27] risk factor for balance impairment reduced in intervention group at 1 year ($P = .001$), impairment in toilet transfers reduced ($P = .05$)	

Psychosocial	Self-Rated Health	Mortality	Health Care Utilization	Other
Health related quality of life using the 15D,[153, 154] Zung Questionnaire		No significant difference	Health care resource utilization, hospitalizations, permanent institutionalization	
GDS,[13] extent of social network and quality of social support[157]			Costs, significantly more visits to general practitioner among intervention group patients(P = .007), nursing home admission higher among control group patients (P = .02)	Medications, environmental hazards, percentage of ideal body weight[158]
GDS[13]	Self perceived general health,[160] self reported chronic conditions		Nursing home admission was higher in high-risk intervention group (P = .02)	Medication use[15]
		No significant difference	Source of admission, placement at discharge, location 6 months post admission, location of patient after discharge, mean duration of stay was significantly longer in intervention group (P < .001)	
FAI: psychological and social scale[163]		Significantly more patients died in control group at 6 months (P = .01)	Referrals to community service, number of post discharge general practitioner visits, discharge destination, number of days in institution, control group had significantly more readmissions (P = .02)	FAI: economic scale[163]
				Medication
Depressive symptoms[169]			Costs	Room-by-room number of hazards for falling, Falls Efficacy Scale,[170] at 1 year, control group fell significantly more (P = .04), intervention group significantly reduced number of medications (P = .009)

(Continued)

Appendix Table 1. Randomized Controlled Trials of Geriatric Interventions and Associated Outcome Measures—Cont'd

OUTCOME MEASURES

Study	Setting	Study Description	Physical Function	Cognitive Function
Toseland et al, 1997[171]	OAS USA	2 years N = 160 Investigated the effectiveness of an outpatient GEM team by examining changes in health status, health care utilization and costs	SF-20,[172] Functional Independence Measure (FIM)[173–175]	
Tucker et al, 1984[176]	OAS New Zealand	5 months N = 120 Assessed the effectiveness of a day hospital in the geriatric service	Significant increase in Northwick Park ADL Index[177] at 6 weeks for intervention group (P = .002)	Cognitive function[178]
Tulloch & Moore, 1979[179]	OAS UK	2 years N = 295 Evaluated the effects of a geriatric screening and surveillance program on health status of elderly people	Screening for medical disorders found significantly greater incidence in the study group compared to controls (P < .01); greater proportion of medical problems unrecognized in control group (P < .001)	
van Haastregt et al, 2000[180]	HAS Netherlands	18 months N = 316 Assessed whether a multifactorial program of home visits reduces falls and mobility impairments in the elderly	Physical health, mobility, control scale and mobility range scale of SIP68,[181, 182] number of physical complaints, Frenchay daily activities[183, 184]	Mental health section of RAND-36[10, 15]
van Rossum et al, 1993[190]	HAS Netherlands	3 years N = 580 Tested the effectiveness of preventive home visits to elderly people	Self-rated functional state, hearing and vision problems	Memory disturbances[178]
Vetter et al, 1984[193]	HAS UK	2 years N = 1286 Evaluated the effectiveness of health visitors on elderly population of an urban (Gwent) and a rural (Powys) town	Townsend Score[123]	
Vetter et al, 1992[196]	HAS UK	4 years N = 674 Assessed whether health visitors reduced the incidence of fractures in the elderly	Townsend Score,[123] medical condition, assessment and improvement of general muscle tone	

Psychosocial	Self-Rated Health	Mortality	Health Care Utilization	Other
		No significant difference	Outpatient utilization (visitation of UPC/GEM clinic, medicine clinic, surgery clinic, emergency room, and total clinic visits), inpatient utilization (number of hospital admissions, hospital days of care, nursing home admissions and nursing home days of care); GEM patients used significantly fewer emergency room services ($P < .05$), GEM patients used significantly more total outpatient clinic services ($P < .01$), Costs (total inpatient costs, total outpatient costs, nursing home costs, institutional costs, total health care costs); significantly more outpatient cost in GEM patients over 2 years ($P < .05$)	
Zung Index,[68] intervention group showed improved mood at 5 months ($P = .011$)			Domiciliary services, day hospital costs 1/3 greater than alternative	
			Rate of hospital admission, outpatient referrals was significantly higher in study group ($P < .01$), time spent in hospital was less for the study group than controls ($P < .01$)	Socio-economic problems
Social functioning,[185] psychosocial functioning	Perceived health by RAND-36,[186, 187] perceived gait problems			Falls efficacy scale,[170, 188] falls, medications, environmental hazards[190]
Self-rated well-being,[191] loneliness,[192] modified Zung Index[68]	Self-rated health	No significant difference	Costs, use of community and institutional care	
Mental disability,[194, 195] use of social contacts, self-rated quality of life		Significantly more deaths in Powys ($P < .01$)	Use of medical and social services, Gwent intervention group used chiropody significantly more than Powys ($P = .02$), significantly more home visits from Gwent intervention group ($P = .005$)	Availability of caregiver, composition of household, type and quality of housing, participants in Gwent attended more lunch clubs than Powys ($P < .05$)
				Falls and fractures, nutrition, medications, environmental hazards

(Continued)

Appendix Table 1. Randomized Controlled Trials of Geriatric Interventions and Associated Outcome Measures—Cont'd

OUTCOME MEASURES

Study	Setting	Study Description	Physical Function	Cognitive Function
Wagner et al, 1994[197]	HAS USA	2 years N = 1559 Tested a multicomponent program to prevent disability and falls in older adults	Fitness test, physical limitations scale,[198] hearing and vision, control group worsened in RAS ($P < .05$), BBD[131] ($P < .01$) and MOS[199, 200] ($P = .05$) at 1 year follow-up	
Williams et al, 1987[201]	OAS USA	1 year N = 117 Evaluated whether team-oriented assessment can improve traditional health care approaches	Functional status and medical diagnoses[202, 203]	
Winograd et al, 1991[204]	IGCS USA	1 year N = 197 Studied the effect of an inpatient multidisciplinary GCS on health care utilization, functional and mental status	Physical Self-Maintenance Scale, ADLs, IADLs	MMSE[19]
Yeo et al, 1987[205]	OAS USA	18 months N = 205 Compared the effects of two models of outpatient care on functional health and subjective well-being	SIP[57] showed significantly less functional decline in intervention patients ($P = .029$) and its physical dimension ($P = .011$)	

GEMU, geriatric and evaluation management unit, HAS, home assessment service, HHAS, hospital home assessment service, IGCS, inpatient geriatric consultation service, OAS, outpatient assessment service.

Psychosocial	Self-Rated Health	Mortality	Health Care Utilization	Other
	Self-rated health and practices questionnaire			Environmental hazards, alcohol consumption, medications, significantly fewer members of intervention group reported falling than of control group (*difference* = 9.3%, 95% *CI* = 4.1 to 14.5%) at 1 year follow-up
Social supports[202, 203]			Health care utilization, degree of client satisfaction with evaluation, health service utilization behaviours	
Philadelphia Geriatric Morale Scale[113]			Health care utilization	
Zung Self-Rating Depression Scale (SDS),[68, 206] Life Satisfaction Index A (LSI),[207] Affect Balance Scale (ABS),[208] psychosocial dimension of SIP[57]	Self-rated health measure[209, 210]	No significant difference		

Appendix Table 2. Summary of Outcome Measures Used in Randomized Controlled Trials of Geriatric Interventions

OUTCOME MEASURES	Physical Function	Cognitive Function	Psychosocial
Tests Used	• Acute Physiology and Chronic Health Evaluation APACHE II[20] (1) • Barthel Index[70,94] (6) • Berg Balance Scale[162] (1) • Bed disability days and restricted activity days[26,131] (3) • DiffTUG[106] (1) • Functional Autonomy Assessment System (SMAF)[86] (1) • Functional Independence Measure (FIM)[173-175] (1) • Functional and problem evaluation interview[112] (1) • Functional Status Questionnaire [128] (1) • General functional assessment [11,17,151] (5) • General gait and balance assessment[10,63, 156] (4) • Hearing and vision tests[9,99,167,168] (9) • Katz Index of Independence in Activities of Daily Living[2,64-66,92,115,116] (13) • Level of Rehabilitation Scale (LORS)[71] (1) • McMaster health index[111] (1) • Mobility Index[49,140] (2) • Mobility Interaction Fall Chart[105] (1) • NIA lower extremity battery[127] (1) • Older American's Resources and Services Inventory (OARS)[3,56]/Functional Assessment Inventory (FAI)[163] (4) • Oral health assessment[8] (2) • Other (40) • Personal self-maintenance scale[31] (1) • Physical assessment[18, 47] (12) • Physical limitations scale[198] (1) • Physical Performance and Mobility Examination (PPME)[50] (1) • Physical Self-Maintenance Scale (1) • RAND Medical Outcomes Study Short Form General Health Survey (MOS SF-36)[32,44,45,129,130,172, 199-200] (5) • Sickness Impact Profile (SIP): Physical Functioning Dimension[27,57, 181,182] (4) • Townsend Score[123] (3) • Unspecified ADLs[11,31,38,84, 177,183,184] (12) • Unspecified IADLs[11,31, 46,92, 117, 118] (10) • Winchester Disability Rating Scale[36] (1)	• Blessed Dementia Rating Scale[101,102] (1) • Consortium to Establish a Registry for Alzheimer's Disease tool (CERAD)[152] (1) • Clinical Dementia Rating Scale (CDR)[145] (1) • Confusion Assessment Method[98] (1) • Digit Span Test[100] (1) • Folstein Mini Mental State Examination (MMSE)[19,52,56,67,119] (16) • General mental function[73,74,95, 178] (10) • Kahn-Goldfarb Mental Status Questionnaire [12] (3) • Pfeiffer Short Portable Mental Status Questionnaire[4, 52] (4) • RAND MOS SF-36, mental health section[10,15] (1) • Unspecified dementia screening tool[39] (1)	• Affect Balance Scale (ABS)[208] (1) • Center for Epidemiological Studies Depression Scale (CES-D)[5,53,169] (4) • Diagnostic Interview Schedule (DIS), depression and anxiety sections[147,148] (1) • General depression[169] (2) • General Well-being Schedule[87,88] (1) • General social functioning[185] (3) • General social support[157,202,203] (6) • Geriatric Depression Scale (GDS)[13,28] (6) • Global life satisfaction scale (GLS)[33-35] (1) • Global social activity (GSA)[33-35] (1) • Life Satisfaction Index (LSI-Z)[124,138,207] (3) • Memorial University Happiness Scale[77] (1) • Nottingham health profile[112] (2) • OARS/FAI: Psychological and social scale[163] (1) • Other (17) • Patient-Physician Interaction scale[133] (1) • Patient Satisfaction Questionnaire[132] (1) • Philadelphia Geriatric Morale Scale [41,113] (4) • Quality of life (3) • RAND MOS SF-36 emotional health questions [59] (1), quality of life questions[121] (1) • Self-Rating Depression Scale[68] (1) • SIP: psychological deminsion[57] (1) • Social contact score[42] (1) • Social Provisions Scale[89] (1) • Social Readjustment Rating Scale[79] (1) • UCLA Loneliness Scale[78] (1) • Wenger's Scale[40] (measure of support networks) (1) • Zung Questionnaire[68, 206] (5) • 15D (Health-Related Quality of Life)[153, 154] (1)
Conclusions	Of 56 studies described, 54 measured physical function, using 32 different measures, and of which 23 studies reported statistical significance.	Of 56 studies described, 33 measured cognitive function, using 11 different measures, and of which 6 studies reported statistical significance.	Of 56 studies described, 37 measures psychosocial function, using 29 different measures, and of which 12 studies reported statistical significance.

*Numbers in bold denote the frequency of instruments used within the collective studies.

**Instruments categorized in terms of reported use within each study (e.g. SF-36 may be used as a measure of physical function, self-rated health or quality of life)

For a complete list of references, please visit online only at www.expertconsult.com

Self-Rated Health	Mortality	Health Care Utilization	Other
• APACHE II[20,23] (2) • Global health perception[33-35] (1) • Health Locus of Control (HLC)[81] (1) • MacMillan Health Opinion Index[80] (1) • OARS/FAI[56] (1) • Other (2) • RAND MOS SF-36[61,129,186,187] (2) • Unspecified measure of perceived health[29,160] (11)		• Admitting service used (2) • Application for physical restraints (1) • Client satisfaction (1) • Costs (15) • General health and support services utilization (25) • Housing (2) • Institutionalization (20) • Number of days in institution (19) • Number of days in rehabilitation (1) • Number of readmissions (3) • Number of referrals (3) • Other (7) • Place of residence at admission (1) • Place of residence at discharge (6) • Practical help received (1) • Primary health care team contacts (1) • Reason for hospitalization (1) • Relocations (1) • Use of diagnostic tests (2)	• Abbreviated Injury Scale[107] (1) • Alcohol consumption (3) • Bleeding Severity Index[24] (1) • Compliance rates (5) • Environmental assessment (10) • FAI: Economic Scale[163] (1) • Falls Efficacy Scale[170,188] (2) • Immunization rates (2) • Medication Review[15] (2) • Nutrition (4) • Other (17) • Percentage of ideal body weight[14,158] (2) • Tobacco use (2) • Veterans Alcohol Screening Test[6] (1) • Unspecified measure of falls (12) • Unspecified measure of medications (19)
Of 56 studies described, 18 measured self-rated health, using 8 different measures, and of which 4 studies reported statistical significance.	Of 56 studies described, 35 measured mortality, and of which 9 studies reported statistical significance.	Of 56 studies described, 45 measured health care utilization, using 19 different measures, and of which 24 studies reported statistical significance.	Of 56 studies described, 32 measured "other" outcomes, using 16 different measures, and of which 13 studies reported statistical significance.

Appendix References

1. Allen CM, Becker PM, McVey LJ, et al. A randomized, controlled clinical trial of a geriatric consultation team: compliance with recommendations. JAMA 1986;255:2617–21.
2. Katz S, Ford AB, Moskowitz RW, et al. Studies of illness in the aged: the index of ADL: a standardized measure of biological and psychosocial function. JAMA 1963;185:914–9.
3. Pfeiffer E. Multidimensional Functional Assessment: The OARS Methodology. Durham, NC: Center for the Study of Aging and Human Development, Duke University; 1975.
4. Pfeiffer E. A short portable mental status questionnaire for the assessment of organic brain deficit in elderly patients. J Am Geriatr Soc 1975;23:433.
5. Radloff LS. The CES-D scale: a self-report depression scale, for research in the general population. Appl Psychol Meas 1977;1:385–401.
6. Magruder-Habib K. Validation of the Veteras Alcoholism Screening Test. J Stud Alcohol 1982;43:910–26.
7. Alessi CA, Stuck AE, Aronow HU, et al. The process of care in preventive in-home comprehensive geriatric assessment. J Am Geriatr Soc 1997;45:1044–50.
8. Atchinson KA, Dolan TA. Development of a geriatric oral health assessment index. J Dent Educ 1990;54:680–7.
9. Lachs MS, Feinstein AR, Cooney LM, et al. A simple procedure for general screening for functional disability in elderly patients. Ann Intern Med 1990;112:699–706.
10. Tenetti ME. Performance-oriented assessment of mobility problems in elderly patients. J Am Geriatr Soc 1986;34:119–26.
11. Lawton MP, Moss M, Fulcomer M, et al. A research and service oriented multilevel assessment instrument. J Gerontol 1982;37:91–9.
12. Kahn RL, Goldfarb AI, Pollack M, et al. A brief objective measure for the determination of mental status in the aged. Am J Psychiatry 1960;117:326–8.
13. Sheikh JI, Yesavage JA. Geriatric Depression Scale (GDS): recent evidence and development of a shorter version. Clin Gerontol 1986;5:122–5.
14. Master AM, Lasser RP, Beckman G. Tables of average weight and height of Americans aged 65 to 94 years. JAMA 1960;172:658–63.
15. Stuck AE, Beers MH, Steiner A, et al. Inappropriate medication use in community-residing older persons. Arch Intern Med 1994;154:2195–200.
16. Applegate WB, Miller ST, Graney MJ, et al. A randomized controlled trial of a geriatric assessment unit in a community rehabilitation hospital. N Engl J Med 1990;322:1572–8.
17. Jette AM, Branch LG. The Framingham disability study. II. Physical disability among the aging. Am J Public Health 1982;71:1211–6.
18. Williams ME, Hadler NM, Earp JAL. Manual ability as a marker of dependency in geriatric women. J Chronic Dis 1981;35:115–22.
19. Folstein M, Folstein S, McHugh PR. Mini-mental state: a practical method for grading the cognitive state of patients for the clinician. J Psychiatr Res 1975;12:189–98.
20. Knaus WA, Draper EA, Wagner DP, et al. APACHE II: a severity of disease classification system. Crit Care Med 1985;13:818–29.
21. Beyth RJ, Quinn L, Landefeld CS. A multicomponent intervention to prevent major bleeding complications in older patients receiving warfarin: a randomized controlled trial. Ann Intern Med 2000;133:687–95.
22. Landefeld CS, Anderson PA, Goodnough LT, et al. The Bleeding Severity Index: validation and comparison to other methods for classifying bleeding complications of medical therapy. J Clin Epidemiol 1989;42:711–8.
23. Rosendaal FR, Cannegieter SC, van der Meer FJM, et al. A method to determine the optimal intensity of oral anticoagulant therapy. J Thromb Haemost 1993;69:236–9.
24. Hirch J, Dalen JE, Deykin D, et al. Oral anticoagulants. Mechanism of action, clinical effectiveness, and optimal therapeutic range. Chest 1995;108(Suppl 4):231S–46S.
25. Boult C, Boult LB, Morishita L, et al. A randomized clinical trial of outpatient geriatric evaluation and management. J Am Geriatr Soc 2001;49:351–9.
26. Kovar MG, Poe G. The design (1973-84) and procedures (1975-83) of the national health interview survey. Vital Health Stat 1987;1:1–15.
27. Bergner M, Bobbitt RA, Carter WB, et al. The sickness impact profile: development and final revision of a health status measure. Med Care 1981;9:787–805.
28. Yesavage JA, Brink TL. Development and validation of a geriatric depression screening scale: a preliminary report. J Psychiatr Res 1982;17:37–49.
29. Kovar MG, Fitti JE, Chyba MM. The longitudinal study of aging. Vital Health Stat 1992;1:1–248.
30. Burns R, Nicols LO, Martindale-Adams J, et al. Interdisciplinary geriatric primary care evaluation and management: two-year outcomes. J Am Geriatr Soc 2000;48:8–13.
31. Lawton MP, Brody EM. Assessment of older people: self-maintaining and instrumental activities of daily living. Gerontologist 1969;9:179–86.
32. Brook RH, Ware JE, Davies-Avery A, et al. Overview of adult health status measures fielded in Rand's health insurance study. Med Care 1979;17(Suppl 17):1–131.
33. Applegate WB, Phillips HL, Schnaper H, et al. A randomized controlled trial of the effects of three antihypertensive agents on blood pressure control and quality of life in older women. Arch Intern Med 1991;151:1817–23.
34. Engle VF, Graney MJ. Self-assessed and functional health of older women. Int J Aging Hum Dev 1986;22:301–13.
35. Cantril H. The Pattern of Human Concerns. Piscataway, NJ: Rutgers University Press; 1965.
36. Carpenter GI, Demopoulos GR. Screening the elderly in the community. Br Med J 1990;300:1253–6.
37. Clarke M, Clarke SJ, Jagger C. Social intervention and the elderly. Am J Epidemiol 1992;136:1517–23.
38. Jagger C, Clarke M, Davies RA. The elderly at home: indices of disability. J Epidemiol Community Health 1984;40:139–42.
39. Clarke M, Jagger C, Anderson J, et al. The prevalence of dementia in a total population: a comparison of two screening instruments. Age Ageing 1991;20:396–403.
40. Wegner GC. The Supportive Network. London: Allen & Unwin; 1984.
41. Morris JN, Sherwood S. A retesting and modification of the Philadelphia Geriatric Center Morale Scale. J Gerontol 1975;30:77–84.
42. Tunstall J. Old and Alone: A Sociological Study of Old People. London: Routledge & Kegan Paul; 1966.
43. Cohen HJ, Feussner JR, Weinberger M, et al. A controlled trial of inpatient and outpatient geriatric evaluation and management. N Engl J Med 2002;346:905–12.
44. Tarlow AR, Ware JE, Greenfield S, et al. The Medical Outcomes Study: an application of methods for monitoring the results of medical care. JAMA 1989;262:925–30.
45. Weinberger M, Oddone EZ, Henderson WG. Does increased access to primary care reduce hospital readmission? N Engl J Med 1996;334:1441–7.
46. Fillenbaum G. Screening the elderly: a brief instrumental activities of daily living measure. J Am Geriatr Soc 1985;33:698–706.
47. Rueben DB, Siu AL. An objective measure of physical function of elderly outpatients: the Physical Performance Test. J Am Geriatr Soc 1990;38:1105–12.
48. Counsell SR, Holder CM, Liebnauer LL, et al. Effects of a mulitcomponent intervention on functional outcomes and process of care in hospitalized older patients: a randomized controlled trial of acute care for elders (ACE) in a community hospital. J Am Geriatr Soc 2000;48:1572–81.
49. Stewart AL, Ware JE, Brook RH. Advances in the measurement of functional status: construction of aggregate indexes. Med Care 1981;19:473–88.
50. Winograd CH, Lemsky CM, Nevitt MC, et al. Development of a physical performance and mobility examination. J Am Geriatr Soc 1994;42:743–9.
51. Charlson ME, Pompei P, Ales KL, et al. A new method of classifying prognostic comorbidity in longitudinal studies: development and validation. J Chronic Dis 1987;40:373–83.
52. Pfeiffer E. A short portable mental status questionnaire for the assessment of organic brain deficit in elderly patients. J Am Geriatr Soc 1975;23:433–41.
53. Kohout FJ, Berkman L, Evans DA, et al. Two shorter forms of the CES-D depression symptoms index. J Aging Health 1993;5:179–93.
54. Ware JE, Hays RD. Methods for measuring patient satisfaction with specific medical encounters. Med Care 1988;26:393–402.
55. Epstein AM, Hall JA, Fretwell M, et al. Consultative geriatric assessment for ambulatory patients. A randomized trial in a health maintenance organization. JAMA 1990;263:538–44.
56. Duke University Center for the Study of Aging and Human Development. Multidimensional Functional Assessment: The OARS Methodology. Durham, NC: Duke University; 1978.
57. Bergner M, Bobbitt RA, Pollard WE, et al. The sickness impact profile: reliability of a health measure. Med Care 1976;4:57–67.
58. Wan TTH. Stressful Life Events, Social-Support Networks, and Gerontological Health: A Prospective Study. Lexington, Mass: Lexington Books; 1982.
59. Ware JE, Johnston SA, Davies-Avery A, et al. Conceptualization and Measurement of Health for Adults in the Health Insurance Study, vol. III, Mental Health. Santa Monica, Calif: RAND Corp; 1979.
60. DiMatteo MR, Hays R. The significance of patients' perceptions of physician conduct: a study of patient satisfaction in a family practice center. J Community Health 1980;6:18.

61. Ware JE, Davis-Avery A, Donald CA. Conceptualization and Measurement of Health Insurance Study, Vol. V. General Health Perceptions. Santa Monica, Calif: RAND Corp; 1978.
62. Fabacher D, Josephson K, Pietruszka F, et al. An in-home preventive assessment program for independent older adults. J Am Geriatr Soc 1994;42:630–8.
63. Tinetti ME, Williams TF, Mayewski R. Fall index for elderly patients based on number of chronic disabilities. Am J Med 1986;80:429–34.
64. Katz S, Downs TD, Cash HR, et al. Progress in the development of the index of ADL. Gerontologist 1970;10:20–30.
65. Fretwell MD, Raymond PM, McGarvey ST, et al. The senior care study. A controlled trial of a consultative/unit-based geriatric assessment program in acute care. J Am Geriatr Soc 1990;38:1073–81.
66. Katz S, Akpom CA. A measure of primary sociobiological functions. Int J Health Serv 1976;6:493–508.
67. Klein LE, Roca RP, McArthur J, et al. Diagnosing dementia: univariate and multivariate analyses of the mental status examination. J Am Geriatr Soc 1985;33:483.
68. Zung WWK. A self-rating depression scale. Arch Gen Psychiatry 1965;12:63–70.
69. Gayton D, Wood-Dauphinee S, de Lorimer M, et al. Trial of a geriatric consultation team in an acute care hospital. J Am Geriatr Soc 1987;35:726–36.
70. Mahoney FI, Barthel DW. Functional evaluation: the Barthel index. Md Med J 1965;4:61–5.
71. Carey GC, Posavac EH. Program evaluation of a physical medicine and rehabilitation unit. Arch Phys Med Rehabil 1978;59:330.
72. Gilchrist WJ, Newman RJ, Hamblen DL, et al. Prospective randomized study of an orthopaedic geriatric inpatient service. BMJ 1988;297:1116–8.
73. Still CN, Goldschmidt TJ, Mallin R. Mini object test: a new brief clinical assessment for aphasia-apraxia-agnosia. South Med J 1983;76:52–4.
74. Hughes AM, Gray RF, Downie IV D. Brief cognitive assessments of the elderly-the mini object test and the Clifton assessment procedures for the elderly. Br J Clin Psychol 1985;3:81–3.
75. Gunner-Svensson F, Ipsen J, Olsen J, et al. Prevention of relocation of the aged in nursing homes. Scand J Prim Health Care 1984;2:49–56.
76. Hall N, De Beck P, Johnson D, et al. Randomized trial of a health promotion program for frail elders. Can J Aging 1992;11:72–91.
77. Kozma A, Stones MS. The measurement of happiness: development of the Memorial University of Newfoundland Scale of Happiness (MUNSH). J Gerontol 1980;35:906–12.
78. Russell D, Peplau LA, Cutrona CE. The revised UCLA Loneliness Scale: concurrent and discriminant validity evidence. J Pers Soc Psychol 1980;39:472–80.
79. Holmes TH, Rahe RS. The Social Readjustment Scale. J Psychosom Res 1967;11:219–25.
80. MacMillan AM. The health opinion survey: technique for estimating prevalence of psychoneurotic and related types of disorders in communities. Psychol Rep 1957;3:325–39.
81. Wallston BS, Wallston KA, Kaplan GD, et al. Development and validation of the Health Locus of Control (HLC) Scale. J Consult Clin Psychol 1976;44:580–5.
82. Hansen FR, Spedtsperg K, Schroll M. Geriatric follow-up by home visits after discharge from hospital: a randomized controlled trial. Age Aging 1992;21:445–50.
83. Harris RD, Henschke PJ, Popplewell PY, et al. A randomised study of outcomes in a defined group of acutely ill elderly patients managed in a geriatric assessment unit or a general medical unit. Aust NZ J Med 1991;21:230–4.
84. Sheikh K, Smith DS, Meade TW, et al. Repeatability and validity of modified activities of daily living (ADL) index in studies of chronic disability. Int Rehabil Med 1979;1:51–8.
85. Hébert R, Robichaud L, Roy PM, et al. Efficacy of a nurse-led multidimensional preventive programme for older people at risk of functional decline. Age Ageing 2001;30:147–53.
86. Hébert R, Carrier R, Bilodeau A. The Functional Autonomy Measurement System (SMAF): description and validation of an instrument for the measurement of handicaps. Age Ageing 1988;17:293–302.
87. Dupuy HJ: Self-representation of general psychological well-being of American adults. Paper presented at the American Public Health Association meeting. Los Angeles, Oct 17, 1978.
88. Bravo G, Gaulin P, Dubois MF. Validation d'une échelle de bien-être général auprès d'une population francophone âgée de 50 à 75 ans. Can J Aging 1996;15:112–8.
89. Cutrona C, Russell DW. The provisions of social support and adaptation to stress. Adv Pers Relationships 1987;1:37–67.
90. Hendriksen C, Lund E, Stromgard E. Consequences of assessment and intervention among elderly people. BMJ 1984;289:1522–4.
91. Hjort Sorensen K, Sivertsen J. Follow-up three years after intervention to relieve unmet medical and social needs of old people. Compr Gerontol B 1988;2:85–91.
92. Katz S. Assessing self maintenance. J Am Geriatr Soc 1983;31:721–7.
93. Hogan DB, Fox RA. A prospective controlled trial of a geriatric consultation team in an acute-care hospital. Age Ageing 1990;19:107–13.
94. Granger CV, Albrecht GL, Hamilton BB. Outcome of comprehensive medical rehabilitation: measurement by PULSES profile and the Barthel index. Arch Phys Med Rehabil 1979;60:145–54.
95. Hodkinson HM. Evaluation of a mental test score for assessment of mental impairment in the elderly. Age Ageing 1972;1:233–8.
96. Hogan DB, Fox RA, Badley BWD, et al. Effect of a geriatric consultation service on management of patients in an acute care hospital. Can Med Assoc J 1987;136:713–7.
97. Inouye SK, Bogardus ST, Charpentier PA, et al. A multicomponent intervention to prevent delirium in hospitalized older patients. N Engl J Med 1999;340:669–76.
98. MacPhee GJ, Cowther JA, McAlpine CH. A simple screening test for hearing impairment in elderly patients. Age Ageing 1988;17(5):347–51.
99. Inouye SK, van Dyck CH, Alessi CA, et al. Clarifying confusion: the confusion assessment method: a new method for detection of delirium. Ann Intern Med 1990;113:941–8.
100. Cummings JL. Clinical Neuropsychiatry. Orlando, Fla: Grune & Stratton; 1985.
101. Blessed G, Tomlinson BE, Roth M. The association between quantitative measures of dementia and of senile change in the cerebral grey matter of elderly subjects. Br J Psychiatry 1968;114:797–811.
102. Ulhmann RF, Larson EB, Buchner DM. Correlations of mini-mental state and modified Dementia Rating Scale to measures of transitional health status in dementia. J Gerontol 1987;42:33–6.
103. Jensen J, Nyberg L, Gustafson Y, et al. Fall and injury prevention in residential care—effects in residents with higher and lower levels of cognition. J Am Geriatr Soc 2003;51:627–35.
104. Wade DT, Collin C. The Barthel ADL index. A standard measure of physical disability? Int Disabil Stud 1988;10:64–7.
105. Lundin-Olsson L, Nyberg L, Gustafson Y. The mobility interaction fall chart. Physiother Res Int 2000;5:190–201.
106. Lundin-Olsson L, Nyberg L, Gustafson Y. Attention, frailty, and falls: the effect of a manual task on basic mobility. J Am Geriatr Soc 1988;46: 758–61.
107. Committee on Injury Scaling. The Abbreviated Injury Scale. Morton Grove, Ill: American Association for Automotive Medicine; 1990.
108. Kennie DC, Reid J, Richardson IR, et al. Effectiveness of geriatric rehabilitative care after fractures of the proximal femur in elderly women: a randomised clinical trial. BMJ 1988;297:1083–6.
109. McEwen RT, Davison N, Forster DP, et al. Screening elderly people in primary care. Br J Gen Pract 1990;40:94–7.
110. Hunt SM, McEwan J, McKenna P. Measuring Health Status. London: Croom Helm; 1986.
111. Chambers LW, MacDonald LA, Tugwell P, et al. The McMaster health index questionnaire as a measure of the quality of life. J Rheumatol 1982;9:780–4.
112. Weed LA. Medical Records, Medical Education and Patient Care. Cleveland: The Press of Case Western Reserve University; 1974.
113. Lawton MP. The Philadelphia Geriatric Center Morale Scale: a revision. J Gerontol 1975;30:85–9.
114. Melin AL, Bygren LO. Efficacy of the rehabilitation of elderly primary health care patients after short-stay hospital treatment. Med Care 1992;30:1004–15.
115. The Staff of the Benjamin Rose Hospital. Multi-disciplinary studies of illness in aged persons. II. A new classification of functional studies in activities of daily living. J Chronic Dis 1959;9:55.
116. Brorsson B, Hulter Asberg K. Katz index of independence in ADL. Reliability and validity in short-term care. Scand J Rehabil Med 1984;16:125.
117. Spector WD, Katz S, Murphy JB, et al. The hierarchical relationship between activities of daily living and instrumental activities of daily living. J Chronic Dis 1987;40:481.
118. Kane RA, Kane RL. Assessing the Elderly. A Practical Guide to Measurement. Lexington, Mass: Lexington Books; 1986.
119. Galasko D, Klauber MR, Hofstetter R, et al. The Mini-Mental State Examination in the early diagnosis of Alzheimer's disease. Arch Neurol 1990;47:49.
120. Newbury JW, Marley JE, Beilby JJ. A randomized controlled trial of the outcome of health assessment of people aged 75 years and over. Med J Aust 2001;175:104–7.
121. SF-36 Health Survey: Scoring Manual for English Language Adaptations: Australia/New Zealand, Canada, United Kingdom. Boston: Medical Outcomes Trust; 1994.

122. Pathy MSJ, Bayer A, Harding K, et al. Randomised trial of case finding and surveillance of elderly people at home. Lancet 1992;340:890–3.
123. Townsend P. Poverty in the United Kingdom. Harmondsworth, UK: Penguin; 1979.
124. Neugarten BL, Navighurst RJ, Tobin SS. The measurement of life satisfaction. J Gerontol 1961;16:134–43.
125. Powell C, Montgomery P. The age study: the admission of geriatric patients through emergency. J Am Geriatr Soc 1990;38:A35.
126. Reuben DB, Frank JC, Hirsch SH, et al. A randomized clinical trial of outpatient comprehensive geriatric assessment coupled with an intervention to increase adherence to recommendations. J Am Geriatr Soc 1999;47:269–76.
127. Guralnik JM, Simonsick EM, Ferrucci L, et al. A short performance battery assessing lower extremity function: association with self-reported disability and prediction of mortality and nursing home admission. J Gerontol 1994;49:M85–94.
128. Jette AM, Davies AR, Cleary PD, et al. The functional status questionnaire: reliability and validity when used in primary care. J Gen Intern Med 1986;1:143–9.
129. Ware JE, Sherbourne CD. The MOS 36-Item Short-Form Health Survey (SF-36):1. conceptual framework and item selection. Med Care 1992;30:473–83.
130. Hays RD, Sherbourne CD, Mazel RM. The RAND 36-item health survey 1.0. Health Econ 1993;2:217–27.
131. National Center for Health Statistics. Current estimates from the national health interview survey: United States 1986. Vital Health Stat 1986;10:160.
132. Ware JE, Snyder MK, Wright WR, et al. Defining and measuring patient satisfaction with medical care. Eval Program Plann 1982;6:247–63.
133. Maly RC, Frank JC, Marshall GN. Perceived Efficacy in Patient-Physician Interactions (PEPPI): validation of an instrument in older persons. J Am Geriatr Soc 1998;46:889–99.
134. Rubenstein LZ, Josephson KR, Wieland GD, et al. Effectiveness of a geriatric evaluation unit: a randomized clinical trial. N Engl J Med 1984;311:1664–70.
135. Rubin CD, Sizemore MT, Loftis PA, et al. The effect of geriatric evaluation and management on medicate reimbursement in a large public hospital: a randomized clinical trial. J Am Geriatr Soc 1992;40: 989–95.
136. National Center for Health Statistics. Long Term Health Care: Minimum Data Set. Washington, DC: US Government Printing Office; 1978.
137. Rubin CD, Sizemore MT, Loftis PA, et al. A randomized, controlled trial of outpatient geriatric evaluation and management in a large public hospital. J Am Geriatr Soc 1993;41:1023–8.
138. Wood V, Wylie ML, Sheafor B. An analysis of a short self-report measure of life satisfaction: correlation with rater judgment. J Gerontol 1969;24:265–469.
139. Shaw FE, Bond J, Richard DA, et al. Multifactorial intervention after a fall in older people with cognitive impairment and dementia presenting to the accident and emergency department: randomized controlled trial. BMJ 2003;326:73–8.
140. Tinetti ME. Performance-oriented assessment of mobility problems in elderly patients. J Am Geriatr Soc 1986;34:119–26.
141. Koch M, Gottschalk M, Baker DI, et al. An impairment and disability assessment and treatment protocol for community-living elderly persons. Phys Ther 1994;74:286–98.
142. Tidelksaar R. Preventing falls: home hazard checklists to help older people protect themselves. Geriatrics 1986;41:26–8.
143. Silverman M, Musa D, Martin DC, et al. Evaluation of outpatient geriatric assessment: a randomized multi-site trial. J Am Geriatr Soc 1995;43: 733–40.
144. George LK, Fillenbaum GG. OARS methodology. A decade of experience in geriatric assessment. J Am Geriatr Soc 1985;33:607–15.
145. Berg L, Hughes CP, Coben LA. Mild senile dementia of the Alzheimer's type: research diagnostic criteria, recruitment, and description of a study population. J Neurol Neurosurg Psychiatry 1982;45:962–8.
146. McCusker J. Development of scales to measure satisfaction and preferences regarding long-term and terminal care. Med Care 1984;22:476–93.
147. Helzer JE, Robins LN. The diagnostic interview schedule: its development, evolution, and use. Soc Psychiatry Psychiatr Epidemiol 1988;23:6–16.
148. Robins LN, Helzer JE, Croughan J, et al. National Institute of Mental Health diagnostic interview schedule: its history, characteristics, and validity. Arch Gen Psychiatry 1981;38:381–9.
149. Moryсz RK. Caregiving strain and the desire to institutionalize family members with Alzheimer's disease. Res Aging 1985;7:329–61.
150. Strandberg TE, Pitkala K, Berglind S, et al. Multifactorial cardiovascular disease prevention in patients aged 75 years and older. A randomized controlled trial. Am Heart J 2001;142:945–51.
151. Ettinger WH, Fried LP, Harris T, et al. Self-reported causes of physical disability in older people: the cardiovascular health study. J Am Geriatr Soc 1994;42:1035–44.
152. Heyman A, Fillenbaum G, Nash F, et al. Consortium to Establish a Registry for Alzheimer's Disease: the CERAD experience. Neurology 1997;49(Suppl. 3):S1–23.
153. Sintonen H: 15D. NCHPE working papers 41 and 42. Available at http://www.chpe.buseco.monash.edu.au.
154. Rissan P, Sogaard J, Sintonen H, et al. Do QOL instruments agree? A comparison of the 15D (health-related quality of life) and NHP (Nottingham Health Profile) in hip and knee replacements. Int J Technol Assess Health Care 2000;16:696–705.
155. Stuck AE, Aronow HU, Steiner A, et al. A trial of annual in-home comprehensive geriatric assessments for elderly people living in the community. N Engl J Med 1995;333:1184–9.
156. Tinetti ME, Baker DI, McAvay G, et al. A multifactorial intervention to reduce the risk of falling among elderly people living in the community. N Engl J Med 1994;331:821–7.
157. Rubenstein LZ, Aronow HU, Schloe M, et al. A home-based geriatric assessment, follow-up and health promotion program: design, methods and baseline findings from a 3-year randomised clinical trial. Aging Clin Exp Res 1994;6:105–20.
158. Master AM, Lasser RP, Beckman G. Tables on average weight and height of Americans aged 65 to 94 years. JAMA 1960;172:658–63.
159. Stuck AE, Minder CE, Peter-Wuest I, et al. A randomized trial of in-home visits for disability prevention in community-dwelling older people at low and at high risk for nursing home admission. Arch Intern Med 2000;160:977–86.
160. Nelson EC, Landgraf JM, Hays RD, et al. The functional status of patients: how can it be measured in physicians' offices? Med Care 1990;28:1111–6.
161. Teasdale TA, Shuman L, Snow E, et al. A comparison of outcomes of geriatric cohorts receiving care in a geriatric assessment unit and on general medicine floors. J Am Geriatr Soc 1983;31:529–34.
162. Thomas DR, Brahan MD, Haywood ACSW. Inpatient community-based geriatric assessment reduces subsequent mortality. J Am Geriatr Soc 1993;41:101–4.
163. Pfeiffer E, Johnson T, Chiofolo R. Functional assessment of elderly subjects in four service settings. J Am Geriatr Soc 1981;29:433.
164. Timonen L, Rantanen T, Ryynänen OP, et al. A randomized controlled trial of rehabilitation after hospitalization in frail older women: effects on strength, balance, and mobility. Scand J Med Sports 2002;12:186–92.
165. Berg KO, Wood-Dauphinee SL, Williams JI, et al. Measuring balance in the elderly. Validation of an instrument. Can J Public Health 1992;83(Suppl 2):S7–S11.
166. Tinetti ME, Baker DI, McAvay G, et al. A multifactorial intervention to reduce the risk of falling among elderly people living in the community. N Engl J Med 1994;331:821–7.
167. Spaeth EB, Fralick FB, Hughes WF. Estimation of loss of visual efficiency. Arch Ophthalmol 1955;54:462–8.
168. Macphee GJA, Crowther JA, McAlpine CH. A simple screening test for hearing impairment in elderly patients. Age Ageing 1988;17:347–51.
169. Radloff LS. The CES-D Scale: A self-report depression scale for research in the general population. Appl Psychol Meas 1977;1:385–401.
170. Buchner DM, Hornbrook MC, Kutner NG, et al. Development of the common data base for the FICSIT trials. J Am Geriatr Soc 1993;41: 297–308.
171. Toseland RW, O'Donnell JC, Engelhardt JB, et al. Outpatient geriatric evaluation and management: is there an investment effect? Gerontologist 1997;37:324–32.
172. Stewart AL, Hays RD, Ware JE. The MOS short-form general health survey: reliability and validity in a patient population. Med Care 1988;26:724–35.
173. Granger CV, Hamilton BB. UDS report: the Uniform Data System for Medical Rehabilitation report of first admissions for 1990. Am J Phys Med Rehabil 1992;71:108–13.
174. Granger CV, Hamilton BB, Keith RA, et al. Advances in functional assessment for medical rehabilitation. Topics Geriatr Rehabil 1986;1: 59–74.
175. Linacre JM, Heinemann AW, Wright BD, et al. The structure and stability of the functional independence measure. Arch Psychol Med Rehabil 1994;75:127–32.
176. Tucker MA, Davison JG, Ogle SJ. Day hospital rehabilitation—effectiveness and cost in the elderly: a randomised controlled trial. BMJ 1984;289:1209–12.
177. Benjamin J. The Northwick Park ADL Index. Br J Occup Ther 1976;12:301–6.
178. Qureshi KM, Hodkinson HM. Evaluation of a 10 question mental test in the institutionalised elderly. Age Ageing 1974;3:152–7.
179. Tulloch AJ, Moore V. A randomized controlled trial of geriatric screening and surveillance in general practice. J R Coll Gen Pract 1979;29:733–42.

180. van Haastregt JCM, Diederiks JPM, van Rossum E, et al. Effects of a programme of multifactorial home visits on falls and mobility impairments in elderly people at risk: Randomized controlled trial. BMJ 2000;321:994–8.
181. De Bruin AF, Diederiks JPM, de Witte LP, et al. The development of a short generic version of the sickness impact profile. J Clin Epidemiol 1994;47:407–18.
182. De Bruin AF, Buys M, de Witte LP, et al. The sickness impact profile: SIP68, a short generic version; first evaluation of the reliability and the reproducibility. J Clin Epidemiol 1994;47:368–71.
183. Holbrook M, Skilbeck CE. An activities index for use with stroke patients. Age Ageing 1983;12:166–70.
184. Schuling J, de Haan R, Limburg M, et al. The Frenchay activities index: assessment of functional status in stroke patients. Stroke 1993;24:1173–7.
185. Donald CA, Ware JE, Brook RH, et al. Conceptualization and Measurement of Health for Adults in the Health Insurance Study. Santa Monica, Calif: RAND Corp; 1978.
186. RAND 36-Item Health Survey: RAND Health Science Program. Santa Monica, Calif: RAND Corp; 1992.
187. Van der Zee I, Sanderman R. Het meten van de algemene gezondheidstoestand met de RAND-36: een handleiding. Groningen, Netherlands: Noordelijk Centrum voor Gezondheidsvraagstukken; 1993.
188. Tinetti ME, Richman D, Powell L. Falls efficacy as a measure of fear of falling. J Gerontol 1990;45:239P–43P.
189. Stalenhoef P, Diederiks J, Knottnerus A, et al. How predictive is a home-safety checklist of indoor fall risk for the elderly living in the community? Eur J Gen Pract 1998;4:114–20.
190. van Rossum E, Frederiks CMA, Philipsen H, et al. Effects of preventative home visits to elderly people. BMJ 1993;307:27–32.
191. Templeman CJJ. Welbevinden bij ouderen. Konstruktie van een meetinstrument. Groningen, Netherlands: University of Groningen (PhD thesis); 1987.
192. Jong-Gierveld J, Kamphius FH. The development of a Rasch-type loneliness scale. Appl Psychol Meas 1985;9:289–99.
193. Vetter NJ, Jones DA, Victor CR. Effect of health visitors working with elderly patients in general practice. BMJ 1984;288:369–72.
194. Foulds GA, Bedford A. Manual of the Delusions, Symptoms States Inventory. Windsor: NFER Publishing; 1979.
195. McNab A, Philip AE. Screening an elderly population for psychological well-being. Health Bull (Edinb) 1980;38:160.
196. Vetter NJ, Lewis PA, Ford D. Can health visitors prevent fractures in elderly people? BMJ 1992;304:888–90.
197. Wagner EH, LaCroix AZ, Grothaus L, et al. Preventing disability and falls in older adults: a population based randomised trial. Am J Public Health 1994;84:1800–6.
198. Scholes D, LaCroix AZ, Wagner EH, et al. Tracking progress toward national health objectives in the elderly: what do restricted activity days signify? Am J Public Health 1991;8:485–8.
199. Ware JE. Reliability and Validity of General Health Measures. Santa Monica, Calif: RAND Corp; 1976.
200. Ware JE, Sherbourne CD, Davis A, et al. The MOS Short-Form General Health Survey: Development and Test in a General Population. Santa Monica, Calif: RAND Corp; 1988.
201. Williams ME, Williams TF, Zimmer JG, et al. How does the team approach to outpatient geriatric compare with traditional care: a report of a randomized control trial. J Am Geriatr Soc 1987;35:1071–8.
202. Eggert GM, Brodows BS. The ACCESS program: assuring quality in long-term care. QRB Qual Rev Bull 1982:9–15.
203. Eggert GM, Bowlyow JE, Nichols CW. Gaining control of the long-term care system: first returns from the ACCESS experiment. Gerontologist 1980;20:356–63.
204. Winograd CH, Gerety M, Lai N. Another negative trial of geriatric consultation: is it time to say it doesn't work? J Am Geriatr Soc 1991;39:A13.
205. Yeo G, Ingram L, Skurnick J, et al. Effects of a geriatric clinic on functional health and well being of elders. J Gerontol 1987;42:252–8.
206. Zung WW. Depression in the normal aged. Psychosomatics 1967;8:287–92.
207. Adams DL. Analysis of a life satisfaction index. J Gerontol 1969;24:470–4.
208. Bradburn NM. The Structure of Psychological Well-Being. Chicago: Aldine; 1969.
209. Blazer D, Houpt J. Perception of poor health in the healthy older adult. J Am Geriatr Soc 1979;27:330–4.
210. Mossey JM, Shapiro E. Self-rated health: a predictor of mortality among the elderly. Am J Public Health 1982;72:800–6.

CHAPTER 40

Chronic Cardiac Failure

Neil D. Gillespie
Miles D. Witham
Allan D. Struthers

Cardiac failure increases in both prevalence and incidence with age.[1] It is a disease of middle and old age, although the underlying causes differ considerably with age.[2] In younger patients with cardiac failure, the cause is frequently coronary artery disease, whereas in the older patient valvular disease and hypertension are more often implicated. Most epidemiologic studies are based on symptoms and signs of cardiac failure, but more recent data include objective assessments of ventricular function, which is more senistive.[3]

The prevalence of heart failure continues to rise as more patients survive myocardial infarction as a result of fibrinolytic therapy. In addition, patients with hypertension are surviving longer as a result of continued improvements in the prevention of strokes.[4] Fortunately, it appears that the effective treatment of hypertension may in fact prevent the onset of heart failure even in the very old.[5] The HYVET study of nearly 4000 hypertensive patients aged 80 and over showed a significant reduction in any cardiovascular event, including the development of any heart failure, in the group treated for hypertension.

When considering the epidemiology of heart failure, note that it is defined as the presence of symptoms and signs of cardiac decompensation, together with objective evidence of underlying structural heart disease. These are the definitions used by the European Society of Cardiology[6] and the American Heart Association[7] who have recently independently reached a consensus on the diagnosis of heart failure. This is an important step because it has resulted in a more focused approach when considering precisely what disease entity is being treated in individual patients. Heart failure is of major economic significance; in the United Kingdom it accounts for up to 5% of hospital admissions,[8] and in the rest of Europe hospitalization for heart failure is a significant financial burden for a number of countries.[9] Many older adults with heart failure also have multiple pathologies and coexistent diseases, including cognitive impairment, which make the diagnosis more difficult to confirm.[10]

EPIDEMIOLOGY

Relatively few studies report the incidence and prevalence of heart failure in the older patient population. Much of the epidemiologic data comes from Scandinavia[11] and the Framingham study,[12] although recently new data have come from the United Kingdom from a relatively young population.[3] The early data collected from studies were predominantly from medical record analysis and patient questionnaires. This type of data collection has its limitations.

In a West London study,[13] the prevalence of heart failure in those aged under 65 was reported as 0.06%, compared with 2.8% in those over 65. This study likely underestimated the severity of the problem as only patients who had been prescribed as diuretic were included; others with relatively mild disease might have been missed. Many earlier epidemiologic studies were performed on populations that were inadequately described and give no information on the population at risk. The precise prevalence of left ventricular dysfunction in the whole population has been obscure until recent years. Studies in the late 1950s revealed a prevalence of 0.2% in the 45 to 64 year age group[14] and 1.9% in those over the age of 65. Another U.S. study demonstrated prevalence rates of 1% and 6.5% in corresponding age groups.[15]

The criteria for heart failure used in the Framingham Heart Study population[12] were more strictly defined and the baseline prevalence was 0.3% of the population aged 62 or less. However, over a 34-year follow-up period the prevalence rate was 0.8% in ages 50 to 59 and 9.1% in the over 80s age group.[16] By contrast, more recent estimates from North Glasgow, Scotland, estimated the prevalence of left ventricular systolic dysfunction based on echocardiographic criteria to be about 2.9%.[3] This figure was obtained from a population of 1640 patients between the ages of 25 and 74. The systolic dysfunction was symptomatic in 1.5% of patients and asymptomatic in 1.4%. In this study it therefore appears that systolic dysfunction was at least twice as common as symptomatic heart failure defined by clinical criteria.

The longitudinal Framingham study suggested that prevalence rates doubled every decade and reached approximately 10% for people in their 80s.

Prescribing data also highlight the extent of the problem; in the United States, up to 1 in 5 elderly patients were being treated for chronic cardiac failure.[17] In the United Kingdom, echocardiographic data in patients over 75 years of age suggest that prevalence may be around 10% of patients being managed in the community.[18]

Information on the incidence of heart failure also reveals a sharp increase over the age of 75 years. The best available incidence data are from the Framingham Heart Study[19] and the study of men born in 1913.[20] In the Framingham study, 5200 individuals have been followed since 1948 and the incidence rises markedly with age. The annual incidence was 2% per thousand in men and 1% per thousand in women under the age of 54, and 14% per thousand in men and 13% per thousand in women between the ages of 75 and 84. The Framingham study data probably underestimate the incidence because the entry criteria did not include the milder forms of heart failure.

In the Scandinavian study of men born in 1913, the annual incidence for those in the 50 to 54 year age group was 1.5 per thousand per year, which increased to 10.2 per thousand per year at ages 61 to 67.

The Hillingdon Heart Failure Study[21] was a population-based surveillance system in which patients first developing heart failure were identified. Over a 20-month period, 220 patients fulfilled the criteria for heart failure and the incidence of the condition increased steeply with age and was higher in men than in women at all ages. Newer studies using echocardiography show not just that many patients have asymptomatic left ventricular dysfunction, but that heart failure with normal systolic function is increasingly recognized.[22]

Hospitalizations for chronic heart failure are frequent; but this may relate mainly to approaches to treatment and assessment, together with awareness of the condition, rather than being a reflection of the incidence or prevalence. The number of hospital discharges where a diagnosis of heart failure has been coded has increased in recent years both in Holland[23] and in Scotland.[24] In the United States in 1991, congestive heart failure was the primary discharge diagnosis in around 790,000 hospitalizations.[25]

DISEASE COURSE AND PROGNOSIS

Heart failure has a variable disease progress but in general, patients with impaired left ventricular systolic function have a poorer prognosis, whereas patients with normal systolic function heart failure tend to fare better. These patients are more likely to be hypertensive, have mild coronary artery disease, and be prone to deterioration in renal function during hospitalization.[26] Among older adults hospitalized with heart failure, mean survival time is about 2.5 years. However, there is considerable heterogeneity in survival.[27] In one study, the presence of chronic heart failure in older patients resulted in an approximate 50% reduction in life expectancy.

The increased numbers of patients hospitalized for heart failure may reflect improved survival following myocardial infarction, but also an improvement in heart failure management. As a result patients with heart failure are living longer, with more episodes of decompensation requiring hospital admission. Data from North America suggest that there is a high rate of readmission in heart failure patients.[28] Evidence suggests that a multidisciplinary approach to the treatment of heart failure may reduce the need for hospitalization in elderly patients with the condition.[29] Such an approach is crucial in the older patient where issues such as adherence, cognition, and continence figure prominently in the clinical decision-making process.

The prognosis for heart failure, although improved in recent years by drug treatment, is nevertheless still poor. The majority of patients with New York Heart Association Class IV disease (Table 40-1) will be unlikely to survive a year.

A study of elderly men admitted as inpatients with heart failure revealed that the 1-year mortality was in the region of 50%.[30] It is thus clear that heart failure is a relatively malignant condition and, although newer treatments have been shown to improve the prognosis for many patients, alleviation of symptoms and improved morbidity is as important as any potential mortality benefits in the older patient.[31]

PATHOPHYSIOLOGY

As noted, the pathophysiology of heart failure is multifactorial, especially in older patients in whom hypertensive heart disease and valvular heart disease are more common. There may be structural abnormalities within the heart together with overcompensatory mechanisms in the renin-angiotensin system, the sympathetic nervous system, and the peripheral vasculature. Although there are specific changes in the cardiovascular system with age, (see Chapter 14) such as increased calcification, increased myocardial fibrosis, and reduced ventricular compliance,[32] most elderly patients with heart failure have additional pathology to explain their symptoms. In patients with heart failure due to ischemia, remodeling can result in alterations in the shape and morphology of the left ventricle with ultimate left ventricular dilatation and a large end-diastolic volume.[33] In addition to changes in the structure of the left ventricle, many elderly patients have associated calcific degeneration of both the aortic and mitral valves, with functional and hemodynamically significant consequences.[34] The cardiomyopathies[35] are also a small but significant cause of heart failure in older patients, although the widely seen asymmetrical septal hypertrophy itself is not of great significance.[36] In hypertensive patients with left ventricular hypertrophy, the increase in collagen content of the ventricular wall and associated myocardial fibrosis may lead to diastolic filling abnormalities,[37] which may contribute to the symptoms of heart failure, and represent a major pathophysiologic substrate for the phenomenon of heart failure with preserved systolic function (HPSF). In addition, loss of atrial contraction can result in significant hemodynamic deteriorations as atrial systole has an increased importance in the older patients when left ventricular wall stiffness is increased.[38]

In a healthy person, cardiac output is influenced directly by stroke volume and heart rate. In the failing heart, stroke volume is maintained by increasing the left ventricular end-diastolic pressure and volume, which is the basis of Starling's law of the heart. However, eventually at very high left ventricular end-diastolic volumes there will be no subsequent compensatory increase in cardiac output. One of the aims of heart failure treatment is to minimize increases in left ventricular end-diastolic pressure, so that cardiac output can be maintained and so that subsequent tissue oxygenation is adequate for perfusion of the vital organs.

The autonomic nervous system and the neuroendocrine systems initially support the failing heart, but ultimately the compensatory mechanisms may themselves prove harmful. Activation of the renin-angiotensin-aldosterone system can result in increased levels of angiotensin and aldosterone in the heart, kidney, brain, and vascular system, with undesirable consequences.[39] Furthermore, the associated high levels of plasma adrenaline and noradrenaline (epinephrine and norepinephrine) are associated with a poor prognosis due to deleterious effects on myocardial function, autonomic balance, and peripheral vascular function.[40]

Much of the fluid overload and edema in heart failure is a result of the effects of the renin-angiotensin system on the kidney, and reduced bradykinin may be associated with increased vasoconstriction. Changes in the morphology of skeletal muscle may explain the fatigability seen in heart failure patients over and above that expected with reduced tissue blood supply.[41] Disruption of the microvasculature is also seen with impaired endothelial function.[42] These changes are usually consequences of the disease process

Table 40-1. New York Heart Association Classification of Heart Failure

Class I	No symptoms
Class II	Symptoms with ordinary activity
Class III	Symptoms with less than ordinary activity
Class IV	Symptoms at rest

and not merely related to age, although in extremely old patients with mild symptoms of cardiac failure, true pathologic processes and age-related processes may be difficult to differentiate.

Such age-related changes include a reduction of cardiac output on exercise, an increase in end-systolic volume, a decrease in ejection fraction with exercise, and a reduced heart rate with exercise.[43] It is important to note, however, that heart failure is a disease with systemic effects; derangements of immune function cause a proinflammatory response that may in itself be cardiotoxic and contributes to the development of anemia; circulating cytokines may also help to drive the prominent skeletal myopathy that accompanies heart failure and is in fact the major cause of tiredness and breathlessness in heart failure patients. This skeletal myopathy in turn causes abnormalities of ergoreceptor function that drive further sympathetic nervous system activation. Disturbance of lung architecture and gas exchange are seen in the lungs of heart failure patients even in the absence of overt fluid overload—a further contributor to the symptoms of heart failure.

Most of the established treatments for heart failure are in patients with systolic dysfunction. Even so, there are many elderly patients with normal systolic function who have symptoms and signs compatible with heart failure. Conversely, many elderly patients have these "diastolic abnormalities" on echocardiography but no symptoms of heart failure. The relative clinical significance of the diastolic abnormalities in these patients is unclear. They may go on to develop subsequent heart failure as a result of atrial fibrillation or systolic dysfunction, or may have intermittent episodes of mild cardiac decompensation possibly as a result of silent myocardial ischemia. Furthermore, echocardiographically determined measures of diastolic dysfunction are critically dependent on the degree of activation of the sympathetic nervous system. Such variables include transmitral flow velocities (the E to A ratio), the isovolumic relaxation time.[44] Further work is needed to establish the clinical usefulness of these measures and newer echocardiographic indices such as measures of longitudinal systolic function.

THE ETIOLOGY OF HEART FAILURE

Heart failure has been described as a syndrome rather than a diagnosis or disease, and the underlying cause must always be sought in patients having the syndrome. The most frequent cause of heart failure is left ventricular systolic dysfunction, usually as a consequence of ischemic heart disease, especially myocardial infarction. However, in elderly patients, valvular heart disease frequently contributes to the symptoms.

Less frequently, heart failure in the older patient may be caused by one of the cardiomyopathies, amyloidosis, storage diseases (e.g., hemochromatosis), secondary to chemotherapy or vitamin B deficiencies. In the over-80s, aortic or mitral valve disease frequently contributes to heart failure and many elderly patients in long-term care have background cardiac valvular disease.[45] Furthermore, as already noted, it is increasingly recognized that many patients have symptoms associated with heart failure in the presence of normal systolic function and no evident valvular disease. This is often called diastolic heart failure or more commonly heart failure with preserved systolic function (HPSF). HPSF may be responsible for as much as 30% to 50% of heart failure in the elderly population.[46] The etiology of this heart failure is unclear, but it is more likely to be present in patients with hypertension and left ventricular hypertrophy. It is less clear how these patients should be managed, as most of the major studies have addressed patients with left ventricular systolic dysfunction as a cause of their heart failure.[47–50]

Patients in heart failure with systolic dysfunction have a poorer prognosis than those with normal systolic function. It is also well established that patients with an increased left ventricular end-diastolic volume secondary to myocardial dilatation have a poor prognosis.[51] Not infrequently heart failure will be precipitated by anemia, alcohol, and a number of other factors[52] (Table 40-2).

DIAGNOSIS OF HEART FAILURE

It is fairly easy to recognize heart failure in its more severe versions when the patient has pronounced symptoms and signs accompanied by echocardiographic evidence of left ventricular dysfunction.[53] Even so, diagnostic difficulties arise in its milder forms.

The European Society of Cardiology (ESC) has developed guidelines for the diagnosis of heart failure[6] (Table 40-3). However, with any guidelines there is a degree of vagueness, and in particular there is no specific definition of precisely what is meant by cardiac dysfunction. An example to highlight some of the difficulties is the case of the elderly lady whose echocardiogram shows preserved systolic function and who has swollen ankles with no breathlessness and mild fatigue. Does this type of patient have heart failure? Nonetheless, the ESC guidelines have generally clarified the situation even if there are still a few areas of ambiguity.

Table 40-2. Factors Which May Precipitate Heart Failure in the Elderly Person

Anemia
Alcohol
Intercurrent infection, including endocarditis
Fluid overload (often postoperatively)
Thyrotoxicosis
Drugs (e.g., NSAIDs)
Atrial fibrillation
Altered drug compliance
Pulmonary emboli

Table 40-3. European Society of Cardiology Guidelines for the Diagnosis of Heart Failure

Essential Features
• Symptoms of heart failure (for example, breathlessness, fatigue, ankle swelling)
• Objective evidence of cardiac dysfunction (at rest)
Nonessential Features
In cases where the diagnosis is in doubt, there is a response to treatment directed toward heart failure.

Table 40-4. Symptoms of Heart Failure in Elderly Patients, and Differential Diagnoses

Classic Symptoms	Atypical Features	Differential Diagnoses
Dyspnea	Lethargy	Anemia
Orthopnea	Confusion	COPD
Peripheral edema	Falls	Depression or anxiety
	Dizziness	Hypothyroidism
	Syncope	Hypoalbuminemia
	Immobility	Malnutrition
		Renal disease
		Neoplasm
		Lymphedema

COPD, chronic obstructive pulmonary disease.

For the clinician who is faced with an elderly patient with suspected heart failure, two questions should be considered before further assessment:

1. Are the patient's symptoms at least partly cardiac in origin?
2. If so, what kind of cardiac disease is producing these symptoms?[54]

Table 40-4 lists the typical and atypical symptoms in the elderly patient with suspected heart failure and potential differential diagnoses.

The diagnosis of heart failure is especially difficult because it is not defined by an absolute level of any one parameter, as is the case with a number of other diseases. Consequently the diagnosis is a judgment based on a careful history and examination, chest radiology, electrocardiography, echocardiography, and other routine baseline investigations, such as full blood count, serum biochemistry, and thyroid function.

Clinical history

The most classic symptom of heart failure is exertional breathlessness. However, this is a common symptom and is often a result of chronic obstructive pulmonary disease (COPD), deconditioning, obesity, or interstitial lung disease.[55] Most people will experience some breathlessness with moderate exertion and, during exercise, the stage at which breathlessness is experienced depends on the overall level of fitness.

Anemia and obesity are confounding factors that make exertional dyspnea a very nonspecific symptom. Orthopnea is a more specific symptom that does not occur in normal patients and is not usually a feature in respiratory disease. However, the disease process has to be relatively advanced before orthopnea occurs; and even if it is present, diuretics have often been instituted by the patient's general practitioner to relieve this symptom. Likewise, paroxysmal dyspnea (PND) is a more extreme version of dyspnea and is a result of fluid redistribution which increases the left ventricular end-diastolic pressure. Again, PND is specific but an insensitive symptom because it signifies fairly severe heart failure, which should have been noted and previously treated.

Fatigue and lethargy are other common problems in heart failure, but they are probably even harder to define and assess than dyspnea, particularly in elderly patients. Fatigue is common in people who are ill and more common still in older adults who are frail.

Ankle edema is a common presenting feature, but again there are many alternative causes, such as cor pulmonale, deep venous thrombosis, dependent edema, or hypoalbuminemia. Elderly women often have ankle edema, which is not caused by heart failure. Its precise cause is unknown, although venous insufficiency accompanied by pelvic obstruction to venous blood flow are commonly blamed. Indeed, it is elderly women with swollen ankles who most commonly cause false positives for heart failure when assessed subsequently by echocardiography.

Probably the best indication of underlying heart failure comes from the history, with a history of previous myocardial infarction or hypertension being useful indicators.[56] It should be remembered, however, that many elderly patients have silent myocardial ischemia or infarctions. In addition, many are unsure whether a previous hospitalization for chest pain was for a myocardial infarction or angina. Additional features that may suggest the diagnosis of heart failure include excessive alcohol intake, a history of rheumatic fever, and the use of drugs such as nonsteroidals, which might precipitate heart failure. Note too, however, that heart failure is associated with cognitive impairment, including memory impairment and frontal systems dysfunction that often manifests with slowness and decreased initiative.[10] In consequence, it is easy in a busy clinical practice to be misled by incomplete or seemingly vague answers; both false-positive and false-negative responses can put the history off track.

Physical signs

Many of the physical signs of heart failure are nonspecific and of relatively low predictive value. These include tachycardia, pulmonary crepitations, and peripheral edema. Equally, many of the physical signs that are specific to heart failure are insensitive because they occur only once the heart failure has become severe. These include elevation of the jugular venous pressure, a gallop rhythm, and displacement of the cardiac apex beat. The situation is further compounded by the variable ability of doctors to detect these clinical signs.[57] As a result, few of the symptoms and signs are of any value on their own. The probability of the diagnosis of heart failure is weighed up by the individual clinician making full use of clinical judgment together with the findings on examination and careful history taking.[58]

Investigations

The SIGN guidelines used in Scotland[59] for the diagnosis and treatment of heart failure due to left ventricular systolic dysfunction, although not specifically written for the elderly patient, provide a useful framework for investigations.

CHEST X-RAY

Chest x-ray is performed routinely and can produce useful information for patients with suspected heart failure. Cardiac enlargement (cardiothoracic ratio greater than 50%) implies cardiomegaly, and if present is a good guide to heart failure.[60] However, many heart failure patients do not exhibit cardiomegaly, so it tends to be a specific but insensitive test which identifies severe heart failure only. Other helpful chest x-ray findings are pulmonary edema, upper lobe diversion, fluid in the horizontal fissure, and Kerly-B-lines in the costophrenic angles. In extreme cases, pleural effusions may be present, although clearly there are alternative explanations for them such as bronchial carcinoma, pneumonia, or pulmonary emboli. In a meta-analysis of 29 studies,[61] Bayesian analysis found that chest radiography can only exclude heart failure (posttest probability less than 5%) and a decreased ejection fraction in patients who are asymptomatic can never confirm heart failure (posttest probability greater than 95%). However, it is likely that cardiomegaly represents underlying structural cardiac disease and in many patients heart failure will develop at some stage.

A chest x-ray can reveal other clues as to noncardiac disease that might be causing breathlessness. A lung tumor might be obvious, and emphysema may also be present. Nevertheless, the chest x-ray should be seen as a whole. For example, the finding of cardiomegaly plus bilateral pleural effusions with no other parenchymal lung disease makes heart failure extremely likely (although the presence of structural heart disease should still be confirmed by echocardiography).

ELECTROCARDIOGRAM

The 12-lead electrocardiogram (ECG) should be performed routinely. Left ventricular systolic dysfunction is rare in the presence of a completely normal 12-lead ECG, making it a useful "rule out" test. Recent data[62] suggest that an abnormal resting ECG is sensitive (94%) with excellent negative predictive value (98%) but is much less specific (61%) and has poor positive predictive value (35%). Most studies suggest that this is the case; where there is doubt, an echocardiogram should be performed.

Other abnormalities on the ECG may be useful in the assessment of patients. For example, the presence of atrial fibrillation may be useful in concluding whether the patient should receive additional anticoagulation.

ECHOCARDIOGRAPHY

The optimum investigation in the elderly patient with suspected heart failure is echocardiography.[63] Both qualitative and quantitative assessment can be useful. However, the degree of left ventricular systolic dysfunction can be assessed by a number of indices. Fractional shortening is usually sufficient in most instances.[64] Left ventricular ejection fraction,[65] and more recently a regional motion index,[66] have been shown to provide accurate assessments of left ventricular systolic function; global assessment of function by an experienced operator is another valid approach, which correlates well with measured ejection fraction.[67] Echocardiography can clearly distinguish whether the left ventricle is dilated or not; this approach to assessing left ventricular dimensions is preferable to chest x-ray. Left ventricular dilatation and left ventricular systolic dysfunction usually accompany each other, but occasionally the left ventricle is dilated despite the presence of normal systolic function. Nevertheless, left ventricular dilatation implies impending left ventricular systolic dysfunction and should probably be treated as such.

Echocardiography can also identify patients with mitral valve disease or aortic stenosis who may benefit from surgery. It can also assess diastolic dysfunction, although there is some controversy over this.[68] The problem relates to the fact that the left ventricle becomes stiffer as it ages, and it is difficult to define consistently when the stiff ventricle constitutes diastolic dysfunction. At the time of this writing, no echocardiographic criteria are fully accepted as measures of diastolic dysfunction.

However, there is one extreme version of diastolic dysfunction that can cause severe pulmonary edema. This occurs when the left ventricle is so stiff that left atrial pressure increases and leads to fast atrial fibrillation with profound breathlessness. In the short term, treatment is to reverse the abnormal rhythm, but longer-term strategies are required to prevent LV stiffness, which leads to atrial fibrillation. Echocardiography also provides information about left ventricular hypertrophy if present; such a finding provides evidence of structural heart disease to support a diagnosis of heart failure even if LV systolic function is normal.

Figure 40-1 suggests an approach for diagnosing heart failure in practice.

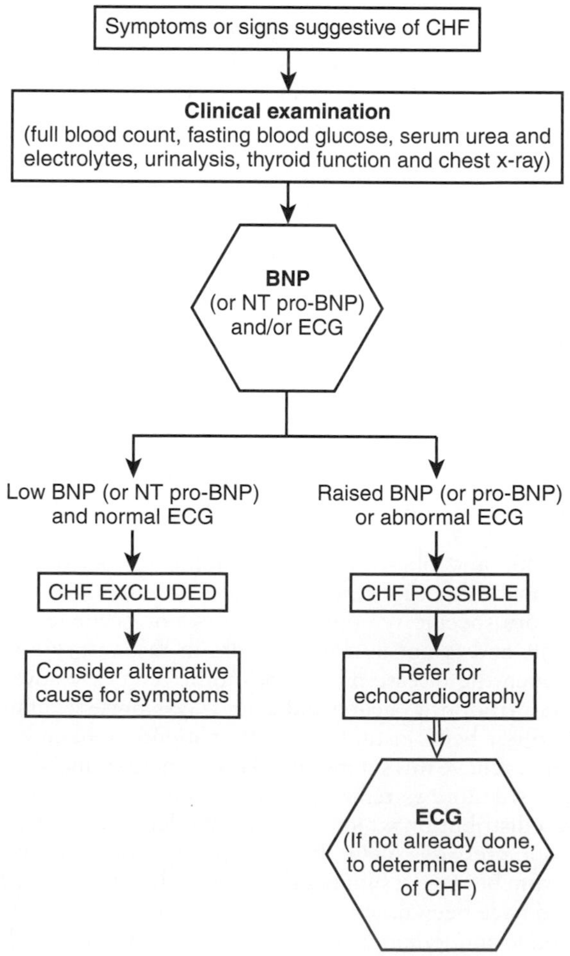

Figure 40-1. Diagnostic algorithm for patients with suspected chronic heart failure (CHF).

Natriuretic peptides

The natriuretic peptides (NPs) that are released from the atrium and ventricles have a variety of cellular effects, act as vasodilators, and cause a natriuresis. They have been shown to reflect left ventricular function, and levels correlate reasonably well with quantitative assessments of left ventricular function.[69] There is emerging evidence that the natriuretic peptides—and in particular BNP—have a role in identifying patients with left ventricular systolic dysfunction.[70,71] These agents may have a role in the preselection of patients for echocardiography when it is not always available. In patients following myocardial infarction, it appears that the levels of B-type natriuretic peptide closely relate to ejection fraction.[72] It has also been shown that in patients with acute dyspnea, plasma levels of BNP reflect left ventricular function.[71] Testing is now possible with newer patient tests comparable to stick testing for blood sugar. In a community study, natriuretic peptides were effective in detecting patients with left ventricular systolic dysfunction.[73] Many other studies also demonstrate the role of BNP and ANP in the assessment of patients with heart disease, including their potentially prognostic role. One of the major challenges is now to make these tests more routinely available in clinical practice. Figure 40-1 shows a diagnostic algorithm for patients with suspected chronic heart failure.

In summary, the diagnosis of heart failure is a sequential one which relies on a clear clinical history and examination followed by either electrocardiography, chest radiology, or echocardiography. Echocardiography is desirable in all cases although it may not be always available, particularly in older patients.[74] Nevertheless, it is probably more important in the elderly patient to obtain an echocardiogram before instigating treatment because structural abnormalities are more common and optimum treatment requires as accurate a diagnosis as possible so that adverse effects may be kept to a minimum.

When echocardiography proves to be technically difficult, objective assessments of left ventricular function may be made by radionuclide ventriculography. In the older patient, functional capacity can be assessed by performing a 6-minute walking test.[75] This can provide useful prognostic information.

TREATMENT OF HEART FAILURE

General issues

Since the 1960s, when loop diuretics were introduced,[76] treatments for heart failure have diversified. As the pathophysiology of heart failure has become clearer, treatment options have broadened and a number of agents, including ACE inhibitors and β-blockers, have been shown to improve prognosis. It is now known that the impairments in left ventricular function and the peripheral circulation can be treated, with consequent hemodynamic improvement. Neurohumoral activation can be blocked and left ventricular remodeling can be reduced.[77] These adverse consequences of heart failure are the targets of drug treatment. As a result, patients may require multiple-drug treatment and priorities need to be established. It is important that patients and their caregivers understand the implications of their treatment.

In the frail elderly patient, quality of life and alleviation of symptoms are especially important. The major clinical trials of heart failure have generally excluded older patients, so that most patients enrolled in studies are in the age range 50 to 70 years, favoring single system and single cause disease. Frail patients, by contrast, typically have many active illnesses resulting in co-morbidity which may require management itself.

Such complex patients require multidimensional evaluation and management both in hospital and in the community.[78] This ensures that a full picture of the patient's abilities, needs, and wishes is obtained, so that the goals of treatment are fully aligned with what the patient requires. It is clearly of little use to treat heart failure with all of the recommended therapies but to further impair function and quality of life through intolerable side effects.

It is worth remembering and reemphasizing that the different treatments are mediated by different mechanisms. Diuretics relieve the symptoms of fluid retention, and there is now evidence from a meta-analysis showing reduced rates of hospitalization and a mortality benefit.[79]

ACE inhibitors improve symptoms and exercise tolerance as well as prognosis in patients with heart failure.[47–49] This should be contrasted with β-blockers,[50,80–82] where symptomatic benefit may be mild and even deleterious in the early stages of treatment. It is therefore important to carefully guide a patient through treatment, making sure that he or she understands the process of the disease. The key point is that, in the long term, β-blockers slow progression and improve prognosis dramatically. More recently the angiotensin antagonists have been shown to be tolerated[83–85] and improve symptoms in patients with heart failure already taking diuretic treatment; there is good evidence that they are a useful substitute for ACE inhibitors in some patients, but they may not improve outcomes when added to ACE inhibitors.[86–89] In the last few years digoxin[90] has been shown convincingly to improve symptoms and reduce hospitalizations in patients with severe heart failure refractory to standard treatments, although it appears that it does not alter mortality in patients who are in sinus rhythm with heart failure and carries significant risks of cardiac toxicity and confusion.

Nonpharmacologic management of the patient is particularly important, but also susceptible to problems with adherence, particularly in older people with cognitive impairment. Where possible, patients should be given advice about monitoring their weight, about the nature and relevance of their symptoms, and about the dosages of their drugs and the opportunity for flexible dosing dependent on symptoms. In general, patients should be advised to perform moderate exercise and stop smoking. Patients who drink alcohol to excess should be advised to cut back. Often patient caregivers have a vital role to play in the successful management of heart failure.

As with all medication use in older people, a drug should be started at a low dose and titrated in relation to the response, especially since patients may be taking over-the-counter preparations and the potential for drug interactions is considerable.[91] Each of the aforementioned drug classes will be considered in more detail; but in addition to the main therapeutic options, mention will be made of drugs that have less proven efficacy.

Summary of Treatment Options

Chronic Heart Failure

Diuretics
- For symptoms of fluid overload and edema.
- Loop diuretic (furosemide or bumetanide) at appropriate dose. Also consider thiazide.

ACE inhibitor
- Symptomatic and mortality benefit for systolic dysfunction following confirmation of diagnosis by echocardiography.
- Options include enalapril, lisinopril, captopril, perindopril, ramipril. Dose should be titrated.

β-Blocker
- Should be considered for symptomatic and mortality benefit in mild, moderate, and even severe heart failure under close hospital supervision.
- Beneficial effects may not be immediate.
- Options include carvedilol, metoprolol, bisoprolol. Dose should be titrated.

Spironolactone
- Adjunctive treatment with a mortality benefit.

Digoxin
- As adjunctive treatment for symptomatic benefit and control of atrial fibrillation. Also provides symptomatic improvement in sinus rhythm but no clear mortality benefit.

Nitrates
- As adjunctive treatment for symptomatic benefit and control of associated angina.

Other options
- Amlodipine, ferrous sulfate, erythropoietin, warfarin, and amiodarone.

Nonpharmacologic
- Weight loss; low-salt diet; cessation of smoking; exercise; compliance aids.
- Multidisciplinary management.

Diuretics

Diuretics are fundamental to the treatment of chronic heart failure. The loop diuretics introduced in the 1960s were shown to be very effective in reducing symptoms associated with fluid retention and they had a clear hemodynamic benefit. Studies have shown deterioration in symptomatic heart failure when diuretics are withdrawn, and diuretics have been shown to reduce mortality and hospitalization in chronic heart failure.[92]

The loop diuretics (which include furosemide and bumetanide) block the sodium-potassium-chloride transport exchange in the ascending limb of the loop of Henle.[93] Thiazides have a different site of action and work in the distal convoluted tubule.[94] Spironolactone has a yet different mode of action, antagonizing the aldosterone-mediated sodium exchange with potassium and hydrogen in the collecting ducts.[95] In older patients with heart failure, the rate of absorption of loop diuretics and time to peak plasma concentration are reduced as renal function is often impaired. High doses of diuretics may need to be used to produce a diuresis as the coexisting relative acidosis results in increased competition for the organic acid transport pathway at the proximal tubule. The bioavailability of furosemide can be very variable, from 20% to 80%, but is more consistent with bumetanide.[96] Most of the loop diuretics have a fairly short half-life, in the region of 1 to 2 hours. In contrast, the thiazide and potassium-sparing diuretics have longer half-lives, which allow once-daily doses. Tolerance can occur to diuretics and this has clinical relevance. The natriuretic response diminishes after the first dose, but this can be reversed by restoring intravascular volume. Long-term administration of a loop diuretic can also result in tolerance, which can be combated by combining loop and thiazide diuretics together.[97]

In patients with acute left ventricular failure, intravenous furosemide is effective, but prolonged use can result in a reduction in right-sided heart pressure with a consequent fall in cardiac output and increase in peripheral vascular resistance.[98] This can often be combated by treatment with a concomitant vasodilator such as a nitrate.[99] When furosemide is given to patients with severe acutely decompensating heart failure, high doses should be used until symptoms and signs of fluid overload have been controlled. An intravenous dose of 40 to 50 mg is often sufficient to control the symptoms; but when resistance to loop diuretics occurs, up to 250 to 500 mg per day may be required. In resistant cases, furosemide can be given by a continuous infusion of up to 4 g per day.

Metolazone[100] is a thiazide that can be used for resistant edema and heart failure. It blocks sodium reabsorption in the proximal convoluted tubule along with having thiazide effects on the distal convoluted tubule. It is given orally at a dose between 1.25 mg and 10 mg per day. It can result in a profound diuresis and postural hypotension may be significant. Close monitoring of electrolytes is essential.

When patients with heart failure are being treated with a diuretic, it is essential to monitor plasma biochemistry regularly. Particular electrolyte disturbances include hypokalemia,[101] which may precipitate cardiac arrhythmias; hyponatremia,[102] which may cause drowsiness and fits; and hypomagnesemia,[103] which may cause a number of cellular effects including muscle weakness and arrhythmias. Hypokalemia may be alleviated by the concomitant use of potassium-sparing diuretics such as spironolactone or by using an ACE inhibitor (see later discussion). Diuretic treatment can also result in disturbances of lipid metabolism, glucose intolerance, and hyperuricemia.[104]

In addition to the above diuretic side effects, older patients are prone to difficulties with urinary incontinence, immobility, postural hypotension, dehydration, and confusion. These problems should be prominent in the prescriber's mind when instigating treatment in an individual patient. It is also important not to administer intravenous furosemide rapidly as this may precipitate an irreversible hearing loss.[105]

A Dutch study of older adults[106] assessed the impact of discontinuing diuretic therapy for relatively mild symptoms of heart failure (patients with severe symptoms and acute heart failure, and those requiring intravenous diuretics, were excluded). In the follow-up period, diuretic therapy had to be reintroduced in half of the patients in whom it had been withdrawn, owing to symptomatic deterioration. Even though the patients in whom diuretic therapy had to be restarted were relatively well, this study highlights the likelihood of a recurrence of symptoms if diuretics are discontinued in an elderly population.

Angiotensin-converting enzyme inhibitors

Angiotensin-converting enzyme (ACE) inhibitors have been available since the early 1980s, and evidence accumulated since then confirms their considerable efficacy in the treatment of heart failure. ACE inhibitors block overactivity of the renin-angiotensin system and the sympathetic nervous system.[107] In addition to these effects, ACE inhibitors seem to enhance the bradykinin-nitric oxide system in the vascular endothelium.[108] They may also have an influence outside the circulation in various tissues.[109] In patients with mild to moderate heart failure and even asymptomatic left ventricular dysfunction, they reduce morbidity and mortality.[47–49] Mechanistically, ACE inhibitors are vasodilators with subsequent reduction in cardiac preload and afterload, resulting in hemodynamic and symptomatic improvement for patients with heart failure. In addition to reducing the overcompensatory activity of the renin-angiotensin system together with beneficial effects on the endothelium, ACE inhibitors may also have anti-ischemic effects[110] and have an influence on the deleterious effects of the remodeling of the left ventricle following myocardial infarction.

The first study that demonstrated a benefit was in patients with severe heart failure (New York Heart Association class IV). In the CONSENSUS study,[47] patients were randomized to treatment with enalapril 2.5 mg titrated to 10 mg twice daily if tolerated, or a placebo. At 1-year follow-up, mortality was 52% in the placebo group and 36% in the enalapril group. There were also significant reductions in hospital admissions in the treatment group. In the SOLVD study,[48] patients with mild to moderate heart failure treated with enalapril 10 mg twice daily obtained a mortality benefit. This benefit also extended to patients in a prevention group of the SOLVD study as well as those in the treatment group. The trials not only demonstrated a mortality and symptomatic benefit, but also confirmed that, in general, treatment was well tolerated. The patients in these studies were middle-aged, so it may not be possible to extrapolate the findings directly to frail elderly patients. Nonetheless, most physicians would probably treat the older patient who had systolic dysfunction with an ACE inhibitor. Treatment with an ACE inhibitor also reduces the likelihood of myocardial ischemic events. In the SAVE study,[49] patients with asymptomatic left ventricular dysfunction (LVEF <40%) following myocardial infarction were treated with titrated doses of captopril up to 50 mg three times daily. There was a risk reduction of 19% in mortality compared with patients treated by placebo.

Further evidence for the efficacy of ACE inhibitors in patients with heart failure following myocardial infarction was obtained by the AIRE study.[111] Patients were randomized to treatment with ramipril 2.5 mg twice daily, increased to 5 mg twice daily if tolerated. In the 15-month follow-up the mortality rate in those treated with ramipril was 17%, compared with 23% in the placebo group.

As a result of the findings of all these trials, the use of ACE inhibitors has become increasingly widespread in patients with left ventricular systolic dysfunction. Subgroup analysis from large trials suggests that ACE inhibitors reduce mortality in older and younger patients, and even very old heart failure patients tolerate ACE inhibitors well and show an improvement in exercise capacity relative to a placebo.[112] Care is still required to ensure that renal dysfunction and orthostatic hypotension do not result from ACE inhibitor use in older patients.[113]

The main contraindications to treatment with ACE inhibitors are obstructive valvular disease and renal impairment. Patients who are volume-depleted, particularly those with hyponatremia, are more likely to experience hypotension with initial dosage. However, this may be less marked with some ACE inhibitors than others.[114] Treatment should be gradually titrated in divided doses until the maximum achievable dose is obtained. In general terms the optimal benefit is obtained at the top end of the dose range. The recent ATLAS study[115] compared low and high doses of lisinopril in heart failure and patients with higher dosages fared better. Ideally, the diuretic dose should be reduced or curtailed to optimize intravascular volume at the time of initiation of therapy. This reduces the likelihood of hypotension. Renal function and electrolytes should be monitored at regular intervals, initially every few days or weekly and then every 3 to 6 months. It may be possible to reduce the dose of maintenance diuretic therapy once the patient has been established on ACE inhibition.

The effects of ACE inhibitors on heart failure appear to be a class effect. Individual drugs currently used include captopril, enalapril, lisinopril, perindopril, and quinapril. The main side effects of ACE inhibitors include cough, hypotension, hyperkalemia, and, rarely, angioneurotic edema. The occurrence of a cough with ACE inhibitors should prompt a switch to an angiotensin receptor blocker (ARB).

The role of ACE inhibition in patients in heart failure with normal systolic function is less clear. The recent PEP-CHF study[116] compared perindopril with a placebo in older patients with preserved systolic function heart failure. There was no significant reduction in mortality, but symptoms and hospitalization were improved in the perindopril group. In practice, many older people with heart failure and preserved systolic function will require an ACE inhibitor for another indication, such as myocardial infarction, angina, hypertension, or stroke disease.

β-Blockers

It has become increasingly clear in the last few years that β-blockade is beneficial for patients with left ventricular systolic dysfunction and heart failure. A role for β-blockers was suggested as far back as the early 1970s.[117] Part of the rationale behind their use relates to reducing the adverse consequences of overstimulation of the sympathetic nervous system in patients with heart failure.

The main historical concerns relate to the negative inotropic effects of β-blockers with the potential for hypotension, fatigue, and acute worsening of decompensated heart failure. However, the results of randomized trials now suggest that, after mild intolerance associated with starting treatment in some patients, the benefits of longer-term therapy are significant and worth pursuing. Improved understanding of the pathophysiology of heart failure has highlighted the potential role for β-blockers in reducing the effects of vasoconstriction and fluid retention associated with heart failure. Indeed it is the case that blockade of the sympathetic nervous system by β-blockers complements the beneficial effects of ACE inhibitors on the renin-angiotensin system. Beta-blockers also have an antiarrhythmic effect and additionally facilitate coronary blood flow by prolonging diastole. Blockade of the adrenergic system may reduce both adrenaline (epinephrine)-mediated myocyte cell loss and myocyte dysfunction, thus reducing associated left ventricular systolic dysfunction.[118] Furthermore, the promotion of cellular growth and ventricular remodeling which is mediated by noradrenaline (norepinephrine) is blocked by β-blockers. It also appears that β-blockade may reduce some of the uncoupling of the B-receptors from their G protein at a cellular level, preventing further deterioration in systolic function.[119]

In the last few years it has been confirmed that treatment with β-blockade initially in small dosages, with a number of agents, can result in significant mortality benefits for patients with heart failure.[79–81] It is important that the dose be carefully titrated, with a close evaluation following each up-titration in order to detect worsening heart failure or associated hypotension. Up-titration of the dose should occur only when the patient is stable. Although most patients will show some improvement in their clinical condition and the progression of heart failure is reduced, exercise capacity may be only partially improved by treatment. However, hospital admissions for decompensated heart failure are overall less frequent.

Although the evidence for the use of β-blockade in heart failure is strengthening, some earlier studies in the late 1980s and early 1990s showed only a mild benefit following treatment.[120] It is only with the MERIT Heart Failure study,[83] the CIBIS II,[84] and the US COPERNICUS Heart Failure study[50] that the evidence base for the use of β-blockers in heart failure has become robust.

- In the MERIT study, nearly 4000 patients with New York Heart Association class II-IV heart failure were treated with long-acting metoprolol in divided and increasing doses. The treatment group started on a dose between 12.5 and 25 mg daily which was titrated to a target dose of 200 mg daily. Those patients treated had a reduced mortality rate of 34% in the 1-year follow-up period, the absolute mortality rate being reduced from 11% to 7.2%. Deaths from worsening heart failure and sudden deaths were both reduced significantly.
- In the CIBIS II study, the findings are similar with patients in New York Association class III-IV on standard treatment with diuretics and ACE inhibitors deriving additional benefit by treatment with bisoprolol, a β_1 selective adrenoceptor blocker. The dose of bisoprolol was titrated up to 10 mg daily, with the mortality rate being reduced from 13.2% to 8.8% in the treatment group. Carvedilol is a nonselective β-blocker with antioxidant, β-blocking, and vasodilator activity.[121] Following treatment with titrated doses of carvedilol, patients with chronic heart failure, including those with severe heart failure, derived benefit following a 6.5-month follow-up period.
- In the COPERNICUS trial,[50] a 35% reduction in analyzed mortality was obtained in patients treated with carvedilol compared to placebo. The benefit was also significant in patients with NYHA class IV heart failure, with an annual mortality rate of 18.5% in the placebo group compared with 11.4% in the carvedilol group.

These landmark trials have convincingly demonstrated that β-blockers improve mortality in patients with chronic heart failure. The precise role of β-blockers in frailer older patients with associated cognitive impairment and more frequent postural hypotension and comorbidity is unclear. However, there is a compelling case for β-blockade in patients with no contraindications, especially for those beta-blockers that do not cross the blood-brain barrier.

Contraindications include bradycardia, AV block, hypotension, asthma, or chronic obstructive pulmonary disease with significant reversibility; it is worth noting that many patients with COPD can tolerate β-blockade, and such patients were successfully enrolled in the CIBIS II trial of bisoprolol in heart failure. Problems with tolerability may be accentuated if the patient is taking other cardioactive medications. Patients with peripheral vascular disease may also find β-blockers difficult to tolerate.

Until recently, data on the tolerability of β-blockade in older heart failure patients was lacking. Recent studies have suggested that β-blockers are tolerated by a majority of older heart failure patients,[122] and the recent SENIORS trial[123] specifically evaluated a cohort of older patients with heart failure, mean age 76. In this study nebivolol had a significant effect on reducing hospital admissions, although the impact on all-cause mortality did not reach significance, and the effects in patients aged over 75 appeared less than in the younger old. Also of note was the fact that a significant proportion of patients in the SENIORS study had preserved left ventricular function, suggesting that β-blockade may provide some benefits in this understudied group of heart failure patients.

Spironolactone

In the RALES study,[124] the effectiveness of spironolactone added to an ACE inhibitor and a loop diuretic for severe chronic heart failure was assessed. This was a randomized double-blind placebo-controlled trial in which 1633 patients with New York Heart Association class III-IV heart failure, and ejection fraction of less than 30% and established on full ACE inhibitor and diuretic therapy with or without digoxin, were included. Small doses of spironolactone (25 to 50 mg/day) were well tolerated and reduced total mortality by 30% in the treatment group. Deaths from progressive heart failure and sudden deaths were reduced equally, and the incidence of severe hyperkalemia was low in both arms of the study.

Clinical experience of spironolactone in older people with heart failure suggests the need for great caution, however. The incidence of renal dysfunction and hyperkalemia in practice is up to 10 times that seen in the RALES trial and inappropriate use of spironolactone outside the indications used in the RALES trial may lead to a high incidence of side effects.[125]

Digoxin

Digoxin has been used in the treatment of heart failure for over 200 years. It is a positive inotrope and the effects of digoxin are mediated by inhibition of the Na^+, K^+-ATPase, which influences intracellular sodium with resultant influences on sodium/calcium exchange across the sarcolemmal membrane.[126] It has a relatively narrow therapeutic window, with the result that side effects are common, particularly in the elderly with renal impairment and hypokalemia.

In addition to its effects on the myocardium, digoxin is a weak diuretic and can cause gastric irritation[127] and has a mild estrogenic effect.[128] Digoxin improves the cardiac output and the stroke volume index with a resultant improvement in hemodynamic status in heart failure patients. The side effects of digoxin are more pronounced in patients with hypokalemia because potassium competes for the binding site at the site of action.

Until recently there has been considerable controversy over the role of digoxin in patients with heart failure. Its role in patients with sinus rhythm was particularly unclear. In the DIG trial,[90] nearly 8000 patients were assessed in over 300 centers. Patients were randomized to digoxin or placebo and followed for an average of 3 years. The patients had clinical heart failure but were in sinus rhythm. In the majority of patients, the cause of heart failure was ischemic heart disease and the average ejection fraction was 32%. Total mortality was no different between the digoxin and placebo groups. Heart failure deaths were reduced in the digoxin group, but there was a trend toward an increase in deaths because of arrhythmias or myocardial infarction. Hospital admissions were significantly reduced. Thus digoxin can now be recommended to patients with heart failure and sinus rhythm who remain symptomatic despite the use of diuretics and ACE inhibitors, and β-blockers.

Clearly in older patients close monitoring of therapy is essential. Two relatively recent withdrawal studies[129,130] indicate that digoxin is a useful adjunct to treatment in patients on ACE inhibitors and diuretics. With impaired renal function and reduced clearance of the drug, symptomatic nausea and fatigue are probably the most frequent complication together with bradycardia. A number of therapeutically important drug interactions also exist with digoxin, particularly with quinidine and amiodarone.[131] It is also sometimes difficult to distinguish between digoxin toxicity and the underlying symptoms of cardiac failure; digoxin is also capable of worsening confusion in older people. Digoxin is the third most commonly implicated drug in admissions precipitated by medication side effects; the balance between potential benefits for patients with refractory heart failure must always be carefully weighed against this side effect profile.

Digoxin remains useful in controlling ventricular rate in patients with fast atrial fibrillation and decompensated heart failure. The recent Scottish Intercollegiate Guideline Network has suggested that patients with heart failure and atrial fibrillation who need control of their ventricular rate should be considered for treatment with digoxin. Others to be considered include patients with moderately severe or severely symptomatic heart failure; those who remain symptomatic despite diuretic and ACE inhibitor therapy; those who have had more than one hospital admission for heart failure; and those who have had poor left ventricular systolic function and persisting cardiomegaly.

The maintenance dose of digoxin in heart failure should be in the region of 125 μg/day, but smaller doses may be necessary in some patients. Although additional therapeutic benefit may be obtained at higher doses, toxicity becomes increasingly likely.

Angiotensin antagonists

Attention recently has been directed toward angiotensin receptor blockade as a means of modifying the symptoms of heart failure. It appears that there are at least two angiotensin receptors: AT I and AT II. Stimulation of the former results in vasoconstriction, whereas stimulation of the latter results in vasodilatation. Angiotensin I receptor antagonists are effective in hypertension and their use is becoming more widespread.

The effects of these agents in elderly patients with heart failure were clarified in the ELITE, CHARM and Val HeFT[85–89] studies. In the first, where mortality was the primary endpoint, no mortality difference was seen between patients treated with losartan or captopril. In the Val HeFT study, there appeared to be no improvement in mortality in patients with heart failure treated with valsartan on top of an ACE inhibitor. However, symptomatic improvement was demonstrated and the need for hospital admission was reduced by valsartan on top of an ACE inhibitor.

These agents are generally well tolerated and should certainly be used in patients who are intolerant of ACE inhibition because of cough. They are, however, licensed in the United Kingdom currently only as a treatment for hypertension. The most recent data are presented in the CHARM studies, which evaluated candesartan in three different groupings of patients. In the CHARM "alternative" study, comparing candesartan with a placebo in patients intolerant of ACE inhibitors, there was a significant reduction in hospital admission and cardiovascular death for those patients treated with candesartan. In the CHARM "preserved" study, which compared candesartan with a placebo in patients with heart failure and preserved LV systolic function, addition of candesartan to standard treatments reduced hospital admissions but had no impact on mortality. In the CHARM "added" study, candesartan further reduced death and hospitalization for patients already taking an ACE inhibitor when compared with a placebo. Concern exists, however, that multiple blockade of the renin-angiotensin system may lead to an increased incidence of side effects, particularly renal impairment, which may limit the usefulness of this approach in older people with heart failure.

Other pharmacologic agents

Nitrates have a well-established role in the treatment of angina, but they also have a role in the management of cardiac failure. They act predominantly through stimulation of intracellular guanylate cyclase with subsequent sequestration of intracellular calcium and resultant vasodilatation. Beneficial hemodynamic effects include a reduction in blood pressure together with decreased pulmonary artery wedge pressure.[132] These favor an increase in cardiac output by reducing the preload on the left ventricle.[133] Tolerance to nitrate therapy is well recognized, but this can be reduced by nitrate-free periods.

A study of intravenous nitrate therapy showed that this treatment is effective in the treatment of acute pulmonary edema with reduction in symptoms of breathlessness and discomfort.[134] In one trial of acute left ventricular failure, intravenous isosorbide dinitrate appeared better than intravenous furosemide as a first-line therapy.[135]

In the first Veterans Administration Cooperative Heart Failure trial (V-HeFT 1), isosorbide dinitrate and hydralazine[136] were compared with prazosin and placebo in patients with New York Heart Association class II-III heart failure. There was a mild improvement in mortality in the nitrate and hydralazine group and ejection fraction and exercise performance also improved. The most notable effect was seen in patients of African extraction, and these findings were confirmed in patients with severe heart failure in the more recent A-HeFT study.[137] This highlights the potential value of nitrates and hydralazine as an intervention for patients unable to tolerate ACE inhibition who remain severely symptomatic. In addition to nitrates, other vasodilators such as calcium antagonists may have a role in heart failure. However, the PRAISE trial[138] showed that amlodipine has a neutral effect on mortality, which means that amlodipine can be used for its anti-ischemic effect in heart failure patients without worsening their heart failure.

Other agents have been evaluated in patients with cardiac failure but the above-mentioned drugs are currently the conventional treatment. In general terms, positive inotropes have been largely unhelpful and phosphodiesterase inhibitors have merely increased mortality.[139,140] Flosequinan is also associated with increased mortality.[141] Short-term use of intravenous positive inotropes may be useful in occasional patients, but their overall benefit is limited. Other simple measures may be useful. In a patient with a mild anemia, treatment of the anemia may improve tissue oxygenation and subsequent cardiac performance. This may require ferrous sulfate given intravenously, erythropoietin, or both. In patients with nutritional deficiencies, vitamin B supplementation may also be useful. There has been some recent concern that treatment with aspirin may negate the beneficial effects of ACE inhibitors in patients with left ventricular systolic dysfunction.[142] The evidence for this is not strong and such patients with left ventricular systolic dysfunction should still be treated with an ACE inhibitor where possible. There is currently no strong evidence that anticoagulation for patients with heart failure in sinus rhythm is of any benefit. Patients with atrial fibrillation should receive treatment with warfarin if not contraindicated.

Cardiac arrhythmias are relatively common in patients with heart failure. Patients with atrial fibrillation should be managed with anticoagulation where possible, although it should be remembered that the risks of hemorrhagic side effects are likely to be greater in the older patient and tight control of the INR is mandatory. Anticoagulation should be avoided in patients who are frequent fallers. Rapid ventricular rates associated with fast atrial fibrillation can be controlled by digoxin and/or β-blockers. Conversion to sinus rhythm can prove difficult as often the atrial fibrillation is longstanding. However, as atrial systole has increased importance in the older patient, attempts to maintain sinus rhythm should be made if symptoms are severe, either electrically or pharmacologically with β-blockers or amiodarone. Recent studies have suggested that there is little prognostic benefit in cardioversion to sinus rhythm compared with a rate control strategy for patients with an ejection fraction of 35% or less, symptoms of congestive heart failure and a history of atrial fibrillation.[143] Ventricular arrhythmias are also relatively common in patients with heart failure. These ventricular arrhythmias may cause considerable hypotension and may even be fatal. Amiodarone is often used in the context of symptomatic ventricular arrhythmias, but it has a number of noncardiac side effects including pulmonary fibrosis, liver function abnormalities, thyroid dysfunction, and peripheral neuropathy. In a trial in South America,[144] 500 patients with heart failure were randomized to amiodarone or placebo at a relatively low dose and followed up at 13 months. The mortality in the amiodarone group was 33.5%, compared with 41.4% in the placebo group—a risk reduction of 28%. In the CHF-STAT trial,[145] a higher dosage of amiodarone was used in a similar number of patients. At the higher dose, no mortality benefit was seen, although there was a reduced mortality trend in patients with a nonischemic cause. These studies would tend to suggest that amiodarone should be the antiarrhythmic of choice in patients with heart failure and symptomatic ventricular arrhythmias, but there is no role for widespread use of prophylactic amiodarone.

Drug interactions are frequently a problem in the elderly population and there are a number of significant interactions with amiodarone. The most significant of these is with warfarin and treatment should be carefully monitored. Patients with heart failure who have associated angina and myocardial ischemia should be treated for their ischemic heart disease by conventional means. Patients may require treatment with aspirin, β-blockade, statins, oral nitrates, calcium antagonists or other, nondrug, measures.

In patients with ischemic heart disease and mild to moderate impairment of left ventricular systolic functions, left ventricular performance may be improved by coronary bypass surgery. Such patients may have a hibernating area of myocardium, which could potentially be salvaged following bypass surgery.

Role of the heart failure nurse

Heart failure nurses have a critical role to play in coordinating heart failure care, monitoring patients symptoms, educating patients and caregivers, and up-titrating medications. They are therefore a pivotal member of the multidisciplinary team. Older heart failure patients, with their complex care needs, are particularly well placed to benefit from the skills that the heart failure nurse brings to bear. Trial evidence confirms that heart failure nurse intervention leads to lower levels of death and readmission in heart failure patients.[146]

Multidisciplinary team interventions

Similarly, there is evidence to support multidisciplinary intervention in older heart failure patients; the combination of nurse specialist intervention, pharmacist medication review, and education plus physician intervention led to reduced hospitalization and improved symptom control and quality of life in a U.S. trial.[29]

Both clinic-based and home-based MDT models have been used successfully; the addition of telemonitoring—for example, of weight and symptoms—or using more sophisticated invasive measures of hemodynamic function, is a potentially exciting adjunct to these models of care. Trials will be required in older, frail individuals to see whether such telemonitoring approaches are feasible and add to the quality of care.

Exercise in CHF

There is good evidence that at least for younger heart failure patients, regular submaximal aerobic or resistance exercise training leads to important improvements in symptoms, quality of life, reduces hospitalizations, and leads to a reduction in mortality.[147] There are few studies in older heart failure patients to guide the type, duration, and intensity of exercise intervention best suited to older heart failure patients.

In younger old patients, group circuit exercise in cardiac rehabilitation classes[148] appears successful, but in older, frailer patients, gentle seated exercise does not appear efficacious and a more vigorous alternative may be needed.[149]

Patients with uncontrolled atrial fibrillation, active sepsis, decompensated fluid overload, severe aortic stenosis, or malignant ventricular arrhythmias (unless an implantable cardioverter defibrillator [ICD] is fitted) should probably not participate in exercise, but for other patients, exercise appears remarkably safe. An exercise intensity of up to 80% of maximal should be the aim; in practical terms this is a level at which patients can still talk. The optimal session frequency and length have yet to be determined, but will depend on symptoms and the practicalities such as a suitable venue and transportation. It is important to note that exercise training needs to be continued for sustained benefit; improvements in exercise capacity are lost rapidly on cessation of exercise. Exercise programs should therefore be capable of being continued at home unsupervised rather than being confined to supervised sessions in hospital or outpatient settings.

Smoking

Smoking increases the chance of further myocardial ischemic events, and directly worsens tissue oxygenation. Smoking should always be actively discouraged in patients with heart failure, however old. Counseling remains the cornerstone of intervention for those prepared to quit; nicotine replacement may be used with care in patients with stable coronary artery disease and no history of malignant ventricular arrhythmias, and bupropion may be useful in carefully selected patients without other contraindications.

Alcohol

Alcohol has depressant effects on the myocardium, and also interacts with common comorbid diseases, particularly urinary incontinence, where the excess of fluid and decreased sensation caused by alcohol may worsen incontinence. Consumption in older people should therefore be limited to one or two units per day. Patients with alcoholic cardiomyopathy should be strongly encouraged to abstain totally.

Diet

Surprisingly little data exist to guide practice regarding diet in heart failure. Many older people with heart failure are overweight, and although obesity may reduce exercise tolerance still further, cohort studies suggest that overweight heart failure patients survive longer than patients of normal weight. The value of calorie restriction in heart failure has not been subjected to randomized controlled trials, and caution thus seems appropriate in recommending this, even in obese patients.

Cardiac cachexia is less common in heart failure, but is associated with advanced disease and a particularly poor prognosis. Dietary approaches to reversing cardiac cachexia have not been subjected to randomized trials; nevertheless, a pragmatic approach to dietetic intervention in underweight heart failure patients is probably merited, given the overlap with other chronic causes of frailty and undernutrition seen in older people.

Although salt and fluid restriction has long been promoted as beneficial in controlling symptoms in heart failure, practical issues limit the applicability of this advice. Efforts should be made to avoid excessive fluid consumption, but salt restriction below the recommended 6 g/day limit is often difficult in older patients who may have deeply ingrained cooking habits, a reliance on preprepared foods, and for whom the flavor-enhancing properties of salt are important in stimulating appetite and food intake.

PROBLEMATIC DISEASE INTERACTIONS — COPD, INCONTINENCE, COGNITIVE IMPAIRMENT, DEPRESSION

Heart failure in older people never exists in isolation, and the art of good care of older people with heart failure is to balance the management of their heart failure with management of their comorbid diseases, taking into account their physical and psychological state, quality of life, and treatment preferences. The following comorbid conditions often give rise to particular problems in patients with heart failure.

COPD

As smoking is a risk factor for both heart failure and COPD, the syndromes often coexist. This may make diagnosis more challenging; in older people experiencing breathlessness, it is often necessary to investigate for both syndromes. Severe COPD may also lead to right heart dysfunction as the underlying cause of the heart failure syndrome.

Management of heart failure in the presence of COPD still involves ACE inhibitors and diuretics; overdiuresis may cause a precipitous drop in cardiac output and blood pressure if the right ventricle is impaired because the impaired ventricle requires high filling pressures. B-blockers can be used in many patients with COPD unless significant reversible airway obstruction is present. There are theoretical advantages to using β_1-selective agents. In many patients, only an empirical trial of β-blockers will show if they are tolerated.

Exercise, in the form of pulmonary rehabilitation, is an important component of therapy for COPD, and exercise training should thus be encouraged when both conditions exist. Smoking, needless to say, should be firmly discouraged.

Urinary incontinence

Incontinence, always a prevalent problem in older people, is a particular problem in patients with heart failure. Reduced mobility and exercise capacity mean that reaching a toilet in time may be difficult, and the use of diuretics may lead to large urine volumes accumulating with little warning. This in turn leads to activity restriction because patients are worried about leaving the house after taking diuretics, or worse, patients deliberately miss diuretics, leading to decompensation of heart failure. Nocturia may also be a problem in patients with heart failure; lying flat causes excess fluid to redistribute from the lower extremities, increasing renal blood flow and urine excretion.

Careful adjustment of the dose and timing of diuretics is needed to circumvent these problems. Dividing doses, avoiding diuretics late in the day, or using diuretics with a slower onset of action such as torsemide[150] may all help. Use of interventions such as ACE inhibitors and exercise may help to improve exercise capacity, thus allowing patients to reach the toilet more easily.

Cognitive impairment

Cognitive impairment is common in older patients with heart failure, almost certainly a result of the two major causes of cognitive impairment sharing vascular risk factors with heart failure.[10] The presence of marked cognitive impairment may cause problems with adherence to medication, the ability to undertake self-monitoring (e.g., weight), and the ability to understand and retain information about the illness, medications, and prognosis.

Such problems should be anticipated, and strategies to manage medication (e.g., dosette boxes), close involvement of caregivers in education, fluid management, meal preparation, and medication administration are vital. Heart failure itself is not necessarily a contraindication to anticholinesterase inhibitor therapies, but care is needed to ensure that there is no evidence of underlying AV or SA node disease or that other rate-limiting drugs do not cause heart block.

Depression

Depression is common in heart failure patients, as is the case in many older people with chronic disease. Debate continues as to whether depression is truly an independent risk factor for death in heart failure, but there is no doubt that it exacerbates symptoms and worsens an already poor quality of life.

As with all unwell older people, depression should be sought whenever a comprehensive assessment is performed, preferably using a screening tool such as the Geriatric Depression Score or the Hospital Anxiety and Depression Scale. Psychological interventions remain the cornerstone of treatment for mild to moderate depression; more severe depression may require drug treatment. Although there are no randomized controlled trials to guide treatment of depression in heart failure, the known cardiotoxic side effects of tricyclic antidepressants mean that this class should be avoided. Anecdotal evidence suggests that SSRIs and related classes are relatively safe for use in heart failure.

Rationalizing the drug burden

Heart failure as a disease entity often entails a large number of extra medications. Added to the medications that patients often need to take for their comorbid diseases, this presents a substantial burden (including financial) to patients, increases the chances of drug interactions, and makes adherence to therapy less likely.[151]

It is possible to use heart failure treatments for multiple indications, especially for multiple vascular diseases, which may help to reduce the burden of therapy. ACE inhibitors will help to treat hypertension and reduce the risk of myocardial infarction; β-blockers can be used for rate control in AF, reducing blood pressure and treating angina. If further antianginals are needed, using nitrates can have further beneficial effects on blood pressure and heart failure. Such approaches may provide a way of reducing the number of vascularly active medications that a patient takes. In some patients, sodium restriction and use of ACE inhibitors may even allow diuretics to be withdrawn, with consequent improvement in urinary continence and urge symptoms. Such an approach may then allow other medications aimed at the urinary tract to be reduced or stopped.

Device therapy

Two major advances in device therapy for heart failure have become commonplace in recent years: implantable cardioverter-defibrillators (ICDs) and cardiac resynchronization therapy (CRT), also known as a biventricular pacemaker. The two devices can also be combined into a single unit (ICD-CRT).

In patients with significantly impaired ejection fractions, ICDs are known to reduce death rates by providing timely treatment of ventricular arrhythmias.[152] However, considerable discussion is required before using such devices in older heart failure patients with multiple comorbid diseases; such devices do not improve physical function or quality of life, may cause significant psychological distress—not to mention physical discomfort from defibrillation shocks—and will not prolong life in the face of the multiple system failures that are the hallmark of frailty.

Cardiac resynchronization on the other hand may dramatically improve cardiac function, exercise capacity, symptoms, and quality of life in carefully selected patients with advanced heart failure and significant dyssynchrony between the left ventricular septum and free wall.[153] Such devices may additionally allow sufficient hemodynamic improvement for other medications, such as ACE inhibitors and β-blockers, to be tolerated.

Palliative care for CHF

For patients with end-stage heart failure, there is good evidence to suggest that control of symptoms can be effectively managed by palliative care teams. The emphasis of most medical efforts in heart failure is directed to extending the duration of life, and sadly there are many patients with heart failure who do not have the opportunity to die a good death.

Communication is key; patients need to appreciate the prognosis in heart failure, which is worse than for breast and colorectal cancer. As the illness advances, sensitive discussions should take place to explore whether patients wish for life-prolonging therapy, including hospital admission, intubation, and inotropic support during exacerbations, and whether they wish to undergo cardiopulmonary resuscitation in the event of cardiac arrest. Involvement of caregivers as wished by patients, together with meticulous documentation of such discussions, can go a long way toward preparing the patients and their loved ones for the day when further efforts to prolong life become futile.

Near the end of life, some medications may be withdrawn if they are not contributing to symptom management. Intractable breathlessness may be alleviated by small doses of opiates; older patients with end-stage heart failure commonly also have pain, which is underreported.[154] Good palliative care involves the provision of support for all the patient's needs, including psychosocial and spiritual, and thus the narrow medical model used to manage heart failure or other chronic disease early in the course of the disease becomes less and less relevant as the illness progresses.[155]

CONCLUSIONS

Chronic heart failure is a major cause of morbidity and mortality in older patients. Optimum treatment requires an accurate diagnosis. In the older patient, the cause of heart failure is often heterogeneous and the clinical and examination findings should be confirmed by more objective assessments including chest radiology, electrocardiography, and particularly echocardiography. Elderly patients often have limited access to echocardiography, but it is essential given the high prevalence of background valvular disease and structural heart disease.

Once an accurate diagnosis has been established, treatment of left ventricular systolic dysfunction should follow the recent guidelines of the European Society of Cardiology and the American Heart Association where possible, with consideration of the specific requirements of the individual patient. Close supervision of treatment is mandatory particularly with ACE inhibitors and β-blockers where the possibility of short-term side effects is significant. Specific drug interventions should be tailored to individual patients, with cognitive impairment and additional pathology restricting the choice of agents available.

The prognosis for chronic heart failure is poor and at all times when treating the older patient emphasis should be on improving the patient's quality of life and symptom control, rather than merely delaying death.

Many of the major multicenter clinical trials have excluded older patients from analysis, but evidence should emerge about drug tolerability in patients over the age of 75. However, when there is evidence of fluid retention patients should be treated with a diuretic, and once evidence of left ventricular systolic dysfunction is confirmed they should be treated with an ACE inhibitor. Strong consideration should be given to treatment with a β-blocker. If the patient has severe heart failure, spironolactone (25 mg/day) should be added to the furosemide, ACE inhibitor, and β-blocker, but it is crucial to monitor the serum electrolytes carefully in the first month of therapy. If the patient is in atrial fibrillation and control of the ventricular rate is an issue, digoxin should be used. Other agents should be chosen in the light of contraindications to these major treatments. Digoxin and nitrates improve symptoms, and spironolactone may improve mortality. As in any illness, the response to treatment should be carefully monitored by the physician.

Multidisciplinary care is crucial, as with all older patients, and staff skilled in the care of older people should be closely involved in teams caring for heart failure patients. Exercise training, smoking cessation, and avoidance of excessive fluid and salt are important adjuncts to pharmacologic therapy. In carefully selected patients, device therapy such as cardiac resynchronization therapy may provide additional significant improvements.

KEY POINTS

Chronic Cardiac Failure

- Chronic heart failure is a major cause of morbidity and mortality in elderly patients.
- The optimum treatment requires an accurate diagnosis. In the older patient, the cause of heart failure is often heterogeneous, so the clinical and examination findings should be confirmed by more objective assessments, including chest radiology, electrocardiography, and, particularly, echocardiography.
- Once an accurate diagnosis has been established, treatment of left ventricular systolic dysfunction should follow the recent guidelines of the European Society of Cardiology and the American Heart Association where possible, with consideration of the specific requirements of the individual patient.
- Close supervision of treatment is mandatory, particularly with ACE inhibitors and β-blockers, where the possibility of short-term side effects is significant.
- The prognosis for chronic heart failure is poor. Emphasis should be on improving the patient's quality of life and symptom control, although new treatments may also improve mortality.
- Many of the major multicenter clinical trials have excluded older patients from analysis, but evidence should emerge in the next few years about drug tolerability in patients over the age of 75.
- When there is evidence of fluid retention, patients should be treated with a diuretic. Once evidence of left ventricular systolic dysfunction is confirmed, they should be treated with an ACE inhibitor.
- Strong consideration should be given to treatment with a β-blocker. If the patient has severe heart failure, spironolactone (25 mg/day) should be added to the furosemide.
- If the patient is in atrial fibrillation and control of the ventricular rate is an issue, digoxin should be used.
- Other agents should be chosen in the light of contraindications to these major treatments. Digoxin and nitrates improve symptoms and spironolactone may improve mortality.

For a complete list of references, please visit online only at www.expertconsult.com

CHAPTER 41

Diagnosis and Management of Coronary Artery Disease

Wilbert S. Aronow

The most common cause of death in elderly persons is coronary artery disease (CAD). Coronary atherosclerosis is very common in the elderly, with autopsy studies demonstrating a prevalence of at least 70% in persons older than 70 years. The prevalence of CAD is similar in elderly women and men.[1] In one study, clinical CAD was present in 502 of 1160 men (43%), mean age 80 years, and in 1019 of 2,464 women (41%), mean age 81 years.[1] At 46-month follow-up, the incidence of new coronary events (myocardial infarction or sudden cardiac death) was 46% in the elderly men and 44% in the elderly women.[1]

CAD is diagnosed in elderly persons if they have either coronary angiographic evidence of significant CAD, a documented myocardial infarction (MI), a typical history of angina pectoris with myocardial ischemia diagnosed by stress testing, or sudden cardiac death. The incidence of sudden cardiac death as the first clinical manifestation of CAD increases with age.

CLINICAL MANIFESTATIONS

Dyspnea on exertion is a more common clinical manifestation of CAD in elderly persons than is the typical chest pain of angina pectoris. The dyspnea is usually exertional and is related to a transient rise in left ventricular (LV) end-diastolic pressure caused by ischemia superimposed on reduced LV compliance. Because elderly persons are more limited in their activities, angina pectoris in elderly persons is less often associated with exertion. Elderly persons with angina pectoris are less likely to have substernal chest pain, and they describe their anginal pain as less severe and of shorter duration than do younger persons. Angina pectoris in elderly persons may occur as a burning postprandial epigastric pain or as pain in the back or shoulders. Acute pulmonary edema unassociated with an acute MI may be a clinical manifestation of unstable angina pectoris due to extensive CAD in elderly persons.[2]

Myocardial ischemia, appearing as shoulder or back pain in elderly persons, may be misdiagnosed as degenerative joint disease. Myocardial ischemia, appearing as epigastric pain, may be misdiagnosed as peptic ulcer disease. Nocturnal or postprandial epigastric discomfort that is burning in quality may be misdiagnosed as hiatus hernia or esophageal reflux instead of myocardial ischemia because of CAD. The presence of comorbid conditions in elderly persons may also lead to misdiagnosis of symptoms as a result of myocardial ischemia.

Elderly persons with CAD may have silent or asymptomatic myocardial ischemia.[3–5] In a prospective study, 133 of 195 men (68%), mean age 80 years, with CAD and 256 of 771 women (33%), mean age 81 years, with CAD had silent myocardial ischemia detected by 24-hour ambulatory electrocardiograms (ECGs).[5] At 45-month follow-up, the incidence of new coronary events in elderly men with CAD was 90% in those with silent myocardial ischemia versus 44% in men without silent ischemia.[5] At 47-month follow-up, the incidence of new coronary events in elderly women with CAD was 88% in those with silent ischemia versus 43% in women without silent ischemia.[5]

The reason for the frequent absence of chest pain in elderly patients with CAD is unclear.

RECOGNIZED AND UNRECOGNIZED MI

Pathy[6] reported that in 387 elderly patients with acute MI, 19% had chest pain, 56% had dyspnea or neurologic symptoms or gastrointestinal symptoms, 8% had sudden death, and 17% had other symptoms. Another study showed that in 110 elderly patients with acute MI, 21% had no symptoms, 22% had chest pain, 35% had dyspnea, 18% had neurologic symptoms, and 4% had gastrointestinal symptoms (Table 41-1).[7] Other studies have also shown a high prevalence of dyspnea and neurologic symptoms in elderly patients with acute MI.[8–10] In these studies, dyspnea was present in 22% of 87 patients,[8] in 42% of 777 patients,[9] and in 57% of 96 patients.[10] Neurologic symptoms were present in 16% of 87 patients,[8] 30% of 777 patients,[9] and 34% of 96 patients.[10]

As with myocardial ischemia, some patients with acute MI may be completely asymptomatic or the symptoms may be so vague that they are unrecognized by the patient or physician as an acute MI. Studies have reported that 21% to 68% of MIs in elderly patients are unrecognized or silent.[7,11–17] These studies also found that the incidence of new coronary events including recurrent myocardial infarction, ventricular fibrillation, and sudden death in patients with unrecognized MI is similar to[11,14–16,18] or higher[19] than in patients with recognized MI.

Elderly patients with acute MI have a higher prevalence of non-ST-segment elevation MI (NSTEMI) with absence of pathologic Q-waves than ST-segment elevation MI (STEMI) with pathologic Q-waves.[20,21] Of 91 consecutive patients aged 70 years and older, mean age 78 years with acute MI, 61 (75%) had NSTEMI.[21]

DIAGNOSTIC TECHNIQUES

Resting ECG

In addition to diagnosing recent or prior MI, the resting ECG may show ischemic ST-segment depression, arrhythmias, conduction defects, and LV hypertrophy that are

Table 41-1. Presenting Symptoms in 110 Elderly Patients with Acute Myocardial Infarction

Dyspnea was present in 35% of patients
Chest pain was present in 22% of patients
Neurologic symptoms were present in 18% of patients
Gastrointestinal symptoms were present in 4% of patients
No symptoms were present in 21% of patients

Adapted from Aronow WS. Prevalence of presenting symptoms of recognized acute myocardial infarction and of unrecognized healed myocardial infarction in elderly patients. Am J Cardiol 1987;60:1182.

related to subsequent coronary events. At 37-month mean follow-up, elderly patients with ischemic ST-segment depression 1 mm or greater on the resting ECG were 3.1 times more likely to develop new coronary events than were elderly patients with no significant ST-segment depression.[22] Elderly patients with ischemic ST-segment depression 0.5 to 0.9 mm on the resting ECG were 1.9 times more likely to develop new coronary events during 37-month follow-up than were elderly patients with no significant ST-segment depression.[22] At 45-month mean follow-up, pacemaker rhythm, atrial fibrillation, premature ventricular complexes, left bundle branch block, intraventricular conduction defect, and type II second-degree atrioventricular block were associated with a higher incidence of new coronary events in elderly patients.[23] Numerous studies have also demonstrated that elderly patients with ECG LV hypertrophy have an increased incidence of new coronary events.[24–26]

Numerous studies have found that complex ventricular arrhythmias in elderly persons with CAD are associated with an increased incidence of new coronary events including sudden cardiac death.[27–30] The incidence of new coronary events is especially increased in elderly persons with complex ventricular arrhythmias and abnormal LV ejection fraction[27] or LV hypertrophy.[28] At 45-month follow-up of 395 men, mean age 80 years, with CAD, complex ventricular arrhythmias detected by 24-hour ambulatory ECGs significantly increased the incidence of new coronary events 2.4 times.[29] At 47-month follow-up of 771 women, mean age 81 years, with CAD, complex ventricular arrhythmias detected by 24-hour ambulatory ECGs significantly increased the incidence of new coronary events 2.5 times.[29]

Exercise stress testing

Hlatky et al[31] found the exercise ECG to have a sensitivity of 84% and a specificity of 70% for the diagnosis of CAD in persons older than 60 years of age. Newman and Phillips[32] found a sensitivity of 85%, a specificity of 56%, and a positive predictive value of 86% for the exercise ECG in diagnosing CAD. The increased sensitivity of the exercise ECG with increasing age found in these two treadmill exercise studies was probably due to the increased prevalence and severity of CAD in elderly persons.

Exercise stress testing also has prognostic value in elderly patients with CAD.[33–35] Deckers et al[35] demonstrated that the 1-year mortality was 4% for 48 patients 65 years of age or older who were able to do an exercise stress test after acute MI and 37% for the 63 elderly patients unable to do the exercise stress test after acute MI.

Exercise stress testing using thallium perfusion scintigraphy, radionuclide ventriculography, and echocardiography is also useful in the diagnosis and prognosis of CAD.[36–38] Iskandirian et al[36] showed that exercise thallium-201 imaging can be used for risk stratification of elderly patients with CAD. The risk for cardiac death or nonfatal MI at 25-month follow-up in 449 patients 60 years of age or older was less than 1% in patients with normal images, 5% in patients with single-vessel thallium-201 abnormality, and 13% in patients with multivessel thallium-201 abnormality.

Pharmacologic stress testing

Intravenous dipyridamole-thallium imaging may be used to determine the presence of CAD in elderly patients who are unable to undergo treadmill or bicycle exercise stress testing.[39] In patients 70 years of age or older, the sensitivity of intravenous dipyridamole-thallium imaging for diagnosing significant CAD was 86%, and the specificity was 75%.[39] In 120 patients older than 70 years, adenosine echocardiography had a 66% sensitivity and a 90% specificity in diagnosing CAD.[40] An abnormal adenosine echocardiogram predicted a threefold risk of future coronary events, independent of coronary risk factors.[40] In 120 patients older than 70 years, dobutamine echocardiography had a 87% sensitivity and a 84% specificity in diagnosing CAD.[40] An abnormal dobutamine echocardiogram predicted a 7.3-fold risk of future coronary events.[40]

Ambulatory electrocardiography

Ambulatory ECGs performed for 24 hours is also useful in detecting myocardial ischemia in elderly persons with suspected CAD who cannot perform treadmill or bicycle exercise stress testing because of advanced age, intermittent claudication, musculoskeletal disorders, heart failure, or pulmonary disease. Ischemic ST-segment changes demonstrated on 24-hour ambulatory ECGs correlate with transient abnormalities in myocardial perfusion and LV systolic dysfunction. The changes may be associated with symptoms, or symptoms may be completely absent, which is referred to as silent myocardial ischemia. Silent myocardial ischemia is predictive of future coronary events, including cardiovascular mortality in elderly persons with CAD.[3–5,30,41–43] The incidence of new coronary events is especially increased in elderly persons with silent myocardial ischemia plus complex ventricular arrhythmias,[30] abnormal LV ejection fraction,[41] or echocardiographic LV hypertrophy.[43]

Signal-averaged electrocardiography

Signal-averaged electrocardiography (SAECG) was performed in 121 elderly postinfarction patients with asymptomatic complex ventricular arrhythmias detected by 24-hour ambulatory ECGs and a LV ejection fraction of 40% or higher.[44] At 29-month follow-up, the sensitivity, specificity, positive predictive value, and negative predictive value for predicting sudden cardiac death were 52%, 68%, 32%, and 83%, respectively, for a positive SAECG; 63%, 70%, 38%, and 87%, respectively, for nonsustained ventricular tachycardia; and 26%, 89%, 41%, and 81%, respectively, for a positive SAECG plus nonsustained ventricular tachycardia.[44]

Multislice computed tomography and magnetic resonance imaging

A direct comparison of multislice computed tomography angiography (MSCTA) with magnetic resonance imaging (MRI) for noninvasive coronary arteriography was performed in 129 patients, mean age 64 years, with suspected CAD.[45] Sensitivity for coronary stenoses greater than 50% of luminal diameter was 82% for MSCTA versus 54% for MRI; the respective specificities were 90% and 87%. The negative predictive value was slightly higher for MSCTA (95% versus 90%). In this study, 74% of patients preferred MSCTA over MRI. The greater diagnostic accuracy of MSCTA over MRI in this study is consistent with meta-analyses of both tests.[46,47]

64-MSCTA and coronary angiography were performed in 145 patients, mean age 67 years, and stress testing in 47 of these patients to determine the sensitivity, specificity, positive predictive value, and negative predictive value of these tests in diagnosing obstructive CAD in patients with suspected CAD.[48] Of 145 patients, 64-MSCTA had a 98% sensitivity, a 74% specificity, a 90% positive predictive value, and a 94% negative predictive value in diagnosing obstructive CAD. Of 47 patients, stress testing had a 69% sensitivity, a 36% specificity, a 78% positive predictive value, and a 27% negative predictive value for diagnosing obstructive CAD, whereas 64-MSCTA had a 100% sensitivity, a 73% specificity, a 92% positive predictive value, and a 100% negative predictive value for diagnosing obstructive CAD. 64-MSCTA has a better sensitivity, specificity, positive predictive value, and negative predictive value than stress testing in diagnosing obstructive CAD.[48]

CORONARY RISK FACTORS

Cigarette smoking

The Cardiovascular Health Study demonstrated in 5201 men and women 65 years of age or older that greater than 50 pack-years of smoking increased 5-year mortality 1.6 times.[49] The Systolic Hypertension in the Elderly Program pilot project showed that smoking was a predictor of first cardiovascular event and MI/sudden death.[50] At 5-year follow-up of 7178 persons 65 years of age or older in three communities, the relative risk for cardiovascular disease mortality was 2.0 for male smokers and 1.6 for female smokers.[51] The incidence of cardiovascular disease mortality in former smokers was similar to that in those who had never smoked.[51] At 40-month follow-up of 664 men, mean age 80 years, and at 48-month follow-up of 1488 women, mean age 82 years, current cigarette smoking increased the relative risk of new coronary events 2.2 times in men and 2.0 times in women.[52] At 6-year follow-up of older men and women in the Coronary Artery Surgery Study registry, the relative risk of MI or death was 1.5 for persons 65 to 69 years of age and 2.9 for persons 70 years of age and older who continued smoking compared with quitters during the year before study enrollment.[53]

Elderly men and women who smoke cigarettes should be strongly encouraged to stop smoking to reduce the development of CAD and other cardiovascular diseases. Smoking cessation will decrease mortality from CAD, other cardiovascular diseases, and all-cause mortality in elderly men and women. A smoking cessation program should be instituted.[54]

Hypertension

Systolic hypertension in elderly persons is diagnosed if the systolic blood pressure is 140 mm Hg or higher from two or more readings on two or more visits.[55] Diastolic hypertension in elderly persons is similarly diagnosed if the diastolic blood pressure is 90 mm Hg or higher.[55] In a study of 1819 persons, mean age 80 years, living in the community, the prevalence of hypertension was 71% in elderly African Americans, 64% in elderly Asians, 62% in elderly Hispanics, and 52% in elderly whites.[56]

Isolated systolic hypertension in elderly persons is diagnosed if the systolic blood pressure is 140 mm Hg or higher with a diastolic blood pressure of less than 90 mm Hg.[55] Approximately two thirds of elderly persons with hypertension have isolated systolic hypertension.[56]

Isolated systolic hypertension and diastolic hypertension are both associated with increased CAD morbidity and mortality in elderly persons.[57] Increased systolic blood pressure is a greater risk factor for CAD morbidity and mortality than is increased diastolic blood pressure.[57] The higher the systolic or diastolic blood pressure, the greater the morbidity and mortality from CAD in elderly women and men. The Cardiovascular Health Study demonstrated in 5202 elderly men and women that a brachial systolic blood pressure greater than 169 mm Hg was associated with a 2.4-fold greater 5-year mortality.[49]

At 30-year follow-up of persons 65 years of age and older in the Framingham Heart Study, systolic hypertension was related to a greater incidence of CAD in elderly men and women.[58] Diastolic hypertension correlated with the incidence of CAD in elderly men but not in elderly women.[58] At 40-month follow-up of 664 elderly men and 48-month follow-up of 1488 elderly women, systolic or diastolic hypertension was associated with a relative risk of new coronary events of 2.0 in men and 1.6 in women.[52] Recent data from Framingham also suggest the importance of increased pulse pressure, a measure of large artery stiffness. Among 1924 men and women aged 50 to 79 years, at any given level of systolic blood pressure of 120 mm Hg or greater, the risk of CAD over 20 years rose with lower diastolic blood pressure, suggesting that higher pulse pressure was an important component of risk.[59] Among 1061 men and women aged 60 to 79 years in the Framingham Heart Study, the strongest predictor of CAD risk was pulse pressure (hazard ratio = 1.24).[60]

Elderly persons with hypertension should be treated with salt restriction, weight reduction if necessary, cessation of drugs that increase blood pressure, avoidance of alcohol and tobacco, increase in physical activity, decrease of dietary saturated fat and cholesterol, and maintenance of adequate dietary potassium, calcium, and magnesium intake. In addition, antihypertensive drugs have been shown to reduce CAD events in elderly men and in elderly women with hypertension.[61–69]

The Hypertension in the Very Elderly Trial (HYVET) randomized 3845 patients aged 80 years and older, mean age 84 years, with a sitting mean blood pressure of 173/90 mm Hg to indapamide plus perindopril if needed versus a double-blind placebo.[69] The study was prematurely stopped at 2 years (median follow-up was 1.8 years) because antihypertensive drug therapy reduced fatal or nonfatal stroke by 30%, fatal stroke by 39%, all-cause mortality by 21%, death from cardiovascular causes by 23%, and heart failure by 64%.[69]

Elderly persons with CAD should have their blood pressure reduced to less than 135/85 mm Hg and to less than 130/80 mm Hg if diabetes mellitus or chronic renal disease is present.[55] JNC 7 pointed out that most patients with hypertension will require two or more antihypertensive drugs to achieve this blood pressure goal.[55] The drugs of choice for treating CAD with hypertension are β-blockers and angiotensin-converting enzyme (ACE) inhibitors.[55,70] If a third antihypertensive drug is needed, a thiazide diuretic should be administered.[55]

Left ventricular hypertrophy

Elderly men and women with ECG LV hypertrophy[24–26] and echocardiographic LV hypertrophy[25,26,28,71] have an increased risk of developing new coronary events. At 4-year follow-up of 406 elderly men and 735 elderly women in the Framingham study, echocardiographic LV hypertrophy was 15.3 times more sensitive in predicting new coronary events in elderly men and 4.3 times more sensitive in predicting new coronary events in elderly women than was electrocardiographic LV hypertrophy.[71] At 37-month follow-up of 360 men and women, mean age 82 years, with hypertension or CAD, echocardiographic LV hypertrophy was 4.3 times more sensitive in predicting new coronary events than was electrocardiographic LV hypertrophy.[25]

Physicians should try to prevent LV hypertrophy from developing or progressing in elderly men and women with CAD. A meta-analysis of 109 treatment studies found that ACE inhibitors were more effective than other antihypertensive drugs in decreasing LV mass.[72]

Dyslipidemia

Numerous studies have demonstrated that a high serum total cholesterol is a risk factor for new or recurrent coronary events in elderly men and women.[52,73–75] At 40-month follow-up of 664 elderly men and at 48-month follow-up of 1488 elderly women, an increment of 10 mg/dL of serum total cholesterol was associated with an increase in the relative risk of 1.12 for new coronary events in both men and in women.[52]

A low-serum high-density lipoprotein (HDL) cholesterol is a risk factor for new coronary events in elderly men and women.[52,73,76–78] In the Framingham study,[73] in the Established Populations for Epidemiologic Studies of the Elderly study,[76] and in a large cohort of nursing home patients,[52] a low serum HDL cholesterol was a more powerful predictor of new coronary events than was serum total cholesterol. At 40-month follow-up of 664 elderly men and at 48-month follow-up of 1488 elderly women, a decrement of 10 mg/dL of serum HDL cholesterol increased the relative risk of new coronary events 1.70 times in men and 1.95 times in women.[52]

Hypertriglyceridemia is a risk factor for new coronary events in elderly women but not in elderly men.[52,73] At 40-month follow-up of elderly men and at 48-month follow-up of elderly women, the level of serum triglycerides was not a risk factor for new coronary events in men and was a very weak risk factor for new coronary events in women.[41]

Numerous studies have demonstrated that statins reduce new coronary events in elderly men and in elderly women with CAD.[79–92] The absolute reduction in new coronary events in these studies is greater for elderly persons than for younger persons. In an observational prospective study of 488 men and 922 women, mean age 81 years, with prior MI and a serum low-density lipoprotein (LDL) cholesterol of 125 mg/dL or higher, 48% of persons were treated with statins.[83] At 3-year follow-up, statins reduced new coronary events by 50%.[83] The lower the LDL cholesterol level achieved in this study, the greater the reduction in new coronary events.[83]

In the 1263 persons aged 75 to 80 years at study entry and 80 to 85 years at follow-up in the Heart Protection Study, any major vascular event was significantly reduced 28% by simvastatin. Lowering serum LDL cholesterol from less than 116 mg/dL to less than 77 mg/dL by simvastatin caused a 25% significant reduction in vascular events.[82]

In the Heart Protection Study, 3500 persons had initial serum LDL cholesterol levels less than 100 mg/dL.[82] Decrease of serum LDL cholesterol from 97 mg/dL to 65 mg/dL by simvastatin in these persons caused a similar decrease in risk as did treating patients with higher serum LDL cholesterol levels. The Heart Protection Study investigators recommended treating persons at high risk for cardiovascular events with statins, regardless of the initial levels of serum lipids, age, or gender.[82]

On the basis of these and other data,[83,89–92] the American College of Cardiology (ACC)/American Heart Association (AHA) guidelines[54] and the updated National Cholesterol Education Program III guidelines[93] state that in very high-risk persons, a serum LDL cholesterol level of less than 70 mg/dL is a reasonable clinical strategy. When a high-risk person has hypertriglyceridemia or low HDL cholesterol, consideration can be given to combining a fibrate or nicotinic acid with an LDL cholesterol-lowering drug.[54,93]

Diabetes mellitus

Diabetes mellitus is a risk factor for new coronary events in elderly men and women.[52,73,94] In the Cardiovascular Health Study, an elevated fasting glucose level (>130 mg/dL) increased 5-year mortality 1.9 times.[49] At 40-month follow-up of 664 elderly men and at 48-month follow-up of 1488 elderly women, diabetes mellitus increased the relative risk of new coronary events 1.9 times in men and 1.8 times in women.[52] Elderly diabetics without CAD have a higher incidence of new coronary events than elderly nondiabetics with CAD.[95]

Persons with diabetes mellitus are more often obese and have higher serum LDL cholesterol and triglyceride levels and lower serum HDL cholesterol levels than do nondiabetics. Diabetics also have a higher prevalence of hypertension and LV hypertrophy than do nondiabetics. These risk factors contribute to the increased incidence of new CAD events in diabetics compared to nondiabetics. Increased age can further amplify these risk factor differences and contribute to greater CAD risk.

Diabetics with microalbuminuria have more severe angiographic CAD than diabetics without microalbuminuria.[96] Diabetics also have a significant increasing trend of HbA_{1c} levels over the increasing number of vessels with CAD.[97]

Elderly persons with diabetes mellitus should be treated with dietary therapy, weight reduction if necessary, and appropriate drugs if necessary to control hyperglycemia. The HbA_{1c} level should be maintained at less than 7%.[54,98] Other risk factors such as smoking, hypertension, dyslipidemia, obesity, and physical inactivity should be controlled. The serum LDL cholesterol level should be reduced to less than 70 mg/dL.[54,93] The blood pressure should be reduced to less than 130/80 mm Hg.[55] Sulfonylureas should be avoided in person with CAD.[99,100]

Obesity

Obesity was an independent risk factor for new CAD events in elderly men and women in the Framingham Heart Study.[101] Disproportionate distribution of fat to the abdomen assessed by the waist-to-hip circumference ratio has also been shown to be a risk factor for cardiovascular disease, mortality from CAD, and total mortality in elderly men and women.[102,103]

Obese men and women with CAD must undergo weight reduction. Weight reduction is also a first approach to controlling mild hypertension, hyperglycemia, and dyslipidemia. Regular aerobic exercise should be used in addition to diet to treat obesity. The body mass index should be reduced to 18.5 to 24.9 kg/m^2.[54]

Physical inactivity

Physical inactivity is associated with obesity, hypertension, hyperglycemia, and dyslipidemia. At 12-year follow-up in the Honolulu Heart Program, physically active men 65 years of age or older had a relative risk of 0.43 for CAD compared with inactive men.[104] Lack of moderate or vigorous exercise increased 5-year mortality in elderly men and women in the Cardiovascular Heart Study.[49]

Moderate exercise programs suitable for elderly persons include walking, climbing stairs, swimming, or bicycling. However, care must be taken in prescribing any exercise program because of the high risk of injury in this age group. Group or supervised sessions, including aerobic classes, offered by senior health care plans are especially appealing. Exercise training programs are not only beneficial in preventing CHD[105] but have also been found to improve endurance and functional capacity in elderly persons after MI.[105,106]

THERAPY OF STABLE ANGINA

Nitroglycerin is used for relief of the acute anginal attack. It is given either as a sublingual tablet or as a sublingual spray.[107] Long-acting nitrates prevent recurrent anginal attacks, improve exercise time until the onset of angina, and reduce exercise-induced ischemic ST-segment depression.[108,109] To prevent nitrate tolerance, it is recommended that a 12- to 14-hour nitrate-free interval be established when using long-acting nitrate preparations. During the nitrate-free interval, the use of another antianginal drug will be necessary.

β-blockers prevent recurrent anginal attacks and are the drug of choice to prevent new coronary events.[110] β-blockers also improve exercise time until the onset of angina and reduce exercise-induced ischemic ST-segment depression.[110] β-blockers should be administered along with long-acting nitrates to all patients with angina unless there are contraindications to the use of these drugs. Antiplatelet drugs such as aspirin or clopidogrel should also be administered to all patients with angina to reduce new coronary events.[111–113]

There are no class I indications for the use of calcium channel blockers in the treatment of patients with CAD.[54] However, if angina pectoris persists despite the use of β-blockers and nitrates, long-acting calcium channel blockers such as diltiazem or verapamil should be used in elderly patients with CAD and normal LV systolic function and amlodipine or felodipine in patients with CAD and abnormal LV systolic function as antianginal agents.[107]

Ranolazine reduces frequency of angina episodes and nitroglycerin consumption and improves exercise duration and time to anginal attacks without clinically significant effects on heart rate or blood pressure.[114,115] Ranolazine was approved for use as combination therapy when angina is not adequately controlled with other antianginal drugs. The recommended dose of sustained release ranolazine is 750 mg or 1000 mg twice daily.

If angina persists despite intensive medical management, coronary revascularization with either coronary angioplasty or coronary artery bypass surgery should be considered.[116,117] The use of other approaches to manage stable angina pectoris, which persists despite antianginal drugs and coronary revascularization, is discussed elsewhere.[107]

ACUTE CORONARY SYNDROMES

Unstable angina pectoris is a transitory syndrome that results from disruption of a coronary atherosclerotic plaque that critically decreases coronary blood flow causing new onset angina pectoris or exacerbation of angina pectoris.[118] Transient episodes of coronary artery occlusion or near occlusion by thrombus at the site of plaque injury may occur and cause angina pectoris at rest. The thrombus may be labile and cause temporary obstruction to flow. Release of vasoconstriction substances by platelets and vasoconstriction due to endothelial vasodilator dysfunction contribute to a further reduction in coronary blood flow, and in some patients, myocardial necrosis with NSTEMI occurs. Elevation of serum cardiospecific troponin I or T or creatine kinase-MB levels occur in patients with NSTEMI but not in patients with unstable angina.

Older patients with unstable angina pectoris should be hospitalized, and depending on their risk stratification, may need monitoring in an intensive care unit.[118] In a prospective study of 177 consecutive unselected patients hospitalized for an acute coronary syndrome (91 women and 86 men) aged 70 to 94 years, unstable angina was diagnosed in 54%, NSTEMI in 34%, and STEMI in 12%[119–121]. Obstructive CAD was diagnosed by coronary angiography in 94% of elderly men and in 80% of elderly women.[119]

Therapy

Treatment of patients with unstable angina pectoris/NSTEMI should be initiated in the emergency department. Reversible factors precipitating unstable angina pectoris should be identified and corrected. Oxygen should be administered to patients who have cyanosis, respiratory distress, congestive heart failure, or high-risk features. Oxygen therapy should be guided by arterial oxygen saturation and should not be given if the arterial oxygen saturation is more than 94%. Morphine sulfate should be administered intravenously when anginal chest pain is not immediately relieved with nitroglycerin or when acute pulmonary congestion and/or severe agitation is present.

Aspirin should be administered to all patients with unstable angina pectoris/NSTEMI unless contraindicated and continued indefinitely.[122] The first dose of aspirin should be chewed rather than swallowed to ensure rapid absorption.

The American College of Cardiology (ACC)/American Heart Association (AHA) 2002 guidelines update states that clopidogrel should be administered for up to 9 months in addition to indefinite use of aspirin in hospitalized patients with unstable angina pectoris/NSTEMI in whom an early noninterventional approach is planned or in whom a percutaneous coronary intervention (PCI) is planned. Clopidogrel should be withheld for 5 to 7 days in patients in whom elective coronary artery surgery is planned.[122] On the basis of data from the Clopidogrel in Unstable Angina to Prevent Recurrent Events (CURE) trial[123,124] and from the Clopidogrel for the Reduction of Events During Observation (CREDO) trial,[125] 81 mg of aspirin daily plus 75 mg of clopidogrel daily should be administered to patients with unstable angina/NSTEMI for at least 1 year.

Nitrates should be administered immediately in the emergency department to patients with unstable angina/NSTEMI.[126] Patients whose symptoms are not fully relieved with three 0.4 mg sublingual nitroglycerin tablets or a spray taken 5 minutes apart and the initiation of an intravenous β-blocker should be treated with continuous intravenous nitroglycerin.[126] Topical or oral nitrates are alternatives for patients without ongoing refractory symptoms.[126]

β-blockers should be administered intravenously in the emergency department, unless there are contraindications to their use, followed by oral administration and continued indefinitely.[126] Metoprolol may be given intravenously in 5 mg increments over 1 to 2 minutes and repeated every 5 minutes until 15 mg has been given followed by oral metoprolol 100 mg twice daily. The target resting heart rate is 50 to 60 beats per minute.

An oral ACE inhibitor should also be given unless there are contraindications to its use and continued indefinitely.[126] In patients with continuing or frequently recurring myocardial ischemia despite nitrates and β-blockers, verapamil or diltiazem should be added to their therapeutic regimen in the absence of LV systolic dysfunction (class IIa indication).[126] The benefit of calcium channel blockers in the treatment of unstable angina pectoris is limited to symptom control.[126] Intra-aortic balloon pump counterpulsation should be used for severe myocardial ischemia that is continuing or occurs frequently despite intensive medical therapy or for hemodynamic instability in patients before or after coronary angiography.[126]

A platelet glycoprotein IIb/IIIa inhibitor should also be administered in addition to aspirin and clopidogrel and heparin in patients in whom coronary angioplasty is planned.[122] Abciximab can be used for 12 to 24 hours in patients with unstable angina/NSTEMI in whom coronary angioplasty is planned within the next 24 hours.[122] Eptifibatide or tirofiban should be administered in addition to aspirin and low-molecular-weight heparin or unfractionated heparin to patients with continuing myocardial ischemia, an elevated cardiospecific troponin I or T, or with other high-risk features in whom an invasive management is not planned.[122]

Intravenous thrombolytic therapy is not recommended for the treatment of unstable angina/NSTEMI.[122] Prompt coronary angiography should be performed without noninvasive risk stratification in patients who fail to stabilize with intensive medical treatment.[126] Coronary revascularization should be performed in patients with high-risk features to reduce coronary events and mortality.[122,126–128]

On the basis of the available data, the ACC/AHA 2002 guidelines recommend the use of statins in patients with acute coronary syndromes and a serum LDL cholesterol of 100 mg/dL or higher 24 to 96 hours after hospitalization.[122] Statins should be continued indefinitely after hospital discharge.[89,93,122] The ACC/AHA 2002 guidelines also recommend use of a fibrate or nicotinic acid if the serum HDL cholesterol is less than 40 mg/dL, occurring as an isolated finding or in combination with other lipid abnormalities.[122]

Patients should be discharged on aspirin plus clopidogrel, β-blockers, and on ACE inhibitors in the absence of contraindications. Nitrates should be given for ischemic symptoms. A long-acting nondihydropyridine calcium channel blocker may be given for ischemic symptoms that occur despite treatment with nitrates plus β-blockers. Hormonal therapy should not be administered to postmenopausal women.[129,130]

THERAPY OF STEMI

Chest pain due to acute MI should be treated with morphine, nitroglycerin, and β-blockers.[131] If arterial saturation is lower than 94%, oxygen should be administered. Aspirin should be given on day one of an acute MI and continued indefinitely to reduce coronary events and mortality.[70,111,112,132,133] The first dose of aspirin should be chewed rather than swallowed. The addition of clopidogrel to aspirin is also beneficial in reducing coronary events and mortality.[134,135] Early intravenous β-blockade should be used during acute MI and oral β-blockers continued indefinitely to reduce coronary events and mortality.[70,136–143] ACE inhibitors should be given within 24 hours of acute MI and continued indefinitely to reduce coronary events and mortality.[70,143–149] Statins should be given to patients with acute MI and a serum LDL cholesterol of 100 mg/dL or higher 24 to 96 hours after hospitalization.[70] Statins should be continued indefinitely after hospital discharge to reduce coronary events and mortality.[78,86,87,93]

The ACC/AHA guidelines state there are no class I indications for the use of calcium channel blockers during or after acute MI.[70] However, if older persons have persistent angina after MI despite treatment with β-blockers and nitrates and are not suitable candidates for coronary revascularization, or if they have hypertension inadequately controlled by other drugs, a nondihydropyridine calcium channel blocker such as verapamil or diltiazem should be added to the therapeutic regimen if the LV ejection fraction is normal. If the LV ejection fraction is abnormal, amlodipine or felodipine should be added to the therapeutic regimen.

The ACC/AHA guidelines recommend using intravenous heparin in persons with acute MI undergoing primary coronary angioplasty or surgical coronary revascularization and in persons with acute MI at high risk for systemic embolization, such as persons with a large or anterior MI, atrial fibrillation, history of pulmonary or systemic embolus, or LV thrombus.[70] In persons with acute MI not receiving intravenous heparin, the ACC/AHA guidelines recommend using subcutaneous heparin 7500 U twice daily for 24 to 48 hours to decrease the incidence of deep venous thrombosis.[70]

Thrombolytic therapy is beneficial in the treatment of STEMI in patients younger than 75 years of age.[70,132,150–153] From the available data, one cannot conclude whether thrombolytic therapy is beneficial or harmful in patients older than 75 years with acute MI.[153] However, the data favor the use of primary coronary angioplasty in eligible patients both younger and older than 75 years with acute MI to reduce coronary events and mortality.[153–158]

THERAPY AFTER MI

Elderly persons after MI should have their modifiable coronary risk factors intensively treated as discussed previously in this chapter. Aspirin or clopidogrel should be given indefinitely to reduce new coronary events and mortality.[70,111–113,159,160] The ACC/AHA guidelines recommend as class I indications for long-term oral anticoagulant therapy after MI: (1) secondary prevention of MI in post-MI patients unable to tolerate daily aspirin or clopidogrel; (2) post-MI patients with persistent atrial fibrillation; and (3) post-MI patients with LV thrombus.[70] Long-term warfarin should be given in a dose to achieve an INR between 2.0 and 3.0.[160]

β-blockers (Table 41-2)[70,136–143] and ACE inhibitors (Table 41-3)[70,143–149,161–163] should be given indefinitely unless contraindications exist to the use of these drugs to reduce new coronary events and mortality. Long-acting nitrates are effective antianginal and antiischemic drugs.[107–109]

There are no class I indications for the use of calcium channel blockers after MI.[70]

Teo et al[164] analyzed randomized controlled trials comprising 20,342 persons that investigated the use of calcium channel blockers after MI. Mortality was 4% insignificantly higher in persons treated with calcium channel blockers.[164] In this study, β-blockers significantly reduced mortality by 19% in 53,268 persons.[164] In another study, elderly persons who were treated with β-blockers after MI had a 43% decrease in 2-year mortality and a 22% decrease in 2-year cardiac hospital readmissions than in elderly persons who were not treated with β-blockers.[165] Use of a calcium channel blocker instead of a β-blocker after MI doubled the risk of mortality.[165]

Aldosterone antagonists

At 16-month follow-up of 6632 patients after MI with a LV ejection fraction of 40% or less and either heart failure or diabetes mellitus treated with ACE inhibitors or angiotensin receptor blockers and 75% with β-blockers, compared with the placebo, patients randomized to 50 mg of eplerenone daily had a significant 15% reduction in mortality and a 13% significant reduction in death from cardiovascular causes or hospitalization for cardiovascular events.[166] The ACC/AHA guidelines recommend an aldosterone antagonist in patients after MI treated with ACE inhibitors plus β-blockers if they have a LV ejection fraction of 40% or less with either heart failure or diabetes mellitus if they do not have significant renal dysfunction or hyperkalemia.[54]

Antiarrhythmic therapy after MI

A meta-analysis of 59 randomized controlled trials comprising 23,229 persons that investigated the use of class I antiarrhythmic drugs after MI showed that mortality was 14% significantly higher in persons receiving class I antiarrhythmic drugs than in persons receiving no antiarrhythmic drugs.[164] None of the 59 studies showed a reduction in mortality by class I antiarrhythmic drugs.[164]

In the Cardiac Arrhythmia Suppression Trials I and II, older age also increased the likelihood of adverse effects including death in persons after MI receiving encainide,

Table 41-2. Effect of β-Blockers on Mortality in Elderly Patients after Myocardial Infarction

Study	Follow-Up	Results
Goteborg Trial[136]	90 day	Compared with placebo, metoprolol caused a 45% significant decrease in mortality in patients aged 65–74 years.
Norwegian Multicenter Study[137]	17 mo (up to 33 mo)	Compared with placebo, timolol caused a 43% significant reduction in mortality in patients aged 65–74 years.
Norwegian Multicenter Study[138]	61 mo (up to 72 mo)	Compared with placebo, timolol caused a 19% significant decrease in mortality in patients aged 65–74 years.
Beta Blocker Heart Attack Trial[139]	25 mo (up to 36 mo)	Compared with placebo, propranolol caused a 33% significant decrease in mortality in patients aged 60–69 years.
Carvedilol Post-Infarct Survival Control in Left Ventricular Dysfunction Trial[140]	1.3 yr	Compared with placebo, carvedilol caused a 23% significant reduction in mortality, a 24% significant reduction in cardiovascular mortality, a 40% significant reduction in nonfatal myocardial infarction, and a 30% significant decrease in all-cause mortality or nonfatal myocardial infarction in patients, mean age 63 years.

Table 41-3. Effect of Angiotensin-Converting Enzyme Inhibitors on Mortality in Elderly Patients after Myocardial Infarction

Study	Follow-Up	Results
Survival and Ventricular Enlargement Trial[147]	42 mo (up to 60 mo)	In patients with MI and LVEF ≤ 40%, compared with placebo, captopril reduced mortality 25% in patients aged ≥ 65 years.
Acute Infarction Ramipril Efficacy Study[148]	15 mo	In patients with MI and clinical evidence of heart failure, compared with placebo, ramipril decreased mortality 36% in patients aged ≥ 65 years.
Survival of Myocardial Infarction Long-Term Evaluation Trial[149]	1 yr	In patients with anterior MI, compared with placebo, zofenopril reduced mortality or severe heart failure 39% in patients aged ≥ 65 years.
Trandolapril Cardiac Evaluation Study[161]	24 to 50 mo	In patients, mean age 68 years, with LVEF ≤ 35%, compared with placebo, trandolapril reduced mortality 33% in patients with anterior MI and 14% in patients without anterior MI.
Heart Outcomes Prevention Evaluation Study[162]	4.5 yr (up to 6 yr)	In patients aged ≥ 55 years with MI (53%), cardiovascular disease (88%), or diabetes (38%) but no heart failure or abnormal LVEF, ramipril reduced MI, stroke, and cardiovascular death 22%.
European trial on reduction of cardiac events with perindopril in patients with stable coronary artery disease[163]	4.2 yr	In patients, mean age 60 years, with coronary artery disease and no heart failure, compared with placebo, perindopril reduced cardiovascular death, MI, or cardiac arrest 20%.

MI, myocardial infarction; *LVEF*, left ventricular ejection fraction.

flecainide, or moricizine.[167] Compared with no antiarrhythmic drug, quinidine or procainamide did not reduce mortality in elderly persons with CAD, normal or abnormal LV ejection fraction, and presence versus absence of ventricular tachycardia.[168]

Compared with placebo, D,L-sotalol did not reduce mortality in post-MI persons followed for 1 year.[169] Mortality was also significantly higher at 148-day follow-up in persons treated with D-sotalol (5.0%) than in persons treated with a placebo.[170] On the basis of the available data, persons after MI should not receive class I antiarrhythmic drugs or sotalol.

In the European Myocardial Infarction Amiodarone Trial, 1486 survivors of MI with an LV ejection fraction of 40% or less were randomized to amiodarone (743 patients) or to a placebo (743 patients).[171] At 2-year follow-up, 103 patients treated with amiodarone and 102 patients treated with a placebo had died.[171] In the Canadian Amiodarone Myocardial Infarction Arrhythmia Trial, 1202 survivors of MI with nonsustained ventricular tachycardia or complex ventricular arrhythmias were randomized to amiodarone or to a placebo.[172] Amiodarone was very effective in suppressing ventricular tachycardia and complex ventricular arrhythmias. However, the mortality rate at 1.8-year follow-up was not significantly different in the persons treated with amiodarone or a placebo.[172] In addition, early permanent discontinuation of drug for reasons other than outcome events occurred in 36% of persons taking amiodarone.

In the Cardiac Arrest in Seattle: Conventional Versus Amiodarone Drug Evaluation Study, the incidence of pulmonary toxicity was 10% at 2 years in persons receiving amiodarone in a mean dose of 158 mg daily.[173] The incidence of adverse effects for amiodarone also approached 90% after 5 years of treatment.[174] On the basis of the available data, amiodarone should not be used in the treatment of persons after MI.

However, β-blockers have been shown to reduce mortality in persons with nonsustained ventricular tachycardia or complex ventricular arrhythmias after MI in patients with normal or abnormal LV ejection fraction.[175–178] On the basis of the available data, β-blockers should be used in the treatment of elderly persons after MI, especially if nonsustained ventricular tachycardia or complex ventricular arrhythmias are present, unless there are specific contraindications to their use.

In the Antiarrhythmics Versus Implantable Defibrillators (AVID) trial, 1016 persons, mean age 65 years, with a history of ventricular fibrillation or serious sustained ventricular tachycardia were randomized to an automatic implantable cardioverter-defibrillator (AICD) or to drug therapy with amiodarone or D,L-sotalol.[179] Persons treated with an AICD had a 39% reduction in mortality at 1 year, a 27% reduction in mortality at 2 years, and a 31% reduction in mortality at 3 years.[179] If persons after MI have life-threatening ventricular tachycardia or ventricular fibrillation, an AICD should be inserted.

The Multicenter Automatic Defibrillator Implantation Trial (MADIT)

II randomized 1232 persons, mean age 64 years, with a prior MI and a LVEF of 30% or less to an AICD or to conventional medical therapy.[180] At 20-month follow-up, compared with conventional medical therapy, the AICD significantly decreased all-cause mortality 31% from 19.8% to 14.2%.[180] The effect of AICD therapy in improving survival was similar in persons stratified according to age, sex, LV ejection fraction, New York Heart Association class, and QRS interval.[180]

In MADIT II, the reduction in sudden cardiac death in patients treated with an AICD was significantly reduced by 68% in 574 patients aged less than 65 years, by 65% in 455 patients aged 65 to 74 years, and by 68% in 204 patients aged 75 years.[181] The median survival in 348 octogenarians treated with AICD therapy was greater than 4 years.[182] These data favor considering the prophylactic implantation of an AICD in elderly postinfarction patients with a LVEF of 30% or lower.

HORMONE REPLACEMENT THERAPY

The Heart Estrogen/Progestin Replacement Study (HERS) investigated the effect of hormonal therapy versus a double-blind placebo on coronary events in 2763 women with documented CAD.[183] At 4.1-year follow-up, there were no significant differences between hormonal therapy and the placebo in the primary outcome (nonfatal MI or CAD death) or in any of the secondary cardiovascular outcomes. However, there was a 52% significantly higher incidence of nonfatal MI or death from CAD in the first year in persons treated with hormonal therapy than in persons treated with the placebo.[183] Women on hormonal therapy had a 289% significantly higher incidence of venous thromboembolic events and a 38% significantly higher incidence of gallbladder disease requiring surgery than women on the placebo.

At 6.8-year follow-up in the HERS trial, hormonal therapy did not reduce the risk of cardiovascular events in women with CAD.[184] The investigators concluded that hormonal therapy should not be used to decrease the risk of coronary events in women with IHD.[184] At 6.8-year follow-up in the HERS trial, all-cause mortality was insignificantly increased 10% by hormonal therapy.[184] The overall incidence of

Table 41-4. Medical Approach to Elderly Patients after Myocardial Infarction

1. Stop cigarette smoking.
2. Treat hypertension with β-blockers and angiotensin-converting enzyme (ACE) inhibitors; the blood pressure should be reduced to <140/85 mm Hg and to <130/80 mm Hg in persons with diabetes mellitus or renal insufficiency.
3. The serum low-density lipoprotein cholesterol should be reduced to <70 mg/dL with statins if necessary and at least 30% to 40%.
4. Diabetes mellitus, obesity, and physical inactivity should be treated.
5. Aspirin or clopidogrel, β-blockers, and ACE inhibitors should be given indefinitely unless contraindications exist to the use of these drugs.
6. Long-acting nitrates are effective antianginal and anti-ischemic drugs.
7. There are no class I indications for the use of calcium channel blockers after myocardial infarction (MI).
8. Postinfarction patients should not receive class I antiarrhythmic drugs, sotalol, or amiodarone.
9. An automatic implantable cardioverter-defibrillator should be implanted in postinfarction patients at very high risk for sudden cardiac death.
10. Hormone replacement therapy should not be administered to postmenopausal women after MI.
11. The two indications for coronary revascularization in elderly persons after MI are prolongation of life and relief of unacceptable symptoms despite optimal medical management.

venous thromboembolism at 6.8-year follow-up was significantly increased 208% by hormonal therapy.[184] At 6.8-year follow-up, the overall incidence of biliary tract surgery was significantly increased (48%), the overall incidence for any cancer was insignificantly increased (19%), and the overall incidence for any fracture was insignificantly increased (4%).[184]

CORONARY REVASCULARIZATION

Medical therapy alone is the preferred treatment in elderly persons after MI (Table 41-4). The two indications for revascularization in elderly persons after MI are prolongation of life and relief of unacceptable symptoms despite optimal medical management. In a prospective study of 305 patients aged 75 years and older with chest pain refractory to at least two antianginal drugs, 150 patients were randomized to optimal medical therapy and 155 patients to invasive therapy.[116,117] In the invasive group, 74% had coronary revascularization (54% coronary angioplasty and 20% coronary artery bypass surgery). During the 6-month follow-up, one third of the medically treated group needed coronary revascularization for uncontrollable symptoms. At 6-month follow-up, death, nonfatal MI, or hospital admission for an acute coronary syndrome was significantly higher in the medically treated group (49%) than in the invasive group (19%).[116] Revascularization by coronary angioplasty[185] or by coronary artery bypass surgery[186] in elderly persons is extensively discussed elsewhere. If coronary revascularization is performed, aggressive medical therapy must be continued.

For a complete list of references, please visit online only at www.expertconsult.com

CHAPTER 42

The Frail Elderly Patient with Heart Disease

George A. Heckman
Kenneth Rockwood

INTRODUCTION

Despite a decline during recent decades in overall cardiovascular mortality in developed countries, the burden of cardiovascular disease remains substantial.[1] The prevalence of coronary artery disease (CAD) and heart failure (HF) increases with age, largely as a result of better survival of patients with acute cardiac events in the context of population aging.[2] The lifetime risk for symptomatic CAD after the age of 40 years is 49% in men and 32% in women.[2] The average age of patients suffering a first myocardial infarction is 64.5 years in men and 70.4 years in women.[2] Similarly, the prevalence of HF also rises sharply with age, and patients reaching the age of 80 years face a 20% lifetime risk of developing HF.[3]

Although the burden of heart disease is greatest among older patients, therapeutic recommendations are usually extrapolated from clinical trials conducted on relatively younger and healthier patients. Historically, a significant majority of potential candidates for these trials has been excluded because of multiple medical and age-associated comorbidities.[4] Furthermore, clinical trials have generally measured "hard outcomes," such as rates of death, mortality, or other cardiovascular events, outcomes that may not be as important to some older patients as quality of life, preserving cognition, or maintaining functional independence in the community. The recent publication of the Hypertension in the Very Elderly Trial (HYVET) illustrates some recent progress made in this regard and the significant gaps that remain.[5] In this multicenter randomized controlled trial of 3845 patients aged 80 years and over, treatment of hypertension with indapamide with or without perindopril for 2 years was well tolerated and reduced the risk of stroke, death, and HF. In contrast to most prior cardiovascular trials, HYVET specifically targeted older patients, with the average age of trial participants being almost 84 years, thus filling an important gap in hypertension management literature. However, compared with the general population, HYVET participants had fewer comorbid conditions, were not demented, and outcomes such as functional decline, caregiver burden, or institutionalization have not been reported. What is more, the recent report on dementia prevention in HYVET illustrates some of the pragmatic difficulties to be faced.[6] The early and significant benefits of treatment meant that the main trial was stopped early. In consequence, there was no significant difference in the proportion on active treatment versus placebo that developed dementia. Even so, when the data from HYVET-Cog were combined with that of other antihypertension trials, a statistically significant reduction in dementia was seen.[6] As the accompanying editorial made clear, though this is not entirely satisfactory, it is hard to imagine that mounting a placebo controlled trial to definitively address that question would be ethically permissible.[7] Thus much of the question about generalizing studies on fit elderly people to frail elderly people comes down to this: At what price should the evidence come? When is extrapolation justified? How do we distinguish between therapeutic adventurism and therapeutic nihilism? Here we aim to provide a framework to assist clinicians in the process of determining the most appropriate courses of action for frail older cardiac patients.

MAKING TREATMENT DECISIONS: SHOULD AGE MATTER?

Older patients with CAD are less likely to receive ACE-inhibitors, β-blockers, lipid-lowering agents, or antiplatelet agents.[8,9] Similarly, older age in HF patients continues to be associated with a lower likelihood of receiving the recommended standard of care.[10] Underlying these findings appears to be the assumption that aging is a homogenous phenomenon and that all older cardiac patients require the same clinical approach. Clearly, this is unjustified; chronologic age alone is an inadequate criterion upon which treatment decisions are made.

Some of the heterogeneity seen in aging can be accounted for by the development of chronic illnesses. According to the Canadian National Population Health Survey, the proportion of persons with no chronic illness declines with increasing age, from 44% of those aged 40 to 59 years, to 12% of those 80 or above.[11] In contrast, the proportion of persons with three or more chronic conditions in the same age brackets rises from 12% to 41%, respectively. However, the difference between successful and unsuccessful aging reflects more than just the burden of chronic disease, and is a manifestation of underlying frailty. Though consensus on a definition of frailty has yet to be achieved, frailty can be understood as a state of increased vulnerability due to reduced physiologic reserve and that is most often, but not exclusively, found in older persons.[12] In the Cardiovascular Health Study, prior myocardial infarction, angina, or HF were all associated with a greater risk of frailty.[13] In a cohort of 309 patients aged 77 ± 5 years and hospitalized with CAD, frailty, as assessed by decreased gait velocity, was associated with an almost fourfold increased risk of mortality at 6 months.[14] However, frailty is not invariably associated with chronic disease: although some older persons with chronic illness are frail, many are not.[15]

Assessing frailty can be considered akin to estimating a person's biologic age. Several reports show that biologic age can be inferred from a frailty index.[16–18] Given that the mean values of a frailty index typically correlate very highly ($r^2 > 0.9$) with chronologic age, biologic age can be inferred for an individual based on their observed frailty index, in relation to the age at which that value is seen on average. In each study, an individual's frailty index value (i.e., that person's biologic age) was a more important predictor of mortality than chronologic age. These data suggest that chronologic age *per se* may not be an adequate factor for making treatment decisions for older persons, but rather that a comprehensive assessment of frailty may provide more valid information upon which to base therapeutic recommendations.

The following clinical vignettes are provided to illustrate how assessing frailty can be incorporated into clinical decision making when considering interventions for older patients with cardiovascular disease.

Case 1: Ludwig B. is a bright, relatively healthy retired engineer with a history of hypertension controlled with hydrochlorothiazide, 12.5 mg daily. He is fully independent in performing his basic and instrumental activities of daily living and passed a driving test the year before. He stopped playing golf last year to look after his 75-year-old wife who has moderately severe Alzheimer's disease. He experiences a 1 hour episode of retrosternal chest pressure radiating to his left shoulder, but does not seek medical attention as he has to look after his wife. When he finally sees his family physician a week later, an ECG demonstrates new inferior Q waves and an echocardiogram demonstrates an ejection fraction of 55% with hypokinesis of the inferior wall of the left ventricle, consistent with a recent myocardial infarction. His family physician prescribes enteric-coated acetylsalicylic acid, an angiotensin-converting-enzyme inhibitor, and a β-blocker, all of which are well tolerated. Ludwig declines further investigations as he now feels well and must look after his wife. A cholesterol profile demonstrates an LDL of 145 mg/dL and an HDL of 35 mg/dL. Should Ludwig be prescribed a statin for secondary prevention of cardiovascular events?

Clinical trials have demonstrated that in patients who have suffered a myocardial infarction, statins reduce the risk of subsequent coronary events and mortality. However, inclusion criteria for the most recent trials have only included patients up to the age of 82.[19,20] The family physician must consider whether the results of these trials are applicable to Ludwig, who is 87 years old. Using the CSHA Clinical Frailty Scale (Table 42-1), the family physician determines that Ludwig falls in category 3 (well, with treated comorbid disease), which is associated with a relatively good prognosis.[21] The arguments for and against treating Ludwig with a statin are presented in Table 42-2. In this situation, the balance of arguments weighs in favor of offering Ludwig a statin.

Table 42-1. The Canadian Study of Health and Aging Clinical Frailty Scale

Frailty Level	Description
1. Very fit	Robust, active, energetic, well motivated, and fit; these people commonly exercise regularly and are in the fittest group for their age
2. Well	Without active disease but less fit than people in category 1
3. Well, with treated comorbid disease	Disease symptoms are well controlled compared with those in category 4
4. Apparently vulnerable	Although not frankly dependent, these people commonly complain of being "slowed up" or having disease symptoms
5. Mildly frail	With limited dependence on others for instrumental activities of daily living
6. Moderately frail	Help is needed with both instrumental and noninstrumental activities of daily living
7. Severely frail	Completely dependent on others for activities of daily living, or terminally ill

From Rockwood K, Song X, MacKnight C, et al. A global measure of fitness and frailty in elderly people. CMAJ 2005;173:489–95.

Case 2: Ludwig's 75-year-old wife Thelma has moderately severe Alzheimer's disease. She requires assistance for all instrumental activities of daily living, and with washing, grooming and dressing. She has episodes of urinary incontinence because she cannot always find her way to the washroom. She has had falls, requires a walker, and cannot leave the house unattended. Otherwise, she has no cardiovascular risk factors or other comorbid conditions and has never sustained a cardiovascular event. Routine cholesterol profile reveals an LDL of 145 mg/dL and an HDL of 35 mg/dL. Should Thelma be prescribed a statin for the primary prevention of cardiovascular events?

Statins are often recommended in the primary prevention of cardiovascular events, though the benefits may be marginal in patients with no other concomitant cardiovascular risk factors.[23] The family physician determines that Thelma falls within category 6 (moderately frail) of the CSHA Clinical Frailty Scale, which is associated with a poor prognosis over the medium term.[21] Furthermore, the family physician considers the results of the NHANES 1 study, which found that high cholesterol was associated with CAD only in active individuals aged 65 to 74 years.[24] The arguments for and against treating Thelma with a statin are presented in Table 42-3 below. In this situation, the balance of arguments weighs against offering Thelma a statin.

Table 42-2. Arguments For and Against Treating Ludwig with a Statin

Arguments Favoring Statin Therapy	Arguments Against Statin Therapy
Ludwig is not very frail. He may be chronologically old, but not as old biologically	Ludwig's age exceeds clinical trial inclusion criteria and he is thus too old
No compelling evidence that atherosclerosis is substantially different in an 87-year-old person than it is in a 77-year-old person	Potential risk for adverse events[22]
Ludwig is otherwise healthy, has no other competing comorbidities, and therefore has a remaining life expectancy of approximately 5 years	
In the PROSPER trial, benefits of statin therapy became apparent after 1 year	
Ludwig is at high risk for a recurrent event, which might leave him unable to care for his wife	

Table 42-3. Arguments For and Against Treating Thelma with a Statin

Arguments Favoring Statin Therapy	Arguments Against Statin Therapy
Possible but unconfirmed benefits of statins in Alzheimer disease[25]	Thelma is frail. Her biologic age is greater than her chronologic age
Even a remotely small reduction in the risk of a cardiovascular event might permit Ludwig to look after his wife at home as long as possible	Thelma is inactive according to the NHANES 1 definition and therefore her cholesterol level is unlikely to be a risk factor for a coronary event
	Marginal benefit of statins in persons at low cardiovascular risk[23]
	Increased polypharmacy
	Potential risk for adverse events[22]

In summary, using chronologic age to determine whether to offer a particular therapy to an older patient may be an inadequate strategy. In the absence of reliable evidence from clinical trials in truly representative populations of older persons, clinical decision making needs to be individualized, consider patient and caregiver preferences, and may be facilitated by assessing a patient's degree of frailty.

Does treatment of heart disease improve outcomes of importance of older persons?

The majority of clinical trials in cardiology have focused on outcomes such as rates of mortality, hospitalization, coronary interventions, and other objective assessments of cardiovascular events. Older persons often have other goals and priorities: for example, compared with physicians, older patients with atrial fibrillation place more importance on avoiding disability from a stroke than on the risks of bleeding associated with anticoagulation.[26] Though a few recent trials have examined whether control of vascular risk factors has beneficial effects on cognitive decline, outcomes of interest to older persons, such as preventing functional, caregiver stress, and institutionalization are considered infrequently if at all.

Nurse-led HF management programs may be more successful when patient goals are taken into account.[27] Evidence from smaller trials and observational data support the benefits of HF therapies for older patients, which may include the preservation of function and cognition.[28] In a randomized placebo-controlled trial of 60 NYHA class II-III patients with HF from LV systolic dysfunction aged 81 ± 6 years, perindopril over 10 weeks was associated with a 37-meter increase in 6-minute walking distance compared to baseline, versus no significant change in the control group ($p < 0.001$).[29] A supervised exercise program over 18 weeks in 20 NYHA class III HF patients aged 63 ± 13 years and LV EF 35% or less, resulted in improvements in psychomotor speed and general attention.[30] Numerous observational studies suggest that ACE inhibitors prescribed to older HF patients result in slower functional decline, improved cognition, and less depression.[31–34] Although these data require confirmation by larger clinical trials, they do support the notion that standard HF therapies have the potential to address outcomes of importance to frail older persons.

Few trials have addressed outcomes of interest to frail older patients with CAD. There is evidence to suggest that cognitive decline may develop up to 5 years after coronary artery bypass surgery.[35–38] Even so, data on the mechanism of the decline or the impact of revascularization on function in older patients are sparse. In the Trial of Invasive versus Medical therapy in Elderly patients with chronic symptomatic CAD (TIME), 305 patients aged 75 years and older, 78% of whom had chronic CCS class III or IV angina despite being given at least two antianginal drugs, were randomized either to optimal medical therapy (148 patients) or early invasive therapy (153 patients).[39,40] In the early invasive therapy group, 72% of patients underwent revascularization, which was associated with a significant early mortality hazard. However, after 1 year there were no statistically significant mortality differences between the two groups. In the first 6 months of follow-up, patients in the early invasive group experienced greater improvements in quality of life and functional capacity. During the second 6 months of follow-up, patients in the optimal medical therapy group experienced more adverse cardiovascular events than those in the early invasive group. After 1 year, differences in quality of life between both groups disappeared, likely due to the 46% of patients in the optimal medical therapy group who underwent revascularization due to intolerable symptoms in the latter half of the year. In short, older patients with intolerable angina who proceed with an early invasive approach to treatment appear to face an early mortality hazard, which, should they survive, is offset by earlier improvement in quality of life and functional capacity, fewer cardiovascular events, and lower mortality over the subsequent year. Patients able to tolerate their angina may choose to undergo revascularization at a later date, at the expense of a greater risk of cardiovascular events over the subsequent year (Case 3).

Case 3: Following his myocardial infarction, Ludwig does well for 6 months. However, he subsequently develops angina. Despite optimal medical therapy with an ACE inhibitor, acetylsalicylic acid, a statin, a β-blocker, nitrates, and a calcium channel blocker, his chest pain continues to be brought on by climbing six steps and occasionally when he helps his wife dress. Clinical evaluation and investigations reveal no new ECG changes or evidence of HF. Ludwig expresses the wish to continue looking after his wife Thelma, whose cognition has remained relatively stable, for as long as possible. Should he undergo revascularization?

Recent data suggests that while adverse events related to percutaneous coronary interventions are more common in octogenarians than in younger patients, overall complication rates remain relatively low and have been improving over time.[41] Arguments for and against submitting Ludwig to a coronary intervention are summarized in Table 42-4 below.

Ludwig undergoes percutaneous revascularization with resolution of his angina. His procedure is complicated by a false aneurysm of the right femoral artery, treated conservatively. He also experiences a transient ischemic attack affecting his speech, but with no permanent sequelae. His acetylsalicylic acid is replaced by clopidogrel. He is able to continue caring for his wife, who eventually dies at home from pneumonia 6 months later.

In summary, most clinical trials in cardiology do not consider all outcomes of importance to frail older persons. However, limited evidence exists to highlight the importance of considering these outcomes when considering interventions and therapies for older adults with heart disease.

Table 42-4. Arguments For and Against Submitting Ludwig to a Coronary Intervention

Arguments Favoring Intervention	Arguments Against Intervention
Successful intervention would allow him to more fully resume caring for his wife	Risk of complications such as stroke or death that would preclude him from looking after his wife
Delaying the intervention increases the likelihood of adverse coronary events in the near future	He can always undergo the procedure at a later date
He may as well undergo the procedure now, as there is a high likelihood that he will require one in the near future	

Are the manifestations of cardiac disease different in older persons?

The manifestations of heart disease in frail older persons are often at variance with the classical syndromes of angina pectoris due to CAD, or exertional dyspnea, orthopnea, paroxysmal nocturnal dyspnea and edema as a result of HF.[42,43] Though such manifestations are often referred to as *atypical disease presentations*, they are so common—especially among frail patients—that they might more properly be referred to as *nonclassical*.

Nonclassical illness presentation is more likely to occur in older patients with concomitant functional impairment and/or frailty.[42] Patients who are sedentary from other comorbidities may not experience exertional symptoms. In bed-bound patients, edema may accumulate over the sacrum rather than in the legs, and may reflect venous insufficiency, treatment with calcium-channel blockers, reduced oncotic pressure, or pulmonary disease, rather than HF.[43] Nonspecific sleep disturbances may be atypical manifestations of orthopnea, paroxysmal nocturnal dyspnea, or nocturia due to the mobilization of peripheral edema in the recumbent position.[44,45] Psychiatric symptoms, such as anxiety or depressed mood, may be associated with symptomatic or undertreated HF in frail older persons.[34]

In a cross-sectional cohort of 1939 persons aged 67 ± 11 years and hospitalized with an acute coronary syndrome, presenting symptoms included weakness and fatigue in more than 50%, anxiety in 34%, and vertigo or presyncope in 26%.[46] In a cross-sectional analysis of 247 older patients aged 76 ± 6 years hospitalized after an acute MI, only 22% had classic chest pain.[47] Almost 30% had a symptom complex of fatigue, sleep disturbance, psychological distress, dyspnea, and moderate pain, whereas almost half had multiple mild respiratory and gastrointestinal symptoms, fatigue, sleep disturbances, and pain. Delirium is one of the most common complications of myocardial infarction in persons aged 90 years and over.[48,49]

The consequences of delayed or missed diagnoses as a result of nonclassical presentations can be significant. Hospitalized patients having nonclassical symptoms are more likely to suffer adverse consequences such as being restrained or institutionalized.[42] Unrecognized myocardial infarctions in older persons not having classical angina or clinical evidence of HF are very common[50–52] and are associated with a similar prognosis to recognized myocardial infarctions.[53]

HEART DISEASE, POLYPHARMACY, AND COGNITIVE IMPAIRMENT

The prescription of multiple therapies to older cardiac patients, many of whom often suffer from multiple comorbidities, often leads to inappropriate polypharmacy. As a result, these patients may be at greater risk for adverse drug events, drug interactions, and nonadherence to therapy, especially when their cardiovascular illness is seen with concomitant cognitive impairment.

Older patients with heart disease are often prescribed diuretics and medications affecting the renin-angiotensin-aldosterone system, and should be followed closely for changes in renal function and the development of fluid and electrolyte abnormalities.[28] Older persons are more susceptible to dehydration, particularly in the setting of an acute illness. If dehydration is suspected, serum electrolytes, creatinine, and urea should be measured without delay, and spironolactone temporarily withheld because of the risk of hyperkalemia.[54] The importance of appropriate prescribing and monitoring is underscored by the occurrence in 2001 in Ontario, Canada, of an estimated 560 additional hospitalizations and 73 deaths from hyperkalemia following more widespread use of spironolactone for HF after publication of the Randomized Aldactone Evaluation Study.[55]

A number of cardiac medications have measurable anticholinergic activity, including commonly prescribed drugs such as warfarin, isosorbide dinitrate, hydrochlorothiazide, chlorthalidone, hydralazine, furosemide, nifedipine, and digoxin.[56,57] Advanced age is a risk factor for digoxin toxicity, which can occur at serum concentrations generally considered normal (1.4 to 2.0 ng/mL).[58] The cumulative anticholinergic burden associated with prescribed medications can adversely affect cognition in older patients, including a greater predisposition to delirium, more severe delirium, and may possibly accelerate cognitive decline in patients with Alzheimer's disease.[59–61]

Polypharmacy has been associated with an increased risk for falls.[62] Recommendations to aggressively lower blood pressure in older patients can lead in some older patients, particularly those who are frail, to orthostatic and/or postprandial hypotension, resulting in falls, fracture, angina or strokes.[63,64] In a cohort study of 4071 patients aged 83 years on average, excessive blood pressure lowering was associated with an increased mortality risk.[65] The highest survival rate was for systolic pressure of 130 to 139 and diastolic pressure of 80 to 89, with lower values associated with higher mortality. Prescribing physicians should monitor patients for orthostatic and postprandial hypotension and exercise caution when escalating doses of antihypertensive drugs.

The management of polypharmacy in older cardiac patients may often be complicated by concomitant, and often unsuspected, cognitive impairment. The same risk factors for heart disease are also risk factors for cognitive impairment.[66] Patients with HF in particular are prone to cognitive impairment through additional mechanisms, including hypoperfusion, hypercoagulability and other rheologic abnormalities, and concurrent depression.[68,71] In HF patients, cognitive impairment has been associated with nonadherence to prescribed therapy, rehospitalization, functional decline, and mortality.[72–75]

A variety of cognitive domains can be impaired in patients with heart disease, including difficulties learning new tasks as well as executive dysfunction.[67] Cognitive impairment is particularly common and problematic for patients with HF, who may have impaired memory, attention, processing speed, learning, and executive function deficits.[68] These deficits have the potential to interfere with adherence to lifestyle and dietary prescriptions, medications, regular weighing, and the recognition of early symptoms of decompensated HF.[69,70] Rehospitalization for HF has been associated with medication mismanagement, and failure to recognize HF symptoms and take corrective action or seek medical attention in a timely manner.[76–79]

Assessment of mood and cognition should be considered by clinicians prescribing new medications to older cardiac patients, particularly those with recurrent hospitalizations, multiple functional deficits, polypharmacy, limited social support systems, or poorly controlled cardiovascular risk factors.[28,80,81] Preliminary evidence suggests that treating depression may improve cognition in HF patients.[71] Care should be taken to simplify medication regiments, preferably with once daily medications. Adherence to prescribed therapy may be improved through the use of aids, such as weekly dosettes or blister packs; close supervision by a pharmacist or caregiver; and ensuring adequate social support through family members or visiting nurses.[82] Although referral of frail cardiac patients to chronic disease management programs or specialized geriatric services should be considered, the continued involvement of their primary care physicians is essential.[28] Transitional care programs based on Advanced Practice Nurse (APN)-led interventions to enhance self-management skills of older cardiac patients have been shown to decrease rates of adverse outcomes for up to 1 year following the intervention and are cost-effective.[83,84]

CONCLUSION

Assessing frailty, cognition, and patient goals are essential to the appropriate management of heart disease in older persons. Although the use of some standard cardiac therapies may be beneficial for outcomes and goals of importance to frail older cardiac patients, clinicians must weigh these potential benefits against their potential risks, which include not only the possibility of adverse drug events, but also of falls and other geriatric syndromes. Clinical trials of cardiovascular therapies in representative populations of older cardiac patients and which assess all relevant outcomes are urgently required.

For a complete list of references, please visit online only at www.expertconsult.com

CHAPTER 43

Hypertension

John F. Potter

Coronary heart disease and stroke remain the major causes of death in people aged over 65 years in westernized societies, with an elevated blood pressure (BP) level being the biggest treatable risk factor. With the ever-increasing number of elderly people in the population, hypertension is preeminent as a public health problem. It is perhaps surprising to realize that it was only in 1985 that the first large trial of blood pressure reduction in the elderly population was published, demonstrating the benefits of treatment in terms of reducing cardiovascular complications.[1] Prior to this, a general reluctance to treat hypertension in older people prevailed, based it would seem on a few case reports of the adverse effects of antihypertensive drugs. This chapter deals with some of the more important aspects of hypertension in elderly people, while highlighting areas where important questions remain unanswered.

EPIDEMIOLOGY

Blood pressure increases with age. This has been shown in both cross-sectional and longitudinal studies in nearly all industrialized cultures. The rise in systolic blood pressure (SBP) is almost linear up to age 80 years, values tending to plateau thereafter. Diastolic blood pressure (DBP) levels plateau earlier, at 50 to 60 years, and then fall.[2] These changes herald the important age-related changes that occur in pulse pressure (PP) and mean arterial pressure (MAP). PP tends to rise steeply after the age of 60 years irrespective of the SBP levels when young; whereas MAP shows a much greater increase with age in those with high values in their 30s and 40s and reaches a plateau after the age of 50 to 60 years.

There are many factors governing these changes, both environmental and genetic. For example, blacks tend to have a greater age-related rise than whites, especially in women. Important sex differences in the BP changes with age are also found when comparing the results from cross-sectional and longitudinal studies, with the former showing women to have higher SBP and DBP values than men after 50 years of age. Cohort studies show a different pattern, with SBP increasing to the same degree in both sexes with little difference in age-related values; whereas DBP levels for women are consistently lower than for men, of the order of 5 mm Hg. It is possible that some of these differences in cross-sectional studies are due to selective mortality differences (such as death rates being higher in those with higher BP levels) resulting in an underrepresentation of those with initially high BP levels in the older age groups. Lifestyle differences probably account for some of these age-related alterations, little change in BP being seen with advancing years in some nonwesternized cultures.

Prevalence and incidence

The prevalence of hypertension is dependent on the definition used. Classically the threshold is the BP levels at which treatment appears to offer benefit over nontreatment, but the actual BP levels taken for defining hypertension have changed considerably recently. Definite hypertension, as originally defined in the Framingham Heart Study (SBP = 160 mm Hg and/or DBP = 95 mm Hg or on antihypertensive treatment), was present in 39% of men and 48% of women in those aged 65–94 years.[2] In the United Kingdom, higher overall prevalence rates for hypertension have been reported, using the more liberal criteria (160/90 mm Hg) 61% of men and 63% of women aged 65 and over had hypertension, which rose to 78% and 83%, respectively, using a 140/90 mm Hg cut-off point.[3] There are, however, marked differences in prevalence rates between countries (e.g., North American rates being about 50% for those aged 65 to 74 years compared with 80% for Germany).[4] In the majority of these studies, these rates are based on two or three recordings at a single visit and, given the increased BP variability in older people, the estimates are probably too high and the rates based on repeated measurements are about 30% less than those quoted. For example, in a U.K. study of people aged 65 years and over, 52.2% had hypertension at first screening compared with 10.3% at the third visit 6 to 12 weeks later.[5]

As the systolic BP tends to increase to a greater extent than the diastolic BP with advancing years, isolated systolic hypertension (ISH) is the commonest form of hypertension in older people. Prevalence rates for ISH in the BIRNH Study were 9.9% in men and 11.7% in women aged 65 to 74 years, compared with rates for diastolic hypertension (DBP = 95 mm Hg) of 15.8% and 10.6%.[6] For those aged 75 to 89, ISH rates increased to 15.3% and 17.4% in men and women, whereas diastolic hypertension (DH) fell to 7.7% in men but increased slightly to 11.2% in women. Interestingly, 84% of all female hypertensives in the study were aware of their diagnosis, compared with less than 70% of men, highlighting the need for BP screening in this age group. Other studies using multiple BP recordings made on several visits have found prevalence rates for ISH of 4.2%, combined hypertension (CH) in 3.9%, and isolated DH of 1% in those aged 65 to 84 years.[5]

Favorable trends in terms of decreasing hypertension prevalence are being reported. In the United States, rates have declined progressively since 1971. For example, in the NHANES study, rates of hypertension in men aged 60 to 74 fell from 37.9% in 1971–1974 to 35.4% in 1988–1991, and for women from 64.7% in 1971–1974 to 51.1% in 1988–1991.[3] Incidence rates have changed little, being of the order of 9% and 6% per 2 years for men and women, respectively, in those aged 70 to 79 years.[7] However, reliable incidence data are relatively scarce, particularly in the very elderly population.

Blood pressure and risk

Framingham data have shown that elderly hypertensives have three times the risk of a cardiovascular (CV)-related death than age- and sex-matched normotensives.[8] There has been much discussion as to whether this relationship between BP and CV mortality is linear, U-shaped, or J-shaped, giving rise to the opinion that there may be an optimum level to which elevated BP values should be reduced. Intervention studies have suggested that reducing

BP levels too much may paradoxically increase cardiovascular and noncardiovascular risk. However, a U- or J-shaped relationship between BP and CV mortality has been reported in the placebo arms of these studies, so this could not be an effect of treatment per se.

Many of the studies suggesting an increased risk with lower BP levels were of relatively short duration and did not control for potentially confounding variables. The largest meta-analysis of prospective observational studies to date, involving nearly 1 million adults with no previous history of CV disease, has clearly shown a log-linear relation between increasing BP levels and CV mortality at least up to the age of 89 years with no evidence of a J- or U-shaped effect down to SBP levels of 115 mm Hg and DBP values of 75 mm Hg. A reduction in SBP of 20 mmHg would reduce risk of stroke mortality by 74% in those aged 40–49 years but only by 33% in those aged 80–89 years; for CHD the figures were 0.49 and 0.67 respectively. However, as the absolute risk of stroke and CHD events is much greater in the elderly, a 20 mm Hg lower SBP or a 10 mm Hg lower DBP would result in an annual difference in absolute risk that is almost 10 times greater in those aged 80 to 89 years compared with the 50- to 59-year-old group.[9] For the very elderly, blood prospective observational studies have suggested high BP is not a risk factor for mortality and low values are associated with excess mortality.[10]

SBP, DBP, and risk

Systolic blood pressure is a bigger risk factor than DBP for cardiovascular disease in older people. In the Copenhagen heart study,[11] the risk ratio (RR) for stroke due to ISH (SBP = 160 mm Hg, DBP <90 mm Hg) in men was 2.7, but for diastolic hypertension (DBP = 90 mm Hg irrespective of SBP) it was 1.7 compared with normotensives. For myocardial infarction no such difference was seen in the relative risk between ISH and diastolic hypertension. More important, borderline ISH (SBP 140 to 159, DBP <90 mm Hg) in the Physicians Health Study[12] was associated with a 32% increase in CV events compared with normotensives, and a 56% increase in CV deaths. If future studies show that treatment of borderline ISH reduces CV risk, this will have enormous implications because over 20% of those aged over 70 years fall into this BP category.

Pulse pressure and risk

Pulse pressure increases greatly after the age of 50 years as a result of arterial wall stiffening with the associated increase in SBP and fall in DBP. In older age groups in the Framingham study,[13] coronary heart disease was found to be inversely related to DBP at any given level of SBP =120 mm Hg, suggesting that higher pulse pressure is as important, if not more so, than any other component of BP in predicting CHD risk (Figure 43-1). Pulse pressure was a better predictor than SBP, independent of DBP levels, for estimating the development of congestive heart failure (CHF); for each 10 mm Hg increase in pulse pressure there was a 14% increased risk of CHF, compared with a 9% increase for the same change in SBP.

Although SBP and PP are the best predictors of coronary heart disease, the same is not necessarily true for stroke. Mean arterial pressure has been found, in some studies at least, to be a better predictor of stroke than either SBP or PP. In the Systolic Hypertension in the Elderly Programme,[14] a 10 mm Hg increase in PP was associated with a relative risk of stroke of 1.11 (1.01 to 1.22) compared with 1.20 (1.02 to 1.42) for a similar MAP rise.

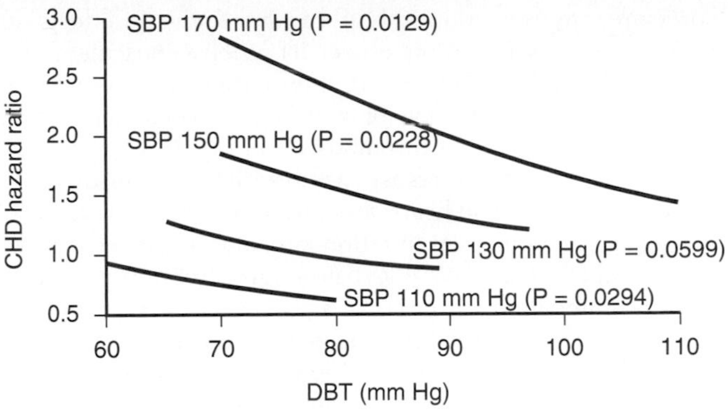

Figure 43-1. Influence of systolic and diastolic blood pressure on CHD risk in 50- to 79-year-olds. CHD hazard ratios are determined from the level of DBP within SBP groups. Hazard ratios are set to a reference value of 1.0 for an SBP of 130 and a DBP of 80 mm Hg. All estimates are adjusted for age, sex, body mass index, smoking, glucose tolerance, and total/HDL cholesterol. *(Data from the Framingham study, reprinted from Franklin et al. [1999].[13])*

The finding that PP is as good a predictor of coronary heart disease as SBP has potential implications for treating hypertension because there seems little point in lowering SBP and DBP to the same extent, (keeping PP unchanged) because this may contribute to maintaining some degree of CV risk. It would thus appear that, in elderly people, CHD events are more closely related to pulsatile load than steady-state components of blood pressure. This may explain why, overall, 30% to 60% of all CV events in the elderly population are attributable to mild or moderate hypertension.

PATHOGENESIS

Mean arterial pressure (MAP) is determined by cardiac output and peripheral vascular resistance (PVR) and is the steady-state component of blood pressure. The dynamic component, pulse pressure (PP), is the variation around the mean state and is influenced by large artery stiffness, early pulse-wave reflection, left ventricular ejection, and heart rate. A rise in PVR and large artery stiffness will increase the systolic BP component, whereas a decrease in PVR or an increase in large artery stiffness will result in a fall in diastolic BP, the latter being the dominant change in older hypertensives.

The main cardiovascular pathophysiologic changes associated with aging are arterial dilation and a decrease in large artery compliance, especially in the aorta, because of the loss of elastic fibers in the vessel wall and a concomitant increase in collagen. Arterial stiffening leads to enhanced pulse-wave velocity and early reflected waves augmenting the late systolic aortic pressure wave, resulting in a systolic increase and diastolic fall. The rise in mean aortic pressure is augmented by the rise in PVR, seen particularly in older women, enhanced by impaired endothelial release of nitric oxide, especially in older hypertensives. The increase in systolic load puts excess mechanical strain on the left ventricle, leading to concentric wall thickening. Because coronary artery perfusion is primarily dependent on the diastolic pressure, any reduction in DBP can have adverse effects on coronary artery perfusion, especially as left ventricular myocardial demands are increased in hypertension. Intimal wall damage results in the development of atherosclerosis and an increased likelihood of thrombosis.

The other main features associated with hypertension in old age are a reduction in heart rate, cardiac output, intravascular volume, and glomerular filtration rate, and decreased cardiac baroreceptor sensitivity (BRS) although cerebral autoregulation is unimpaired with normal aging and hypertension.[15,16] This decrease in cardiac BRS accounts for the increase in BP variability found in older hypertensives, and it perhaps plays a role in the increased susceptibility to postural hypotension. Both renal plasma flow and plasma renin activity (PRA) levels decrease with age, the fall in PRA being more marked in elderly hypertensives than in normotensives. Plasma noradrenaline (norepinephrine) levels increase with age and are associated with a decrease in β-adrenoreceptor sensitivity. The effect of age and hypertension on α-adrenoreceptor sensitivity is still unclear.

OTHER CARDIOVASCULAR RISK FACTORS

Hypertension should not be considered in isolation. Irrespective of the age of the patient, it is important that overall cardiovascular risk be assessed, taking into account other important risk elements such as cholesterol levels, smoking habits, and the presence or absence of diabetes.

Lipid abnormalities

Early data suggested that serum total cholesterol (TC) levels increase with age and remain a significant independent predictor for CHD in men. The effect in women is less clear because the number studied has been too small to draw firm conclusions. The SHEP study[14] found that TC and LDL cholesterol remained significant indicators of risk in both sexes, such that a 1 mmol/L increase in TC was associated with a 30% to 35% higher CHD event rate. More recently the Prospective Studies Collaboration meta-analysis of prospective observational studies involving more than 900,000 adults has shown increasing TC levels to be a risk factor for CV mortality even in the very old, though the risk is attenuated with age such that a 1 mmol/L lower TC was linked to a significant reduction in the HR for CHD to 0.57 in those aged 50 to 59 years compared with 0.85 in the 80- to 89-year-old group.[17] As in previous studies the effect was greater in men than women in the older age groups, but the effect was seen in both sexes up to 90 years. However, for stroke, the link with TC was not as strong as for CHD. For a similar TC reduction, there was a significant lowering of the HR for stroke by 9% in 50- to 59-year-olds compared with a nonsignificant 5% increase in the HR in those aged 80 to 89 years. For CHD, but not stroke, the ratio of TC to HDL-cholesterol was a better predictor than TC alone but the predictive power fell with age, a 1.33 lower ratio being related to a 31% decrease in CHD mortality in the age 70- to 89-year-group compared with a 44% reduction in 40- to 59-year-olds. For stroke in those aged 70 to 89 years and with a SBP greater than 145 mm Hg, TC was negatively correlated with hemorrhagic and total stroke mortality, a 1 mmol/L lower TC.

Diabetes mellitus

Up to 10% of elderly people with hypertension will have impaired glucose tolerance, and diabetes doubles the risk of developing coronary heart disease and stroke in those aged 65 to 94 years. Like total cholesterol, however, its impact on CV events falls with age: women remain slightly more at risk than men, though the absolute risk from diabetes is greater in the elderly than the young.

Body mass index

Increasing body mass index (BMI) is associated with an elevation in blood pressure, but the risk of obesity-related hypertension declines with age, there being a threefold increase in hypertension in obese 20- to 45-year-olds compared with a 1.5 increase in 65- to 94-year-olds. For each unit of BMI increase (kg/m^2), SBP can be expected to increase by 1.2 mm Hg and DBP by 0.7 mm Hg.

Interestingly, for elderly hypertensive men, CV relative risk increases from 1.8 to 2.9 between the lowest and highest tertiles of BMI, whereas the reverse is true for women. Even so, hypertension still more than doubles the risk of developing CV disease in both sexes. In the European Working Party on Hypertension in the Elderly (EWPHE) study,[18] those with the lowest total mortality and CV terminating events were found in the moderately obese group with a BMI of 28 to 29 kg/m^2, whereas those with a BMI of 26 to 27 had the lowest cardiovascular mortality. Truncal obesity (reflected in an increased waist to hip ratio) is more strongly related to hypertension and is a better predictor for coronary heart disease and stroke than BMI alone.

Smoking

Although the number of smokers decreases with age, smoking remains a significant risk factor for CV mortality in older persons (the relative risk is 2.0 for males and 1.6 for females). The relative risk of stroke among older hypertensive smokers is five times that of normotensives but 20 times that of normotensive nonsmokers. The benefits of stopping smoking in terms of reducing coronary heart disease and stroke mortality are still present even in the 70- and over age group, with the excess risk of mortality declining within 1 to 5 years of quitting. Older smokers should therefore be encouraged to stop. Hypertensive cigarette smokers have an increased relative risk of stroke nearly quadruple that of hypertensive nonsmokers (pipe/cigar use still increases the risk threefold). Encouragingly, hypertensive exsmokers of less than 20 cigarettes per day have, after only a few years of quitting, a similar risk to that of hypertensive nonsmokers.

Atrial fibrillation and left ventricular hypertrophy

In patients with atrial fibrillation, hypertension doubles the stroke risk compared with normotensives. Electrocardiographically diagnosed left ventricular hypertrophy (LVH) increases with age, reported prevalence rates being 6% in men and 5% in women aged 65 to 74 years, compared with 9.4% and 10.8%, respectively, in those aged over 85. LVH has a significant effect on CV risk. Its presence in those aged 65 to 94 years nearly triples the risk for men and quadruples that in women, but this effect is less than that seen in younger age groups with a similar blood pressure.

Alcohol and diet

ALCOHOL

The association between high alcohol consumption and blood pressure has been known for a very long time, although the relationship is not linear in most epidemiologic studies. It takes on a J- or U-shaped form, with the lowest incidence of hypertension being seen in those consuming around 5 to 10 units of alcohol per week. Large falls in BP (19/10 mm Hg) have been recorded with abstention in those aged 70 to 74 years who had a long history of heavy alcohol intake. Excessive alcohol intake has been directly related to stroke risk. It is unknown whether this is due to its direct pressor effect or to some other mechanisms, such as alcohol-induced cerebral vasoconstriction or cardiac dysrhythmia, particularly atrial fibrillation. As there appears to be a mild protective effect of a small amount of alcohol in older people, two units per day would seem a reasonable upper limit to recommend.

DIET

The relationship between dietary sodium intake and hypertension strengthens with age. For a 100 mmol/day increase, mean BP rises by 5 mm Hg in those aged 20 years but this more than doubles in those aged 60 to 69 years. Conversely, increasing potassium intake by 60 mmol per day reduces BP in older people by as much as 10/6 mm Hg. Increasing potassium dietary intake may also reduce stroke risk independently of its hypotensive effect. The average daily potassium intake in elderly people in the United Kingdom is around 60 to 70 mmol. This could be raised to over 100 mmol simply by increasing consumption of vegetables and fruit.

Physical exercise

Even mild-to-moderate physical exercise such as walking for 30 minutes three to four times a week has a hypotensive effect. Vigorous exercise in young to middle-aged persons prevents stroke in later life. Whether these effects are mediated solely through BP-lowering or are a result of other mechanisms, such as exercise-induced decreases in fibrinogen levels or an increase in HDL cholesterol, is unknown.

Hormone replacement

There has been considerable controversy over the benefits or otherwise of hormone replacement therapy (HRT) in CV disease prevention. A recent overview has suggested treatment has no significant effect on all-cause mortality, nonfatal myocardial infarction rates, or CHD death but a significant 29% increase in stroke risk and therefore cannot be recommended to reduce CV disease.[19] The effect of HRT in hypertensives is unknown and data are insufficient to see if the general increased risk of stroke is further increased in this group.

COMPLICATIONS OF HYPERTENSION

Stroke

Hypertension remains the major treatable risk factor for stroke, although the attributable risk for increasing BP levels decreases with age. For a 10 mm Hg increase in usual diastolic BP, the risk of stroke is almost doubled. A reduction of 9/5 mm Hg can be expected to produce about a 30% reduction in stroke incidence, whereas a fall of 18/10 mm Hg halves the risk; these expectations are irrespective of baseline BP levels.

The relative risk of cerebral infarction varies depending on the hypertension type in older age groups.[20] Isolated systolic hypertension (ISH) is a bigger risk factor (ratio 2.3) than is combined systolic and diastolic hypertension (ratio 1.5). The population attributable risk for stroke in those aged 70 to 79 years with ISH is about 21% for women and 17% for men, whereas for those aged 50 to 59 years the figures are 5% for women and 4% for men. Although the relative risk of stroke from raised BP decreases with age, this is not because hypertension per se loses its effect as a risk factor, but that more strokes occur in those with "normal" blood pressure. Intracerebral hemorrhage is also closely related to hypertension, the relative risk varying from 2.0 to 9.0 between studies—being greater for combined hypertension than ISH, particularly in younger patients.

Raised BP levels are common in the first days to weeks after stroke, and BP levels tend to settle spontaneously. There is, however, increasing evidence that raised BP levels following acute stroke are associated with a poor outcome in terms of death and dependency.[21] There is a small but convincing body of evidence to suggest an almost linear relationship between increased BP values in the poststroke period and stroke recurrence rate.

BP and asymptomatic cerebrovascular disease

Deep white matter lesions (leukoaraiosis) in asymptomatic hypertensive elderly patients are frequently found on magnetic resonance scanning. Whether these lesions account for the age-related cognitive impairment seen with hypertension that has been reported in many studies is unknown. It is also uncertain whether they increase the risk of subsequent cerebral infarction or hemorrhage. Isolated systolic hypertension, in particular, is associated with these subcortical lesions, and good BP control appears to have a protective effect. Large diurnal falls in BP are associated with silent subcortical white matter lesions and lacunar infarcts, but these are found also in those who have marked nocturnal rises in BP.

Cognitive impairment

The influence of blood pressure on cognitive decline and psychomotor function, over and above its association with vascular dementia, has been much debated. Some studies show no such relationship whereas others report a strong positive correlation with both vascular and Alzheimer-type dementia. A recent overview has suggested that increasing BP levels in midlife are a risk factor for cognitive impairment and dementia in old age, but that there is an inverse correlation between BP measured in old age and dementia in cross-sectional studies. The results of longitudinal studies of BP and cognition in later life are inconsistent, as are those for BP and dementia, though the majority suggest a low BP is common in those with severe cognitive impairment.[22] Treating hypertension even with small falls in BP is associated with improvements in MMSE scores and immediate and delayed memory scores.[23] A recent meta-analysis showed treating hypertension in the very elderly significantly reduced the risk of dementia by 13%.[24] The pathogenesis of hypertension-related cognitive impairment is unclear. It could be linked to a decrease in cerebral blood flow with increasing BP levels and alteration in the cerebral metabolism over and above the changes associated with leukoaraiosis.

Cardiac disease

The relationship between coronary heart disease and hypertension is discussed in Chapter 34. Hypertension accelerates the development of coronary artery atheroma through many mechanisms, particularly in association with metabolic abnormalities as in the insulin-resistance syndrome. Increased blood glucose and insulin levels, and changes in total cholesterol, HDL and LDL levels, and endothelial dysfunction result in impaired endothelial-dependent relaxation and increased leukocyte adherence, smooth muscle proliferation, intimal macrophagic accumulation, fibrosis, and arterial medial wall thickening. These changes, along with increased vascular oxidative stress and free radical production (see Chapter 32), result in inflammatory changes in the arterial wall, monocyte migration into the intima, and plaque formation.

DIAGNOSIS AND EVALUATION

General issues

Assessment of blood pressure levels in elderly people can pose particular problems, but it is essential that accurate measurements be made if patients are not to receive unnecessary or inadequate treatment. Minute-to-minute BP variations occur with respiratory and vasomotor changes. During the 24-hour period, BP fluctuations are related to mental and physical activity, sleep, and postprandial changes. Seasonal variations are also seen, with BP levels being higher during the winter months. Hypertensive patients have a greater absolute BP variability than normotensives, but when corrected for baseline values little difference exists. Clinically important differences are frequently found between individual readings at a single visit and between visits. Large falls in BP with repeated measurements in elderly hypertensives have been reported in nearly every placebo-controlled interventional trial, the effect increasing with age and amounting to as much as a 10/5 mm Hg decrease. The tendency for BP levels to decrease with time is related in part to regression to the mean and familiarity with the procedure of BP measurement. The British Hypertension Society (BHS) guidelines recommend that in uncomplicated cases an average of two readings be taken sitting on four occasions over a 2- to 3-month period during initial assessment.[25] It is particularly important to measure BP levels 1 and 3 minutes after standing to assess postural BP change in view of the frequency of orthostatic hypotension in this age group.

Measuring blood pressure

With the expected phasing out of mercury sphygmomanometers and their replacement by semiautomatic devices, it is important that manufacturers provide accurate equipment validated in the elderly. A list of BP measuring devices that have been validated for use in young and elderly persons is constantly updated on the British Hypertension Society Web site (www.bhsoc.org). Cuff size is important as undercuffing gives falsely high BP values. Cuff width should be equal to two thirds of the distance between axilla and antecubital fossa, and when the bladder is placed over the brachial artery, it should cover at least 80% of the arm's circumference—which should be kept supported at heart level. Clinicians should obtain both standard and large cuffs and ensure they are used appropriately.

The measurement should be taken in both arms initially because more than 10% of elderly people have at least a 10 mm Hg difference between arms. The arm with the highest reading should be used for subsequent measurements. All elderly people should have their BP measured every 5 years up to age 80 years at least, and in those with high normal BP (135 to 139/85 to 89 mm Hg) it should be assessed annually.

Ambulatory blood pressure monitoring

The role of ambulatory monitoring (ABPM) in the assessment of elderly people with hypertension is still being defined. Twenty-four-hour monitoring reduces the variability and the alerting response to measurement, so that 75% of elderly hypertensives will have lower ABPM measurements than clinic values. Casual measurements tend to be in the order of 20/10 mm Hg higher than 24-hour values. Daytime BP values are the best predictor of target organ damage.

The value of other information that the 24-hour ABPM profile can provide, such as day-night differences, is unknown. The Syst-Eur study[26] has emphasized that ABPM is a significantly better predictor of CV risk than are casual measurements. ABPM could be recommended in the following cases:

- To diagnose white-coat hypertension (persistently elevated clinic BP levels while normotensive on ABPM)
- When BP appears resistant to therapy (using three or more agents)
- In those with symptoms of postural hypotension and postprandial hypotension

However, there is little justification as yet to use it routinely in all elderly hypertensive patients because it is expensive and time-consuming, though generally well tolerated.

Suggested normal values are: daytime ≤135/85 mm Hg; nighttime <120/70 mm Hg; and 24-hour ≤130/80 mm Hg. Abnormal values are: daytime >140/90 mm Hg; nighttime >125/75 mm Hg; and 24-hour >135/85 mm Hg.[27]

Cuff measurements tend to underestimate intra-arterial levels of systolic BP by up to 5 to 10 mm Hg, and to overestimate diastolic BP by about 5 to 15 mm Hg. "Pseudohypertension" refers to falsely high noninvasive recordings caused by arterial rigidity, which prevents the vessel collapsing during cuff inflation. The prevalence of this condition in an unselected elderly population is probably very low, of the order of 1% to 2%. Unfortunately there is no accurate way of predicting the condition. Osler's maneuver (said to be positive when the radial artery is still palpable following the occlusion of the brachial artery) is unreliable.

Clinical assessment and investigations

One common feature of hypertension in young and elderly people alike is that it is very often asymptomatic. Complaints often attributed to increased BP levels, such as headache, are in fact unrelated in most cases. History and examination should include assessment for the presence of important CV risk factors (such as diabetes), for symptoms and signs of secondary causes of hypertension, and for evidence of target organ damage. Other important factors to be considered are the presence of confusion, urinary incontinence, decreased mobility, other medication use (for possible drug interactions which will affect the need for and type of antihypertensive agent)— all of which will influence treatment decisions. Examination should focus on evidence of target organ damage, including peripheral pulses and bruits (renal or carotid), and cardiac murmurs. Ophthalmoscopy is used for possible malignant-phase and diabetic changes, and a neurologic examination for signs of cerebrovascular disease and vascular dementia.

Initial investigations should include height, weight, blood samples for urea and electrolytes, creatinine and glucose estimations, and a 12-lead ECG (to exclude ischemic change, dysrhythmias, and left ventricular hypertrophy). In those aged $\leq$70 years for primary prevention, and in those $\leq$75 years for secondary prevention, total cholesterol and HDL cholesterol levels along with urine analysis for protein and blood should be included. Chest x-ray is of doubtful benefit, except in those who may have heart failure or chest disease. Plasma calcium and uric acid levels may also be useful to look for primary hyperparathyroidism (which is more frequent in elderly people with hypertension) and to check for gout. Echocardiography is rarely needed.

Renal artery stenosis is the only major secondary cause of hypertension in this age group. It should be considered:

- When there is a sudden onset or rapid progression of hypertension
- If BP control suddenly becomes difficult, particularly in those at greater risk of atherosclerotic renal artery stenosis, diabetics, smokers, and those with peripheral vascular disease
- In those developing malignant phase hypertension
- Where there is rapid deterioration of renal function, particularly after starting angiotensin-converting enzyme inhibitors

Renal ultrasound is not reliable for making the diagnosis of renal artery stenosis, although a significant difference in renal size may be suggestive. Captopril renography is not always helpful, and imaging techniques—either duplex ultrasonography or MR angiography—are the mainstays of diagnosis.[28]

MANAGEMENT OF HYPERTENSION

This section summarizes briefly the results of the important trials of drug therapy on outcome in elderly people. Space does not allow a full description of each trial.

Several recent large intervention studies have assessed the effects of antihypertensive drug treatment on outcome in elderly people, all of which have shown a positive benefit for active treatment. This is perhaps surprising given the heterogeneity of the patients included in the trials (those with combined hypertension, combined and ISH, or ISH alone, the presence or absence of target organ damage, and varying CV risk factors), the differences in antihypertensive drugs used, and the varying length of follow-up.

Published trials

TRIALS IN COMBINED HYPERTENSION

The first large trial solely in elderly patients, which awoke widespread interest, was the European Working Party Hypertension in the Elderly (EWPHE) trial published in 1985.[1] The results suggested that, for every 1000 elderly patients treated for 1 year initially with a diuretic, 11 fatal cardiac events, 6 fatal and 11 nonfatal strokes, and 8 cases of congestive cardiac failure would be prevented. Other randomized controlled trials that have enrolled hypertensive patients over 70 years include: that reported by Kuramoto et al[29] using thiazide diuretics as first-line therapy; the Hypertension in Elderly People trial,[30] using β-blockers; the MRC elderly study,[31] using thiazides or β-blockers; and the STOP-Hypertension trial,[32] again using thiazides or β-blockers as first-line agents. These have all shown the benefits of treatment in reducing cardiovascular disease (Table 43-1).

MORTALITY. Of the five studies noted above, only the STOP-Hypertension trial reported a significant reduction in all-cause mortality following treatment (relative risk 0.57; 95% CI = 0.37 to 0.87). A meta-analysis of these five trials demonstrates an insignificant overall reduction in total mortality (odds ratio [OR] 0.90; 0.79 to 1.02), but overall

Table 43-1. Compelling and Possible Indications, Contraindications, and Cautions for Use of the Major Classes of Antihypertensive Drugs in Elderly People

Class of Drug	Compelling Indications	Possible Indications	Compelling Contraindications	Possible Contraindications
A. ACE inhibitors	Heart failure	Chronic renal disease Left ventricular dysfunction Type 1 diabetic neuropathy	Renovascular Type 2 diabetic neuropathy	Renal impairment disease PVD
B. Beta-blockers	Myocardial infarction Angina	Heart failure	Asthma/COPD Heart block	Heart failure Dyslipidemia PVD
C. Calcium antagonists (dihydropyridine)	Elderly ISH	Elderly angina	—	—
D. Thiazide diuretics	Elderly		Gout	Dyslipidemia
Others				
Alpha-blockers	Prostatism	Dyslipidemia	Urinary incontinence	Postural hypotension
All antagonists	ACE-inhibitor-induced cough	Heart failure Intolerance of other antihypertensive drugs	Renovascular disease	PVD
Calcium antagonists with (rate-limiting)	Angina	Myocardial infarction	Heart block Heart failure	Combination with blockade

See text for explanation of ABCD classification.
Abbreviations: *ACE*, angiotensin-converting enzyme; *ISH*, isolated systolic hypertension; *COPD*, chronic obstructive pulmonary disease; *PVD*, peripheral vascular disease.
Adapted from Ramsey LE, Williams B, Johnston GD, et al. Guidelines for the management of hypertension: Report of the third working party of the British Hypertension Society. J Hum Hypertens 1999;9:569–92.

cardiovascular deaths were significantly reduced (OR 0.78; 0.66 to 0.92), as were CHD deaths (OR 0.73; 0.59 to 0.91) and stroke deaths (OR 0.68; 0.50 to 0.94).

NONFATAL EVENTS. An overall picture of treatment effects on nonfatal events is difficult to formulate because different trials used different criteria for defining nonfatal events; for example, "cerebrovascular events" may have included or excluded transient ischemic attacks or minor strokes. With these provisos in mind, nonfatal stroke events were significantly reduced (OR 0.69; 0.54 to 0.87), as were CV events (OR 0.72; 0.60 to 0.88), but with considerable variation between trials. For example, nonfatal stroke events in the STOP-Hypertension trial were reduced by 38% and in the HEP trial by 27%, and nonfatal coronary events by 20% in HEP and by 9% in EWPHE.[33] The benefits of treatment in terms of proportional risk reduction were similar between studies (a 35% to 40% decrease in all stroke events), but the absolute benefit seen was related to the underlying patient risk. In the MRC study,[31] strokes prevented per 1000 patient years of treatment were approximately 2.5, compared with approximately 14 in the STOP-Hypertension trial.[32] Drug therapy reduced the risk of hemorrhagic stroke within just 1 year of starting treatment, and within 2 years for ischemic stroke.

TRIALS IN ISOLATED SYSTOLIC HYPERTENSION

Trials involving ISH patients only (SHEP,[34] Syst-Eur,[35] and Syst-China[36]) have shown similar reductions in stroke and, to a lesser extent, coronary heart disease. Syst-Eur and Syst-China were unique in their time because they were the first to use calcium channel blockers (CCBs) as first-line antihypertensive treatment. Concerns had been raised about decreasing diastolic pressure further in patients with ISH because low DBP levels in cross-sectional longitudinal studies have been shown to be associated with an adverse prognosis in this age group. However, these worries do not seem justified because in the SHEP study treatment reduced DBP from 77.5 mm Hg to 68 mm Hg and yet significant reductions were seen in fatal and nonfatal stroke and myocardial infarct rates. Overall for the ISH studies there were significant reductions in total mortality by 17%, in CV mortality by 25%, and in fatal and nonfatal stroke by 37%. These benefits are similar to those seen in non-ISH trials.

COMBINED RESULTS

The combined results of the CH and ISH trials are shown in Figure 43-2. They suggest that only 45 elderly people with hypertension would need to be treated for 5 years to prevent one CHD event, compared with 180 younger hypertensives. For stroke the benefits are even greater, with only 22 elderly patients needing treatment to prevent a cerebrovascular event compared with 113 under 65 years. These benefits were achieved with relatively modest reductions in BP of about 20/10 mm Hg. Drug compliance among elderly hypertensives is generally as good as that for younger patients despite numerous factors that can affect this, including poor eyesight and hearing, confusion, etc. Simple once-daily drug regimens, and perhaps increased use of combined preparations, will improve compliance and therefore blood pressure control.

There is now convincing evidence that antihypertensive treatment should be introduced in nearly all patients up to

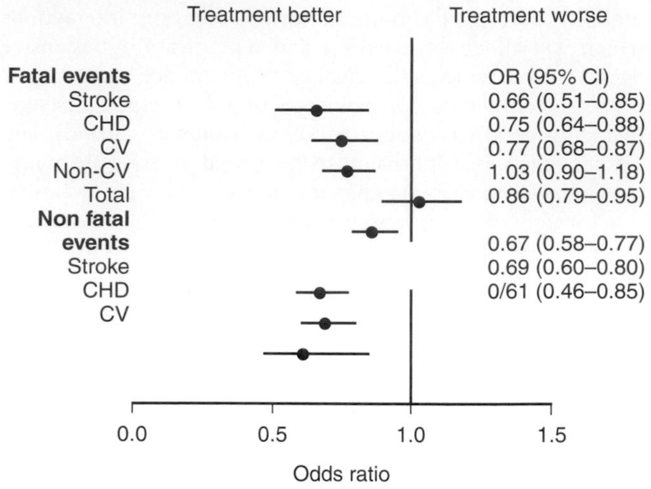

Figure 43-2. Effects of treatment on fatal and nonfatal events. Data from randomized outcome trials involving hypertensive patients aged 70 years and over.[1,29–36]

the age of 80 years if they have a systolic BP equal to 160 mm Hg and/or a diastolic BP equal to 100 mm Hg despite nonpharmacologic measures (see later discussion). Treatment should also be introduced in those patients with an SBP of 140 to 159 mm Hg and/or DBP equal to 90 to 99 mm Hg if target organ damage or other CV risk factors such as diabetes are present and their 10-year CHD risk is 15% (equivalent to a 20% CV risk). This risk can now be easily calculated using the Joint British Societies Coronary Risk Prediction Chart[24] or a similar computer program. This chart cannot be used to predict risk in those aged over 75 years or those on treatment, but it can be used for assessing the need for statin therapy based on the TC:HDL-cholesterol ratio and for the introduction of aspirin (see later discussion).

Target BP levels for treatment

Target blood pressure levels in trials have varied considerably and have also fallen considerably with time; for instance, target levels in the HEP study were 170/105 mm Hg, compared with less than 140 mm Hg for systolic BP in SHEP. The fact that the degree of CV risk reduction was so similar between studies is even more remarkable. However, with the concern still present about a potential U- or J-shaped relationship between BP levels on treatment and outcome, it was unclear how far BP should be reduced because no trial had specifically looked at this aspect in elderly patients, or in those with ISH. Results from the EWPHE trial[1] suggested that all-cause mortality was lower in those with an SBP on treatment of 150 mm Hg compared with those who achieved an SBP of 130 mm Hg.

The HOT study has gone some way to answering questions.[37] This recruited 18,790 patients aged 50 to 80 years (mean 61.5 years) with a diastolic BP of 100 to 115 mm Hg who were randomized to three target DBP groups: ≤ 80 mm Hg; ≤ 85 mm Hg; or ≤ 90 mm Hg. All patients received initial therapy with the dihydropyridine calcium-channel blocker felodipine. In addition, patients were randomized to low-dose aspirin (75 mg daily) or no aspirin. Unfortunately it proved difficult to reach target BPs, particularly in the two lowest groups of DBP, despite triple therapy in the majority of patients. No differences were seen in outcome measures between the three target BP groups, apart from a borderline-significant reduction in myocardial infarctions in the less than 80 mm Hg group compared with the less than 90 mm Hg group. However, combining all patient groups showed that the lowest risk point for major cardiovascular events was a mean achieved SBP of 138.5 mm Hg and a DBP of 82.6 mm Hg, and CV mortality was lowest with a BP of 138.8/86.5 mm Hg. For stroke, the lowest estimated incidence was with an SBP of 142 mm Hg with no definite minimum DBP level. In a diabetic subgroup, however, major CV events were highly significantly reduced, the risk being halved for those in the ≤ 80 mm Hg group compared with the ≤ 90 mm Hg group. There seems to be little to be gained in reducing the diastolic BP below 80 mm Hg except in diabetic patients.

Based on these results, the British Hypertension Society guidelines recommend that clinic BP levels for optimal control should be SBP less than 140 mm Hg and DBP less than 85 mm Hg, and in diabetics less than 130/80 mm Hg, with minimum recommended levels for BP control of less than 150/90 mm Hg and 140/85 mm Hg, respectively.[25]

It is important to bear in mind that introducing antihypertensive treatment is only part of the risk-reduction process. It is the level of blood pressure while on treatment that is a much better predictor of subsequent events than baseline values—hence the need to achieve these target levels. This will mean three or more different antihypertensive agents in 20% to 30% of elderly hypertensives. It is also important that other CV risk factors be dealt with simultaneously, such as raised lipid levels and smoking.

Prophylaxis

ASPIRIN USE

Although aspirin reduces deaths following myocardial infarction and stroke, its routine use in patients with uncomplicated hypertension has been unclear. In the HOT study,[37] those randomized to 75 mg of aspirin had a 15% (1% to 27%) reduction in major CV events, and MIs were reduced by 36% (15% to 51%); but stroke, total, and CV mortality rates were unaffected by treatment. Similar results were seen in a thrombosis prevention trial of men aged 45 to 69 years at high risk of CHD.[38] Both studies emphasized that if any benefit from aspirin were to be achieved, BP levels must be controlled (i.e., <150/90 mm Hg before aspirin is started in patients with uncomplicated hypertension).

For elderly patients matters are less clear because the benefits of prophylactic aspirin use appear to decrease with age. There was a 52% risk reduction with aspirin for CHD in those aged 45 to 49, compared with 29% increase in those aged 60 to 69 years. Those least likely to benefit were patients with a systolic BP greater than 145 mm Hg compared with those with SBP less than 130 mm Hg.

Elderly hypertensive patients should receive low-dose aspirin (75 mg daily) only if BP levels are well controlled and their 10-year CV risk is equal to 15%, unless there are other specific indications (i.e., after stroke or MI, with diabetes, or other evidence of target organ damage). Even then, good BP control should be the aim.

Statin use

No studies of statin use have specifically targeted people with hypertension, young or old. Conclusions drawn are therefore based on subgroup analysis of the large trials.

Insufficient data exist to support lipid-lowering therapy for primary prevention in patients aged over 75 years, and so routine lipid screening over this age is unnecessary. With regard to those at high CV risk and in secondary prevention, there have been just three large studies of statin use in patients up to the age of 82 years.[39,40] The results suggest that a much more proactive stance should be taken. Evidence indicates that 65- to 82-year-olds with risk factors for, or established, CV disease and a TC level equal to 3.5 to 4.0 mmol/L will benefit from statin therapy in terms of reducing subsequent major CV events by about 20% to 25%, although the results for stroke were inconsistent ranging from no benefit to a 25% reduction over 5 years. Stroke patients in the nonacute phase with a mean TC of 5.5 mmol/L also benefit from cholesterol reduction with a statin, subsequent stroke events being reduced by 16% and CV events by 20%.[41]

There are no long-term studies of the effects of diet on lipid levels and CV events. Such measures are likely to reduce TC only by 10%. Effective reductions will therefore require potentially expensive statin treatment. Evidence suggests statin therapy could be justified in those with a 10-year CHD risk of 6%, which would mean that nearly two thirds of the elderly population should be on treatment! This is unlikely to be possible, so guidelines recommend that patients up to the age of 75 years with CHD or overt atherosclerotic diseases should be considered for secondary prevention with a view to reducing TC to ≤ 5 mmol/L or by 25%, whichever is greater (or LDL cholesterol to ≤ 3mmol/L or by 30%). For primary prevention, those up to the age of 70 years with TC equal to 5 mmol/L and a 10-year CHD risk greater than 30% should be considered for treatment.

Nonpharmacologic methods

There is a general lack of enthusiasm for nondrug measures to reduce BP in elderly patients, despite the evidence of their efficacy (see later discussion). Various guidelines have emphasized their importance as first-line treatment in trying to achieve normotension and in reducing other CV risk factors.

WEIGHT LOSS

A 2-kg weight loss over a 6-month period will reduce blood pressure by about 4/5 mm Hg in elderly hypertensive subjects.[42] However, constant encouragement is needed to maintain this weight loss if the long-term benefit is to be seen. A body weight within 10% of ideal (or a BMI <26 kg/m^2) should be encouraged, not just for its hypotensive effects but also to improve glycemic control and lipid profiles, and to improve mobility and respiratory and cardiac function.

SALT RESTRICTION

The hypotensive effect of reducing sodium intake increases with age. In elderly people with hypertension, an 80 mmol/day decrease in sodium intake will result in an 8 mm Hg fall in SBP.[43] This level of sodium reduction can be achieved simply by avoiding salty foods and not adding salt while cooking or at the table. Reducing salt added to processed food would make even greater reductions possible.

INCREASING POTASSIUM INTAKE

Increasing potassium intake by 40 mmol/day will have a significant hypotensive action, reducing clinic BP by 10/6 mm Hg and 24-hour BP levels by 6/2 mm Hg.[44] In addition, increasing dietary potassium intake may reduce stroke rates over and above any hypotensive action. The average intake of potassium in the United Kingdom is about 60 to 70 mmol/day, and an intake of 100 to 110 mmol/day can be achieved by encouraging greater consumption of fresh fruit and vegetables. Potassium supplements are not routinely recommended for their hypotensive action, and care must obviously be taken in those with renal impairment.

REDUCING ALCOHOL INTAKE

The alcohol-hypertension link has been firmly established, but the relationship is nonlinear. Most epidemiologic studies have shown a J-shaped curve, with the lowest incidence of hypertension in those drinking about 1 unit (10 g) of alcohol per day.[45] Low levels of alcohol intake also appear to have a protective effect with regard to the development of coronary heart disease, even in older individuals, by raising HDL levels and having an antithrombotic effect.

OTHER MEASURES

Changing magnesium and calcium intake have not been found to have a significant effect on BP in the elderly population, although increasing vitamin C intake does have a mild hypotensive action and a positive effect on the lipid profile in older hypertensives.[46] Caffeine may have an acute pressor effect in caffeine-naïve persons, but regular caffeine intake does not have a pressor effect (although some studies have shown increasing consumption is associated with an increased CHD risk). Mild aerobic exercise (walking 30 minutes a day three to four times a week) results in important reductions in BP (approximately 20/10 mm Hg) in older hypertensives. It also decreases stroke risk independently of its hypotensive action, and improves glucose profiles, reduces weight, and improves general well-being.[47]

COMBINED EFFECTS

The combined effect of dietary interventions has been investigated in two important studies. The Dietary Approaches to Stop Hypertension (DASH) trial[48] studied the effects of a special diet rich in vegetables and fruit and low in dairy products. It compared this to a standard diet, while varying levels of sodium intake in persons with and without hypertension. The DASH diet with a low sodium intake resulted in a BP fall of 7 mm Hg in normotensives and 11.5 mm Hg in hypertensives—similar effects to those that might be seen with a thiazide diuretic (see later). However, the duration of the trial was only 30 days.

The Trial of Non-pharmacologic intervention in the Elderly (TONE) study[42] randomized elderly hypertensives who were normotensive on monotherapy to drug treatment withdrawal and either sodium reduction (and, if obese, sodium reduction or weight loss or the combination) or usual care with a 30-month follow-up. End points of restarting hypotensive drug treatment or developing a CV event were significantly reduced by all the interventions, with a 53% risk reduction in the obese on the combined sodium-restriction and weight-loss diet. The study was underpowered to find a significant decrease in CV events alone, but the nutritional interventions were well tolerated.

Approximately 25% of elderly people with mild hypertension could remain off drug treatment for 12 months or more using nonpharmacologic measures. Predictors of those who will remain normotensive include the absence of ECG evidence of LVH, obesity, and patients with well-controlled SBP levels prior to withdrawal of treatment. In general, nonpharmacologic methods should be tried initially in all patients and given time to work, although constant encouragement will be needed. In the majority of patients drug therapy will also be needed. Important synergistic effects between nonpharmacologic and drug treatments are found, such as in sodium restriction with those patients treated with ACE inhibitors.

Drug treatments

THIAZIDES

Low-dose thiazide diuretics remain the first-choice antihypertensive agents in elderly patients for combined or isolated systolic hypertension.[24] Their mode of action has not been fully resolved, but is in part due to a reduction in peripheral vascular resistance. Although there are concerns that thiazides may induce postural hypotension, this is not a significant side effect. Mild hypokalemia, hyponatremia, and hyperuricemia can occur but are not normally clinically significant if low doses are used. Impotence can still be a problem with these agents in all age groups. Serum electrolytes should be checked before and a few weeks after starting treatment to assess the need for additional potassium supplementation.

B-ADRENORECEPTOR BLOCKERS

β-blockers, such as thiazide diuretics, have been used as first-line therapy in several large intervention trials in the elderly. There are, however, theoretical reasons why they may not be the most obvious choice in elderly patients with hypertension because they reduce cardiac output and renin levels that are already reduced, and increase peripheral resistance. Although they can effectively reduce BP in this age group, they do not have a good side effect profile. For instance, in the MRC study in the elderly,[31] 30% of the β-blocker group were withdrawn because of major side effects, compared with 15% in the diuretic limb and 4% of those on a placebo. There were also significant differences between treatment limbs in outcome measures in the trial. The β-blocker group showed no significant reduction in coronary events, unlike the diuretic group.

A recent meta-analysis of all trials in elderly patients with hypertension using diuretics and/or β-blockers as first-line agents showed that, although β-blockers prevented all stroke events, they did not reduce stroke mortality; nor did they reduce CHD events, CV, or all-cause mortality, whereas diuretics showed a positive and significant advantage in all these outcome measures.[49]

In view of these findings, patient compliance and economic factors, thiazides are the drug of first choice for initial therapy. However, as over half of such patients will require two or more agents, β-blockers should still be considered as additional therapy but probably more as fourth-line agents except in certain elderly patient groups where β-blockers may still be considered as first-line agents (e.g., those who have had a previous myocardial infarction or have angina).

CALCIUM-CHANNEL BLOCKERS

Recent intervention studies involving elderly people with hypertension—the Syst-Eur,[34] Syst-China,[35] and HOT[37] studies—have used members of the dihydropyridine CCB group as first-line therapy. There has been considerable debate about the safety of the dihydropyridines, and various meta analyses have arrived at diametrically opposite conclusions. It is clear that the placebo-controlled intervention studies in the elderly using dihydropyridine CCBs as first-line treatment have shown significant benefits, particularly in terms of stroke and CV risk reduction. We still need the security of long-term safety data, but trial evidence indicates that these agents are generally well tolerated and effective, so are recommended as first-line agents in patients with isolated systolic hypertension in whom thiazide diuretics cannot be tolerated.[23] Short-acting calcium-channel blockers have no role in the treatment of hypertension.

ANGIOTENSIN-CONVERTING ENZYME INHIBITORS AND ANGIOTENSIN RECEPTOR BLOCKERS

ACE inhibitors (ACEIs) are effective antihypertensive agents in young and old alike. First-dose hypotension may occur, especially in patients who are on large-dose diuretics, so it is usually recommended that these agents be stopped for a few days before initiating ACEI therapy. Hyperkalemia can be a problem, so potassium-sparing diuretics should be stopped with the introduction of these drugs. Problems with renal impairment have been reported in older patients taking NSAIDs and those with preexisting renal impairment. Renal failure may be precipitated in those with occult renal artery stenosis, so it is recommended that urea and electrolytes be checked before and 1 to 2 weeks after starting treatment. Cough can be a problem in about 10% of patients, so an AII antagonist may be a suitable alternative. There are theoretical reasons to suggest that the combination of ACE and AII inhibitors could be potentially synergistic in their hypotensive actions, although it is too early to recommend this combination.

There are now several outcome studies using ACEIs as first-line therapy in the elderly. STOP-2 trial[50] compared the newer antihypertensive agents—a dihydropyridine CCB and an ACEI—against standard therapy with β-blockers and diuretics. Overall there was little difference in terms of outcome measures between the new and old agents. A comparison of the ACEI and CCB groups showed a greater reduction in myocardial infarction and congestive heart failure in the ACEI group (by 23% and 22%, respectively) but a greater decrease in stroke mortality with CCBs. Overall CV mortality, total mortality, and all major CV events were similar in the ACEI and CCB groups, with CV mortality being 20.5 per 1000 patient years in the ACEI group and 19.2 per 1000 patient years in the CCB group. There have been no large outcome studies using ACEIs as first-line therapy in elderly people with hypertension. Angiotensin receptor blockers (ARBs) have also been shown to be highly effective agents in the elderly hypertensive patient and do not have the troublesome side effect of cough seen with ACEIs.

OTHER AGENTS

α-Blockers still have a minor role in treating elderly people with hypertension and are usually used as additional, rather than first-line, therapy. The withdrawal of doxazosin as initial therapy in the ALLHAT study[51] because of increased risks of heart failure and stroke compared with chlorthalidone supports this policy. α-Blockers may have a role in men with prostatic symptoms, and they can be used in renal failure, although postural hypotension and urinary incontinence remain a drawback in a significant number of patients.

Methyldopa, hydralazine, and centrally acting agents are rarely used because of their adverse side effect profiles. The former two agents need to be taken more than once a day, which does not aid compliance. There seems little reason to use agents that do not have a 24-hour hypotensive action when taken once daily.

COMBINATION THERAPY

More than 50% of these patients will need two or more agents if adequate blood pressure control is to be achieved.[37] Not all agents have a synergistic effect. For example, the addition of a calcium-channel blocker to a thiazide diuretic in most studies has a minimal additional hypotensive effect. Adoption of the British Hypertension Society's "ACD strategy" will help form logical combinations, such that antihypertensive combinations are likely to have an additional hypotensive effect if their mechanisms of action are complementary.

The first-line agents in the elderly should be a thiazide diuretic (D) or, if that is not tolerated, a calcium-channel blocker (C). If control is not achieved, a first-line agent of the other group (i.e., ACEIs (A) or ARB) could be tried. If good control is still not obtained, an additional agent from the other group is added along the following lines in the elderly: (C or D) add (A) add (D or C) add to combination (A+C+D) fourth-line agent (e.g. alpha-blocker, or beta-blocker or speronolactone or amiloride) (see Table 43-1). It has been suggested the protective effect of blood pressure lowering is not substantially affected by the type of drug class given but is more dependent on the level of BP lowering achieved.[52]

SPECIAL CASES

The 80 and over age group

Several trials have included patients over the age of 80, but it has been unclear whether they benefit from treatment. Longitudinal studies have shown that raised blood pressure in the very old (aged 75 to 80+ years) is not as big a risk factor as in younger people. However, the SHEP study[34] showed that only the 80 and over age group had a significant reduction in CV risk with active treatment compared with placebo, although there were similar trends in the 60 and over and 70 and over age groups. A meta-analysis of these trials[53] that included all the patients aged 80 and over showed that treatment prevented 34% (18% to 52%) of strokes, with a reduction in major CV events (23%) and heart failure (42%). However, total mortality was increased by 15% in the actively treated group, leaving physicians with a considerable dilemma as what is best for very old hypertensive patients.

The Hypertension in the Very Elderly Trial (HYVET)[54] was specifically designed to assess if lowering BP (with a diuretic ± ACEI regime) reduced CV events in the 80 and over age group. After a relatively short follow-up period of 1.8 years, active treatment significantly lowered BP by 15/6 mm Hg and reduced the risk of fatal and nonfatal stroke by 30%, heart failure by 64%, and total mortality by 21%, and there were less side effects than in the placebo group. Given these important findings, patients aged 80 and over with newly diagnosed hypertension and who are generally fit with a reasonable life expectancy should be considered for treatment whether they have evidence of target organ damage or not. Those who reach 80 years of age already on treatment this should be continued.

Type II diabetes

Hypertension is common in elderly type II diabetics. Nearly two thirds will have raised BP levels that require treatment. Elderly diabetics as much as their younger counterparts should be treated aggressively in terms of BP reduction. The UK Prospective Diabetes Study[55] showed that strict BP control reduces stroke by 44% (11% to 65%) and death related to diabetes by 32% (6% to 51%). A subgroup of elderly diabetics in the SHEP study[34] did similarly well, with a 5-year reduction of major CV events of 34% (6% to 54%) compared with placebo, and a reduction of nonfatal and fatal CHD events by 54% (12% to 76%). The HOT study[37] also included a group of diabetics and only this group showed a significantly better outcome in those in whom diastolic BP was reduced to less than 80 mm Hg compared with less than 90 mm Hg on treatment, with a 50% reduction in CV end points in the lowest BP group. Diabetics in the STOP-2 study showed no difference in outcome between those on conventional therapy (low-dose thiazide diuretic or β-blocker) and those on the newer agents (ACE inhibitors and CCBs). This again highlights how it is the degree of BP reduction and not the agent used that predicts CV risk, and diabetics require lower target BP levels as evidenced by the HOT study. Hence, in diabetics, BP levels for the introduction of therapy should be equal to 140/90 mm Hg (lower starting BP levels than for nondiabetics) with optimum control levels set at less than 140/80 mm Hg. No one group of antihypertensive agents appears more efficacious than another.

Cognitive function, dementia, and quality of life

Although increased blood pressure has been associated with impaired cognitive function, this does not mean that antihypertensive treatment will reduce this decline. Indeed, it has been suggested that antihypertensive treatment may actually hasten it. Reassuringly, the MRC study in the elderly found no difference in the changes in cognitive function between β-blocker- or diuretic-treated patients compared with the placebo over a 54-month follow-up.[56]

Since hypertension is associated with both vascular dementia and Alzheimer's disease, it might be hoped that treatment could slow down or prevent cognitive decline. The Syst-Eur study,[35] encouragingly for a relatively short follow-up period of 2 years, found that active treatment reduced the incidence of dementia by 50% (though the numbers actually involved were very small) and improved the Mini Mental State score slightly, whereas in the placebo group scores deteriorated significantly. However, the SHEP study[34] failed to find a decrease in the incidence of dementia with active treatment. The cognitive arm of the HYVET study[24] did not find BP lowering in the very elderly reduced dementia but the follow-up period was probably too short to see any benefit. Combining all trials assessing the effects of BP lowering in elderly hypertensives on dementia found a 13% reduction with active treatment.[24]

Although there are relatively limited numbers of studies assessing the long-term effects of antihypertensives on quality-of-life measures, most have shown a long-term benefit. Quality of life should be an essential part of the overall patient assessment, but it does not necessarily require a lengthy or complex questionnaire. Simple clinical assessment of possible changes in physical function (e.g., mobility and balance, and ability for self-care), sexual function, energy levels and mood, cognitive function, life satisfaction, and social interaction is sufficient. Of particular importance are the effects of treatment on cognitive function, mood, and mobility. Thiazide diuretics appear to be the "cleanest" in terms of effects on quality-of-life factors, but there are at present too few data on the newer agents to assess whether some of the positive qualities of these agents (e.g., improved mood with ACEI use) are borne out in large clinical trials.

Stroke

Antihypertensive treatment helps to prevent primary stroke, but in the acute stroke and poststroke situation, the evidence for reducing an elevated BP is less clear. Acutely postictus, BP is frequently raised but the few antihypertensive intervention studies have been disappointing. β-blockers and calcium-channel blockers given orally or intravenously have been shown either to have no effect on prognosis or to be associated with an adverse outcome. The numbers of patients studied have been small and the study design often questionable, so there is a desperate need for a suitable trial to assess whether lowering of BP in the acute situation is of benefit. Until such evidence is available, in the majority of cases raised blood pressure is probably best left untreated, at least for the first 2 weeks.

Trials of BP reduction in the weeks and months following stroke have also been disappointing. There have been only two randomized intervention trials that have specifically recruited patients with raised BP levels following stroke, and only three others that have included both normotensive and hypertensive individuals. Overall these studies have shown that treatment does not reduce stroke recurrence or total

KEY POINTS
Hypertension

- Hypertension is the main treatable risk factor for cerebrovascular and coronary artery disease in elderly people, although significant numbers of elderly hypertensives remain inadequately treated.
- Those aged up to at least 90 years with sustained systolic BP ≥160 mm Hg and/or diastolic BP ≥100 mm Hg should be treated. Those with an SBP of 140–159 mm Hg and/or a DBP of 90–99 mm Hg, evidence of target organ damage (TOD), or a CVD risk of ≥20% over 10 years (nearly all those aged 70 years plus), should also receive antihypertensive treatment.
- Hypertension should not be treated in isolation; other cardiovascular risk factors (e.g., cholesterol levels, smoking, and diabetes) should also be treated and aspirin added if the 10-year CV risk is >20%.
- Lifestyle changes (e.g., salt restriction, increasing exercise) should be considered before, and in conjunction with, antihypertensive drug therapy.
- Thiazide diuretics remain the preferred first-line therapy, although dihydropyridine calcium-channel blockers may be useful alternative agents in those with isolated systolic hypertension. Target clinic BP levels on treatment should be <140/85 mm Hg in nondiabetics and <140/80 mm Hg in diabetics. The majority of patients will require two or more antihypertensive drugs to achieve these levels.

mortality, but it does reduce the number of nonfatal strokes by 19% (5% to 32%) and all major CV events by 18% (5% to 28%). The PROGRESS Trial taking patients with controlled BP levels several weeks to months after stroke has shown the benefits of the combination of perindopril and indapamide in reducing stroke recurrence by 43% and major vascular events by 40%.[57]

SUMMARY

Hypertension is the biggest single treatable risk factor for stroke and cardiovascular disease in the elderly, but it is becoming increasingly appreciated that other elements that dictate cardiovascular risk in older people—such as diabetes and abnormal lipid profiles—also require active management. Nonpharmacologic methods of BP reduction should initially be tried in all patients. Thiazide diuretics are the first-choice antihypertensive in the vast majority of patients, there being no evidence to date that any of the newer antihypertensive agents are more efficacious. It is the level of BP reduction rather than any specific treatment that is important in reducing event rates, and the majority of patients will need two or more antihypertensive agents to obtain adequate BP control. Effective treatment leads to a substantial reduction in cerebrovascular and coronary heart disease events within a short time of starting treatment, without producing adverse side effects or compromising quality of life. Statin therapy and prophylactic aspirin use (when BP levels are controlled) are warranted in patients at the appropriate level of cardiovascular risk.

Although we have come a long way in a short time in terms of evidence-based management of the older hypertensive patient, there is still no room for complacency. Too many elderly patients remain undiagnosed or inadequately treated, in terms of BP reduction and management of other cardiovascular risk factors, for the full benefits of treatment to be realized.

For a complete list of references, please visit online only at www.expertconsult.com

CHAPTER 44

Valvular Heart Disease

Wilbert S. Aronow

AORTIC STENOSIS

Etiology and prevalence

Valvular aortic stenosis (AS) in older persons is usually due to stiffening, scarring, and calcification of the aortic valve leaflets. The commissures are not fused as in rheumatic AS. Calcific deposits in the aortic valve are common in older persons and may lead to valvular AS.[1–7] Aortic cuspal calcium was present in 295 of 752 men (36%), mean age 80 years, and in 672 of 1663 women (40%), mean age 82 years.[6] Of 2358 persons, mean age 81 years, 378 (16%) had valvular AS, 981 (42%) had valvular aortic sclerosis (thickening of or calcific deposits on the aortic valve cusps with a peak flow velocity across the aortic valve ≤ 1.5 m/sec), and 999 (42%) had no valvular AS or aortic sclerosis.[7] Calcific deposits in the aortic valve were present in 22 of 40 necropsy patients (55%) aged 90 to103 years.[2] Calcium of the aortic valve and mitral annulus may coexist.[1–3,8,9]

In the Helsinki Aging Study, calcification of the aortic valve was diagnosed by Doppler echocardiography in 28% of 76 persons aged 55 to 71 years, in 48% of 197 persons aged 75 to 76 years, in 55% of 155 persons aged 80 to 81 years, and in 75% of 124 persons aged 85 to 86 years.[5] Aortic valve calcification, aortic sclerosis, and mitral annular calcium (MAC) are degenerative processes,[1,2,10–12] accounting for their high prevalence in an elderly population.

Otto et al[11] showed that the early lesion of degenerative AS is an active inflammatory process with some similarities to atherosclerosis, including lipid deposition, macrophage and T-cell infiltration, and basement membrane disruption. In a study of 571 persons, mean age 82 years, 292 persons (51%) had calcified or thickened aortic cusps or root.[13] A serum total cholesterol ≥ 200 mg/dL, a history of hypertension, diabetes mellitus, and a serum high-density lipoprotein cholesterol less than 35 mg/dL were more prevalent in older persons with calcified or thickened aortic cusps or root than in older persons with normal aortic cusps and root.[13]

In the Helsinki Aging Study, age, hypertension, and a low body mass index were independent predictors of aortic valve calcification.[14] In 5201 persons older than 65 years of age in the Cardiovascular Health Study, independent clinical factors associated with degenerative aortic valve disease included age, male gender, smoking, history of hypertension, height, and high lipoprotein(a) and low-density lipoprotein (LDL) cholesterol levels.[12] In 1275 older persons, mean age 81 years, AS was present in 52 of 202 persons (26%) with 40% to 100% extracranial carotid arterial disease (ECAD) and in 162 of 1073 persons (15%) with 0% to 39% ECAD.[15] In 2987 persons, mean age 81 years, symptomatic peripheral arterial disease occurred in 193 of 462 persons (42%) with AS and in 639 of 2525 persons (25%) without AS.[16]

In 290 persons, mean age 79 years, with valvular AS who had follow-up Doppler echocardiograms, older persons with MAC had a greater reduction in aortic valve area/year than older persons without MAC.[17] Significant independent risk factors for progression of valvular AS in 102 persons, mean age 76 years, who had follow-up Doppler echocardiograms were cigarette smoking and hypercholesterolemia.[18] Palta et al[19] also showed that cigarette smoking and hypercholesterolemia accelerate the progression of AS. These and other data suggest that aortic valve calcium, MAC, and coronary atherosclerosis in older persons have similar predisposing factors.[11–21]

A retrospective analysis of 180 elderly patients with mild AS who had follow-up Doppler echocardiograms at 2 or more years showed that significant independent predictors of the progression of AS were male gender, cigarette smoking, hypertension, diabetes mellitus, a serum low-density lipoprotein cholesterol equal to 125 mg/dL at follow-up, a serum high-density lipoprotein cholesterol less than 35 mg/dL at follow-up, and use of statins (inverse association).[22] A retrospective analysis of 174 patients, mean age 68 years, with mild to moderate AS showed that statin therapy reduced the progression of AS.[23] In a retrospective study of 156 patients, mean age 77 years, with AS, at 3.7-year follow-up, statin therapy decreased the progression of AS by 54%.[24]

In a prospective open-label study of 121 patients with an aortic valve area between 1.0 and 1.5 cm^2, 61 patients with a serum LDL cholesterol greater than 130 mg/dL were treated with rosuvastatin and 60 patients with a serum LDL cholesterol less than 130 mg/dL did not receive statins.[25] At 73-week follow-up, patients treated with rosuvastatin had significantly less progression of AS. These data differ from the results reported in 155 patients in the Scottish Aortic Stenosis and Lipid Lowering Trial, Impact on Regression Study, which included patients with extensive aortic valve calcification.[26] Two trials are in progress investigating the effect of statins on AS.

The frequency of AS increases with age. Valvular AS diagnosed by Doppler echocardiography was present in 141 of 924 men (15%), mean age 80 years, and in 322 of 1881 women (17%), mean age 81 years.[27] Severe valvular AS (peak gradient across aortic valve of ≥ 50 mm Hg or aortic valve area <0.75 cm^2) was diagnosed in 62 of 2805 older persons (2%).[27] Moderate valvular AS (peak gradient across aortic valve of 26 to 49 mm Hg or aortic valve area of 0.75 to 1.49 cm^2) was present in 149 of 2805 older persons (5%).[27] Mild valvular AS (peak gradient across aortic valve of 10 to 25 mm Hg or aortic valve area ≥ 1.50 cm^2) occurred in 250 of 2805 older persons (9%).[27] In 501 unselected persons aged 75 to 86 years in the Helsinki Aging Study, critical AS was present in 3% and moderate-to-severe AS in 5% of the 501 older persons.[5]

Pathophysiology

In valvular AS, there is resistance to ejection of blood from the left ventricle (LV) into the aorta, with a pressure gradient across the aortic valve during systole and an increase in LV systolic pressure. The pressure overload on the LV leads to concentric LV hypertrophy, with an increase in LV wall thickness and mass, normalizing systolic wall stress, and maintenance of normal LV ejection fraction and cardiac output.[28,29] A compensated hyperdynamic response is common in older women.[30] Older persons with a comparable degree of AS have more impairment of LV diastolic function than do younger persons.[31] Coronary vasodilator reserve is more severely impaired in the subendocardium in patients with LV hypertrophy caused by severe AS.[32]

The compensatory concentric LV hypertrophy leads to abnormal LV compliance, LV diastolic dysfunction with decreased LV diastolic filling, and increased LV end-diastolic pressure, further increased by left atrial systole. Left atrial enlargement develops. Atrial systole plays an important role in diastolic filling of the LV in persons with AS.[33] Loss of effective atrial contraction may cause immediate clinical deterioration in persons with severe AS.

Sustained LV hypertrophy eventually leads to LV chamber dilatation with reduced LV ejection fraction and ultimately congestive heart failure (CHF). The stroke volume and cardiac output decrease, the mean left atrial and pulmonary capillary pressures increase, and pulmonary hypertension occurs. Older persons with both obstructive and nonobstructive coronary artery disease have an increased incidence of LV enlargement and LV systolic dysfunction.[34] In a percentage of older persons with AS, the LV ejection fraction will remain normal and LV diastolic dysfunction will be the main problem.

In 48 older persons with CHF associated with unoperated severe valvular AS, the LV ejection fraction was normal in 30 persons (63%).[35] The prognosis of persons with AS and LV diastolic dysfunction is usually better than that of persons with AS and LV systolic dysfunction, but is worse than that of persons without LV diastolic dysfunction.[35,36]

Symptoms

Angina pectoris, syncope or near syncope, and CHF are the three classic manifestations of severe AS. Angina pectoris is the most common symptom associated with AS in older persons. Coexistent coronary artery disease (CAD) is frequently present in these persons. However, angina pectoris may occur in the absence of CAD as a result of an increase in myocardial oxygen demand with a decrease in myocardial oxygen supply at the subendocardial level. Myocardial ischemia in persons with severe AS and normal coronary arteries is due to inadequate LV hypertrophy with increased LV systolic and diastolic wall stresses causing reduced coronary flow reserve.[37]

Syncope in persons with AS may be caused by decreased cerebral perfusion following exertion when arterial pressure falls because of systemic vasodilatation in the presence of a fixed cardiac output. LV failure with a reduction in cardiac output may also cause syncope. In addition, syncope at rest may be caused by a marked decrease in cardiac output secondary to transient ventricular fibrillation or transient atrial fibrillation or transient atrioventricular block related to extension of the valve calcification into the conduction system. Coexistent cerebrovascular disease with transient cerebral ischemia may contribute to syncope in older persons with AS.

Exertional dyspnea, paroxysmal nocturnal dyspnea, orthopnea, and pulmonary edema may be caused by pulmonary venous hypertension associated with AS. Coexistent CAD and hypertension may contribute to CHF in older persons with AS. Atrial fibrillation may also precipitate CHF in these persons.

CHF, syncope, or angina pectoris was present in 36 of 40 older persons (90%) with severe AS, in 66 of 96 older persons (69%) with moderate valvular AS, and in 45 of 165 older persons (27%) with mild valvular AS.[38]

Sudden death occurs mainly in symptomatic AS persons.[35,38–41] It may also occur in 3% to 5% of asymptomatic persons with AS.[39,42] Marked fatigue and peripheral cyanosis in persons with AS may be caused by a low cardiac output. Cerebral emboli causing stroke or transient cerebral ischemic attack, bacterial endocarditis, and gastrointestinal bleeding may also occur in older persons with AS.

Signs

A systolic ejection murmur heard in the second right intercostal space, down the left sternal border toward the apex, or at the apex is classified as an aortic systolic ejection murmur (ASEM).[3,4,42,43] An ASEM is commonly heard in older persons[1,3,42] occurring in 265 of 565 unselected older persons (47%).[3] Of 220 older persons with an ASEM and technically adequate M-mode and two-dimensional echocardiograms of the aortic valve, 207 (94%) had aortic cuspal or root calcification or thickening.[3] Of 75 older persons with an ASEM, valvular AS was diagnosed by continuous-wave Doppler echocardiography in 42 persons (56%).[43]

Table 44-1 shows that an ASEM was heard in 100% of 19 older persons with severe AS, in 100% of 49 older persons with moderate AS, and in 95% of 74 older persons with mild AS.[4] However, the ASEM may become softer or absent in persons with CHF associated with severe AS because of a low cardiac output. The intensity and maximal location of the ASEM and transmission of the ASEM to the right carotid artery do not differentiate among mild, moderate, and severe AS.[3,4,43] The ASEM may be heard only at the apex in some older persons with AS. The apical systolic ejection murmur may also be louder and more musical than the basal systolic ejection murmur in some older persons with AS. The intensity of the ASEM in valvular AS increases with squatting and by inhalation of amyl nitrite and decreases during the Valsalva maneuver.

Prolonged duration of the ASEM and late peaking of the ASEM best differentiate severe AS from mild AS.[3,4,43] However, the physical signs do not distinguish between severe and moderate AS (see Table 44-1).[4,43]

Table 44-1. Correlation of Physical Signs of Aortic Stenosis With Severity of Aortic Stenosis in Older Persons

	SEVERITY OF AORTIC STENOSIS		
	Mild (n = 74) (%)	Moderate (n = 49) (%)	Severe (n = 19) (%)
Aortic systolic ejection murmur	95	100	100
Prolonged duration aortic systolic ejection murmur	3	63	84
Late-peaking aortic systolic ejection murmur	3	63	84
Prolonged carotid upstroke time	3	33	53
A_2 absent	0	10	16
A_2 reduced or absent	5	49	74

A_2, aortic component of second heart sound
Adapted from Aronow WS et al.[4]

A prolonged carotid upstroke time does not differentiate between severe and moderate AS in older persons.[4,43] A prolonged carotid upstroke time was palpable in 3% of older persons with mild AS, in 33% of older persons with moderate AS, and in 53% of older persons with severe AS (see Table 44-1).[4] Stiff noncompliant arteries may mask a prolonged carotid upstroke time in older persons with severe AS. The pulse pressure may also be normal or wide rather than narrow in older persons with severe AS because of loss of vascular elasticity. An aortic ejection click is rare in older persons with severe AS because of loss of vascular elasticity. An aortic ejection click is rare in older persons with AS because the valve cusps are immobile.[4,43]

An absent or reduced A_2 occurs more frequently in older persons with severe or moderate AS than in persons with mild AS (see Table 44-1). However, an absent or decreased A_2 does not differentiate between severe and moderate AS.[4,43] The presence of atrial fibrillation, reversed splitting of S_2, or an audible fourth heart sound at the apex also does not differentiate between severe and moderate AS in older persons.[43] The presence of a third heart sound in older persons with AS usually indicates the presence of LV systolic dysfunction and elevated LV filling pressure.[44]

Electrocardiography and chest roentgenography

Echocardiography is more sensitive than electrocardiography in diagnosing LV hypertrophy in an older person with AS.[4] In 19 older persons with severe valvular AS, LV hypertrophy was diagnosed by electrocardiography in 58% of persons and by echocardiography in 100% of persons.[4] In 49 older persons with moderate AS, LV hypertrophy was diagnosed by electrocardiography in 31% of persons and by echocardiography in 96% of persons. In 74 older persons with mild valvular AS, LV hypertrophy was diagnosed by electrocardiography in 11% of persons and by echocardiography in 74% of persons.[4] Rounding of the LV border and apex may occur as a result of concentric LV hypertrophy. Poststenotic dilatation of the ascending aorta is commonly seen. Calcification of the aortic valve is best seen by echocardiography or fluoroscopy.

Involvement of the conduction system by calcific deposits may occur in older persons with AS. In a study of 51 older persons with AS who underwent aortic valve replacement, conduction defects occurred in 58% of 31 persons with MAC and in 25% of 20 persons without MAC.[9] In another study of 77 older persons with AS, first-degree atrioventricular block occurred in 18% of persons, left bundle branch block in 10% of persons, intraventricular conduction defect in 6% of persons, right bundle branch block in 4% of persons, and left axis deviation in 17% of persons.[45]

Complex ventricular arrhythmias may be detected by 24-hour ambulatory electrocardiograms in persons with AS. Older persons with complex ventricular arrhythmias associated with AS have a higher incidence of new coronary events than older persons with AS and no complex ventricular arrhythmias.[46]

Echocardiography and Doppler echocardiography

M-mode and two-dimensional echocardiography and Doppler echocardiography are very useful in the diagnosis of AS. Of 83 persons with CHF or angina pectoris and a systolic precordial murmur in whom severe AS was diagnosed by Doppler echocardiography, AS was not clinically diagnosed in 28 persons (34%).[47] Echocardiography can detect thickening, calcification, and reduced excursion of aortic valve leaflets.[3] LV hypertrophy is best diagnosed by echocardiography.[4] Chamber dimensions and measurements of LV end-systolic and end-diastolic volumes, LV ejection fraction, and assessment of global and regional LV wall motion give important information on LV systolic function.

Doppler echocardiography is used to measure peak and mean transvalvular gradients across the aortic valve and to identify associated valve lesions. Aortic valve area can be calculated by the continuity equation using pulsed Doppler echocardiography to measure LV outflow tract velocity, continuous-wave Doppler echocardiography to measure transvalvular flow velocity, and two-dimensional long-axis view to measure LV outflow tract area.[48,49] Aortic valve area can be detected reliably by the continuity equation in older persons with AS.[49]

Shah and Graham[50] reported that the agreement in quantitation of the severity of AS between Doppler echocardiography and cardiac catheterization was greater than 95%. Persons with a peak jet velocity greater than 4.5 m/sec had critical AS, and those with a peak jet velocity less than 3.0 m/ssec had noncritical AS. Slater et al[51] demonstrated a concordance between Doppler echocardiography and cardiac catheterization in the decision to operate or not to operate in 61 of 73 persons (84%) with valvular AS. In 75 persons, mean age 76 years, with valvular AS, the Bland-Altman plot showed that 4 of the 75 persons (5%) had disagreement between cardiac catheterization and Doppler echocardiography that was outside the 95% confidence limits.[52]

Cardiac catheterization was performed in 105 persons in which Doppler echocardiography demonstrated an aortic valve area $\leq$ 0.75 cm^2 or a peak jet velocity $\geq$ 4.5 m/sec, consistent with critical AS.[53] Doppler echocardiography was 97% accurate in this subgroup. Cardiac catheterization was performed in this study in 133 persons with noncritical AS. Doppler echocardiography was 95% accurate in this subgroup. Although most older persons do not require cardiac catheterization before aortic valve surgery, they require selective coronary arteriography before aortic valve surgery. Persons in whom Doppler echocardiography shows a peak jet velocity between 3.6 and 4.4 m/sec and an aortic valve area greater than 0.8 cm^2 should undergo cardiac catheterization if they have cardiac symptoms attributable to AS.[49] Persons with a peak jet velocity between 3.0 and 3.5 m/sec and a LV ejection fraction less than 50% may have severe AS, requiring aortic valve replacement, and should undergo cardiac catheterization.[50] Persons with a peak jet velocity between 3.0 and 3.5 m/sec and a LV ejection fraction greater than 50% probably do not need aortic valve replacement but should undergo cardiac catheterization if they have symptoms of severe AS.[50]

Natural history

Ross and Braunwald[39] demonstrated that the average survival rate was 3 years after the onset of angina pectoris in persons with severe AS. Ross and Braunwald[39] reported that the average survival rate after the onset of syncope in persons with severe AS was 3 years and showed that the average survival rate after the onset of CHF in persons with severe AS was 1.5 to 2 years.

Persons with symptomatic severe valvular AS have a poor prognosis.[38–41,54] At the National Institutes of Health, 52% of persons with symptomatic severe valvular AS not operated on were dead at 5 years.[40,41] At 10-year follow-up, 90% of these persons were dead.

At 4-year follow-up of patients aged 75 to 86 years in the Helsinki Aging Study, the incidence of cardiovascular mortality was 62% in persons with severe AS and 35% in persons with moderate AS.[55] At 4-year follow-up, the incidence of total mortality was 76% in persons with severe AS and 50% in persons with moderate AS.[55]

In a prospective study, at 19-month follow-up (range 2 to 36 months), 90% of 30 persons with CHF associated with unoperated severe AS and a normal LV ejection fraction were dead.[35] At 13-month follow-up (range 2 to 24 months), 100% of 18 persons with CHF associated with unoperated severe AS and an abnormal LV ejection fraction were dead.[35]

Table 44-2 shows the incidence of new coronary events in older persons with no, mild, moderate, and severe AS. Independent risk factors for new coronary events in this study were prior myocardial infarction, AS, male gender, and increasing age.[38] In this prospective study, at 20-month follow-up of 40 older persons with severe AS, CHF, syncope, or angina pectoris was present in 36 of 37 persons (97%) who developed new coronary events and in none of 3 persons (0%) without new coronary events.[38] At 32-month follow-up of 96 older persons with moderate valvular AS, CHF, syncope, or angina pectoris was present in 65 of 77 persons (84%) who developed new coronary events and in 1 of 19 persons (5%) without new coronary events.[38] At 52-month follow-up of 165 older persons with mild AS, CHF, syncope, or angina pectoris was present in 40 of 103 persons (39%) who developed new coronary events and in 5 of 62 persons (8%) without new coronary events.[38]

In a prospective study of 981 persons, mean age 82 years, with aortic sclerosis and of 999 persons, mean age 80 years, without valvular aortic sclerosis, older persons with aortic sclerosis had at 46-month follow-up at 1.8 times higher chance of developing a new coronary event than those without valvular aortic sclerosis.[7] Otto et al[56] also reported in 5621 men and women $\geq$ 65 years of age that AS and aortic sclerosis increased cardiovascular morbidity and mortality.

Kennedy et al[57] followed 66 persons with moderate AS diagnosed by cardiac catheterization (aortic valve area 0.7 to 1.2 cm^2). In 38 persons with symptomatic moderate AS and 28 persons with minimally symptomatic moderate AS, the probabilities of avoiding death from AS were 0.86 for persons and 1.0 for persons with minimally symptomatic moderate AS at 1-year follow-up, 0.77 for persons with symptomatic AS and 1.0 for persons with minimally symptomatic AS at 2 years, 0.77 for persons with symptomatic AS and 0.96 for persons with minimally symptomatic AS at 3 years, and 0.70 for persons with symptomatic AS and 0.90 for persons with minimally symptomatic AS at 4 years.[57] During 35-month mean follow-up in this study, 21 persons underwent aortic valve replacement.

Hammermeister et al[58] followed 106 persons with unoperated AS in the Veterans Administration Cooperative Study on Valvular Heart Disease for 5 years. During follow-up, 60 of 106 persons (57%) died. Multivariate analysis demonstrated that measures of the severity of the AS, the presence of CAD, and the presence of CHF were the important predictors of survival in unoperated persons.

Studies have shown that patients with asymptomatic severe AS are at low risk for death and can be followed until symptoms develop.[59–62] Turina et al[59] followed 17 persons with asymptomatic or mildly symptomatic AS. During the first 2 years, none died or had aortic valve surgery. At 5-year follow-up, 94% were alive and 75% were free of cardiac events. Kelly et al[60] followed 51 asymptomatic persons with severe AS. During 17-month follow-up, 21 (41%) of the persons became symptomatic. Only 2 of the 51 persons (4%) died of cardiac causes. In both persons, death was preceded by the development of angina pectoris or CHF. Pellikka et al[61] showed that 113 of 143 persons (79%), mean age 72 years, with asymptomatic severe AS were not initially referred for aortic valve replacement or percutaneous aortic balloon valvuloplasty. During 20-month follow-up, 37 of 113 persons (33%) became symptomatic. The actuarial probability of remaining free of cardiac events associated with AS, including cardiac death and aortic valve surgery, was 95% at 6 months, 93% at 1 year, and 74% at 2 years. No asymptomatic person with severe AS developed sudden death while asymptomatic.

Rosenheck et al[62] followed 126 persons with asymptomatic severe AS for 22 months. Eight persons died and 59 persons developed symptoms necessitating aortic valve replacement. Event-free survival was 67% at 1 year, 56% at 2 years, and 33% at 4 years. Five of the 6 deaths from cardiac disease were preceded by symptoms. Of the persons with moderately or severely calcified aortic valves whose aortic jet velocity increased by 0.3 m/sec or more within 1 year, 79% underwent aortic valve replacement or died within 2 years of the observed increase.

However, recent data have demonstrated that asymptomatic severe AS should be considered for aortic valve replacement (AVR).[63,64] Of 338 patients with severe asymptomatic AS, mean age 71 years, 99 (29%) had AVR during a mean follow-up of 3.5 years.[63] Survival at 1, 2, and 5 years in the nonoperated patients was 67%, 56%, and 38%, respectively, compared with 94%, 93%, and 90%, respectively, in those who underwent AVR ($p < 0.0001$).[63] In this study, unoperated patients had a 48% significant reduction in mortality if they were treated with statins and a significant 48% reduction in mortality if they were treated with β-blockers.[63]

Table 44-2. Incidence of New Coronary Events in Older Persons With No, Mild, Moderate, and Severe Aortic Stenosis (AS)

	No AS (n = 1496)	Mild AS (n = 165)	Moderate AS (n = 96)	Severe AS (n = 40)
Age (yr)	81	84	85	85
Follow-up (mo)	49	52	32	20
New coronary events (%)	41	62	80	93

Adapted from Aronow WS, et al.[38]

Data were analyzed for 622 patients, mean age 72 years, with asymptomatic severe AS at the Mayo Clinic.[64] After the initial diagnosis, 166 patients (27%) developed chest pain, shortness of breath, or syncope and had AVR. Another 97 patients (16%) had AVR in the absence of symptoms. The operative mortality was 2% for the symptomatic patients and 1% for the asymptomatic patients. The survival of the 263 patients who had AVR was not significantly different from an age- and sex-matched population. The 10-year survival was 64% for symptomatic patients and 64% for asymptomatic patients who had AVR.[64] At 3 years after the diagnosis of severe AS, 52% of the 622 patients had had symptoms develop, undergone AVR, or died.[64] Absence of AVR was an independent risk factor for mortality with a hazard ratio of 3.53.

Medical management

Prophylactic antibiotics should not be used to prevent bacterial endocarditis in persons with AS regardless of severity, according to current American Heart Association (AHA) guidelines.[65] Persons with CHF, exertional syncope, or angina pectoris associated with moderate or severe AS should undergo AVR promptly. Valvular surgery is the only definitive therapy in these older persons.[66] Medical therapy does not relieve the mechanical obstruction to left ventricular outflow and does not relieve symptoms or progression of the disorder. Persons with asymptomatic AS should report the development of symptoms possibly related to AS immediately to the physician. If significant AS is present in asymptomatic older persons, clinical examination and an electrocardiogram and Doppler echocardiogram should be performed at 6-month intervals if AVR is not being considered. Nitrates should be used with caution in persons with angina pectoris and AS to prevent the occurrence of orthostatic hypotension and syncope. Diuretics should be used with caution in persons with CHF to prevent a decrease in cardiac output and hypotension. Vasodilators should be avoided. Digitalis should not be used in persons with CHF and a normal LV ejection fraction unless needed to control a rapid ventricular rate associated with atrial fibrillation.

Aortic valve replacement

Table 44-3 lists four class I indications and one class IIa indication for performing AVR in elderly patients with AS.[67] AVR is the procedure of choice for symptomatic elderly patients with severe AS. Other class I indications for AVR in elderly patients with severe AS include patients undergoing coronary artery bypass surgery (CABS), undergoing surgery on the aorta or other heart valves, and patients with a LV ejection fraction less than 50%.[67] Patients with moderate AS undergoing CABS or surgery on the aorta or other heart valves have a class IIa indication for AVR.[67]

Although the American College of Cardiology (ACC)/AHA guidelines do not recommend AVR in patients with asymptomatic severe AS and normal LV ejection fraction, there are recent data suggesting otherwise.[63,64] The data from these two recent studies favor AVR in patients with a diagnosis of asymptomatic severe AS when there is a low institutional perioperative mortality.

Echocardiography is recommended in asymptomatic patients with AS every 1 year for severe AS, every 1 to 2 years for moderate AS, and every 3 to 5 years for mild AS.[64] AVR is the procedure of choice for symptomatic older persons with severe AS. The bioprosthesis has less structural failure in older persons than in younger persons and may be preferable to the mechanical prosthetic valve for AS replacement in the elderly due to the anticoagulation issue.[68,69] Persons with mechanical prostheses need anticoagulant therapy indefinitely. Patients with porcine bioprostheses may be treated with aspirin in a dose of 75 to 100 mg daily unless the patient has atrial fibrillation, abnormal LV ejection fraction, previous thromboembolism, or a hypercoagulable condition.[67,70] Table 44-4 lists four class I indications and two class IIa indications for antithrombotic therapy in patients with AVR.[67]

Arom et al[71] performed aortic valve replacement in 273 persons aged 70 to 89 years (mean age 75 years), 162 with AVR alone, and 111 with AVR plus CABS. Operative mortality was 5%. Late mortality at 33-month follow-up was 18%. Actuarial analysis showed at 5-year follow-up that overall survival was 66% for persons with AVR alone, 76% for persons with AVR plus CABS, and 74% for a similar age group in the general population.

Culliford et al[70] performed AVR in 71 persons aged ≥ 80 years, 35 with AVR alone, and 36 with AVR plus CABS. Hospital mortality was 6% in persons with AVR alone and 19% in persons with both AVR plus CABS. At 1-year

Table 44-3. American College of Cardiology/American Heart Association Indications for Aortic Valve Replacement in Persons With Severe Aortic Stenosis (AS)

1. Patients with symptomatic severe AS (class I indication)
2. Patients with severe AS undergoing coronary artery bypass surgery (class I indication)
3. Patients with severe AS undergoing surgery on the aorta or other heart valves (class I indication)
4. Patients with severe AS and a left ventricular ejection fraction <50% (class I indication)
5. Patients with moderate AS undergoing coronary artery bypass surgery or surgery on the aorta or other heart valves (class IIa indication)

Adapted from Bonow RO, et al.[67]

Table 44-4. Indications for Antithrombotic Therapy in Patients With Aortic Valve Replacement (AVR)

1. After AVR with bileaflet mechanical or Medtronic Hall prostheses, if no risk factors, administer warfarin to maintain INR between 2.0–3.0; if risk factors are present, the INR should be maintained between 2.5–3.5 (class I indication).
2. After AVR with Starr-Edwards valves or mechanical disc valves (other than Medtronic Hall prostheses), in patients with no risk factors, warfarin should be administered to maintain INR between 2.5–3.5 (class I indication).
3. After AVR with a bioprosthesis and no risk factors, administer aspirin in a dose of 75–100 mg daily (class I indication).
4. After AVR with a bioprosthesis and risk factors, administer warfarin to maintain an INR between 2.0–3.0 (class I indication).
5. During the first 3 months after AVR with a mechanical prosthesis, it is reasonable to give warfarin to maintain an INR between 2.5–3.5 (class II_a indication).
6. During the first 3 months after AVR with a bioprosthesis in patients with no risk factors, it is reasonable to give warfarin to maintain an INR between 2.0–3.0 (class IIa indication).

Risk factors include atrial fibrillation, prior thromboembolism, left ventricular systolic dysfunction, and hypercoagulable condition.
Modified from Bonow RO, et al.[67]

follow-up, survival from late cardiac death was 100% for persons who had AVR alone and 96% for persons who had AVR plus CABS. At 3-year follow-up, survival from late cardiac death was 100% for persons who had AVR alone and 91% for persons who had AVR plus CABS. Freedom from all valve-related complications (thromboembolism, anticoagulant-related complications, endocarditis, and reoperation or prosthetic failure) was 93% at 1-year follow-up and 80% at 3-year follow-up. At follow-up, 65% of survivors were in New York Heart Association (NYHA) functional class I or II, 31% in NYHA functional class III, and 4% in NYHA functional class IV.

Levinson et al[72] performed AVR in 71 octogenarians, mean age 82 years. The operative mortality was 9% in these older persons. At 28-month follow-up, 100% of the survivors were in NYHA functional class I or II. Actuarial 1-, 5-, and 10-year survival rates were 83%, 67%, and 49%, respectively. A United Kingdom heart valve registry showed in 1100 persons aged ≥ 80 years (56% women) who underwent AVR that the 30-day mortality was 6.6%.[73] The actuarial survival was 89% at 1 year, 79% at 3 years, 69% at 5 years, and 46% at 8 years.

AVR is associated with a reduction in LV mass and in improvement of LV diastolic filling.[74,75] Hoffman and Burckhardt[76] performed a prospective study in 100 persons who had AVR. At 41-month follow-up, the yearly cardiac mortality rate was 8% in persons with electrocardiographic LV hypertrophy and repetitive ventricular premature complexes ≥ 2 couplets per 24 hours during 24-hour ambulatory monitoring and 0.6% in persons without either of these findings.

If LV systolic dysfunction in persons with severe AS is associated with critical narrowing of the aortic valve rather than myocardial fibrosis, it often improves after successful AVR.[77] In 154 persons, mean age 73 years, with AS and a LV ejection fraction ≤ 35% who underwent AVR, the 30-day mortality was 9%. The 5-year survival was 69% in persons without significant CAD and 39% in persons with significant CAD. NYHA functional class III or IV was present in 58% of persons before surgery versus 7% of persons after surgery. Postoperative LV ejection fraction was measured in 76% of survivors at a mean of 14 months after surgery. Improvement in LV ejection fraction was found in 76% of persons.[77]

Balloon aortic valvuloplasty

AVR is the procedure of choice for symptomatic older persons with severe AS. In a Mayo Clinic study, the actuarial survival of 50 older persons, mean age 77 years, with symptomatic severe AS in whom AVR was refused (45 persons) or deferred (5 persons) was 57% at 1 year, 37% at 2 years, and 25% at 3 years.[78] Because of the poor survival in this group of persons, balloon aortic valvuloplasty should be considered when operative intervention is refused or deferred.

Balloon aortic valvuloplasty is effective palliative therapy for some older persons with symptomatic AS, although restenosis with recurrence of symptoms is common.[79–88] Rodriguez et al[85] found that in 42 older persons, mean age 78 years, undergoing aortic valvuloplasty that the 2-year survival was 36% in persons with LV ejection fractions less than 40% and 80% in persons with LV ejection fractions greater than 40%. The 2-year event-free survival (freedom from aortic valve surgery or severe CHF) was 0% in persons with LV ejection fractions less than 40% and 34% in persons with LV ejection fractions greater than 40%.[85] Block and Palacios[80] showed recurrence of symptoms, death, or hemodynamic evidence of restenosis in 56% of 90 older persons, mean age 79 years, an average of 5.5 months after aortic valvuloplasty. Kuntz et al[86] found immediate clinical improvement after successful aortic valvuloplasty in the majority of 205 older persons, mean age 78 years, but restenosis in more than 50% of the persons within 1 to 2 years. On the basis of the available data, balloon aortic valvuloplasty should be considered for older persons with symptomatic severe AS who are not candidates for aortic valve surgery and possibly for persons with severe LV dysfunction as a bridge to subsequent valve surgery.[86–88]

Percutaneous transcatheter implantation of aortic valve prostheses

Percutaneous heart valve implantation may be performed in nonsurgical patients with end-stage calcific AS.[89,90] Ongoing trials will define the clinical role for this therapy.

Eighteen high-risk patients, mean age 76 years, with severe AS and moderate CAD amenable to percutaneous coronary intervention (PCI) had combined PCI followed by minimally invasive AVR.[91] One of 18 patients (6%) died postoperatively with no late mortality after a mean follow-up of 19 months.[91] This hybrid strategy may be a new therapeutic approach for elderly high-risk patients with combined CAD and severe AS.

AORTIC REGURGITATION

Etiology and prevalence

Acute aortic regurgitation (AR) in older persons may be due to infective endocarditis, rheumatic fever, aortic dissection, trauma following prosthetic valve surgery, or rupture of the sinus of Valsalva, and causes sudden severe LV failure. Chronic AR in older persons may be caused by valve leaflet disease (secondary to any cause of AS, infective endocarditis, rheumatic fever, congenital heart disease, rheumatoid arthritis, ankylosing spondylitis, following prosthetic valve surgery, or myxomatous degeneration of the valve), or by aortic root disease. Examples of aortic root disease causing chronic AR in older persons include association with systemic hypertension, syphilitic aortitis, cystic medial necrosis of the aorta, ankylosing spondylitis, rheumatoid arthritis, Reiter's disease, systemic lupus erythematosus, Ehler-Danlos syndrome, and pseudoxanthoma elasticum. Mild or moderate AR was also diagnosed by Doppler echocardiography in 9 of 29 persons (31%) with hypertrophic cardiomyopathy,[92] Margonato et al[93] linked the increased prevalence of AR with age to aortic valve thickening.

The prevalence of AR increases with age.[93–95] In a prospective study of 450 unselected persons, mean age 82 years, AR was diagnosed by pulsed Doppler echocardiography in 39 of 114 men (34%) and in 92 of 336 women (27%).[95] Severe or moderate AR was diagnosed in 74 of 450 older persons (16%). Mild AR was diagnosed in 57 of 450 older persons (13%). In a prospective study of 924 men, mean age 80 years, and 1881 women, mean age 82 years, valvular AR was diagnosed by pulsed Doppler recordings of the aortic valve in 282 of 924 men (31%) and in 542 of 1881 women (29%).[27]

Pathophysiology

The primary determinants of AR volume are the regurgitant orifice area, the transvalvular pressure gradient, and the duration of diastole.[96] Chronic AR increases LV ventricular end-diastolic volume. The largest LV end-diastolic volumes are seen in persons with chronic severe AR. LV stroke volume increases to maintain the forward stroke volume. The increased preload causes an increase in LV diastolic stress and the addition of sarcomeres in series. This results in an increase in the ratio of the LV chamber size to wall thickness. This pattern of LV hypertrophy is called eccentric LV hypertrophy.

Primary myocardial abnormalities or ischemia due to coexistent CAD decrease the contractile state. LV diastolic compliance decreases, LV end-systolic volume increases, LV end-diastolic pressure rises, left atrial pressure increases, and pulmonary venous hypertension results. When the LV end-diastolic radius-to-wall thickness ratio rises, LV systolic wall stress increases abnormally because of the preload and afterload mismatch.[29,97] Additional stress then decreases the LV ejection fraction response to exercise.[98] Eventually, the LV ejection fraction, forward stroke volume, and effective cardiac output are decreased at rest. We demonstrated that an abnormal resting LV ejection fraction occurred in 8 of 25 older persons (32%) with CHF associated with chronic severe AR.[99]

In persons with acute severe AR, the LV cannot adapt to the increased volume overload. Forward stroke volume falls, LV end-diastolic pressure increases rapidly to high levels,[100] and pulmonary hypertension and pulmonary edema result. The rapid rise of the LV end-diastolic pressure to exceed the left atrial pressure in early diastole causes premature closure of the mitral valve.[101] This prevents backward transmission of the elevated LV end-diastolic pressure to the pulmonary venous bed.

Symptoms

Persons with acute AR develop symptoms due to the sudden onset of CHF, with marked dyspnea and weakness. Persons with chronic AR may remain asymptomatic for many years. Mild dyspnea on exertion and palpitations, especially on lying down, may occur. Exertional dyspnea, orthopnea, paroxysmal nocturnal dyspnea, fatigue, and edema are common clinical symptoms when LV failure occurs. Syncope is rare. Angina pectoris occurs less often in persons with AR than in persons with AS and may be due to coexistent CAD. However, nocturnal angina pectoris, often accompanied by flushing, diaphoresis, and palpitations, may develop when the heart rate slows and the arterial diastolic pressure falls to very low levels. Most persons with severe AR who do not have surgery die within 2 years after CHD develops.[102]

Signs

The AR murmur is typically a high-pitched blowing diastolic murmur that begins immediately after A_2. The diastolic murmur is best heard along the left sternal border in the third and fourth intercostal spaces when AR is due to valvular disease. The murmur is best heard along the right sternal border when AR is due to dilatation of the ascending aorta. The diastolic murmur is best heard with the diaphragm of the stethoscope with the person sitting up, leaning forward, and holding the breath in deep expiration. The severity of AR correlates with the duration of the diastolic murmur, not with the intensity of the murmur.

Grayburn et al[103] heard an AR murmur in 73% of 82 persons with AR and in 8% of 24 persons without AR. Saal et al[104] heard an AR murmur in 80% of 35 persons with AR and in 10% of 10 persons without AR. Meyers et al[105] heard an AR murmur in 73% of 66 persons with AR and in 22% of 9 persons without AR. An AR murmur was heard in 95% of 74 older persons with severe or moderate AR diagnosed by pulsed Doppler echocardiography, in 61% of 57 older persons with mild AR, and in 3% of 319 older persons with no AR.[95]

In persons with chronic severe AR, the LV apical impulse is diffuse, hyperdynamic, and displaced laterally and inferiorly. A rumbling diastolic murmur (Austin Flint) may be heard at the apex, with its intensity reduced by inhalation of amyl nitrite. A short basal systolic ejection murmur is heard. A palpable LV rapid filling wave and an audible S_3 at the apex are usually found. Physical findings due to a large LV stroke volume and a rapid diastolic runoff in persons with severe AR include a wide pulse pressure with an increased systolic arterial pressure and an abnormally low diastolic arterial pressure, an arterial pulse that abruptly rises and collapses, a bisferiens pulse, bobbing of the head with each heart beat, booming systolic and diastolic sounds heard over the femoral artery, capillary pulsations, and systolic and diastolic murmurs heard over the femoral artery when compressing it proximally and distally.

Electrocardiography and chest roentgenography

The electrocardiogram may initially be normal in persons with acute severe AR. Roberts and Day[106] demonstrated in 30 necropsy persons with chronic severe AR that the electrocardiogram did not accurately predict the severity of AR or cardiac weight. Using various electrocardiographic criteria, the prevalence of LV hypertrophy varied from 30% ($RV_6 > RV_5$) to 90% (total 12-lead QRS voltage >175 mm). The P-R interval was prolonged in 28% of persons, and the QRS duration was ≥ 0.12 second in 20% of persons.[106]

The chest x-ray in persons with acute severe AR may show a normal heart size and pulmonary edema. The chest x-ray in persons with chronic severe AR usually shows a dilated LV, with elongation of the apex inferiorly and posteriorly and a dilated aorta. Aneurysmal dilatation of the aorta suggests that aortic root disease is causing the AR. Linear calcifications in the wall of the ascending aorta are seen in syphilitic AR and in degenerative disease.

Echocardiography and Doppler echocardiography

M-mode and two-dimensional echocardiography and Doppler echocardiography are very useful in the diagnosis of AR. Two-dimensional echocardiography can provide information showing the cause of the AR and measurements of LV function. Eccentric LV hypertrophy is diagnosed by echocardiography if the LV mass index is increased with a relative wall thickness less than 0.45.[107–109] Echocardiographic measurements reported to predict an unfavorable response to aortic valve replacement in persons with chronic AR include a LV end-systolic dimension greater than 55 mm,[110] a LV shortening fraction less than 25%,[110] a LV diastolic radius-to-wall thickness ratio greater than 3.8,[111] a LV end-diastolic dimension index greater than 38 mm/m^2,[111] and a LV ventricular end-systolic dimension index greater than 26 mm/m.[111]

Grayburn et al[103] found that pulsed Doppler echocardiography correctly identified the presence of AR in 57 of 57 persons (100%) with ≥ 2+ AR and in 22 of 25 persons (88%) with 1+ AR. Saal et al[104] showed that pulsed Doppler echocardiography identified the presence of AR in 34 of 35 persons (97%) with documented AR. Continuous-wave Doppler echocardiography has also been demonstrated to be very useful in diagnosing and quantitating AR.[112,113] AR is best assessed by color flow Doppler imaging.[114]

Natural history

The natural history of chronic AR is significantly different than the natural history of acute AR. Persons with acute AR should have immediate aortic valve replacement because death may occur within hours to days. In one study of persons with hemodynamically significant chronic AR treated medically, 75% were alive at 5 years after diagnosis.[54,115] Of persons with moderate-to-severe chronic AR, 50% were alive at 10 years after diagnosis.[54,115] The 10-year survival rate for persons with mild-to-moderate chronic AR was 85% to 95%.[54,116]

In another study of 14 persons with chronic severe AR who did not have surgery, 13 (93%) died within 2 years of developing CHF.[102] The mean survival time after the onset of angina pectoris is 5 years.[115]

During 8-year follow-up of 104 asymptomatic persons with chronic severe AR and normal LV ejection fraction, 2 persons (2%) died suddenly, and 23 persons (22%) had aortic valve replacement.[117] Of the 104 persons, 19 (18%) had aortic valve replacement because of cardiac symptoms and 4 persons (4%) had aortic valve replacement because of the development of LV systolic dysfunction in the absence of cardiac symptoms. Multivariate analysis showed that age, initial end-systolic dimension, and rate of change in end-systolic dimension and resting LV ejection fraction during serial studies predicted the outcome.

In a prospective study, at 24-month follow-up (range 7 to 55 months) of 17 persons, mean age 83 years, with CHF associated with unoperated severe chronic AR and a normal LV ejection fraction, 15 persons (88%) were dead.[99] At 15-month follow-up (range 8 to 21 months) of eight persons, mean age 85 years, with CHF associated with unoperated severe chronic AR and an abnormal LV ejection fraction, eight persons (100%) were dead.[99]

Medical and surgical management

Asymptomatic persons with mild or moderate AR do not require therapy. Prophylactic antibiotics should not be used to prevent bacterial endocarditis in persons with AR, according to current AHA guidelines.[65] Echocardiographic evaluation of LV end-systolic dimension should be performed yearly if the measurement is less than 50 mm but every 3 to 6 months if the LV end-systolic dimension is 50 to 54 mm. Aortic valve replacement should also be considered when the LV ejection fraction approaches 50% before the decompensated state.[111]

Persons with asymptomatic, chronic severe AR should be treated with hydralazine,[118] nifedipine,[119] or preferably angiotensin-converting enzyme therapy[120] to decrease the LV volume overload. Infections should be treated promptly. Systemic hypertension increases the regurgitant flow and should be treated. Drugs that reduce LV function should not be used. Arrhythmias should be treated. Persons with AR due to syphilitic aortitis should receive a course of penicillin therapy. Prophylactic resection should be considered in persons with Marfan's syndrome when the aortic root diameter exceeds 55 mm.[121]

Bacterial endocarditis should be treated with intravenous antibiotics. Indications for AVR in persons with AR due to bacterial endocarditis are CHF, uncontrolled infection, myocardial or valvular ring abscess, prosthetic valve dysfunction or dehiscence, and multiple embolic episodes.[122–124]

CHF should be treated with sodium restriction, diuretics, digoxin if the LV ejection fraction is abnormal, vasodilator therapy, and aortic valve replacement. Angina pectoris should be treated with nitrates.

Persons with acute severe AR should undergo AVR immediately. Persons with chronic severe AR should have aortic valve repair if they develop symptoms of CHF, angina pectoris, or syncope.[67,117] AVR should also be performed in asymptomatic persons with chronic severe AR if they develop LV systolic dysfunction.[67,117] ACC/AHA indications for performing AVR in elderly patients with severe chronic AR are listed in Table 44-5.

Older persons undergoing aortic valve replacement for severe AR have an excellent postoperative survival if the preoperative LV ejection fraction is normal.[112–114] If LV systolic dysfunction was present for less than 1 year, persons also did well postoperatively. However, if the person with severe AR has an abnormal LV ejection fraction and impaired exercise tolerance and/or the presence of LV systolic dysfunction for longer than 1 year, the postoperative survival is poor.[125–127] After AVR, women exhibit an excess late mortality, suggesting that surgical correction of severe chronic AR should be considered at an earlier stage in women.[128]

The operative mortality for AVR in older persons with severe AR is similar to that in older persons with AVR for valvular AS. The mortality rate is slightly increased in persons with infective endocarditis and in those persons needing replacement of the ascending aorta plus AVR. The bioprosthesis is preferable to the mechanical prosthetic valve for AVR in older persons as in older persons with valvular AS.[68,69] Persons with porcine bioprostheses may be treated with antiplatelet therapy alone unless they have atrial fibrillation, abnormal LV ejection fraction, previous thromboembolism, or a hypercoagulable state.[67]

Table 44-5. American College of Cardiology/ American Heart Association Indications for Aortic Valve Replacement in Persons With Chronic Severe Aortic Regurgitation (AR)

1. Symptomatic patients with severe AR and normal or abnormal left ventricular (LV) ejection fraction (class I indication)
2. Asymptomatic patients with severe AR and LV ejection fraction ≤ 50% at rest (class I indication)
3. Patients with severe AR undergoing coronary artery bypass surgery or surgery on the aorta or other heart valves (class I indication)
4. Asymptomatic patients with severe AR with LV ejection fraction >50% but a LV end-diastolic dimension >75 mm or a LV end-systolic dimension >55 mm (class IIa indication)

Adapted from Bonow RO, et al.[67]

Of 450 patients with severe AR, 273 (61%) had a LV ejection fraction equal to 50%, 134 (30%) had a LV ejection fraction of 35% to 50%, and 43 patients (10%) had a LV ejection fraction less than 35%.[129] The operative mortality was 3.7% for patients with a normal LV ejection fraction, 6.7% for patients with a LV ejection fraction of 35% to 50%, and 14% for patients with a LV ejection fraction less than 35%.[129] At 10-year follow-up, survival rates were 70% for patients with a normal LV ejection fraction, 56% for patients with a LV ejection fraction of 35% to 50%, and 41% for patients with a LV ejection fraction less than 35%.

In a prospective study, AVR in 38 persons with severe AR normalized LV chamber size and mass in two thirds of persons undergoing surgery.[130] At 9-month follow-up after AVR, 58% of persons had a normal LV end-diastolic dimension and 50% of persons had a normal LV mass. During further follow-up (18 to 56 months postoperatively) 66% of persons had a normal LV end-diastolic dimension and 68% of persons had a normal LV mass. The LV end-diastolic dimension normalized in 86% of persons with a preoperative LV end-systolic dimension ≤ 55 mm. A preoperative LV end-systolic dimension greater than 55 mm was present in 81% of persons with postoperative persistent LV dilatation.

MITRAL ANNULAR CALCIUM

MAC is a chronic degenerative process that is common in older persons, especially women. The amount of calcium may vary from a few spicules to a large mass behind the posterior cusp, often extending to form a ridge or ring encircling the mitral leaflets, occasionally lifting the leaflets toward the left atrium. Sphincter function loss of the mitral annulus and mechanical stretching of the mitral leaflets can cause improper coaptation of the leaflets during systole, resulting in mitral regurgitation (MR).[8]

Although the calcific mass may immobilize the mitral valve, actual calcification of the leaflets is rare. In persons with severe MAC, the calcification may extend inward to involve the underside of the leaflets. Mitral stenosis (MS) may result from severe calcific deposits within the mitral annulus protruding into the orifice.[131,132] Calcific deposits may extend from the mitral annulus into the membranous portions of the ventricular septum, involving the conduction system and causing rhythm and conduction disturbances.[9,133,134] Although the annular calcium is covered with a layer of endothelium, ulceration of this lining can expose the underlying calcific deposits, which may serve as a nidus for platelet-fibrin aggregation and subsequent thromboembolic (TE) episodes.[135–137] In persons with endocarditis associated with MAC, the avascular nature of the mitral annulus predisposes to periannular and myocardial abscesses.[138–141]

Prevalence

MAC is a degenerative process that increases with age and occurs more frequently in women than in men.* MAC was present in 298 of 924 men (36%), mean age 80 years, and in 985 of 1881 women (52%), mean age 81 years.[27]

*References 2, 3, 10, 20, 27, 121, 135, 142–147.

Predisposing factors

Because calcific deposits in the mitral annulus, in the aortic valve cusps, and in the epicardial coronary arteries are commonly associated in older persons and have similar predisposing factors, Roberts[20] suggested that MAC and aortic cuspal calcium are a form of atherosclerosis. MAC and aortic cuspal calcium may coexist.* The prevalence of CAD is higher in men and women with aortic valve calcium[6] and with MAC[6,150–152] than in men and women without aortic valve calcium and MAC.

Breakdown of lipid deposits on the ventricular surface of the posterior mitral leaflet at or below the mitral annulus and on the aortic surfaces of the aortic valve cusps is probably responsible for the calcification.[8] Increased LV systolic pressure due to AS increases stress on the mitral apparatus and may accelerate development of MAC.[2,3,8,135,149] Tricuspid annular calcium and MAC may also coexist and have similar predisposing factors.[153]

Systemic hypertension increases with age and predisposes to MAC.† Persons with diabetes mellitus also have a higher prevalence of MAC than nondiabetic persons.[2,8,21,148] MAC occurs in the teens in persons with serum total cholesterol levels greater than 500 mg/dL.[155] Waller and Roberts[2] suggested that hypercholesterolemia predisposes to MAC. The prevalence of hypercholesterolemia with a serum total cholesterol ≥ 200 mg/dL was higher in older persons with MAC than in older persons without MAC.[21]

Roberts and Waller[156] found that chronic hypercalcemia predisposes to MAC. Older persons with chronic renal insufficiency have a higher prevalence of MAC and aortic valve calcium than older persons with normal renal function.[157,158] Persons undergoing dialysis for chronic renal insufficiency have an increased prevalence of MAC.[156–164] MAC has also been found to be a marker of LV dilatation and reduced LV systolic function in persons with end-stage renal disease on peritoneal dialysis.[164] Cardiac calcium in persons with chronic renal failure has been attributed to secondary hyperparathyroidism[161,164] Nair et al[148] found a similar mean serum calcium, a higher mean serum phosphorus, and a higher mean product of serum calcium and phosphorus in persons younger than 60 years with MAC than in a control group. However, Aronow et al[21] demonstrated no significant difference in mean serum calcium, serum phosphorus, or product of serum calcium and phosphorus between elderly persons with and without MAC.

By accelerating LV systolic pressure, hypertrophic cardiomyopathy predisposes to MAC.[8] Kronzon and Glassman[165] diagnosed MAC in 12 of 18 persons (67%) older than 55 years with hypertrophic cardiomyopathy and in 4 of 28 persons (14%) younger than 55 years with hypertrophic cardiomyopathy. Nair et al[166] observed MAC in 12 of 42 persons (27%) with hypertrophic cardiomyopathy. Their persons with both MAC and hypertrophic cardiomyopathy were older than their persons with hypertrophic cardiomyopathy and no MAC. Motamed and Roberts[167] demonstrated MAC in 30 of 100 autopsy persons (30%) with hypertrophic cardiomyopathy older than 40 years and in none of 100 autopsy persons (0%) younger than 40 years with hypertrophic cardiomyopathy. Aronow and Kronzon[168] diagnosed MAC in

*References 2, 8, 20, 21, 135, 144, 148, 149.
†References 2, 8, 21, 135, 144, 154.

13 of 17 older persons (76%) with hypertrophic cardiomyopathy and in 176 of 362 older persons (49%) without hypertrophic cardiomyopathy.

Diagnosis

Calcific deposits in the mitral annulus are J, C, U, or O shaped and are seen in the posterior third of the heart shadow.[135,143,159,169–175] MAC may be diagnosed by chest x-ray films or by fluoroscopy.[175] However, the procedures of choice for diagnosing MAC are M-mode and two-dimensional echocardiography.

Posterior MAC is diagnosed by M-mode echocardiography when a band of dense echoes is recorded anterior to the LV posterior wall and moving parallel with it.[176] These echoes end at the atrioventricular junction and merge with the LV posterior wall on echocardiographic sweep from the aortic root to the LV apex. Anterior MAC is diagnosed by M-mode echocardiography when a continuous band of dense echoes is observed at the level of the anterior mitral leaflet in both systole and diastole.[176] These echoes are contiguous with the posterior wall of the aortic root. Calcification may extend from the mitral annulus throughout the base of the heart and into the mitral and aortic valves.

Using multiple echocardiographic views, MAC may be classified as mild, moderate, or severe.[151,177] The echo densities in mild MAC involve less than one third of the annular circumference (<3 mm in width) and are usually restricted to the angle between the posterior leaflet of the mitral valve and the LV posterior wall. The echo densities in moderate MAC involve less than two thirds of the annular circumference (3 to 5 mm in width). The echo densities in severe MAC involve more than two thirds of the annular circumference (>5 mm in width), usually extending beneath the entire posterior mitral leaflet with or without making a complete circle.

MAC was diagnosed in the original chest x-ray report in three of eight persons (38%) with MAC diagnosed at autopsy.[143] Schott et al[159] diagnosed MAC by chest x-ray films in 2 of 41 persons (5%) with MAC diagnosed by echocardiography. Dashkoff et al[178] detected MAC by chest x-ray films in five of eight persons (63%) with MAC diagnosed by echocardiography.

In a blinded prospective study, MAC was diagnosed by M-mode and two-dimensional echocardiography in 55% of 604 older persons.[175] The diagnosis of MAC by chest x-ray films using a lateral chest x-ray in addition to the posterior-anterior or anterior-posterior chest x-ray had a sensitivity of 12%, a specificity of 99%, a positive predictive value of 95%, and a negative predictive value of 47%. Persons with radiographic MAC were more likely than persons without radiographic MAC to have a more severe form of the disease, with significant MR, functional MS, or conduction defects. However, persons with echocardiographically severe MAC and significant MR, functional MS, or conduction defects may have no evidence of MAC on chest x-ray films.

Chamber size

Persons with MAC have a higher prevalence of left atrial enlargement* and LV enlargement[143,144,148,177,179] than persons without MAC. In a prospective study of 976 older persons (526 with MAC and 450 without MAC), left atrial enlargement was 2.4 times more prevalent in persons with MAC than in the group without MAC.[180]

*References 135, 143–145, 147, 148, 177, 179.

Table 44-6. Prevalence of Apical Systolic Murmurs of Mitral Regurgitation (MR) and of Mitral Stenosis (MS) in Persons With Mitral Annular Calcium

PREVALENCE OF MR MURMUR		PREVALENCE OF MS MURMUR	
No.	%	No.	%
14/14	100,143	3/14	21,143
10/14	71,159	2/14	14,159
2/4	50,131	1/4	25,131
72/80	90,135	5/59	8,171
26/132	12,144	2/132	2,144
17/104	16,176	7/104	7,176
129/293	44,146	28/293	10,146
43/100	43,182	6/100	6,182

Atrial fibrillation

Persons with MAC also have a higher prevalence of atrial fibrillation than persons without MAC.* The prevalence of atrial fibrillation was increased 12 times,[144] 5 times,[177] and 2.8 times[181] more in persons with MAC than in persons without MAC.

Conduction defects

Because of the close proximity of the mitral annulus to the atrioventricular node and the bundle of His, persons with MAC have a higher prevalence of conduction defects, such as sinoatrial disease, atrioventricular block, bundle branch block, left anterior fascicular block, and intraventricular conduction defect, than persons without MAC.[9,133–135,149,177] The calcific deposits may also extend into the membranous portions of the interventricular septum involving the conduction system, or may even extend to the left atrium, interrupting interatrial and intra-atrial conduction. In addition, MAC may be associated with a sclerodegenerative process in the conduction system. Nair et al[177] showed in their study that persons with MAC had a higher incidence of permanent pacemaker implantation because of both atrioventricular block and sinoatrial disease than persons without MAC.

Mitral regurgitation

MAC is thought to generate systolic murmurs by the sphincter action loss of the annulus and the mechanical stretching of the mitral leaflets causing MR and from vibration of the calcified ring or vortex formation around the annulus. Table 44-6 shows that the prevalence of apical systolic murmurs of MR in persons with MAC ranged from 12% to 100% in different studies.† Table 44-7 states the prevalence of MR diagnosed by Doppler echocardiography in persons with MAC.[179,182,183] The prevalence of mitral regurgitation associated with MAC ranged from 54% to 97% in the Doppler echocardiographic studies.[179,182,183]

The greater the severity of MAC, the greater the severity of MR associated with MAC. Moderate to severe MR was diagnosed by Doppler echocardiography in 33% of 51 persons

*References 135, 143–145, 147, 177, 180, 181.
†References 131, 135, 143, 144, 146, 159, 176, 182.

Table 44-7. Prevalence of Mitral Regurgitation (MR) and of Mitral Stenosis (MS) Diagnosed by Doppler Echocardiography in Persons With Mitral Annular Calcium

PREVALENCE OF MR		PREVALENCE OF MS	
No.	%	No.	%
28/51	55,183	4/51	8,183
54/100	54,182	6/100	6,182
28/29	97,179	83/1028	8,181

with MAC by Labovitz et al[183] and in 22% of 1028 older persons with MAC by Aronow et al.[181] Kaul et al[179] diagnosed severe MR in 7% of their 29 persons with MAC. Kaul et al[179] also concluded from their study that MR in persons with MAC is caused by a decreased sphincteric action of the mitral annulus, with MAC preventing the posterior annulus from contracting and assuming a flatter shape during systole.

Mitral stenosis

An apical diastolic murmur may be heard in persons with MAC as a result of turbulent flow across the calcified and narrowed annulus (annular stenosis). Table 44-6 shows that the prevalence of apical diastolic murmurs of MS in persons with MAC ranged from 0% to 25% in different studies.* Table 44-7 indicates that MS associated with MAC was diagnosed by Doppler echocardiography in 8% of 51 persons by Labovitz et al,[183] in 6% of 100 persons by Aronow and Kronzon,[182] and in 8% of 1028 persons by Aronow et al.[181]

The decrease of mitral valve orifice in persons with MAC is due to the annular calcium and to decreased mitral excursion and mobility secondary to calcium at the base of the leaflets.[182] The commissures are fused in rheumatic MS but are not fused in MS associated with MAC. The mitral leaflet margins in MAC may be thin and mobile, and the posterior mitral leaflet may move normally during diastole. However, Doppler echocardiographic recordings show increased transvalvular flow velocity and prolonged pressure halftime and, therefore, smaller mitral valve orifice in persons with MS, regardless of the cause.

Bacterial endocarditis

Bacterial endocarditis, with a high incidence of *Staphylococcus aureus* endocarditis, may complicate MAC.[135,138–141,147] Persons with MAC associated with chronic renal failure are especially at increased risk for developing bacterial endocarditis.[156] The calcific mass erodes the endothelium under the mitral valve, which is exposed to transient bacteremia. The avascular nature of the mitral annulus interferes with antibiotics reaching a nidus of bacteria, predisposing to periannular and myocardial abscesses and, consequently, to a poor prognosis.[138–141] Therefore Burnside and DeSanctis[138] recommended prophylactic antibiotics to prevent bacterial endocarditis in persons with MAC.

Nair et al[177] observed at 4.4-year follow-up no significant difference in incidence of bacterial endocarditis in

*References 131, 132, 143, 144, 146, 171, 176, 182.

Table 44-8. Incidence of New Cardiac Events in Persons With and Without Mitral Annular Calcium (MAC)

	CARDIAC EVENTS		
	MAC (%)	No MAC (%)	Relative Risk
Nair et al[177] (99 with MAC, 101 without MAC)			
Total cardiac death	31	2	15.5
Sudden cardiac death	12	1	12.0
Congestive heart failure	41	6	6.8
Mitral or aortic valve replacement	9	0	—
Aronow et al[147]			
Cardiac events*, if Atrial fibrillation (90 with MAC, 41 without MAC)	69	54	1.3
Sinus rhythm (436 with MAC, 409 without MAC)	36	26	1.4
All persons (526 with MAC, 450 without MAC)	42	28	1.5

*Myocardial infarction, primary ventricular fibrillation, or sudden cardiac death.

99 persons younger than 61 years with MAC compared with a control group of 101 persons. However, Aronow et al[147] demonstrated at 39-month follow-up a 3% incidence of bacterial endocarditis in 526 older persons with MAC and a 1% incidence of bacterial endocarditis in 450 elderly persons without MAC. On the basis of these data, we recommend using prophylactic antibiotics to prevent bacterial endocarditis in persons with MAC.

Cardiac events

In a prospective study of 107 persons (8 lost to follow-up) younger than 61 years of age with MAC and 107 (6 lost to follow-up) age- and sex-matched control subjects, Nair et al[177] observed at 4.4-year follow-up that persons with MAC had a higher incidence of new cardiac events than control subjects (Table 44-8). In a prospective study of 526 older persons with MAC and 450 older persons without MAC, Aronow et al[147] found at 39-month follow-up that the incidence of new cardiac events (myocardial infarction, primary ventricular fibrillation, or sudden cardiac death) was also higher in older persons with MAC than in older persons without MAC.

Mitral valve replacement

Nair et al[184] reported that mitral valve replacement can be accomplished in persons with MAC with morbidity and mortality similar to those in persons without MAC. Following mitral valve replacement, subsequent morbidity and mortality during 4.4-year follow-up were also similar in persons with and without MAC.

Cerebrovascular events

Although the increased prevalence of atrial fibrillation, MS, MR, left atrial enlargement, and CHF predisposes persons with MAC to TE stroke, some investigators consider MAC a marker of other vascular disease causing stroke rather than the primary embolic source.[185] However, the prevalence of prior stroke was higher in 280 African-American, Hispanic, and white men with MAC (40%) than in 484 African-American, Hispanic, and white men without MAC (27%) and in 876 African-American, Hispanic, and white women with MAC (36%) than in 799 African-American, Hispanic, and white women without MAC (22%).[186] In addition, six prospective studies have demonstrated an increased incidence of new cerebrovascular events in persons with MAC than in persons without MAC.[151,177,181,187–189]

Nair et al[177] showed at 4.4-year follow-up in 107 persons (8 lost to follow-up) younger than 61 years with MAC and 107 (6 lost to follow-up) age- and sex-matched control subjects that persons with MAC had a five times higher incidence of new TE cerebrovascular events than persons without MAC. The Framingham Heart Study observed at 8 years follow-up in 160 persons with MAC and 999 persons without MAC that the incidence of stroke was increased 2.7 times more in persons with MAC than in persons without MAC.[187] At 39-month follow-up of 526 older persons with MAC and 450 older persons without MAC, Aronow et al[147] observed a 1.5 times higher incidence of new TE stroke in persons with MAC than in persons without MAC if atrial fibrillation was present, a 1.6 times higher incidence of new TE stroke in persons with MAC than in persons without MAC if sinus rhythm was present, and a 1.7 times higher incidence of new TE stroke in all persons with MAC than in all persons without MAC. The Boston Area Anticoagulation Trial for Atrial Fibrillation study demonstrated at 2.2 years follow-up in 129 persons with atrial fibrillation and MAC, and 291 persons with atrial fibrillation without MAC, a four times higher incidence of ischemic stroke in persons with MAC than in persons without MAC.[188] At 45-month follow-up, Aronow et al[189] showed that the incidence of TE stroke was 1.5 times higher in 101 persons with 40% to 100% ECAD and MAC than in 49 persons with 40% to 100% ECAD and no MAC, and 2.2 times higher in 365 persons with MAC and 0% to 39% ECAD than in 413 persons with no MAC and 0% to 39% ECAD.

Table 44-9 shows the incidence of new TE stroke at 44-month follow-up in 310 older persons with chronic atrial fibrillation and in 1838 older persons with sinus rhythm, mean age 81 years.[181] MS and the severity of MR were diagnosed by Doppler echocardiography in this study. In older persons with chronic atrial fibrillation, MAC increased the incidence of new TE 2.1 times if MS was associated with MAC, 1.7 times if 2 to 4+ MR was associated with MAC, and 1.4 times if 0 to 1+ MR was present.[181] In older persons with sinus rhythm, MAC increased the incidence of new TE stroke 3.6 times if MS was associated with MAC, 3.1 times if 2 to 4+ MR was associated with MAC, and 2.7 times if 0 to 1 MR was present.[181]

Table 44-9. Incidence of New Thromboembolic (TE) Stroke at 44 Months

	TE Stroke (%)
Atrial fibrillation, no MAC (n = 85)	35
Atrial fibrillation with MS due to MAC (n = 42)	74
Atrial fibrillation with MAC and 2–4+ MR (n = 90)	59
Atrial fibrillation with MAC and 0–1+ MR (n = 93)	48
Sinus rhythm, no MAC (n = 1035)	9
Sinus rhythm with MS due to MAC (n = 41)	32
Sinus rhythm with MAC and 2–4+ MR (n = 134)	28
Sinus rhythm with MAC and 0–1+ MR (n = 625)	24

MAC, mitral annular calcium; *MS*, mitral stenosis; *MR*, mitral regurgitation.
Adapted from Aronow WS et al.[181]

There was a higher prevalence of MAC in older persons with 40% to 100% ECAD (67% of 150 persons) than in older persons with 0% to 39% ECAD (47% of 778 persons).[189] The increased prevalence of significant ECAD contributes to a higher incidence of TE stroke in older persons with MAC. Thrombi of the mitral annulus also contribute to TE stroke in older persons with MAC.[190–192] In addition, MAC is associated with complex intra-aortic debris, which could contribute to TE stroke.[193]

Since persons with MAC and atrial fibrillation or sinus rhythm have a higher incidence of TE stroke than persons without MAC, antithrombotic therapy should be considered in persons with MAC and no contraindications to antithrombotic therapy. In the Boston Area Anticoagulation Trial for Atrial Fibrillation study, warfarin significantly reduced the incidence of TE stroke in persons with MAC by about 90%.[194,195]

Until data from prospective, randomized studies evaluating the efficacy and risk of antithrombotic therapy in persons with MAC are available, we recommend treating persons with MAC associated with either atrial fibrillation, MS, or moderate to severe MR with warfarin treatment if they have no contraindications to anticoagulant therapy. The INR should be maintained between 2.0 and 3.0. The efficacy of antiplatelet treatment in persons with MAC is unknown.

MITRAL STENOSIS

Prevalence and etiology

MS due to rheumatic heart disease was diagnosed by Doppler echocardiography in 3 of 924 men (0.3%), mean age 80 years, and in 34 of 1881 women (2%), mean age 81 years.[27] The most common cause of MS in older persons is MAC. The differentiation of MS due to rheumatic heart disease from MS caused by MAC by echocardiography has been discussed in the section on MAC. In a study of 1699 persons, mean age 81 years, the prevalence of rheumatic MS was 6% in persons with atrial fibrillation versus 0.4% in persons with sinus rhythm.[181]

Pathophysiology

MS leads to an increase in left atrial pressure, pulmonary capillary pressure, and right ventricular and pulmonary artery systolic pressure, causing pulmonary hypertension. Atrial fibrillation predisposes persons with MS to develop stroke, peripheral arterial embolism, and CHF.

Symptoms and signs

If MS is moderate or severe (especially if atrial fibrillation is present), exertional dyspnea, orthopnea, paroxysmal nocturnal dyspnea, and pulmonary edema may develop. Pulmonary hypertension leads to right-sided CHF. Hemoptysis may result from ruptured bronchial veins.

The loud first heart sound and opening snap heard in persons with MS may become softer or disappear if valvular calcification is present. An apical low frequency diastolic murmur heard as a rumble with presystolic accentuation is heard at the point of maximum apical impulse. The low frequency diastolic murmur begins after the opening snap, is prolonged with increasing severity of the MS, and increases in intensity after inhalation of amyl nitrite. The closer the opening snap is heard to A_2, the more severe the MS. If atrial fibrillation develops, the presystolic accentuation usually disappears.

Diagnostic tests

The electrocardiogram and chest x-ray will often show left atrial enlargement in persons with MS. Electrocardiographic right ventricular hypertrophy (RVH) is usually present with severe MS. Documentation of MS and of the severity is made by Doppler echocardiography. Echocardiography will also rule out left atrial myxoma, which can mimic mitral stenosis.

Management of mitral stenosis

A rapid ventricular rate associated with atrial fibrillation is controlled by digoxin and/or β-blockers, verapamil, or diltiazem. Diuretics should be used to control congestive symptoms. Unloading therapy with vasodilators is not beneficial and may cause a significant reduction in cardiac output. Long-term anticoagulation with oral warfarin is indicated in persons with MS and atrial fibrillation (especially) or sinus rhythm to prevent systemic embolization. The INR should be maintained between 2.0 and 3.0. Prophylactic antibiotics should not be used to present bacterial endocarditis in persons with MS, according to recent AHA guidelines.[65]

Interventional therapy is indicated for symptomatic persons with severe MS. A mitral valve area of 1.0 cm^2 or less is considered severe MS. Mitral valve replacement is usually performed because the calcified mitral valve is usually not amenable to open mitral commissurotomy. For the few older persons who have an uncalcified mitral valve or mild calcific deposits, flexible mitral valve leaflets, and no or mild MR, percutaneous balloon valvuloplasty is the procedure of choice.[196]

ACUTE MITRAL REGURGITATION

Acute severe MR in older persons may be caused by ruptured chordae tendineae or development of a flail mitral valve secondary to acute myocardial infarction, infective endocarditis, papillary muscle rupture, or mucoid degeneration of the mitral valve cusps. Acute severe MR usually results in severe CHF with pulmonary edema and right-sided CHF.

Signs

The MR murmur associated with acute severe MR is characteristically a harsh systolic murmur (with an associated palpable thrill) heard at the apex, which begins with the first heart sound but ends early when the noncompliant left atrium can no longer accept the large regurgitant volume. The first heart sound is soft, and the pulmonic component of the second heart sound is increased. A left ventricular third heart sound gallop and an atrial fourth heart sound gallop are heard at the apex.

Diagnosis and management

Doppler echocardiography confirms the diagnosis of severe MR. Transesophageal echocardiography provides a highly accurate anatomic assessment of the cause of the acute MR and assists in determining whether the mitral valve can be repaired or must be replaced.[197] CHF needs to be managed medically. Infective endocarditis should be treated with appropriate antibiotics. Mitral valve surgery should be performed urgently.

CHRONIC MITRAL REGURGITATION

Prevalence and etiology

Chronic MR was present in 298 of 924 men (32%), mean age 80 years, and in 630 of 1881 women (33%), mean age 81 years.[27] MR 2 to 4+ was present in 10% of 2148 persons, mean age 81 years.[164] The commonest cause of MR in older persons is MAC.[146] Other causes of chronic MR in older persons include papillary muscle dysfunction after myocardial infarction, rheumatic heart disease, myxomatous degeneration of the mitral valve leaflets and chordae tendineae with mitral valve prolapse (MVP), ruptured chordae tendineae, and following endocarditis. MR may also result from alteration in the geometry of the mitral annulus occurring with dilatation of the LV and CHF.

Pathophysiology

The regurgitant volume gradually increases in chronic MR, increasing the left atrial volume during systole and the LV volume during diastole. Eccentric LV hypertrophy occurs. Atrial fibrillation develops, and the LV cannot maintain an effective forward stroke volume because of depressed LV contractility. Left-sided CHF develops, resulting in increased pulmonary artery and right ventricular systolic pressure, and eventually right-sided CHF. Decreased LV systolic and diastolic function in persons with chronic MR contribute to the clinical manifestations of CHF.[198] Unrecognized MR may contribute to acute pulmonary edema in persons with normal or abnormal LV systolic function.[199]

Symptoms and signs

Older persons with chronic MR may be asymptomatic or have a reduction in exercise tolerance with easy fatigability. Dyspnea on exertion will develop with significant MR and progress to orthopnea, paroxysmal nocturnal dyspnea, and dyspnea at rest caused by left-sided CHF. Right-sided CHF will cause ankle swelling, anorexia, and right upper abdominal tenderness from hepatic congestion. Symptoms may also result from the development of atrial fibrillation. Atypical chest pain, palpitations, or syncope due to arrhythmias may be associated with MVP. In some persons, acute pulmonary edema may be the initial manifestation of severe MR from MVP.[200]

The heart murmur associated with chronic MR is heard as an apical holosystolic, late systolic, or early systolic murmur beginning with the first heart sound but ending in midsystole. The holosystolic murmur may radiate to the left axilla, to the back, and over the entire precordium. A nonejection systolic click may precede the mid-to-late systolic apical murmur associated with MVP. With severe MR, the first heart sound becomes decreased, and a LV third heart sound is heard at the apex.

Diagnosis

Doppler echocardiography can quantitate the severity of MR and assess LV size and function. Doppler echocardiography and especially transesophageal echocardiography can also determine the cause of the MR. Vegetations are seen with infective endocarditis. MVP and thickening of the mitral valve leaflets suggest myxomatous degeneration. MAC can be diagnosed. Thickened retracted leaflets and chordal fusion suggest rheumatic heart disease as the cause of MR. A flail mitral valve and ruptured chordae tendineae can be diagnosed. The sensitivity of transesophageal echocardiography in diagnosing specific causes of MR was 82% for vegetations, 99% for MVP, 100% for a flail mitral valve, and 84% for ruptured chordae tendineae.[197] In persons with severe chronic MR, the electrocardiogram may show atrial fibrillation or left atrial enlargement, LV hypertrophy in about 50% of persons, and RVH in approximately 15% of persons.

Management

Older persons with chronic MR should have Doppler echocardiograms every 6 to 12 months. There are no long-term studies supporting the use of vasodilator therapy in asymptomatic persons with chronic MR. Angiotensin-converting enzyme inhibitors should be used in treating persons with symptomatic chronic MR.[201] Persons with atrial fibrillation should be treated with long-term oral warfarin therapy to maintain the INR between 2.0 and 3.0. CHF should be treated with standard medical therapy. Prophylactic antibiotics should not be used to prevent bacterial endocarditis in persons with MR, according to current AHA guidelines.[65]

Timing of surgery

Of 478 persons with nonischemic chronic severe MR undergoing surgery, the cause of MR was MVP in 79%, rheumatic in 8%, endocarditis in 8%, and miscellaneous in 4%.[202] Surgical repair of the mitral valve was performed in 68% of persons and mitral valve replacement in 32% of persons. CABS was performed in 27% of persons in association with mitral valve surgery.[202]

The operative mortality was 0% for persons younger than 75 years of age. In persons 75 years of age and older, the operative mortality was 3.6% in persons with NYHA class I or II symptoms and 12.7% in persons with severe symptoms.[202] In persons with a LV ejection fraction ≥ 60%, the 10-year survival was 79% in persons with class I or II symptoms versus 49% in persons with class III or IV symptoms.[202] In persons with a LV ejection fraction less than 60%, the 10-year survival was 75% in persons with class I or II symptoms versus 41% in persons with class III or IV symptoms.[202]

Table 44-10 lists the ACC/AHA class indications for performing mitral valve surgery in persons with nonischemic severe MR.[67] Older persons with chronic nonischemic MR who have NYHA class I symptoms and normal LV function should be followed at 3- to 6-month intervals.[67] If LV dysfunction, atrial fibrillation, or pulmonary hypertension develops, the person should be considered for cardiac catheterization and possible mitral valve surgery, especially if it is thought that the mitral valve can be repaired.[67]

The prognosis for the person with ischemic MR is worse than that for MR from other causes. CABS may improve LV function and decrease ischemic MR.[67] The best operation for ischemic MR is controversial.[67]

Table 44-10. Indications for Mitral Valve Surgery in Persons With Nonischemic Severe Mitral Regurgitation

1. Acute symptomatic MR (class I indication)
2. Persons with NYHA class II, III, or IV symptoms in the absence of severe LV dysfunction defined as a LV ejection fraction <30% and/or LV end-systolic dimension >55 mm (class I indication)
3. Asymptomatic persons with mild to moderate LV dysfunction defined as a LV ejection fraction of 30% to 60% and/or a LV end-systolic dimension of 40 to 55 mm (class I indication)
4. Mitral valve repair is recommended over mitral valve replacement in the majority of patients with severe chronic MR who require surgery (class I indication)
5. Mitral valve repair is reasonable for asymptomatic patients if the likelihood of successful repair without residual MR is >90% (class IIa indication)
6. Mitral valve surgery is reasonable for asymptomatic patients , normal LV function, and new onset of atrial fibrillation (class IIa indication)
7. Mitral valve surgery is reasonable for asymptomatic patients, normal LV function, and a pulmonary artery pressure >50 mm Hg at rest or >60 mm Hg with exercise (class IIa indication)
8. Mitral valve surgery is reasonable in patients with a primary abnormality of the mitral apparatus, NYHA class III or IV symptoms, and severe LV dysfunction in whom mitral valve repair is highly likely (class IIa indication)

MR, mitral regurgitation; *NYHA*, New York Heart Association; *LV*, left ventricular.
Adapted from Bonow RO et al.[67]

TRICUSPID REGURGITATION

In older persons, tricuspid regurgitation (TR) is usually caused by dilatation of the right ventricle and tricuspid annulus associated with right-sided heart failure resulting from left-sided heart failure or pulmonary hypertension associated with pulmonary vascular disease. The murmur of TR is usually high-pitched and holosystolic heard in the third or fourth intercostal space at the left sternal border and occasionally in the subxiphoid area, and increases with inspiration in 50% of persons. When TR is mild, the systolic murmur may be a short ejection murmur or absent. P_2 is increased with pulmonary hypertension. If TR is severe, a prominent large V wave is seen in the jugular venous pulse. Systolic pulsation of an enlarged tender liver is commonly present. Ascites and peripheral edema are frequent. Diagnosis of TR is confirmed by Doppler echocardiography. Medical treatment of CHF is indicated. Surgery is rarely necessary

TRICUSPID STENOSIS

Tricuspid stenosis (TS) in older persons is rare and due to multivalvular rheumatic heart disease or the carcinoid syndrome. Symptoms of right-sided heart failure occur. A low-frequency diastolic rumble is heard in the third or fourth intercostal space at the left sternal border, which increases with intensity with inspiration. A prominent A wave with poor or absent Y descent is seen in the jugular venous pulse. The electrocardiogram shows tall right atrial P waves and no RVH. The chest x-ray shows a dilated right atrium without an enlarged pulmonary artery segment. Diagnosis of TS is confirmed by Doppler echocardiography.

Medical therapy is indicated for mild TS. Balloon valvotomy is recommended for persons with TS with signs of right-sided heart failure or with a marked reduction in exercise tolerance due to an inability to increase cardiac output. If the tricuspid valve is calcified (rarely), tricuspid valve replacement is indicated. A porcine bioprosthetic heart valve is recommended in the tricuspid position.

PULMONIC REGURGITATION

In older persons, pulmonic regurgitation (PR) is almost always due to pulmonary hypertension resulting from left-sided heart failure or pulmonary vascular disease. A high-pitched, blowing decrescendo murmur beginning immediately after P_2 is heard in the second and third intercostal space to the left of the sternum. Diagnosis of PR is confined by Doppler echocardiography. Management of PR is directed at treating the underlying disorder and trying to reduce pulmonary artery pressure.

For a complete list of references, please visit online only at www.expertconsult.com

CHAPTER 45

Cardiac Arrhythmias

Wilbert S. Aronow

VENTRICULAR ARRHYTHMIAS

The presence of three or more consecutive ventricular premature complexes (VPCs) on an electrocardiogram (ECG) is diagnosed as ventricular tachycardia (VT).[1,2] VT is considered sustained if it lasts (30 seconds and nonsustained if it lasts <30 seconds).[2] Complex ventricular arrhythmias (VA) include VT or paired, multiform, or frequent VPCs. I consider frequent VPCs an average of 30/hr on a 24-hour ambulatory ECG or 6/min on a 1-minute rhythm strip of an ECG.[2,3] Simple VA include infrequent VPCs and no complex forms.

The prevalence of nonsustained VT diagnosed by 24-hour ambulatory ECGs in older persons without cardiovascular disease was 4%,[1,4,5] 2%,[6] and 4% in 729 elderly women and 13% in 643 elderly men in the Cardiovascular Health Study.[7] The prevalence of nonsustained VT detected by 24-hour ambulatory ECGs was 9% in elderly persons with hypertension, valvular heart disease, or cardiomyopathies and 16% in elderly persons with coronary artery disease (CAD).[5]

The prevalence of complex VA in elderly persons without cardiovascular disease detected by 24-hour ambulatory ECGs was 50%,[1] 31%,[4] 30%,[5] 20%,[6] 16% in women, and 28% in men,[7] and 33%.[3] The prevalence of complex VA detected by 24-hour ambulatory ECGs was 55% in elderly persons with hypertension, valvular heart disease, or cardiomyopathies,[5] 68% in elderly persons with CAD,[5] and 55% in 843 elderly persons with heart disease.[3] Complex VA were present on a 1-minute strip of an ECG in 2% of 104 elderly persons without cardiovascular disease and 4% of 843 elderly persons with cardiovascular disease.[3] In elderly persons with cardiovascular disease, there is a higher prevalence of VT and of complex VA in persons who have an abnormal left ventricular (LV) ejection fraction,[8] echocardiographic LV hypertrophy,[9] or silent myocardial ischemia.[10]

Prognosis of ventricular arrhythmias

NO HEART DISEASE

Nonsustained VT or complex VA diagnosed by 24-hour ambulatory ECGs,[5,11,12] or by 12-lead ECGs with 1-minute rhythm strips[3] in elderly persons with no clinical evidence of heart disease were not associated with an increased incidence of new coronary events. Exercise-induced nonsustained VT[13] or complex VA,[14] in elderly persons with no clinical evidence of heart disease also were not associated with an increased incidence of new coronary events. Therefore asymptomatic nonsustained VA or complex VA in elderly persons without heart disease should not be treated with antiarrhythmic drugs.

HEART DISEASE

In elderly persons with heart disease, nonsustained VT[5,10,12] or complex VA[3,5,10,12] increased the incidence of new coronary events. At 2-year follow-up of 391 elderly persons with heart disease, the incidence of new coronary events was increased 6.8 times in elderly persons with VT plus an abnormal LV ejection fraction and 7.6 times in elderly persons with complex VA plus an abnormal LV ejection fraction.[5] At 27-month follow-up of 468 elderly persons with heart disease, the incidence of primary ventricular fibrillation or sudden cardiac death was increased 7.1 times in elderly persons with VT plus echocardiographic LV hypertrophy and 7.3 times in persons with complex VA plus echocardiographic LV hypertrophy.[12] At 37-month follow-up of 404 elderly persons with heart disease, the incidence of new coronary events was increased 2.5 times in elderly persons with VT plus silent ischemia and 4.0 times in elderly persons with complex VA plus silent ischemia.[10]

General therapy

Underlying causes of complex VA should be treated when possible. Treatment of congestive heart failure (CHF), LV dysfunction, digitalis toxicity, hypokalemia, hypomagnesemia, myocardial ischemia by antiischemic drugs such as β-blockers or by coronary revascularization, hypertension, LV hypertrophy, hypoxia, and other conditions may abolish or reduce complex VA. The person should not smoke or drink alcohol and should avoid drugs that may cause or increase complex VA.

All elderly persons with CAD should be treated with aspirin,[15–17] with β-blockers,[16–22] with angiotensin-converting enzyme (ACE) inhibitors,[16,17,23–28] and with statins[16,17,29–34] unless there are contraindications to these drugs.

Age-related physiologic changes may affect absorption, distribution, metabolism, and excretion of cardiovascular drugs.[35] Numerous physiologic changes occur with aging that affect pharmacodynamics, resulting in changes in end-organ responsiveness to cardiovascular drugs.[35] Drug interactions between antiarrhythmic drugs and other cardiovascular drugs are common, especially in elderly persons.[35] Important drug-disease interactions also occur in elderly persons.[35] Class I antiarrhythmic drugs are more proarrhythmic than class III antiarrhythmic drugs. Except for β-blockers, all antiarrhythmic drugs can cause torsades des pointes VT (polymorphous appearance associated with a prolonged QT interval).

Class I antiarrhythmic drugs

Class I antiarrhythmic drugs are sodium channel blockers. Class Ia antiarrhythmic drugs have intermediate channel kinetics and prolong repolarization. These drugs include disopyramide, procainamide, and quinidine. Class Ib antiarrhythmic drugs have rapid channel kinetics and shorten repolarization slightly. These drugs include lidocaine, mexiletine, phenytoin, and tocainide. Class Ic antiarrhythmic drugs have slow channel kinetics and have little effect on repolarization. These drugs include encainide, flecainide, lorcainide, moricizine, and propafenone. None of the class I antiarrhythmic drugs have been demonstrated in controlled, clinical trials to decrease sudden cardiac death, total cardiac death, or total mortality.

Table 45-1 shows the effect of class I antiarrhythmic drugs on mortality in persons with heart disease and complex VA.[36–42] A meta-analysis of six double-blind studies of persons with chronic atrial fibrillation (AF) who underwent direct-current cardioversion to sinus rhythm showed that the mortality at

Table 45-1. Effect of Class I Antiarrhythmic Drugs on Mortality in Persons With Heart Disease and Complex Ventricular Arrhythmias

Study	Results
International Mexiletine and Placebo Antiarrhythmic Coronary Trial[36]	At 1-year follow-up, mortality was 7.6% for mexiletine and 4.8% for the placebo
Cardiac Arrhythmia Suppression Trial I[37,38]	At 10-month follow-up, mortality for arrhythmia or cardiac arrest was 4.5% for encainide or flecainide versus 1.2% for the placebo; mortality was 7.7% for encainide or flecainide versus 3.0% for the placebo; adverse events including death were more frequent in elderly persons taking encainide or flecainide
Cardiac Arrhythmia Suppression Trial II[38,39]	At 18-month follow-up, mortality for arrhythmia or cardiac arrest was 8.4% for moricizine versus 7.3% for the placebo; 2-year survival rate was 81.7% for moricizine versus 85.6% for the placebo; adverse events including death were more frequent in elderly persons taking moricizine
Aronow et al[40]	At 2-year follow-up, mortality was 65% for quinidine or procainamide versus 63% for no antiarrhythmic drug; quinidine or procainamide did not reduce sudden death, total cardiac death, or total mortality in elderly persons with ischemic or nonischemic heart disease, abnormal or normal LV ejection fraction, and presence or absence of VT
Moosvi et al[41]	2-year sudden death survival was 69% for quinidine, 69% for procainamide, and 89% for no antiarrhythmic drug; 2-year total survival was 61% for quinidine, 57% for procainamide, and 71% for no antiarrhythmic drug
Hallstrom et al[42]	At 108-month follow-up, the adjusted relative risk of death or recurrent cardiac arrest on quinidine or procainamide versus no antiarrhythmic drug was 1.17

LV, left ventricular; *VT*, ventricular tachycardia.

Table 45-2. Effect of β-blockers on Mortality in Persons With Heart Disease and Complex Ventricular Arrhythmias

Study	Results
Hallstrom et al[42]	At 108-month follow-up, the adjusted relative risk of death or recurrent cardiac arrest for β-blockers versus no antiarrhythmic drug was 0.62
Beta Blocker Heart Attack Trial[46–48]	At 25-month follow-up, propranolol reduced sudden cardiac death by 28% in persons with complex VA and by 16% in persons without VA; propranolol decreased total mortality by 34% in persons aged 60–69 years
Norwegian Propranolol Study[49]	High-risk survivors of acute MI treated with propranolol for 1 year had a 52% decrease in sudden cardiac death
Aronow et al[50]	At 29-month follow-up, compared with no antiarrhythmic drug, propranolol caused a 47% reduction in sudden cardiac death, a 37% decrease in total cardiac death, and a 20% borderline significant decrease in total death
Cardiac Arrhythmia Suppression Trial[51]	Persons on β-blockers had a reduction in all-cause mortality of 43% at 30 days, of 46% at 1 year, and of 33% at 2 years and a decrease in arrhythmic death or cardiac arrest of 66% at 30 days, of 53% at 1 year, and of 36% at 2 years; β-blockers were an independent factor for reduced arrhythmic death or cardiac arrest by 40% and for decreased all-cause mortality by 33%

VA, ventricular arrhythmias; *MI*, myocardial infarction.

1 year was higher in persons treated with quinidine (2.9%) than in persons treated with a placebo (0.8%).[43]

Of 1330 patients in the Stroke Prevention in Atrial Fibrillation Study, 127 were treated with quinidine, 57 with procainamide, 34 with flecainide, 20 with encainide, and 7 with amiodarone.[44] The adjusted relative risk of cardiac mortality was increased 1.8 times and the adjusted relative risk of arrhythmic death was increased 2.1 times in persons receiving antiarrhythmic drugs versus no antiarrhythmic drugs.[44] In persons with a history of CHF, the adjusted relative risk of cardiac death was increased 3.3 times and the adjusted relative risk of arrhythmic death was increased 5.8 times in persons taking antiarrhythmic drugs versus no antiarrhythmic drugs.[44]

An analysis was made of 59 randomized, controlled clinical trials including 23,229 patients that investigated the use of class I antiarrhythmic drugs after myocardial infarction (MI).[45] The class I antiarrhythmic drugs investigated included aprindine, disopyramide, encainide, flecainide, imipramine, lidocaine, mexiletine, moricizine, phenytoin, procainamide, quinidine, and tocainide. Mortality was increased in persons receiving class I antiarrhythmic drugs versus persons receiving no antiarrhythmic drugs (odds ratio = 1.14).[45] None of the 59 studies showed that the use of a class I antiarrhythmic drug decreased mortality in persons after MI.[45]

On the basis of the available data, none of the class I antiarrhythmic drugs should be used to treat VT or complex VA in elderly or younger persons with heart disease.

Calcium channel blockers

Calcium channel blockers are not useful in the therapy of complex VA. Although verapamil can terminate a left septal VT, hemodynamic collapse can occur if intravenous verapamil is given to persons with the more common forms of VT. An analysis was made of randomized, controlled clinical trials including 20,342 patients that investigated the use of calcium channel blockers after MI.[45] Mortality was insignificantly increased in persons receiving calcium channel blockers than in persons receiving no antiarrhythmic drugs (odds ratio = 1.04).[45]

On the basis of the available data, none of the calcium channel blockers should be used to treat VT or complex VA in elderly or younger persons with heart disease.

β-blockers

An analysis of 55 randomized, controlled clinical trials including 53,268 persons that investigated the use of β-blockers after MI showed that mortality was decreased in persons receiving β-blockers versus a placebo (odds ratio = 0.81).[45] β-blockers caused a greater decrease in mortality in older persons than in younger persons.[18–21,46] Table 45-2 indicates the effect of β-blockers on mortality in persons with heart disease and complex VA.[42,46–51]

The decrease in mortality by β-blockers in elderly persons with heart disease and complex VA is due more to an antiischemic effect than to an antiarrhythmic effect.[52]

β-blockers also abolish the circadian distribution of sudden cardiac death or fatal MI,[53] markedly decrease the circadian variation of complex VA,[54] and abolish the circadian variation of myocardial ischemia.[55]

On the basis of the available data, β-blockers should be used to treat older and younger persons with heart disease and complex VA if there are no contraindications to the use of β-blockers.

Angiotensin-converting enzyme inhibitors

ACE inhibitors have been demonstrated to reduce sudden cardiac death in some studies of persons with CHF.[24,56] ACE inhibitors should be used to reduce total mortality in older and younger persons with CHF,[24,26,56,57] an anterior MI,[25] and a LV ejection fraction (40% after MI).[23,26,58] ACE inhibitors should be administered to treat elderly and younger persons with CHF with abnormal LV ejection fraction[24,26,56,57] or with normal LV ejection fraction.[59,60]

On the basis of the available data, ACE inhibitors should be used to treat older and younger persons with VT or complex VA associated with CHF, an anterior MI, or a LV ejection fraction (40% after MI if there are no contraindications to the use of ACE inhibitors. β-blockers should be administered in addition to ACE inhibitors in treating these persons.[58]

Class III antiarrhythmic drugs

Class III antiarrhythmic drugs are potassium channel blockers, which prolong repolarization manifested by an increase in QT interval on the ECG. These drugs are effective in suppressing complex VA, including nonsustained VT by increasing the refractory period. However, antiarrhythmic aggravation can occur, especially torsades des pointes.

Table 45-3 shows the effect of class III antiarrhythmic drugs on mortality in persons with heart disease.[61–66] None of the class III antiarrhythmic drugs has been found in a double-blind, randomized, placebo-controlled clinical trial to decrease mortality in persons with heart disease and complex VA.

Table 45-3. Effect of Class III Antiarrhythmic Drugs on Mortality in Persons With Heart Disease

Study	Results
Julien et al[61]	At 1-year follow-up, mortality was not different in persons after MI on d,l-sotalol versus a placebo
Waldo et al[62]	At 148-day follow-up, mortality in persons after MI was increased by d-sotalol (5.0%) versus a placebo (3.1%)
Singh et al[63]	At 2-year follow-up of persons with CHF and complex VA, survival was not different for amiodarone versus a placebo
Canadian Amiodarone MI Arrhythmia Trial[64]	At 1.8-year follow-up of persons after MI with complex VA, mortality was not different for amiodarone versus a placebo
European MI Amiodarone Trial[65]	At 21-month follow-up of persons after MI, mortality was not different for amiodarone (13.9%) versus a placebo (13.7%)
Sudden Cardiac Death in Heart Failure Trial[66]	At 45.5-month follow-up, compared with a placebo, amiodarone caused an insignificant (6%) increase in mortality, and implantable cardioverter-defibrillator therapy significantly reduced mortality by 23%

MI, myocardial infarction; *CHF*, congestive heart failure; *VA*, ventricular arrhythmias.

In 481 persons with VT, d,l-sotalol caused torsades des pointes (12 persons) or an increase in VT episodes (11 persons) in 23 persons (5%).[67] On the basis of the available data, β-blockers are preferred to the use of d,l-sotalol in treating elderly and younger persons with heart disease and VT or complex VA.

Amiodarone is very effective in suppressing VT and complex VA associated with heart disease.[63,64,66,68] However, the incidence of adverse effects from amiodarone approaches 90% after 5 years of therapy.[69] In the Cardiac Arrest in Seattle: Conventional Versus Amiodarone Drug Evaluation study, the incidence of pulmonary toxicity was 10% at 2 years in persons receiving 158 mg of amiodarone daily.[68] Amiodarone can also cause hyperthyroidism, hypothyroidism, and cardiac, dermatologic, gastrointestinal, hepatic, neurologic, and ophthalmologic adverse effects.

Because amiodarone has not been demonstrated to reduce mortality in elderly or younger persons with VT or complex VA associated with prior MI or CHF and has a very high incidence of toxicity, β-blockers are preferred to the use of amiodarone in treating these persons. There are some data suggesting that persons receiving amiodarone plus β-blockers had a better survival time than persons receiving amiodarone.[70]

Invasive intervention

If persons have life-threatening VT or ventricular fibrillation resistant to antiarrhythmic drugs, invasive intervention should be conducted. Persons with critical CAD and severe myocardial ischemia should undergo coronary artery bypass graft surgery to reduce mortality.[71]

Surgical ablation of the arrhythmogenic focus in persons with life-threatening ventricular tachyarrhythmias can be curative. This treatment includes aneurysmectomy or infarctectomy and endocardial resection with or without adjunctive cryoablation based on activation mapping in the operating room.[72–74] However, the perioperative mortality rate is high. Endoaneurysmorrhaphy with a pericardial patch combined with mapping-guided subendocardial resection frequently cures recurrent VT with a low operative mortality and improvement of LV systolic function.[75] Radiofrequency catheter ablation of VT has also been beneficial in the management of selected persons with arrhythmogenic foci of monomorphic VT.[76–78]

Automatic implantable cardioverter-defibrillator

The automatic implantable cardioverter-defibrillator (AICD) is the most effective treatment for persons with life-threatening VT or ventricular fibrillation. Table 45-4 indicates the effect of the AICD on mortality in persons with ventricular tachyarrhythmias.[79–85] Tresch et al[73,74] showed in retrospective studies that the AICD was very effective in treating life-threatening VT in elderly and younger persons. The Canadian Implantable Defibrillator Study found that persons most likely to benefit from an AICD were those with two of the following factors: age (70 years), LV ejection fraction (35%), and New York Heart Association function class III or IV.[86]

In MADIT-II, the reduction in sudden cardiac death in patients treated with an AICD was significantly reduced: by

Table 45-4. Effect of the Automatic Implantable Cardioverter-Defibrillator on Mortality in Persons With Ventricular Tachyarrhythmias

Study	Results
Multicenter Automatic Defibrillator Implantation Trial[79]	At 27-month follow-up, the AICD caused a 54% reduction in mortality
Antiarrhythmics Versus Implantable Defibrillators Trial[80]	Compared with drug therapy, the AICD caused a 39% decrease in mortality at 1 year, a 27% reduction in mortality at 2 years, and a 31% decrease in mortality at 3 years
Canadian Implantable Defibrillator Study[81]	Compared with amiodarone, at 3 years, total mortality rate was insignificantly decreased by 20% and the arrhythmic mortality was insignificantly reduced by 33%
Cardiac Arrest Study Hamburg[82]	Propafenone was stopped at 11 months because mortality from sudden death and cardiac arrest recurrence was 23% for propafenone versus 0% for an AICD
Cardiac Arrest Study Hamburg[83]	Compared with amiodarone or metoprolol, the 2- year mortality was decreased 37% by an AICD
Multicenter Unsustained Tachycardia Trial[84]	Compared with electrophysiologic guided antiarrhythmic drug therapy, the 5-year total mortality was borderline significantly decreased 20% by an AICD and the 5-year risk of cardiac arrest or death from arrhythmia was decreased 76% by an AICD
Multicenter Automatic Defibrillator Implantation Trial II[85]	At 20-month follow-up, compared with medical therapy, the AICD caused a 31% significant reduction in mortality

68% in 574 patients aged less than 65 years, by 65% in 455 patients aged 65 to 74 years, and by 68% in 204 patients aged 75 years.[87] The median survival in 348 octogenarians treated with AICD therapy was greater than 4 years.[88]

At 26-month follow-up, survival was 91% for persons treated with metoprolol plus an AICD versus 83% for persons treated with d,l-sotalol plus an AICD.[89] An observational study in 78 persons with CAD and life-threatening VA treated with an AICD showed at 490-days follow-up that the use of lipid-lowering drugs reduced recurrences of life-threatening VA.[90] During 33-month follow-up of 1038 patients, mean age 70 years, who had AICDs, use of β-blockers significantly reduced the frequency of appropriate AICD shocks.[91] At 32-month follow-up of 965 of these patients, all-cause mortality was significantly reduced 46% by use of β-blockers, 42% by use of statins, and 29% by use of ACE inhibitors or angiotensin receptor blockers.[92] These data favor using β-blockers, statins, and ACE inhibitors or angiotensin receptor blockers in the treatment of persons with AICDs.

The ACC/AHA guidelines recommend that class I indications for treatment with an AICD are (1) cardiac arrest due to VT or ventricular fibrillation not caused by a transient or reversible cause; (2) spontaneous sustained VT; (3) syncope of undetermined origin with clinically relevant, hemodynamically significant sustained VT or ventricular fibrillation induced at electrophysiologic study when drug therapy is ineffective, not tolerated, or not preferred; and (4) nonsustained VT with CAD, prior MI, LV systolic dysfunction, and inducible ventricular fibrillation or sustained VT at electrophysiologic study that is not suppressed by a class I antiarrhythmic drug.[93]

The updated ACC/AHA guidelines for treatment of CHF with a class I indication recommend use of an AICD in (1) patients with current or prior symptoms of CHF and reduced LV ejection fraction with a history of cardiac arrest, VF, or hemodynamically destabilizing VT; (2) in patients with CAD at least 40 days after MI, a LV ejection fraction equal to 30%, NYHA class II or III symptoms on optimal medical therapy, and an expected survival greater than 1 year; (3) in patients with nonischemic cardiomyopathy, a LV ejection fraction equal to 30%, NYHA class II or III symptoms on optimal medical therapy, and an expected survival greater than 1 year; and (4) with a class IIa indication in patients with a LV ejection fraction of 30% to 35% of any origin with NYHA class II or III symptoms on optimal medical therapy, and an expected survival greater than 1 year.[94] An AICD should also be used in patients with CHF requiring cardiac resynchronization therapy.[95]

ATRIAL FIBRILLATION

Atrial fibrillation (AF) is the most common sustained cardiac arrhythmia. The prevalence of AF increases with age.[96–99] The prevalence of AF in 2101 persons, mean age 81 years, was 5% in persons aged 60 to 70 years, 13% in persons aged 71 to 90 years, and 22% in persons aged 91 to 103 years.[97] Chronic AF was present in 16% of elderly men and in 13% of elderly women.[97] The prevalence of chronic AF in a study of 1563 persons, mean age 80 years, living in the community and seen in an academic geriatrics practice was 9%.[99]

AF may be paroxysmal or chronic. Episodes of paroxysmal AF may last from a few seconds to several weeks. Spontaneous conversion of paroxysmal AF to sinus rhythm occurs in 68% of persons having AF of less than 72 hours duration.[100]

Predisposing factors

Factors predisposing to AF include alcohol, atrial myxoma, atrial septal defect, cardiomyopathies, chronic lung disease, conduction system disease, CHF, CAD, diabetes mellitus, drugs, emotional stress, excessive coffee, hypertension, hyperthyroidism, hypoglycemia, hypokalemia, hypovolemia, hypoxia, myocarditis, neoplastic disease, pericarditis, pneumonia, postoperative state, pulmonary embolism, systemic infection, and valvular heart disease. Table 45-5 lists the increased prevalence of echocardiographic findings in 254 older persons with chronic AF compared with 1445 older persons with sinus rhythm, mean age 81 years.[101] In the Framingham Heart Study, low serum thyrotropin levels were independently associated with a 3.1 times increase in the development of new AF in elderly persons.[102]

Associated risks

The Framingham study showed that the incidence of death from cardiovascular causes was 2.0 times higher in men and 2.7 times higher in women with chronic AF than in men and

Table 45-5. Echocardiographic Findings in 254 Persons With Chronic Atrial Fibrillation and 1,445 Persons With Sinus Rhythm, Mean Age 81 Years

Variable	Higher Prevalence in Atrial Fibrillation
Rheumatic mitral stenosis	times
Left atrial enlargement	times
Abnormal LV ejection fraction	times
Aortic stenosis	times
≥ 1+ mitral regurgitation	times
≥ 1+ aortic regurgitation	times
LV hypertrophy	times
Mitral annular calcium	1.7 times

Adapted from Aronow WS et al.[101]
LV, left ventricular.

women with sinus rhythm.[103] The Framingham study also demonstrated that after adjustment for preexisting cardiovascular conditions, the odds ratio for mortality in persons with AF was 1.5 in men and 1.9 in women.[104] At 42-month follow-up of 1359 persons, mean age 81 years, with heart disease, persons with AF had a 2.2 times higher probability of developing new coronary events than those with sinus rhythm after controlling for other prognostic variables.[105] In 106,780 Medicare beneficiaries (65 years of age from the Cooperative Cardiovascular Project treated for acute MI, AF was present in 22%.[106] Compared with sinus rhythm, elderly persons with AF had a higher in-hospital mortality (25% versus 16%), 30-day mortality (29% versus 19%), and 1-year mortality (48% versus 33%).[106] AF was an independent predictor of in-hospital mortality (odds ratio = 1.2), 30-day mortality (odds ratio = 1.2), and 1-year mortality (odds ratio = 1.3).[106] Elderly persons developing AF during hospitalization had a worse prognosis than elderly persons who had AF.[106]

AF is an independent risk factor for thromboembolic (TE) stroke, especially in older persons.[96,97] In the Framingham study, the relative risk of stroke in persons with nonrheumatic AF compared with persons in sinus rhythm was 2.6 times higher in persons aged 60 to 69 years, 3.3 times higher in persons aged 70 to 79 years, and 4.5 times higher in persons aged 80 to 89 years.[96] AF was an independent risk factor for TE stroke in 2101 persons, mean age 81 years, with a relative risk of 3.3.[97] The 3-year incidence of TE stroke was 38% in persons with AF and 11% in persons with sinus rhythm.[97] The 5-year incidence of TE stroke was 72% in persons with AF and 24% in persons with sinus rhythm.[97]

AF was present in 313 of 2384 persons (13%), mean age 81 years.[107] AF was present in 201 of 1024 persons (17%) with LV hypertrophy and in 112 of 1360 persons (8%) without LV hypertrophy.[107] At 44-month follow-up, both AF (risk ratio = 3.2) and LV hypertrophy (risk ratio = 2.8) were independent risk factors for new TE stroke. The higher prevalence of LV hypertrophy in elderly persons with chronic AF contributes to the higher incidence of TE stroke in elderly persons with AF.

At 45-month follow-up of 1846 persons, mean age 81 years, both AF (risk ratio = 3.3) and 40% to 100% extracranial carotid arterial disease (ECAD) (risk ratio = 2.5) were independent risk factors for new TE stroke.[108] Elderly persons with both chronic AF and 40% to 100% ECAD had a 6.9 times higher probability of developing new TE stroke than those with sinus rhythm and no significant ECAD.[108]

Symptomatic cerebral infarctions were present in 22% of 54 autopsied patients aged 70 years or older with paroxysmal AF.[109] Symptomatic cerebral infarction was 2.4 times more common in older persons with paroxysmal AF than in older persons with sinus rhythm.[109] AF also causes silent cerebral infarction.[110]

AF is a predisposing factor for CHF in older persons. As much as 30% to 40% of LV end-diastolic volume may be attributable to left atrial contraction in older persons. Absence of a coordinated left atrial contraction decreases late diastolic filling of the LV because of loss of the atrial kick. A fast ventricular rate associated with AF also shortens the diastolic filling period, which further decreases LV filling.

A retrospective analysis of the Studies of Left Ventricular Dysfunction Prevention and Treatment Trials found that AF was an independent risk factor for all-cause mortality (relative risk = 1.3), progressive pump failure death (relative risk = 1.4), and death or hospitalization for CHF (relative risk = 1.3).[111]

AF was present in 132 of 355 persons (37%), mean age 80 years, with prior MI, CHF, and an abnormal LV ejection fraction.[112] AF was present in 98 of 296 persons (33%), mean age 82 years, with prior MI, CHF, and a normal LV ejection fraction.[112] In this study, AF was an independent risk factor for mortality with a risk ratio of 1.5.[112]

A fast ventricular rate associated with chronic or paroxysmal AF may cause a tachycardia-related cardiomyopathy, which may be an unrecognized curable cause of CHF.[113,114] Control of a fast ventricular rate by radiofrequency ablation of the atrioventricular (AV) node with permanent pacing caused an improvement in LV ejection fraction in persons with medically refractory AF.[115]

Clinical symptoms

Elderly persons with AF may be symptomatic or asymptomatic with their arrhythmia detected by physical examination or by an ECG. Examination of a person after a stroke may lead to the diagnosis of AF. Symptoms may include palpitations, skips in heartbeat, fatigue on exertion, exercise intolerance, cough, dizziness, chest pain, and syncope. A fast ventricular rate associated with loss of atrial contraction reduces cardiac output and may cause hypotension, angina pectoris, CHF, acute pulmonary edema, and syncope, especially in elderly persons with mitral stenosis, aortic stenosis, or hypertrophic cardiomyopathy.

Diagnostic tests

When AF is suspected, a 12-lead ECG with a 1-minute rhythm strip should be obtained to confirm the diagnosis. If paroxysmal AF is suspected, a 24-hour AECG should be obtained. All persons with AF should have an M-mode, 2-dimensional, and Doppler echocardiogram to determine the presence and severity of cardiac abnormalities causing AF and to identify risk factors for stroke. Appropriate tests for noncardiac causes of AF should be performed when clinically indicated. Thyroid function tests should be performed as AF or CHF may be the only clinical manifestations of apathetic hyperthyroidism in elderly persons.

General treatment measures

Along with drug therapy, treatment of AF should include therapy of the underlying disorder (such as hyperthyroidism, pneumonia, or pulmonary embolism) when possible.

Surgical candidates for mitral valve replacement should undergo surgery if it is clinically indicated. If mitral valve replacement is not performed in persons with significant mitral valve disease, elective cardioversion should not be performed in persons with AF. Precipitating factors such as CHF, hypoxia, hypokalemia, hypoglycemia, hypovolemia, and infection should be treated immediately. Alcohol, coffee, and drugs (especially sympathomimetics) that precipitate AF should be avoided. Paroxysmal AF associated with the tachycardia-bradycardia (sick sinus) syndrome should be treated with permanent pacing in combination with the use of drugs to slow a fast ventricular rate associated with AF.[116]

Control of very fast rapid ventricular rate

Immediate direct-current cardioversion should be performed in persons who have paroxysmal AF with a very fast ventricular rate associated with an acute MI, chest pain caused by myocardial ischemia, hypotension, severe CHF, or syncope. Intravenous verapamil,[117] diltiazem,[118] or β-blockers[119–122] may be used to immediately slow a very fast ventricular rate associated with AF.

Control of fast ventricular rate

Digitalis glycosides are ineffective in converting AF to sinus rhythm.[123] Digoxin is also ineffective in slowing a fast ventricular rate associated with AF if there is associated hyperthyroidism, fever, hypoxia, acute blood loss, or any condition involving increased sympathetic tone.[124] However, digoxin should be used for slowing a fast ventricular rate in AF unassociated with increased sympathetic tone, the Wolff-Parkinson-White syndrome, or hypertrophic obstructive cardiomyopathy, especially if there is LV systolic dysfunction. The usual maintenance oral dose of digoxin administered to persons with AF is 0.25 mg to 0.5 mg daily, with the dose decreased to 0.125 mg to 0.25 mg daily for elderly persons who are more susceptible to digitalis toxicity.[125]

Oral verapamil,[126] diltiazem,[127] or a β-blocker[128] should be added to the therapeutic regimen if a fast ventricular rate associated with AF occurs at rest or during exercise despite digoxin. These drugs act synergistically with digoxin to depress conduction through the AV junction. In a study of digoxin 0.25 mg daily, diltiazem-CD 240 mg daily, atenolol 50 mg daily, digoxin 0.25 mg plus diltiazem-CD 240 mg daily, and digoxin 0.25 mg plus atenolol 50 mg daily, digoxin and diltiazem as single drugs were least effective and digoxin plus atenolol was most effective in controlling ventricular rate in AF during daily activity.[129]

Amiodarone is the most effective drug for slowing a fast ventricular rate associated with AF.[130,131] However, its adverse effect profile limits its use in the treatment of AF. Oral doses of 200 mg to 400 mg of amiodarone daily may be administered to selected persons with symptomatic life-threatening AF refractory to other drug therapy.

Therapeutic concentrations of digoxin do not decrease the frequency of episodes of paroxysmal AF or the duration of episodes of paroxysmal AF detected by 24-hour AECGs.[132,133] In fact, digoxin has been demonstrated to increase the duration of episodes of paroxysmal AF, a result consistent with its action in reducing the atrial refractory period.[132] Therapeutic concentrations of digoxin also do not prevent a rapid ventricular rate from developing in persons with paroxysmal AF.[132–134] Therefore digoxin should be avoided in persons with sinus rhythm with a history of paroxysmal AF.

Nondrug therapies

Radiofrequency catheter modification of AV conduction should be performed in persons with symptomatic AF in whom a fast ventricular rate cannot be slowed by drug therapy.[135,136] If this procedure does not control the fast ventricular rate associated with AF, complete AV block produced by radiofrequency catheter ablation followed by permanent pacemaker implantation should be performed.[137,138] In 44 patients, mean age 78 years, radiofrequency catheter ablation followed by pacemaker implantation was successful in ablating the AV junction in 43 of 44 patients (98%) with AF and a rapid ventricular rate not controlled by drug therapy.[138]

In persons with CHF and chronic AF, AV junction ablation with implantation of a VVIR pacemaker was superior to drug therapy in controlling symptoms in a randomized, controlled study of 66 persons.[139] Surgical techniques have also been developed for use in persons with AF in whom a rapid ventricular rate cannot be slowed by drug treatment.[140–142] Appropriate indications for using an implantable Atrioverter in the treatment of AF need further investigation.[143]

Tachycardia-bradycardia syndrome

Paroxysmal AF associated with the tachycardia-bradycardia (sick sinus) syndrome should be treated with a permanent pacemaker in combination with drugs to decrease a rapid ventricular rate associated with AF.[116] Ventricular pacing is an independent risk factor for the development of chronic AF in persons with paroxysmal AF associated with the tachycardia-bradycardia syndrome.[144] Persons with paroxysmal AF associated with the tachycardia-bradycardia syndrome and no signs of AV conduction abnormalities should be treated with atrial pacing or dual-chamber pacing rather than with ventricular pacing because atrial pacing is associated with less AF, less TE complications, and a lower risk of AV block than is ventricular pacing.[145]

Wolff-Parkinson-White syndrome

Direct-current cardioversion should be performed if a fast ventricular rate in paroxysmal AF associated with the Wolff-Parkinson-White syndrome is life-threatening or fails to respond to drug treatment. Drug treatment for paroxysmal AF associated with the Wolff-Parkinson-White syndrome includes propranolol plus procainamide, disopyramide, or quinidine.[146] Digoxin, verapamil, and diltiazem are contraindicated in persons with AF associated with the Wolff-Parkinson-White syndrome because these drugs shorten the refractory period of the accessory AV pathway, causing faster conduction down the accessory pathway. This results in a marked increase in ventricular rate. Radiofrequency catheter ablation or surgical ablation of the accessory conduction pathway should be considered in persons with AF and fast AV conduction over the accessory pathway.[147]

Slow ventricular rate

Many elderly persons are able to tolerate AF without the need for treatment because the ventricular rate is slow as a result of concomitant AV nodal disease. These persons should not be treated with a drug that depresses AV conduction.

A permanent pacemaker should be implanted in persons with AF who develop cerebral symptoms such as dizziness or syncope associated with ventricular pauses greater than 3 seconds that are not drug-induced, as documented by a 24-hour AECG. If persons with AF have drug-induced symptomatic bradycardia and the causative drug cannot be discontinued, a permanent pacemaker must be implanted.

Elective cardioversion

Elective direct-current cardioversion has a higher success rate of converting AF to sinus rhythm than does medical cardioversion.[148] Unfavorable conditions for elective cardioversion of chronic AF to sinus rhythm include duration of AF greater than 1 year, moderate to severe cardiomegaly, echocardiographic left atrial dimension greater than 45 mm, digitalis toxicity (contraindication), slow ventricular rate (contraindication), sick sinus syndrome (contraindication), mitral valve disease, CHF, chronic obstructive lung disease, recurrent AF despite antiarrhythmic drugs, and inability to tolerate antiarrhythmic drugs. Elective cardioversion of AF either by direct current or by antiarrhythmic drugs should not be performed in asymptomatic elderly persons with chronic AF.

Antiarrhythmic drugs that have been used to convert AF to sinus rhythm include amiodarone, disopyramide, dofetilide, encainide, flecainide, ibutilide, procainamide, propafenone, quinidine, and sotalol. None of these drugs are as successful as direct-current cardioversion (which is 80% to 90% successful) in converting AF to sinus rhythm. All of these drugs are proarrhythmic and may aggravate or cause cardiac arrhythmias.

Encainide and flecainide caused atrial proarrhythmic effects in 6 of 60 persons (10%).[149] The proarrhythmic effects included conversion of AF to atrial flutter with a 1-to-1 AV conduction response and a very fast ventricular rate.[149] Flecainide has induced VT and ventricular fibrillation in persons with chronic AF.[150] Antiarrhythmic drugs including amiodarone, disopyramide, flecainide, procainamide, propafenone, quinidine, and sotalol caused cardiac adverse effects in 73 of 417 patients (18%) hospitalized for AF.[151] Class IC drugs such as encainide, flecainide, and propafenone should be avoided in persons with prior MI or LV systolic dysfunction because these drugs may cause life-threatening ventricular tachyarrhythmias in these persons.[38]

Ibutilide and dofetilide are class III antiarrhythmic drugs that have recently been used to try to convert AF to sinus rhythm. Twenty-three of 79 persons (29%) with AF treated with intravenous ibutilide converted to sinus rhythm.[152] Polymorphic ventricular tachycardia developed in 4% of persons taking ibutilide in this study.[152] All of these persons had abnormal LV systolic function. Eleven of 75 persons (15%) with AF treated with intravenous dofetilide converted to sinus rhythm.[153] Torsade de pointes occurred in 3% of persons treated with intravenous dofetilide.[154] After 1 month, 22 of 190 patients (12%) with CHF and AF had sinus rhythm restored with dofetilide compared with 3 of 201 patients (1%) treated with a placebo.[154] Torsade de pointes developed in 25 patients (3%) treated with dofetilide and in none of the patients (0%) treated with a placebo.[154] Direct-current cardioversion of AF has a higher success rate in converting AF to sinus rhythm and a lower incidence of cardiac adverse effects than any antiarrhythmic drug. However, pretreatment with ibutilide has been shown to facilitate transthoracic cardioversion of AF.[155]

Unless transesophageal echocardiography has shown no thrombus in the left atrial appendage before cardioversion,[156] oral warfarin therapy should be administered for 3 weeks before elective direct-current cardioversion or drug cardioversion of persons with AF to sinus rhythm.[157] Anticoagulant therapy should be administered at the time of cardioversion and continued until sinus rhythm has been maintained for 4 weeks.[157] After direct-current or drug cardioversion of AF to sinus rhythm, the left atrium becomes stunned and contracts poorly for 3 to 4 weeks, predisposing to TE stroke unless the patient is receiving oral warfarin.[158,159] The maintenance dose of oral warfarin should be titrated by serial prothrombin times so that the INR is 2.0 to 3.0.[157] A controlled, randomized, prospective clinical trial is needed to compare conventional anticoagulant treatment before cardioversion of AF with a transesophageal echocardiography-guided strategy.[160]

Use of antiarrhythmic drugs to maintain sinus rhythm

The efficacy and safety of antiarrhythmic drugs after cardioversion of AF to maintain sinus rhythm has been questioned. It has not been demonstrated that persons cardioverted from AF to sinus rhythm will have a decreased incidence of subsequent TE stroke. A meta-analysis of six double-blind, placebo-controlled studies of quinidine involving 808 persons who had direct-current cardioversion of chronic AF to sinus rhythm found that 50% of persons receiving quinidine and 25% of persons receiving a placebo were in sinus rhythm at 1 year.[43] However, the mortality was higher in persons treated with quinidine (2.9%) than in persons treated with a placebo (0.8%).[43] In a study of 406 persons, mean age 82 years, with heart disease and complex VA, the incidence of adverse effects causing drug cessation was 48% for quinidine and 55% for procainamide.[40] The incidence of total mortality at 2-year follow-up was insignificantly higher in persons receiving quinidine or procainamide than in persons not receiving an antiarrhythmic drug.[40]

In another study, 98 persons were randomized to sotalol and 85 persons to quinidine after direct-current cardioversion of AF to sinus rhythm.[161] At 6-month follow-up, 52% of sotalol-treated persons and 48% of quinidine-treated persons were in sinus rhythm.[161] At 1-year follow-up of 100 persons with AF cardioverted to sinus rhythm, 30% of 50 persons randomized to propafenone and 37% of 50 persons randomized to sotalol remained in sinus rhythm.[162]

Of 1330 persons in the Stroke Prevention in Atrial Fibrillation (SPAF) Study, 127 persons were receiving quinidine, 57 procainamide, 34 flecainide, 20 encainide, 15 disopyramide, and 7 amiodarone.[44] Patients taking an antiarrhythmic drug had a 2.7 times increased adjusted relative risk of cardiac mortality and a 2.3 times increased adjusted relative risk of arrhythmic death compared with persons not taking an antiarrhythmic drug.[44] Persons with a history of CHF taking an antiarrhythmic drug had a 4.7 times increased relative risk of cardiac death and a 3.7 times higher relative risk of arrhythmic death than persons with a history of CHF not taking an antiarrhythmic drug.[44]

A meta-analysis of 59 randomized, controlled studies comprising 23,229 persons, including elderly persons, that investigated the use of aprindine, disopyramide, encainide, flecainide, imipramine, lidocaine, mexiletine, moricizine, phenytoin, procainamide, quinidine, and tocainide after MI showed that the mortality was higher in persons receiving class I antiarrhythmic drugs (odds ratio = 1.14) than in persons not receiving an antiarrhythmic drug.[45] None of the 59 studies demonstrated a decrease in mortality by class I antiarrhythmic drugs.[45]

Ventricular rate control

Because maintenance of sinus rhythm with antiarrhythmic drugs may need serial cardioversions; exposes persons to the risks of proarrhythmia, sudden cardiac death, and other adverse effects; and needs the use of anticoagulant treatment in persons in sinus rhythm who have a high risk of recurrence of AF, many cardiologists, including myself, prefer the treatment strategy, especially in elderly persons, of ventricular rate control plus anticoagulant treatment in persons with AF. β-blockers such as propranolol (10 mg to 30 mg, three to four times daily) can be administered to control ventricular arrhythmias[50] and following conversion of AF to sinus rhythm. Should AF recur, β-blockers have the additional advantage of slowing the ventricular rate. β-blockers are also the most effective drugs in preventing and treating AF after coronary artery bypass graft surgery.[163] In a double-blind, randomized placebo-controlled study of 394 persons receiving metoprolol CR/XL or a placebo after cardioversion of persistent AF, metoprolol was more effective than a placebo in preventing recurrence of AF and in decreasing the ventricular heart rate if AF recurred.[164]

The Atrial Fibrillation Follow-Up Investigation of Rhythm Management (AFFIRM) Study randomized 4060 patients, mean age 70 years (39% women), with paroxysmal or chronic AF of less than 6 months duration and with high risk for stroke to either maintenance of AF with ventricular rate control or to an attempt to maintain sinus rhythm with antiarrhythmic drugs after cardioversion.[165] Patients in both arms of this study were treated with warfarin. All-cause mortality at 5 years was insignificantly increased (15%) in the maintenance of sinus rhythm group compared with the ventricular rate control group (24% vs. 21%).[165] TE stroke was insignificantly reduced in the ventricular rate control group (5.5% vs. 7.1%), and all-cause hospitalization was significantly reduced in the ventricular rate control group (73% vs. 80%).[165] In both groups, the majority of strokes occurred after warfarin was stopped or when the INR was subtherapeutic. There was no significant difference in quality of life or functional status between the two treatment groups.[165]

The Rate Control Versus Electrical Cardioversion for Persistent Atrial Fibrillation Study Group randomized 522 patients with persistent AF after a previous electrical cardioversion to receive treatment aimed at ventricular rate control or rhythm control.[166] Both groups were treated with oral anticoagulants. At 2.3-year follow-up, the composite end point of death from cardiovascular causes, heart failure, TE complications, bleeding, implantation of a pacemaker, and severe adverse effects of drugs was 17.2% in the ventricular rate control group versus 22.6% in the rhythm control group.[166] In this study, women randomized to rhythm control had a 3.1 times significant increase in cardiovascular morbidity or mortality versus women randomized to ventricular rate control.[167]

Table 45-6. Risk Factors for New Thromboembolic Stroke in 312 Elderly Persons With Chronic Atrial Fibrillation

Variable	Risk Ratio
Age	1.03/yr increase
Prior stroke	1.6
Abnormal LV ejection fraction	1.8
Mitral stenosis	2.0
LV hypertrophy	2.8
Abnormal LV ejection fraction	1.8
Serum total cholesterol	1.01 per 1 mg/dL increase
Serum high-density lipoprotein cholesterol	1.04 per 1 mg/dL decrease

Adapted from Aronow WS et al.[173]
LV, left ventricular.

The 2-year mortality was similar in 1009 patients with AF and CHF treated with rate control or rhythm control.[168] During 19-month follow-up of 110 patients with a history of AF treated with antiarrhythmic drug therapy, recurrent AF was diagnosed by ECG recordings in 46% of the patients and by an implantable monitoring device in 88% of the patients.[169] AF lasting longer than 48 hours was detected by the monitoring device in 50 of the 110 patients (46%). Nineteen of these 50 patients (38%) were completely asymptomatic.[169]

RISK FACTORS FOR THROMBOEMBOLIC STROKE

Risk factors for TE stroke in persons with AF include age,[96,170–173] diabetes mellitus,[171] echocardiographic left atrial enlargement,[174,175] echocardiographic LV systolic dysfunction,[173,175,176] echocardiographic LV hypertrophy,[173,174] ECAD,[108] history of CHF,[171,176,177] prior MI,[170,171,174,178] hypertension,[171,174,176,177] mitral annular calcium,[170,179] prior arterial thromboembolism,* rheumatic mitral stenosis,[173,174] and women older than 75 years.[176] Table 45-6 lists independent risk factors for new TE stroke in 312 persons with chronic AF, mean age 84 years.

In the SPAF Study involving persons, mean age 67 years, with nonrheumatic AF, recent CHF (within 3 months), a history of hypertension, prior arterial thromboembolism, echocardiographic LV systolic dysfunction, and echocardiographic left atrial enlargement were independently associated with new TE events.[175,177] The incidence of new TE events was 18.6% per year if three or more risk factors were present, 6.0% per year if 1 or 2 risk factors were present, and 1.0% per year if none of these risk factors was present.[175] In the SPAF III Study, persons, mean age 72 years, were considered to be at high risk for developing TE stroke if they had either a previous thromboembolism, CHF, or abnormal LV systolic function, a systolic blood pressure higher than 160 mm Hg, or the person was a woman older than 75 years of age.[176]

Antithrombotic therapy

Prospective, randomized studies have shown that warfarin was effective in reducing the incidence of TE stroke in persons with nonvalvular AF.[171,176,180–186] Analysis of pooled

*References 97, 103, 171–173, 176, 177, 180.

data from five randomized controlled trials demonstrated that warfarin decreased the incidence of new TE stroke by 68% and was more effective than aspirin in decreasing TE stroke.[171] Nonrandomized observational data from an elderly population mean age 83 years, found that 141 persons with chronic AF treated with oral warfarin to achieve an INR between 2.0 and 3.0 (mean INR was 2.4) had a 67% decrease in new TE stroke compared with 209 persons with chronic AF treated with oral aspirin.[187] Compared with aspirin, warfarin caused a 40% decrease in new TE stroke in persons with prior stroke, a 31% reduction in new TE stroke in persons with no prior stroke, a 45% decrease in new TE stroke in persons with an abnormal LV ejection fraction, and a 36% reduction in new TE stroke in persons with a normal LV ejection fraction.[187]

At 1.1-year follow-up in the SPAF III Study, persons with nonvalvular AF considered to be at high risk for developing TE stroke randomized to therapy with oral warfarin to achieve an INR between 2.0 and 3.0 had a 72% decrease in ischemic stroke or systemic embolism compared with persons randomized to therapy with oral aspirin 325 mg daily plus oral warfarin to achieve an INR between 1.2 to 1.5.[176] Adjusted-dose warfarin caused an absolute decrease in ischemic stroke or systemic embolism of 6.0% per year.[176] In the Second Copenhagen Atrial Fibrillation, Aspirin, Anticoagulation (AFASK) Study, low-dose warfarin plus aspirin was also less effective in decreasing stroke or a systemic TE event in persons with AF (7.2% after 1 year) than was adjusted-dose warfarin to achieve an INR between 2.0 to 3.0 (2.8% after 1 year).[188]

Analysis of pooled data from five randomized controlled trials showed that the annual rate of major hemorrhage was 1.0% for the control group, 1.0% for the aspirin group, and 1.3% for the warfarin group.[171] The incidence of major hemorrhage in persons taking adjusted-dose warfarin to achieve an INR of 2.0 to 3.0 in the SPAF III Study (mean age 72 years) was 2.1%.[176] In the Second Copenhagen AFASK Study, the incidence of major hemorrhage in persons, mean age 73 years, was 0.8% per year for persons taking adjusted-dose warfarin to achieve an INR between 2.0 and 3.0 and 1.0% per year for persons treated with aspirin, 300 mg daily.[188] The incidence of major hemorrhage in elderly persons, mean age 83 years, was 4.3% (1.4% per year) for persons with chronic AF taking warfarin to maintain an INR between 2.0 and 3.0 and 2.9% (1.0% per year) for persons with chronic AF treated with aspirin, 325 mg daily.[187]

In the SPAF III Study, 892 persons, mean age 67 years, at low risk for developing new TE stroke were treated with oral aspirin, 325 mg daily.[189] Mean follow-up was 2 years. The incidence of new ischemic stroke or systemic embolism (primary events) was 2.2% per year.[189] The incidence of new ischemic stroke or systemic embolism was 3.6% in persons with a history of hypertension and 1.1% in persons without a history of hypertension.[189]

In the Anticoagulation and Risk Factor in Atrial Fibrillation Study, women off warfarin had significantly higher annual rates of thromboembolism (3.5%) than men (1.8%).[190] Warfarin was associated with significantly lower adjusted TE rates for both women (60% reduction) and men (40% reduction) with similar annual rates of major bleeding (1.0% and 1.1%, respectively).[190]

The Atrial Fibrillation Clopidogrel Trial with Irbersartan for the Prevention of Vascular Events (ACTIVE W) demonstrated in patients with AF that the annual risk of first occurrence of stroke, noncentral nervous system systemic embolus, MI, or vascular death was 3.93% in 3371 patients randomized to warfarin to maintain an INR between 2.0 and 3.0, and 5.60% in 3335 patients randomized to clopidogrel 75 mg daily plus aspirin 75 to 100 mg daily, with a 44% significant decrease in the primary outcome attributed to warfarin.[191] The incidence of major bleeding was insignificantly (10%) higher in patients treated with clopidogrel plus aspirin than in persons treated with warfarin.[191]

On the basis of the available data, elderly persons with chronic or paroxysmal AF who are at high risk for developing TE stroke or who have a history of hypertension and who have no contraindications to anticoagulation therapy should receive long-term oral warfarin to achieve an INR of 2.0 to 3.0.[157,192] Hypertension must be controlled. Whenever the person has a prothrombin time taken, the blood pressure should also be checked. The physician prescribing the dose of oral warfarin should be aware of the numerous drugs that potentiate the effect of warfarin causing an increased prothrombin time and risk of bleeding.[35] Elderly persons with AF who are at low risk for developing TE stroke or who have contraindications to therapy with long-term oral warfarin should be treated with aspirin 325 mg orally daily.

ATRIAL FLUTTER

Atrial flutter is usually paroxysmal and only rarely chronic. Untreated persons with atrial flutter and no disease of the AV junction usually have a 2:1 AV conduction response with an atrial rate of about 300 beats/min and a ventricular rate of 150 beats/min. Over time, atrial flutter usually degenerates into AF.

Management of atrial flutter is similar to management of AF. Direct-current cardioversion is the treatment of choice for converting atrial flutter to sinus rhythm.[193] Atrial flutter treated with intravenous ibutilide in 38% of 78 persons converted to sinus rhythm.[150] Atrial flutter treated with intravenous dofetilide in 54% of 16 persons converted to sinus rhythm.[151] Atrial pacing may also be used to try to convert atrial flutter to sinus rhythm.[194]

Intravenous verapamil,[117] diltiazem,[118] or β-blockers[119–122] may be used to immediately slow a very rapid ventricular rate associated with atrial flutter. Oral verapamil,[126] diltiazem,[127] or a β-blocker[128] should be added to the therapeutic regimen if a rapid ventricular rate associated with atrial flutter occurs at rest or during exercise despite digoxin. Amiodarone is the most effective drug for slowing a rapid ventricular rate associated with atrial flutter.[131] Digoxin, verapamil, and diltiazem are contraindicated in persons with atrial flutter associated with the Wolff-Parkinson-White syndrome because these drugs shorten the refractory period of the accessory AV pathway, causing more rapid conduction down the accessory pathway. Drugs such as quinidine should never be used to treat persons with atrial flutter who are not being treated with digoxin, a β-blocker, verapamil, or diltiazem as a 1:1 AV conduction response may develop.

Persons with atrial flutter are at increased risk for developing new TE stroke.[195,196] Anticoagulant therapy should be administered before direct-current cardioversion or drug cardioversion of persons with atrial flutter to sinus rhythm using the same guidelines as for converting AF.[157–160,192] Persons with chronic atrial flutter should be treated with oral warfarin with the INR maintained between 2.0 and 3.0.[157,192]

Radiofrequency catheter ablation of atrial flutter is a highly successful procedure, especially when the right atrial isthmus is incorporated in the atrial flutter circuit.[197,198] Demonstration of bi-directional isthmus block after catheter ablation predicts a high long-term success rate.[198] A second radiofrequency catheter ablation may be needed in up to one third of patients, especially in those with right atrial enlargement.[197] Radiofrequency catheter ablation was successful in converting 63 of 70 patients (90%), mean age 78 years, with atrial flutter to sinus rhythm.[138]

ATRIAL PREMATURE COMPLEXES

The prevalence of frequent atrial premature complexes (APCs) diagnosed by 24-hour AECGs in older persons was 18% in 729 older women and 28% in 643 older men in the Cardiovascular Health Study[7] and 28% in 407 persons, mean age 82 years.[8] Although frequent APCs may trigger a paroxysm of AF, atrial flutter, or supraventricular tachycardia (SVT), they are of no clinical significance when found incidentally and should not be treated. If a supraventricular tachyarrhythmia is triggered by frequent APCs, a β-blocker should be administered.

SUPRAVENTRICULAR TACHYCARDIA

The ventricular rate in paroxysmal SVT usually ranges between 140 and 220 beats per minute and is extremely regular. The prevalence of short bursts of paroxysmal SVT diagnosed by 24-hour AECGs in 1476 persons, mean age 81 years, with heart disease was 33%.[172] At 42-month follow-up of 1359 persons, mean age 81 years, with heart disease, paroxysmal SVT was not associated with an increased incidence of new coronary events.[105] At 43-month follow-up of 1476 persons, mean age 81 years, paroxysmal SVT was not associated with an increased incidence of new TE stroke.[172]

Sustained episodes of SVT should first be treated by increasing vagal tone by carotid sinus massage or the Valsalva maneuver. If vagal maneuvers are unsuccessful, intravenous adenosine is the drug of choice.[199] Intravenous verapamil, diltiazem, or β-blockers may also be used. If these measures do not convert SVT to sinus rhythm, direct-current cardioversion should be used.

Most persons with paroxysmal SVT do not require long-term therapy. If long-term therapy is required because of symptoms due to frequent episodes of SVT, digoxin, propranolol, or verapamil may be administered.[200] These drugs are the initial drug of choice for AV nodal reentrant and AV reentrant SVT, the commonest forms of SVT. For SVT associated with the Wolff-Parkinson-White syndrome, flecainide or propafenone may be used if there is no associated heart disease.[201] If heart disease is present, quinidine, procainamide, or disopyramide plus a β-blocker or verapamil should be used.[201] Radiofrequency catheter ablation should be used to treat older persons with symptomatic, drug-resistant SVT and should be considered an early treatment option.[138,202]

Radiofrequency catheter ablation was successful in converting 60 of 66 patients, mean age 78 years, with SVT to sinus rhythm.[138]

ACCELERATED ATRIOVENTRICULAR RHYTHM

Accelerated AV junctional rhythm also called nonparoxysmal AV junctional tachycardia (NPJT) is a form of SVT and is caused by enhanced impulse formation within the AV junction rather than by reentry.[203] This arrhythmia is usually due to recent aortic or mitral valve surgery, acute MI, or digitalis toxicity. The ventricular rate usually ranges between 70 and 130 beats/min. Treatment of NPJT is directed toward correction of the underlying disorder. Hypokalemia, if present, should be treated with potassium. Digitalis should be stopped if digitalis toxicity is present. β-blockers may be given cautiously if this is warranted by clinical circumstances.

PAROXYSMAL ATRIAL TACHYCARDIA WITH ATRIOVENTRICULAR BLOCK

Digitalis toxicity causes 70% of cases of paroxysmal atrial tachycardia (PAT) with AV block. Digoxin and diuretics causing hypokalemia should be stopped in these persons. If the serum potassium is low or low-normal, potassium chloride is the treatment of choice. Intravenous propranolol will cause conversion to sinus rhythm in about 85% of persons with digitalis-induced PAT with AV block and in about 35% of persons with PAT with AV block not induced by digitalis.[204] By increasing AV block, propranolol may also be beneficial in slowing a rapid ventricular rate in PAT with AV block.

MULTIFOCAL ATRIAL TACHYCARDIA

Multifocal atrial tachycardia (MAT) is usually associated with acute illness, especially in older persons with pulmonary disease. MAT is best managed by treatment of the underlying disorder. Intravenous verapamil has been reported to be effective in controlling the ventricular rate in MAT, with occasional conversion to sinus rhythm.[205] However, the author found intravenous verapamil not very effective in treating MAT.[206] The tendency of intravenous verapamil to aggravate preexisting arterial hypoxemia also limits its use in the group of persons most likely to develop MAT.[205]

BRADYARRHYTHMIAS

With aging, there is a loss of specialized muscle cells (called P cells) within the sinus node, which are responsible for initiating impulse formation. By age 75 years, the sinus node may consist of less than 10% P cells.[207] A progressive increase in the amount of collagen within the sinus node also occurs with aging.[208] There is an age-related reduction in conducting cells in the His bundle and both bundle branches, which are the distal parts of the cardiac conduction system. Diseases associated with aging such as CAD, hypertension, and valvular heart disease also adversely affect the cardiac conduction system.

Numerous drugs can cause bradyarrhythmias and conduction disturbances. Hypothyroidism, hyperkalemia, hypokalemia, and hypoxia can also depress cardiac impulse formation and conduction. Drugs and endocrine and metabolic disorders causing reversible cardiac impulse formation and conduction abnormalities must be considered before deciding to implant a permanent pacemaker.

A 12-lead ECG with a 1-minute strip may detect bradyarrhythmias caused by a sick sinus syndrome, AV block, right and left bundle branch block, bifascicular block, and trifascicular block. ECG manifestations of sick sinus syndrome include severe sinus bradycardia, sinus pause or arrest, sinus exit block, sinus node reentrant rhythm, AF or atrial flutter with a slow ventricular rate not drug-induced, failure of restoration of sinus rhythm after cardioversion for tachyarrhythmias, a longer than 3-second pause after carotid sinus massage, and a tachycardia-bradycardia syndrome. The tachycardia-bradycardia syndrome is characterized by paroxysmal AF, atrial flutter, or SVT followed by periods of sinus bradycardia, sinus arrest, or sinoatrial block.

Dyspnea, weakness, fatigue, falls, angina pectoris, CHF, episodic pulmonary edema, dizziness, faintness, slurred speech, personality changes, paresis, and convulsions in older persons may be caused by bradyarrhythmias. Death may result from prolonged ventricular asystole. Older persons with symptoms that may be due to bradyarrhythmias should have a 12-lead ECG with a 1-minute rhythm strip. Since ECG abnormalities may be intermittent, a 24-hour AECG may need to be performed.

In a prospective study of 148 persons, mean age 82 years, with unexplained syncope, 24-hour AECGs diagnosed bradyarrhythmias with pauses greater than 3 seconds requiring permanent pacemaker implantation in 21 persons (14%).[2] Of these 21 persons, 8 had sinus arrest, 7 had advanced second-degree AV block, and 6 had AF with a slow ventricular rate not drug-induced. At 38-month follow-up after pacemaker implantation, recurrent syncope developed in only 3 of the 21 older persons (14%).[2]

In some older persons without clinical evidence of heart disease and recurrent episodes of unexplained syncope, a patient-activated memory loop event recorder may be used to capture the ECG tracings preceding and during syncope.[209] Older persons with unexplained syncope and heart disease should undergo an electrophysiologic study.[209] Table 45-7 shows class I indications for permanent pacemaker implantation.[93] Modes of pacing, pacemaker codes, and pacemaker follow-up are discussed in detail elsewhere.[210]

Table 45-7. Class I Indications for Permanent Pacing

A. Third-degree atrioventricular (AV) block with:
   1. Symptomatic bradycardia
   2. Arrhythmias and other medical conditions that require drugs that cause symptomatic bradycardia
   3. Pauses ≥ 3.0 seconds or any escape ventricular rate <40 beats per minute in awake, symptom-free patients
   4. After catheter ablation of AV junction
   5. Postoperative AV block not expected to resolve after surgery
   6. Neuromuscular diseases with AV block

B. Second-degree AV block with symptomatic bradycardia

C. Chronic bifascicular and trifascicular block with:
   1. Intermittent third-degree AV block
   2. Type II second-degree AV block
   3. Alternating bundle branch block

D. After acute myocardial infarction with:
   1. Persistent second-degree AV block in His-Purkinje system with bilateral bundle branch block or third-degree AV block within or below His-Purkinje system
   2. Transient second- or third-degree infranodal AV block and associated bundle branch block
   3. Persistent and symptomatic second- or third-degree AV block

E. Sinus node dysfunction
   1. Sinus node dysfunction with symptomatic bradycardia
   2. Symptomatic chronotropic incompetence

F. Prevention and termination of tachyarrhythmias
   1. Symptomatic recurrent supraventricular tachycardia terminated by pacing after drugs and catheter ablation fail to control arrhythmia or cause intolerable side effects (downgraded to class IIa indication)
   2. Symptomatic recurrent sustained ventricular tachycardia as part of an automatic defibrillator system

G. Prevention of tachycardia
   1. Sustained pause-dependent ventricular tachycardia, with or without prolonged QT, in which efficacy of pacing is documented

H. Hypersensitive carotid sinus and neurally mediated syncope
   1. Recurrent syncope caused by carotid sinus stimulation; minimal carotid sinus pressure induces asystole >3 seconds in absence of any drug that depresses sinus node or AV conduction

Adapted from Gregoratos G et al.[93]

For a complete list of references, please visit online only at www.expertconsult.com

CHAPTER 46

Syncope

Rose Anne Kenny

DEFINITION

Syncope (derived from the Greek words, "syn" meaning "with" and the verb "koptein" meaning "to cut" or more appropriately in this case "to interrupt") is a symptom, defined as a transient, self-limited loss of consciousness, usually leading to falling. The onset of syncope is relatively rapid, and the subsequent recovery is spontaneous, complete, and usually prompt.

EPIDEMIOLOGY

Syncope is a common symptom, experienced by up to 30% of healthy adults at least once in their life time.[1,2] Syncope accounts for 3% of emergency department visits and 1% of medical admissions to a general hospital.[3] Syncope is the seventh most common reason for emergency admission of patients over 65 years of age.[4] The cumulative incidence of syncope in a chronic care facility is close to 23% over a 10-year period with an annual incidence of 6% and recurrence rate of 30% over 2 years. The age of first faint, a commonly used term for syncope, is less than 25 years in 60% of persons but 10% to 15% of individuals have their first faint after age 65 years.[5,6]

Syncope due to a cardiac cause is associated with higher mortality rates irrespective of age. In patients with a noncardiac or unknown cause of syncope, older age, a history of congestive cardiac failure, and male sex are important prognostic factors of mortality.[7] It remains undetermined whether syncope is directly associated with mortality or is merely a marker of more severe underlying disease.[2] Figure 46-1 details the age-related difference in prevalence of benign vasovagal syncope compared with other causes of syncope.

PATHOPHYSIOLOGY

The temporary cessation of cerebral function that causes syncope results from transient and sudden reduction of blood flow to parts of the brain (brain stem reticular activating system) responsible for consciousness. The predisposition to vasovagal syncope starts early and lasts for decades. Other causes of syncope are uncommon in young adults, but much more common as persons age.[8,9]

Regardless of the cause, the underlying mechanism responsible for syncope is a drop in cerebral oxygen delivery below the threshold for consciousness. Cerebral oxygen delivery, in turn, depends on both cerebral blood flow and oxygen content. Any combination of chronic or acute processes that lowers cerebral oxygen delivery below the "consciousness" threshold may cause syncope. Age-related physiologic impairments in heart rate, blood pressure, cerebral blood flow, and blood volume control, in combination with comorbid conditions and concurrent medications account for the increased incidence of syncope in the older person. Blunted baroreflex sensitivity with aging is manifested as a reduction in the heart rate response to hypotensive stimuli. Older adults are prone to reduced blood volume because of excessive salt wasting by the kidneys as a result of a decline in plasma renin and aldosterone, a rise in atrial natriuretic peptide, and concurrent diuretic therapy.[8] Low blood volume together with age-related diastolic dysfunction can lead to a low cardiac output, which increases susceptibility to orthostatic hypotension and vasovagal syncope.[10] Cerebral autoregulation, which maintains a constant cerebral circulation over a wide range of blood pressure changes, is altered in the presence of hypertension and possibly by aging; the latter is still controversial.[11] In general it is agreed that sudden mild to moderate declines in blood pressure can affect cerebral blood flow greatly and render an older person particularly vulnerable to presyncope and syncope. Syncope may thus result either from a single process that markedly and abruptly decreases cerebral oxygen delivery or from the accumulated effect of multiple processes, each of which contributes to the reduced oxygen delivery.[12]

Multifactorial causes

Previously up to 40% of patients with recurrent syncope remained undiagnosed despite extensive investigations, particularly older patients who have marginal cognitive impairment and for whom a witnessed account of events is often unavailable. More recently, diagnostic yield for all ages has improved with application of guidelines.[13] Although diagnostic investigations are available, the high frequency of unidentified causes in clinical studies may occur because patients failed to recall important diagnostic details[14,15] because of the stringent diagnostic criteria used in clinical studies or, probably most often, because the syncopal episode resulted from a combination of chronic and acute factors rather than from a single obvious disease process.[16] Indeed, a multifactorial cause likely explains the majority of cases of syncope in older persons who are predisposed because of multiple chronic diseases and medication effects superimposed on the age-related physiologic changes described above.[17] Common factors that in combination may predispose to, or precipitate, syncope include anemia, chronic lung disease, congestive heart failure, and dehydration. Medications that may contribute to, or cause, syncope are listed in Table 46-1.

Individual causes of syncope

Common causes of syncope are listed in Table 46-2. The most frequent individual causes of syncope in older patients are neurally mediated syndromes, including carotid sinus syndrome, orthostatic hypotension, and postprandial hypotension and arrhythmias, including both tachyarrhythmias and bradyarrhythmias. These disease processes are described in the next section. Disorders that may be confused with syncope and which may, or may not, be associated with loss of consciousness are listed in Table 46-3. In older patients, 75% of syncope is due to noncardiac causes and 15% is due to cardiac causes.[18]

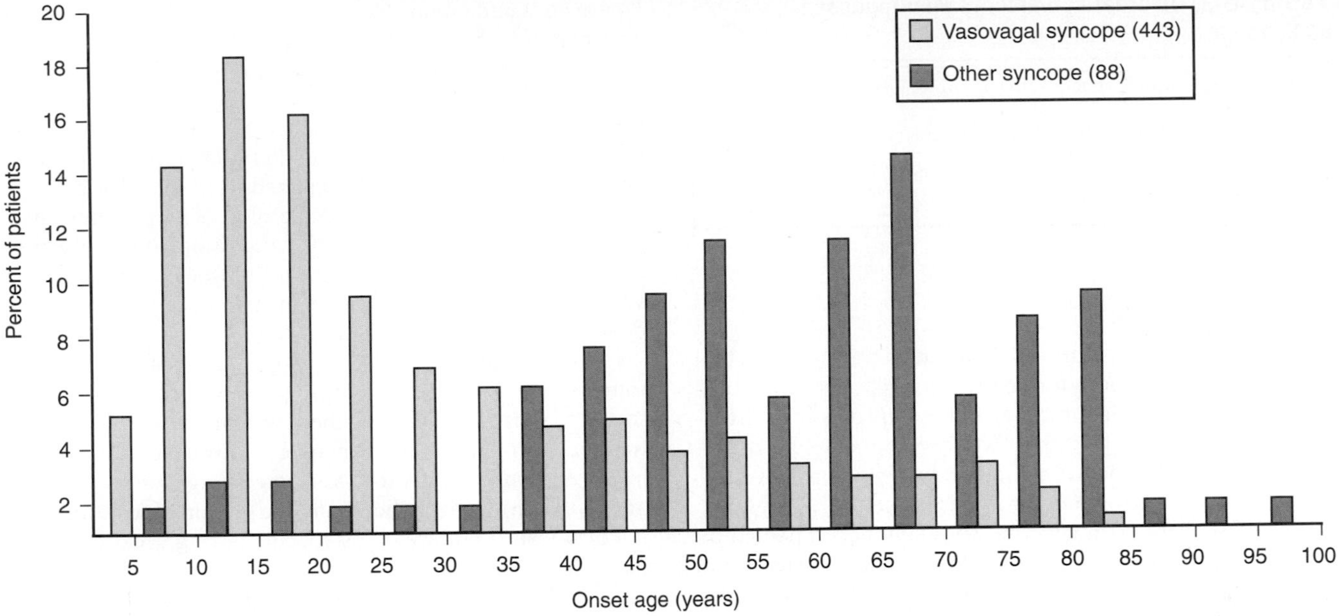

Figure 46-1. Comparison of ages of first syncope in 443 patients with vasovagal syncope and 88 patients with syncope of other known cause.

Table 46-1. Drugs That Can Cause or Contribute to Syncope

Drug	Mechanism
Diuretics	Volume depletion
Vasodilators	Reduction in systemic vascular resistance and venodilation
Angiotensin-converting enzyme inhibitors	
Calcium channel blockers	
Hydralazine	
Nitrates	
Alpha adrenergic blockers	
Prazosin	
Other antihypertensive drugs	Centrally acting antihypertensives
Alpha methyldopa	
Clonidine	
Guanethidine	
Hexamethonium	
Labetalol	
Mecamylamine	
Phenoxybenzamine	
Drugs associated with torsades de pointes	Ventricular tachycardia associated with a prolonged QT interval
Amiodarone	
Disopyramide	
Encainide	
Flecainide	
Quinidine	
Procainamide	
Sotalol	
Digoxin	Cardiac arrhythmias
Psychoactive drugs	Central nervous effects causing hypotension; cardiac arrhythmias
Tricyclic antidepressants	
Phenothiazines	
Monamine oxidase inhibitors	
Barbiturates	
Alcohol	Central nervous system effects causing hypotension; cardiac arrhythmias

Table 46-2. Causes of Syncope

Reflex Syncopal Syndromes
- Vasovagal faint (common faint)
- Carotid sinus syncope
- Situational faint
  - Acute hemorrhage
  - Cough, sneeze
  - Gastrointestinal stimulation (swallow, defecation, visceral pain)
  - Micturition (postmicturition)
  - Postexercise
  - Pain, anxiety
- Glossopharyngeal and trigeminal neuralgia

Orthostatic
- Aging
- Antihypertensives
- Autonomic failure
  - Primary autonomic failure syndromes (e.g., pure autonomic failure, multiple system atrophy, Parkinson's disease with autonomic failure)
  - Secondary autonomic failure syndromes (e.g., diabetic neuropathy, amyloid neuropathy)
- Medications (see Table 46-1)
- Volume depletion
  - Hemorrhage, diarrhea, Addison's disease, diuretics, febrile illness, hot weather

Cardiac Arrhythmias
- Sinus node dysfunction (including bradycardia/tachycardia syndrome)
- Atrioventricular conduction system disease
- Paroxysmal supraventricular and ventricular tachycardias
- Implanted device (pacemaker, ICD) malfunction, drug-induced proarrhythmias

Structural Cardiac or Cardiopulmonary Disease
- Cardiac valvular disease
- Acute myocardial infarction/ischemia
- Obstructive cardiomyopathy
- Atrial myxoma
- Acute aortic dissection
- Pericardial disease/tamponade
- Pulmonary embolus/pulmonary hypertension

Cerebrovascular
- Vascular steal syndromes

Multifactorial

Table 46-3. Disorders Commonly Misdiagnosed as Syncope

- Transient ischemic attacks (TIA) of carotid or vertebro-basilar origin
- Hypoglycemia and other metabolic disorders
- Some forms of epilepsy
- Alcohol and other intoxications
- Hyperventilation with hypocapnia

PRESENTATION

The underlying mechanism of syncope is transient cerebral hypoperfusion. In some forms of syncope, there may be a premonitory period in which various symptoms (e.g., light-headedness, nausea, sweating, weakness, and visual disturbances) offer warning of an impending syncopal event.[18] Often, however, loss of consciousness occurs without warning.[14,15] Recovery from syncope is usually accompanied by almost immediate restoration of appropriate behavior and orientation. Amnesia for loss of consciousness occurs in many older individuals and in those with cognitive impairment. The postrecovery period may be associated with fatigue of varying duration. In young patients, nausea, blurred vision, and sweating predict noncardiac syncope; only dyspnea predicts cardiac syncope in older patients.[18]

Syncope and falls are often considered two separate entities with different causes. Recent evidence suggests, however, that these conditions may not always distinctly be separate.[19] In older adults, determining whether patients who have fallen have had a syncopal event can be difficult. Half of syncopal episodes are unwitnessed and older patients may have amnesia for loss of consciousness.[15] Amnesia for loss of consciousness has been observed in half of patients with carotid sinus syndrome who experience falls and a quarter of all patients with carotid sinus syndrome irrespective of presentation.[20] Emerging evidence suggests a high incidence of falls in addition to traditional syncopal symptoms in older patients with sick sinus syndrome and atrioventricular conduction disorders. Thus syncope and falls may be indistinguishable and may, in some cases, be manifestations of similar pathophysiologic processes. The presentation of specific causes of syncope is presented in the following sections.

EVALUATION

The initial step in the evaluation of syncope is to consider whether there is a specific cardiac or neurologic cause or whether the cause is likely multifactorial.[21–23] The starting point for the evaluation of syncope is a careful history and physical examination. A witness account of events is important to ascertain when possible.[24,25] Three key questions should be addressed during the initial evaluation: (1) Is loss of consciousness attributable to syncope? (2) Is heart disease present or absent? and (3) Are there important clinical features in the history and physical examination that suggest the cause?

Differentiating true syncope from other "nonsyncopal" conditions associated with real or apparent loss of consciousness is generally the first diagnostic challenge and influences the subsequent diagnostic strategy. A strategy for differentiating true syncope and nonsyncope is outlined in Figure 46-2 and Figure 46-3. The presence of heart disease is an independent predictor of a cardiac cause of syncope, with a sensitivity of 95% and a specificity of 45%.[26]

Patients frequently complain of dizziness alone or as a prodrome to syncope and unexplained falls. Four categories of dizzy symptoms—vertigo, dysequilibrium, light-headedness and others—have been recognized. The categories have neither the sensitivity nor specificity in older patients, as in younger ones. Dizziness, however, may more likely be attributable to a cardiovascular diagnosis if associated with pallor, syncope, prolonged standing, palpitations, or the need to lie down or sit down when symptoms occur.

Initial evaluation may lead to a diagnosis based on symptoms, signs, or electrocardiograph (ECG) findings. Under such circumstances, no further evaluation is needed and treatment, if any, can be planned. More commonly, the initial evaluation leads to a suspected diagnosis (see Figure 46-3), which needs to be confirmed by directed testing.[1,27] If a diagnosis is confirmed by specific testing, treatment may be initiated. On the other hand, if the diagnosis is not confirmed, then patients are considered to have unexplained syncope and should be evaluated following a strategy such as that outlined in Figure 46-3. It is important to attribute a diagnosis, if possible, rather than assume that an abnormality known to produce syncope or hypotensive symptoms is the cause. To attribute a diagnosis, patients should have symptom reproduction during investigation and preferably alleviation of symptoms with specific intervention. It is not uncommon for more than one predisposing disorder to coexist in older patients, rendering a precise diagnosis difficult. In older persons treatment of possible causes without clear verification of attributable diagnosis may often be the only option.

An important issue in patients with unexplained syncope is the presence of structural heart disease or an abnormal ECG. These findings are associated with a higher risk of arrhythmias and a higher mortality at 1 year.[28] In these patients, cardiac evaluation consisting of echocardiography, stress testing, and tests for arrhythmia detection, such as prolonged electrocardiographic and loop monitoring or electrophysiologic study are recommended. The most alarming ECG sign in a patient with syncope is probably alternating complete left and right bundle branch block, or alternating right bundle branch block with left anterior or posterior fascicular block, suggesting trifascicular conduction system disease and intermittent or impending high-degree AV block. Patients with bifascicular block (right bundle branch block plus left anterior or left posterior fascicular block, or left bundle branch block) are at high risk of developing high-degree AV block. A significant problem in the evaluation of syncope and bifascicular block is the transient nature of high degree AV block and therefore the long periods required to document it by ECG.

In patients without structural heart disease and a normal ECG, evaluation for neurally mediated syncope should be considered. The tests for neurally mediated syncope consist of tilt testing and carotid sinus massage.

The majority of older patients with syncope are likely have a multifactorial cause and thus both predisposing and precipitating causes should be sought in the history, examination, and laboratory evaluation, particularly if the initial evaluation does not suggest an obvious single cause.

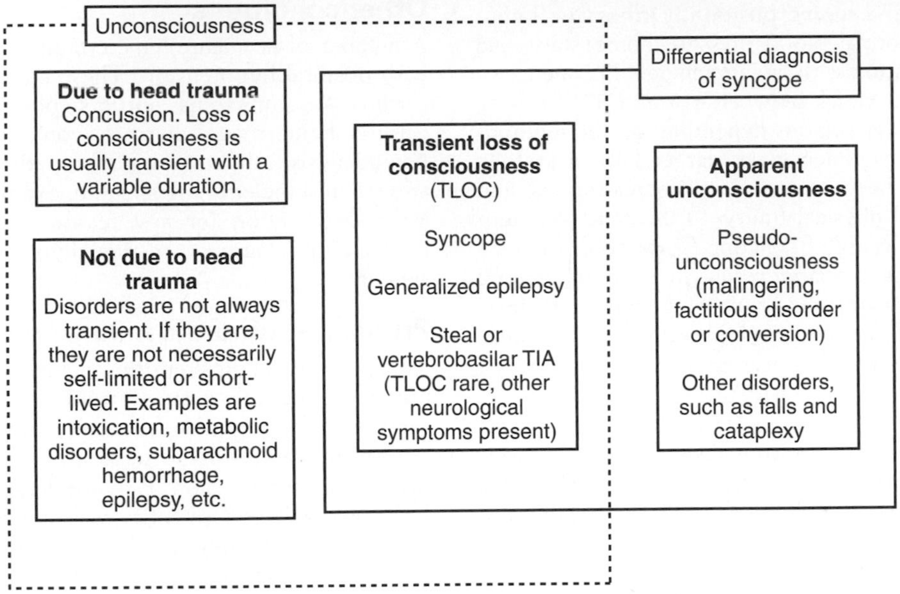

Figure 46-2. Syncope in relation to real and apparent loss of consciousness.

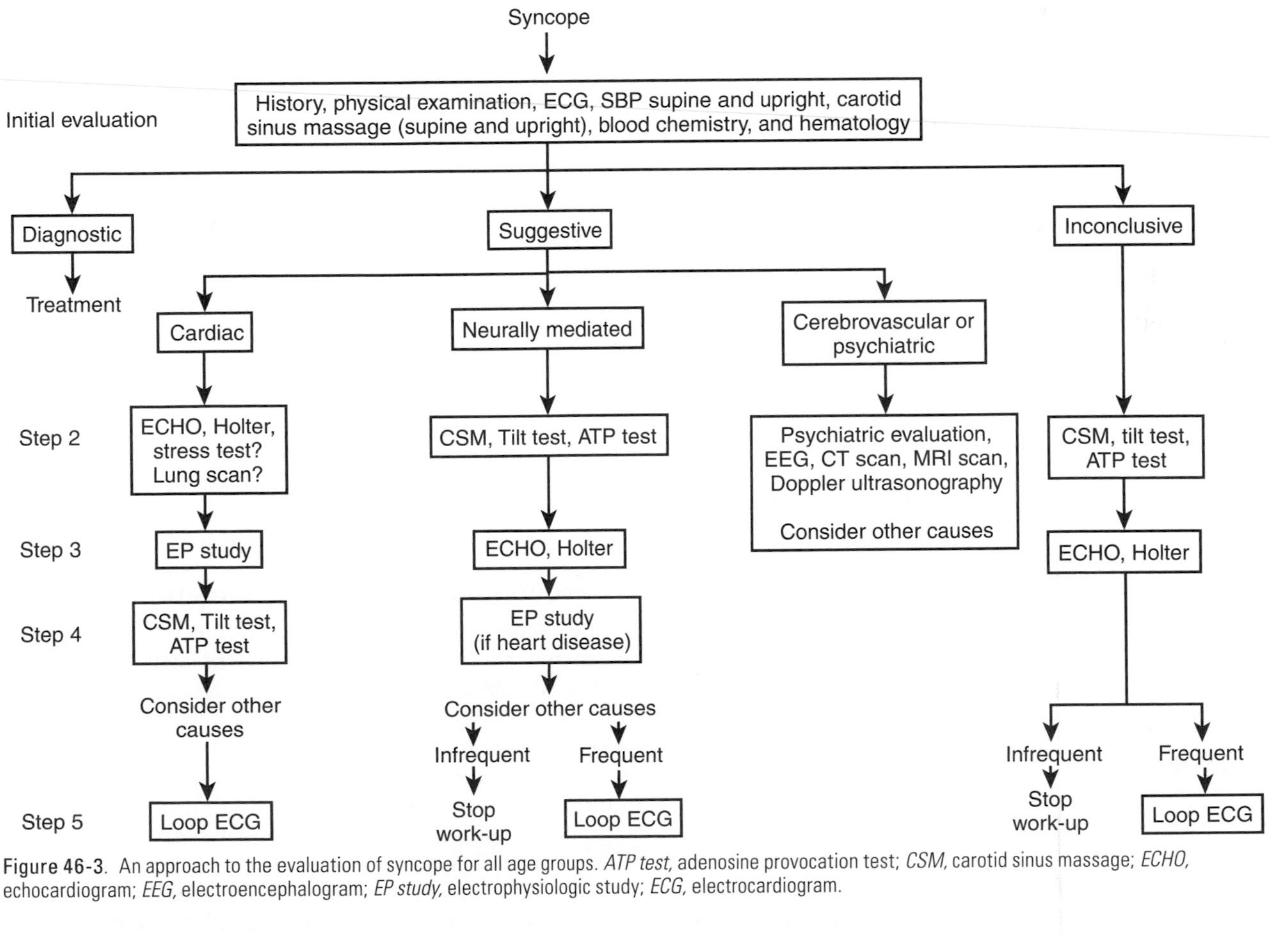

Figure 46-3. An approach to the evaluation of syncope for all age groups. *ATP test,* adenosine provocation test; *CSM,* carotid sinus massage; *ECHO,* echocardiogram; *EEG,* electroencephalogram; *EP study,* electrophysiologic study; *ECG,* electrocardiogram.

The presentation, evaluation, and management of other common causes of syncope are presented in the following sections. These causes may occur as the sole cause of a syncopal episode or as one of multiple contributing causes.

ORTHOSTATIC HYPOTENSION

Pathophysiology

Orthostatic or postural hypotension is arbitrarily defined as either a 20 mm Hg fall in systolic blood pressure or a 10 mm Hg fall in diastolic blood pressure on assuming an upright posture from a supine position. Orthostatic hypotension implies abnormal blood pressure homeostasis and is a frequent observation with advancing age. Prevalence of postural hypotension varies between 4% and 33% among community living older persons depending on the methodology used. Higher prevalence and larger falls in systolic blood pressure have been reported with increasing age and often signify general physical frailty. Orthostatic hypotension is an important cause of syncope, accounting for 14% of all diagnosed cases in a large series. In a tertiary referral clinic dealing with unexplained syncope, dizziness, and falls, 32% of patients over age 65 years had orthostatic hypotension as a possible attributable cause of symptoms.

Aging

The heart rate and blood pressure responses to orthostasis occur in three phases: (1) an initial heart rate and blood pressure response, (2) an early phase of stabilization, and (3) a phase of prolonged standing. All three phases are influenced by aging. The maximum rise in heart rate and the ratio between the maximum and the minimum heart rate in the initial phase decline with age, implying a relatively fixed heart rate irrespective of posture. Despite a blunted heart rate response, blood pressure and cardiac output are adequately maintained on standing in active, healthy, well-hydrated, and normotensive older persons because of decreased vasodilation and reduced venous pooling during the initial phases and increased peripheral vascular resistance after prolonged standing. However, in older persons with hypertension and cardiovascular disease receiving vasoactive drugs, these circulatory adjustments to orthostatic stress are disturbed, rendering them vulnerable to postural hypotension.[29]

Hypertension

Hypertension further increases the risk of hypotension by impairing baroreflex sensitivity and reducing ventricular compliance. A strong relationship between supine hypertension and orthostatic hypotension has been reported among unmedicated institutionalized older persons. Hypertension increases the risk of cerebral ischemia from sudden declines in blood pressure. Older persons with hypertension are more vulnerable to cerebral ischemic symptoms even with modest and short-term postural hypotension because the threshold for cerebral autoregulation is altered by prolonged elevation of blood pressure. In addition, antihypertensive agents impair cardiovascular reflexes and further increase the risk of orthostatic hypotension.

Medications

Drugs (Table 46-1) are important causes of orthostatic hypotension. Ideally establishing a causal relationship between a drug and orthostatic hypotension requires identification of the culprit medicine, abolition of symptoms by withdrawal of the drug, and rechallenge with the drug to reproduce symptoms. Rechallenge is often omitted in clinical practice in view of the potential serious consequences. In the presence of polypharmacy, which is common in the older person, it becomes difficult to identify a single culprit drug because of the synergistic effect of different drugs and drug interactions. Thus all drugs should be considered as possible contributors to orthostasis.

Other conditions

A number of nonneurogenic conditions are also associated with postural hypotension. These conditions include myocarditis, atrial myxoma, aortic stenosis,[30] constrictive pericarditis, hemorrhage, diarrhea, vomiting, ileostomy, burns, hemodialysis, salt loosing nephropathy, diabetes insipidus, adrenal insufficiency, fever, and extensive varicose veins. Volume depletion for any reason is a common sole, or contributing, cause of postural hypotension, and, in turn, syncope.

Primary autonomic failure syndromes

Three distinct clinical entities, namely pure autonomic failure (PAF), multiple system atrophy (MSA), or Shy-Drager syndrome (SDS), and autonomic failure associated with idiopathic Parkinson's disease (IPD) are associated with orthostatic hypotension. PAF, the least common condition and a relatively benign entity, was previously known as idiopathic orthostatic hypotension. Symptoms of this condition include orthostatic dizziness, defective sweating, impotence, and bowel disturbances. No other neurologic deficits are found and resting plasma noradrenaline levels are low. MSA is the most common and has the poorest prognosis. Clinical manifestations include features of dysautonomia and motor disturbances due to striatonigral degeneration, cerebellar atrophy, or pyramidal lesions. Additional neurologic deficits include muscle atrophy, distal sensory-motor neuropathy, pupillary abnormalities, restriction of ocular movements, disturbances in rhythm and control of breathing, life-threatening laryngeal stridor, and bladder disturbances. Psychiatric manifestations and cognitive defects are usually absent. Resting plasma noradrenaline levels are usually within the normal range but fail to rise on standing or tilting.

The prevalence of orthostatic hypotension in Parkinson's disease rises with advancing years and with the number of medications prescribed. Cognitive impairment, in particular abnormal attention and executive function, is more common in Parkinson's disease with orthostatic hypotension, suggesting a possible causal association with hypotension including watershed lesions. Orthostatic hypotension in Parkinson's disease can also be due to autonomic failure and or to side effects of anti-Parkinsonian medications.

Secondary autonomic dysfunction

Autonomic nervous system involvement is seen in several systemic diseases. A large number of neurologic disorders are also complicated by autonomic dysfunction, which may involve several organs leading to a variety of symptoms in addition to orthostatic dizziness, including anhidrosis, constipation, diarrhea, impotence, retention of urine, urinary incontinence, stridor, apneic episodes, and Horner's syndrome. Among the most serious and prevalent conditions associated with a orthostasis due to autonomic dysfunction are diabetes, multiple sclerosis, brain stem lesions, compressive and noncompressive spinal cord lesions, demyelinating polyneuropathies (Guillain-Barré's syndrome), chronic renal failure, chronic liver disease, and connective tissue disorders.

Presentation

The clinical manifestations of orthostatic hypotension are due to hypoperfusion of the brain and other organs. Depending on the degree of fall in blood pressure, symptoms can vary from dizziness to syncope associated with a variety of visual defects, from blurred vision to blackout. Other reported ischemic symptoms are nonspecific lethargy and weakness, suboccipital and paravertebral muscle pain, low back ache, calf claudication, and angina. Several precipitating factors for orthostatic hypotension have been identified including speed of positional change, prolonged recumbency, warm environment, raised intrathoracic pressure (coughing, defecation, micturition), physical exertion, and vasoactive drugs.[31]

Evaluation

The diagnosis of orthostatic hypotension involves a demonstration of a postural fall in blood pressure after active standing. Reproducibility of orthostatic hypotension depends on the time of measurement and on autonomic function. The diagnosis may be missed on casual measurement during the afternoon. The procedure should be repeated during the morning after maintaining supine posture for at least 10 minutes. Sphygmomanometer measurement will detect hypotension which is sustained. Phasic blood pressure measurements are more sensitive for detection of transient falls in blood pressure. Active standing is more appropriate than head-up tilt because the former more readily represents the physiologic alpha adrenergic vasodilation due to calf muscle activation. Once a diagnosis of postural hypotension is made, the evaluation involves identifying the cause or causes of orthostasis mentioned above.

Management (Table 46-4)

The goal of therapy for symptomatic orthostatic hypotension is to improve cerebral perfusion. There are several nonpharmacologic interventions that should be tried in the first instance. These interventions include avoidance of precipitating factors for low blood pressure, elevation of the head of the bed at night by at least 20 degrees, and application of graduated pressure from an abdominal support garment or from stockings. Medications known to contribute to postural hypotension should be eliminated or reduced. There are reports to suggest benefit from implantation of cardiac pacemakers, in a small number of patients, by increasing heart rate during postural change. However, the benefits of tachypacing on cardiac output in patients with maximal vasodilation are short lived, probably because venous pooling and vasodilation dominate. A large number of drugs have been used to raise blood pressure in orthostatic hypotension, including fludrocortisone, midodrine, ephedrine, desmopressin (DDAVP), octreotide, erythropoietin, and nonsteroidal antiinflammatory agents. Fludrocortisone (9-alpha fluohydrocortisone) in a dose of 0.1 to 0.2 mg, causes volume expansion, reduces natriuresis, and sensitizes alpha adrenoceptors to noradrenaline. In older people, the drug can be poorly tolerated in high doses and for long periods. Adverse effects include hypertension, cardiac failure, depression, edema, and hypokalemia. Midodrine is a directly acting sympathomimetic vasoconstrictor of resistance vessels. Treatment is started at a dose of 2.5 mg three times daily and requires gradual titration to a maximum dose of 45 mg/day. Adverse effects include hypertension, pilomotor erection, gastrointestinal symptoms, and central nervous system toxicity. Side effects are usually controlled by dose reduction. Midodrine can be used in combination with low dose fludrocortisone with good effect. DDAVP has potent antidiuretic and mild pressor effects. Intranasal doses of 5 to 40 microgram at bed time are useful. The main side effect is water retention. This agent can also be combined with fludrocortisone with synergistic effect. The drug treatment for orthostatic hypotension in older persons requires frequent monitoring for supine hypertension, electrolyte imbalance, and congestive heart failure. One option for treating supine hypertension, which is most prominent at night, is to apply a GTN patch after going to bed, remove it in the morning, and take midodrine +/− fludrocortisone 20 minutes before rising. This is effective provided that the older person remains in bed throughout the night. Nocturia is therefore an important consideration. To capture these coexistent diurnal BP variations of supine hypertension and morning orthostasis, 24-hour ambulatory BP monitoring is the preferred investigation for the management of postural hypotension. Postprandial hypotension, due to splanchnic vascular pooling, often co-exists with orthostatic hypotension in older patients.

Table 46-4. Management of Orthostatic Hypotension in Older Persons

Identify and Treat Correctable Causes
Reduce or eliminate drugs causing orthostatic hypotension (see Table 46-2)
Avoid situations that may exacerbate orthostatic hypotension:
Standing motionless
Prolonged recumbency
Large meals
Hot weather
Hot showers
Straining at stool or with voiding
Isometric exercise
Ingesting alcohol
Hyperventilation
Dehydration
Raise the head of the bed to a 5- to 20-degree angle
Wear waist-high custom-fitted elastic stockings and an abdominal binder
Participate in physical conditioning exercises, i.e.,
Controlled postural exercises using the tilt table
Avoid diuretics and eat salt-containing fluids (unless congestive heart failure is present)
Caffeine
Drug therapy
Fludrocortisone
Midodrine
Desmopressin
Erythropoietin

CAROTID SINUS SYNDROME AND CAROTID SINUS HYPERSENSITIVITY

Pathophysiology

Carotid sinus syndrome is an important but frequently overlooked cause of syncope and presyncope in older persons.[9] Episodic bradycardia and/or hypotension resulting from exaggerated baroreceptor mediated reflexes or carotid sinus hypersensitivity characterize the syndrome. The syndrome is diagnosed in persons with otherwise unexplained recurrent syncope who have carotid sinus hypersensitivity. The latter is considered present if carotid sinus massage produces asystole exceeding 3 seconds (cardioinhibitory), or a fall in systolic blood pressure exceeding 50 mm Hg in the absence of cardioinhibition (vasodepressor) or a combination of the two (mixed).[13,32]

Epidemiology

Up to 30% of the healthy aged population have carotid sinus hypersensitivity. The prevalence is higher in the presence of coronary artery disease or hypertension. Abnormal responses to carotid sinus massage are more likely to be observed in individuals with coronary artery disease and in those on vasoactive drugs known to influence carotid sinus reflex sensitivity such as digoxin, beta blockers, and alpha methyl dopa. Other hypotensive disorders such as vasovagal syncope and orthostatic hypotension coexist in one third of patients with carotid sinus hypersensitivity. In centers which routinely perform carotid sinus massage in all older patients with syncope, carotid sinus syndrome is the attributable cause of syncope in 30%.[33] This frequency needs to be interpreted within the context that these centers evaluate a preselected group of patients who have a higher likelihood of carotid sinus syndrome than the general population of older persons with syncope. The prevalence in all older persons with syncope is unknown.

Carotid sinus syndrome is virtually unknown before the age of 50 years; its incidence increases with age thereafter. Males are more commonly affected than females and the majority have either coronary artery disease or hypertension. Carotid sinus syndrome is associated with appreciable morbidity. Approximately half of patients sustain an injury, including a fracture, during symptomatic episodes. In a prospective study of falls in nursing home residents, a threefold increase in the fracture rate in those with carotid sinus hypersensitivity was observed. Indeed, carotid sinus hypersensitivity can be considered as a modifiable risk factor for fractures of the femoral neck. Carotid sinus syndrome is not associated with an increased risk of death. The mortality rate in patients with the syndrome is similar to that of patients with unexplained syncope and the general population matched for age and sex. Mortality rates are similar for the three subtypes of the syndrome.

The natural history of carotid sinus hypersensitivity has not been well investigated. In one study, the majority (90%) of persons with abnormal hemodynamic responses but without syncopal symptoms, remained symptom free during an average follow-up of 20 months while half of those who had syncope had symptom recurrence. More recent neuropathologic research suggests that carotid sinus hypersensitivity is associated with neurodegenerative pathology at the cardiovascular center in the brain stem. Why some persons with carotid sinus hypersensitivity develop syncope as a consequence and others remain asymptomatic is not clear.

Presentation

The syncopal symptoms are usually precipitated by mechanical stimulation of the carotid sinus, such as head turning, tight neckwear, neck pathology, and by vagal stimuli such as prolonged standing. Other recognized triggers for symptoms are the postprandial state, straining, looking or stretching upwards, exertion, defecation, and micturition. In a significant number of patients, no triggering event can be identified. Abnormal response to carotid sinus massage (see later discussion) may not always be reproducible, necessitating repetition of the procedure if the diagnosis is strongly suspected.

Evaluation

CAROTID SINUS MASSAGE

Carotid sinus reflex sensitivity is assessed by measuring heart rate and blood pressure responses to carotid sinus massage (Figure 46-4). Cardioinhibition and vasodepression are more common on the right side. In patients with cardioinhibitory carotid sinus syndrome, more than 70% have a positive response to right-sided carotid sinus massage either alone or in combination with left-sided carotid sinus massage. There is no fixed relationship between the degree of heart rate slowing and the degree of fall in blood pressure.

Carotid sinus massage is a crude and unquantifiable technique and is prone to intraobserver and interobserver variation. More scientific diagnostic methods using neck chamber suction or drug-induced changes in blood pressure can be used for carotid baroreceptor activation, but are not validated for routine clinical use. The recommended duration of carotid sinus massage is from 5 to 10 seconds. The maximum fall in heart rate usually occurs within 5 seconds of the onset of massage (Figure 46-2).

Complications resulting from carotid sinus massage include cardiac arrhythmias and neurologic sequelae. Fatal arrhythmias are extremely uncommon and have generally only occurred in patients with underlying heart disease undergoing therapeutic rather than diagnostic massage. Digoxin toxicity has been implicated in most cases of ventricular fibrillation. Neurologic complications result from either occlusion of, or embolization from, the carotid artery. Several authors have reported cases of hemiplegia following

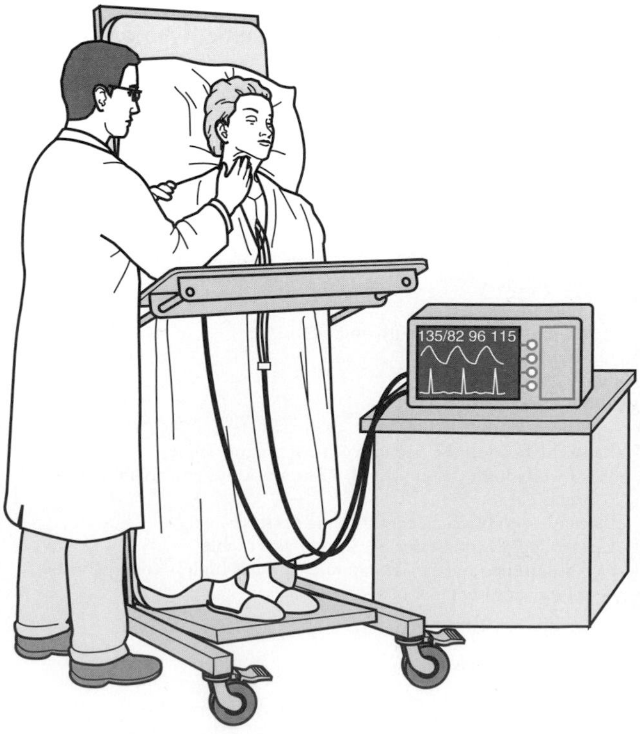

Figure 46-4. Procedure for carotid sinus massage while upright.

carotid sinus stimulation, often in the absence of hemodynamic changes. Complications from carotid sinus massage, however, are uncommon. In a prospective series of 1000 consecutive cases, no patient had cardiac complications and 1% had transient neurologic symptoms, which resolved. Persistent neurologic complications were uncommon, occurring in 0.04% of cases.[34] Carotid sinus massage should not be performed in patients who have had a recent cerebrovascular event or myocardial infarction.

Symptom reproduction during carotid sinus massage is preferable for a diagnosis of carotid sinus syndrome. Symptoms reproduction may not be possible for older patients with amnesia for loss of consciousness. Spontaneous symptoms usually occur in the upright position. It may thus be worth repeating the procedure, with the patient upright on a tilt table, even after demonstrating a positive response when supine. This reproduction of symptoms aids in attributing the episodes to carotid sinus hypersensitivity, especially in patients with unexplained falls who deny loss of consciousness. In one third of patients, a diagnostic response is only achieved during upright carotid sinus massage.

Management

No treatment is necessary in persons with asymptomatic carotid sinus hypersensitivity.[35] There is no consensus, however, on the timing of therapeutic intervention in the presence of symptoms. Considering the high rate of injury in symptomatic episodes in older persons and the low recurrence rate of symptoms, it is prudent to treat all patients with a history of two or more symptomatic episodes. The need for intervention in those individuals with a solitary event should be assessed on an individual basis, taking into consideration the severity of the event and the patient's comorbidity.

Treatment strategies in the past included carotid sinus denervation achieved either surgically or by radioablation. Both procedures have largely been abandoned. Dual chamber cardiac pacing is the treatment of choice in patients with symptomatic cardioinhibitory carotid sinus syndrome. Atrial pacing is contraindicated in view of the high prevalence of both sinoatrial and atrioventricular block in patients with carotid sinus hypersensitivity. Ventricular pacing abolishes cardioinhibition but fails to alleviate symptoms in a significant number of patients because of aggravation of a coexisting vasodepressor response or the development of pacemaker-induced hypotension, referred to as pacemaker syndrome. The latter occurs when ventriculo-atrial conduction is intact as is the case for up to 80% of patients with the syndrome. Atrioventricular sequential pacing (dual chamber) is thus the treatment of choice and because this maintains atrioventricular synchrony, there is no risk of pacemaker syndrome. With appropriate pacing, syncope is abolished in 85% to 90% of patients with cardioinhibition.

In a recent report of cardiac pacing in older fallers, (mean age of 74 years) who had cardioinhibitory carotid sinus hypersensitivity, falls during 1 year of follow up were reduced by two thirds in patients who received dual chamber systems.[33] Syncopal episodes were reduced by half. Over half of the patients in the aforementioned series had gait abnormalities and three quarters had balance abnormalities, which would render individuals more susceptible to falls under hemodynamic circumstances, thus further suggesting the multifactorial nature of many falls and syncopal episodes.[22]

Treatment of vasodepressor carotid sinus syndrome is less successful because of a poor understanding of its pathophysiology. Ephedrine has been reported to be useful, but long-term use is limited by side effects. Dihydroergotamine is effective but poorly tolerated. Fludrocortisone, a mineralocorticoid widely used in the treatment of orthostatic hypotension, is used in the treatment of vasodepressor carotid sinus syndrome with good results but its use is limited in the longer term by adverse effects. A recent small randomized controlled trial suggests good benefit with midodrine (an alpha agonist). Surgical denervation of the carotid artery may be a valid treatment option.[36,37]

VASOVAGAL SYNCOPE

Pathophysiology

The normal physiologic responses to orthostasis, as described earlier, are an increase in heart rate, rise in peripheral vascular resistance (increase in diastolic blood pressure), and minimal decline in systolic blood pressure to maintain an adequate cardiac output. In patients with vasovagal syncope, these responses to prolonged orthostasis are paradoxical. The precise sequence of events leading to vasovagal syncope is not fully understood. The possible mechanism involves a sudden fall in venous return to the heart, rapid fall in ventricular volume, and virtual collapse of the ventricle due to vigorous ventricular contraction. The net result of these events is stimulation of ventricular mechano-receptors and activation of Bezold-Jarisch reflex leading to peripheral vasodilatation (hypotension) and bradycardia. Several neurotransmitters, including serotonin, endorphins, and arginine vasopressin, play an important role in the pathogenesis of vasovagal syncope possibly by central sympathetic inhibition, although their exact role is not yet well understood.[38]

Healthy older persons are not as prone to vasovagal syncope as younger adults. Due to an age-related decline in baroreceptor sensitivity, the paradoxical responses to orthostasis (as in vasovagal syncope) are possibly less marked in older persons. However hypertension, atherosclerotic cerebrovascular disease, cardiovascular medications, and impaired baroreflex sensitivity can cause dysautonomic responses during prolonged orthostasis (in which blood pressure and the heart decline steadily over time) and render older persons susceptible to vasovagal syncope. Diuretic or age-related contraction of blood volume further increases the risk of vasovagal syncope.[39]

Presentation

The hallmark of vasovagal syncope is hypotension and/or bradycardia sufficiently profound to produce cerebral ischemia and loss of neural function. Vasovagal syncope has been classified into cardioinhibitory (bradycardia), vasodepressor (hypotension), and mixed (both) subtypes depending on the blood pressure and heart rate response. In most patients, the manifestations occur in three distinct phases: a prodrome or aura, loss of consciousness, and postsyncopal phase. A precipitating factor or situation is identifiable in most patients. Common precipitating factors include extreme emotional stress, anxiety, mental anguish, trauma, physical pain, or anticipation of physical pain (e.g., anticipation of venesection), warm environment, air travel and prolonged standing. The commonest triggers in older individuals are prolonged standing and vasodilator medication. Some patients experience symptoms in specific situations, such as micturition, defecation, and coughing. Prodromal symptoms include extreme fatigue, weakness, diaphoresis, nausea, visual defects, visual and auditory hallucinations, dizziness, vertigo, headache, abdominal discomfort, dysarthria, and paresthesia. The duration of prodrome varies greatly from seconds to several minutes, during which some patients take actions such as lying down to avoid an episode. Older patients may have poor recall for prodromal symptoms. The syncopal period is usually brief during which some patients develop involuntary movements, usually myoclonic jerks but tonic clonic movements also occur. Thus vasovagal syncope may masquerade as a seizure. Recovery is usually rapid but older patients can experience protracted symptoms, such as confusion, disorientation, nausea, headache, dizziness, and a general sense of ill health.

Evaluation

Several methods have evolved to determine an individual's susceptibility to vasovagal syncope, such as Valsalva maneuvers, hyperventilation, ocular compression, and immersion of the face in cold water. However, these methods are poorly reproducible and lack correlation with clinical events. Using the strong orthostatic stimulus of head-upright tilting and maximal venous pooling, vasovagal syncope can be reproduced in a susceptible individual.[40] Head-up tilting as a diagnostic tool was first reported in 1986[41] and since then validity of this technique in identifying susceptibility to neurocardiogenic syncope has been established. Subjects are tilted head up for 40 minutes at 70 degrees. Heart rate and blood pressure are measured continuously throughout the test. A test is diagnostic or positive if symptoms are reproduced with a decline in blood pressure of greater than 50 mm Hg or to less than 90 mm Hg. This may be in addition to significant heart rate slowing. As with carotid sinus syndrome, the hemodynamic responses are classified as vasodepressor, cardioinhibitory, or mixed. The cardioinhibitory response is defined as asystole in excess of 3 seconds or heart rate slowing to less than 40 beats/min for a minimum of 10 seconds. Orthostatic hypotension, vasovagal syncope, and carotid sinus hypersensitivity may overlap particularly in older patients.[42]

The sensitivity of head-up tilting can be further improved by provocative agents, which accentuate the physiologic events leading to vasovagal syncope. One agent is intravenous isoprenaline, which enhances myocardial contractility by stimulating β-adreno-receptors. Isoprenaline is infused, before head-up tilting, at a dose of 1 mcg per minute and gradually increased to a maximum dose of 3 mcg per minute to achieve a heart rate increase of 25%. Though the sensitivity of head-up tilt testing improves by about 15%, the specificity is reduced. In addition as a result of the decline in β-receptor sensitivity with age, isoprenaline is less well tolerated, less diagnostic, and has a much higher incidence of side effects. The other agent that can be used as a provocative agent and is better tolerated in older persons is sublingual nitroglycerin, which, by reducing venous return due to vasodilation can enhance the vasovagal reaction in susceptible individuals. Nitroglycerin provocation during head-up tilt testing is thus preferable to other provocative tests in older patients.[40,43] The duration of testing is less, cannulation is not required, and the sensitivity and specificity are better than for isoprenaline.

Because syncopal episodes are intermittent, external loop recording will not capture events unless they occur approximately every 2 to 3 weeks. Implantable loop recorders (Reveal; Medtronic) can aid diagnosis by tracking bradyarrhythmias or tachyarrhythmias, causing less frequent syncope. To date no implantable BP monitors are available with the exception of intracardiac monitors, which are not recommended for diagnosis of a benign condition such as vasovagal syncope.[44,45]

Management

Avoidance of precipitating factors and evasive actions, such as lying down during prodromal symptoms, have great value in preventing episodes of vasovagal syncope. Withdrawal or modification of culprit medications is often the only necessary intervention in older persons. Doses and frequency of antihypertensive medications can be tailored by information from 24-hour ambulatory monitoring. Older patients with hypertension who develop syncope—either orthostatic or vasovagal—while taking antihypertensive drugs, present a difficult therapeutic dilemma and should be treated on an individual basis.

Many patients experience symptoms without warning, necessitating drug therapy. A number of drugs are reported to be useful in alleviating symptoms. Fludrocortisone (100 to 200 mcg/day) works by its volume expanding effect. Recent reports suggest that serotonin antagonists, such as fluoxetine (20 mg/day) and sertraline hydrochloride (25 mg/day), are also effective although further trials are necessary to validate this finding. Midodrine acts by reducing peripheral venous pooling and thereby improving cardiac output and can be used either alone or in combination with fludrocortisone but with caution. Elastic support hose, relaxation techniques (biofeedback), and conditioning using repeated head-up tilt as therapy have been adjuvant therapies. Permanent cardiac pacing is beneficial in some patients who have recurrent syncope due to cardioinhibitory responses.[46]

POSTPRANDIAL HYPOTENSION

The effect of meals on the cardiovascular system was appreciated from postprandial exaggeration of angina, which was demonstrated objectively by deterioration of exercise tolerance following food. Postprandial reductions in blood pressure manifesting as syncope and dizziness were subsequently reported, leading to extensive investigation of this phenomenon. In healthy older subjects, systolic blood pressure falls by 11 to 16 mm Hg, and the heart rate rises by 5 to 7 beats/min 60 minutes after meals of varying compositions and energy content. However the change in diastolic blood pressure is not as consistent. In older persons with hypertension, orthostatic hypotension and autonomic failure, the postprandial blood pressure fall is much greater and without the corresponding rise in heart rate.[47] These responses are marked if the energy and simple carbohydrate content of the meal is high. In the majority of fit and frail older persons, most postprandial hypotensive episodes go unnoticed.[48] When systematically evaluated, postprandial hypotension was found in over one third of nursing home residents.

Postprandial physiologic changes include increased splanchnic and superior mesenteric artery blood flow at the expense of peripheral circulation and a rise in plasma insulin levels without corresponding rises in sympathetic nervous system activity. Vasodilator effects of insulin and other gut peptides, including neurotensin and VIP contribute to hypotension. The clinical significance of a fall in blood pressure after meals is difficult to quantify. However, postprandial hypotension is causally related to recurrent syncope and falls in older persons. A reduction in simple carbohydrate content of food, its replacement with complex carbohydrates or high protein, high fat, and frequent small meals are effective interventions for postprandial hypotension. Drugs useful in the treatment of postprandial hypotension include fludrocortisone and indomethacin, octreotide, and caffeine. Given orally along with food, caffeine prevents hypotensive symptoms in fit and frail older persons but should preferably be given in the mornings as tolerance develops if it is taken throughout the day.[49,50]

SUMMARY

Syncope is a common symptom in older adults due to age-related neurohumoral and physiologic changes plus chronic diseases and medications, which reduce cerebral oxygen delivery through multiple mechanisms. Common individual causes of syncope encountered by the geriatrician are orthostatic hypotension, carotid sinus syndrome, vasovagal syncope, postprandial syncope, sinus node disease, atrioventricular block, and ventricular tachycardia. Algorithms for the assessment of syncope are similar to those for young adults, but the prevalence of ischemic and hypertensive disorders and cardiac conduction disease is higher in older adults and the cause is more often multifactorial. A systematic approach to syncope is needed with the goal being to identify either a single likely cause or multiple treatable contributing factors. Management is then based on removing or reducing the predisposing or precipitating factors through various combinations of medication adjustments, behavioral strategies, and more invasive interventions in select cases, such as cardiac pacing, cardiac stenting, and intracardiac defibrillators. It is often not possible to clearly attribute a cause of syncope in older persons who frequently have more than one possible cause and pragmatic management of each diagnosis is recommended.

For a complete list of references, please visit online only at www.expertconsult.com

CHAPTER 47

Vascular Surgery

Arnab Bhowmick
Charles N. McCollum

The prevalence of atherosclerosis increases with advancing age, so it is hardly surprising that the majority of a vascular surgeon's patients are elderly and have a full range of concomitant diseases typical of such patients. Equally, specialists in geriatric medicine frequently find vascular disease in the patients they treat. Decisions regarding treatment need to be balanced against quality of life and cardiac and respiratory risk factors. In many patients neither invasive investigation by arteriography nor vascular surgery will be indicated. However, vascular surgery is now being performed with increasing safety in patients who have longer life expectancies. The principle of balancing benefit against risk of treatment is emphasized repeatedly throughout this chapter.

Elderly people suffer a range of vascular conditions, but this chapter covers the three most common problems presenting to vascular surgeons: (1) vascular disease of the limb, either acute or chronic; (2) carotid disease; and (3) abdominal aortic aneurysm. New techniques are rapidly changing our approach to the management of vascular conditions; for example, the use of percutaneous transluminal angioplasty as the sole treatment for lower-limb critical ischemia,[1] and the introduction of endovascular stent-grafts for the treatment of abdominal aortic aneurysms.[2]

ARTERIAL DISEASE OF THE LIMB

Most patients with peripheral vascular disease have symptoms of chronic ischemia. This ranges from intermittent claudication with a benign prognosis, to critical ischemia having rest pain, gangrene, ischemic ulceration, and the threat of amputation.

Acute ischemia of a limb may be due to emboli, but it is now more usually secondary to thrombosis in diseased arteries. The majority of emboli lodge at the bifurcation of a main vessel, giving rise to distal dysfunction. Acute ischemia may have some or all of the classic symptoms such as pain, pallor, paresthesia, paralysis, and lack of pulse.

Chronic peripheral vascular disease

PREVALENCE

Atherosclerosis is the most common disease affecting peripheral arteries in the elderly population and may severely limit mobility and quality of life.[3] Amputation for peripheral vascular disease or gangrene is the second most common operation in patients aged over 90 years.[4] At least one third of patients with arterial stenosis or arterial occlusion, particularly involving the superficial femoral artery at the adductor canal, are asymptomatic.[5] However, approximately 50% of patients having intermittent claudication have a superficial femoral artery occlusion.[6] The prevalence of claudication is only 1.0% to 1.5% in men aged under 50 years, but it rises substantially thereafter—up to 20% to 25% in those over 85.[7,8]

PROGNOSIS

Only 10% of individuals with intermittent claudication consult a doctor and only a minority of these will ever come to surgery.[9] The outlook for the legs in patients with claudication is good, but peripheral vascular disease is a strong predictor of subsequent mortality, which more than doubles that of nonclaudicants.[10–12] The majority of claudicants die from associated cardiovascular events, in particular stroke and myocardial infarction, and this high mortality risk is only partly explained by the expected association of peripheral vascular disease with coronary artery disease owing to the generalized nature of atherosclerosis.[13–15] In the Speedwell prospective heart disease study,[15] men with intermittent claudication had a 30%, 5-year mortality compared with 6% in men without intermittent claudication. The increased risk of cardiovascular death may stem from repeated ischemia/reperfusion injury in the leg muscle, leading to leukocyte and platelet activation and increased thrombogenicity.[16]

INVESTIGATIONS

Investigation of patients with intermittent claudication should concentrate on identifying risk factors for cardiac and cerebrovascular events. Smoking is strongly associated with intermittent claudication, as are diabetes, hypertension, and abnormal lipid levels.[10,15,17] In diabetic patients, there is increased involvement of small vessels with distal artery occlusion, which carries a poor prognosis.[11]

The ankle brachial pressure index (ABPI) may be helpful in quantifying the severity of peripheral vascular disease, but only a minority of patients with abnormal APBIs are symptomatic.[18] As a general rule, patients with a mean ABPI of less than 0.6 who have symptoms or leg ulcers need vascular surgical assessment.[19]

Rest pain, ischemic ulceration, or gangrene is an absolute indication for investigation with a view to treatment. Duplex imaging or angiography may be used to identify the sites of stenotic or occlusive disease, but they are indicated only if surgery or angioplasty is being considered. Duplex imaging has become increasingly important in the diagnosis and follow-up of arterial lesions because it is noninvasive and can be repeated on many occasions to monitor disease progress, graft patency, and the need for intervention. It identifies arterial occlusions and hemodynamically significant stenoses with a sensitivity and specificity of 92% and 97%, respectively, and has the potential to replace angiography. The presence of multiple stenoses is the main limitation on diagnostic accuracy.[20–22] Duplex imaging alone can be used to predict the indication for percutaneous transluminal angioplasty.[23]

TREATMENT

Treatment is directed at control of risk factors for cardiovascular and cerebrovascular mortality, such as hypertension, hyperlipidemia, and diabetes. Surgery or angioplasty for peripheral vascular disease is rarely indicated for intermittent claudication, but it may be offered to those whose symptoms are intolerable for their lifestyle despite a period of conservative care. The best advice for patients with claudication is to stop smoking, lose weight if appropriate, and keep walking. Exercise training can improve claudication distances significantly.[24]

The treatment for rest pain, ischemic ulceration, or gangrene depends on the state of the peripheral circulation. New treatment modalities have revolutionized the revascularization of lower-limb ischemia. Percutaneous transluminal angioplasty is becoming the most frequent option in the treatment of both claudication and revascularization for critical ischemia. If there is a lesion amenable to angioplasty, then this should be treated. Alternatively, whether reconstructive surgery is indicated depends on the level and length of arterial occlusions and the severity of disease distally in the limb.

Acute limb ischemia

The clinical distinction between arterial thrombosis or embolism can be difficult, but errors in diagnosis lead to a higher surgical failure rate and higher hospital mortality.[25,26] Acute ischemia of the lower limb may occur due to embolization into a previously patent arterial tree, but it is now more likely to be due to thrombosis in diseased arteries. The most frequent site of origin for an arterial embolus is the heart, resulting from poor atrial emptying in atrial fibrillation or from a mural thrombus following myocardial infarction. Alternatively, an embolus may originate from a previously undiscovered ventricular or aortic aneurysm.

Arterial emboli to the arm are infrequent and usually seen only in elderly patients. Approximately two thirds of emboli are of cardiac origin, although peripheral aneurysm may account for up to 20% of cases.[27,28] Conservative management is appropriate for many of these patients if the hand is viable and the pressure index (relative to the opposite normal arm) is greater than 0.6.[29,30] Surgical embolectomy can be performed under local anesthetic and achieves excellent results. However, there is an associated mortality of greater than 10%, related predominantly to the underlying cardiac condition.[27]

Management of femoral embolism

Early femoral embolectomy is the standard for acute leg ischemia in patients with a strong clinical suspicion of an embolus, such as those with a short history of ischemia (less than 72 hours), an embolic source such as atrial fibrillation, and no past history of intermittent claudication.[31] Embolectomy using a Fogarty catheter will usually restore limb perfusion, but it has been associated with a 16% to 26% mortality due predominantly to coexisting cardiac disease.[31–33] Following embolectomy, the patient should be given long-term anticoagulant therapy, initially by heparin infusion and then with oral anticoagulants. Investigation by full blood count, echocardiography, and duplex imaging of the arterial supply to the leg is essential.

Management of acute thrombosis

In contrast, the management of acute critical ischemia due to arterial thrombosis is one of the more demanding surgical emergencies and should be dealt with only by an experienced vascular team. There is usually a little more time to make the diagnosis and arrange treatment as a collateral circulation offers some protection. Heparin should be given as soon as possible to reduce extension of the thrombus. If the limb is not completely anesthetic or paralyzed there should be sufficient time for adequate preoperative investigations by urgent duplex imaging and angiography if indicated to assess the distal arterial tree.

Intra-arterial thrombolysis achieves lysis of such thrombi (or emboli) in approximately two thirds of cases.[34] Accelerated techniques of lysis, such as clot suction and the pulse-spray method, may be undertaken in as little as 30 minutes, but higher doses of thrombolytic agents tend to increase the risk of hemorrhagic complications.[35] Following lysis, the underlying arterial disease should be treated either by transluminal angioplasty or by arterial reconstruction. In patients requiring urgent surgery, "on table" operative angiography may be performed (Figure 47-1) to assess the extent of the occlusion and the quality of the distal arteries. This should be repeated on completion of surgery to check the reconstruction and give an indication of prognosis.

Outcome of limb salvage for severe ischemia

An aggressive policy of revascularization achieves limb and patient survival rates of approximately 75% at 1 year, even in the elderly population.[36] Almost all patients with severe leg ischemia should be offered a limb salvage procedure because this is associated with a better quality of life (Figure 47-2).[37] The availability of specialist vascular surgeons reduces the frequency of major lower limb amputations, with a concomitant increase in the number of distal reconstructions.[38] Arterial reconstruction to save the leg and alleviate pain is preferable to an amputation, particularly as few elderly patients regain mobility and independence after lower-limb amputation and most require institutional care or at least homes adapted for wheelchair use.[32] Although the initial operative costs of reconstructive surgery are higher than those of amputation, this cost is more than offset by the duration of inpatient stay and the high community costs of rehabilitating amputees.[33]

CAROTID DISEASE

Diagnosis and investigations

DIAGNOSIS

Carotid disease may be asymptomatic or may occur with stroke, transient ischemic attacks (TIAs), or possibly with vague symptoms such as dizziness. Carotid artery stenosis may cause stroke by hypoperfusion or by emboli; indeed many strokes are preceded by TIAs that are ignored by the patient and the doctor.

Carotid bruits can occur in the absence of significant internal carotid artery disease, and severe carotid disease may not produce a bruit. Thus a bruit is not a reliable indicator of underlying carotid disease.[39,40] In a study examining the predisposing factors for acute cerebral infarction, only 14% had cervical bruits.[41] All patients presenting with either TIAs, or who recover from an appropriate stroke and are fit for surgery, should undergo carotid imaging; significant carotid artery disease is found in just over 30% of those with anterior circulation infarcts as classified by the Oxford Community Stroke Project Classification.[42,43]

INVESTIGATIONS

Noninvasive techniques to assess carotid disease include color duplex Doppler imaging, which incorporates continuous-wave Doppler to estimate blood velocity, and B-mode ultrasound to image the whole vessel. High-resolution B-mode scanning has also been shown to give prognostic information:

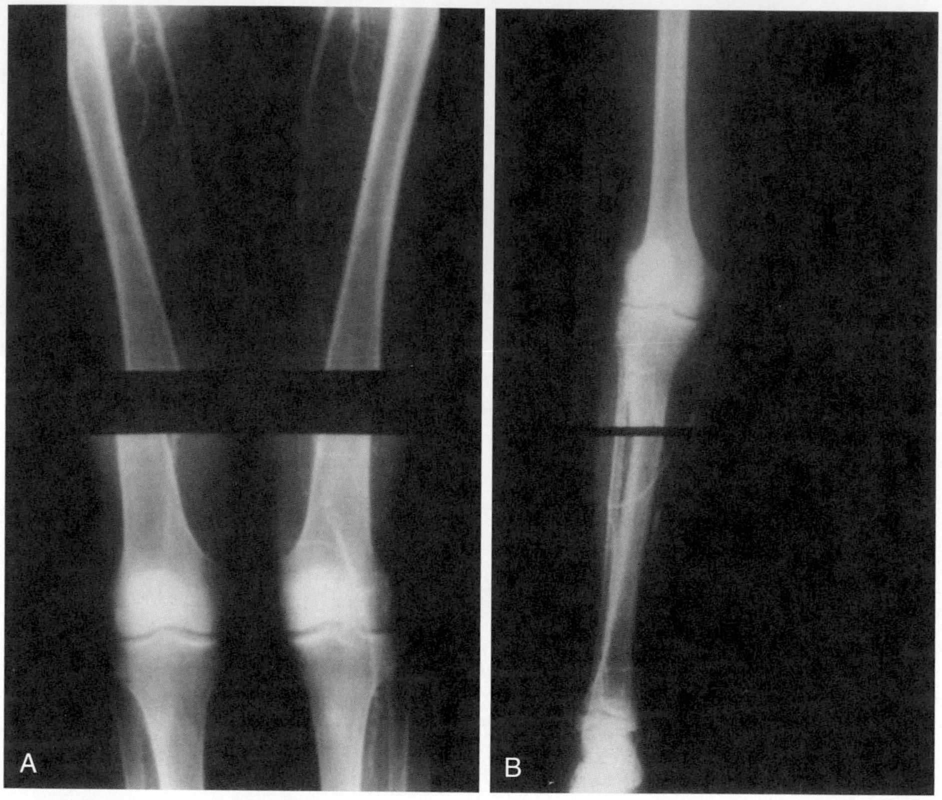

Figure 47-1. A sequence of arteriograms from a patient with acute right lower limb ischemia. In **A**, there is no visualization of "run-off" below a recent occlusion in the proximal popliteal artery. Subsequent on-table angiogram using the distal popliteal artery revealed a patent anterior tibial artery. In **B**, the completed bypass (with reversed saphenous vein) is shown.

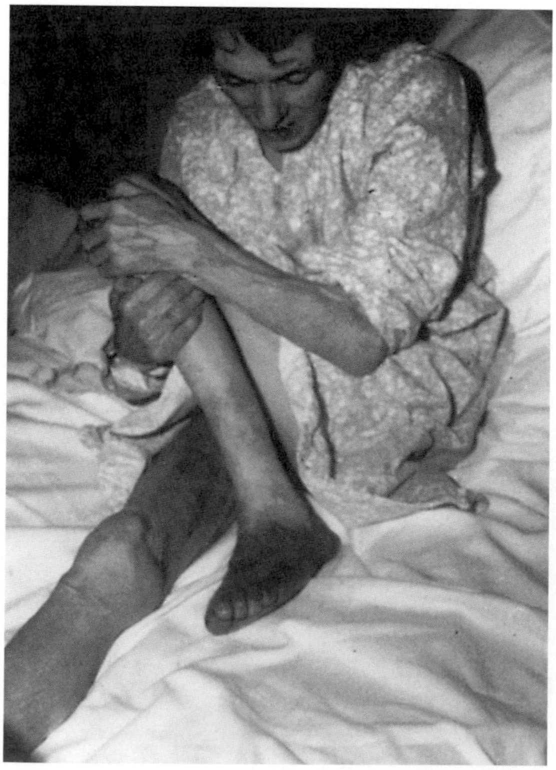

Figure 47-2. Prolonged rest ischemia, often requiring opiates, leads to distress, malaise, and general disability. Physiotherapy should be started immediately to release the flexion contracture of the knee.

echo-lucent (soft) plaque may have a greater propensity for embolization than echo-dense (hard) plaque.[44]

Portable continuous-wave Doppler (Figure 47-3) can be used to assess the blood flow at the bifurcation and in both the internal and external carotid arteries as far as the mandible. An experienced vascular technologist can readily distinguish the waveforms from each of these three vessels. Those from the internal carotid artery have a high diastolic component caused by low peripheral resistance from the cerebral circulation. In comparison, the external signal is more pulsatile with a sharp initial peak and usually a characteristic small second peak resembling the flow signals from the peripheral arteries. Increased blood velocity through a stenotic area is detected by increased frequency in the Doppler shift so that the grade of stenoses more than 50% may be easily detected. As stenoses less than 50% have little or no hemodynamic significance, diagnostic accuracy and the value of the investigation improves as the degree of stenosis increases.

Although this method is simple, quick, and accurate for detecting stenoses of greater than 50%, mistakes can be made in heavily calcified vessels that may appear occluded if calcification prevents ultrasound penetration. In these circumstances, and where there are clinical symptoms relevant to carotid artery disease, duplex Doppler (Figure 47-4) should be used to guide therapy. Occasionally, even duplex imaging may be difficult to interpret; in particular, total occlusion may be falsely diagnosed as trickles of blood flow through a very tight stenosis. In these cases digital subtraction angiography is indicated.

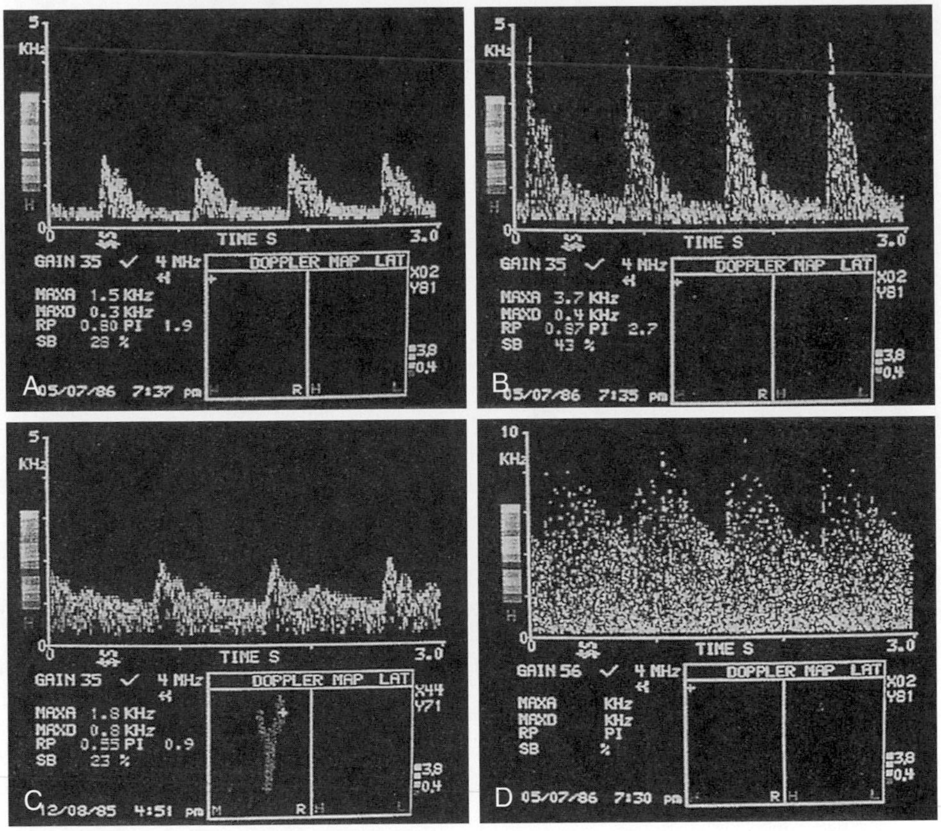

Figure 47-3. Doppler spectral analysis flow signals in normal (A) common carotid artery; (B) external carotid artery; and (C) internal carotid artery. (D) A stenosed internal carotid artery demonstrating increased Doppler frequencies.

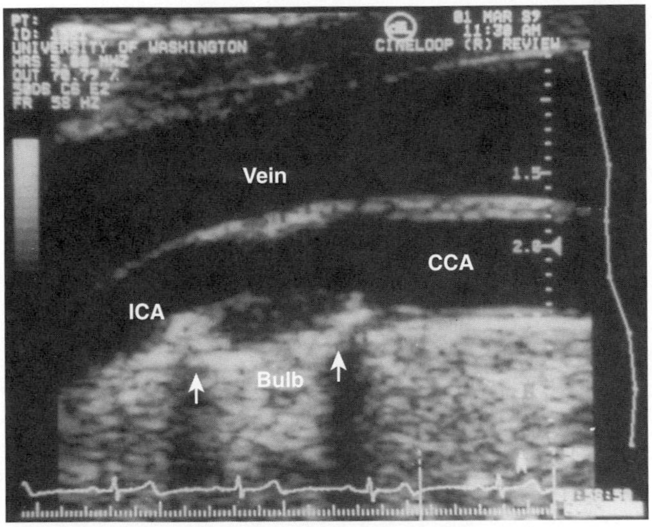

Figure 47-4. B-mode image of the carotid bifurcation demonstrating the jugular vein, common carotid (CCA), and internal carotid (ICA) arteries. An ulcerated, calcified plaque is seen at the origin of the internal carotid.

The most important risk of angiography is transient or permanent neurologic deficits, with estimates in the ranges 0.5% to 4% and 0.09% to 1.3%, respectively. Local complications include hematoma, dissection of the femoral artery, and embolism. Systemic complications such as allergic reactions and renal failure also occur. The overall complication rate is in the range 0.9% to 10%.[45,46]

In contrast, color duplex ultrasound is noninvasive and risk-free and has a positive predictive value of more than 95% for significant stenosis.[47] The controversial issue of whether ultrasound alone is adequate as the definitive investigation before surgery is now resolving. Both magnetic resonance and digital subtraction angiography may well underestimate or overestimate the degree of carotid stenosis if a large plaque is situated asymmetrically within the vessel lumen.[48,49] It is also argued that angiography is necessary to exclude additional stenotic lesions elsewhere in the cerebral circulation, typically in the carotid siphon, or coincidental cerebral aneurysms, but the relevance of these so-called "tandem lesions" is uncertain.[50] Computed tomography (CT) angiography provides another noninvasive alternative in carotid assessment, but has yet to gain widespread acceptance.[51] In patients with a recent acute stroke, a cerebral CT scan (Figure 47-5) should be performed to exclude intracerebral hemorrhage.

The risks and cost of angiography do not justify its routine use before carotid surgery. Exceptions to this policy are if the duplex imaging is inconclusive, or if the artery appears to be occluded on ultrasound when it is important to exclude the possibility of "trickle flow" through a very tight stenosis.

Carotid surgery

BENEFITS

The role of carotid surgery in the prevention of stroke in symptomatic patients with severe stenosis (70% to 99%) of the internal carotid artery is now well established. In the North American Carotid Surgery Trial,[52] covering 50

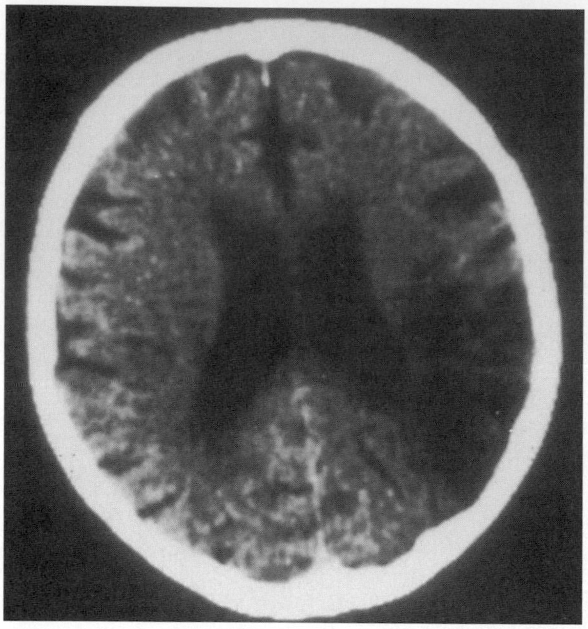

Figure 47-5. CT brain imaging of a large cerebral infarct in the left parietal region.

clinical centers, patients with internal carotid stenosis and a history of a hemispheric or retinal transient ischemic attack or nondisabling stroke within 120 days of onset were randomized to surgery or best medical care. In patients with 70% to 99% stenosis (diameter reduction on angiography) of the symptomatic artery, the cumulative estimated risk at 2 years of an ipsilateral stroke was 26% in the 331 medical patients and 9% in the 328 surgical patients. For a major or fatal ipsilateral stroke, the corresponding rates were 13.1% and 2%. The perioperative stroke and death rate was 5.8%, but only 2.1% for major stroke and death.

In the European Carotid Surgery Trial,[53] patients with a stenosis of the relevant carotid artery who after a carotid territory nondisabling ischemic stroke, a transient ischemic attack, or amaurosis fugax were also randomized to surgery or best medical care. In patients with mild carotid stenosis (less than 69%), there was low 3-year risk of ipsilateral stroke, so any benefit from surgery was outweighed by the risks. In patients with severe carotid stenosis (greater than 70%), there was a 7.5% risk of stroke or death within 30 days of surgery. However, during the next 3 years the risks of ipsilateral stroke were only 2.8% for surgery patients and 16.8% for control patients. At 3 years, the total risk of death or any stroke was 12.3% for surgery and 21.9% for control patients.

Asymptomatic carotid artery stenosis

The role of carotid endarterectomy in patients with asymptomatic carotid artery disease remains unanswered. The Asymptomatic Carotid Atherosclerosis Study[54] suggested that endarterectomy halved the risk of stroke in patients with greater than 70% carotid stenosis. However, there were methodological anomalies and this is the first large randomized study to reach such a conclusion. This finding would also have massive cost implications as the rate of stroke was only 4% to 5% each year without surgery. The European equivalent, the asymptomatic Carotid Surgery Trial, is ongoing and so a conservative approach is recommended until the results of that study are known.

Mortality from carotid surgery

Current mortality and complication rates for carotid endarterectomy in the United Kingdom and Ireland are low: there is a 1.3% mortality and 2.1% stroke rate by 30 days postoperatively.[55] Over half of all perioperative strokes are caused by intraoperative or postoperative thrombosis and embolization.[56] Studies have confirmed that carotid endarterectomy can be performed safely in the elderly population, including nonagenarians, but outcome is dependent on the individual surgeon.[57–60] Clearly, the key issues in the decision to offer carotid surgery are the risk of stroke, the quality of life enjoyed by the patient, and life expectancy.

Timing of carotid surgery after stroke

Traditionally, surgery is delayed for 2 months following acute stroke. In the 1960s, several studies of the role of urgent carotid surgery were published. The results were poor, and postmortem studies often demonstrated intracerebral hemorrhage.[61,62] It was concluded that urgent surgery precipitated hemorrhage within the infarct. However, CT was not available then to exclude a primary intracerebral hemorrhage, where surgery would be clearly inappropriate. Furthermore, many of the patients in those early studies had dense neurologic deficits and were in "coma, semicoma or stupor."[63]

Interest in the role of urgent carotid surgery following acute stroke was renewed by reports of improvement in neurologic deficits in patients with progressing stroke and limited deficit.[64] The rationale for carotid surgery in such patients is twofold: first to restore cerebral perfusion and limit neuronal death; and second, to reduce early recurrence or progression of stroke as a result of further emboli from the diseased carotid. Urgent surgery in patients with progressing strokes and acute stable strokes have shown better results than the natural history of acute stroke in small studies, but there has been no adequate trial on carotid surgery in acute stroke since CT scans were introduced.[65,66] A recent feasibility study concluded that trials of urgent carotid surgery should focus on partial anterior circulation infarcts and yet would still need large numbers of patients to be randomized.[67]

Carotid angioplasty and stenting

A future alternative in the treatment of carotid stenosis may lie in angioplasty and stenting. A recent multicenter randomized trial comparing these techniques with endarterectomy showed similar rates of disabling stroke or death in the two groups, at around 6%.[68] Concern has been raised, however, that lower complication rates than demonstrated in this study should be achievable by surgery.

ABDOMINAL AORTIC ANEURYSM

Prevalence and natural history

PREVALENCE

Abdominal aortic aneurysms are common. Mortality statistics from the U.K. Office of Population Censuses and Surveys show that each year approximately 10,000 deaths are due to aortic aneurysm in England and Wales. However, quoted statistics may vastly underestimate the number of deaths related to aortic aneurysms as most aneurysms remain undiagnosed and may be certified as myocardial infarction following sudden unexplained death in an elderly person. The true figure is estimated at nearer 25,000. Deaths from rupture are rare below the age of 50 years; deaths from rupture peak in men aged 75 to 79 years.[69]

The prevalence of aortic aneurysms is increasing, though some would argue that this finding merely reflects improved diagnosis, changing patterns of referral, and an increased awareness of the disease.[70,71] Difficulties arise in estimating the prevalence and mortality of aneurysms because of varying definitions of aneurysm and operative mortality, especially because an aneurysm is still most frequently diagnosed on postmortem examination.

The Vascular Surgery Society proposed that an aneurysm was by definition 50% dilated above normal, "normal" being an estimate taken from the literature and adjusted for gender and radiologic modality.[72] Collin[73] suggested that an abdominal aortic aneurysm was present by definition when the infrarenal aorta was at least 4 cm in diameter or exceeded the maximum diameter of the aorta between the origin of the superior mesenteric and left renal arteries by at least 0.5 cm. Sterpetti[74] has suggested that an abdominal aneurysm is present when the ratio of infrarenal to suprarenal measurements is 1.5 or greater. Screening of 4237 men and women aged 65 to 80 years around Chichester, U.K., yielded aneurysms of 3 cm or more in 4.3% of cases and aneurysmal changes can be detected in 10.7% of men in the eighth decade of life.[75,76] The prevalence of aneurysms is higher in men over the age of 50, in first-degree male relatives of patients with proven aneurysms, and inpatients with hypertension or peripheral vascular disease.[77–79]

Natural history

Aneurysms less than 5 cm in diameter seldom rupture, but the outlook for larger aneurysms is grim without surgery; the 2-year mortality for aneurysms greater than 6 cm may be 72%, though this high mortality does reflect a bias against operating on patients who are unfit at diagnosis. However, the majority of deaths in patients with large aneurysms are due to rupture.[80,81] The expansion rate of aortic aneurysms depends on aneurysm size and in small aneurysms is approximately 2 mm per year, but growth is neither consistent, steady, or predictable.[82] Smoking may increase the rate of aneurysm growth.[83] Growth rates tend to accelerate as the aneurysm size increases, and the only reliable predictor of aneurysm rupture is aneurysm size and female sex.[74,80,84] Irrespective of size, symptomatic or tender aneurysms should be investigated with a view to surgery as soon as possible because more than 25% of these will rupture in the next year.

Clinical presentation and diagnosis

PRESENTATION

Although most aortic aneurysms are asymptomatic or occur with a rupture, they may cause back or abdominal pain. This is not always classic lumbar back pain, and all abdominal or back pain in patients with an abdominal aortic aneurysm should be attributed to the aneurysm unless another diagnosis is obvious. Alternatively, the first presentation may be that of acute leg ischemia due to distal emboli from the aneurysm, although this is surprisingly rare considering the frequency of thrombus within the aneurysm sac.

When an aortic aneurysm ruptures, the vast majority of patients die immediately and without reaching a hospital. The early survivors have severe back or abdominal pain and hemorrhagic shock. Patients with retroperitoneal rupture, where the bleed is contained by the pressure of surrounding tissues, are more likely to reach the hospital alive, but still the majority of patients die before reaching a hospital.[85] Less common presentations include rupture of the aneurysm into the vena cava (leading to a massive arteriovenous fistula and high-output cardiac failure) or into the gastrointestinal tract (hematemesis and melena) because of an aortoduodenal fistula.

DIAGNOSIS

Most aneurysms are detected incidentally, usually either on physical examination or on abdominal ultrasound (Figure 47-6). Physical examination tends to overestimate aneurysm size by about 20% owing to overlying retroperitoneal tissue and the thickness of the abdominal wall.[86] Although ultrasound is the most cost-effective imaging method for diagnosis and follow-up, further information should be obtained before elective repair. The relationship to the origin of the renal arteries should be defined, and patency and diameter of the iliac arteries confirmed. Most aortic aneurysms are infrarenal. If there is suprarenal extension of the aneurysm, the operative difficulty increases, as does the operative mortality because of the need to cross-clamp above the renal arteries with subsequent increased risk of renal embolization and renal failure. Specialist centers favor either computed tomography (Figure 47-7) or nuclear magnetic resonance imaging (MRI) for this assessment. Both are noninvasive and are sensitive to the level of the renal arteries.[87] Neither provides adequate information on occlusive arterial disease, either viscerally or peripherally, although MR angiography is an option. Arteriography has been found to be unhelpful as it underestimates the size and extent of the aneurysm owing to luminal thrombus.

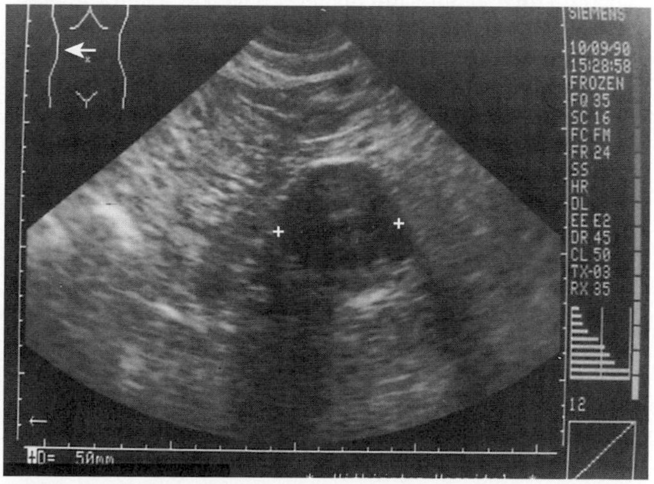

Figure 47-6. Abdominal ultrasound image demonstrating a large abdominal aortic aneurysm in transverse section.

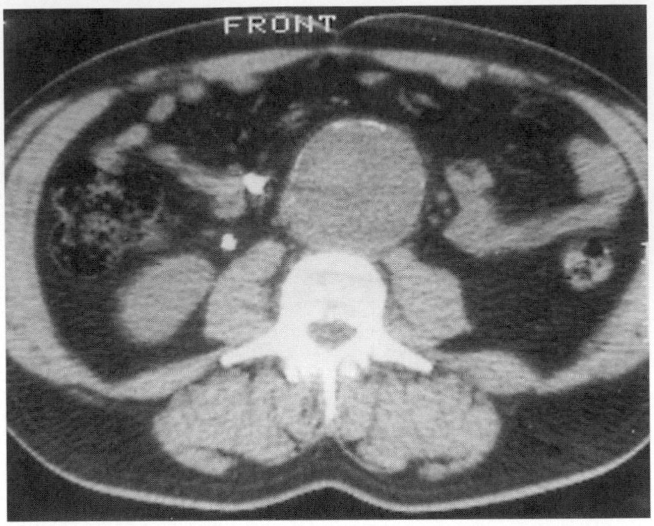

Figure 47-7. An 8-cm abdominal aortic aneurysm with calcified wall on CT imaging.

Complications of aneurysm surgery

MORTALITY FROM RUPTURE

The operative mortality for a ruptured aneurysm varies between centers, from 31% to more than 75%.[88,89] However, this represents only the tip of the iceberg because the overall mortality is greater than 80% because only a minority of patients reach the hospital alive.[85] Mortality rates for emergency surgery have improved very little over the years, with an overall rate in the United Kingdom of around 70% but with lower rates in specialized vascular centers.[90]

OPERATIVE MORTALITY

The 30-day mortality for elective aneurysm surgery has been quoted from zero to 8.4% depending on the series of patients and the center.[91,92] However, independently assessed mortality in clinical trials is invariably much higher, at around 10% to 12%. Generally, in the United Kingdom mortality rates for elective surgery should be around 5%.

In a recent study of more than 16,000 patients, operative mortality was increased by cerebral vascular occlusive arterial disease, chronic pulmonary disease, and impaired renal function.[93] Cardiac failure and diabetes have also been shown to adversely affect outcome.[94] Intraoperative hypotension, left renal vein ligation, and blood loss greater than 4 units are known to be associated with increased mortality,[95] and postoperative renal failure is the strongest predictor of death.[89] Following successful aneurysm repair, prognosis is excellent, with a life expectancy comparable to that of an age- and sex-matched population.[93]

Cardiac complications

Aneurysm patients tend to have increased operative risk owing to concomitant cardiac and pulmonary disease. Just under half of these patients have electrocardiographic evidence of ischemic heart disease.[96] Myocardial infarction is the most frequent cause of death in patients undergoing elective aneurysm repair. If there is a history of significant angina, coronary angiography should be considered to define the coronary disease before elective surgery. An echocardiogram may be of some value in identifying segmental wall motion abnormalities indicative of underlying ventricular dysfunction, and in providing an estimate of the left ventricular ejection fraction. Patients with an ejection fraction greater than 60% are unlikely to experience significant cardiac problems postoperatively, but a low ejection fraction is a poor predictor of complications.

Respiratory complications

Severe pulmonary insufficiency with dyspnea at rest is a contraindication to surgery. A simple clinical assessment based on ability to walk or climb a flight of stairs without needing to rest identifies most "problem" patients, but arterial blood gases and pulmonary function tests may be useful in defining the severity of pulmonary insufficiency. Patients with obstructive lung disease require careful preoperative physiotherapy and bronchodilators to increase pulmonary capacity, thereby reducing postoperative morbidity and mortality.

Surgical approach may also influence outcome. Abdominal aortic aneurysm repair has traditionally been performed via a transperitoneal approach, but an extended retroperitoneal approach may be less stressful for elderly patients and those with limited pulmonary reserve.[97]

Renal complications

After cardiac causes, renal insufficiency is the next most frequent cause of death following aortic aneurysm repair. Elevated preoperative serum creatinine is significantly associated with postoperative mortality risk.[98] This preexisting renal insufficiency may be caused by repeated embolization from an atheromatous aorta, coexisting atheroma of the renal arteries, or concomitant disease such as hypertension or diabetes. It is especially important to avoid perioperative hypovolemia in these patients.

Cerebrovascular complications

Stroke is an infrequent complication of aneurysm repair.[94] Noninvasive duplex Doppler investigation reliably identifies potentially treatable carotid artery stenosis, but carotid surgery is of proven benefit only in patients with appropriate symptoms in the relevant carotid territory.

Decreasing operative mortality

There are many ways to improve the outcome for patients undergoing elective abdominal aortic surgery. Patients should have the benefit of standard intensive monitoring including, electrocardiography (ECG), arterial pressure monitoring, and pulse oximetry. Intensive or high-dependency facilities must be available for postoperative care, ventilation, and monitoring as required. This type of monitoring has led to a progressive decrease in morbidity and mortality, and a decrease in the incidence of renal complications, by minimizing periods of hypotension.[99] Perioperative β-blockade reduces cardiovascular mortality significantly in patients with preexisting cardiac disease.[100,101]

Modern vascular surgery should also include a strategy for managing blood transfusion. Techniques such as preoperative donation, perioperative hemodilution, and the use of salvage autotransfusion result in an appreciable saving of bank blood transfusion and a reduction in systemic inflammatory response. The many risks inherent in blood transfusions are obviated.[102]

The osmotic diuretic mannitol has been used sporadically in aortic surgery for the last 30 years to maintain urine output during aortic cross-clamping.[103] More recently, mannitol has been shown to scavenge oxygen-free radicals produced by restoration of blood flow to ischemic tissues, and these are important in the development of ischemia/reperfusion injury. A prospective randomized clinical trial in elective aortic aneurysm repair has shown a significant benefit in postoperative pulmonary function in patients who received mannitol before cross-clamping.[104]

Aortic aneurysm repair in the elderly population

Aneurysm surgery can be well tolerated in octogenarians, but mortality for aneurysm repair is undoubtedly increased in those aged over 75, mainly owing to comorbid conditions.[95] Regrettably, in a recent British survey nearly 50% of general practitioners would not refer to a specialist an 80-year-old with a palpable aneurysm.[105] Clearly, we should take advantage of the current enthusiasm for continued medical education to ensure that appropriately selected patients are offered elective repair before rupture occurs.

ENDOVASCULAR TECHNIQUES

Endovascular stent-grafts have been used successfully to exclude abdominal aortic aneurysms in selected patients. Currently, endovascular aneurysm repair (EVAR) is offered in the United Kingdom only as part of randomized controlled trials comparing this technique either to surgery or, in those unfit for surgery, to best medical care. The results of this study will not be available before 2003, but national audit data from the United Kingdom suggest a 1%, 30-day mortality from EVAR if the patient is considered fit for surgery and a 17% mortality in those considered unfit.[106]

The stent-graft is assembled within the aorta via the femoral artery at operation. This avoids a laparotomy with its associated cardiac and respiratory morbidity in these high-risk patients. However, only a minority of patients are suitable for this technique because a widely patent and not too tortuous iliac system is required through which the graft can reach its destination. A suitable length of nonaneurysmal aorta below the renal arteries is essential, as is a normal aorta above the bifurcation or acceptable iliac arteries for stent attachment.[2] These measurements are all taken during spiral CT or MR imaging.

MANAGEMENT OF SMALL ANEURYSMS

For many years it remained unclear how to manage aortic aneurysms less than 5.5 cm in diameter. The UK Small Aneurysm Trial[107] randomized 1090 patients with aneurysms 4 to 5.5 cm in diameter to either surgery or regular surveillance by ultrasonography. No significant difference in survival was found between the two groups despite follow-up of up to 6 years. Hence surgery should now be reserved for aneurysms greater than 5.5 cm and smaller aneurysms monitored with regular ultrasound imaging. The cost-effectiveness of screening for aortic aneurysm compares favorably with breast and cervical cancer screening, provided surgery is offered only for asymptomatic aortic aneurysms greater than 5.5 cm in diameter.[108]

CONCLUSIONS

Informed consent for surgery in elderly people is especially important because of the concomitant risks but surgical intervention in selected patients is well tolerated.

Carotid endarterectomy or revascularization for peripheral vascular disease is intended primarily to enhance quality of life. Without such treatments the elderly patient may lose independence through a stroke or limb amputation. The loss of independence and long-term care costs after limb amputation or stroke argue for the cost-effectiveness of an aggressive policy of early revascularization for limb salvage or carotid disease.

KEY POINTS
Vascular Surgery

- Intermittent claudication should be managed by lifestyle advice, exercise, and antiplatelet agents such as aspirin. Angioplasty/stenting and surgery are usually reserved for severe symptoms sufficient to impair quality of life or ischemic rest pain.
- Cardiorespiratory comorbidity indicates the risk of mortality after vascular surgery.
- Carotid endarterectomy is appropriate for symptomatic internal carotid artery stenosis of greater than 70%, provided the quality of life is good. Lesser symptomatic stenoses should be managed medically.
- Aortic aneurysms greater than 5.5 cm in diameter require open or endovascular repair. Below this diameter, regular ultrasonographic surveillance is indicated.

For a complete list of references, please visit online only at www.expertconsult.com

CHAPTER 48

Venous Thromboembolism in the Elderly

Hamsaraj G. M. Shetty
Ian A. Campbell
Philip A. Routledge

INTRODUCTION

Venous thromboembolism (VTE) causes 25,000 to 32,000 deaths in hospitalized patients in the United Kingdom. It accounts for 10% of all hospital deaths. This, however, is likely to be an underestimate because many hospital deaths are not followed by a postmortem examination. The cost of managing VTE in the United Kingdom is estimated to be approximately £640 million. About 25% of patients treated for deep vein thrombosis (DVT) subsequently develop debilitating venous leg ulceration, treatment of which is estimated to cost £400 million in the United Kingdom. The most serious complication of VTE is pulmonary embolism (PE), which untreated has a mortality of 30%. With appropriate treatment, mortality is reduced to 2%.[1] The diagnosis of VTE is often delayed until the occurrence of a clinically obvious (and occasionally fatal) PE.

VTE is more common in older adults. The incidence of DVT and PE increases with increasing age. Between 65 and 69 years of age, annual incidence rates per 1000 for DVT and PE are 1.3 and 1.8, respectively, and rise to 2.8 and 3.1 in individuals aged between 85 and 89 years. Older men are more likely than women of similar age to develop pulmonary embolism. About 2% develop PE and 8% develop recurrent PE within 1 year of treatment for DVT.[2] The diagnosis of PE is more often missed in elderly people and is sometimes made only at postmortem.[3]

The Virchow's triad (named after Rudolf Virchow, 1821–1902) describes the three main predisposing factors for development of thrombosis. The first is alteration in blood flow, which may be reduced in heart failure—a common problem in the elderly, less mobile individual. The second factor (injury to the vascular endothelium) is more relevant to arterial thromboembolism than to VTE. The third factor (hypercoagulability) is important since increases in clotting factor concentration, platelet and clotting factor activation, and a decline in fibrinolytic activity have all been reported in the elderly.[4]

Risk factors

The risk factors for VTE are well recognized (Table 48-1). Many of these (e.g., poor mobility, hip fractures, stroke, and cancer) are more frequently present in the elderly, who are also more likely to be hospitalized and to have orthopedic surgery. Hospitalization itself is associated with an increased risk of VTE (the incidence is 135 times greater in hospitalized patients than in the community). The risk of VTE is greatest in "medical" inpatients. It is estimated that 70% to 80% of hospital-acquired VTEs occur in this group. Without prophylaxis, 45% to 51% of orthopedic patients develop DVT. It is estimated that in Europe approximately 5000 patients per year are likely to die of VTE following hip or knee replacement, when prophylactic treatments are not given. About a third of all surgical patients developed VTE before the introduction of prophylactic treatments.[1]

Clinical presentation and diagnosis

DEEP VEIN THROMBOSIS

Unilateral swelling of a leg is the most common feature in elderly patients having DVT. Calf pain may sometimes be present. Normally there is a history of recent hospitalization for orthopedic surgery, stroke, or for some other illness. There may occasionally be a history of anorexia, weight loss, or other symptoms suggestive of an underlying neoplasm. However, the patient is often otherwise asymptomatic.

It is well recognized that the clinical diagnosis of DVT can be difficult because the physical signs may often be subtle, and diagnosis may be more difficult in the elderly. Some individuals may be unable to complain about a swollen leg because of dementia or dysphasia. In addition, other conditions mimicking DVT, such as a ruptured Baker's cyst, are also more likely to occur in this age group. The clinical diagnosis of DVT relies on observing a swollen, warm, lower limb, which may sometimes be associated with engorged superficial veins. Calf tenderness may also be present. If there is a difference of more than 2 cm in circumference between the two lower limbs, DVT must be excluded by appropriate investigations, unless there is another obvious explanation.

Doppler ultrasonography has a sensitivity of 96% and specificity of 98% for proximal DVT and so it is the investigation of first choice to diagnose DVT.

Contrast venography may be necessary in selected patients, especially if clinical suspicion is high and the Doppler scan

Table 48-1. Risk Factors for VTE

Low Risk
• Minor surgery (<30 min) + no risk factors other than age
• Minor trauma or medical illness
Moderate Risk
• Major general, urologic, gynecologic, cardiothoracic, vascular, or neurologic surgery + age >40 yr or other risk factor
• Major medical illness or malignancy
• Major trauma or burn
• Minor surgery, trauma, or illness in patients with previous DVT or PE or thrombophilia
High Risk
• Prolonged immobilization
• Age over 60 years
• Previous DVT or PE
• Active cancer
• Chronic cardiac failure
• Acute infections (e.g., pneumonia)
• Chronic lung disease
• Lower limb paralysis (excluding stroke)
• BMI >30 kg/m^2
• Fracture or major orthopedic surgery of pelvis, hip, or lower limb
• Major pelvic or abdominal surgery for cancer
• Major surgery, trauma, or illness in patients with previous DVT, PE, or thrombophilia
• Major lower limb amputation

Modified from references 1 and 42.

is negative. Estimation of the concentration D-dimer levels (a fibrin degradation product of thrombolysis), especially when combined with a clinical probability score, has a good negative predictive value but poor positive predictive value.[5] Other investigations such as magnetic resonance imaging are currently being evaluated.

PULMONARY EMBOLISM

Sudden onset of dyspnea is the most common presenting feature of PE in the elderly. Sudden onset of a pleuritic chest pain, cough, syncope, and hemoptysis are other common presenting symptoms. In an elderly patient with stroke or recent orthopedic surgery, onset of any of these symptoms should greatly increase the suspicion of underlying PE. Because of high incidence of cardiovascular disease and age-related decline in cardiovascular function in general, the elderly are less likely to tolerate cardiovascular decompensation because of moderate or severe pulmonary embolism. They are, therefore, more likely to have syncope after a PE.[6] Patients with smaller PEs may present with very nonspecific symptoms and the diagnosis is often missed in this group.

Clinical features will depend on the severity of the PE. In patients with moderate to severe PE, tachycardia, hypotension, cyanosis, elevated jugular venous pressure, right parasternal heave, loud delayed pulmonary component of the second heart sound, tricuspid regurgitation murmur, and pleural rub may be present. However, in patients with smaller PEs, clinical examination may be normal, except possibly for a sinus tachycardia. Unexplained tachycardia in a patient who is potentially at risk for VTE should alert the clinician to the possibility of PE.

Arterial blood gas analysis is a useful initial test in patients with suspected PE. Presence of hypoxia or worsening of preexisting hypoxia makes the diagnosis more likely, unless there are other comorbid conditions to account for it.

An ECG may show sinus tachycardia, S wave in lead I, Q wave and T inversion in lead III, right bundle branch block or a right ventricular strain pattern. In patients with severe PE, a P *"pulmonale"* may be seen. New onset of atrial fibrillation may also be a feature of PE.

A chest radiograph may show elevated hemidiaphragm, atelectasis, focal oligemia, an enlarged right descending pulmonary artery, or a pleural effusion. Many elderly patients have coexistent cardiac failure or chronic pulmonary diseases, which may also cause some of the radiographic abnormalities associated with PE.

At present, ventilation perfusion (V/Q) scans are still widely used in the United Kingdom for diagnosing PE. A medium or high probability scan is diagnostic, whereas a low probability scan virtually rules out PE.

Computed tomography pulmonary angiography (CTPA) is increasingly being used as the diagnostic test for detecting PE. A meta-analysis has indicated that the rate of subsequent VTE after a negative CTPA is similar to that following conventional pulmonary angiography.[7] One randomized single blind noninferiority trial has demonstrated that CTPA is equivalent to a V/Q scan in ruling out PE. In the study, CTPA also diagnosed PE in significantly more patients.[8] Although this study was conducted in younger patients, CTPA is likely to replace the V/Q scan as the investigation of first choice in elderly patients because of its greater ability to detect PE even in patients with coexistent cardiac and respiratory disease. The British Thoracic Society has recommended CTPA as the initial lung imaging modality of choice for nonmassive PE.[9]

Although the measurement of D-dimer concentration has high sensitivity and negative predictive value in the elderly patient with PE, it has a very poor specificity and positive predictive value and therefore cannot be recommended for routine diagnostic use.[10]

Contrast enhanced magnetic resonance imaging appears to be a promising imaging technique for detecting PEs. An echocardiogram is also particularly useful in evaluating the severity of PE. Invasive investigations such as pulmonary angiography are very rarely performed in the elderly patients.

Treatment

Anticoagulant therapy is the most widely used treatment for VTE. Other less frequently used treatments and interventions include thrombolytic therapy, thromboembolectomy, and the use of vena caval filters.

For initial treatment of both DVT and PE, low molecular weight heparins (LMWHs) are the drugs of first choice. Because they produce predictable anticoagulation with a weight-based (per kg body weight), once daily dose by subcutaneous route—and do not require routine laboratory monitoring (except for grossly overweight or underweight patients and those with renal failure)—they have almost replaced unfractionated heparin (UFH), which is now generally used only in special circumstances such as during the perioperative period. Randomized clinical trials have shown that LMWHs are as effective as UFH for treatment of both DVTs and PEs.[11,12] LMWHs appear to cause less hemorrhagic complications and for the reasons described earlier, are much more convenient to use. With the widespread use of LWMHs in hospitals within the United Kingdom, many patients with DVT can now be treated as outpatients.

Once the diagnosis of DVT or PE is confirmed, warfarin therapy is commenced immediately and LMWHs are continued for at least 5 days or until therapeutic international normalized ratios (INRs) have been maintained for 48 hours. The recommended target INR for treatment of VTE is 2.5 (range 2 to 3).[13] A higher intensity of 3.5 (range 3 to 4) is recommended for treating patients who develop recurrent VTE while in a therapeutic INR range between 2 and 3.[14]

As elderly patients are more sensitive to the effects of warfarin, they are much more likely to be over-anticoagulated during initiation of the treatment. Use of a tailored induction dosing regime is likely to reduce this possibility. One such regimen[15] uses a first dose of 10 mg and subsequent doses are adjusted daily thereafter, depending on the INR (Table 48-2). Another induction regimen that has been shown to be safe and accurate in elderly hospitalized patients (over 70 years) involves giving 4 mg of warfarin daily for 3 successive days.[16]

The various recommendations with regard to the duration of warfarin therapy following VTE have generated a considerable amount of debate. One guideline recommended a minimum of 6 months of treatment.[14] However, a randomized trial has shown that 3 months of anticoagulation is adequate for patients with a first episode of VTE (idiopathic or otherwise) and is less likely to be associated with serious hemorrhages.[17] It is now being increasingly recognized that the duration of warfarin therapy should depend on the risk of recurrent VTE in an individual patient. If the

Table 48-2. Warfarin Initiation Schedule

Day	INR (9–11 AM)	Warfarin Dose
Day 1	<1.4	10
Day 2	<1.8	10.0
	1.8	1.0
	>1.8	0.5
Day 3	<2.0	10.0
	2.0–2.1	5.0
	2.2–2.3	4.5
	2.4–2.5	4.0
	2.6–2.7	3.5
	2.8–2.9	3.0
	3.0–3.1	2.5
	3.2–3.3	2.0
	3.4	1.5
	3.5	1.0
	3.6–4.0	0.5
	>4.0	0.0
		Predicted Maintenance Dose
Day 4	<1.4	>8.0
	1.4	8.0
	1.5	7.5
	1.6–1.7	7.0
	1.8	6.5
	1.9	6.0
	2.0–2.1	5.5
	2.2–2.3	5.0
	2.4–2.6	4.5
	2.7–3.0	4.0
	3.1–3.5	3.5
	3.6–4.0	3.0
	4.1–4.5	Miss out next day's dose, then give 2 mg
	>4.5	Miss out 2 days' doses, then give 1 mg

Adapted from Fennerty A, Dolben J, Thomas P et al. Flexible induction dose regimen for warfarin and prediction of maintenance dose. Br Med J 1984;288:1268–70.

VTE occurred following surgery, the risk of recurrence after 1 year of stopping anticoagulant therapy is approximately 3% and in such a situation it is safe to discontinue warfarin therapy after 6 weeks if there are no persistent risk factors. In patients with minor reversible risk factors (e.g., soft tissue leg injury), who have a recurrence risk of 5%, anticoagulants can be stopped within 3 months. On the other hand, patients who have a major, nonreversible risk factor such as cancer are at high risk of recurrence, and therefore should be considered for long-term anticoagulant therapy.[18] One author has recently recommended long-term anticoagulation after unprovoked (idiopathic) VTE,[19] but a recent study does not support this view and the BTS guideline recommends 3 months of anticoagulation after the first episode.[9,17]

Practical aspects of oral anticoagulant therapy in the elderly

Older people are more sensitive to the anticoagulant effect of warfarin. This is probably due to a combination of pharmacodynamic and pharmacokinetic factors.[20,21] Warfarin dose requirement declines with age and in one study patients aged less than 35 years required a mean of 8.1 mg/day, more than twice as much to maintain the same INR as in those older than 75 years.[21] The relationship between age and warfarin requirements is, however, rather weak.[21] Warfarin clearance (wholly by metabolism since no warfarin is excreted unchanged in the urine) has been shown to decline with age in one study.[22]

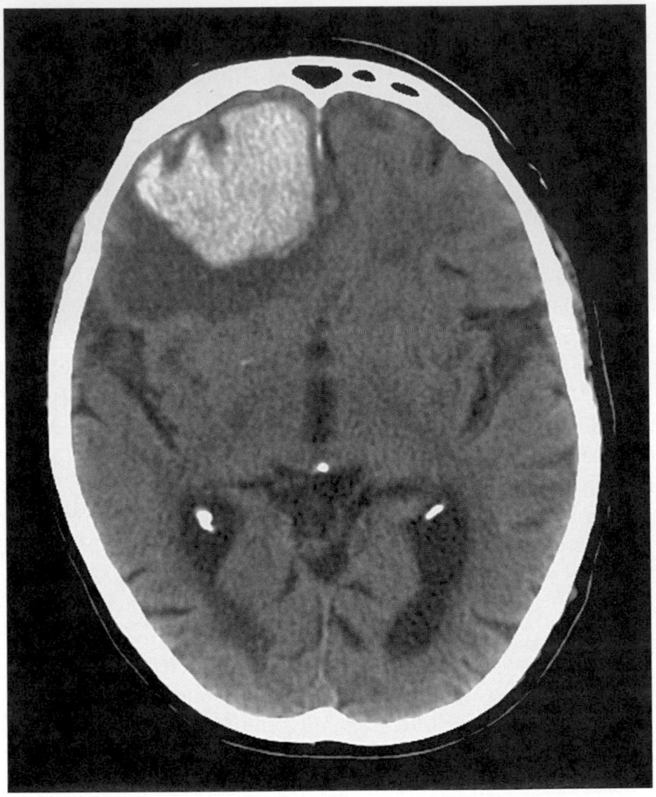

Figure 48-1. CT head showing intracerebral hemorrhage.

Chronologic age does not appear to be a risk factor for bleeding with warfarin therapy, except possibly in those older than 80 years.[23] Hemorrhagic complications due to warfarin are more likely to occur in the first 90 days of anticoagulant therapy (especially in the first month), either because of poor control of anticoagulation or the unmasking of an underlying lesion, such as a peptic ulcer or malignancy. High INRs (>4.5), poor control of anticoagulation, and inadequate patient education regarding anticoagulant therapy are likely to increase the risk of bleeding.

Studies have reported a log-linear relationship between the intensity of anticoagulation and the risk of bleeding.[24] The risk of bleeding rises threefold between INRs 2 and 3 and further threefold between 3 and 4.[25] As a high INR is one of the most important risk factors for bleeding in the elderly, the aim of treatment should be to maintain the lowest intensity of anticoagulation consistent with effective treatment or prophylaxis.

Polypharmacy is very common in the elderly and it increases the chances of drug interactions, which may result in overanticoagulation. Using medicines that are well known to enhance anticoagulant effect (e.g., antibiotics [particularly macrolides], amiodarone, etc.) with care and adjusting the dose of warfarin appropriately will reduce the likelihood of overanticoagulation and consequent bleeding.

Fatal hemorrhages tend to be intracranial and are more likely to occur in older people.[25] (Figure 48-1). The elderly are more predisposed to intracranial bleeding because of the increased prevalence of leukoaraiosis and other cerebrovascular diseases. Older people are also more likely to have falls and so are at a greater risk of developing subdural hematomas.

An outpatient bleeding risk index included four risk factors for major bleeding (attracting 1 point each): age over 65 years, history of gastrointestinal bleeding, history of stroke, and one or more specific comorbid conditions (recent myocardial infarction, hematocrit of less than 30%, presence of diabetes mellitus, and serum creatinine of greater than 1.5 mg/dL). The authors indicated that a score of zero was associated with low risk, 1 to 2 with medium risk, and 3 to 4 with high risk (23% in 3 months and 48% in 12 months).[26] The drawback of this clinical tool is that it places all people aged over 65 years in the medium risk category for bleeding, which may not necessarily be the case.

Hemorrhage associated with anticoagulant therapy should always be investigated to exclude an underlying pathology, even if the bleeding occurred when the INR was high. Unexplained anemia in an anticoagulated patient may well be due to occult bleeding (e.g., retroperitoneal hemorrhage). Sometimes atypical bleeding sites and presenting symptoms may pose diagnostic difficulties (e.g., alveolar hemorrhage [having unexplained anemia or dyspnea]).

Management of overanticoagulation and bleeding

Because of the high risk of bleeding associated with overanticoagulation, measures to bring the INR down to the therapeutic range should be instituted as soon as possible. If the INR is less than 8 (and depending on the indication for anticoagulation), warfarin is temporarily discontinued and reinstituted once the INR has fallen to less than 5, providing there is no bleeding or only minor bleeding.[14] If the INR is over 8 and there is no bleeding or minor bleeding, temporary discontinuation of warfarin is also recommended, but if the patient has other risk factors for bleeding, low dose vitamin K either orally (0.5 to 2.5 mg) or intravenously (0.5 mg) will help to bring it within the therapeutic range in the majority of patients.[13,27] Anaphylactoid reactions with intravenous vitamin K have rarely been reported, but their incidence seems to be lower with newer preparations, and when the dose is administered very slowly. In patients with major bleeding, warfarin should be discontinued and anticoagulation reversed urgently with prothrombin complex concentrate (factors II, VII, IX, and X) or fresh frozen plasma if the concentrate is not available. In addition, vitamin K_1, 5 to 10 mg by slow intravenous injection is recommended to sustain the reversal. Urgent reversal of anticoagulation is particularly important in patients with intracerebral bleeding as it will prevent the continued expansion of the hematoma (the latter is associated with an even poorer outcome).

Monitoring warfarin therapy

Close monitoring of warfarin therapy will reduce the likelihood of over- or under-anticoagulation. Currently, most patients are either monitored by their general practitioners or in a hospital-based anticoagulation clinic. With appropriate training, patient self-management of anticoagulation has been shown to be feasible, effective, and safe. A randomized controlled trial, which compared routine care with patient self-management (with twice weekly use by patients, at home, of an INR measurement device and a simple dosing chart), showed that percentage of time in therapeutic range and serious adverse events were similar between the two groups. Patients who had poor control before the study showed an improvement with self-management.[28] At present, the point of care INR measurement devices are quite expensive. They are, nevertheless, particularly useful for patients living in remote areas or those who have difficulty in accessing services of an anticoagulation service in primary or secondary care.

Inferior vena caval filters

In patients who have contraindications for anticoagulation, and those who bleed or continue to have thromboembolism during anticoagulant therapy, placement of an inferior vena caval (IVC) filter can be lifesaving. The PREPIC study, which included 400 patients with proximal DVT, with or without PE, followed up for 8 years, reported a significant reduction in the incidence of symptomatic PE, but an increase in the incidence of DVT in patients treated with filter compared with those who received standard anticoagulant therapy. There was no significant difference in the development of postphlebitic syndrome or mortality between the two groups.[29] Complications of IVC filters include misplacement or embolization of the filter, vascular injury or thrombosis, pneumothorax, and air embolus.

A limited number of small studies have reported no inferior vena caval thrombosis with the use of retrievable inferior vena caval filters.[30] Further studies are needed to confirm these encouraging initial findings.

Treatment of PE with hemodynamic instability

Massive PE may have acute cor pulmonale or cardiogenic shock. Elderly patients are much more likely to develop right heart failure and shock with massive PE. Such patients should be managed in an intensive therapy unit unless they have a terminal illness or have previously had a very poor quality of life. In addition to cardiovascular and respiratory resuscitation, treatment options include thrombolysis or thromboembolectomy. The most commonly used thrombolytic agent is recombinant tissue plasminogen activator (rt-PA). Intracranial hemorrhage occurs in about 3% of patients treated with thrombolytic agents. In patients with massive PE who have contraindications for thrombolysis, or when it has failed, pulmonary embolectomy can be attempted. Despite these measures, mortality is very high in patients with PE having cardiogenic shock.

Prevention

Many hospitalized elderly patients are at risk for VTE. Those with stroke, hip fractures, and those who have had orthopedic surgery are at particularly high risk. In such patients, prophylaxis implementation rates have been reported to range between 13% and 64%. Prophylactic treatments are particularly underused in medical patients. A very large multinational cross-sectional survey, designed to assess the VTE risk in an acute hospital setting, found 51.8% to be at risk (64.4% surgical, mean age 60 years and 41.5% medical patients, mean age 70 years); of these 58.5% of surgical and only 39.5% of medical patients received appropriate thromboprophylaxis.[31]

A meta-analysis of thromboprophylaxis in hospitalized medical patients showed that, compared with controls, treatment with low dose UFH or LMWH reduced the risk of DVT (risk ratio 0.33 and 0.56, respectively) and PE (risk ratio 0.64 and 0.37, respectively). Treatment with LMWH was associated with a greater reduction in DVT risk (relative risk: 0.68) compared with UFH. There was no difference in the risk of bleeding or thrombocytopenia between the two drugs and neither of them reduced mortality.[32]

The American College of Chest Physicians (ACCP) recommends LMWH, low-dose UFH, or fondaparinux for thromboprophylaxis in hospitalized, acutely ill, medical patients. In those who have contraindications for anticoagulant use, graduated compression stockings or intermittent pneumatic compression can be used.[13]

A meta-analysis involving 9 studies compared extended thromboprophyaxis (for 30 to 42 days) with heparin (8/9 studies used LMWH) or warfarin with a placebo or untreated controls after total hip replacement (THR) and total knee replacement (TKR). It showed a significant reduction in symptomatic VTE (equivalent to 20 symptomatic VTEs per 1000 patients treated) without an associated increase in major hemorrhage in the treatment group.[33]

A number of new anticoagulants are currently being investigated for thromboprophylaxis. Orally administered factor Xa inhibitors and direct thrombin inhibitors have already been investigated in randomized clinical trials in patients undergoing THR and TKR.

A randomized, double-blind study compared subcutaneous, once daily, preoperative enoxaparin, with postoperative fondaparinux in patients undergoing elective THR (age range: 24 to 97 years; mean age 67 years). The risk of VTE was significantly reduced in those receiving fondaparinux (relative risk reduction 55.9%, CI 33.1 to 72.8). Frequency of deaths and clinically relevant bleeding were similar in the two groups.[34]

Another double-blind, randomized study compared postoperative oral dabigatran etexilate with preoperative enoxaparin in patients undergoing THR (mean age range: 63 to 65 years). In this study, oral dabigatran was found to be as effective as enoxaparin in reducing VTE risk and there was no difference in the risk of major bleeding between the two drugs.[35]

The randomized, double-blind studies, Regulation of Coagulation in Orthopaedic Surgery to Prevent Deep Vein Thrombosis and Pulmonary Embolism 1 (RECORD 1)[36] and RECORD 3,[37] compared a 10-mg once-daily dose of rivaroxaban, an oral direct factor Xa inhibitor, with 40 mg of enoxaparin, for extended thromboprophylaxis in patients undergoing THR and those undergoing TKR, respectively. Rivaroxaban was significantly more effective in reducing DVT (symptomatic and asymptomatic), nonfatal PE, and death from any cause (at 36 days for THR patients and within 13 to 17 days for TKR patients). There was no significant difference in the risk of major bleeding.

The RECORD 2 study compared oral rivaroxaban 10-mg dose once daily given for 31 to 39 days with subcutaneous enoxaparin 40-mg dose once daily given for 10 to 14 days in patients undergoing elective THR. Extended thromboprophylaxis with rivaroxaban significantly reduced VTE, including symptomatic events.[38]

Although these studies are encouraging, LMWH and warfarin presently remain the most frequently used agents for thromboprophylaxis in most circumstances in elderly people.

Graduated compression stockings

Graduated compression stockings (GCS) reduce the risk of VTE in surgical patients, but they are not superior to LMWHs. Ideally, they should be used along with LMWHs. In patients who are at high risk of bleeding, they can be used on their own. As most elderly patients have peripheral vascular disease, the GCS should be used with extreme caution: inappropriate use has been known to cause ischemic complications.

The role of GCS in medical patients needs further investigation. A large multicenter clinical trial (the CLOTS trial) is currently investigating its role in stroke patients.

After proximal DVT, approximately 60% of patients develop postphlebitic syndrome. A randomized trial has shown that, when sized-to-fit, GCS reduce the incidence by about 50%.[39] Patients with proximal DVT should start wearing GCS as soon as possible after the diagnosis and continue to wear them for at least 2 years.[39]

Prognosis

A population-based cohort study of patients with VTE found that the overall probable and definite (in parentheses) cumulative percentage of VTE recurrence at 7, 30, and 180 days and 1 and 10 years was 1.6% (0.2%), 5.2% (1.4%), 10.1% (4.1%), 12.9% (5.6%), and 30.4% (17.6%), respectively.

KEY POINTS
Venous Thromboembolism in the Elderly

- Venous Thromboembolism (VTE) is an important cause of mortality in hospitalized patients and is more common in the elderly.
- Risk factors for VTE, such as immobility, hip fracture, and stroke are more common in older people.
- In an elderly patient with stroke or recent orthopedic surgery, sudden onset of dyspnea, chest pain or syncope should markedly increase the suspicion of underlying PE.
- Computed tomography pulmonary angiography (CTPA) is the initial lung imaging modality of choice for nonmassive PE.
- For prevention and initial treatment of both DVT and PE, low molecular weight heparins are the drugs of first choice.
- Older people are more sensitive to the anticoagulant effect of warfarin.
- Studies have reported a log-linear relationship between the intensity of anticoagulation and the risk of bleeding.
- In patients with massive pulmonary embolism, treatment options include thrombolysis or thromboembolectomy.
- Orally administered factor Xa inhibitors and direct thrombin inhibitors are being investigated in randomized clinical trials for treatment of VTE.
- Prompt clinical diagnosis and carefully monitored institution of therapy will reduce morbidity and mortality from VTE in the aging population.

The risk of recurrence was greatest in the first 6 to 12 months after the initial VTE. Independent predictors of first overall VTE recurrence included increasing age and body mass index, neurologic disease with paresis, malignant neoplasm, and neurosurgery.[40]

A prospective international registry, which studied clinical predictors for fatal PE in patients with VTE, has reported 3-month mortality and fatal PE rates of 8.65% and 1.68%, respectively. Patients with symptomatic nonmassive PE at presentation were found to have a 5.42-fold higher risk of fatal PE compared with patients with DVT without symptomatic PE ($P < 0.001$). The risk of fatal PE was 17.5 times higher in patients having a symptomatic massive PE. Other independent risk factors for fatal PE were immobilization for neurologic disease, age greater than 75 years, and cancer.[41]

Long-term complications of VTE include postphlebitic syndrome and chronic thromboembolic pulmonary hypertension.

CONCLUSION

VTE continues to be an important cause of morbidity and mortality in older people. There have been major advances in its diagnosis and treatment over the past 15 to 20 years. A number of new antithrombotic drugs (e.g., orally administered factor Xa inhibitors and direct thrombin inhibitors) are currently being investigated and may provide an alternative to warfarin therapy. Whatever treatment is advocated in the future, prompt clinical diagnosis and carefully monitored institution of therapy will reduce morbidity and mortality from VTE in the aging population.

For a complete list of references, please visit online only at www.expertconsult.com

CHAPTER 49

Asthma and Chronic Obstructive Pulmonary Disease

Sidney S. Braman
Muhanned Abu-Hijleh

DISEASES OF AIRFLOW OBSTRUCTION

There are three common airway diseases of older adults that cause limitation of airflow: chronic bronchitis, emphysema, and asthma. All have in common a reduction of maximum expiratory flow and a slow forced emptying of the lung on spirometric testing. Chronic bronchitis and emphysema share common clinical and pathologic abnormalities. Most patients with these conditions have a significant smoking history and attempts were made to incorporate both conditions under the term chronic obstructive lung disease (COPD). As asthma became recognized as an inflammatory disease with a different cellular and inflammatory mediator profile, it was no longer considered under the term COPD. This was also justified by the fact that asthma is felt to be distinct because airflow obstruction is predominantly reversible and the airways of asthmatics are notably hyperresponsive to a variety of specific (aeroallergens) and/or nonspecific (methacholine, histamine, cold air) inhaled substances. Current definitions of these diseases of the airways are presented in Table 49-1.

Although it is still clinically useful to distinguish asthma from COPD (chronic bronchitis and emphysema), it is important to recognize three problems with this nosology:

- Remission rates for adults with asthma are much less than those seen in children and this probability increases with age. As a result, most asthmatics, even those who have never smoked, who are at the age when COPD is most often recognized (over age 60), have evidence of poorly reversible airflow obstruction on pulmonary function testing. This is thought to be caused by a structural remodeling of the airways with what may be permanent changes. This is supported by data from longitudinal studies that the average FEV_1 in asthmatics declines over a period of years. Despite these findings, there are many patients who show no correlation between their FEV_1 and the duration of their disease.
- Bronchial hyperresponsiveness—the exaggerated bronchoconstrictive response to nonspecific agonists such as methacholine is a constant feature in asthmatics that is so important to its pathogenesis. On the other hand, increased responsiveness to constrictors such as methacholine and histamine (but not indirect bronchoconstrictors such as cold air and bradykinin, which do not act directly on airway smooth muscle) is seen in the majority of older smokers with COPD. This was shown to be a strong predictor of progression of airway obstruction in younger smokers who continue to smoke. In asthma, bronchial hyperresponsiveness is not related to baseline airway caliber, whereas in COPD the increased responsiveness to bronchoconstrictors can be explained entirely by the geometric effect of fixed airway narrowing.
- Unfortunately, many adult patients with asthma are current or former smokers. It is likely that such patients have more than one pathologic process with several pathways of inflammation. Although studies on the effects of smoking on the rate of decline of FEV_1 in asthma have given conflicting results, most smoking asthmatics will have some degree of fixed airflow obstruction. This has raised a complexity of semantic issues that have not been solved. One attempt has been to combine two of the major pathologic processes and describe such patients using the term "asthmatic bronchitis" but this has not been widely accepted.

Although there are distinct differences between asthma and COPD in older patients, the clinical differentiation in some individuals is quite problematic. Fortunately, although the pathologic mechanisms leading to asthma and COPD differ, the pharmacologic and nonpharmacologic therapeutic approaches to these two conditions are quite similar as described later in this chapter, making clinical decisions less problematic. An overview of the distinguishing clinical features of these conditions is seen in Table 49-2.

ASTHMA IN THE ELDERLY

Introduction

Asthma is a common debilitating disease that affects 300 million people globally with a 50% increase in the prevalence every decade, in addition to climbing morbidity and mortality. In response to these alarming statistics of the twentieth century, the National Asthma Education and Prevention Program (NAEPP) commissioned an expert panel that would help bridge the gap between current knowledge and clinical practice. The panel was charged to develop guidelines for the care of asthma that would raise public awareness, improve physician recognition that asthma is a growing health problem, and improve asthma control. The first expert panel report was offered in 1991. Based on new evidence from the medical literature, updates were published in 1997 and 2002. The most recent update was made available in 2007 as the Expert Panel Report 3, entitled "Guidelines for the Diagnosis and Management of Asthma" www.nhlbi.nih.gov/guidelines/asthma.[1]

The NAEPP guidelines offered a new definition of asthma (see Table 49-1) that is now widely accepted and appropriate for any age. This description of asthma clearly established it as an inflammatory disease and provided the basis for anti-inflammatory therapy. This has been the foundation of treatment for asthma over the last 2 decades.[2] In fact, there is strong evidence linking anti-inflammatory therapy with inhaled corticosteroids to a reduction in asthma mortality.[3]

Epidemiology: prevalence

The prevalence of asthma has risen over the last several decades with recent data showing that 22 million Americans are affected by this disease. The overall prevalence of asthma

Table 49-1. Definitions of Obstructive Lung Diseases

- Asthma: a chronic inflammatory disease of the airways in which many cells play a role, in particular, mast cells, eosinophils, and T-lymphocytes. In susceptible individuals, this inflammation causes recurrent episodes of wheezing, breathlessness, chest tightness, and cough, particularly at night and/or in the early morning. These symptoms are usually associated with widespread but variable airflow limitation that is at least partially reversible either spontaneously or with treatment. This inflammation also causes an associated increase in airway hyperresponsiveness to a variety of stimuli. Reversibility of airflow limitation may be incomplete in some patients with asthma.
- COPD: a preventable and treatable disease state characterized by airflow obstruction that is no longer fully reversible. The airflow limitation is usually progressive and is associated with an abnormal inflammatory response of the lungs to noxious particles and gases, primarily caused by cigarette smoking. Although COPD affects the lungs, it also produces considerable systemic consequences:
  - o Chronic bronchitis: a condition characterized by the presence of chronic cough and sputum expectoration that is present for most days for a minimum of 3 months per year, for at least 2 successive years and not attributable to other pulmonary or cardiac causes
  - o Emphysema: a condition defined anatomically by enlargement of air spaces distal to the terminal bronchiole, accompanied by destruction of their walls and capillaries, without obvious fibrosis

Table 49-2. Distinguishing Clinical Features of Asthma and COPD in Elderly Patients

Asthma	COPD
History of allergy is common	Normal prevalence of allergy
Smoking history in some patients	90% have smoked cigarettes
Episodic attacks of dyspnea	Progressive dyspnea over years
Nocturnal attacks of dyspnea	Daytime exertional dyspnea
Reversible airflow obstruction	Minimal or no reversibility
Good QOL	Progressively poor QOL

QOL, Quality of life.

in the U.S. population is approximately 6% to 7%.[4] Although the diagnosis and treatment of asthma are often focused on younger population, it is estimated that more than 1 million adults older than 65 years of age in the United States carry a diagnosis of asthma.

In a survey of the elderly in the United States, the prevalence of physician-diagnosed asthma was 4%, with an additional 4% having probable asthma (symptoms of asthma without a diagnosis).[5] Other estimates of prevalence have shown a broad range from 4% to 9%. In many older patients, it is not possible to distinguish asthma from chronic bronchitis or COPD, especially in current or former cigarette smokers. In population surveys that inquire about asthma and COPD, subjects frequently reported more than one disease. In an investigation of two databases[6] from the United States and the United Kingdom, 8.5% of the participants from the U.S. population reported asthma, chronic bronchitis, or emphysema. Of these subjects, the asthma-only group was the largest, accounting for 50.3% and 79.4% of these patients in the United States and United Kingdom, respectively. This number decreased with increasing age. Overall, 17% and 19% of patients in the United States and in the United Kingdom, respectively, reported more than one condition, and this percentage increased with age. In those over 50 years of age in the U.K. cohort, individuals with more than one condition accounted for as many as 50% of the patients with obstructive lung disease. This proportion was 25% in a 45- to 69-year age group in another study from Australia.[7]

Community surveys in which a physician diagnosis of asthma was required have provided data on asthma in the general population. The prevalence of active asthma in one study, which represented new cases excluding those in remission, peaked in early childhood at about 8% to 10%, declined to approximately 5.5% during late adolescence and then rose again to about 7% to 9% during late adulthood (over age 70). In 1987, data from the National Center for Health Statistics showed that in the 65- to 74-year age group, the rate of active asthma or wheeze was 10.4% compared to 5.7% in teenagers, 6.9% in the 18- to 44-year-old age group, and 9.6% in the 45- to 64-year-old age group. In another report from a population-based cohort of elderly individuals living in Rochester, Minnesota, a group of asthmatics were identified with the onset of asthma after age 65. The age-specific incidence of asthma in those aged 65 to 74 years of age was 103/100,000; it was 81/100,000 in those aged 75 to 84 years, and 58/100,000 in those older than 85 years.

Epidemiology: morbidity and mortality

Asthma in the elderly is associated with a significant number of hospitalizations and emergency department visits, which leads to substantial health care cost. In 1999, the United States rate for asthma hospitalization for patients older than 65 years of age was 21.1/10,000.[4] Elderly patients with asthma are more likely to die from their disease than younger individuals and although mortality rates in some age groups have decreased, this is not the case in the elderly, especially women.[8]

According to the U.S. Centers for Disease Control and Prevention (CDC), asthma deaths in the elderly account for more than 50% of asthma fatalities annually with an approximately 5.8 asthma deaths per 100,000 in this group reported in the years 2001–2003.[4,9] In a U.S. study of asthma deaths of patients who had died in hospitals or nursing homes, 80% of the deaths occurred in patients age 55 and older. Seventy-five percent of these patients were known to be smokers or ex-smokers. A careful analysis of these cases revealed that many younger asthmatics did clearly have asthma and had died of a severe sudden attack. In those over age 55, confounding factors were much more prevalent. These patients frequently had underlying chronic bronchitis or COPD, were admitted to the hospital for nonrespiratory problems, and died of chronic respiratory failure. Less aggressive therapy was given to these elderly patients, both in the outpatient setting and during hospitalization. This study suggested that many elderly patients with asthmalike symptoms and a history of previous smoking have COPD as an underlying or even dominant feature of their disease. This undoubtedly overestimated the true mortality from asthma in this age group. Factors that may increase risk of death in the elderly include the delay in seeking diagnosis and treatment, poor cardiopulmonary reserve, impaired perception of increasing airway obstruction, blunted hypoxic ventilatory drive, and psychosocial and cognitive problems, which are very common in this age group.

Pathogenesis

Asthma is caused by a complex interaction of cells, mediators, and cytokines that result in airway inflammation,[10] which results in a number of typical histopathologic findings in the airways. This inflammation results in the three cardinal features described in the definition of asthma that are involved in the pathogenesis of the disease: airflow obstruction, reversibility of obstruction, and bronchial hyperresponsiveness.

Histopathologic findings

Infiltration of the airways by inflammatory cells such as mast cells, eosinophils, activated T-lymphocytes, and neutrophils was demonstrated on biopsies and bronchoalveolar lavage. The number of activated lymphocytes found in bronchial biopsies has been correlated with the number of local activated eosinophils and the severity of asthma. Specific cytokines, most of which are products of lymphocytes and macrophages, appear to direct the movement of cells to the site of airway inflammation. Mast cells, usually as a result of IgE-mediated stimulation, also release preformed mediators, such as histamine and proteases, and further act as a regulator of inflammation by producing cytokines that promote eosinophil infiltration and activation. Several mast cell products induce bronchoconstriction and cause increased mucus secretion.

Edema of the airway mucosa occurs as a result of increased capillary permeability with leakage of serum proteins into the interstitium. Denudation of the airway epithelium can lead to airway edema and loss of substances in the mucosa that protect the airway. Epithelial damage promotes bronchial hyperresponsiveness since access by irritating substances to sensory nerve endings is increased. Another characteristic finding in severe asthma is the presence of tenacious mucus plugs in the airways. Death from asthma usually occurs from blockage of the airways by diffuse mucus plugging.

Thickening of the reticular basement membrane, the lamina reticularis, is a constant feature of asthma. There is evidence of increased bronchial smooth muscle mass that contributes considerably to the thickness of the airway wall. The airway architecture is also changed by the deposition of type III and V collagen and fibronectin beneath the basement membrane (referred to as "subepithelial fibrosis"). The architectural changes seen in and beneath the basement membrane and in the bronchial smooth muscle are referred to as airway remodeling and are thought to cause permanent changes that result in fixed airflow obstruction.

Histopathologic findings in elderly asthmatics

Sputum, bronchoalveolar lavage, and bronchial mucosal biopsy specimens from elderly stable asthmatics have confirmed the presence of prominent eosinophilia, and CD4+ T lymphocytes, as seen with younger asthmatics.[11] Thickening of the reticular basement membrane and disruption of the epithelial lining has also been described. Pathologic findings have been compared in young and older subjects who have died of fatal asthma attacks.[12] Both old and young patients with asthma have thickened airway smooth muscle compared with normal subjects. However, older asthmatics with a longer duration of disease demonstrate an increase in airway wall thickness predominantly due to an increase in the adventitial area. Greater postmortem reduction in airway lumen is also found in elderly asthmatics. The luminal content and subepithelial collagen deposition are similar in both asthma groups. This supports the concept that aging and/or asthma duration result in airway remodeling, causing "fixed" or irreversible airflow obstruction in this population.

Airflow obstruction

Airflow obstruction is a cardinal feature of asthma. Objective measures of lung function such as spirometry and peak flow measurements are generally underutilized in elderly patients, which contributes to the delay or absence of diagnosis.[13] Lung function testing is especially important in this age group since there is an age-related reduction in the perception of dyspnea seen in the elderly. However, spirometry may be difficult to perform in some situations because of physical or poor cognitive impairments. In addition, it is hard to define the lower limits of predicted normal values in this age group, which may vary considerably.

During an acute asthma attack, lung hyperinflation occurs, protecting airway narrowing. This happens because of the interdependence of lung volume and airway caliber since parenchymal attachments cause greater tethering of the airways at higher lung volumes. Inflammation of the bronchial wall, however, may uncouple the mechanical linkage between the parenchyma and the airway. This may contribute to airway narrowing and also to bronchial hyperresponsiveness. During an acute attack of asthma, airway resistance increases and all measures of airflow (peak expiratory flow rate [PEFR], forced expiratory volume in 1 second [FEV_1], forced expiratory volume in 1 second as a fraction of the forced vital capacity [FEV_1/FVC %], airway resistance [R_A], etc.) are abnormal. During remission, these tests may normalize, and yet considerable dysfunction may be present in peripheral airways. Studies using bronchoscopic measurements have shown that peripheral resistance can be tenfold higher than in normal subjects.

Reversibility of airflow obstruction

Another hallmark of asthma is that the airflow obstruction reverses to normal or toward normal after treatment. This may occur rapidly, after treatment with a short-acting inhaled β-agonist, or after weeks or months of intense anti-inflammatory therapy. Although complete reversibility is frequently seen with young asthmatics, most elderly asthmatics, and those of any age group with more severe and persistent symptoms, show only partial reversibility despite continuous intense anti-inflammatory and bronchodilator therapy. In one random survey of 1200 elderly asthmatics older than 65 years from the Mayo Clinic, only one in five patients had normal pulmonary function (FEV_1 >80% predicted) whereas a similar number showed moderate to severe airflow obstruction (FEV_1 <50% predicted) even after administration of an inhaled short-acting bronchodilator.[14] There is growing evidence that the airway function of young and middle age asthmatics declines at a greater rate than normal subjects. The rate of decline increases with increasing age and in those who smoke cigarettes. However, these effects on asthmatics are variable since not all individuals show a steep rate of decline. The precise reasons for this individual variability have not been defined, although there is evidence that atopy and marked bronchial hyperresponsiveness are two important risk factors for airflow obstruction.

In addition, the long duration and severity of previous disease are also important factors.[15] On the other hand, for those who develop asthma at an advanced age, there is evidence that lung function is reduced, even before a diagnosis is made, and declines rapidly shortly after diagnosis. Thereafter, it remains fairly stable. Hence, many elderly asthmatics with severe airflow obstruction report a short duration of symptoms for months to a few years. The cause of chronic persistent airflow obstruction in older asthmatics with longstanding disease or with recently acquired asthma has not been explained, and airway remodeling is thought to be the main cause.

Diagnostic tests for reversible airflow obstruction

The presence of airflow obstruction can be easily confirmed by simple office spirometry. A reduced FEV_1 and ratio of FEV_1/FVC is demonstrated with the timed vital capacity maneuver or by the flow volume loop. The loop is produced by the simultaneous measurement of airflow and lung volume during forced exhalation and inhalation (Figure 49-1). The configuration of the flow volume loop can be helpful in the differential diagnosis of airflow obstruction in the elderly. Traditionally, an FEV1/FVC ratio of less than 70% increases the probability of asthma in an elderly patient with asthma symptoms. A brisk response to a short-acting bronchodilator may demonstrate the second cardinal feature of asthma, reversible airflow obstruction ("a responder"). Evidence of reversibility (postbronchodilator FEV_1 or FVC increases more than 12% and 200 mL) increases the probability of asthma. However, many patients with COPD will also meet the reversibility criteria on any given testing day although the response to an inhaled bronchodilator is generally greater with asthma (16% asthma vs. 11% COPD). A positive response in a patient with COPD may not persist over time; over 50% of patients will change "responder" status between visits. This makes the test less than reliable to confirm the diagnosis of asthma especially in the elderly. In general, when complete reversibility of airflow obstruction is documented, COPD, a disease of fixed airway obstruction becomes less likely. As noted above, many patients with asthma will not meet the reversibility criteria and airway remodeling may be the cause. Additionally, reduced β_2-adrenoreceptor responsiveness has been demonstrated in normal elderly men and women, and asthmatics. When compared to young and elderly normal subjects, elderly late-onset asthmatics have been shown to have reductions in β-adrenergic receptor affinity while maintaining normal receptor density. There is also evidence that post receptor events are impaired in the aged as cyclic AMP production by pathways that are independent of adrenergic receptor stimulation is depressed. Although the bronchodilator response to inhaled β-agonists declines with age, this is not the case with anticholinergic agents.

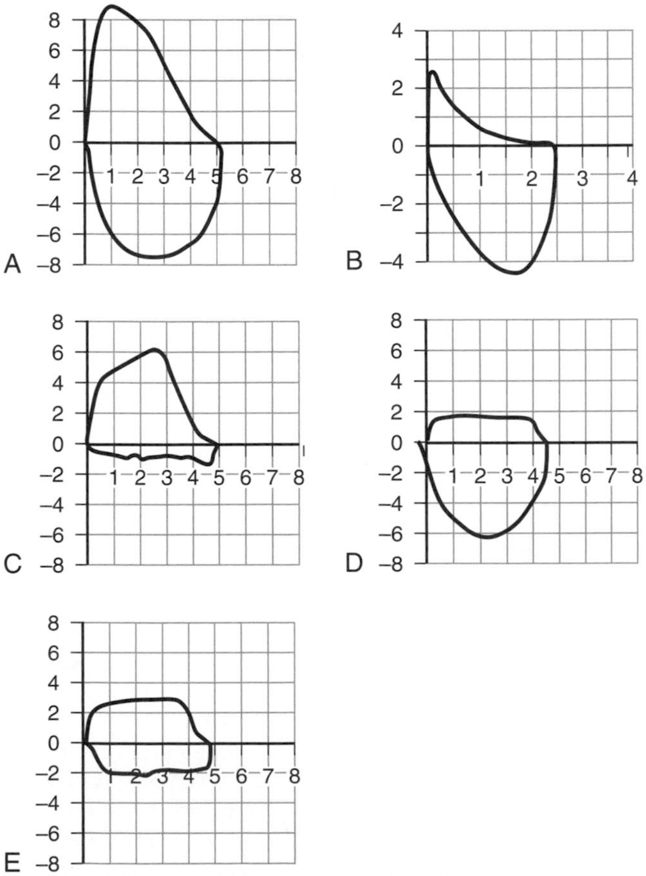

Figure 49-1. Flow-volume loops in a normal subject (A), a patient with COPD (B), extrathoracic dynamic airway obstruction with airflow limitation during inspiration (C), intrathoracic dynamic airway obstruction with airflow limitation during expiration (D) and fixed airway obstruction with airflow limitation during inspiration and expiration (E).

Bronchial hyperresponsiveness

Airway inflammation is thought to be a key factor in producing the third cardinal feature of asthma, BHR. This can be described as an exaggerated bronchoconstrictive response by the airways to a variety of stimuli, such as aeroallergens, histamine, methacholine, cold air, and environmental irritants. It is not clear whether BHR is acquired or is present at birth and genetically determined to appear with the appropriate stimulus, such as during allergen exposure, respiratory viral illness, or the inhalation of noxious agents, such as ozone or sulfur dioxide. Anti-inflammatory agents such as inhaled corticosteroids are effective in reducing bronchial hyperactivity.

The degree of bronchial hyperresponsiveness can be determined in the pulmonary function laboratory by standard inhalation bronchoprovocation challenge testing. The methacholine inhalation challenge is the most frequently used clinical tool to determine the presence and degree of bronchial hyperresponsiveness. When the patient has asthma symptoms, and the tests looking for airflow obstruction are normal, the methacholine challenge can be used for diagnosis. A positive test is not specific for asthma. A strongly positive test coupled with a high pretest probability offers a high likelihood of asthma. A negative bronchoprovocation test rules out asthma as a cause of pulmonary symptoms. Bronchoprovocation testing is a safe and effective method to uncover asthma in the elderly.

There is evidence that some sympathetic and parasympathetic nervous system functions are diminished with age. This decline in autonomic nervous system function is consistent with a generalized diminution of peripheral somatic nerve function with aging. However, although the protective laryngeal gag reflex appears diminished in normal elderly subjects, there is evidence that the cholinergically mediated cough reflex may not be similarly affected. Measurements of cholinergic bronchoconstrictive reflexes have shown mixed results although most studies have shown a positive correlation between aging and airway hyperresponsiveness.[16] There is also a relationship between the degree of bronchial hyperresponsiveness and prechallenge pulmonary function; a low FEV_1 predicts heightened responsiveness. Although this may explain why some studies have shown that bronchial responsiveness is heightened in the elderly, aging may be an independent factor influencing airway responsiveness. Other factors that may contribute to heightened airway responsiveness in the older population are atopy and current or previous smoking history.

Atopic asthma

Allergic or atopic reactions in the upper (nose, sinuses) and lower airways are both important in the pathogenesis of asthma in childhood and young adulthood. Their role in the elderly is less clear. Atopy is defined by the presence of abnormal amounts of IgE antibodies in response to contact with environmental antigens. This can be demonstrated clinically by elevated total or specific serum IgE levels in the blood or by positive skin prick tests to a variety of standardized aeroallergens. In elderly patients with or without asthma, an elevated level of IgE may be an important risk factor for the development of chronic airflow obstruction. This is especially true in current smokers, but also seen in former smokers.

Atopy is an age-related phenomenon; in community surveys the peak prevalence of immediate skin test reactivity occurs during the third decade and falls rapidly after age 50. The proportion of asthmatics that are atopic varies with age; in childhood about 80%; between ages 20 to 40, 50%; and after age 50, less than 20%. Elevated serum IgE levels are closely related to the likelihood of a subsequent asthma diagnosis in younger asthmatics and this may be seen with elderly asthmatics. More likely, those that acquire asthma after age 60 are nonatopic. In the Cardiovascular Health Study,[5] many elderly asthmatics reported respiratory problems that started in childhood and half stated that wheezing was triggered by contact with plants, animals, or pollens and that it was seasonal. Elderly urban dwelling patients with asthma may show evidence of cockroach-specific IgE antibody and are more likely to have more severe asthma and airflow obstruction.[17] IgE specific antibodies to cat and dog dander, cockroach, and dust mite can also be present in elderly asthmatics with atopy.[18] A history of atopy is the strongest predictor of asthma in the elderly.[19] Those who are capable of becoming sensitized will usually have done so by the time they are older adults. Avoidance of potential allergens in the environment of the elderly asthmatic should be advised.

Clinical features

The distinctive features of asthma in older adults have been described in an NIH consensus conference[20] and also the subject of a comprehensive clinical review.[21] In adulthood, there is a steady incidence of new-onset asthma through all ages, even in the elderly. Many patients begin with symptoms following respiratory viral infections. This pattern may gradually or abruptly develop into persistent symptoms and often severe, poorly responsive disease. Classic symptoms of asthma, including episodic wheezing, shortness of breath, and chest tightness, are typical of elderly and young asthmatics. These symptoms are generally worse at night and with exertion and are often precipitated by an upper respiratory tract infection. These symptoms of asthma in the elderly are nonspecific and may be caused by a variety of other conditions. Shortness of breath, especially on exertion, is a common symptom and may be attributed to different underlying diseases, including heart or lung diseases. Many elderly patients limit their activity to avoid experiencing shortness of breath, and others assume that their dyspnea is resulting from their aging process and, thus, avoid seeking early medical attention. However, aging per se does not cause dyspnea, and a cause always needs to be pursued in assessing an elderly patient with breathlessness. Underreporting of symptoms in the elderly may have many causes, including depression, cognitive impairment, social isolation, denial, and confusing symptoms with those of other comorbid illnesses. On the other hand, elderly patients have been shown to have a reduced perception of bronchoconstriction and this also may delay medical intervention. Cough is another prominent symptom of asthma and may occasionally be the only presenting symptom.[20] The presence of wheezing is not very specific and does not correlate with the severity of airflow obstruction. Asthma symptoms are often triggered by environmental exposures and can also be provoked by medications, such as aspirin, nonsteroidal anti-inflammatory agents, or β-blockers, commonly used by this population; this fact emphasizes the need for the physician to perform a comprehensive review of medications upon presentation.

Physical examination in elderly patients with asthma is usually nonspecific and may misguide the diagnosis. During an acute attack of asthma, tachypnea and tachycardia are present. Sinus tachycardia is also a complication of asthma therapy with such drugs as sympathomimetics and theophylline. As airway function improves with sympathomimetic treatment, sinus tachycardia usually improves rather than worsens. In acute asthma, premature ventricular contractions occur occasionally, whereas atrial arrhythmias are extremely uncommon. Other abnormalities seen in acute severe asthma include P pulmonale, right axis shift, right bundle branch block, and right ventricular strain. Diffuse musical wheezes are characteristic of asthma, but their presence or intensity does not reliably predict the severity of asthma. By the time wheezing can be detected by the stethoscope, peak flow rates may be decreased by as much as 25% or more. In general, wheezing during inspiration and expiration, loud wheezing, and high-pitched wheezing are associated with greater airway obstruction. In very severe cases, wheezing may be absent. This suggests very poor air movement and impending respiratory failure. A prolonged phase of exhalation is typically seen, as is chest hyperinflation. These are due to airflow obstruction and air trapping, respectively. Accessory muscle use, pulsus paradoxus, and diaphoresis are associated with severe airflow obstruction, although their absence does not rule out a severe attack. Cyanosis and signs of acute hypercarbic acidosis, such as mental obtundation, can be observed in extreme cases.

Table 49-3. NAEPP Goals of Asthma Care

Control chronic and nocturnal symptoms
Maintain normal activity levels, including exercise
Prevent acute episodes of asthma
Minimize emergency room visits and hospitalizations
Minimal need for reliever medications
Maintain near-normal lung function
Avoid adverse effects of medications

Management

The NAEPP guidelines have set goals to care for asthmatics.[1] The goals of asthma therapy are seen in Table 49-3. Short-term objectives are the control of immediate symptoms and response to falling peak flow rate measurements. Long-term objectives are those directed at disease prevention since there are now well-proven strategies to avoid serious exacerbations of acute bronchospasm that often lead to emergency room visits or hospitalization. To meet these therapeutic objectives, four components of asthma care should be addressed:

1. Environmental control measures to avoid or eliminate factors that precipitate asthma symptoms or exacerbations: Symptoms may be minimal or nonexistent at any time and can appear suddenly with no apparent cause. They may result from specific (aeroallergens) or nonspecific (dust, cigarette smoke, fumes, cold air, exercise, etc.) exposures. For those patients that have persistent asthma symptoms, the clinician should evaluate the patient for environmental causes, particularly indoor inhalant allergens such as house-dust mites, indoor pets and cockroaches, household products, medications, and passive exposure to tobacco smoke.
2. Use of objective measures of lung function to assess the severity of asthma and to monitor the course of therapy: It is recommended to monitor lung function before and after treatment to insure adequate response. The degree of reversibility in a "responder" correlates with the degree of airway inflammation. Patients with a high degree of reversibility have a greater risk of hospitalization and mortality, and a greater chance of developing irreversible airflow obstruction in subsequent years. The test can, therefore, be useful in identifying high-risk patients who need close monitoring.
3. Comprehensive pharmacologic therapy for long-term management designed to reverse and prevent airway inflammation: Therapeutic approach to asthma in elderly patients does not differ from what is recommended for young patients. The medications used to treat asthma are listed in Table 49-4. Treatment protocols in the NAEPP guidelines use step-care pharmacologic therapy based on the intensity of asthma symptoms and the clinical response to these interventions. As symptoms and lung function worsen, step-up or add-on therapy is given. As symptoms improve, therapy can be "stepped down." When disease is well controlled and symptoms are infrequent a short-acting β-agonist can be used for symptom relief. When this agent is used two or more times a week, anti-inflammatory therapy is needed and inhaled corticosteroids are the preferred agents. Several considerations have to be taken into account when choosing appropriate pharmacologic therapy in elderly patients with asthma (Table 49-5).

Table 49-4. Medications Used to Treat Asthma

Controller Medications

These are agents that are capable of reducing airway inflammation and thus improve lung function, decreasing bronchial hyperreactivity, reduce symptoms, and improve the overall quality of life.

Corticosteroids are the most useful anti-inflammatory agents.

- Inhaled corticosteroids are safe and effective
- Prevent migration and activation of inflammatory cells
- Reduce microvascular leakage
- Enhance the action of smooth muscle β_2-adrenergic receptors
- They are recommended for persistent asthma
- High doses (>1000 μg/d) may suppress hypothalamic-pituitary axis
- Local adverse effects are hoarseness and dysphonia
- Oral candidiasis can be avoided by rinsing mouth
- Poorly controlled asthma may require oral therapy

Long-acting β-agonists are effective bronchodilators

- Available in different formulations
- May be helpful for long-term maintenance therapy
- Useful when added to inhaled corticosteroids
- Should not be used as single agents

Leukotriene pathway modifiers

- 5-lipoxygenase inhibitors (zileuton)
- Cysteinyl leukotriene antagonists (montelukast, zafirlukast)
- Less effective in older asthmatics

Omalizumab: a humanized murine monoclonal antibody that inhibits the binding of IgE to mast cells by forming complexes with circulating free IgE

- Effective in patients with atopic asthma
- Available for parental use twice a month
- For moderate to severe asthma
- Reduce asthma exacerbation rates and corticosteroid use
- Not useful in older adults who are nonatopic

Theophylline: an effective bronchodilator with some anti-inflammatory properties

- Available as a sustained-release oral preparation
- Monitor theophylline blood levels to avoid toxicity
- Elderly asthmatics more susceptible to adverse effects
- GI side effects are seen with mild toxicity (20 to 30 μg/mL)
- Serious cardiac arrhythmias and seizures with blood level in excess of this range
- A range of 8–15 μg/mL is generally considered therapeutic

Rescue Medications

Inhaled short-acting β-adrenergic agonists

- The treatment of choice for the acute exacerbation of asthma symptoms
- Inhaled agents can be delivered by metered-dose inhaler, dry-powder capsules, and compressor-driven nebulizers

Parenteral corticosteroids

- Useful for acute exacerbations of asthma
  - o Intravenous corticosteroids every 6 to 8 hours
  - o Oral prednisone in doses of 40 to 60 mg/day
  - o Therapy can be slowly tapered after response
- Associated with many side effects
- Risk of osteoporosis, cataracts, and diabetes mellitus
- May rarely depress immunity to infection

Table 49-5. Special Considerations for the Pharmacologic Therapy of Asthma and COPD in the Elderly

Consideration	Contributing Factor(s)
Delivery of medication	Poor inhaler technique is common in the elderly and should be recognized.
Effectiveness of medication	Different pharmacodynamics and pharmacokinetics from younger population, diminished response. to β_2-agonists may occur and comorbidities such as cardiac disease may increase side effects.
Compliance with medication	Complex regimens, prohibitive cost, poor memory, and delivery technique may lead to poor adherence to recommendations and inadequate response.
Safety of medication	Increased risk from comorbid conditions (cardiac, osteoporosis) and interaction with other medications should be monitored.

Table 49-6. Levels of Asthma Control

Characteristic	Controlled (all of the following)	Partly Controlled (any measure present in any week)	Uncontrolled
Daytime symptoms	None (twice or less/wk)	More than twice/week	Three or more features of partly controlled asthma present in any week
Limitation of activities	None	Any	
Nocturnal symptoms/awakening	None	Any	
Need for reliever/rescue treatment	None (twice or less/week)	More than twice/week	
Lung function (PEF or FEV_1)‡	Normal	<80% predicted or personal best (if known)	
Exacerbations	None	One or more/year*	One in any week†

*Any exacerbation should prompt review of maintenance treatment to ensure that it is adequate.
†By definition, an exacerbation in any week makes that an uncontrolled asthma week.
‡Lung function is not a reliable test for children 5 years and younger.

In previous years, treatment decisions have been based on assessing the disease severity and its intrinsic intensity. A severity classification of mild intermittent, mild persistent, moderate persistent, and severe persistent disease encouraged the application of a step-care approach for asthma. The use of the severity scale is advocated in the 2007 NAEPP guidelines, but only during the initial assessment of the asthmatic before initiating therapy. A major difference in the new 2007 guidelines is the focus on the assessment of asthma control rather than severity. Control is defined as the degree to which the manifestations of asthma are minimized by therapeutic interventions and the goals of asthma therapy are adequately met. Table 49-6 shows the NAEPP levels of asthma control. A number of measures of asthma control have been offered in the medical literature. Some are more suited for research and others, such as the Asthma Control Test (ACT), are more suited for clinical use but have not been validated in an elderly population.[22]

4. Patient education that fosters a partnership among the patient, his or her family, and clinicians: Asthma self-management education is essential to provide patients with the skills necessary to control asthma and improve outcomes. The goals of asthma care should be discussed and agreed upon by the patient and all members of the health care team. Sites for self-management education outside the usual office setting should be explored. The actions of the medications should be discussed and the potential complications should be understood. Action plans should be written down and used as guidelines for daily care. An action plan for the acute exacerbation of asthma is essential, including when to use oral corticosteroids, when to call the physician, and when to use emergency services. For asthmatics that have frequent symptoms and exacerbations or those who poorly perceive their symptoms, the use of hand-held peak flow meters may be useful to monitor daily lung function. An action plan for worsening lung function may be extremely helpful in avoiding emergency room visits and near-fatal attacks.

Outcomes

Elderly asthmatics with severe symptoms, long-standing disease, reduced pulmonary function, or a concomitant diagnosis of COPD are much less likely to have a remission. Like other chronic diseases in this age group, asthma in the elderly population has a major impact on patient well-being and is a cause of significant impairment in overall health status. Patients with asthma may consequently suffer from poor general health, symptoms of depression, and significant limitation of daily activity.[20,23]

The number of unscheduled ambulatory visits, emergency visits, and hospitalizations are high in elderly asthmatics, confirming the high degree of morbidity in this age group.[25,26] Quality of life scores are also low in patients with persistent asthma when compared with elderly patients with mild asthma or no asthma at all.[5] The prevalence of comorbidities, such as sinusitis, heartburn, chronic bronchitis, emphysema, and congestive heart failure, was also higher in older compared with younger asthmatics.

These conditions can cause respiratory symptoms and can obscure the diagnosis of asthma or enhance asthmatic symptoms. Despite at times severe symptoms and physiologic impairment, most elderly patients with asthma can lead active productive lives if their asthma is detected early and is appropriately managed. In fact, if elderly patients with severe or difficult to treat asthma have been identified by physician assessment, they appear to do better than younger patients. In the Epidemiology and Natural History of Asthma: Outcomes and Treatment Regimens (TENOR) study, despite lower lung function, older asthmatics (mean age 72 years) had lower rates of unscheduled office visits, emergency department visits, and corticosteroid bursts.[27] Patients reported in this study received more aggressive care than younger adults, including higher use of inhaled and oral corticosteroids, and this undoubtedly had an impact on outcomes.

COPD IN THE ELDERLY

Introduction

Cigarette smoking is the major cause of chronic obstructive pulmonary disease (COPD) in the developed world. Cigarettes cause widespread lung injury and destruction that occur over many years. Yet, clinical manifestations usually do not become apparent in the smoker or ex-smoker until many decades have passed. Unfortunately, when the disease does become apparent, the clinical course persists for a considerable period of time, even many decades. Therefore COPD is a disease seen predominantly in the geriatric population in our society and one that causes considerable morbidity and mortality. During the latter part of the twentieth century, smoking increased dramatically among American women. This has resulted in a dramatic demographic change. The prevalence of the disease is now greater in women and in 2000, for the first time, more women died of COPD than men.

The smoking epidemic of the twentieth century has resulted in a large number of adults with COPD, a largely preventable disease. It is estimated that 24 million U.S. adults have COPD and only 12 million have been diagnosed by a physician.[28] Based on lung function testing, it is believed that an additional 12 million COPD patients are undiagnosed.[29] COPD has risen to become the fourth leading cause of death in the United States. It is projected to become the third leading cause of death in the United States and worldwide, and will rank fifth as a worldwide health burden within the next 20 years.

COPD is associated with significant comorbidities, such as cardiovascular disease and cancer. It has a tremendous impact as a comorbid condition, often as a silent partner until a serious complication arises. What may begin as a simple elective surgical procedure in an elderly patient may result in a prolonged complicated hospital admission as a result of postoperative pneumonia or respiratory failure because of unrecognized COPD.

The statistics of COPD have caused considerable alarm around the world.[30] To address this growing problem, the Global Initiative for Chronic Obstructive Lung Disease (GOLD) was established. In 2001 this offered a global strategy to increase awareness of the disease and guidelines for disease prevention and treatment (GOLD Guidelines), which was frequently updated.[31] These guidelines and the evidence-based guidelines published by the American Thoracic Society (ATS) and European Respiratory Society (ERS) will be incorporated into this chapter.[32] The term COPD defined by GOLD differs from previous consensus statements. It does not incorporate the terms chronic bronchitis and emphysema into the definition but rather highlights the major physiologic consequence of this disease—airflow obstruction—that is no longer fully reversible and is usually progressive over years. In this description, it was first acknowledged that the pathology of COPD, and the symptoms, the pulmonary function abnormalities, and complications all could be explained on the basis of the underlying inflammation. In 2006 the ATS and ERS added to the definition of COPD the phrase "preventable and treatable" to emphasize these two important aspects of the disease (see Table 49-1). This was done to encourage a positive outlook for patients and the health care community toward COPD and to stimulate effective management programs to treat patients with this disease.

Epidemiology of COPD

The National Health Interview Survey (NHIS) is an annually conducted, nationally representative survey of about 40,000 U.S. households. In 2000, it was estimated that 10 million U.S. adults reported "physician-diagnosed COPD." By adding spirometry testing, it was possible to determine the presence of airway obstruction, the prevalence of diagnosed COPD, and the estimated prevalence of COPD in the population. By including anyone with airflow obstruction by spirometry, it was estimated that 23.6 million adults (13.9%) have COPD; the majority of the subjects had evidence of mild to moderate airflow obstruction and only 1.4% of the population suffered from more advanced disease. International COPD prevalence rates in adult populations have been reported to be in the 5% to 10% range.

Another manifestation of the importance of COPD is its burden determined by using disability-adjusted life-years (DALY). In 1996 COPD was estimated to be the eighth leading cause of DALY among men and the seventh leading cause of DALY among women. Worldwide, COPD is expected to move up from the 12th leading cause of DALY in 1990 to the 5th leading cause in 2020. In 2000, COPD was responsible for 8 million physician office and hospital outpatient visits, 1.5 million emergency department visits, 726,000 hospitalizations, and 119,000 deaths.[30]

COPD is also associated with significant comorbid disease.[30,33,34] In a nationally representative sample of 47 million hospitalizations from 1979 to 2001, hospital discharges with a diagnosis of COPD were more likely to be re-admitted to the hospital with pneumonia, hypertension, heart failure, ischemic heart disease, pulmonary vascular disease, thoracic malignancies, and ventilatory failure, when compared with age-adjusted discharges without COPD. Further, having a diagnosis of COPD was associated with higher age-adjusted in-hospital mortality for pneumonia, hypertension, heart failure, ventilatory failure, and thoracic malignancies, when compared with hospital discharges with these co-morbidities who did not have a COPD diagnosis.[5] These results suggest that the burden of disease associated with COPD is largely underestimated since having a diagnosis of COPD is associated with increased risk for hospitalization and in-hospital mortality from other common diagnoses.

During the period 1980–2000, the most substantial change was the increase in the COPD death rate for women, from 20.1/100,000 in 1980 to 56.7/100,000 in 2000, compared with the more modest increase in the death rate for men, from 73.0/100,000 in 1980 to 82.6/100,000 in 2000. The number of women dying from COPD surpassed the number of men dying from COPD in 2000. Progressive respiratory failure accounts for approximately one third of the COPD-related mortality, therefore factors other than progression of lung disease must play a substantial role.[30]

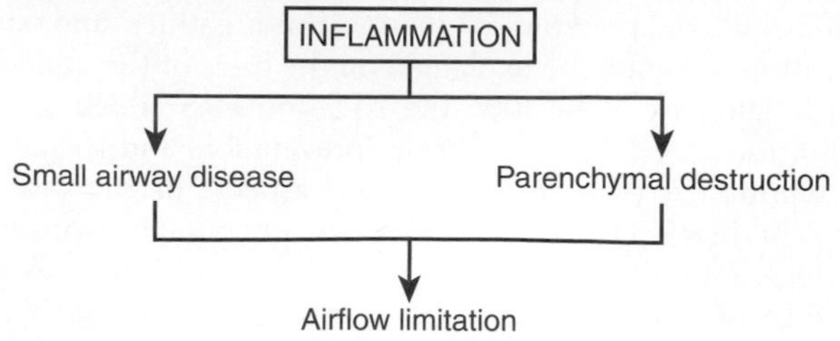

Figure 49-2. Mechanisms underlying airflow limitation in chronic obstructive pulmonary disease. *(From NIH/NHLBI: Global Initiative for Chronic Obstructive Lung Disease. NHLBI/WHO Workshop Report 2001. Available at:* http://www.goldcopd.com/workshop.html *(accessed Sept. 8, 2008).)*

Pathogenesis of COPD

The pathologic changes in COPD are found in the large and small (<2 mm) airways and in the lung parenchyma[34,36] (Figure 49-2). In advanced stages, there are also changes in the pulmonary circulation, the heart, and the respiratory muscles. Alveolar hypoxia causes medial hypertrophy of vascular smooth muscle with extension of the muscularis layer into distal vessels that do not ordinarily contain smooth muscle. Intimal hyperplasia also occurs in advanced stages. These latter changes are associated with the development of pulmonary hypertension and its consequences—right ventricular hypertrophy and dilation. Loss of vascular bed also occurs with emphysema in association with the destructive alveolar processes. In some patients with advanced COPD, there is atrophy of diaphragmatic muscle, loss of skeletal muscle, and wasting of limb muscles.

Changes in the airways of smokers

Early structural changes have been described in otherwise healthy smokers even as young as 20 to 30 years old. The burden of gases and particles that are inhaled into the lungs results in inflammatory and immune responses. Inflammatory cells migrate into the epithelial layer including polymorphonuclear cells, eosinophils, macrophages, natural killer cells, and mast cells. Uncommitted B cells and CD4 and CD8 lymphocytes also participate in the inflammatory response.

Cigarette smokers have an increase in the number of neutrophils and macrophages. Macrophages likely play an important role in perpetuating the inflammatory process of COPD. They may release neutrophil chemotactic factors and proteolytic enzymes such as matrix metalloproteinases (MMPs) that damage the epithelial barrier. Neutrophils are also thought to be important in causing the tissue damage of COPD. They release a number of mediators including proteases, such as neutrophil elastase and MMPs; oxidants, such as the oxygen free radical H_2O_2; and toxic peptides, such as defensins. The repair process that ensues includes the secretion of antiproteases to regulate the proteolytic process. Although $CD4^+$ lymphocytes are found in the airways of atopic asthmatics, the T lymphocytes of patients with cigarette-induced COPD are $CD8^+$ cells. These cells are also thought to cause cell damage. Eosinophilic inflammation is a hallmark of asthma and not usually seen in chronic bronchitis. However, the number of tissue and sputum eosinophils is greatly increased during attacks of acute bronchitis. Bronchial biopsies from former smokers show similar inflammatory changes to the active smokers, suggesting that inflammation may persist in the airway once established.

Progression to COPD

Other structural changes in the airways of smokers include mucus hypersecretion, bronchiolar edema, smooth muscle hypertrophy, and peribronchiolar fibrosis. These changes result in narrowing of the small airways (<2 mm). As the inflammation and peribronchiolar fibrosis progress, lung function and the symptoms of COPD become progressively worse.[38]

In addition to the structural abnormalities seen in the small airways, there is also a loss of alveolar attachments to the airway perimeter and there is permanent enlargement of the gas-exchanging units of the lungs (acini).[36] This impairs elastic recoil and favors increased tortuosity and early closure of the small airways during expiration. The pathogenesis of COPD that targets the airways (chronic bronchitis) and lung parenchyma (emphysema) is thought to occur because of a complex interaction between extracellular signaling proteins, oxidative stress, and proteolytic digestion of connective tissue.

Smokers with chronic bronchitis produce larger amounts of sputum each day, averaging about 20 to 30 mL/day and even as high as 100 mL/day. This occurs as a result of an increase in the size and number of the submucosal glands and an increase in the number of goblet cells on the surface epithelium.

Pulmonary function testing in COPD

Early in the course of COPD, the expiratory flow-volume curve shows a scooped-out lower part of the expiratory limb as a result of abnormal flow at low lung volume. In later stages there is decreased expiratory flow at all lung volumes (see Figure 49-1). Nonuniform ventilation of the lungs is seen even in the earlier stages of COPD and this leads to low ventilation/perfusion ratios. This type of mismatch causes arterial hypoxemia. Lung and thoracic wall hyperinflation occur as a consequence of the loss of elastic recoil. Airway obstruction and hyperinflation, especially during exertion (dynamic hyperinflation), increases the work of breathing and contributes to the sensation of dyspnea.

Pulmonary function studies are important for the diagnosis and staging of COPD.[31,32] The FEV_1 has been shown to correlate with morbidity, mortality, and severity scoring on the basis of the degree of airflow obstruction. The GOLD guidelines include four stages based on the spirometric severity of airflow obstruction (Figure 49-3).

Natural history of COPD

Cigarette smoking is the agent causing COPD in at least 85% to 90% of cases. Other factors linked to the development of COPD include occupational or environmental exposures to dusts, gases, vapors or fumes,[39] exposure to biomass smoke, malnutrition, early life infections, increased airways responsiveness, and asthma.[30,31] As only 15% to 20% of heavy smokers will develop an accelerated decline of lung function over time and clinically evident COPD, a genetic predisposition is also an important factor. One genetic abnormality that has been known and well studied is α_1-antitrypsin (AAT) deficiency, which accounts for less than 1% of COPD in the United States. Cigarette smoking is the most

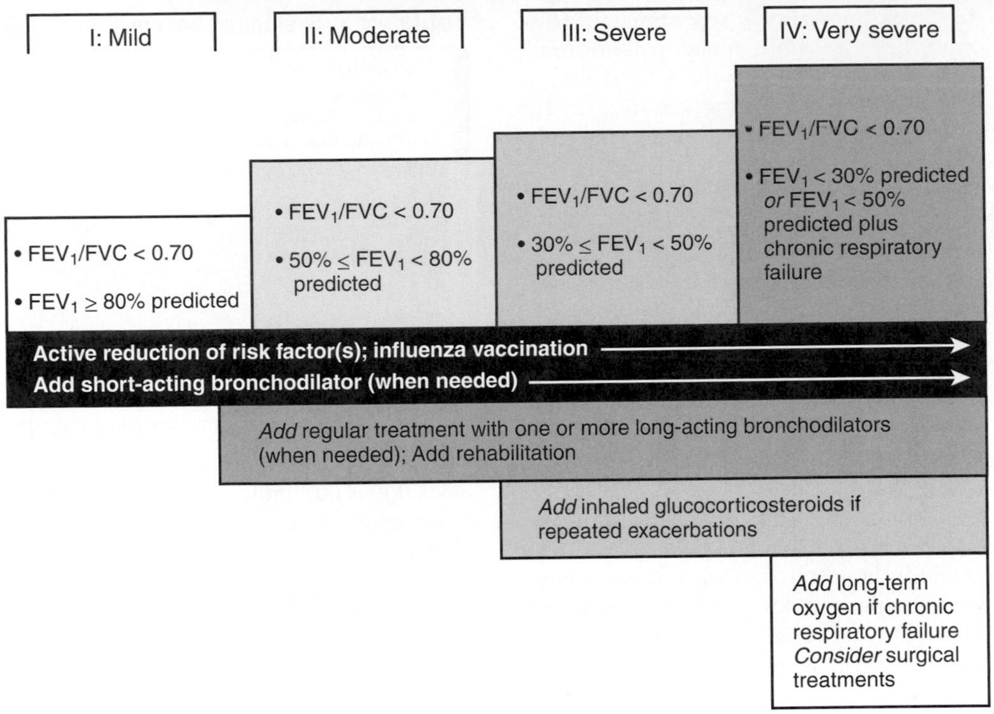

Figure 49-3. GOLD severity scale based on symptoms and lung function with treatment algorithm based on severity (accessed on Sept. 8, 2008). *(Adapted from Global Initiative for Chronic Obstructive Lung Disease [GOLD], www.goldcopd.org.)*

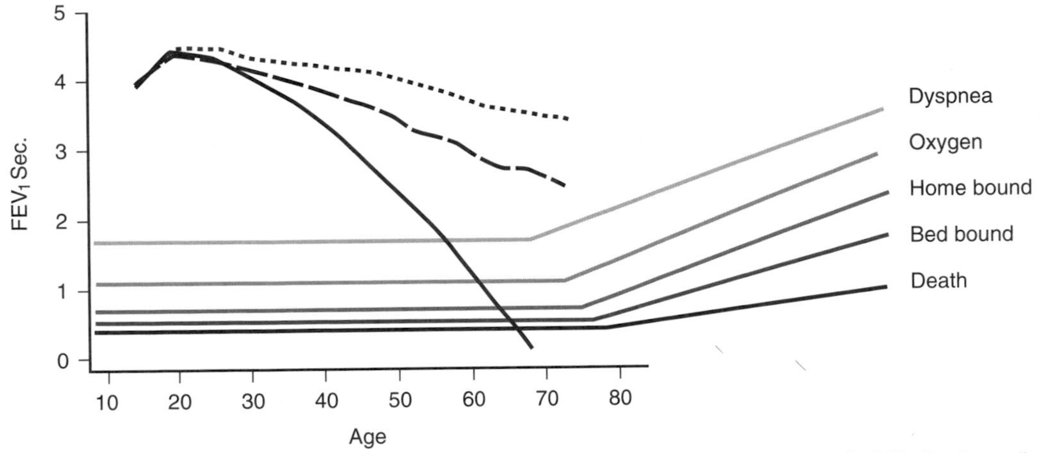

Figure 49-4. Natural history of COPD. A rapid decline in lung function (FEV_1) occurs over decades in the patient with COPD *(solid line)* leading to disability and death. This is compared with a slow decline in normal aging *(dotted line)*. The smoker who does not develop COPD has a greater decline than normal but does not become disabled *(dashed line)*. *(Adapted from Fletcher C, Peto R. BMJ 1977;1:1645–48.)*

important risk factor for the development of COPD in patients with AAT deficiency. Symptoms begin early in adult life in cigarette smokers. Patients with this deficiency who do not smoke may develop COPD; their age at onset of dyspnea is 48 to 54 years compared with 32 to 40 years in smokers. In older patients with COPD and no previous smoking history, especially those with a strong family history, a blood test to determine the level of AAT should be considered.

Patients who develop COPD have a prolonged preclinical period of approximately 20 to 40 years (Figure 49-4). During this asymptomatic period, there is deterioration of lung function in marked excess of the normal age-related decline. Nonsmokers, without respiratory disease, can expect to lose 25 to 30 mL of lung function per year after age 35. The rate of decline appears to accelerate slightly with aging, but sudden large irreversible falls are uncommon. Although nonsmokers lose FEV_1 slowly, they never develop significant airflow obstruction; this is also true of the nonsusceptible smokers. Susceptible smokers on the other hand develop varying degrees of airflow obstruction as they often demonstrate a decline in lung function of 60 mL or more per year. This ultimately causes exertional dyspnea when the FEV_1 is between 40% and 59% of its predicted value and becomes disabling when the FEV_1 declines by about 70%. Such an inexorable decline may lead to fatality. When the FEV_1

falls below 1 L, the 5-year mortality is approximately 50%. Smoking cessation in the susceptible smoker will not result in recovery of lost FEV_1, but will slow the rate of decline to similar rates of nonsmokers. Smoking cessation in the patient with early changes of COPD at age 45 can make the difference between a normal life span and premature death.

Clinical features of COPD

SYMPTOMS OF COPD

The symptoms that are associated with COPD are usually not present until the patient has been smoking a pack of cigarettes a day for at least 20 years.[30,31] The patient usually presents in the fifth decade with chronic cough often worsened after a viral respiratory infection. Dyspnea, the second major symptom, usually does not present until the sixth or seventh decade. Over the last several decades, as a result of an intense antismoking campaign, the rate of smoking in the United States has been reduced from about a third of the adult population to its current level of about 22%. Since there is a slow decline in lung function with normal aging, COPD patients who stopped smoking in midlife may only delay the onset of COPD symptoms until late in life. It is not unusual to see a former smoker with COPD present for the first time with symptoms at age 75 and beyond.

PHYSICAL EXAM AND LABORATORY TESTS

The signs of COPD are well known: slow and prolonged expiration, wheezing, chest wall hyperinflation, limited diaphragmatic motion on auscultation, distant breath sounds and heart sounds, and often coarse early inspiratory crackles. The accessory muscles of respiration may be in use and the patient may be using pursed-lip breathing. Signs of cor pulmonale include pedal edema, a tender congested liver, and neck vein distention. Cyanosis may be present, and asterixis that is associated with severe hypercapnia may be observed. The roentgenographic signs of COPD include a low flat diaphragm, an increased retrosternal airspace, and a tear-drop shaped heart. Pruning of the pulmonary arterial vessels and bullae are seen in emphysema. The high resolution CT scan has a much better sensitivity and specificity, but is not recommended for routine use.

COPD EXACERBATION

The slowly progressive course of COPD is often interrupted by a sudden change in symptoms and lung function requiring a change in management, including medication and sometimes hospital admission.[32] These acute respiratory illnesses or exacerbations are usually caused by viral or bacterial infections and are heralded by an increase in symptoms and associated with an increase in pulmonary and systemic signs of inflammation. Patients with mild and moderate stages of COPD may develop one to two exacerbations per year; those with more severe disease could possibly have many more. Risk factors for hospitalization include admissions for COPD in the previous year, a low FEV_1, under-prescription of long-term oxygen therapy, current smoking and systemic inflammation as evidenced by nonspecific markers of inflammation such as serum fibrinogen.[39,41] The exacerbations usually cause a modest decrease in lung function for up to 90 days. COPD exacerbations have been associated with a poor quality of life and an accelerated decline of airflow obstruction.

Table 49-7. Systemic Consequences of COPD

Cardiovascular disease
Osteoporosis
Metabolic disease (diabetes mellitus)
Gastrointestinal disease
Anorexia
Weight loss
Skeletal muscle dysfunction
Anemia of chronic disease
Generalized fatigue
Depression
Altered sleep
Cor pulmonale

SYSTEMIC INFLAMMATION AND COPD

There is growing evidence that the inflammatory response of COPD is not limited to the lungs.[33,42] There are a number of systemic consequences of the disease that are considered related to systemic inflammation (Table 49-7). Individuals with stable COPD have significantly raised blood levels of C-reactive protein (CRP), fibrinogen, TNF-α, endothelin-1, interleukin 6, and circulating leukocytes and vascular endothelial growth factor (VEGF), compared with normal. Elevated levels of inflammatory cytokines in the blood of COPD patients suggest a persistent level of systemic inflammation, possibly caused by a "spill over" from lung inflammation. This latter theory, however, has not been proven.

Management of COPD

Once the diagnosis of COPD is established, pulmonary function testing can be helpful to stage the disease. Pharmacologic intervention is offered according to disease severity and the patient's tolerance for specific drugs (see Figure 49-4). The goals of therapy are to induce bronchodilation, decrease airway inflammation, and improve mucociliary transport. The patient who still smokes should be encouraged to quit. Preventive therapy with a pneumococcal vaccine and a yearly influenza vaccine is recommended. Vaccination with the flu shot has been shown to result in 52% fewer hospitalizations for pneumonia and influenza in patients with COPD. Vaccinated patients also have fewer outpatient visits for respiratory symptoms. Current COPD guidelines are evidence-based and offer treatment algorithms.[30,31] Evidence-based medical reviews are also available to guide treatment of stable COPD[44] and COPD exacerbations.[45]

SMOKING CESSATION

Cigarette smoking compromises airway function: it damages airway epithelial cells, increases mucous viscosity, and slows mucociliary clearance. There is a greater bacterial adherence to oropharyngeal epithelial cells in smokers compared with nonsmokers. Smokers are prone to acute exacerbations of COPD. As a result, they show increased rates of unexpected office visits, use of emergency services, work absenteeism, and medication use. Smokers also show greater decline in lung function, worsening of respiratory symptoms, and lower quality of life scores than a comparable group of nonsmoking patients with COPD. Unfortunately most studies have shown that the presence of respiratory illness such as COPD is not a motivator for smoking cessation. Physician-delivered smoking cessation interventions can significantly increase smoking abstinence rates. Smoking cessation interventions for COPD include physician intervention, group smoking cessation programs, and pharmacologic therapy, which may be needed in highly dependent smokers who smoke a pack a day or more, require their first cigarette within 30 minutes of arising in the morning, and find it difficult refraining from smoking in places where it is forbidden. Therapy with nicotine replacement modalities, the antidepressant bupropion hydrochloride, and with varenicline (a partial agonist of nicotinic acetylcholine receptors) has been shown to be effective.

PHARMACOLOGIC THERAPY

Short-acting β_2-agonists achieve variable degrees of bronchodilation, relieve acute dyspnea, and improve exercise capacity. They have a rapid onset of action with duration of 4 to 6 hours. The use of these agents by metered dose inhaler as β_2-selective agents is safe when given three or four times a day. Higher doses may cause hypokalemia, cardiac arrhythmias, and reduced arterial oxygen tension. Long-acting β_2-agonists have a maximal effect comparable to the short-acting β_2-agonists but have a longer duration of action (12 hours or longer). Agents such as salmeterol and formoterol have been shown to improve symptoms and quality-of-life measures and reduce COPD exacerbations over time. They have a good safety profile with recommended doses and no tachyphylaxis with chronic use.[46] Occasional tremor is seen but it usually improves after several days of use. Nonbronchodilating effects, such as inflammatory mediator release, stimulation of mucociliary transport, and cytoprotection of the respiratory mucosa, have also been reported.[47]

The short-acting anticholinergic ipratropium offers bronchodilation and relief of symptoms for 4 to 6 hours. The long-acting anticholinergic tiotropium offers improved bronchodilation and has a duration of 24 hours. It has the advantage of a once-daily dosage. These agents have not been associated with tachyphylaxis. Tiotropium has been shown to reduce exacerbation rates and hospitalizations due to exacerbations.[48,49] The side effects are usually mild and include occasional dry mouth. Because of the anticholinergic effects, the drug should be used with caution in patients with narrow-angle glaucoma, myasthenia gravis, bladder neck obstruction, prostatic hyperplasia, and moderate to severe renal impairment. The use of a short-acting and long-acting anticholinergic together is discouraged. The combination of ipratropium and albuterol is available by metered dose inhaler or nebulizer. They provide a small additional benefit to either drug alone with no additional side effects.

The use of theophylline for COPD was very popular before other safer and more effective agents became available. This agent can produce small improvements in FEV_1, relieve symptoms, and improve exercise capacity with chronic use. It can be used safely in elderly adults when additional agents are needed for symptom relief.[50] Frequent adverse effects are seen even with therapeutic blood levels (nausea, diarrhea, headache, and irritability). Seizures and cardiac arrhythmias are considerably (10 to 15 times) more common in the elderly with toxic blood levels. Frequent close monitoring is mandatory to insure therapeutic blood levels when theophylline is used in the elderly.

Twenty to thirty percent of patients with COPD report improvement in symptoms if given oral steroid therapy. Responders have more eosinophils in induced sputum and bronchial biopsies and likely have concomitant asthma. Long-term treatment with oral corticosteroids is not recommended for patients with COPD. Treatment of hospitalized patients with an acute exacerbation of COPD results in fewer treatment failures and shorter hospital stays.[45] Two weeks of therapy is sufficient and longer treatment programs can be associated with more side effects. Complications of therapy include cataracts, osteoporosis, secondary infection, diabetes, and skin damage. Milder exacerbations of COPD can be managed with a short course of oral corticosteroids.

Inhaled corticosteroids have been shown to provide small but significant improvements in lung function, reduce exacerbation rates, and improve the quality-of-life indices. The benefits of inhaled corticosteroids are enhanced when coupled with long-acting β-agonist treatment. Combination agents are available with favorable effects like improved lung function and symptoms, fewer exacerbations, and better quality of life.[51] COPD practice guidelines recommend starting inhaled corticosteroids when the FEV_1 percent predicted is less than 50% (Stage III and IV) and the patient is having repeated exacerbations.

Mucoactive drugs are agents that can modify mucus production and secretion or can change the nature and composition of the mucus. Examples include expectorants that may induce cough or increase the volume of secretions and mucolytics that reduce the viscosity of mucus. There is little evidence that oral expectorants such as guaifenesin improve lung function or objective measures of well-being in COPD, although some patients do report subjective improvement. Guaifenesin is available without a prescription and has minimal side effects at recommended doses. Mucolytics such as acetylcysteine are not approved for this indication in the United States. The results of multiple trials favor the use of antibiotics for acute exacerbations of COPD that include worsening dyspnea, increased sputum volume, sputum viscosity, and purulence. There is no evidence to support prophylactic use.

Several controlled studies of oxygen use in COPD have been completed: oxygen verses no oxygen (Medical Research Council [MRC]) and continuous versus nocturnal oxygen (Nocturnal Oxygen Therapy Trial [NOTT]). In patients with hypoxemia and congestive heart failure, death rates are significantly lower and quality of life indices are improved when oxygen is chronically used. Patients who use oxygen for at least 15 hours per day have a significant fall in pulmonary artery pressures and an increase in cardiac output. Oxygen should be prescribed when: (1) the arterial PaO_2 is less than 55 mm Hg or SaO_2 is less than 88%; (2) PaO_2 is 56 to 59 mm Hg with ECG evidence of pulmonary hypertension, pedal edema, and/or secondary erythrocytosis. Long-term oxygen therapy does not improve survival in patients with moderate hypoxemia (PaO_2 56 to 65 mm Hg) or in patients with isolated nocturnal hypoxemia.

PULMONARY REHABILITATION

Pulmonary rehabilitation is a multidisciplinary program that attempts to return the patient to the highest functional capacity possible. Evidence supports the use of lower-extremity exercise training as it improves exercise tolerance. Upper-extremity strength and endurance training is also recommended. Pulmonary rehabilitation improves dyspnea, improves quality of life scores, and reduces the number of hospitalizations and days in the hospital; the effects on survival are not proven.[52]

Surgery for COPD

Lung volume reduction surgery (LVRS) has emerged as a treatment for far-advanced COPD due to emphysema.[53] It involves resection of functionless areas of emphysematous lung to improve lung elastic recoil in addition to lung and chest wall hyperinflation. Overall mortality with the procedure is less than 3% within 30 days of surgery and less than 6% within 90 days. In patients with very severe degrees of airflow obstruction (FEV_1<20% of predicted with evidence of homogeneous emphysema and/or very severe impairment in the diffusion capacity [<20% of predicted]), the rates are significantly higher and prohibitive. Significant surgery-related morbidity remains as a major concern when considering this approach. LVRS could be considered for patients with severe upper lobe predominant emphysema with significant impairment in baseline exercise capacity with potential overall mortality and morbidity benefit. Patients with homogeneous (nonupper lobe predominant disease) and high baseline exercise capacity should not be considered for this approach because of higher expected morbidity and mortality when compared with medical management alone. Emphysema patients within the spectrum between the two mentioned groups could have functional and symptomatic benefits from LVRS without overall mortality advantage. In appropriate candidates, improvement in the FEV_1, dyspnea scores, and distance walked on the 6-minute walk test were reported. Oxygen requirements can improve in responders. Resection of large bullae is occasionally beneficial. The best results occur when the bullae occupy more than one third of the hemithorax. Lung transplantation can be life-saving in end-stage disease but is not offered to those of advanced age. Several bronchoscopic approaches with various goals, including volume reduction, improvement in dynamic hyperinflation, redistribution of ventilation from the emphysematous areas to the relatively spared areas, improving ventilation/perfusion ratio, and influencing collateral ventilation, are undergoing clinical trials with promising early results.

Weight loss and malnutrition

Malnutrition occurs in one quarter to one third of patients with moderate to severe COPD and is an independent risk factor for mortality.[54] Both fat mass and fat-free mass are depleted; the latter caused by depressed protein synthesis. It is believed that weight loss, and, particularly, skeletal muscle mass loss, is associated with a systemic inflammatory response in malnourished patients with COPD as the proinflammatory cytokines IL-6 and TNF-α have been shown to be elevated. Recent studies have shown that leptin, an adipocyte-derived hormone involved in the control of body weight, is decreased in patients with COPD. Serum leptin levels have been correlated with TNF-α levels, thus creating a link between nutritional status and systemic inflammation in COPD. Resting energy expenditure is elevated and contributes to the negative energy balance. Nutritional supplements alone do not reverse the loss but some early evidence suggests that it may when coupled with a pulmonary rehabilitation programs.

Prognosis of COPD

Traditionally, the FEV_1 has been used as the main indicator of clinical outcomes including mortality in COPD. A composite of predictors, the body-mass index, the degree of airflow obstruction, the degree of dyspnea, and a measure of exercise capacity offer an index of severity, the BODE index, that offers a superior grading system for COPD mortality.[55] The two-year mortality among patients with severe COPD (FEV_1 in the range of 27%) that received medical or surgical treatment was almost 26% for both groups in the National Emphysema Treatment Trial (NETT).[53]

Differential diagnosis of asthma and COPD

A number of studies have shown that symptoms of obstructive lung disease, whether asthma or COPD, are underreported by elderly patients and underdiagnosed or misdiagnosed by their physicians. Several factors contribute to this problem. The symptoms of these two diseases are similar to other diseases seen in this age group. The hallmark symptoms of asthma and COPD, including shortness of breath, wheezing, and cough, are nonspecific in the elderly and are mimicked by and often confused with such diseases as congestive heart failure, chronic aspiration, gastroesophageal reflux (GERD), and upper airway obstruction.

Upper airway obstruction (UAO) can occur at any level of the central airways and can involve the extrathoracic portion of the airway above the thoracic inlet or the intrathoracic portion, with dynamic (functional) or anatomical (fixed) obstruction. The integrity and tone of the upper airway are important to maintain a functional lumen. The loss of airway tone (e.g., weakness of the airway structure or loss of muscle tone), extrinsic compression, or intraluminal pathology can result in dynamic obstruction that occurs when the functional lumen of the upper airway is compromised in response to changes in the transmural pressures during inspiration and/or expiration. Fixed obstruction is usually not responsive to changes in the transmural pressures. The incidence of UAO in the elderly is unknown. However, this appears to be increasingly recognized because of the higher incidence of malignancy and airway instrumentation (e.g., endotracheal intubation and tracheostomy) in this age group, in addition to advances in thoracic imaging, physiologic evaluation, and endoscopic techniques.[56,57]

The signs and symptoms of UAO are usually nonspecific, develop after significant obstruction, and considerably overlap with those of the more common small airway disorders (COPD and asthma). This leads to significant delays in the appropriate diagnosis and management. UAO symptoms can be exacerbated by activity that is also nonspecific. Symptoms usually develop with activity when the airway lumen is compromised to the range of 8 mm, whereas dyspnea at rest and stridor develop when the airway lumen is in the range of 5 mm. Positional exacerbation of symptoms, especially in the supine position with sleep disordered breathing, is one of the clues to the diagnosis of UAO. Thus daytime sleepiness and fatigue can be a prominent feature. Chronic respiratory failure and cor pulmonale can also develop. Additional signs and symptoms related to the specific UAO cause (e.g., hemoptysis and hoarseness) can suggest a diagnosis other than small airway disease. The configuration of the

Table 49-8. An Overview of the Potential Causes of Upper Airway Obstruction

- Malignancy:
  - Primary head and neck cancer
  - Primary tracheal malignancies
  - Metastatic malignancy to the airway
  - Direct extension to the airway
- Tracheomalacia (and tracheobronchomalacia):
  - Localized
  - Diffuse

  Other classification:
  - Saber-sheath trachea (lateral): in patients with COPD
  - Crescent (anteroposterior)
- Laryngeal and tracheal stenosis:
  - Endotracheal intubation
  - Tracheostomy
  - Airway instrumentation
  - Posttraumatic
  - Inhalational injuries
  - Radiation therapy
  - Infection
  - Inflammatory and postinflammatory:
    - Wegener's granulomatosis
    - Relapsing polychondritis
    - Polyarteritis
    - Sarcoidosis
    - Scleroderma
    - Primary or secondary amyloidosis
    - Inflammatory bowel disease
    - Idiopathic progressive subglottic stenosis
- Infection:
  - Deep cervical space infections
  - Supraglottitis
  - Laryngotracheobronchitis
  - Bacterial tracheitis
  - Tuberculosis
  - Other infections (e.g., histoplasmosis, papillomatosis, rhinoscleroma)
- Neuromuscular disorders:
  - Vocal cord paralysis or paresis
  - Bulbar muscle dysfunction
  - Vocal cord dysfunction
- Foreign body aspiration
- Trauma:
  - Blunt trauma
  - Penetrating injuries
  - Postintubation (e.g., stenosis, vocal cord paralysis, contact granuloma, arytenoid dislocation)
  - Inhalational injuries
- Extrinsic compression:
  - Mediastinal masses and adenopathy
  - Esophageal pathology
  - Thyromegaly
  - Cervical osteophytes
  - Parathyroid cysts
  - Fibrosing mediastinitis
  - Laryngoceles
  - Saccular cysts
  - Hematomas
  - Aneurysms and pseudoaneurysms
  - Vascular anomalies
- Other causes:
  - Tracheobronchopathia osteochondroplastica
  - Laryngo-pharyngeal reflux; can contribute to the symptoms and severity of UAO
  - Postpneumonectomy syndrome
  - Mucous balls (with transtracheal oxygen catheters)

KEY POINTS
Asthma and Chronic Obstructive Pulmonary Disease

- Asthma and COPD are common disorders associated with significant morbidity and mortality in the elderly.
- The NAEPP and GOLD guidelines are valuable in the management of asthma and COPD in the elderly.
- Recognizing the role of inflammation in the pathogenesis of asthma and COPD is important in the management of both disorders.
- COPD is a systemic disease associated with extrapulmonary manifestations, including muscle wasting and systemic inflammatory response.
- The symptoms and signs of airway disease in the elderly can be nonspecific and overlap considerably with other common disorders in this age group.
- Upper airway obstruction in the elderly can mimic asthma and COPD. Special vigilance is necessary to diagnose upper airway obstruction in the elderly.

flow volume loops can be helpful to diagnose upper airway obstruction (see Figure 49-2).

UAO can be related to a variety of airway and systemic disorders.[58,59] Common causes of UAO include malignancy, infection, inflammatory disorders, trauma, and extrinsic compression related to enlargement or pathology of adjacent structures. It appears that malignancy and benign strictures related to airway interventions are becoming more prevalent. Table 49-8 provides an overview of the potential causes of UAO in the elderly.

For a complete list of references, please visit online only at www.expertconsult.com

CHAPTER 50

Nonobstructive Lung Disease and Thoracic Tumors

Katie Pink
Ben Hope-Gill

Respiratory disease is a major cause of morbidity and mortality, affecting 1 in 10 of the population over 65 years old.[1] The presentation and management of respiratory disease often differs in the elderly and this chapter aims to provide some insight into these differences while reviewing current evidence.

RESPIRATORY INFECTIONS

Respiratory infection is common in the elderly. This is explained by a number of factors. A decline in lung function and structural changes to the chest wall and muscles result in a loss of chest wall compliance.[2] In addition, mucociliary function declines with age and the immune system can be depressed. With increasing age there is an increase in oropharyngeal colonisation with potential respiratory pathogens as well as an increased incidence of microaspiration. Comorbid conditions resulting in dysphagia or a reduced conscious level may increase the risk of aspiration.[3] Malnutrition, in particular hypoalbuminaemia, has also been associated with an increased risk of infection in the elderly.[4] Finally, institutionalisation leads to increased exposure to respiratory pathogens.

INFLUENZA

Influenza tends to occur in seasonal epidemics each winter. In the United States, influenza causes 20,000 to 40,000 deaths per year. Although 60% of cases of influenza occur in adults less than 65 years old, more than 80% of deaths as a result of seasonal influenza occur in adults aged over 65.[5–7] The elderly are more likely to be hospitalized[8] and to experience significant functional decline.[9] Complications such as infective bronchitis and secondary bacterial pneumonia also occur more frequently in the elderly, most commonly because of *Staphylococcus aureus* and *Streptococcus pneumoniae* infection.[10] In addition, cerebrovascular and cardiovascular deaths may be precipitated by influenza infection.[11]

Vaccination

National guidelines in the United Kingdom recommend influenza vaccination for all adults aged over 65 years and those in long-term care. Influenza vaccination is effective in long-term care facilities. It has been shown to prevent 45% of pneumonia episodes and reduce hospital admissions and influenza-related deaths.[12] In one study the vaccine was less effective in elderly populations living in the community; however, a 25% reduction in the proportion of people hospitalized from influenza or related illness was achieved.[12] There is some evidence that vaccination of health care workers in long-term care institutions is also associated with a reduction in influenza-related mortality among patients.[13] However, a recent Cochrane review concluded that further studies were required.[12,14]

In the United States national vaccination uptake is only 65%[15] and in the United Kingdom and Europe only a minority of those eligible for vaccination receive it.[16,17] Possible explanations include patient concerns regarding side effects, frustration that previous vaccination has not prevented influenza-like illness, and the deferment of vaccination by doctors when patients have a mild upper respiratory tract infection.[15]

Treatment

Neuraminidase inhibitors (zanamivir, oseltamivir) are effective at preventing and treating influenza.[18] These agents must be taken within 48 hours of the onset of symptoms. United Kingdom guidelines recommend their use for at-risk groups, including adults aged over 65 years.[19] Clinical trials have shown that these agents reduce symptom duration by 1 to 2 days and decrease hospitalization and death rates in the elderly.[18,20,21] The neuraminidase inhibitors are well tolerated and the safety profile among the elderly is similar to that in younger adults. The most common adverse effects are nausea, vomiting, and abdominal pain. Zanamivir may cause bronchospasm.[22] Amantadine and rimantadine are only effective against influenza A and are associated with toxic side effects and with rapid emergence of drug-resistant variants.[22,23] Routine use of these agents is not recommended.[19,23]

In the United Kingdom the National Institute for Clinical Excellence (NICE) guidelines recommend that postexposure prophylaxis with oseltamivir is given to all adults living in residential care facilities, regardless of vaccination status. When given within 48 hours, this has been shown to reduce influenza rates by 92%.[24] In the community setting, postexposure prophylaxis is only recommended to high-risk adults (including those over 65 years) if they have not been vaccinated or if the circulating strain of influenza is known to be different than the vaccination strain. Amantadine is not recommended for postexposure prophylaxis.[25]

PNEUMONIA

Community-acquired pneumonia has an incidence of 5 to 11/1000 adult population.[3,26,27] The incidence is higher in the elderly, with those over 75 having six times greater risk compared with those less than 60 years.[27–30] Older adults in residential care are particularly vulnerable.[3,31] This is largely explained by the increase in comorbidities in this population. Chronic obstructive pulmonary disease (COPD), diabetes, heart failure, malnutrition, malignancy, and dysphagia are all risk factors for pneumonia in the elderly.[3,32] Mortality is 5.7% to 14% and increases with age. In the United States lower respiratory tract infection is the eighth leading cause of death.[26,33–36]

The most common causative organism is *S. pneumoniae*. Other pathogens include *Haemophilus influenzae*, viruses, gram-negative bacilli and *S. aureus*. In the elderly infections with "atypical" organisms, such as *Mycoplasma* and *Legionella*, are less common.[33,34] Infection with gram-negative bacilli and anaerobic organisms may occur after aspiration.[3,37] There is no evidence that the pathogens associated with nursing home–acquired pneumonia are different from other older adults in the United Kingdom, although studies in

Table 50-1. Pneumonia Severity Prediction; CURB-65 Score

- Confusion of new onset. (or worsening of existing state for those with background cognitive impairment)
- Serum urea >7 mmol/L
- Respiratory rate ≥ 30/min
- Blood pressure (systolic BP <90 mm Hg or diastolic BP ≤ 60 mm Hg)
- Age ≥ 65 years

A score is awarded for each variable present. A score ≥ 3 represents severe pneumonia.

North America have reported an increased incidence of gram-negative bacilli and *S. aureus*.[38–40]

Presentation in the elderly is frequently nonspecific and the classic symptoms and signs of pneumonia may not be present. Confusion, lethargy, anorexia, and falls are common presenting symptoms.[3] For example, a chest x-ray will demonstrate pneumonia in nearly a quarter of elderly patients having acute confusion and no clinical signs.[41] Fever is less likely to be present in elderly patients.[3,26,42] An important clinical sign in the elderly is the presence of tachypnea.[42]

A number of scoring systems can be used to assess severity in community-acquired pneumonia, including the Pneumonia Severity Index and the CURB-65 score.[43,44] Current BTS[26,45] and ATS[46] guidelines recommend the use of the CURB-65 score (Table 50-1) because of its simplicity and strong predictive power for severe pneumonia, particularly in the elderly. Those patients with a low score (0 to 2) have a low mortality risk and may be suitable for outpatient treatment with oral antibiotics.[44] However, in the elderly this may not be appropriate because of comorbidities and psychosocial concerns.

Management

The investigation and management of community-acquired pneumonia is discussed in guidelines published by both the British and the American Thoracic Societies.[26,45,46] Initial empirical treatment is with broad-spectrum antibiotic therapy with activity against *Pneumococcus* and "atypical" organisms. Current recommendations suggest the combination of β-lactam plus macrolide antibiotics for patients requiring admission to hospital. An alternative in penicillin-allergic patients is a fluoroquinolone with enhanced pneumococcal activity, such as levofloxacin.[45] Local antibiotic resistance patterns will need to be taken into account. Intravenous antibiotic therapy is only required in severe pneumonia or in patients who are unable to take oral preparations. In the elderly antibiotic associated colitis and *Clostridium difficile* infection is a particular concern with intravenous antibiotics.[47–49] There is evidence that in severe pneumonia delay in the administration of the first antibiotic is associated with increased mortality.[50–52]

Following an episode of pneumonia it is important to ensure that radiologic changes resolve, particularly in the elderly and in smokers who are at increased risk of an underlying malignancy. Radiologic clearance is slower in the elderly.[26,34]

Nosocomial pneumonia

The incidence of hospital-acquired pneumonia increases significantly with age[53] and the mortality rate can be 50%.[3] Treatment regimes should cover gram-negative anaerobic bacteria and *Pseudomonas* sp. Methicillin-resistant *S. aureus* (MRSA) should also be considered.

Vaccination

Polysaccharide pneumococcal vaccination is recommended for all adults over 65 years.[26,46] There is no need for reimmunization. A recent meta-analysis concluded that there was insufficient evidence to support the routine use of pneumococcal vaccination to prevent all-cause pneumonia or mortality.[54] However, vaccination did prevent invasive pneumococcal disease in the elderly.

TUBERCULOSIS

The incidence of tuberculosis is now declining in the Western world, although it continues to rise in Africa because of the HIV epidemic. WHO surveillance data from 2006 showed an incidence of 4 cases/100,000 population in the United States and 15 cases/100,000 population in the United Kingdom.[55] In those born in either the United Kingdom or the United States, the incidence of active TB increases with age, with a doubling of the incidence in adults over 80 years old.[56] The reason for this is multifactorial. Most cases of TB in the elderly represent reactivation of previous disease.[56] This may be precipitated by an age-related reduction in cell-mediated immunity or secondary to other factors such as malnutrition, alcoholism, cancer, diabetes mellitus, HIV infection, and treatment with corticosteroids.[2]

TB is particularly common among care home residents in the United States[57] with the incidence of active TB being two to three times higher than in the community-dwelling elderly[58,59] because of reactivation of disease and institutional outbreaks.[60]

Presentation

Presentation in the elderly may be insidious and nonspecific; weight loss, weakness, or a change in cognitive function may be the only manifestation.[2,61] Dyspnea is often present, whereas hemoptysis and fevers are observed less frequently in the elderly.[57] It is important to consider TB if a patient has a cough or pneumonia that incompletely responds to conventional treatment.

The chest radiographic changes of TB are similar in all age groups although in the elderly there is a greater prevalence of mid and lower zone shadowing.[2] In addition, cavitating disease is less common.[57] Miliary TB is likely in older adults, although the diagnosis is frequently missed.[2] The presence of radiographic manifestations of previous TB infection in an elderly patient with nonspecific infective symptoms should alert physicians to exclude reactivation. Extrapulmonary TB is uncommon and is often difficult to diagnose. Sites involved include the genitourinary tract, the central nervous system, the lymphatics, and bone. Extrapulmonary TB is more common in children and the elderly.[62]

Investigation

Pulmonary TB is usually diagnosed by culturing *Mycobacterium tuberculosis* from sputum. Guidelines suggest that three sputum samples should be sent for culture.[63] In elderly patients it may be difficult to obtain spontaneous sputum samples, and sputum induction or bronchoscopy with bronchial washings may be required. The presence of acid-fast bacilli (AFB) on Ziehl-Neelsen staining (smear positive) suggests the diagnosis; however, *Mycobacterium tuberculosis* can take up to 6 weeks to be cultured using conventional techniques. It is important to remember that AFB smear positivity alone does not distinguish *M. tuberculosis* from nontuberculous mycobacterial infection (NTM). Rapid culture techniques, including polymerase chain reaction (PCR) or gene probe analyses allow earlier diagnosis. Once a patient is diagnosed with TB, consideration should be given to HIV testing.

Patients with suspected TB are usually investigated as outpatients; however, smear-positive elderly care home residents may benefit from isolation to prevent transmission.[59] If admitted to the hospital, patients should be isolated until their sputum status is known. If multidrug-resistant tuberculosis (MDR-TB) is suspected, patients should be managed in a negative air pressure room. Patients who are smear-positive need to remain isolated until they have completed 2 weeks of antituberculous treatment.[59,63]

Tuberculin skin test

The tuberculin skin test measures cell-mediated immunity against TB. It is positive in both active and latent disease and also individuals that have received BCG immunization. False negatives can occur in immunocompromised patients because of anergy. Anergy is more prevalent among the elderly because of a decline in cellular immunity, and the value of the tuberculin skin test is therefore reduced.[56] It is mainly used in the diagnosis of latent TB.

Gamma interferon tests

Gamma interferon tests are a recent development. A blood test can detect tuberculosis infection by measuring interferon-gamma release from T cells in response to antigens that are highly specific to *M. tuberculosis*, but are absent from BCG vaccine. In the United Kingdom they are primarily used to confirm the diagnosis of latent TB in the presence of a positive tuberculin skin test.[63] It is likely that their role will increase in the future.

Management

Recommendations for antituberculous therapy do not differ in the elderly. Initial empirical therapy should consist of a four-drug regimen for 2 months (rifampicin, isoniazid, pyrazinamide, ethambutol), followed by a two-drug regimen for 4 months (rifampicin and isoniazid). Extrapulmonary TB is treated in the same way, with the exception of TB meningitis, which requires 12 months' treatment.[63] Directly observed therapy may be useful in selected individuals who are at risk of poor compliance. Contact tracing is an important aspect of management and current recommendations are available in national and international guidelines.[63]

Multidrug-resistant TB (resistance to rifampicin and isoniazid) is uncommon in the elderly population at present in the United Kingdom and United States. This is probably because active TB in the elderly usually results from reactivation of latent infection that was acquired when there was no effective antituberculous chemotherapy.[56]

Drug toxicity and intolerance is more common in the elderly. Older adults are more likely to be coprescribed other medication and this increases the likelihood of drug interactions. Rifampicin in particular may reduce the levels of many medications through induction of the cytochrome P450 system. The use of isoniazid has been associated with increased levels of some anticonvulsants and benzodiazepines.[60]

Rifampicin, isoniazid, and pyrazinamide are all associated with gastrointestinal side effects and hepatotoxicity. Hepatic toxicity is increased in elderly patients.[64] Ethambutol can cause a loss of visual acuity and color discrimination and close monitoring is required in elderly patients whose visual acuity may already be impaired. Isoniazid can cause peripheral neuropathy, particularly in patients with coexisting renal failure. This can be prevented by pyridoxine. Finally, rifampicin may cause bodily fluids to become discolored orange.

Latent TB

Latent TB is defined as a positive tuberculin skin test, with a normal CXR and no symptoms of TB. Individuals who are identified as having latent TB through contact screening should be offered chemoprophylaxis. In the United States all residents of care homes are screened for latent TB on admission. Those with latent TB are treated with chemoprophylaxis. Treatment regimens comprise either isoniazid alone for 6 months or isoniazid and rifampicin combined for 3 months.[59]

Prognosis

Tuberculosis-related deaths are more common in the elderly. In 2004 in the United Kingdom there were 328 deaths from active TB, 68% of which occurred in adults aged over 65 years.[1] Many elderly patients will have long-term sequelae from tuberculous infection. Pulmonary fibrosis is a recognized complication as is pleural thickening and restrictive lung disease from pleural infection. Historical surgical techniques can also lead to chest wall deformities.

NONTUBERCULOUS MYCOBACTERIAL INFECTION

Pulmonary infection with nontuberculous mycobacteria has become increasingly recognized in the elderly population over recent years.[65] Predisposing factors include chronic lung diseases, such as COPD and bronchiectasis, along with immunosuppression, particularly HIV infection. Clinical and radiologic features are similar to pulmonary tuberculosis. Treatment in the elderly can be difficult because of drug intolerance. Guidelines on the diagnosis and treatment of nontuberculous mycobacteria have been published by both the British and the American Thoracic Societies.[66,67]

BRONCHIECTASIS

Bronchiectasis is characterized by the permanent dilation of bronchi, with chronic airway inflammation and excess sputum production. Bronchiectasis is a relatively rare condition affecting 1 to 2/100,000. A Finnish study suggested a prevalence of 39 cases per million population rising to 104 cases per million in those over 65.[68] However, the advent of high-resolution computed tomography (HRCT) scanning means milder forms of bronchiectasis are now being identified.

In the elderly population bronchiectasis is often a sequela of childhood infections such as pertussis, measles, tuberculosis, and severe pneumonia.[69] Bronchiectasis is increasingly being recognized as a complication of COPD. A causative

Table 50-2. Causes and Investigation of Bronchiectasis

All-Age Causes of Bronchiectasis	(% prevalence)
Idiopathic	(53%)
Postinfectious	(29%)
Allergic bronchopulmonary aspergillosis	(11%)
Immune deficiency	
- Total humoral	(11%)
- Total neutrophil function	(1%)
Rheumatoid arthritis	(4%)
Ulcerative colitis	(2%)
Ciliary dysfunction	(3%)
Young syndrome	(5%)
Cystic fibrosis	(3%)
Aspiration/gastroesophageal reflux	(4%)
Panbronchiolitis	(<1%)
Congenital	(<1%)
Investigation of Bronchiectasis	
HRCT	
Spirometry with bronchodilator reversibility	
Sputum culture and AFB culture	
Total IgE, *Aspergillus* specific IgE and IgG	
Serum Igs	
Antipneumococcal antibody titers	
Rheumatoid factor	
CF genotype, sweat test	
Serum α_1-antitrypsin levels	

Adapted from Pasteur MC et al. Am J Respir Crit Care Med 2000;162:1277–84.

Table 50-3. Causes of Unilateral Pleural Effusion

Transudative Effusions	Exudative Effusions
Very Common	Common
- Left ventricular failure	- Malignancy
- Liver cirrhosis	- Parapneumonic effusion
- Hypoalbuminemia	
- Peritoneal dialysis	Less common
	- Pulmonary infarction
Less common	- Rheumatoid arthritis
- Hypothyroidism	- Autoimmune disease
- Nephrotic syndrome	- Benign asbestos effusion
- Mitral stenosis	- Pancreatitis
- Pulmonary embolus	- Post-MI syndrome
Rare	Rare
- Constrictive pericarditis	- Yellow nail syndrome
- Urinothorax	- Drugs
- Superior vena cava obstruction	- Fungal infections

factor cannot be identified in many cases and these are termed idiopathic bronchiectasis. Causes and investigation of bronchiectasis are outlined in Table 50-2.

Management

The aims of treatment are to reduce symptoms, promptly treat exacerbations, and prevent disease progression. A multidisciplinary approach with input from physiotherapists, respiratory nurses, and dietitians is particularly important for elderly patients. Bronchodilators are effective in treating associated airflow obstruction and mucolytics are useful to aid sputum clearance.[70] Daily physiotherapy with postural drainage or cough augmentation is important, particularly during exacerbations. Inhaled corticosteroids may be useful in improving lung function and reducing exacerbation infrequency.[71,72] Surgery remains an option for selected patients with localized disease or those with troublesome hemoptysis.

Table 50-4. Light's Criteria for Classification of Unilateral Pleural Effusion

The pleural fluid is an exudate if one or both of the following criteria are met:
Pleural fluid protein divided by serum protein >0.5
Pleural fluid LDH divided by serum LDH >0.6

Acute exacerbations should be treated promptly with antibiotics. Regular oral or nebulized antibiotics may be necessary for those individuals who have frequent exacerbations. Azithromycin twice weekly has anti-inflammatory and antimicrobial properties and has shown promise in reducing exacerbation frequency in bronchiectasis.[73] The results of microbiologic investigations may be difficult to interpret because most patients are chronically colonized by a variety of organisms, most commonly *H. influenzae*. *Pseudomonas aeruginosa* infection is often difficult to treat and may require more prolonged courses of combination intravenous antibiotics.[72]

PLEURAL EFFUSION

The investigation and management of pleural effusions are summarized in guidelines from the British Thoracic Society and are beyond the scope of this chapter.[73] Investigation in the elderly does not differ from younger individuals. A diagnostic pleural tap will differentiate exudative from transudative effusions and will often ascertain the cause (Table 50-3). Light's criteria should be used to classify effusions with pleural fluid total protein content between 25 and 35 g/dL, particularly in the elderly in whom a single pleural fluid protein value is less reliable (Table 50-4). Other parameters that may be diagnostically useful include pleural fluid cytology, culture and sensitivity, glucose, pH and cell profile, depending upon the clinical scenario.[74] If the cause of an exudative effusion remains unclear after pleural fluid analysis, a CT scan of the thorax is advised. This is most useful if performed before drainage of the effusion. If diagnostic uncertainty still remains following a CT scan, then medical thoracoscopy should be considered. Thoracoscopy is more sensitive than the Abram's blind pleural biopsy and is well tolerated in all ages. It is a useful diagnostic technique, allowing direct visualization of the pleura and has the added advantage of offering fluid drainage and in a single procedure.[73]

PNEUMOTHORAX

The incidence of pneumothorax in the United Kingdom is 24/100,000 per year for men and 9.8/100,000 per year for women. There is a biphasic age distribution with peaks seen in the 20 to 24 and 80 to 84 year age groups[75] and is attributed to primary and secondary spontaneous pneumothorax, respectively. Elderly patients tend to have secondary pneumothorax related to underlying chronic lung disease, most commonly COPD.

Pneumothorax in the elderly usually presents with acute dyspnea, which is often out of proportion to the size of the pneumothorax. Pleuritic chest pain occurs less frequently than in younger patients.[76] The diagnosis is usually confirmed on a chest radiograph; however, in rare cases a CT scan of the thorax may be necessary to differentiate a pneumothorax from complex bullous lung disease.[77]

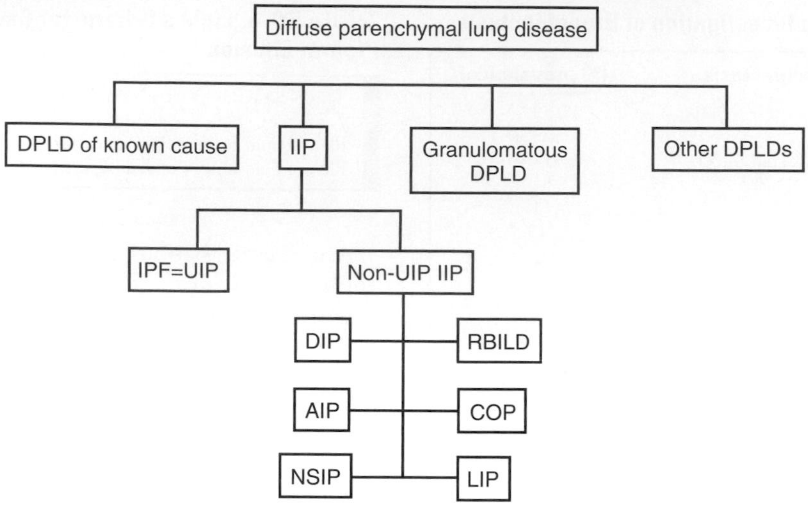

Figure 50-1. Classification of diffuse parenchymal lung disease. (*IIP,* idiopathic interstitial pneumonia; *UIP,* usual interstitial pneumonia; *DIP,* desquamative interstitial pneumonia; *AIP,* acute interstitial pneumonia; *RBILD,* respiratory bronchiolitis associated ILD; *NSIP,* nonspecific interstitial pneumonia; *COP,* cryptogenic organizing pneumonia; *LIP,* lymphocytic interstitial pneumonia.)

The treatment of secondary pneumothorax in the elderly involves hospital admission and intercostal drain insertion. Simple aspiration is unlikely to succeed and is not recommended.[77] Small asymptomatic pneumothoraces (<1 cm) can be managed by close observation.

Indications for surgical intervention include persistent air leak, second ipsilateral pneumothorax, and first contralateral pneumothorax. The aims of surgery are to resect or suture the bleb that caused the pneumothorax and to perform pleurodesis to prevent recurrence. Thoracoscopy and VATS (video-assisted thoracic surgery) can be performed safely in the elderly population with a low morbidity and mortality.[78,79] In those patients who are either unable or unwilling to undergo surgery, chemical pleurodesis can be attempted; however, recurrence rates are high with this approach.[77]

DIFFUSE PARENCHYMAL LUNG DISEASE

Diffuse parenchymal lung disease (DPLD) is a term used to describe a heterogeneous group of disorders characterized by damage to the lung parenchyma by varying patterns of inflammation and fibrosis.[80] The most important distinction among the idiopathic pneumonias is between idiopathic pulmonary fibrosis (IPF) and the other interstitial pneumonias.[80] Figure 50-1 outlines the current classification system.

The diagnosis of DPLD is complex and elderly patients with suspicious features should be referred for a specialist respiratory opinion. Clinical, radiologic, and pathologic features frequently overlap, making accurate diagnosis difficult. Therefore diagnosis should be undertaken in the context of a multidisciplinary team meeting comprising respiratory clinicians, thoracic radiologists, and pathologists with expertise in the evaluation of DPLDs. The diagnostic process requires a comprehensive clinical and physiologic evaluation followed by HRCT scanning in most cases. Surgical biopsy is recommended if clinical or radiologic features are not typical and preclude accurate diagnosis. Surgical lung biopsy is well tolerated; however, specific studies in the elderly are lacking.[81] Video-assisted thoracoscopic biopsy is increasingly being performed in place of open lung biopsy. Transbronchial biopsy is less invasive although, with the exception of sarcoidosis, samples are usually nondiagnostic. A history of systemic involvement (eye, joint, skin) or the presence of serum auto-antibodies may suggest an underlying connective tissue disorder. It is particularly important to distinguish UIP from other idiopathic interstitial pneumonias (IIP) because survival is significantly worse in this condition.[82] In addition, these other IIPs have a better response to immunosuppressive therapy.

IDIOPATHIC PULMONARY FIBROSIS

Idiopathic pulmonary fibrosis (previously termed cryptogenic fibrosing alveolitis) is the commonest of the idiopathic interstitial pneumonias. The diagnosis requires either a radiologic or pathologic diagnosis of usual interstitial pneumonia (UIP). The prevalence of IPF is estimated to be between 4/100,000 for persons aged 18 to 34 to 227/100,000 for those 75 years or older.[83] It is therefore a disease of the elderly with the age at symptom onset usually greater than 50 years.

Patients typically have progressive breathlessness and an irritating dry cough. Clinical examination will reveal digital clubbing in 25% to 50% of patients and fine end-inspiratory crackles, usually in a posterobasal distribution, on auscultation of the chest.[80,84] Lung function tests typically show a restrictive deficit with a reduction in vital capacity, total lung capacity, and transfer factor. Chest radiograph changes include reticulonodular shadowing with reduced lung volumes. High resolution computed tomography scan appearance is pivotal to establishing the diagnosis. Typical HRCT features of UIP include subpleural reticulation with honeycombing and traction bronchiectasis with basal predominance. Surgical lung biopsy is not required in patients with typical clinical and radiologic features of UIP, but should be considered in the presence of atypical features.[80]

The prognosis in UIP is poor. Median survival from diagnosis is less than 3 years.[80] However, the course of the disease can be highly variable in individual patients, with some declining rapidly whereas others remain stable.

Management

There is no good evidence that any treatment alters the course of idiopathic pulmonary fibrosis. Corticosteroids have traditionally been the mainstay of treatment; however, there have been no controlled trials comparing them to placebo, and no data to show that they improve either survival or quality of life.[85,86] Previous studies suggesting a favorable response to steroid treatment included patients with conditions other than UIP that are associated with a better treatment response and prognosis (e.g., nonspecific interstitial pneumonia). Significant adverse effects with oral corticosteroids are more prevalent in the elderly.[87]

Immunosuppressant therapy, in particular azathioprine, has been used in combination with corticosteroids in idiopathic pulmonary fibrosis. However, a recent meta-analysis concluded that there was little evidence to justify their use.[88] One controlled trial did show a nonsignificant trend toward improvement in lung function with azathioprine, and when adjusted for age, a statistically significant improvement in survival.[89] It is on this basis that azathioprine is used; however, patient numbers were small. Other agents such as cyclophosphamide, methotrexate, and mycophenolate mofetil have been tried; however, evidence regarding their efficacy is lacking. Immunosuppressant therapy is associated with significant toxicity including myelosuppression and hepatic toxicity. In the elderly population drug interactions are also a particular problem because of frequent comorbidities and polypharmacy. For example, the concomitant use of allopurinol with azathioprine leads to increased azathioprine levels.[90]

A recent trial suggests that treatment with oral N-acetylcysteine may slow decline in vital capacity and transfer factor in patients with UIP when added to prednisolone and azathioprine.[91]

Current management guidelines suggest withholding treatment unless there is advanced disease (FVC <50%, TLCO <40%) or evidence of significant disease progression.[92] Standard treatment includes combination therapy using prednisolone plus azathioprine with N-acetylcysteine. Patients younger than 65 years should also be considered for referral for lung transplantation.[93] Best supportive care includes oxygen therapy, pulmonary rehabilitation, and palliative care.

DRUG-INDUCED INTERSTITIAL LUNG DISEASE

Drug-induced interstitial lung disease is most prevalent in the elderly by virtue of their increased exposure to multiple drugs. The most commonly prescribed causative agents are amiodarone, methotrexate, ACE inhibitors, and nitrofurantoin. Treatment involves withdrawal of the causative agent and immunosuppressive therapy in some cases.

CONNECTIVE TISSUE DISEASE

Autoimmune disorders including rheumatoid arthritis, Sjögren syndrome, SLE, systemic sclerosis, and polymyositis are all associated with lung fibrosis. Respiratory symptoms may precede other manifestations of the disease. The association between rheumatoid and interstitial fibrosis is strongest in the elderly and has a mean age of onset in the fifth or sixth decade. The incidence, clinical presentation, prognosis, and response to therapy vary depending on the underlying disorder and the histologic pattern of disease. In general interstitial lung disease associated with the collagen vascular disorders has a better prognosis and response to treatment than IPF.[94]

SARCOIDOSIS

Sarcoidosis is a multisystem disorder that most frequently affects the lungs. It occurs less commonly in the elderly, with case series suggesting older adults represent between 7.8% (adults >65 years) and 17% (adults >50 years) of cases.[95,96] Presentation is usually with breathlessness and cough, although symptoms may be nonspecific, with a decline in general health.[97] Löfgren syndrome is rarely seen in adults aged over 50 years.[98] Serum angiotensin-converting enzyme (ACE) levels are of limited value diagnostically, particularly in the elderly who have an increased incidence of renal failure and diabetes (which are associated with raised serum ACE levels).[97,98] Diagnosis should be confirmed histologically if possible.[99] The course of disease seems to be similar in younger and older patients.[97] Corticosteroids are used to treat selected patients with pulmonary involvement and should be supervised by clinicians with expertise in the management of sarcoidosis. Other indications for systemic corticosteroid use in sarcoidosis include hypercalcemia, ocular disease, and cardiac, neurologic, or renal involvement.

PULMONARY VASCULITIS

The vasculitides are broadly subclassified according to size of vessel involvement, clinical features, and associated conditions. Small vessel vasculitis is further subdivided according to the presence or absence of antineutrophil cytoplasmic antibodies (ANCA). The incidence of ANCA-associated vasculitis is increasing. Wegener granulomatosis is a small vessel, systemic necrotizing vasculitis with a peak age of onset at 55 years. Clinical presentation in the elderly is similar to that seen in younger adults although ear, nose, and throat involvement is observed less frequently.[100–102] Some studies suggest elderly patients have an increased incidence of renal and neurologic involvement at diagnosis,[102] although other studies dispute this.[100,101] Diagnosis may be difficult because of the presence of coexistent disease such as COPD that influences clinical and radiologic features.[90] Circulating ANCA levels are positive in the majority of patients with renal involvement but are frequently negative in more limited disease. Biopsy of affected organs is recommended to confirm the diagnosis. Therapy is subdivided into phases with different treatment regimens for remission induction and maintenance therapy. There have recently been several large scale multicenter trials, which have provided clarification regarding the most appropriate treatment regimens. The combination of oral corticosteroids and cyclophosphamide will induce remission in 90% of patients. However, relapse rates are high and survival is worse in those over 60 years of age.[100–102] Renal involvement is also associated with a poorer prognosis. Death usually results from uncontrolled vasculitis or systemic infection.

HYPERSENSITIVITY PNEUMONITIS

Hypersensitivity pneumonitis is caused by an immunologic reaction to the inhalation of organic antigens. It is often associated with the formation of systemic precipitating antibodies. Common precipitating antigens include bird proteins (bird fancier's lung) and thermophilic actinomycetes (farmer's lung). Most commonly it presents as a chronic illness related to repeated exposure but an acute form is recognized. Management centers on antigen avoidance although in some patients the disease will progress despite this. Corticosteroids can be used to improve lung function, although their effect on long-term outcome is unclear.

OCCUPATIONAL LUNG DISEASE

Pneumoconiosis

Pneumoconioses are pulmonary diseases caused by the inhalation of mineral dusts. Common causative mineral dusts include coal dust, silica, beryllium, and asbestos. The incidence of pneumoconiosis appears to be decreasing in the United Kingdom with a 5.7% reduction in reported cases between 1999 and 2005.[103] In 2004 there were 3000 deaths from pneumoconiosis of which 90% occurred in adults over 65 years of age.[1]

Coal workers pneumoconiosis

There has been a steady reduction in the numbers of underground coal miners in Western Europe and the United States, with a consequential fall in the incidence of coal workers pneumoconiosis. Other countries still employ large numbers of miners. Dust exposure results in inflammation and fibrosis of the lung parenchyma. Coexistent COPD is common. Simple pneumoconiosis is usually asymptomatic and is identified as nodular shadowing on a chest x-ray. Progressive massive fibrosis is associated with exertional breathlessness and a cough (often productive of black sputum) and may lead to cor pulmonale and respiratory failure. Chest x-ray features include fibrotic masses, usually in the upper zones, on a background of simple coal workers pneumoconiosis.

Asbestosis

Asbestosis is a fibrotic lung disease caused by exposure to asbestos dust. Diagnosis depends on a reliable history of significant asbestos exposure (usually a 10 to 20 year exposure period). Markers of exposure, such as pleural plaque or pleural thickening, are invariably present. Occupations at greatest risk include shipyard workers, asbestos factory workers, plumbers, insulation workers, electricians, and builders. There is a latency period of at least 15 to 20 years between exposure and the development of asbestosis, hence it is predominantly a disease of middle to old age. The incidence of asbestosis has increased over the last 10 years in both the United Kingdom and United States.[104,105] Treatment is supportive and patients should be informed of their eligibility for compensation.

LUNG CANCER

Lung cancer is the commonest malignancy in developed countries and is the leading cause of cancer deaths. It is predominantly a disease of the elderly with more than 50% of cases being diagnosed in patients over the age of 65, and about 30% of cases being diagnosed in patients over the age of 70.[106] Most patients have advanced disease at presentation and as a result the 5-year survival rate is poor. In the United Kingdom, the 1-year survival rate is ~21%, with a 5-year survival rate of only 5.5%.[107] In the United States, the 5-year survival rate is higher (13% to 17%).[108] Guidelines on the diagnosis and management of lung cancer have been published by the American College of Chest Physicians.[109]

Presentation and investigation

Most cases of lung cancer have symptoms of breathlessness, recurrent chest infections, chest pain, hemoptysis, or weight loss. Other cases may be diagnosed as an incidental finding on routine chest x-ray. The aims of investigation are to make a definitive diagnosis and to stage the cancer appropriately, facilitating treatment decisions. A staging computed tomography (CT) scan of the thorax, followed by bronchoscopy, is the usual approach. In patients with peripheral tumors, a percutaneous CT-guided biopsy will be more likely to obtain a histologic diagnosis. Bronchoscopy is well tolerated in all age groups, with a low risk of significant complications. In very frail patients, invasive investigation may not be appropriate and a clinical diagnosis of lung cancer may suffice. Positive emission tomography (PET) scanning is indicated for any patients who are being considered for potentially curative treatment. It also has a role in the investigation of the solitary pulmonary nodule. The specificity of PET is not high and many benign inflammatory lesions produce false-positive results.[107]

Non–small cell lung cancer (NSCLC) (including adenocarcinoma, squamous cell carcinoma, and large cell carcinoma) accounts for 85% of all new diagnoses. Small cell lung cancer accounts for the remaining 15%.[110] Non–small cell lung cancer is staged using the TNM system. This staging system is currently under review. Small cell lung cancer is staged as limited disease if the tumor is confined to one hemithorax (including ipsilateral mediastinal and supraclavicular nodes). Spread beyond the hemithorax is staged as extensive disease.

Management

Treatment decisions in lung cancer are based on the stage of disease, histology, the presence of co-morbid diseases, and on performance status (Table 50-5). They should not be based on chronologic age. Despite this there is evidence that the elderly are undertreated and are underrepresented in clinical trials, making evidence-based decision making difficult.[111,112] When assessing patients it is useful to perform a comprehensive geriatric assessment including measures of functional status, comorbidity, cognitive state, and nutritional status. Aging is associated with a physiologic decline

Table 50-5. WHO Performance Status Score

Asymptomatic	
1.	Symptomatic but ambulatory (able to perform light work)
2.	In bed <50% of day (unable to work but able to live at home with some assistance)
3.	In bed >50% of day (unable to care for self)
4.	Bedridden

in organ function and a number of changes in drug pharmokinetics and pharmodynamics. This results in differences in treatment tolerance between older and younger patients.[110] Clinical trials specifically designed for the elderly population are needed.

NON–SMALL CELL LUNG CANCER

Surgery

Surgery is the treatment of choice for all patients with stage I/II NSCLC who are fit enough for the procedure. Improvements in surgery and perioperative care mean that an increasing number of elderly patients are eligible for curative treatment. Video-assisted thoracic surgical techniques (VATS) are increasingly useful.[78] Age has no influence on long-term survival after surgery.[113]

Adjuvant chemotherapy

Adjuvant treatment of NSCLC in elderly patients is controversial because of a lack of prospective trials. Randomized trials suggest that postoperative chemotherapy improves survival in the general population with stage II to IIIA NSCLC. There is no evidence that any group of patients specified by age benefited more or less from adjuvant therapy.[114]

Radical radiotherapy

Elderly patients with stage I/II disease are frequently unable to undergo surgery because of comorbidities or reluctance to proceed. In these cases radical radiotherapy is effective with reported mean survival times of 20 to 27 months and 5-year survival rates of 15% to 34% in patients over 70 years old. Treatment outcomes and toxicity rates do not differ with age.[113] Continuous hyperfractionated accelerated radiotherapy (CHART) is high-dose radiotherapy given three times a day for 12 days. A large randomized trial has shown an improvement in 2-year survival from 20% with conventional radiotherapy to 29% with CHART.[115]

Locally advanced disease

Patients presenting with locally advanced NSCLC (stage III) are usually treated with radiotherapy or combined chemo/radiotherapy. Combined treatment may offer a chance of cure although conflicting evidence exists regarding this approach in elderly patients. Treatment outcomes are comparable to younger patients; however, there is a higher risk of toxicity. For patients with an impaired performance status or severe comorbidity, radiotherapy alone is an alternative.[116,117]

Palliative chemotherapy

Chemotherapy is the mainstay of treatment for patients with advanced disease at presentation.[107] A standard regimen would include a platinum-based chemotherapy agent with a single third generation agent (e.g., carboplatin/cisplatin plus vinorelbine/gemcitabine/paclitaxel/docetaxel). This has a modest survival benefit (increase in median survival by 1.5 months, 10% improvement in 1-year survival) compared with supportive care alone.[107,108] Platinum-based chemotherapy is efficacious in older individuals; however, it is associated with significant toxicity (nephrotoxicity, ototoxicity, neurotoxicity).[106] Furthermore, the survival benefit of chemotherapy is limited to patients with a good performance status (WHO 0–1).[117] It is therefore only an option in fit elderly patients.

In elderly patients who are unable to tolerate a platinum combination, a single third generation drug can be used. The ELVIS trial showed that single agent vinorelbine significantly improved both survival and quality of life when compared with supportive care alone (mean survival time 27 vs. 21 weeks).[118] The MILES study demonstrated that combination treatment has no advantage over single-agent therapy.[119]

Palliative radiotherapy

Radiotherapy can be used to improve symptoms, particularly hemoptysis, chest pain, dyspnea, and cough. Elderly patients tolerate radiotherapy well and gain equivalent palliation to their younger counterparts.[120] Performance status does not influence benefit from radiotherapy.

New therapies

Knowledge of cancer biology has enabled the development of new agents that specifically block pathways involved in oncogenesis. Gefitinib and erlotinib are selective inhibitors of epidermal growth factor receptors that have demonstrated activity in patients with NSCLC.[121] These agents are well tolerated in the elderly and may have a role in the future.

SMALL CELL LUNG CANCER

Small cell lung cancer is an aggressive form of cancer that tends to metastasize early. As a result chemotherapy is the mainstay of treatment. Two thirds of patients have extensive disease at presentation. The median survival is only 2 to 4 months without treatment.[122]

Limited disease

In limited disease, response rates to chemotherapy are between 70% and 80%, with a median survival of 12 to 16 months. Only 4% to 5% of patients can be considered cured.[121] The standard treatment for limited disease SCLC is four to six cycles of a platinum-based chemotherapy regimen (commonly etoposide plus carboplatin) combined with thoracic radiotherapy. In patients that achieve complete remission, prophylactic cranial irradiation is offered. Prophylactic cranial radiotherapy has been shown to reduce the incidence of brain metastases and is associated with a slight survival benefit (5.4% at 3 years).[122]

Many trials have looked at chemotherapy regimens for elderly patients with SCLC. Standard regimens remain the most effective, and therefore the treatment of choice despite their significant toxicity. For those with significant comorbidity, less aggressive regimens can be used. Such regimens include dose reduction, shortened treatment duration, and single-agent chemotherapy. At present the optimal treatment is not established.[123,124]

Thoracic radiotherapy is associated with considerable toxicity (bone marrow and esophageal), particularly in elderly patients. Sequential chemoradiotherapy is less toxic than a standard concurrent approach. A meta-analysis looking at thoracic radiotherapy showed a small but significant survival benefit (5.4% ± 1.4% at 3 years) for the use of thoracic radiotherapy. However, this effect was lost in patients over 70 years old.[125]

Extensive disease

Response rates to chemotherapy are between 60% to 70%, with a median survival of 7 to 11 months. Virtually no patients survive to 5 years.[123] Chemotherapy alone is the standard treatment of extensive disease as radiotherapy only has a palliative role. Dual-agent platinum-based regimens are the most effective and usually six cycles are given. Quality of life should be the goal. There is evidence that prophylactic cranial radiotherapy in extensive SCLC reduces the incidence of symptomatic brain metastasis and improves overall survival (1-year survival rate 27.1% vs. 13.3%).[126]

Palliative care

Supportive care is particularly important in lung cancer as most patients have incurable disease. Symptom control, psychological support, and social requirements all should be addressed. A multidisciplinary approach is recommended involving the respiratory physicians, palliative care teams, oncologists, physiotherapists, occupational therapists, and dieticians.[125]

MALIGNANT MESOTHELIOMA

Pleural mesothelioma has been increasing in incidence in the United Kingdom since the 1960s. The annual number of deaths from mesothelioma is predicted to peak at between 1950 and 2450 between 2011 and 2015.[127] Asbestos exposure is the cause of 85% of cases of mesothelioma.[128,129] The latency period is typically long with a mean of 41 years (range 15 to 67).[129] As a result mesothelioma is typically a disease of older men. The prognosis is poor with a median survival of 14 months from symptom onset.[129] Patients with mesothelioma may be eligible for compensation if they are able to verify occupational exposure to asbestos.

Presentation is classically with chest pain and dyspnea, which is related to pleural fluid or thickening. Mesothelioma of the peritoneal cavity can also occur. A CT scan of the thorax may identify pleural nodules or diffuse thickening. Pathologic diagnosis can be made by examination of pleural fluid cytology (sensitivity of 60% to 76%[74,128]); however, a pleural biopsy is usually required. Thoracoscopy is increasingly used to diagnose mesothelioma because of its superior sensitivity compared with blind Abram's needle biopsy (90% vs. 43%).[130,131]

Management

The management of mesothelioma is largely palliative. Dyspnea is relieved by drainage of pleural fluid and pleurodesis. Palliative chemotherapy can be given to patients who have a good performance status although there is no randomized control trial evidence to show that chemotherapy confers better quality of life and survival than active supportive care alone.[128] Pemetrexed in combination with cisplatin is licensed for treatment of malignant mesothelioma after a randomized controlled trial showed a survival benefit compared with cisplatin alone (median survival time 13.2 vs. 9.3 months).[132] Combination treatment was associated with a higher incidence of significant toxicity. Pemetrexed has been shown to be efficacious and well tolerated in elderly patients,[133] although trials have not specifically addressed this treatment in elderly patients with mesothelioma.

The role of surgery in mesothelioma remains controversial. Radical surgical resection (extrapleural pneumonectomy) is associated with a relatively high risk of morbidity and mortality and does have a significant beneficial impact on survival.[131] Debulking surgery is effective in preventing fluid recurrence and may be associated with increased survival although it has not yet been tested in a randomized control trial.

Radiotherapy can be used as a palliative treatment to provide pain relief and is also used as part of the management strategy when extrapleural pneumonectomy is performed. Prophylactic radiotherapy is administered to scars produced by biopsy and/or pleural drainage. A randomized trial has shown that this prevents the risk of seeding of malignant cells[134] although more recent trials have questioned this.[135]

KEY POINTS
Nonobstructive Lung Disease and Thoracic Tumors

- Age-related changes to the lungs predispose the elderly to higher rates of respiratory disease.
- Respiratory infections, diffuse parenchymal lung disease, and thoracic tumors are common in the elderly.
- Most respiratory illness in the elderly requires a multidisciplinary approach to care including care of the elderly and respiratory physicians.
- Management strategies require a careful evaluation of performance status, comorbidity, and concurrent medication.
- Respiratory disease is diverse and frequently presents nonspecifically in the elderly. Accurate diagnosis usually requires careful systematic evaluation.

For a complete list of references, please visit online only at www.expertconsult.com

CHAPTER 51

Dementia Diagnosis

Richard Camicioli
Kenneth Rockwood

OVERVIEW

Dementia is a critical public health problem worldwide, especially as populations age. In consequence, physicians dealing with a range of other age-associated problems can expect to see them in patients with dementia. Dementia diagnosis is evolving. Here, we build on a recent review to highlight aspects of the differential diagnosis of dementia.[1] Generally defined in terms of multifocal cognitive impairment sufficient to impair function, dementia is distinguished from cognitive decline of lesser severity and impact. This distinction might have a quantitative rather than a qualitative basis since pathologic changes consistent with pathologically defined entities, including Alzheimer's disease (plaque and tangles), Parkinson's disease (Lewy bodies), and cerebrovascular disease (large and small vessel strokes, white matter changes) can be seen in patients with cognitive decline short of dementia. Individuals can also have clinical dementia without clear pathologic markers. Recent developments in frontotemporal dementia highlight the fact that novel pathologic markers are continually being identified.[2] Less common but clinically distinguishable entities can sometimes be seen, alerting physicians to the need for careful consideration of presenting features in patients with cognitive impairment.

LIMITATIONS OF CURRENT CLASSIFICATION

Most people, as they age, find that their memory is not as good as it used to be. Many fewer actually have dementia.[3] Where to draw the line between memory complaints and dementia—and how many lines to draw—is controversial, highlighting the artificiality of the definition.[4] In addition, other aspects of behavior such as psychiatric problems (including depression) and mobility difficulties precede dementia and are associated with cognitive decline, highlighting the restrictive nature of current classifications based mainly on cognitive criteria.[5] Nevertheless, the recognition of severity of cognitive impairment and significant impact on activities of daily living has practical implications in terms of care needs and assists with specificity in terms of linking cognitive and behavioral syndromes to pathology. Another limitation of the current nosology for dementia surrounds the issue of onset. Delirium is considered a syndrome of acute onset with fluctuating attention and an identifiable cause. Delirium does not always reverse. Whether this is because the delirium causes the chronic cognitive impairment or simply because the delirium occurred in the setting of dementia is not clear. Nevertheless acute onset of dementia can occur and needs to be put in the context of delirium.[6] Another issue to consider is that of overlapping pathology, which may be more the rule in the elderly where Alzheimer pathology can overlap with vascular or Lewy bodies, findings which are complicated by the fact that all of these pathologies can be present in patients who are apparently cognitively intact and that older people can decline cognitively without obvious brain changes, by current techniques. Patients with dementia can have other comorbid conditions contributing to cerebral dysfunction, which are difficult to diagnose in life.[7] This can complicate diagnostic classifications based on pure syndromes. In the future, although biomarkers may increase the certainty of a certain type of pathology, which may assist with diagnosis and treatment decisions, it will have to be kept in mind that in vivo tests will most likely not have 100% accuracy and that gold standards may evolve.[8]

DEMENTIA DEFINITIONS

General criteria for dementia include the DSM-IV criteria and ICD-10 criteria; each features the requirements of both cognitive impairment (in more than one domain of cognition) and functional impairment. Memory impairment is specified as a domain for both DSM-IV and ICD-10. The NINCDS-ADRDA criteria for Alzheimer's disease and those of NINCDS-AIREN for vascular dementia have standardized definitions, but in the case of criteria for vascular dementia other criteria such as the California and Mayo clinic criteria exist.[9] In general, although specific, these vascular dementia criteria may be insensitive.[10] Dementia with Lewy bodies has had revision of criteria, recently acknowledging the presence of distinctive clinical features, such as REM sleep behavior disorder, and laboratory findings such as decreased dopamine transporter binding.[11] The definition of Parkinson's dementia has been addressed,[12] although its main distinction in relation to Lewy body dementia (how long motor symptoms preceded cognitive ones) is artificial. Criteria for frontotemporal lobar degeneration that predict pathologic findings have also been put forward.[13,14]

RISK FACTORS

Age

Age is the most potent risk factor for most dementias.[15] These include Alzheimer's disease, dementia with Lewy bodies, and Parkinson's disease with dementia and vascular cognitive impairment/dementia. Since age is associated with each of these, overlapping pathology is common.[16] Despite the obvious relationship with age, the NINCDS-ADRD criteria place age limits, with a lower limit of 40 years of age and upper limit of 90 years of age for a diagnosis of Alzheimer's disease.[17] In familial Alzheimer's disease, onset in the 30s is not unheard of and even though more unusual disorders such as childhood metabolic disorders become more common, Alzheimer's remains an important consideration in younger cases. Although a number of genetic and metabolic conditions cause dementia in younger people, these will not be covered.[18] Practically, in very old age, both Alzheimer's disease pathology and cerebrovascular disease are common and often contribute to dementia.

Frontotemporal dementias (FTDs) are a group of clinically defined syndromes associated with dementia, typically with onset younger than age 65.[19] However, many patients with FTLD syndromes, including frontotemporal degeneration, progressive nonfluent aphasia, semantic dementia, corticobasalganglionic degeneration, frontotemporal dementia with motor neuron disease, have onset in old age, where clinical features, such as memory loss and visuospatial impairment, may be confused with Alzheimer's disease,[20] which itself can have focal presentations.[21]

Distinct pathologic entities, including argyrophilic grain disease[22] and hippocampal sclerosis,[23] have been recognized as entities that overlap phenotypically with more common dementias. Given their predilection for medial temporal lobe involvement, not surprisingly, memory impairment is evident, which leads to confusion with Alzheimer's disease.[24] Their distinction from other pathologic disorders such as the FTD syndromes is not clear.

Family history and genetics

Young onset dementia is more often associated with a strong family history consistent with autosomal dominance. As examples, familial Alzheimer's disease, frontotemporal dementia, and Huntington's disease typically occur in the younger age range but late onset individuals are not that unusual in practice. Patients with frontotemporal dementias are more likely to have a family history.[25] The range in age of onset can vary within a family with a genetic family history, and sometimes family history might not be known.[26] In Alzheimer's disease, mutations in the *presenilin-1* gene predominate among patients who are less than 60 years of age, but can have a range in age of onset.[27] Occasional families with late onset dementia occur. A family history, with dementia occuring more than one first degree relative is not uncommon, even in old age. A history of more than one first-degree relative is more common in young onset dementia than in those with onset in the oldest old age range (>80 years). Although the apolipoprotein E4 (*ApoE4*) allele is a risk factor for Alzheimer's dementia, it does not account for all of the increased risk associated with family history.[28]

Gender is a factor that affects the differential diagnosis on an epidemiologic basis, with men more likely to have vascular dementia and dementia with Lewy bodies and women more likely to have Alzheimer's disease.[29] More than a genetic factor, gender influences behavior (i.e., exposure to environmental risk factors) and hormonal levels, which could influence dementia risk. Moreover, women may be at greater risk for autoimmune disorders.

Psychiatric disorders

As noted, neuropsychiatric symptoms may precede a dementia diagnosis and are more common in people with mild cognitive impairment than in cognitively intact elderly people.[30] Depression has been identified as a risk factor for dementia and a depression syndrome of dementia has been identified.[31] Even so, disentangling the two can be complicated. Reactive depression can occur as a consequence of a dementia diagnosis. Given that depression is common in the elderly, occurrence of dementia with depression might occur by chance. However, common causes (i.e., cerebrovascular disease, dementia with Lewy bodies, and Alzheimer's disease) can lead to both depression and dementia and, in several studies, depression precedes dementia.[32]

Psychosis, specifically visual hallucinations, are part of the core criteria for dementia with Lewy bodies and commonly occur in Parkinson's disease, where such symptoms can precede dementia or occur in the setting of dementia.[33,34] Delusions, notably paranoia, are commonly seen in Alzheimer's disease and impaired insight and judgment are part of the spectrum of symptoms of frontotemporal dementia and are seen in vascular dementia.[35]

Other risk factors

Cardiovascular disease–related risk factors (i.e., hypertension, diabetes, smoking, hypercholesterolemia) increase the risk of late life dementia.[36] It is not clear if vascular risk factors cause damage via stroke or ischemia that lowers cognitive reserve or if they incite a pathologic cascade that leads to accelerated cognitive decline. Related risk factors are educational attainment and physical activity level, which have been associated with dementia risk, but are confounded by socioeconomic status, which in turn affects general health, especially cardiovascular health.[37]

Head trauma is another fairly consistently identified risk factor for late life dementia, which may similarly affect brain function.[38] Both acute cerebrovascular events and head injury in older people can be associated with global cognitive decline and can accelerate the course of an established dementia. Data regarding mild cognitive impairment are less clear.

DEMENTIA ASSOCIATED WITH OTHER DISORDERS

Numerous disorders can cause dementia because of effects on brain function and about 7% to 10% of dementia can come on suddenly, often indicating a cerebrovascular event or other medical problem.[39] When onset is abrupt, it is possible that the onset marks a delirium, and investigations and interventions should proceed accordingly. Although the differential diagnosis of delirium can overlap with that of dementia, and people with dementia are at risk for delirium, they should be considered distinct. The disorders discussed in this section can give rise to prolonged illness that can lead to confusion with degenerative disorders. In some cases they are treatable and can potentially be cured, although this is unusual.[40,41] Strictly speaking such disorders are among issues that should be excluded for a patient to meet criteria for a degenerative dementia; however, sometimes they can cause irreversible change in the absence of a neurodegenerative disorder.

Alcohol/drugs/toxins

Alcohol is an important covert cause of dementia worldwide. Abuse of alcohol is underrecognized in general, and it should be screened for.[42] Direct effects of alcohol on central nervous system function can produce syndromes, such as Wernicke encephalopathy (nystagmus, restricted extraocular movements, ataxia) and Korsakoff syndrome (with persistent executive and memory dysfunction), which are recognizable causes of cognitive impairment since they often present in association with other examination features in the setting of alcohol abuse.[43] This clinical picture can also occur in the absence of alcohol exposure with severe malnutrition where similar imaging and clinical changes are present, with involvement of the medial thalami and the periventricular region of the third ventricle, the periaqueductal area, the mamillary bodies, the tectal plate, and rarely the dorsal medulla.[44] It can be difficult to separate effects of chronic exposure of alcohol from other effects, such as effects on vascular risk and brain injuries. Associated lifestyle habits, such as smoking, and socioeconomic status can also compound risk for dementia in a population prone to alcohol abuse. Lower levels of intake of alcohol are reported to be protective, but it is difficult to separate this from other risk factors.

Although alcohol is a common cause of hepatic disease, including cirrhosis, hepatic dysfunction from any cause can lead to an encephalopathy and cognitive impairment. Although in principle reversal of liver damage will lead to normalization of cognitive function, this may not always be the case. Direct effects of toxins such as manganese accumulation and unmeasured substances may be responsible for neurologic dysfunction in the setting of hepatic dysfunction.[45]

Medications for various conditions have been associated with chronic cognitive impairment. Particular drugs include corticosteroids, anticholinergic medications, benzodiazepines, psychiatric medications, and antiepileptic medications, among others. Drugs should be discontinued if they might be temporally associated with cognitive decline. Aging is associated with pharmacokinetic and pharmacodynamic changes that might lead to a chronic medication becoming toxic without clearly being temporally associated with cognitive decline. Accidental overdosing due to forgetfulness can also contribute to amplified effects of medications.[46]

Other toxins, especially metals such as aluminum, mercury, bismuth, and lead, have been associated with chronic cognitive dysfunction. Toxins affecting cholinergic or mitochondrial function (i.e., pesticides) or those causing white matter damage (i.e., solvents) can be related to chronic cognitive impairment. Metals such as copper, zinc, and iron are involved in normal cellular processing and have been examined in relation to dementia.

Autoimmune/inflammatory disorders

Autoimmune and inflammatory causes are rare but treatable causes of dementia in the elderly. Vasculitis can cause dementia through ischemic damage. All forms of vasculitis (i.e., small vessel or large vessel) can lead to progressive neurologic dysfunction. There are often clues to the diagnosis, such as systemic complaints, headache, and sometimes evidence for an associated autoimmune disease. Large vessel vasculitis such as giant cell (temporal) arteritis, Churg-Strauss syndrome, polyarteritis nodosa, Wegener's granulomatosis, and Bechet's and Sjögren syndromes often show evidence for systemic disease and inflammatory markers (increased C-reactive protein and sedimentation rate). Serological investigations can identify vasculitis associated with other autoimmune disorders; however, primary central nervous system vasculitis can cause progressive cognitive decline unassociated with other markers.[47] Angiography and brain biopsy may be necessary to diagnose inflammatory disorders causing dementia,[48] although evidence for an inflammatory process can often be identified by examining spinal fluid (elevated cell count, increased immunoglobulin synthesis, elevated protein level).

Inflammatory disorders can also lead to a hypercoagulable state, which can be seen in association with anticardiolipin or antiphospholipid antibodies, sometimes with evidence for a lupus anticoagulant. Sneddon syndrome is characterized by livedo reticularis associated with hypercoagulability, which typically occurs in younger people but can also occur in older people.[49]

Nonvasculitic autoimmune meningoencephalitis is a relatively recently recognized cause of dementia, sometimes, but not necessarily, associated with collagen vascular disorders such as Sjögren syndrome, antiphospholipid antibody syndrome, systemic lupus erythematosus, mixed connective tissue disease, or Hashimoto encephalitis.[50] In some patients brain biopsy may be warranted, which may be justifiable given that it is treatable.[51] Drugs, notably nonsteroidal anti-inflammatory medications, can be associated with a meningoencephalitis, which can mimic a subacutely progressive dementia.[52]

Multiple sclerosis (MS), which typically begins in younger people, can have onset in old age and can manifest as dementia. Although often relapsing and remitting early in its course, MS can be gradually progressive and primary progressive MS can also occur. Typical patients with onset of MS accumulate deficits and can have strategic lesions that can lead to cognitive impairment. White matter changes are nonspecific and can be associated with a number of disorders and in older people suggest ischemic disease. Hence the diagnosis of white matter disease such as MS can be difficult.

Sarcoidosis is a great mimicker among inflammatory disorders. It can have ocular, central, and peripheral nervous system involvement. Since it can present at any age, it should be considered in the differential diagnosis of dementia in older people.[53]

Endocrine disorders

Metabolic and endocrine dysfunction are common, but occasionally are associated with potentially treatable causes of dementia.[54] Thyroid disorders, including hyperthyroidism and hypothyroidism, are associated with chronic cognitive impairment, and hence screening for thyroid dysfunction is recommended by most consensus guidelines. Autoimmune thyroid disease is associated with Hashimoto encephalitis, which is a treatable cause of dementia, with an abrupt or insidious onset, elevated antithyroid antibodies, and response to steroids.[55] Thyroid disease has also been identified as a risk factor for dementia.

Hyper- and hypoparathyroidism have been associated with cognitive impairment. Hyperparathyroidism is associated with hypercalcemia, which itself can lead to cognitive dysfunction. Hypoparathyrodism is commonly caused by surgical removal of the parathyroid glands, and treatment with calcium replacement and vitamin D are necessary. Parathyroid dysfunction is common in renal failure. Parathyroid disorders can be associated with brain calcification.

Secondary or primary adrenal dysfunction can lead to cognitive dysfunction. Clues such as a history of steroid treatment or electrolyte abnormalities are often present. Assessment of adrenal function and possibly empirical therapy should be considered.

Diabetes is diagnosed by the presence of sustained hyperglycemia, which increases risk for cerebrovascular disease, but it may also lead to cognitive dysfunction without intervening cerebrovascular events.[56] Other secondary consequences include hyperlipidemia. Moreover, treatment of diabetes can lead to hypoglycemic episodes. Whether recurrent mild hypoglycemia causes direct nervous system damage is not clear, but severe and prolonged episodes clearly can cause permanent brain dysfunction.

The metabolic syndrome defined by the presence of truncal obesity, hyperglycemia, high triglycerides, low HDL, and hypertension may increase the risk of cognitive impairment, but separating the effects of each component and elucidating direct from indirect (i.e., via strokes or accelerating progression of Alzheimer pathology) may be challenging.[57] Nevertheless, given a proven association and treatment targets, it may become prudent to treat metabolic syndrome.

Head trauma and dementia in older adults

Head injury is a risk factor for dementia. Although profound head trauma can clearly cause cognitive impairment, and repeated severe injury can lead to a dementia (i.e., dementia pugilistica), the mechanism by which (and if) less severe head injury leads to cognitive impairment is not as clear.[58] Whether minor head injuries can trigger dementia also is not clear.

In older people, subdural hematoma is a consequence of head injury, but can occur spontaneously.[59] Anticoagulant use is a risk factor for hemorrhage and is a clear indication for brain imaging in patients with cognitive decline. Other states, such as renal failure should be kept in mind. Relatively rapid progression and focal signs are indicators that should prompt imaging. The decision to image can be challenging in patients with an existing dementia, but intervention can lead to improvement in function and should be considered in the case of superimposed subdural hematoma.

Infectious disorders

Acute infections of any kind can lead to delirium, for which dementia is an important risk factor, and which in turn is a risk for dementia.[60] Chronic infection of the nervous system can be associated with progressive cognitive decline without obvious systemic manifestations. Among these HIV and syphilis are diseases for which serologic testing is diagnostic, although cerebrospinal fluid examination is needed to confirm central nervous system involvement.[61] Although these disorders are more likely considerations in younger patients, it is important to realize that they can occur at any age. Given successful chronic treatment for HIV infection, more people will be living into old age and hence at risk for dementia.[62] In addition, HIV has a worldwide reach and is an important contributor to cognitive dysfunction on a global scale.

Other chronic central nervous system infections such as cryptococcus and tuberculosis should be considered in atypical patients with dementia. Although these often occur in the setting of immunosuppression, where other opportunistic infections occur (i.e., toxoplasmosis, *Nocardia*, aspergillosis), they can occur without obvious predisposing factors. Another progressive infection that can cause insidious cognitive decline in a setting of immunoincompetence is primary multifocal leukoencephalopathy (PML). This generally presents as a patchy white matter disease.

Viral encephalitis can present insidiously and cause sufficient brain damage to lead to dementia. These often have additional clinical features and risk factors (including exposures), which raises one's index of suspicion.

Whipple disease, Lyme disease, West Nile virus, and listeriosis are unusual infectious disorders with central nervous system predilection. Both Whipple disease and Lyme disease can be associated with a chronic course. West Nile and other viral encephalopathies generally occur as an acute illness. Whipple disease is associated with other neurologic findings (see later discussion) on examination, such as vertical gaze palsy and parkinsonism, and is important to consider in unusual subacute central nervous system disorders since it is treatable.[63]

Prion disease can occur at any age. It can occur in sporadic, genetic, and iatrogenic or infectious forms. Although sporadic Creutzfeld-Jakob disease (CJD) is common in the elderly, some genetic mutations associated with CJD can have late life onset and specific polymorphisms can affect the clinical presentation. Clinically CJD leads to a rapidly progressive dementia, usually with other clinical findings, including myoclonus, visuospatial impairment, and cerebellar ataxia, parkinsonism/pyramidal signs, and akinetic mutism being features of the diagnosis.[64] Laboratory evidence for CJD includes EEG findings of periodic sharp waves, MRI changes on T2, FLAIR or diffusion weighted scans, and CSF evidence for elevation of the 14-3-3 protein. MRI changes are both sensitive and specific, whereas EEG changes are not sensitive, but in the appropriate clinical setting are highly suggestive, and, like elevated 14-3-3 protein levels are not specific. EEG and CSF examinations remain useful in ruling out other clinical mimics such as nonconvulsive seizures or chronic infections. Mimics include lithium toxicity, dementia with Lewy bodies, and vasculitis of the central nervous system and nonvasculitic autoimmune encephalopathy.

Metabolic disorders and nutritional deficiencies

Most guidelines recommend assessment of metabolic conditions in the setting of dementia. Although criteria for degenerative conditions require exclusion of a potentially contributory condition, a common scenario is the co-occurrence of metabolic and degenerative conditions. With this in mind, assessment of complete blood count, glucose, electrolytes, renal function, liver function, vitamin B_{12}, and thyroid-stimulating hormone (TSH) is commonly recommended. Including calcium, magnesium, and phosphates among electrolyte assessment may uncover abnormalities contributing to cognitive impairment. Similarly, folate levels and those of other B vitamins, such as thiamine, riboflavin, and niacin, can sometimes be associated with cognitive impairment, but are usually normal. A sedimentation rate or C-reactive protein can be associated with a chronic inflammatory process of any cause, but also specifically with giant cell arteritis. Testing for syphilis was recommended routinely in the past, but should be considered when appropriate. A search for chronic systemic infections by chest x-ray, urinalysis, and spinal fluid examination should be done if there are clinical clues or rapid onset. Immunoglobulins are elevated in inflammatory disorders, but monoclonal elevation can be associated with multiple myeloma.

Hepatic and renal dysfunction can be associated with delirium, but also with a chronic picture of cognitive impairment. Although conditions leading to dysfunction in these organs, such as alcohol in the case of hepatic dysfunction or diabetes in the case of renal dysfunction, can also lead to cognitive impairment, toxin accumulation as a consequence of hepatic or renal dysfunction can directly affect cognition.

Hepatic dysfunction can lead to manganese accumulation, which is associated with parkinsonism and cognitive impairment. Hyperammonemia on the basis of hepatic dysfunction can be associated with a chronic encephalopathy, even in the absence of elevated transaminases or bilirubin. It is increasingly recognized that patients with renal failure on dialysis can have dementia, which has important implications in terms of decision making.[65] In dialysis patients, cognitive impairment can be a consequence of secondary hyperparathyroidism in addition to other factors, such as elevated creatine.[66]

Neoplastic and paraneoplastic disorders

Direct effects of central nervous system neoplasms are usually self-evident and would be sought out using imaging if there are systemic clues or a history of a malignancy. Signs of physical examination generally progress along with cognitive dysfunction. Occasionally patients do not have a prior history, making this possibility one of the important reasons for brain imaging. Some primary central nervous system neoplasms, such as lymphomas or gliomas, can present relatively insidiously, and imaging might not declare their presence or can be nonspecific. Angiocentric lymphomatosis is an example where proliferating cells are perivascular and imaging may be normal.[67] Although CNS lymphomas are often seen in the setting of immunosuppression on the basis of medications or HIV, they can occur independent of these risk factors.

Indirect effects of malignancy can be associated with paraneoplastic syndromes that include dementia-like presentations. Limbic encephalitis is associated with CNS directed antibodies, which can occur in the absence of a neoplasm.[68]

Chemotherapy and central nervous system radiation therapy for malignancy can complicate the picture by causing central nervous system effects that can be immediate and direct, or delayed. Radiation-induced leukoencephalopathy can sometimes be confused with recurrence or emergence of central nervous system malignancy.

Respiratory and sleep disorders

Hypoxemia and hypercarbia have direct effects on cognitive function, hence pulmonary problems such as chronic obstructive pulmonary disease should be considered in the assessment of both acute and chronic cognitive decline. Acute anoxic injury is a well-recognized form of brain damage, and selective vulnerability of specific cell groups such as hippocampal neurons is recognized.

Disruption of sleep is common in dementia. Increased sleep fragmentation is common in aging and exaggerated in Alzheimer's disease. Insomnia and hypersomnolence can occur in the course of a number of dementias. Familial fatal insomnia is a prion disease associated with dementia that can also present sporadically. A specific problem such as REM sleep behavior disorder is a common symptom in synucleinopathies such as dementia with Lewy bodies. Sleep apnea is another sleep problem that should be considered in the differential diagnosis of patients with day-to-day fluctuations in cognitive complaints. Sleep apnea alone is associated with problems on cognitive test performance. Recent studies have shown sleep apnea to be a risk factor for cerebrovascular disease, which provides another mechanism for causing cognitive impairment.

Structural lesions/normal pressure hydrocephalus

Structural lesions of all types provide deficits that are localization related. The presence of rapid progression, focal features (including gait impairment and incontinence, which suggest frontal-striatal damage), and risk factors for structural lesions (i.e., evidence for systemic malignancy, anticoagulation, or renal disease) merit cerebral imaging. In patients with existing cognitive impairment, the search for an additional structural cause may be necessary in cases of rapid decline. One consequence of structural problems near sites of ventricular drainage is hydrocephalus, which should be differentiated from normal pressure hydrocephalus (NPH).

Normal pressure hydrocephalus is a specific entity where hydrocephalus is present in the setting of the clinical triad of dementia, gait difficulty, and urinary urgency and incontinence. Since these clinical symptoms/signs are each common in older people for various reasons, it is plausible to have all three occur by chance. Moreover, cerebrovascular disease can affect the same frontostriatal circuits affected in NPH. The presence of comorbid CNS disease does not preclude improvement from shunting in individual patients. Currently the presence of the clinical triad with imaging evidence for hydrocephalus is necessary for the diagnosis. Improvement with lumbar puncture removal of a large volume of CSF, continuous external lumbar drain, or increased compliance on infusion into the lumbar space may be helpful in predicting patients who will improve from shunting. Clinical features such as longstanding clinical features, especially dementia, and the presence of verbal memory impairment make improvement less likely.[69]

CLINICAL EXAMINATION FEATURES IN DIFFERENTIAL DIAGNOSIS

Aging is associated with physical changes that need to be differentiated from those of age-related disease. Features on the neurologic examination can assist in the differential diagnosis of degenerative dementias, as well. Although patients with Alzheimer's disease and frontotemporal dementia often have normal basic neurologic examinations, subtle findings such as slowing are often present early on. Over time and in subsets of patients, features such as extrapyramidal signs (bradykinesia and rigidity, often without resting tremor) can develop. Cerebrovascular disease commonly coexists with Alzheimer disease; hence focal pyramidal findings (including the Babinski sign) and gait impairment can confound the diagnosis.

AUTONOMIC DYSFUNCTION

Older people can have autonomic problems such as postprandial hypotension, which can be exaggerated in the setting of systemic disorders such as diabetes. Autonomic dysfunction is more commonly seen in dementia with Lewy bodies and in Parkinson's disease with or without dementia.[70] This can be identified by history and confirmed by autonomic testing. Cardiac MIBG nuclear medicine scans can be seen in dementia with Lewy bodies and Parkinson's disease. This can also occur in vascular dementia, where it might be, in part, related to risk factors such as diabetes. Multiple system atrophy, which is characterized by autonomic dysfunction, parkinsonism, and cerebellar dysfunction, is associated with executive dysfunction, which if severe enough can lead to dementia. Prion disease has also been associated with autonomic dysfunction.

OCULAR AND VISUAL FINDINGS

Pupillary irregularities and abnormalities in accommodation, impaired pursuit movements, and diminished upgaze are seen in aging. Dementing disorders associated with eye movement abnormalities include Huntington's disease, which is associated with an inability to perform saccades. Patients need to move their head (head thrusts) during saccades. Impaired downgaze, which can be overcome with oculocephalic head maneuvers, is characteristic of progressive supranuclear palsy. Dementias affecting the frontal lobes, including PSP, can affect initiation of saccades.[71] Opsoclonus (rapid nonstereotyped irregular involuntary eye movements) is seen in postviral encephalitis and as a paraneoplastic syndrome. Rhythmic eye movements associated with jaw and palate movements (oculomasticatory myorhythmia) is characteristic of Whipple disease. Nystagmus is characteristic of multiple system atrophy.

Visuospatial impairment is common in Alzheimer's disease and marks a clinical feature seen in CJD. This can occur early in the course of Alzheimer's disease and indicates a phenotypic variant with some (but not absolute) diagnostic confidence.[72,73]

PYRAMIDAL DISORDERS

Pyramidal (upper motor neuron) signs (decreased fine motor function, spastic increase tone, brisk reflexes, upgoing plantar responses) are common with cerebrovascular disease affecting the grey or white matter as well as in amyotrophic lateral sclerosis (motor neuron disease), which is also associated with lower motor neuron signs (weakness, wasting, fasciculations, which can be associated with progressive cognitive decline. Motor neurone disease can also be seen in frontotemporal dementia. Upper motor neuron signs are also seen in multiple system atrophy. Structural lesions of the nervous system often cause upper motor neuron signs.

PARKINSONIAN DISORDERS

Parkinsonism is defined by two signs among rest tremor, rigidity, and bradykinesia. These signs are nonspecific, but are seen in Parkinson's disease, dementia with Lewy bodies, progressive supranuclear palsy, multiple system atrophy, vascular parkinsonism, and normal pressure hydrocephalus and occur in late Alzheimer's disease and frontotemporal dementias. Thus parkinsonian features are very helpful in the differential diagnosis of dementia. Although gait impairment can occur early in Parkinson's disease, it is more common in the other parkinsonian disorders noted and, if present at the time of diagnosis, provides a diagnostic trigger that the diagnosis is not Parkinson's disease.

CEREBELLAR SIGNS

Cerebellar dysfunction can also lead to gait ataxia. It is prominent in alcohol-related dementia and along with parkinsonism can be seen in CJD. The cerebellar variant of multiple system atrophy, which can be associated with executive dysfunction, is also characterised by nystagmus on extraocular motility testing, appendicular dysmetria, and gait ataxia along with autonomic features.

NEUROPATHY AND OTHER LOWER MOTOR NEURON FINDINGS

Evidence of neuropathy can be seen in a number of systemic problems associated with dementia, such as alcoholism, diabetes, renal dysfunction, and vitamin B_{12} deficiency. More ominously, rapidly progressive lower motor neuron problems can indicate a process involving the subarachnoid space (i.e., infection, carcinomatous meningitis). Neuropathy can be seen in paraneoplastic syndromes.

GAIT IMPAIRMENT

Balance and gait are integrated functions that involve all levels of the nervous system and require intact musculoskeletal and cardiorespiratory function, therefore impaired balance or gait in the setting of dementia provides important clues to the differential diagnosis and raises concern for systemic disorders that might be contributing to cognitive dysfunction. Obviously gait and balance impairment impact mobility and safety and need to be addressed if they are causing functional impairment. Dementias associated with gait impairment include Parkinson's disease with dementia, vascular dementia, dementia with Lewy bodies, and normal pressure hydrocephalus.[74]

SEIZURES AND MYOCLONUS

Seizures increase in frequency with aging, often in association with central nervous system disease and metabolic insults. It is always important to consider reversible causes of seizures. Intermittent nonconvulsive seizures can mimic dementia by affecting cognitive function. Conversely, drugs used to treat seizures can themselves affect cognitive function.

Myoclonus is defined as rapid jerking movements associated with motor activation (positive myoclonus) or loss of activation (negative myoclonus). Myoclonus is common in CJD, but can be seen in other disorders associated with cognitive dysfunction such as Alzheimer's disease and corticobasalganglionic degeneration. Asymmetric apraxia and overlapping features with primary progressive aphasia and frontotemporal dementia are characteristic of corticobasalganglionic degeneration. Jerking movements can be clues to the presence of seizures as well.

LABORATORY INVESTIGATIONS IN DEMENTIA

Laboratory investigations in dementia can be looked at from two perspectives; one is to obtain positive evidence for a diagnosis. A brain biopsy can provide proof of the presence of an entity associated with dementia.[75] This must be kept in clinical context since the diagnosis is based on the presence of a clinical picture accompanied by pathologic evidence. In living patients, other laboratory tests can provide strong evidence for the cause of dementia in an individual.

An example is vascular dementia caused by an acute stroke in a location that makes sense with the clinical picture. Another example is identification of a potentially reversible metabolic or infectious problem, which when reversed leads to reversal of dementia. Although reversible dementia was emphasized until the 1990s, since the publication of reviews drawing attention to the relative rarity of reversible dementia, enthusiasm for reversible dementia has been tempered.[76,77] This too came about with the move from the long tradition of seeing Alzheimer's disease as a "diagnosis of exclusion" in which a long list of competing diagnoses must be "ruled out" to the recognition of more characteristic staging. Covert causes of cognitive impairment form the basis for recommendation of laboratory testing formed by consensus groups.[3,78] In many cases disorders so identified do not account for the full clinical picture in a patient with dementia, yet it still can help with improving a patient's function and, hence, quality of life. This highlights the importance of identifying and considering treatment of "treatable" conditions even in a patient in whom a degenerative dementia might be considered. Treatments need to be addressed in the context of a patient's overall prognosis.

SUMMARY

In summary, dementia is a syndrome with a range of causes and contributing conditions. A framework for diagnosing degenerative dementias (discussed in other chapters) must take into consideration the possibility of other coexisting conditions that can contribute to cognitive dysfunction in the elderly. To do this one must not only understand the natural history of degenerative dementias, including atypical presentations, but the ways in which systemic problems interact with older people with and without dementia.

KEY POINTS
Dementia Diagnosis

- Dementia is generally defined as multifocal cognitive impairment which is sufficient to impair function. It is distinguished, though not always without arbitrariness, from cognitive decline of lesser severity and impact.
- The differential diagnosis of dementia is long, but as people age, a diagnosis of Alzheimer's disease, commonly in the presence of cerebrovascular disease, becomes more likely.
- This approach of starting with what is common, and looking for features that make this diagnosis less likely is distinct from the long tradition of seeing Alzheimer disease as a "diagnosis of exclusion" in which a long list of competing diagnoses must be "ruled out."

For a complete list of references, please visit online only at www.expertconsult.com

CHAPTER 52

Presentation and Clinical Management of Dementia

Antony Bayer

Dementia is a syndrome, especially common in old age, describing a characteristic pattern of symptoms that can result from many different brain diseases. It is not a diagnosis, nor can it be identified neuropathologically or by neuroimaging, nor is it the result of normal aging. Once recognized, it requires further assessment to identify the likely subtype (e.g., Alzheimer's disease, vascular dementia, dementia with Lewy bodies, Parkinson's disease, or frontotemporal dementia). This discussion will help the medical professional to indicate prognosis and guide best management.

The word *dementia* is derived from the Latin "demens" meaning without mind. In lay use, it can have a pejorative meaning, and this negative connotation impacts on public and professional attitudes. Chronic brain failure (to parallel heart failure, kidney failure, liver failure, etc.) is an alternative, first suggested by Bernard Isaacs and Francis Caird longer than 30 years ago,[1] but does not seem to have gained favor. More recently it has been suggested that alternative umbrella terms of cognitive impairment or neurocognitive impairment are clear and less stigmatizing and may be preferred when dealing with patients and families.[2] When there is a need to distinguish the illness before and after age 65, the terms young- and late-onset dementia are preferable to the old terminology of presenile and senile dementia.

Too great an emphasis on the biomedical aspects of dementia can detract from the human impact of the condition and management can cease to be person centered.[3] In contrast to the more usual clinical terminology, Keady and Nolan for example have described the dementia process as one of slipping, suspecting, covering up, revealing, confirming, surviving (or maximizing), disorganization, declining, and finally death.[4] Social models view the disability of dementia not as an intrinsic characteristic of the individual but as an outcome produced by social processes of exclusion and therefore greatly influenced by factors such as culture, income, housing, and environment.[5] The biomedical and social models are not mutually exclusive, and best practice should incorporate evidence from both traditions.[6]

PRESENTATION

Diagnostic criteria

Dementia is defined in the Diagnostic and Statistical Manual of Mental Disorders (DSM-IV-TR) of the American Psychiatric Association[7] and in the International Classification of Diseases, 10th Edition (ICD-10) of the World Health Organization.[8] Both operational definitions are broadly similar and are based primarily on clinical criteria of multiple cognitive deficits, including memory impairment, associated with a decline in ability to carry out daily activities and often personality and behavioral changes. The deficits must represent a decline from a previous level of functioning (to distinguish from learning disability) and occur in the absence of disturbed or clouded consciousness (to distinguish from delirium). The condition is usually (but not always) irreversible and progressive and of chronic duration (ICD-10 requires deficits to have been present for at least 6 months). The criteria identify similar groups of patients.[9]

Although these criteria are generally accepted, the essential requirement for presentation with memory impairment means that they are closely tied to Alzheimer's disease and may exclude cases of frontotemporal dementia and vascular cognitive impairment until late in their course. Fluctuations of consciousness may be seen in dementia with Lewy bodies and in vascular dementia and are characteristic of delirium, a syndrome that often develops in association with underlying dementia. Thus, discussions around revisions of the criteria for DSM-V and ICD-10 have concluded that the definition of dementia should be reconfigured to not require memory impairment but to be based on a decline in two or more cognitive abilities lasting at least 1 year. There may also be greater emphasis on impairment of instrumental activities of daily living (ADL) and on positive indicators of Alzheimer's disease, rather than regarding it mainly as a diagnosis by exclusion. Genetic, imaging, and biomarkers are considered to have tremendous research promise but are not yet ready for clinical diagnostic use.[10]

The main subtypes of dementia each have standardized diagnostic criteria. The NINCDS-ADRDA criteria have long been the diagnostic standards for research in Alzheimer's disease,[11] although revised criteria incorporating biomarkers have recently been suggested.[12] The consensus diagnostic criteria for dementia with Lewy bodies are widely accepted,[13] as are criteria for dementia associated with Parkinson's disease[14] and frontotemporal dementia.[15]

The NINDS-AIREN criteria[16] or ADDTC criteria[17] are used for vascular dementia, but mainly only in research studies as their sensitivity is only about 50%.[18] The Hachinski Ischemic Score has been used clinically for longer than 30 years to differentiate between multi-infarct dementia and Alzheimer's disease.[19] A low score (4 or less) makes a vascular etiology unlikely. The higher the score, the greater is the likelihood of stroke disease. Despite reservations about its reliability and validity,[20] the simplicity of the Ischemic Score means that it remains useful in the absence of anything better. There are no evidence-based clinical diagnostic criteria for the common neuropathologic finding of mixed dementia.[21]

Clinical presentation

Regardless of the cause, the clinical syndrome of dementia is manifested by cognitive and functional deficits, often associated with behavioral and psychological symptoms (Table 52-1). Poor performance on formal cognitive testing, but without significant impairment of activities of daily living is not sufficient for diagnosis of dementia. However, it may suggest a predementia state and justifies follow-up with repeated assessments. Early recognition and intervention reduces risk of misdiagnosis of dementia and inappropriate management, facilitates optimal care, and delays the morbidity associated with progressive deterioration.[22]

Table 52-1. Aspects of Cognition, Daily Living Activities, and Behavior Affected by Dementia

Cognition	Daily Living Activities	Behavioral and Psychological Symptoms
Working memory	Handling financial affairs/money	Agitation/restlessness
Episodic (anterograde) memory	Managing medication	Eating behavior
Remote memory	Maintaining hobbies/interests	Aggression/rage/violence
Semantic memory	Using public transport	Anxiety/phobias/fears
Language	Driving safety	Apathy
Orientation	Using telephone	Compulsive behaviors
Praxis	Traveling away from home	Delusions/illusions/misidentifications
Recognition/agnosia	Shopping	Depression
Visuospatial ability	Housekeeping	Disinhibition
Calculation	Preparing meals	Hallucinations
Attention/concentration	Dressing/undressing	Personality change
Planning/organization/sequencing	Grooming	Sexual behaviors
Abstract thinking	Bathing/showering	Shouting/screaming
Judgment	Continence	Social awareness
Writing/reading	Feeding	Sleep-wake disturbance
	Mobility/falls	Sundowning

Predominantly cortical or subcortical patterns of impairment can be described.[23,24] Cortical dementias present with impaired memory, language, praxis, and visuospatial abilities with relatively preserved attention and executive function, as is characteristic in Alzheimer's disease. Subcortical dementia is characterized by cognitive slowing (bradyphrenia), with deficits of attention and retrieval of information from memory, apathy, personality change, reduced spontaneous speech, and often associated gait disturbance and slowing of movement (bradykinesia). The prototypical subcortical dementias are progressive supranuclear palsy and Huntington's disease. A mixed cortical and subcortical picture is most often seen in vascular dementia and dementia with Lewy bodies, reflecting pathology in the deep white matter and basal ganglia, as well as the cortex.

It is characteristic of dementia, especially when the result of Alzheimer's disease, that patients themselves tend to deny any significant difficulties and do not present themselves to clinicians. Rather, concerned relatives or caretakers who have noticed a change in the person's ability to cope with everyday life or are frustrated by repetitiveness and unreliability bring them to the attention of health or social care professionals. Sometimes the abrupt loss of support from a caretaker who has been quietly compensating for the person's cognitive deficits will suddenly reveal the presence of dementia.

COGNITIVE SYMPTOMS

The cognitive or neuropsychological symptoms of dementia reflect the location of brain pathology, and particular patterns of symptoms are characteristic of particular underlying diseases. Alzheimer's disease, for example, usually develops in the hippocampus and temporal lobe and the typical presentation is with an amnesic syndrome, frontotemporal dementia will be associated with impairment of executive or language abilities, and dementia with Lewy bodies is associated with visuospatial deficits. Vascular disease may affect any part of the brain and so is not associated with any typical clustering of cognitive deficits, but focal cognitive deficits or executive dysfunction are the most common presentations. Eliciting a history of the cognitive deficit that was first recognized, as well as the nature of its onset and subsequent progression, is therefore very important. The patient's recall and insight will often be compromised by the underlying illness; when addressed with any questions directly, the patient will turn his or her head toward a relative looking for the relative to answer.

Typical complaints initially reported by patients with early dementia include problem-solving difficulties, poor concentration, thought block, inability to quickly recall names, losing track of conversations, a feeling of disassociation from surroundings, feeling and becoming lost in familiar surroundings, not being able to fully coordinate and control speech and actions, and writing block,[25] although there is considerable overlap with the everyday cognitive deficits of "normal aging."[26]

ACTIVITIES OF DAILY LIVING

The consequence of cognitive impairment is to interfere with ability to carry out activities of daily living (ADL), initially higher-level skills such as handling finances, coping with medication and driving (instrumental ADL [IADL]), and subsequently personal care skills such as dressing and bathing (basic ADL [BADL]).[27] This progressive loss of functional ability is a reversal of the pattern observed in normal human development, with the early loss of complex activities followed by later deterioration in simpler overlearned tasks leading to increasing dependency and caregiver burden.

Assessment of IADL and BADL is necessary before a diagnosis of dementia can be made and subsequently will guide provision of appropriate advice and care and input from practical support services. The ICD-10 criteria are perhaps easiest to operationalize, requiring "interference with everyday living" so that "complicated daily tasks or recreational activities cannot be undertaken." The DSM-IV criteria specify "cognitive deficits ... (that) each cause significant impairment in social or occupational functioning and ... a significant decline from a previous level of functioning." This may be more difficult to interpret in elderly people whose opportunity to continue an active occupational and social life may be already compromised by comorbid medical and psychiatric illness, sensory deficits, retirement, and shrinking social networks.

Functional ability is assessed generally by history rather than by completion of the many available formal measurement scales, which are most commonly used to evaluate treatment efficacy in research studies. A large number of scales have been adapted or developed for use in dementia, but some have problems of gender bias or are not culturally sensitive. The most widely used scales that are sensitive to clinically significant change are the Disability Assessment for Dementia scale (DAD), the Bristol Activities of Daily Living scale (BADL), [28] and the Alzheimer's Disease Cooperative Study–Activities of Daily Living (ADCS-ADL).[29] The Functional Assessment Staging (FAST) is a seven-stage scale that reflects the hierarchical pattern of gradual functional loss from normal aging to severe Alzheimer's disease (further broken into 11 substages) and is valuable in characterizing the severity and sequence of functional loss.[30]

In familiar surroundings and with a regular routine, people may cope surprisingly well with usual day-to-day activities until dementia is well established. However, if there is a change in circumstances, such as a bereavement or an overnight stay away from home, then the developing functional impairment can be unmasked. This may suggest erroneously that the problems are of sudden onset, but a careful history is likely to reveal a background of minor lapses and gradual decline over the previous few months, the significance of which had not been appreciated.

In younger people with dementia, impairment may first become apparent in performance at work, whereas in the majority it will concern maintaining the household to their normal standard, keeping up interest in hobbies and social activities, remembering appointments, using the telephone, dealing efficiently with financial affairs, taking medication reliably, getting from place to place in unfamiliar environments, and driving safely. Gradually independent living becomes compromised, with problems handling money, shopping, navigating even in familiar surroundings, and meal preparation. Finally problems with basic ADL emerge, initially choosing appropriate clothing and grooming and then with dressing, bathing, and toileting and finally urinary and fecal incontinence, immobility, and total dependency.

Behavioral and psychological symptoms

The noncognitive symptoms of dementia have been grouped together by the International Psychogeriatric Association under the term *behavioral and psychological symptoms* (BPSDs),[31] although many of those working in mental health settings prefer to talk about "challenging behaviors." A division can be made between observed behaviors (physical aggression, screaming, restlessness, agitation, wandering, sexual disinhibition, hoarding, swearing, and shadowing) and psychological symptoms elicited by interview with the patient or caretakers (anxiety, depression, hallucinations, and delusions). An alternative classification distinguishes between behavioral excesses (e.g., screaming, wandering, physical and verbal aggression) and deficits (e.g., excess dependency, lack of social interaction/communication).[32] However, symptoms from different groups can overlap (e.g., depression in dementia may be diagnosed on the basis of observed behavior as much as elicited symptoms) and some symptoms tend to cluster together (e.g., restlessness and agitation with anxiety, and hallucinations, delusions, and misidentifications as the "psychosis of Alzheimer's disease and related dementias").[33] A factor analysis of a large sample of patients from the European Alzheimer's Disease Consortium identified four neuropsychiatric subsyndromes: hyperactivity, psychosis, affective symptoms, and apathy.[34]

Although BPSDs are not features of the diagnostic criteria of dementia, most patients will demonstrate at least one noncognitive symptom at any time. Different symptoms tend to be more common at different phases of the illness. Mood disturbances are more likely to occur early and agitation, wandering, and psychotic symptoms later, although BPSDs become less evident in the advanced stages of dementia. Symptoms are often transient, persisting for a few days to months. Wandering and agitation, however, tend to be more enduring.[35] Frontal dementia is dominated by BPSDs, and visual hallucinations can be persistent in patients with dementia with Lewy bodies. Caretakers find BPSDs especially burdensome, and they are often the trigger for referral to specialist services.

DIFFERENTIAL DIAGNOSIS

Cognitive problems or any suggestion of "confusion" (an ill-defined and unhelpful term) in someone over the age of 50 is too often assumed to indicate dementia, without sufficient effort being made to confirm that it is indeed the cause. Mild cognitive impairment (MCI) or cognitive impairment not dementia (CIND) is about twice as common as dementia and may evolve into a dementing illness, although this is not inevitable. The commonest mental health problem in older people in the community is depression, and the commonest cause of cognitive impairment in hospital patients is delirium. The major differential diagnosis of dementia is therefore from these two D's, whereas drugs, deafness, and isolated dysphasia or dyspraxia should not be overlooked. A careful history will be of most value in reaching the correct diagnosis, although the presence of one condition superimposed on another is common and may complicate the clinical presentation.

Delirium will be of relatively abrupt onset and brief duration (hours or days) and characterized by fluctuating disturbance of attention, behavior, and wakefulness, as well as cognitive impairment. An underlying physical cause of the delirium will often be evident, such as infection, pain, metabolic disturbance, or dehydration. Most cases of delirium will rapidly and completely resolve with appropriate management. The fluctuating performance and not infrequent visual hallucinations associated with delirium will need to be distinguished from the symptoms of Lewy body disease.

Subjective memory complaint may be a prominent feature of depression in older people, especially in the "young old," whereas severe depression may be associated with objective cognitive impairment, particularly on complex tasks and timed tests. Cerebrovascular disease is often responsible. Questions on cognitive testing are more likely to be answered by "don't know" or refusals, rather than guesses or near misses, and performance may be inconsistent, with the subjects typically highlighting their failings. In contrast to dementia, sense of time and direction is often relatively intact; there is an absence of rapid forgetting and improvement with practice.

Major depressive illness presenting with the clinical picture of dementia has been termed *pseudodementia,* although mild dementia presenting with depressive symptoms (which might be termed *pseudodepression*) is more common. The true diagnosis is perhaps most often established only in retrospect, after the depressive symptoms have been treated successfully.[36] However, up to 50% of elderly patients presenting with depression and cognitive impairment develop full-blown dementia within 3 to 5 years,[37] and depression often precedes the dementia syndrome in vascular dementia, dementia with Lewy bodies, and other subcortical dementias.[38]

The reduced cognitive reserve of the aging brain means that it is especially sensitive to the adverse effects on higher mental functions of many prescribed and over-the-counter drugs. Sedative medication and anticholinergics are the most common culprits, but any drug with central nervous system activity may be implicated. Symptoms generally respond rapidly to drug withdrawal or dose reduction.[39] Identification of reversible causes of dementia will ensure that appropriate interventions can be mobilized that may stabilize, improve, or even cure the underlying condition.

Reaching a diagnosis

There is no quick and simple way to reliably diagnose dementia and its subtypes, particularly in the early stages. The NICE Guidelines[6] summarize the process as depending on "pattern recognition, deductive reasoning and accumulation of diagnostic evidence from multiple sources. These processes tend to be iterative and may be relatively prolonged." An adequate assessment should consist of a detailed history from both patient and someone who knows the patient well, a physical examination, a mental state and cognitive assessment, and appropriate investigations, including laboratory tests and neuroimaging (Figure 52-1). This may be best carried out in a memory clinic setting.[40]

HISTORY TAKING

Independent histories should be obtained from patient and informant, ideally out of earshot of each other. The priorities should be to establish the nature, onset, evolution, and impact of the presenting symptoms. Areas to investigate include ability to find their way around independently and use public transport, driving, taking medication, using the telephone, interest in hobbies, dealing with financial affairs, shopping, housework and meal preparation, social behavior, relationships and self-care skills (bathing, grooming, dressing, toileting).

Establishing the very earliest symptom, its onset, and its subsequent course is especially valuable. A slow, insidious decline of working memory is typical of Alzheimer's disease, whereas a fluctuating course is suggestive of dementia with Lewy bodies. Frontotemporal dementia will present with progressive change in personality and social conduct and language. A more acute onset of cognitive impairment with a stepwise progression is characteristic of vascular dementia.

Other important areas of the history include psychiatric and behavioral symptomatology, education, employment and premorbid functional ability, past and present medical problems (especially stroke, Parkinson's disease, head injury, and diabetes mellitus), medication (prescribed and nonprescribed, especially centrally acting drugs and those with anticholinergic effects), past and present alcohol intake, family history, and social support. Specific attention also should be given to the caretakers' emotional and physical state, how much practical care and supervision they need to undertake, and how much they understand about the nature of the patient's condition.

A structured interview schedule covering the essential elements of the history forms the first two parts of the CAMDEX (Cambridge Examination for Mental Disorders of the Elderly).[41] The Informant Questionnaire on Cognitive Decline in the Elderly (IQCODE) may be used to document an informant's report of changes in the everyday cognitive function of an elderly person compared with 10 years earlier.[42]

PHYSICAL EXAMINATION AND MENTAL STATE ASSESSMENT

The medical examination of the person with possible dementia may help to elucidate the cause of the illness, identify physical consequences of the condition, or identify important coexisting morbidities. Especially relevant are the neurologic examination (for focal motor and sensory signs, primitive frontal reflexes, involuntary movements, and gait disturbance, especially parkinsonism), cardiovascular system examination, assessment of vision and hearing, and recognition of signs of self-neglect or injury, either unintentional or related to possible physical abuse. A mental state examination should look for presence of BPSD and psychiatric conditions that may cause diagnostic confusion.

COGNITIVE TESTING

Testing cognitive function can start with a brief screening assessment and proceed to more detailed neuropsychological testing if necessary. The Mini Mental State Examination (MMSE)[43] is probably the most widely used cognitive screening test, taking about 5 to 10 minutes to complete and covering orientation, attention, memory, language, and visuoconstructional skills. It yields a score from 0 to 30, with cutoff below about 23 or 24 said to be indicative of dementia. However, total scores need to be interpreted cautiously and the nature and pattern of deficits is more instructive than the total score. As well as acquired cognitive impairment, performance will be influenced by premorbid ability, education, language, culture, sensory deficits, and motivation. Other short tests include the Abbreviated Mental Test Score (AMT),[44] the 7-minute screen,[45] and the 6-CIT.[46] Clock-drawing[47] is quick and nonthreatening, testing comprehension, planning, visuospatial skills, and memory, but it is difficult to score. Verbal fluency (naming animals or words starting with a particular letter of the alphabet in one minute) is a quick screening measure of frontal lobe function.

More comprehensive standardized cognitive tests are used routinely in specialist dementia services, such as memory clinics. The Addenbrooke's Cognitive Examination (ACE-R)[48] includes the MMSE, clock drawing, and verbal fluency and consists of 26 tasks divided into five domains: attention and orientation, memory, verbal fluency, language, and visuospatial skills. It takes about 15 minutes to administer and has value in distinguishing dementia from affective disorders and mild cognitive impairment and that because of Alzheimer's disease from frontotemporal dementia and atypical parkinsonian syndromes. Other more detailed tests that are commonly used include the Cambridge Cognitive Examination (CAMCOG-R)[41,49] and the Repeatable Battery for the Assessment of Neuropsychological Status (RBANS).[50]

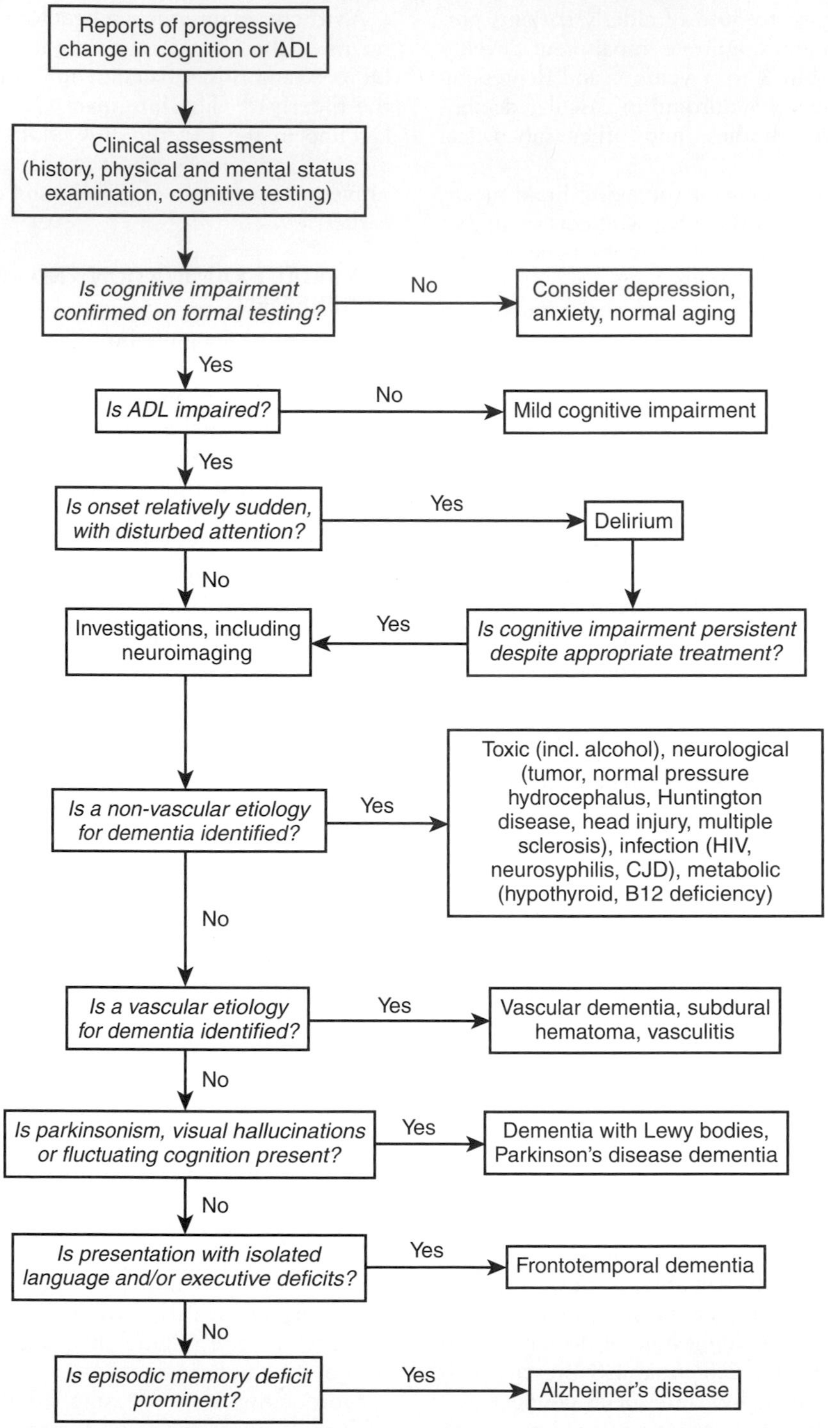

Figure 52-1. Diagnostic process for dementia. This simplified diagram ignores the possibility that dementia might have a mixed etiology—a common finding in practice.

LABORATORY TESTING

Recommended laboratory investigations include full blood count, urea and electrolytes, liver function, calcium, blood glucose, thyroid function, vitamin B12, folate, and C-reactive protein (CRP). Syphilis serology, lipids, and HIV testing are not necessary routinely but should be undertaken if indicated by the clinical circumstances. An electrocardiogram may be indicated if vascular disease is suspected. Other tests are appropriate if delirium is a possibility, such as a midstream urine sample, blood cultures, and chest x-ray.[6]

NEUROIMAGING

Structural neuroimaging with magnetic resonance imaging (MRI) or computed tomography (CT) is a necessary part of the dementia workup in most patients.[51] They will rule out potentially treatable intracerebral lesions causing dementia, such as subdural hematoma or normal pressure hydrocephalus and rule in cortical and subcortical infarcts and white matter changes indicative of vascular disease and localized atrophy characteristic of particular neurodegenerative dementias. For example, atrophy of the hippocampus and medial temporal lobe is an early and sensitive marker for Alzheimer's disease and atrophy of the frontal or anterior temporal lobe may be seen in frontotemporal dementia. The choice of MRI or CT will depend on local availability, cost considerations, patient acceptability, and contraindications, but MRI is generally more sensitive and is the preferred modality.[6,52]

Functional imaging with single-photon emission computed tomography (SPECT) or positron emission tomography (PET) shows regionally distinct patterns of underperfusion or hypometabolism and can help to differentiate Alzheimer's disease from frontotemporal dementia or vascular dementia.[53,54] PET scanning remains largely a research tool because of its high cost and lack of general availability. Study of the dopamine transporter (DaTSCAN) can be used to distinguish dementia with Lewy bodies from Alzheimer's disease.[55]

Recent neuroimaging advances, such as the Pittsburgh Compound-B (PIB) ligand for positron emission tomography imaging in Alzheimer's disease, look to have a major future role in differentiating among the neurodegenerative dementias and monitoring treatment effects.[56] Other studies are under way to identify specific imaging markers for different types of dementia, including cerebral volumetric measurements, diffusion weighted MRI, MR spectroscopy, and very-high-field MRI scans of senile plaques in Alzheimer's disease.

OTHER INVESTIGATIONS

Examination of cerebrospinal fluid (CSF) is diagnostically valuable in patients with suspected infectious, inflammatory, autoimmune, or demyelinating disease. In normal pressure hydrocephalus, it may help to predict response to surgery. The presence of the CSF 14-3-3 protein confirms the diagnosis of Creutzfeldt-Jakob disease. CSF markers of Alzheimer's disease (reduced beta amyloid 1–42 and elevated total tau and phosphorylated tau) may also allow earlier and more accurate diagnosis, but problems with patient acceptability of lumbar puncture and of standardization of laboratory assays limit their routine use.[57]

Studies of plasma biomarkers of Alzheimer's disease have shown significant overlap with control cases, but plasma concentrations of beta amyloid40 and low plasma concentrations of beta amyloid42 indicate an increased risk of dementia and may have a future role in therapeutic monitoring.[57,58] Genetic testing is rarely indicated and should only be undertaken after appropriate counseling, preferably in a specialist genetics clinic. Testing may be indicated in suspected Huntington's disease (Huntington gene), cerebral autosomal dominant arteriopathy with subcortical infarcts and leukoencephalopathy or CADASIL (notch 3 gene mutation), familial Alzheimer's disease (presenilin and amyloid precursor protein gene mutations), or frontotemporal dementia (tau gene mutations). Determination of apolipoprotein genotype is not diagnostically useful, the e4 allele being neither sufficient nor necessary for development of Alzheimer's disease, although it may have a role in predicting therapeutic response.[59]

The electroencephalogram (EEG) is usually diffusely abnormal in dementia but may be normal in frontotemporal dementia and the presence of triphasic spikes is helpful diagnostically in prion disease.[60] Brain biopsy may be indicated very rarely when a treatable disorder is thought to underlie dementia.[61]

TELLING THE DIAGNOSIS

Sharing the diagnosis of dementia can be challenging and the practice of diagnosis disclosure among dementia specialists is changing. In the 1990s, less than a third of old age psychiatrists and geriatricians usually told people with mild dementia their diagnosis, but more recent studies report that half or more of specialists now regularly disclose diagnosis, with few still seeing no benefit in doing so.[62]

It is now established good practice that, in most cases, it is best for the person with dementia to be told sensitively what is wrong, what the implications are, and what can be done (Table 52-2).[63,64] Certainly, all should be given the opportunity to learn as much or as little as they want to know, and people should routinely be asked if they wish to know the diagnosis and with whom this should be shared.[6] Reactions of patients to being told their diagnosis include relief (as it provides an explanation for their difficulties), disbelief (as they may lack insight and do not feel ill), loss (grieving for failing intellectual abilities), and fear (of becoming a burden and of limitations in the future).[65] Family members and caretakers also need to understand the diagnosis, with specific attention given to comprehensible and practical information about coping strategies, care services, likely course of the disease, available treatment, and plans for follow-up.

Communication of the diagnosis should ordinarily occur in a joint meeting with patient and family.[66] Sufficient time needs to be allowed for an adequate discussion, perhaps outside the standard clinic schedule. Simple language should be used, avoiding technical jargon that may conceal the truth, but including the specific medical diagnosis (e.g., Alzheimer's disease) rather than just dementia. Both terms will need to be explained. The bad news can be mellowed with information about available therapeutic approaches to maintain quality of life and care must be taken to avoid conveying the feeling that nothing more can be done. A graded approach to disclosure and information provision can be adopted, which is patient-led and ensures that what is said answers what the patient wants to know. At the end of the discussion, the patient and family's understanding should be assessed and

Table 52-2. Arguments for and against Disclosure of a Diagnosis of Dementia

Against Disclosure
- Making an accurate diagnosis is complex and uncertain in the absence of neuropathology.
- There is no curative intervention.
- Giving such a diagnosis may cause avoidable anxiety and depression.
- People with dementia will not be able to understand or retain the information given to them.

For Disclosure
- Maximizes individual autonomy and choice by providing information necessary for decision-making and advance planning
- Increases opportunities for accessing appropriate and specialist support services and symptomatic treatments
- Demonstrates respect for individual rights, especially the "right to know" and avoids paternalism
- Relieves the anxiety of uncertainty
- Provides an explanation for cognitive failures and problems in everyday life, allowing the person to make sense of them
- Promotes positive coping strategies and fulfillment of short-term goals

follow-up arranged, to reinforce information provided, clarify misunderstandings, and answer questions that are outstanding. A telephone call or a home visit by an informed professional a few days later will be helpful.

Verbal information should be backed up by written information,[67] with recommendations for further reading and trustworthy Web sites and mention made of local support groups and meetings, with contact details of local Alzheimer associations. Postdiagnostic counseling, individually or in a group setting, can be of great value.[68]

MANAGEMENT

Treatment goals in early dementia center on improving or stabilizing cognitive ability and mood, maintaining or reestablishing independence, promoting autonomy, and effective planning for the future. As the condition progresses, emphasis shifts to facilitating mental and physical stimulation, managing behavioral disturbances, and providing practical care for patients and respite for their families. Finally there should be the timely introduction of appropriate end-of-life care.[69]

The concept of personhood and person-centered dementia care, pioneered by Kitwood[70] in the late 1980s, is central to best management. Brooker[3] has identified the key components as valuing people with dementia and those who care for them, treating people as individuals, looking at the world from the perspective of the person with dementia, and promoting a positive social environment in which the person living with dementia can experience relative well-being. The technique of Dementia Care Mapping (DCM)[71] is closely linked to person-centered care and is an attempt to help professionals to take the standpoint of the person with dementia when evaluating the quality of care, using a combination of empathy and observational skills. This information can be used to plan more person-centered care on an individual, group, and organizational level.

Good practice requires clinicians to try nonpharmacologic approaches to managing problems related to dementia before pharmacologic treatment,[6] although disease-modifying drugs, should they become available, would be required to be used from an early stage. Often a combination of interventions tailored to the needs of the individual is most appropriate (Figure 52-2). Although the professional's primary responsibility will always be to the patient, addressing caretakers' needs as well will often result in a better outcome for all. However, sometimes the patient's and caretaker's wishes can conflict (for example, a patient not wishing to attend day center, although the caretaker is in need of respite), and in these circumstances decisions about best management can be especially difficult. Disagreements within families can also cause conflict, commonly involving accusations of neglect, exploitation, lack of communication, or sequestration of the person with dementia.[72]

Safety and risk

Impaired judgment and insight, perceptual problems, deficits of attention, slow reaction time, and impaired memory will all contribute to the person with dementia being at increased risk of accidents and unwanted outcomes. Caretakers often use concern about people being "at risk" as the justification for management decisions, from the need for regular uninvited home visits, whether by family or professionals, to the need for admission to institutional care. However, there is a need to balance the desire to reduce risk as much as possible, against that of encouraging the person's continuing independence and dignity. An emphasis on total safety and risk prevention is likely to erode people's personhood and autonomy. Everyone, whether or not they have dementia, has a right to reasonable freedom of choice, as long as they do not put others at significant risk. A stimulating environment and positive and interesting activities are incompatible with total safety and some occasional minor accidents are inevitable. Good risk management will involve a carefully considered trade-off between efforts to maximize environmental and emotional security and the promotion of individual and community rights.[73]

The commonest unsafe behaviors reported by relatives of demented patients living at home are wandering and problems in the kitchen and with driving. The most common accidents are falls, injuries arising from sharp objects, and getting lost. Examples of simple measures to improve safety include use of personal identification bracelets, keeping a spare set of house keys with a neighbor, installing smoke alarms, providing community alarm systems so that help can be summoned immediately if needed, ensuring good

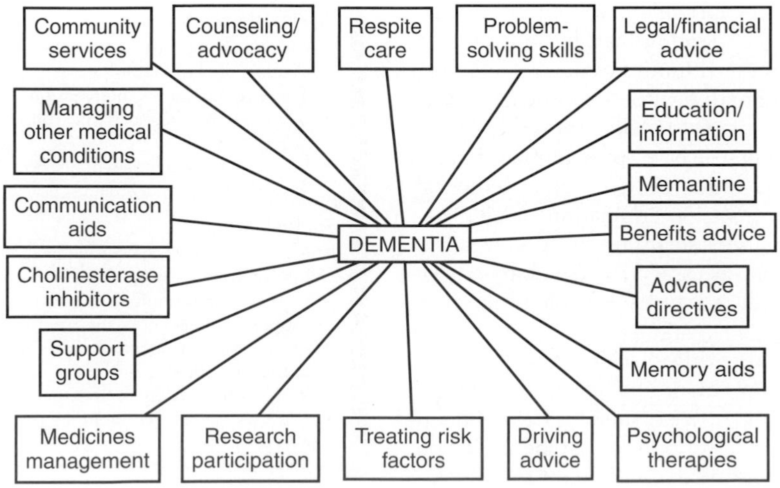

Figure 52-2. Potential interventions in management of dementia.

lighting, fitting a gas detector, or disconnecting supplies and installing hot water thermostats. Simplifying drug regimens, dispensing medication in prepacked pillboxes and ensuring unused medication is stored safely out of reach will help to improve compliance and reduce risk of overdose. Alarms on front doors can immediately alert caretakers that someone is leaving the building, or unfamiliar locks or difficult-to-use door handles on exits can act as an effective barrier. A pressure mat placed next to the bed or in doorways can be used to alert caretakers when a patient is up and about. There is a growing industry developing electronic aids and "smart homes" that make use of new technologies to monitor patients' activities, but empirical evidence of their value is so far lacking.[74]

Driving is an especially difficult issue as safety will be inevitably lost as dementia progresses. Clinicians and family members can help patients realize when it is no longer safe for them to drive, but sometimes close relatives have selfish motives for minimizing driving difficulties. It has been suggested that the risk of crashes is acceptably low for up to 3 years after onset of Alzheimer's disease, but this varies between people.[75] Cognitive testing cannot determine whether individuals with dementia are able to drive safely.[76] Regulations on driving and dementia differ from country to country, with mandatory reporting to licensing authorities in many, but not all. The clinician must make an immediate decision on safety to drive, ensure that the licensing agency is notified as appropriate, and help patients and their families to accept and adapt to the new limitations in mobility if driving must stop.

Loss of mental capacity will place people at risk of being unable to cope with everyday decisions and open to abuse. Arranging a power of attorney allows the person with dementia (the donor), while still capable, to delegate to another (the attorney) the ability (power) to act on their behalf in relation to financial, property, and legal affairs. It can also be extended to include welfare and health decisions. An advanced directive or living will allows the person to state his or her wishes about future treatment and potentially life-saving interventions, such as artificial feeding and resuscitation in the event of cardiorespiratory arrest. Powers of attorney are widely regarded as good practice in dementia care and are widely used, although fewer people currently arrange an advanced directive.[77]

Memory aids and cognitive training

The most simple and effective methods of helping patients (other than asking other people to remember things for them) are the establishment of everyday routines and careful planning of daily activities, allowing sufficient time and avoiding unnecessary overcomplication. Use of environmental cues, such as labeling or color coding of switches and doors, can be useful, as may systematic use of external memory aids such as diaries and checklists and strategically positioned notes as reminders. Electronic aids and smart house technology can also be used to generate prompts. None of these approaches requires the patient to learn new strategies of thinking or remembering and may thus be useful for most people with mild to moderate dementia.[78] Personal memory albums are a visual record of the key facts of a person's life, both past and present, and can serve as a valuable orientation and reminiscence aid in people with more severe dementia. They stimulate conversation and provide opportunity for life review, allowing patient and caretakers to focus on the good times and help raise confidence and self-esteem. Optimizing communication, using both verbal and nonverbal techniques, will help patients to maintain a sense of control and minimize misunderstandings that can lead to BPSD. Efforts should also be made to compensate for any hearing and visual deficits. Professionals should always introduce themselves face-to-face and fully explain what they are doing using a clear, relaxed, and normal speech rhythm and simple, concrete language.[79]

Formal cognitive training programs may have some benefits in improving, retaining, or regaining skills in motivated individuals with mild dementia, although empirical evidence in support is limited.[80] Any advantage is not sustained for long and gains in one particular skill tend not to generalize to other areas. Specific approaches to memory training have included relaxation techniques, regular and repeated practice sessions (using spaced retrieval to rehearse information), organization of material (e.g., use of categorization or mnemonics), techniques for improving visual imagery (e.g., pegword methods, face-name association, etc.), verbal strategies (rhymes, first letter cueing, alphabet searching, etc.), and most recently computer-aided cognitive training.[81] Training in groups with other people with memory impairment or with family members and caretakers may provide opportunities for mutual support and education.

Nonpharmacologic therapies

A number of psychological and complementary therapeutic approaches have been developed for use in dementia.[82,83] No one approach is suitable for all patients or is likely to continue to suit any single patient throughout the course of his or her illness.

Reminiscence[84] involves recall of events in a person's life, in conversation with another, in a group, or alone. Relevant pictures, music, objects, and sounds are used to trigger the store of memories. It can be an enjoyable diversionary activity for patients and encourages those involved in care to get to know more about patients as individuals. Proponents have reported benefits to include an increase in interaction, improved orientation, and a reduction in behavioral disturbance.

Reality orientation (RO)[85] provides information about the time, place, or person to give the person with dementia a greater understanding of his or her situation, with the aim of improving sense of control and self-esteem. The currently favored approach, especially in care homes, is to provide 24-hour RO by providing clocks, clear signposting, large notice boards, and consistent information in all interactions. Sustained improvement in verbal and spatial orientation has been claimed, but it needs to be employed skillfully to avoid confrontation.

Cognitive stimulation therapy (CST)[86] aims to promote cognitive function through regular sessions of themed activities, using quizzes, word and number games, and everyday objects to actively stimulate and engage people with mild to moderate dementia. When undertaken in a group setting, there are both learning and social benefits.

Validation therapy[87] emphasizes the importance of relating to the inner reality of the patient rather than encouraging the patient to be concerned with external factors as with

RO. The therapist acknowledges and empathizes with the patient's feelings, whether or not they are based on reality. The emphasis is on accepting and validating feelings rather than factual content. Validation can be delivered individually in formal sessions, as group therapy, or as 24-hour informal therapy.

Animal-assisted therapy[88] involves introducing pets, such as resident cats or visits by a dog, to institutionalized patients (provided that they do not scare people). It can significantly increase the number of interactions while the therapy dog is present, producing longer conversations and increased rates of touch, as well as promoting a homely environment and facilitating the expression of emotions. Installation of fish tanks in the dining area of specialized dementia units has even been reported to increase nutritional intake and weight gain.

Music therapy[89] can be undertaken, either individually using recorded tapes or simple instruments or in groups using old songs or dance music. People respond best when they listen to music they prefer. Group music therapy can significantly improve speech content and fluency and some severely impaired patients may respond to music, even when other forms of communication have been lost. Individualized music therapy can significantly decrease agitation.

Physical exercise[90] may be undertaken either through informal walks or using structured exercise sessions. Walking combined with conversation in nursing home residents with dementia helps to maintain functional mobility, and student-led one-to-one exercise sessions can result in significant fitness gains, is inexpensive, and gives family caretakers some respite.

Relaxation therapy[91] can take various forms. Progressive muscle relaxation, in those who can learn the technique, can decrease behavioral disturbance and improve memory in people with mild to moderate dementia. Interventions incorporating aspects of touch may also help some people. Hand massage and intermittent gentle touch on the arm and shoulder, accompanied by calm soothing talk, were shown to have a temporary benefit on disturbed behavior in one study. Rocking chairs can also improve emotions and relaxation.

Bright light therapy[92] has been claimed to improve cognition and behavior in people with Alzheimer disease, eventhough the exposure must be for several hours each day for several weeks and the light must be of high intensity. Low-intensity dawn-dusk simulation, a naturalistic form of light therapy, was ineffective.

Snoezelen therapy[93] involves multisensory stimulation using a variety of lights, gently stimulating music, aromas, and tactile objects. Regular snoezelen sessions may improve behavior and mood in people with moderate to severe dementia.

Aromatherapy[94] may also prove to be beneficial. Studies have shown reduction in agitation associated with regular application of *Melissa officinalis* (lemon balm) oil applied to the hands, with lavender oil via an aromatherapy stream and with a course of aromatherapy combined with massage. There were no major adverse effects.

Creative activities[95] encourage normalization, provide mental stimulation, and enable the person with dementia to recognize an ability to achieve, lessening the feeling of helplessness. Care must be taken to ensure that the activity is of interest to the patient rather than to the helper and, whatever the activity, the emphasis should always be on enjoyment while taking part, not on what is finally produced. Suitable activities might include painting and collage, pottery, flower arranging, indoor gardening, traditional games, and puzzles.

Drug management

As the etiology of dementia is so varied, no one drug is likely to be beneficial in all patients. The choice of medication should clearly relate to the underlying condition or the specific symptom that is to be treated. A small minority of dementing conditions can be effectively halted or reversed by specific drug treatment; for example, hypothyroidism by levothyroxine, pernicious anemia by parenteral vitamin B_{12}, neurosyphilis by penicillin, cerebral vasculitis by corticosteroids or immunosuppressants, and Wernicke-Korsakoff's syndrome and possibly alcoholic dementia by thiamine. However, truly reversible dementia is probably rare.

Of the many drugs that have been claimed to be of more general benefit in the prevention and management of dementia, few have withstood the critical test of large, prospective, randomized, placebo-controlled trials. Thus, over the years, vasodilator drugs, nootropics, cholinergic supplementation with lecithin and choline, antioxidants (notably vitamin E and gingko biloba), anti-inflammatory drugs, and estrogen have all been shown ineffective.

The association of cardiovascular risk factors with Alzheimer's disease as well as vascular dementia suggests a potential value of vascular preventive treatment,[96] and there is some evidence of benefit for antihypertensive drugs.[97] However, despite strong epidemiologic support, randomized controlled trials of statin drugs have so far not shown positive effects on cognition when used for primary prevention[98] or treatment of established Alzheimer's disease.[99] Likewise, low-dose aspirin is ineffective in preventing cognitive decline in asymptomatic middle-aged to elderly adults.[100,101]

Available drugs of proven efficacy in Alzheimer's disease are the acetylcholinesterase inhibitors (AChEIs), donepezil, galantamine, and rivastigmine, and the *N*-methyl-D-aspartate (NMDA) receptor antagonist, memantine. The three AChEIs differ in their pharmacologic properties but have broadly similar efficacy and safety. They work by blocking the enzyme acetylcholinesterase and so inhibit the breakdown of the neurotransmitter acetylcholine. Numerous placebo-controlled clinical trials have shown consistent, if modest, benefits on cognitive and global measures in a majority of patients with mild to moderate Alzheimer's disease and most studies show improvement (or less deterioration) in activities of daily living, behavior, caretaker burden, and use of resources.[102,103] Side effects are generally mild and dose-related, typically nausea, vomiting, and diarrhea. The effects of AChEIs are also seen in patients with severe dementia, although trial evidence is limited.[104] Despite their clinical efficacy and safety in Alzheimer's disease, the cost-effectiveness of AChEIs has been questioned and, in the United Kingdom, the NICE appraisal process controversially recommended their use only in moderate dementia.[105] In vascular dementia there is also some evidence of limited benefit,[106] and rivastigmine is the drug of first choice for treating cognitive impairment in dementia with Lewy bodies and Parkinson's disease dementia.[107]

Memantine blocks pathologically elevated glutamate and consequent calcium overload while still allowing physiologic receptor activation. It is available for treatment of moderately severe and severe Alzheimer's disease, either given alone or in combination with an AChEI. In systematic reviews, memantine shows benefit on cognitive and global function of the same order of magnitude as seen for the AChEIs,[108] and it also seems to have specific benefit against agitation.[109] It is very well tolerated.

Neuroleptic drugs were for many years commonly used to treat BPSD, but their efficacy is limited and it is now recommended that their use is restricted to the short-term (e.g., not more than 3 months) treatment of aggression or psychotic symptoms associated with serious distress or risk when other therapies have proven ineffective.[110] The evidence is best for the atypical drugs, risperidone and aripiprazole. Adverse effects can be significant and include excessive sedation, parkinsonism, falls, hastening of cognitive decline, increased stroke risk,[111] and premature death.[112] In dementia with Lewy bodies and Parkinson's disease dementia, neuroleptics may precipitate severe sensitivity reactions in up to 50% of patients treated and should only be used with particular caution.[113]

Non-neuroleptic drugs to treat BPSD have not been studied extensively in clinical trials, but there is some evidence for benefit from carbamazepine, sodium valproate, trazodone, and citalopram to treat aggression and agitation.[114] Depressive symptoms are best treated with a selective serotonin reuptake inhibitor (SSRI) antidepressant such as citalopram or sertraline, or mirtazapine or trazodone if sleep is disturbed.

There is a lot of activity investigating novel therapeutic strategies that aim to fundamentally alter the natural history of dementia by targeting the underlying pathologic process. The main area of interest has been interfering with the deposition of beta amyloid protein in Alzheimer's disease. In animal models, immunization with beta amyloid reduces plaque formation and protects against learning and memory impairment. Initial human trials of active immunization in Alzheimer's patients were discontinued because of meningoencephalitis in about 1 in 20 patients treated, although some cognitive, functional and biochemical outcomes proved promising.[115,116] Subsequent clinical trials are focusing on passive immunization with monoclonal antibodies against amyloid, which are thought unlikely to generate an inflammatory response. Long-term follow-up of early trial patients has confirmed the clearance of amyloid plaques from the brain, although patients are still dying with severe dementia.[117]

Alternative antiamyloid approaches involve secretase inhibitor drugs that target its production and those that inhibit its aggregation, but initial large-scale human trials in established Alzheimer's disease have been disappointing. Other approaches in Alzheimer's disease include drugs targeting the abnormally phosphorylated tau protein, neurotrophic agents, and drugs impacting on multiple neurotransmitters. There remain many unanswered questions.[118]

KEY POINTS

Presentation and Clinical Management of Dementia

- Dementia is a syndrome (not a diagnosis) describing a characteristic pattern of multiple cognitive deficits, usually including memory impairment, associated with a progressive decline in the ability to carry out daily activities and often associated with personality and behavioral changes.
- The diagnostic process requires confirmation from history and cognitive testing of the presence of dementia and then identification of the likely subtype (e.g., Alzheimer's disease, vascular dementia, dementia with Lewy bodies, Parkinson's disease, frontotemporal dementia, etc.). This may be best carried out in a memory clinic setting.
- Early recognition and intervention reduces risk of misdiagnosis of dementia and inappropriate management, facilitates optimal care, and can delay morbidity associated with progressive deterioration.
- Sharing the diagnosis can be challenging, but in most cases people with dementia benefit from being told sensitively what is wrong with them, what the implications are, and what can be done for them. Caretakers need to understand the diagnosis and be given comprehensible and practical information about coping strategies, care services, likely course of the disease, available treatment, and plans for follow-up.
- Both pharmacologic and nonpharmacologic treatments are effective. Management goals in early dementia center on improving or stabilizing cognitive ability and mood, maintaining or reestablishing independence, promoting autonomy, and effective planning for the future. As the condition progresses, emphasis shifts to facilitating mental and physical stimulation, managing behavioral disturbances, and providing practical care for patients and respite for their families.

For a complete list of references, please visit online only at www.expertconsult.com

CHAPTER 53

Neuropsychology in the Diagnosis and Treatment of Dementia

Margaret C. Sewell
Andrew Vigario
Mary Sano

INTRODUCTION

The aging of the United States population has given rise to a significant increase in the prevalence of Alzheimer's disease with estimates of 10.3% of those over 65 and 47.2% of those over 85.[1] It is estimated that in the next 50 years 1 in 45 Americans will have Alzheimer's disease.[2] Dementia represents significant impairment in cognitive functioning, defined as a decline in memory and at least one other cognitive domain (most commonly executive function, aphasia, or agnosia) serious enough to interfere with daily life, and not accounted for by other medical conditions. Many cases remain undiagnosed and untreated, an estimated half of elderly primary care patients[3], in part because health care providers may not regularly use screening instruments or refer for comprehensive evaluations. Neuropsychologists can assist in characterizing cognitive loss, its causes and consequences, and aid in the determination of decisional capacity.

This chapter will (1) outline why a neuropsychological evaluation may be needed, what it entails for the patient, and identify challenges to assessment of elderly patients, (2) explain the role of neuropsychology in the development of pharmacologic treatment for dementia, (3) describe screening instruments and common neuropsychological tests, and (4) review recent research that has identified typical patterns of impairment that distinguish one dementia from another, including depression.

REASONS FOR NEUROPSYCHOLOGICAL ASSESSMENT

A geriatric neuropsychological evaluation, unlike a brief cognitive screening or clinical interview, can distinguish the cognitive changes associated with normal aging from mild cognitive impairment (MCI) or dementia (both cortical and subcortical), distinguish dementia from depression, and arguably, differentiate one form of dementia from another.

A common referral question regards differentiating MCI or preclinical Alzheimer's disease from normal aging. Since cognitive changes with aging are well documented, including reduced processing speed, mental flexibility, and psychomotor slowing, cognitive complaints may be difficult to distinguish from changes attributed to aging or medical problems that may be associated with aging. This is important in individuals with particularly high or low levels of formal education and when other aspects of the medical or psychosocial history may leave doubt about how to interpret cognitive complaints. Well-established normative data on cognitive tests can provide a method for evaluating cognitive performance.

In the presence of clear cognitive impairment, however, neuropsychological assessment may be of value in distinguishing underlying causes. Historically, the pattern of neuropsychological deficit has been used to pinpoint deficit and to identify impairment in local neural networks. Longitudinal samples of well-characterized disease groups provide signature patterns of cognitive strengths and weaknesses, which may be used to support the diagnosis of specific types of dementia.

Neuropsychological assessment can also be useful to predict course or progression of cognitive disease. The characterization of syndromes such as mild cognitive impairment (MCI) allows prediction of future diagnoses with fair reliability. This can help determine the need for present and future assistance and support.

Neuropsychologists are also called upon to determine functional abilities, including decisional capacity, which is task specific. Neuropsychological evaluation of memory and executive functions (e.g., planning, reasoning) are important in this area as they document the cognitive strengths and weaknesses that can help determine a patient's current ability to drive, make medical decisions, live alone, or manage finances. There are also several measures available, including the widely used structured interview, the MacCAT-T,[4] which can aid in the direct assessment of specific decisional capacities.

In the research setting, cognitive testing is used to assess the effectiveness of treatments for dementia and in particular for Alzheimer's disease, the most common type of dementia. In this setting performance, differences between active and placebo conditions are used to assess efficacy of agents in combination with other global and functional measures (e.g., activities of daily living, behavioral symptoms). Baseline neuropsychological performance may also be used to assess an intervention or the cognitive impact of a medical procedure or treatment.

A comprehensive neuropsychological battery to determine the presence and nature of a dementia can be accomplished in several hours. The battery consists primarily of paper and pencil type of tests, with a few that can be administered on a computer—though the wisdom of using a computer with elderly patients needs to be determined on a case by case basis. Typically the assessment includes a clinical interview, and well-normed tests of memory, language, attention, visuospatial function, motor function, executive function, and depression. Because of beliefs that psychological testing of any kind is necessarily lengthy and expensive, it may be useful to reassure family members that the testing is relatively brief and is covered by Medicare.

CHALLENGES TO NEUROPSYCHOLOGICAL ASSESSMENT IN THE ELDERLY

There are several challenges to neuropsychological assessment, particularly in the elderly, which should be kept in mind as one selects tests and interprets results. First sensory impairment, common in elders, may interfere with testing. Since many tests present stimuli, visually or orally, serious hearing and visual loss can make interpretation of test performance difficult. However, these can be addressed by direct assessment, and sample items are often used to ensure sensory capacity is adequate for the test. Another challenge is mobility limitations as arthritis in hand joints may slow performance on timed tests and limit the validity of such procedures. This can be overcome in some cases by measuring differences in time for low and high cognitive demand tests rather than depending on the absolute time of a single test.

Low literacy, defined as not reading in any language, due to low levels of formal education or life-long disability can also impede testing but can be addressed by selecting assessment tools that use oral presentation, pictures, or other stimuli that do not require reading or knowledge of the alphabet. In this situation, it is important to rely on normative data of comparable individuals in order to have confidence about deficits. When this is not available, one must depend on clinical experience.

Language and culture can also challenge selection and interpretation of testing. Ideally a patient should be assessed in the language in which they are most competent by an evaluator who is equally competent in the language. Translation can be used but adequate normative samples against which to compare performance are sparse. Cultural specificity may figure into test items that can also compromise scoring. For example, literal translations may not provide the same complex meaning as demonstrated in the original version but experienced translators can help overcome these pitfalls.

Brief cognitive screening tools

Because of the increasing elderly population and subsequent demand on the primary care provider to screen for dementia, there has been a proliferation of screening tools developed in the past 15 years. There is no shortage of brief and easy screens, with reasonable reliability, sensitivity, and specificity. The challenge is in persuading physicians and health care providers of the value of using them. The goal of these instruments is to provide a quick and reliable method of identifying cognitive impairment that is easy to administer and score and may be used as part of routine care in those over 65 years old. The advantage of them, as a group, is the opportunity to distinguish patients with normal age-related changes in cognition from those who may need a thorough diagnostic neuropsychological work-up. The disadvantages include poor normative data, and varying levels of sensitivity/specificity. Below, several of the most popular screening tools are described.

Mini-Mental Status Examination (MMSE)[5]: The MMSE was intended to be a brief, easy to use tool for grading cognitive impairments. A major advantage of the MMSE is that most health care providers use the instrument in daily practice, thus facilitating communication among various clinicians.[6] This 30-point, 10-minute screening instrument is particularly useful when used repeatedly to measure change in cognitive status. The MMSE has been criticized for its limited usefulness among those with low levels of English literacy or formal education.[7] To address this, different cut-off points for an abnormal result have been created for those of differing ages and educational levels.[8] Overall, the MMSE's ability to detect dementia ranges from 71% to 92% sensitivity and 56% to 98% specificity.[7] In a meta-analysis conducted by Mitchell, the MMSE had very limited ability to distinguish MCI from either normal controls or those with Alzheimer's disease.[9]

Clock Drawing Test (CDT): The CDT, a simple task of drawing a clock face set to a particular time, is an easy to administer and frequently used screening measure that taps visuospatial and constructional abilities along with executive function (planning, abstract thinking)—areas frequently compromised in early dementia and is free of some of the biases inherent in other tests (e.g., non-English speaking). The test has been used to distinguish normal aging from dementia,[10] and track progress over time,[11] though it has not been as useful in distinguishing normal aging from MCI.[12,13] There are numerous methods of scoring, some simple, some complex, and some researchers suggest that with more comprehensive scoring systems, the clock can be useful in identifying MCI patients at high risk for progressing to dementia.[14] Naïve raters have been shown to judge the normalcy of a clock and most rating systems in healthy elders or moderate/severe demented patients, but not in those with mild dementia.[15]

Mini-Cog: The Mini-Cog[16] consists of a three-word recall task and a clock drawing. The results designate someone as demented or not demented, and while useful in distinguishing demented patients from normal elderly,[17] it has not been as useful in identifying those with MCI.[18]

The Montreal Cognitive Assessment (MoCA)[19]: This brief screening instrument which requires same training is a relatively new measure that takes approximately 10 minutes to administer and was designed for those suspected of mild cognitive dysfunction. It assesses orientation, attention and concentration, executive function, memory, visuospatial skills, language, conceptual ability, and calculation. It has been shown in those with a MMSE of at least 26, to detect MCI with 90% sensitivity, and early AD with 100% sensitivity.

The Telephone Interview for Cognitive Status (TICS)[20]: This 11-item test takes approximately 10 minutes to administer on the telephone and is a brief cognitive screen that measures global cognitive functioning. It is normed on those 60 to 98, and because it is given on the telephone, and therefore not reliant on visual ability, may be useful for visually impaired patients. Patients are classified as unimpaired, ambiguous, mildly impaired, and moderately to severely impaired. There are two sets of norm groups for those with less and greater than 12 years of education.

In summary, these screening measures as a group can be useful "quick and dirty" measures that can be administered by those with a minimal amount of training and serve as useful "red flags" to identify those in need of further evaluation. Because we lack reliable biologic markers to identify Alzheimer's disease, neuropsychological testing remains the most accurate method to identify and characterize very early symptoms and distinguish them from other types of cognitive impairment.

NEUROPSYCHOLOGICAL TESTS: DOMAINS OF ASSESSMENT AND NORMATIVE DATA

Most neuropsychologists do not use ready-made batteries but rather select specific tests or sets of tests that assess the major domains of cognition affected in dementia, namely verbal and visual memory, attention, naming, fluency, executive function, visuospatial function, motor function, and depression. A summary of commonly used tests may be found in Table 53-1. All test results are compared to normative data based on age, often education, and sometimes gender. Results are then examined for typical patterns that may suggest different types of cognitive impairments. Additionally, the neuropsychologist will determine the presence of neuropsychiatric symptoms and level of independence with ADL and IADL. The presence of a caregiver for the interview portion of the evaluation is critical.

Premorbid functioning estimates

To determine whether someone has significantly declined from a previous level of cognitive functioning, it is necessary to estimate premorbid level of functioning. This can be accomplished through a careful review of someone's educational and occupational history, tests of vocabulary that tend not to decline even in the presence of dementia, or, for those with at least 8 years of formal education, word reading tests that use a formula taking into account education, and number of reading errors to provide a crude estimate of premorbid verbal IQ.[21]

Alzheimer's disease. Though postmortem diagnosis is still the gold standard, Alzheimer's, the most common form of dementia in those over 65, can be accurately clinically diagnosed greater than 90% of the time.[22] The two standard sets of criteria for Alzheimer's disease (AD) include the Diagnostic and Statistical Manual of Mental Disorders, fourth edition (DSM-IV-TR)[23] and the National Institute of Neurological Disorders and Stroke-Alzheimer's Disease Related Disorders (NINCDS-ADRDA).[24] The DSM-IV-TR criteria require impairment in memory and in one other area of cognition (e.g., apraxia, aphasia, agnosia, executive function, attention, visuospatial ability), with concomitant functional impairment (either social or vocational). The NINCDS-ADRDA also includes criteria that the progression is insidious and that other diseases that could cause cognitive decline have been ruled out.

AD, characterized by damage (plaque and neurofibrillary tangles, synapse loss, atrophy) beginning in the medial temporal lobe (hippocampus and entorhinal cortex), is usually marked by a slow and steady progression. The dementia associated with these neuropathologic changes includes significant memory loss as the central core, with other impairments in language (semantic and phonemic fluency, naming), executive function (parallel processing, planning, switching cognitive sets, abstraction), and later in the illness, attention, and visuospatial function.

Recent neuropsychological research has focused on identifying the very earliest cognitive impairments associated with AD, usually episodic memory. Verbal memory is most commonly assessed with either word lists (e.g., CVLT, RAVLT) or stories (e.g., logical memory), and normative data for initial and delayed recall along with recognition is well-established on these tests across age and education categories well into the ninth decade. A substantial amount of research has indicated that AD is associated with a particular pattern of cognitive deficits that distinguish it from normal aging,[25] and, in some cases, from other forms of dementia.

The ability to learn and retain verbal information distinguishes between those with mild AD and healthy elders.[26–31] Neuropsychological performance on verbal memory tests is marked by difficulty not only in the free recall of recently learned information, but in the aided retrieval of that information with cues.[32] In very early AD, initial learning may be relatively well-preserved, though, compared to normal controls, deficits in both acquisition and consolidation of information may still be present, along with evidence of a shallower learning curve.[33,34] Deficits in both encoding and delayed recall become more severe as the disease progresses.[35]

Examination of specific patterns of responses on delayed recall suggests that normal controls tend to recall words equally from the beginning and end of a list but AD patients rely heavily on words only from the end of the list (recency effect), arguing that the AD patient, not having transferred the information from primary to secondary memory, has not really "learned" the words at all.[36,37] AD patients are sensitive to interference,[38] and this is evidenced by a high number (relative to normal controls) of intrusions (e.g., when words from a second list of words appears while the patient

Table 53-1. Neuropsychological Tests

Domains to be Assessed	Commonly Used Tests Used with Age-Corrected and/or Education Norms for Those >65
Premorbid ability	North American Reading Test *(NART)*
	Vocabulary *(WAIS-III)*
Verbal memory	Rey Auditory Verbal Learning Test *(RAVLT)*
	California Verbal Learning Test *(CVLT)*
	Logical Memory Test *(from WMS)*
	CERAD Word List Test
Visual memory	Visual Reproduction *(from WMS-III)*
	Rey Osterrieth Figure Drawing Test *(RFDT)*
Simple attention	Digit Span *(from WAIS-III)*
	Trail-Making Part A
Language	Animal Naming Test *(ANT)*
	Controlled Oral Word Association Test *(COWAT)*
	Boston Naming Test
Executive function	Trail-Making Part B
	Wisconsin Card Sort Test *(WCST)*
	Stroop
	Similarities *(from WAIS-III)*
Visuospatial	Digit Symbol Test *(from WAIS-III)*
	Rey Osterrieth Figure Drawing Test *(RFDT)*
	Clock Drawing Test
Motor	Grooved Pegboard Test
	Finger Tapping Test
Depression	Geriatric Depression Scale *(GDS)*
	Hamilton Depression Rating Scale *(HDRS)*

WAIS-III. Wechsler Adult Intelligence Scale, ed 3; WMS-III: Wechsler Memory Scale, ed 3.

is attempting to recall words from a previously learned list), and repetitions.[39] This finding is observed on tests of both word lists and stories.[40]

Very recent research has focused on clarifying other aspects of episodic memory problems, highlighting the attentional and organizational skills required that may help better characterize the deficits in very mildly impaired patients.[41]

Visual memory may also be assessed, although there is some evidence that visuospatial skills naturally deteriorate with age, making these tasks less discriminatory. However, some recent studies have identified nonverbal memory impairments in very mildly impaired AD patients compared with normal controls. For example, performance on the recall portion of the Rey-Osterrieth Complex Figure Test (RCFT) has been shown to be impaired even in very mild AD patients.[42]

Difficulties with executive functioning may be the first symptom to appear after episodic memory impairments.[43] Those with AD exhibit marked difficulty relative to normal controls with various executive functions including cognitive flexibility, problem solving, parallel processing, planning, set shifting, and abstract thinking. These deficits, which worsen as the disease progresses, are observed on lower than expected performance on common tests of executive function including phonemic fluency, card sorting, and trail-making. The careful measurement of various executive abilities is important in those with early AD because deficits in this area have been consistently related to poorer functional ability,[44] ability to manage finances,[45] and higher need for care.[46]

Language abilities are also impaired in early AD. Important language domains include naming, commonly assessed with a picture naming task such as the Boston Naming Test (a test of 60 pictures covering high and low frequency words), and fluency, which is assessed by assessing the rate of production of words beginning with a given letter (phonemic fluency) or within a given category (semantic fluency).

Confrontation naming is impaired early,[47] and unlike healthy elders who also have benign "senior moments," those with AD often do not benefit from cues, either semantic (giving hints about what the object is) or phonemic (saying the beginning of the sound of the word). A considerable amount of research indicates that scores on the BNT can effectively discriminate among normal controls, MCI, and AD patients.[48,49] Difficulties with naming and fluency worsen as AD progresses.[50] However, in early AD patients, basic comprehension and verbal expression are intact.

Semantic fluency test performance (e.g., naming as many animals as possible in 60 seconds) is impaired very early in AD, relative to phonemic fluency.[51,52] Some suggest[53] that animal naming is more difficult due to impairment of semantic knowledge and executive function required for any category test.

Simple attention (measured, for example, by Digit Span) is usually preserved in early AD. However, tasks that require divided attention (Trails B) or selective attention (the Stroop Test) are usually difficult for the AD patient[43] and may reflect problems with working memory, which involves the ability to process and respond to several pieces of information simultaneously. Some researchers have observed relatively intact divided attention ability in very mild AD patients,[41,35] though problems are more significant at the moderate stages of the illness.[54]

Visuospatial functioning may be preserved, relative to memory, language, and executive function. However, deficits may be seen on visuoconstructional tests, such as clock drawing and complex geometric figure drawing.[55] Deficits in visuospatial abilities have been associated with wandering and driving difficulties.[56] Performance on tests of visuospatial functioning (e.g., the copy portion of the Rey Osterrieth Drawing Test) may be confounded by cognitive demands that are more executive than visuospatial, namely planning and organization, and difficulties with these abilities may artificially lower test scores. Other tests of visuospatial function that do not have a high executive demand, such as the Judgment of Line Orientation Test, may be a more accurate measure of pure visuospatial ability.

In summary, a typical early AD profile, in the absence of significant depression, might reveal (1) moderately impaired initial learning with significantly impaired delayed recall on tests of verbal memory, (2) relatively well-preserved performance on phonemic fluency in context of impaired semantic fluency and naming, (3) intact simple attention, (4) impaired performance on executive functioning tests measuring cognitive flexibility and planning through abstraction may be well-preserved, and (5) mildly impaired performance on tests of visuospatial and visuoconstructional ability.

Mild cognitive impairment

Mild cognitive impairment (MCI) has been characterized as a transitional phase between the cognitive changes associated with normal aging and dementia.[49] Though there are no universally accepted criteria for the diagnosis of MCI,[57] criteria include memory complaint and objective memory impairment compared to age-matched elders with other cognitive domains and daily function relatively intact. Conversion rates for this group of MCI patients to AD may range 12% to 15% a year[58] and up to 80% at 6 years[57] (Petersen, 2004). Furthermore, a group of MCI patients with multiple cognitive domain impairments including memory impairment (but who do not meet criteria for dementia) have been shown to convert to AD at a rate of 50% at 3-year follow-up,[59] suggesting that this group may represent the highest conversion risk.

Recently, the MCI criteria have expanded to include nonamnestic MCI, representing impairments in nonmemory domains (e.g., language, executive function), that may place one at a high risk for developing another form of dementia, such as vascular or frontotemporal dementia.[60,61] One large study[62] observed that those with nonamnestic multidomain MCI were in fact more likely to develop a non-Alzheimer's type dementia.

Recent studies[63] have observed that neuropsychological testing can identify those at highest risk for progressing to dementia within 5 years, even among these patients with very mild cognitive impairments who do not meet formal research criteria for MCI. A review by Twamley and colleagues[64] highlighted the importance of the role of attention in context of memory, language, executive function, and processing speed regarding those who later developed dementia.

There is intense interest in neuropsychological measures that can identify impairment in its earliest stages and in better understanding the cognitive decline evident years before a diagnosis of dementia,[65,66] as this could allow the development of useful clinical trials and earlier intervention.[67] Poor performance (usually defined as >1.5 standard deviations below age-adjusted norms) on standardized tests of verbal memory (e.g., delayed recall of word lists) or executive ability (e.g., Trails B, Stroop Interference Test) have been shown in numerous studies to be sensitive predictors of progression to AD in those with amnestic MCI[68–72] and in discriminating MCI from AD.[73] In some studies[59] but not all,[69] naming and semantic fluency tests have also distinguished between amnestic MCI patients who convert to AD and those who do not.

Efforts have been made to identify simple screening tests that could be conducted in the primary care office to diagnose MCI, with limited success. Mitchell[9] reported in his meta-analysis of eight studies examining the ability of the MMSE to distinguish AD from MCI or MCI from healthy controls, that overall, the measure did not discriminate well between either normal aging and MCI or MCI and early dementia. Some have suggested[74] that examining specific scores of the MMSE, rather than the total score, may help better distinguish amnestic and non-amnestic MCI patients from normal controls. Among those with non-amnestic MCI, neither the MMSE nor the Mini-Cog had adequate sensitivity as screening instruments.[18] However, the Montreal Cognitive Assessment (MoCA) has shown some promise in its ability, in those with a MMSE of at least 26, to distinguish normal controls from MCI and MCI from early AD with a high degree of accuracy[19] and has been used with those with Parkinson's disease to identify MCI in patients whose MMSE scores were in the normal range.[75]

To identify the largest group of at-risk patients (including amnestic, nonamnestic, and multi-domain MCI), a thorough neuropsychological evaluation that includes measures of delayed recall, executive function, and language still remains the most effective way to identify MCI.[76]

In summary, patients with MCI may have cognitive complaints but no significant functional decline; neuropsychological testing can identify significant memory impairment relative to normal controls in those with amnestic-MCI, with a significant number ultimately converting to AD. Those who have cognitive complaint and a nonamnestic area of decline (e.g., language, executive function) may be at greater risk of developing a non-Alzheimer's dementia.

Vascular dementia

Vascular dementia is the most common cause of dementia after Alzheimer's disease and it is estimated to account for approximately a third of all dementia cases. Many diagnostic classification schemes exist for vascular dementia and vascular cognitive impairment but most exclude the focal cognitive deficits of stroke and consider those conditions with impairment in multiple cognitive domains. The diagnosis is largely dependent on the history or presence of clinical stroke or radiologic findings of infarct. The diagnostic problem is further complicated by the fact that vascular disease and cerebrovascular disease often co-occur with Alzheimer's disease and other dementias. Critical issues related to the criteria for diagnosis of vascular dementia include the definition of the cognitive syndrome (i.e., the type, extent, and combination of cognitive impairments), attention to additive effects on cognitive impairment in the presence of comorbidity, and temporal occurrence of symptoms and deficits.

Accurately identifying vascular dementia requires careful attention to historical information. The onset may be both rapid and temporally related to a strokelike event, or it may be gradual with a progression that is described as stepwise. Reports of an accumulation of cognitive worsening and functional incapacity are common.

Wiederkehr and colleagues[77] examined diagnostic criteria for eight cognitive syndromes in vascular disease. Although DSM-IV VaD criteria require memory impairment,[78] the widely used NINDS-AIREN criteria for vascular dementia (VaD) include memory impairment (either in anterograde or retrograde memory) along with deficits in two or more other cognitive domains, which are sufficient to interfere with activities of daily living.[79] In clinical practice, among those with a history of stroke, the cognitive criteria may be assessed by the report of cognitive deficit in the absence of formal testing. However, several studies suggest that when these individuals are diagnosed clinically, group comparisons with AD subjects often find the VAD group to have less severe memory impairment. The pattern that is often reported within VaD is one in which working memory is more likely to be impaired than delayed recall, a pattern which is the opposite of AD.[80] Cued recall and recognition of previously learned material is generally intact, unlike AD.

Executive function is commonly impaired in VaD and the deficit may be disproportional to other cognitive deficits such as memory.[81] Executive function deficit is also more commonly reported in VaD than in AD, at least at the mild and early forms of dementia.

Regarding language, naming and verbal fluency impairments are common particularly with subcortical and thalamic infarcts. Verbal fluency is usually impaired, though the distinctive pattern of preserved phonemic fluency and impaired semantic fluency so often seen in AD, is uncommon.[82] In fact, some studies suggest that in contrast to AD, patients with VaD have worse phonemic fluency scores relative to semantic fluency,[83,84] which may reflect an executive function impairment severe enough such that even the structure of the alphabet is not sufficient to organise the patient's responses.

Another area reported to be impaired in VaD is psychomotor speed and measures of attention. Although focal deficits can be responsible for some such impairments, they may be exacerbated by depression, which is a common concomitant of VaD.[85]

A prodromal condition of vascular cognitive impairment (VCI) has been described. This condition, characterized by cognitive complaints observed by the patient or others, is associated with impairment in any of a wide range of neuropsychological functions.[86,87] Recent longitudinal data suggests that the presence of multiple cognitive impairments is predictive of the transition from VCI to VaD.[87]

In summary, VaD and VCI may have a less robust episodic memory deficit with the possibility of a range of impairments. The likelihood of executive function deficit and depression are higher than in AD. Although the precision of diagnosing VaD and other cognitive syndromes is hampered by the breadth of the possible deficits, it is important to consider vascular condition and risks because many may be controlled, hopefully stabilising cognition.

Frontotemporal dementia

Frontotemporal dementia (FTD) is a common cause of dementia in those under 65 years old[88] and may account for 20% of dementia cases in those 45 to 65 years old.[89] It is important to distinguish AD and FTD because treatment and prognosis may differ, yet efforts to distinguish the two clinically have been met with limited success. The efficacy of cholinesterase inhibitors is perceived to be highest in AD and poorest in FTD. Perceived efficacy is affected more by whom is treated than by what is used.[90] In the past several decades, numerous terms have been proposed to describe this complex group of related but distinct conditions associated with pathology in the frontal and anterior temporal areas, including dementia of the frontal lobe type,[91] frontotemporal lobar degeneration,[92] Pick's disease,[93] and familial chromosome 17-linked frontal lobe dementia,[94] among others.

Currently, the term frontotemporal dementia (FTD) is frequently used with two variations, semantic dementia (SD) and progressive nonfluent aphasia (PNFA). Typically, the primary characteristics of FTD are early age of onset (45 to 65) relative to AD, a more precipitous course, and early behavioral changes including disinhibition, apathy, hyperorality, and inappropriate social interaction.[26] The striking and early behavioral symptoms necessitate a differential diagnosis not just among dementias, but between dementia and psychiatric illness.[95]

Neuropsychological profiles in FTD patients are, compared with AD patients, characterized by poor executive and language function and relatively spared memory function, particularly early in the illness. Efforts to distinguish FTD from AD patients using neuropsychological tests have been inconsistent, in part due to small sample sizes, different stages of illness, and varying diagnostic criteria.

Regarding memory function, performance on the delayed recall and retention portion of word list tests is better preserved in FTD patients relative to those with AD.[96] Overall better memory performance (compared with other cognitive functions) has been noted in other studies as well regarding both delayed recall and the ability to use cues.[97]

On language tests, studies have suggested that those with FTD are more impaired than those with AD on tests of verbal fluency. Specifically, Rascovsky and colleagues[96] found that compared with AD patients, those with autopsy-confirmed FTD exhibited more impairment on verbal fluency tests (both semantic and phonemic) perhaps due to the significant executive demand of search strategies. Some have observed more impaired phonemic fluency compared with semantic fluency in those with FTD,[98,52] the reverse of the pattern typically observed in AD.

On tests of executive function, FTD patients may be proportionately worse on tests of cognitive set switching and cognitive flexibility than memory tests.[99] FTD patients may have difficulty with selective and divided attention, but these results are not consistent.[100]

Visuospatial skills are relatively intact relative to other cognitive deficits,[101] though visuospatial tasks that include significant executive ability such as organization and planning (e.g., the Rey Osterrieth Copy Test) may prove difficult. Clock drawing and block design may be better measures of visuospatial ability in FTD.

In summary, early behavioral change is the "red flag" of FTD, accompanied by relatively spared memory and visuospatial skills, but impaired language and executive function.

PRIMARY PROGRESSIVE APHASIAS: SEMANTIC DEMENTIA (SD) AND PROGRESSIVE NONFLUENT APHASIA (PNFA)

Semantic dementia

Semantic dementia (SD), characterized by atrophy in the left anterior temporal lobe, is associated with severe and progressive problems with naming, category fluency, picture naming, and comprehension.[102] Language problems begin first and by definition, one must have had a 2-year period of language impairment in the relative absence of other cognitive difficulties. Scores on category fluency may be worse than letter fluency, and naming may be worse than comprehension.[103] Later in the illness, despite profound deficits in semantic memory and meaning, expressive language may retain its fluency (e.g., normal prosody and volume), but often grows increasingly empty.

Early in the illness, visuospatial, attentional, and executive abilities generally remain relatively intact, and the significant behavioral symptoms associated with FTD absent. Regarding memory function, one study observed poor delayed recall, but normal new learning in those with semantic dementia.[98]

Progressive Nonfluent Aphasia (PNFA)

Progressive nonfluent aphasia (PNFA), associated with damage in the left perisylvian language areas, is characterized by preserved comprehension, but poor expressive language. Speech may be hesitant, accompanied by poor articulation, dysarthria, and profound word finding difficulty not accounted for by stroke. The behavioral problems associated with FTD are generally not present.

Performance is poor on tests of verbal fluency. Some researchers[104] argue that category and letter fluency tests can help distinguish among SD, PNFA and AD, with AD patients least impaired and PNFA patients most impaired on letter fluency. However, others have found that fluency tests do not distinguish among FTD, PNFA, and SD patients.[98] This may be because many cognitive abilities are involved in this test. However, Hodges and colleagues[105] observed that a simple "Repeat and Point" test was effective in distinguishing semantic dementia from PNFA, with poor performance by SD patients on pointing (comprehension), and poor performance by PNFA patients on repeating.

There is evidence of slower executive functioning performance compared with patients with either semantic dementia or AD.[98] However, compared with patients with FTD, executive function and attention may be relatively well-preserved.[106] Episodic memory scores are generally intact early in the illness,[104] though due to the nature of the illness (poor expressive language), nonverbal tests of memory may be more useful.

Parkinson's disease dementia (PDD) and dementia with Lewy bodies (DLB)

The dementia associated with Parkinson's disease, which may develop in 20% to 40% of Parkinson's patients,[107] is consistent with a typical subcortical pattern, namely impairments in attention (including working memory and divided attention), executive function (particularly planning and set shifting), and visuospatial function. The onset is typically insidious, with variable rates of progression, and the dementia must follow onset of motor symptoms by at least 1 year.[108] The cognitive deficits are in the context of a mildly impaired episodic memory, with problems with delayed recall but intact cued recognition. Compared with other impairments, language function is relatively well-preserved.[109] Neuropsychiatric symptoms, including hallucinations and depression, are frequent.[110]

Most research concurs that episodic memory deficits are milder in PDD than in AD, and that the problems are due more to deficits in retrieval than encoding and storage.[111–113] This is illustrated by the ability to recall previously learned information when provided cues.

Compared with AD, PDD patients exhibit poor executive functioning[114,115] noted by poor performance on tests of initiation/perseveration and card sorting.[106] Deficits on attention tests distinguish PDD from AD,[116] particularly on tasks that require divided attention.[117]

Visuospatial task performance may be more impaired in PDD than AD, including pentagon copy.[118] Patients with PDD exhibit cognitive slowing, but measuring this is often complicated by the fact that most tests have some motor component,[119] making it difficult to distinguish the physical from the cognitive.

It is important to measure depression as it occurs in up to 50% of Parkinson's patients, and its presence may exacerbate poor neuropsychological test performance.[120] Furthermore, the presence of depression is associated with more significant cognitive impairment, even in those Parkinson's patients without dementia.[121]

There is a long literature describing cognitive deficit in PD patients without dementia. Recently, these deficits have been labeled mild cognitive impairment (MCI) with the observation that it frequently progresses to dementia.[122,123] This notion is controversial and still being developed. One study[124] found that single and multiple nonmemory domain PD-MCI patients were more likely to convert to dementia than the PD-MCI amnestic group.

In summary, the dementia associated with PDD is characterized by high rates of depression and by a subcortical pattern of poor attention, visuospatial and executive functioning, slowed processing speed with relatively spared memory and language abilities.

Dementia with Lewy bodies

The complex role of Lewy body pathology in dementia with Lewy bodies (DLB) and its relationship to PDD is not fully understood.[118] The primary triad of symptoms associated with DLB includes fluctuating cognition (e.g., attention and alertness that vary noticeably day to day), Parkinson-like symptoms (e.g., bradykinesia, rigidity, and gait disturbance) and visual hallucinations. Other symptoms may include rapid eye movement sleep disorders, and frequent falls. Accurate diagnosis of DLB is critical because DLB is associated with a dangerous sensitivity to neuroleptic medications.[125] The cognitive changes observed in PDD and DLB are so similar that the two disorders are clinically distinguished by the timing of the onset of symptoms: the motor symptoms in DLB patients occur no more than 1 year before the onset of dementia and frequently after the onset of dementia in contrast to PDD, where motor symptoms must precede dementia by at least a year.[107]

Characterizing DLB with neuropsychological testing can be difficult, as the cognitive deficits often overlap with those of AD and PDD, but most closely resemble PDD.[111] Memory is impaired, though not as severely as in AD, and, as in PDD, the problem is more one of retrieval than encoding.[124] Taken together, studies suggest that DLB patients, compared with AD patients, exhibit more severe deficits in executive functioning, visuospatial functioning, and attentional abilities.[111,126,127] Poor visuospatial function appears to be a predictor of further cognitive decline in those with DLB but not AD.[128] In DLB, the poor performance on tests of visuoperceptual and spatial functions may be related to the fact they are vulnerable to visual hallucinations.[121] Though it is difficult to distinguish DLB from PDD with neuropsychological testing, a handful of studies have observed poorer performance by DLB patients on tests of attention, visuoperceptual skills, and executive function, controlling for illness severity.[111,129]

In summary, DLB is difficult to distinguish from PDD and AD with neuropsychological testing, though the cognitive impairments, which usually precede any Parkinsonian symptoms, are more likely to resemble PDD and be accompanied by fluctuating attention and visual hallucinations.

Mood: distinguishing depression from dementia

Older adults may have symptoms of forgetfulness and apathy that relate to depression, dementia, or both. Distinguishing dementia from depression is critical because of the comparative success with which depression can be treated. Patterns on test performance emerge that suggest depression or early dementia, and in conjunction with clinical history, results may help in predicting which nondemented depressed patients are at high risk for developing dementia.

In the past, the term "pseudodementia"[130] was used to describe the presence of forgetfulness and confusion in the presence of depression. However, recent research shows that even after depressive symptoms are successfully treated, for many the cognitive deficits remain.[131]

In elderly patients with depression, significant cognitive impairment is common[132] and the severity of impairment on tests of memory, executive function, processing speed, attention and language generally falls somewhere between normal controls and those with early AD. Among depressed nondemented patients, difficulties with attention and executive function may be the primary cognitive complaints. Elderly patients experiencing a first-time depression exhibit problems with executive function and attention, with less relative memory impairment, compared with either those with recurrent depression or normal controls.[133] Older depressed adults without dementia perform poorly on tests of psychomotor speed and various aspects of executive function compared to those without depression.[134,135]

Some have observed[136] that the cognitive deficits associated with depression fit a more subcortical than cortical pattern, with the relative preservation of language, memory, and praxis relative to AD patients. On tests of verbal memory, depressed patients perform better than AD patients with less impairment in retention and recognition of previously learned material.[137]

Regarding language, a meta-analysis of fluency in depressed elderly patients observed that AD patients were more impaired on both phonemic and semantic fluency than depressed patients, though the relative severity of semantic fluency impairment in AD patients remained.[138]

Some research suggests that specific neuropsychological profiles may predict which depressed patients are at high risk for developing dementia. In a small retrospective study, Jean and colleagues[139] observed in a group of elderly depressed patients that baseline performance on tests of attention and memory were more impaired in those with subsequent dementia—with additional deficits in orientation in those who went on to develop AD, and in executive and visuospatial function in those who developed Lewy body or vascular dementia. Repeated neuropsychological evaluations may be useful in those with depression with cognitive complaints, as one large prospective study[140] suggests that cognitive functioning will continue to decline in depressed patients who eventually develop dementia, and that baseline neuropsychological test performance (including executive function, visuospatial ability, and delayed recall) was lower at baseline in those depressed patients who went on to develop dementia. These studies underscore the usefulness of neuropsychological evaluation in depressed patients who also have cognitive complaints.

The relationship between depression and AD is complex.[141] The issue centers on whether depression in late life (whether recurrent or initial onset) may herald incipient dementia.[142,143] or whether the presence of depression is a risk factor for the later development of dementia.[144,145] A considerable amount of recent research has examined factors that may affect this distinction, including the proximity of depression and dementia,[146] whether the depression onset is early or late,[138] the presence of vascular illness,[147] and gender.[148]

In summary, though the relationship between depression and dementia is complex and not fully understood, a clinical presentation of depression, particularly with symptoms of apathy and cognitive complaints, warrant neuropsychological evaluation. The results, particularly if measured on more than one occasion, may help in determining whether the patient has depression, dementia, or both. A summary of the pattern of cognitive deficits associated with different dementias and depression may be found in Table 53-2.

Other areas that may be measured

Level of independence with activities of daily living (ADL) and instrumental activities of daily living (IADL) should always be evaluated, either informally or with standard measures. Impairment in these areas has a dramatic impact on both the patient and caregiver regarding quality of life, caregiver burden, and decisions regarding nursing home placement. Activities of daily living include highly overlearned tasks, such as dressing, toileting, and grooming, whereas

Table 53-2. Patterns of Cognitive Impairment by Domain and Dementia

	Episodic Memory	Attention	Language	Executive	Visuospatial	Behavioral Symptoms
Alzheimer's disease	(I)	Simple (P) Divided (I)	Phonemic (P) Semantic (I) Naming (I)	(I)	Simple (P) Complex (I)	Early apathy; Late psychotic symptoms
Mild cognitive impairment—amnestic	Immediate and delayed recall (I) Recognition (I)	Simple (P) Divided (P)	(P)	(P)	(P)	(P)
Vascular dementia	Immediate and delayed recall (V) Recognition (P)	Simple (P) Divided (I)	(I)	(I)	(P)	Depression
Frontotemporal dementia	(V)	Simple (P) Divided (I)	(I)	(I)	(P)	Disinhibition, apathy, hyperorality, inappropriate social interaction
Semantic dementia	(P)	(P)	(I) Comprehension (I) fluency	(P)	(P) (I) Visual agnosia	(P)
Progressive non-fluent aphasia	(P)	(P)	(I) fluency (P) comprehension, (I) expressive speech	(P)	(P)	(P)
Parkinson's disease dementia	(V) Immediate and delayed recall (P) Recognition	(I)	(P)	(I)	(I)	Depression, possible hallucinations, psychomotor slowing
Dementia with Lewy bodies	(V) Immediate and delayed recall (P) Recognition	(V)	(V)	(I)	(I)	Hallucinations, delusions
Depression	(V) Immediate and delayed recall (P) Recognition +	(V)	(V) fluency (P) Naming	I/V	(P)	Psychomotor slowing, apathy

P, Preserved; V, Variable; I, Impaired.

instrumental activities of daily living refer to more complex tasks with greater cognitive demand such as managing money, cooking, and shopping. Decline in ability to manage IADL may happen relatively early in AD, and is related to deficits in memory, sustained attention, and problem-solving. Most patients in the mild to moderate stages of AD evidence some difficulty with medication, cooking, and shopping.[149]

SUMMARY

Neuropsychological testing is a valuable tool in the identification and description of many cognitive disorders and can aid in the differential diagnosis of normal aging, MCI, AD, and other dementias, including depression. Screening tools are useful for quick assessment of those who may be in need of further evaluation.

The variability among neuropsychological profiles is most apparent in the first several years of the illness, underscoring the importance of early evaluation, diagnosis, and treatment. Knowledge of a dementia diagnosis early on can improve health outcomes in several ways: by initiating pharmacologic treatment during the time of illness in which it works best, by providing clinical research opportunities to families that could lead to better treatment, and by giving the patient the opportunity, while they still retain decisional capacity, to prepare for the future by creating advance directives, and making decisions about finances and other family matters.

A frank and empathic discussion may also help alleviate the guilt and blame that occurs when the patient or caregiver has been under the erroneous impression that the cognitive deficits would disappear if only one "tried harder." The role of the caregiver cannot be underestimated, and as psychosocial interventions for caregivers are effective,[150] an early and accurate diagnosis of a loved one may open the door for the caregiver to seek both support and education.

KEY POINTS

Neuropsychology in the Diagnosis and Treatment of Dementia

- Neuropsychological testing is an effective way of identifying very early cognitive impairments and distinguishing them from normal aging, MCI, and various types of dementia using relatively brief batteries of tests.
- Neuropsychologists can assist in characterizing cognitive loss, its causes and consequences, distinguish between dementia and comorbidities such as depression, and determine decisional capacity.
- Patients who have cognitive impairments in context of either motor symptoms (e.g., gait changes) or behavioral symptoms (disinhibition) should be referred for a neuropsychiatric evaluation.
- Early diagnosis of a dementia or depression is critical in terms of treatment effectiveness, future planning, and quality of life.
- Screening measures (e.g., MMSE, clock drawing) are useful tools to monitor changes in functioning over time and to identify "red flags" that may warrant referral to a neuropsychologist or other specialist, though they lack diagnostic reliability.
- Comprehensive assessment of memory loss is the core feature of a dementia evaluation. Non-Alzheimer's dementias may be characterized by other cognitive or behavioral impairments, such as language (SD, PNFA), executive function (PDD, VD), personality changes (FTD), and psychotic symptoms (DLB).
- A clinical presentation of depression, particularly with symptoms of apathy and other cognitive complaints, warrants neuropsychological evaluation.

For a complete list of references, please visit online only at www.expertconsult.com

CHAPTER 54

Alzheimer's Disease

Martin R. Farlow

Alzheimer's disease (AD) is the most common cause for dementia afflicting older adults. The illness was first described by Alois Alzheimer in 1906 in a 51-year-old woman with well-described features of dementia. After death her brain was examined and found to have numerous cortical plaques and tangles, characteristic of the illness.[1] The disease was thought to be rare for six decades until its clinical and neuropathologic features were recognized to be largely identical to those occurring in elderly dementia patients.[2]

The illness is by far the most frequent cause of dementia in the United States, currently afflicting as many as 5.2 million mostly elderly individuals.[3] The incidence doubles every 6 years after the age of 50. As the over-age-80 population has rapidly grown, with improved health care leading to longer survival, it is estimated that the prevalence of AD in the United States by 2050 will almost triple to 11 million to 16 million Americans.[4] This disabling disease is by far the most common cause of neurodegeneration and the major condition leading to nursing home placement. The economic costs are huge with direct health care, nursing home costs, and caregiving costs at home globally totaling greater than $315 billion.[5] Only symptomatic therapies are currently available, but no known therapy delays or halts disease progression. If a drug or lifestyle alteration (e.g., diet, exercise) could be found that delayed functional deterioration by as little as 1 to 2 years, it would substantially reduce the costs to both families and society.

PATHOLOGY AND MECHANISMS OF DISEASE

In AD, the illness begins with atrophy in the entorhinal cortex and hippocampus, and as clinical symptoms worsen, there is spread to, more generally, most areas of the cortex, excepting only the occipital lobes.[6]

Microscopic examination of cortical sections from the brain of a patient with AD reveals global loss of neurons and increased numbers of extracellular amyloid plaques.[7] The amyloid plaques are both "diffuse," possibly benign, since similar deposits may be found in normal elderly individuals, and "compact," often associated with neuritic changes, possibly caused by the effects of the deposited amyloid or by smaller oligimers of the β-amyloid protein on surrounding dendrites and axons (Figure 54-1). β-Amyloid proteins are also frequently found deposited diffusely in cerebral blood vessel walls. In addition to β-amyloid plaques, intracellular lacy fibrillar accumulations of material are present in neurons, called neurofibrillary tangles (NFTs)[8] (Figure 54-2). NFTs are composed of paired helical filaments largely consisting of abnormally hyperphosphorylated tau. These are the defining features originally described by Alzheimer 102 years ago.

The amyloid plaques are made of β-amyloid proteins of various lengths from 39 to 42 amino acids long.[9] The β-amyloid 1–40 amino acid type is in plasma and CSF, but the 1–42 form comprises the major component of the cores of these amyloid plaques. The β-amyloid proteins are derived from a larger widely present transmembrane protein in the brain called the amyloid precursor protein (APP). They are cleaved from APP by the β-secretase and γ-secretase enzymes, which have been recently characterized and are active targets for drug therapy.[10]

Mutations have been found to be associated with familial AD, as will be described later in this chapter, in both the genes coding for the β-amyloid proteins and for the presenilins, which likely are a component of γ-secretase.[11] Studies of the effects of these mutations in cell lines and transgenic animals that develop amyloid deposits and plaques in their brains similar to patients with AD have provided insights into how these proteins normally function and how, when disturbed by mutation, their functions are altered, leading to dementia. Those findings should give insights into sporadic AD, and, using these models, several drugs have been developed to reduce production of the amyloid β proteins or speed their metabolism and clearance. It is hoped that these drugs will also be effective for sporadic AD.

Interestingly, although considerable evidence suggests that β-amyloid and its toxic effects on the brain may initiate the cascade of pathophysiologic processes that leads to AD, progression of dementia correlates more closely to numbers of NFTs or number of synapses lost.

Clearly a cascade of processes involving different mechanisms, including inflammation and disturbed calcium homeostasis, occurs as AD progresses (Figure 54-3). Neurotransmitter systems are differentially affected. The cholinergic system is susceptible to early dysfunction, and increasing cholinergic deficiency has been correlated with clinical progression. As AD progresses, the glutaminergic, noradrenergic, and serotonergic systems deteriorate, causing further cognitive losses and often behavioral abnormalities. Therapeutic research since the late 1980s has focused on correcting these neurotransmitter deficits, with some modest success and resulting clinical benefits.

Extracellular amyloid plaques and intraneuronal NFTs in the cortex are the cardinal features of AD. Stereotypic spread of the NFTs, as originally described by Braak and Braak (1991),[6] defined a basis for neuropathologic criteria for AD staging that still is useful today. NFTs are found in the entorhinal cortex and adjacent areas of the hippocampus. Braak stages I and II typically are not associated with clinical symptoms. In stages III and IV, NFTs have spread to the limbic regions, and cognitive deficits are present. By stages V and VI, NFTs have spread to other regions of the cortex excepting the occipital cortices, and the severity of the dementia is worse.

Substantial evidence suggests, however, that plaques and tangles can be found in substantial numbers in many elderly individuals with normal cognitive functioning and that considerable overlap exists in plaque and tangle pathology between very elderly normals (over age 90) and those in this age range with dementia, reemphasizing the necessity for clinicopathologic correlation in diagnosis.[12] Newer criteria assessing both plaque and tangle densities have been developed. Khachaturian criteria count numbers of amyloid plaques in a 1 mm^2 field of the neocortex with numbers adjusted for age.[13] The Consortium to Establish a Registry for Alzheimer's Disease criteria count plaques in three designated brain regions using defined stains.[14] More recently the Reagan criteria assess both plaques and tangle numbers in a highly specified way and appear to have generally high correlation in confirming the diagnosis of AD and in assessing disease stage.[15]

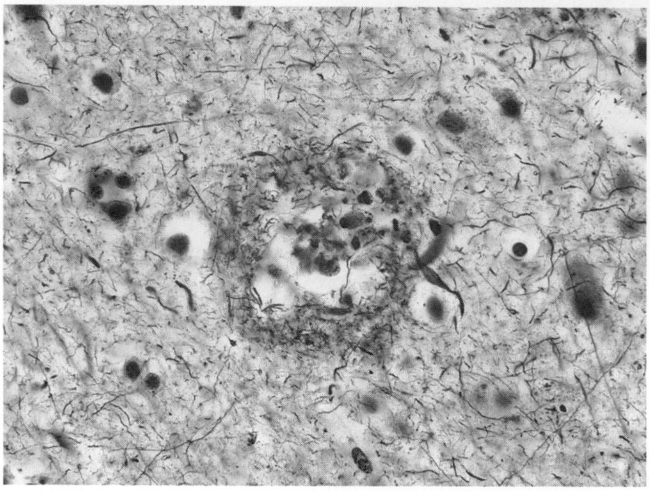

Figure 54-1. Neuritic plaques revealed by silver stain from cortex of patient with Alzheimer's disease.

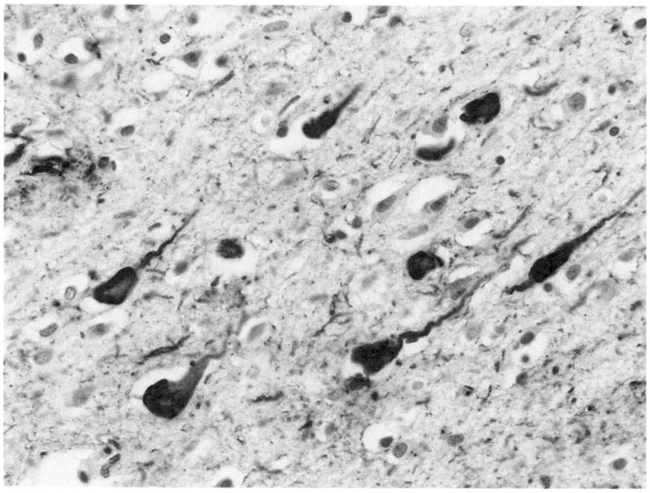

Figure 54-2. Neurofibrillary tangles in cortical section of brain from patient with Alzheimer's disease.

EPIDEMIOLOGY AND GENETICS OF ALZHEIMER'S DISEASE

Aging is the biggest risk factor for Alzheimer's disease. Rarely patients in their 20s and 30s have been reported to have AD, but onset of clinical symptoms is uncommon until the 50s with yearly probability of incidence rapidly increasing to age 65 to 75, when 1% to 5% of the general population is affected. By age 75, the prevalence is as high as 15% in the United States, and by age 85 it has been estimated to afflict 35% to 50% in the very old age range.[16] Studies suggest the prevalence continues to climb, with the majority of individuals by their 90s showing clinical signs of at least early dementia. However, in these oldest old with dementia, underlying brain pathology may differ little from age-matched normal subjects other than demented patients have greater neuronal losses, and their rate of disease progression may be relatively slow. Therefore, even though these patients meet current clinical criteria for AD, it is unclear that these individuals really have the same illness. The second most common risk factor for AD is family history, with approximately 20% of patients with AD having two or more first-degree relatives affected. The pattern of inheritance is typically autosomal dominance.

In families with AD, several genetic mutations have been identified that are causative for the disease. Almost all of the known mutations cause presenile forms of the disease. A few dozen families with onset of AD predominantly in the 40s and 50s have mutations in the APP gene, usually in the region of the gene that codes for the β-amyloid proteins. It is thought that these mutations result in abnormal

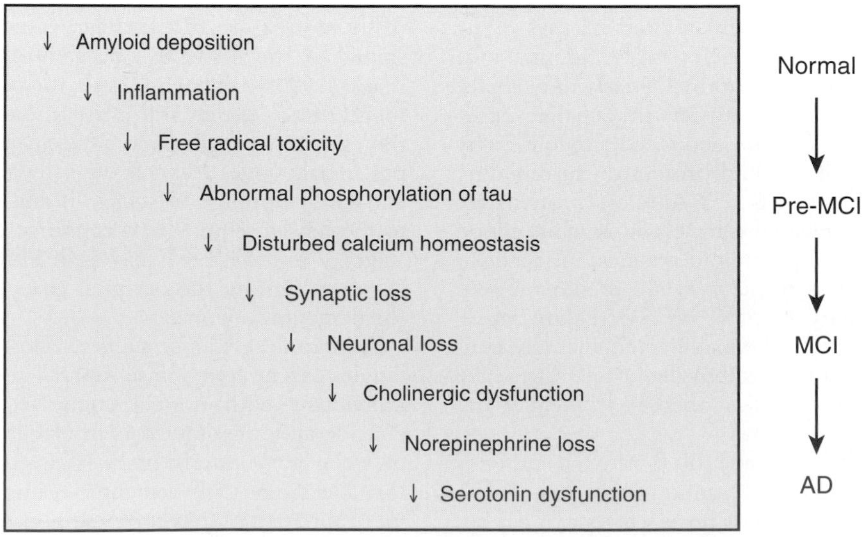

Figure 54-3. The cascade of mechanisms in Alzheimer's disease. Hypothetical cascade of processes occurring as Alzheimer's disease progresses. The specific abnormalities are well established, but their order with regard to causality remains controversial. MCI = mild cognitive impairment; AD = Alzheimer's disease.

β-amyloid metabolism with resultant chronically higher levels of amyloid β proteins leading to AD.[17]

The other mutations causing early onset familial disease have been localized to the presenilin-1 (PS-1) gene on chromosome 14 and the presenilin-2 (PS-2) gene on chromosome 1. Again, only a few dozen families have been found in which PS-2 gene mutations are associated with AD, whereas more than 160 different mutations in the PS-1 have been found in several hundred families to cause AD and occasionally other symptoms such as spasticity or seizures.[18] The presenilins are part of a complex that acts functionally as γ-secretase.[11] As previously mentioned, γ-secretase slices APP to produce β-amyloid.

Increased levels of β-amyloid are also found in AD patients with PS-1 or PS-2 mutations.[17] These mutations are the most commonly known cause of autosomal dominant familial AD, but they still cause less than 1% of all cases of AD. Even in patients with family history of onset of dementia under the age of 65, these mutations are causative in less than 10%. An early-onset patient with AD is more likely to have one of these mutations if there is family history of multiple other affected family members having similar early age of onset. Rather than aid in confirming the diagnosis or risk for AD in a limited number of these relatively rare families, the major importance of these mutations has been to create transgenic animals that have been useful in unraveling disease mechanisms and to speed development of new drugs and testing and other novel therapeutic approaches, such as targeted immunologic stimulation by β-amyloid vaccination or administering monoclonal antibodies targeted to the β-amyloid proteins to accelerate their degradation.

The major genetic risk factor identified for AD in both late onset, sporadic and familial patients is the ε4 polymorphism of the APOE4 gene.[19] APOE is one of the major cholesterol- and lipid-carrying proteins in peripheral blood. In the brain and spinal fluid compartments, it is the only significant lipid transport protein and also functions as a transport protein for β-amyloid. It comes in types ε2, ε3, and ε4, with the ε2 allele being relatively uncommon. The ε4 allele is carried by 15% to 20% of the general population, and the ε3 allele by almost everyone else. The 1% to 2% of individuals who are homozygous for the ε4 have a 50% risk of developing AD by their mid to late 60s. Those who are heterozygous for the ε4 allele have a 50% risk of developing AD by their mid to late 70s.[19] Women heterozygous for ε4 are more likely to develop AD at an earlier age than men. Individuals who carry only the ε3 or ε2 alleles are likely not to develop AD in their 80s or not at all. Some evidence suggests inheriting the ε2 allele may be protective, reducing risk for AD. Inheritance of the ε4 allele confers similar risk for AD regardless of whether or not there is family history. Determination of APOE genotype in a patient with dementia does improve diagnostic specificity in the subset of subjects with the ε4 genotype, but it is arguable whether diagnostic accuracy is improved enough to be clinically helpful. If subjects who are homozygous or heterozygous for ε4 and do not develop dementia in their at-risk age range, current evidence suggests their future risk of dementia is no greater than that of an age-matched non-ε4 carrier in the general population for developing AD. Therefore, presymptomatic APOE4 genotyping for future risk for AD is currently not recommended. Recently, it has been found that in individuals with mild cognitive impairment (MCI), the APOE ε4 genotype is associated with a significantly greater risk for conversion to AD,[20] and that ε4-carrying patients with MCI were more responsive to donepezil therapy.[21] Clinical disease progression after conversion to AD is not influenced by APOE genotype, so the ApOE4 protein may be more influential in the earlier biologic stages of the illness, but once disease spreads and the cascade of destructive pathophysiologic processes begin, APOE genotype no longer influences rate of progression. Considerable evidence suggests in late onset Alzheimer's disease other, as yet unidentified, genetic polymorphisms play a role in increasing their risk for developing the disease.

Other factors that influence risk for AD are gender and education. Women are at greater risk for AD, even with adjustment for their greater survival to older ages. In the past, this greater risk for AD has been suggested by several epidemiologic studies to be due to postmenopausal estrogen deficiency, and estrogen replacement was believed to be a primary prevention for AD. However, the Women's Health Initiative Memory Study of estrogen in elderly women has shown that estrogen replacement may increase, rather than decrease, the risk for dementia.[22,23]

In several studies, increased education has been associated with reduced overall risk for AD and/or later onset of the illness. It has been hypothesized that better-educated individuals have a greater cognitive reserve, so the underlying biologic process disease for the must progress further for clinical symptoms to develop.[24,25] However, the protective effects of cognitive training and mental exercises have not demonstrated convincing benefits in delaying disease onset. Interestingly, several studies have suggested that physical exercise may be protective and decrease brain atrophy and/or delay disease progression.[26]

Epidemiologic studies and small pilot trials have suggested that nonsteroidal anti-inflammatory drugs (NSAIDs) prevented or delayed progression in AD.[27] However, several large double-blind, placebo-controlled trials have indicated no significant reduction in risk for AD with NSAIDs and, rather, a significant increased risk for gastrointestinal symptoms, such as hemorrhage, and cardiovascular disease including stroke.[28,29]

Head trauma has been suggested as a risk factor for AD, but studies have been muddled by wide differences in reported series in the criteria used for defining what constitutes significant previous head trauma history. Further, APOE ε4 patients have been demonstrated to recover less completely from head trauma, so a more prominent history of head trauma may be a pseudomarker for carrying the APOE ε4 polymorphism, which is a risk factor for AD.[30]

More recently, a number of studies and trials have suggested the metabolic syndrome increases risk for AD.[31] Specifically the main features of the metabolic syndrome; diabetes mellitus or insulin resistance, high cholesterol, hypertension, and obesity are all suggested risk factors for AD. Several prospective are investigating whether improving or treating these factors individually will reduce conversion of normal or MCI individuals to AD and/or delay progression of AD in subjects already affected. It remains to be determined whether these approaches: such as treating hypertension such as treating insulin resistance with glitazones, and statins to reduce cholesterol, are effective. In a related therapeutic approach, some recent studies have suggested exercise may delay progressive brain atrophy in patients with AD.

CLINICAL DIAGNOSTIC CRITERIA FOR ALZHEIMER'S DISEASE

Criteria for the clinical diagnosis of AD have been developed and are widely used to diagnose this form of dementia. These are the *Diagnostic and Statistical Manual of Mental Disorders, Fourth Edition* (DSM-IV)[32] and consensus criteria developed by the National Institute of Neurological and Communicative Disorders and Stroke and the Alzheimer's Disease and Related Disorders Association (NINCDS-ADRDA).[33]

The DSM-IV criteria are more general, essentially requiring insidious and progressive memory and cognitive impairments where other potential causes have been excluded (Table 54-1).

NINCDS-ADRDA criteria for "definite AD" require clinical features for probable AD and autopsy confirmation. A diagnosis of "probable AD" requires deficits in two or more areas of cognition, including memory, that are progressively worsening, confirmed by clinical and neuropsychological evaluations, and not caused by either delirium or other brain or systemic illnesses. Onset is between 40 and 90 years of age (Table 54-2). The diagnosis is further supported by impaired function in activities of daily living (ADLs) and altered patterns of behavior and family history (particularly if supported by previous neuropathology). Other features include supportive laboratory results. A diagnosis of "possible AD" includes cases where there is either a single progressively more severe cognitive deficit, or a second brain or systemic cause for their dementia, or an atypical onset (early or with unusual symptoms or course [unusually rapid or stuttering]). Both DSM-IV and NINCDS-ADRDA criteria rely heavily on history and the neurologic examination, and recent evidence suggests that both sets of criteria exclude broad populations of patients in very early stages of the illness who arguably may be more likely to respond to future disease progression–delaying therapeutic approaches. These patients typically have isolated amnesia with minimal impairment in function in ADLs and are labeled as having mild cognitive impairment (MCI). However, there has been resistance to this entity largely related to lack of consensus regarding the defining criteria, by various regulatory authorities. These or similar more expansive criteria will likely facilitate not just research studies with diagnosis but clinical care for such patients in general practice.

Table 54-1. DSM-IV Criteria for Dementia

Multiple Cognitive Deficits Criteria

Criterion A
- Memory impairment
- One or more of the following:
  - Aphasia (language disturbance)
  - Apraxia (impaired motor activity)
  - Agnosia (impaired recognition)
  - Disturbed executive function (planning, organization, etc.)

Criterion B
- Cognitive deficits in criteria A1 and A2 each cause:
  - Impairment in social or occupational functioning
  - Are not due to a CNS disease
  - Are not due to a medical disorder
  - Do not occur solely during the course of delirium
- **Criterion C**: Gradual and continued cognitive decline
- **Criterion D**: Other systemic neurologic and psychiatric illnesses should be eliminated
- **Criterion E**: AD should not be diagnosed in the presence of delirium

Criteria adapted from American Psychiatric Association: Diagnosis and Statistical Manual of Mental Disorders (DSM-IV-TR), 4th ed. Washington DC: American Psychiatric Association; 2000.

Table 54-2. NINCDS-ADRDA Criteria for AD

I. Criteria for the Clinical Diagnosis of Probable AD
- Dementia established by clinical examination and documented by the Mini-Mental State Test, Blessed Dementia Scale, or some similar exam, and confirmed by neuropsychological tests
- Deficits in two or more areas of cognition
- Progressive worsening of memory and other cognitive functions
- No disturbance of consciousness
- Onset between ages 40 and 90, most often after age 65
- Absence of systemic disorders or other brain diseases that could account for the dementia

II. Conditions That Support a Probable Alzheimer's Disease Diagnosis
- Progressive deterioration of specific cognitive functions such as language (aphasia), motor skills (apraxia), and perception (agnosia)
- Impaired activities of daily living and altered patterns of behavior
- Family history of similar disorders, particularly if confirmed neuropathologically
- Laboratory results of: normal lumbar puncture as evaluated by standard techniques; normal pattern or nonspecific changes in EEG, such as increased slow-wave activity; and evidence of cerebral atrophy on CT with progression documented by serial observation

III. Other Clinical Features Consistent with the Diagnosis of Probable Alzheimer's Disease
- Plateaus in the course of the illness
- Associated symptoms: depression, insomnia, incontinence, delusions, illusions, hallucinations, catastrophic verbal, emotional, or physical outbursts, sexual disorders, weight loss; other neurologic abnormalities present in some patients, especially with more advanced disease may include motor signs such as increased muscle tone, myoclonus, or gait disorders
- Seizures in advanced disease and structural imaging study (CT or MRI) normal for age

IV. Features that Make the Diagnosis of Probable AD Uncertain or Unlikely
- Sudden, apoplectic onset
- Focal neurologic findings such as hemiparesis, sensory loss, visual field deficits, and incoordination early in the course of the illness
- Seizures or gait disturbances at the onset or very early in the course of the illness

V. Some Criteria for Possible AD
- Dementia syndrome, in the absence of other neurologic, psychiatric, or systemic disorders sufficient to cause dementia, and in presence of variations in onset, in the presentation, or in clinical course
- Presence of second systemic or brain disorder sufficient to produce dementia, which is not considered to be the cause of the dementia
- A single, gradually progressive severe cognitive deficit identified in the absence of other identifiable causes

VI. Criteria for Diagnosis of Definite Alzheimer's Disease
- The clinical criteria for probable Alzheimer's disease
- Histopathologic evidence obtained from a biopsy or autopsy

Dubois et al[34] have proposed consensus criteria that define the earliest stage of AD as an isolated amnestic deficit, not requiring significant functional impairment in ADLs, but rather biomarker or other objective test results specifically supporting the diagnosis of AD; CSF with low amyloid β and high tau; abnormalities on PET; and mutations associated with autosomal dominant familial AD.

CLINICAL EVALUATION FOR ALZHEIMER'S DISEASE

Questioning a patient with Alzheimer's disease directly about his or her illness and past medical history may be either misleading or unproductive. When asked for their chief complaint, the patient may say nothing is wrong or discuss some other unrelated health problem. It is often necessary for a family member, caregiver, or friend with knowledge of the patient's general cognitive functioning and function in ADLs to confirm or give the history. Insidious onset of short-term memory problems is key for the diagnosis of AD. Patients often repeat themselves in conversation and forget appointments. Typically, they may read the newspaper and watch TV but remember little or nothing of what they have read or seen. Memory impairment becomes broader to include poor recall of past events as the illness worsens. A number of cognitive deficits beyond memory impairment differentiate AD from normal aging. Language deficits including inability to name family or friends and word finding difficulties in conversation may be present. This advances with decreased fluency as the illness progresses to a more severe stage with the patient eventually becoming mute.

Visuospatial impairments are common. An affected individual may get lost trying to find their car at the mall or go off route by many miles while driving from what should be a short trip near home. Important items such as a wallet, purse, checkbook, or keys may be mislaid in the home. Calculation difficulties are often present with the patient unable to figure a tip or balance his or her checkbook. Patients with executive functioning difficulties are unable to follow a recipe, plan trips, or manage their financial affairs. Dyspraxia may be present such that they cannot dress themselves or operate kitchen appliances.

Behavioral disturbances in AD occur in a large majority of patients as the illness progresses. Apathy typically occurs early in the illness causing marked loss of initiative and reduced interest in the surroundings. As many as 30% of patients in the early stages of AD will have significant depression, including loss of energy, appetite, or sleep disturbances such as insomnia.[35] However, insomnia in AD patients may also be caused by sleep apnea, myoclonus, or side effects of various medications. Other behavioral symptoms include anxiety, particularly when family members leave them at home alone or when they are forced to interact with larger groups of unfamiliar people. As AD progresses from moderate to severe stages, paranoia and delusions become more frequent. A common delusion is the belief that their spouse is having an affair with someone else or that neighbors, friends, or family are stealing from them. Misidentification and visual hallucinations may occur with a daughter or another individual thought to be their spouse or the patient may see other people in the house or just outside who are not really present. As AD progresses, agitation occurs eventually in up to 75% of patients, with typical symptoms including verbal or physical aggression toward a family member, wandering, or repetitive motor symptoms such as pacing.[36,37] Patients may develop disinhibition and inappropriate behaviors with examples being; off-color jokes in inappropriate venues, rough play with children, or sexual advances directed toward family members, including children, or even strangers.

The ideal history should document any cognitive deficits, impairment in ADLs, and behavioral abnormalities. Rate of progression over time should be globally assessed. Risk factors should be determined including previous cardiovascular disease or stroke, hypertension, lipid disorders, diabetes mellitus, head trauma, or family history of dementia.

NEUROLOGIC EXAMINATION

Both general physical and neurologic examinations are important to the evaluation of a dementia patients to look for signs that might suggest other causes of dementia, as well as to document any findings that may relate directly to AD. A mental status exam is needed to document presence of cognitive deficits supporting the dementia diagnosis and to begin staging the illness.

The differential diagnosis process for dementia still very much remains a diagnosis of exclusion. The focus is to exclude reversible causes of cognitive impairment and the other irreversible dementias. The physical examination provides a brief screen to exclude organ system problems as the source of the patient's cognitive impairment. The general neurologic examination may often be normal in the demented patient with AD, but the presence of focal deficits (e.g., visual field deficits, weakness, or spasticity in an arm or leg) suggests a vascular etiology for dementia. Older series have reported signs of Parkinson's disease such as rigidity, bradykinesia, and tremor, in as many as 10% to 30% of patients with AD. With recent inclusion of immunohistochemistry in neuropathologic studies in a large series of patients with previous history of dementia, and clinicopathologic correlation, it has become clear that many, if not most, of these patients have diffuse Lewy body disease (DLBD) or Parkinson's disease with dementia.

Gait or balance impairment may also indicate Binswanger's disease (a form of vascular dementia associated with multiple lacunar subcortical strokes), normal pressure hydrocephalus, or progressive supranuclear palsy. Continuing gait problems can also occur in more severe stages of AD leading to substantially increased risk for falls. Myoclonus in early-stage dementia is worrisome for Creutzfeldt-Jacob disease (CJD) or other prion diseases whereas it may be found later in the disease course in 5% to 10% of patients with AD. The list of neurologic findings that may suggest possible, if rarer, etiologies for a patient's dementia is quite lengthy. In general, clues from the history and physical examination guide any additional laboratory testing outside the standard dementia evaluation.

Mental status testing varies in its breadth and depth according to the preferences of the individual physician. In general, assessment should include level of alertness or attention, orientation (person, place, time), short-term and remote memory (remembering three words for 5 minutes and knowledge of their birth date and high school), language, visuospatial functioning (copying figures), calculation, and executive functioning or judgment. The Mini-Mental State Examination (MMSE) is most widely used to screen for cognitive dysfunction to support the diagnosis of dementia and to stage the dementia (Table 54-3).[38] A significant limitation is that it does not assess executive function, a major feature of AD and other dementias. Also, education, as well as ethnicity, familiarity with the English language, and other factors, may influence MMSE scores. It is also relatively insensitive to measuring change in the dementia patient. It is widely familiar to physicians, but its future use may be limited as recently the copyright is being enforced and payment may be demanded for its use.

Clock drawing is a similarly useful very short screen for dementia.[39] It is easy for physicians to administer and score. Surprisingly, for such a simple test, at least a dozen different ways to score performance on clock drawing have been proposed, and all appear to be valid, correlating well with other tests assessing cognition in dementia.

LABORATORY STUDIES

It has been estimated that more than 95% of dementia in elderly persons is caused by neurodegenerative or ischemic diseases that are not reversible. The focus of laboratory evaluations has been to first and primarily identify the small minority of patients who have reversible causes for their dementia (Table 54-4).[37,40] In reality, a potentially reversible cause may be identified in 25% to 40% of patients, but when the laboratory abnormality is corrected or an offending drug (anticholinergic, pain medication) is withdrawn, only transient mild improvement or stabilization in cognitive functioning occurs. The patient still has progressive dementia, most often AD. Nonetheless, any improvement in cognition or function in ADLs, even if limited or transient, is greatly appreciated by patients and their caregivers, and the benefits fully justify doing an evaluation for reversible conditions.

Table 54-3. Instruments Used to Monitor Response to Pharmacologic Therapy in Clinical Practice

Mini-Mental State Examination
- Global measure of cognition widely used by physicians and third-party caregivers
- Assesses orientation, registration, recall, language, and attention
- Uses a 30-point scale
- Requires approximately 5 to 10 minutes to complete
- Sensitivity 80% to 90% and specificity 80%
- Administered by psychometricians, nurses and physicians
- AD typically advances by 3 points per year

Clock Drawing
- Global measure of cognition widely used by physicians
- Multiple scoring systems with proven validity, sensitivity 59%, and specificity 90%
- Assesses in a single test multiple cognitive domains
- 1 to 2 minutes to complete
- Minimal training to administer

Geriatric Depression Scale
- Evaluates depressive symptoms in patients
- Requires 5 minutes to complete
- Very useful in assessing depression in both new patients and in follow-up
- Minimal training to administer
- East of administration is leading to rapid spread in its use

A second purpose of the laboratory evaluation is to aid differential diagnosis among the neurodegenerative and vascular dementias (AD, dementia with Lewy bodies or Parkinson's dementia, vascular dementia, frontotemporal dementias [FTDs]). Accurate diagnosis about the cause of dementia can guide counseling patients, families, and caregivers regarding course and prognosis. Accurate diagnosis of dementia is also important in guiding therapeutic choices. There is evidence from double-blind, placebo-controlled trials suggesting some efficacy for available drugs in all of the irreversible dementias mentioned above except FTD.

In evaluating for potentially reversible causes of dementia, space-occupying masses or other structural abnormalities in the brain may be identified by brain imaging with techniques such as computed tomography (CT) or magnetic resonance imaging (MRI). Most frequent abnormalities identified might include ischemic changes including strokes, normal pressure hydrocephalus, subdural hematomas and hygromas, tumors such as large meningiomas, and gliomas or brain metastases from unidentified primary tumors.

Selective frontal or temporal atrophy on MRI or CT may suggest FTD, and multiple large vessel strokes or smaller subcortical strokes may suggest vascular dementia. Discrimination of FTD from AD in individual patients may be difficult using clinical examination and CT or MRI. Functional imaging measuring blood flow or metabolism by single-photon emission computed tomography (SPECT) or positron emission tomography (PET) may be better able to discriminate FTD from AD and other forms of dementia.

With regard to reversible causes of dementia, metabolic abnormalities worsen cognitive deficits. Relatively minor deviations out of the normal range can exacerbate mental impairment in elderly individuals, particularly those with some other preexisting cause for these cognitive impairments or dementia. Metabolic and endocrine causes are all potentially reversible.

Hyperkalemia may occur in many patients taking diuretics for treatment of hypertension or with congestive heart failure, as well as in individuals taking steroids; hypernatremia may be found in patients with dehydration, which can occur in impaired elderly patients who are dependent on others for fluid intake; hyponatremia may occur in association with

Table 54-4. Laboratory Evaluation of Patients with Dementia

Basic studies excluding reversible with specific indication from history causes of dementia or examination	
Complete blood count (CBC)	Sedimentation rate
Chemistry or metabolic panel (SM-17)	HgbA-IC
Thyroid function tests (TSH)	Urinalysis
Vitamin B12, folate levels	Urine or plasma for drugs or heavy metals
Computerized tomography (CAT) or	
Magnetic resonance imaging (MRI)	Chest X-ray
HIV testing	
Adjuvant Studies to Aid Diagnosis	
Other tests as indicated by history or physical or neurologic examinations	
Single photon emission computed tomography (SPECT)	
Positron emission tomography (PET)	
Lumbar puncture with cerebrospinal fluid for Aβ and tau levels	

a variety of chronic illnesses or medications; hypocalcemia and hypercalcemia are found more rarely but also can affect cognitive functioning and should be screened for.

The most common reversible endocrine cause for dementia in older adults is hypothyroidism. Diabetes mellitus, which is increasing rapidly in the United States, is another cause that has both reversible and irreversible aspects. Unrecognized intermittent hyperglycemia or hypoglycemia may cause cognitive impairment, which is reversible. The longer-term effects of diabetes mellitus on vessel walls may cause subcortical ischemic vascular disease, directly causing vascular dementia and also being a risk factor for AD.

Chronic diseases of the major organ systems may all secondarily cause cognitive impairment. These chronic illnesses include acute and chronic pulmonary diseases such as asthma, chronic obstructive pulmonary disease and pulmonary fibrosis, liver diseases such as hepatitis and cirrhosis, cardiac diseases such as congestive heart failure and arrhythmias, chronic CNS infections (including tuberculosis, *Cryptococcus*, and other fungal infections), HIV, Creutzfeldt-Jacob disease, Whipple's disease, and syphilis. Most will have other symptoms or signs and lumbar puncture to obtain cerebrospinal fluid for testing is most often required for diagnosis. Elderly patients with urinary tract infections, as well as upper respiratory infections, may also have reversible cognitive impairments. Subclinical or partial seizures may mimic dementia, with intermittent worsening confusion or automatisms such as lip smacking suggesting the diagnosis.

Polypharmacy in older adults is arguably the most common reversible cause of cognitive impairment. A partial list of the drug categories that are the biggest offenders includes anticholinergics, antihypertensives, antidepressants, antianxiety drugs, antipsychotics, analgesics, and hypnotics. If suspected, use may be eliminated or the lowest dosage necessary to control symptoms should be used.

BEHAVIORAL SYMPTOMS IN ALZHEIMER'S DISEASE

Behavioral disturbances are common in AD and increase as the illness declines to the more severe stages. Dysfunctions in the cholinergic and glutaminergic systems are associated with cognitive impairment in AD, but with disease progression, abnormalities in multiple other neurotransmitter systems can be demonstrated that likely underlie the onset of behavioral or psychiatric symptoms.[41] For example, aggressiveness has been associated with dysregulation in the γ-aminobutyric acid-ergic, serotonergic, and noradrenergic systems. Similarly depressive symptoms have been associated with loss of neurons in both the medium raphe nuclei and locus ceruleus and consequent depletion of serotonin and noradrenalin. Treatment approaches have been guided by these observations. Major therapeutic targets in patients with AD include agitation, depression, anxiety, and insomnia or disturbances in day-night sleep cycles. Treatment of these symptoms may be difficult and none of the drugs currently used to treat these symptoms is approved by the U.S. Food and Drug Administration for treating behavioral symptoms in AD.

Double-blind, placebo-controlled trials are limited, but available data suggest that substantial placebo effects occur with therapy of most of these symptoms and that many commonly used drugs have modest real effects. Treatment of behavioral symptoms is of great importance to family members and caregivers because they are difficult to manage and are one of the principal factors for nursing home placement.

Aggressive or assaultive behaviors are relatively common in AD with roughly 20% of patients in the community and up to 50% of nursing home patients committing physical assaults. Verbal attacks are reported to occur in 50% of patients with AD. Hallucinations occur in as many as 30% of patients at home and in 50% of nursing home patients. Changes in the environment, such as being moved to a new locale, having a new caregiver, or simply as the result of disease progression, may precipitate all of the previously listed symptoms. A recent comparative study suggests limited efficacy for the most commonly used drugs for agitation.[42] The atypical neuroleptics, despite recent evidence suggesting some increased risk for stroke with chronic use, are still most useful in patients with AD for treating agitation.[43,44]

In the absence of approved drugs or a convincing clinical trials evidence base for treating patients with behavioral symptoms, the following general therapeutic approach should be followed.

Target symptoms for treatment should be identified before therapy begins. Typical symptoms include wandering, physical aggression, restlessness, agitation, pacing, screaming, disinhibition, delusions, hallucinations, misidentification, sleep disturbances, and very frequently depression.

Iatrogenic causes such as anticholinergic and pain medications should be excluded and infections and other new illnesses should be eliminated, and potential sources of pain in the patient eliminated and possible changes in his or her environment should be investigated. For the identified target symptoms, drug therapies should be started slowly and advance slowly. When the symptoms are controlled, periodic attempts should be made to wean the medications.

BIOLOGIC MARKERS OF DIAGNOSIS OF DISEASE PROGRESSION

No biomarkers are currently sensitive and specific enough to reliably establish the diagnosis of AD, but some have potential utility as adjuncts to the clinical evaluation. None of these surrogate disease markers have enough utility as of yet to be broadly used in clinical practice. Structural MRI is the most thoroughly validated of the potentially available surrogate markers. Progressive atrophy in the hippocampus and loss of whole brain volumes have had high correlation with progression of clinical symptoms.[45] This methodology is widely used as a secondary assessment to support efficacy claims for antidementia drugs in clinical trials (Figure 54-4). Serial MRIs may be more widely used clinically to assess disease progression if one of the investigational drugs currently under study delays disease progression. Both MRI spectroscopy and 18-fluorodeoxyglucose PET detect metabolism changes associated with AD (Figure 54-5), but lack of longitudinal data and high cost have limited their broad adoption.

An agent labeling amyloid, PIB, has been demonstrated to reliably label amyloid deposits in the brains of patients with AD (Figure 54-6). Unfortunately 10% to 20% of normal elderly by age 65 show PIB positivity, and the percentage of normals with significant PIB positivity progressively increases to 50% for normal patients in their mid-80s.[46] However, in subjects with amnestic MCI, PIB positivity appears to predict earlier conversion to dementia, and absence of PIB positivity appears to be strong evidence against progression to AD.[47] Short half-life and the need for an outside cyclotron to produce the Carbon[14]-label of PIB has limited its use. Very similar amyloid-labeling compounds using radioactive fluorine, which has a longer half-life, may have broader future potential to aid clinical imaging in Alzheimer's disease; particularly if drugs in development that reduce amyloid in the brain become more widely available.

Aβ1–42 protein levels in CSF from patients with AD are lower than in age-matched controls.[48] Similarly, tau protein levels and phospho-tau levels are significantly higher in AD than in normal elderly patients.[49] Unfortunately, abnormal Aβ and tau levels occur in other neurodegenerative diseases such as CJD and DLBD, and some overlap occurs with normal aging. Combining these two measures improves accuracy of diagnosis, but it is unclear that CSF Aβ and tau measurements improve specificity of clinical diagnosis enough to justify lumbar puncture in most patients. In general, biologic markers for AD and disease progression have

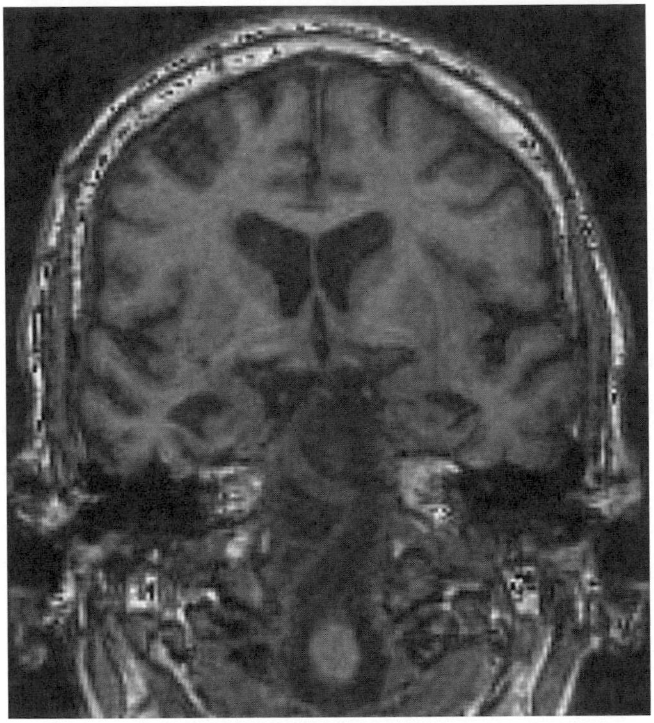

Figure 54-4. MRI study with coronal view through the hippocampal region illustrating moderately severe medical temporal atrophy and milder global atrophy typical for Alzheimer's disease.

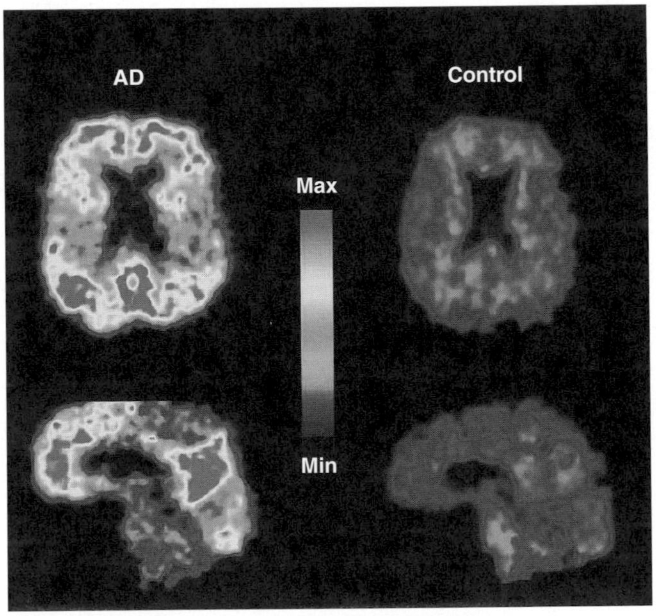

Figure 54-6. Agent labeling amyloid, PIB illustrating significant uptake in frontal and parietal regions.

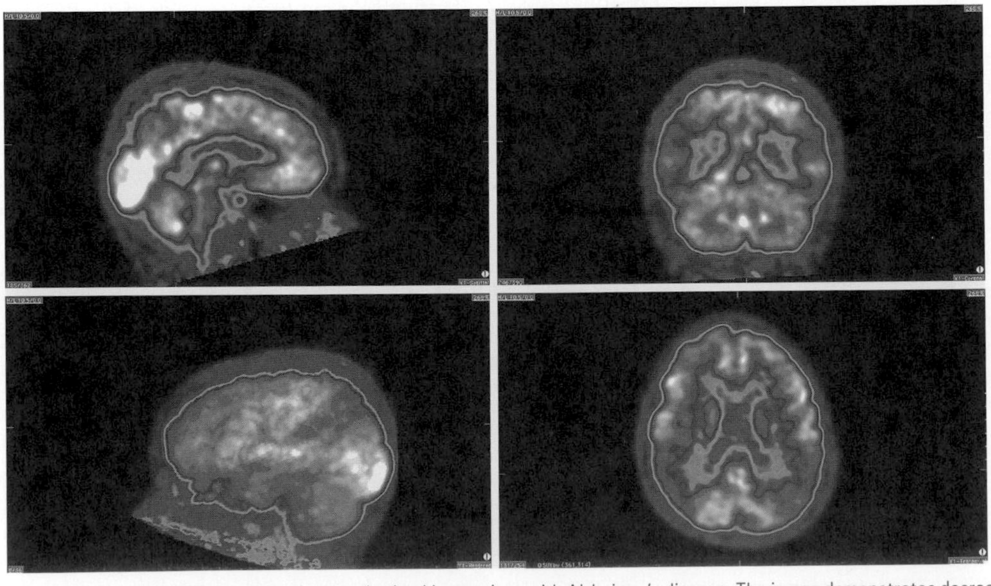

Figure 54-5. Views from PET study using 18-fluorodeoxyglucose obtained in a patient with Alzheimer's disease. The image demonstrates decreased signal or metabolism in the posterior parietal regions as may characteristically be seen with this illness.

had limitations that have limited their adoption in clinical practice.[50] Ultimately, investigation of a number of markers in plasma and CSF in large prospective longitudinal studies, such as the Alzheimer's Disease Neuroimaging Initiative, may yield more sensitive and specific biologic markers for AD.

TREATMENT

Current therapies for AD treat either cognitive or behavioral symptoms but have not been shown to delay biologic progression of disease. The development of a therapy to delay or prevent onset of dementia and to delay disease progression remains an actively pursued but so far elusive goal. Currently available drugs for AD modestly improve some aspects of cognition and function in ADLs as well as less well-established beneficial effects on behavioral disturbances (Table 54-5). Significant benefits are seen only in a minority of patients, and stabilization and temporary reduction of symptomatic decline are the best results achieved in most others. Families and caregivers need to be cautioned against unrealistic expectations. Benefits always need to be weighed against adverse effects when deciding whether a drug dose should be increased or whether the antidementia medication should be continued at all.

Recognition that cholinergic deficiency, including progressive loss of cholinergic neurons in a brain region known to be involved in learning and memory, led to the development of the cholinesterase inhibitors. Tacrine, the first cholinesterase inhibitor successfully developed to treat AD, caused frequent liver toxicity, thus requiring frequent blood testing to monitor lever functions and had a very short half-life, which made four times per day dosing necessary, which was very difficult for AD patients and their caregivers to comply with. It never was broadly used in clinical practice. Donepezil is a cholinesterase inhibitor more selective for acetylcholinesterase; rivastigmine inhibits both acetylcholinesterase and butyrylcholinesterase; and galantamine inhibits cholinesterase but also modulates acetylcholine effects on nicotinic receptors. The clinical significance of these differences in the cholinesterase inhibitor is unknown. Double-blind, placebo-controlled trials have demonstrated that donepezil, rivastigmine, and galantamine mildly improve cognition, function in ADLs, and behavior in some patients with mild to moderate-stage AD for periods of between 6 and 18 months.[56] Donepezil also has proven effective in treating patients with moderate- to severe-stage dementia (see Table 54-5).[57]

When therapy is initiated, all cholinesterase inhibitors need to be titrated to decrease adverse effects and to achieve the maximum-tolerated dose to optimize benefits. If adverse effects occur, doses may be skipped or the dosage reduced until they abate or lessen, and higher dosages may again be tried at a later time. In general, the effects on cognition, function in ADLs, and behavior potentially may be accompanied by and weighed against adverse effects such as nausea, vomiting, and diarrhea, which also increase with dose. Finding the best balance between adverse and beneficial drug effects in the individual patient is the goal. If patients are intolerant of one cholinesterase inhibitor, they may tolerate another, so a trial of switching to an alternative medication sometimes is appropriate. Both the AD 2000 Collaborative Group study and the Alzheimer's Disease Cooperative Studies–Mild Cognitive Impairment Trial suggested that donepezil, and by implication the other cholinesterase inhibitors, may be less effective after 18 to 24 months.[21,58] Neuropathologic studies, however, suggest that central cholinergic deficits in MCI may be less than in AD,[59] and the AD 2000 study design included periodic withdrawal, suggesting that the conclusion from each of these studies, that efficacy of cholinesterase inhibitor therapy waned after 18 to 24 months, may not be generalizable. Substantial open-label follow-up data are available for all of the cholinesterase inhibitors suggesting, but not proving, continued beneficial effects for 5 years or longer. However, these data are uncontrolled and biased by selective dropouts.

When to withdraw these drugs is a major concern. As a general principle, these drugs should be stopped when the patient is no longer benefiting from their use, but this may be difficult to assess in late-stage individuals. In severely affected patients, the drugs should be withdrawn when patients are no longer able to meaningfully interact with family or caregivers.

Memantine belongs to a second class of drugs that works by partially antagonizing glutamate at the NMDA receptor, which may improve symptoms in AD by two different mechanisms of action. First the regulation of glutamate effects improves signal transmission improving the efficiency of neurotransmission and presumably at a clinical level improves cognitive symptoms. Second, memantine may prevents excess calcium entrance into the neurons following glutamate stimulation, thus potentially having neuroprotective effects. In patients with moderate- to severe-stage disease, as demonstrated in previous clinical trials, memantine mildly improves cognitive deficits, function in ADLs, and behavior. Adverse clinical effects with memantine are fewer than with the cholinesterase inhibitors, and one large double-blind, placebo-controlled trial in AD patients on

Table 54-5. Clinical Trials Evidence for Drugs Approved for Treatment of Alzheimer's Disease

Study	Treatment/ Dose Placebo	Number of Subjects	Treatment, Effect
Donepezil	Placebo	153	
Rogers et al,	5 mg	152	2.5
1998[51]	10 mg	150	2.9
Rivastigmine	Placebo	235	
Corey-Bloom	1–4 mg	233	21
et al, 1998[52]	6–12 mg	231	3.8
Galantamine	Placebo	213	
Raskind et al,	24 mg	212	1.6
2000[53]	32 mg	211	3.4
			SIB
Memantine	Placebo	126	
Reisberg et al,	20 mg	126	5.7
2003[54]			
Memantine +	Placebo	201	
Donepezil	10 mg D +	203	3.3
Tariot et al,	20 mg M		
2004[55]			

*Severe Impairment Battery (1-100), Alzheimer's Disease Assessment Scale Cognitive Component (1-70).

established donepezil suggested that there may be fewer rather than more side effects when memantine was added, as well as an additive symptomatic benefit. Trials in patients with milder-stage AD have demonstrated less consistent benefits. Memantine is currently not recommended for use in this population. With memantine, as with the cholinesterase inhibitors, symptomatic benefits may be difficult for caregivers to judge in some patients and so they should be counseled about realistic expectations regarding the potential magnitude of benefits with this therapy. As with the cholinesterase inhibitors, memantine should be continued until patients are judged to be no longer benefiting or until the patients have no meaningful personal interactions.

PREVIOUSLY ACCEPTED THERAPIES MAY BE INEFFECTIVE

Vitamin E was reported to delay functional deterioration, nursing home placement, and death by approximately 25% in moderate- to severe-stage AD in a large double-blind, placebo-controlled trial.[60] However, these results were obtained only after adjusting for group differences in cognitive functioning at baseline, and no cognitive benefits were seen in the group taking vitamin E. Recently, the vitamin E group in the Alzheimer's Disease Cooperative Study Group–Mild Cognitive Impairment study showed no benefit versus placebo,[21] and other studies have also suggested risks concerning thrombosis with the 2000 U vitamin E dose used in the above studies. Vitamin E is no longer broadly recommended as a therapy for AD.

Similarly, several epidemiology studies have suggested that estrogens and nonsteroidal anti-inflammatory drug (NSAIDs) may delay the onset of AD.[27] However, several recent large double-blind, placebo-controlled studies have suggested both estrogens and NSAIDs used as preventatives in normal elderly individuals and in patients with AD may have greater risks than benefit.[29,61–63]

MORE TARGETED THERAPEUTIC APPROACHES IN ALZHEIMER'S DISEASE THERAPY

Broad acceptance of the amyloid hypothesis as a target for therapy and the availability of transgenic animal models known to develop amyloid plaques has made reducing amyloid the major focus in developing drugs to delay disease progression. More detailed understanding of AD's metabolism has led to the development of β- and γ-secretase inhibitors that block the formation of Aβ from the amyloid precursor protein (APP) by interfering with the enzymes that slice it from the larger APP. Despite concerns regarding potentially an adverse side effect of γ -secretase inhibitors on notch signaling that may cause severe gastrointestinal toxicity[64] and concerns about the potential for β-secretase inhibition to adversely affect central or peripheral myelinization,[65] both types of secretase inhibitors are in phase II or III AD therapeutic trials.

An entirely different approach, vaccination using the β-amyloid protein, has proved effective initially in reducing β-amyloid plaques in transgenic animals, and a similar vaccine has been tested in a large phase II trial.[66] This large vaccination study was suspended when several subjects developed encephalitis.[69] Some evidence has suggested cell-mediated immunity may have been involved in these adverse reactions. However, autopsy in patients who later died showed apparent clearance of β-amyloid plaques from broad areas, particularly the frontal lobes of the cortex. Vaccinated patients were followed and clinically appeared to have less than expected clinical deterioration but greater cortical atrophy. The dichotomy between clinical and structural effects has yet to be adequately explained. However, several groups have resumed clinical trials in AD patients with more targeted approaches using revised protein targets and adjuvants monoclonal antibodies to Aβ have been developed that are being passively infused into AD patients. One of these Aβ antibodies recently was shown to reduce progression versus placebo over 1 year at low doses but to cause frequent vasogenic edema at higher doses.[68] Patients with the APOE4 genotype appear more likely to develop vasogenic edema at lower doses than those without this allele. It remains unclear; however, whether these newer vaccination or antibody infusion approaches will stabilize or reverse clinical symptoms of AD or rather these patients will continue to deteriorate despite reduced plaque formation and/or burden. If this proves true, other approaches, possibly focusing on the tau protein, will need to be pursued for developing future therapies.

ACKNOWLEDGMENT

This work was supported in part by PHS P30 AG10133 from the National Institutes of Health/National Institute of Aging.

KEY POINTS

Alzheimer's Disease

- The diagnosis of probable Alzheimer's disease is determined by a clinical process rather than a laboratory test.
- The major risk factors for Alzheimer's disease are older age, APOE4 genotype, and lifestyle (metabolic syndrome).
- It is unclear whether determination of APOE4 genotype in a patient with dementia improves diagnostic specificity enough to be clinically useful.
- Several different disease mechanisms associated with Alzheimer's disease have been identified that are targets for drug therapy.
- Symptomatic treatment with cholinesterase inhibitors is effective in patients with mild-, moderate-, and severe-stage Alzheimer's disease.
- Symptomatic treatment with memantine is effective in moderate- to severe-stage Alzheimer's disease and benefits are seen with memantine additive to cholinesterase inhibitors.
- Mutations associated with familial Alzheimer's disease have led to the creation of transgenic animals that have greatly facilitated therapeutic research.
- Amyloid-labeling agents using PET imaging research are being evaluated for their predictive, diagnostic, and risk factor utility regarding Alzheimer's disease.
- Behavioral symptoms in Alzheimer's disease are common, and most therapies are unapproved and at best marginally effective.
- Several promising treatments for Alzheimer's disease identified in epidemiology studies have failed in clinical trials.

For a complete list of references, please visit online only at www.expertconsult.com

CHAPTER 55

Vascular Cognitive Impairment

Paige A. Moorhouse
Kenneth Rockwood

Vascular cognitive impairment (VCI) is a global diagnostic category applied to a heterogeneous group of cognitive disorders that share a presumed vascular cause. Note that it is an umbrella term, which includes several syndromes, and is not simply the vascular counterpart of mild cognitive impairment (MCI). Specifically, VCI includes vascular dementia (including poststroke and multi-infarct dementia), mixed primary neurodegenerative disease and vascular dementia, and cognitive impairment of vascular origin that does not meet dementia criteria (VCI-ND). VCI may be preventable, although the evidence for this is not as complete as it is for the prevention of stroke. Beyond prevention, specific treatment has shown limited efficacy. Updated clinical diagnostic criteria for VCI are needed, and clinical investigators now emphasize harmonized standards to study the clinical, neuropathologic, and neuroimaging manifestations of VCI in daily practice. This chapter builds on a recent review[1] to outline the evolution of the VCI construct, presents current thinking regarding clinical diagnosis and the supportive role of neuroimaging, and addresses the challenges that will shape future developments in this area.

HISTORICAL OVERVIEW

The conceptual prototype for VCI was "multi-infarct dementia" (MID),[2] itself an improvement over "senile dementia due to hardening of the arteries."[3] Like many prototypes, MID was constructed with inefficient tools: neuropsychological testing based on the Alzheimer's disease paradigm and (initially) no or rudimentary neuroimaging. This construct defined MID as dementia arising as a consequence of multiple strokes and was said to account for 15% of dementias.[4] As neuroimaging techniques evolved, the array of vascular pathologies outgrew the MID construct, so the vascular dementia (VaD) construct (of which MID became a subtype) was created to allow more flexibility in the size and distribution of neuroimaging abnormalities (from single strategic infarcts to leukoaraiosis) related to the diagnosis.[5,6]

Like its forerunner, the VaD construct was soon outgrown due to at least three key developments. First, growing neuropathologic evidence indicated that most dementias have both neurodegenerative (most commonly Alzheimer disease [AD]) and vascular features[7] and that these features appear to act synergistically.[8,9] Second, existing diagnostic criteria all required that memory impairment be present to diagnose VaD and this was at odds with clinical experience.[5,6,10,11] Finally, with improved clinical recognition of earlier stages of cognitive impairment and increasing emphasis on prevention, the VaD construct was not sensitive to the clinical phenotype of cognitive impairment of a presumed vascular cause that was not severe enough to meet the criteria for dementia. The VCI construct therefore includes a broader spectrum of clinical profiles. These range from individuals with cognitive impairment not dementia, individuals who meet the criteria for VaD (poststroke dementia, MID, etc.) and individuals in whom cognitive impairment shows mixed "primary" neurodegenerative (PND) and vascular features (mixed PND/VaD).[12]

The development of the VCI construct represents advances in how we understand cognitive impairment that is related to cerebrovascular disease. It recognizes that in addition to single strategic infarcts, multiple infarcts, and leukoaraiosis, there are other mechanisms of cerebrovascular disease, such as chronic hypoperfusion, which may account for the pattern of cognitive deficits (another old idea that has become modern again). It also affords greater attention to opportunities for primary and secondary prevention.[13] The VCI construct also recognizes that more than one cause of dementia might exist in the same patient. Even so, the formulation of the VCI construct is not entirely settled. In consequence, the ongoing debate regarding the precision of the construct[14,15] and the ever-changing terminology have posed significant challenges to ongoing research in the area. For example, estimates of incidence and prevalence of VCI rely on varied definitions. Similarly inclusion criteria for research studies vary according to the diagnostic criteria used and hamper meta-analyses and external validity. Incomplete agreement on terminology has also undermined development of standardized language and criteria for vascular lesions in neuropathology and neuroimaging.[16]

EPIDEMIOLOGY

VCI is common. Approximately one third of dementia cases show significant vascular pathology on autopsy,[7,17] although this does not indicate the clinical relevance of such pathology. Depending on how cerebrovascular mechanisms are understood, VCI can be considered the most common form of cognitive impairment[14] but it is most commonly referred to as the second most common form of cognitive impairment (after Alzheimer's disease).

The novelty and the heterogeneity of the VCI construct (particularly the inclusion of those with VCI-ND) create challenges for descriptive epidemiology, much of which still relies on vascular dementia terminology. In the Canadian Study of Health and Aging, it was estimated that approximately 5% of people over the age of 65 had VCI, with 2.4% having VCI-ND, 0.9% having mixed dementia, and 1.5% having VaD.[18] The incidence of vascular dementia ranges from 6 to 12 cases per 1000 over the age of 70 per year.[19]

SUBTYPES OF VCI

As argued elsewhere,[1] given the considerable heterogeneity within VCI, subgroup classification is necessary. Proposed subgroup schemata have distinguished subtypes on the basis of neuropathology, risk factors, and treatment response,[20] but in practice VCI is a clinical diagnosis, often supported by neuroimaging, therefore subgroups will be described here on the basis of their clinical presentation. Clinical subgroups include VCI-ND, mixed PND/VaD, and VaD. In this classification system, disorders originally included in the VaD construct, such as poststroke dementia, multi-infarct dementia, subcortical dementia, and leukoaraiosis remain in the VaD subtype. This system is not universally agreed upon.

Poststroke dementia has been proposed as separate from these subgroups but is limited as a standalone subgroup by the omission of poststroke VCI-ND[21,22] and incomplete overlap of clinical and neuroimaging findings. Similarly, cerebral autosomal dominant arteriopathy with subcortical infarcts and leukoencephalopathy (CADASIL)[23] does not easily fit into this subgroup classification scheme but remains a relatively infrequent (albeit possibly underdiagnosed[24]) cause of VCI.

The neuropathologic relationship between AD and VaD is incompletely understood, but their coexistence is well recognized[25] with mixed dementia emerging as one of the most common forms of dementia in neuropathologic studies.[7] Neuropathologic features of vascular disease (atherosclerosis, endothelial proliferation, and neovascularization) have been described in those with AD since Alois Alzheimer's first case of AD,[25] but the two processes were conceptually distinguished from one another for most of the twentieth century on the basis of clinical and neuroimaging features.[2,26] With the emergence of increasingly sensitive neuroimaging techniques and emphasis on earlier detection and prevention of cognitive impairment, the pendulum has swung back to embrace the interactions between vascular and neurodegenerative pathologies. Some have even considered AD to be a primary vascular disorder, but this has not been confirmed with epidemiologic, clinicopathologic, or animal model studies to date.[16] Alternatively, structural changes in actin and deposition of beta amyloid in AD may lead to vascular reactivity and impaired cerebral autoregulation, thereby potentiating cerebral vessel damage.[27]

What is well accepted is that vascular risk factors are associated with late-life cognitive impairment, including Alzheimer's disease (see Prevention and Treatment). In addition, it seems clear that when both neurodegenerative lesions and vascular ones are present, they interact synergistically, to the detriment of cognition. The Nun Study[9] indicated an additive effect of vascular lesion burden and neurodegenerative pathology on cognitive impairment, but it may be that the interaction is dependent on lesion type,[28] location,[29] and dementia stage.[16] Lesion thresholds have been discussed but remain controversial.[28] Infarction in the frontal subcortical tracts may be responsible for clinical presentation with neurodegenerative changes being incidental.[30]

ETIOLOGY AND PATHOPHYSIOLOGY OF VCI

VCI comprises many heterogeneous syndromes, each with its own array of causes and clinical manifestations. A mechanistic approach to pathophysiology divides cognitive impairment associated with large vessel disease from small vessel disease (including subcortical ischemic vascular disease) and noninfarct ischemic changes. Neuropathologic lesions associated with VCI include large and small vessel infarcts, white matter changes, hemorrhage, gliosis, and in mixed dementia, neuropathologic changes of AD.[31]

Large vessel disease

Poststroke dementia is the clinical archetype for VCI associated with large vessel disease. Poststroke dementia (PSD) is defined as cognitive impairment from any cause following stroke that is significant enough to impact daily function. The prevalence of PSD varies depending on diagnostic criteria used, age of the study population, and delay between stroke and cognitive evaluation[32] but ranges from 14% to 32%, with incident poststroke dementia ranging from 20% at 3 months to 33% at 5 years.[33,34] Poststroke cognitive impairment—that is, inclusion of cases in which cognitive impairment without dementia is diagnosed following stroke—may be even more common.[35,36] In the Framingham study the rate of dementia in people with a history of stroke is approximately double that of the nonstroke population.[37]

Risk factors for PSD may be patient related or stroke related. Vascular risk factors such as hypertension, diabetes, hyperlipidemia, and smoking have shown inconsistent association with PSD,[35,36] whereas age, low education, and preexisting cognitive impairment or dependency have shown more consistent association.[32,36,38] The relationship between preexisting cognitive impairment and the risk of poststroke dementia had been seen as robust, likely reflecting some combination of the effects of stroke, the effects of chronic ischemia, and the presence of preexisting neurodegenerative impairment. A report from the large and carefully conducted Rotterdam study has brought this into question, however.[39] It may be that the number of vascular risk factors is more important than any one individual factor in predicting PSD.[35] Neuroimaging features such as global cerebral atrophy and medial-temporal lobe atrophy are associated with a higher risk of PSD.[40] Although medial-temporal atrophy has been proposed as a marker of preexisting neurodegenerative disease in these cases,[41] it is also present in VaD and in patients without preexisting clinical evidence of dementia.

Single strategic infarcts in the cortex (hippocampus, angular gyrus) or subcortex (thalamus, caudate, globus pallidus, basal forebrain, fornix, and genu of the internal capsule) can result in characteristic PSD cognitive syndromes. For example, angular gyrus infarction is associated with an acute onset of fluent dysphasia, visuospatial disorientation, agraphia, and memory loss that can be mistaken for AD.[42] Large vessel disease seldom occurs in isolation, as neuroimaging evidence of small vessel disease is ubiquitous in the older population with varying degrees of clinical significance. Most often, cognitive impairment in association with vascular disease results from the cumulative effects of several cortical infarcts of varying size and number—the basis of cortical MID as described by Hachinski in 1974.[2] The infarcts of MID occur predominantly in the cortical and subcortical arterial territories and distal fields.

Small vessel disease

Small vessel disease includes leukoaraiosis, subcortical infarcts, and incomplete infarction. It is more common by far than large vessel disease[43] and may be the most common cause of VCI.[44,45]

Leukoaraiosis describes diffuse, confluent white matter abnormalities (low density on computed tomography [CT] and hyperintense on T2-weighted magnetic resonance imaging [MRI] and FLAIR). Increasing sensitivity of MRI has resulted in less specificity and predictive validity of leukoaraiosis, which can now be detected in more than 90% of older people.[46] Just as the term *leukoaraiosis* does not presuppose pathology, white matter changes are not specific to infarcts but may also occur with leukodystrophies, metastases, and other inflammatory conditions.[47] Leukoaraiosis may be present at varying degrees from small punctate hyperintensities to large confluent lesions. The major neuropathologic features found in leukoaraiosis in association with VCI include axonal loss, enlargement of perivascular spaces, gliosis, and myelin pallor.[47] Whether periventricular and deep white matter lesions are distinct in their etiologies, presentations, or rates of progression is not well understood.[48]

The association between leukoaraiosis and cognitive and functional decline appears robust,[49] but the cognitive domains affected are not clearly established. The Framingham study indicates association between presence of leukoaraiosis and executive functions, new learning, and visual organization.[50] In general, confluent lesions appear to have a worse prognosis than punctate ones, but decline is more consistently related to measures of atrophy.[35] Visual and volumetric quantitative measurement scales for leukoaraiosis have been developed[51] but are limited in their utility as outcome measures by ceiling effects.[52]

Subcortical ischemic vascular disease

The term *subcortical ischemic vascular disease* (SIVD) was proposed to characterize a clinical profile of a dysexecutive syndrome, with no (or minimal) memory impairment, commonly accompanied by psychomotor slowing, which was seen in the presence of subcortical—including white matter—injury. Subcortical vascular injury occurs through small vessel infarct, ischemia or incomplete ischemia within the cerebral white matter, basal ganglia, and brain stem, especially the prefrontal subcortical circuit and the thalamocortical circuit. Lacunes are infarcts < 15 mm in diameter in the cortical white matter or in the corona radiata, internal capsule, centrum semiovale, thalamus, basal ganglia, or pons.[45]

It is clear that lesions in the prefrontal subcortical circuit (including the prefrontal cortex, caudate, pallidum, and thalamus) or thalamocortical circuit may manifest as the "subcortical syndrome" as described previously. Commonly, however, the profile is accompanied by memory impairment that is more than "minimal."[53] In any case, these lesions are also associated with increased risk of stroke and dementia. Although it has been held that this profile is associated with more rapid cognitive decline even when controlling for other vascular risk factors, this view has been disputed.[54]

Subcortical lesions are often associated with impairments of executive function,[50,55,56] which is broadly defined as the ability to sequence, plan, organize, initiate, and shift between tasks. Even so, there are several distinct frontal lobe syndromes, so that to say a given patient has executive dysfunction is not always to give a precise account of what is wrong. Each of the major three frontal syndromes has been described in people with cerebral ischemia/infarction: dorsolateral (executive function and impaired recall), orbitofrontal (behavioral and emotional changes), and anterior cingulate (abulia and akinetic mutism).[57] Clinically, however, mixed syndromes are common. The importance of executive dysfunction in VCI[58–62] is unclear, but it is unlikely to be unique to VCI at any stage.[30,63,64] Strong support for this contention comes from a recent prospective neuropsychological/autopsy-based study.[65]

Cerebral autosomal dominant arteriopathy with subcortical infarcts and leukoencephalopathy (CADASIL) is a hereditary microangiopathy associated with mutation in the *Notch* 3 gene on chromosome 19.[23] Clinical presentation consists of migraine with aura, mood disturbance, recurrent subcortical strokes, and progressive cognitive decline.[24] Although a comparatively rare cause of VCI, it deserves special mention for two reasons. First, it is generally considered to be a model of pure VaD because generally onset occurs between the ages of 40 and 50, when comorbid AD pathology is rare. Second, the use of cholinesterase inhibitors in those with CADASIL has shown statistically significant improvement in some measures of executive function. This provides a basis for cholinergic therapy in VCI. Cholinergic mechanisms appear to play a critical role in cerebral perfusion.[66] The best diagnostic criteria for CADASIL are the NINDS-AIREN criteria for subcortical ischemic VaD.[67]

Noninfarct ischemic changes and atrophy

Noninfarct ischemia is an integral part of the pathophysiology of VCI, affecting both clinical presentation and outcomes.[68] Diffusion tensor MRI techniques can detect abnormalities that extend beyond the visible borders of leukoaraiosis and that show more robust association with cognition than leukoaraiosis alone.[69] Ischemia also may contribute to mixed dementia by promoting the neuropathologic changes of AD. In animal models, ischemic changes in vascular endothelium increase amyloid precursor protein cleavage, promote tau phosphorylation, and inhibit clearance of extracellular amyloid.[70–72] Hypoperfusive hypoxic changes are associated with concurrent AD neuropathology[73] and might explain poor outcomes in people with VCI who have no lesions on neuroimaging.[74]

Gray matter atrophy may show stronger association with cognitive impairment than strategic infarcts and subcortical vascular disease.[75] Cortical atrophy predicts cognitive decline independent of vascular burden on neuroimaging.[76] In particular, medial-temporal atrophy (MTA) shows association with cognitive dysfunction (including executive dysfunction).[62] MTA was initially thought to indicate underlying neurodegenerative pathology because of the predilection of amyloid plaques in the medial-temporal lobes of those with AD. However, MTA may also result from vascular pathology.[62] Thalamic volume has also shown association with the degree of cognitive impairment.[77]

Cerebral amyloid angiopathy

Cerebral amyloid angiopathy (CAA) is a heterogeneous group of sporadic and (more rarely) hereditary diseases in which amyloid proteins aggregate in the vessel walls of leptomeningeal and cortical arteries, arterioles, capillaries, and, less commonly, veins.[78] CAA is associated with a spectrum of clinical presentations including TIAs, stroke, seizures, migraine, and cognitive impairment and behavioral symptoms. Clinical presentations include lobar hemorrhage, subarachnoid hemorrhage, cortical infarction, and cognitive profiles similar to subcortical ischemic vascular disease. CAA is a prevalent finding in dementia with vascular and neurodegenerative pathology[2,16] but is also found in clinically asymptomatic patients in autopsy studies.[2] T2-weighted MRI often reveals evidence of prior cerebral microhemorrhage, but its significance in a given patient with cognitive impairment is unclear and needs to be correlated with other clinical and imaging characteristics.[79] Positron emission tomography (PET) scans using Pittsburgh Compound B allows labeling of vascular and parenchymal amyloid. The number of cerebral microbleeds has been shown to be an independent predictor of cognitive impairment and dementia.[80]

DIAGNOSIS

Diagnostic criteria for VCI *writ large* are lacking. Current VaD include the National Institute of Neurological Disorders and Stroke Association Internationale Pour la Recherche et l'Enseignement en Neurosciences (NINDS-AIREN) criteria,[6] the Alzheimer's Disease Diagnostic and Treatment Centers (ADDTC) criteria,[5] the *Diagnostic and Statistical Manual of Mental Disorders,* fourth edition (DSM-IV) criteria,[10] and the International Classification of Diseases (ICD-10) criteria[11] (Table 55-1). These diagnostic criteria show low associations with each other, making comparisons difficult,[81–83] and do not include VCI-ND, which may account for up to half of people with VCI.[81,84] Further, the timelines for temporal association have not been reflected by empirical data. In a Mayo Clinic population-based neuropathologic study in which 13% had "pure" VaD without major evidence of AD, requiring that dementia follow a known stroke resulted in high specificity but low sensitivity of autopsy-verified cases.[85] The recently developed Harmonization Standards are consensus recommendations from the NINDS and the Canadian Stroke Network (CSN)[71] that aim to establish screening protocols and datasets for clinical practice and research.[86]

Clinical evaluation

VCI is a clinical diagnosis. A detailed account from the patient and informant of the onset and progression of cognitive domains affected (such as memory, speed of thinking or acting, mood, and function), vascular risk factors (such as hypertension, hyperlipidemia, diabetes mellitus, alcohol or tobacco use, and physical activity), gait disturbance, and urinary incontinence should be sought.[47,86,87] History of atrial fibrillation, coronary artery bypass surgery or angioplasty stenting, angina, congestive heart failure, peripheral vascular disease, transient ischemic attacks or strokes, and endarterectomy is also important. Other elements of medical history including hypercoagulable states, migraine, and depression may also be helpful.[86] Physical examination should include blood pressure, pulse, body mass index (BMI), waist circumference, and examination of the cardiovascular system for evidence of arrhythmias or peripheral vascular disease, neurologic examination for focal neurologic signs, and assessment of gait initiation and speed.[88]

Cognitive assessment

The pattern of cognitive deficit in VCI is as broad as the construct itself. Single strategic infarcts can have characteristic cognitive profiles, whereas subcortical lesions (and less commonly cortical lesions[89]) are often associated with a cluster of features termed *the subcortical syndrome,* which includes abnormalities of information processing speed, executive function, and emotional lability that are not recognized by standard cognitive assessments such as the Mini-Mental State Examination (MMSE).[90] Screening with subsets of tests such as the five-word immediate and delayed recall, six-item orientation task, and phonemic fluency tests from the Montreal Cognitive Assessment (MoCA)[91] is currently recommended[86] with administration of the entire MoCA, the Trail Making Test,[82] or a semantic fluency test if time allows.[86] Although executive dysfunction has proven useful and sensitive for the evaluation and even prediction of disease progression, this is not specific to VCI.[65,74] Even though clinicians who evaluate patients for VCI and for executive dysfunction more generally are justly skeptical about relying on the MMSE as a global screening measure of cognition, tests of executive function are not adequate, in isolation, for

Table 55-1. Comparison of Diagnostic Criteria for Vascular Dementia

Diagnostic Criteria	Requirements for Diagnosis	Criticism
DSM-IV [10]	Course characterized by stepwise decline in cognition and function. Focal neurologic signs and symptoms or laboratory evidence of focal neurologic damage judged to be related to the clinical presentation.	Requires memory impairment as one of the cognitive domains affected. Definitions lack detail. No information regarding neuroimaging features. Does not include VCI-ND.
ADDTC [5] Criteria for ischemic vascular dementia	At least one infarct outside the cerebellum. Evidence of two or more strokes by history, neurologic signs, or neuroimaging. *Or*, in the case of a single stroke, a clear demonstration of a temporal relationship between the stroke and cognitive presentation.	Temporal relationship not defined. Requirement for neuroimaging evidence of stroke is too confined: small vessel disease including leukoaraiosis not included.
ICD-10 [11]	Patchy distribution of cognitive deficits and focal neurologic signs. Cerebrovascular disease must be judged to be etiologically related to the dementia.	Definitions lack detail. Does not include VCI-ND.
NINDS-AIREN [6]	Cognitive decline in memory *and* two other cognitive domains severe enough to interfere with activities of daily living *and* Clinical and radiographic evidence of cerebrovascular disease *and* A relationship between neuroimaging and clinical presentation (onset of dementia within 3 months following a stroke or abrupt onset of cognitive impairment or fluctuating stepwise progression of cognitive decline.	Requirement for cognitive domains affected is less permissive compared with ADDTC criteria. Requirement for neuroimaging evidence of CVD is more strict. Does not include VCI-ND Temporal relationship with cerebrovascular event is strict.

DSM, *Diagnostic and Statistical Manual of Mental Disorders,* 4th ed.; ADDTC, Alzheimer's Disease Diagnostic and Treatment Centers; ICD-10, International Classification of Diseases-10th version; NINDS-AIREN, National Institute of Neurological Disorders and Stroke Association Internationale Pour la Recherche et l'Enseignement en Neurosciences.

evaluation of VCI.[92] The problem appears to be both one of specificity; highly educated people with dementia, for example, might appear to have "memory sparing" on screening tests—and one of sensitivity—the sorts of behaviors that are troublesome failures of judgment are not always captured by the ability to draw a clock or to copy a motor sequence.

Neuropsychiatric profiles

Unsurprisingly, given how common injury to the prefrontal circuitry is, neuropsychiatric symptoms are common in people with VCI.[93] Depression is the most extensively studied affective syndrome in VCI.[53,74] In addition, criteria for a so-called "vascular depression" have been proposed, but they have yet to be fully accepted.[94] As noted, distinct frontal lobe syndromes have been described in patients with VCI. A host of poststroke cognitive syndromes also are well known.[32]

Neuropathology

Many researchers believe that neuropathology is the gold standard for a diagnosis of VCI, even though a considerable body of evidence appears to undermine its standard as a test "of 100% sensitivity and specificity."[7,9,17,95] This is because neuropathology (on autopsy) does not inform the relationship between vascular lesions and clinical presentation[96] nor has a neuropathologic threshold of cerebrovascular disease reliably distinguished between NCI and dementia.[7] Instead, the role of neuropathology is to identify the type and extent of lesions present (especially those that are not visible with neuroimaging), as well as other coincident pathologies.[16]

Neuroimaging

Neuroimaging studies remain subordinate to clinical assessment; there are no pathognomonic neuroimaging features for VCI, and infarct location often does not correlate with the cognitive profile (Figure 55-1). At present, neuroimaging cannot reliably confirm the chronology of lesions or inform the relative contribution to the clinical presentation of neurodegenerative versus ischemic processes. Increasing recognition of the importance of incomplete infarction and hypoperfusion inform the understanding that VCI may be present in the absence of neuroimaging abnormalities because of incomplete infarction and hypoperfusion, and absence of neuroimaging lesions in those with VCI is associated with a particularly poor prognosis.[74] However, advances in neuroimaging technology, especially MRI-based techniques, have begun to allow improved understanding of the lesion type and location.

Clinically significant white matter disease is associated with loss of neuronal integrity leading to higher mean diffusivity and lower fractional anisotropy.[97] Diffusion tensor MRI studies (DTI) allow mapping of white matter fiber pathways (tractography), thereby enhancing the understanding of lesion location and volume in relation to clinical presentation.[69] DTI such as fractional anisotropy have been helpful in differentiating clinically significant leukoaraiosis (that associated with lower FA). Semiquantitative methods such as the Cholinergic Pathways Hyperintensities Scale (CHIPS scale) allow assessment of the degree to which cholinergic pathways are affected in those with mixed AD/leukoaraiosis

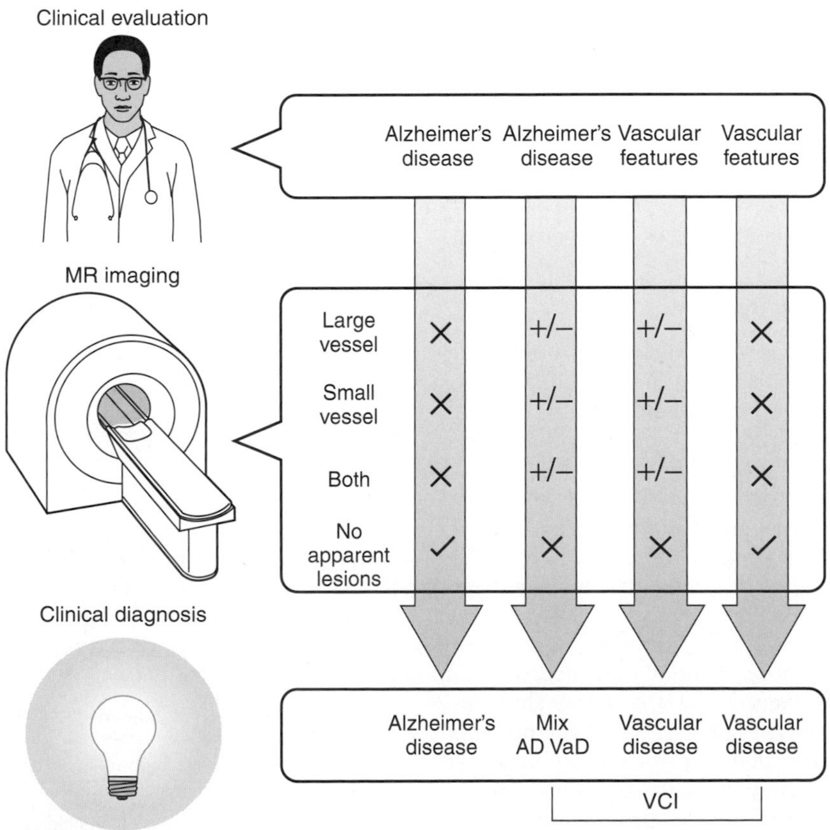

Figure 55-1. Clinical and neuroimaging profiles inform the clinical diagnosis of vascular cognitive impairment. VCI, vascular cognitive impairment; mix AD VaD, mixed neurodegenerative (AD); and vascular dementia (VaD).

pathology,[98] and this has been shown to correlate with response to anticholinergic medications.[99] MRI also allows more detailed assessment of leukoaraiosis, which has clinical importance. For example, individuals with punctate leukoaraiosis on MRI show a lower tendency toward progression over time compared with those who have confluent lesions, but this association is likely modulated by other factors such as atrophy.[100]

The clinical importance of atrophy in VCI is increasingly recognized and may show a stronger association with disease progression and depressive symptoms than white matter change.[84] Medial temporal atrophy is emerging as an important correlate of cognitive dysfunction, including executive dysfunction.[62]

Biomarkers

In addition to neuroimaging biomarkers, molecular biomarkers are indicators that may or may not be on the causal pathway of disease and correlate with disease process and progress. Biomarkers for VCI could aid in early detection, discrimination of neuropathology, estimation of prognosis, and monitoring of disease progression or treatment response. However, the presence of pathology (such as white matter hyperintensities) in normal individuals as well as the high prevalence of mixed dementia in VCI poses challenges for the development of biomarkers. Biomarkers cannot be expected to take the place of clinical diagnosis, and their contribution to our understanding of VCI requires significant empirical data and standardized measurement techniques.

To date, no single molecular biomarker has shown consistent discriminative ability in VCI, and it is more likely that profiles consisting of an array of biomarkers will be necessary. Candidate biomarkers include the cerebrospinal fluid (CSF) blood-brain albumin index (which is compromised in many types of dementia)[101] and matrix metalloproteinases.[102,103] Higher CSF concentrations of molecules found in normal myelin have been found in people with subcortical vessel disease compared to AD[104] and may be markers of demyelination.[105] CSF tau and phospho-tau are elevated in nonvascular dementias and may be useful as negative biomarkers.[106]

DISEASE PROGRESSION

Within the VCI construct, the parallel condition to MCI is VCI-ND, although the term *vascular pre-dementia MCI* is sometimes used in the MCI literature rather than VCI-ND.[107] However, VCI-ND should not be used interchangeably with nonamnestic MCI because other types of MCI also show progression to VCI.[108,109] Like MCI, VCI-ND may exist in a spectrum between normal cognition and VaD,[61] but little is known about the progression of VCI-ND. VCI-ND does not always progress to dementia, and improvement is common.[110] VCI-ND is common after stroke, but here too a substantial proportion of patients show cognitive improvement, especially those without evidence of prior frontal-subcortical involvement.[111] VCI-ND may show less progression than other subtypes of VCI,[74] but the presence of certain baseline features such as prior history of stroke and memory impairment coupled with functional impairment may indicate an increased risk of progression to incident dementia.[59,112] Medial temporal atrophy and thalamic atrophy appear to be more important than white matter hyperintensities in predicting cognitive impairment and dementia after stroke.[113]

Similar to VCI-ND, progression of poststroke dementia shows considerable variability, with up to one third of people having a change in their diagnostic category (NCI, CIND, dementia) within 1 year after stroke.[114] Risk factors for progression and functional decline include age, previous cognitive impairment, polypharmacy, hypotension during acute stroke,[115] depression,[116] and medial temporal atrophy.[61,113]

Most people with VCI show clinical progression that is readily detectable. Current cognitive and functional assessments such as the MMSE, Disability Assessment for Dementia (DAD), and the Functional Rating Scale (FRS) may be less responsive to deterioration in the severe stages of VCI.[74] Compared with AD, those with VCI may show more prominent progression of affective symptoms such as depression.[74]

PREVENTION AND TREATMENT

Data on prevention of VCI through treatment of vascular risk factors had shown largely equivocal support for primary and secondary prevention, although this may be changing.[117] In the Hypertension in the Very Elderly Trial–Cognitive Function Assessment study, patients assigned to indapamide +/− perindorpil had a lower risk of developing dementia than those on placebo (33/1000 patient years versus 38/1000 patient years). Although this difference was not statistically significant, the trial was stopped early because of less all-cause mortality and stroke in the treatment arm. An accompanying editorial pointed out that this may be the best data available, given that it would no longer be ethical to conduct a placebo-controlled study of this question.[118] The authors combined the data from their trial with others to show a net benefit for blood pressure dementia treatment on the prevention of dementia. In a secondary analysis of the Study on Cognition and Prognosis in the Elderly trial, patients treated with the angiotensin receptor blocker (ARB) candesartan showed a reduced risk of white matter hyperintensities,[113] possibly related to blockage of AT1 and activation of AT2 receptors.[119] Benefits of primary prevention of stroke or general cognitive decline through blood pressure lowering have not yet been shown in meta-analysis.[104] Additionally, one meta-analysis showed benefit of blood pressure lowering

KEY POINTS

Vascular Cognitive Impairment

- Vascular cognitive impairment (VCI) is an umbrella term that includes vascular dementia (including poststroke and multi-infarct dementia), mixed primary neurodegenerative disease and vascular dementia, and cognitive impairment of vascular origin that does not meet the criteria for dementia.
- The clinical diagnostic criteria for VCI are evolving.
- VCI is a clinical diagnosis, with neuroimaging and neuropathology having a supportive role.
- Treatment of VCI is often unsatisfactory. Cholinesterase inhibitors and N-methyl-D-aspartate (NMDA) antagonists have only limited evidence for use, although some of this may represent underrecognition of mixed dementia in Alzheimer disease trials.
- Preventive strategies for VCI include exercise and vascular risk factor control.

for some cognitive outcomes but detrimental effects for others.[120] Consideration of composite end points including cognition, stroke, macular degeneration, renal, and heart disease may make a more convincing case for primary prevention through blood pressure control.[121]

Diabetes has been associated with risk of stroke, cognitive decline and dementia in several population studies.[122–124] A large-scale prospective study is now examining the effects of glycemic control on incident cognitive function and structural brain changes.[125] Hypercholesterolemia (especially in midlife)[126] is a well-recognized risk factor for stroke, and the Stroke Prevention by Aggressive Reduction in Cholesterol Levels (SPARCL) study found a reduction in recurrent stroke for those with a history of stroke or transient ischemic attack, treated with statins.[127] Individuals with poststroke dementia show a slow decline in the absence of further cerebrovascular disease.[89] Beyond controlling established vascular risk factors for stroke, prevention of VCI may be possible through physical activity,[128] but physical activity has not been associated with a decreased rate of progression of white matter changes on MRI.[129]

The effects of treatment in VaD are modest. A meta-analysis concluded that only small benefits of uncertain clinical meaningfulness were available from cholinesterase inhibitors or memantine.[130] Although some patients experience clinical benefit, no clinical features predicting treatment response have been found. The case for cholinergic inhibition is mixed. On one hand, the use of cholinesterase inhibitors in those with CADASIL has shown statistically significant improvement in some measures of executive function, and cholinergic mechanisms appear to play a critical role in cerebral perfusion.[66] However, the studies that most persuasively assembled groups of "pure" VaD patients[131] had small effect sizes, no dose response, limited evidence for convergence of treatment effects within and across trials, and no clear translation into what physicians might look for in usual care.[132]

For a complete list of references, please visit online only at www.expertconsult.com

CHAPTER 56

Frontotemporal Dementia

Kristel Sleegers
Christine Van Broeckhoven

Frontotemporal dementia (FTD) is the most frequent and well-recognized clinical presentation of frontotemporal lobar degeneration (FTLD). FTD typically presents with changes in personality, behavior, and social comportment and is associated with atrophy of the prefrontal and anterotemporal cortex. The other two clinical manifestations of FTLD, semantic dementia (SD) and progressive nonfluent aphasia (PNFA), mainly exhibit language dysfunction.[1] PNFA is characterized by dysfunction of expressive language and is associated with asymmetric atrophy of the left frontal and temporal cortices. On the other hand, the pattern of atrophy in SD is bilateral, affecting the middle and inferotemporal cortex, and language dysfunction mainly consists of impaired word comprehension. Notwithstanding clear distinctions, considerable clinical overlap exists between these disorders, likely reflecting the expanding distribution of pathologic changes in different brain regions.

Scientific progress in recent years has greatly improved the characterization of these disorders, most notably in terms of the dissimilar pathomechanisms that may underlie similar clinical phenotypes. The increasing understanding of this etiologic heterogeneity is causing a shift in perspective from one that focuses on differences in clinical manifestation to one that is based on distinct proteinopathies. This distinction will be crucial in the diagnosis and management of these diseases, as well as for development of biomarkers and a curative treatment where none currently exists.

ETIOLOGY

It is now more than a century ago since Arnold Pick, a Czechoslovakian neurologist and psychiatrist, first published a report on frontotemporal dementia, describing a 71-year-old man who developed dementia with sensory aphasia and behavioral symptoms.[2] Autopsy demonstrated severe atrophy of the frontotemporal lobes, swollen ("ballooned") achromatic neurons and argyrophilic inclusions within frontal neurons consisting of insoluble filaments of the microtubule associated protein tau, a protein crucial for intraneuronal transport and structural integrity of the cell. These tau-positive inclusions were later referred to as Pick bodies, and their presence was necessary for pathologists to come to a diagnosis of Pick's disease. Gradually, the eponym was taken over by clinicians to diagnose patients with a dementia syndrome with disinhibited behavior, even though at autopsy a substantial number of patients appeared not to have Pick bodies or even tau pathology. The importance of tau in FTLD was lent further support by the discovery that mutations in the gene encoding the microtubule associated protein tau (*MAPT*)[3] caused an autosomal dominantly inherited form of FTLD. At present, 43 mutations in *MAPT* have been described in 127 families with FTLD or related disorders (http://www.molgen.ua.ac.be/FTDMutations). Yet abnormal aggregation of tau is not necessary for a clinical manifestation of FTLD. Over 50% of autopsies do not display a tauopathy but rather show ubiquitin immunoreactive neuronal inclusions that are tau negative.[4] A majority of these inclusions was recently shown to consist mainly of ubiquitinated, hyperphosphorylated TAR DNA-binding protein 43 (TDP-43),[5] leading to the notion of TDP-43 proteinopathy as opposed to tauopathy. In recent years, mutations in three different genes have been found to give rise to tau-negative, ubiquitin-positive FTLD, progranulin (*PGRN*, also known as *GRN*),[6,7] valosin-containing protein (*VCP*),[8] and chromatin-modifying protein 2B (*CHMP2B*).[9]

Ever since the discovery of loss-of-function mutations in *PGRN* in autosomal dominant FTLD in 2006,[6,7] the number of FTLD patients in whom a *PGRN* mutation is detected has risen dramatically (currently 57 different mutations in 160 unrelated patients), revealing that *PGRN* is at least as important as *MAPT* in the genetic etiology of FTLD (http://www.molgen.ua.ac.be/FTDMutations). Frequency estimates vary, depending on source population and ascertainment, but are around 5% in unselected groups of patients and up to 25% in patients with a positive family history.[10] Progranulin is a widely expressed secreted precursor protein with functions ranging from cell growth to inflammatory response. Given the reduction in functional progranulin protein in loss-of-function mutation carriers, progranulin is postulated to have a role in neuronal survival or neuroinflammation as well. Mutations in *VCP* and *CHMP2B* are infrequent (<1%) causes of tau-negative FTLD. Mutations in *VCP* cause a rare autosomal dominant syndrome of inclusion body myopathy associated with Paget's disease of the bone and frontotemporal dementia (IBMPFD).[8] Mutations in *CHMP2B* disrupt the endosomal secretory complex, because of accumulation of mutant protein on the surface of enlarged vesicular structures. Of interest, whereas both *PGRN* and *VCP* mutations are associated with TDP-43 positive inclusions, the inclusions observed in *CHMP2B* carriers are TDP-43 negative,[4] suggesting another distinct pathomechanism (Table 56-1).

Not all patients with a positive family history can be explained by mutations in one of the genes. In a Belgian study, for example, 37% of the 43 patients with a positive family history is explained by mutations in *MAPT* (N = 2), *PGRN* (N = 11), *VCP* (N = 2) and *CHMP2B* (N = 1).[11] The contribution of these four genes to familial FTLD might be somewhat underestimated because more complex mutations, such as large deletions, duplications or mutations in distant regulatory elements, are not readily detected in standard mutation screening, although this is unlikely to fully explain the remaining portion of familial FTLD patients. Rather, other as yet unknown genes play a role in FTLD, but they are missed in genetic studies because of reduced penetrance. Genetic linkage of families with FTLD and amyotrophic lateral sclerosis (ALS) to a chromosomal region on chromosome 9 suggests at least one other gene involved in the etiology of FTLD.[12,13] Further, extensive clinical heterogeneity can be observed in families with a known mutation in *MAPT* or *PGRN*, suggesting the existence of other genes modifying the clinical phenotype.[14,15] A plausible candidate gene was *TARDBP*, encoding TDP-43, but no mutations have been found in FTLD patients.[16] In contrast, mutations in *TARDBP* do appear to play a role in the etiology of ALS,

Table 56-1. Genes Involved in FTLD with Associated Clinical and Pathologic Phenotypes

Gene	Protein	Chromosome	Mutations (Families)*	Clinical Phenotype	Pathologic Phenotype
MAPT	Microtubule associated protein tau	17q21.31	43 (127)	FTLD	FTLD-tau
PGRN	Progranulin	17q21.31	57 (160)	FTLD	FTLD-U/TDP-43 +
VCP	Valosin containing protein	9p13.3	11 (25)	IBMPFD	FTLD-U/TDP-43 +
CHMP2B	Charged multivesicular body protein 2B	3p11.2	4 (4)	FTLD	FTLD-U/TDP-43 –

*http://www.molgen.ua.ac.be/FTDMutations (accessed July 1, 2008).
FTLD, frontotemporal lobar degeneration; IBMPFD, inclusion body myopathy associated with Paget disease of the bone and frontotemporal dementia; FTD-MND, frontotemporal dementia with motor neuron disease; TDP-43, TAR-DNA binding protein.

a disorder that has a similar TDP43-opathy as the majority of FTLD-U patients.[17,18]

CLINICAL PRESENTATION

Of the clinical variants of FTLD, FTD is the most common, with an estimated frequency of 57% among FTLD patients. PNFA is estimated to occur in 24% and SD in 19% of all FTLD patients.[19]

FTD, sometimes referred to as frontal variant FTD or behavioral variant FTD, typically presents with an insidious change of personality and behavioral abnormalities, such as loss of social awareness, poor insight, and blunting of affect. Other prominent symptoms include disinhibition, antisocial behavior, poor impulse control, and stereotypical or ritualized behavior, such as foot tapping, or more complex behavioral routines, or repetitive use of a phrase,[20,21] reflecting the topography of neurodegeneration. Behavioral symptoms seem to be most severe in patients with right-hemisphere involvement.[22] Cognitive impairment may be less prominent initially and mainly involves working memory and executive function. Cognitive changes include impaired attention, abstraction, problem solving, planning and organization, and perseveration. Visuospatial skills are remarkably spared until late stages of the disease. Frequently, dietary changes are reported, such as cravings for sweets and gluttony, leading to weight gain in many patients. Apathy can be another prominent feature, often reflecting involvement of the medial frontal and anterior cingulate regions. Language changes may include echolalia, perseveration and eventually mutism.[21] During the course of the disease, motor symptoms may develop such as parkinsonian signs (akinesia and rigidity; in ~14%) or symptoms of MND (4–17%).[23]

SD most often presents with fluent aphasia. Communication is mainly impaired by difficulties in recognizing and understanding the meaning of words. Use of substitute words and semantic paraphasias is frequent in otherwise grammatically flawless speech.[24] Loss of word comprehension is part of a more widespread loss of semantic knowledge of faces and emotions, facts and objects. This puts additional strain on daily activities (e.g. by inability to recognize ordinary household objects).[20] SD patients often display disinhibited or compulsive behavior, which may be more prominent than in FTD.[20] Episodic memory is relatively spared, but memory for autobiographical events is often affected.

In contrast to SD, patients with PNFA present with decreased fluency of speech, whereas comprehension of single words is usually intact. Symptoms include word-finding difficulties, changes in pronunciation, grammatical errors, anomia, phonemic paraphasias, stuttering, and apraxia of speech.[20] Semantic and episodic memories are preserved. Awareness of language deficits may explain socially withdrawn behavior and depression. Changes in behavior tend to occur later in the disease, and numerous patients eventually develop corticobasal syndrome (CBS) or progressive supranuclear palsy (PSP).

Although FTLD may clearly present with one of the three disorders, in the natural course of the disease patients will invariably develop symptoms of the other FTLD syndromes. Moreover, overlap with symptoms of Parkinson's disease (PD), CBS, PSP, ALS, or Alzheimer's disease (AD) is not exceptional.[25] This may be due to progressive involvement of other brain regions in the disease process, but it also results from comorbidity, especially in elderly patients.

EPIDEMIOLOGY

FTD is the third most common cause of neurodegenerative dementia, after AD and dementia with Lewy bodies (DLB).[4] FTD is mostly thought of as an early onset dementia, and indeed, the majority of patients develop symptoms before 65 years, with an estimated age-specific prevalence of 4 to 15 per 100,000 for people aged 45 to 65 years.[23,26] Epidemiologic data on FTD in the elderly are sparse, but a population-based survey in the Netherlands suggested that almost 1 out of 4 patients have an onset after 65 years. Of those, over one third were older than 70 years when they developed first symptoms of FTD.[23] Even in families with a known pathogenic mutation, onset age can be highly variable and may range from the third to eighth decade. Onset age for patients with a mutation in *MAPT* tends to be younger (mean onset age 47.9 ± 10 years) than for patients carrying a *PGRN* mutation (mean onset age 60.6 ± 8.6 years), but both *MAPT* and *PGRN* mutation carriers may be asymptomatic until late in life.[10] Disease duration is generally shorter than for other neurodegenerative diseases like AD[27] and is estimated to be on average 6 to 7 years but may be as long as 35 years.[10] Concomitant symptoms of MND are associated with a shorter survival,[28] whereas a clinical phenotype of SD[27] or a *MAPT* mutation[10] is associated with a longer survival. Variability is considerable, however, so prognosis should not be based on absence or presence of any of these factors.

Although data on risk factors for FTLD are sparse, positive family history has long been recognized as a major risk factor for FTLD. About 40% of FTLD patients have a positive family history, and in 20% to 30% the mode of inheritance is autosomal dominant.[10] Most likely, in some patients without a clear mode of inheritance, age-dependent or incomplete penetrance of a pathogenic mutation obscures a clear inheritance pattern, but other genetic factors probably exist (see also Etiology). First-degree relatives of patients with FTD have a 3.5 times increased risk of developing FTD.[29]

DIAGNOSIS

It can be quite challenging to come to a clinical diagnosis of FTLD; diagnostic delay is estimated to be between 3 to 4 years.[28] Because of insidious changes in behavior and personality, patients are often initially referred to a psychiatrist. A neurologic examination, with emphasis on detailed cognitive and behavioral assessment, combined with neuropsychological testing and neuroimaging, provide the foundations for a clinical diagnosis of FTLD. It is important to exclude other (potentially reversible) causes of cognitive and behavioral deficits, such as normal pressure hydrocephalus, tumors, hypothyroidism, alcohol abuse, and large or small vessel disease.

Clinical criteria

In 1998, consensus clinical criteria were established to serve as a guideline in the diagnosis of FTD.[1] In an overall clinical profile dominated by change of character and social conduct, several core features are required to come to a diagnosis of FTD. These core features include an insidious onset and gradual progression of symptoms, early decline in social interpersonal behavior, early impairment in regulation of personal conduct, blunting of affect, and loss of insight. Supportive diagnostic features include behavioral disorders (decline in decorum, mental rigidity, distractibility, dietary changes, perseverative or stereotyped behavior, and utilization behavior), disorders of speech and language (economy of speech, stereotypy, echolalia, perseveration, and eventually mutism), and physical signs (most notably parkinsonism). Using these guidelines, a good diagnostic accuracy can be obtained, with sensitivity and specificity greater than 85%.[21]

For general physicians, a simpler set of criteria is available,[30] consisting of six items: early and progressive change in personality or language, impairment in social and occupational functioning, gradual and progressive course, exclusion of other causes, presence of deficits in the absence of delirium, and exclusion of psychiatric causes. Whereas sensitivity of these criteria will be high, specificity will be reduced, but they may serve well to expedite referral to specialized centers.[21]

Neuropsychological testing

Mini-Mental State Examination (MMSE)[31] has limited use in diagnosing FTLD. In patients with the behavioral variant FTD, MMSE scores may be normal even when the patient already requires nursing home care.[32] On the other hand, language may be impaired, hindering a proper MMSE test of patients with SD or PNFA.[20] But also other neuropsychological test results should be interpreted with caution, especially when only the (quantitative) test scores are considered. Failure to perform on a neuropsychological test may have various reasons, which are not reflected in the overall score. Especially in FTD, behavioral abnormalities such as impulsive behavior and perseveration may affect test performance[21] such that the neuropsychological test scores would not differentiate from other neurodegenerative disorders such as AD. However, when taking into account the qualitative errors during testing, diagnostic accuracy for FTD may increase from 71% to 96%.[33] A large meta-analysis of cognitive tests discriminating between AD and FTD showed that measures of orientation, memory, language, visuomotor function, and general cognitive ability discriminated best, but that overlap in test performance was still considerable, indicating that a differential diagnosis should not be based on neuropsychological tests alone.[34]

Several more easily applicable clinical and behavioral assessment scales exist that are not (or less) burdensome to the patient, such as the Middelheim Frontality Score,[35] the Philadelphia Brief Assessment of Cognition,[36] or the Frontal Behavioral Inventory (for caregivers),[37] and that perform relatively well in distinguishing patients with FTLD from other neurodegenerative diseases.

Neuroimaging

Neuroimaging may further help in the differential diagnosis. The three clinical FTLD syndromes show different patterns of atrophy on structural MRI, which can also be distinguished from AD and other related disorders, such as PSP and CBS.[25] Further, other structural causes of behavioral abnormalities, such as tumors or small or large vessel disease, can be excluded. In the early stages of disease, MRI may show cortical volumina within normal limits. Functional neuroimaging with positron emission tomography or single photon emission computed tomography might already reveal a pattern of hypoperfusion in frontal or temporal lobes.[38] At present it is not clear if the underlying pathology (tau positive or not) can be distinguished based on existing neuroimaging techniques.[39] Large multicenter collaborations will likely address these issues in the near future.

Postmortem diagnosis

A definite diagnosis can only be established postmortem, unless a pathogenic mutation in one of the known genes has been found. It should be noted, however, that neuropathology does not always shed light on the underlying etiology. Rare instances are known of mutations in genes typically involved in one neurodegenerative disease to give rise to a different pathology. A mutation in presenilin 1 (*PSEN1*) (e.g., a gene usually involved in AD) has been found in a patient with a clinical phenotype of FTD and a pathologic diagnosis of Pick's disease.[40]

Based on the most recent insights, renewed neuropathologic criteria for FTLD have been formulated[4] distinguishing seven broad classes, including three distinct types of tauopathy, three types defined by the presence of tau-negative ubiquitin-immunoreactive (Ub-ir) inclusions, and one class lacking distinctive histology.

The three types of tauopathy are defined by the occurrence of specific tau isoforms in the intraneuronal inclusions. In adult brain, six isoforms of tau exist, three of which contain three microtubule-binding domains (3R), and the other three contain four binding domains (4R), at a 1:1 ratio. Different mutations in *MAPT* may bring about changes in this ratio in both directions, leading to a predominance of either 3R or 4R or equal presence of both in the insoluble tau aggregates typical for tauopathy, but different isoform signatures are also found in absence of a *MAPT* mutation. When the 3R isoforms are predominantly hyperphosphorylated, the diagnosis most likely is FTLD with Pick bodies or *MAPT* mutation. Predominance of 4R isoforms points toward corticobasal degeneration, PSP, FTLD with a *MAPT* mutation, or less frequently, multisystem tauopathy or argyrophilic grain disease, dependent on clinicopathological correlations. FTLD with a *MAPT* mutation may also be the underlying diagnosis when both 3R and 4R isoforms are present, but presence of 3R and 4R isoforms may also indicate neurofibrillary tangle dementia (in absence of amyloid beta plaques) or AD.[4]

Four types of nontauopathies can be found, three of which are characterized by Ub-ir neuronal inclusions in the nucleus or cytoplasm. The presence of a TDP-43 proteinopathy (when the inclusions contain TDP-43) points toward FTLD with *PGRN* or *VCP* mutations. In absence of a known mutation, the diagnostic criteria propose a diagnosis of FTLD-U (where U stands for ubiquitin-positive) with or without MND. Diagnoses in this category will likely be subject to change when novel causes for TDP-43 proteinopathy are identified. FTLD-U, but without TDP-43 positive inclusions, is typical for FTLD caused by a *CHMP2B* mutation or may indicate basophilic inclusion body disease, but it could also include other as yet unknown disease causes. When alpha-internexin-positive inclusions are found in addition to FTLD-U, the most likely diagnosis is neuronal intermediate filament inclusion disease (NIFID).[4]

The seventh category, of frontotemporal neuronal loss and gliosis without any signature inclusions, currently is called dementia lacking distinctive histologic features (DLDH) but may in future years reveal a distinct phenotype. Of note, several cases of DLDH are now known, because of the use of immunohistochemistry and discovery of novel disease entities, to have FTLD-U.[4] Immunohistochemistry of other inclusions such as amyloid beta, alpha synuclein will allow distinction from other neurodegenerative diseases, but overlap between different proteopathies is not infrequent, especially in elderly patients. It should further be noted that the density and distribution of protein aggregates do not always correlate well with the clinical symptoms.[4]

Genetic testing

The only way to obtain certainty regarding the underlying disease entity during life is when a mutation screening of the genes implicated in FTLD reveals a pathogenic mutation. *MAPT* and *PGRN* mutations are both found in approximately 5% of referred patients, whereas mutations in *CHMP2B* and *VCP* are rare. Moreover, *VCP* is associated with other clear clinical features, as part of IBMPFD, suggesting an initial screening in an FTLD patient should be targeted to *MAPT* and *PGRN*. In specialized genetic diagnostic centers genetic testing is available, for *MAPT* exons known to harbor mutations and for the coding regions of *PGRN*. No clinical distinctions exist that may point toward one specific gene, although it has been suggested that primary progressive aphasia (PPA) is frequent in *PGRN* mutation carriers.[10,41] Moreover, *PGRN* mutations have, so far, not been found in FTLD with concomitant MND. *MAPT* mutations are highly penetrant, so arguably these need not be screened for in sporadic patients,[42] whereas *PGRN* mutations have been identified in sporadic patients as well.[43] A caveat here is that both mutations in *PGRN* and *MAPT* show considerable clinical heterogeneity, so the presence of ALS or PD may be misinterpreted when examining family history. Further, because of the high variability in onset age, an autosomal dominant pattern of inheritance may be obscured.

Genetic testing should always be paired with genetic counseling, as it does not only serve to give diagnostic certainty but also has a profound impact on family members, especially in the current absence of a targeted cure for tau-positive or tau-negative FTLD. Reduced penetrance complicates the interpretation of a positive test, incomplete knowledge of the causes of FTLD complicates the interpretation of a negative test, and it is possible that mutations of questionable pathogenic significance are found.

BIOMARKERS

The availability of biomarkers for FTLD is still limited, but development of proteinopathy-specific biomarkers will increasingly be important. Because tau has long been the only recognized protein to be involved in FTLD, focus in the development of biomarkers has been on tau. Commercial tests are available to measure levels of total tau, hyperphosphorylated tau, and amyloid beta simultaneously in cerebrospinal fluid, which may add to the differential diagnosis between AD, DLB and FTLD. Levels of total tau have been found to be lower in FTLD compared to AD,[44] but they have also been found to be higher or normal.[39] Levels of hyperphosphorylated tau appear to be increased in AD patients compared to FTLD and DLB. The level of tau has also been correlated with cortical volume of the right frontal and left ventral temporal brain regions.[44] The inconsistency of the results might be explained by the fact that until now, study populations of FTLD contained a large proportion of unrecognized FTLD-U patients, obscuring a correlation between CSF-tau levels and tau-positive FTLD. Sufficiently large studies correlating CSF tau levels with neuropathologic phenotype are unfortunately still lacking.

The discovery of PGRN loss-of-function mutations as an important cause of tau-negative FTLD,[6,7] and the identification of TDP-43 as a major constituent of the characteristic inclusions in the majority of FTLD-U patients[5] will likely allow antemortem distinction between tau-positive and tau-negative FTLD in the very near future. Because loss-of-function mutations in *PGRN* leads to a loss of functional PGRN protein, levels of circulating PGRN will probably be reduced in mutation carriers versus nonmutation carriers. Indeed, evidence exists that a reduction of PGRN because of a loss-of-function mutation is detectable in CSF[45] and serum[46] by means of Enzyme-linked immunosorbent assay (ELISA). Another group recently reported on an ELISA to measure TDP-43 in plasma.[47] Elevated plasma levels of TDP-43 were detected in 46% of FTLD patients, which is close to the expected frequency of FTLD-U. Unfortunately, correlation of plasma levels with TDP-43 pathology in the brain could not be assessed. Variability of TDP-43 levels was considerable, even in healthy individuals, suggesting the usefulness as predictor of disease may be limited.

The advent of biomarkers specific for these molecular entities will add to the ability to reliably diagnose the different

FTLD syndromes. Moreover, it will facilitate the development of etiologically based medication. Inclusion criteria for drug trials can be more stringent based on biomarker profiles, and the biomarkers can be used to monitor efficacy of treatment accurately. Once a preventive strategy becomes available, these biomarkers may even be measured as predictors of disease, to guarantee intervention in the preclinical stage of the disease.

TREATMENT AND STRATEGIES

Although currently no etiologically based curative treatment exists for FTD, treatment options exist to diminish the burdensome (behavioral) symptoms associated with the disease, to significantly improve patient care and quality of life. Both pharmacologic and nonpharmacologic symptomatic approaches exist. Strategies for symptomatic treatment of FTLD are derived from other disorders with behavioral disturbances, such as AD. Studies addressing the efficacy and safety of these symptomatic medications in FTLD are limited. Most evidence comes from case reports and open-label studies of small patient groups. The decision to prescribe any of these medications should be carefully considered for each patient, but especially in the elderly, in light of interaction with other medications and comorbidity.

Selective serotonin reuptake inhibitors (SSRIs: fluoxetine, fluvoxamine, sertraline and paroxetine) may counteract social abnormalities (such as depression, anxiety, disinhibition, impulsivity, and sexually inappropriate and stereotyped behavior), but they are also reported to suppress eating abnormalities (such as decreased satiety and food cravings).[20,48] Although the use of SSRIs in FTLD is plausible given the association of these behavioral abnormalities changes in cortical serotonin levels,[48] the results of the few existing trials have been inconsistent.[49,50]

Other behavioral features such as agitation and psychosis are often treated with neuroleptic medication, but the traditional neuroleptic agents have undesirable side effects, such as parkinsonism or somnolence, particularly in the older patient. Extrapyramidal side effects may be less pronounced when prescribing atypical antipsychotic drugs, but increased mortality during use of atypical antipsychotics was reported in the elderly.[48] On the other hand, a study specifically addressing this issue suggested these drugs are well tolerated by the elderly.[51] Anticonvulsant drugs are sometimes given to treat aggression, but side effects (including confusion) limit their use in the elderly.[52] No placebo-controlled trials exist.[48]

With the availability of acetylcholinesterase inhibitors (rivastigmine, donepezil, galantamine) for symptomatic treatment of AD, these are also being examined in FTLD patients, even though the cholinergic system seems to be relatively unaffected in FTLD compared to AD.[48] Studies on the efficacy of cholinesterase inhibitors give inconsistent results.[20,48] Overall, cholinesterase inhibitors appear not to have an effect on cognition. Memantine, a drug targeting the glutamatergic system in AD, has been tested in a trial; it resulted in no changes in behavior and a worsening of cognitive performance.[53]

Behavioral symptoms tend to be more distressful early in the disease, also for those surrounding the patient. But as the pathologic process progresses, patients gradually display more apathy and less behavioral disturbances, allowing withdrawal of symptomatic treatment in advanced stages.[20]

Like the pharmacologic treatments, the nonpharmacologic management of a patient should be tailored to his or her specific symptoms and should be adapted when needed along the course of the disease. Interventions may include structuring of the environment and the establishment of daily schedules to reduce the chance of agitation, controlled access to food for patients with food cravings, and help in planning and avoiding of complex multistep activities for patients with executive dysfunction.[52]

When language dysfunction is prominent, focus should be on optimizing communication, for example, by speaking slowly in short sentences in case of impaired comprehension and by employing picture cards or computer-assisted devices in case of reduced fluency.[52] Other nonpharmacologic approaches should be targeted to reduce physical discomfort, such as reducing the risk of falls, physical therapy, prevention of decubitus ulcers in bed-ridden patients, and prevention of aspiration pneumonia, especially in patients with gorging behavior.[52] Special attention should also be given to caregivers of FTLD patients. The symptoms of FTLD (inappropriate behavior, agitation, and psychosis) may cause considerable distress for the caregiver and are unknown to many people, so community support for caregivers may fall short. Studies have shown that caregivers experienced most distress in the initial stages of the disease, especially when a patient was institutionalized after short dementia duration,[54] suggesting there may be adaptation over time.

Ultimately, management should be fitted to the underlying disease entity, because this will be the only possibility to cure the disease. Ideally, targeted therapy should be commenced in the early stages of disease, before the disease becomes clinically manifest, even allowing prevention of FTLD. The discovery of novel FTLD genes has not only been instrumental in identifying novel molecular targets for drug development, it also presents researchers with the possibility of developing biomarkers that will help in early detection. This in turn will allow more efficiently organized drug trials that are not confounded by etiologic heterogeneity.

KEY POINTS
Frontotemporal Dementia

- Main presenting symptoms of FTLD are changes in personality and behavior, or language dysfunction.
- Currently only symptomatic treatment exists, which may increase quality of life but can have adverse side effects, so their use in elderly patients should be carefully considered.
- FTLD has a strong genetic component, with two major genetic causes (*MAPT* and *PGRN*) and two rare genetic causes (*CHMP2B* and *VCP*) currently known.
- FTLD is a clinically, genetically, and pathologically heterogeneous disorder.
- Distinction of the different molecular entities (tauopathy, TDP43-opathy, or other) will increasingly be important when etiology-based medicine becomes available.
- Biomarkers specific for the different molecular entities are in early stages of development.

For a complete list of references, please visit online only at www.expertconsult.com

CHAPTER 57

Functional Psychiatric Illness in Old Age

Cornelius Katona
Gill Livingston
Claudia Cooper

Older people may suffer a wide range of psychiatric difficulties in late life, and those who have a concurrent physical illness are particularly vulnerable. Although these conditions tend to be underdetected and undertreated, their outcome with appropriate management is often excellent. This chapter discusses in some detail the clinical presentation, epidemiology, management, and outcome of depression; the schizophrenia-like psychoses and delusional disorders; mania; the anxiety disorders; alcohol-related problems; and disorders of personality in old age, with briefer discussions of obsessive-compulsive disorder, somatoform disorders, and posttraumatic stress disorder.

DEPRESSION

By 2020, depression will be second only to heart disease as a contributor to global disability and a major public health problem in older people.[1] Despite this, depression is often missed, ignored, or not managed adequately, especially in this age group. Patients present needing help but with presenting complaints other than low mood. This is in part a consequence of widely held "agist" assumptions that depression is intrinsic to the aging process and that treatment is inappropriate, excessively risky, or unlikely to be effective. These assumptions are demonstrably untrue: the majority of older people are not clinically depressed (despite their increased risk of loss and of adversity); those that are respond as well to the range of pharmacologic and psychological treatment as do younger depressed patients.

Epidemiology

The prevalence of depression in older people varies widely depending on sample selection, instruments used, and "caseness" criteria. The clinical features of depressive disorder may be complicated by its less than obvious presentation as well as by coexisting medical problems or cognitive impairment. Older subjects in the community appear to have a lower prevalence of *major* depression [as defined within the *Diagnostic and Statistical Manual of Mental Disorders* (DSM) system] than their younger counterparts.[2] An early United Kingdom community study found a 10% prevalence for depression in community residents, but only 1.3% met criteria for major depression.[3] In an Australian study,[4] which included individuals living in both community and institutional settings, the rate for depressive episodes was 3.3% using ICD-10,[5] compared to 11% using DSM-III-R criteria.[6] Within DSM criteria, rates for dysthymia (chronic mild depression) are far from consistent; for example, in the U.S. Epidemiologic Catchment Area Study, the prevalence was 1% to 1.5% in those aged over 65,[7] whereas in a Finnish study,[8] the rate was 23%. More consistent results have been achieved using semistructured interviews and diagnostic algorithms.[9,10] Studies using these instruments have found prevalences of 14.2% for moderate to severe depression in Tasmania,[11] 11.3% in Liverpool,[12] 16.2% in New York City, and 19.5% in London.[13] An inner London community-based study[14] reported a 15.9% rate of depression and an annual new incidence rate of 3.8%.

In these studies, the overall depression prevalence rates for women were about 50% greater than for men, but for severe depression they were similar in male and female subjects. A comprehensive review[15] reported an average prevalence of 13.5%. Rates for women and for people who were socioeconomically disadvantaged were consistently higher. Similarly, a review comparing nine European community studies[16] found an overall prevalence of 12.3% (women 14.2%, men 8.6%).

The prevalence of depressive illness appears higher among older GP attenders, with reported rates as high as 31%,[17] although others give a prevalence of about 15%.[18] There is an established interrelationship between increased depression, physical disability, and more contact with services including GP attendance,[14,19] suggesting that frequent attendance may be a "marker" of depression.

In the hospitalized elderly, the prevalence of depression is also high, with a reported range between 12% and 45%.[20,21] Similarly, the prevalence of depressive disorders among elderly people in long-term institutional care is in excess of 20%.[22]

Depression in old age may be complicated by underlying cerebral pathologies. Rates of depression of 20% to 30% are found in people with Alzheimer's disease.[23,24] Studies that screen out individuals with cognitive impairment may miss cases of clinically significant depression, although such depression may be relatively likely to remit spontaneously.[25]

Etiology

Demographic, social, and biologic factors have all been implicated in the etiology of depression in old age.

Gender and age

Most community studies find significantly higher rates for depression in women than in men—this is particularly clear in a recent meta-analysis.[16] The relationship between depression and age itself within the elderly population is not clear-cut; some studies find depression to be more common in the very old,[11] whereas others find the reverse to be true.[26]

Genetic susceptibility

Genetic factors are generally reported to be less important in elderly patients with depression than in their younger counterparts.[27] However, some studies have found a positive family history for depression in about one third of patients with first onset of depression after the age of 60.[28]

Neurobiologic risk factors

In both depression and aging, there may be decreased nonadrenergic responsiveness with compensatory increases in postsynaptic receptor number. A positive correlation has been noted between age and platelet α_2 adrenergic binding capacity in controls but not in subjects with depression.[29] Aging may enhance depression-associated changes in serotonergic responsiveness as evidenced by reduced platelet ^{3}H-imipramine binding[30] and blunted prolactin responses to the 5HT precursor L-tryptophan.[31] It has been hypothesized that cholesterol might be an important factor in the relationship between serotonergic dysfunction and depression, through alterations in synaptosomal membrane properties. However, a meta-analysis of the outcome of older patients participating in clinical trials of cholesterol-lowering agents revealed no significant associations between low cholesterol concentration and severity of depressive symptoms.[32]

Imaging techniques have been widely used in the study of depression in old age. Abnormalities of the amygdala might predispose to depression with patients having a larger amygdala volume than controls. Increased activity of the amygdala combined with inadequate corticoregulation of its emotional output probably contributes to depressive symptoms.[33] Ventricular enlargement and ischemic changes are more frequently found in patients whose first onset of depression was after the age of 60.[34] Older patients with depression have lower regional cerebral blood flow (rCBF) than controls, particularly in the left hemisphere.[35] However, rCBF failed to correlate with severity of depressed mood. In another study, reduced anterior frontal and temporal blood flow, an increase in occipital flow,[36] and a reduction in whole brain glucose metabolic rate were associated with depression.

Physical health

Depression is more common in physically ill than in healthy older people. As physical illness and depression both often present with physical features (such as sleep disturbance, loss of appetite, and pain), then the use of screening tests that utilize biologic symptoms can lead to false positives. The prevalence range varies from 6% to 25% when diagnostic interviews validated among elderly people are used.[37,38] The main risk factors for depression appear to be the severity of physical illness, the degree of disability, pain, coexisting cognitive impairment, and a positive past psychiatric history.

Although illness in general is a risk factor for depression, stroke and Parkinson's disease have been associated with a particularly high likelihood of developing depression. The 1-year prevalence of depression following a stroke is 20% to 50%, with an apparent peak within the first 6 months.[39] Reported relationships with lesion size and site in stroke have been inconsistent. Rates of 40% to 50% have been reported in people with Parkinson's disease.[40] Among people who have had a myocardial infarction or undergone cardiac catheterization, a quarter have major depression and a further quarter minor depression.[33] Physical disability seems to be particularly strongly associated with depression in institutional settings.[22]

Depression in elderly medical patients frequently becomes chronic and in turn appears to have an adverse effect on the physical prognosis, especially in terms of likelihood of successful rehabilitation.[41] In addition, older medical patients with depression consume more health care resources, have longer admissions, have a higher mortality, and are more likely to be transferred to residential care.[42] However, medical staff members frequently overlook depression in elderly medical patients, despite high rates of depressive symptomatology.[43] Its detection may be facilitated by simple screening tests such as the Geriatric Depression Scale (GDS).[44] The five-item version of the GDS has the best psychometric properties for use in medically ill people, with a sensitivity of 97% and specificity of 85%.[45] The following questions are included in the five-item GDS: "Are you basically satisfied with your life?" "Do you often get bored?" "Do you often feel helpless?" "Do you prefer to stay at home rather than going out and doing new things?" and "Do you feel pretty worthless the way you are now?" Positive answers for depression screening are no to the first question and yes to the other questions, with at least two positive answers denoting a screen positive result. The Patient Health Questionnaire Depression module (PHQ-9) is increasingly used in general practice as a depression screen, and it has also been validated in older people. This scale acts both as a brief self-reported diagnostic screen and as a measure of the severity of major depression.[46] Several studies support its validity, feasibility, and capacity to detect changes in depressive symptoms over time.

Personality and social factors

Those individuals with late-onset depressive illness appear to have more robust personalities than those with recurrent depression arising earlier.[47] Dependent, anxious, and avoidant personality traits have, however, been reported to be associated with late life depression.[48]

Life events often precipitate depression in old age.[49] Several community studies have shown the importance of loss in the depressions of old age. Illness, chronic disability, social isolation, bereavement, and poverty are all correlates of depressive symptoms.[50,51] The importance of physical illness has already been discussed. People who are separated, divorced, or widowed (and have therefore lost a partner) are more likely to have a depressive illness than those who are married or cohabiting.[52] Similarly, depression is associated with recent deaths and accidents in near relatives.[53] Being a caregiver for someone with dementia or depression is associated with an increased risk of depression in the caregiver; this is particularly marked in women, in spouse-caregivers, where the premorbid relationship was poor, and where there are prominent behavioral problems such as aggression.[54,55] A confidant may act as a buffer against such loss-related depression, particularly in women.[51] The direction of causality is unclear as poor support may render persons liable to depression, or the depression may lead to the loss of support. Personality variables are likely to be important mediators.

Clinical features

Depression often presents in a less typical fashion in old age. This clearly has implications for the under- or misdiagnosis of depression in the elderly. Older patients tend to have an increase in somatic complaints, sleep disturbance (initial insomnia), and agitation.[53] There are two main symptom clusters: *affective suffering,* which included low mood, tearfulness and occasionally hopelessness, seeing the future as bleak, and the wish to die, and a *motivational cluster,* comprising loss of interest, poor concentration, and lack of enjoyment.[56] Depressed mood, guilt, anxiety, and diurnal mood variation are more common in women than in men with depression.[57] People whose first episode of depression occurred in late life are less likely to display psychotic features and are also more likely to display cognitive impairment.[58]

Depression and dementia

Cognitive impairment is frequently found in association with depression in older people. Its presence may be important not only in terms of hindering diagnosis but, more positively, as an etiologic and prognostic pointer and an element in a possible specific approach to the subtyping of depression in old age. Prominent cognitive dysfunction that initially reverses with successful antidepressant treatment is the essential clinical feature in the minority of elderly depressed patients with *depressive pseudodementia*.[59] Subtle cognitive impairment may, however, be present in a broad spectrum of the elderly depressed and may in any case not be as consistently reversible as had been thought.[60] Although depression is increased in those with dementia, the risk of depression is not related either to insight or to severity. It is, however, less common in those who take exercise.[61]

A recent thoughtful review suggests that there may be clinically distinct subtypes of depression within dementia. In particular, apathy may be prominent, as may executive dysfunction and disinhibition.[62] Physically aggressive behavior in people with dementia may in particular be depression driven. Apathy may also be an important presenting feature.

The evolution of cognitive and depressive symptoms in people in whom these coexist is not always straightforward.[63] Lack of motivation increased sharply with decreasing cognitive function, and increasing disability may be associated with deterioration in both mood and motivation symptoms. This depression-executive dysfunction syndrome has retardation, reduced interest, limited insight, and poor self-care as predominant features. The closely related concept of *vascular depression* is characterized clinically by apathy, psychomotor retardation, loss of verbal fluency, and generalized cognitive impairment with radiologic evidence of cerebrovascular disease and high rates of progression full-blown dementia.[33]

The detection of depression in people with severe dementia is difficult. People find it difficult as dementia progresses to articulate emotional distress or remember their symptom pattern. There are, however, rating scales specifically designed to detect depression in subjects with dementia; the best of these is probably the Cornell Scale.[64]

The Geriatric Depression Scale[45] is sensitive and specific in hospital settings, is quick to administer, and is highly acceptable to patients.

The management of depression in old age

The management of depression in physically ill elderly patients is essentially the same as for depression in general. Antidepressant and psychological therapy are equally effective in older and younger adults,[33] although in pharmacotherapy, medical comorbidities, and the possibility of adverse consequences or interactions between antidepressants and other drug treatments must be considered carefully.

Certain drugs are associated with depression. These include propranolol, beta-blockers, antiparkinson drugs, cimetidine, clonidine, estrogens and progesterone, tamoxifen, and dextropropoxyphene. Depression is also associated with malignant and cerebrovascular disease, myocardial infarction, thyroid, parathyroid, and adrenal endocrine disturbance.[33] Removal of depression-causing medication and treatment of illnesses associated with depression may improve mood. Antidepressants should be given at adequate doses for a minimum of 4 weeks before concluding they are ineffective and changing to a different class. If response is poor, consider whether the patient is adhering to the treatment and increase to a higher dose.[33]

A recent Cochrane review found 29 trials of antidepressant therapy in people aged 55 and over; selective serotonin reuptake inhibitors (SSRIs) and tricyclic antidepressants were equally efficacious, although tricyclics were associated with more withdrawals because of side effects.[65] Patients with depression may make different decisions about life-sustaining therapy after their depression is treated, so wherever possible such decisions should be postponed until they have recovered. Serotonin-norepinephrine reuptake inhibitors (SNRIs) (venlafaxine and duloxetine) have also been demonstrated to be effective treatment for depression in older people.[66,67]

Depression in old age frequently fails to respond to initial treatment. Pharmacologic strategies for treatment-resistant depression may be useful despite the toxicity risk. Nortriptyline, lithium, and bupropion were found to be useful additive treatments where an SSRI is the initial treatment.[33] People with dementia are at an increased risk of developing depression. In people with Alzheimer's disease, the findings from controlled trials of antidepressants (reviewed by Lyketsos et al)[68] are inconsistent, though sertraline was efficacious in a recent RCT.[69]

Antidepressant prescribing for depressed older people appears to have increased in recent years, perhaps because of the perceivably superior safety profile of SSRIs.[70] Pathologic crying, or more rarely pathologic laughing, may develop poststroke in 7% to 48.5% of stroke survivors, and there is evidence that SSRIs can be efficacious in reducing symptoms within days of commencing therapy [Number Needed to Treat 1.5 (NNT 1.5)].[71]

The safety profile of electroconvulsive therapy (ECT) in older patients with depression is very good.[72] A wide spectrum of clinical responses has been demonstrated, including reduction of anxiety symptoms. A meta-analysis of published studies revealed 62% recovery and 21% substantial improvement rates.[73] Although much of the evidence base for ECT is from studies of predominantly younger adults, reanalysis of these studies indicates that ECT is at least as effective in adults aged 60 and older and may positively influence outcome.[74] Unilateral electrode placement appears as effective as bilateral in older patients, but there is clearer evidence that unilateral electrode placement is associated with fewer memory-related side effects in this age group.[75] A study comparing an SSRI (paroxetine) to ECT in resistant depression in elderly has reported a dramatic difference in the results, with a low response rate of 28% in the paroxetine group compared to 71% in the ECT group.[76]

Psychological treatments are underused in old age. This is partly because their availability is often limited. There is also a misconception that older people lack the psychological flexibility to benefit from psychotherapeutic interventions.[77]

Elderly people appear to respond particularly well to cognitive therapy for depression; this is effective both in an individual setting and (more economically) in groups. The focus is often on real or threatened losses (bereavement, physical health, financial security) and on fears of impending death. Brief, highly focused cognitive-behavioral therapies such as problem-solving therapy are being advocated increasingly for older people, including those with some degree of cognitive dysfunction,[78] and they may be effective when used in people at high risk to prevent as well as treat depression in old age.[79] Another brief talking therapy, interpersonal psychotherapy, has also been shown to be effective in older people.[80]

Community and primary care studies suggest that only a small minority of older patients with depression receive treatment. A community study found that only 13% of subjects with depression were being treated with antidepressants; at follow-up, the figure remained virtually the same at 14%.[14] Similarly, only 10% of patients with depression identified from consecutive primary care attenders were receiving treatment for depression.[17] However, their general practitioners were aware of depression in 95% of cases. This suggests that GPs may conceptualize depression in old age as a legitimate and unavoidable consequence of aging and associated adversity, which is recognizable but not seen as treatable. Collaborative care has emerged as a helpful approach toward integrating primary and secondary care teams and combining the use of a range of treatment modalities. Tailored collaborative care was associated with substantial benefits (compared with treatment as usual) in terms of improvement in depressive symptoms, better physical functioning, and an enhanced quality of life.[81]

Suicide and depression in old age

Suicide in old age is almost twice as common in North American older people than in the rest of the population[82]; similarly, suicide rates in most countries are highest in the elderly.[83] In the United Kingdom, the rate in those over 65 years is approximately three times that in the 15-to-24-year age group. Older people are more likely to die in a suicide attempt than younger people, and in men, the rate continues to rise into the ninth decade. Deaths are usually by overdose, but men more frequently use violent means (hanging, firearms, etc.).[84] Suicide is much more closely associated with depression in older than in younger subjects, and the best predictor of suicidality is the current severity of depression. The increased rate of suicide in those experiencing physical ill health is mediated by depression.[85] Other factors associated with suicide in old age include bereavement, substance misuse, increasing social isolation, deteriorating physical health, and pain.

Attempted suicide closely resembles completed suicide in the elderly.[85,86] Psychiatric illness, particularly depression, is prominent in most cases. Minor depression and personality dysfunction are associated with suicide attempts of relatively low intent and higher levels of psychosocial stresses. Hopelessness persisting after remission of other depressive symptoms is associated with suicide attempts and completed suicide.[87]

The close association between depression and deliberate self-harm in old age carries a clear message that all such behavior in older patients should be taken seriously with particular attention to the exclusion or treatment of underlying depressive illness.

The prognosis of depression in old age

Treatment is generally as effective for older adults as for younger ones if depression is recognized and treated,[33] although patients often have recurrences. The mortality rate is considerably higher in elderly patients with depression than in age- and sex-matched controls.[88] Although this in large part reflects preexisting health problems that are significantly more common in depressed patients, they have a worse outcome than those with the same degree of physical illness who are not depressed.

The prognostic significance of cognitive impairment within elderly depressed patients remains unclear. However, in patients presenting with "pseudodementia," not only do computed tomography (CT) scan abnormalities seem to be significantly more common but this subgroup of patients has a poorer prognosis and 40% of them develop dementia within 3 years of follow-up.[89]

In older people with depression, physical illness, cognitive impairment, and severe depressive symptoms rather than social factors are markers of a less optimistic prognosis.[90] Family problems including psychiatric symptoms in the spouse or adult child and poor physical health also adversely influence prognosis.[91] Chronic health problems and acute new physical illness predict poor outcome, with the combination of depressive symptoms and physical disability together initiating a spiraling decline in physical and psychological health.

Continuing treatment appears to have a protective effect against relapse. This has been shown most clearly for maintenance antidepressant drugs,[92] but the efficacy of supportive group psychotherapy has also been shown.[93]

LATE LIFE PSYCHOSIS

The onset of schizophrenia-like psychotic illness later in life not due to an organic or affective disorder has been referred to as *paraphrenia*, *late paraphrenia*, and *late-onset schizophrenia*. In 2000, the International Late-Onset Schizophrenia Group defined the terms *late-onset schizophrenia* and *very late-onset schizophrenia* for schizophrenia-like illnesses with onsets between age 40 and 60 and after age 60, respectively. The term *late-onset schizophrenia* is used to describe these conditions within this chapter. More circumscribed delusional disorders also occur in late life; these are referred to later as *late life delusional disorders*. In addition, the challenges posed by patients with long-standing psychotic illness (usually schizophrenia) who "graduate" to old age are also considered within this section.

Late-onset schizophrenia

The original concept of late-onset schizophrenia referred to the first onset of persecutory delusions and associated hallucinations after the age of 60 years in the absence of an affective or organic psychosis.[94] It may thus be viewed as schizophrenia or a schizophrenia-like illness in old age.

Epidemiology

Although the incidence of schizophrenia is highest in people aged 16 to 25, there is a second peak in incidence in those aged ≥65.[95] The prevalence of nonaffective psychosis in people aged ≥65 years has been reported as 2.3% in women and 1.7% in men.[96] Data from GP practices regarding patients with treated schizophrenia (1997–1998) indicate that prevalence peaks in women in the 65-to-74 age group compared with the 45-to-54 age group in men, reflecting the higher prevalence of late-onset schizophrenia in women. The incidence of late-onset schizophrenia has been reported at 12.6 per 100,000 population per year.[97] Incidence is positively correlated with age, with first admission data suggesting an increase of 11% for every 5-year increase in age.[98] In the United Kingdom, African-Caribbean older people are more likely than white British older people to be in contact with services for a new diagnosis of psychosis.[99] Prevalence of late-onset schizophrenia is likely to be underestimated by community surveys and treatment data as those affected are far less likely than the rest of the population to cooperate with survey investigators and often refuse treatment. They may only be treated compulsorily and in the context of particularly severe behavioral disturbance or when the illness affects their physical health.

Etiology

About 10% of the relatives of patients developing schizophrenia in middle age also have the disease; this is similar to the proportion for patients with early-onset schizophrenia.[100] In family studies of late-onset schizophrenia, however, the rate of schizophrenia in first-degree relatives is much lower.[101] Standardized instruments were not used in the late-onset schizophrenia studies, however, so the data are not directly comparable to those from fully operationalized family studies of younger subjects.

The influence of personality, social, and environmental factors in association with genetic predisposition is clearly complex.[102] Patients with late-onset schizophrenia are often socially isolated and live alone.[103] They are more likely to have paranoid or schizoid premorbid personalities that are characterized by suspicion, sensitivity to setback and disappointment, and preoccupation with what others may think about them.[104] Their isolation is often longstanding and may well be secondary to personality traits. They are predominantly unmarried women without close family or personal attachments. Those who do marry often end up divorced or separated. However, premorbid educational, occupational, and psychosocial functioning is less impaired in late-onset than early-onset schizophrenia.[104] Fertility seems markedly reduced. This social isolation, which is often increased by sensory isolation and retirement in older people, creates an environment allowing the individual to become preoccupied with his or her own internal world.

In terms of sensory impairment, there is a confirmed association between deafness and very-late-onset schizophrenia in particular.[104] Many of those patients have conductive hearing loss contracted in early life to such a degree as to impair social interaction resulting in "social deafness."[105] Visual impairment may be present but is probably no more common than in normal elderly people.[94] Patients with late-onset schizophrenia have been found to come from the lower social classes or socioeconomic groups[103]; this may result from social deterioration secondary to the disease, as also occurs in younger people with schizophrenia.

Presentation and clinical features

Patients often come to the attention of services because they complain to the police and neighbors with bizarre accusations over a period of time or because of neighborly concern triggered by extreme self-neglect. On mental state assessment, there are no qualitative differences between the positive symptoms of early-onset schizophrenia and of late-onset schizophrenia. The clinical presentation of late-onset schizophrenia is quite varied. Patients are in clear consciousness. Usually their affective state is normal although occasionally a secondary depressive mood is found. The history may be difficult to elicit from patients with late-onset schizophrenia who tend to be distrustful and hostile.

Delusions are central. Persecutory delusions are particularly common. Sexual themes are common in women. The patient may accuse a man or men of entering her bed at night and molesting her sexually. Delusions of influence and passivity phenomena are frequently reported.[106] Patients may describe their bodies as being controlled, or complain that some power affects them and they are made to do things against their will. Thought insertion, withdrawal, and broadcasting are, however, fairly rare, and formal thought disorder is almost nonexistent.

Hallucinations are frequently experienced.[103] Those with late-onset schizophrenia experience a great number of different types of hallucinations. Auditory hallucinations are the most common and usually have an accusatory and/or insulting content. The voices speak in the second or the third person with "running commentary" occasionally encountered. Hallucinations of bodily sensation are also found. Patients complain of being vibrated, raped, or forced to have sexual intercourse. Olfactory hallucinations often relating to poisonous gas are encountered. Visual hallucinations are rare in late-onset schizophrenia and if present should raise the strong suspicion of an underlying organic state. Comorbid depression and suicidal ideation are common.

It is not only social and sensory isolation that may make people vulnerable to psychosis but also a more vulnerable brain. Their cognitive function is often mildly impaired at initial presentation, to a much lesser degree than found in dementia, but significantly more than in psychiatrically healthy age-matched controls.[105] Decline is usually slowly progressive, with only a small group of patients entering the dementia range at 3-year follow-up.

Studies of older adults with psychosis have found lower quality of life to be associated with depression, positive and negative symptoms, cognitive deficits, physical disorders, and poorer perceived health, as well as social factors including loneliness and financial strain.[107]

Brain imaging studies

Structural neuroimaging findings in later onset illness are similar to those found in patients with early onset schizophrenia. A representative computed tomography (CT) study has reported increased mean ventricle to brain ratio with cortical sulcal appearances remaining within normal limits.[105] Single-photon emission computed tomography (SPECT) studies have found reduced rCBF in late-onset psychotic patients compared to controls, which also appear similar to those found in early onset schizophrenia.[108] Magnetic resonance imaging (MRI) has demonstrated increased periventricular hyperintensities and thalamic signal hyperintensities in late-onset schizophrenia, which have led to the suggestion that cerebrovascular disease may be significant in the pathogenesis of the condition,[109,110] although these findings have not been consistently replicated[111] and may have reflected the overrepresentation of individuals with cerebrovascular disease risk factors.

A number of studies using PET have shown increased basal ganglia dopamine D2 receptors in late-onset schizophrenia.[114] However, these findings have not been consistently replicated, particularly in drug-naïve subjects, suggesting that some of the differences initially reported may have reflected treatment rather than disease-induced receptor alteration.

Neuropsychological testing

Patients with late-onset schizophrenia have been shown to perform less well on the Mental Test Score and Digit Copying Test than age-matched controls. Deficiencies have also been shown on full-scale IQ tests, tests of frontal lobe function, and verbal memory tasks.[105] The presence of brain abnormalities was not associated with particularly low neuropsychological test scores. When patients with late life schizophrenia are compared to those with young onset disease, they have less neuropsychological deficits in abstraction and cognitive flexibility but more global impairment.

Assessment, treatment, and course

The initial management of late late-onset schizophrenia involves evaluation and engagement.[103] Patients should be assessed at home (rather than in a clinic) both because they are unlikely to comply with outpatient appointments and because their psychopathology may be strongly triggered by cues within their normal environment and less obvious away from it. It is also not surprising on this basis that hospital admission commonly results in an apparent complete remission followed by relapse on return home. Health workers may initially find it difficult to gain access to the home of a patient with late-onset schizophrenia. Once initial access is gained, patients often engage and are willing to discuss their delusional beliefs.

Late-onset schizophrenia may run a chronic course,[112] but recent studies have shown remission rates with treatment of 48% to 60%. Attempts at treatment should begin in the community wherever possible, with hospital admission reserved for patients with particularly severe or dangerous behavioral disturbance or poor self-care. Medication, psychosocial intervention, and ECT have all been reported to produce temporary remission. Adequate antipsychotic treatment produces improvement in psychotic symptoms but not much improvement to the patient's pretreatment level of social functioning. Dosages are much lower than those used in younger patients with schizophrenia; people with late-onset schizophrenia are often very sensitive to extrapyramidal side effects.[113] Patients do better in terms of side effects, efficacy, and negative symptoms with atypical antipsychotics, but risperidone and olanzapine are relatively contraindicated in those with cardiovascular morbidity or diabetes. Patients are often not adherent to medication, particularly as they usually live alone and do not have any insight into treatment necessity. Even when compliance is assured, many patients with late-onset schizophrenia remain psychotic, although they may be less distressed by their symptoms and less disturbed in their behavior.[114,115] Community psychiatric nurses are most likely to ensure a favorable response. There is conflicting evidence regarding whether depot medication improves adherence.[99]

An attempt should be made to correct remediable physical or environmental contributory factors, particularly through alleviating sensory or social isolation. A flexible approach is required, and patients' characteristic insistence on remaining isolated (as they have often been for much of their lives) must be respected. Patients' importuning requests for rehousing should be resisted if they are secondary to delusional beliefs; although if symptoms improve or even abate in a new home setting this is usually only a temporary respite. Old "tormentors" reemerge, and new ones may be acquired. Antipsychotic medication is a vital component of the total therapeutic package but is far from the whole answer; improvisation and ingenuity in engaging these patients and then retaining them in long-term follow-up is crucial to maintain both compliance and an optimal level of social functioning and to reduce risk of symptomatic relapse.

Late-life delusional (paranoid) disorder

It has been estimated that 4% of a community-living elderly population experience some persecutory delusions.[116] Such beliefs are commonly associated with a neuropsychiatric disorder. A primary delusional disorder is present when there is evidence of persistent, nonbizarre delusions that are not attributable to another psychiatric disorder or any organic cause.[117] Delusional disorder refers to persistent delusions without evidence of schizophrenia, schizophreniform, or mood disorders. Hallucinations are not prominent. There is no evidence of organic dysfunction. The distinction between such disorders and late-onset schizophrenia reflects the relative absence of schizophrenia-like features other than delusions in the late-life delusional group. Delusional disorder occurs in middle as well as late life. Men tend to be affected earlier than women (40 to 49 years versus 60 to 69 years).

Pathogenesis and etiology

An increased prevalence of schizophrenia has been observed in families of patients with late-life delusional sorder.[118] Individuals with avoidant, paranoid, or schizoid personality disorders may be more susceptible to developing a delusional disorder. There is an association between hearing loss and delusional disorder in the elderly.[119] Immigration or low socioeconomic status may also predispose individuals to delusional disorder.[120] There is an increased frequency of women, immigrants, or children of immigrants with somatic delusions diagnosed as part of a delusional disorder. There may be a possible association of early life trauma and the failure to reproduce progeny with the development of delusions in later life.[121]

Management and outcome

The optimal approach encompasses drug treatment, psychotherapy, and environmental change.[122] Antipsychotics may be effective in decreasing the intensity of the delusions, but (as in late-onset schizophrenia) nonadherence is a common problem and allocation of a community mental health worker may be important if the person is willing to engage with services. Intramuscular depot neuroleptics may be preferable. Antidepressant drugs and ECT have been used with variable success in delusional patients, particularly those with coexistent depressive symptoms. The provision of alternative explanations for patients' delusional beliefs may be a useful psychotherapeutic approach. There are few outcome data available, but the overall outcome is often poor.[117]

Graduates

The term *graduates* is used to refer to patients with long-standing mental illness who have "graduated" to elderly status.[123] Many graduates entered a mental hospital when relatively young and remained in institutional care for much of their lives, only returning to the community to live independently or in group homes when the large psychiatric hospitals closed in the 1990s.

The largest subgroup is composed of graduates who have schizophrenia. Most of the remainder have primary diagnoses of affective psychoses, learning disability, or personality disorder. Disability in the graduate population is varied. Some patients may require total nursing care, whereas others remain physically fit and relatively competent in daily living skills. Many have some degree of cognitive impairment. There are associations between negative symptoms (social withdrawal, slowness, underactivity, poverty of speech, lack of interest, and poor self-care), cognitive deficit, and structural brain abnormality. This highlights the issue of the long-term cognitive effects of schizophrenic illness. Some of the deficits of chronic schizophrenia are probably integral to the illness process and may manifest at a relatively early stage in the evolution of the illness over time. In addition, increasing social disability may be secondary to the deleterious effects of institutional care on the capacity to return to independent living. It has been suggested that in some patients a phenomenon of "burnout" in schizophrenia (an amelioration of positive symptoms after the age of 55) may occur, but this is still disputed.[124] The lowered prevalence of positive symptoms in this group may be due to reduced exposure to the stresses and strains of everyday life rather than either the effects of medication or the natural history of schizophrenia.

Patients with schizophrenia have high rates of obesity, hypertension, diabetes, cigarette smoking—and therefore cardiovascular and respiratory disease—compared to the nonschizophrenic population, and consequent to this and higher rates of suicide their life expectancy is reduced by 20%.[125] Among those living in institutional settings, there is a high prevalence of physical disability and handicap. This increases with age but is not confined to elderly patients or those with the longest duration of stay. The presence of neurologic abnormalities referred to as "soft" neurologic signs—including disorders of posture and tone, motor performance, inappropriate activity, abnormal movements, automatic movements, and speech production—seem to be intrinsic to the schizophrenic process and cannot be attributed to hospitalization, physical treatment, or undiagnosed neurologic illness.[126]

The care of graduate patients encompasses elements of good practice within old age psychiatry, psychiatric rehabilitation, and medicine of the elderly.[123] The needs of graduates are very different from those of patients with severe dementia, and they should not be cared for in the same settings. Patients' skills should be identified and cultivated as part of a rehabilitative process, in the context of working toward an improved quality of life by improving the physical and social environment. Residential options in the community are varied and should be determined by the individual's present and likely future physical and mental health needs. Medication regimens often need review, and many patients benefit from cautious reduction or withdrawal of antipsychotic drugs that have often been prescribed in substantial amounts over the years.

MANIA

Epidemiology

A recent community 35-year incidence survey in the United Kingdom found that the incidence of mania peaks in early adult life, with a tenth of new onset cases of mania occurring above the age of 60.[127] This contrasts with studies based on psychiatric admission data, which suggested a stable incidence rate across age bands. Bipolar affective disorder is not uncommon in the elderly; prevalence rates range from 0.1% to 0.4%. However, it accounts for 5% of patients admitted to geropsychiatric inpatient units.[128]

Older patients with mania typically had their first manic episode in their mid- to late 50s.[129] People with mania of earlier onset are underrepresented in these hospitalized samples; possible explanations for this include effective treatment with lithium, burnout after many years, and higher mortality rates among younger patients with bipolar disorder. In about half of elderly patients with mania, the first episode of mental illness is depression,[130] with many years of latency before mania becomes manifest.

Clinical features

Many of the clinical features of mania are similar to those found in younger patients, but dramatic physical overactivity, violence, criminal behavior, infectious euphoria, and grandiosity are less common.[131] Clinical experience suggests that mixed mood states are more commonly found in older subjects, but this has not been substantiated in a controlled study.[132] Adverse life events, particularly episodes of illness, more commonly appeared to precipitate mania in older subjects. Subjective confusion or perplexity is relatively prominent in the elderly. First episode mania in very late life with no previous psychiatric history is often associated with comorbid neurologic disorder.

Secondary mania

This concept refers to an episode of mania causally associated with medical illness, exogenous substances, and organic cerebral dysfunction.[131] First-onset mania in old age should be considered to have an underlying organic cause until proven otherwise. The frequent presence of some degree of nonprogressive cognitive impairment in secondary mania reflects its heterogeneous etiology. Even if no acute cause is discovered, there is still a greater prevalence of coexisting neurologic illness. Stroke is the most characteristic precipitant of secondary mania, and long-standing cerebrovascular disease is also overrepresented, with white matter hyperintensities often found on MRI scanning. Family history and prior psychiatric disturbance are uncommon in secondary mania.

The treatment of mania in old age

The drug treatment of elderly people with mania is similar to that in younger patients. However, drug doses will generally be smaller. Neuroleptics are the mainstay of acute treatment. In secondary mania, treatment is also directed at the underlying medical cause. First-line prophylactic treatment is with lithium, although the risks of neurotoxicity are higher, even at relatively low serum lithium levels. The acute antimanic effect may also be useful in older people. The anticonvulsants carbamazepine, sodium divalproate, and atypical antipsychotics are increasingly widely used for their mood-stabilizing effects, but few data have been reported in older people with mania. Olanzapine and risperidone are contraindicated in people with dementia because of increased risk of stroke. Family involvement is important in ongoing management. The risk of marital and family breakup is high. The range of skills available within a multidisciplinary team is often needed to deal with the complexities of managing bipolar disorder in old age.

Outcome

The acute and long-term outcome is similar to that in younger patients. Mania with first onset in old age may, however, have a poorer prognosis than mania recurring in old age, perhaps because of the greater likelihood of comorbid physical disease or cognitive impairment.[132]

ANXIETY DISORDERS

Epidemiology

Several studies have examined the prevalence of anxiety disorders in community-based populations.[133–135] The prevalence rates for phobias range between less than 1% to 11.7%; for generalized anxiety, the range is between 1.4% and 7.1%. The variability in these findings probably reflects the use in some of specific case-finding instruments designed for older people and also whether a hierarchical approach is used in which those who have depression are not counted as anxious. Anxiety is frequently comorbid with depression. There is consensus that panic disorder is extremely rare in old age.

Specific groups of people may be likely to become anxious as they are in stressful situations and these include carers and the physically ill. As well as changing the situation (which is not always possible), psychological strategies such as the use of appropriate coping strategies may be helpful. Cognitive-behavioral treatment (CBT) and other psychological treatments are first line, although the only randomized controlled trial comparing antidepressants (sertraline) to CBT showed that sertraline had a larger effect size (0.94 versus 0.42 at 3 months) for all anxiety disorders.[136]

Phobic disorders

Phobic disorders consist of persistent or recurrent irrational fear of an object, activity, or situation that results in the compelling desire to avoid the phobic stimulus.[137] In old age they are associated with higher rates of medical and of other psychiatric morbidity but are frequently found in the absence of other psychiatric disorder.[133] Agoraphobia is often triggered by the traumatic experience or acute physical ill health.[137]

The longitudinal course of phobic disorders in old age is unclear. Individuals with one phobia may develop another. Fear of crime is particularly common in old age, leading to fear of going out and to nighttime fearfulness. Social phobias in old age have usually developed earlier in life and persisted; they tend to be chronic and unremitting.[138] Comorbidity with agoraphobia, specific phobia, depression, and alcohol abuse is common.[139] Older people rarely seek treatment but change their life to accommodate their avoidance. Anxiolytics provide only symptomatic relief and are best avoided because of their dependency potential.[137]

Generalized anxiety disorder

Generalized anxiety disorder consists of generalized, persistent anxiety, with motor tension, autonomic symptoms, apprehensiveness, and hypervigilance.[140] It usually runs a chronic course.[139] It is hard to diagnose in the elderly because of its high degree of comorbidity with depression. Coexistent medical conditions can complicate the situation. Benzodiazepines have been the mainstay of treatment, but dependence and adverse effects should limit their use to very short-term management only. Antidepressants may be useful, and cognitive-behavioral strategies may be effective.

Panic disorder

Panic disorder is characterized by recurrent attacks of panic, with sudden, discrete periods of intense fear accompanied by severe somatic anxiety symptoms, usually lasting for 1 to 10 minutes. The disorder usually runs a chronic course[141] but may remit spontaneously or become less disabling secondary to reduced rates of social interaction in old age. It may, albeit rarely, occur de novo in older people.[142] Panic disorder with onset earlier in life is associated with depression,[143] alcohol abuse,[144] increased suicide risk,[145] and higher cardiovascular morbidity.[146] Panic disorder becomes less rare as people age. Part of the explanation for the low prevalence in the elderly may be that sufferers may not survive into old age. Physical limitations in daily activities as well as the presence of other psychiatric disorders (major depression and social phobia) are significantly associated with panic disorder.[147] Antidepressants are the pharmacologic antipanic agents of choice with SSRIs increasingly used in preference to tricyclics.[139] Benzodiazepines are efficacious for symptom control but can only be used very short term because of undesirable side effects and dependence. Cognitive-behavioral therapy is often effective. Long-term outcome is improved by combination drug and cognitive-behavioral approach.

Posttraumatic stress disorder and bereavement

Posttraumatic stress disorder (PTSD) occurs in response to a catastrophic event. Symptoms usually start after a month but always within 6 months. Traumatic events in old age can trigger similar PTSD reactions to those occurring in younger victims.[139] PTSD is still present is some aging survivors of combat and can arise again when a person ages and becomes vulnerable again. In one study of Holocaust survivors in older age, experience of more severe trauma, use of immature defense mechanisms, and higher neuroticism were associated with significant PTSD and psychological morbidity.[148] The intensity of the physiologic response to the original trauma may be the most significant predictor of a poor outcome. Further stressful life events can slow recovery, which may also be hindered by drug and alcohol abuse, which may themselves be triggered by PTSD.[149] Busuttil[150] provided an overview of treatment in older people. Treatment outcome studies are lacking in older people. Therefore, treatment follows the principles used in younger adults. These include medications and psychotherapy separately or in combination. Stabilization using medication first may be indicated. Useful medications for treating PTSD include antidepressants. SSRIs are usually first line, which help for reexperiencing and hyperarousal. Psychotherapeutic interventions include behavioral, cognitive, cognitive-behavioral therapies and eye movement desensitization and reprocessing (EMDR). Several trials have demonstrated highly significant reductions in PTSD symptomatology.

Bereavement is, sadly, an all-too-common experience for older people. Although depressive symptoms are common in the weeks immediately after bereavement, this is normal and most people experience a gradual diminution of these symptoms without developing a full-blown depressive illness. Persistence and severity of symptoms are what differentiates depression and normal grieving following bereavement. Postbereavement depression is most strongly associated with a past history of depression. Surprisingly, only weak statistical associations are found with quality of the relationship with the lost partner or with level of postbereavement social support.[151]

Obsessive-compulsive disorder

Obsessions are intrusive thoughts, images, or impulses that are unpleasant, consciously resisted, which the patient is aware arise from his or her own mind. A compulsion is a behavior that causes anxiety when resisted and is usually repeated and recognized as purposeless. The diagnosis is only made when the problem interferes with normal functioning. Obsessive-compulsive disorder (OCD) has a prevalence rate of 1.5% in older people.[134] The onset is usually earlier in life, with persistence into old age.[139] OCD is often resistant to treatment, but the use of serotonin enhancers (clomipramine, SSRIs) and cognitive-behavioral techniques has improved the outlook.[152] In the elderly, it is important to bear in mind that obsessive-compulsive phenomena frequently occur within a primary depressive illness, and the development of obsessional orderliness may indicate the onset of dementia or an affective disorder.[153]

SOMATOFORM DISORDERS

Somatoform disorders are those in which physical symptoms occur in the absence of any or sufficient organic pathology to account for them and include conversion disorder, somatization disorder, pain disorder, and hypochondriasis. They are not due to malingering or fabricated symptoms and the patient experiences the symptoms presented. Psychological contributory factors can usually be identified.

Although somatoform disorders—in particular syndromes of chronic fatigue, irritable bowel syndrome, and fibromyalgia—have received considerable attention recently in psychiatry and relevant consumer groups, this has not been true for older people, and health practitioners are less likely to recognize these disorders.[154] This may be because somatoform disorders present differently in older people; this has significant implications for their measurement and validation in older people. For example, such disorders are masked by physical comorbidity, and practitioners may be more likely to perceive associated mental distress as appropriate in older people.[154] Somatizing presentations are common among older primary care attendees.[155] Older people often develop exaggerated bodily complaints in the context of physical illness. Physically ill patients may also present with generalized anxiety or panic symptoms. The common medical disorders producing anxiety symptoms are endocrine, cardiovascular, pulmonary, and neurologic conditions. A thorough history should help to establish the temporal relationship of psychiatric symptomatology and the onset of medical illness.

Although the onset of somatoform disorder is usually in early life and runs a chronic course, somatizing patients avoid psychiatrists in youth and adulthood and so not uncommonly present to them for the first time in old age.[153] The epidemiologic catchment area studies from the United States suggest the prevalence is the same and rare (0.1%) throughout adult life when the disorder is defined as having 12 or more unexplained medical symptoms. Rates of persistent fatigue are also similar across age groups and occur in more than a quarter of adults of all ages.[154] Such patients usually have clear symptoms of depression or anxiety; their bodily complaints tend to be restricted to one or two body organs or systems. They are preoccupied with the possibility of serious physical illness. They demand investigation rather than treatment. In contrast, hypochondriacal preoccupation presenting for the first time in old age is unlikely to be secondary to anxiety and depression. Hypochondriasis is a persistent, unrealistic preoccupation with the possibility of having at least one serious disease in which normal sensations and appearances are often misinterpreted as abnormal and signs of disease, and the patient cannot accept reassurances of doctors. Elderly patients only rarely present with conversion reactions (e.g., paralysis) or dissociative amnesia in response to stressful experience. Treatment of associated psychiatric conditions may lead to improvement in somatic attributions.[155] There have been no specific trials in older people, but cognitive approaches are effective among younger patients[156] and so may also be helpful in older people.

ALCOHOL

The average alcohol intake of older people is less than that of younger adults. Fewer drink regularly,[157] and abstinence is more common.[158] Social and psychological factors may contribute to a decrease in alcohol intake with age, including reduced social opportunities and financial constraints. Moderate drinking rather than abstinence seems to be better in terms of mortality and cognition.[159,160] Older people are, however, more vulnerable to the effects of alcohol because of physiologic changes and the increased presence of pathologic processes. Despite the general downward trend, drinking is an important contributor to mental and physical ill health in some old people.[161]

Epidemiology and etiology

Studies in the United States suggest that the prevalence of abusive or dependent drinking is about 5% in the population aged 65 years and over, with a male preponderance of about 4:1.[162] A British community study reported a 1% prevalence of problem drinking.[163] In the hospital setting, elderly patients who abuse alcohol are concentrated in general medical settings; one study[164] identified 14% of elderly emergency admissions as having current alcohol abuse. Cultural, ethnic, and socioeconomic factors; differences between countries; and regional variation may influence drinking behavior and related problems resulting in variable prevalence.

The rates of alcohol abuse in the elderly are related to the levels of consumption by the community as a whole.[165] The surveys, which are cross-sectional, do not take into account that drinking less may be a cohort rather than an age effect, whereby those who are currently older may always have had a relatively low intake. New cohorts of older people may drink more than those who started drinking in the 1920s.[166] Psychiatric disorder and personality attributes predispose to alcohol abuse. In particular, those older people with a late onset of alcohol abuse tend to have a past history of harmless drinking patterns, with consumption increased in the context of depression, bereavement, lack of social support, or deteriorating physical health.[161,167] Elderly people with insomnia or chronic pain, those previously dependent on alcohol, and those with current depression or dementia seem particularly vulnerable to developing alcohol-related problems in old age.[168] Persisting social problems perpetuate the cycle of loneliness and further drinking.[165]

Clinical features

The diagnosis of alcohol abuse may be difficult because the presentation may be masked, unsuspected, or atypical.[169] In a general medical setting the prevalence is higher and the index of suspicion should be raised.[170] In particular, alcohol abuse should be suspected in the assessment of otherwise unexplained falls. Alcohol abuse may present with a wide range of neuropsychiatric complications.[157] Patients can present with cognitive impairment, problems related to mixed intoxication with drugs, or unrecognized withdrawal states. Alcohol abuse is also associated with functional psychiatric disorder, particularly depression.[171] Up to one third of elderly persons who break the law either abuse alcohol or are dependent on it.[172] They are often under the influence of alcohol when the crime is committed.

There is little information regarding the clinical course and prognosis. Light to moderate use of alcohol is associated with a decreased mortality in the elderly. The benign course of "normal" drinking seems very different, however, from that of the problem drinkers in old age, who often present when brain damage or social breakdown supervenes. A past history of alcohol-related problems is associated with both depression and dementia in later life. Depression and anxiety are major comorbid diagnoses.

Management

Alcohol abuse in older people is probably often undetected,[173] particularly in patients presenting with medical conditions. Screening at-risk groups[168] may identify individuals at risk of alcohol abuse. Screening instruments used for younger people are probably of limited value in the elderly; a review by Beresford[162] presents one such screening test designed for older people, the Michigan Alcoholism Screening Test—Geriatric Version, although this has yet to be extensively validated.

When an individual is recognized as having an alcohol-related problem, several services may need to be involved. Home visits are often invaluable in the initial assessment.[174] Hospital admission may be needed to break the drinking routine, reduce risks associated with acute alcohol withdrawal,[175] and allow for full physical and psychiatric assessment. Alcohol withdrawal symptoms become more severe with age, and detoxification is more likely to be complicated by intercurrent illness. Withdrawal seizures occur within 24 hours if at all. Tremor, tachycardia, hypertension, anxiety, nausea, and insomnia are prominent features of the alcohol withdrawal syndrome in old age. The patient should be nursed in a calm, well-lit environment. Shorter acting benzodiazepines are preferred for sedation. The dosage for older patients undergoing detoxification should begin at about one third of that used for a fit younger person and should then be titrated against the clinical response.

A long-term management plan needs to be formulated with either abstinence or controlled drinking as a goal. Older people respond better to social intervention than to intensive confrontation. Alcohol is often an occupation, and drinkers' social contact may be entirely with other drinkers. Thus, part of the plan has to involve consideration of where and how someone who wishes to be an ex-drinker will spend the day. Amelioration of social stresses, group socialization, family work, medical treatment, and management of depression are all part of the approach needed. Cognitive therapy, sometimes delivered through alcohol services, is often used. Those who wish to continue to drink and are eating little will often take thiamine and this may help protect them form Korsakov's syndrome. Disulfiram is not recommended in older people because of increasing medical risks involved with ingesting alcohol while taking the drug.[176]

PERSONALITY DISORDERS IN OLD AGE

Personality disorders are generally recognizable by adolescence or earlier and continue throughout most of adult life, although they become less obvious in middle or old age and as in younger people the diagnosis is only applicable to those who have long-standing dysfunction from the beginning of their adult life.[177] Some lifelong obsessive or schizoid personality traits may worsen in old age, possibly as a result of experiencing increasing stress and adversity or as a way of adapting to losses in old age[178] and may present for the first time possibly as a person who has interpersonal difficulties becomes dependent on others. Global well-being, life satisfaction, and capacity to cope with illness and loss in old age are also critically influenced by personality and its adaption to old age.[179] Personality traits may be critical in adapting to the adverse life events all too often encountered by older people.

Epidemiology

An individual's personality is essentially stable over time.[179] Introversion has, however, been shown to increase with age,[180] whereas extraversion, neuroticism, and openness to experience decrease.[181] Older people tend to have higher scores on scales for orderliness, social conformity, and emotional stability and lower scores for activity and energy.[182] A decline in sociopathy and criminality has been documented.[183] Few large-scale studies of personality disorder in old age have been performed. An early epidemiologic survey[3] reported a prevalence of 3.6% to 10.6% for personality disorders in people aged 65 years and older. More recent surveys of older community-living individuals using standardized diagnostic schedules have found lifetime prevalence rates for personality disorders ranging between 2.1% and 18%; a more recent meta-analysis reported an overall prevalence of 10% of those over 50 years old.[184,185] The mental health of older male prisoners is reported to be worse than that of younger prisoners, with 45% having a psychiatric illness with a prevalence of personality disorders of 30%.[186]

Comorbidity

People with personality disorders are vulnerable to other psychiatric illnesses as there is a particular association between personality disorders and affective illness, although the first episodes of depression or anxiety disorders usually occur before old age. People with late-onset schizophrenia often have premorbid schizoid or paranoid traits.

Senile self-neglect (Diogenes syndrome)

Patients with this syndrome (also known as senile self-neglect or senile squalor syndrome) often present to units for medicine of the elderly. There is usually gross self and domestic neglect, often with hoarding and social withdrawal. Although the most common diagnosis is dementia, others are depressed, have a paranoid psychosis, or abuse alcohol. Rarely patients have an obsessional disorder. Several studies have reported that about a third to a half have no psychiatric illness and tend to have higher than average intelligence.[187] For others, the syndrome can be understood as an expression of abnormal personality traits, in reaction to stress and loneliness or as the end stage of long-standing reclusiveness. It may be, however, as some authors have suggested, that frontal lobe degeneration or obsessive compulsive disorder tends to be present if those patients are investigated thoroughly, although this is usually difficult as patients are uncooperative.[188] The clinical picture is of very gross self-neglect. Most people live alone but a number of cases of folie à deux have been reported. The prognosis of such cases is not good. Compulsory hospitalization is difficult to accomplish, and mortality is high; apparently successful rehabilitation is usually followed by relapse.[189] Daycare might maintain an individual, but some form of institutional care usually becomes necessary. The recent Mental Capacity Act may prove helpful.

Outcome of personality disorder in old age

Clinical experience suggests that patients with personality disorders do not cause as much trouble for themselves, their families, and health care professionals by the time they reach old age.[177] Formal long-term follow-up studies are, however, sparse. Immature personality disorders including antisocial, impulsive, histrionic, dependent, and narcissistic usually improve with time. Mature personality disorders, including anancastic, paranoid, schizoid, and schizotypal, tend to persist into later life. Deterioration may become evident in the obsessive-compulsive patient as increased rigidity, in the paranoid patient as more suspiciousness and isolation, and in the schizotypal/schizoid patient as more social withdrawal and anxiety.

Patients with borderline personality tend to improve (or not survive) as they age and thus rarely present in older age. Good global outcome in such patients is associated with high intelligence, attractiveness, artistic talent, and coexisting obsessive-compulsive traits.[190] The highly subjective "likeability" seems also to confer good prognosis. Poor outcome is associated with a history of parental brutality, impulsivity, poor premorbid functioning, and coexistent schizotypal/antisocial personality disorder.[191]

In patients with antisocial personality disorder, there is a tendency toward spontaneous remission so that these individuals are rarely encountered over the age of 60.[177] Patients with schizotypal and schizoid personality disorder rarely seek treatment, so little is reported on their long-term outcome but the outlook is probably poor.[192] There is also little information on the outcome of histrionic, narcissistic, obsessive-compulsive, and depressive personality disorders.[177]

KEY POINTS

Functional Psychiatric Illness in Old Age

- By 2020, depression will be second only to heart disease as a contributor to global disability and a major public health problem in older people.
- The management of depression in physically ill elderly patients is essentially the same as for depression in general. Antidepressant and psychological therapy are equally effective in older and younger adults, although there is a need for increased caution with medication because of medical comorbidities and the greater possibility of adverse effects and drug interactions.
- Occasionally the age onset of schizophrenia is over 60. New psychotic symptoms in older people are more often due to delirium, dementia, or depression.
- The initial approach to late-life paranoid illnesses encompasses drug treatment and managing sensory impairment and isolation. Olanzapine and risperidone are contraindicated in people with dementia because of increased risk of stroke.
- A tenth of new onset cases of mania occur in individuals above the age of 60. The drug treatment of elderly people with mania is similar to that prescribed for younger patients.
- Bereavement is a common experience for older people. Although depressive symptoms are prevalent in the weeks immediately after, this is normal and most people experience a gradual diminution of these symptoms. Postbereavement depression is most strongly associated with a past history of depression and should be suspected if symptoms are severe or persist.

Management of personality disorder in old age

There has been little formal study of treatment approaches to personality disorders in old age.[177] The management of coexisting psychiatric illness is as discussed previously, and many of the traits are less expressed in behavior when these are treated. The psychotherapeutic treatment of elderly patients may be unpromising for individuals with long-standing personality disorders who may have particular difficulty in resolving a lifetime of failed relationships and missed opportunities. Cognitive analytic therapy, which is about interpersonal understanding rather than using an illness model, is a therapy used to search for the meaning behind symptoms and offers a narrative reconstruction of an individual's life story.[193] It is used to generate a written reformulation and diagrams and has been used to help older people with narcissistic and borderline traits.[193] The use of medication in old age personality disorders has not been formally studied.

For a complete list of references, please visit online only at www.expertconsult.com

CHAPTER 58

The Older Adult with Intellectual Disability

John M. Starr

DEFINITIONS AND ETIOLOGY

Intellectual disability (ID) is the current term used to describe what in the United Kingdom has been known as *learning disability* and in the United States as *mental retardation*. In Australia, the 1986 Victorian Act of Parliament, which established the basis on which services to people with intellectual disabilities or significant delay in their development are provided, defines intellectual disability as follows:

> *Intellectual disability in relation to a person over the age of five years means a significant subaverage general intellectual functioning existing concurrently with deficits in adaptive behaviour and manifested during the developmental period.*
>
> (Intellectually Disabled Persons Services Act, 1986)

The threshold at which general intellectual functioning is considered "subaverage" is often fixed at an IQ of 70, two standard deviations below the mean IQ. Controversially, in 1992 the American Association on Intellectual and Developmental Disabilities (AAIDD) loosened this threshold to include people with IQs in the range of 70 to 75. The AAIDD also required 2 out of 10 areas of adaptive functioning to be assessed to have deficits. This definition was adapted by the American Psychiatric Association's *Diagnostic and Statistical Manual of Mental Disorders*, fourth edition (DSM-IV). In 2002, the AAIDD reinstated the IQ 70 threshold and required deficits in conceptual, social, and practical adaptive skills to be present. These changes in definition have implications for epidemiologic data collection, but the key concept of ID remains. An IQ of less than 70 is necessary, but this in itself is inadequate for the diagnosis to be made. There has to be evidence of both a developmental disorder, that is onset during childhood, and deficits in adaptive behavior for the diagnosis to be made.

Further classification of ID can be made within the broad definition. The Diagnostic Criteria for Psychiatric Disorders for Use with Adults with Learning [Intellectual] Disabilities (DC-LD)[1] describes a person with ID's mental health in terms of ID severity, ID etiology, and related mental disorders (developmental disorders, psychiatric illness, personality disorders, problem behaviors, and other disorders). Severity is grouped according to IQ as 50-69 mild ID, 35-49 moderate, 20-34 severe, and less than 20 profound. The Swedish model of ID classification developed by Kylen[2] is often helpful in clinical situations where IQ is not known:

- Severe: Communication is based on simple nonverbal signs, no verbal communication, no concept of time or space. Equivalent to IQ <10.
- Moderate: Limited verbal skills. Limited understanding of local space. Can structure thoughts in relation to individual experiences. Equivalent to IQ 10 to 40.
- Mild: Basic literacy and mathematical skills present. Can rearrange, structure, and perform concrete cognitive operations. Equivalent to IQ 41 to 70.

In addition, the DC-LD includes appendices that relate to medical factors influencing health status and contact with health services. The latter are highly relevant because developmental disorders that affect the brain, giving rise to ID, often affect other body systems also.

The etiology of ID is frequently unknown in older adults, but it can be considered along conventional lines of external causes (infection, injury, poisoning), internal disorders (endocrine, metabolic), perinatal insults, and congenital conditions (chromosomal abnormalities, gene mutations). The latter are of particular relevance to the health of older adults with ID, as specific syndromes are associated with risk of particular physical disorders and diseases. Common syndromes seen in older adults include Down syndrome (DS), Angelman syndrome, fragile X syndrome, Klinefelter syndrome, Turner syndrome, and Williams syndrome. Table 58-1 provides a brief description of these syndromes. It is worth noting that, given the preceding definition of ID, by no means does everyone with one of these syndromes fulfill the diagnostic criteria for ID; this is particularly true of women with Turner syndrome who have a tendency for nonverbal cognitive deficits but are often of average intelligence.

Just as there is a considerable overlap between congenital syndromes, such as DS and ID, there is a similar overlap between ID and autism. The diagnosis of autism depends on (1) abnormal social development, (2) communication deficits, and (3) restricted and repetitive interests and behavior. Around three quarters of people with autism have a nonverbal IQ less than 70 and hence also fulfill diagnostic criteria for ID; but in autism, social and communication skills are worse than expected for any given nonverbal IQ.

EPIDEMIOLOGY OF INTELLECTUAL DISABILITY AND AGING

Prevalence

In 2001, the World Health Organization reported the following:

> *The prevalence figures [of ID] vary considerably because of the varying criteria and methods used in the surveys, as well as differences in the age range of the samples. The overall prevalence of mental retardation is believed to be between 1% and 3%, with the rate for moderate, severe and profound retardation being 0.3%.*[3]

Extrapolating these figures to the United Kingdom provides estimates of around 175,800 people with moderate-to-profound

Table 58-1. Characteristics of Common Syndromes Associated with Intellectual Disability

The phenotypic features are "typical" and may not be evident in all people with the syndrome. Similarly, many phenotypic features are found in unaffected individuals.

Syndrome Name	Chromosomal Abnormality	Phenotypic Appearance
Angelman syndrome	15q11-q13 in the maternally contributed chromosome (cf Prader-Willi has same deletion in paternal chromosome); a few cases are due to paternal chromosome 15 disomy and a few are due to putative single gene mutation on chromosome 15	Microcephaly, ataxic gait, strabismus, scoliosis
Down syndrome (DS)	Vast majority trisomy of chromosome 21; a few have trisomy 21 mosaicism. Small proportion translocation of chromosome 21	Flat facial profile, epicanthic fold, relative hyperglossia, single palmar crease
Fragile X syndrome	X-linked, semi-dominant disorder with reduced penetrance. Number of fragile sites on X-chromosome identified, two important for ID around X27.3.	Broad forehead with long face, large ears, strabismus, high arched palate, macro-orchidism, scoliosis, joint hyperextensibility
Klinefelter syndrome	XXY and XXY mosaicism with variants XXXY or XXYY	Taller than average, microorchidism, youthful appearance, gynecomastia
Turner syndrome	XO, partial deletion of second X chromosome, XO mosaicism	Short stature, premature ovarian failure, high arched palate, low set ears, webbed neck, strabismus, cubitus valgus, scoliosis, short fourth metacarpals
Williams syndrome	Deletion of *CLIP2*, *GTF2I*, *GTF2IRD1*, *LIMK1*, and other genes from chromosome 7	'Elfin features' of upturned nose, widely spaced eyes, wide mouth with full lips, small chin, high levels of empathy and anxiety

ID with mild ID ranging from 586,000 to 1,465,000.[4] For Finland, the equivalent estimates are 15,300, 51,000 and 127,500 respectively. Population-based surveys in Finland have estimated moderate-to-profound ID prevalence at no more than 0.2% and overall ID prevalence at just over 1%.[4] The situation is similar for the United Kingdom.[4] Notably, Finnish prevalence rates estimated from national registers is a little lower at 0.7%, perhaps indicating that not all people with ID are known to Finnish health or social services.[5] Within overall prevalence figures there is considerable variation by age. In the Finnish national register survey, the rates were 0.53% for individuals 0 to 15 years of age, 0.70% for those 16 to 39 years, 0.92% for those 40 to 64 years, and 0.38% for those 65 years and older.[5] Variation in Finland between age groups was attributed to changes in incidence, mortality, diagnostic practices, and benefit provision. Changes in diagnostic practices have been discussed in the previous section and benefit provision is specific to Finland, but changes in ID incidence and mortality have been tracked across the world.

Incidence

Estimation of ID incidence is problematic given that ID is, by definition, a developmental disorder and thus there is no single point at which it is recognized. In view of this reality, Down syndrome is often used as a proxy because it is the largest single cause of ID. However, its use as a proxy is far from ideal because risk is clearly associated with maternal age and prenatal screening has been widely introduced. Table 58-2 summarizes secular trends in DS incidence from various countries. Overall DS incidence appears to have been rising before the introduction of prenatal screening. This resulted in a decrease that is projected to be offset by increasing mean maternal age. Overall, there seems little to indicate a great change in ID incidence and numbers of people with ID may track the overall birth rates in different countries.

Mortality

Mortality has had the greatest impact on ID prevalence, especially in older age groups. In 1900, a child with DS would expect to survive to around 9 years of age. In the United States, the median age at death increased from 25 years in 1983 to 49 years in 1997.[6] The improvement is likely to reflect improved socioeconomic circumstances, improved correction of congenital cardiac abnormalities, and perhaps changing attitudes to treating people with ID. There is little difference in life expectancy for people with DS compared with other causes of ID.[7] Identification of common causes of death in people with ID is made difficult by poor death certificate completion. For example, many people in the United States had either ID or DS listed as a primary cause of death, which is inappropriate.[7] However, as the ID population ages, the causes of death are thought to resemble those in the general population more and more closely. Those with mild ID survive

Table 58-2. Secular Trends in Down Syndrome Incidence

Study	Country	Dates	Incidence Changes (per 10,000 Live Births)
Krivchenia et al. Am J Epidemiol 1993;137:815–28	United States	1970–1989	Increase in all groups except urban white population where incidence decreased due to terminations of pregnancy; 11.7 average over whole period
Carothers et al. J Med Genet 1999;36:386–93	Scotland	1990–1994	Decrease from 10.8 to 7.7
Merrick J. Down Syndrome Res Practice 2001;6:128–30	Israel	1964–1997	Decrease from 24.3 to 10, but unchanged when terminations of pregnancy included
Verloes et al. Eur J Hum Genet 2001;9:1–4	Belgium	1984–1998	Decrease following, but not fully explained by, prenatal screening from 12.6 to 6.2 live births
Nazer et al. Rev Med Chile 2006;134:1549–57	Chile	1972–2005	Increase, 3.36 average over whole period

longer, and there is some equivalence to this observation in the general population where people with low IQs within the normal range suffer premature mortality largely attributable to cardiovascular disease.[8] Current trends suggest that people with ID can expect to survive to 60 to 65 years and an increasing proportion will survive beyond this age.

BIOLOGIC AGING IN ID: SYNDROMIC AND NONSYNDROMIC

Even with recent improvements, life expectancy of people with ID is considerably less than that of the non-ID population. This raises the question as to whether ID is associated with accelerated biologic aging. The measurement of biologic age usually depends on identifying suitable biomarkers of aging. Criteria for such biomarkers have been proposed[9]:

1. They must reflect some basic biologic process of aging rather than disease.
2. They must have high cross-species reproducibility.
3. They must change independently of chronologic time.
4. They must be obtainable antemortem.
5. They must be measurable over a short period compared to the life span of the organism.

One such biomarker is telomere length.[10] There is a paucity of data on telomere length in ID in general, but there is evidence for telomere shortening in DS[11] although this appears to be downstream from cellular redox status[12] as is also likely in the general population.[13] In cri-du-chat syndrome, there is often a deletion of the short arm of chromosome 5 where the telomerase reverse transcriptase (*hTERT*) gene is localized (5p15.33). Reconstitution of telomerase activity by ectopic expression of *hTERT* extends telomere length, increases population doublings, and prevents the end-to-end fusion of chromosomes.[14] It may thus be one element contributing to the syndrome's phenotypic features. Whether this is the case or not, accelerated telomere shortening occurs with aging in this syndrome.[15] At least a further 5% of ID is attributable to similar subtelomeric deletions or copy number variations,[16] and these too may influence telomere length. Telomere length is thus a potentially useful index of accelerated biologic aging in ID, but whether it contributes to aging itself or is only a correlate remains unclear. Moreover, telomere shortening is subject to syndrome-specific effects. Beyond the cellular level, various physiologic biomarkers are also affected in ID. Physiologic variables are long recognized as indices of biologic age.[17] The limited data available indicate that people with DS had accelerated biologic aging, but that people with nonsyndromic ID do not.[18,19] In summary, the evidence suggests that syndromic biologic aging dominates over any accelerated biologic aging that might be associated with ID in general and that different ID syndromes are likely to have different aging profiles depending on the specific genetic changes underlying them.

AGE-RELATED DISEASE: SYNDROMIC AND NONSYNDROMIC PATTERNS

People with ID exhibit considerable morbidity. A study of 346 people aged 20 to 50 years in North Sydney found they had a mean 2.5 major problems and 2.9 minor problems each with 42% of these undiagnosed before the study and, of the 58% already known, only 49% were being managed adequately.[20] A study of 1371 adults aged 40 years and over in New York State found that increased age was associated with higher prevalence of cardiovascular disease, cancer, respiratory disease, musculoskeletal disorders, infections, and visual and hearing impairments; gastrointestinal disease was not associated with age but with being male, more severe ID, cerebral palsy, and obesity.[21] Compared with the non-ID population, there was less cardiovascular disease and musculoskeletal disease, except osteoarthritis, and people with DS did not have solid neoplasias. However, these data may reflect underdiagnosis and lifestyle factors such as the low rate of cigarette smoking among people with ID. A similar age-related pattern of disease was found in Southern Holland.[22] The pattern may change as fewer people with ID live in institutions: there is evidence from the United Kingdom that poor diet, reduced physical activity, and obesity risk factors are greater in women with ID who are more able and independent.[23] In addition to the general tendency for high levels of morbidity, which is associated with both age and degree of ID severity, specific syndromes carry their own particular risks (Table 58-3). The

Table 58-3. Common Adult Medical Problems in Various ID Syndromes

Syndrome	Cardiovascular Problems	Neurologic Problems	Sensory Problems	Other Problems
Angelmann	Septal defects, valvular disease	Seizures common, ataxia, absence of speech	Otitis media	Respiratory infections, obesity
Down	Septal defects, valvular disease	Seizures in around 10%, Alzheimer-type dementia	Cataracts, hearing loss	Osteoporosis, hypothyroidism, blood dyscrasias, atlantoaxial instability
Fragile X	Septal defects, valvular disease	Seizures may occur	Cataracts, coloboma	Joint instability, hernias
Myotonic dystrophy		Myotonia with muscle weakness		
Rubinstein-Taybi	Septal defects, valvular disease	Seizures may occur	Cataracts, optic nerve abnormalities, hearing loss	Renal abnormalities (absent/extra kidneys, etc.), cryptorchidism
Smith-Lemli-Opitz	Septal defects, valvular disease		Visual and hearing loss	Low cholesterol levels, multiple organ abnormalities
Smith-Magenis	Septal defects, valvular disease, hypertension	Sleep disturbance, self-injury, aggression, peripheral neuropathy	Hyperacusis, wax buildup	Multiple organ abnormalities, hypothyroidism, immunoglobulin deficiency
Williams	Septal defects, valvular disease, hypertension	Cerebrovascular disease		Multiple organ abnormalities, hoarse voice, hypothyroidism, constipation

most common syndrome in older adults with ID is DS, and discussion of the various problems in people with DS can provide a general approach to such problems in other syndromes.

Down syndrome: effects on systems

CARDIOVASCULAR: LATE EFFECTS OF CONGENITAL HEART DISEASE AND HYPERLIPIDEMIA

Congenital heart disease is common in many ID syndromes as multiple genes contribute to its etiology; DS is a common cause of ID-associated congenital heart disease. Nowadays there is no reason why children with DS and congenital heart defects should not have surgical correction.[24] Complications of uncorrected congenital heart disease, such as Eisenmenger's syndrome and infective endocarditis, are thus becoming rare. In addition, persistent atrial septal defects are associated with increased risk of cerebral embolic events. However, many people with DS are not under regular follow-up once they become adults and may continue to have problems with arrhythmias. In particular, right bundle branch block is not uncommon after surgery. This is usually of no relevance until some form of left bundle branch block occurs when progression to complete heart block becomes more likely. There may also be residual hypoxemia because of persisting right-to-left shunts. Again this generally is of no consequence until some extra stress to the system occurs such as a general anesthetic. Some residual shunts may also be associated with a degree of pulmonary hypertension. Lifestyle factors and associated obesity put adults with DS at increased risk of hyperlipidemia. It is unclear how much impact this has on cardiovascular disease risk in this population, but there is evidence for a deleterious effect on cognition (see the next section).

NEUROLOGIC: DEMENTIA, EPILEPSY, VISION, AND HEARING LOSS

Dementia is three to four times more prevalent among adults with ID than the similarly aged general population.[25] The prevalence in DS is substantially higher. Forty percent of those over 50 years acquire an Alzheimer-type dementia with the typical neuropathologic features present in nearly everyone by the age of 40 years.[26] Dementia incidence over 50 is 18%,[27] indicating the very short survival once the condition is diagnosed. Despite similar neuropathologic features, clinical manifestation of dementia often differs in DS with frontal lobe symptoms, such as deficits in executive functioning characterized by planning problems, personality changes, and development of problem behaviors, being present at an early stage. It is natural to attribute any such changes to the onset of a dementing illness in DS because dementia is so common, but other conditions, even something as simple as constipation, may also present with similarly atypical symptoms. A full health assessment, paying attention to physical factors, is therefore necessary. Epilepsy is common in ID, including DS, and may signal the onset of dementia in older adults, and this may be especially the case for late-onset myoclonic epilepsy. People with more severe ID are at increased risk of seizures. Seizures are usually controllable with monotherapy. In other syndromes, seizures can be far more difficult to control.

Visual problems in DS may be associated with development; around 60% of children require glasses, for instance. People with DS have a flat nasal bridge and this can result in their glasses slipping. Strabismus is also common. In later life, cataracts are highly prevalent, nearly 30% in those aged 65 and older.[28] Hearing impairment is also common and, like visual impairment, may date from childhood. This may result from a buildup of earwax, but hearing aids are often needed for both conductive and sensorineural deficits.

GASTROINTESTINAL: DENTITION, GASTROESOPHAGEAL REFLUX, AND CONSTIPATION

Although not associated with either aging or mortality, gastrointestinal complaints are frequent in DS. In the general population, dental status is an index of socioeconomic status and so poor dentition may reflect this in DS where conventional socioeconomic measures are often unhelpful. It may also reflect both severity of ID, affecting oral hygiene, and age. Chronic gingivitis and especially periodontitis is highly prevalent in DS and is associated with cardiovascular disease, respiratory disease, and diabetes. Gingival hyperplasia is sometimes found in people who are taking phenytoin for epilepsy. Obesity is common in DS and is associated with gastroesophageal reflux disease (GERD) and cholelithiasis. A Dutch study of 77 adults with ID aged 60 years or over found 9% had GERD, 10% symptomatic cholelithiasis, and 57% had chronic constipation; the latter was far more common in those with mild ID compared to moderate or severe ID.[29] Only the minority of adults with GERD complained of typical symptoms; most presented with insomnia or behavioral changes.

ENDOCRINOLOGY: HYPOTHYROIDISM, TESTOSTERONE, AND ESTROGEN DEFICIENCY

Around one quarter of people with DS develop hypothyroidism, many in childhood or early adulthood. Other forms of endocrine failure are also more common. Women with DS are twice as likely to experience an early menopause as the general population[30] with a median age around 46 years. Those women who experience menopause earlier were also at increased risk of developing dementia at a younger age.[31] This may reflect some general biologic aging phenomenon or be associated with a specific lack of estrogen. It is unclear whether age at menopause relates to IQ, as is the situation in the general population.[32] Men with DS tend to have elevated follicle-stimulating hormone (FSH) and luteinizing hormone (LH) with low testosterone levels. There is a lack of trials of testosterone replacement therapy in men with DS, so it is unclear whether testing gonadal hormone levels is useful.

MUSCULOSKELETAL SYSTEM: ARTHRITIS, METABOLIC BONE DISEASE

Osteoarthritis is common in DS and, like other conditions, may be associated with obesity. Osteoporosis is also common and may, in part, relate to hypothyroidism and gonadal hormone failure. In people with ID, in general ages 40 to 60 years, and who were community residents, 21% had osteoporosis and 34% osteopenia.[33] People with DS appear to benefit from vitamin D and calcium treatment as much as the general population.[34]

DERMATOLOGY: ECZEMA, ACNE, AND DISEASES OF THE SCALP

Eczema, acne, and yeast-associated folliculitis are all common in DS. The latter may reflect some subtle deficiency of cellular immunity as also reflected by increased prevalence of fungal infections of the nails.[35] There is evidence of altered T-cell function, especially in older men with DS.[36] An immune etiology may also underpin the increased incidence of alopecia as suggested by the high prevalence of autoimmune thyroid disease. Adults with DS may have low neutrophil counts with a tendency of lymphocyte counts also to be on the low side.[35]

ASSESSMENT OF THE HEALTH OF OLDER ADULTS WITH ID

The preceding sections indicate that older people with ID have an increased disease load and usually suffer from multiple pathologies. Disease load increases with ID severity; hence it particularly affects those people with more communication problems. Partly for this reason, the disease often goes undetected. When assessing the health of someone with ID it is worth recalling the North Sydney experience where half of the major medical problems were unknown and of the half that were already known, half were inadequately managed.

The multidisciplinary setting of assessment

People with ID are usually at the center of a complex support system. It is usually worth taking time to elucidate this together with identifying all the health and social care professionals involved, as this often provides useful information. Typical professional contacts might include social work, clinical psychology, speech and language therapy, community nurses, psychiatrists with an interest in ID, occupational therapists, audiology services, community dentistry, and so on. In some countries, there may be a formal legal representative of the person with ID; for example, in Scotland a welfare guardian may have been appointed under the Adults with Incapacity Act. Although information gathering is important, such information may not always be reliable. For example, when 589 adults with ID were being discharged from a large Scottish institution, the nurses who had been looking after them thought 49% of the adults had perfect vision, whereas an actual ophthalmologic assessment showed that only 0.8% did.[37] Similarly, the nurses thought 74% of the adults had perfect hearing, whereas an audiologic assessment found this was the case for only 11%.

Brief physical health screening tools

A number of brief physical health screening tools have been developed. These are often designed to be administered by nurses. They are usually based on making medical diagnoses and are not designed to assess atypical presentation of disease. Wilson and Haire provided the prototype for this kind of assessment, largely by applying methods of examination used in the non-ID population, which, like other studies, noted the large number of health problems that had been undetected prior to screening.[38] These assessments were originally designed to detect threats to health. For example, routine physical examination of the chest is performed because respiratory infection is a major cause of death in people with intellectual disabilities.[39–41] However, even in the general population chest examination[42] has poor sensitivity and specificity. The same can be said for many aspects of routine physical examination, such as abdominal examination[43] and musculoskeletal examination.[44] In addition, older adults with ID do not always find conventional medical examinations easy to tolerate. It may be difficult to explain the relevance of various elements, such as chest percussion, and there may have been experiences of physical or sexual abuse, recall of which is cued by a physical examination. Screening tools are therefore best used to provide a checklist for information gathering as a background for fuller assessment.

User-led physical health assessments

One way to find a workable way to assess the health of older people with ID is to find out what they consider to be health and what kinds of assessment they find acceptable. The comprehensive health assessment program (CHAP) is one such example developed in Australia and validated by randomized control trial with its acceptability to participants assessed.[45,46] The CHAP is, itself, a development from the Cardiff health check that was also subject to a randomized controlled trial[47]; its validation is thus reassuring as to the validity of caregiver-answered items, because other assessments have found caregiver responses to be unreliable as noted previously. Although acceptable to people with ID, the CHAP was not designed to align with their particular priorities for health. This alignment is essential because at present people with ID feel that the partnership between them and their doctor is far from equal.[48] Moreover government policies are beginning to require this as, for example, NHS Scotland directives, which recommended attention to these "critical factors":

- Component parts of the health screen which must be relevant to the particular health needs of persons with learning disabilities (rather than the general population).
- The acceptability of the health screen to persons with learning disabilities and their caregivers.[49]

When older adults are asked about their understanding of health three key themes emerge:

1. Being able to do things and participate in activities
2. Nutrition
3. Hygiene/self-care[50]

Moreover, their concept of health is much closer to the World Health Organization's definition in that it incorporates aspects of well-being beyond the mere absence of disease.[51] Appropriate health assessments need to capture these positive aspects, therefore, by asking questions related to the key health themes in addition to the standard medical checklists designed to identify disease. Similarly, examination needs to incorporate measures germane to the health themes rather than merely aiming to identify disease. Unsurprisingly, adults with ID welcome such aspects of assessment,[50] and several have been validated in this population. Figure 58-1 provides a template user-led health assessment that includes independently validated items that are both generally acceptable and feasible.[52] In practice it takes an average of 20 to 30 minutes to complete, and this tends to be a little quicker in those with more severe ID who find some of the items very difficult (e.g., peak flow). Indeed, it is sensible to note the severity of ID in conjunction with the assessment and, where this is unknown, use the Swedish classification developed by Kylen (discussed earlier). The assessment provides a good baseline against which changes in health status can be assessed. To work out foot size to which shoe size can be compared, the chart in Table 58-4 can be used by measuring foot length (draw a line on a piece of paper at the heel and toes); allow one half size either way. It is not uncommon for older adults with ID to have shoes larger than their measured size because their feet are often disproportionately wide.

Medical information

Age ______ Sex ______ Cause of LD __________

Known medical problems

1 __________ 2 __________
3 __________ 4 __________
5 __________ 6 __________

Medication

1 __________ 2 __________
3 __________ 4 __________
5 __________ 6 __________

Allergies __________

Smoking __________ **Alcohol** __________

Residence and support __________

Hobbies/interests __________

Systems enquiry

Respiratory SOBOE Wheeze Cough ____

GI GORD symptoms Constipation Weight loss ____

Fecal incontinence never / occasional / frequent / always

GU urinary incontinence never / occasional / frequent / always

Menstruation Previous pregnancies ______

Trauma/falls in the last year __________

Vision

Recognizes parents, staff, etc.	Y/N
Recognizes shapes	Y/N
Names/matches colors	Y/N
Gets lost in house, street, etc.	Y/N
Can climb stairs, see curbstone	Y/N
Can walk in the dusk	Y/N
Recognizes houses, cars, etc. when moving	Y/N
Can find small object on patterned tablecloth	Y/N
Gazes at lights	Y/N
Is visual attention fleeting	Y/N

Sleep

Hours per night Wakes at night During day ____

Physical activity

Hours of moderate/severe per week __________

Socioeconomic

Number of pairs of outdoor shoes __________

Townsend disability scale

Are you able to... Score (0, no difficulty; 1 with difficulty; 2 unable)

1 Cut your own toenails? __________
2 Wash all over or bathe? __________
3 Get on a bus? __________
4 Go up and down stairs? __________
5 Do the heavy housework? __________
6 Shop and carry heavy bags? __________
7 Prepare and cook a hot meal? __________
8 Reach an overhead shelf? __________
9 Tie a good knot in a piece of string? __________

TOTAL __________

Physical assessment

Height cm Pubis-feet cm

Weight kg Waist cm Hip cm

Teeth Missing Decayed Filled

Vision Range of EOM's normal / abnormal

Funduscopy

Hearing (End expiratory whisper out of direct view 1m from ear)

Objects	Left	Right
Key		
Ball		
Pen		
Comb		
Bag		
Tape		

Otoscopy Normal / Abnormal

Cardiovascular

Pulse BP sitting BP standing

Heart sounds pp's edema

Respiratory

Cervical lymphadenopathy Thoracic kyphoscoliosis Yes / No

PEFR l/min

Neurological

Grip strength Sit / stands 20 secs

Resting tremor Yes / No Foot vibration sense Left Right

Feet Size Size of footwear

Nails in good condition

Figure 58-1. A template health user–led assessment for older adults with ID.

Table 58-4. Foot Size Chart Giving Various Sizes (United States, United Kingdom, Europe, Mondo Point Sizing) Depending on Foot Length (Biggest Foot with Sock On)

Inches	cm	Men	Women	United Kingdom	Europe	Mondo
8	20.3	2	3	1	33.0	21.3
8⅙	20.7	2½	3½	1½	33.6	21.7
8⅓	21.2	3	4	2	34.3	22.2
8½	21.6	3½	4½	2½	34.9	22.6
8⅔	22.0	4	5	3	35.5	23.0
8⅔	22.4	4½	5½	3½	36.2	23.4
9	22.9	5	6	4	36.8	23.9
9⅙	23.3	5½	6½	4½	37.5	24.3
9⅓	23.7	6	7	5	38.1	24.7
9½	24.1	6½	7½	5½	38.7	25.1
9⅔	24.6	7	8	6	39.4	25.6
9⅚	25.0	7½	8½	6½	40.0	26.0
10	25.4	8	9	7	40.6	26.4

Mental health assessment

Assessing mental health may fall to specialists in the psychiatry of ID. However, it is useful for physicians to be able to diagnose delirium and dementia in older adults with ID. The principles of diagnosing delirium in people with ID are no different from those in the general population. The ICD-10 diagnostic criteria are made up of the following: (1) impairment of consciousness and attention, (2) global disturbance of cognition, (3) psychomotor disturbance, (4) sleep/wake cycle disturbance, and (5) emotional disturbance. Generally the diagnosis applies to symptom duration of less than 6 months. The challenge is being able to make the diagnosis in people with severe or profound ID where there is usually a background disturbance of all five criteria. Here a fluctuating course can be a helpful indicator of the presence of delirium. Similarly, psychomotor disturbance, unexplained hypo- or hyperactivity is also a useful pointer. Emotional disturbance is likely to be expressed nonverbally by changes in behavior.

Similarly, the diagnosis of dementia in people with ID can also require considerable clinical skill. Often decline in function or change in behavior can be useful signs. Change in new learning ability and the presence of repetitive questioning can be helpful pointers in the history. The key diagnostic criterion is demonstrating cognitive decline from baseline, and this usually requires two detailed clinical psychology assessments. Several assessment tools are available; one that spans the general and ID population is the Severe Impairment Battery.[53] Having demonstrated cognitive decline, a hierarchical approach can be adopted to determine etiology.[25] This comprises considering (1) physical illness, (2) effects of medication, (3) sensory loss, (4) environmental change or life events, and (5) mental illness.[25] This is not to say that the diagnosis of dementia cannot be made in the presence of any of these five possible contributors to cognitive decline; indeed, not infrequently such potential contributors coexist with dementia. Nevertheless, it is generally worthwhile addressing reversible causes of cognitive decline (e.g., sensory loss) where possible. As noted earlier, behavioral changes may predate any clinically evident cognitive decline.

COMMUNICATION

The General Medical Council's *Tomorrow's Doctors*[54] lists 14 basic duties of a doctor, the first 8 of which are especially pertinent when caring for older adults with ID:

- Make the care of your patient your first concern.
- Treat every patient politely and considerately.
- Respect patients' dignity and privacy.
- Listen to patients and respect their views.
- Give patients information in a way they can understand.
- Respect the rights of patients to be fully involved in decisions about their care.
- Keep your professional knowledge and skills up to date.
- Recognize the limits of your professional competence.

Caregivers and other members of the multidisciplinary team, such as nurses and speech language therapists, can be particularly helpful if you feel you are reaching the limits of your own professional competence in communicating with people with ID. Most older adults with ID will lie in the mild end of the spectrum and thus be able to communicate verbally. It is important to take account of any sensory loss, which is common, and to provide an appropriate environment to facilitate communication. Plenty of time should be available. It is good practice to keep sentences short with just one idea per sentence and to use plain language. Conditional sentences are best avoided. It is also helpful to use concrete rather than abstract terms, supporting this with nonverbal aids whenever possible. If you are drawing a body part, remember to put this in context of the external human figure. Pictures of sunrises or beds may help with eliciting duration of symptoms. Just as with other communication, it is sensible to check what has been understood by asking people with ID to explain things in their own words. Various organizations produce easy-to-read information on common health topics, which can be helpful. For example, the Royal College of Psychiatrists has produced a "Books Beyond Words" series.

HEALTH PROMOTION

Health promotion is predicated on having appropriate health targets. Typically targets aim for equity with the non-ID population based on evidence for effective interventions[55] and cover these areas:

- Dental health
- Hearing and vision
- Nutrition and growth
- Prevention and treatment of chronic constipation
- Epilepsy review

- Thyroid screening
- Identification and treatment of mental health problems
- GERD and *H. pylori* eradication
- Osteoporosis
- Medication review
- Vaccination
- Provision of exercise opportunities
- Regular physical assessment and review
- Breast and cervical cancer screening

In addition to these general recommendations, there may be syndrome-specific actions to be considered. User-led concepts of health (functional ability and participation, nutrition, self-care, and hygiene) are likely to be useful in structuring health promotion for older adults with ID. Communication is key to good health promotion. For example, if a health promotion campaign endorses a negative stereotype of obesity, people with ID may identify with the stereotype and feel unhealthy as a consequence. It would be preferable to deliver a clear positive message about healthy eating and exercise instead. Perhaps the most important task of health promotion is to communicate with caregivers and any social or health care professionals involved in the care of an older adult with ID the importance of enhancing functional abilities, participation, and self-care.

KEY POINTS

The Older Adult with Intellectual Disability

- There is a rapid increase in the number of adults with intellectual disability surviving into old age.
- Diagnosis requires an IQ <70 together with both evidence of a developmental disorder and deficits in adaptive behavior.
- Severity of intellectual disability can be estimated according to verbal skills.
- Health status is influenced by the degree of intellectual severity and specific syndromic associations.
- Older adults with intellectual disability envisage health in terms of (1) being able to do things and participate in activities, (2) nutrition, (3) hygiene/self-care.
- User-led health assessments are feasible and relate closely to conventional health outcomes.
- Dementia is common in older adults with intellectual disability. Diagnosis is aided by a hierarchical approach considering (1) physical illness, (2) effects of medication, (3) sensory loss, (4) environmental change or life events, and (5) mental illness.

For a complete list of references, please visit online only at www.expertconsult.com

CHAPTER 59

Epilepsy

Khalid Hamandi

INTRODUCTION

Epilepsy is a common cause of morbidity and mortality. Epilepsy is not thought of as a disease of old age in the same way as cerebrovascular or neurodegenerative conditions, probably because of the presence of other comorbidities and complex etiologic factors and a less visible socioeconomic burden compared to adults of working age. Epilepsy in the elderly presents greater diagnostic difficulty than in the young. Management considerations include the presence of concomitant disease, altered drug handling, polypharmacy, social isolation, and lack of access to specialist investigation or treatment.

Epileptic seizures are typically brief and transitory. They cause disability because of the unpredictable nature of attacks, the risk of injury they bring, and the neurologic impairment from repeated seizures and adverse effects of treatment.[1] Driving is restricted, and there is social embarrassment, stigma, and impact on employment.[2–4] Fundamental questions regarding the neurobiology of epilepsy, reasons for its development, what makes a seizure start and stop, and the variable responses to treatments remain unanswered.

Epilepsy in the elderly needs special consideration.[5] The older person presenting with attacks that might be epilepsy can present a considerable clinical challenge.[6] Diagnosis rests on the history of events obtained from the patient and a reliable witness. There are rarely clinical signs that can be elicited in clinic to support the diagnosis, and tests can be normal or show nonspecific abnormalities that catch the unwary. The differential diagnosis of collapse or altered consciousness in the elderly is wide. A previous diagnosis of epilepsy made earlier in life, either as a child or an adult, should not be assumed to explain new or ongoing attacks and the term *known epileptic* should be avoided.

Older people with a diagnosis of epilepsy can be considered as falling into four groups:

1. Those with new onset seizures in late life
2. Those with an established diagnosis of epilepsy with seizures persisting or recurring in late life
3. Those with new onset attacks in late life that have been misdiagnosed as epilepsy
4. Those with an established diagnosis of epilepsy with new or ongoing attacks that are not due to epilepsy

DEFINITION

An epileptic seizure is the clinical manifestation of an abnormal synchronous neuronal discharge. Epilepsy is defined as a tendency to recurrent epileptic seizures. A diagnosis of epilepsy is not appropriate after a single event.[7] In the elderly, the likelihood of further seizures after a first is more likely as a result of a higher incidence of seizures resulting from a structural brain lesion.[8–10] The ability to predict the individual who will develop epilepsy after a first seizure still remains insufficient to warrant the label or treatment.

EPIDEMIOLOGY

Epilepsy is the third most common neurologic condition in old age after dementia and stroke.[11] The incidence is two to three times higher than that seen in childhood.[6] A community study, the United Kingdom General Practice Survey of Epilepsy and Epileptic Seizures, found that 24% of newly diagnosed cases of definite epilepsy occurred in patients over 60 years old.[9,12] A significant rise in incidence with increasing age has been confirmed by a number of studies, from an overall incidence of 50/100000 to 70 to 80 per 100,000 in the over 60s and 160 per 100,000 in the over 80s[13–18] (Figure 59-1). The prevalence of epilepsy is generally taken as between 5 and 10 cases per 1000 persons, with a lifetime prevalence of 2% to 5%.[19] Rates are dependent on case ascertainment and agreement on definitions used, for example, definite active epilepsy (ongoing seizures) versus those on treatment.[20]

In light of these figures, there would appear to be relative under provision in specialist care for the elderly with epilepsy, in research and in treatment trials. The reasons are unclear, whether they relate to a lesser perceived impact on lifestyle compared to younger patients with epilepsy or that associated or unrelated comorbidities leave epilepsy low down on a list of other medical conditions.[21]

CLASSIFICATION

Epilepsy classification is often thought of as complex and hard to follow. This need not be the case if the principles behind the classification are understood. The current classification of epilepsy was developed by the Commission on Classification and Terminology of the International League against Epilepsy (ILAE).

There are two parallel schemes, one for epileptic seizures[22] and another for epilepsy syndromes.[23]

There are a number of areas of confusion in classification encountered in the nonspecialist setting. Typically these arise from the use of outdated terminology or failing to distinguish between terms intended to describe seizure types and those intended to designate epilepsy syndromes or some etiologic substrate. Accurate syndromic classification helps direct treatment decisions and inform on prognosis. Classification is also important for epidemiologic studies and service needs assessments. Furthermore, rigorous attempts at classification benefit the whole diagnostic process and reduce or identify previous epilepsy misdiagnoses. A good understanding of epilepsy syndromes that present in childhood or early adult life remain useful when dealing with elderly patients in that seizures risk can persist throughout life, patients may carry a diagnostic label that may not be correct, and questions regarding the continuation of long-standing medication may be raised.

Epilepsy is not a specific disease but a heterogeneous group of disorders manifesting the neuroanatomic and pathophysiologic substrate causing the seizures.

The latest proposals from the ILAE suggest five parts or "axes," organized in a hierarchical fashion allowing the

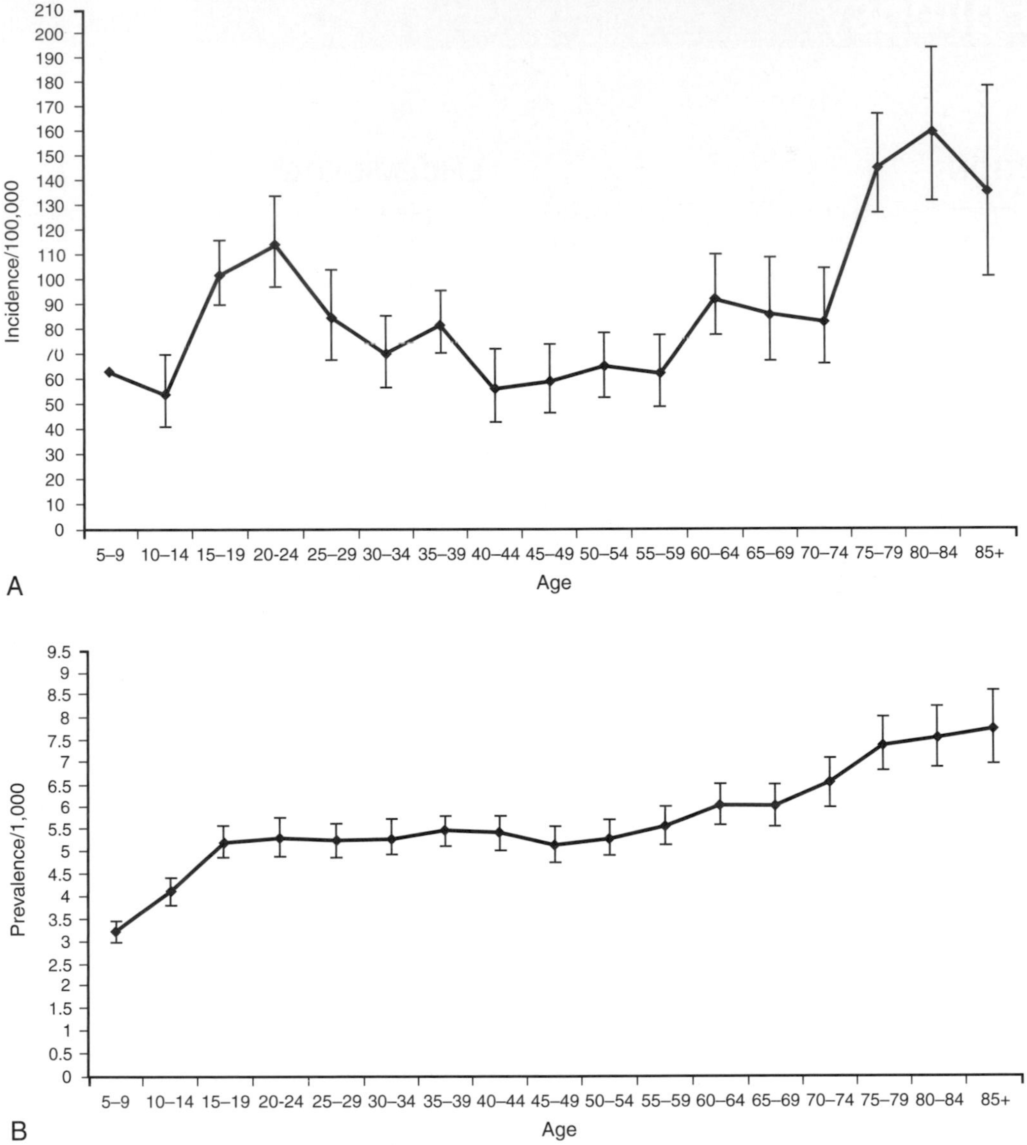

Figure 59-1. **A,** Age-specific incidence of treated epilepsy per 100,000 persons. **B,** Age-specific prevalence of treated epilepsy per 1000 persons. *(From Wallace H, Shorvon S, Tallis R. Age-specific incidence and prevalence rates of treated* epilepsy *in an unselected population of 2,052,922 and age-specific fertility rates of women with epilepsy. Lancet 1998;352:19–26, with permission.)*

integration of available and new information. The five axes are as follows:

Axis 1: Ictal phenomenology. Describing in detail the ictal event (Table 59-1).

Axis 2: Seizure type. Localization within the brain and precipitating stimuli for reflex seizures should be specified when appropriate.

Axis 3: Syndrome. With the understanding that a syndromic diagnosis may not always be possible.

Axis 4: Etiology. This includes a specific disease, genetic defects, or pathologic substrates causing seizures.

Axis 5: Impairment. This optional but often useful additional diagnostic parameter can be derived from an impairment classification adapted from the World Health Organization International Classification of Disease (WHO ICD10).

It remains to be seen whether this five axis scheme will be widely adopted and other axes have already been proposed.[24] The long-running debate of how best to classify epilepsy continues.[25]

Shortcomings of the classification scheme

Changing lists of descriptive entities inevitably cause confusion. A simplified system based on etiology rather than descriptive terminology is suggested by some, particularly with advances in imaging and genetics.[26] Perhaps the main shortcomings of the ILAE classification schemes are its poor dissemination among nonepilepsy specialist health care professionals. Revisions in the classification scheme and the

Table 59-1. ILAE Task Force Seizure Classification

Generalized Seizures
- Tonic-clonic seizures (includes variations beginning with a clonic or myoclonic phase)
- Clonic seizures
  - Without tonic features
  - With tonic features
- Typical absence seizures
- Atypical absence seizures
- Myoclonic absence seizures
- Tonic seizures
- Spasms
- Myoclonic seizures
- Massive bilateral myoclonus
- Eyelid myoclonia
  - Without absences
  - With absences
- Myoclonic atonic seizures
- Negative myoclonus
- Atonic seizures
- Reflex seizures in generalized epilepsy syndromes
- Seizures of the posterior neocortex
- Neocortical temporal lobe seizures

Focal Seizures
- Focal sensory seizures
  - With elementary sensory symptoms (e.g., occipital and parietal lobe seizures)
  - With experiential sensory symptoms (e.g., temporo parieto occipital junction seizures)
- Focal motor seizures
  - With elementary clonic motor signs
  - With asymmetrical tonic motor seizures (e.g., supplementary motor seizures)
  - With typical (temporal lobe) automatisms (e.g., mesial temporal lobe seizures)
  - With hyperkinetic automatisms
  - With focal negative myoclonus
  - With inhibitory motor seizures
- Gelastic seizures
- Hemiclonic seizures
- Secondary generalized seizures
- Reflex seizures in focal epilepsy syndromes

rationale behind them tend to be published in specialist journals and as such remain relatively inaccessible to the nonepilepsy specialist. Given that epilepsy is so commonly encountered, this is one area that should be addressed.

The terms *grand mal* and *petit mal* are still commonly heard. Although they may provide a vague reference to a seizure type, they give little indication of the true seizure semiology, the possible pathophysiology, or even a secure diagnosis. Patients may use the term *grand mal* to refer to either a complex partial seizure or a generalized tonic clonic seizure. Similarly, *petit mal* can be used to refer to any brief alteration of consciousness, without further appropriate history to attempt to define the event further.

Despite the shortcomings in epilepsy classification, those involved in the care of patients with epilepsy or episodes that might be attributed to epilepsy should familiarize themselves with the current scheme and in particular the principles behind it.

EPILEPTIC SEIZURES

The international classification of epileptic seizures (ICES) was developed by a panel of international experts examining video recordings of clinical and electroencephalographic seizures.[22] As such it is based on a consensus of opinions. Table 59-1 shows the current recommended classification of epileptic seizures. By design, the categories are descriptive. The first level of this system distinguishes between generalized seizures, a seizure whose initial semiology indicates, or is consistent with, involvement of entire cerebral hemispheres, and focal onset seizures, a seizure whose initial semiology indicates, or is consistent with, initial activation of only part of one cerebral hemisphere.

Generalized seizures

Generalized seizures are divided into absence, myoclonic, tonic, clonic, or tonic-clonic events. Absence seizures can be divided into typical absence and atypical absences. Typical absences are seen in idiopathic generalized epilepsy (discussed later). They occur in childhood onset syndromes but can persist into old age. Typical absence seizures of childhood used to be referred to as *petit mal*; however, this term should now be considered obsolete. They consist of an alteration of consciousness, occasionally there is associated eye flickering but other motor manifestations are rare; attacks are brief, usually less than 30 seconds. Characteristic electroencephalography (EEG) findings are of generalized spike wave discharges of 3 to 5 Hz. Myoclonic jerks are brief muscular jerks affecting limbs and less commonly trunk. The term *myoclonic jerk* comes under the heading of generalized seizures; however, myoclonic jerks do occur in focal epilepsy, affecting one limb or side; strictly following the ILAE scheme would classify these as focal motor seizures.

Focal seizures

Focal seizures are separated into motor, somatosensory or special sensory, autonomic, and psychic. The term *localization related*, previously proposed for focal seizures, is cumbersome and not widely adopted; the terms *focal* or *partial* remain in more common use. For the past few decades, focal seizures have been separated into simple partial seizures (consciousness is preserved, with maintained awareness) or complex partial seizures (consciousness is lost). The preservation or loss of consciousness is very relevant in the clinical setting, indicating a level of impairment caused by seizures. A seizure aura, often taken to be the warning before a seizure, is a simple partial seizure that may immediately precede a complex partial seizure or secondary generalization. Auras can occur in isolation (i.e., a simple partial seizure). Auras are typically short lived—over a few seconds to minutes but rarely longer.

TEMPORAL LOBE SEIZURES

Temporal lobe seizures are perhaps the most familiar of all focal seizure types. Seizures either arise from mesial temporal structures, part of the limbic system (e.g., the hippocampus), or from the temporal neocortex. Symptoms at onset include epigastric discomfort, "butterflies" or a rising sensation, abnormal taste, experiential phenomena such as déjà vu, and psychic features, fear, or euphoria; these symptoms are usually short lived of a few seconds to minutes and can occur in isolation without progression to loss of awareness of secondary generalization. Patients will often recall these initial symptoms as seizure auras. A complex partial seizure of temporal origin will typically manifest with orofacial automatism—lip smacking or repeated swallowing. This is an extremely useful piece of history from a witness and specific inquiry is helpful. In addition, there may be limb automatisms and typically there is dystonic posturing. Patients typically feel tired with the need to sleep after an attack.

FRONTAL LOBE SEIZURES

Frontal lobe seizures vary greatly because of the size of the frontal lobe and widespread functions it subserves. The semiology of frontal lobe seizures depends on the origin and spread of the epileptogenic focus.[27] The frontal lobe contains the primary motor cortex, supplementary motor cortex, prefrontal cortex, and limbic and paralimbic cortices.

In general, frontal lobe seizures manifest with prominent motor manifestations. There may be forced head version or forced eye deviation. Limb involvement can include tonic, clonic, or postural movements or bilateral vigorous motor automatisms—for example, bicycling. Sometimes bizarre motor movements are seen; occasionally patients can retain consciousness even with jerking in all four limbs; these features can lead to an incorrect diagnosis of nonepileptic seizures. A "Jacksonian march" refers to a march or spread of the focal motor seizure in a predictable and sequential manner from a distal limb to proximal areas or from leg to arm. The term *Todd paresis* refers to a transient hemiparesis that can last a day or more occurring after a secondary generalized focal motor seizure.

OCCIPITAL SEIZURES

Occipital onset seizures manifest as would be expected with visual phenomena. Typically these are vivid or formed hallucinations. They are distinct from migraine aura in that colors are vivid and they evolve over seconds rather than the several minutes of a migraine aura. They may involve flashing balls of light or revolving bright colors. Other manifestation include well-formed hallucinations, again these are short lived of seconds to minutes and may evolve to secondary generalized seizures.

PARIETAL SEIZURES

Parietal lobe seizures are rare. For a review see reference.[28] The parietal lobes are involved in the processing and integration of sensory and visual information. Stereotyped episodes that involve pain, numbness and tingling, heat, or pressure sensations suggest parietal lobe seizures.

EPILEPSY SYNDROMES

The international classification of epilepsy syndromes and epilepsies (ICEES)[23] supplements the ICES. Some epilepsy categories represent pure disease entities, whereas others represent a spectrum of clinical forms (e.g., idiopathic generalized epilepsy).

The dichotomy between generalized and focal is retained in the syndrome classification. The next classification level takes into account known or suspected etiology: symptomatic, with a known underlying cause; idiopathic, occurring without known underlying disease. Two further categories are recognized, one of epilepsies and epilepsy syndromes where categorization into focal or generalized is not possible because of a lack of clearly distinguishing features often the case with nocturnal seizures, and another for seizures associated with a specific situation, fever, drugs, and metabolic disturbance (i.e., provoked seizures).

Idiopathic generalized epilepsy

Idiopathic generalized epilepsy (IGE) is characterized by one or more of the following seizure types: typical absences, myoclonic jerks, and generalized tonic-clonic seizures (GTCS); interical and ictal generalized spike or polyspike; and wave on EEG. Further syndromic subclassification of IGE is made on the prevalence of the different seizure types and EEG features. Some propose the inclusion of age of onset and diurnal seizure patterns. The main subgroups seen in adults with epilepsy are as follows:

- Juvenile myoclonic epilepsy (JME)
- Juvenile absence epilepsy (JAE)
- Epilepsy with generalized tonic clonic seizures on awakening (EGTC)

It remains debated whether different clinical manifestations represent different ends of a biologic continuum or a group of distinct syndromes.[29] The typical onset age of onset of IGE is childhood or in early adult life; however, a later onset form is recognized;[30,31] and there are case reports of classical IGE presenting for the first time in the elderly.[32,33]

The term *idiopathic* refers to a disorder unto itself, *sui generis* (i.e., without other neurologic abnormality) and *not* etiology unknown. The risk of seizures in IGE usually continues into old age. A late presentation of absence status in four patients over age 60 with a prior diagnosis of IGE and absence seizures that resolved in their second decade has been reported.[34] Response to appropriate antiepileptic drug treatment is good in most, but not all. One study of epilepsy patients with IGE over age 60 found a small subgroup who experience an exacerbation of seizures in old age.[35]

Idiopathic focal epilepsy

The idiopathic focal epilepsies are restricted to childhood and rarely if at all persist into adult life. They are mentioned here for completeness. They are typically benign. It would be highly unusual and probably indicate an incorrect diagnosis if seizures persist into late life.

Symptomatic epilepsy

Focal symptomatic epilepsy is the predominant cause of new onset seizures in the elderly.[21,36] Symptomatic epilepsy means a cause is known. In the absence of an imaging abnormality, a history of prior brain injury—for example, from intracranial infection (meningitis or encephalitis) or trauma—can be sufficient to attribute a cause to new onset seizures. The term *remote symptomatic* is used for patients developing seizures some years after a significant brain injury, in contrast to acute symptomatic, where epilepsy is a presentation of new brain dysfunction.

Probably symptomatic (cryptogenic) epilepsy

The term *cryptogenic* was used to classify those with epilepsy of unknown etiology. The ILAE now recommends the term *probably symptomatic*. With advances in brain imaging, the proportion of patients in this group is falling. Younger adults with normal magnetic resonance imaging (MRI) and refractory epilepsy remain a significant health burden. In the elderly, the likelihood of MRI abnormalities is high, particularly leukoaraiosis.[37] The relationship of such abnormalities to epilepsy and why some develop seizures and other not remains unclear.[38]

MAKING THE DIAGNOSIS

Epilepsy can present with disparate manifestations. Similarly, a number of other conditions present with features that may be mistaken for epileptic seizures. The key feature in epilepsy is that episodes are typically stereotyped, unchanged over a long period of time, and usually short lived. The following episodic manifestations occurring in isolation or in combination can be caused by epilepsy:

- Loss of awareness or consciousness
- Generalized convulsive movements
- Drop attacks
- Focal movements—jerks, posturing, semipurposeful movements, rarely thrashing, bicycling or motor agitation
- Sensory episodes—tingling, pain, burning
- Vocalization—formed speech, incomprehensible words, screams, or laughter
- Psychic experiences
- Episodic phenomena from sleep
- Prolonged confusion or fugue state

The importance of a careful history in making a diagnosis of epilepsy cannot be overstated. This should include a description of events from the patient and crucially a first-hand witness description. Overreliance on a secondhand statement of "it looked like a fit" is likely to lead to misdiagnoses. There is no single test to make a diagnosis of epilepsy, and time taken by an experienced clinician in taking a careful history cannot be circumvented. In each case, an account of the circumstances, time of day, situation, prodrome or warning, detailed account the attack, its semiology and duration, the rate and nature of recovery, and associated symptoms or signs—for example, headache or confusion—are needed.

Direct questions about the attack itself and other previous attacks are helpful but care should be taken not to lead the history, and these questions are best left until the patient and witness have given a free account of the event or events in question. Useful features that are worth inquiring about directly if not first offered include head or eye deviation, the nature of limb movements, posturing, jerks, or automatisms, and whether movements are rhythmic or synchronous and how they evolve over time. Asking a witness about repeated swallowing or lip smacking can be revealing. Any changes of color, breathing pattern, or sweating need to be ascertained along with an account of the recovery period, its duration, and any subsequent symptoms such as headache, confusion, or altered behavior. It is always useful to ask about possible prior attacks that the patient may not associate with the current event—for example, a patient presenting after his or her first generalized tonic clonic seizure may not make the link between previously experienced simple partial seizures. Classically tongue biting and incontinence were thought to strongly indicate an epileptic seizure. This is not always the case. Urinary incontinence can occur during syncope. Injury to the tip of the tongue can occur in syncope, although if the sides of the tongue or inner cheek are severely bitten then this usually indicates that a generalized tonic clonic seizure has taken place.[39]

The past medical history should include inquiries about previous history of head injury or intracranial infection, and cardiac history. Family history, medication history, and social history are important as in any other presentation. Specific inquiry should go into living arrangements, driving, occupation, and hobbies or pastimes.

DIFFERENTIAL DIAGNOSIS

The two main differential diagnoses of epileptic seizures to consider are syncope and psychogenic or nonepileptic attacks. Manifestations of both epileptic seizures and syncope may differ in the elderly compared to the young, making diagnosis difficult or increasing misdiagnosis. Other more rare conditions leading to blackouts or altered consciousness to consider are hypoglycemia, other metabolic disorders, structural abnormalities at the skull base affecting the brain stem, and lesions affecting cerebrospinal fluid circulation. Transient cerebral ischemia or transient ischemic attacks (TIAs) are usually easily separated from epileptic events by their frequency and time course. They rarely present with loss of consciousness, and TIAs are typically less frequent and do not remain stereotyped over long periods of time. One exception are focal "seizures" affecting the hand seen in critical cortical ischemia; this is described in more detail later in this chapter.

Syncope

Syncope is the most common cause of episodes of loss of awareness. Syncope is covered in greater detail in Chapter 46. Aspects of an attack should not be taken in isolation and given undue emphasis, as elements of epileptic seizures can occur in syncope. Key features of syncopal episodes versus epileptic seizures are the precipitating factors, warning symptoms, a brief loss of consciousness, and rapid recovery, although there can be greater variation in older people (see Table 59-2). Features that may mimic seizures include head turning, automatisms and urinary incontinence, and relatively minor tongue biting.[40] Injury can occur from a syncopal fall, although this is less common as people tend to crumple to the floor rather than experience the stiff fall of an epileptic seizure.

In cardiac syncope, attacks occur without warning; there is abrupt unprovoked collapse with brief unconsciousness and rapid recovery. The attacks are not situational, and there is less often a prodrome than in vasovagal syncope. Cardiac syncope should be strongly suspected in those with a history of structural heart disease, previous myocardial infarction, rheumatic fever, or heart murmur.

Psychogenic attacks

Episodes that outwardly appear similar to epileptic seizures but are not caused by ictal electrical discharges in the brain are referred to by a number of terms: nonepileptic attacks (NEA), nonepileptic seizure (NES), psychogenic nonepileptic attacks or seizures (PNEA) or (PNES), or the less favored pseudoseizures.[41] The prevalence of PNEA appears less in the elderly, although no studies have looked at ascertainment or reporting bias. In a study of video-EEG monitoring in the elderly (>60), PNEA was diagnosed in 10 of 34 patients who had recoded events during the monitoring period;[42] this series came from 71 patients over 60 years of age who had

Table 59-2. Features that Help Distinguish Syncope from Epileptic Seizures

	USUAL DIFFERENCE		
Features	**Faints**	**Fits**	**Modification in Older Patients**
Posture	Usually occur in the upright position	Not position dependent	Faints in older people are not always position dependent because they are often the result of significant, position-independent pathology
Onset	Gradual	Sudden	Loss of consciousness may be quite abrupt in syncope in an older person; complex partial seizures may have a gradual onset
Injury	Rare	More common	A syncopal attack may be associated with significant soft tissue or bony injury in an older person
Incontinence	Rare	Common	An individual prone to incontinence may be wet during a faint; partial seizures will not usually be associated with incontinence
Recovery	Rapid	Slow	A fit may take the form of a brief (temporal lobe) absence; a faint associated with a serious arrhythmia may be prolonged
Postevent confusion	Little	Marked	A prolonged hypoxic episode as the result of a faint may be associated with prolonged postevent confusion
Frequency	Usually infrequent with a clear precipitating cause	May be frequent and usually without precipitating cause	Faints associated with cardiac arrhythmias, low cardiac output, postural hypotension, or carotid sinus sensitivity may be frequent

undergone video EEG monitoring out of a total of 440 over a 7-year period. Another study[43] found a diagnosis of PNEA was made 7 of 16 patients over 60 years of age undergoing video-EEG monitoring, this from a total of 834 admitted for long-term video-EEG monitoring. Further study of long-term video EEG monitoring over an 8-year period identified 39 patients over the age of 60 who were admitted for evaluation, 13 of whom were diagnosed with PNEA on the basis of video EEG.[44] Nevertheless PNEA remains an important differential diagnosis in the elderly, particularly when apparent medically refractory epilepsy is encountered.[45]

PNEA probably arises as a result of patients responding to psychosocial stress with unexplained somatic symptoms that come to medical attention,[46] and PNEA is associated with a number of distinct pathologic personality profiles that could be used to tailor therapy.[47] Somatoform disorders, anxiety disorders, mood disorders, and reinforced behavior pattern are all features associated with PNEA. In one study, a subgroup of elderly patients were described who had PNEA that presented over the age of 55; they were more likely to be male and more likely to have a history of traumatic experience related to ill health.[48] Suspicion of PNEA should be raised where there are unusual features to attacks, associated physical or mental ill health, adverse social circumstances, or bereavement before presentation. Confidently securing a diagnosis of PNEA usually requires long-term video-EEG monitoring, an investigation that would appear to be of limited access to the elderly population in most centers.

The Cochrane database review in 2007 found insufficient evidence to recommend specific treatments for PNEA and stressed the need for randomized trials to assess treatment interventions.[49] One of the first aims of treatment once a diagnosis is made should be to reduce unnecessary medical interventions or hospital admissions.

Transient epileptic amnesia

Transient epileptic amnesia (TEA) has been used to describe recurrent episodes of transient amnesia in the absence of overt seizures.[50] TEA needs to be distinguished from transient global amnesia (TGA) (discussed later). In TEA, there is evidence for a diagnosis of epilepsy based on one or more of EEG abnormalities, co-occurrence of other clinical features of epilepsy (for example, automatisms or olfactory hallucinations), and clear-cut response to antiepileptic medications.[51] Other features include interictal memory disturbance manifest by accelerated forgetting, remote autobiographic amnesia (i.e., patients demonstrate a patchy but dense loss of memories for important personal events from the remote past), and topographical amnesia (i.e., patients have difficulty navigating their way around new or familiar routes).[52,53] It is not clear whether episodes of TEA represent ongoing ictal activity or a postictal phenomenon. Whether TEA is a sufficient diagnostic entity to be regarded as a distinct syndrome[50] or another manifestation of temporal lobe seizures in the elderly remains to be seen.

Transient global amnesia

Transient global amnesia (TGA) is a condition of transient loss of memory function that has been described for over 40 years.[54,55] It is most common in middle to late life. Episodes of TGA have a characteristic presentation. There is usually, but not always, a history of provoking factors; these can include one or more of the following: vigorous exercise, acute emotional stress, or change in temperature. During an attack, patients appear mildly agitated and repeatedly question or engage in searching behavior. Attacks typically last several hours, but less than 24 hours. During an attack, patients retain self-awareness and long-term memory and can perform familiar task or navigate a familiar environment but appear unable to lay down any new memories and appear amnesic of all recent events during the attack. Once an attack is over, patients regain some memory around the event but remain amnesic for the central period of the episode. Attacks are usually isolated, but there is a 6% recurrence rate. The clinical presentation is usually so characteristic that once seen it is not easily mistaken for epilepsy. There is no evidence to support an epileptic etiology or transient arterial ischemic events.[56] A popular hypothesis is that of venous congestion in bilateral temporal lobes as a result of internal jugular vein valve insufficiency and sudden rises in intrathoracic pressure.[57]

If attacks are recurrent, have associated features (e.g., automatisms), and symptoms of memory impairment outside an attack, the diagnosis of transient epileptic amnesia should be considered.

Psychogenic amnesia

Psychogenic amnesia or dissociative fugue is rare and typically triggered by stressful or adverse life events. Careful clinical evaluation may reveal inconsistencies in the presentation that alert the practitioner to a conversion disorder. Features include extensive loss of autobiographic memories, including self-identity, in the context of preserved new learning and absence of repetitive questioning, and the ability to continue normal activities of daily living.

Parasomnias

Parasomnias are disorders that manifest around or during sleep. They are sometimes mistaken for epileptic seizures. The classification of parasomnias is changing as new information emerges.[58] They include REM parasomnias and periodic limb movements. An accurate history is usually sufficient to distinguish these form epilepsy, and occasionally video monitoring can be helpful.

Transient ischemic attacks

TIA symptoms tend to be negative (i.e., a loss of function). Epileptic seizures invariably produce positive symptoms. One rare exception is that of apparent focal motor seizures caused by critical cortical ischemia from carotid artery stenosis, or shaking limb TIA (SLTIA) (Figure 59-2). First described in 1962,[59] a handful of cases of SLTIA are reported in the literature.[60–62] Events involve shaking of usually the upper limb that does not spread to the face. Episodes can be short lived or prolonged. They are typically provoked by maneuvers that appear to decrease cerebral perfusion, such as rising from a bed or a chair, or hyperextending the neck. Shaking does not respond to antiepileptic medication or benzodiazepines. The EEG during attacks is normal. The abnormal movements respond to measures that restore adequate cerebral perfusion (i.e., carotid endarterectomy or correcting relative hypotension). Single photon emission tomography studies (SPECT) support the hypothesis that SLTIAs are due to hypoperfusion rather than recurrent thromboembolic events.[63]

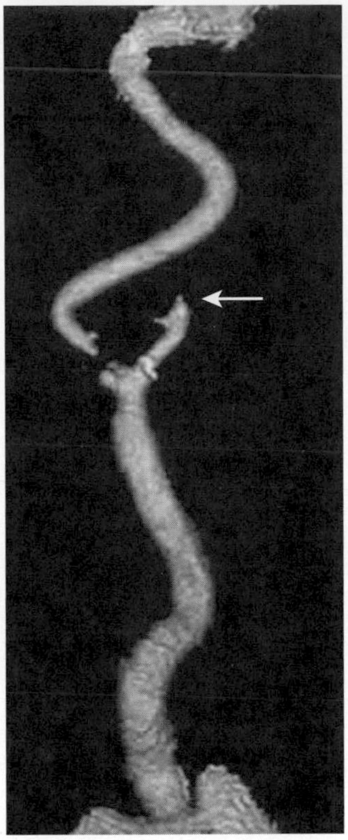

Figure 59-2. A CT angiogram in a 79-year-old patient with recurrent episodes of right arm shaking, worse on standing; shows occlusion of the left internal carotid artery.

OTHER CONSIDERATIONS

Convulsive status epilepticus

Convulsive status epilepticus (CSE) is defined as ≥30 minutes of either continuous seizure activity or consecutive seizures without regaining consciousness between them. CSE has a bimodal distribution with highest rates in infants and the elderly. It is associated with a significant morbidity and mortality. Increasing age and underlying etiology are predictors of higher mortality.[64–66] Acute or remote stroke is a common cause of status epilepticus (SE) in the elderly.[67,68]

CSE is a medical emergency. Treatment algorithms for CSE are the same for the elderly as for younger adults.[69] There may be local variation on treatment algorithms, but general principles are similar. Those treating medical patients in the acute setting should familiarize themselves with local guidelines. Initially, general resuscitation measures are required; drug treatment should start as soon as the diagnosis is suspected with intravenous benzodiazepines; care should be taken to avoid respiratory depression, particularly in the elderly. If there is no response to intravenous benzodiazepines, the next drug of choice is usually phenytoin, given as an infusion, with an initial loading dose. If there is a failure to respond to phenytoin, sedation with an anesthetic agent is necessary. Concurrent EEG monitoring is essential, in conjunction with a search for an underlying cause. Sedation is usually maintained for at least 24 hours while therapeutic levels of an anticonvulsant are instigated.

Nonconvulsive status epilepticus

Nonconvulsive status epilepticus (NCSE) is relatively common, making up a third of all cases with SE. It increases in incidence with age.[70] In the elderly it also more difficult to diagnose, presenting as an acute or subacute prolonged confusional state. The presentation can be subtle. A high index of suspicion is required, and EEG essential to make the diagnosis.[71] In the absence of coma, aggressive treatment should be avoided. A prospective study of 25 elderly patients with NCSE found that treatment with intravenous benzodiazepines was associated with an increased risk of death, and admission to the intensive care unit prolonged hospital stays without improving the outcome.[72] NCSE should be considered in those who suffer neurologic deterioration after a stroke or subarachnoid hemorrhage.[73,74] NCSE is an EEG diagnosis. EEG criteria for NCSE continue to be developed.[75]

Sudden unexplained death in epilepsy (SUDEP)

Sudden unexplained death in epilepsy (SUDEP) is a term used when sudden death occurs in someone with epilepsy with no obvious cause of death found at postmortem.[76] It accounts for 7% to 17% of epilepsy deaths.[77] It seems likely that either cardiac or respiratory arrest in the context of a generalized tonic clonic seizure causes SUDEP, with the etiology being patient and seizure dependent.[77]

Risk factors for SUDEP include the presence of generalized tonic clonic seizures, being alone in bed during a seizure, severe epilepsy, structural brain lesion, and younger onset of epilepsy and young age.[78] Reporting bias might explain the last two factors. Sudden death in the elderly is not necessarily an unusual occurrence. By definition SUDEP requires that no other cause of death is found at postmortem. Attributing sudden death in the elderly to SUDEP is unlikely in the presence of other comorbidities, whereas sudden death in the otherwise healthy young with epilepsy is a matter that generates the fullest investigation. It is not known whether the same mechanisms for SUDEP operate across all age groups, with the elderly equally susceptible, or that the elderly are somehow immune from this condition. How to measure its occurrence in the elderly may prove difficult.

ETIOLOGY

Cerebrovascular disease

Cerebrovascular disease is the most common cause for epilepsy in the elderly;[79] it accounts for 30% to 50% of epilepsy cases in the elderly[36] and 75% of symptomatic epilepsies. Poststroke seizures and epilepsy are considered as early, occurring within 2 weeks of stroke, or late, occurring after 2 weeks. A large study of 6044 hospital admissions with acute stroke found 3.1% had epileptic seizures within 24 hours of the stroke and 8.4% had seizures within the first 24 hours after subarachnoid hemorrhage (SAH) or intracerebral hemorrhage (ICH).[80] In the United Kingdom national general practice study of epilepsy and epileptic seizures (NGPSE), the standard mortality ratio was highest for those with epilepsy and cerebrovascular disease.[81]

Cortical involvement of infarct is predilection for developing seizures, and there may be an association with the site of infarction and development of epilepsy.[82] In a large multicenter study, a worse outcome and increased in-hospital complication rate was associated with prophylactic antiepileptic drug use after SAH.[83] Patients who suffer status epilepticus (SE) of cerebrovascular etiology were found to have twice the risk of death at 6 months than patients with stroke and not SE,[84] although the independent effect of SE on mortality after stroke is controversial.[85]

Cerebral tumors

The elderly patient with new onset seizures should have cerebral imaging to exclude a structural cause (see Figure 59-3). Benign tumors (e.g., meningiomas) can also present with epilepsy. Surgery for these tumors depends on their location and the age of the patient. Typically, meningiomas are indolent; however, they can be slow growing and there is a small risk of malignant transformation of benign meningiomas that favors surgery in younger patients with peripheral lesions. Epilepsy from malignant tumors is rarely seen in the specialist setting, although seizures can be particularly refractory to treatment.

Neurodegenerative disease

Alzheimer's disease is associated with a six-fold increase in unprovoked seizures.[86] The history of seizures in these cases invariably needs to be form the caregiver. A further study found that 21% of a patients developed seizures after a diagnosis of dementia of Alzheimer type.[87]

Other causes

Any structural, inflammatory, immune, or vascular intracerebral process can lead to epileptic seizures. Other causes include trauma; intracranial infection, in particular herpes simplex encephalitis and pneumococcal meningitis; subdural hematoma, paraneoplastic syndromes; limbic encephalitis; and malformations of cortical development (see Figure 59-3).

Provoked seizures

One or even more provoked seizures do not require a diagnosis of epilepsy. Provoked seizures can be caused by metabolic or toxic disturbance. It is important to recognize provoked seizures, as these typically do not warrant treatment with antiepileptic drugs and driving eligibility may vary.

INVESTIGATION

In the elderly, routine hematology, biochemistry, plasma glucose, calcium, and liver function should be checked. The mainstay of investigation includes the ECG, EEG, and neuroimaging. Particular attention should be paid to the effect of "normal" aging on brain imaging and neurophysiology. This includes atrophy on computed tomography (CT), atrophy and nonspecific white matter change on MRI, and EEG slowing.

Electrocardiography

Electrocardiography (ECG) is a simple, quick, inexpensive, and noninvasive test. It should be performed in all patients presenting for the first time with an episode of loss of consciousness, even if the history is strongly suggestive of an epileptic seizure The ECG should be examined in detail for evidence of conduction abnormalities.[88] More advanced investigation for cardiac or vasovagal syncope should also be considered depending on the history (see Chapter 46).

Electroencephalography

The EEG should be used judiciously. It is a primary tool in the investigation of epilepsy. Nevertheless, the diagnosis of epilepsy remains a clinical one with EEG playing a supporting role. It is not appropriate as a screening tool or means of excluding epilepsy in those with suspected syncope.[89] The indiscriminate use of the EEG and its reporting and can lead to an overdiagnosis of epilepsy.[90] The interpretation of EEG requires a skilled neurophysiologist. Nonspecific findings can catch the unwary (Figure 59-4). The gold standard for classifying seizure is simultaneous video-EEG monitoring. Facilities for this monitoring are rarely available in the elderly care setting.

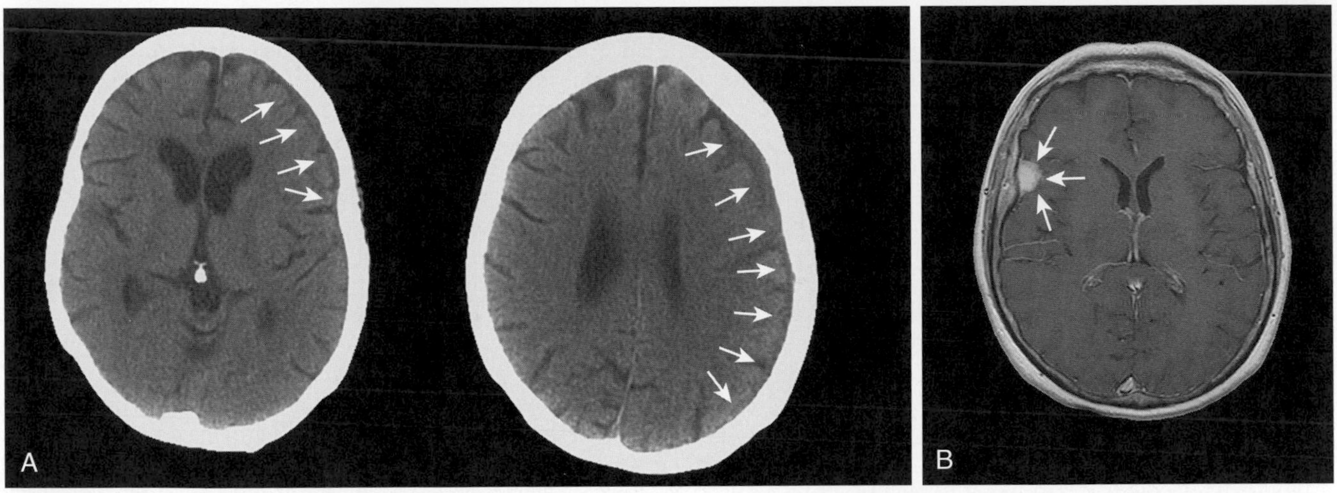

Figure 59-3. Causes of epilepsy. **A,** CT head showing a subdural hematoma in a 68-year-old woman presenting with focal motor seizures affecting her left hand. **B,** Gadolinium enhanced T1-weighted axial MRI showing right temporal meningioma presenting with simple partial seizures in a 60-year-old woman.

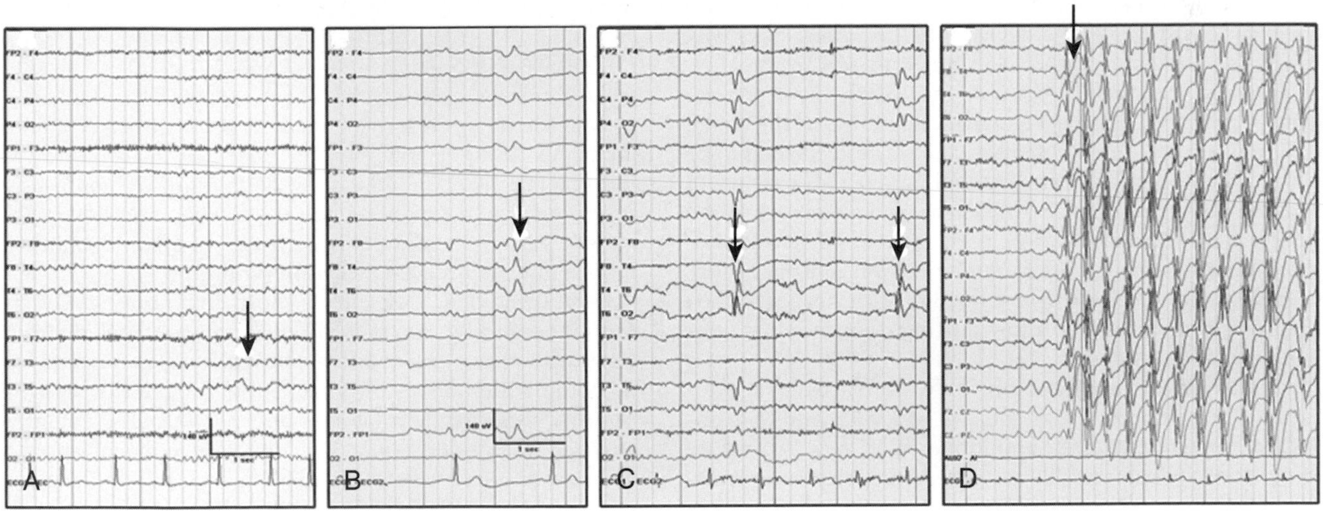

Figure 59-4, EEG features. **A,** Left temporal slow activity, a nonspecific feature. **B,** Right temporal sharp waves in 78-year-old man supporting a diagnosis of complex partial seizures. **C,** Focal spikes in a teenager with Benign epilepsy with centrotemporal spikes. **D,** Generalized spike wave activity in a young adult with IGE, an unequivocal "epileptiform" discharge.

Long-term video-EEG is useful tool in the investigation of epilepsy in all ages.[91–94] It is primarily used for the following indications:

- Diagnostic clarification of epilepsy versus nonepileptic attacks
- Localization of seizure onset (of practical utility only in younger patients being considered for epilepsy surgery)
- Determination of seizure frequency in suspected partial or nocturnal seizures

It is notable that in published series on the utility of video-EEG on the elderly from large epilepsy centers, patients over the age of 60 make up only 2% to 17% of adult admissions to the monitoring units.[92–95]

Neuroimaging

The two standard neuroimaging modalities used in epilepsy are computerized tomography (CT) and magnetic resonance imaging (MRI). All cases of new onset seizures in adults should have brain imaging to exclude a structural lesion. The choice of CT or MRI rests on the cost and practicalities of each technique versus the expected yield leading to a change in management.

CT involves the reconstruction of X-rays taken in multiple planes to produce an image, and as such involves a radiation dose. Modern CT scanners are quick and brain images are acquired within a matter of minutes. The CT bore is relatively open and only the head needs enter. CT is therefore most appropriate in the acute or emergency setting, particularly if the patient is unwell and needs close monitoring, and for patients with claustrophobia or who have difficulty lying flat. CT is superior to MRI for identifying intracranial hemorrhage and for identifying areas of calcification. MRI involves the subject lying in a strong magnetic field with superimposed time-varying magnetic field gradients. It takes longer to administer an MRI than a CT, typically 10 to 20 minutes for a full series of brain images. The subject needs to lie still for the duration of the scan as images are degraded by even a small amount of motion. The scanner bore is relatively narrow and long; patients enter the bore head first, and it covers most of the patient's body. Patients with claustrophobia or those unable to lie flat will not tolerate MRI. The advantage of MRI over CT is its much higher image resolution and tissue contrast, hence the ability to detect subtle abnormalities that might cause epilepsy; this is perhaps of more relevance in young adults with medically refractory seizures being considered for epilepsy surgery. Surgical resection of a benign lesion to treat epilepsy is rarely advantageous in the elderly, and the pursuit of subtle benign lesions causing epilepsy is unlikely to alter management in the elderly.

ANTIEPILEPTIC DRUG THERAPY

To the nonspecialist, there can be a bewildering array of new drugs to treat epilepsy. Twelve antiepileptic drugs (AEDs) have been developed and licensed worldwide since 1989. By convention, drugs that were available before this time are known as standard AEDs and those that became available after 1990 are called new AEDs. A number of further AEDs are in various stages of the development pipeline, some well advanced in phase 3 trials[96] and likely to add to the ever-growing list. Studies of AEDs in the elderly, however, are scant,[36] and those that exist tend to concentrate on the young elderly (aged 65 to 74).[97] Benefits and side effects tend to be extrapolated from studies in younger patients. Key points to consider when prescribing AEDs in the elderly are increased risk of side effects; drug-drug interactions; and altered protein binding, hepatic metabolism, and renal clearance; also, a careful review of already prescribed drugs is needed. When commencing a new AED, a low starting dose and slow titration are recommended.

Standard AEDs are acetazolamide, carbamazepine, clobazam, clonazepam, ethosuximide, valproic acid, phenobarbital, phenytoin, and primidone. The new AEDs are gabapentin, felbamate, lamotrigine, levetiracetam, oxcarbazepine, pregabalin, rufinamide, tiagabine, topiramate, vigabatrin, and zonisamide. Of these, felbamate and vigabatrin should not be used because of the risk of severe adverse effects, namely, potentially fatal liver failure or aplastic anamia with felbamate and retinal damage with irreversible visual field constriction with vigabatrin. These adverse effects were not recognized until a few years following the drugs' widespread use and highlight the need for postmarketing surveillance and adverse reaction reporting in all new drugs. Standard and new AEDs commonly used in adults are summarized in Table 59-3.

The currently recommended first-line AEDs are valproic acid for generalized epilepsy and carbamazepine or lamotrigine for focal epilepsy. For many elderly patients, phenytoin still forms the mainstay of treatment.[98,99] Some elderly patients with lifelong epilepsy may still be taking phenobarbital or primidone; it is not appropriate to change these for newer AEDs in patients who are stable.

The new AEDs are typically licensed as add-on therapy after randomized trials against placebo. Direct head-to-head comparisons of standard and new AEDs are lacking. Recent efforts to address this imbalance include the U.K. study of the Standard and New Antiepileptic drugs (SANAD) study, comparing sodium valproate against new AEDs in generalized seizures and carbamazepine against new AEDs in focal epilepsies. Valproic acid was found to be most effective in IGE,[100] whereas lamotrigine was favored over carbamazepine for focal epilepsies.[101] The trial did not include a number of later but now important AEDs—levetiracetam, zonisamide, and pregabalin—and further ongoing studies are needed.

A large multicenter study comparing lamotrigine, gabapentin, and carbamazepine in 593 elderly patients with newly diagnosed epilepsy found lower adverse events in those randomized to lamotrigine or gabapentin compared to carbamazepine, without significant difference in seizure-free rates at 12 months.[102] A subsequent study comparing lamotrigine and sustained release carbamazepine in 185 patients over the age of 65 did not find a significant difference between lamotrigine and carbamazepine, but there was a trend toward greater efficacy with carbamazepine and lower adverse effects with lamotrigine.[103] A smaller study found similar efficacy but better tolerability of lamotrigine over carbamazepine in poststroke epilepsy,[104] and another study found switching to lamotrigine was associated with an improvement on the side-effect profile.[105]

Adverse effects

All AEDs have side effects. These can be dose dependent or idiosyncratic. Dose-dependent side effects can be minimized by using a low starting dose with slow titration. Idiosyncratic side effects cannot be minimized, and usually necessitate rapid drug withdrawal. Idiosyncratic side effects include rash, blood dyscrasias, bone marrow impairment, liver failure, and Stevens-Johnson syndrome.

Dose-dependent side effects most commonly affect the central nervous system (CNS). They typically include dizziness; drowsiness; lack of energy or weakness; unsteadiness or incoordination; mood disturbance that includes depression, hostility, anger and irritability, and nervousness; cognitive effects that include confusion, difficulty concentrating or paying attention, abnormal thinking, speech or language problems; and difficulty falling asleep or staying asleep. Gastrointestinal side effects include nausea, abdominal pain, and diarrhea. Side effects can include frequency or urgency of micturition and effects on sexual function. Dose-dependent side effects are typically worsened by polytherapy,[106] and the lowest dose of AED that controls seizures should be the aim. Taking more than three AEDs in combination is rarely helpful, and those on several AEDs should have medication rationalized as best as possible.

Patients should be cautioned specifically regarding common or potentially serious side effects (see Table 59-3). It is helpful if patients have a rapid access point or contact number for advice should side effects develop so that drugs are not either stopped suddenly or continued with potentially harmful consequences. Some side effects occur when starting or raising the dose of an AED, but these wear off after a few days. Recurrent or unpleasant side effects need to be identified and addressed early.

Long-term adverse effects include osteoporosis. Osteoporosis is more common in women taking AEDs. Measuring calcium and vitamin D levels in women taking enzyme-inducing AEDs every 2 to 5 years and bone densitometry can be used to assess the risk of osteoporosis. Vitamin D and calcium supplementation can be taken in an attempt to correct any deficiencies. Bone fracture rates in epilepsy are two

Table 59-3. Main Antiepileptic Drugs Used for Epilepsy in the Elderly and Their Key Features

	Putative Mode of Action	Metabolism and Kinetics	Usual Starting and (Daily Maintenance Dose)	Adverse Events	Key Points
Carbamazepine* (1963)	Sodium channel inhibition	Hepatic metabolism; active metabolite	100–200 mg (400–1800 mg)	Idiosyncratic rash	First line for focal seizures can worsen MJ and absences in IGE Wide drug interaction including warfarin and other AEDs
Clobazam	GABA augmentation	Hepatic metabolism; active metabolite	10 mg (10–30 mg)	Rarely idiosyncratic rash	More commonly used as short-term adjunct
Clonazepam	GABA augmentation	Hepatic metabolism	0·5 mg (1–6 mg)	Rarely idiosyncratic rash	More commonly used as short term adjunct
Gabapentin (1993)	Calcium channel modulation	Not metabolized, urinary excretion unchanged	300 mg (1800–3600 mg)	Weight gain	Can worsen MJ and absences in IGE impaired cognition at higher doses
Lamotrigine (1991)	Sodium channel inhibition	50% protein bound, hepatic metabolism	25 mg (100–400 mg)	Idiosyncratic rash Rarely Stevens Johnson Syndrome	First line for focal seizures. Rapidly withdraw if rash occurs
Levetiracetam (1999)	Synaptic vesicle protein modulation	Urinary excretion	250 mg (750–3000 mg)	Tiredness, mood disturbance	Mood disturbance includes irritability, short temper
Phenobarbital* (1912)	GABA augmentation	Hepatic metabolism; 25% excreted unchanged	30 mg (30–180 mg)	Drowsiness, mood change, osteomalacia	Rarely initiated today; if withdrawal considered, needs to be slow
Pregabalin (2004)	Calcium channel modulation	Hepatic metabolism (saturation kinetics) 90% protein bound	50 mg (100–600 mg)	Drowsiness Weight gain	Can worsen MJ and absences in IGE dose-dependent side effects
Primidone* (1952)	GABA augmentation	Hepatic metabolism	125 mg (500–1500 mg)	Idiosyncratic rash	Rarely initiated; if withdrawal considered, needs to be slow
Oxcarbazepine* (1990)	Sodium-channel inhibition	Hepatic metabolism	150–300 mg (900–2400 mg)	Idiosyncratic rash; hyponatremia	Similar structure to carbamazepine
Tiagabine (1996)	GABA augmentation	Hepatic metabolism	5 mg (30–45 mg)	Increased seizures; nonconvulsive status	
Topiramate* (1995)	Glutamate reduction; sodium-channel modulation; calcium-channel modification	Mostly hepatic metabolism, with renal excretion	25 mg (75–200 mg)	Weight loss; kidney stones; impaired cognition; word finding difficulty	Dose-dependent side effects
Valproic acid (1968)	GABA augmentation	Hepatic metabolism; active metabolites	200 mg (400–2000 mg)	Rare hepatotoxicity or encephalopathy	First line for generalized seizures
Zonisamide (1990)	Calcium channel inhibition	Urinary excretion	50–100 mg (200–600 mg)	Idiosyncratic rash	Newly licensed in United Kingdom

*Induces hepatic enzymes and therefore affect plasma levels of other drugs undergoing hepatic metabolism (e.g., warfarin).

to three times that for the general population,[107] and screening for bone health in epilepsy is recommended.[108]

Drug-drug interactions

Drugs that undergo hepatic metabolism are altered by hepatic enzyme-inducing AEDs (see Table 59-3). Those with the least risk for interactions are levetiracetam, gabapentin, and pregabalin,[109] although it remains to be seen how this translates in clinical practice. Enzyme-inducing AEDs should be considered carefully in patients already on medication, all prescribed drugs should be reviewed, and warfarin can be a particular concern.

There is a long-held belief that antidepressants lower the seizure threshold and are proconvulsant. There is in fact little evidence to support this view.[110] Depression is common in patients with epilepsy and where present should be treated appropriately. The risk of seizures is dose dependent, and new antidepressants particularly at low doses are considered safe in most cases. Antidepressants least likely to affect AED levels are citalopram, escitalopram, venlafaxine, duloxetine, and mirtazapine.[111]

Therapeutic plasma monitoring

With the exception being phenytoin, monitoring plasma drug levels is generally not helpful in managing AED therapy. Laboratory reference ranges are of little value in dose adjustments, which should be done according to clinical response and dose-related side effects. A cross-sectional study of 92 nursing home residents in the United States found lower serum carbamazepine doses and concentrations than those used for young adults. The daily dose was significantly lower for the oldest age group (>85),[112] supporting this view. A recent review suggests situations in which therapeutic drug monitoring can be helpful.[19]

Withdrawing AEDs

Should AEDs be withdrawn in patients with elderly-onset seizures that have been seizure free for a period of time? What about those who have taken AEDs most of their lives with seizure freedom entering old age? Studies that address drug withdrawal have been done in a younger population.[113,114] Conditions that lead to an increased risk of relapse after drug withdrawal include focal epilepsy, generalized tonic clonic seizures, the presence of cerebral pathology, and an abnormal EEG. Many of these conditions apply to the elderly with new onset seizures. The severity and frequency of seizures and the patient's view on taking medication can influence decisions to withdraw AEDs. It is difficult to extrapolate recurrence risk from population studies to the individual presenting in clinic.

Worthy of special note is the older person who has been on lifelong treatment with phenobarbital or primidone. Both are barbiturates and very difficult to withdraw without potential dangerous recurrence of seizures. If withdrawal of one of these agents is being considered, then it should be with the advice of a specialist and the drug slowly titrated down over many months—for instance, 10% of the initial daily dose every 6 weeks.

THE IMPACT OF EPILEPSY

Epilepsy is a chronic disease. It is associated with stigma and public misconceptions. There is no single test to confirm or refute a diagnosis of epilepsy, and misdiagnosis is a problem. Comprehensive and systematic investigation on the impact of epilepsy are lacking; however, a number issues are well characterized. A questionnaire-based survey in a small number of elderly patients with epilepsy found their main concerns to be the impact on driving and transportation and concerns about medication side effects.[115] Other concerns included personal safety, social embarrassment, employment, and memory loss (Table 59-4).

In a study of more than 1000 adults with epilepsy in the United States and comparison with the U.S. Census Bureau, respondents received less education, were less likely to be employed or married, and came from lower-income households.[116] Uncertainty and fear of having a seizure were listed as the worst things about having epilepsy. Lifestyle, school, driving, and employment limits were also listed as major problems, and when asked to rank a list of problems, cognitive impairment was ranked highest. A study using a health-related, quality-of-life questionnaire in the elderly found lower scores in those with epilepsy compared to those without. AED side effects and depression were felt to be the main reasons,[117] whereas another study concluded that fear of even infrequent seizures could affect quality of life in the elderly.[4] Cognitive impairment is a major concern and is higher in those on more than one antiepileptic drug.[118,119]

For patients with epilepsy, motor vehicle licensing is usually restricted until a defined seizure-free interval has passed.[120] This varies from country to country. Medical practitioners need to be familiar with their own licensing authority regulations.[121]

Beyond driving restrictions, a commonsense approach should be taken to further restrictions on activity. Day-to-day activities should otherwise not be limited. Patients with severe or frequent seizures may develop a fear of public places or of being left alone. The physician should be mindful of this reaction.

Table 59-4. The Impact of Epilepsy

Seizures
Time lost
Injury
Social disruption/embarrassment
Hospital admission
Cognitive decline
Driving
Hobbies
Social interactions
Grand parenting
Diagnosis
Stigma
Misconceptions
Fear
Medication
Acute adverse events
Long-term side effects
Drug-drug interactions
Underlying disorder
Neurologic decline

SERVICES FOR PATIENTS WITH EPILEPSY

Elderly patients with epilepsy or presenting with blackouts should be seen by a specialist with an interest in the condition. Not all elderly patients will have access to specialist services. Syncope is the main differential diagnosis, and all physicians, not only epilepsy specialists and geriatricians, who treat patients with blackout should be aware of different presentations. An epilepsy service should work closely with cardiologists as well as with representative of the investigative specialties, neuroradiology and neurophysiology. One area that appears lacking is access to video-EEG. Epilepsy nurse specialists have not only taken some of the roles in long-term follow-up but also fill an important role in information giving and rapid access to specialist advice.[122–125] The role of a wider multidisciplinary team dedicated to epilepsy, which includes input on all aspects of social care (such as social and occupational services), has not been well characterized.

AREAS FOR RESEARCH

Raymond Tallis wrote in the last edition of this book, "The observation made in previous editions of this textbook that geriatric epileptology is a relatively underdeveloped and under-researched field remains true. The outstanding research agenda is substantially the same."

There remains much to be learned about how and why seizures start and stop. Research in this area is predominantly in the young, usually those undergoing detailed investigation for epilepsy surgery, and in animal experimentation. Are there differences in seizure mechanisms in the elderly? Why is there such a disparity between idiopathic generalized epilepsy and symptomatic epilepsy across the extremes of age? How common is misdiagnosis? How common is PNEA? It is easily missed without an index of suspicion and access to apporpriate investigation.

Do seizures have more adverse physical effects in old people, or is the converse true? Is there such a thing as SUDEP in the eldelry? How frequent are fractures and other significant injuries? What cognitive imapirments are associated with repeated seizures? Is this cause or effect? The main themes of many social epilepsy review articles are women with epilepsy, preganacy, driving, and lifestle issues. What are the information needs of the older person with epilepsy?

When to use AEDs

Should one treat a single unprovoked tonic–clonic seizure in old age or wait for two or more seizures? The ongoing MESS study referred to earlier should help. What are the chances of recurrence where there is no overt cause? How easy are seizures to control in old age? More prospective studies are needed to answer these questions.

The role of the newer generation of AEDs

What is the place of the new generation of anticonvulsants in the de novo treatment of elderly-onset seizures? Studies addressing these questions should focus not simply on the traditional end points such as seizure control. The importance of newer AEDs may lie more in reducing subtle adverse effects on gait and mobility than in improved seizure control, especially as "minor" effects of this sort may, in a frail elderly person, translate into significant dysfunction.

The organization of epilepsy services

How best should we provide a service for elderly people with seizures? What are the elements of an optimal overall comprehensive service? Who should provide it? How should we evaluate it? If we had answers to these questions, our management of seizures in old age would be considerably better than it is now.

KEY POINTS
Epilepsy

- The most important step in the management of a person with suspected seizures is to determine whether or not the events are indeed epileptic fits.
- All adult patients with new onset or suspected seizures should have a brain scan.
- About 80% of people with elderly-onset seizures will be controlled with the first-choice drug. Drug-drug interactions are an important consideration in older people.
- The management of established epilepsy goes far beyond drug treatment. Key elements are reassurance, education, information, and support.
- Aside from phenytoin treatment, anticonvulsant blood level monitoring is not routinely indicated and for most antiepileptic drugs.
- Elderly patients with seizures require an initial specialist assessment and should have access to continuing specialist services, in line with recommendations for younger people.

For a complete list of references, please visit online only at www.expertconsult.com

CHAPTER 60

Headache and Facial Pain

Gerry J. F. Saldanha

INTRODUCTION

Headache remains the commonest neurologic disorder worldwide, yet only since the late 1980s has research, clinical diagnosis and management, and interest in the field been stimulated by the publication of *The International Classification of Headache Disorders,* the first edition (1988) and the second edition (2004).[1] Improved diagnostic criteria has led to better quality studies and more robust data from clinical trials, and it has engendered a more rigorous approach to headache diagnosis in the clinic, with inevitable improvements in management. Although this has obviously benefited the sufferers of headache, most published data are from younger cohorts, and few clinical trials recruit older people. This is pertinent as the populations of the developed world age, increasing the strain on the national health economy. In 1980, the World Health Organization (WHO) European demographic returns indicated that the proportion of the European Union population over 65 years of age was 13.22%, a figure that had increased to 16.47% by 2005 with every likelihood that this trend will increase.

Few epidemiologic studies have been carried out to estimate the size of the headache problem. In 1 year in the United States, 70% of the general population had a headache, 5% of whom sought medical attention.[2] Less is known about the frequency of headache in the elderly population, although in a large population-based study carried out in East Boston,[3] some 17% of patients over 65 years of age reported frequent headache, with 53% of women and 36% of men reporting headache in the previous year. Headache prevalence in the elderly age group ranged from 5% to 50%.[4,5] Overall, headache appears to be less frequently reported in the elderly population.[6] and shows a decline with age.[3,7] Most studies agree that the prevalence of primary headache syndromes declines with increasing age.[7–10] One obvious limitation of these studies is that none is longitudinal and so may not differentiate an effect of aging from cohort or period effects. In addition, elderly patients may be less complaining, or the emergence of other more serious problems may have suppressed reporting of a benign symptom such as headache.

In elderly people headache is more likely to represent organic pathology.[11] A clinic-based retrospective case record study[12] concluded that, although it was less likely that elderly people would attend a hospital outpatients clinic for diagnosis of headache, there was a 10-fold increase in the likelihood of finding organic pathology. Recruitment bias is a problem in these studies. Nevertheless it is likely that headache is a more serious complaint from the elderly patient.

A large lifetime prevalence study[13] utilizing a population-based questionnaire found that although migraine and tension-type headache appeared to decrease with increasing age, chronic tension headache has significantly higher prevalence rates in the elderly population. Medication overuse remains an important factor in the etiology of chronic daily headache in the elderly, especially in patients who have been subject to frequent migraine headache.[14]

The author concludes that headache remains an extremely common condition of elderly people; much of it has benign origin, but more care needs to be taken with older patients to rule out underlying pathology, especially when they present for the first time.

PRIMARY HEADACHE DISORDERS

Migraine

Migraine is an episodic disorder that is diagnosed from the history, commonly starts around puberty, but may start at *any* age.[15] Epidemiologic studies are difficult to carry out and are dogged by numerous problems.[16] Only 5% of migraineurs consult specialists,[17] so clinic-based studies will suffer from referral bias. It is clear that a significant proportion of the burden of migraine headache is undiagnosed and untreated, more so in the elderly. A number of population-based studies have been carried out.[9,17–28]

Rasmussen et al[26] did not find a decrease in migraine prevalence with increasing age, in contrast to the findings of Stewart et al[24] who also showed that it is uncommon for migraine to start in a person's later years.[9] The female preponderance of migraineurs persists in this age group.[17] Migraine headaches tend to improve with increasing age.[29]

Symptoms and diagnosis of migraine

Migraine is classified into two main forms, migraine with aura (formerly "classic migraine") and migraine without aura (formerly "common migraine"), based on criteria of the International Headache Society.[1] Other varieties of migraine include ophthalmoplegic, retinal, basilar, and familial hemiplegic, complications of migraine such as migrainous infarction (a neurologic deficit not reversible in 7 days) and status migrainosus (an attack of headache or aura lasting more than 72 hours). Migraine aura can exist without headache, and the same patient may at different times experience headache with aura, headache without aura, or aura without headache.[30,31]

To diagnose migraine without aura, five attacks are needed, each lasting 4 to 72 hours and having two of the following four characteristics: unilateral location, pulsating quality, moderate or severe intensity, and aggravation by routine physical activity. In addition, the attacks must have at least one of the following: nausea or vomiting or photophobia and phonophobia. Migraine without aura is more common than migraine with aura and is usually more disabling.

Migraine with aura is diagnosed when there have been at least two attacks with any three of the following features:

- One or more fully reversible aura symptoms
- Aura developing over more than 4 minutes
- Aura lasting less than 60 minutes
- Headache following aura with a free interval of less than 60 minutes

A simpler working definition for the clinical diagnosis of migraine was proposed by Solomon and Lipton.[32] A positive diagnosis could be made on any two of the following four symptoms:

- Unilateral headache
- Pulsating quality
- Nausea
- Photophobia and phonophobia

A similar headache must have occurred in the past and structural disease excluded. Migraine attacks may generally be divided into five phases: the prodrome (hours or days before the headache), the aura (migraine with aura), the headache, the headache termination, and the postdrome phase.[30] Symptoms of the prodrome may include mental, neurologic, or general (constitutional, autonomic) symptoms. Individuals may experience depression, euphoria, irritability, restlessness, mental slowness, hyperactivity, and drowsiness. General symptoms may include a feeling of coldness, sluggishness, thirst, anorexia, diarrhea, constipation, fluid retention, and food cravings. Photophobia and phonophobia may also occur.

The aura is a group of neurologic symptoms that precedes or accompanies the attack. They may be visual, sensory, or motor and may also cause language or brainstem disturbance. Headache usually occurs within 60 minutes of the end of the aura,[1] but it may begin with the aura. Most patients may have more than one type of aura and progress from one type to another in subsequent attacks. Common visual symptoms are the positive phenomena such as hemianopic photopsia (flashes of light) and teichopsia or fortification spectra. Scotomata may follow. Complex visual distortions and hallucinations are reported but are more common in younger people.[33] Somatosensory phenomena, typically paresthesias with anatomic march of symptoms, may occur and motor disturbance may result in hemiparesis. Aphasia has also been reported.[7,34] Migraine aura symptoms may therefore be characterized by both positive and negative symptoms. Acephalgic migraine is an entity characterized by the neurologic dysfunction of the aura but without headache. This is strictly a diagnosis of exclusion especially in elderly people. These so-called migraine accompaniments may occur for the first time in the older age group[35,36] and can be easily confused with transient ischemic attacks (TIAs) except in the most classic of cases. Migraine with aura and acephalgic migraine can both be confused with TIAs, and vice versa. Headache occurred with 36% of TIAs in one series[37] and is more common in vertebrobasilar ischemia.[38,39] Migrainous aura in the elderly person presents a particularly difficult diagnostic dilemma. Transient hemiparetic or hemisensory symptoms occurring in elderly people for the first time should be assumed to be vascular (i.e., TIA) in etiology until proved otherwise. Alternating hemisensory/paretic symptoms are more likely to be migrainous but still could have an embolic cause. Investigation including carotid Doppler studies and echocardiography will be necessary to manage potentially treatable embolic sources. Visual disturbance is more likely to be helpful as fortification spectra and colored zigzag lines are unlikely to occur in straightforward TIAs and are almost always migrainous in origin. Migraine with aura may occur for the first time in the elderly person, although in general new onset migraine in the older age group is unusual[12,40] and may reflect the development of vascular change. It is often helpful in these cases to elicit a previous history of common migraine earlier in life.

The headache of migraine is typically throbbing in nature and exacerbated by exercise.[41] The pain may be unilateral in 60% of cases but bilateral at the outset in up to 40%.[7] Unilateral headache may later become bilateral during the attack. The intensity is moderate to severe and pain may radiate down the neck to the shoulder. Some 40% of migraineurs report short-lived jabs of pain lasting seconds and having a needle-like quality, the so-called "ice-pick" pains.[42]

The common accompanying symptoms of nausea and vomiting may make it difficult for the patient to take oral medication. There is usually photophobia and phonophobia; many patients retire to a dark and quiet room for rest. Constitutional, mood, and mental changes are universal,[7] and the patient is usually left feeling lethargic for a period after the attack.

Basilar migraine is a variant characterized by brain stem dysfunction such as ataxia, dysarthria, diplopia, vertigo, nausea and vomiting, and alteration in cognition and consciousness. Headache is invariable. In the elderly person these symptoms should be assumed to be of vascular origin until proven otherwise.

Ophthalmoplegic migraine is rare and can be confused with the presentation of Berry aneurysm. Attacks of migraine-like pain occur around the eye with oculomotor nerve dysfunction and dilation of the pupil. The ophthalmoplegia may last from hours to months. The differential diagnosis includes orbital inflammatory disease and diabetic mononeuropathy.

Migraine attacks may vary in frequency from a few a year to several a week. Trigger factors include certain foods, red wine,[43] hormone replacement treatment in postmenopausal women,[44] irregular meals, and a change in sleep habit.[45] Environmental triggers include flickering lights, noise, rapidly altering visual stimuli, and even certain types of weather. Head injury and stress may lead to migraine attacks.

TREATMENT OF MIGRAINE

Once the diagnosis has been established, reassuring the patient may suffice. Any obvious precipitating cause such as diet, lack of sleep, or environmental factors should be discussed. Relaxation therapy may be helpful, but special diets have little place in management.

Pharmacotherapy includes treatment of the acute attack and consideration of prophylactic therapy. It should be remembered that changing biology in the elderly will influence response to medication.[46] Thus, gastric emptying slows, delaying absorption of medication; hepatic blood flow is reduced and so is glomerular filtration rate, affecting drug metabolism, usually leading to increased half life. In general, therefore, pharmacotherapy should be started with caution in the elderly who are often taking medications for other comorbidities. Acute treatment should be started by the patient at the outset of an attack and is best limited to simple soluble analgesics such as paracetamol or aspirin (Table 60-1). Combination analgesics such as co-proxamol should be avoided, if possible, because of side effects and risk of medication overuse leading to so-called transformed migraine. For a more severe headache, nonsteroidal anti-inflammatory drugs are used.[47] Ibuprofen (200 mg three times daily) may be obtained in the United Kingdom without prescription, or naproxen (250 mg t.d.s.) by prescription,

Table 60-1. Drugs for Use in the Treatment of Migraine*

Migraine Attack Treatments	Migraine Prophylaxsis
Soluble aspirin	Propranolol and other β-blockers
Soluble paracetamol	Tricyclic antidepressants
Antiemetics such as domperidone	Pizotifen
Suppositories	Topiramate
Nonsteroidal anti-inflammatory drugs	Calcium channel antagonists
Sumatriptan (subcutaneous or oral)	Methysergide
Other triptans	Sodium valproate
Medihaler ergotamine and other ergotamine preparations	
Combination analgesia	

*Care must be taken with possible interactions with preexistent treatments and conditions such as asthma (if β-blockers are to be prescribed). The table lists medication in order of preference.

or diclofenac (75 mg twice-daily). This group of drugs should be administered with caution in the elderly population because of the increased risk of gastrointestinal hemorrhage, especially when there is a past history of peptic ulceration[48,49] or renal insufficiency.

For moderate to severe migraine not responding to simple analgesia, sumatriptan can be tried. The initial dose is 50 mg orally and can be increased to 100 mg if there is no response. Subcutaneous self-administration is the preferred route when there is significant nausea or vomiting. Sumatriptan is a $5HT_1$ agonist and is thought to act as a selective cerebral vasoconstrictor. Up to 80% of patients obtain relief from headache within 2 hours after an injection[50] and up to 65% after a tablet dose.[51] The advantage is that the drug may be administered at any point during an attack and repeated if necessary. Flushing, tingling in the neck and head, and chest tightness can occur in up to 5% of patients.[52] Because sumatriptan may cause coronary vasoconstriction, it is contraindicated in patients with ischemic heart disease or uncontrolled hypertension. Special care in the elderly person is required because the loss of subcutaneous fat may lead to intramuscular injection and more rapid absorption. A recent study failed to demonstrate increased risk of stroke, myocardial infarction, cardiovascular death, ischemic heart disease, and overall mortality in the elderly.[53] Pharmacotherapy should be combined with rest and sleep. A number of newer triptans have been licensed for use in migraine treatment and may be selected for the individual patient.[54]

Ergotamine preparations are best reserved for occasional (>1 month interval) severe headaches. They are potent vasoconstrictors and are best avoided in patients with a history of vaso-occlusive disease, peripheral vascular disease, or hypertension, and those receiving β-blockers or with a history of Raynaud's phenomenon. Patients should be strongly encouraged to avoid overuse of these drugs, because this can lead to resistant medication-misuse headache. Admission for drug withdrawal may be required when this occurs.

The accompanying symptoms of nausea and vomiting are often as disabling as the headache and require treatment in their own right. Metoclopramide is the most commonly used antiemetic, and by promoting gastric emptying, it aids absorption of coadministered medication. It can cause extrapyramidal side effects, especially in the elderly person. Domperidone is less likely to cause this problem as it does not cross the blood–brain barrier but does not aid gastric emptying.

Prophylactic therapy is indicated when there is severe recurrent headache causing disruption to daily life—as a guide, more than two severe headaches per month. Various drugs are used including β-blockers, antidepressants, serotonin antagonists, calcium-channel blockers, and occasionally anticonvulsants. Treatment is started at a low dose and built to maintenance. Possible side effects should be discussed and the regimen kept as simple as possible as many patients in this age group are likely to have coexistent medication. Patients should be weaned from therapy every 4 to 6 months.

Of the β-blockers, propranolol, metoprolol, and atenolol have all been shown to be effective in up to 60% to 80% of patients producing a greater than 50% reduction in attack frequency.[55,56] Atenolol (50 to 100 mg daily) has a better side-effect profile than propranolol (20 to 160 mg daily). Patients may complain of fatigue, dizziness, nightmares, and cold extremities. Care should be taken when there is peripheral vascular disease and in combination with ergotamine.

The tricyclic antidepressants have been used in migraine prophylaxis, although the evidence for their efficacy is largely based on anecdotal reports or uncontrolled trials. Their effect in headache may be independent of their antidepressant effect.[55,57] Amitriptyline is most commonly used, although fluoxetine has fewer anticholinergic side effects and causes less weight gain.[58] Paroxetine may be a suitable alternative where anxiety is a factor.[59] Because of their common side effect of drowsiness, the tricyclics are administered at the lowest effective dose at bedtime and slowly increased as necessary. Elderly people are more vulnerable to the muscarinic side effects. The typical starting dose for amitriptyline should be 10 mg, increasing to 150 mg if needed.[60]

Sodium valproate (0.6 to 2.5 g daily) is well tolerated and there is clinical trial evidence of efficacy.[61] Side effects of valproate include tremor, ataxia, and less commonly an extrapyramidal syndrome. Topiramate now has a license for use in migraine prophylaxis; the use of anticonvulsants for migraine prophylaxis has been reviewed recently.[62]

Calcium-channel antagonists are not licensed for migraine prophylaxis in the United Kingdom but have been shown to be of benefit.[55] The mechanism of action of these compounds in migraine is uncertain and side effects are common, including edema, flushing, dizziness, and not infrequently an initial increase in headache frequency. Improvement of headache may require several weeks of treatment.[63]

Of the serotonin antagonists, the two most commonly prescribed are pizotifen and methysergide. Pizotifen is a $5HT_2$ antagonist that is usually commenced in a dose of 0.5 mg at night and increased in stepwise manner to a dose of 4.5 mg. It has mild antidepressant activity but unfortunately stimulates appetite and leads to weight gain if diet is not controlled. It can produce beneficial effects in 40% to 79% of patients.[64] Methysergide is also a $5HT_2$ antagonist with some affinity for the $5HT_1$ receptor. It is effective prophylaxis in up to 60% of migraineurs, possibly with better results in those with migraine with aura.[65] Side effects are common and include myalgia, weight gain, nausea, and hallucinations (especially after the first dose). The complication of retroperitoneal, endocardial, and pulmonary fibrosis is rare and prevented by stopping treatment for 3 to 4 weeks every 4 to 6 months. The starting dose is 1 mg at night but may be increased to 6 mg daily in divided dosage.

Feverfew (*Tenacetum parthenium*) is a herbal remedy long used for headache treatment. It has limited effect, and the side effects include mouth ulceration and loss of taste.[66,67]

Tension headache

Tension-type headache may be broadly classified into infrequent episodic tension-type headache, frequent episodic tension-type headache (at least 10 episodes occurring between 1 and 15 days a month), and chronic tension-type headache (headache occurring on more than 15 days per month).[1] The clinical features include the following:

- Pressing/tightening (nonpulsating) quality
- Mild or moderate intensity
- Bilateral location
- No aggravation on walking up or down stairs or similar routine physical activity

There should *not* be photophobia and phonophobia, although either alone is permitted within the definition. Patients should *not* experience nausea or vomiting (although the International Headache Society (IHS) criteria allow for nausea but not vomiting in the diagnosis of chronic tension-type headache).

In both types of headache, there may be pericranial muscle tenderness with or without increased electromyographic activity, although this does not assume that muscle tension is the cause of the headache.[68] In all age groups, tension-type headache is the most common form of headache, peaking in the 30s and 40s.[69] Chronic tension-type headache is more common in the older age groups than episodic tension-type headache, and only 5% of patients with chronic tension-type headache report onset after the age of 60 years.[70] Within all age groups, tension headache remains most common in females with a 1-year period prevalence of 27.1% in females and 25.6% in males in one large telephone-based study.[26,69]

The pain of tension-type headache is usually described as a constant ache, which is infrequently pulsatile. Patients may describe a tight band about the head or a sensation of wearing a tight cap. There may be associated stiffness of the neck and upper back; in contrast to migraine, the pain is usually of lesser intensity. Scalp tenderness may lead to avoidance of hair brushing. This symptom is also recorded in migraineurs, and it may persist for some days after the headache has subsided.[71]

The headache may be unilateral or bilateral, commonly occipital or frontal, but may involve any site. It can be relieved by changing position.

Patients with episodic tension headache may experience pericranial muscle tenderness with palpable nodules.[72] Depression, anxiety, and other psychological factors are important in the pathogenesis of tension headache, although not infrequently patients may initially deny any role.

Depression is common in the community at large, and in an average family practice in the United Kingdom it is the fourth most commonly diagnosed disorder.[73] The headache associated with depression can have features described for tension-type headache, and the headaches are often present for years or even throughout the patient's life. The headache is typically diurnal, usually worse in the morning and in the evening. There may be identifiable emotional, physical, and psychic complaints. These problems merit attention in their own right, especially in the elderly person when organic pathology is more likely anyway. The presence of severe depression in elderly people may be easily overlooked. Other headaches associated with depression can be described more bizarrely with almost a delusional tone. Such headaches may indicate a serious psychiatric disorder and should lead to urgent psychiatric referral.

Treatment includes reassurance, simple analgesia as abortive treatment for the acute attack, and treatment of any psychopathology that may be present. Simple analgesia such as paracetamol should be used for acute attacks of pain. Nonsteroidals are more likely to be associated with side effects in the elderly such as gastric erosions and renal and hepatic complications.[74] Frequent episodic tension-type headache and chronic tension-type headache may require the use of prophylaxis—tricyclics such as amitriptyline remain the most useful drugs, especially when there is sleep disorder. The latter is especially useful when sleep disturbance is a prominent symptom.[75] Fluoxitene (20 mg daily) is less sedating. Paroxetine (10 mg daily) may be helpful where there are additional anxiety symptoms. Monoamine oxidase inhibitors should be avoided if possible. Psychiatric help may be appropriate, although patients often initially reject this suggestion. Relaxation therapy and biofeedback may also have a role.

The mixed headache syndrome—migraine and tension-type headache in the same patient—usually responds to treatment with tricyclic antidepressants with the addition of analgesia for acute episodes. There are no specific data on the prognosis of tension-type headache in the elderly, although there is a tendency for improvement with increasing age.[76] It is important to continually bear in mind that secondary headache is more common in the older patient and that careful evaluation of the history and examination and a lower threshold for investigation should be applied in the elderly presenting with apparent nonspecific headache.

Chronic daily headache

The syndrome of chronic daily headache (CDH) accounts for 40% of patients seen in headache clinics[77] and worldwide is estimated to affect 3% to 5% of the population.[78] Only 5% reported their chronic headache as starting after 60 years of age.[70] Chronic daily headache is defined as 15 or more headache days a month for 3 moths or more.

There are several subtypes of CDH (Table 60-2), with chronic migraine presenting five times more commonly than chronic tension-type headache to the specialist headache clinic.[79] The features of tension-type headache are discussed elsewhere in this section. Medication overuse is probably the third most common form of chronic headache after chronic tension-type headache and chronic migraine and is thought to affect up to 1% of the world population.[80,81] The free availability of analgesics containing caffeine, codeine, barbiturates, and tranquilizers over the counter has been implicated as one cause of this syndrome.[82,83] The management of this syndrome can be particularly challenging and hinges on the discontinuation of analgesic overuse, the possibility of going "cold turkey," and the use of suitable alternatives for weaning and prophylaxis.[84] In a proportion of patients the headache may revert to its original episodic form, but in the remainder the avoidance of analgesic overuse will

Table 60-2. Chronic Daily Headache Subtypes

Chronic tension-type headache
Transformed migraine
Drug induced
Nondrug related
Chronic tension-type headache
Medication overuse headache
New daily persistent headache
Posttraumatic headache

require the initiation of prophylaxis.[85] Suitable prophylactic treatment such as amitriptyline in an initial dose of 10 mg at night increased to 75 mg as tolerated is effective, with improvement seen at 2 to 14 days. The drug should be continued at an effective dose for 6 months and then withdrawn slowly over 3 months. Caution should be exercised in those with glaucoma and prostatism. Anticonvulsant drugs used in migraine prophylaxis may be effective, and sodium valproate, gadapentin, and more recently topiramate have been used with favorable results.[86,87] Patient and physician education is especially important in prevention and management of this difficult headache syndrome.

Episodic migraine may evolve into CDH. In one study, 489 of 630 patients (78%) with CDH had a clear preceding history of episodic migraine.[88] This so-called transformed migraine may be caused by excessive use of opioid and simple analgesics, barbiturates, ergot compounds, caffeine, and frequent use of triptans. Headaches are often more severe on waking owing to a drug-free withdrawal period overnight effectively causing rebound. Hemicrania continua is side-locked headache that often has autonomic symptoms and shows an exquisite response to indomethacin.[89,90]

The differential diagnosis includes headaches arising from the neck, temporal arteritis, mass lesions, and visual acuity problems. Because tension-type headache is often associated with depression, sleep disorder, and situational life events, especially in the elderly population, the treatment of CDH must include behavioral, psychological, and social aspects.

Cluster headache

This condition, although most common in young adults, may have its onset in the seventh decade[91,92] The International Headache Society classification divides the condition into episodic and chronic cluster headache, the latter being more common in the elderly population.[93] A review of the literature suggests a lifetime prevalence of 124 per 100,000,[94] with a higher male preponderance in the young but more females over 60 years affected than males.[95]

Cluster headache is characterized by bouts of severe pain often described as "boring." The pain is constant, and patients walk around trying to find relief—in contrast to those with migraine who lie quietly. The pain is often centered around one eye, and there may be ipsilateral lacrimation, nasal stuffiness, and rhinorrhea. There is usually conjunctival injection, and there may be an associated ptosis, meiosis, and eyelid edema. The pain may spread to the whole side of the face. Bouts of pain occur one to three times per day with alarm-clock regularity, commonly an hour or so after going to sleep, and last from 15 minutes to a few hours (with a usual duration of 45 to 90 minutes). The headache may start and end abruptly, and in a few patients there may be interictal discomfort.[96] The cluster period typically lasts for 1 to 2 months and then subsides. During the cluster attacks, alcohol is a potent precipitant, usually setting off an attack within an hour of ingestion, as are vasodilator drugs such as nitrates. The chronic form continues without remission often for many years.

Treatment is symptomatic. Oxygen at 100% is useful in the casualty department and can be given at home. It is important that a high flow valve is used with a nonrebreather mask capable of delivering 7 to 10 liters per minute. More practically, sumatriptan by subcutaneous injection is the drug of choice for acute attacks.[97] Nasal sumatriptan may be used but appears to be less effective.[98] Preventive treatments may be considered in terms of short-term measures and longer duration treatment for those with a more chronic course to their clusters. Steroids (prednisolone 1 mg/kg daily for a week and reducing by 10 mg a week) may shorten a cluster period, but relapse often occurs and so they may be used with other forms of prophylaxis.[99] Verapamil is the drug of choice for all forms of cluster headache prophylaxis[100] and compares favorably with lithium,[101] particularly in view of the plethora of potential neuropsychiatric side effects of the latter. Doses of verapamil range from 240 mg to 960 mg twice daily in divided dose. As this drug may cause heart block, a baseline electrocardiogram (ECG) should be taken, an initial dose of 80 mg three times daily commenced, and then every 10 days or so the dose should be increased in 80 mg increments until attacks are suppressed or side effects prevent further titration. An ECG should be done after each increment. Sodium valproate may be tried in resistant cases.[102] Lithium carbonate given in standard psychiatric doses (600 to 1200 mg) and monitored accordingly is useful in *chronic* cluster, but less so in episodic cluster headache.

Rarely, surgical intervention is attempted. Percutaneous radiofrequency trigeminal gangliorhizolysis or posterior fossa trigeminal sensory rhizolysis have been performed but are of unproven benefit. Operation can cause a reduction in facial sensation and corneal hypoesthesia with increased risk of corneal ulceration.[103]

Cluster headache is an underdiagnosed cause of recurrent paroxysmal cranial pain in the elderly population. It may not have the usual classic features in this age group. Treatment may need to be given empirically when there is doubt.

Chronic paroxysmal hemicrania (Sjaastad headache), a rare variant of cluster headache, differs in the brevity (3 to 45 minutes) and frequency (up to 40 times a day) of the attacks. The invariable response to indomethacin now forms part of the diagnostic criteria.[104]

FACIAL NEURALGIAS

Trigeminal neuralgia

DIAGNOSIS

Trigeminal neuralgia is diagnosed clinically. It rarely begins before the age of 30 years,[105,106] has a prevalence of 0.1 to 0.2 per 1000 and an incidence of up to 20/100,000/year after the age of 60 years, and the female-to-male ratio is 3:2.[107] The symptoms are pathognomonic. The pain is periodic, of high intensity, and lancinating, lasting from 20 to 30 seconds followed by a period of relief lasting a few seconds to a minute, which may be followed by further paroxysms of pain. The pain usually commences in the maxillary and mandibular divisions of the trigeminal nerve, and in fewer than 5% of cases it begins in the ophthalmic division. In some 10% to 15% of cases, all the divisions are involved and the symptoms may be bilateral in 3% to 5%.[96] Apart from the quality and characteristic site of pain, the patient can usually identify trigger factors such as brushing the teeth, washing the face, shaving, biting, chewing, or even a gust of cold wind on the face. Avoidance behavior is common.

The pain may occur daily for weeks or months followed by remission of varying periods. Unfortunately there is a tendency for the disorder to deteriorate, with increased frequency of attacks increasingly resistant to treatment. Clinical examination should be normal, and any loss of facial sensation should be promptly investigated, preferably with gadolinium-enhanced magnetic resonance imaging (MRI) of the brain and trigeminal system, to rule out a compressive lesion of the nerve.

ETIOLOGY

The presence of chronic irritation of the roots of the trigeminal nerve has been demonstrated to cause neuralgia, and it is believed that in the majority of patients, demyelination of the proximal nerve roots is causative. The proximal nerve roots lie within central nervous system (CNS) nerve tissue, which extends several millimeters from the surface of the pons. Animal laboratory data, however, are more consistent with a central mechanism mediated by the loss of segmental inhibition within the spinal trigeminal sensory nucleus. To reconcile these observations, Fromm et al[108] proposed that spontaneous peripheral activity from the irritated nerve, in the presence of the failure of the normal central inhibitory mechanisms, may cause paroxysmal bursts of neuronal activity within the trigeminal nucleus and its thalamic relays, perceived as neuralgia by the patient. This has been likened to a form of "sensory reflex epilepsy."[109] Some evidence for the peripheral component of this hypothesis comes from the common finding of vascular loops (arterial or venous) in association with the nerve root in a majority of symptomatic patients.[110,111] Other compressive pathology should be considered including schwannoma, lymphoma, meningioma, and a variety of other tumors and infiltrative lesions. Pathologic specimens reveal focal demyelination within the proximal, CNS part of the root. It is proposed that ephaptic transmission of spontaneously generated ectopic impulses results in symptoms.[112] Because vessels tend to become more ectatic with age, this may explain why the condition is more common in the elderly population.

TREATMENT

The treatment of this condition is initially medical.[113–115] Occasionally the symptoms are so severe that hospital admission is required to control symptoms and prevent a downward spiral of increasing pain, dehydration, and depression. This is particularly the case for the elderly and infirm individual.

A recent review confirmed that carbamazepine remains the first choice drug, and pain relief is usually obtained within 4 to 24 hours.[116] The initial dose of 100 mg three times daily is increased every 48 hours in a stepwise manner until symptom relief or side effects occur. Patients should be warned of the potential for drowsiness, rash, and unsteadiness. A baseline full blood count is recommended because leukopenia does occur commonly and agranulocytosis rarely; treatment should be stopped immediately if the latter occurs. Although carbamazepine is usually effective at blood levels of 25 to 50 mg/L, the dose can be titrated to the maximum tolerated in resistant cases. Therapy should be maintained until the patient has been free of pain for at least 4 weeks, after which slow reduction of dose by decrements of 100 mg of carbamazepine each week may allow for complete withdrawal of the drug. For patients who experience limited efficacy or side effects, oxcarbazepine should be tried.

If adequate pain relief is not obtained with standard doses of carbamazepine, a second drug such as baclofen (10 mg three times daily up to 1.03 mg/kg daily) can be added. This may aggravate drowsiness. Alternatively, phenytoin, clonazepam, or sodium valproate can be added. Polypharmacy should be avoided if possible because of additional side effects and problems with compliance.

Surgical intervention should be considered if medical treatment fails. Up to 50% of patients may eventually require some form of surgical treatment. There are two main options, rhizotomy or microvascular decompression.

Radiofrequency rhizotomy or alternatively glycerol rhizolysis is relatively safe and simple. Patients require only light anesthesia, and the procedure is carried out under radiographic screening control. Selective root lesioning is achieved if a stimulating electrode is employed, and this reduces the side effects (discussed later). Acute pain relief can be accomplished in over 90% of patients, and this can be maintained in the long term with repeated treatments if necessary.[117] Glycerol injection into Meckel's cave acts as a neurotoxin.

The main side effect is sensory loss (usually less with glycerol injection). Corneal hypoesthesia is a problem and may result in ulceration. Rarely there may be masseter weakness. Both forms of treatment have about 90% success, and the patient can be discharged home within 24 hours. Unfortunately, the reported recurrence rates are about 25%. In a study comparing glycerol rhizolysis and posterior fossa exploration, freedom from pain at 5 years was 59% and 68%, respectively.[118]

Microvascular decompression involves major neurosurgery with a posterior fossa approach. This procedure was pioneered by Jannetta.[119] If a blood vessel is found in close association with the trigeminal root or deforming it, it is mobilized and a small sponge of polyvinyl chloride interposed between the nerve and the vessel. This procedure is generally well tolerated by elderly patients who are otherwise medically fit for surgery. Recurrence rates of up to 24% at 30 months after the procedure were reported in one study.[120] Overall the recurrence of pain after any surgical procedure was 19% with a minimum 5-year follow-up, with microvascular decompression providing the greatest relief and patient satisfaction.[121]

Glossopharyngeal neuralgia

This syndrome has the same symptom characteristics as trigeminal neuralgia but the pain is felt in the region of the tonsil and ear. Trigger factors include swallowing, coughing, and talking, and the distribution of the pain is in the sensory territory of the glossopharyngeal nerve and the auricular and pharyngeal branches of the vagus nerve. Rarely the patient may become unconscious during an attack because of asystole.[33] Neurologic examination is normal unless the syndrome is secondary to pathology such as neoplasm, infection, or inflammatory disease.

Treatment is the same as for trigeminal neuralgia with carbamazepine and other drugs. The medical treatment of this condition is less successful than in the case of trigeminal neuralgia and surgery is more often undertaken.[122] If there is no improvement, microvascular dissection of the intracranial section of the glossopharyngeal nerve and upper two rootlets of the vagus can be undertaken.[123,124]

Postherpetic neuralgia

Postherpetic neuralgia occurs following 10% of attacks of shingles, but this figure rises to 50% in the over-60 age group.[125] The most common site is the ophthalmic division of the trigeminal nerve. The virus has a predilection for the trigeminal (23% of cases[126]) and upper cervical ganglia, and in the acute stages the herpetic eruption is seen in the appropriate distribution. The Ramsay Hunt syndrome is due to herpetic infection of the facial nerve. Excruciating pain may precede the eruption of vesicles by 1 to 3 days. The latter are seen over the external auditory meatus and mastoid process and may occur with edema and redness of the ear, making examination difficult. Occasionally, other cranial nerves may be affected with involvement of the trigeminal nerve, leading to loss of sensation on the face and numbness of the palate occurring when the 9th nerve is affected. A careful search for vesicles around the ear and in the mouth will make the diagnosis clear. There may also be involvement of the 4th, 6th, and oculomotor nerves,[127] with the possibility of long-term paralysis.

The syndrome of postherpetic neuralgia is characterized by a constant burning or aching pain with occasional stabbing components and occurs following healing of the rash. It may take several weeks or months to emerge. There is sensory loss over the affected area, and invariably allodynia develops.

Treatment is symptomatic.[128] Antiviral therapy such as acyclovir was shown to provide marginal evidence for reduction of pain incidence at 1 to 3 months following zoster onset. Famciclovir reduced the duration of the neuralgia but not its incidence, as did valacyclovir. Steroids had no effect on postherpetic neuralgia.[129,130] Amitriptyline taken at the onset may reduce the incidence of postherpetic neuralgia, but more trials need to be undertaken.[129] Acyclovir (800 mg five times daily) may be prescribed if the rash is extensive or if there is a threat to eyesight. Opiate analgesia may be required. Once neuralgia is established, amitriptyline is of proven benefit,[131,132] and carbamazepine may help to control the stabbing component of the pain. Relief of pain may be gained in up to 80% of cases. Nortriptyline and desimipramine may be better tolerated, causing less sedation; the former has been shown to be as effective as amitriptyline.[133] Transcutaneous electrical nerve stimulation (TENS) may sometimes be useful. Topical capsaicin cream has had variable success.[134,135] Both gabapentin and pregabalin are licensed for the treatment of this condition,[136,137] which is notoriously difficult to treat, but presently there is no role for surgery.

ATYPICAL FACIAL PAIN

More correctly defined as idiopathic persistent facial pain, this syndrome is rare in the elderly population. It is characterized by a continuous, chronic head or facial pain that does not follow dermatomal boundaries or conform to any of the known patterns of headache or cranial neuralgia. The diagnosis can be made only after the exclusion of organic pathology, including dental and sinus disease.[138] Many patients are believed to be depressed[37] and receive tricyclic antidepressants, generally with a good result.[139] Lance and Goadsby[96] have proposed an organic basis to this syndrome. However, tricyclics remain the treatment of choice, together with the judicious use of baclofen. Occasionally the pain may have a throbbing vascular nature, and when intermittent it is worth considering a diagnosis of facial or "lower half" migraine.[140] In this case, a trial of a β-blocker or sumatriptan may be useful.

HEADACHE ARISING FROM THE NECK

Cervical spondylosis, affecting the neck vertebrae, has a strong association with aging.[141] Degenerative changes lead to a loss of intervertebral height with narrowing of the central canal and the intervertebral foramina. Spondylotic changes may compress cervical nerves or the spinal cord to produce a syndrome of cervical spondyloradiculopathy with or without myelopathy. Symptomatic cervical spondylosis is more common in men than in women and produces symptoms typically in the fifth and sixth decades. Neck pain and headache may result; and although most of the population over the age of 40 years has radiologic changes consistent with cervical spondylosis without symptoms, in those with symptomatic disease (brachialgia or myelopathy), 40% reported headache as a chief symptom and 25% reported it as a major symptom.[142] The mechanism of cervicogenic headache remains uncertain and is hotly debated.[143] It may be defined as headache arising from the structures of the neck, is unilateral, and may be exacerbated by neck movement. It is proposed that the convergence of sensory afferents form cervical structures with descending trigeminal pathways in the upper cervical segments of the spinal cord allow for bidirectional referral of pain between the neck and trigeminal receptive fields of the face and head.[144] However, overall cervical spondylosis is an uncommon cause of headache.

The head pain resulting from cervical degenerative disease is frequently occipital in distribution but may radiate to the vertex or even the frontal area. The greater occipital nerve (C2) provides much of the sensory input from the back of the head, and irritation of this nerve typically causes occipital headache. The pain is usually described as constant, not throbbing, and of moderate intensity. Associated muscle tenderness, perhaps secondary to spasm, may be present, and this may make differentiation from tension headache difficult. It is disputed whether the cervical spine itself gives rise to headache per se, but headache may arise as a secondary phenomenon because of muscle spasm in the neck.[141] Movements of the cervical spine may aggravate the headache, and examination will reveal reduced range of movement and suboccipital tenderness with muscle spasm.

Treatment is usually conservative with nonsteroidal drugs or simple analgesics. Cervical collars are of uncertain worth and anyway should be combined with referral to a physiotherapist for neck exercises. Surgery is considered when there is myelopathy or radiculopathy, especially when it is progressive.

Lesions of the bones of the upper cervical spine and base of skull can give rise to occipital ache by pressure on the cervical nerves. Myeloma, osteomyelitis, metastatic tumor, and erosive inflammatory disease such as rheumatoid arthritis may all cause headache and neurologic deficit. Paget's disease can cause basilar invagination with traction on the upper cervical nerves and or hydrocephalus, both of which may result in headache.[142] A plain skull x-ray will usually rule out these possibilities if suspected.

SINUS DISEASE AND DENTAL DISEASE

Head and facial pain may be referred from the cranial sinuses. Experiments have shown that inflammation of the sinus lining is rarely painful,[145] but that pain arises from inflammation of the ducts and ostia of the sinuses or inflammation of the nasal turbinates.[33] Disease of the frontal sinuses causes ache localized over these sinuses; that of the antrum is usually referred to the maxillary region and into the zygomatic or temporal areas. Headache associated with sphenoidal and ethmoidal disease is mainly felt behind the eyes and over the vertex of the skull. Sinus headache is frequently overdiagnosed in the primary care setting, and many patients satisfy criteria for tension-type headache and migraine.[146] A sensible approach is to carefully elicit a history of symptoms compatible with nasal *acute* sinus inflammation (purulent nasal discharge, local pain over the relevant sinus) in addition to headache. Chronic sinusitis rarely causes headache.

The pain of sinus disease is usually deep-seated and dull, aching, and nonpulsatile. Adopting a recumbent position may relieve the headache of sinus disease, so these headaches are less prominent at night than during the day. Pain may be exacerbated by shaking the head or adopting a head-down position. Coughing or straining also exacerbates the pain by raising intracranial venous pressure.

The treatment of sinusitis is symptomatic with decongestants and analgesia, but unremitting pain may indicate a more sinister cause and merits further investigation.

Dental disease is referred to the distribution of the trigeminal nerve. In general, upper jaw disease is referred to the maxillary division and lower jaw disease to the mandibular division. The etiology of such pain is usually obvious, but continued facial pain may merit referral to a maxillofacial surgeon. Examination of the patient with facial pain includes assessment of the teeth and a search for tooth sensitivity with percussion.

VASCULAR DISORDERS AND HEADACHE

Giant cell arteritis

(See also Chapter 72)

This condition is rare below the age of 50 years, with incidence rising 10-fold between the sixth and ninth decades. The reported incidence of the condition has risen in recent decades, possibly because of raised awareness. Population-based studies suggest that up to 40% to 60% of patients have polymyalgia rheumatica in addition to giant cell arteritis.[147] The female-to-male ratio is approximately 4:1, and the prevalence varies from 7 per 100,000 in 50-year-olds to 70 per 100,000 in octogenarians.[148] The reported rates are highest in Scandinavian countries and lower in Mediterranean and Asian countries, and there is an association of HLA-DRB1*04.[149] Headache is the most common symptom (85% at some point in the disease).[150] It is usually severe, *persistent*, may throb, and disturbs sleep. The pain is usually bitemporal but may be unilateral, frontal, or generalized. Scalp tenderness is common, and patients may avoid grooming the hair. Jaw claudication (facial pain when chewing) is virtually pathognomonic of this condition and may affect up to half of patients,[151] and infarction of the tongue can follow. Vascular claudication may affect the arms and even the muscles of deglutition. Patients may report a number of constitutional symptoms such as fatigue and malaise, lethargy, anorexia, and a low-grade fever. Weight loss and sweating are common.

Sudden visual loss may affect up to 20% of cases and is an early manifestation.[152,153] This is a result of ischemia of the posterior ciliary arteries (and less commonly ischemia of the retinal artery) and secondary ischemic optic neuropathy, or infarction of the choroid. Patients may complain of nonpainful amaurosis fugax, a shade covering the eye, sudden total visual loss, or transient diplopia. Left untreated, the second eye usually becomes affected within 1 to 2 weeks. Interestingly, patients with optic complications had lower clinical and laboratory markers of inflammation, were less likely to be anemic, and were more likely to be HLA-DRB1*04 positive.[154] Patients who have other ischemic complications were more likely to experience retinal ischemia.

Giant cell arteritis affects the proximal aorta and its extracranial arteries (i.e., large and medium-sized muscular arteries with a prominent internal elastic membrane and vasa vasorum. The inflammation is most severe at the junction of the intima and media of vessels, disrupting the elastic lamina. Intradural vessels do not have a lamina, so intracranial inflammation is rarely seen.[155] The affected vessels become nodular, tortuous, and swollen. The superficial temporal artery may become palpable, tender, and pulseless. There is medial necrosis with formation of granulomatous tissue and invasion of lymphocytes and giant cells. Often there is thrombosis of the lumen.

Although temporal artery biopsy remains the gold standard, unfortunately the pathology is not continuous, and "skip lesions" mean that there is a good chance that a temporal artery biopsy will be negative. A minimum biopsy length of 1 cm can help to minimize the risk of false negatives.[156] Although a biopsy is desirable, treatment should not be delayed in clinically suspicious cases; biopsy specimens may show changes even 2 weeks after initiation of steroid treatment.[157]

The sedimentation rate is a vital diagnostic test but can be normal in up to 10% of cases.[158–160] C-reactive protein is believed to be a more sensitive indicator of disease activity in giant cell arteritis, although ESR remains the time-honored marker.[161] Nonspecific abnormalities include a mild normochromic normocytic anemia and leukocytosis. Plasma fibrinogen levels are elevated, as are other acute-phase proteins. Liver function tests are often abnormal, with an elevated alkaline phosphatase and elevated transaminases. An elevated creatine phosphokinase does not occur and should lead to a search for an alternative diagnosis.

If clinical suspicion is high, the patient should be commenced on high-dose corticosteroids immediately because failure to act may cost the patient loss of vision. Prednisolone (60 to 80 mg) is given usually with rapid clinical effect. Failure of the symptoms to respond within 24 to 48 hours should lead to review of the diagnosis. This high dose is maintained for 2 to 4 weeks and then tapered gradually (by a maximum of 10% of the total daily dose every 2 weeks) depending on the sedimentation rate and the patient's symptoms. Alternate day steroid regimens are associated with a higher treatment failure rate and should be avoided.[162] The addition of nonsteroidal anti-inflammatory drugs (NSAIDs) can reduce minor recurrent symptoms.[163] Patients will need treatment for many months and most for several years; relapse is most common in the first year after stopping steroids, especially when the dose is reduced to 5 to 10 mg daily.[164,165] After stopping treatment, the patient's sedimentation rate and symptoms should be monitored for at least 6 months to a year in case of relapse. Visual loss because of a relapse is unusual after a lengthy course of steroids. Osteoporosis prophylaxis may be necessary. There is some evidence from retrospective studies that combining low-dose aspirin with steroid therapy (where there is no contraindication, and with a proton-pump inhibitor) may lower the risk of ischemic complications, even though thromboembolic occlusion is not thought to be the cause.[166,167]

Any elderly person with malaise, arthralgia, depression, and vague headache should be considered a possible case until proven otherwise.

Cerebrovascular disease and hypertension

Headache is a common accompaniment to cerebrovascular disease[168,169] and may occur before, during, or after transient ischemic attack or stroke. The pain is often throbbing in nature and exacerbated with effort. Usually it is lateralized to the side of ischemia. It occurs most frequently when there is parenchymal hemorrhage (57%) but also with TIAs (36%), thromboembolic infarct (29%), and lacunar infarction (17%). It appeared that posterior circulation events (44%) were more frequently associated with headache than anterior circulation events (31%).[170] This study was before the computed tomography (CT) era, so it may be that hemorrhagic strokes were included in the data. A more recent study, however, reached similar conclusions.[171]

Headache does not occur more frequently in the hypertensive than in the normotensive general population unless it is of extreme degree or associated with rapid rises of blood pressure, as in pheochromocytoma.[172] Occasionally, however, migraine has undoubtedly been aggravated by the occurrence of hypertension.

Carotid and vertebral artery dissection

Extracranial arterial dissection is a more common cause of stroke and headache in younger persons, but it remains a cause of headache and cerebrovascular ischemia in the elderly. The anterior circulation is more commonly affected.[173] Carotid artery dissection and occlusion give rise to ipsilateral pain involving the face and forehead and occasionally the neck. The pain is described as burning or throbbing but can be sudden and stabbing and may be mistaken for subarachnoid hemorrhage (discussed later). A Horner's syndrome may be present ipsilateral to the involved artery, with contralateral neurologic signs. Occasionally there are no associated neurologic signs.

Vertebral artery dissection is associated with neck and occipital pain[174] and may occur more commonly than is thought in patients diagnosed with so-called vertebrobasilar insufficiency. The occipital headache associated with this form of dissection is almost always associated with neurologic deficits from the brain stem. The treatment of arterial dissection remains controversial as there is yet no solid evidence base to favor either antiplatelet or anticoagulant treatment, and in the elderly the risks of treatment are more prescient.[175]

Subarachnoid hemorrhage

Intracerebral aneurysms are usually silent except when aneurysms cause compression of neural structures to produce focal signs and headache or when they rupture. The sudden, severe catastrophic headache of subarachnoid hemorrhage is easily diagnosed, and in the elderly patient the prognosis is usually poo.[176] Patients with thunderclap headache should be investigated for the possibility of aneurysmal bleed. An early CT scan should be undertaken; if that is negative, a lumbar puncture delayed to 12 hours after the ictus should be undertaken to exclude xanthochromia. Elderly patients respond potentially well to endovascular treatment.[177,178]

Chronic subdural hemorrhage

This condition usually presents in an insidious manner and a history of head trauma may be absent or forgotten. The history may be one of fluctuating awareness, headache, memory disturbance, gait and balance problems, focal weakness, and a host of other nonspecific symptoms. Coagulopathy, particularly with a background of excessive alcohol consumption, is a well-recognized predisposing factor. Particular attention to the possibility of this diagnosis should be paid to those taking anticoagulants and, to a lesser extent, antiplatelet drugs. Brain imaging, either CT or MRI, is undertaken, and large symptomatic hematomas are usually evacuated, but smaller hematomas may be left and the patient's neurologic state monitored clinically. The resolution of the hematoma is reviewed by serial scans.

Headache associated with trauma

Between 9% and 14% of those admitted to head injury units are over 65 years of age, and this group has the worst prognosis.[179] Headache after injury, sometimes apparently trivial, is a common complaint, but persistence of headache usually indicates a psychogenic component. CT brain scan should be reserved for those with focal signs or fluctuating consciousness. Simple analgesia should be used, but resistant headache may require psychological management and the use of psychotropic drugs.

INTRACRANIAL TUMORS

(See also Chapter 55)

Although headache is present in 60% of those with an intracranial tumor,[180] it has to be reported as the sole presenting symptom in only 8% to 20% of patients of all age groups,[181,182] and only 10% of elderly patients had headache in one series.[183] In a retrospective study from a large neurosurgical cohort of patients with primary and secondary headache, only 2% had headache without any other symptoms.[180] As in most age groups, the most common intracranial mass lesions in the elderly population are secondary tumors. Some tumors may grow to a large size in the elderly before symptoms and signs are evident; this is attributed to the increased space within the cranium secondary to cerebral atrophy. The mechanism of headache in brain tumors is thought to be due to rises in intracranial pressure.

The typical features of raised intracranial pressure are the same in the elderly population as in all age groups: morning headache, vomiting, visual obscurations, or gradual visual loss. Coughing, straining, or bending forward may exacerbate the headache. There may be incontinence, gait disturbance, and cognitive decline. Papilledema is often absent. Stretching of pain-sensitive structures such as the dura may cause persistent focal headache; only infratentorial tumors seemed to be more likely to cause localized headache (occipital headache). Most supratentorial parenchymal tumors tend to produce poorly localized headache and not infrequently can mimic primary headache such as tension headache and migraine. Indeed, headache was more likely to be present with tumor if there was a history of preexisting headache (e.g., tension-type headache).[180] Thus, further investigation including a brain scan may be indicated in an elderly patient whenever there is recent onset of head pain syndrome or a change in pattern of preexistent headache.[184] Headache persisting for more than 6 months is unlikely to have a structural cause. However, rarely, pituitary tumors, which distort the sella turcica, can cause long-term headache, which is often deep-seated and retro-orbital.

The most common benign primary brain tumors are meningiomas, which are usually operable with good result in the otherwise fit elderly patient where there is headache or other symptoms and signs referable to the tumor. Asymptomatic meningiomas can be managed conservatively if monitored regularly.

LOW-PRESSURE HEADACHE SYNDROME

Orthostatic headache is most commonly seen after lumbar puncture, but the syndrome of spontaneous cerebrospinal fluid (CSF) leak and low-pressure headache is well recognized if often clinically overlooked. It may be a cause of chronic daily headache, especially when the initial orthostatic headache pattern has either evolved or been forgotten. It is less common in the elderly population[185–191] and may be associated with a variety of symptoms, including pain or stiffness of the neck, nausea, emesis, change in hearing, visual blurring, interscapular pain, and occasionally facial numbness or weakness and upper limb radicular symptoms.[192] The most common site of the leak is in the spine around the point at which the spinal nerve roots pierce the dura, usually in the thoracic and cervicothoracic regions. Magnetic resonance imaging (MRI) may show diffuse pachymeningeal enhancement; subdural and epidural collections may be seen. The management is conservative in the first instance; rarely, blood patches may be required to provide relief.

DRUG-INDUCED HEADACHE

Drugs causing headache

A large number of the drugs prescribed for elderly people cause headache (Table 60-3). The pain is usually described as involving the whole head, but it may be occipital or frontal.

Table 60-3. Drugs That Can Cause Headache

Calcium-channel blockers	Nitrates
Indomethacin	Dipyridamole
Lithium	Corticosteroids
Hydralazine	Sympathomimetics
Monoamine oxidase inhibitors	Cimetidine
Ranitidine	Theophyllines

Medication-misuse headache

Medication overuse headache is the third most common form of headache worldwide after tension-type headache and migraine, affecting up to 1% of the world's population and accounting for 5% to 10% of patients attending headache clinics.[193–195] The overuse of analgesics—particularly codeine-containing compounds and ergotamine—can lead to the development of chronic refractory headache, which then increases dependence on medication. Patients with initially intermittent migraine or tension-type headache may develop chronic daily headache because of analgesic abuse. These patients have higher depression scores, and attempted discontinuation leads to withdrawal symptoms and a refractoriness to prophylactic treatments.[196] Side effects of the medication are also more likely—such as ergotism, analgesic nephropathy, and gastrointestinal problems. Patients with migraine and tension-type headache who take analgesics for other conditions such as arthritis are more likely to develop rebound headache.[197]

The only option is to stop the analgesics, although this almost inevitably precipitates a temporary worsening of the headaches. Prevention of the syndrome in the first place should involve patient and physician education.[83] Patients with severe headache may need to be admitted for drug withdrawal and given temporary cover with opiates and steroids along with instigation of antidepressant therapy and consideration of migraine prophylaxis.[198,199]

HEADACHE AND THE EYE

The eye and orbit derive a rich innervation from the first division of the trigeminal nerve, and these structures are common causes of pain around the eye and of headache.[200]

In the elderly population, glaucoma can be an important cause of eye pain and headache. Although the condition may be acute or chronic, it is the acute closed-angle glaucoma that causes sudden onset of severe constant pain, centered on the affected eye. This may spread to give a generalized headache, and there are visual symptoms such as colored haloes in the visual field and misting of vision. There may be photophobia and nausea or vomiting. Patients may be diagnosed as suffering from subarachnoid hemorrhage unless the history or signs of eye disease are discovered. Clinically there is limbic injection, corneal edema (hazy appearance), and the globe will be hard and tender to palpation. This condition is an emergency that requires immediate referral to an ophthalmic casualty department for further treatment. Opiate analgesia will be necessary.

Proptosis, ophthalmoplegia, and pain can be caused by orbital pseudotumor.[201,202] Often there is an elevated sedimentation rate and a rapid response to high-dose corticosteroids. The differential diagnosis includes dysthyroid eye disease, or orbital neoplasia (secondary spread from, for example, melanoma). Superior orbital fissuritis (Tolosa-Hunt syndrome)[203] is one end of the spectrum of orbital inflammatory disease. MRI of the skull or CT of the skull should differentiate between these conditions, but often the response to steroids aids the diagnosis.[204–206]

Painful oculomotor paresis with retro-orbital pain is usually due to one of two main pathologies. If the pupil is fixed and dilated, then a surgical cause is likely, with aneurysm of the posterior communicating artery being the most common cause. If the pupil reacts to light, then the cause is likely to be nonsurgical and diabetes is the most likely cause. Angiography may still be necessary to rule out aneurysm even if the blood sugar is elevated.

Anterior uveitis and posterior uveitis are also causes of eye pain and visual disturbance. There may be evidence of coexistent systemic pathology, and the presence of local ocular changes help aid the diagnosis. Refractive disorders (so-called eye strain) rarely cause headache. Orbital pain may arise from entrapment of the greater occipital nerve as it emerges from between the occiput and first cervical vertebra. Pain usually starts in the occipital region and radiates forward to the eye, although it may be isolated to the orbit. Treatment is symptomatic and should include physiotherapy, appropriate use of analgesia, and limited use of a soft collar.

MISCELLANEOUS CAUSES OF HEAD PAIN

The hypnic headache syndrome was first described by Raskin[207] and reviewed by Evers and Goadsby.[208] It is an uncommon form of headache occurring only in the elderly population. Headaches wake the patient from sleep at a regular time each night. The headaches are usually ill defined, may have a pulsating quality, and may occur several times a month. They may last from half an hour to a few hours and recur the same night. There are no associated autonomic symptoms. Diagnostic criteria have been proposed.[208] Polysomnography has shown that this is a REM sleep disorder. This disorder is rarely associated with secondary pathology,[209] but the differential diagnosis includes mass lesions, temporal arteritis, and cluster headache, although the latter is characterized by additional autonomic features. Lithium carbonate has the best efficacy but is limited by its pronounced side effects in the elderly.[208] Caffeine, flunarizine, and indomethacin may also be useful, as so may low-dose topiramate.[210]

The *exploding head syndrome*[211] is another benign cause of disturbance experienced more commonly by elderly people but that may affect any age group.[212] It is not a pain or headache but a loud noise occurring in sleep or drowsiness and waking the patient. It may occur for a short period of weeks or months on an infrequent basis or recur irregularly. The noise is deep in the center or back of the head and causes fear in the patient. Some may describe momentary difficulty in breathing, tachycardia, or sweating. There are no sequelae, and usually patients do not have a preceding illness or history of neurologic disease. The etiology of the condition is unknown, and it is almost certainly underreported. Reassurance is usually all that is required. There is a limited report of successful use of clomipramine in three cases.[213]

About a third of patients with Parkinson's disease report occipital headache, usually dull in nature. The cause of this is not clear, and it is not associated with nuchal rigidity.[214] Amitriptyline in low doses may be effective.[215]

Infections, whether bacterial or viral, may be associated with headache. Chronic meningitis may cause headache and be associated with gait disorder secondary to hydrocephalus. Multiple cranial nerve involvement may be associated with basal meningeal involvement as seen in carcinomatous meningitis, tuberculosis, and sarcoidosis. Systemic metabolic causes of headache include hypoglycemia of less than 2.2 mmol/L, renal dialysis, hypercalcemia, and severe anemia.[216] Carbon monoxide poisoning from poorly ventilated gas appliances may be an insidious cause of chronic headache and nonspecific symptoms.[217,218] Sleep-disordered breathing may be associated with headache, commonly on waking.

Headaches associated with sleep may arise because of a medical comorbidity such as obstructive sleep apnea syndrome and can be evaluated with an appropriate history from a sleeping partner and polysomnography.[219,220] Primary headache disorders such as migraine, cluster headache and chronic paroxysmal hemicrania may also cause sleep-related headache and headache on waking, but a careful history will identify these and exclude complicating factors such as medication overuse and mood disorder. Such conditions are easily treated with appropriate medication.[221]

THE DIAGNOSTIC APPROACH TO HEADACHE

As in any branch of medicine, the diagnosis rests heavily on the history of the complaint and use of appropriate investigations after a thorough physical examination. The duration of symptoms and their mode of onset together with the tempo of their development provide valuable diagnostic clues. Quality of headache is a less useful feature, but patients should be asked about position and intensity together with radiation of the pain and the presence of exacerbating and relieving factors. A complete drug history should be obtained, and appraisal of the patient's mood, sleep, and vegetative functions are helpful for discerning the impact of the illness and possible psychological background.

Although the vast majority of headaches in all age groups are benign, in the elderly population the risk of organic pathology is increased.[12] The diversity of symptoms of temporal arteritis can often lead to a delay in diagnosis. Chronic malaise, myalgia, and arthralgia are frequently seen in giant cell arteritis but easily dismissed as nonspecific symptoms and resulting from the aging process. Severe pain of sudden onset, pain that is persistent and progressively worsening with time, early morning headache with vomiting, and exacerbation by coughing, straining, and bending forward all suggest underlying organic disease. Migraine can be identified when there is a long history or classic symptoms, but complicated migraine may be difficult to differentiate from TIAs[35] and complete investigation is warranted. This is particularly because migrainous accompaniments are more common in the older age group. The presence of other symptoms such as drowsiness, confusion, and memory loss will raise the index of suspicion. Other worrying symptoms include progressive visual disturbance, weakness, clumsiness, and loss of balance. It is important to realize that the cranial neuralgias are not associated in their simple form with neurologic deficits and have a strict definition for a positive diagnosis. The description of bands of pain or a tight cap on the head is more likely to result from muscle tension as seen in a tension-type headache or disease of the neck, but it can be a symptom of a more serious disease. Injury to the head may precede the formation of a subdural hematoma, which is more likely with coagulopathy or chronic alcohol abuse. Brachialgia together with myelopathy should point to the neck as the source of headache.

A normal neurologic examination will often help rule out serious underlying disease and avoid unnecessary investigations. A lower threshold for investigation should apply in the case of the elderly patient complaining of headache.

Summary of Management Algorithm Headache

Indications for Investigation

New headache with:

- Abnormal neurologic signs
- A history suggesting raised intracranial pressure
- Impairment of memory
- Impairment of consciousness
- Worsening pain which may disturb sleep
- Headache on waking and associated with vomiting

Apparent "late-onset" migraine
Atypical facial pain

- Migraine

Avoid easily identified triggers
Bedrest
Analgesia

- Paracetamol or aspirin
- NSAIDs (beware peptic and renal side effects)
- Triptans for moderate to severe headache
- Antiemetics if required

Prophylaxis

- β-blockers
- Tricyclic antidepressants
- Topirimate/valproate
- Serotonin antagonists (e.g., pizotifen)
- Tension-type headache

  Reassurance after careful clinical assessment.
  Simple analgesia.
  Address possible psychological issues.
  Treat depression if identified (tricyclics useful).
  Question relaxation therapy and biofeedback.
  Avoid chronic analgesic use, which can lead to the syndrome of chronic daily headache.

- Trigeminal neuralgia

This is diagnosed only on strict criteria.
Carbamazepine is still first line treatment.
Alternatives include baclofen, phenytoin, sodium valproate, clonazepam, gabapentin, and lamotrigine.
Up to 50% of patients may require surgical treatment.

- Postherpetic neuralgia

Up to 50% of elderly patients may develop this syndrome.
Amitriptyline and carbamazepine are both of proven benefit.
Gabapentin and pregabalin are licensed to treat this condition.

- Giant cell arteritis

This medical emergency requires swift initiation of steroids.
Jaw claudication is virtually pathognomonic.
Constitutional symptoms are common.
In up to 10% of cases, the sedimentation rate may be normal.

KEY POINTS

Headache and Facial Pain

- Headache is a common problem in the whole population. However, it is less often reported by elderly people in whom there is a decline in prevalence, although the symptom is more likely to represent serious pathology.
- Management of the common primary headache conditions is the same as for younger patients. Elderly people are more likely to have comorbidity that may limit their ability to tolerate medication or side effects resulting from drug interactions.
- A careful history of analgesic use, including proprietary analgesics, should be elicited in patients presenting with a chronic daily headache syndrome, as medication-overuse headache is common.
- Giant cell arteritis is a medical emergency and should be treated without delay if suspected.

For a complete list of references, please visit online only at www.expertconsult.com

CHAPTER 61

Stroke: Epidemiology and Pathology

Amanda G. Thrift
Velandai K. Srikanth

STROKE EPIDEMIOLOGY

The World Health Organization (WHO) defined stroke as "rapidly developing clinical signs of focal disturbance of cerebral function lasting more than 24 hours (unless interrupted by surgery or death) with no apparent cause other than of vascular origin." The major types of stroke are ischemic stroke (caused by a cerebral vessel occlusion) and hemorrhagic stroke (caused by bleeding from the cerebral vessel). Stroke epidemiology is concerned with the study of patterns and risk factors associated with stroke. This is important because it enables one to determine efficient strategies for stroke prevention. It also enables one to make predictions about the future burden of stroke. This can then be used for planning of future health care requirements.

In the following sections, we summarize the current knowledge about the epidemiology of stroke. In particular, we have focused on the burden of stroke including mortality, incidence, and prevalence, as well as known risk factors and prevention strategies. The pathology underlying strokes is briefly described.

Burden of stroke

From a population level, the burden of stroke can be measured in three different ways, each method having advantages and limitations (Table 61-1). Stroke mortality figures usually include all individuals with stroke recorded as the primary cause of death on their death certificates. Systematic and long-term collection of these data allows assessment of trends over time and comparisons between countries. Mortality figures are subject to some limitations including imprecision in death certification and incomplete assessment of the overall burden of stroke; between 45% and 60% of people with stroke survive beyond 5 years.[1–3] Prevalence studies can be used to assess burden in stroke survivors. Using methods such as door-to-door surveys, one can estimate the impact of stroke on survivors and assists with the planning of community health care resources.

Carefully conducted stroke incidence studies provide the best source of information on the burden of stroke at an individual and societal level. These allow a better understanding of the empirical relation between incidence, mortality, and survival. For example, changes in stroke mortality may be attributable to changes in stroke incidence, case-fatality, or a combination of both. Comparison between two identically conducted stroke incidence studies will help to determine where the changes have occurred. Worldwide, few of these studies have been conducted, largely because of the expense and labor-intensive nature in undertaking them using the strict "ideal" criteria for stroke incidence studies.[4–7] Because of this restraint, most of the incidence studies conducted using these criteria have been undertaken in developed countries.

It is estimated that more than 55 million people worldwide are survivors of stroke,[8] and more than half of these individuals are expected to have some form of stroke-related disability. This burden is likely to increase rapidly in the coming years, largely because of the increasing life expectancy.[9] This is because there is a strong positive relationship between age and stroke incidence.

Stroke mortality

There is some disagreement about whether stroke is the second or third most common cause of death worldwide. According to WHO, stroke is the second most common single cause of death in the world after ischemic heart disease.[10] However, if all cancers were grouped together, they would occupy second place. Regardless of the ranking, in 2002 an estimated 5.5 million deaths from stroke occurred worldwide; these deaths comprising approximately 9.7% of all deaths.[10] Approximately one third of these deaths occurred in developed countries; the remainder occurring in developing countries. The large number of stroke deaths occurring in developing countries is largely attributable to their large population (approximately 3.5-fold that of the population in developed countries). This is despite the fact that the mortality rate (number of deaths per 100,000 population per year) is lesser in developing countries (76.7/100,000/year) than in developed ones (130.5/100,000/year).[10,11]

The best data about changes in stroke mortality come from developed countries. Stroke mortality declined in many of these nations between the 1960s and the early 1990s,[12] although there was evidence of a leveling off of this decline in the 5-year period to 1994.[12–14] Countries with the lowest mortality rates, such as the United States, Canada, Switzerland, France, and Australia, tended to have the steepest declines. In contrast, in all countries that previously belonged to the former Soviet Union, stroke mortality increased among both men and women.[12] These differences in geographic variations are likely to reflect an influence of environmental factors on mortality. An example is the particularly large increase in mortality rate observed in the countries of the former Soviet Union during the 1990s, this being

Table 61-1. Methods for Assessing Stroke Burden

Method	Advantages	Limitations
Mortality	Allows study of time trends Allows comparisons between regions	Imprecision in death certification Only part of the overall burden
Prevalence	Assists in study of impact of stroke in survivors Enables health care resources planning for survivors	Time-consuming and expensive Only part of the overall burden
Incidence	Allows study of relation between incidence, prevalence, and mortality	Expensive Labor-intensive

a time of great political upheaval and economic uncertainty in this region.[12]

Changes in stroke mortality may reflect changes in incidence, case-fatality, or a combination of the two. In their analysis of time trend data from the World Health Organization Monitoring Trends and Determinants in Cardiovascular Disease (WHO MONICA) project, Sarti and colleagues provide preliminary evidence that case-fatality may underlie the observed changes in mortality.[15] They reported that in countries with increasing mortality from stroke, the increase was almost entirely attributable to an increase in case-fatality, whereas in countries where stroke mortality was declining, approximately two thirds were explained by a reduced case-fatality, the remainder being attributable to reduced stroke occurrence.[15] This analysis was limited to people aged 35 to 64 years, so it may not necessarily reflect what occurs among those in older age groups.

Stroke prevalence

A number of well-designed stroke prevalence studies have been conducted around the world. Stroke prevalence (per 100,000 population standardized to the world population aged more than 65 years) appears least in rural South Africa (1539/100,000), the United States (4536/100,000), and New Zealand (4872/100,000), whereas greater prevalence was evident in L'Aquila (Italy; 6812/100,000), Newcastle (United Kingdom; > 7000/100,000), and Singapore (7337/100,000).[16–19] Interestingly in Singapore, prevalence rates among Malays (5396/100,000) appeared less than those of Chinese (7829/100,000) or Indian (6,871/100,000) descent, although this was not statistically different.[19] Importantly, about half of these survivors of stroke are likely to require assistance in everyday activities. This places a great burden on family caregivers of stroke survivors and the health care system. Because a decline in case-fatality has been reported to account for two thirds of the decline in mortality in those countries where mortality is declining,[15] prevalence must be increasing. This increase in prevalence will result in an increase in the burden of stroke to those communities affected.

INCIDENCE OF STROKE AND STROKE SUBTYPES

Most incidence studies of stroke that have been conducted according to "ideal" criteria have been undertaken in developed nations, largely coming from Europe, Australia, and the Americas,[16,20–29] with Barbados being the only exception.[30] After adjusting to a common standard to eliminate variation attributable to demographic differences, there do appear to be some regional differences. When comparing incidence rates between regions, adjusted to the European population aged 45 to 84 years, the lowest incidence rates occurred in Dijon (238 per 100,000 population per year), whereas the greatest were in Russia (626/100,000/year) and the Ukraine (938/100,000/year).[31–33] The remaining studies exhibited similar incidence rates. There is a lack of studies from regions such as Africa and Asia.

Longitudinal trends in stroke incidence can be examined when ideal incidence studies have been repeated over successive time points using the same methods. Upon examination of these data, stroke incidence has declined significantly over the past few decades, particularly in the 1970s and 1980s,[25, 34–39] with some notable exceptions in Denmark, the United States, and Estonia.[40–42]

HETEROGENEITY OF STROKE

Stroke is a heterogeneous condition with three main subtypes each with differing incidence rates, risk factors, and outcomes. The most common, ischemic stroke (IS), accounts for between 63% to 84% of all strokes.[16] Depending on the study region, intracerebral hemorrhage (ICH) accounts for between 7% and 20% of all strokes, whereas subarachnoid hemorrhage (SAH) accounts for between 1% and 13% of all strokes.[16] The proportion of strokes that are hemorrhagic appear to be greater in nonwhite populations and among those living in developing countries compared with white populations in developed countries.[23,43–45] This suggests that there may be differences in risk factor prevalence or indeed genetic differences between white and nonwhite populations. Within the category of ischemic stroke, there are further subtypes that are based on clinical signs or have a mechanistic basis.[46,47] The most robust classification system for use in population-based epidemiologic studies is a system based on clinical findings devised by the investigators of the Oxfordshire Community Stroke Project.[47] The advantage of this classification system is that it is based on clinical findings, and there is no need to rely on expensive investigations that may be unavailable in some regions.

COSTS OF STROKE

On a societal level, stroke is responsible for a significant portion of formal health care costs; globally approximately 2% to 4% of total health care costs are attributable to stroke. The cost of stroke has been estimated by using a variety of "bottom up" and "top down" approaches in a number of Western countries. Using a bottom-up approach, the estimated 12-month cost of stroke in Australia in 1997 was US$420 million.[48] Acute hospitalization (28%) and inpatient rehabilitation (27%) comprised the majority of these costs. The average cost per case was US$14,361 during the first 12 months and US$33,658 over a lifetime, with overall lifetime costs being greater for ischemic stroke than for ICH.[48,49] With the expected increase in overall number of strokes, there is likely to be increased strain on health care systems.

There are also significant economic costs attributable to informal caregiving. Dewey et al[50] undertook an economic analysis to determine the total 12-month costs associated with informal care for first-ever strokes. They estimated that the total costs of informal care for first-ever strokes comprised between 4% and 7% of total stroke-related costs during the first year and between 14% and 23% of costs over a lifetime. This demonstrates the considerable burden placed on the families of people with stroke.

Risk factors for stroke

During the last half of the past century, a large number of major stroke risk factors were identified. These risk factors, and protective factors, may be modifiable or nonmodifiable (Table 61-2). There are some indications that the stroke risk factor profile in developing nations is not the same as in developed nations.[51] With this in mind, the following discussion relates to risk factors in developed nations.

Table 61-2. Risk Factors for Ischemic Stroke

Nonmodifiable Risk Factors	Modifiable Individual Risk Factors: Known	Modifiable Individual Risk Factors: Possible
Age	Hypertension	Physical inactivity
Gender	Smoking	Obesity
Heart disease	Diabetes	Dietary factors
Family history	Atrial fibrillation	Oral contraceptive use
Ethnicity	Hypercholesterolemia	Lack of hormone replacement therapy
Socioeconomic status	Prior transient ischemic attack or stroke	Infection
	Heavy alcohol consumption	Stress
	Prothrombotic factors	Air pollution
	Hyperhomocysteinemia	Depression
	C-reactive protein (inflammation)	Subclinical atherosclerosis

NONMODIFIABLE RISK FACTORS

Nonmodifiable risk factors are those that cannot be altered by intervention. These include factors such as advancing age, male gender, ethnicity, socioeconomic status, family history and genetic conditions. Age is strongly associated with stroke incidence, with incidence rising from between 10 to 30 per 100,000 person-years aged less than 45, to 1200 to 2000 per 100,000 person-years in those aged 75 to 84 years.[16] Within each age group, stroke incidence is greater among men than women.[20,52] In the older age groups, however, the overall number of strokes is often greater in women than men simply because of the larger number of women surviving to these ages. People living in more disadvantaged regions have been reported to have a greater incidence of stroke. Those living in the most disadvantaged areas of Melbourne, Australia, had incidence rates of stroke that were almost double (366/100,000/year) that of those living in the least disadvantaged areas (200/100,000/year).[53] Similar differences have been seen in other parts of the world, including Sweden[54] and the United Kingdom,[55,56] although in some studies it is unclear whether differences are attributable to ethnicity rather than socioeconomic status.

MODIFIABLE RISK FACTORS

Modifiable risk factors are those factors that can be altered through either treatment or by changes in behavior. By reducing the prevalence of these risk factors, it is therefore possible to reduce the incidence or reoccurrence of the disease. Such established and modifiable risk factors include hypertension, smoking, diabetes, and atrial fibrillation. There are also other less well-established risk factors and protective factors including alcohol consumption, regular exercise, obesity, oral contraception, hormone replacement, and illicit drug use. It is possible that such risk factors interact with each other in many different ways in contributing to the risk of stroke rather than being independent of each other. Such interactions may be different between different age groups.

Hypertension, a condition that is highly prevalent with increasing age, is one of the most clearly recognized and probably the most important risk factor for stroke at a population level. In a meta-analysis of about 13,000 strokes in 450,000 people, prospective cohorts undertaken to assess the influence of diastolic blood pressure on the risk of stroke, the authors showed that for each 10 mm Hg increase in diastolic blood pressure the risk of stroke increased almost two fold with a relative risk of 1.84 (95% confidence interval [CI] 1.80–1.90).[57] In the same collaborative study, the strength of the association between usual blood pressure and risk of death from stroke was shown to decline to some extent with increasing age. However, stroke is so much more common in old age than in middle age that the absolute annual difference in stroke death associated with a given difference in blood pressure increases with increasing age. Atrial fibrillation is associated with a high stroke risk and accounts for a major part of the population-attributable risk of stroke, particularly in older age. In the Framingham study, the risk attributable to atrial fibrillation increased significantly from 1.5% for those aged 50 to 59 years to 23.5% for those aged 80 to 89 years.[58] Diabetes mellitus may be responsible for up to 20% of the population-attributable risk fraction in the developed world.[58] However, it is uncertain whether the risk attributable to diabetes mellitus or other factors such as dyslipidemia changes significantly with increasing age.

Numerous studies have been undertaken to assess the association between smoking and stroke.[59] Evidence for an association between smoking and the risk of stroke is strengthened by the demonstration of a positive dose-response relationship. In addition, smoking cessation is associated with a reduced risk of stroke when compared with current smoking. In the Honolulu Heart Program, smokers who continued to smoke at the sixth year of follow-up were at an increased risk of stroke, whereas those who had ceased smoking at the sixth year of follow-up showed a reduced risk of stroke.[60] This provides some further support that smokers can reduce their risk of ischemic stroke after ceasing smoking.

People at high risk of stroke often have multiple risk factors. This is important because some risk factors interact, resulting in greatly increased risk of stroke. Important interactions have been shown to occur between transient ischemic attacks and age, hypertension and age, and cigarette smoking and age; all risk factors have shown a declining risk of stroke with increasing age. An interaction has also been observed between atrial fibrillation, hypertension, and age: hypertension potentiated the risk of stroke among those with intermittent atrial fibrillation, and this declined with age.[61] People with hypertension who also smoke have also shown a potentiation in the risk of stroke.[62]

The increasing burden of stroke

Current projections support the notion of a large increase in the future number of strokes occurring in both developed and developing countries. In Australia, it is estimated that the number of stroke occurring in Australia will more than double over the next 25 years, even assuming that incidence remains the same.[63] In developed countries, this increase is largely attributable to an aging population. In developing countries, the population is also aging; however, an epidemiologic transition is also occurring.[64] With an increased availability of clean water, food, shelter, and medical care, life expectancy increased from 41.2 years in 1951–1961 to 61.4 years in 1991–1996.[65] Thus, more individuals are now reaching ages where stroke more commonly occurs. In parallel, there is rapid industrialization and urbanization, which has resulted in significant dietary changes and increases in

Table 61-3. Relative Population Impact of Treating Selected Risk Factors for Ischemic Stroke

Risk Factor	Prevalence	Relative Risk (range)	Relative Impact
Hypertension	~ 20% men ~ 15% women	2.5–8.0	High
Atrial fibrillation:			
aged ≥ 40 years	~ 2.0%	2.0–6.0	High in older age groups with additional risk factors
aged ≥ 65 years	~ 5.0%		
men aged ≥ 75 years	~ 10%		
women aged ≥ 75 years	~ 6.0%		
Smoking	~ 25% men ~ 20% women	1.5–6.0	High
Hypercholesterolemia*	~ 15% men ~ 15% women	1.5	Low
Diabetes	~ 5%	1.5–4.0	Low
Heavy alcohol consumption†	~ 2.5%	2.0–2.5	Low

*Hypercholesterolemia is defined as a plasma cholesterol level of ≥ 6.5 mmol/liter.
†Heavy alcohol consumption is defined as drinking on average ≥ 5 standard drinks per day.

smoking prevalence.[66–69] Diets containing more meat and dairy products, processed grains, and added sugar are associated with increases in blood pressure, serum cholesterol levels, and body weight. Combined, these factors are likely to result in increases in stroke incidence in the future.

Prevention of stroke

If the impending increase in burden of stroke is to be minimized, or even reduced, prevention strategies must be improved considerably. The main aim of primary and secondary prevention strategies for stroke is to reduce stroke incidence and reoccurrence. The effectiveness of prevention strategies is influenced by three important characteristics of each risk factor for stroke: whether the risk factor is modifiable, the strength of the association, and the prevalence of the risk factor in the population. The strength of the association is indicated by the relative risk or odds ratio of the exposure variable. Higher relative risks indicate stronger associations. The prevalence of a risk factor is the proportion of people within the population in whom the factor is present. The more common the risk factor within the population, the greater is its prevalence. Together, the relative risk and prevalence give an indication of how useful these factors are as targets for prevention strategies (Table 61-3).

Declines in stroke incidence and mortality have largely been attributed to improvements in the primary prevention of stroke. Both the introduction of blood pressure lowering agents with increasing efficacy and improvement in living standards provide plausible explanations for these declines. The Oxford Vascular Study investigators reported significant decreases in systolic and diastolic blood pressure, cholesterol levels, and prevalence of smoking during the 20-year interval in which incidence rates of stroke were seen to decline by 29%.[25] More modest declines in incidence among more recent studies may reflect the fact that other risk factors, such as an aging population, obesity, and diabetes mellitus, may be on the rise despite aggressive approaches to reducing hypertension, hypercholesterolemia, and smoking.[39]

Mass approach

The mass or population approach to prevention involves changing risk factors at a population level. This may involve media and education campaigns to alter risky behaviors on a population basis, or it may involve the use of government legislation. This approach may result in an overall small reduction in the risk factor on an individual basis, but it may have a significant impact on the whole population.

Reducing blood pressure levels within the population is an important strategy for reducing stroke risk. This could be achieved by a number of means including reducing salt intake and promoting exercise. It is estimated that people consume on average approximately two to three times more salt than is recommended.[70] Reducing salt intake by half would reduce blood pressure in both hypertensive and normotensive individuals[71] and is also estimated to reduce stroke incidence by 22%[72] and stroke mortality by up to 25%.[73] Eighty percent of the salt we consume is hidden within processed foods, thus reducing the amount of salt added to food during manufacture would have an enormous public health impact.[74] A reduction in only 20% of the salt content of processed foods could lead to a significant drop in blood pressure levels in the population. Encouraging governments to legislate such changes within the food industry remains a major barrier. Other cost-effective population-wide prevention strategies may be tobacco and alcohol control via increased taxation and the regulation of accessibility, and promotion of healthy diets and exercise. Because geriatricians, more than many other specialties, are used to taking a population perspective and to patient advocacy, they—and their specialty societies—may find a role in advocating for changes in food processing or better city and building design to come easily.

High-risk approach

The high-risk individual approach involves identifying people at high risk of stroke and either introducing treatment strategies or minimizing risky behaviors. People may be identified through mass screening campaigns or through opportunistic screening during other health consultations. People could be encouraged to cease smoking, introduce exercise, or reduce alcohol or fat intake. Risk factors could also be modified in high-risk individuals by treatment with medications, such as antihypertensive agents to reduce blood pressure levels or use of lipid lowering drugs to reduce cholesterol levels.

In a meta-analysis conducted by the Blood Pressure Lowering Treatment Trialists' Collaboration, people treated with antihypertensive medication had a 28% to 38% lower incidence of stroke, depending on the medication used.[75] Although improvements have been made in the identification and treatment of hypertension, significant improvements in both of these areas still need to be made, particularly in developing regions.[76]

Another high-risk approach is to target people who have already had a stroke, as these individuals are at increased risk of stroke recurrence. Among those who survive an initial stroke, up to 20% suffer another event within 5 years.[77] Controlling hypertension can reduce the incidence of recurrent stroke by up to 28%.[78] Furthermore, this reduction in risk has been observed in both normotensive and hypertensive individuals with stroke.[79] Other prevention strategies that have demonstrated effectiveness in those with a previous stroke include the use of antiplatelet agents, such as aspirin, dipyridamole, ticlopidine, or clopidogrel, and the use of anticoagulants in people with atrial fibrillation.

COMBINED APPROACH TO PREVENTION

To maximize the prevention of stroke, a combined approach to prevention should be used. This includes population and high-risk primary prevention approaches, as well as targeting those who have already had a stroke (secondary stroke prevention). The high-risk approach may involve screening patients for particular risk factors opportunistically and then providing treatment for those individuals at high risk. To complement this strategy, the population approach should also be utilized. This might be achieved by educating people via mass media campaigns or by government legislation.

PATHOLOGIC MECHANISMS UNDERLYING STROKE

Ischemic stroke

CEREBRAL VESSEL OCCLUSION

Atherosclerosis is by far the most common cause of cerebral infarction caused by large and medium vessel disease and is mediated by thrombotic and embolic complications. Atherosclerosis is an almost universal feature of large and medium-sized arteries in elderly people and is most severe in the aortic arch and at points of bifurcation (e.g., carotid bifurcation) and confluence (e.g., basilar artery). At least in large extracranial vessels, thrombus tends to complicate the ruptured or eroded "unstable" atherosclerotic plaque.[80] Such plaques are characterized by a large necrotic core covered by a thin, inflamed fibrous cap similar to coronary arterial plaque.[81] Exposure of the thrombogenic plaque core causes activation of platelets and triggering of the coagulation cascade. The resulting thrombus either occludes the vessel in situ or, more commonly, probably dislodges as embolus and occludes a distal smaller vessel. Rupture of unstable plaques appears to be less common in intracranial vessels, where atherosclerosis may more commonly mediate stroke by low-flow effects or by acting as luminal narrowings at which emboli impact. On occasion, intracranial or extracranial vessel occlusion may occur as a result of dissection of the lumen, the most commonly seen sites being the vertebral and the carotid arteries.

Small, deep (lacunar) infarcts are likely to be due to two important causes.[82] The first is small vessel arteriolosclerosis, and the second is a complex destructive lesion of small arteries ("lipohyalinosis") characterized in the acute phase by fibrinoid necrosis and a healed phase characterised by loss of wall architecture, collagenous sclerosis, and mural foam cells.[82] The pathogenesis of lipohyalinosis is uncertain, but it may be linked to inherited and acquired disorders of small vessel tone.[83]

Ischemic strokes crossing arterial boundaries may occur because of cerebral venous sinus thromboses. Cerebral veins and venous sinuses may become thrombosed when a variety of constitutive and acquired factors, both local and systemic, promote hypercoagulability or venous stasis.[84] However, in many cases the pathogenesis is uncertain.

CONSEQUENCES OF VESSEL OCCLUSION

The size, shape, and location of occlusive arterial infarcts conform more or less to individual arterial supply zones, variations dependent on interindividual differences in vascular anatomy, adequacy of collaterals, preexisting vascular disease, and other factors. Hemorrhagic transformation of initially pale ischemic infarcts is relatively common following lysis, either spontaneous or therapeutic, of thromboemboli.[85] Bleeding may be severe enough to mimic a primary intracerebral hemorrhage.[86] The distribution of infarction in global cerebral circulatory insufficiency is diverse but commonly involves spinal as well as cerebral arterial border zones and selectively vulnerable brain regions such as the CA1 zone of the hippocampus, neocortical layers 3, 5, and 6, cerebellar Purkinje cells, and basal ganglia.[86,87] Venous infarcts characteristically do not conform to arterial supply zones and are often accompanied by subarachnoid and intracerebral hemorrhage and massive brain swelling.

Irrespective of size or location, brain infarcts are areas of ischemic coagulative necrosis of all cellular elements, ultimately becoming fluid-filled cavities.[88] Temporary or less severe ischemia may produce areas of so-called incomplete infarction,[89] characterized by death of only the most vulnerable cells, in particular neurons, representing perhaps a neuropathologic substrate of transient ischemic attacks.[90] The ultimate fate of affected brain depends not only on the severity and duration of ischemia but also on how selectively vulnerable is the region and its component neurons and on the degree and duration of reperfusion ("delayed neuronal death").[91] In humans, cerebral blood flow must fall from an average normal value of about 50 mL 100 g^{-1} min^{-1} to 18 to 20 mL 100 g^{-1} min^{-1} before neurons become electrically silent and to 8–9 mL 100 g^{-1} min^{-1} before neuronal ion pumps fail.[92] The marginal zone of brain around the doomed ischemic core has cerebral blood flow levels between these thresholds of synaptic transmission and membrane failure. This "penumbra," nonfunctional yet viable, is the focus of potential therapeutic salvage.[93] Better understanding of the cascade of ischemic neuronal damage[94] may yet provide effective stroke therapy targets, and it is increasingly speculated that the future of stroke treatment lies in rapidly instituted combination therapy with thrombolytic, neuroprotective, and ultimately perhaps regenerative/trophic agents.

Hemorrhagic stroke

CAUSES OF VESSEL RUPTURE

The most common type of hemorrhagic stroke remains the classic spontaneous "hypertensive" hemorrhage, characteristically in basal ganglia, thalamus, lobar white matter, cerebellum, and pons, in approximate descending order of frequency.[95] Their pathogenesis has been difficult to study, but circumstantial evidence points to the same, or closely related, lesion as that causing lacunar infarction[31] with which it colocalizes and shares a common risk factor profile. Thus, a destructive lesion characterized by fibrinoid necrosis and associated with hypertension is considered by many to be the underlying vascular lesion in most cases.[96] In elderly people, an increasingly recognized form of spontaneous brain hemorrhage is due to cerebral amyloid angiopathy, in which bleeds are classically lobar, superficial, and multiple.[97] The mechanism of amyloid-related bleeds, their relation to classic "hypertensive" bleeds, and the contribution of amyloid angiopathy to cognitive decline in Alzheimer's disease are ill understood.

The most common cause of isolated, spontaneous subarachnoid hemorrhage is rupture of a berry aneurysm, about 85% of which in adults occur at proximal arterial bifurcations on the anterior circle of Willis.[98] Their pathogenesis is disputed but appears to involve acquired degenerative tunica media defects at arterial branch points, sometimes in genetically predisposed individuals.

CONSEQUENCES OF VESSEL RUPTURE

Intracerebral hemorrhage is more often acutely fatal than ischemic stroke, largely because of its mass effect and the consequent potential for raised intracranial pressure and reduced cerebral perfusion. Hematomas, however, tend to dissect and separate brain tissue, with relatively less direct parenchymal damage. Therefore, should the patient survive and the hematoma be cleared by phagocytic cells to leave a blood-stained slit-like cavity, the prognosis for recovery may potentially be better than that for cerebral infarcts of similar size and location.

For a complete list of references, please visit online only at www.expertconsult.com

CHAPTER 62

Stroke: Clinical Presentation, Management and Organization of Services

Velandai K. Srikanth
Thanh G. Phan

INTRODUCTION

Stroke is the most common clinical manifestation of disease of cerebral blood vessels and thus falls under the broad category of *cerebrovascular disease*. Transient ischemic attacks (TIA) are harbingers of a particular type of stroke known as ischemic stroke. Other common subclinical manifestations of cerebrovascular disease include cerebral white matter lesions (WML) and "silent" brain infarcts. This chapter will primarily focus on stroke and TIA, with some emphasis on WML and silent infarcts, the management of which are uncertain at the present time.

Stroke and TIA are the leading cause of acute neurologic admissions to hospitals throughout the world, and tend to predominantly affect older people. The seriousness of stroke is underlined by the fact that it is the second leading single cause of death worldwide.[1] Approximately a third of stroke patients die within the first 6 months, and approximately 60% by 5 years after stroke.[2] Stroke also ranks as the sixth most important cause of disability among survivors.[3] With aging populations, it has been estimated that stroke will rank as the fourth most important cause of disability in the western world by the year 2030.[3] Older people are at greater risk of accumulating other age-related diseases and consequently greater frailty.[4] The impact of a stroke on such people with preexisting disability can be particularly devastating, often leading to a move from their home environment to residential care facilities.

Stroke is also an expensive disease in monetary and societal terms. In Australia, during the year 1997, the average cost per stroke patient was estimated as A$18,956 during the first 12 months and A$44,428 over a lifetime.[5] Overall, the most important categories of cost during the first year were acute hospitalization A$154 million, inpatient rehabilitation A$150 million, and nursing home care A$63 million.[5] There are also significant costs for caregivers of stroke patients, with much of the informal care provided by family members leading to loss of earnings, family time, or leisure time.[6] Although it is ideal to prevent strokes from occurring in the first place, it is equally important to adopt a cohesive and multidisciplinary approach toward clinical management and rehabilitation of stroke patient to minimize long-term stroke-related disability. Although stroke care has been regarded by many physicians with a sense of pessimism in the past, there have been remarkable advances in the last decade that have led to significant improvements in stroke care and measurable reductions in mortality and disability. The advent of multidisciplinary Stroke Care Units (SCUs) and more specific treatments based largely on evidence from randomized controlled trials have led to an exciting transformation in the attitude of physicians and the general medical community toward stroke management.

DEFINITIONS

Stroke - The World Health Organization (WHO) defined stroke as "rapidly developing clinical signs of focal disturbance of cerebral function lasting more than 24 hours (unless interrupted by surgery or death) with no apparent cause other than of vascular origin."[7] The emphasis of this definition is on the *focal nature* of the clinical signs, implying that stroke is a disease causing focal brain injury, and the *acute onset* which is identified by the patient's ability to specifically describe what he or she may have been doing when the first symptoms occurred. This definition excludes cases of primary cerebral tumor, cerebral metastases, subdural hematoma, postseizure paralysis, and brain trauma. Although it is a predominantly clinical definition, it still holds validity in the current era of medical imaging because of the differences in the temporal and clinical presentations of other differential diagnoses mentioned earlier. For example, the time of onset of symptoms in patients with brain tumor may be difficult to pin down compared with stroke, and other conditions such as subdural hematoma and postictal paralysis are usually associated with a history of injury or seizures. However, brain imaging has assumed an important role in excluding other diagnoses, determining whether a hemorrhagic stroke may have occurred, and more recently is also of interest in trying to establish the occurrence of infarction in patients with suspected TIA.

Transient Ischemic Attack (TIA) - TIA refers to the transient occurrence of symptoms of ischemic stroke. The classic definition for a TIA differs from that for stroke primarily in the duration of symptoms. By this definition, TIA is considered as a diagnosis if there is a focal disturbance of cerebral function of sudden onset, lasting less than 24 hours and with no apparent cause other than of vascular origin. This emphasis on the 24-hour criterion evolved in the 1950s, was adopted at the Fourth Princeton Conference in 1965,[8] and reinforced by the National Institutes of Health (NIH) in 1975.[9] However, the majority of data at the time, and even at present, indicate that symptoms of TIA last less than an hour in most patients.[10] Therefore it is now being increasingly considered that the 24-hour cutoff is out of date. Moreover, changes of infarction have been detected on MRI in a significant proportion of patients with suspected TIA.[11,12] These issues have led to further debate on whether the definition of TIA should be altered to incorporate changing views on the typical duration of symptoms and imaging findings.[10] At this point, the traditional definition of TIA remains widely in use and is important particularly in the context of epidemiologic studies of TIA that require standard definitions to compare incidence or prevalence rates over time and between populations. Older terms such as reversible ischemic neurologic deficit (RIND) and cerebral infarction with transient symptoms (CITS) have been discarded because they do not assist any further in disease phenotyping, understanding mechanisms, or clinical management. The presence of symptoms such as faintness, dizziness, confusion, or falls is highly unlikely to be because of a TIA unless they are accompanied by focal neurologic symptoms.[13] Transient global amnesia (TGA), a self-limited anterograde memory loss, is often mistaken to be a TIA. However, there is little evidence to suggest that it has a vascular mechanism.[14] Similarly the occurrence of transient isolated neurologic symptoms, such as double vision, vertigo, or dysphagia, are more likely to be due to nonvascular causes. Acute delirium is unlikely to last only a few hours and is almost always not secondary to a TIA, although it can be an uncommon presentation of stroke.

Cerebral White Matter Lesions - These are radiologically defined and are visible as hyperintensities (bright signals) seen on T2 or fluid attenuated inversion recovery (FLAIR) sequences of MRI scans.[15] They are seen to some degree in most people over the age of 65 years[16] and are often considered to be "subclinical" manifestations of chronic occlusive disease affecting small cerebral blood vessels, although they can be nonspecific. Although chronic arterial hypertension is a consistent risk factor,[17] the histopathology of WML is heterogeneous, showing a number of changes, including ischemia, demyelination, and chronic inflammation.[18]

Silent Brain Infarcts - These are small areas of typical infarction that are detected radiologically as areas of reduced intensity on T2 or FLAIR sequences of MRI in the absence of obvious acute stroke symptoms.[19] They are detected in the subcortical regions of the brain in about 20% of healthy elderly and up to 50% in selected clinical samples.[19] They increase in prevalence with age and are also associated with risk factors for small vessel disease, such as hypertension, smoking, hypercholesterolemia, and diabetes mellitus.[19]

STROKE TYPES

Strokes are either ischemic or hemorrhagic, with each having different pathophysiologic mechanisms and treatments. Approximately 80% of all strokes are ischemic, caused by an acute occlusion of a cerebral blood vessel. Increasing age, history of TIA or stroke, hypertension, atrial fibrillation, cigarette smoking, diabetes mellitus, and hypercholesterolemia are important risk factors for ischemic stroke.[1] The mechanisms of arterial occlusion are predominantly those of artery-to-artery embolism and cardioembolism, rather than in situ vessel thrombosis. Hemorrhagic strokes (primary intracerebral hemorrhage [PICH]) occur in approximately 15% of all cases and most often result from chronic hypertensive small vessel disease, leading to vessel wall lipohyalinosis, microaneurysm formation, and rupture, and less commonly in relation to other conditions such as amyloid angiopathy.[20] Subarachnoid hemorrhage (SAH) is also classified as a type of stroke within the WHO definition, occurring in about 5% of all strokes and caused by the rupture of larger saccular intracerebral aneurysms within the subarachnoid space. Cigarette smoking, hypertension, female gender, and heavy alcohol intake have been identified as important risk factors for SAH, and these may interact with genetic susceptibility to aneurysm formation and rupture.[21,22]

The distinction between ischemic and hemorrhagic stroke is important as their treatments are quite different (Figure 62-1). For example, thrombolysis is an acute treatment for ischemic stroke, but contraindicated for hemorrhagic stroke for obvious risks of worsening the hemorrhage. Computed tomography (CT) or MRI are both established methods for effectively excluding hemorrhagic stroke in the acute setting.[23]

Ischemic stroke subtypes

The classification of ischemic strokes into further subtypes has been driven by the needs of observational epidemiologic studies and clinical trials in stroke. The most commonly used classification in observational epidemiology is the Oxfordshire Community Stroke Project Classification (OCSP).[24] In clinical trials and in situations that require an understanding of the mechanisms underlying

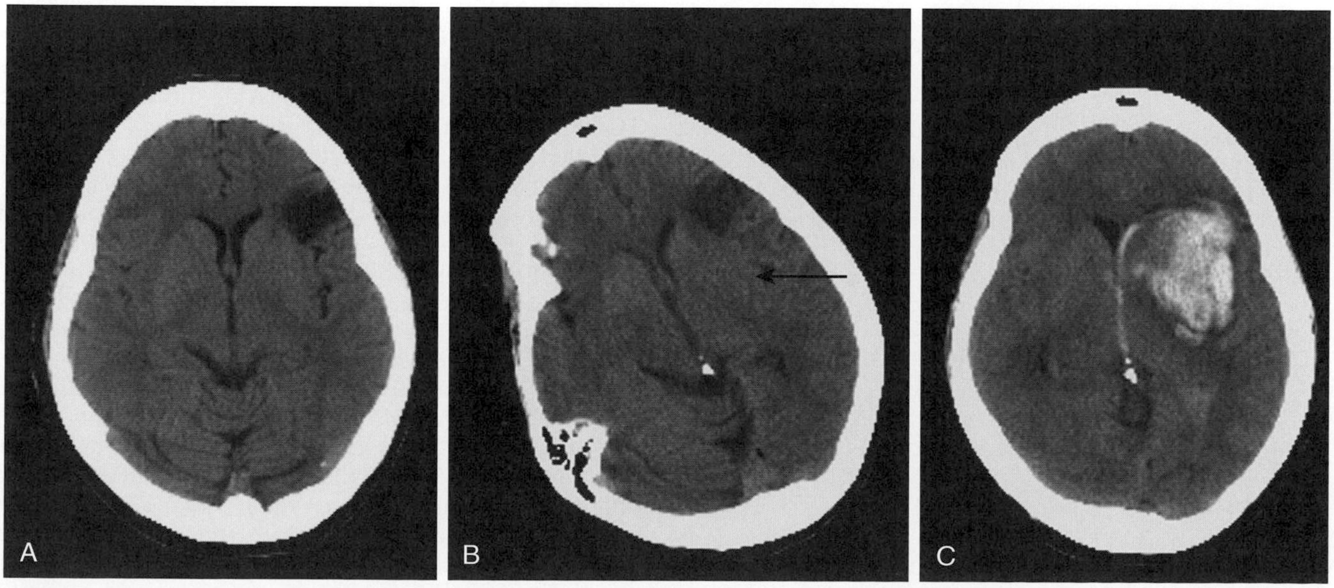

Figure 62-1. Hemorrhagic infarct and not primary intracerebral hemorrhage. 83 year old female had resolving right hemiparesis but residual right hemianesthesia (**A**). Twelve hours later she redeveloped right hemiparesis with obscuration of the left lentiform nucleus (*solid arrow* in **B**). Her blood pressure was elevated at 230/120 mm Hg. She deteriorated overnight with the final CT performed 24 hours (**C**) after admission, looking indistinguishable from a primary intracerebral hemorrhage.

the stroke, the most commonly used criteria for classification are the Trial of Org 10172 in Acute Stroke Treatment (TOAST) criteria.[25]

Oxfordshire Community Project Classification (OCSP) According to the OCSP classification, ischemic strokes are classified as one of four subtypes by their clinical presentation: Total Anterior Circulation Infarcts (TACI), Partial Anterior Circulation Infarcts (PACI), Posterior Circulation Infarcts (POCI), and Lacunar Infarcts (LACI) (Table 62-1). In a recent population-based study of stroke incidence, the annual incidence rates per 100,000 persons adjusted to the "world" population were 11 (95% confidence interval or CI, 4–18) for TACI, 25 (95% CI, 15–35) for PACI, 17 (95% CI, 9–25) for POCI, and 18 (95% CI, 10–26) for LACI. It is important to note that the OCSP classification is a syndromic classification based on the constellation of clinical signs and symptoms at stroke onset. Although this type of classification may be useful in studying risk factors and outcomes, or assigning prognosis, it does not allow a definitive understanding of the actual mechanism underlying the stroke in an individual patient without further investigations.

TACI usually involves a major portion of the carotid artery territory and may occur as a result of occlusion of the internal carotid artery or proximal stem of the middle cerebral artery (MCA), with or without involvement of the anterior cerebral artery (ACA). Given the extensive nature of infarction, TACI is associated with a very high case-fatality (approximately 35% die within the first 28 days).[26] Survivors of TACI are usually left with severe generalized neurologic deficits attributable to the affected hemisphere, consequent immobility, and high levels of disability or handicap.[26,27] PACI probably occurs as a result of occlusion of more distal branches of the MCA and is associated with a lesser degree of, but nonetheless significant, neurologic impairment including higher cortical deficits. PACI carries the highest rate of early stroke recurrence among the OCSP subtypes (approximately 17% in the first year),[26] necessitating a comprehensive assessment and management of modifiable risk factors. POCI refers to ischemic strokes occurring in the vertebrobasilar artery territory and generally has an intermediate level of case-fatality, lower than TACI but higher than LACI.[26] LACI refers to the different presentations of ischemic strokes with mainly motor or sensory deficits in the absence of signs and symptoms attributable to the cerebral cortex or the posterior circulation. They are generally milder and have a relatively good prognosis compared with the other OCSP subtypes.[26] Although it is assumed that LACI occurs because of the occlusion of small deep cerebral blood vessels, this cannot be definitively ascertained without further investigation.

Trial of Org 10172 in Acute Stroke Treatment (TOAST) Criteria - This is a classification of subtypes using a combination of clinical features and results of ancillary diagnostic studies, and is extremely important for use in trials of stroke treatment or prevention. "Possible" and "probable" diagnoses can be made based on the physician's certainty of diagnosis based on all available clinical information. Apart from use in trials, it allows the clinician to focus on disease mechanisms underlying the stroke and therefore a better framework for clinical decision-making for treatment. The TOAST classification was first developed in 1993 as part of a clinical trial and denotes five categories of ischemic stroke: (1) large-artery atherosclerosis, (2) cardioembolism, (3) small-vessel occlusion, (4) stroke of other determined cause, and (5) stroke of undetermined cause.[25] These were developed using available diagnostic and clinical information at the time, and given the limitations of these diagnostic tests, may have led to many cases placed in the category of undetermined cause. A more recent adaptation is the SSS-TOAST (Stop Stroke Study-TOAST), which takes into account recent advances in diagnostic technologies, particularly neuroimaging and cardiac imaging, to further specify the level of confidence (evident, probable, and possible) for assigning ischemic stroke subtype.[28] This classification scheme also allows for the possibility that there may be more than one mechanism involved in causing the stroke. The SSS-TOAST criteria can now even be applied in a web-based algorithm allowing for standardization in multicenter studies of stroke.[29]

Table 62-1. Oxfordshire Community Stroke Project Classification (OCSP)

Total Anterior Circulation Infarct (TACI)
- Unilateral motor deficit of at least two areas of the face, arm, and leg
- Homonymous hemianopia
- Higher cerebral dysfunction (for example, aphasia, neglect, dyscalculia, visuospatial disorder)
- If the conscious level was impaired and formal testing of higher cerebral function *or* the visual fields was not possible, a deficit is assumed

Partial Anterior Circulation Infarct (PACI)
One of:
- Any *two* of the features listed above for TACI
- Higher cerebral dysfunction alone
- Motor and/or sensory deficit more restricted than those classified as LACI (for example, confined to one limb, or to face and hand but not to whole arm)

Posterior Circulation Infarct (POCI)
One or more of:
- Bilateral motor or sensory signs not secondary to brainstem compression by a large supratentorial lesion
- Cerebellar signs, unless accompanied by ipsilateral motor deficit (see ataxic hemiparesis)
- Unequivocal diplopia with or without external ocular muscle palsy
- Crossed signs, for example, left facial and right limb weakness
- Hemianopia, alone or with any of the four items above
- Ipsilateral cranial nerve palsy with contralateral motor and sensory deficit

Lacunar Infarction (LACI)
Pure Motor Stroke (PMS)
- Unilateral, pure motor deficit
- Clearly involving two of three areas (face, arm and leg)
- With the whole of any limb being involved

Pure Sensory Stroke (PSS)
- Unilateral purely sensory symptoms (± signs)
- Clearly involving two of three areas (face, arm, and leg)
- With the whole of any limb being involved

Ataxic Hemiparesis (AH)
- Ipsilateral cerebellar and corticospinal tract signs
- With or without dysarthria
- In the absence of higher cerebral dysfunction or a visual field defect

Sensory-Motor Stroke (SMS)
- PMS and PSS combined (i.e., unilateral motor and sensory signs and symptoms)
- In the absence of higher cerebral dysfunction or a visual field deficit

CLINICAL PRESENTATION

The patterns of clinical presentations for stroke vary and cannot be exhaustively dealt with in this chapter alone. For a detailed examination of this topic, readers are referred to the authoritative text titled "Stroke Syndromes," edited by Bogousslavsky and Caplan.[30] However, in the following section, the most commonly encountered clinical features associated with stroke will be presented.

Stroke

Clinical presentations of ischemic stroke, PICH and TIA, can most often be ascribed to specific brain locations that are affected. Stroke and TIA, being part of the same clinical spectrum of disease, have very similar presentations except for the transient nature of symptoms in the latter. It is also unusual to have a TIA with purely sensory symptoms. The most commonly encountered clinical manifestations of stroke are as below:

1. Motor weakness - Hemiparesis or other motor weakness is the most common presenting abnormality in stroke, usually seen in more than 80% of patients.[31] This is possibly because of the large extent of the corticospinal pathways in the brain making it susceptible to the effects of stroke almost anywhere in the brain. Motor weakness leads to obvious difficulty in mobility and consequent disability. Apart from the predictable nature of large superficial MCA stroke, there is not a strong correlation between the location of stroke and severity of motor weakness.[32] Hemiparesis uniformly affecting the upper and lower limbs is the most frequently encountered motor deficit in about two thirds of cases, followed much less frequently by monoparesis, paraparesis, or quadriparesis.[31] The pattern of weakness may provide clues toward the topography of the stroke, although recent advances in MR imaging provide this information with far greater accuracy. Weakness of the face, arm, and leg usually indicates the involvement of the MCA territory, whereas predominant weakness of the lower limb is commonly seen in cases of anterior cerebral artery stroke. On occasion, proximal posterior cerebral artery occlusion can produce a pattern of weakness combined with deficits in higher cortical function that mimics MCA infarction.[33] The presence of a pure motor hemiparesis involving face, arm, and leg in the absence of cortical signs is the most common manifestation of lacunar infarction, resulting from a deep penetrating artery occlusion in the internal capsule or the base of the pons.[30] Care has to be taken to differentiate between true motor weakness and other deficits that may mimic weakness; for example, an apraxia of movement may be mistaken for motor weakness. Apraxia refers is a higher cortical disorder of initiation of movement in the absence of motor weakness, either for whole limb movement or more skilled movement. Motor weakness of the articulatory apparatus or the muscles involved in chewing and swallowing may lead to dysarthria and swallowing difficulties.
2. Sensory dysfunction - More than 60% of stroke patients admitted to the hospital suffer some form of tactile sensory impairment, and smaller proportions either suffer loss of proprioception or cortical sensory impairment.[34] The true prevalence of sensory abnormalities after stroke may well be underestimated given the usual laxity in sensory examination and the lack of sensitive clinical tools for detecting abnormalities. Protopathic sensory loss (involving peripheral perception of pain, temperature, vibration) may lead to problems with daily function, such as when coming into contact with hot and cold temperatures and using utensils or instruments, and also with mobility in case of significant proprioceptive loss. Severe sensory loss may lead to a difficulty in performing complex tasks in the affected limb causing a "pseudoparesis," and on occasion result in motor incoordination or involuntary movements. Strokes involving the brain stem (medulla, pons, midbrain), the thalamus and occasionally thalamocortical radiation may all lead to varying degrees of impairment in touch, pain, temperature, and vibration. The exact location of the stroke will dictate the modalities that are impaired and the pattern of co-occurrence of other neurologic deficits. Examples of cortical sensory impairments include loss of discrimination sense, difficulty in localizing touch and pain (topagnosia), failure to recognize numbers or letters drawn on the skin (graphesthesia), and failure to recognize texture, size, or shape of objects by palpation (astereognosis). These signs are usually seen with parietal cortical strokes in the MCA territory in combination with other features, such as hemiparesis, hemianopia, aphasia, or hemineglect. Sensory abnormalities may be associated with poststroke pain syndromes, which can be very debilitating to the patient. Poststroke pain may occur in up to 10% of stroke patients and usually has a delayed onset.[35] The symptoms are variable and may include burning, aching, lacerating, and cold sensations among others. Dysesthesia and allodynia are also commonly present. The pathophysiology underlying central poststroke pain is poorly understood.
3. Higher cortical dysfunction - There are several types of cortical dysfunction that can occur after stroke depending on the location of the lesion. The cortical deficits that have the most important adverse impact on stroke outcome are dysphasia (usually dominant hemisphere stroke) and hemineglect (usually right hemisphere stroke). Language is served by several sites in the brain that are part of a network, and hence disruption of this network at any site may produce several types of language deficits. Broca's aphasia (also termed expressive aphasia or motor aphasia) is most commonly caused by strokes involving the left frontal opercular and central cortex, with or without involvement of the subcortical striatocapsular region. It is characterized by effortful speech, word-finding difficulty, phonemic errors, and agrammatism, but with relatively preserved comprehension. Global aphasia refers to severe impairment of motor

speech and comprehension and is usually a consequence of a major left MCA stroke. Verbal apraxia (also termed as pure motor aphasia) is characterized by an inability to position the articulation apparatus to produce words because of a loss of programming of skilled motor movements, and is commonly seen in conjunction with Broca's aphasia. Transcortical aphasia is a disorder of spontaneous speech but with preserved repetition and comprehension, generally because of stroke involving the dominant mesial frontal cortex or the supplementary speech area. Sensory aphasia with relatively fluent speech but poor language comprehension is usually associated with strokes involving the superior temporal lobe and includes Wernicke's aphasia and conduction aphasia, among others.

Hemineglect is characterized by a reduction in attention to stimuli and events on one side of the body. This is usually seen in right hemisphere stroke, although it can be seen in varying degrees in up to 20% of left hemisphere strokes.[36] Hemineglect may affect visual, auditory, and somatosensory perceptual systems. Clinically, it can be detected using tests of cancellation or copying, simultaneous sensory testing or dichotic listening, or from clinical observation of the fact that the patient may ignore stimuli arising from the affected side, not eat food on the plate on the affected side, or ignore personal hygiene on the affected side. The presence of significant hemineglect is associated with greater dependence in function[37] and hence requires significant effort in rehabilitation. Other perceptual disorders associated with hemispherical strokes include impaired topographical recognition (disorientation to previously known surroundings), visual agnosia (impaired recognition of visual material in the presence of normal acuity), prosopagnosia (inability to recognize previously known faces), anosognosia (lack of concern for deficits on affected side), and occasionally auditory or visual hallucinations.

4. Visual dysfunction and eye movements - Visual symptoms may arise from lesions affecting the visual pathway anywhere from the retina to the occipital cortex. Retinal or ophthalmic artery occlusion occurs because of embolism from the carotid system and may lead to monocular blindness. When monocular visual loss is acute and transient, then it represents a TIA, warranting urgent investigation of the carotid circulation to identify and treat internal carotid artery stenosis that may be the source of the embolus. Visual field defects are a common visual manifestation that occurs as a result of stroke affecting the optic radiation fibers, leading to either hemianopia or quadrantanopia depending on the site of the lesion and the extent of damage to the optic radiation. Middle cerebral artery and posterior cerebral artery strokes can lead to visual field defects, the former affecting the parietal and occipital optic radiation and the latter the more distal occipital radiation fibers. Strokes affecting the striate cortex may lead to visual agnosia, color perception defects in addition to visual field defects. Less commonly, bilateral striate cortex infarction may lead to complete cortical blindness that may be distinguished from ocular disease by the presence of normal papillary light response and fundus examination. Some patients with cortical blindness may deny their visual problems and claim normal vision, and this has been termed Anton's syndrome. A further common feature in stroke is visual hemineglect (also termed as visual inattention) in which the patient may fail to attend to visual stimuli on the side of the body contralateral to the stroke lesion. Detection of visual neglect can be clinically extremely difficult in the presence of a hemianopia. Ocular movement abnormalities are commonly seen in stroke affecting the brainstem, but also less commonly seen with cerebellar and cerebral lesions. Diplopia is usually associated with eye movement abnormality and can be quite disabling. The importance of detection and characterizing visual deficits in stroke patients is of extreme importance, given their potential impact on daily life and complex activities such as driving.
5. Posterior fossa syndromes - Vertigo, or a disordered perception of motion of either the patient or the environment, can be caused by strokes involving the vertebrobasilar circulation and is often accompanied by nystagmus. Ataxia of the trunk or limbs may be caused by strokes affecting the cerebellum and adjacent brainstem. Ataxic hemiparesis is a condition that is characterized by the presence of mild hemiparesis and ipsilateral limb ataxia without sensory loss. It may be caused by stroke involving the base of pons, crus cerebri, thalamus, or internal capsule by affecting projection fibers in the corticopontocerebellar or the dentate-thalamic pathways. Several auditory symptoms may also be associated with brainstem strokes including hearing loss, hyperacusis, tinnitus, and auditory hallucinations. Sudden stroke-related hearing loss is uncommon and usually occurs in conjunction with other brainstem signs. However, it has been described on occasion in patients with vertigo and nausea without additional brainstem signs.[38]
6. Neurocognitive syndromes - Stroke is very commonly associated with alteration in cognitive status at acute presentation and in the medium to long term.[39] About 25% of stroke patients have an acute confusional state.[40] It is important to exclude other causes of acute confusion in the hospitalized stroke patient, such as infection, hypoxia, or alterations in biochemical profile. Close to 50% of survivors have some form of cognitive impairment at 3 months after stroke.[41] Stroke is strongly associated with a twofold increase in the risk of dementia after stroke, with the presence of prestroke cognitive decline explaining a large proportion of these cases.[42] This suggests that the majority of cases of dementia diagnosed after stroke are likely to be due to a combination of stroke-related cognitive impairment and preexisting neurodegenerative disease such as Alzheimer's disease. In most cases of stroke-related cognitive impairment, the deficit may be explained

by the location of the lesion. For example, medial temporal or left thalamic strokes are strategically placed to cause memory impairments by disrupting the limbic pathways.[43] Thalamic and caudate strokes can produce several other cognitive deficits in addition to memory impairment, such as reduced problem-solving capacity and attention. Frontal lobe strokes may lead to several cognitive sequelae, such as lack of initiation, apathy, and poor planning. Such strategic cognitive syndromes may be associated with some improvement with time, but many patients are left with some residual cognitive deficits. In many situations, however, stroke patients suffer nonspecific reductions in attentional capacity and working memory, representing a more widespread disorder of fundamental cognitive abilities irrespective of the location of the lesion. Much of the cognitive burden associated with strokes may go unrecognized, particularly in those with so-called "silent" brain infarcts (SBI) that usually are not associated with the classic motor or sensory symptoms seen in the average stroke patient. Care must be taken to look for cognitive loss in people with SBI. SBI may have important effects on future cognitive outcome, particularly in increasing the risk of incident dementia.[19] Up to 30% of patients may also suffer from depressed mood in the medium to long term after stroke,[44] with disability and history of depression being important predictors of long-term depression.[45] Patients with frontal or temporal lobe involvement may also display emotional outbursts (poststroke emotionalism). Such nonspecific neurocognitive syndromes may impact significantly with their functional status and quality of life irrespective of physical recovery.[46] Cognitive and mood examination is therefore extremely important in stroke patients to allow clear plans to be made for rehabilitation or supported care, more so in the very elderly who are at higher risk of other causes of cognitive impairment.

Apart from the manifestations mentioned above, stroke may less commonly have other clinical presentations. These include extrapyramidal features such as tremor, hemiballismus or dystonia (due to lesions affecting the basal ganglia), seizures, and disorders of wakefulness and sleep.

7. Incontinence - Urinary and fecal incontinence are common and disabling effects of stroke. The prevalence of urinary incontinence among survivors of stroke has been shown to range from 36%[47] to 83%[48] within the first 3 months. The incidence of urinary incontinence has been reported to be 29/1000 persons per month in a hospital-based sample of post-acute stroke patients.[49] Increasing stroke severity is a predictor of the presence of incontinence independent of age. Incontinence may be a direct consequence of loss of neurogenic control or because of functional incapacitation secondary to immobility or cognitive loss. Urinary incontinence is a marker for increased mortality after stroke and overall poor outcome among survivors. Fecal incontinence is also common after stroke. In a community-based postal survey, 5% of stroke survivors reported major fecal incontinence, with 4.3% reporting fecal and urinary incontinence and 0.8% reporting isolated fecal incontinence.[50]

Effects of cerebral white matter lesions

Cerebral white matter lesions (WML) have been linked to cognitive and noncognitive effects. Most commonly, they are associated with reductions in fundamental cognitive abilities, such as attention, speed of processing, and executive function, presumably secondary to the disconnection of white matter association tracts that enable brain networks.[51,52] They have also been associated with poorer gait and balance because of a general disruption of motor control.[53] It is likely that these effects may be clinically most evident when there are very large volumes of WML in the brain, as may have been found in very early descriptions of Binswanger's disease[54] characterized by abnormal gait, dementia, incontinence, and motor deficits.

INVESTIGATIONS

Brain imaging

DIAGNOSIS OF HEMORRHAGE

Computed tomography (CT) should be performed to exclude intracranial hemorrhage. On rare occasions, a subdural hematoma may have transient symptoms mimicking a TIA. Hemorrhage in the basal ganglia and pons suggests that hypertension may be the likely cause, whereas hemorrhage in cortical (lobar) locations suggests the possibility of amyloid angiopathy as the primary causal mechanism. In some cases, primary intracerebral hemorrhage and hemorrhagic infarcts are indistinguishable on CT unless a series of CT scans have been obtained to record the evolution of hemorrhage into the infarct (see Figure 62-1).

RECOGNITION OF ISCHEMIC CHANGES ON CT

It was only recently recognized that early ischemic changes are present in the first 6 hours in approximately a half to three quarters of patients with MCA territory infarction.[55] Significant early ischemic changes include parenchymal hypoattenuation and diffuse swelling of the hemisphere.[56] The definition of parenchymal hypoattenuation is a decrease in tissue density below that of white matter but greater than that of cerebrospinal fluid. This definition excludes old cerebral infarction in which the tissue density is similar to that of cerebrospinal fluid. Lacunar strokes resulting from small vessel disease are not easily seen in the first 24 hours after stroke.

MRI FINDINGS IN STROKE

Signal change on MRI diffusion-weighted imaging (DWI) reflecting altered water diffusion can reveal abnormalities within minutes of ischemia in the majority of patients with ischemic stroke.[57] This change is seen earlier than on conventional MR imaging sequences such as T2-weighted images. The bright signal change on DWI becomes less bright after 10 days.[58] Hemorrhage on the other hand contains paramagnetic material and has a dark signal on T2-weighted images. The evolution of MR signal changes in intracerebral hemorrhage is quite complex and the reader is referred to the excellent description by Atlas and Thulborn.[59]

In older people, focal areas of signal loss on gradient echo (GE) MR imaging pathologically represent focal hemosiderin deposition associated with previous hemorrhagic events. These are usually cerebral microhemorrhages and have been found in patients with previous ischemic stroke, intracerebral hemorrhage (ICH), cerebral amyloid angiopathy (CAA), and cerebral autosomal dominant arteriopathy with subcortical infarcts and leukoencephalopathy (CADASIL). In patients with CAA, such microhemorrhages may predict the risk of recurrent lobar ICH.[60]

EVALUATING TISSUE AT RISK

Stroke pathophysiology can now be inferred from dynamic scanning by tracking a bolus of intravenous contrast with sequential acquisition of CT or MR images (Figure 62-2). These CT or MR perfusion images enable analysis of cerebral perfusion deficit. For MR images, the salvageable tissue is represented by the difference of the poorly perfused region and the region of restricted diffusion (infarct core).[61] For CT scan, the infarct core is represented by the most poorly perfused region on CT perfusion images. These dynamic scanning methods are being tested as guides to therapy in trials of thrombolysis therapy beyond 3 hours after stroke onset.[62]

Diagnosis of stroke mechanism

EXTRACRANIAL ARTERY ULTRASOUND

Ultrasound is traditionally performed to screen for carotid artery atherosclerosis. It can provide evidence of vertebral artery disease as well. There are a few caveats to interpreting ultrasound results: firstly, the result is dependent on the operator; secondly, assignment of degree of carotid artery stenosis is to a large extent dependent on the velocity of flowing blood in that artery. Consequently, a critically narrow artery on one side may lead to compensatory elevation of velocity in the contralateral artery leading to erroneous misclassification of the contralateral artery as critically stenosed; thirdly, ultrasound assignment of carotid artery stenosis as moderate (50% to 70% stenosis) can either mean that the artery is 50% to 70% stenosed or greater than 70% stenosed; finally, near occlusion on ultrasound can mean near occlusion, complete occlusion, or critical stenosis. A rule of thumb is that when the ultrasound suggests more than 50% stenosis and the patient is fit for carotid endarterectomy, a second test such as CT angiography or contrast enhanced MR angiography may be necessary to clarify the exact degree and nature of the stenosis.

CT ANGIOGRAPHY

CT angiography is performed by rapid injection of contrast bolus and acquiring the images during the arterial phase of contrast arrival in the brain. CT angiography can provide coverage from the aortic arch to the circle of Willis. This method has excellent correlation with digital subtraction angiography[63] and together with MR angiography has largely replaced the latter for investigating carotid artery disease.

MR ANGIOGRAPHY

MR angiography techniques are divided into those designated as "bright blood" and "black blood" techniques depending on the signal intensity of blood. In bright blood techniques, voxels within a blood vessel have bright signal. Hence, very slowly moving parts (very tight stenosis) or stationary parts (occluded) of the blood vessel will experience a loss of signal. Hence this "time of flight" MRA sequence cannot reliably distinguish between complete occlusion or a critically stenosed carotid artery. Phase contrast MR angiogram, on the other hand, provides information on direction of flow and velocity of flowing blood in that vessel and is more often used for research purposes. Contrast-enhanced MR angiography (CEMRA) is performed by fast injection of an intravascular contrast agent (gadolinium) and acquiring images during the arterial phase of contrast arrival. Unlike the time of flight MRA, this method relies on contrast with the lumen to depict the arterial lumen size and thus provide similar findings as digital subtraction angiography. Likc CT angiography, this method has largely replaced digital subtraction angiography for investigation of carotid artery disease.[63,64]

STROKE PATTERNS

The stroke patterns on CT and MR images can also be used to infer stroke mechanism. DWI-MRI has been advocated to be better than CT because it may reveal smaller strokes not seen on CT images.[65] A small deep lacunar infarct may indicate the presence of small vessel disease. Bilateral hemispheric (MCA) strokes imply cardiac embolism or artery-to-artery embolism from an aortic arch atheroma. However, bilateral anterior cerebral artery strokes may occur in the absence of a central embolic source. In this situation, the mechanism may be due to distal artery-to-artery embolism to a single proximal anterior cerebral artery that gives rise to the two distal anterior cerebral arteries (an anatomic variant). This situation can also occur in the case of bilateral thalamic infarction because of occlusion of the artery of Percheron, a solitary arterial trunk that arises from one of the proximal segments of a posterior cerebral artery, and on occasion supplies both thalami.[66] Strokes involving both posterior cerebral arteries may be due to artery-to-artery embolism from a vertebrobasilar source and do not necessarily indicate a cardiac mechanism.

ECHOCARDIOGRAPHY

Echocardiography can assist in clarifying the mechanism of ischemic stroke. However, the routine use of echocardiography for determining stroke mechanism is controversial. It is rare to find an abnormality on echocardiography that would lead to anticoagulation in patients with a normal electrocardiogram and cardiovascular examination. The need for routine echocardiography in ischemic stroke needs to be supported by strong evidence for a benefit from therapy, namely prophylactic anticoagulation. At present, there is level I evidence that anticoagulation prevents stroke in patients with atrial fibrillation.[67] There is no evidence at present to support routine anticoagulation for stroke prophylaxis in people with sinus rhythm even among high-risk patients with heart failure.[68] This lack of level I evidence may have been the reason why the current stroke guidelines have not emphasized the role of echocardiography in stroke. Routine echocardiography may lead to the chance finding of patent foramen ovale or valvular strand, which may further confuse clinical decisions, as the evidence is lacking for anticoagulation or surgical therapy in such situations.[69,70] On the other hand, echocardiography may prove to be useful in detecting aortic arch atheroma. Complex aortic arch atheroma confers a fourfold increased risk

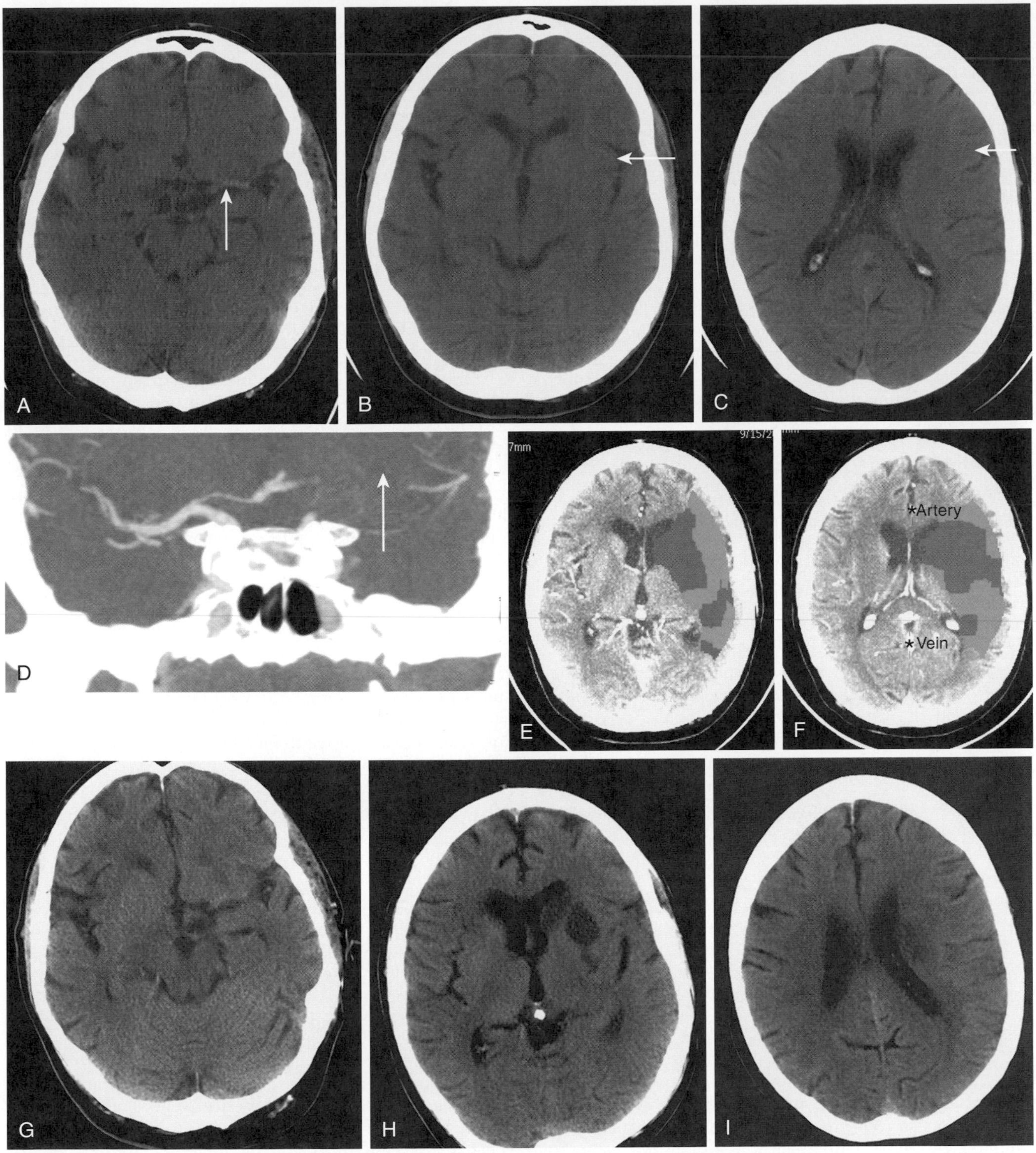

Figure 62-2. CT imaging revealing salvageable tissue in acute ischemic stroke. An 84-year-old man had acute left MCA occlusion resulting in aphasia and dense right hemiparesis while playing golf. This man was known to have AF and not on warfarin. The acute CT scan (**A**) showed the hyperdense MCA sign, which corresponded with CT angiography (**D**) evidence of left MCA occlusion. There is obscuration of the lentiform nucleus and edema in the left frontal cortex (**B** and **C**). The CT perfusion pictures (**E** and **F**) showed that the striatocapsular region was likely to be infarcted, whereas the surrounding area was at risk of infarction. He was treated with tissue plasminogen activator and the CT scans performed (**G–I**) 2 days later showed infarction of **only** the left striatocapsular region.

of stroke.[71] Although emboli from aortic arch atheroma do not strictly originate from the heart, the stroke syndromes they cause are similar. Transesophageal echocardiography is superior to transthoracic echocardiography for the detection of aortic arch atheroma.[72] However, there is no evidence at this time whether warfarin may be more useful than routine antiplatelet therapy in patients with arch atheroma as the predominant mechanism, reducing the urgency to pursue this stroke mechanism at the present time.[71]

Blood tests for the diagnosis of stroke risk factors

SERUM CHOLESTEROL

Measuring fasting serum cholesterol has taken on greater importance with the recent success of statins in secondary stroke prevention.[73] When measuring serum cholesterol, it is important to realize that the levels dip acutely after stroke and return to "true" value approximately 12 weeks after stroke onset.[74] Consequently, a "normal" result within 1 week of stroke may represent a falsely low result.

SERUM GLUCOSE

Measurement of fasting glucose is essential to exclude diabetes mellitus, which can often surface as a diagnosis after stroke. To avoid the confounding of results by acute phase hyperglycemia, it is often advisable to conduct definitive testing with fasting glucose or glucose tolerance testing a few weeks after stroke.

INFLAMMATORY MARKERS

Erythrocyte sedimentation rate (ESR) and high sensitivity C-reactive protein (CRP) can be performed to examine the possibility of temporal arteritis or subacute bacterial endocarditis as unusual causes of stroke. Recently, high-sensitivity C-reactive protein has been recognized as a marker of stroke prognosis and active atherosclerotic disease.[75]

ANTIPHOSPHOLIPID ANTIBODY SYNDROME

The relationship between antiphospholipid antibody and stroke is not as straightforward as previously thought since this antibody has a high prevalence in people above the age of 40.[76] It is recognized that this antibody is a marker of increased risk of stroke, peripheral vascular disease, and ischemic heart disease.[76,77] It is often difficult to ascribe a causal role for the antibody in contributing to the stroke mechanism in an individual patient. It appears that identifying the presence of antiphospholipid antibody in stroke patients may not assist in deciding whether to treat with antiplatelet agents or anticoagulants. Patients with this antibody do reasonably well when treated with aspirin, whereas those treated with warfarin have a similar reduction in stroke risk, but with a potentially higher risk of intracranial hemorrhage.[78] Routine testing for this antibody is generally not recommended.

THROMBOTIC RISK FACTORS

The contribution of hypercoagulable states to arterial occlusion in ischemic stroke is controversial despite its recognized role in causing cerebral venous thrombosis.[79] Coagulation abnormalities have been described in stroke patients, but often concurrently with other well-established causes of stroke.[80] In elderly patients, a full blood count can be helpful to exclude rare cases of thrombocythemia or polycythemia rubra vera. It is unlikely that a search for other rare causes of stroke would be useful in elderly patients in the absence of clinical pointers.

Management of stroke patients

ACUTE TREATMENT OF ISCHEMIC STROKE

Acute stroke treatments may involve either stroke-specific therapies or more general treatments aimed at optimizing the overall medical state. Three specific interventions have been shown to be effective in randomized trials for the acute treatment of ischemic stroke. These include antiplatelet agents,[81] tissue plasminogen activator (tPA),[82,83] and organized stroke units.[84] The latter is particularly important because it provides the framework for ensuring appropriate overall management of a patient. Recently, there have been limited data on the usefulness of decompressive hemicraniectomy in patients with malignant MCA infarction.[85] The role of other medications (such as antihypertensive drugs and statins) in the acute phase of ischemic stroke is uncertain and remains to be clarified. Neuroprotective agents have largely failed to show benefits in acute stroke therapy.

ORGANIZED STROKE UNIT CARE

The implementation of organized stroke units has been the most important advance in acute stroke management. A collaboration of stroke unit trial lists demonstrated that organized stroke units result in long-term reductions in the odds of death (14%), death or institutionalized care (18%), and death and dependency (18%) regardless of age, sex, or stroke severity.[86,87] This translates to having to treat approximately 25 patients (number need to treat [NNT]) to prevent one from dying or being dependent. Outcomes were also found to be better in patients admitted to a discrete ward under the care of a dedicated multidisciplinary team, compared with a roving stroke service visiting patients on general medical wards.[88] Furthermore, there were no indications that stroke unit care resulted in longer hospital length of stay.[86,87] It has been proposed that stroke units work by reducing secondary complications of stroke and reducing disability through the use of a dedicated team of nurses and allied health members and implementation of stroke protocols. The consistent characteristics of effective stroke units appear to be (1) a comprehensive approach to medical problems, impairments, and disabilities, (2) active and careful management of physiologic abnormalities, (3) early mobilization, (4) skilled nursing care, (5) early setting of rehabilitation plans, and (6) early assessment and planning of discharge needs with involvement of caregivers.[89] Appropriate fluid and nutritional support in the acute phase with either intravenous fluids or nasogastric feeding are also important in those with significant dysphagia and risk of aspiration. The use of percutaneous endoscopic gastrostomy (PEG) in the acute phase is generally not recommended because it is associated with an increased risk of death or poor outcome at 6 months.[90] The early detection and treatment of pyrexia and infectious complications is a major contributor to the effectiveness of stroke unit care.[91] A protocol driven approach in stroke units may also enable the standard use of low-molecular weight heparin to prevent venous thromboembolism, with recent evidence supporting their superiority in ischemic stroke patients compared with standard unfractionated heparin.[92] Nursing care should incorporate avoidance of pressure areas, urinary catheters, and bed rest because these contribute significantly to the development of complications, such as sepsis and deep venous thromboses. Blood pressure reduction should be generally avoided in the acute phase (except in selected situations, such as before thrombolysis or in people with hemorrhagic strokes and mass effect) because of concerns about interfering with cerebral autoregulation, and if performed should be done cautiously and in well-monitored situations. A very important component of stroke unit care is the conduct of regular (weekly) formal multidisciplinary meetings that serve as forums for the entire team to discuss various aspects of individual patient care and set early plans for rehabilitation and discharge.[89] Among the established acute stroke therapies, it has been estimated that stroke unit care has the greatest ability to prevent disability or death (approximately 50 patients for every 1000 strokes) compared with aspirin (4 patients per 1000) and tPA (6 per 1000).[93]

ANTIPLATELET THERAPY

The International Stroke Trial (IST) and Chinese Aspirin Stroke Trial (CAST) clearly demonstrated the efficacy of aspirin (160 to 300 mg) as an acute stroke therapy for ischemic stroke,[81,94] with approximately 80 people (NNT) needing treatment to prevent one from dying or being dependent. In both studies, heparin was not found to be superior to aspirin. There have been several trials of the efficacy of low molecular weight heparin in acute ischemic stroke, with none showing superiority over aspirin but with increased risk of intracranial hemorrhage.[95] The benefit of aspirin in the acute phase of stroke is relatively small, with about four patients saved from death or disability per 1000 treated. However, it is an inexpensive therapy, is widely available, and should be used in acute ischemic stroke treatment in the absence of a significant contraindication.

THROMBOLYSIS FOR ACUTE ISCHEMIC STROKE

Until recently, stroke therapy had largely been confined to secondary ischemic stroke prevention and rehabilitation because reversal of neurologic deficit and salvage of ischemic tissue was thought not possible. The introduction of recombinant tissue plasminogen activator (tPA) has led to new found optimism for reversing the neurologic deficit because of ischemic stroke.[82,83] It is postulated that the mechanism of action of tPA is lysis of the thrombus/embolus leading to recanalization of the arterial lumen and salvage of the ischemic brain tissue. In a pivotal randomized controlled trial (the NINDS trial), tPA given within 3 hours of symptom onset led to a 12% increase in the number of patients discharged home with no neurologic deficit.[82] Approximately 18 patients (NNT) will need to be treated with tPA to prevent one from dying or being dependent. These results were duplicated in a large phase IV study involving 6483 patients treated with tPA across Europe.[96] There have been several smaller phase IV studies examining the safety of thrombolysis in patients over the age of 80.[97] With the advent of tPA, there have been significant efforts to enable more patients to have access to the therapy, with improved ambulance response and emergency department triaging being important to reduce the "door-to-needle time" and allow treatment to be given within the 3-hour time window. The most important adverse effect of tPA is symptomatic intracerebral hemorrhage in about 6% of cases. The risk of symptomatic intracerebral hemorrhage rises with age, high blood pressure, and very severe neurologic deficits.[1] Although there have been concerns regarding an increased risk of bleeding in older people, the majority of available data indicate that the benefit is also seen in the older patient with ischemic stroke who meets the strict inclusion criteria used in the NINDS trial.[82] However, there are some important caveats to using tPA in elderly patients. Those patients with extensive cerebral white matter lesions on CT scan are more likely to develop thrombolysis-related intracranial hemorrhage.[98] The presence of a significant preexisting dementia or extreme frailty (particularly in those already living in high-level residential care) may be a cause for concern and be relative contraindications to thrombolysis. At this point, there is insufficient evidence to support the use of tPA when the 3-hour time window has passed.

EMERGING TREATMENTS

Decompressive hemicraniectomy may be considered in the occasional patient who has a rapidly declining neurologic state and a large MCA infarct with mass-effect (malignant infarction), with a pooled analysis from three trials that indicate a benefit in survival but not necessarily a large reduction in disability, with the majority of survivors having a modified Rankin score of 4 indicating severe disability.[85] There are several other approaches that are being studied to improve the acute treatment of ischemic stroke. These include ways to extend the time window for thrombolysis, using transcranial ultrasound to assist in clot lysis during thrombolysis, acute blood pressure lowering, and invasive procedures such as thrombectomy.

Acute treatment of intracranial hemorrhage

At present, there are no specific treatment options with proven efficacy for intracerebral hemorrhage. Trials of recombinant factor VII[99] and neuroprotective agents in intracerebral hemorrhage have met without success. Surgical intervention for decompression may also be considered in patients with cerebellar hematoma at risk of brainstem herniation.

RECOVERY AND REHABILITATION

Stroke recovery

Most patients who survive a stroke make some functional recovery. Recovery is of two types: intrinsic, which involves a degree of return of neural control, and adaptive, in which alternative strategies are used to overcome disability. Although the exact neural mechanisms underlying stroke recovery are still poorly understood, there is emerging evidence that the plasticity of the adult brain may play a role. It is postulated that recovery from brain injury occurs because of restoration of function in damaged neural structures (restitution), and by the development of new pathways in the unaffected areas of brain, which take over the lost function (substitution).[100] The process of reorganization of neural activity has been demonstrated in stroke patients.[101] It is now believed that there are multiple motor circuits in the brain that serve similar functions. Conventional pathways dominate in healthy subjects and inhibit the activity of alternative pathways in other areas of the brain. Disruption of traditional pathways in cerebral ischemia reduces or eliminates the inhibition normally exerted by these pathways and allows activation of alternate pathways in the premotor areas of the affected side and primary motor areas on the unaffected side. Hence, the paradigm for function has shifted from strict cerebral localization to that of interactive functioning of brain networks. It is conceivable that interventions in rehabilitation may act by modifying the process of reorganization and recovery in stroke patients. With the advent of neuroimaging techniques such as functional magnetic resonance imaging (fMRI) and transcranial magnetic stimulation (TMS), there has been considerable recent interest in the study of neural activation that may be facilitated by sensory stimulation,[102] repetitive movement of the affected limbs,[103] or the use of drugs which modify neurotransmitter release.[104]

The highest rate of recovery usually occurs in the first few weeks after stroke, with lesser amounts occurring over the next 12 months.[105] Measurable recovery seldom occurs after 12 months, although there are the occasional exceptions to this rule. The degree of recovery depends largely on the severity of the initial deficit, with the likelihood of complete recovery lower in those with severe initial deficit. There is also considerable variation in rates or patterns of recovery between patients and it is often difficult to make predictions of recovery in individual patients except those with very mild stroke. Recovery may be affected adversely by the development of stroke-related complications and importantly by the presence of comorbidity and frailty.[106]

Rates of recovery may vary for different types of impairments. Some problems such as homonymous hemianopia, dysphagia, lower extremity weakness, and sitting balance may resolve more rapidly in stroke survivors, whereas arm paralysis, perceptual disorders, and language impairment recover more slowly and less completely. Although minor cognitive deficits have the potential to recover, most patients with poststroke cognitive impairment early after stroke will have some persisting deficit at 2 years.[107] Urinary incontinence also tends to persist in many stroke survivors, with the Erlangen Stroke Project reporting a prevalence of 53% immediately after stroke decreasing to 32% at 1 year,[108] whereas the South London Stroke Register reported an initial prevalence of approximately 48%, which decreased to 10% at 2 years.[109]

Overall functional recovery, which is probably more relevant than the recovery of individual impairments, depends on the level of initial disability and the level of prestroke disability. Mild to moderately disabled patients with little preexisting disability usually make good improvements in the first 3 months. The older, more frail patient with significant preexisting physical or cognitive disability, on the other hand, faces an uphill task in functional improvement. Anecdotally, some patients with severe stroke attain relative independence after a prolonged rehabilitation, some continuing to show functional improvement beyond 3 months.

Rehabilitation

There is mounting evidence showing that functional recovery can be influenced by coordinated rehabilitation.[110] Rehabilitation techniques in stroke are now being examined in light of their potential ability to modify brain plasticity and thus influence recovery.[111] Rehabilitation is not simply a matter of being treated by a therapist or a group of therapists but involves a whole range of approaches to managing disability provided by a coordinated multidisciplinary team and tailored to restore patients to their fullest possible physical, mental, and social capability.[112] It is now recognized that the best models of rehabilitation may be those that emphasize commencement of active therapy very early after stroke with acute care and rehabilitation being provided in a seamless fashion preferable at the same location.[113] The goals of rehabilitation are not always easy to define because it deals with many aspects of human performance. In general, rehabilitation should aim to maximize patients' role fulfillment and independence in their environment within the limitations imposed by underlying impairment and availability of resources. It should help them to make the best adaptation possible to any difference between the roles desired and the roles achieved following stroke.

According to the revised World Health Organization International Classification of Impairments, Disabilities, and Handicaps, the major areas of concern in rehabilitation are limitation of activity (disability) and restriction of participation (handicap).[114] *Disability* is defined as "restriction, or lack of ability, to perform an activity in the manner or within the range considered to be normal." Disability relates to function, and the ability to undertake basic activities of self-care is fundamental to any physical rehabilitation program. *Handicap*, the social consequence of disability, is defined as "limitations faced by stroke patients in fulfilling their normal role in the society." It is not always possible to differentiate handicap from disability, and most pragmatic approaches tend to combine these two dimensions, referring to them as social disability.

Rehabilitation in stroke is essentially a multidisciplinary activity that has been described as a problem-solving process focusing on disability and intended to reduce handicap.[114] The basic principles that should be applied throughout rehabilitation of stroke patients are the following: Documentation of impairments, disabilities, and handicaps and, where possible, measuring them using simple, valid scales; maximization of independence and minimization of learned dependency; and a holistic approach to patients, taking into account their physical and psychosocial background, their environment, and their caregivers. It is accepted that goals of rehabilitation vary according to the expectations of the parties involved. The goal of hospitals may be to discharge patients as soon as possible, whereas the goal of patients may be to return to their previous functional status even if this is unattainable. There is good evidence to suggest that early supported discharge works well with regard to patient outcomes including quality of life provided that such a program is well resourced.[115] The goal of caregivers may be to minimize the level of input they need to provide even at the cost of institutionalization. Many of the difficulties ultimately faced in managing patients and in evaluating the effectiveness of interventions can be traced back to conflicts between the goals and objectives of different parties.

Studies on specific therapeutic interventions in stroke rehabilitation are limited but growing in number. Techniques that are being investigated for efficacy include device-assisted gait or locomotion training, functional intramuscular stimulation, constraint-induced therapy, mirror therapy, and even transcranial magnetic stimulation.[116–120] There is, however, no evidence supporting any specific treatment technique for stroke patients. A pragmatic functional approach individualized for each patient's needs is recommended.

The amount of formal therapy received by stroke patients may be small even in organized stroke units with only 13%

of patients shown to receive mobility-improving therapy within the first 14 days after stroke in a recent study.[121] There have been many misconceptions about the risks of early mobilization of stroke patients, but consensus is emerging that immobilization is more likely to be harmful.[122,123] Evidence may soon become available about the efficacy of early mobilization (within 24 hours) after stroke from randomized controlled trials.[123] The effects of intensive therapeutic input on recovery from stroke have been investigated in well-designed controlled studies.[124–126] These investigations have shown a small but definite relationship between the amount of therapy given and the amount of improvement in functional ability, which is independent of the nonspecific effects of changes in attention or adaptive mechanisms.

The impact of premorbid cognitive status, age, and frailty are also important issues to consider in the selection of patients for rehabilitation. Unless there is clear evidence of severe preexisting cognitive impairment (such as a severe dementia) that may interfere with the process of rehabilitation, there is no good argument to exclude stroke patients from rehabilitation on the grounds of cognition or age alone. In fact, one may argue that such a patient may require more specialized attention in a rehabilitation setting to ensure a return to his or her usual living environment.[127] There are extremely limited data demonstrating the efficacy of rehabilitation following stroke in the oldest old (85+ years) and it may be that the effort invested in rehabilitating patients in this group is no less justified than in younger elderly patients.[128] Specific clinical issues requiring medical input in a rehabilitation setting include poststroke spasticity, neuropathic pain, shoulder pain, incontinence, and depression, all of which can significantly impede recovery and need specialized medical therapies such as botulinum toxin, neural pain modulators, continence management, and antidepressant therapy.

SECONDARY STROKE PREVENTION

Secondary prevention refers to the treatments that may be used to prevent a recurrent stroke, or a first stroke after a TIA. There have been significant advances in secondary prevention in the last decade with the conduct of several large scale randomized controlled trials.

Antiplatelet therapy

These form the cornerstone for secondary stroke prevention. There are a variety of antiplatelet drugs on the market. These range from prostaglandin inhibitors such as aspirin, to adenosine diphosphate inhibitors such as clopidogrel. Older adenosine diphosphate inhibitors such as ticlopidine are now superseded by clopidogrel. Aspirin appears to be the drug of choice for arterial noncardioembolic ischemic stroke and is as effective as warfarin in this setting.[129,130] A collaborative meta-analysis showed that aspirin was effective even at the low dose of 75 mg/day with recommendation that the loading dose be at least 150 mg.[131] The addition of dipyridamole (200 mg twice a day) to aspirin provided an additional stroke reduction of 1% per year over aspirin alone.[132,133] Contrary to the theoretical concern regarding the potential for dipyridamole to exacerbate ischemic heart disease, this combination also reduced the risk of nonfatal myocardial infarction and vascular death.[134] The drawback to the aspirin-dipyridamole combination is that up to 18% of people may drop out of therapy because of vasodilatory headache caused by dipyridamole.[132,133] Very recently, it was also shown that the combination of aspirin-dipyridamole appears to have equivalent efficacy to clopidogrel alone.[135] Although the combination of aspirin and clopidogrel provides additive benefit in acute coronary syndrome, this combination does not offer better stroke protection than clopidogrel alone.[136]

Warfarin

Warfarin has clearly been shown to be effective for secondary prevention in patients with atrial fibrillation (AF)[137] but not in cases of intracranial artery stenosis.[138] The optimal INR for stroke prevention is 2-3.[139] The annual risk of intracranial hemorrhage associated with warfarin is relatively low at approximately 2%.[140] The risk of hemorrhage with warfarin is higher in patients with renal or liver impairment or history of bleeding. The risk of falling is often cited as the reason for not starting warfarin in very elderly people, although the benefits of stroke prevention in this high risk group may still outweigh the risk of bleeding in older patients.[141] Recent application of a computerized clinical decision-making tool was successful in identifying nonvalvular AF patients who were potentially at a higher risk of hemorrhagic complications.[142] Such tools if validated in different settings may become extremely useful in secondary prevention of stroke related to AF. Aspirin is mildly effective in preventing stroke in people with AF compared with warfarin,[140] and should be considered when warfarin is contraindicated. Following intracerebral hemorrhage, it is relatively safe to discontinue warfarin for approximately 1 week even in patients at high risk of embolism (prosthetic heart valve). Warfarin's effect needs to be reversed aggressively with fresh frozen plasma, vitamin K, and prothrombinex. Reversal of warfarin is always necessary in intracerebral hemorrhage but may not be necessary in patients with hemorrhagic infarct.

Blood pressure reduction

Blood pressure reduction has assumed great importance in secondary stroke prevention. The paradigm for the management of blood pressure has changed with a trial involving the combination of the Angiotensin Converting Enzyme Inhibitor (ACE-I) perindopril and the diuretic indapamide, showing a significant reduction in the risk of stroke among both hypertensive and nonhypertensive individuals with a history of stroke or transient ischemic attack.[143] In this study the combination therapy arm produced larger blood pressure reductions and larger risk reductions than did single drug therapy with perindopril alone. This finding regarding the benefit of perindopril with or without indapamide has been confirmed in patients over the age of 80 years,[144] suggesting that there needs to be a very good reason why older, more frail people should not be given blood pressure lowering therapy for stroke prevention. There is no evidence that the effect is limited to the angiotensin-converting enzyme inhibitor with a recent trial showing that angiotensin receptor blocker (telmisartan) is as effective.[145] In this study, telmisartan had a higher incidence of symptomatic hypotension but lower risk of angioedema and cough compared with the ACE-I ramipril.[145] Overall, successful secondary prevention hinges heavily on blood pressure control, whether it is achieved with lifestyle modifications or medication, with the latter often being required.

Lipid lowering agents

A role for hydroxymethylglutaryl coenzyme A (HMG-CoA) reductase inhibitors (statins) in lipid lowering and stroke prevention was initially suggested by the observed risk reduction for ischemic stroke in trials involving simvastatin (40 mg) and pravastatin (40 mg) for prevention of coronary heart disease. Recently, the first trial specifically examining their effects in stroke prevention showed that atorvastatin (80 mg) provided an absolute risk reduction of approximately 2% over 5 years.[73] Despite this trial focusing on patients 75 years or less, data from secondary prevention trials involving statins in heart disease suggest a benefit in patients above the age of 80.[146] There is a small increase in the risk of hemorrhagic stroke with statins that is outweighed by the overall benefit, and this increased risk is associated with having an initial hemorrhagic stroke, being older, having poorly controlled blood pressure, but not with low cholesterol levels.[147] The use of statins for stroke prevention in the very old must be cautious and preferably at lower doses. The mechanism by which statins provide benefit against stroke is likely multifactorial, involving both the low-density lipoprotein cholesterol-lowering effect with stabilization of vulnerable plaque, and other effects such as improvement of endothelial function, increased nitric oxide bioavailability, antioxidant properties, and inhibition of inflammatory responses.[148]

Carotid endarterectomy

Carotid endarterectomy is one of the most effective secondary measures for the prevention of recurrent ischemic stroke in patients with 70% to 99% symptomatic internal carotid artery stenosis,[149,150] with seven patients needing to be treated to prevent one ischemic stroke. In a pooled analysis of large trials, the benefit of carotid endarterectomy appeared to be magnified in elderly patients given their greater overall risk of stroke.[151] There is no justification for withholding carotid endarterectomy for patients older than 75 years who are deemed medically fit to undergo surgery. The benefit is likely to be greatest in this group because of their high risk of stroke on medical treatment, although it should be noted that the trials included very few patients older than 80 years. Approximately 5 patients aged 75 years or older with symptomatic internal carotid stenosis need to be treated to prevent one ipsilateral stroke over 5 years.

Endovascular therapy

The role of endovascular therapy (angioplasty and stenting) of the carotid artery is evolving. Two European trials in patients with symptomatic carotid stenosis suggested that angioplasty and stenting were less effective than endarterectomy.[152,153] By contrast, a U.S. trial consisting of symptomatic and asymptomatic patients has shown equivalence between the two modes of therapy.[154] There is evidence suggesting that perioperative risk of stroke and other complications such as restenosis are higher with angioplasty and stenting than endarterectomy.[155] Such endovascular procedures may have to be used with extreme caution and not preferred as first line treatment for symptomatic carotid stenosis.

Patent foramen ovale (PFO) has been linked with stroke in the young rather than elderly patient but is present in 15% to 20% of normal individuals. In a randomized trial, treatment with warfarin did not confer an advantage over aspirin for these patients.[69] At present, randomized clinical trial evidence demonstrating benefit for endovascular closure of a PFO is not yet available.

TIA clinics

TIA clinics are a relatively new advance in secondary stroke prevention. These are clinics that are aimed to attend quickly to patients having a TIA with the knowledge that the risk of stroke is highest in the first few days after a TIA.[156] Recent studies have shown that such urgent evaluation of patients with TIA or minor stroke leads to a dramatic reduction in the risk of recurrent ischemic event at 90 days by up to 80%.[156,157] The principal focus of the clinic would be to assess and institute appropriate secondary prevention strategies, such as antiplatelet therapy, blood pressure control, and lipid lowering, keeping in mind that patients with atrial fibrillation and carotid stenosis may need special and rapid attention. Such clinics, if well organized, may have the potential to prevent unnecessary admission of TIA patients to the hospital.

PRIMARY STROKE PREVENTION

Primary prevention refers to efforts to prevent a first stroke or a TIA and may adopt the population or mass approach, or a high-risk individual approach. There have been several proposed population primary prevention strategies to reduce hypertension, which in turn will reduce the incidence of stroke. The relationship between excessive salt intake and the risk of hypertension has been firmly established.[158] Reducing salt intake by half would not only reduce blood pressure in hypertensive and normotensive individuals,[159] but is also estimated to reduce stroke incidence by 22%.[158] Eighty percent of the salt we consume is hidden within processed food, thus reducing the amount of salt added to food during manufacture would have an enormous public health impact. Reductions in salt content of processed food by 10% to 20%, an amount imperceptible to salt taste receptors, could result in reductions in daily salt intake of about 6 grams. This could lead to a significant drop in blood pressure levels in the population without requiring any lifestyle changes—the latter generally being associated with poor compliance. The major difficulty, however, lies in moving governments to legislate such drastic changes within the food industry. Other potentially cost-effective population-wide prevention strategies may be tobacco control via the regulation of tobacco accessibility and taxation, and promotion of healthy diets and exercise.

The high-risk individual approach involves identifying and treating those with hypertension, atrial fibrillation, and diabetes mellitus, these disorders potentially contributing to a large proportion of population-attributable risk of stroke, given their high prevalence and strong association with stroke risk. A meta-analysis conducted by the Blood Pressure Lowering Treatment Trialists' Collaboration demonstrated that treatment with antihypertensive medication reduces the incidence of stroke by 28% to 38%, depending on the medication used.[160] The efficacy of warfarin for stroke prevention in atrial fibrillation is well established.[161] The combination of aspirin and clopidogrel is inferior to warfarin in reducing stroke recurrence and carries the same risk of intracranial hemorrhage.[162] A large trial of intensive blood sugar lowering in type 2 diabetes mellitus was not associated with a reduction of macrovascular outcomes, and hence its role in primary stroke prevention is uncertain at the present time.[163]

ORGANIZATION OF STROKE SERVICES

Given the rapid advances in stroke care in the past decade, it is now recognized that there needs to be a well-organized network of stroke services to deliver such care effectively to stroke patients, and this often requires integration of hospital and community services. There is much debate about how such services must be organized within hospitals, and it is clear that different systems will operate in different countries and regions.[164] Most evidence for benefit from organized stroke units in hospitals is seen for comprehensive stroke units, which are those combining acute care and rehabilitation.[165] Pure rehabilitation units also confer some benefit for patients, whereas the evidence is weakest for mobile stroke teams roving within general wards and for purely acute units.[165] The core requirements of a comprehensive stroke unit are a well-staffed multidisciplinary team of physicians, nurses, and therapists whose work is coordinated through regular meetings, and the presence of protocol-guided care pathways.[165] The physician who is associated with a stroke unit must have a significant passion for stroke care. In addition to neurologists, geriatricians, internists, and rehabilitation specialists may each have the ability to manage stroke units provided they have appropriate training in acute and subacute care. Nursing, in particular, is an integral part of any stroke service, particularly given the constancy of nursing provision in any phase of stroke care. A key person within a stroke service is the "stroke nurse manager," whose role involves acute triaging and delivery of acute treatment; coordination of care on the ward; liaison between the stroke team, patients, and their caregivers; and external organizations involved in stroke care. There needs to be greater emphasis on improving communication with caregivers and closely involving them in the care of patients, particularly in ensuring adequate support for them on discharge. The development of community-based support networks and rehabilitation services (home-based or outpatient) are important to develop in the context of an integrated stroke care service. Such community services will enable early supported discharge from hospitals and ongoing support for patients after leaving the hospital. Obviously, key factors in developing such services include cost-effectiveness analyses and regional resources and needs. Such systems have been established and tested in developed nations, but the challenge of providing stroke care in developing nations remain enormous. In populous developing nations such as China and India, urban hospital stroke care is emerging, but the vast majority of the populations in these countries may need to be serviced by region-specific modifications of community-based stroke care.

For a complete list of references, please visit online only at www.expertconsult.com

CHAPTER 63

Disorders of the Autonomic Nervous System

Horacio Kaufmann
Italo Biaggioni

We will focus on the consequences of aging on autonomic cardiovascular control. The neurobiology of aging and the effects of aging on gastrointestinal and urinary tract function are detailed in other sections in this book.

We will first provide a brief summary of autonomic pathways involved in cardiovascular control, and the methods used to assess their function. We will then review the effect of aging on the different components involved in autonomic cardiovascular control, namely, alterations in afferent and efferent function, and in end-organ responsiveness. We will then discuss the integrated effect of these changes on the response of elderly people to daily stresses of life (i.e., response to upright posture and to food ingestion). We conclude by discussing pathologic disorders of the autonomic nervous system that are present clinically in elderly people, such as orthostatic hypotension, syncope, pure autonomic failure, and multiple system atrophy.

BASIC CONCEPTS OF AUTONOMIC PHYSIOLOGY

Autonomic pathways

Autonomic regulation depends on three main components. Afferent fibers continuously sense changes in blood pressure (baroreceptors), blood content of oxygen, and other chemical signals (chemoreceptors), pain (sensory afferents), and cortical stimulation. These signals are integrated in brainstem centers that ultimately modulate sympathetic and parasympathetic outflows, which are transmitted to target organs via efferent fibers. The baroreflex provides an example of these pathways (Figure 63-1). This is a redundant system, with input from multiple independent afferent pathways that ensure maintenance of cardiovascular regulation even after partial damage.[1] The afferent limb of this reflex includes pressure-sensitive receptors located in the walls of cardiopulmonary veins, the right atrium, and within almost every large artery of the neck and thorax, but particularly within the carotid and aortic arteries. Stimulated by stretch, these low- and high-pressure baroreceptors monitor venous and arterial pressures, respectively, and relay that information to brainstem centers. Information both from the venous and the aortic arch baroreceptors is carried centrally via fibers that course within the vagus nerve (X cranial nerve). Carotid sinus baroreceptor nerve activity is relayed centrally by passage first through the carotid sinus (Hering's) nerve, then through the glossopharyngeal nerve (IX cranial nerve) before arriving at the same brainstem centers.

Afferent fibers from these multiple baroreceptors have their first synapse in the nucleus tractus solitarii (NTS) of the medulla oblongata.[2] This nucleus inhibits sympathetic tone and is crucial to baroreflex function. Its destruction (e.g., by experimental lesion[3] or neurologic damage)[4] leads to loss of baroreflex function, resulting in episodes of hypertension and tachycardia.[5] In addition to the afferent input arising from the baroreceptors, the NTS also receives modulating input from many other cardiovascular brain centers, such as the area postrema. The NTS provides excitatory inputs to the caudal ventrolateral medulla (CVLM), which in turn inhibits the rostral ventrolateral medulla (RVLM),[6,7] where the pacemaker neurons that originate sympathetic tone are believed to be located.[8] RVLM neurons project to the preganglionic sympathetic neurons in the intermediolateral column of the spinal cord that send fibers outside the CNS. Parasympathetic activity is also modulated by the NTS, through projections to preganglionic parasympathetic neurons in the nucleus ambiguus and the motor nucleus of the vagus (Figure 63-1).

The importance of autonomic mechanisms in the regulation of blood pressure is most evident when they fail. Damage of baroreflex afferents (e.g., as consequence of radiation or surgery, leads to labile blood pressure that is very difficult to control).[5] At the other extreme, degeneration of central or efferent structures, as seen in patients with primary autonomic failure, leads to disabling orthostatic hypotension.[9] In the most severe cases, patients are unable to stand but for few seconds before profound orthostatic hypotension and loss of consciousness ensues. These disorders are described later in this chapter.

Methods used to test autonomic function

POSTURE (ORTHOSTATIC) TEST

Perhaps the most informative and simplest autonomic evaluation is the posture test. The patient's blood pressure and heart rate are measured after 5 to 10 minutes in the supine position, and repeated after the subject stands motionless for 3 to 5 minutes. There is some value in repeating measurements at each of these time points, but just one measurement is informative. Virtually all patients with severe autonomic failure will have an immediate fall in blood pressure on standing. Other autonomic conditions associated with delayed orthostatic hypotension require a 30-minute stand test for their diagnosis,[10] but these are usually not associated with widespread autonomic neuropathy. Heart rate is crucial in interpreting blood pressure changes. Patients with severe autonomic failure characteristically have no or little (about 10–15 beats/min) increase in heart rate despite profound orthostatic hypotension. A greater increase in heart rate usually indicates that other conditions (e.g., volume depletion or medications) are contributing to orthostatic hypotension.

NONINVASIVE AUTONOMIC TESTS

Heart rate responses to deep breathing (i.e., respiratory sinus arrhythmia) and to the Valsalva maneuver are simple yet informative autonomic tests. They require real-time monitoring of heart rate. Respiratory sinus arrhythmia is assessed during controlled breathing at a rate of six deep breaths per minute (Figure 63-2). The sinus arrhythmia ratio is calculated by dividing the longest to the shortest R-R interval. This expiratory/inspiratory (E/I) ratio decreases progressively with age. Subjects younger than 40 usually have a ratio

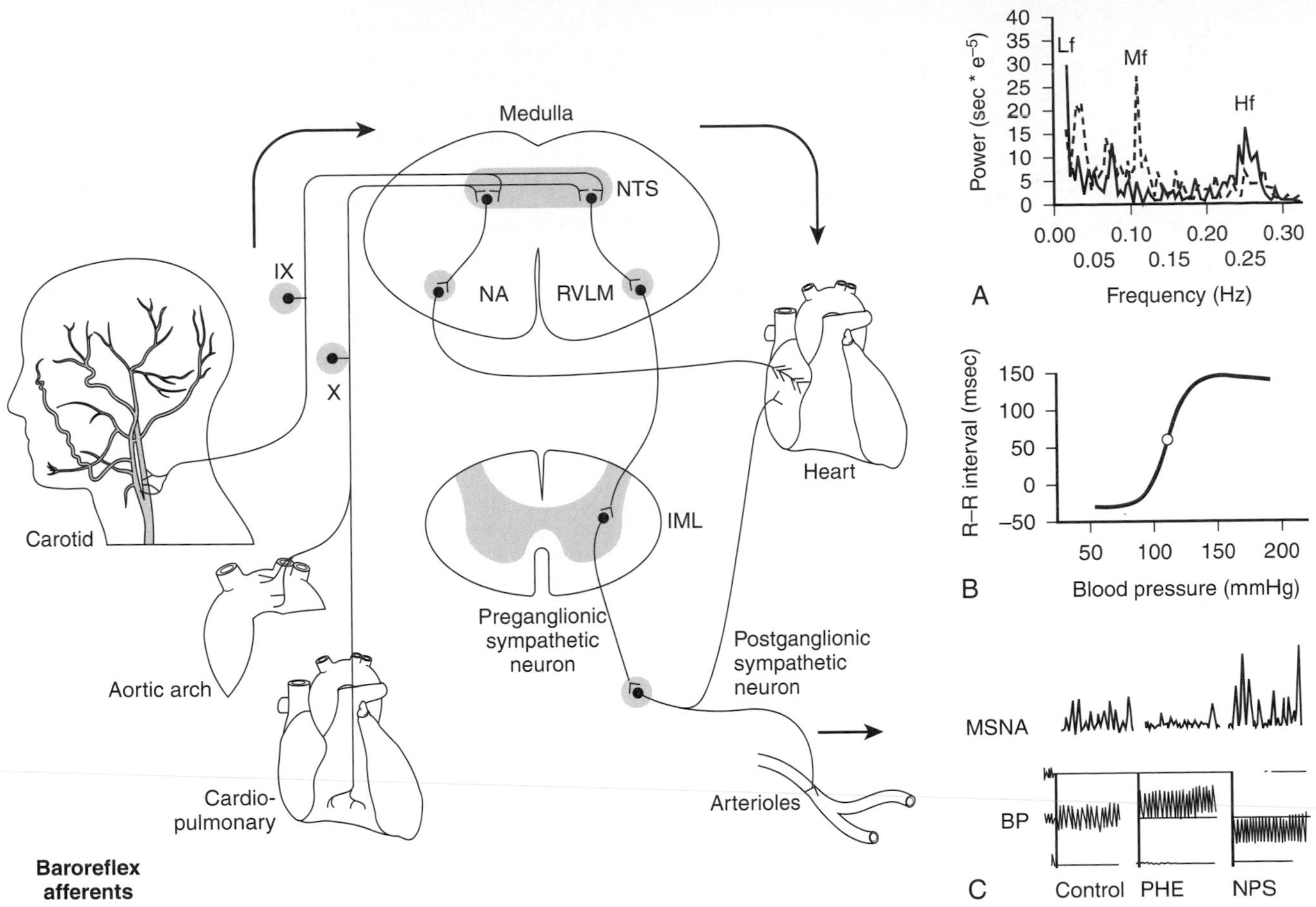

Figure 63-1. Simplified anatomic/functional scheme of baroreflex function. Afferent fibers located in the right atrium and in the cardiopulmonary veins (low-pressure baroreceptors), and in the aortic arch and carotid sinus (high-pressure baroreceptors) are activated by stretch, and relay this information through the vagus (X) or glossopharyngeal (IX) nerves to the nucleus tractus solitarii (NTS) of the brainstem. The NTS provides excitatory inputs to the caudal ventrolateral medulla, which in turn inhibits the rostral ventrolateral medulla (RVLM)[6,7] (for simplicity the NTS is shown as projecting direct inhibitory pathways to the RVLM), where pacemaker neurons that originate sympathetic tone are believed to be located. These cell bodies send their efferent projections through the intermediolateral column of the spinal cord (IML). Baroreflex function can be simplified as follows: an increase in blood pressure is detected by arterial baroreceptors, which increase their firing into the NTS; activation of the NTS leads to a greater inhibitory output to the RVLM; inhibition of pacemaker cells in the RVLM results in a compensatory reduction in sympathetic tone. Conversely, a decrease in blood pressure results in decreased firing in the NTS, withdrawal of the inhibitory influence of this nuclei on the RVLM, and a compensatory increase in sympathetic tone. Parasympathetic activity is also modulated by the NTS, through projections to the nucleus ambiguus (NA). An increase in blood pressure will lead to activation of the NTS and of the NA, with increased parasympathetic activity. Methods to assess baroreflex function include (**A**) spectral analysis, by correlating spontaneous changes in blood pressure and heart rate, and (**B**) by the neck barocuff method. Results obtained by these methods are influenced by afferent baroreceptor input, brainstem pathways, and end-organ responsiveness. Baroreflex modulation of sympathetic activity can be assessed with (**C**) microelectrode recording of postganglionic efferent sympathetic nerve activity (MSNA). In this example, blood pressure increment with phenylephrine (PHE) produced a baroreflex-mediated decrease in MSNA and blood pressure reduction with nitroprusside (NPS) produces a baroreflex-mediated increase in MSNA.

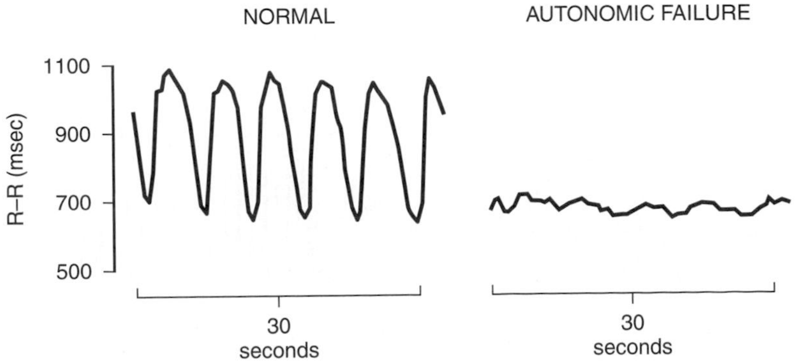

Figure 63-2. Successive electrocardiographic R-R intervals during paced breathing in a normal subject (*left*) and in a patient with autonomic failure (*right*).

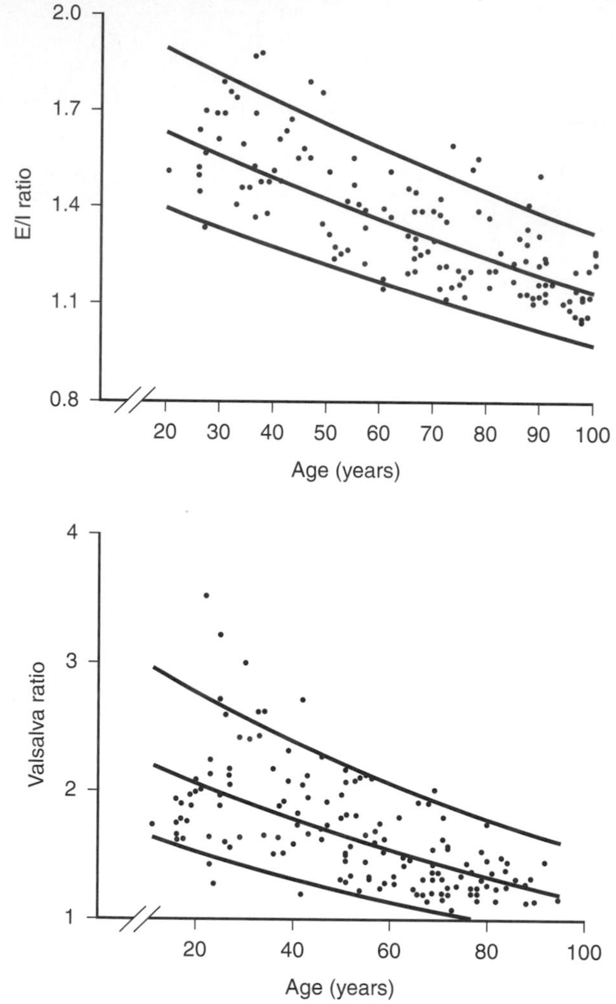

Figure 63-3. (*Top*) Expiratory/inspiratory (E/I) ratio during paced breathing in normal subjects according to age. Linear regression and confidence limits are shown. (*Bottom*) Valsalva ratio in normal subjects according to age. Linear regression and confidence limits are shown.

less than 1.2 (Figure 63-3). A Valsalva maneuver is induced by having the subject blow against a 40 mm Hg pressure for 12 seconds. A 5 to 10 cc syringe can be used as a mouthpiece and can be connected to a sphygmomanometer to monitor pressure. A small leak should be introduced into the system to ensure the subject uses thoracic effort. The increase in intrathoracic pressure produces a transient fall in blood pressure with narrowing of pulse pressure during phase II (strain), whereas blood pressure overshoots above baseline values during phase IV (after release) (Figure 63-4). In autonomic failure blood pressure continues to fall during phase II and the normal overshoot is absent during phase IV. Thus appropriate evaluation of the Valsalva response requires continuous recording of blood pressure, which can be accomplished noninvasively with finger plethysmography (Finapress, Portapress) or tonometry of the radial artery (Colin). Even if blood pressure cannot be monitored, however, heart rate responses are useful. The blood pressure changes described previously produce reciprocal baroreflex-mediated changes in heart rate; heart rate increases during the hypotensive phase II of the Valsalva maneuver, and decreases during the blood pressure overshoot of phase IV. The Valsalva ratio is calculated by dividing the fastest heart rate during phase II by the slowest heart rate during phase IV. As with the E/I ratio, the Valsalva ratio decreases with age and results should be interpreted accordingly (see Figure 63-3).

SPECTRAL ANALYSIS OF HEART RATE AND BLOOD PRESSURE

Blood pressure and heart rate are kept within a relatively narrow range because of autonomic baroreflex mechanisms. Within this narrow range, however, blood pressure shows substantial variability. Most of this variability is not random, but follows natural rhythmic patterns, which can be studied using spectral analysis techniques. These patterns are importantly modulated by the respiratory frequency. In particular, respiration frequency influences heart rate variability, and this interaction is under baroreflex control via the vagus

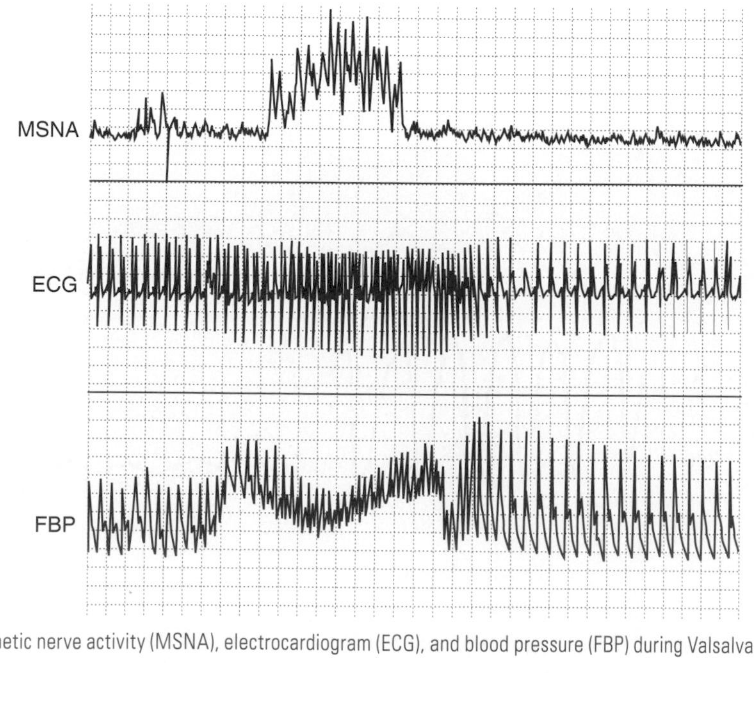

Figure 63-4. Muscle sympathetic nerve activity (MSNA), electrocardiogram (ECG), and blood pressure (FBP) during Valsalva maneuver in a normal subject.

nerves. The "respiratory peak" of heart rate variability, evident in the high-frequency spectrum, can be used to assess cardiac parasympathetic function. Respirations also modulate blood pressure, but this is mediated through mechanical events and does not reflect autonomic mechanisms and is not affected by autonomic blockade.[11] In contrast, blood pressure shows a lower frequency rhythm (Mayer waves). This is mediated in part by sympathetic modulation of vascular tone. There is substantial interindividual variability in the spectral analysis of heart rate and blood pressure, making these methods less suitable for the diagnosis of individual patients with less than severe autonomic impairment. Nonetheless, population studies have shown that impaired heart rate variability as shown by spectral analysis of heart rate is an independent predictor of mortality in patients after myocardial infarction, and in patients with diabetes mellitus.

Assessment of baroreflex function

Several methods can be used to quantify the changes in heart rate (or R-R interval) produced by unit change of blood pressure. These methods require the simultaneous monitoring of blood pressure and heart rate. Baroreflex function can be assessed by measuring the reciprocal changes in blood pressure and heart rate that occur spontaneously, or during the phase IV of the Valsalva maneuver. Blood pressure can be increased with phenylephrine or decreased with nitroprusside and the gain of the baroreflex expressed as the change in R-R interval per unit of blood pressure (expressed in msec/mm Hg) during the linear portion of this relationship. Each of these methods provides slightly different normative values of baroreflex gain. It is important to note that changes in blood pressure affect all baroreflex afferents, including carotid sinus and aortic high-pressure receptors and low-pressure receptors located in the venous circulation. The carotid sinus reflex can be selectively investigated by producing positive and negative pressure to the neck, to simulate decreases and increases in intracarotid pressure, respectively. All of the methods described above rely on instantaneous changes in heart rate, which depend exclusively on the parasympathetic limb of the baroreflex. The sympathetic limb of the baroreflex can be assessed by relating changes in blood pressure to reciprocal changes in muscle sympathetic nerve activity (see later discussion).

BIOCHEMICAL ASSESSMENT OF SYMPATHETIC FUNCTION

Plasma norepinephrine provides a useful measure of sympathetic activity. It is particularly useful when measuring acute changes to standard stimuli. For example, upright posture induces a doubling of plasma norepinephrine. Patients with autonomic impairment have a blunted response. Basal norepinephrine, however, is different depending on the underlying pathology. It is low in patients with PAF and normal or slightly decreased in patients with MSA (see later discussion). In contrast, patients with volume depletion will have enhanced norepinephrine response to upright posture.

ESTIMATION OF NOREPINEPHRINE SPILLOVER

Despite the usefulness of plasma norepinephrine measurements, it is noteworthy that only a small percentage of the norepinephrine released by noradrenergic nerves actually reaches the circulation. Most of it is taken back into nerve terminals by the norepinephrine transporter (i.e., reuptake) or is metabolized. Norepinephrine clearance can be measured by infusing a known amount of titrated norepinephrine. During steady-state infusion, it is assumed that clearance of titrated norepinephrine reflects clearance of endogenous norepinephrine. Once clearance is calculated, the norepinephrine appearance rate into the circulation (spillover) can be estimated. A comprehensive review of the advantages and limitations of this technique is beyond the scope of this chapter and can be found elsewhere.[12]

MUSCLE SYMPATHETIC NERVE ACTIVITY

Nerve activity can be recorded directly by introducing a recording electrode into an accessible peripheral nerve. Afferent and efferent fibers can be recorded using this technique. Sympathetic efferent activity can be selectively recorded by careful placement of the electrode. The peroneal nerve at the level of the knee is commonly used to measure postganglionic sympathetic nerve activity. Although there is considerable interindividual variability in muscle sympathetic nerve activity, baseline recordings expressed as sympathetic bursts per minute are highly reproducible in a single individual between different recording sites, and when measured on different occasions. Muscle sympathetic nerve activity effectively monitors central sympathetic outflow and is tightly modulated by the baroreflex. Stimuli that increases blood pressure by activating central sympathetic outflow will be reflected as an increase in muscle sympathetic nerve activity. Conversely, stimuli that increase blood pressure directly (e.g., an injection of phenylephrine), will produce baroreflex-modulated suppression of muscle sympathetic nerve activity. This recording is also exquisitely sensitive to sympathetic withdrawal. For example, sympathetic activity disappears during neurogenic syncope.[13]

EFFECT OF AGING ON THE DIFFERENT COMPONENTS OF AUTONOMIC CARDIOVASCULAR CONTROL

Baroreflex function

There is a progressive decline in baroreflex sensitivity with aging[14] due to both vascular and neural deficits. Cardiovagal baroreflex gain (i.e., the reciprocal heart rate changes produced by changes in arterial pressure) declines with age, but the ability of the cardiopulmonary baroreflex to inhibit sympathetic nerve traffic has been reported to be well preserved with age in healthy adults. Hence, vagal, but not sympathetic baroreflex gains vary inversely with subjects' ages and their baseline arterial pressures. There is no correlation between sympathetic and vagal baroreflex gains.[15]

Cardiac parasympathetic function

Cardiac vagal innervation decreases with age as clearly shown by a progressive reduction in respiratory sinus arrhythmia (see Figure 63-3). Experimental evidence suggests that long-term physical activity attenuates the decline in cardiovagal baroreflex gain by maintaining neural vagal control,[16] but among older adults, the level of fitness does not prevent the decrease in cardiac vagal function, suggesting that the age decline in cardiac vagal function cannot be completely prevented by physical activity.[17]

Systemic sympathetic function

Muscle sympathetic nerve activity (MSNA) increases progressively with age likely because of increased central nervous system drive (Figure 63-5). Sympathetic nerve traffic increases in a region-specific manner; however, outflow to skeletal muscle and the gut increases, but not to the kidney.[18] The increase in central sympathetic outflow results in higher levels of plasma norepinephrine with age, but reduced norepinephrine clearance appears to play a role as well.[19,20] It is suggested that age-related elevations in whole-body and abdominal adiposity can explain the increase in basal MSNA with age in healthy humans.[21] The relation between body fat and MSNA is observed in both young and older populations.[22] Tanaka et al[21] showed that although body mass index (BMI) was similar in groups of younger and older subjects, both total body fatness and abdominal adiposity were greater in the older subjects and were directly related to baseline levels of MSNA. Preliminary data[23] indicate that circulating concentrations of leptin are related to both adiposity and MSNA. Thus age-associated elevations in total and abdominal adiposity may be linked to increases in MSNA, at least in part, via elevations in leptin levels.[18] In contrast to sympathetic neuronal activity, adrenaline secretion from the adrenal medulla is greatly reduced with age, and adrenaline release in response to acute stress is attenuated in older men. Plasma adrenaline concentration remains normal, however, because of reduced plasma clearance.

End-organ responsiveness

Despite the number of β-adrenergic receptors in lymphocytes being unaltered with age[24] and higher neurotransmitter levels, β-adrenergic responses to norepinephrine are blunted with progressive aging, probably because of β-adrenergic receptor downregulation in response to higher circulating levels of norepinephrine and a defect in G-protein receptor complexes and reduced adenyl cyclase activity.[25,26] Depressed β_1 responses lead to impaired cardioacceleration and reduced cardiac contractility. Reduced β_2 responses are manifested by increased vascular tone because α_1 vasoconstriction ability remains unchanged. The combination of age-related vascular stiffening and depressed β-adrenergic function result in reduced arterial baroreflex sensitivity[27] in elderly subjects.[28–30] This reduces cardioacceleration during hypotension.[31] Reduced postural cardioacceleration, and decreased baroreceptor gain with age, increases the risk for orthostatic hypotension in elderly people.[32,33] Blood pressure in older subjects is sustained by increased peripheral vascular tone, despite depressed cardioacceleration. Due to a higher reliance on vascular resistance, dehydration and vasodilator medications pose a high risk for hypotension and syncope in older subjects. On the other hand, vasovagal syncope is reportedly less frequent in elderly subjects.[34] Postjunctional α-mediated vasoconstriction is also impaired in older adults.[35]

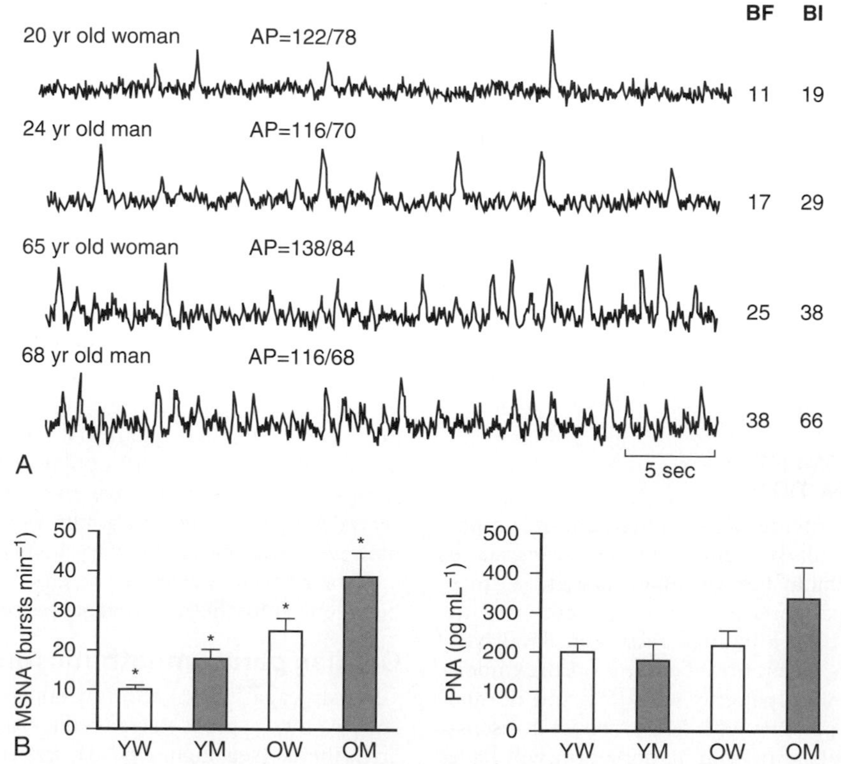

Figure 63-5. Age-associated increases in muscle sympathetic nerve activity. (A) Muscle sympathetic nerve activity (MSNA) from four healthy adult humans under supine resting conditions (*top to bottom*): young female, young male, older female, older male. MSNA burst frequency (BF; bursts min^{-1}) and burst incidence (BI; bursts $(100 \text{ heart beats})^{-1}$) are higher in the neurograms of the older adults in both sexes. However, the female subjects demonstrate lower MSNA than the males at each age. *AP,* arterial blood pressure. (B) Mean ± SEM; values for MSNA in four groups of subjects: young women (YW), young men (YM), older women (OW), and older men (OM). MSNA was at least twice as great in the older compared with the young subjects of the same sex. At each age, however, MSNA was significantly lower in the women. These age and sex differences in MSNA were not reflected in the corresponding antecubital venous plasma noradrenaline concentrations. *PNA,* plasma noradrenaline concentration; $^*P < 0.05$ versus all other groups. *(Reproduced from Seals and Esler.[18])*

Vascular changes

Aging stiffens blood vessels[36] and alters vasomotor function. In elderly subjects, coronary vasodilation capacity is reduced because of reduced nitric oxide release by the senescent endothelium. Conversely, endothelin release by the endothelium is increased in elderly people, promoting vasoconstriction.[37] These alterations increase susceptibility to myocardial ischemia, particularly during increased demand stresses such as tachyarrhythmias[38] and may also impair cerebral autoregulation, increasing susceptibility to syncope. Other age-dependent cardiovascular alterations that may increase predisposition to syncope are increased left ventricular afterload, and myocyte hypertrophy. These alterations lead to impaired diastolic filling and chronic ischemia that may predispose subjects to cardiac arrhythmias and decrease ventricular volume that may manifest as syncope. Decreased preload volume precipitated by vasodilators, dehydration, or blood pooling can dramatically reduce cardiac output and precipitate syncope. Susceptibility to atrial fibrillation increases with age because of reductions in pacemaker cells, progressive fibrosis of the cardiac conduction system, and concomitant cardiovascular diseases that alter atrial morphology. In older patients, impaired diastolic filling and a reduction of up to 50% in cardiac output may develop during atrial fibrillation and lead to syncope.

Neuroendocrine changes

Plasma renin and aldosterone levels fall with age[39,40] and atrial natriuretic peptide increases fivefold to ninefold.[41] The vasopressin response to hypotension may also be reduced.[42] These changes make sodium and water conservation less effective and intravascular volume depletion more frequent, thus increasing the tendency for syncope. In addition, many elderly people have an impaired thirst response to increases in osmolality and do not consume sufficient fluids to prevent hypovolemia.

EFFECT OF AGING ON AUTONOMIC RESPONSE TO STRESS

The most frequent autonomic stress is the cardiovascular adaptation to upright posture and other physiologically induced changes in intravascular volume. Vascular and neurogenic dysfunction, and a host of medications, can cause orthostatic hypotension in the elderly. In the Cardiovascular Health study,[43] the prevalence of orthostatic hypotension was 18% in subjects age 65 years or older, although only 2% of the subjects reported dizziness with standing. There was a modest association with systolic hypertension when supine, carotid stenosis greater than 50%, and with the use of oral hypoglycemic agents, but only a weak association with the use of β-blockers and no association with other antihypertensive drugs. In other reports, however, as expected, the use of antihypertensive medications was significantly related to postural hypotension in elderly people[44] and discontinuing antihypertensive medications led to an improvement of orthostatic hypotension.

Orthostatic hypotension

Elderly people have impaired defenses against the fluid shifts that normally accompany upright posture. Their threshold to develop symptomatic orthostatic hypotension is, therefore, lower compared with younger subjects. A variety of symptoms develop with a reduction in blood flow to the brain. Typically, patients will complain of visual disturbances (e.g., blurring, tunneling, or darkening of vision), dizziness, light-headedness, giddiness, feeling faint, and a dull neck and shoulder ache (coat hanger pain). When orthostatic hypotension is pronounced and cerebral blood flow decreases below a critical level (approximately 25 mL/min per 100 grams), syncope (i.e., loss of consciousness) occurs. A decrease in baroreceptor sensitivity is probably involved in the mild, frequent postural hypotension seen in elderly people. One study, for example, showed a diminished response to tilt (a baroreceptor-mediated response) but not to non–baroreceptor-mediated stimuli, such as the cold pressor test or isometric exercise.[45] The reduced baroreceptor response in elderly people (when compared with younger controls) was seen in both hypertensive and normotensive subjects. Insults that would be compensated for in the young may induce symptomatic hypotension in elderly people. For example, drug-induced orthostatic hypotension is the cause of recurrent dizzy spells or syncope in 12% to 15% of elderly patients and should always be suspected.[46] Diuretics, calcium antagonists, angiotensin-converting enzyme (ACE) inhibitors, and nitrates are frequently prescribed in elderly patients for the management of hypertension, congestive heart failure, and ischemic heart disease. Other pharmacologic agents frequently associated with orthostatic hypotension include phenothiazines, antidepressants, sedatives, and narcotics. Similarly, prolonged bed rest is frequent in elderly people and an important cause of cardiovascular deconditioning. Several mechanisms contribute to decreased orthostatic tolerance and syncope after prolonged bed rest.[47] Bed rest reduces extracellular fluid volume, and the skeletal muscle deconditioning impairs the lower limb muscle pump that facilitates venous return in the upright posture. Under normal conditions, important mechanical adjustments to counteract orthostatic pooling of the blood are the muscle and respiratory pumps. Skeletal muscle tone has critical bearing on the volume of blood displaced into the legs when standing. Because intramuscular pressure is decreased after prolonged bed rest, venous pooling augments and venous return to the heart is easily compromised in the standing posture. Thus skeletal muscle atrophy due to prolonged bed rest should be considered as a primary or aggravating factor in any patient with symptoms of light-headedness on standing or documented orthostatic hypotension. If the problem persists after adequate measures are taken, a pathologic impairment of autonomic function should be considered. The occurrence of orthostatic hypotension in elderly people is predictive of mortality.[48] A study of 3522 Japanese-American men, age 71 to 93 years, found that orthostatic hypotension, defined as a decrease in systolic blood pressure by 20 mm Hg or in diastolic blood pressure by 10 mm Hg, was present in 7% and increased with age.

Postprandial and heat-induced hypotension

A frequent reason for falls and syncope in elderly people is postprandial and heat-induced hypotension.[49,50] In normal subjects, eating, especially carbohydrates, is accompanied by splanchnic vasodilation, and hot weather produces cutaneous vasodilation but there is little change in arterial pressure because of a compensatory increase in sympathetic vasoconstrictor outflow. In elderly people, however, similarly to what occurs in patients with autonomic failure, both eating and hot weather significantly lower blood pressure (even in the supine position) because these subjects cannot compensate for the vasodilation with an appropriate increase in sympathetic outflow.[51,52] Among elderly residents of nursing homes, for example, 24% to 36% have a 20 mm Hg or greater fall in systolic blood pressure within 75 minutes after eating a meal.[53] In patients with autonomic failure, postprandial hypotension occurs within 30 minutes of meal ingestion, lasts about 1.5 to 2 hours, and can be profound; blood pressure falls of as much as 50 to 70 mmHg can be observed. This is not only a useful diagnostic test, but it is important to consider the timing of meals when measuring blood pressure in these patients. The initial syncopal episode in patients with chronic autonomic failure is frequently triggered by postprandial hypotension.

DISORDERS OF THE AUTONOMIC NERVOUS SYSTEM IN ELDERLY PEOPLE

Neurally mediated syncopal syndromes

The most frequent cause of hypotension and syncope in otherwise normal subjects is neurally mediated syncope, also referred to as vasovagal, vasodepressor, or reflex syncope. Vasovagal syncope is generally, although not exclusively, observed in patients with no evidence of structural heart disease. Prodromal symptoms include dizziness, blurred vision, nausea, and diaphoresis. This syncope results from acute vasodilation and bradycardia. According to the apparent trigger mechanism, neurally mediated syncope can be classified in several distinct syndromes: emotional faint, carotid sinus syncope, micturition or gastrointestinal syncope, glossopharyngeal or trigeminal syncope, ventricular or neurocardiogenic syncope, and exercise syncope (commonly seen in aortic stenosis).

Neurally mediated syncope is an acute hemodynamic reaction produced by a sudden change in autonomic nervous system activity.[54] The normal pattern of autonomic outflow that maintains blood pressure in the standing position (increase sympathetic and decreased parasympathetic activity) is acutely reversed. Parasympathetic outflow to the sinus node of the heart increases, producing bradycardia, while sympathetic outflow to blood vessels is reduced, resulting in profound vasodilation.

Classic neurally mediated syncopal syndromes are triggered after compression of carotid baroreceptors in the neck (carotid sinus syncope),[13] following rapid emptying of a distended bladder (micturition syncope)[56] or distention of the gastrointestinal tract.[55] Glossopharyngeal or trigeminal neuralgia can induce syncope by a similar mechanism.[57,58] In several clinical types of neurally mediated syncope the trigger locus is easily identified, but frequently neurally mediated syncope occurs with no obvious trigger. Although in these cases the source of abnormal afferent signals was believed to be sensory receptors in the heart (i.e., neurocardiogenic or "ventricular" syncope,[59,60] neurally mediated syncope has recently been induced in patients with heart transplants in whom the ventricle is likely to be denervated.[61] Perhaps sensory receptors in the heart transplant patients are in the arterial tree rather than the ventricle. Similarly, the threshold to trigger neurally mediated syncope can be lowered by a reduction in cardiac preload caused by reduced intravascular volume or excessive venous pooling. Intravascular volume depletion is common in elderly people because sodium and water conservation are less effective, renin and aldosterone levels fall, atrial natriuretic peptide increases, and the vasopressin response to hypotension may be reduced. Moreover, many elderly subjects have an impaired thirst response to increases in osmolality and are prone to hypovolemia, particularly during febrile illnesses. Excessive venous pooling occurs postprandially in the splanchnic circulation, in the skin during exposure to heat, and in the lower limbs because of muscle atrophy when standing after prolonged periods of bed rest, significantly increasing susceptibility to syncope.

Despite the diverse trigger mechanisms of these different types of neurally mediated syncope, the efferent reflex response is remarkably similar. There is an increase in parasympathetic efferent activity to the sinus node producing bradycardia or even a few seconds of sinus arrest, and a decrease in sympathetic activity responsible, at least in part, for the fall in blood pressure. Bradycardia is not the only or even the main cause of hypotension because neither atropine nor a ventricular pacemaker, which prevent bradycardia, is able to prevent hypotension and syncope. Blood pressure falls mainly because of vasodilation. The mechanisms responsible for vasodilation are not completely understood. Sympathetic efferent activity decreases as shown by studies using microneurography and measurements of circulating norepinephrine.[62–64] Sympathetic "withdrawal," however, seems an incomplete explanation for profound vasodilation. Norepinephrine fails to increase but vasopressin, endothelin-1, and angiotensin II vasoconstrictor peptides, important to maintain blood pressure—which should partially compensate for the fall in sympathetic activity—increase normally during neurally mediated syncope.[63] To explain the profound fall in blood pressure, β-mediated vasodilation induced by a rise in adrenaline has been postulated.[65] Nitric oxide–mediated vasodilation due to a rise in cholinergic activity may be involved.[54,66] In summary, current understanding of neurally mediated syncope shows inappropriate reduction in sympathetic nerve activity and norepinephrine release. There is an appropriate increase in epinephrine, angiotensin II, vasopressin, and endothelin release, and preliminary evidence suggests that nitric oxide synthesis is activated.

Baroreflex failure

The most common cause of baroreflex failure is iatrogenic damage during neck surgery or radiation therapy of neural structures that carry afferent input from the baroreceptors. Neurologic disorders involving the nucleus tractus solitarii, where these afferents have their first synapse, can also produce baroreflex failure.[4] In a few cases, the underlying cause is not found. Baroreflex function is impaired in essential hypertension, and may be transmitted as a genetic trait.[67] It is not clear if these cases of baroreflex failure of unknown etiology represent the extreme of the spectrum of baroreflex impairment in essential hypertension. Baroreflex failure patients have severe labile hypertension and hypotension, often accompanied by headache, diaphoresis, and emotional instability. Wide fluctuations of blood pressure are observed, with systolic blood pressure ranging from 50 to 280 mm Hg. The hypertensive crises are accompanied by tachycardia, and are due to sympathetic surges, as documented by notable increases in plasma norepinephrine. Treatment with sympatholytics may provide some benefit, attenuating these surges of hypertension and tachycardia, but adequate blood pressure regulation is seldom achieved in the absence of functional baroreflexes. Of interest is that virtually all reported cases are due to bilateral lesions, whereas unilateral lesions are usually clinically silent. This clinical observation underscores the redundancy of the baroreflex system and its importance in cardiovascular regulation.

Chronic autonomic failure

Autonomic failure is divided into primary and secondary forms. Primary autonomic failure is caused by a degenerative process affecting central autonomic pathways (multiple system atrophy [MSA]), or peripheral autonomic neurons (pure autonomic failure). Secondary autonomic failure results from destruction of peripheral autonomic neurons in disorders, such as diabetes, amyloidosis, and other neuropathies, and very rarely by an enzymatic defect in catecholamine synthesis (dopamine β-hydroxylase deficiency). In chronic autonomic failure, orthostatic hypotension and syncope are caused by impaired vasoconstriction and reduced intravascular volume. Vasoconstriction is deficient because of reduced baroreflex-mediated norepinephrine release from postganglionic sympathetic nerve terminals and low circulating levels of angiotensin II caused by impaired secretion of renin.[68] In patients with autonomic failure and central nervous system dysfunction (i.e., MSA), impaired endothelin and vasopressin release also contribute to deficient vasoconstriction in the standing position.[63,69]

Primary autonomic failure

Primary autonomic failure includes several neurodegenerative diseases of unknown cause: pure autonomic failure (PAF), in which autonomic impairment (i.e., orthostatic hypotension, bladder, and sexual dysfunction) occurs alone; MSA (also called Shy-Drager syndrome) in which autonomic failure is combined with an extrapyramidal and/or cerebellar movement disorder; Parkinson's disease (PD) in which autonomic failure is combined with an extrapyramidal movement disorder; and diffuse Lewy body disease (DLB), in which autonomic failure is combined with an extrapyramidal movement disorder and severe cognitive impairment.

Recent findings suggest that the same neurodegenerative process underlies MSA, PD, DLB, and PAF, as accumulation of α-synuclein in neuronal cytoplasmic inclusions occurs in all these disorders. A gene encoding for α-synuclein, a neuronal protein of unknown function, is mutated in autosomal dominant PD.[70] Nonfamilial PD does not have the mutation but α-synuclein accumulates in Lewy bodies in these patients, suggesting a toxic role for aggregates of this protein.[71] Interestingly, cytoplasmic inclusions in MSA also stain positive for α-synuclein,[72] and Lewy bodies in PAF[73] are strongly synuclein positive. Thus abnormalities in the expression or structure of α-synuclein or associated proteins may cause degeneration of catecholamine-containing neurons. α-Synuclein, therefore, is an important component of intraneuronal inclusions in PAF, PD, DLB, and MSA neurodegenerative disorders, all of which affect the autonomic nervous system to a variable degree. Thus these disorders are best classified as α-synucleinopathies. It is not surprising, therefore, that there is overlap in the clinical presentation of these disorders, and the clinical differences may reflect the type of deposits (forming Lewy bodies or not) and the localization of these deposits within the nervous system. These similarities and differences are discussed later.

PURE AUTONOMIC FAILURE (PAF)

Pure autonomic failure, a disorder first described by Bradbury and Eggleston is a sporadic, adult onset, slowly progressive degeneration of the autonomic nervous system characterized by orthostatic hypotension, bladder and sexual dysfunction, and no other neurologic deficits. Neuropathologic reports of patients with pure autonomic failure showed α-synuclein-positive intraneuronal cytoplasmic inclusions (Lewy bodies) in brainstem nuclei and peripheral autonomic ganglia.[73,74] These patients are otherwise normal and their prognosis is relatively good. Complications are usually those related to falls and associated disorders.

MULTIPLE SYSTEM ATROPHY

Multiple system atrophy (MSA) is a term introduced by Graham and Oppenheimer in 1969 to describe a group of patients with a disorder of unknown cause affecting extrapyramidal, pyramidal, cerebellar, and autonomic pathways. MSA includes the disorders previously called striatonigral degeneration (SND), sporadic olivopontocerebellar atrophy (OPCA), and the Shy-Drager syndrome (SDS). The discovery in 1989 of glial cytoplasmic inclusions in the brain of patients with MSA provided a pathologic marker for the disorder (akin to Lewy bodies in Parkinson's disease), and confirmed that SND, OPCA, and SDS are the same disease with different clinical expression.[75] MSA is a progressive neurodegenerative disease of undetermined cause that occurs sporadically and causes parkinsonism, cerebellar, pyramidal autonomic, and urologic dysfunction in any combination.[76]

Because parkinsonism is the most frequent motor deficit in MSA, these patients are regularly misdiagnosed as suffering from PD. Data from PD brain banks showed how frequently the diagnosis of PD was incorrect; up to 10% of these brains turn out to have MSA.[77] Indeed, even case 1 of James Parkinson's original description (1817), upon which much of his description of paralysis agitans was based, was probably suffering from MSA.

Life expectancy in MSA is shorter than in PD. Ben-Shlomo et al[78] analyzed 433 published cases of pathologically proven MSA over a 100-year period. Mean age of onset was 54 years (range 31–78) and survival 6 years (range 0.5–24). Survival was unaffected by gender, parkinsonian, or pyramidal features, or whether the patient was classified as SND or OPCA. Survival analysis showed a secular trend from a median duration of 5 years for publications between 1887 and 1970, to 7 years between 1991 and 1994. These figures may be biased toward the worst cases, however.

PARKINSON'S DISEASE

Autonomic dysfunction in Parkinson's disease is rarely as severe as in patients with MSA. There is a subgroup of patients with PD, however, with severe autonomic failure even early in the course of the disease. In most cases, autonomic failure occurs late in the course of the illness and is associated with levodopa and dopamine agonist therapy. In patients with PD, Lewy bodies are found in central and in peripheral autonomic neurons, and autonomic dysfunction in this disorder may be caused by both preganglionic and postganglionic neuronal dysfunction.

DIFFUSE LEWY BODY DISEASE

The clinical presentation of these patients is that of PD, but dementia often dominates the clinical picture. Autonomic failure is frequently associated with this disorder.

DIFFERENTIAL DIAGNOSIS AMONG THE α-SYNUCLEINOPATHIES

During the early stages of MSA, autonomic deficits may be the sole clinical manifestation, thus resembling PAF, but after a variable period of time, sometimes several years, extrapyramidal or cerebellar deficits or both invariably develop. In PD, extrapyramidal motor problems are the presenting feature, but later in the disease process, patients may suffer severe autonomic failure, making the clinical distinction with MSA difficult. Complicating the distinction further, similar to what occurs in PD, some MSA cases display motor deficits before autonomic failure is apparent. In clinical practice all these possibilities lead to two main diagnostic problems. First, it cannot be determined whether a patient who has autonomic failure as the only clinical finding and is believed to have PAF, will develop more widespread nonautonomic neuronal damage and turn out to have MSA. Second, it may be difficult to establish if a patient with autonomic failure and a parkinsonian movement disorder has PD or MSA. Clinically, the classic parkinsonian resting tremor of unilateral predominance is rarely seen in patients with MSA, in whom bradykinesia and rigidity predominate. Also, with rare exceptions, patients with MSA do not respond as well to antiparkinsonian medications and the progression of disease is faster.

In addition to clinical criteria, several tests have been used to distinguish between PD, PAF, and MSA. For example, vasopressin release in response to hypotension and growth hormone secretion in response to clonidine are blunted in MSA but preserved in PAF and PD, because brainstem-hypothalamic-pituitary pathways are only affected in MSA.[69,79] Plasma norepinephrine concentration while supine is frequently normal in MSA but low in PAF because postganglionic neurons are normal in MSA.[80] Sphincter EMG shows denervation in MSA because the Onuf's nucleus in segments S2-S4 of the spinal cord is affected in MSA but is normal in PD.[81]

There are also important differences in cardiovascular control between MSA, PAF, and PD with autonomic failure. Although patients with MSA have substantial CNS degeneration, the brainstem centers where sympathetic tone originates (most likely the rostroventrolateral medulla) and distal pathways are intact. In support of this postulate, supine plasma norepinephrine is normal or slightly decreased in MSA, but this residual sympathetic activity is not baroreflex-responsive, hence their inability to maintain upright blood pressure. Furthermore, interruption of this residual sympathetic activity with the ganglion blocker trimethaphan leads to a profound decrease in supine blood pressure in MSA. In contrast, supine plasma norepinephrine is very low in PAF and treatment with trimethaphan produces small or no changes in blood pressure, indicating that the lesion is distal to brainstem centers.[82]

Similarly, sympathetic cardiac innervation is selectively affected in PD and PAF but is intact in MSA. Several studies using single photon emission computed tomography (SPECT) imaging with ^{123}I metaiodobenzylguanidine (MIBG),[83–85] and positron emission tomography (PET) with 6-[^{18}F] fluorodopamine[86] have shown abnormal cardiac sympathetic innervation in patients with PD, while it was normal in patients with MSA.[87] This may turn out to be a useful diagnostic test to distinguish between PD and MSA because sympathetic innervation of the heart is impaired in PD, and not in MSA. Moreover, in a patient with presumed PAF, finding normal sympathetic cardiac innervation indicates a likely development of MSA.

AUTONOMIC AND NEUROENDOCRINE TESTING

Numerous studies have described abnormal cardiovascular reflexes in MSA patients. A characteristic of MSA is that afferent and central autonomic and neuroendocrine reflex pathways are selectively affected, whereas postganglionic autonomic fibers are spared.[69] Baroreceptor-mediated vasopressin release—a measurement of afferent baroreceptor function—is spared in PAF, and presumably in PD, but is blunted in MSA.[69] Intravenous clonidine, a centrally active α_2-adrenoceptor agonist that stimulates growth hormone (GH) secretion, also tests the function of hypothalamic-pituitary pathways. Clonidine raised serum growth hormone in patients with PD and patients with pure autonomic failure but did not in those with MSA. This finding suggests that the growth hormone responses to IV clonidine can differentiate MSA from PD and pure autonomic failure, and suggests a specific α_2-adrenoceptor-hypothalamic deficit in MSA.[79]

Brain imaging

In patients with MSA, magnetic resonance imaging (MRI) of the brain can frequently detect abnormalities of striatum, cerebellum, and brainstem.[88-92] Striatal abnormalities in MSA include putaminal atrophy and putaminal hypointensity (relative to pallidum) on T2-weighted images, and slitlike signal change at the posterolateral putaminal margin. The striking slitlike signal change in the lateral putamen corresponds to the area showing the most pronounced microgliosis and astrogliosis, and the highest amount of ferric iron, at necropsy. This abnormal intensity is frequently asymmetric (Figure 63-6).

Infratentorial abnormalities in patients with MSA seen on MRI include atrophy and signal change in the pons and middle cerebellar peduncle. The pontine base and the middle cerebellar peduncle may appear as high signal intensity on T2-weighted images and as low intensity on T1, suggesting degeneration and demyelination.

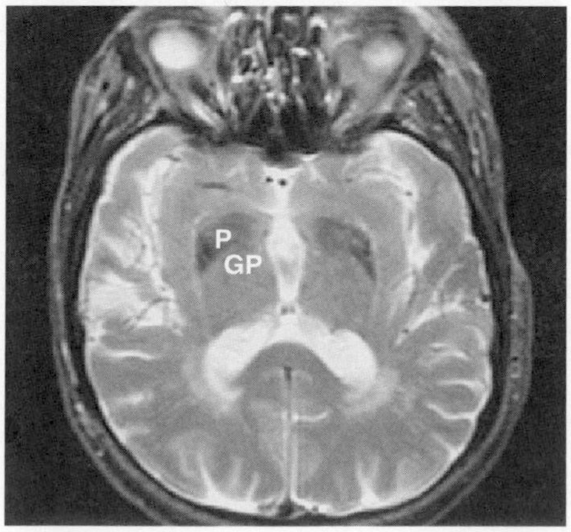

Figure 63-6. Moderate putaminal (P) hypointensity relative to the globus pallidum (GP) in a patient with parkinsonian multiple system atrophy (MSA-P), axial T2 weighting, 1.5 tesla MRI.

Most if not all these tests are frequently ambiguous and accurate methods to distinguish PD from other diseases with extrapyramidal involvement, particularly MSA, are needed. It is argued that because the diagnosis of MSA during life is based on clinical features, it can only be made with possible or probable certainty, and that definite diagnosis requires pathologic confirmation.

TREATMENT

There are no known treatments targeted at the underlying degenerative disorder or therapies that will modify the course of any of these disorders. Treatment outcomes of the motor abnormalities in MSA patients remain dismal. As mentioned before, these patients often do not respond to antiparkinsonian medications. Of the autonomic abnormalities, orthostatic hypotension is often treated successfully. An outline of treatment strategies is included later in this chapter.

Secondary autonomic failure

CHOLINERGIC FAILURE

Botulism and the Lambert-Eaton myasthenic syndrome (LEMS) impair the release of acetylcholine in both somatic and autonomic nerves, producing muscle weakness and cholinergic dysautonomia. Botulism presents as an ascending, predominantly motor polyneuropathy with cranial nerve involvement, beginning 12 to 36 hours after ingesting food contaminated with the neurotoxins of the anaerobic bacteria *Clostridium botulinum*. The toxin impairs the presynaptic calcium-associated release of acetylcholine leading to symptoms of cholinergic failure: dry eyes, dry mouth, blurred vision, dizziness, paralytic ileus, urinary retention, and anhidrosis. Treatment is supportive; respiratory failure and cardiac arrhythmia can occur. Recovery is often protracted with autonomic dysfunction lasting as long as 6 months after onset.

LEMS is an autoimmune disorder, most commonly paraneoplastic, associated with small-cell lung carcinoma. Autoantibodies to voltage-gated calcium channels, most commonly the P/Q type, have been found in these patients. Electrophysiologic and pharmacologic studies have reproduced the functional effects of LEMS in passively immunized mice, and confirmed that anti-P/Q-type calcium channel antibodies inhibit transmitter release from autonomic neurons and are likely to be responsible for the autonomic dysfunction in this syndrome.

Dry mouth, erectile dysfunction, proximal muscle weakness, and depressed tendon reflexes are characteristic.[93–95] The risk of developing cancer is estimated to be 62% over the next 2 years following diagnosis; this risk decreases over time.[93,96] Autonomic dysfunction is worse in older patients with a carcinoma[94] but improves with treatment of the underlying carcinoma.[95]

PANDYSAUTONOMIAS

Pandysautonomias involve both sympathetic and parasympathetic neurons. Pandysautonomic neuropathies can be divided into preganglionic (most frequently demyelinating) and postganglionic (most frequently axonopathic).[97] These neuropathies are acute or subacute with gradual but often incomplete recovery of autonomic function.[97,98] Patients have blurred vision, dry eyes and mouth, nausea, vomiting, abdominal pain, diarrhea, constipation, and loss of sweating.

The acute pandysautonomias are uncommon in elderly people and affect almost exclusively healthy young individuals. Those with a protracted course and incomplete recovery are, more frequently, postganglionic axonal.[97,99] The preganglionic demyelinating pandysautonomia with variable involvement of the somatic nervous system is part of a spectrum ranging from pure pandysautonomia—with minimal somatic deficits—to classic Guillain-Barré syndrome (GBS)[100] and profound muscle weakness and may have a better outcome than the postganglionic axonopathic pandysautonomia.[97] The cause of these pandysautonomias is unknown but a postinfectious or other immune-mediated process is postulated. In some cases they are paraneoplastic,[101,102] and many patients have autoantibodies to ganglionic acetylcholine receptors (see later discussion). Patients with anti-Hu antibody-related paraneoplastic syndrome having progressive dysautonomia have also been described, both with acute onset and a subacute course of neurologic symptoms. Autonomic symptoms may improve with treatment of the underlying cancer.

Signs of autonomic hyperactivity or hypoactivity are present in one third to two thirds of patients with the acute inflammatory demyelinating polyradiculoneuropathy (AIDP) or GBS.[103,104] In the majority of cases, there is mild autonomic hypoactivity with resting tachycardia because of decreased parasympathetic activity and ileus. Urinary retention is less common. With autonomic hyperactivity, sweating is excessive and there can be alternating hypertension or hypotension and alternating bradycardia or tachycardia. Mortality is increased with significant dysautonomia.[105]

Chronic small fiber (postganglionic) neuropathies can be metabolic (e.g., diabetes or amyloidosis), inherited (e.g., Fabry's disease), or infectious (e.g., HIV). Autonomic dysfunction in both amyloid and diabetes tends to involve all organs. Autonomic failure (orthostatic hypotension and a fixed heart rate) may be the presenting feature. More frequently, patients show a mixed pattern of distal small fiber autonomic and sensory neuropathy or predominantly small fiber sensory neuropathy with only mild autonomic involvement.[101,106] The autonomic symptoms may accompany, precede, or follow the somatic neuropathy.[107,108] Alternating diarrhea and constipation, explosive diarrhea, urinary retention, anhidrosis or gustatory hyperhidrosis may be present. Erectile dysfunction is the most common autonomic symptom in diabetes[109,110] and sudomotor changes may be the earliest sign in diabetic neuropathy.[111–114]

Pandysautonomias are commonly associated with the acquired immunodeficiency syndrome (AIDS),[115–117] often combined with a distal sensory polyneuropathy.[118,119] Autonomic symptoms such as bladder and sexual dysfunction are present in up to 60% of patients.

Mild, chronic (or subacute) autonomic neuropathies or ganglionopathies, affecting both sympathetic and parasympathetic fibers, are sometimes associated with Sjögren's syndrome.[101,102] Tonic pupils, sudomotor dysfunction, and cases of severe pandysautonomia have been reported.[120]

AUTOIMMUNE AUTONOMIC GANGLIONOPATHY

Acetylcholine is the neurotransmitter in sympathetic and parasympathetic autonomic ganglia, activating nicotinic receptors. Antibodies against ganglionic nicotinic receptors have recently been identified and proposed to play an causal role in cases of dysautonomia.[121] Clinical presentation can be that of classic acute pandysautonomic following a viral type of illness, or can be indistinguishable of pure autonomic failure. Recent reports show complete (but in some cases transient) recovery in a few patients with acute pandysautonomic that were treated early with intravenous immunoglobulin therapy[122] or plasma exchange.[123] Although encouraging, it is difficult to establish a definitive treatment of this condition based on case reports, and it is likely that some form of immunosuppression will be needed to manage these patients. Nonetheless, they do provide preliminary evidence of the causal role of these antibodies in causing autonomic impairment.

MANAGEMENT OF ORTHOSTATIC HYPOTENSION

Pathophysiology-guided therapy

Maintenance of blood pressure in the standing position requires a sustained increase in peripheral vascular resistance (i.e., vasoconstriction) and adequate intravascular volume. In patients with chronic autonomic failure, orthostatic hypotension is due to deficient baroreflex-mediated vasoconstriction and also because of reduced intravascular volume and reduced venous return.

DEFICIENT VASOCONSTRICTION

In autonomic failure, vasoconstriction is mainly deficient because of reduced baroreflex-mediated norepinephrine release from postganglionic sympathetic nerve terminals and lack of activation of postsynaptic α-adrenergic receptors in the vascular wall.[68] Also contributing to blunted orthostatic vasoconstriction in these patients are low circulating levels of angiotensin II resulting from deficient renal sympathetic innervation and reduced secretion of renin.[9,124] In patients with autonomic failure and central nervous system dysfunction (i.e., MSA), impaired endothelin and vasopressin release are also likely to contribute to the deficient vasoconstriction.[63,69]

Summary of Management Algorithm

Stepwise approach to the management of orthostatic hypotension in elderly people

- Remove aggravating factors:
  - Volume depletion
  - Drugs (e.g., diuretics, tricyclic antidepressants, venodilators, antihypertensives, insulin in diabetics with autonomic impairment)
  - Inactivity/prolonged bed rest/deconditioning
  - Alcohol
- Nonpharmacologic treatment:
  - Liberalized salt intake
  - Head-up tilt during the night
  - Waist-high support stockings
  - Exercise/physical activity as tolerated
- Pharmacologic treatment:
  - Sodium chloride 1 g with meals
  - Fludrocortisone (Florinef) 0.1–0.2 mg/day
  - Midodrine (Proamatine) 5–10 mg PRN
  - Yohimbine 5.4 mg PRN
  - Pyridostigmine 30–60 mg PRN
  - Atomoxetine 18 mg PRN

REDUCED INTRAVASCULAR VOLUME

There are several reasons for reduced extracellular fluid volume in patients with autonomic failure. First, impaired sympathetic activation directly decreases sodium reabsorption in the kidney.[125] Second, impaired sympathetic activation inhibits renin secretion so that aldosterone is low and renal sodium reabsorption is decreased.[121] Finally, other hormones involved in fluid homeostasis are also impaired in autonomic failure. For example, hypophyseal vasopressin release in response to hypotension is markedly reduced in patients with autonomic failure caused by CNS lesions (e.g., MSA).[69] Low vasopressin levels prevent water conservation contributing to intravascular volume depletion.

Anemia is a common complication of autonomic failure, likely the result of inadequate erythropoietin levels.[126,127] Although basal erythropoietin synthesis is not reduced in autonomic failure, the increase in erythropoietin synthesis in response to anemic hypoxia appears to be blunted in these patients. The reason for this abnormality is unknown, but in patients with autonomic failure, the lower the plasma norepinephrine levels in the upright posture, the lower the hemoglobin levels, suggesting some relationship between decreased sympathetic activity and reduced erythropoiesis.[126] Similar to what occurs with the secretion of renin, another renal hormone, decreased renal sympathetic nerve activity may be the cause of impaired erythropoietin response to anemia in patients with autonomic failure. The modest decrease in red blood cell mass is another contributing factor to reduced intravascular volume.

Nonpharmacologic treatment

A complete medication history should be obtained to identify and possibly eliminate agents that can cause orthostatic hypotension, such as antihypertensives or diuretics. Levodopa and dopamine agonists exacerbate orthostatic hypotension, especially during the first weeks of treatment. Gradual dosage increases when initiating therapy or dose reductions in established patients can minimize this adverse effect. Dietary sodium and water intake should be maximally increased in these patients. Patients also should be instructed not to lie prone. Lying flat when sleeping at night results in accelerated sodium loss from pressure-natriuresis and reduced renin release leading to loss of intravascular volume. This leads to overnight volume depletion and worsening of orthostatic hypotension in the morning. Elevating the head of the bed by 6 to 9 inches is helpful. The beneficial effect of nocturnal head and torso elevation results from lessening supine hypertension, thus reducing "pressure-natriuresis" by the kidney and, in some patients, by increasing renin secretion. Patients should be educated about the hypotensive effects of food, hot weather, and physical exertion. Isotonic exercise produces less hypotension than isometric exercise, and exercise in a pool prevents blood pressure reductions. In patients with autonomic failure, eating can significantly lower blood pressure because the splanchnic vasodilation induced by food is not appropriately compensated by vasoconstriction in other vascular beds. In some patients, hypotension only occurs postprandially. Thus patients should eat frequent, small meals with a low carbohydrate content and alcohol intake should be minimized. Caffeine taken with breakfast may be helpful. Hot baths should be avoided, and patients should be especially careful during warm weather. This is because heat-induced vasodilation still occurs but sympathetic vasoconstriction is impaired. Straining at stool with a closed glottis (i.e., producing a Valsalva maneuver), playing wind instruments, and singing can be particularly dangerous for patients with hypotension. A high-fiber diet is encouraged to prevent constipation. The use of knee-high compressive stockings is not effective, but waist-high stockings (i.e., Jobst stockings) or abdominal binders may be an effective, albeit poorly tolerated, countermeasure for orthostatic hypotension.

Pharmacologic treatment

Only patients with symptomatic orthostatic hypotension should be treated pharmacologically. Perhaps because of adaptive cerebral autoregulatory changes, some patients with autonomic failure tolerate very low arterial pressures when standing without experiencing symptoms of cerebral hypoperfusion. Blood pressure levels change throughout the day and from one day to another. Thus the patient's normal cycle of blood pressure and orthostatic symptoms should be identified before treatment is initiated. The treatment strategy is based on counteracting the underlying pathophysiology, by increasing intravascular volume (fludrocortisones, desmopressin, erythropoietin), potentiating the pressor effects of endogenous norepinephrine and angiotensin (fludrocortisone), or using short-acting pressor agents to improve upright blood pressure.

Fludrocortisone

Fludrocortisone, a synthetic mineralocorticoid, is practically devoid of glucocorticoid effect.[128] This pharmacologic action leads to sodium and water retention, but this effect is not targeted to the intravascular space and is only transient. It is postulated that its improvement in orthostatic hypotension is due to potentiation of the pressor effects of endogenous vasoconstrictors such as norepinephrine and angiotensin II. Therapy with fludrocortisone (Florinef) is initiated with a dose of 0.1 mg per day. At least 4 to 5 days of treatment are necessary for a therapeutic effect to be evident. Special attention should be given to the development of hypokalemia. Fludrocortisone increases extracellular and intravascular volume by increasing sodium reabsorption by the kidney, thus increasing cardiac output and standing blood pressure. The dose of fludrocortisone should be increased slowly. Body weight, blood pressure, and the possible development of heart failure because of volume overload should be monitored. Weight gain of 2 to 5 pounds is expected. A certain degree of pedal edema should not be of concern. Indeed, it may be necessary to support the venous capacitance bed (water jacket).

Desmopressin

Desmopressin (DDAVP) is a synthetic vasopressin analog, which acts specifically on the V2 receptor (renal tubular cell) responsible for the antidiuretic effect of the hormone. At the dose given, DDAVP has no vasoconstrictor effect because it does not activate the V1 receptor, which is in vascular smooth muscle.[129] Nocturnal intranasal administration of DDAVP reduces nocturnal polyuria and raises standing blood pressure in the morning without worsening supine hypertension.[130] A problem with the use of DDAVP is the potential development of hyponatremia. Treatment with this drug, therefore, should always be started with caution, and serum sodium should be monitored.

Recombinant erythropoietin

Anemia is a common complication of autonomic failure.[126] Because blood pressure in autonomic failure is extremely sensitive to even small changes in intravascular volume, modest decreases in red blood cell mass and blood viscosity may exacerbate orthostatic hypotension. Recent studies in patients with autonomic failure have shown that reversing the anemia using recombinant erythropoietin increases upright blood pressure and ameliorates symptoms of orthostatic hypotension.[126,127,131] Erythropoietin, a polypeptide hormone produced mostly by the kidney, plays a central role in the regulation of red blood cell production. The synthesis of erythropoietin is controlled by a feedback mechanism based on an oxygen sensor.[132] When oxygen delivery to the kidney decreases, as with blood loss or chronic anemia, the synthesis of erythropoietin by renal interstitial cells increases.[133] The hormone is released into the bloodstream and stimulates red cell progenitors in the bone marrow, thereby increasing red cell production. In some patients with autonomic failure, chronic anemia does not produce an adequate increase in serum erythropoietin levels.[126,127,134] This is similar to what occurs in renal disease, malignancy, and other chronic disorders.

A likely mechanism for the increase in blood pressure following erythropoietin treatment is an increase in intravascular volume and blood viscosity because of increased red blood cell mass. In patients with renal failure receiving erythropoietin treatment, however, no correlation was found between increased blood pressure and increased hematocrit[135]; this suggests additional mechanisms for the hypertensive effect of the hormone.

Midodrine

When volume expansion is not sufficient to control symptoms, a pressor agent should be added. The pressor agent of choice is now midodrine, a selective α_1-adrenergic agonist, which is well absorbed after oral administration and does not cross the blood-brain barrier.[9,136] A 10 mg dose of midodrine is effective in increasing orthostatic blood pressure and ameliorating symptoms in patients with orthostatic hypotension.[137] Because this dose increases pressure for only 4 hours, it can be prescribed two or three times daily, depending upon the physical activity of the patient and can be avoided later in the day because it increases supine blood pressure. An advantage of a pressor agent over fludrocortisone is that its blood pressure raising effect lasts only a few hours. Thus it can be administered specifically when the patient needs it; typically before breakfast and before lunch and preceding physical activity.[137] Recumbent hypertension is a common sideeffect but standing up readily lowers blood pressure. The dose of midodrine should be titrated slowly starting with 2.5 mg. The dose can be quickly increased to 10 mg two or three times a day based on the blood pressure response. Most patients with orthostatic hypotension require chronic treatment with fludrocortisone; it is likely that by adding midodrine to fludrocortisone, the dose of the latter can be reduced. This combination treatment may reduce the long-term complications associated with chronic mineralocorticoid administration. Piloerection and scalp itching are frequent side-effects, and may be used as evidence of a pharmacologic effect.

DOPS

DL threo-dihydroxyphenylserine (DL-threo-dops [DOPS] is an unnatural amino acid that is converted to norepinephrine through a single decarboxylation step by the enzyme dopa decarboxylase. In patients with autonomic failure due to congenital dopamine β-hydroxylase deficiency (the enzyme that converts dopamine to norepinephrine), DOPS is extremely efficacious in relieving orthostatic hypotension.[138,139] In patients with other forms of autonomic failure, DOPS[140-142] showed a significant pressor effect and significantly ameliorated postprandial hypotension.

Pyridostigmine

By inhibiting cholinesterase enzymes that degrade acetylcholine, pyridostigmine facilitates neurotransmission at the level of the autonomic ganglia. This results in an increase in blood pressure that is proportional to residual sympathetic tone. Thus pyridostigmine has the advantage of preferentially increasing blood pressure on standing, without worsening supine hypertension.[143] On average, it is not as potent as other short-acting pressor agents, but it can be effective in a given patient.

Atomoxetine

Residual sympathetic tone can also be harnessed in these patients by prolonging the actions of synaptic norepinephrine by inhibiting its reuptake with atomoxetine.[144] In patients with multiple system atrophy and residual sympathetic tone, atomoxetine can be a potent pressor agent even at pediatric doses (18 mg). In contrast, it has little if any effect in patients with pure autonomic failure.

Other agents

Several other agents have been used in the treatment of orthostatic hypotension in autonomic failure. Prostaglandin synthesis inhibitors (indomethacin, ibuprofen),[145,146] and the somatostatin analog octreotide[147,148] are sometimes effective in improving orthostatic hypotension. The dopaminergic blocker metoclopramide increases blood pressure in some patients with autonomic failure,[149,150] but may aggravate or induce extrapyramidal symptoms. Moreover, it was recently reported that metoclopramide infusion acutely lowered blood pressure and worsened orthostatic tolerance in patients with autonomic failure, which should discourage the use of this drug in the treatment of orthostatic hypotension. β-blockers with and without intrinsic sympathomimetic activity (propranolol and pindolol) have been used,[151] but we have not found them consistently effective. Clonidine, an α_2-adrenergic agonist, has been used with occasional success in patients with severe pure autonomic failure by inducing peripheral vasoconstriction.[152] Conversely, the α_2-adrenergic antagonist yohimbine is often useful in less severe patients, by increasing residual sympathetic tone.[153] Ergotamine by nasal inhalation has also been reported effective.[154]

Treatment of related conditions

SUPINE HYPERTENSION AND DIURNAL BLOOD PRESSURE VARIATION

In addition to orthostatic hypotension, two distinct features of autonomic failure are hypertension when the patient is supine and notable diurnal variation in blood pressure. The mechanism responsible for supine hypertension is unclear. It is surprising that despite low norepinephrine and low angiotensin levels, systemic vascular resistance is increased in patients with autonomic failure when they are supine. The nocturnal supine hypertension causes pressure-natriuresis. The subsequent reduction in extracellular fluid volume aggravates orthostatic hypotension in the morning. Patients with chronic autonomic failure frequently have elevated supine blood pressure and may be incorrectly diagnosed with arterial hypertension.

Postprandial hypotension

Although the precise mediators of postprandial hypotension have not been fully characterized, adenosine and insulin are prime suspects. Not surprising, treatment of postprandial hypotension is targeted at these mediators. Caffeine, an adenosine receptor antagonist, and octreotide, which blocks the release of insulin, are effective in preventing postprandial hypotension.[155,156] Octreotide may not be tolerated in patients with diabetic autonomic neuropathy because of gastrointestinal side effects. Acarbose, an α-glucosidase inhibitor, also prevents postprandial hypotension at doses of 50 to 100 mg, likely through its ability to prevent the quick rise in insulin levels that occurs after meals.[157]

SUMMARY

Evaluations of antihypertensive therapy and nonpharmacologic interventions are the first steps in treating orthostatic hypotension. Hypotensive therapy should be discontinued if possible. Salt and fluid intake should be increased, and patients should be instructed to elevate the head of the bed and never to lie flat. Education about the effects of eating, hot weather, bathing, exercise, and rising quickly from a prone position will assist in effective behavior modification. If pharmacotherapy is needed, fludrocortisone, midodrine, and erythropoietin (for anemia) may be helpful in normalizing blood pressure regulation.

KEY POINTS

Disorders of the Autonomic Nervous System

- Dysautonomia is common with age and with a variety of illnesses, which can be grouped as instances of primary autonomic failure (chiefly neurodegenerative) and secondary autonomic failure (paraneoplastic or autoimmune).
- Age-related changes in the autonomic nervous system are not uniform.
- Age-related baroreflex changes can be seen even in older adults who exercise regularly.
- Routine clinical tests of the integrity of the autonomic nervous system rely on orthostatic changes in blood pressure, heart rate responses to deep breathing, and assessment of baroreflex function.
- Orthostatic hypotension and neutrally mediated syncope are the most common manifestations of autonomic impairment in older adults.

For a complete list of references, please visit online only at www.expertconsult.com

CHAPTER 64

Parkinsonism and Other Movement Disorders

Jolyon Meara

Movement disorders can be broadly classified into the akinetic–rigid hypokinetic conditions in which voluntary movement is reduced and hyperkinetic conditions in which excess involuntary movements called dyskinesias are present (Table 64-1). Dyskinesias can be further classified into tremor, dystonia, tics, myoclonus, and chorea. This distinction is not absolute as, for example, in Parkinson's disease (PD), the most common akinetic–rigid syndrome, involuntary movements are often present. Akinetic–rigid syndromes are usually associated with poor mobility and difficulty with walking because of the presence of a gait apraxia.

Movement disorders are common in older age and are a significant cause of impairment, disability, and handicap.[1] Once diagnosed, these disorders can often be effectively treated. These conditions often present medically in older people at an advanced stage. On an average posttake ward round, it is not uncommon in older patients to make the diagnoses of hitherto unrecognized essential tremor, parkinsonism, orofacial dyskinesia, or drug-induced movement disorder.

THE AKINETIC–RIGID SYNDROMES

The akinetic–rigid syndromes are a group of disorders characterized by parkinsonism which results from the combination of akinesia, rigidity, and often, but not always, tremor (Table 64-2). Parkinsonism is often associated with impaired balance, and a gait apraxia leading to falls and impaired mobility. Levodopa-responsive parkinsonism of unknown cause that has particular clinical features, a characteristic clinical progression and Lewy body neuropathology in the substantia nigra (SN) is called *idiopathic parkinsonism* or *PD* and accounts for around 70% of cases of parkinsonism.[2,3] The remaining causes of parkinsonism are due to drug-induced parkinsonism, vascular parkinsonism, and, much less frequently, multisystem degenerative conditions. These include progressive supranuclear palsy, multiple system atrophy, and corticobasal degeneration. With increasing age, not only does the risk of parkinsonism increase, but also the likelihood of parkinsonism being due to a cause other than PD increases.

PARKINSON'S DISEASE

Although PD can present at any age and juvenile-onset forms are well described, it is a rare disorder outside of old age.[4] Cross-sectional prevalence studies of PD and parkinsonism show at least two thirds of subjects to be over the age of 70 years. PD is usually insidious in onset and may have a long symptomatic phase before eventual diagnosis with symptoms being mistakenly attributed by patients and their physicians to the inevitability of "old age." The rate of progression in PD is strongly related to age at onset rather than to disease duration, which explains the often rapidly disabling disease seen in subjects with late-onset disease arbitrarily described as beginning after 70 years of age. Minimal signs of parkinsonism may result from normal aging changes in the basal ganglia, making the diagnosis of PD in the very elderly even more difficult.[5]

Clinical features

Classically PD has been considered a localized disorder of motor control, which in young subjects is a reasonable assumption. However, the increasing realization of the widespread nature of neuropathology in PD, coupled with our increasing recognition of nonmotor symptoms, has now led to the concept of PD being a multisystem disorder.[6] Nonmotor symptoms are increasingly common with disease progression and older age at disease onset and therefore are a major feature of PD in older subjects.[7–9] Cognitive impairment, often progressing to dementia, is the most powerful factor that determines quality of life in older people with PD. Late-onset PD is probably best thought of as being primarily a dementing illness.[10,11]

Table 64-1. Classification of Movement Disorders

Akinetic–Rigid States
Parkinsonism
Hyperkinetic States
Tremor
Chorea
Dystonia
Myoclonus
Complex movement disorders
Drug-induced movement disorders (tardive dyskinesia)

Table 64-2. Causes of Parkinsonism

Primary Parkinsonism
Parkinson's disease (idiopathic/sporadic parkinsonism)
Secondary Parkinsonism
Drug-induced parkinsonism
Neuroleptic drugs
Calcium blocker cinnarizine
Vascular parkinsonism (pseudoparkinsonism)
Multi-infarct states
Single basal ganglia/thalamic infarct
Binswanger's disease
Multisystem degenerative diseases
Progressive supranuclear palsy
Multiple system atrophy (striatonigral type)
Corticobasal degeneration
Alzheimer's disease
Wilson's disease (young-onset parkinsonism)
Dementia with Lewy bodies
Neurofibrillary tangle parkinsonism
Toxins
MPTP
Manganese
Familial parkinsonism
Postinfectious parkinsonism:
Creutzfeldt–Jakob disease
AIDS
Postencephalitis (encephalitis lethargica)
Miscellaneous causes
Hydrocephalus
Posttraumatic
Tumors
Metabolic causes (postanoxic)

Neuropathology

PD is characterized by cell loss and gliosis in the SN and other pigmented brainstem nuclei that is often visible to the naked eye on sectioning the midbrain.[12,13] Aging also results in cell loss in the substantia nigra, although the distribution of cell loss is very different from that seen as a result of PD.[14] Surviving cells in the SN contain typical inclusions in the cytoplasm called Lewy bodies, which are now known to be largely an aggregation of a protein called alpha-synuclein.[15] Most cases of PD diagnosed in life are found to have Lewy bodies in the substantia nigra.[16] However, Lewy body pathology in the substantia nigra does not necessarily lead to the clinical picture of PD and conversely, largely from the studies of familial parkinsonism, other pathologies not involving Lewy bodies can give rise to a clinical picture typical of PD.[17,18] Lewy bodies are also found in other specific brain sites outside the brain stem including the cerebral cortex, olfactory bulb, and enteric plexi.[19,20] Lewy bodies can be found in up to 10% of postmortem examinations in elderly subjects with no apparent history of parkinsonism in life (incidental Lewy body disease). It is unclear whether such individuals, if they had survived, would have developed PD or, because of protective mechanisms, were able to contain the disease process in a subclinical state.[21] The role of the Lewy body in the pathology of PD is still unknown, and it is unclear whether the Lewy body represents a defense mechanism or the result of the primary disease process.

PD also involves the ascending serotonergic, noradrenergic, and cholinergic projections to the cortex and basal ganglia.[22] Clinicopathologic studies have demonstrated that coexisting neuropathology within the striatum and in other areas of the brain is extremely common in elderly subjects with histologically confirmed PD.[23] Braak has proposed that the primary degenerative process in PD, based on the assumption that the presence of Lewy bodies indicates neuronal loss, begins not in the substantia nigra but in the olfactory tracts, lower brain stem, and enteric nervous tissue.[24] This model fits well with the increasing recognition that REM sleep disorders, hyposmia, and constipation may precede the motor symptoms of PD by several years. The proposed pattern of disease progression also indicates the potential for interaction with environmental agents via the olfactory system and gut.

MOTOR FEATURES

Akinesia is the central motor abnormality in PD that refers to a lack of spontaneous voluntary movement, slowness of movement (bradykinesia), and faulty execution of movement.[25] Marsden brilliantly described akinesia as the "failure to execute automatic learned motor plans."[26] Voluntary movements tend to be of low amplitude and to show increased fatigability. There is a particular difficulty with sequential and concurrent self-paced movements. Patients when asked to oppose the index finger to the thumb in a tapping motion often start with reasonably fast, large-amplitude movements but the speed and amplitude then rapidly decrease with the movement fading away. Akinesia in the lower limb is best tested by asking the patient to tap the heel of the foot on the floor as rapidly as possible—in this situation, akinesia can be heard as well as seen. Older patients often find bedside tests for akinesia difficult to execute and may perform poorly because of cognitive impairment, painful arthritis, restricted joint range, and muscle weakness. Action tremor from any cause may interfere with the quality of normal hand and finger movements, and this can make the assessment of akinesia difficult in the presence of essential or dystonic tremor.

Rigidity is an increased resistance of muscle to passive stretch felt by the examiner. Clinically, rigidity is best detected at the wrist joint. The subject is asked to relax as fully as possible while the examiner makes flexion and extension movements of the wrist joint with the subject's forearm supported. Passive movements of the head can be used to detect axial rigidity. Parkinsonian rigidity is not velocity-dependent and is present to the same degree at all joint positions in flexion and extension ("lead-pipe" rigidity). Activation procedures, akin to the Jendrassik maneuver to enhance tendon jerks, can bring out "activated rigidity" that was not present before. Transient activated rigidity may be a normal finding in anxious individuals. Activated rigidity in the neck muscles may be the first sign of rigidity in PD. The presence of tremor in the upper limb due to any cause will result in a ratchet-like quality of intermittent resistance at the wrist joint called *cogwheel rigidity* that is not specific for PD.

Tremor, usually of the hand, is the presenting feature of PD in around 70% of cases. Hand tremor characteristically occurs at rest when the postural muscles are relaxed and has a frequency of around 4 to 6 Hz. In an anxious patient, postural tremor can easily be misidentified as a resting tremor. Most patients with PD manifest a range of resting, postural, and action tremors. A resting tremor of the hand involving the thumb and index finger described as "pill-rolling" and often brought out when the subject is observed walking is very suggestive of PD or drug-induced parkinsonism. Tremor usually begins insidiously in one hand before spreading to the leg on the same side. After a futher delay of sometimes a year or more, the opposite hand and leg become affected. Head and voice tremor, as opposed to jaw tremor, is unusual in PD and suggests a diagnosis of essential tremor. Rest tremor can occur in essential tremor but only when postural and action tremor is prominent. Rarely, PD can present with tremor alone (tremor dominant PD) with variable degrees of mild rigidity and akinesia found on examination. Tremor dominant PD is difficult to distinguish from essential and dystonic tremor. Subjects with a diagnosis of PD recruited into trials of neuroprotection in PD, who are subsequently found to have no evidence of nigrostriatal dysfunction on positron emission tomography (PET) and single-photon emission computed tomography (SPECT) scans, may well have dystonic tremor.

Postural balance can be assessed clinically by asking the patient to stand and then gently pushing the patient forward from behind, with the other hand in front to prevent a fall. Falls or feelings of imbalance strongly suggest the presence of impaired righting reflexes, even if this is not evident at the time of examination. Axial motor disturbances leading to gait disturbance, dysphagia, and dysarthria are a feature of late-onset PD and often respond poorly to drug treatment.

NONMOTOR FEATURES

Nonmotor symptoms, particularly hyposmia, sleep disorder, and constipation, may predate the onset of motor symptoms by many years. Nonmotor features of PD are very varied and with disease progression come to dominate the clinical picture.[9,27] In late-onset PD, nonmotor features are usually advanced by the time of diagnosis and progress more rapidly than in earlier-onset disease. Autonomic system involvement leads to postural hypotension, urinary incontinence, sexual dysfunction, constipation, and abnormalities of sweating.[28] The progression of PD pathology in the cerebral cortex leads to a range of neuropsychiatric and cognitive problems including dementia, psychosis, hallucinations, apathy, and depression.[29,30] Sensory symptoms, usually painful in nature and involving the lower limbs, also occur and are difficult to treat successfully. A rating scale for nonmotor symptoms has recently been developed.[31]

Dementia and cognitive impairment are common problems in the management of PD in older subjects.[32] The cause most frequently appears to be Lewy body pathology in the cerebral cortex.[29] Dementia that develops a year or more after parkinsonian motor symptoms is described as PD dementia (PDD), whereas dementia present at the start of the illness is called dementia with Lewy bodies (DLB). These two conditions are generally thought to represent two ends of a spectrum of Lewy body disease.[33,34] The risk of dementia in older subjects with PD is five times that of age-matched subjects without PD,[11] and after 8 years of follow-up the prevalence of dementia may reach nearly 80%.[10]

Dysthymia, or mild depression, is fairly common in PD,[7,35–37] but major depression is unusual in the absence of previous significant depressive illness. The natural history of depression/depressive symptoms in PD and the response to antidepressant drug treatment has to date been poorly studied.[38] Apathy is also frequently described in subjects with PD and may be mistaken for depression.[39] A range of nocturnal and daytime sleep disorders is now well described in PD and include rapid eye movement (REM) sleep behavior disorder and excessive daytime sleepiness.[40]

Visual hallucinations are common in PD and occur early in late-onset disease.[41] Rather than simply being due to side effects from antiparkinsonian medication, visual hallucinations are now thought to directly be the result of Lewy body pathology in the ventral-temporal brain areas, indicating that the second half of the course of the disease has been reached.[42,43] Visual hallucinations have been suggested as a useful marker to distinguish PD from non–Lewy body parkinsonism.[43]

Psychosis in PD usually occurs in older subjects with established cognitive impairment/dementia and again indicates the presence of significant cortical disease.[44]

Delirium in PD is also common in older subjects with cognitive impairment and is precipitated by the usual suspects commonly invoked in geriatric practice. All antiparkinsonian medications increase the risk of delirium, though this risk is greatest with anticholinergics, dopamine agonists, selegiline, and amantadine. Visual hallucinations commonly occur in conjunction with psychosis/delirium. Delirium has a remarkable but unexplained and little researched effect on motor symptoms in PD. Patients with acute delirium are often hyperactive and wander around the ward despite refusing all antiparkinsonian medication for days at a time. As the delirium lifts and medication is reintroduced, motor function again deteriorates to the previous parkinsonian state of frozen immobility.

Clinical diagnosis

The diagnosis of PD is a two-stage process that is still dependent on clinical skills.[45] First, the symptoms of parkinsonism need to be sought in the history and the signs of parkinsonism established by clinical examination. Progressively small handwriting (micrographia) with the written word disappearing into a shaky line is strongly suggestive of parkinsonism, though it is surprising how few people write letters by hand today. Difficulty turning over in bed is also a good clue to the early development of axial akinesia. A good witness account, usually from a spouse, is very useful in confirming the often rather general and nonspecific slowing down seen in older patients with PD. The gradual inability to keep up with a spouse on daily routine walks is again a useful early indication of gait disturbance and akinesia. Second, if parkinsonism is detected, consideration has to be given to what type of parkinsonism is present by applying validated clinical diagnostic criteria [23,46] (Table 64-3).

In older patients, the diagnosis of parkinsonism can be extremely difficult, even in expert hands, particularly when the clinical picture is complicated by other diseases, cognitive impairment, depression, and atypical features.[47] A confident diagnosis of parkinsonism cannot always be made in older people, and sometimes a trial of levodopa therapy may be required. However, even the results of a 6-week trial of levodopa at adequate dosage (at least 600 mg daily) may be inconclusive. The use of DaTSCAN-SPECT imaging of the nigrostriatal tract using a radiolabeled tracer for the dopamine transporter may help distinguish atypical postural and action tremors in older patients leading to the correct diagnosis of PD, essential tremor, and dystonic tremor.[48,49]

How good are experts at distinguishing PD from other types of parkinsonism? Two important clinicopathologic brain bank studies have addressed this problem and have demonstrated that diagnostic accuracy for PD at death, when diagnostic accuracy is going to be highest, was only around 76%.[23,50] Diagnostic accuracy in more recent cases

Table 64-3. Guideline Diagnostic Criteria for Parkinson's Disease

A progressive usually nonfamilial disorder with bradykinesia (slowness of initiation of voluntary movement, progressive reduction in speed and amplitude of repetitive movement, and difficulty switching smoothly from one motor program to the next) and at least one of the following:

- Muscular rigidity
- Coarse 4 to 6 μHz resting tremor
- Impaired righting reflexes (not caused by primary visual, vestibular, cerebellar, or proprioceptive dysfunction)

Absolute exclusion criteria are the following:

- Exposure to neuroleptic drugs within the year before the onset of symptoms or to MPTP
- Presence of cerebellar or corticospinal tract signs
- Past history of encephalitis lethargica or viral encephalitis with oculogyric crises
- Stepwise progression or a history of multiple strokes
- Presence of communicating hydrocephalus or a supratentorial tumor
- Presence of severe early autonomic failure
- Supranuclear gaze palsy

Modified with permission from Gibb WRG, Lees AJ. A comparison of clinical and pathological features of young and old-onset Parkinson's disease. Neurology 1988;38:1402–6.

Table 64-4. Subtypes of Parkinson's Disease

Early onset < 50 years old versus late onset > 70 years old
Tremor dominant versus postural imbalance and gait disorder
Benign slow progression versus malignant rapid progression
Unilateral with or versus bilateral disease with or without axial disease and without impaired balance
Lewy bodies mainly in brain stem (PD) versus Lewy bodies mainly in cortex (DLB)

Modified from Meara J, Bhowmick BK. Parkinson's disease and parkinsonism in the elderly. In: Meara J, Koller WC, editors. Parkinson's Disease Parkinsonism in the Elderly. Cambridge: Cambridge University Press; 2000, pp. 22–63, with permission of Cambridge University Press.

referred to a brain bank was shown to have improved to around 84%.[51] The use of stringent clinical diagnostic criteria can improve the specificity for correct diagnosis to over 90% but at the expense of a reduced sensitivity of around 70% as true but clincally atypical cases are excluded.

Clinical subtypes

Clinical observation suggests that subtypes of PD exist, though surprisingly little scientific study of this phenomenon has been undertaken (Table 64-4).[46,52,53] Late-onset disease tends to progress more quickly than early-onset disease (symptoms before the age of 40 years) and is more often associated with cognitive impairment.[54] Patients in the longitudinal DATATOP study who were classified as having rapidly progressive disease were older, had more severe postural imbalance and gait disorder (PIGD group), and exhibited less tremor at study entry than the group with slowly progressive disease. Tremor-dominant disease was associated with less disability, less cognitive impairment, and less depression compared to a group with akinetic rigidity and postural imbalance. The DATATOP analysis suggested that cognitive function and motor deterioration were relatively independent once adjustment for age had taken place.[54] However, patients with late-onset disease appear to become demented sooner than patients with early-onset disease of similar duration.[55] The risk of disabling levodopa-induced dyskinesias appears to be much lower in patients with late- compared with early-onset disease. Motor fluctuations are also less evident in late-onset disease with the possible exception of the end-of-dose "wearing off" of drug benefit. A further probable subtype of PD is DLB, though some authorities would still argue that this is a separate disease entity.

The clinical expression and progression of PD with age is likely to reflect the impact of additional neuropathology from vascular or Alzheimer type pathology as well as effects of cell loss because of aging.[56] Indeed, vascular and Alzheimer type changes in the striatum and cortex may protect elderly subjects from levodopa dyskinesia and motor fluctuations but reduce the therapeutic response to levodopa and increase the risk of cognitive impairment/dementia.

Epidemiology

PD has a strong age-associated risk, and both prevalence and incidence increase exponentially with age.[57,58] Whether incidence truly falls in extreme old age is still unclear. The apparent drop in incidence in extreme old age may reflect diagnostic difficulties or limitations of case ascertainment in small populations. PD affects all racial groups and, after adjusting crude rates to a standard population and allowing for differences in study methodologies, has a fairly uniform worldwide distribution of around 110 per 100,000.[57] Differences in adjusted prevalence rates may still be explained by differential survival, diagnostic bias, and variable mortality rates. Population-adjusted prevalence rates for PD in European subjects over the age of 65 years have been reported as 2.3% for parkinsonism and 1.6% for PD.[59] Studies in which all eligible subjects are examined using the total census approach have shown that up to a third or more of subjects ascertained as having PD were medically undiagnosed before the study.[60,61] A longitudinal study of 4341 elderly subjects initially free of parkinsonism reported an average annual incidence rate for parkinsonism of 530 per 100,000 and 326 per 100,000 for PD.[62]

The strong age-associated risk of PD means that over the next few decades the burden of PD worldwide will increase, particularly in the most populous regions of the Far East and China where the greatest increase in older people and incident cases of PD will occur.[63] The number of people over 50 with PD is likely to double in the 10 countries with the biggest populations over the next quarter of a century.[63]

Parkinsonism in institutional care has received little research attention despite the fact that 15 years from diagnosis around 40% of survivors will need long-term care.[9] The prevalence of parkinsonism appears to be high in hospitals, nursing homes, and residential/retirement homes.[64] A survey in the United States of 5000 nursing home residents over the age of 55 years reported a prevalence for medically diagnosed PD of nearly 7%.[65] A European study found that 42% of cases of PD in elderly subjects living in institutions were medically undiagnosed.[66] Nursing home residents with PD tended to be more disorientated, depressed, and functionally disabled than residents without PD.[67,68] Psychosis and dementia are the two main factors increasing the risk of admission to nursing homes of elderly people with PD.[67,68]

Etiology

The cause of sporadic PD is unknown but is likely to represent interaction between environmental agents and genetic susceptibility. Potential mechanisms to explain this interaction are suggested by the Braak hypothesis of disease progression,[24] the existence of environmental neurotoxins such as 1-methyl-4-phenyl-1,2,2,6-tetrahydropyridine (MPTP),[69] and the occurrence of incidental Lewy body disease.

Twin studies suggested that, apart from early-onset disease, genetic mechanisms were relatively unimportant in the etiology of PD.[70] However, since then rare monogenic forms of familial parkinsonism have been described, the most common relating to mutations in the *LRRK2*, *Parkin*, and *PINK1* genes.[71] A total of 13 genetic loci have been reported that result in dominant and recessively inherited parkinsonism usually of early onset and often with clinical features atypical of PD. These genes are most likely to be involved in protein degradation, oxidative stress responses, and mitochondrial function. Neuropathologic findings resulting from these gene mutations are variable but consistently reveal nigral degeneration with or without Lewy bodies. Even when the clinical picture is indistinguishable from PD, as occurs in *LLRK2* mutations, the pathologic findings can be remarkably varied. Mutations at the *LLRK2* locus result in dominantly inherited PD with reduced penetrance causing an age of onset typical of PD that may account for 1% of "sporadic" cases of PD.[72]

Table 64-5. Drugs Used to Treat the Motor Impairment in Parkinson's Disease

Group	Drug	Trade name
Levodopa	Co-careldopa	Sinemet 110
		Sinemet 275
		Sinemet-plus
		Sinemet-S
		Sinemet CR, Half CR
	Co-beneldopa	Madopar 62.5
		Madopar 125
		Madopar 250
		Madopar CR
		Madopar dispersible 62.5/125
COMT inhibitors	Entacapone	Comtess
	Tolcapone	Tasmar
MAO-B inhibitors	Selegiline	Eldypryl
		Zelapar (sublingual)
	Rasagiline	Azilect
Dopamine agonists	Bromocriptine	Parlodel
	Pergolide	Celance
	Ropinirole	Requip
	Cabergoline	Cabasar
	Pramipexole	Mirapexin
	Apomorphine	Britaject
Miscellaneous	Amantadine	Symmetrel
	Anticholinergics	
	Levodopa plus entacapone	Stalevo

Several environmental agents, such as MPTP and manganese, can cause parkinsonism, but no environmental exposure that is widespread enough and persistent enough over thousands of years to cause sporadic PD has yet been found.

TREATMENT OF PD

In the United Kingdom, a wide range of drugs is available to treat the motor symptoms of PD (Table 64-5). Detailed discussion of their use can be found in recent reviews of drug therapy.[72–74] Clinical guidance from the National Institute for Clinical Excellence (NICE) in the United Kingdom has also been issued.[75] Worldwide, many drugs for PD are either unavailable or unaffordable. Levodopa without dopa decarboxylase inhibitors would be a cheap and effective treatment for PD, though it would result in distressing nausea and discomfort for some patients for a time until tolerance developed. No drug treatment appears to delay disease progression. Drug treatment improves, though rarely abolishes, motor impairment.

Considerable interest has been generated by the recent concept of "continuous dopaminergic stimulation" as a strategy to try to replicate physiologic dopaminergic function in the basal ganglia.[76] This has been fostered by the pharmaceutical industry with the development of a range of long-acting dopaminergic drugs. The thrust of this approach is to prevent or delay the future emergence of levodopa-induced dyskinesias and motor fluctuations in at-risk subjects. For elderly people at low risk of these complications, this matter is of far less concern than obtaining the best response to drug therapy possible for the *present* time. A reasoned critique of the thinking behind much of the treatment of younger patients by neurologists has recently been proposed by Nutt.[77]

Naturally, especially in older subjects, drug treatment should be combined with rehabilitative approaches involving physical therapists, occupational therapists, speech and language therapists, and a range of other allied health and welfare professionals.[79–81]

The model of holistic care in PD has been supported by the development of the PD nurse specialist role.[82] Specialist nursing rehabilitative expertise has undoubtably led to significant improvements in the care of older patients with PD, however, possibly because of study design and methodology, the results of a randomized trial of this service were disappointing.[83]

Drug treatment of motor features

LEVODOPA

The most effective and widely available drug treatment for PD remains levodopa combined with dopa decarboxylase inhibitors (co-careldolpa/co-beneldopa), and virtually all people are prescribed these drugs at some stage in their disease. Side effects of levodopa commonly include nausea and vomiting, dizziness on standing, and daytime drowsiness. Confusion and hallucinations are usually only seen in older subjects who already have evidence of cognitive impairment/dementia. Postural hypotension should be assessed before starting levodopa. To avoid falls and injury, care needs to be taken getting out of bed and rising from the table after meals. Many older people will still be driving, so advice should be given about the risk of daytime drowsiness and the need to inform the driving authorities and motor insurers.

To minimize side effects, a "low slow" introduction of levodopa should be adopted. A suggested regime for initiating levodopa treatment in older frail subjects in whom nausea is likely to be an early problem is shown in Table 64-6. Domperidone given half an hour before each levodopa dose is useful in reducing levodopa-induced nausea. In fitter older subjects, domperidone could be omitted and levodopa started at 50 mg daily with food and increased by 50 mg each week until a dose of 200 mg three times daily is reached. Levodopa-induced side effects of disabling dyskinesias and motor fluctuations are of little relevance to older people, and there is no point in delaying levodopa treatment in this group who are often already significantly disabled by PD. Although there is no convincing evidence that levodopa accelerates disease progression, it seems sensible to use the minimum dose of levodopa that leads to an acceptable health-related quality of life for the patient. Unfortunately, many elderly subjects are unable to tolerate a maximally therapeutic dose of levodopa. Conversely, some older people are undertreated with levodopa, and the first stage in management is often to gently increase levodopa dosage and closely monitor the response. In drug-naive subjects, it is important to clearly document the response to a 6-week period of adequate levodopa treatment (ideally if achievable a minimum of 600 mg daily) as this can help to clarify the clinical diagnosis and can also give some indication of the likely degree of the future control of the disease.

Delayed controlled-release (Sinemet-CR/Madopar-CR) and dispersible formulations of levodopa are available and may be useful is selected individuals. Controlled-release preparations may help early sleep disturbance resulting from PD symptoms in the first few hours of the night.[84]

Table 64-6. Starting Levodopa in Frail Older People

Baseline measures of disease state and lying/standing blood pressure
Pretreat for 3 days with domperidone 20 μmg three times daily
Start levodopa 50 μmg as co-careldopa/co-beneldopa with food three times daily, 30 minutes after taking the domperidone
Continue for 4 days before increasing the levodopa by 50 μmg increments in divided doses every 4 days until a total daily dose of 300 μmg levodopa is reached continuing throughout with the domperidone
Review patient to assess motor response, side effects, and postural blood pressure changes
Continue to slowly build the daily dose of levodopa by 50 μmg increments every 4 days in divided doses as before until a total daily dose of 600 μmg is reached
Review to assess motor response and side effects after 4 weeks of 600 μmg levodopa daily
Adjust levodopa dose to obtain optimal benefit with the smallest dose possible
In nonresponders increase levodopa slowly as before until limited by side effects
Failure to respond to a dose of greater than 1.2 μg levodopa daily in the absence of malabsorption makes a diagnosis of Parkinson's disease very unlikely

Unpredictable absorption is a problem with these drugs and may account for the failure of these drugs to reduce levodopa-induced dyskinesias and fluctuations.[85] Dispersible formulations of levodopa (Madopar Dispersible) have a rapid onset of action and may be used to rescue subjects from sudden "off" periods and to provide a "kick start" on getting up in the morning. Subjects with dysphagia may also benefit from dispersible formulations. Sinemet tablets can be crushed and dissolved effectively in fizzy drinks and will readily pass down a fine bore nasogastric tube.

INHIBITION OF LEVODOPA METABOLISM

The effects of levodopa can be boosted by treatment with drugs that inhibit the breakdown of levodopa by the enzymes MAO-B and COMT. Entacapone given at a dose of 200 mg with each daily dose of levodopa prevents the peripheral metabolism of levodopa by COMT and increases the uptake of levodopa in the brain. A combination tablet of levodopa and entacapone (Stalevo) is also now available. Entacapone has been shown to increase the duration of the clinical response to levodopa in patients with and without motor fluctuations.[86–88] Entacapone can cause nausea and vomiting, dyskinesias, discoloration of the urine, and diarrhea. Tolcapone, previously withdrawn because of liver toxicity, is now available again in the United Kingdom for specialist-restricted use under close supervision with careful monitoring of liver function.

Endogenous and exogenous levodopa can also be enhanced by central MAO-B inhibition using selegiline or the newer rasagiline,[89] which, unlike selegiline, is not metabolized to troublesome amphetamine-like metabolites. Both drugs have modest antiparkinsonian effects. The issue of potential neuroprotective effects of both these drugs is unresolved. The combination of selegiline and levodopa in older frail subjects appeared to be associated in one study with increased mortality and falls. Whether this also applies to rasagiline is unknown, but this class of drug may be best avoided in older patients with cognitive impairment or a history of falls and syncope.

LEVODOPA-INDUCED FLUCTUATIONS AND DYSKINESIAS

Chronic levodopa treatment can induce disabling motor fluctuations and dyskinesias.[90,91] Sensory, psychic, cognitive, and autonomic fluctuations can also occur. The mechanisms behind these effects are poorly understood but presumably arise from the abnormal pulsatile stimulation of dopamine receptors resulting from standard drug treatment.[76,92,93] Pulsatile receptor stimulation could lead to dysregulation of basal ganglia genes and proteins, such as preproencephalin and dynorphin, and the induction of abnormal neuronal discharge in the basal ganglia output nuclei. The half-life of levodopa is only 1 to 1.5 hours, and this may explain why levodopa is so commonly associated with these problems. Longer-acting dopaminergic drugs appear to be less likely to cause these problems. Recent clinical studies have shown that motor fluctuations and dyskinesias can be significantly reduced in patients treated with dopamine agonist monotherapy compared with levodopa alone as the initial treatment.[94] Motor complications were also lower in a group of patients in whom levodopa was added to dopamine agonist treatment to improve efficacy compared to levodopa alone.

Clinical impressions suggest that motor fluctuations and dyskinesia are common after 5 years or so of levodopa exposure. The DATATOP study in 352 de novo patients reported a prevalence of 50% for motor fluctuations and 33% for dyskinesia after only a mean of 20 months levodopa exposure.[95] However, a study in 618 patients on levodopa treatment reported motor complications in only 22% of the study group after nearly 5 years of follow-up.[85] This difference may reflect methodologic differences between the two studies in the definitions of motor complications. Factors governing the risk of levodopa-induced complications appear to be the age of the patient at presentation, disease severity, and the dose and duration of levodopa treatment. Young patients presenting before 60 years old appear to be at particular risk of these problems. The risk of these problems, and much more relevantly the risk of *disabling* dyskinesias and motor fluctuations, seems to fall rapidly with increasing age of disease onset.[96] Above a disease onset age of 60 years, disabling dyskinesias as a result of levodopa are rare. Several strategies can be used to treat these problems when they do arise in elderly patients.[93] Amantadine has antidyskinetic effects, and more effective drugs to combat this problem are in development.

DOPAMINE AGONISTS

Dopamine agonist drugs have a limited role in older subjects in whom the risk of disabling levodopa-induced dyskinesias is very low.[97,98] Dopamine agonists, with the exception of apomorphine, are less effective than levodopa, and side effects are more common, especially postural hypotension, confusion, and psychosis. Monotherapy with dopamine agonist drugs in order to delay the use of levodopa is rarely justified in older subjects, though agonists may be useful as adjunctive therapy to levodopa in carefully selected older people.[98] The ergot agonist group (bromocriptine, pergolide, and cabergoline) can rarely cause pleuroperitoneal fibrosis. Pergolide and cabergoline have also recently been linked with an increased risk of regurgitant heart valves.[99] Dopamine agonist treatment probably should now be restricted to nonergot agonists such as pramipexole, ropinirole, or the new transdermal delivery formulation rotigotine. The rotigotine transdermal patch may be particularly useful in patients undergoing planned or emergency surgery to maintain treatment throughout the operation and in patients unable to absorb drugs orally after bowel surgery.[100]

APOMORPHINE

Apomorphine is a particularly valuable but underused dopamine agonist that is administered subcutaneously by intermittent injection or continuous infusion.[101,102] Apomorphine has a rapid onset of action and has a magnitude of effect similar to levodopa but of much shorter duration. Apomorphine by intermittant injection can be used to rescue patients from distressing motor (immobility, rigidity, tremor) and nonmotor (including sleep disturbance, pain, dyspnea, anxiety, depression, panic, dystonia) symptoms refractory to oral medication. Severe nausea and vomiting are commonly induced by apomorphine and can be controlled by pretreatment for a few days with oral or rectal domperidone 20 to 30 mg three times daily. Rotation of injection sites, massage of the skin before and after injection, reduction of apomorphine dose, and good injection technique can reduce the incidence of painful nodules at injection sites. Unfortunately, many older patients are unable to administer apomorphine by injection when they develop an "off" state and then rely on their spouse or partner to help out. Continuous administration by pump over the waking hours can decrease "off" time by around 50% to 70% and can also reduce levodopa-induced dyskinesias [103] and improve neuropsychiatric symptoms. An effective program of apomorphine treatment really requires the expertise and commitment of a PD nurse specialist who can work in both the hospital and the community. The successful use of apomorphine often requires the support of a spouse or partner, which is not often available for single, divorced, or widowed elderly people.

Elderly frail patients with advanced disease who still appear to get reasonable benefit from their oral drugs for at least some period of the day should be considered for a trial of apomorphine therapy.[102] Apomorphine can lead to hypotension and drowsiness, which can limit its use, and nonresponsive features such as dysarthria, freezing, and postural imbalance will continue to progress. After a time, the benefits of apomorphine will become outweighed by side effects, disease progression, and difficulties of administration and will lead to drug withdrawal. In our practice we have successfully managed older patients for up to 5 years on apomorphine therapy with good results over this time.

DRUG TREATMENT OF NONMOTOR FEATURES

The treatment of nonmotor features remains a major challenge, particularly since dopaminergic drugs often make these worse. Cognitive impairment, depression, anxiety, autonomic failure, and sleep disturbance can be improved in some patients by using a wide range of drug and nondrug interventions. Depression can respond well to selective serotonin reuptake inhibitors such as sertraline[104] and citalopram,[38] and low-dose buspirone can help anxiety. Excessive sweating may be controlled by β-blockers in some subjects.[105] Postural hypotension that does not improve after simple measures can be managed by the careful use of fludrocortisone.[106] Domperidone can also be useful in this situation. Levodopa-induced neuropsychiatric complications including hallucinations, delusions, and delirium may respond to atypical neuroleptic drugs such as clozapine and quetiapine started at a very low dose and slowly increased.[107–109] Further research evidence is needed to determine whether acetylcholinesterase inhibitors such as rivastigmine and donepezil are useful to treat cognitive impairment in PD. Daytime drowsiness may respond to modafinil[110,111] and REM sleep behavior disorder to low-dose clonazepam.[112]

DRUG STRATEGIES IN ADVANCED DISEASE AND PALLIATIVE CARE

With time, disabling features of PD dominate the clinical picture and do not respond to dopaminergic drug treatment. These include dementia, postural imbalance, dysarthria, and dysphagia. Falls become increasingly common, drooling is often a major source of embarrassment, and social isolation and difficulties in communication are common. At this stage in the disease, weight loss can be quite marked, appears out of proportion to the difficulties in nutrition caused by dysphagia, and occurs despite apparent adequate nutritional intake. Patients at this stage are less tolerant of dopaminergic drugs, and the insidious onset and development of cognitive impairment results in hallucinations, confusion, and psychosis. A common early sign of intolerance of levodopa is marked drug-induced drowsiness. Drug treatment at this stage is largely limited by the presence and extent of cognitive impairment. All medication needs to be reviewed, and any drugs with anticholinergic activity or known to cause confusion should be slowly withdrawn. Amantadine, selegiline, and dopamine agonist drugs tend to be poorly tolerated at this stage. Finally, if problems persist the dose of levodopa may also have to be reduced and a balance found between mental clarity and mobility.

In advanced stages of the disease, drug regimes often need to be simplified using low doses of standard formulation levodopa to try to maintain mobility as far as possible. Dispersible levodopa can be given by nasogastric tube. Severe rigidity may on occasion respond to intermittent apomorphine used at critical times of the day. Patients approaching the stage of palliative care will often be resident in nursing homes, particularly if cognitive impairment is advanced. The primary care team supported by the PD nurse specialist will need to work closely together to optimize treatment at this time. Pain can be a significant problem in some patients and again may respond to apomorphine. A clear management plan needs to be developed to deal with issues such as the use of antibiotics, the provision of artificial hydration and feeding, cardiopulmonary resuscitation, and the appropriateness of transfer to acute medical facilities.

SURGICAL TREATMENT

Neurosurgery, particularly deep brain stimulation of the subthalamic nucleus, is becoming increasingly used as a treatment option in PD.[113–114] Unfortunately, it is unlikely that older patients will be suitable for neurosurgical interventions as most of these procedures primarily improve drug-induced dyskinesia or improve "off" time in patients with motor fluctuations, neither of which is a common situation in patients with late-onset disease. Additionally, cognitive impairment, which is the major contraindication to neurosurgery, is frequently already present in older patients. Deep brain stimulation also requires a considerable ongoing commitment from both the patient and neurosurgical team. Furthermore, even in older patients with a good initial response, disease progression may result in any benefit from neurosurgery being short-lived.

PROGNOSIS OF PD IN OLDER PATIENTS

Patients and their families faced with the diagnosis of PD are understandably concerned about what the future holds for them in terms of keeping independent and minimizing disability. As with every chronic progressive disease, it is difficult to predict accurately an individual's prognosis. In older people the prognosis may also be determined by concurrent morbidity. Prognosis needs to be based on a detailed clinical assessment, the physician's clinical experience and judgment, and the application of research-based evidence. One large prospective clinical study of drug treatment in PD indicated that disability scores based on clinical assessment scales tended to return to pretreatment levels by 4 years of follow-up.[115] This study recruited 782 patients who mostly had mild disease, though it is unclear how long symptoms had been present before study entry. The mean age of patients in this study was around 62 years old. The unified parkinson's disease rating scale (UPDRS) score of subjects requiring the addition of levodopa in the DATATOP study increased by around 7 points per year over the 3-year follow-up, most of the increase being due to deterioration in the motor subscale.[95] A total of 273 (34%) out of the original 800 patients recruited in this study needed to start levodopa treatment after 1-year follow-up. Clinical features associated with more rapid disease progression and a poor prognosis include older age at onset, impaired cognitive function, dominant akinesia–rigidity, and postural imbalance.[54,55] In the absence of poor prognostic features, most older patients at diagnosis could reasonably be told to expect a period of 5 to 6 years of good disease control. Deteriorating cognitive function is likely to determine health-related quality of life more than advancing motor impairment.

Mortality is significantly increased in older patients with PD despite optimum drug treatment, and age-specific mortality rates appear to be increasing as frailer subjects reach older age. Cognitive impairment/dementia has a powerful influence on the survival of older people with PD.[116]

Other causes of Parkinsonism

Parkinsonism can arise from several causes (see Table 64-2), though these, with the exception of drug-induced parkinsonism, are much rarer than PD. Even though PD is the most common cause of parkinsonism, accounting overall for around 70% of cases, this proportion falls with increasing age.

DRUG-INDUCED PARKINSONISM

The most common form of secondary parkinsonism, largely the result of the use of neuroleptic (dopamine blocking) drugs in the treatment of serious mental illness, is drug-induced parkinsonism (DIP), which may still be frequently overlooked in older patients.[117–119] A total of 32% of a series of patients with parkinsonism referred to a neurology clinic were found to have DIP. Older patients, especially women, have increased risk of DIP and may inadvertently be prescribed neuroleptic drugs to treat dizziness (prochloperazine) and gastric upset (metoclopramide). Other non-neuroleptic drugs such as the calcium channel blocker cinnarazine, tetrabenazine, and very rarely lithium, fluoxetine, paroxetine, and amiodarone can cause DIP. Clinically, DIP is indistinguishable from PD. Over 90% of cases tend to develop within 3 months of starting the offending drug. After withdrawal of the drug, signs of parkinsonism may take several months to resolve. In some older patients the signs never resolve, and careful monitoring reveals the subsequent development of PD. Presumably, subclinical PD was "brought on" by the neuroleptic drug. The treatment of DIP involves whenever possible stopping the causative drug. When this is not possible, anticholinergic medication can help control symptoms, as can amantadine. The value of levodopa is uncertain as it can worsen the mental condition for which the neuroleptic drug may have been originally prescribed and may be ineffective because of the dopamine receptor blockade.

PARKINSONISM-PLUS

Several rare multisystem degenerative conditions, such as progressive supranuclear palsy,[120,121] multiple system atrophy,[122,123] and corticobasal degeneration,[124,125] can present with parkinsonism. Of these, multiple system atrophy can on occasion be impossible to distinguish clinically from sporadic PD for the whole length of the natural history of the disease. The response to treatment can also be misleading as multiple system atrophy can respond well to levodopa. Warning signs suggesting the possibility of parkinsonian-*plus* disease are a poor response to levodopa, poor tolerance of levodopa, striking asymmetry of motor signs, early onset of dementia, the presence of pyramidal or cerebellar signs, early onset of falls, rapidly deteriorating mobility, severe autonomic disturbance, and evidence of progressive supranuclear gaze abnormalities.

VASCULAR PARKINSONISM

Parkinsonism can result from vascular disease of the brain presenting with gait apraxia, truncal ataxia, relative sparing of the upper limb, and absence of tremor.[126,127] A history of hypertension and of other vascular risk factors is often present, and brain imaging usually shows widespread deep white matter ischemic changes. Rarely, strategic infarcts within the basal ganglia can give rise to a condition indistinguishable from PD. The use of DaTSCAN-SPECT may be useful in this situation.

HYPERKINETIC MOVEMENT DISORDERS

Essential tremor

Essential tremor (ET) is the most common involuntary movement disorder and usually presents as a long-standing bilateral persistent postural tremor involving the hands and forearms.[1,128] An action tremor is often also present. The head, voice, and legs may also be involved with decreasing frequency. In around a half of cases, a family history of similar tremor also exists, as does a temporary improvement of tremor after alcohol. Although usually annoying and embarrassing, ET can also result in severe disability and handicap. The prevalence of ET increases with age, reaching a crude figure of 39.2/1000 individuals over the age of 65 years old.[128]

ET is commonly misdiagnosed as PD and is also sometimes confused with dystonic and drug-induced tremor. Dystonic tremor can be easily confused with ET and tremor-dominant PD, though it tends to be more jerky in nature and is often associated with subtle dystonic posturing of the head.[129] Sometimes a trial of treatment is needed to help distinguish between these two conditions. Head tremor is rare in PD, though jaw tremor is not infrequently found. The distinction between ET and PD in older subjects is made more difficult as a resting tremor can occur in ET and tremor-dominant PD can be associated with a postural rather than resting tremor. A trial of drug therapy may again be needed. In this situation, diagnostic difficulty may be resolved by the use of DaTSCAN-SPECT.[48] The prevalence of PD in patients with ET appears to be slightly higher than that expected by chance alone, though this could reflect the diagnostic difficulties in relation to postural tremors.

The treatment of ET is disappointing, though some patients obtain benefit from β-adrenergic drugs such as propranolol or the anticonvulsant primidone. Side effects, especially in older subjects, limit the usefulness of these drugs. Severe cases of ET may respond to repeated botulinum toxin injections or bilateral thalamic stimulation. Primary orthostatic tremor, a fast palpable but not visible tremor of the thigh and calf, should also be recognized as a rare cause of unsteadiness on standing.[130]

Dystonia

In older patients, dystonia most commonly presents as task-specific dystonia such as writer's cramp, blepharospasm, torticollis, dystonic head tremor, laryngeal dystonia, and cranial dystonia. Blepharospasm commonly presents in later life and when severe may respond to botulinum toxin injections. Blepharospasm can also complicate progressive supranuclear palsy and PD. Dystonia can respond to high-dose anticholinergic medication, though older patients tolerate this poorly.

Chorea

The rapid, often jerky, nonrepetitive and dancelike movements that typify chorea are not uncommonly seen in older subjects and require a diagnosis rather than the label of "senile chorea." Drugs are a common cause of this condition, particularly neuroleptics giving rise to tardive chorea. Levodopa also commonly causes choreiform dyskinesias. In older people, chorea can also result from subcortical vascular lesions. Hemiballismus, a high-amplitude form of usually unilateral chorea involving the arm and leg and occasionally the trunk, is seen in older patients as a result of infarction or hemorrhage in the region of the subthalamic nucleus. This movement disorder when severe can be life-threatening but is usually self-limiting and responds to neuroleptic drugs and tetrabenazine. Late-onset Huntington's disease must always be excluded.[131] In this situation, chorea is usually associated with cognitive impairment. The diagnosis can be confirmed by genetic testing for evidence of an expanded cytosine–adenosine–guanine (CAG) repeat sequence on the short arm of chromosome 4.[132] Other rare causes of chorea include systemic lupus erythematosus, neuroacanthocytosis, polycythemia rubra vera, hyperthyroidism, and electrolyte disturbances. Oro-buccal-lingual choreiform dyskinesia is not uncommon in studies of nursing home residents who have never been exposed to neuroleptic drugs, and appears to be related to loss of teeth and failure to wear dentures.[133]

Restless legs syndrome

The condition of unpleasant deep sensory disturbances in the legs associated with irresistible leg movements on trying to get to sleep increases in prevalence with age.[134,135] Subjects with these symptoms usually also have abnormal leg movements in the early stages of pre-REM sleep. Restless legs syndrome occurs in many other neurologic diseases as well as in medical conditions such as anemia and renal failure and in response to certain drugs such as lithium and tricyclic antidepressants. This condition can respond to levodopa, dopamine agonist drugs, clonazepam, and codeine.

Drug-induced movement disorders

Drugs commonly cause involuntary movements, usually as a result of the indiscriminate and inappropriate use of neuroleptic drugs in older people.[136] A wide range of other drugs have been linked usually by isolated case reports in the literature to involuntary movements, though it is often difficult to evaluate the clinical significance of such reports. In addition to parkinsonism and acute dystonic reactions, neuroleptics can also cause a wide range of tardive movement disorders including an intense and distressing motor restlessness called akathisia.[137] Neuroleptic malignant syndrome can result from the introduction or increase in dose of a neuroleptic drug or from sudden reduction in dopaminergic drug treatment for PD.[138] This syndrome consists of fever, intense rigidity, confusion, autonomic disturbance, and involuntary movements. Rigidity elevates the muscle enzyme creatinine phosphokinase, and rhabdomyolysis can develop with associated renal failure. Mortality from this condition can be high. A similar condition, the toxic serotonin syndrome, can result from the combination of a selective serotonin reuptake inhibitor with a monoamine oxidase inhibitor. Many drugs, including lithium, sodium valproate, amiodarone, tetrabenazine, amphetamine, tricyclic antidepressants, and beta agonists, can cause tremor. Chorea can result from the use of estrogens, lithium, and amphetamines, and myoclonus can result from the use of tricyclic antidepressants and chlorambucil.

KEY POINTS

Parkinsonism and Other Movement Disorders

- The prevalence of essential tremor, parkinsonism, and drug-induced movement disorders increases significantly with age.
- Movement disorders in older people often remain undetected and are difficult to diagnose, and individuals in whom such a diagnosis is considered should be referred for specialist assessment.
- Accurate diagnosis, comprehensive assessment, and careful documentation of the response to drug therapy and rehabilitation are key factors in the successful long-term management of these disorders.
- Delaying levodopa treatment in older patients with PD is rarely justified given the disabling nature of the condition and the low incidence of disabling levodopa-induced dyskinesias and motor fluctuations in this age group.
- PD is a multisystem degenerative disease and nonmotor features, particularly dementia and cognitive impairment, dominate the clinical picture in older subjects and largely determine quality of life.

For a complete list of references, please visit online only at www.expertconsult.com

CHAPTER 65

Neuromuscular Disorders*

Timothy J. Doherty
Michael W. Nicolle

Aging is associated with substantial decline in neuromuscular performance.[1] This is perhaps best exemplified by age-associated loss of muscle mass and strength, a phenomenon often referred to as sarcopenia (see Chapter 73 for full review of sarcopenia). Neuromuscular disorders are an important cause of disability at all ages but often result in greater impairment and disability in older adults as they are superimposed on age-related impairment of both motor and sensory function in the peripheral nervous system. For example, it is well established from both anatomic and in vivo electrophysiologic studies that aging alone is associated with significant reductions in the numbers of functioning motor neurons and motor axons.[1–4] This appears true for both distal and proximal muscles in the upper and lower limbs, but it may be more severe in distal lower limb muscles. Moreover, these losses of motor neurons (motor units) approach 70% in distal lower limb muscles by 80 years of age and are a major contributing factor to age-related loss of muscle mass, strength, and power (i.e., assessment of dynamic strength or force at a given velocity).[5,6] In healthy older adults, lower limb strength and power are strongly related to functional indices such as gait speed and balance; these factors become of even greater importance in the frail elderly.[7,8] What is less well appreciated is the substantial impact on function that occurs when a disorder affecting the motor or sensory system is superimposed on the normal aging process. Often this combination results in significant disability and contributes substantially to the frailty syndrome. For example, an 80-year-old woman with preexisting lower limb weakness following a fall and hip fracture who develops a peroneal nerve palsy superimposed on a diabetic neuropathy will experience much greater disability as a result of these combined problems than a younger counterpart with a simple foot-drop from peroneal nerve injury.

The impact of aging on the sensory system is less well established. Postmortem and biopsy studies show that aging results in losses of dorsal root ganglion cells and a decline in the numbers of sensory axons.[9,10] This is apparent in reduced sensory nerve action potential amplitudes from standard nerve conduction studies in older men and women.[11] This likely translates to impaired sensory function that can impact balance and motor control. As with the motor system, any superimposed disorder will have a greater functional impact.

In addition, given these observations, in some cases slowly progressive disorders, such as inclusion body myositis (IBM) or polyradiculopathy, are mistaken for the expected or typical losses of muscle mass, strength, and power associated with aging. Therefore, it is imperative that clinicians appreciate common presenting features of neuromuscular disorders and recognize how they differ from so-called normal aging.

To this end, this chapter focuses on disorders that commonly present in older adults including polyneuropathies, spinal stenosis and neurogenic claudication, myopathies, motor neuron disease, and neuromuscular junction disorders. The general clinical approach is outlined, followed by a discussion of individual disorders and their treatment.

APPROACH TO THE PATIENT WITH NEUROMUSCULAR DISEASE

History

Weakness, fatigue, atrophy, and altered sensation are the most common presenting symptoms of neuromuscular disease (Table 65-1). An accurate history documenting the onset, pattern, and progression of weakness and sensory loss is crucial in differentiating diagnostic possibilities and may require several meetings with the patient and in some cases additional information from a spouse or relatives. In general, most myopathies and disorders of neuromuscular transmission present with proximal weakness and no sensory symptoms. Notable exceptions are myotonic dystrophy type I (DM1) and IBM that may present with predominantly distal weakness. Muscle wasting and loss of reflexes are late manifestations of most myopathies. Alternatively, most neuropathies present primarily with sensory symptoms, earlier loss of reflexes, and distal weakness. Early in the course of polyneuropathies, distal muscle wasting of intrinsic hand and foot muscles is often more impressive than strength loss. Notable exceptions are acute or chronic inflammatory demyelinating polyradiculopathy and diabetic amyotrophy, which may present with mainly proximal weakness.

Table 65-1. Typical Features of Neuromuscular Disorders Based on Their Localization

Motor neuron	Weakness and atrophy in segmental distribution Bulbar/respiratory involvement Fasciculations Upper motor neuron signs in ALS No sensory involvement
Nerve root	Pain and altered sensation in nerve root distribution Reduced or absent reflexes in same distribution Weakness and atrophy in myotomal distribution
Polyneuropathy	Sensory symptoms with distal to proximal progression Depressed or absent reflexes Distally predominant atrophy and weakness Distal sensory deficits
Neuromuscular junction	Proximal fatigue and weakness No atrophy Absence of sensory symptoms Diplopia, ptosis, bulbar involvement Fatigable weakness of proximal muscles
Muscle	Proximal weakness Weakness > atrophy No sensory involvement Retained reflexes

*Material in this chapter contains contributions from the previous edition, and we are grateful to the previous author for the work done.

Inquiries into sporting abilities, hobbies, occupational history, and military service often help establish the onset of symptoms. Many patients initially ascribe their neuromuscular symptoms to normal aging or painful conditions such as arthritis, and directed questioning is often required. Questions include "How far could you walk five years ago?" or "When did you first use a cane?" or "When could you last climb stairs?" More active patients are asked, "When could you last run?" This question is useful because increasing weakness may be present for months, and only the loss or impairment of some well-established task brings it to the patient's attention.

The distribution of weakness is often suggested by the history: difficulties reaching up to a shelf or combing hair suggest upper limb proximal weakness. Proximal lower limb weakness is suggested by difficulty in rising from a low chair or toilet, climbing stairs, and getting in or out of the bathtub. Primary neuromuscular disease rarely presents with falls early in the course, with the exception of inclusion body myositis (IBM), an inflammatory myopathy often associated with asymmetric quadriceps wasting and weakness that may present with "buckling" around the knees and falls. Catching the foot on stairs or difficulty in depressing car pedals, turning a key, or opening a jar suggest distal weakness. In myasthenia gravis (MG), power may be reported as normal at rest, with fatigable weakness developing after exercise or later in the day. Speech and swallowing problems, including coughing and choking after ingestion of solids or liquids, and unexplained recurrent pneumonia may suggest bulbar weakness. Weakness of the cervical muscles may lead to head drop, and some patients will report the need to use the hand to support the head. Some patients with cervical muscle weakness present with neck pain, reflecting prolonged and ineffectual voluntary attempts to keep the head up. The causes of dyspnea are numerous and most often in the elderly not primarily related to neuromuscular disorders. However, many neuromuscular disorders involve respiratory musculature. This may be manifest as shortness of breath on exertion and especially on lying flat, because of diaphragmatic involvement. Inflammatory myopathies, motor neuron disease, and neuromuscular transmission disorders should be considered in this setting. Other symptoms suggestive of neuromuscular hypoventilation include disrupted nocturnal sleep, daytime hypersomnolence, early morning mental clouding, and headache as a result of CO_2 retention with associated cerebral vasodilatation.

Myalgia is a relatively nonspecific feature seen in many patients with progressive muscular disease. Patients often find myalgia hard to describe and differentiate from joint pain. Prominent myalgia is a feature of many inflammatory myopathies, polymyalgia rheumatica, and the metabolic myopathies. However, pain at rest and lack of pain or cramp with exertion is less suggestive of an underlying defect in muscle metabolism and more suggestive of inflammatory muscle disease, referred pain from joint disease or a myofascial pain syndrome. Uncommonly, myalgia is a presenting feature of the muscular dystrophies such as fascioscapulohumeral dystrophy. Proximal myotonic myopathy (PROMM) or DM2, a myotonic disorder with some similarities to myotonic dystrophy (DM1 or Steinert's disease), often presents with muscle pain, stiffness, and proximal weakness. Painful nocturnal muscle cramps can reflect neurogenic diseases including motor neuron disease (MND), polyneuropathies, or chronic lumbosacral nerve root injury. Alcohol and drugs, especially those that induce hypokalemia (e.g., diuretics) or those with a structural effect on muscle (e.g., the statins), may induce myalgia. Finally, myalgia may be a prominent symptom in patients with endocrine dysfunction (especially hypothyroidism and hypocalcemia) and those with connective tissue disorders such as systemic sclerosis.

A wide-ranging systemic inquiry is essential in patients with suspected myopathies, as myositis may be a component of many collagen vascular diseases. Both DM1 and PROMM are multisystem disorders whose manifestations are varied and include diabetes, cataracts, cardiac conduction defects, and muscular weakness and wasting. Cardiac involvement is common in many neuromuscular diseases manifesting with cardiac conduction defects or cardiomyopathy or both. Prominent weight loss is a common feature in MND, reflecting both poor nutritional state and loss of muscle bulk.

Many neuromuscular diseases are inherited, and therefore it is important to inquire specifically about family members and, where appropriate, about consanguinity. Premature cardiac and respiratory deaths in family members may reflect complications of an inherited neuromuscular disease or possible associated malignant hyperthermia, if associated with anesthetic exposure. It is often useful to examine first-degree relatives in a family suspected of having an inherited neuromuscular disorder even when the history does not suggest that the elderly relative is affected, as this can be confirmed by direct examination and has clear genetic implications for the wider family. Myotonic dystrophy, because of its marked variability in expression and the presence of anticipation, may present in older patients with minor manifestations only (e.g., cataracts), compared with major symptoms in siblings. The genetic defect, a trinucleotide repeat expansion, is unstable and may worsen in successive generations particularly via the female line, leading to "anticipation," with earlier onset and more severe disease in successive generations.

Sensory symptoms suggest involvement of the dorsal root ganglion, nerve roots, or sensory fibers (including the central projections such as the dorsal columns). Numbness and paresthesias distally in the toes and feet are the most common presenting symptoms of symmetrical polyneuropathies. Symptoms of burning pain, coldness, tightness, and prickling may suggest predominantly small fiber involvement, whereas numbness and loss of balance may indicate predominantly large fiber involvement. The presence of orthostatic hypotension, gastrointestinal disturbance, dryness of the eyes and mouth, and erectile dysfunction in men indicate autonomic involvement. Sensory loss when patchy or asymmetrical may indicate an underlying vasculitic process or sensory neuronitis. Loss of balance, particularly when in the dark (reducing visual input), may indicate large fiber sensory loss and poor proprioception. Other early clues are difficulty with balance when showering or when walking on uneven surfaces. Again, as with some early motor symptoms, these complaints are often attributed to normal aging and it is not until they are particularly disabling that medical attention is sought or investigation pursued.

Examination

The aim of the examination of the neuromuscular system is to determine the distribution of muscle weakness, sensory loss, and reflex abnormality in order to localize the lesion within the peripheral nervous system (see Table 65-1). Furthermore, it is important to assess the respiratory, cardiovascular, and dermatologic systems for associated abnormalities. The examination may provide clues to the etiology and allows for grading of severity. Most acquired and inherited myopathic disorders present with proximal weakness and wasting (a limb girdle distribution). Selective patterns of muscle involvement may suggest facioscapulohumeral dystrophy (FSHD) or one of the many subtypes of limb girdle muscular dystrophy, but confirmation often relies on DNA analysis or muscle biopsy. A scapuloperoneal distribution of weakness may reflect a myopathic disorder, such as FSHD, or a neurogenic problem, such as spinal muscular atrophy. Myasthenia gravis (MG) presents with fatigable proximal weakness but without wasting. Lambert–Eaton myasthenic syndrome (LEMS) presents with fatigable proximal weakness and wasting that can be hard to distinguish clinically from a myopathy, although the reduction in deep tendon reflexes (DTRs) provides a valuable diagnostic clue. Distal weakness, with involvement of the forearm and hand muscles in the upper limb and the anterior and posterior tibial compartment in the lower limb, is commonly due to a peripheral neuropathy or MND but can also be seen in myotonic dystrophy, IBM, very rare distal forms of spinal muscular atrophy, and in distal myopathies. Weakness of neck flexion and extension (head drop) occurs in myopathic (e.g., DM1, inflammatory myopathy, FSHD), neuromuscular junction (myasthenia gravis), and neurogenic (e.g., MND) disorders. Paradoxical abdominal movements and indrawing of intercostal muscles on inspiration may indicate respiratory muscle and diaphragm weakness.

Having established the pattern of weakness, the symmetry of involvement is often a guide to the underlying etiology. Most myopathic diseases result in symmetric weakness. In addition, around a joint, all of the muscles will be involved to about the same degree. IBM is a noteworthy exception to this as asymmetric quadriceps involvement is common. In some neurogenic diseases, such as MND, asymmetry and unequal involvement around a joint are seen, as the weakness tends to follow a segmental pattern of spinal cord involvement, often starting locally and then progressing.

In primary muscle disorders, tone and reflexes are either normal or mildly reduced. Increased tone and reflexes suggest an upper motor neuron disorder, amyotrophic lateral sclerosis (which ultimately has combined upper and lower motor neuron involvement), or cervical spondylitic myelopathy. Fasciculations are spontaneous, involuntary, visible discrete muscle twitches and reflect motor neuron or motor axon hyperexcitability. Fasciculations are not seen in muscle disease and rather reflect neurogenic disorders such as MND but also peripheral neuropathies and chronic nerve root disease where denervation is a feature. As it is sometimes difficult to differentiate myopathic and neurogenic weakness on symptoms alone, a careful search should be made for fasciculations in all patients presenting with neuromuscular weakness. Fasciculations may be missed if patients are not undressed fully. The back, abdomen, and tongue should be inspected as well as the limbs. Difficulty is often encountered in observing fasciculations in the tongue; these are best seen with the tongue lying at rest in the floor of the mouth. Apparent fasciculation may be seen in the normal individual when the tongue is protruded due to anxiety and tremor.

Myotonia (delayed relaxation) is an uncommon presenting complaint in the older patient, and usually signifies myotonic dystrophy, which usually presents in the second or third decade. Joint contractures are occasionally due to inherited muscle disease, whereas foot deformities such as pes cavus reflect longstanding, often genetic, peripheral neuropathies or a slowly progressive upper motor neuron disorder such as hereditary spastic paraparesis.

Depressed or absent reflexes generally indicate a neuropathic disorder, with reflex loss a late sign in muscle diseases. The combination of muscle wasting, weakness, and hyperreflexia is typical of amyotrophic lateral sclerosis (ALS), but can also be seen with cervical polyradiculopathy and concomitant cervical myelopathy. In these cases, the presence of upper motor neuron signs (e.g., jaw jerk) rostral to the most caudal lower motor neuron signs is a useful observation suggestive of ALS.

Distal, symmetric loss of sensation to pain (pinprick) and temperature are common features of typical, length dependent neuropathies with small fiber involvement. In the elderly, mild loss of vibration sense in the toes is nonspecific, but loss at the ankle or more proximally indicates large fiber involvement, either as a result of a peripheral neuropathy or myelopathy with involvement of the dorsal columns. Loss of proprioception is often a late finding of large fiber sensory loss, as is a positive Romberg's test. Obviously it is important to recognize sensory deficits that follow the distribution of individual peripheral nerves (e.g., median, ulnar or peroneal nerve) or dermatomes as they indicate a focal mononeuropathy or radiculopathy. The combination of intermittent sensory symptoms in the hands and distal sensory loss in the feet may indicate polyneuropathy, but in the elderly carpal tunnel syndrome in combination with multilevel lumbosacral nerve root compression and spinal stenosis should also be considered. As outlined later, electrophysiologic testing is invaluable in sorting these cases out.

Investigations

It is sometimes impossible on the basis of history and examination alone to make an accurate diagnosis in many cases of neuromuscular disease, not least because of the overlap in clinical signs between some neurogenic and myopathic disorders. Confirmation of a neuromuscular diagnosis requires the application of electrophysiologic, pathologic, biochemical, and, increasingly, genetic testing.

With several caveats, measurement of "muscle enzymes" is useful in patients with neuromuscular disease. Serum creatine kinase (CK) appears to be the most sensitive index of muscle necrosis from primary muscle disease and from secondary muscle fiber necrosis because of chronic denervation from neuropathic conditions. The magnitude of CK rise gives some indication of the nature of the pathology: in denervating conditions such as MND, CK levels are commonly mildly elevated in the 200 to 500 IU/L range and rarely above 1000 IU/L, whereas a more significant increase of 10- to 1000-fold suggests a primary muscle (especially inflammatory myopathy). However, CK levels must be interpreted with caution, as "muscle enzymes" are also found in other tissues. CK consists of three separate isoenzymes: MM, derived from skeletal muscle, MB, derived largely from cardiac muscle, and BB, derived mainly from brain. High CK levels may therefore be seen in patients with acute myocardial injury, large strokes, and occasionally with hepatic disease, as well as in patients with muscle disease. Even so, given that the major isoenzyme of CK is MM, a high CK level is most likely to reflect neuromuscular disease. Finally, it is also important to appreciate that mild increases in what are typically thought to be liver enzymes such as AST and ALT can occur in primary muscle disease (ALT proportionally higher is more indicative of hepatic disease).

ELECTROPHYSIOLOGY

Electrophysiologic studies are invaluable in the diagnosis of neuromuscular disorders. A detailed discussion of electrophysiologic (electromyographic, EMG) techniques in the diagnosis of neuromuscular disease is outside the scope of this chapter but can be found in appropriate textbooks.[12] Nerve conduction studies (NCS), in which the conduction velocities and amplitudes of motor and sensory (compound) action potentials in response to electrical stimulation of nerves are measured, are used to detect primary pathology of peripheral nerves. NCS are extremely useful in detecting focal nerve injuries such as median neuropathy at the wrist in the carpal tunnel syndome, or common peroneal nerve injury around the fibular head. Reduced amplitudes of motor and sensory studies with mild conduction velocity slowing in the legs are typical of many of the common axonal, length-dependent polyneuropathies (e.g., drug-related, diabetes, idiopathic). Severe conduction slowing and conduction block in multiple nerve segments are important observations as they indicate an acquired demyelinating, often treatable chronic inflammatory demyelinating polyneuropathy (CIDP).

The most common method for the electrophysiologic assessment of muscle is with concentric or monopolar needle electromyography (NEMG), which detects characteristic patterns that can be used to distinguish neurogenic and myopathic disorders. Normal muscle is electrically silent at rest. In neurogenic disorders resulting in denervation (e.g., ALS), positive sharp waves or fibrillation potentials are seen in NEMG studies, and on voluntary activation a reduced interference pattern of the motor unit potentials is seen, reflecting the loss of motor units. By contrast, in many myopathies NEMG reveals small, short-duration motor unit potentials. Electromyography (EMG) studies may also reveal complex repetitive and myotonic (audible as a "dive bomber" or "revving motorcycle" sound) discharges, useful in confirming myotonic disorders, and may suggest a previously unsuspected diagnosis such as PROMM (DM2) where weakness predominates and myotonia is often subclinical.

Repetitive nerve stimulation studies are useful in neuromuscular transmission disorders. In both MG and LEMS, a decrement in compound muscle action potential response occurs at low frequency (2 to 3 Hz) stimulation, which mirrors the clinical phenomenon of fatigable weakness. In LEMS, a characteristic incremental response occurs with high-frequency stimulation or after brief maximal voluntary contraction, which mirrors the clinical phenomenon of post-tetanic, or post-contraction facilitation. Single-fiber EMG (SFEMG) is useful in confirming a neuromuscular junction disorder, particularly in regional forms of MG. It is important to note that whereas SFEMG is highly sensitive for neuromuscular junction disorders (> 95%), it is, in turn, very nonspecific with abnormal results possible in any chronic neurogenic condition or myopathies.

MUSCLE BIOPSY

Despite advances in biochemistry, neurophysiology, and genetics, the final diagnosis in patients with muscle disease often requires a muscle biopsy. The development of the technique of needle muscle biopsy, which can be undertaken as a simple outpatient procedure, has made possible one-stop diagnostic neuromuscular clinics with combined clinical, neurophysiologic, and muscle sampling. The vastus lateralis and deltoid are commonly biopsied, ideally sampling a muscle that is weak but only moderately affected clinically but not too atrophied, for fear of sampling muscle with only end-stage pathology. Routine histologic stains can be employed on both paraffin-embedded and fresh frozen material and permit assessment of muscle fiber size, fiber morphology, and the presence or absence of inflammation. Other stains allow differentiation of muscle fiber types and can be used to study the distribution of cellular enzymes and metabolic reserves.[13] Immunohistochemistry on frozen muscle using antibodies directed against sarcolemmal muscle proteins, such as dystrophin and the sarcoglycans, is crucial in the diagnostic workup of suspected dystrophinopathies and limb girdle muscular dystrophies and permits a more focused search for genetic abnormalities. Western blotting techniques on muscle are often essential in confirming the suspicion of muscular dystrophies. Direct measurement of enzymic activity in fresh muscle is sometimes useful in diagnosing rare metabolic disease such as acid maltase disease and in mitochondrial myopathies where respiratory chain enzymes can be assayed. Electron microscopy of muscle is useful to confirm suspected mitochondrial abnormalities seen on light microscopy and especially to look for intracellular inclusions, which occur in some inherited and acquired muscle disease. Muscle samples are hard to process, hard to orient, and degrade rapidly—all of which combine to make the technique unsuitable for routine laboratories. Furthermore, interpretation of muscle biopsies and exclusion of artifactual change is difficult, and it is important therefore that muscle samples are sent to special neuromuscular laboratories or to an experienced pathology center. As percutaneous needle and punch biopsies are far less invasive than open procedures, it is possible to follow a patient with a muscle disease and monitor response to treatment in individual patients using sequential biopsies.

PERIPHERAL NEUROPATHIES

Peripheral neuropathies are overall the most common neuromuscular disorders that present in older adults. It is beyond the scope of this text to provide an in-depth review of all peripheral neuropathies, and the reader is directed to a number of excellent texts in this regard.[12] This section provides an overview of peripheral neuropathies and specifically addresses diabetic neuropathy because of its high prevalence in the elderly.

Typical symptoms of peripheral neuropathy include distally predominant weakness, sensory loss, poor balance, and autonomic dysfunction. Weakness in the majority of polyneuropathies follows a length dependent pattern and is therefore often more severe in the lower than upper limbs. Weakness tends to become symptomatic in the extensors of the toes and ankles and evertors of the ankle earlier than in the plantar flexors. In the upper limb, difficulties with fine motor tasks such as fastening buttons or picking up coins can be early indications of weakness.

Sensory symptoms of polyneuropathies can be divided into those that indicate involvement of small, thinly myelinated fibers that subserve pain and temperature and those that suggest involvement of large myelinated fibers that are involved in position sense. Common symptoms of small fiber neuropathies include hypersensitivity to footwear or bedclothes, shooting or stabbing pain, difficulty detecting temperature of bath water, and burning sensation. These symptoms usually predominate in the feet, as most neuropathies are length-dependent. However, when sensory symptoms reach the level of the knees, they often begin in the hands. Small fiber sensory symptoms of burning, prickling, and allodynia are a common cause of sleep disturbance in the elderly. These symptoms should prompt a careful assessment for decreased sensation to pinprick and temperature for consideration of a small fiber–predominant neuropathy.

Large fiber involvement will typically present with loss of balance and gait difficulty because of the loss of proprioception or position sense. These symptoms often result in mobility limitations in the elderly and fear of falling. In particular, patients with balance impairment secondary to peripheral neuropathy tend to avoid crowded areas such as grocery stores and shopping malls. These symptoms should prompt an examination for decreased sensation to light touch, vibration, and position sense as well as loss of deep tendon reflexes.

Autonomic symptoms include urinary retention or incontinence, abnormal sweating, constipation and diarrhea, and symptoms of orthostatic hypotension. These symptoms are often initially overlooked as indicative of a neuropathic disorder and prompt assessment for a primary cardiac or central neurologic disorder cause.

Most neuropathies affect both motor and sensory fibers; however, pure or predominantly sensory involvement can be seen in concert with diabetes, malignancies (paraneoplastic neuropathies), and idiopathic sensory neuropathy in the elderly. Pure motor involvement may indicate multifocal motor neuropathy (MMN), a rare demyelinating disorder that typically presents initially with focal weakness of upper limb muscles, or may suggest motor neuron disease. Along the same lines, most neuropathies present with symmetric, distally predominant features. Asymmetry may indicate mononeuritis multiplex associated with vasculitis, hereditary neuropathy with liability to pressure palsies, or common focal or entrapment neuropathies. Table 65-2 outlines some common presentations based on the predominant fiber population involved.

Once a pattern of small or large sensory fiber predominance has been established, the absence or presence of motor involvement has been defined, and the symptoms and signs have been determined as symmetrical or asymmetric, it is often of considerable value to obtain electrophysiologic studies before other investigations. Most expert clinicians agree that is also useful to obtain a fasting blood sugar, serum creatinine, electrolytes, a complete blood count, vitamin B_{12} level, and serum protein electrophoresis (and immunofixation if indicated) as part of the initial workup. Further, often expensive testing for specific antibodies or genetic testing should await the results of electrophysiologic testing and is often best directed by clinicians and centers with specialized expertise.

Electrophysiologic testing is extremely helpful in tailoring future investigation as it can determine whether the process is predominantly axonal (most common) or demyelinating. The presence of a demyelinating process is extremely important to establish, as these often indicate a treatable acquired neuropathy (CIDP, MMN) or a hereditary neuropathy if there is uniform slowing of conduction velocities. If an axonal neuropathy is present, it is important to determine if it is symmetric (most common) or asymmetrical and multifocal, which may indicate an underlying vasculitic process requiring further investigation and treatment.

It is important to note that standard nerve conduction studies only examine large, myelinated fibers. Therefore, the studies may be normal or only mildly affected in small fiber neuropathies (e.g., diabetes).

Diabetic neuropathy

Diabetic neuropathy is the most common form of peripheral neuropathy in the Western hemisphere with increasing prevalence resulting from the growing prevalence of Type II diabetes. A number of different classification schemes exist for diabetic neuropathy and a common one is outlined in Table 65-3. The commonest form is a mixed but predominantly sensory, motor and autonomic diabetic peripheral neuropathy (DPN) which may comprise up to 70% of cases.[13]

Table 65-2. Peripheral Neuropathies Based on Predominant Symptoms

Motor predominant	Guillain-Barré syndrome, chronic immune demyelinating polyneuropathy, Charcot-Marie-Tooth disease, multifocal motor neuropathy, motor neuron disease
Sensory predominant	Idiopathic, diabetic symmetric polyneuropathy, paraneoplastic (often ganglionopathy), Sjögren's syndrome, paraprotein-associated, vitamin E deficiency (very rare)
Small fiber sensory only	Diabetic neuropathy, idiopathic (acute or chronic), hereditary sensory and autonomic neuropathy (very rare)

Table 65-3. Clinical Classification of Diabetic Neuropathies

Symmetric
- Diabetic polyneuropathy
- Diabetic autonomic neuropathy
- Painful diabetic neuropathy

Asymmetric
- Diabetic radiculoplexopathy
- Diabetic thoracic radiculoneuropathy
- Mononeuropathies
  - Carpal tunnel syndrome
  - Ulnar neuropathy at the elbow
  - Peroneal neuropathy at fibular head
  - Cranial neuropathies

A predominantly sensory, often painful, neuropathy comprises the other largest group. Diabetic neuropathy is common and may be present in up to 50% of type I diabetics and 45% of type II diabetics if comprehensive batteries of testing are used.[14] In patients with only impaired glucose tolerance, the prevalence figures remain controversial.[15] Risk factors for DPN include the duration and severity of hyperglycemia, smoking, and the presence of other complications including retinopathy and nephropathy, and cardiovascular disease. The pathophysiology of DPN remains somewhat controversial but includes axonal injury from polyol flux, particularly sorbitol through the aldose reductase pathway, microangiopathy and hypoxia, oxidative and nitrative stress from free radicals, and deficiency of growth factors.[13]

Symptomatically, patients with DPN typically present with positive neuropathic features such as prickling, tingling, and pins and needles; burning; or occasionally shooting sensations. Negative symptoms such as numbness of the toes or feet can paradoxically occur along with the positive features. Many patients experience symptoms mainly at night and experience painful allodynia (pain in response to nonpainful stimuli) from bed sheets or through the day with walking or footwear. True sensory ataxia is less common but can occur with severe involvement. Symptoms may stay confined to the lower extremity but may advance to the hands as they progress to the level of the knees in the lower limb. Early sensory symptoms in the hands should raise the question of a superimposed carpal tunnel syndrome (CTS), which has a very high prevalence in those with DPN.[16]

Clinical examination in DPN reveals distal, sensory greater than motor deficits to all sensory modalities and often loss of ankle deep tendon reflexes. Motor deficits are less common but patients may have weakness of toe extensors and flexors and in more severe cases weakness of ankle dorsiflexors.

Diabetic foot ulcers are of considerable importance when assessing elderly patients with DPN. Diabetic ulcers occur because of a combination of sensory loss and repetitive pressure on bony prominences such as the metatarsal heads or heel. This in combination with drying and cracking of the skin leads to chronic tissue injury. Further progression may occur as a result of loss of proprioception leading to abnormal foot position and biomechanics. Careful inspection of the feet on a daily basis, screening for early evidence of sensory deficits, proper footwear with adequate height of the toe box or forefoot, and foot orthoses are all useful in terms of preventing the occurrence of ulceration and reducing the risk of amputation.[17]

Diabetic lumbosacral radiculoplexopathy neuropathy (DLRPN), often referred to as diabetic amyotrophy or proximal diabetic neuropathy, requires special mention due to its higher prevalence in the elderly and the severe disability often associated with it. DLRPN is a devastating condition that may affect only about 1% of typically type II diabetics.[18] It typically presents with severe, acute onset of proximal leg pain and weakness. Frequently it occurs in concert with a large concomitant weight loss. In many cases, affected patients have not been diabetic for a long period of time and have no other end organ complications from DM. The symptoms are usually unilateral and involve proximal lower limb segments such as the hip flexors and knee extensors. The condition may spread more distally and to the contralateral side over a few days. Although pain is the most severe initial manifestation, often requiring narcotic analgesia, severe weakness typically develops in the first few days, often severely affecting the hip flexors and knee extensors but also in the more distal muscles including the ankle plantar and dorsiflexors. Gait aids or wheelchairs are often required for mobility.

The cerebrospinal fluid will reveal elevated protein providing evidence that the disease process is proximal at the level of the spinal roots. Electrophysiologic (EMG) testing reveals axonal injury or denervation in affected muscles, including the para-spinals, often with severe loss of recruitment implying substantive loss of axons. Given that axonal loss is the mechanism, the time course of recovery is typically many months. In the authors' experience, most of these patients do well, if provided supportive therapy and then treated later with appropriate physical therapy in the form of resistance exercise and gait retraining.

The pathophysiologic basis of diabetic lumbosacral radiculoplexopathy (DLRP) is ischemic injury possibly secondary to microvasculitis. Given this, immunomodulation may be useful if started early in the course of disease, as has been demonstrated in nondiabetics with idiopathic lumbosacral plexopathy. To date, however, clinical trials in diabetics have not supported this theory.[18]

NEUROGENIC CLAUDICATION AND SPINAL STENOSIS

Lumbosacral radiculopathy and specifically multilevel root disease often associated with lumbosacral spondylosis, and associated spinal stenosis is a common, often debilitating problem that typically affects older adults.[19] Symptoms of neurogenic claudication are often mistaken for polyneuropathy; however, there are specific features on history, physical examination, and electrodiagnostic testing that help distinguish these conditions. The most common symptom of neurogenic claudication secondary to lumbosacral spinal stenosis is back pain and aching pain that refers into the buttocks, hamstrings, thighs, and lower legs worsened with exercise. Often there is associated numbness and weakness that occurs in association with the pain and discomfort. Typically, contrary to most neuropathies, the symptoms of pain, numbness, and weakness improve with rest or when seated. Lumbar extension tends to worsen symptoms, and most patients improve with flexion of the spine (e.g., walking while pushing a shopping cart or riding a bicycle, which may be much easier than walking similar durations). This is in contrast to vascular claudication, which tends to produce more localized pain in the calves, no sensory symptoms, and tends to be unaffected by spinal position.[20,21] The physical examination is often uninformative in patients with features of neurogenic claudication. It may reveal reduced or absent ankle jerks if the S1 roots are affected and distal sensory loss in the L5 and S1 distribution. Fixed weakness is uncommon and usually mild.

Imaging with computed tomography (CT) scanning or magnetic resonance imaging (MRI) typically reveals multilevel degenerative spondylitic disease, foraminal narrowing and encroachment, and central canal narrowing. The latter two are secondary to disk protrusion, thickening of the ligamentum flavum, and facet hypertrophy secondary to degenerative disease. Spondylolisthesis, usually degenerative, also may lead to significant canal narrowing.

Electrodiagnostic testing in patients with neurogenic claudication may reveal reduced distal compound muscle action potentials in the intrinsic foot muscles secondary to chronic axonal injury in the L5 and S1 roots. The sural and superficial peroneal sensory nerve action potentials may be mildly reduced but are typically well preserved given that the injury is proximal to the dorsal root ganglion. This pattern of severe motor involvement and mild sensory involvement is sometimes erroneously interpreted as indicative of a polyneuropathy. However, this is the opposite pattern of that seen in the vast majority of polyneuropathies that present with earlier and more severe sensory involvement on nerve conduction studies with less severe motor involvement. Needle EMG of lower limb muscles (tibialis anterior, gastrocnemius, quadriceps) often reveals mild, chronic denervation, reinnervation changes in the form of large amplitude, long duration motor unit potentials with little or no evidence of active denervation.

Conservative treatment is often undertaken initially and includes physiotherapy mainly focusing on spinal flexion and aerobic exercise such as cycling, which tends to be better tolerated than walking. Pain usually responds to nonsteroidal anti-inflammatory drugs (NSAIDs) or mild narcotic analgesics (e.g., codeine). Patients with severe back and radicular pain may benefit symptomatically from epidural corticosteroid injections.

Surgical intervention should be considered for those who do not respond adequately to nonoperative treatment or if their disability is severe (principally mobility limitations). The typical approach involves laminectomy and partial facetectomy. The role of fusion is less clear but is often recommended when there is stenosis accompanied by spondylolisthesis. There is some evidence from randomized controlled trials supporting surgery over conservative management, at least in the 2 years following surgery,[21] and the surgical outcomes tend to favor those with greater canal narrowing.[22]

INFLAMMATORY MYOPATHY

Inflammatory myopathy, or myositis, is among the most common muscle disorder presenting acutely or subacutely in elderly patients and can be subdivided into infectious and idiopathic categories. Infectious causes, including viral and bacterial pathogens, are the most common causes of myositis worldwide but tend to be transient. Idiopathic inflammatory myopathies are a significant cause of chronic neuromuscular disease and constitute a spectrum that includes polymyositis (PM), dermatomyositis (DM), and inclusion body myositis (IBM). PM and DM are related but distinct conditions and are discussed together first.

Etiology of polymyositis and dermatomyositis

Both PM and DM are autoimmune disorders, though the antigenic targets are ill defined. There is strong circumstantial evidence that PM is an autoimmune (AI) disorder: like most AI disorders, PM is more common in women; PM may arise or fluctuate in pregnancy; PM is often associated with other organ- and nonorgan-specific AI disorders; a PM phenotype can be triggered by viral illnesses (HIV and HTLV-1) or by certain drugs, especially D-penicillamine; PM responds to immunosuppression and modulation; finally, as further discussed later, muscle biopsies provide evidence of T-cell-mediated cytotoxic process directed against unknown muscle antigens. Similarly, DM is more common in women, may arise or fluctuate in pregnancy, is often associated with other AI disorders, can be triggered by D-penicillamine, responds to immune therapies, and muscle biopsies show damage reflecting a humoral-mediated capillary angiopathy.

Clinical features of polymyositis and dermatomyositis

DM presents in childhood or in the elderly with a female predominance, as with many other AI disorders. PM is rare in children and the majority of patients present in the third to fifth decade.[23] PM and DM present with symptomatic proximal weakness causing functional impairment (neck extensors and flexors, shoulder girdle, trunk and abdominal muscles, and hip and knee extensors and flexors), diffuse myalgia in up to a third of patients (especially in DM), or a rash. Examination reveals symmetric proximal weakness and wasting with preserved deep tendon reflexes, and neck and bulbar weakness are common. The pathognomonic rash of DM is a purplish-red butterfly discoloration over the face, often associated with periorbital edema and a heliotrope rash over the eyelids. An additional V-shaped rash may be seen in the sun-exposed areas of the chest. Patients may present with a typical rash of DM without clinically apparent weakness (amyopathic DM), though interestingly these same patients do have subclinical changes evident on muscle biopsy.[24] Polymyalgia rheumatica, sometimes confused for an inflammatory myopathy, causes myalgia that is often worse in the shoulder girdle but without significant weakness.

Symptomatic myoglobinuria may occur in rare, acute presentations of both PM and DM, and can precipitate acute renal failure.

PM and DM are frequently associated with connective tissue disorders: PM with lupus, Sjögren's syndrome, and rheumatoid arthritis; and DM with scleroderma and mixed connective tissue disease.[5] Systemic features including vasculitis of the heart or gut, subcutaneous calcinosis, Gottron's nodules around the knuckles, and nail fold capillary changes are seen in DM.[25]

Respiratory muscle weakness occurs rarely in both PM and DM, but fibrosing alveolitis is relatively common in DM, and it is then often associated with antibodies against Jo-1 (t-histidyl transferase synthase).[26] Aspiration pneumonia can occur in patients with severe bulbar weakness and in DM patients with esophageal involvement.

DM, and perhaps PM, can be associated with an underlying malignancy, though estimates of the frequency of this association vary widely from around 5% to 40% in published series.[27] This disparity in part reflects differences in case ascertainment: many case reports are anecdotal and there are few prospective or retrospective studies. Moreover, diagnostic criteria have also differed between reports, and muscle biopsy has not always been employed to confirm the presence of necrosis. Whatever the true incidence of this association, simple investigations, along with a systemic examination including mammography, a chest radiograph, and an abdominal ultrasound, are appropriate. The underlying malignancies mirror those found in the population of similar age and gender.

Differential diagnosis of polymyositis and dermatomyositis

The clinical diagnosis of DM is usually straightforward, though lupus associated with a facial rash and motor neuropathy might cause confusion. Differential diagnosis of PM is wider, as it may be confused with inclusion body myositis (discussed later), motor neuron disease, or myasthenia. The weakness in MG often affects deltoids and triceps, whereas the inflammatory myopathies more commonly affect deltoid and biceps. Additionally, in myasthenia muscle weakness occurs without significant muscle wasting, and in motor neuron disease both upper and lower motor neuron features are apparent. Finally, as inflammatory myopathies presenting in elderly patients can be confused with muscular dystrophies, it is always prudent to take a family history, particularly in those who have not shown the expected response to immunosuppression.

Investigations of polymyositis and dermatomyositis

Serum creatine kinase (CK) is usually, but not always, elevated, often 10 to 50 times the normal value, and this is almost exclusively due to increases in the CK-MM fraction. However, CK values do not correlate well with either myalgia or weakness in PM and DM patients, and in up to 15% of clinically affected individuals CK values are normal. Although the erythrocyte sedimentation rate (ESR) is also usually elevated, this is nonspecific, and it is not a reliable disease marker. An autoantibody screen is worthwhile given the frequent association with collagen vascular disease. Other appropriate baseline investigations include lung function tests, a chest x-ray, and an electrocardiogram. Particularly in the presence of DM, appropriate screening for malignancy is recommended and includes CT or ultrasound of the abdomen and pelvis, mammogram in women, and colonoscopy if indicated.

Neurophysiologic investigations are crucial in the evaluation of patients with suspected myositis. Concentric or monopolar needle EMG studies in PM and DM patients usually show myopathic features with short-duration myopathic discharges but with additional indications of muscle irritability: increased insertional activity and spontaneous activity (including positive sharp waves and fibrillation potentials), reflecting myogenic denervation secondary to muscle fiber necrosis. To increase the sensitivity of EMG, very proximal muscles should be studied, including the hip flexors, thoracic paraspinals, and proximal shoulder girdle muscles. Nerve conduction and repetitive nerve stimulation studies are useful to exclude motor neuropathy and neuromuscular junction disorders, respectively (however, false positive repetitive stimulation can rarely occur in patients with myositis, with low levels of decrement of less than 20%).

Muscle biopsy is crucial to confirm the diagnosis. As already noted, the biopsy should be performed from a weak but not wasted muscle. Almost invariably the muscle biopsies are abnormal in both PM and DM, but if normal and a strong clinical suspicion remains, a second biopsy should be performed as the pathology can be patchy and sampling errors therefore occur. In PM the pathology consists of a T-cell-mediated cytotoxic necrosis: initially, CD8+ cells and macrophages surround healthy muscle fibers and subsequently invade them. Muscle fibers show increased HLA class I expression (normally minimal or absent).[28,29] Endomysial fibrosis is common in PM, and massive fibrosis may underlie some apparently treatment-resistant cases.[29] In DM, it is thought that circulating antiendothelial antibodies activate complement and C3, triggering further changes in the complement cascade and generating membrane attack complex (MAC), which traverses and destroys endomysial capillaries. With destruction and reduced number of muscle capillaries, ischemia or microinfarcts occurs in the periphery of the muscle fascicle (watershed area). Finally, as a late event, complement-fixing antibodies, B cells, CD4+ T cells, and macrophages traffic to the muscle.[29] There is often a surprising divergence between clinical and pathologic features in DM, and perifascicular atrophy is a useful feature in otherwise bland biopsies.

Treatment of polymyositis and dermatomyositis

Treatment of PM and DM is largely based on clinical practice and experience. Although there have been many studies of immunotherapy in inflammatory myopathies, they often group together adult and childhood DM, PM, and IBM patients. Most studies are retrospective and uncontrolled; and in several studies subjective measures and reduced CK are defined as a response. To date, there have only been a few small randomized trials of intravenous immunoglobulin in PM and DM (see the discussion in Mastalgia).[30]

Oral prednisone remains the drug of first choice for patients with both PM and DM. Patients should be started on oral prednisone 1 mg/kg body weight per day.[30] A clinical response should be evident within 3 months in the majority of patients, with a biochemical response (a reduction in the serum CK level) often preceding clinical improvement. Many now advocate the early use of a second-line immunosuppressive agent such as azathioprine or methotrexate as these have a useful steroid sparing action in the longer term. Intravenous immunoglobulin is useful as a rescue therapy for patients with acute or severe DM, but it has not been proven to work in PM, has been shown not to work in IBM, and is occasionally used at intervals for patients with problems related to steroids. A few patients remain resistant to steroids, and if the diagnosis is secure, cyclophosphamide is a useful alternative agent. It is important to remember that the dose of steroids should be tapered according to the clinical response rather than the CK. It can be difficult for doctor and patient alike to detect subtle improvements, and objective physiotherapy assessments including myometry are useful. Although it is usually possible to taper off the dose of steroids after about 3 months, many patients do require a maintenance dose of steroids. In all cases where prednisone is started and is likely to continue beyond 3 months, but especially in the elderly, osteoporosis prophylaxis with bisphosphonates, calcium, and vitamin D is essential, as is regular screening for diabetes and hypertension.

The prognosis of both DM and PM is generally good, unless associated with an underlying malignancy. Respiratory involvement, and especially fibrosing alveolitis, carries a poor prognosis. If patients fail to respond to steroids, IBM may be the diagnosis. Patients should be reevaluated and sometimes rebiopsied.

INCLUSION BODY MYOSITIS

IBM, initially considered to be a rare inflammatory myopathy in older adults, is emerging as the most common cause of new onset myositis in this age group. The clinical, muscle biopsy, neurophysiologic, and prognostic features of IBM are different from both PM and DM.

The pathogenesis of IBM is unclear, but it is most likely a degenerative condition with a secondary immune attack on muscle. IBM may be an immune disorder as there is a modest association with other autoimmune disorders such as diabetes, and muscle pathology shows inflammatory features similar to PM, with CD8+ cells, macrophages, and increased HLA class I expression. However, IBM may be a degenerative condition involving intracellular muscle protein trafficking as (1) muscle contains increased levels of amyloid, prion protein, and other molecules as seen in Alzheimer's disease and (2) to date there is no evidence of maintained response to immunotherapy in the vast majority of cases.

IBM usually presents as a painless, profound, progressive wasting of quadriceps muscles associated with a characteristic genu recurvatum stance and frequent falls. In a minority of patients, weakness and wasting begins in the arms. It is of note that muscle weakness and wasting is often asymmetric and may develop over many years. Myalgia and myoglobinuria are rare. Between a quarter and a third of patients have profound distal weakness especially in the forearms associated with a wasting of the medial flexor compartment, and weakness of finger flexors, particularly the deep ulnar component. This may be mistaken for ulnar neuropathy or motor neuron disease early in the course of the disease. Deep tendon reflexes are often depressed, out of keeping with the extent of weakness giving rise to confusion with neuropathies. Dysphagia and neck flexion weakness are common in IBM. IBM is not associated with malignancy, and there is a male preponderance.

The differential diagnosis of IBM is wide: upper limb presentations of IBM may be confused with cervical radiculopathies or MND.[31] The depressed reflexes seen in most IBM patients may cause confusion with neuropathies, but the clinical sensory examination is normal. The combination of a weak quadriceps muscle group and a depressed knee reflex may suggest LEMS, but, of course, in IBM no post-tetanic potentiation of reflexes is seen. The indolent history in most patients with IBM may suggest an inherited disorder, but the asymmetric weakness and wasting, as well as the pattern of involvement with IBM, reflect its acquired nature.

Several investigations are helpful in patients with suspected IBM. Nerve conduction studies are usually normal but may show features consistent with a mild axonal neuropathy. On EMG studies, myopathic, neurogenic, or a mixed picture is seen, and a high index of clinical suspicion is therefore necessary if the diagnosis is to be considered. CK may be significantly elevated, but more often it is normal or only mildly elevated reflecting the low turnover of muscle cells in this disorder. Muscle biopsies show inflammatory changes, far more marked than one would expect given the often modest elevation of CK, with an infiltration of CD8+ cells, and macrophages. In addition, muscle fibers may contain eosinophilic inclusions and rimmed vacuoles with basophilic stippling, hinting at a degenerative process. On electron microscopy, characteristic intracellular filamentous inclusions are seen, as in other degenerative conditions. Immunohistochemistry demonstrates an increased expression of "degenerative" proteins including amyloid precursor protein, prion protein, ubiquitin, and alpha-synuclein, prompting comparisons between IBM and Alzheimer's disease.[32] The lack of response to immunotherapy (discussed later) suggests that the inflammatory changes may be secondary to a degenerative process within the muscle, rather than a primary event.

The outcome of treatment of IBM is disappointing and to date all attempts at immunosuppression and immunomodulation have failed to induce a consistent and long-lasting benefit. High-dose steroids, methotrexate, azathioprine, cyclophosphamide, and intravenous immunoglobulin (IVIG) have all been tried separately and in various combinations, with inconsistent and largely negative results.[30] Early studies suggested that some patients might benefit from IVIG, but larger randomized studies failed to substantiate this idea.[33–35] There is some evidence that exercise is of benefit early in the course of the disease, and many patients benefit from the use of canes and walkers. Patients with severe weakness often require wheelchairs or motorized scooters for mobility. Severe dysphagia may require enteral nutrition in the form of a gastrojejunal feeding tube.

DRUG-INDUCED MYALGIA AND MYOPATHY

A large number of drugs induce muscle symptoms, but a simple classification is not possible,[36] and an overview with important examples of each is given. Clinical and neurophysiologic combinations of a myopathy, neuropathy, and neuromuscular junction abnormalities often suggest a drug-related toxic or endocrine cause.

Several drugs, including statins, fibrates, and aminocaproic acid, can induce a painful cramping acute or subacute necrotizing myopathy. Most commonly, statins produce myalgia or a mild asymptomatic elevation of the CK level, with no weakness or electrophysiologic abnormalities. However, statins may cause a painful myopathy a few weeks after starting the drug, and this is more common in patients with diabetes, preexistent renal disease, and hepatic disease, especially if on other P450-inhibiting drugs, multiple lipid-lowering agents, or higher than recommended statin doses. Unfortunately, clofibrate and other fibrates may also induce a myopathy; a useful etiologic clue may be subclinical neurophysiologic evidence of associated neuropathy and myotonia. The underlying mechanisms remain unclear, though secondary mitochondrial dysfunction may be important.[36] Statin- and fibrate-induced myopathies might be confused with inflammatory myopathies; drug-induced myopathies evolve quicker and improve, though often slowly, with cessation of the drug. In the presence of a statin-induced myopathy, the CK level is almost always elevated.

Antimalarial agents (including chloroquine), amiodarone, and perhexiline may all induce a chronic painless proximal myopathy with vacuolar change and lysosomal inclusions on muscle biopsy. Amiodarone-induced neuropathy is more common than a myopathy, though the two may coexist.

Similarly, vincristine commonly induces a neuropathy, though some patients also have a myopathy. Diuretics and laxatives may induce muscle pains and or cramps secondary to hypokalemia and occasionally with very low serum potassium levels can be associated with a painful or painless vacuolar myopathy.

D-Penicillamine may induce an inflammatory myopathy resembling polymyositis, or a drug-induced myasthenia gravis; both conditions tend to improve on withdrawal of the drug.

Critical-illness neuropathy is well recognized and may be associated with a myopathic counterpart. Its pathogenesis is unclear and is likely to reflect a combination of immobility, high-dose steroid treatment, electrolyte imbalance, sepsis, multiorgan failure, and the toxic effects of antibiotics and paralyzing agents, together with vitamin deficiency.

Excessive alcohol consumption is often associated with neuromuscular disease. Alcohol can induce an acute myopathy, often associated with hypokalemia, and possibly a chronic myopathy, though chronic wasting and weakness is more common because of a toxic neuropathy, as is a small fiber neuropathy with painful burning feet.

ENDOCRINE AND METABOLIC MYOPATHIES

Steroid-induced myopathy

The majority of patients with Cushing disease have clinical and neurophysiologic features of a myopathy.[37] The prolonged use of steroids is also often associated with a chronic, painless myopathy and less commonly an acute painful necrotizing (critical-illness) myopathy. Steroid-induced myopathy is typically associated with obesity, moon facies, and other classic stigmata of glucorticoid excess. Steroid myopathy may be difficult to recognize in patients receiving steroids for inflammatory muscle disease, though steroids are unlikely to be the culprit unless used for more than 4 weeks, when patients will have other stigmata of glucocorticoid excess. Proximal leg weakness is the most common clinical manifestation of a steroid myopathy. Needle EMG is usually normal or mildly abnormal, although the presence of fibrillation potentials or positive sharp waves should suggest another etiology. As CK levels may be normal in both steroid-induced and inflammatory myopathies, and EMG findings can occasionally be similar, muscle biopsy is sometimes required to distinguish disease activity from iatrogenic myopathy. The pathogenesis of steroid-induced myopathy is complex and involves hypokalemia and alterations in carbohydrate and protein metabolism. Structural changes on muscle biopsy include type 2 fiber atrophy, although this is nonspecific, lipid deposition, and vacuole formation. Using second-line immunosuppressives such as azathioprine to treat the inflammatory disease in question may facilitate treatment, which consists of slowly withdrawing steroids. Unfortunately, patients recover from steroid-induced myopathy only slowly, and an exercise program may be useful.

Thyroid dysfunction

Muscle weakness is seen in the vast majority of thyrotoxic patients. Hyperthyroid myopathy may be associated with myalgia and fatigue, and thyrotoxic patients may readily overlook it. Weakness may be proximal or generalized and occasionally involves bulbar and respiratory muscles.[38] Ocular involvement (Grave's disease) may occur in patients with hyperthyroidism and reflects both excessive adrenergic activity and inflammatory changes in extraocular muscle and surrounding orbital tissue.[39] Hyperthyroid myopathy is commonly associated with proximal weakness without wasting, resembling that seen in myasthenia gravis. Patients with autoimmune dysthyroid states may have myasthenia and vice versa. Dysthyroid ophthalmopathy, where the extraocular muscles are often enlarged, producing restricted extraocular muscle movement, can be confused with ocular myasthenia and can coexist within the same patient. Recognition of such associations is important in targeting treatment. Patients with thyrotoxicosis may also have alterations in deep tendon reflexes and fasciculations, which may mimic MND and cause diagnostic confusion. Given these potential diagnostic pitfalls, it seems reasonable to recommend initial thyroid function tests, and in some cases screening for autoantibodies against thyroid tissue, in all patients presenting with neuromuscular disease.[40] Investigation of serum CK, EMG, and muscle biopsy is usually unhelpful, because there are no specific diagnostic features of the condition, but it may be useful in rare cases where dual pathology is suspected (e.g., polymyositis and thyroid myopathy). Occasionally, thyrotoxicosis is associated with a neuropathy, though mixed neuropathic and myopathic features are seen in EMG. The pathogenesis of thyroid myopathy is complex and likely to involve alterations in both muscle metabolism and electrical properties, principally through increased Na^+, K^+-ATPase pump activity. Finally, thyrotoxic periodic paralysis[41] is a rare but well-recognized disorder, more common in individuals of Asian descent. (The periodic paralyses are a group of predominantly inherited neuromuscular disorders in which paralysis is related to electrolyte imbalances.)[42]

Hypothyroidism is also frequently associated with neuromuscular manifestations, which may dominate the clinical picture and rarely may predate the development of overt biochemical abnormalities.[38] A recent prospective study underlies the strength of these associations: in patients with recently diagnosed thyroid dysfunction, 79% of hypothyroid patients had neuromuscular complaints including pain and stiffness and 38% had clinical weakness.[43] Symptoms did not correlate with serum CK levels and improved slowly with thyroxine therapy. Muscle biopsy shows glycogen accumulation at the periphery of the muscle fiber. The exact relationship between the muscle biopsy and clinical features remains unexplained. Hypothyroid myopathy may cause diagnostic confusion. First, patients may have delayed relaxation of deep tendon reflexes and occasionally myotonia (Hoffman's syndrome), simulating features of the genetic myotonic disorders. Second, occasionally patients have very high CK levels and marked muscle wasting, simulating an inflammatory or inherited muscle disease.[37]

MOTOR NEURON DISEASE (MND)

MND is a common, fatal, progressive disorder with degeneration of both upper and lower motor neurons of uncertain cause. Death usually occurs as a consequence of respiratory failure. MND has an incidence of 1 to 3 per 100,000 and a prevalence of around 4 to 6 per 100,000.

The etiology of MND is unclear, and a number of potential mechanisms have been suggested: excessive glutamate, an influx of calcium, and a subsequent excitotoxic cascade triggering cell damage and apoptosis are likely to be important. Mutations in the gene for superoxide dismutase (SOD 1) have been found in a minority of patients (fewer than 5%) with the uncommon familial form of MND, suggesting that free-radical damage and excessive oxidative stress are important.[44]

Clinical features of MND reflect upper and lower motor neuron involvement. Nocturnal cramps are an early feature but rarely prompt patients to consult physicians. MND often begins in an asymmetric fashion in a single body region (intrinsic hand muscles, arms, legs, trunk, bulbar musculature) but ultimately involves all four regions; bulbar, cervical, thoracic, and lumbosacral. Lower motor neuron features include asymmetric muscle wasting and weakness, fasciculations, and depressed reflexes. Upper motor neuron features include spastic hypertonia, pyramidal weakness, and brisk deep tendon reflexes with extensor plantar responses. A combination of a wasted, weak quadriceps muscle with a pathologically brisk knee jerk is very suggestive of MND, as is the combination of a wasted and fasciculating tongue but with a pathologically brisk jaw jerk. Neck weakness is common in motor neuron disease and may lead to a head drop. Eye movement disorders, sensory signs (in the absence of entrapment neuropathies), and sphincter involvement are all distinctly rare in motor neuron disease and should suggest another diagnosis.

Investigations in MND (1) provide support for the clinical diagnosis and (2) exclude structural or other potentially treatable pathologies. Serum CK levels may be modestly increased (<1000 IU/mL) but are nonspecific. Neurophysiologic tests are useful in excluding another neurogenic disorder (e.g., multilevel root disease, multifocal motor neuropathy), myopathic process, or neuromuscular transmission disorder; they are also more sensitive than the clinical exam in demonstrating lower motor neuron involvement, with the neurogenic abnormalities reflecting both denervation and chronic reinnervation. A careful search for nerve conduction block is warranted in patients without upper motor neuron signs, who might have multifocal motor neuropathy, a rare but treatable autoimmune neuropathy frequently associated with antibodies against GM1 ganglioside.[45] Structural imaging, ideally MRI scanning, is sometimes useful to exclude pathologies such as degenerative disk disease, which may cause both cord and nerve root compression with consequent mixed upper and lower motor neuron signs. Structural imaging is especially important when signs are confined to the limbs and there are no upper or lower motor neuron signs above the cervical involvement.

Unfortunately, no effective therapies are available, and to date, trials with a variety of nerve growth factors have been disappointing. Riluzole, an antiglutamate agent, produces a moderate prolongation of life and should be considered at an early stage in all patients with possible MND.[46] The lack of curative drug therapy should not be taken to imply that nothing can be done to mitigate the impact of the disease. Rehabilitation utilizing the many different skills of the multidisciplinary team should be available at every stage.[46] Gastrostomy feeding is useful at an early stage both to maintain the patient's nutritional state and to reduce the chance of aspiration in those with significant bulbar weakness. The role of noninvasive and formal ventilation in patients with motor neuron disease remains controversial but overall appears to improve survival and quality of life.[47]

Myasthenia gravis (MG)

Myasthenia gravis is an autoimmune disorder in which neuromuscular transmission is disrupted by antibodies against postsynaptic skeletal muscle proteins, usually the nicotinic acetylcholine receptors (AChR).[48,49] This produces fatigable weakness, characteristically involving extraocular, bulbar, axial, and proximal extremity muscles.[49] Therapies for MG are highly effective, although potentially toxic, and include acetylcholinesterase inhibitors, immunosuppression, and temporary immunomodulation. The clinical features and management of MG in the aged person are similar to that in younger individuals. MG may be more common in the elderly than was thought, and an increased risk of adverse effects of medications as well as increased likelihood of comorbidities in the elderly mandates even more careful monitoring of therapy.[50,51] Thymectomy, though helpful in patients with "early-onset" MG, may not be beneficial for late-onset MG apart from its role in the removal of a thymoma.[52]

Clinical and epidemiologic features of myasthenia gravis

The clinical hallmark of MG is fatigable and fluctuating weakness of skeletal muscles.[49] The initial presentation is often with ocular symptoms: diplopia and ptosis. Most develop generalized weakness subsequently. In 20% to 25% of patients with "ocular MG," the weakness remains restricted to the extraocular muscles.[53,54] In the remainder, generalized weakness can affect bulbar muscles, producing weakness of chewing or facial expression, dysphagia, dysarthria, neck flexion, or extension. Extremity weakness, usually proximal and symmetric, affects arms more than legs. Characteristic in MG is weakness that is worse at day's end and fluctuates in severity over weeks or months.

MG is uncommon, with an estimated prevalence of 80 to $100/10^6$ and an incidence of about $6/10^6$.[55,56] Although myasthenia can present at any age, two peaks of onset define two clinical subgroups.[57–59] In "early-onset" MG, more common in females, onset is between 18 and 50 years. "Late-onset" MG, with onset after 50, is more common in males.[59,60] Epidemiologic evidence suggests that MG is more common in the elderly than was thought, and it may be misdiagnosed more commonly.[9,50,51,60–62] "Seronegative" MG, without detectable anti-AChR antibodies, is clinically similar to seropositive MG, responds to the same treatments, and likely has a similar humoral mediation.[63] In a third of seronegative generalized MG patients, antibodies against muscle-specific kinase (MuSK) are found.[64] Rare nonimmune "congenital myasthenic syndromes" occur when mutations produce a structural abnormality in one of the proteins at the neuromuscular junction.

The Lambert-Eaton myasthenic syndrome (LEMS) is an even more rare disorder, with antibodies against presynaptic nerve terminal voltage-gated calcium channels (VGCC).[65] It is often paraneoplastic, usually secondary to an underlying small-cell lung cancer. The clinical manifestations of LEMS consist of fatigable muscle weakness, mainly affecting the legs and presenting as a gait abnormality, autonomic dysfunction, and depression of the deep tendon reflexes. The diagnosis and treatment of LEMS is similar in many respects to that of MG and will not be discussed further here.

Neuromuscular transmission and the pathophysiology of myasthenia gravis

Depolarization of the nerve terminal at the neuromuscular junction opens presynaptic VGCC, allowing calcium influx and the release of acetylcholine (ACh) from the nerve terminal. ACh binds reversibly to AChRs on the postsynaptic skeletal muscle surface, resulting in muscle fiber depolarization and eventually muscle contraction. Finally, ACh dissociates and is metabolized by acetylcholinesterase (AChE) in the synaptic cleft, or it diffuses away from the neuromuscular junction.[66]

In MG, anti-AChR antibodies impair neuromuscular transmission.[67] If action potential generation fails at enough muscle fibers, the clinical result is weakness. Serum anti-AChR antibodies are found in about 85% of generalized MG patients, although titers may be lower in the elderly.[48,60] The thymus seems to be implicated in the genesis or perpetuation of MG, as most early-onset MG patients have thymic hyperplasia.[68] The other main pathologic alteration, a thymoma, is present in 10% to 20% of all MG patients, in 24% to 38% of late-onset patients, much less commonly in ocular MG, and rarely in seronegative MG.[69,70] When there is a thymoma, MG tends to be more severe, with a higher mortality.[71] In 10% to 20% of MG patients, especially those over 50 years of age, the thymus is atrophic.[62]

Diagnosis

Suspicion for a diagnosis of MG is often delayed as a result of fluctuating weakness.[22] The weakness in MG may be temporarily improved with a "Tensilon test," which involves administering a short-acting acetylcholinesterase inhibitor and assessing for signs of clinical improvement. Routine electrophysiologic studies in myasthenia gravis are usually normal. Repetitive nerve stimulation may reveal a "decrement" in the motor amplitude.[66] Single-fiber EMG (SFEMG) is highly sensitive (>90%) at detecting impaired neuromuscular transmission, but it is less specific.[72,73] Serum anti-AChR antibodies, highly specific for MG, are detected in approximately 85% of patients with generalized MG and in 50% with ocular MG.[48] They are almost always present if there is a thymoma. Approximately 5% of seronegative generalized MG patients have antibodies against a different muscle protein, muscle-specific kinase (MuSK).[64] MuSK antibodies are found more commonly in female MG patients with prominent bulbar weakness and are not found in purely ocular MG.

Treatment

Before effective treatment was available, the mortality from MG was high, even worse in late-onset MG or if a thymoma was present. With treatment, the mortality from MG is less than 5%, although bulbar or respiratory muscle weakness continues to be a major source of morbidity.[74,75]

Treatment options include drugs that mask symptoms and more specific therapies to suppress or modulate the aberrant autoimmune response. The choice of specific therapies is dictated by the need for rapid improvement, convenience, expense, and the frequency of adverse effects.

Mestinon (pyridostigmine) inhibits acetylcholinesterase, increasing ACh at the neuromuscular junction. It does not affect the underlying immune process. Its duration of action is usually 3 to 6 hours but variable, ranging from 2 to 12 hours.[76] A long-acting preparation (Mestinon Supraspan 180 mg) is used at bedtime for patients with significant nocturnal or early morning weakness. Side effects, usually gastrointestinal, are mild. Although usually effective, Mestinon alone is often insufficient, even less so in ocular MG. Most patients eventually require treatment with corticosteroids (CST) or other immunosuppressives.[77]

The efficacy of immunosuppressive agents is similar, and there may be synergism when used in combination. Prednisone is the most commonly used drug after Mestinon. Although highly effective, it has a significant risk of adverse effects. Low doses have fewer side effects but are less effective and take longer. Immediate high dose treatment (50–100 mg/day) may cause transient worsening in weakness, so a gradual increase in dose is preferable.[78] Maximal benefit can take 4 to 9 months. There are numerous adverse effects, especially with prolonged high-dose CST therapy and in the elderly.[69,79] Osteoporosis, more likely in the elderly, can be anticipated and prevented with bisphosphonates, calcium, and vitamin D. Once MG is improved, the dose of prednisone is tapered slowly to lessen the chance of relapse, less likely when other immunosuppressives like azathioprine are also used.[80]

Azathioprine is used as a sole therapy in MG when the situation is less pressing or when there are contraindications to CST. A more common role is as a steroid-sparing agent. Azathioprine is effective with fewer adverse effects than CST. However, its use requires monitoring for hepatic and hematologic toxicity, and it has a long delay (12 to 18 months) before optimal benefit. Cyclosporine is one of the few agents shown in a randomized-controlled trial (RCT) to be of benefit in MG. It is expensive, and has many adverse effects. Therefore, it is used mainly in severe MG not responding to prednisone and azathioprine. Mycophenolate, in widespread use in MG, seems to be effective, although no more so than other available agents, but with less toxicity. Two trials showed no additional benefit to prednisone, probably because prednisone alone is effective in the short term in mild MG. Several other immunosuppressive agents, including cyclophosphamide, tacrolimus, and rituximab, have also been used in MG. None is proven to be superior to the previously mentioned drugs, and they are used mainly when MG is unresponsive to these agents.

Although there is widespread acceptance for thymectomy in MG, the precise indications and surgical approach remain controversial, and a randomized controlled trial is needed to clarify its role in MG.[81] It is generally accepted as effective in early-onset AChR antibody positive patients with generalized MG. Its role is unproven and even more controversial in seronegative patients and in the elderly (in the absence of a thymoma) when the thymus is often atrophic.[82,83] A thymoma is removed to avoid local growth and infiltration of adjacent mediastinal structures, yet it has less effect on the clinical course of MG than removal of a hyperplastic thymus. In MuSK-positive MG patients, the thymus is less pathologically involved, if at all, and the role of thymectomy even more uncertain.[84]

Incomplete benefits or delayed benefits from medical treatment are problematic for patients with moderate or severe MG. Plasma exchange (PE) and intravenous immunoglobulin (IVIg) are both equally useful with significant respiratory and bulbar involvement (a "myasthenic crisis"), as well as before surgery to reduce postoperative complications. Both temporarily improve neuromuscular transmission. Clinical benefit is usually maximal 1 to 2 weeks after treatment begins and lasts for 2 to 8 weeks. Sustained benefit requires immunosuppression. Both are expensive, produce temporary improvement, and are not advisable for the long-term management of most MG patients.[85,86]

Several other drugs may worsen neuromuscular transmission and should be avoided in a patient with MG. However, many myasthenics can take one or more of these medications without any obvious ill effect. It is important to educate the patient and her or his general physician about this possibility and to consider these medications as a cause of otherwise unexplained worsening.

More is known about the pathogenesis of MG than any other autoimmune disorder. As a result, the treatment of MG is highly successful, although the frequency of adverse effects is often a limiting factor. MG may be more common in the elderly, and the aged patient is more susceptible to the adverse effects of medications. Managing a patient with MG is usually a rewarding experience, with most patients responding to treatment and achieving significant improvement in their symptoms, although the adverse effects of long-term treatment can be significant.

KEY POINTS

Neuromuscular Disorders

- Neuromuscular disorders are common in the elderly and may be mistaken for normal biologic aging.
- A careful history and examination is crucial in determining the presence or absence of a neuromuscular disorder superimposed on aging.
- Most acquired and inherited myopathies present with symmetric proximal weakness.
- Most neuropathies present with distal sensory symptoms and weakness as a late manifestation.
- When weakness and fatigue predominate and sensory symptoms are absent, consider a neuromuscular transmission disorder, motor neuron disease, or a myopathy.

For a complete list of references, please visit online only at www.expertconsult.com

CHAPTER 66

Intracranial Tumors

David H. Rosenbaum
Michael L. Gruber
Mary V. MacNeil

Intracranial tumor ("brain tumor") is perhaps the diagnosis most feared by patients presenting for neurologic evaluation. While neoplasms are less common than many of the other conditions that produce neurologic symptomatology, their importance in the elderly population becomes proportionately greater because the incidence of brain tumor increases throughout adult life. Furthermore, the incidence and mortality of primary brain tumor have been increasing since at least the 1970s, and this change has also been most evident in the elderly population.

Although the clinical presentation often suggests the diagnosis, the manifestations of brain tumor are protean. The clinical picture may be even more obscure in an elderly person. The introduction of noninvasive brain imaging modalities—computed x-ray tomography (CT) and magnetic resonance imaging (MRI)—has greatly aided the diagnosis of tumors and intracranial disease in general. Although treatment options and prognosis are less favorable in older adults, recent advances in neurosurgery, radiation treatment, and chemotherapy have to some degree improved this outlook.

CLASSIFICATION

Intracranial brain tumors are neoplasms that arise within the central nervous system (CNS) or spread there from elsewhere (metastatic). Primary brain tumors are a heterogeneous group of neoplasms that arise from a diverse group of cells residing in the CNS. They can be benign or malignant. In 2009, it was estimated that 22,920 people would be diagnosed with a primary malignant brain tumor in the United States, resulting in 12,920 deaths.[1] In keeping with other malignancies, the incidence of brain tumors increases with advancing age.

Metastatic tumors

Metastatic brain tumors have an incidence in the United States of 150,000 each year. Metastatic lesions are more common in the elderly group.[2,3] Of tumors metastatic to the brain, the lung is the most frequent source (50%), and the breast is the second. Renal, gastrointestinal tract, and melanomas account for the majority of remaining metastatic brain tumors.

Primary tumors

Primary brain tumors arise from the brain parenchyma, supporting structures, cranial and spinal nerves, and other specialized structures. Lymphomas can also occur in the brain as the primary site. The latest WHO classification of tumors of the central nervous system includes seven major categories based on tissue of origin and includes tumors of neuroepithelial tissue, tumors of cranial and paraspinal nerves, tumors of the meninges, lymphomas and hematopoietic neoplasms, germ cell tumors, tumors of the sellar region, and metastatic tumors.[4,5] These tumors are further described based on histologic appearance and graded in an attempt to assign biologic behavior, with low grade (I/II) behaving in a more benign fashion and high grade (III/IV) being the most aggressive.

The neuroepithelial derived gliomas and tumors of meningeal origin make up approximately 78% of all incident brain tumors in the geriatric group.[6] Gliomas are made up of astrocytomas, oligodendrogliomas, mixed tumors, and ependymal tumors.[4] The astrocytomas are the most common malignant brain tumor in older adults. They have an infiltrative growth pattern, making a true complete surgical resection impossible. Astrocytomas may be low-grade (I and II), with a favorable behavior, or high-grade anaplastic astrocytomas (grade III) and glioblastoma multiforme (GBM, grade IV) the most aggressive. High-grade tumors predominate in the elderly. Oligodendrogliomas or mixed oligoastrocytomas, and ependymomas, which tend to behave more favorably, occur more often in younger adults. Meningeal derived meningiomas are another common tumor in older adults. These tend to cause less morbidity than gliomas, as most are benign and slow growing with only a small number being malignant. Pituitary-derived adenomas and acoustic neuromas make up most of the remainder, with all other subtypes occurring rarely. Germ cell tumors (neuroepithelial derived) almost never occur in this age group.[6]

Primary CNS lymphomas account for about 1% of parenchymal tumors. They are most often seen in immunocompromised patients (those with AIDS and the transplant population), are uncommon in the immunologically normal, and occur principally in the sixth and seventh decades of life.[7,8] The incidence is increasing in the elderly population.[9]

EPIDEMIOLOGY

As with most cancers, the incidence of tumors of the CNS increases with advancing age. The median age at diagnosis for cancer of the brain and other sites in the nervous system for 2001–2005 was 56 years of age. According to the latest figures from the Surveillance, Epidemiology, and End Results Program (SEER) of the United States covering the period of 2001–2005, children up to 4 years of age have an age-specific incidence rate of 4 cases per 100,000.[1] The rate declines thereafter, reaching its lowest in adolescence, and then climbs again, peaking in the 70-to-74 age group (22 cases/100,000), then slowly declining to 17 cases per 100,000 in those older than 85. Proportionally, this represents approximately 1% of all incident cancers in adults and 23% in children.[1,6,10,11]

Tumor location within the CNS, predominant histologies, behavior, and mortality also vary between young and old.[6] In adults, most brain tumors (malignant and nonmalignant) arise in the cortex or the meninges and only rarely occur in other sites, whereas in children brain tumors primarily arise in the brain stem and cerebellum.[6] Ninety percent of malignant brain tumors in older adults are glial derived, with GBM making up three quarters of these tumors in those 65 to 74, versus 50% in those 45 to 54 years of age. The remaining glial tumors in the elderly are mainly anaplastic astrocytomas. Children most often develop low-grade astrocytomas (e.g., pilocytic) and more primitive types such as primitive neuroectodermal tumors and medulloblastomas.[6,11]

Unfortunately, mortality from brain tumors also increases with age.[6,11] The median age at death for cancer of the brain and other nervous system locations in 2001–2005 was 64 years. The 5-year relative survival rate following the diagnosis of a primary malignant brain tumor for ages <45, 45 to 54, 55 to 64, 65 to 74, and >74 were 63.2%, 28.4%, 13%, 7.4%, and 4%, respectively.[1] This same trend holds true even within histologic subtypes, such as glioblastoma, which has a relative 5-year survival rate of 11% in those 45 to 54 and only 2.7% in those older than 65.[6] Malignant brain tumors make up 2% of all cancer-related deaths in adults, making it among the top 10 malignant causes of death. The strongest prognostic factors for survival therefore remain age and histology. Why tumors such as the malignant gliomas behave more aggressively as one ages is not known. Intensive research into the possible molecular mechanisms is ongoing, with no definitive answers yet.[12]

In the early 1990s, reports surfaced raising concern about the dramatic increase in the incidence of brain tumors in older adults, with rates almost five times higher in 1985 compared to 1973.[13] The rise was seen in both sexes and involved mainly glioblastoma and anaplastic astrocytoma. Similar trends were reported in Canada, Europe, Britain, and Japan, with mortality noted to be increasing as well.[14–16] This raised concern that an as yet unknown etiologic factor might be responsible for the increased incidence.[16] Legler et al, using SEER data to compare age-specific incidence rates from 1977–1995, were able to demonstrate that the increase in age-specific incidence trend was starting to stabilize by 1987 for those 65 years of age and older, and finally by 1995 for those over 85 years of age. They elegantly showed that trends in the use of CT, MRI, and stereotactic biopsy procedures in the elderly over this time period had a similar pattern as the incidence of brain tumors. This offers compelling evidence indicating increases in incidence rates are likely artifactual and may be due in part to physicians adopting more aggressive diagnostic approaches in the elderly. Other factors that may have contributed to this probable artifactual increased incidence rate involve changes in diagnostic classification that have occurred over time, increased availability of neurologists and neurosurgeons, changes in patterns of access to medical care, inaccuracies of data collection, and a changing attitude toward care of the elderly.[11,17–20] Recent reports from the United States and Canada have continued to show that the incidence rates of CNS tumors have leveled off.[21,22]

The main associated causes of brain tumors in all age groups remain hereditary syndromes, prior therapeutic radiation, and immune suppression (predisposing to CNS lymphomas).[17]

CLINICAL PRESENTATION

A brain tumor is a progressively expanding intracranial mass lesion and its clinical hallmark is insidious progression of neurologic deficits. In up to 10% of cases, however, the onset may be abrupt, suggesting a stroke[23]; alternatively, stuttering or paroxysmal symptoms may appear during the course of the illness. These phenomena are occasionally related to intratumoral or peritumoral hemorrhage, secondary vascular compromise, or partial epileptic seizures, but they often remain unexplained. On the other hand, fewer than 1% of those presenting with the clinical picture of stroke will be found to have a tumor.[24]

Typically, brain tumors produce progressive dysfunction related to destruction or compression of areas of cortex and subcortical nuclei. With malignant tumors, symptoms develop over weeks to months, whereas meningiomas may present with insidious progression over months or years.

Primary tumors generally involve the cerebral hemispheres in this age group.[25] Manifestations may include changes in memory, mood, or personality with anterior frontal, deep-seated limbic lesions and temporal tumors; hemiparesis with posterior frontal location; hemisensory loss and hemianopia with parietal lesions; and aphasia with left-sided tumors in the region of the sylvian fissure.

In addition to local effects, because the skull forms a rigid case, the volume increase caused by the tumor and associated edema often raises intracranial pressure. Thalamic tumors may cause obstructive hydrocephalus, leading to the early development of elevated pressure. Intracranial hypertension typically produces both diffuse and remote effects, including headache associated with nausea and vomiting, dizziness, diplopia, gait abnormality, and mental changes—most important and ominously is depressed level of consciousness, suggesting impending brain herniation, which is usually fatal.

Although primary tumors of the brainstem and cerebellum are a rarity in the elderly population, about 20% of metastatic tumors are located in the posterior fossa, more than 75% in the cerebellum.[26] They often present with ataxia or cranial nerve abnormalities.

Acoustic neuromas are very slow-growing Schwann cell tumors of the 8th nerve that produce unilateral hearing loss as the earliest symptom; the adjacent 5th and 7th cranial nerves may be subsequently involved. Only late in their course, with advancing size, do they produce the combination of brainstem and cerebellar signs implicit in their location at the cerebellopontine angle. Audiometric testing (including brainstem auditory potentials) reveals unilateral retrocochlear hearing loss and indicates the need for an imaging study, ideally contrast-enhanced MRI.[27]

Pituitary adenomas may secrete ACTH, growth hormone, or prolactin, but are more commonly nonfunctioning and produce no symptoms.[28] With progressive enlargement, they may cause headache, change in mental status, or change in personality, and they can produce varying degrees of hypopituitarism. If the tumor grows into the suprasellar cistern, it may compress the optic chiasm and result in bitemporal hemianopia, an almost pathognomonic visual-field defect.

Several factors modify the clinical picture of brain tumor in the elderly person, tending to make the diagnosis less readily evident. The loss of brain parenchymal volume that occurs with age allows tumors to grow for a longer time and become larger without producing an increase in cerebrospinal fluid pressure. Consequently, morning headache, with projectile vomiting and papilledema, considered classic signs of brain tumor, is less likely to be prominent in the geriatric patient.[23] Furthermore, elderly individuals are prone to develop mental changes and delirium early in their course, and these changes may be phenomenologically indistinguishable from similar states induced by toxic or metabolic disturbances. The clinical picture may at times be difficult to distinguish from degenerative dementia or depression. Such changes in the absence of detectable motor or sensory abnormalities on examination are more likely to occur with meningiomas, which because of their slow growth and extraaxial location allow neural structures to accommodate to their presence. Focal abnormalities on neurologic examination in a patient presenting with delirium should, of course, raise the suspicion of tumor, as should progression of a deficit that presents as a "stroke." The most frequent clinical manifestations of brain tumor in the elderly population include motor signs in more than one half, mental changes in a third, and sensory changes, hemianopia, or speech abnormalities in one fifth.[23] The incidence and prevalence of seizures (both partial and secondarily generalized) increase progressively with advancing age, and although vascular lesions account for more than half of the cases of epilepsy beginning after the age of 60, a third are caused by brain tumors.[29]

INVESTIGATIONS AND DIAGNOSIS

As in the field of neurology in general, a comprehensive history supplemented by a competent neurologic examination is likely to bring the clinician close to the correct diagnosis and to suggest the most efficient diagnostic plan. In the elderly person, because of the complexities described earlier, it is essential that a high index of suspicion be maintained regarding the possibility of brain tumor, particularly since it is generally a treatable and often curable cause of disability.

Brain imaging

Before CT scanning became widely available in the mid-1970s, a definitive evaluation to exclude or diagnose a brain tumor required hospitalization for invasive, uncomfortable, and relatively high-risk procedures—specifically cerebral arteriography or pneumoencephalography. Clinicians were reluctant to submit patients, particularly the fragile elderly, to such risks in the absence of clear indications, and patients were often followed clinically without definitive testing as "brain tumor suspects." Today, most experienced neurologists would agree that an individual presenting with a new or progressive neurologic deficit or with dementia should, after appropriate clinical evaluation, undergo a definitive brain imaging study. Although CT revolutionized the diagnostic evaluation of these patients, contrast-enhanced MRI has proven to be significantly more sensitive in the detection of focal brain lesions and is currently recognized as the optimal screening technique for the detection of most intracranial neoplasms.[27]

Details of the neuroimaging appearances of different types of tumors are beyond the scope of this chapter, but comprehensive reviews are readily available.[27] A few points are worth making here.

By their nature as growing lesions, tumors generally exert a mass effect and displace surrounding structures. Astrocytomas, in addition, infiltrate and replace normal brain parenchyma. A zone of edema typically surrounds a tumor, with characteristic appearance on CT and MRI, though in the case of gliomas some of this "edema" also consists of "fingers" of infiltrating tumor tissue.[30] Because the blood–brain barrier is defective in most tumors, contrast enhancement is an important diagnostic characteristic, though frequently absent in the low-grade gliomas.[27] None of these features, of course, is pathognomonic, and each finding must be interpreted in its clinical context. Contrast enhancement of a parenchymal tumor suggests a relatively more malignant process, but high-grade pathology can be seen in patients with nonenhancing MRI scans. Multiple lesions, best appreciated with contrast MRI, are typical of metastatic disease but can be seen in 3% of astrocytomas. Primary cerebellar tumors are rare in the elderly population and suggest metastasis.

A primary CNS lymphoma is often seen as a densely enhancing lesion in the deep periventricular white matter.[31] In a third of patients, the lesions are multiple. In 20% of cases, there is either evidence of leptomeningeal spread or concomitant vitreal/retinal disease.[32]

Meningiomas are extra-axial in location and usually have a broad base of attachment to the dura; they show extensive, uniform contrast enhancement and as they enlarge can exert a mass effect.

Functional MRI (perfusion/spectroscopy) is proving helpful in the initial workup of a patient with a nonenhancing mass. In a heterogeneous inoperable glioma it can help the surgeon plan the biopsy target. Functional MRI also is used in treated patients to help determine whether findings on conventional MRI are due to tumor progression or radiation necrosis. In some centers it is used to help assess therapeutic response to chemotherapy and other treatments.

CSF examination

Lumbar puncture is *not* indicated for the diagnosis of brain tumor. While elevation of CSF protein is commonly seen, this is a nonspecific finding whose utility has been eclipsed by the advent of noninvasive imaging. Cytologic examination may reveal malignant cells and aid in pathologic diagnosis, particularly with primary CNS lymphomas, leukemia, or metastases involving the meninges (meningeal lymphomatosis or carcinomatosis).[33] Rarely a glioma will present with a meningeal picture (meningeal gliomatosis) diagnosable by CSF cytology. Since there is a small but real risk that lumbar puncture will cause brain herniation, particularly in the presence of a large tumor and increased intracranial pressure, CT or MR imaging should be performed first to rule out such a situation.

Biopsy

The role of surgery and surgical tumor resection is discussed more fully in the section on treatment. As a rule, a definitive tissue diagnosis should be achieved when practicable. This is both because the particular treatment will depend on the tumor type and because not all space-occupying lesions seen on brain imaging prove to be neoplastic.[34,35] On the other hand, a recent study of 200 patients undergoing stereotactic biopsy concluded that biopsy may not be needed when a clear presumptive diagnosis can be made on the basis of clinical and neuroimaging evidence.[36] Furthermore, the decision to perform a biopsy must be conditioned by the overall clinical context and the patient's medical and psychosocial status. For example, a patient with known malignancy and uncontrolled systemic metastases who presents with brain lesions typical of metastatic disease does not usually require biopsy; nor does a frail patient with end-stage Alzheimer's disease and a large, radiologically malignant brain tumor. In a patient with a single tumor or multiple brain lesions consistent with metastatic disease, workup to identify a primary source beyond complete physical examination (with testing for occult blood in stool) and CT scan of chest is often unrevealing and probably not cost-effective.[37] In this situation, biopsy (or resection, if appropriate—discussed later) would be the logical next step. When biopsy *is* indicated, the procedure of choice is a CT- or MRI-guided stereotactic needle biopsy, which has an overall morbidity of just 2%.[38]

Summary of Management Algorithm

Intracranial Tumors

- Enhanced MRI is the diagnostic test of choice.
- Pathologic diagnosis is mandatory unless the patient is dying from widespread metastatic disease or has a severe, unrelated neurologic or medical condition.
- Older adults should not be denied surgery, radiation therapy, or chemotherapy based on age alone. Even so, precise criteria for which levels of fitness allow surgery and which levels of frailty preclude it are lacking.
- All patients who are eligible for clinical trials should be encouraged to participate.

TREATMENTS

Surgery

The ideal treatment for brain tumor is total surgical resection resulting in cure. As indicated, this is generally possible only for the "benign" lesions: meningioma, acoustic neuroma, and pituitary adenoma. Even here the anatomic location of the tumor or the general health of the patient may preclude aggressive surgery. Age itself is not a contraindication to neurosurgery, and perioperative mortality and morbidity are not necessarily increased after the age of 65.[23] It has also been found that patients over 65 undergoing craniotomy for brain tumor, although sicker and having a higher rate of complications than those under 65, had similar outcomes, including quality-of-life scores.[39] However, because elderly people are more prone to coexisting medical conditions that worsen their prognosis, the approach to treatment is usually balanced toward the less aggressive side, particularly in those who are frail. Even so, precise criteria of who is fit enough for surgery and who is too frail are lacking. A common dilemma in this regard, especially in relation to slower growing tremors, is to know how much of impaired function to attribute to the tumor and how much impaired function reflects underlying frailty. Because the natural history of "benign" tumors is often measured in decades, an incidentally discovered asymptomatic lesion may not require treatment, and partial removal of a tumor that cannot be completely resected may render the patient asymptomatic for the duration of the life span. Stereotactic radiosurgery for unresectable tumors is proving to be an important option (discussed later). Pituitary adenomas can be treated with a high rate of success and low morbidity by transsphenoidal removal,[40] prolactin-secreting tumors are often effectively treated with bromocriptine[41] or other dopaminergic agents, and tumors that are inoperable or incompletely removed should be treated with radiation (discussed later). Radiation therapy may also be useful in preventing recurrence of partially resected meningiomas or in treating recurrences.[42]

For malignant tumors and those that cannot be fully removed, and where the clinical situation does not contraindicate an aggressive approach (see the previous discussion in the section on biopsy), as much of the tumor as is readily accessible should be removed, with care taken not to disturb adjacent brain tissues. Such "debulking" reduces the mass effect, tends to decrease local and diffuse symptoms, often permits a reduction in steroid dose, and may allow the patient to better tolerate the edema that can accompany radiotherapy.[43] Postoperative morbidity is no greater in those undergoing large resections than in those having small resections or biopsies,[44] and large removals, in patients with malignant gliomas, have been shown in some studies to improve survival.[45–47] On the other hand, in the treatment of malignant gliomas many neuro-oncologists feel that resection offers no survival advantage over biopsy, particularly stereotactic serial biopsy.[48] An attempt to study this important question from an evidence-based review of the literature found no qualifying studies.[49]

Primary CNS lymphoma patients should be biopsied for accurate diagnosis. If possible the patient should not be on steroids.

In patients with brain metastasis proven by MRI to be solitary and whose primary cancer is controlled, surgical removal followed by radiation has been shown to increase duration of life (40 vs. 15 weeks) and to greatly prolong the period of functionally independent survival (38 vs. 8 weeks) compared to biopsy plus radiation.[50] Unfortunately, the applicability of this study to older adults is unclear, because the median age of the patients was 60 years and none was over 74. As with gliomas, age is a negative prognostic factor for patients with brain metastases. Of note is that, in this study of 54 patients with known systemic cancer and brain lesions diagnosed by CT or MRI to be consistent with brain metastasis, six patients proved to have lesions that were *not* metastatic. Two were abscesses and one was a nonspecific inflammatory reaction[50]—a compelling argument for tissue confirmation of diagnosis before treatment.

Low-grade gliomas are uncommon in this population and require treatment only when they become symptomatic. This involves maximal feasible resection followed by local radiotherapy.

Adrenal corticosteroids and supportive medications

Malignant glial tumors, metastatic tumors, and some meningiomas are surrounded by edema, which increases the mass effect, accentuates focal deficits, and produces diffuse signs (headache, and mental and gait abnormalities). This "vasogenic" edema is caused by breakdown of blood–brain barrier secondary to abnormal fenestration of vascular endothelium in the tumor, allowing leakage of water and solutes into and around the tumor.[51] Glucocorticosteroids are effective in reversing this leakiness[52] and have been used as palliative and adjunctive therapy since the 1970s. Significant symptomatic improvement occurs within 24 to 48 hours in the majority of patients and may be dramatic. Elderly patients respond as well as the young.[53]

Primary CNS lymphoma may disappear when treated with steroids alone, but it almost invariably recurs. Best results are obtained with chemotherapy followed by whole-brain radiation.[7,31,34]

Dexamethasone is the standard preparation because of its potency, its relatively minimal mineralocorticoid effect, and because it may cause less psychiatric disturbance than other preparations. It has a prolonged biologic half-life that makes it suitable for twice-a-day dosing, and when given with meals, proton pump inhibitors are needed only for patients with a history of peptic ulcer disease. The usual dose is 16 mg a day, with greater doses given if there is not a satisfactory response. One study, however, found that 4 mg a day was as effective as 16 mg (in patients without impending herniation), with significant reduction in toxicity.[55]

The toxicity of glucocorticoids can be quite important, particularly when they are taken for prolonged periods.[56] The most serious relate to immunosuppressive and antipyretic effects, which predispose to infection while masking some of its signs. Weight gain and the development of Cushingoid habitus and facies adversely affect quality of life. Sleep disturbance and emotional lability may occur, the latter to the point of frank psychosis. Hyperglycemia, hypertension, increased gastric acid secretion, and osteoporosis can all lead to major complications. Steroid myopathy, manifesting with proximal muscle weakness, may be quite disabling.[57] The incidence of these toxicities increases with dose and duration of therapy, so that corticosteroids should be used at the lowest effective dose—and tapered, if possible, once definitive therapy has been implemented.

Radiation therapy

Radiotherapy is an important treatment modality in the management of CNS tumors, helping to control tumor growth and improve survival. For elderly patients with malignant gliomas, if no treatment is given after biopsy or resection, median survivals of 1 to 2 months have been reported, whereas radiotherapy administered postoperatively improved median survival to 5 to 10 months.[58–61] These results have been confirmed in a recent randomized trial, where 84 patients with malignant gliomas over the age of 70 years, with a Karnofsky Performance Status (KPS) of >70, were randomized to best supportive care (BSC) after biopsy or surgical resection, versus 50 Gy of radiation for 5 weeks.[62] No chemotherapy was given. Median survival improved from 4 months in the BSC group to 7 months in those receiving radiation. Quality of life and cognitive function declined similarly in both arms over time, indicating radiotherapy did not have an adverse effect on patients. Unfortunately, none of the scales showed improvement in the treatment group relative to BSC.

Appropriate patient selection for treatment is necessary, as there are many factors to consider when treating the elderly.[58] After age, functional status is one of the most important prognostic factors for survival in malignant gliomas. Those patients with a low functional status have poor tolerance for radiation and limited survival of to 1 to 2 months, making supportive care most appropriate.[59,60,63] Few patients experience improvement in neurologic function, as shown in one series where only 20% of elderly patients experienced improved neurologic function after treatment, 13% worsened, and 67% had no change.[59] This has important implications for home support and social functioning. Radiotherapy-induced cognitive decline and fatigue are major problems for the elderly, and some will experience continued global functional decline without signs of tumor progression. Traveling daily for treatment is not manageable for some due to lack of supports and financial issues, not to mention the associated psychological drain and physical fatigue.[64]

Recognizing the limited gains in median survival of 3 months,[62] and the toxicity and inconvenience of daily clinic visits, altered fractionation schemes using higher dose per fraction over shorter time intervals (3 weeks) have shown survival benefits similar to that achieved with longer courses of radiation.[65,66] There is currently no consensus regarding the optimal radiation dose in those older than 70 years, but ongoing studies should help.

"Involved-field" radiation has replaced whole-brain radiation for malignant gliomas. Primary CNS lymphoma is highly sensitive to radiation and is generally treated, as noted earlier, with whole-brain radiation,[13] often preceded by chemotherapy.[31,54]

The remaining CNS tumors that occur in the elderly tend to be infrequent. Radiotherapy is often considered in cases where there has been incomplete surgical excision of the tumor to improve local control, or it can be the primary modality when surgery is not feasible. Discussion of specialized radiotherapy techniques, such as brachytherapy or stereotactic radiotherapy, is beyond the scope of this chapter. These techniques allow a focused beam of radiation to be given, limiting toxicity to surrounding structures, and are used for such things as acoustic neuroma or meningiomas.[4]

Chemotherapy

The role of chemotherapy in the treatment of brain tumors in the elderly is confined mainly to malignant gliomas and primary CNS lymphomas. The usefulness of chemotherapy for benign tumors is limited, as it is in younger adults, where surgery and radiation are the main treatment modalities.

A meta-analysis from 2002, using individual patient data from 12 randomized trials, showed that chemotherapy administered after surgery and radiation (adjuvant therapy) in adults with high-grade gliomas improved median survival by 2 months, with a 1-year survival experienced by 6%.[67] All age groups benefited, including those older than 60 years of age. What is not apparent is how many patients were older than 65. The drugs used in these trials included alkylators such as carmustine or lomustine, which are not easy to administer to older patients as they cause significant neutropenia and thrombocytopenia, even when dose is reduced.[68] There is some evidence that older patients may not respond as well to these alkylators, and the survival benefit in the elderly using these drugs in the adjuvant setting has been questioned.[69]

Fortunately, a newer alkylator, temozolomide, has been developed, showing an improved toxicity profile, with better tolerance, ushering in improvements in the care of patients with glioblastoma multiforme (GBM). A landmark trial from 2005 changed the standard of care for GBM worldwide.[70] This study, which included patients up to the age of 70, compared 6 weeks of radiotherapy (RT) given with daily oral temozolomide (TMZ) chemotherapy, followed by 6 months of adjuvant TMZ versus the same radiotherapy given alone. Treatment was well tolerated in both arms, with combination therapy proving superior, achieving median and 2-year survivals of 14.6 months and 26% versus 12.1 months and 10% in the RT-alone arm. Quality of life was similar between arms.[71] The degree of survival benefit from combined treatment was less in those older than 50 years of age. Patients older than 70 were not included in this trial, so the benefit of adding chemotherapy to radiation in this group is not known. There is evidence, however, from single institutions, showing that RT and TMZ can be given together in patients 65 to 76 years of age with reasonable tolerability, achieving median survivals of 11 to 12 months.[72,73] Degree of surgical resection and performance status (not age) were the most important factors influencing outcome in these series.

Temozolome alone postoperatively has been tried in patients 70 to 80 years of age, achieving median survivals of 5 to 6 months.[74,75] It is unlikely there will be one treatment approach that fits all patients. High functioning older adults with a complete surgical resection might do well and achieve improved survival with more aggressive treatment regimens.[12] The frailer and less fit may be served best with shorter radiation treatments or chemotherapy only. Molecular factors may prove useful in deciding on appropriate therapy, helping determine tumor sensitivity to specific treatments.[76] Future studies should help clarify some of these issues. There are a host of newer drugs specifically designed to attack particular molecular targets that are currently being tested in trials; the hope is that these trials will lead to further improvements in outcome.[77] With recurrent tumors there is currently no accepted standard treatment.

In contrast, chemotherapy does seem to prolong survival in those with primary CNS lymphoma (PCNSL),[54,78,79] although again the prognosis is significantly worse in the elderly population.[80] Attempts to treat PCNSL with chemotherapy alone (methotrexate) have shown some initial success.[79] Avoidance of whole-brain irradiation in elderly people is an important goal.[80]

CONCLUSION

Although the manifestations of a brain tumor in an elderly person can be subtle and nonspecific, careful attention to the neurologic evaluation and appropriate use of brain imaging studies should minimize any delay in diagnosis. It is important to recognize that, ominous as the diagnosis may seem, the majority of primary brain tumors in this population are benign, eminently treatable, and usually curable. Even in the case of malignant tumors, advances in neurosurgical technique, radiation oncology, and chemotherapy have greatly improved the outlook for many elderly patients, in terms of both prolongation of life and enhanced quality of survival. Numerous experimental approaches are currently under investigation, and although a therapeutic breakthrough does not appear imminent, it is to be hoped that in the not-too-distant future more effective treatments for malignant neoplasms of the brain will be found.

KEY POINTS
Intracranial Tumors

- The incidence of all types of brain tumor increases significantly with age.
- Clinical diagnosis in older adults may be more difficult, and a high index of suspicion is appropriate. Although insidious progression of neurologic deficits remains the most common presentation, acute onset-mimicking stroke can occur, together with such "geriatric giant" presentations as delirium, impaired mobility, and falls. Morning headache, projectile vomiting, and papilledema often are less common.
- Neurologic evaluation and MRI scan will nearly always lead to the correct diagnosis.
- Tissue diagnosis is desirable for treatment planning but, depending on clinical context, is not always necessary.
- Benign tumors—meningiomas, pituitary adenomas, and acoustic neuromas—are common in the elderly population, usually have a very good prognosis, and are often surgically curable.
- For malignant growths, surgery may have an important palliative role, but glucocorticoid and radiation therapies are the mainstays. Chemotherapy shows promise as new drugs are developed.

For a complete list of references, please visit online only at www.expertconsult.com

CHAPTER 67

Disorders of the Spinal Cord and Nerve Roots

Sean D. Christie
Richard A. Cowie

The majority of the pathologic processes affecting the spinal cord in elderly people are related to degenerative diseases of the spinal column or to insufficiency of the cord's blood supply. However, old age does not exclude many of the disorders that are more commonly seen in other age groups. In most patients, a definite diagnosis can be made clinically by taking a directed history and performing a careful examination.

Neurologic assessment of an elderly person is sometimes made difficult by failure to obtain a clear history or by the presence of osteoarthritis of the limb joints and consecutive atrophy of the musculature, which masks weakness and reflex changes. Nonetheless, analysis of the way that a neurologic disorder develops and of the pattern of neurologic signs should provide a guide to the location of the lesion along the neural axis. A lesion can usually be localized in the cervical, thoracic, lumbar, or sacral segments before specialized neuroradiologic investigations.

CERVICAL RADICULOPATHY AND MYELOPATHY

General issues

The neuroradiologic sequelae of degenerative disease of the cervical spine were established in the 1950s.[1] The degenerative changes of cervical spondylosis begin with desiccation and fragmentation of the intervertebral disks. As the elasticity of the annulus is reduced, the disk height diminishes. Extremes of movement are less well tolerated, and the vertebral end plates are subjected to greater stress. Secondary osteophytic spurs develop circumferentially around the disk, projecting posteriorly into the spinal canal as bony ridges. Parallel degeneration of the hypophyseal joints combines with spurs from the vertebral bodies to reduce the size of the neural foraminae. In most patients there is progressive loss of movement between vertebrae, although in some cases excessive motion between vertebrae and a degree of subluxation may develop. Pathologic changes in the ligamentum flavum cause lack of elasticity and a tendency to buckle, particularly during extension. The compressive effects of the osteophytic spurs and buckled ligamentum flavum on the spinal cord are greatest when the neck is extended.[2]

These changes bring about restriction of the natural motion of the spinal cord and nerve roots within the spinal canal. Repetitive compression and obstruction of the radicular arteries supplying the cord in the neural foramina may further compromise cord function. This effect is aggravated if there is occlusive vascular disease of the proximal arteries in the neck. Occasionally, acute rupture of a cervical disk can follow sudden twisting or flexion/extension movements of the neck and cause cord or nerve root compression.[3] The same mechanism can also cause hemorrhage into the spinal cord (hematomyelia).

The older the population, the more these degenerative changes increase in severity and extent. It is clear from epidemiologic studies[4,5] that the prevalence of degenerative changes is increased when heavy laboring work has been undertaken.

Atomic and radiologic studies have shown that the neurologic sequelae of cervical spondylosis are more prevalent when the natural size of the spinal canal and neural foramina are restricted.[6] However, the presence of large osteophytic ridges and subluxation of the vertebrae aggravate the situation. The C5–C6 and C6–C7 levels are most commonly affected at the point of transition from the more mobile cervical spine to the relatively fixed section in the upper part of the thoracic spine.[5,7]

Clinically, there is generally loss of lordosis so that the head is held flexed and downward. However, if the natural kyphosis of the thoracic spine is exaggerated, there may be a compensatory extension of the upper cervical spine to maintain forward gaze. Most patients complain of recurrent neck pain and stiffness, together with crepitus on movement. Pain radiates to the occiput, shoulders, and scapula regions.

Radiculopathy

Progressive narrowing of the neural foramina results from osteophytic ridges alongside the intervertebral disks and hypertrophy of the facet joints and causes compression and restriction of movement of the nerve root. Pain radiates down the arm in the distribution of the nerve root(s) with a deep, boring quality, aggravated by activities such as lifting and reaching. The pain is generally accompanied by paresthesiae and some sensory loss in the affected dermatomes. In some patients, sensory symptoms predominate. Muscular weakness is generally mild, but occasionally wasting can occur. The appropriate reflexes are lost.[7]

Cervical myelopathy

Cervical spondylosis is the most frequent cause of chronic cord compression in older adults. The clinical spectrum is wide, depending on many interrelating factors and the pathogenesis of cord damage. Compression leads to atrophy of the anterior horn cells and the lateral and posterior funiculi of the cord.[8] Most commonly the onset of symptoms and signs is insidious, and a clinical history can extend for many months or years before help is sought. Most frequently there is a mixed picture of lower motor neuron features in the arms, together with long tract signs below.[9]

In the upper limbs, complaints of numb, clumsy hands with weakness and loss of dexterity are common. Muscle wasting follows segmental anterior horn cell damage, affecting proximal muscles when compression is high in the neck or the intrinsic muscles of the hand when compression is lower. The tendon reflexes in the arms are usually lost at the segmental level of the cord lesion and are exaggerated below. An inverted radial reflex occurs when the site of compression is above the fifth cervical segment, which has been shown to be the most common in an elderly population.[10]

In contrast, there is commonly a marked lower limb spasticity when the patient complains of a heavy, leaden weakness and a tendency to drag the limb. Some degree of ataxia may be present with reduction of vibration and joint position sense. Many patients complain of paresthesiae and intermittent numbness in the upper and lower limbs.

Occasionally, symptoms may arise abruptly because of severe trauma or sudden extension of the neck such as after a fall. In this situation, a central cord syndrome is common, with marked weakness of the upper limbs because of anterior horn cell damage and a mild spastic weakness of the lower limbs as the peripheral regions of the cord are relatively spared. Frequently this syndrome is accompanied by allodynia in the upper extremities, particularly the hands. Very rarely a Brown–Séquard syndrome can be identified. These neurologic disorders can be associated with vertebrobasilar insufficiency, where symptoms are typically related to rotation and extension of the neck. As the clinical presentation of spondylotic myelopathy varies, it must be distinguished from other conditions with similar symptoms and signs, including multiple sclerosis, cerebrovascular disease, cord tumor or syrinx, normal pressure hydrocephalus, amyotrophic lateral sclerosis, and peripheral neuropathies.

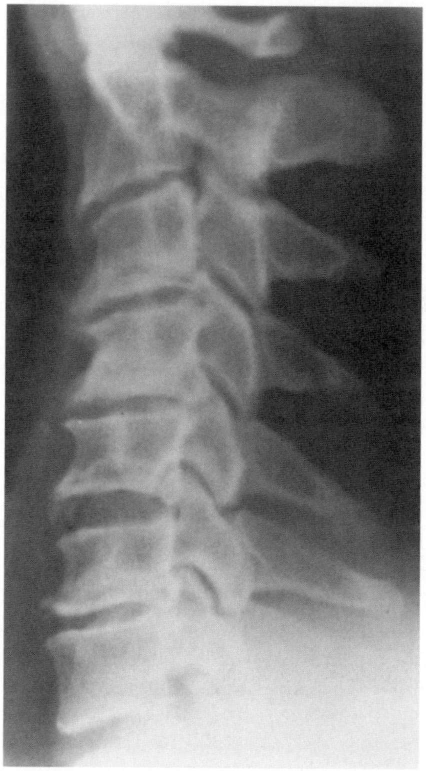

Figure 67-1. Lateral cervical spine radiograph showing widespread spondylosis. Note the loss of disk height and large anterior osteophytes. This patient has a small spinal canal into which project osteophytes at the posterior margin of the C3–C4 of the 4–5 disks.

Investigations

Plain radiographs of the cervical spine reveal narrowing of the intervertebral disk space with sclerosis of adjacent cortical bone. Secondary anterior and posterior osteophytes are demonstrated in Figure 67-1, together with an indication of the size of the spinal canal. Oblique radiographs allow visualization of the neural foramina. However, several authors[11–13] have shown that degenerative changes increase in frequency with age, and that 70% to 90% of those over 65 years of age have radiologic abnormalities. In consequence, there is poor correlation between symptomatic and asymptomatic groups and the structural changes revealed on plain radiographs, with problems of both sensitivity and, especially, of specificity. Rarely, then, do plain radiographs alone dictate therapy.

When the clinical state suggests segmental cord or root compression and surgery is contemplated, then specialized neuroradiologic investigation is required. Magnetic resonance imaging (MRI)—which has largely replaced myelography—reveals degeneration of intervertebral disks, the size of osteophytes, and the presence and degree of cord compression (Figure 67-2). Computed tomography (CT)[14,15] reveals the size and shape of the vertebral canals and the presence of extensive ligamentous calcification, but it cannot give details of vertebral displacements, disk protrusions, and corrugation of the bulging longitudinal ligament unless intrathecal

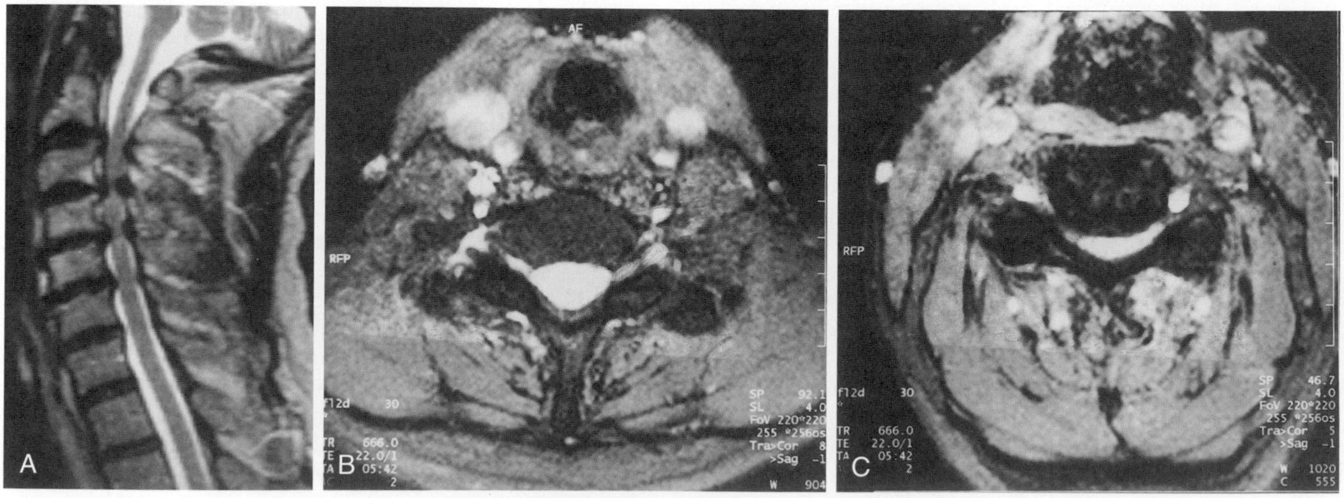

Figure 67-2. A, Lateral magnetic resonance image of the cervical spine showing compression of the spinal cord by posterior osteophytes and buckling of the ligamentum flavum. B, Transverse image of normal cervical spine reveals spinal cord surrounded by cerebrospinal fluid. C, Transverse image of the patient seen in (A) showing severe narrowing of the spinal canal and compression of the cord.

contrast medium has been injected. Myelography is now performed only when MRI is contraindicated, such as in a patient with an implanted pacemaker or neuromodulatory device or in the presence of cerebral aneurysm clips made from materials other than titanium or titanium alloy.[16] Magnetic resonance imaging also allows visualization of intrinsic disorders of the spinal cord (see Figure 67-2).

Management

Patients with neck pain and radiculopathy generally respond to a treatment regimen that may include a supportive collar, restriction of upper limb and shoulder movement, and nonsteroidal antiinflammatory drugs, supplemented by opioid analgesics if necessary.[17] Physical methods of treatment and the application of local heat pads may be soothing. If the symptoms are severe, a brief period of bed rest and cervical traction may provide some relief.[18] Lees and Turner[19] showed that 22 of 51 patients were symptom-free within a few months and generally remained symptom-free during follow-up. These authors showed that patients with radiculopathy rarely progress to a myelopathic state.

Surgery is not generally required unless there is clinical evidence of myelopathy, such as progressive sensorimotor deficits or abnormalities in bladder and bowel control attributable to spinal cord dysfunction. In selected patients, persistent radicular pain that inhibits daily activities and decreases level of function may also be a relative indication. Both anterior and posterior approaches can be used to decompress the nerve roots; each carries a good prognosis for neurologic recovery,[20–22] although recovery of muscle wasting is rarely satisfactory. The decision to operate is made after taking into account the severity of the disability, its effect on the patient's quality of life, and the patient's ability to withstand surgery.

The natural history of myelopathy complicating cervical spondylosis is variable and unpredictable; many patients run a chronic course characterized by episodes of deterioration separated by periods of stability.[9,19] The majority of elderly patients with cervical myelopathy will not need surgical intervention. Surgical treatment is indicated when the myelopathy interferes with daily activities, where there is a short progressive history, or when there is radiologic evidence of severe cord compression or instability. Anterior decompression of disk and osteophytic spurs is usually carried out when one or two intervertebral levels are affected, whereas laminectomy/laminoplasty is indicated for more widespread stenosis and compression of the spinal cord. In general, the prime objective of surgery has been to halt the decline in neurologic function before further damage to the cord has occurred. However, more recently studies suggest that there may be a more reliable improvement in neurologic function than previously appreciated.[23]

There is poor correlation between the presenting severity, the duration of the symptoms, and the outcome.[6] Hukaka et al[24] found that posterior decompression gave better results for more advanced myelopathy and that a short duration of symptoms was associated with better results, although these were not influenced by the age of the patient. Phillips[25] suggested that patients with focal disease who underwent anterior surgery had a better outcome. However, some patients continued to deteriorate, in spite of adequate decompression, possibly because of vascular insufficiency.[9] This may be related to persistent motion across the decompressed segments, and concomitant fusion procedures may reduce the incidence of postoperative neurologic decline.

CORD COMPRESSION IN RHEUMATOID ARTHRITIS

Neck pain and stiffness are common complaints in patients with progressive rheumatoid arthritis (RA). Radiation of pain to the occipital region and cutaneous numbness at the back of the head may occur when the upper cervical nerve roots are compressed. These symptoms may herald the development of atlantoaxial subluxation as a result of destruction of the transverse atlantal ligament by synovitis. There may be rotatory subluxation, and vertical migration of the odontoid into the foramen magnum of the skull (cranial settling). Atlantoaxial subluxation, which occurs in approximately 33% of patients with RA, can be asymptomatic until the slip reaches 8 to 9 mm when cord compression begins. Once myelopathy develops, most patients deteriorate and 50% die within 6 months. Approximately 20% of patients show subaxial subluxation on cervical radiography, often affecting several segments to produce "staircase" deformity of the vertebrae. Compression of the cord is common.

Most patients present with progressive deterioration of upper limb function, accompanied by tingling, numbness, LHermitte's phenomenon, gait disturbance, and possibly bladder and bowel dysfunction. It is common for these symptoms to be attributed to severe peripheral joint disease and muscle atrophy. Abnormality of spinothalamic function, hyperreflexia and hypertonia, and extensor plantar responses help differentiate the cause from peripheral nerve lesions. Compression of the trigeminal nucleus and tract at the craniocervical junction may produce facial numbness or paresthesiae. Lower cranial nerve findings may be present with cranial settling.

Radiologic assessment requires flexion and extension radiographs of the cervical spine followed by MRI, which will reveal compression or distortion of the spinal cord (Figure 67-3).

Surgical management has to be considered when there is progressive or significant atlantoaxial subluxation, or clinical evidence of increasing neurologic morbidity. As most patients have significant medical problems such as pulmonary fibrosis, anemia, atrophic skin, and the effects of prolonged steroid or other immunosuppressive therapies, there is significant risk from surgical intervention that needs to be reviewed with patients and their families. For some patients, particularly the frail, the use of a cervical collar in lieu of surgery may be the best option to manage craniocervical instability, though tolerance of use can be limited.

The surgical approach and procedure may consist of an anterior, transoral, or posterior decompression combined with internal fixation; however, the timing of these inteventions remains controversial.[26]

SPINAL CORD COMPRESSION AND THORACIC DISK PROTRUSION

The central protrusion of a thoracic intervertebral disk is an unusual cause of cord compression, but one that occurs in older age groups as it is associated with degeneration of the

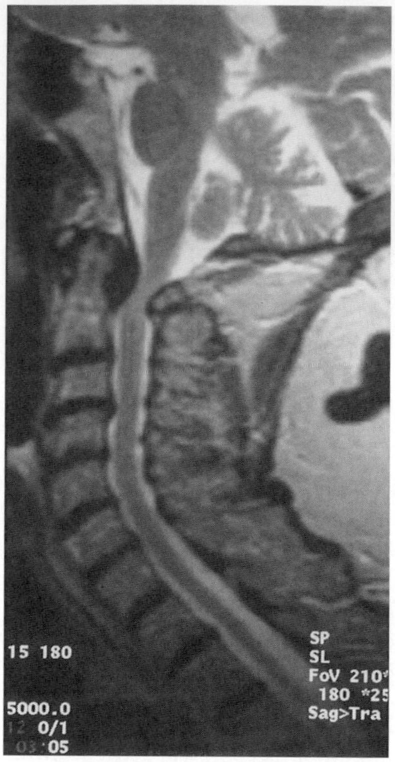

Figure 67-3. Magnetic resonance image of cervical spine, illustrating pathology attributable to rheumatoid arthritis; cranial settling, cevical stenosis, and subaxial instability.

disk annulus. Russell[27] noted that 67% occurred between the eighth and eleventh interspaces. The majority of patients present with a long history of gradually progressive myelopathy where sensory and motor symptoms are equally common. However, 49% of patients complained of radicular symptoms of pain and dysesthesiae. Sometimes the onset is more rapid, leading to a flaccid paraplegia.[28]

The presence of a thoracic disk protrusion is generally recognized when MRI is carried out to investigate the progressive neurologic deficit. Cord compression from this source carries a poor prognosis unless surgery is performed. The results of simple decompressive laminectomy are unsatisfactory; either costotransversectomy, transpedicular, or transthoracic approach is recommended.[27,29] Recent minimal access approaches[30] are better tolerated and may lead to quicker postoperative recovery, particularly in an elderly population.

CORD COMPRESSION FROM INTRADURAL TUMORS

Intradural extramedullary tumors cause local compression of the spinal cord and nerve roots. Meningiomas represent approximately 25% of primary spinal cord tumors, and 80% of them occur in females. They are most commonly seen in the sixth decade, rather later than for neurofibromas; 80% occur in the thoracic spine. The majority of patients complain of local or radicular pain, the significance of which often goes unrecognized for a long period until progressive spastic paraparesis, followed by sensory and bladder dysfunction, develops.[31]

Plain radiographs are rarely helpful, and the condition is diagnosed only by myelography or more commonly MRI.[32] Results of decompressive surgery are generally good. Levy et al[33] reported that one third of paraplegic patients were able to walk after tumor excision. Similar successes have been observed in septagenarians.[34] Neurofibromas are slightly more common than meningiomas, but their peak incidence is in younger age groups, so they are less frequently encountered in an elderly patient.[35] Radicular pain is more common, and enlargement of a neural foramen may be seen on plain radiographs if the tumor extends into the paravertebral tissues. Multiple tumors can be encountered in neurofibromatosis. As with meningiomas, surgical excision should be undertaken and carries a good prognosis for neurologic recovery. However, for the medically unfit radiosurgery is an emerging option that appears to afford long-term clinical stability.[36]

METASTATIC SPINAL TUMORS

The most common extradural and spinal tumors to cause cord compression are those metastasizing from distant carcinomas or primary hematologic tumors. Spread may be hematogenous or via the vertebral venous plexus. Although myeloma and carcinomas of prostate and kidney seem to metastasize preferentially to the spine, in practice the most commonly encountered tumors are those that occur with the greatest frequency in the community. Therefore, primary lung, breast, kidney, and prostate tumors are seen, although in some patients the primary tumor cannot be identified. The thoracic region of the spine is most frequently involved, followed by the lumbosacral and cervical regions.

The majority of patients present with progressive walking difficulty, because of weakness and clumsiness, the significance of which may go unrecognized until the patient is no longer able to bear weight. Many patients have a history of preceding spinal pain, which should always lead to a suspicion of vertebral metastasis in a patient known to have malignant disease. The neurologic deficit may develop very rapidly, with collapse of the vertebra or occlusion of the vascular supply to the cord. An analysis of the level of the sensory deficit helps in assessing the site of the spinal disease and planning the appropriate radiologic investigations. However, plain radiographs of all of the spine and chest should be carried out and may reveal loss of outline of a pedicle, reduction in height of a vertebral body, or a soft tissue mass. MRI of the spine is the investigation of choice. However, CT may reveal evidence of bone destruction and allow percutaneous needle biopsy of the lesion.

There has been considerable debate about the value of decompressive surgery, as laminectomy alone has produced suboptimal results.[37] As a result there has been considerable experience with alternate conservative therapies. Commonly steroids, dexamethasone, are pre-scribed for both their effect on vasogenic edema and to improve tumor-related pain.[38,39] In the 1970s and 1980s, radiotherapy became the mainstay of treatment, and surgical intervention was primarily used as a salvage therapy if patients deteriorated during radiation. In some centers, radiation remains the initial treatment.[39] However, recently there has been a resurgence in surgical interest for these patients. This has been motivated by a randomized controlled trial by Patchell et al.[40] This trial compared radiation alone to surgery (circumferential decompression and stabilization) and radiation. The authors showed that the surgical group had improved bladder control and ambulation status compared to the radiation-alone group, and there was no change in survival. Improvements in ambulation and continence are now felt to be appropriate benefits to offset the risks of surgery in these palliative patients and have been reported by other groups.[41] However, surgery is not indicated for all patients with metastatic epidural compression. Patients with desseminated disease and an expected survival less than 4 months, those with multiple lesions at multiple levels, those medically unfit for surgery, or those with very radiosensitive tumors (lymphoma, myeloma) may not dervive the benefits from surgery.

VASCULAR DISORDERS OF THE SPINAL CORD

The peculiar anatomic arrangement of the arterial blood supply of the spinal cord may protect it from the effects of occlusion of one feeding vessel. The anterior and posterior spinal arteries are fed by radicular arteries, which are branches of vessels arising from either the aorta or the subclavian arteries. There is generally a large feeding artery in the lower thoracic region, most commonly on the left at T10. A watershed lies at the second thoracic segment of the spinal cord, between areas supplied by thoracic vessels and those from the neck. Interruption of supply can occur in atheroma of the aorta,[42] in dissecting aneurysm,[43] or as a complication of aortic open and endovascular surgery.[44] The extent and severity of the spinal cord neurologic deficit varies considerably, probably depending on the anatomic variation of the spinal cord vessels in the individual patient.

The syndrome of the anterior spinal artery arises when this vessel is obstructed by thrombus. The onset is sudden with pain in the back or neck and paresthesias down the arms. The posterior columns receiving a blood supply from the posterior spinal network are preserved, so that proprioception remains intact, whereas thermal and pain appreciation are impaired. In addition, a lower motor paralysis of the arms is associated with spastic paraparesis, or paraplegia. In some cases, the presence of cervical spondylosis and an osteophytic ridge has been implicated in local occlusion of the anterior spinal artery.[45] This phenomenon is also recognized in the setting of thrombophlebitis secondary to epidural abscess.[46]

SPINAL CORD INJURY

Acute spinal cord injury (SCI) is a severe and devastating event for both patients and their families, regardless of age. However, there has been a perception that older adults fare considerably worse than their younger counterparts. A number of authors have observed an increasing proportion of older patients presenting with acute SCI, with falls (often from standing heights) as the leading mechanism of injury in contrast to motor vehicle collisions, which are more common in younger age groups.[47–51] The reasons for these observations are likely multifactorial and include an aging population, alteration in bony structural support secondary to osteopenia/osteoporosis, cervical spondylosis (leading to undiagnosed myelopathic symptoms and predisposing to central cord syndrome), a more fragile ambulation status (because of altered sensory mechanisms), osteoarthritis/decreased mobility, neurologic disorders such as Parkinson's disease or diabetic peripheral neuropathy and the effects of polypharma.[50]

Several authors have endeavored to reassess the outcomes of SCI in the geriatric setting to evaluate whether current treatment modalities have altered clinical outcomes. Furlan and coworkers[51] found, in a retrospective review of a prospective cohort, that patients with SCI 65 years of age and older had a significantly higher mortality rate than younger patients (46.88% vs. 4.86%; $p < 0.001$). However, they also reported that, among survivors, age had no impact on motor or sensory outcomes. This suggests that a significant number of patients (the survivors) could benefit from aggressive treatment and with a better understanding of predictors of outcome, preferably those modifiable, the expected survivors could be identified and treated. Fassett el al[49] conducted a retrospective review 412 patients over the age of 70 years treated between 1978 and 2005. They observed an increase in the incidence from 4.2% to 15.4%, and the elderly cohort as a whole tended to have less severe injuries based on the American Spinal Injury Association (ASIA) grading scale. However, the mortality rate in the elderly patients with severe neurologic impairment was uniformly higher, high enough to yield a statistical difference in mortality between the age groups. Unfortunately their data did not contain information of preinjury medical conditions. Krassioukov and colleagues[47] in a previous study examined the effect that preexisting conditions had on outcomes. In their cohort the ASIA grade was similar between the young and elderly; however, the number of preexisting medical conditions was statistically greater in the geriatric group which correlated to the difference in secondary complications observed between the two groups. When this observation was taken into account there was no statistical difference in complications or mortality reported attributable solely to age. It needs to be borne in mind that this study had relatively small cohorts (28 geriatric, 30 younger) and the conclusions may differ with more statistical power. Despite this the authors advocate for an aggressive multidisciplinary approach to SCI in the elderly and caution against allowing "agism" to bias treatment.

PAGET'S DISEASE

Paget's disease is a generally progressive disorder of bone that causes neurologic sequelae of the brain, spinal cord, or peripheral nerves, depending on which bones are involved. It is important to recognize these complications, as many respond to treatment of the underlying disorder. In the spine, pagetic changes may affect one or several vertebrae. The disease is characterized by bony destruction followed by repair, which leads to flattening and expansion of the diameter of the vertebral bodies, and thickening of the pedicles and laminae. Bony projections in the vertebral canal cause spinal cord and nerve root compression. Neurologic symptoms may develop suddenly if collapse of a vertebral body occurs.

Spinal cord compression is most common in the thoracic region and is generally slowly progressive, causing a spastic weakness of the lower limbs combined with sensory symptoms and signs. Pain may be due to local bony changes, malignant degeneration, or nerve root compression. In some patients progressive myelopathy occurs, yet imaging fails to reveal direct compression of the spinal cord. In these patients, progressive ischemia may be the cause of neurologic deterioration.

When the disease affects the lumbar region, symptoms of single or multiple nerve root compression can develop, producing back pain and sciatica. When the spinal canal is constricted, neurogenic claudication may be the presenting symptom.

Surgical treatment is indicated only when medical treatment fails to control the progression of the neurologic sequelae of the condition. However, control of blood loss from the diseased bone during surgery can be troublesome.[52,53]

NEUROLOGIC COMPLICATIONS OF DEGENERATIVE DISEASE OF THE LUMBAR SPINE

Spondylosis of the lumbar spine increases in severity and extent with advancing age, often occurring simultaneously with disease in the cervical region.[4,54] Biochemical and pathologic changes are similar at both sites. Loss of disk height and the development of traction spurs and osteophytes are associated with sclerosis and enlargement of the vertebral bodies. Simultaneous changes in the facet joints occur, with destruction of articular cartilage, laxity of the joint capsule, and osteophytic enlargement of the joint surfaces.[55] This process may be asymmetric, so that rotational subluxation of one vertebra on the other can develop. The lowest intervertebral disks of the lumbar spine are most commonly affected, at the point of transition from the mobile lumbar spine to the fixed sacrum.

A number of discrete neurologic conditions may complicate lumbar spondylosis.

Acute nerve root entrapment

True herniation of an intervertebral disk can occur in an elderly person and produce a pattern of symptoms and signs similar to that seen in younger patients.[56] However, compared with the average adult population, elderly people have a higher incidence of motor deficits and are more likely to have a sequestrated disk nucleus. Acute root entrapment may also result from compression secondary to rapid expansion of a degenerative spinal cyst.[57]

Chronic nerve root entrapment

Lumbar mono- and polyradiculopathy occur in elderly people, more commonly as a result of nerve root compression in the lateral recess of the spinal canal and in the neural foramen than from disk rupture. As degeneration of the intervertebral disk advances, there is loss of disk height and formation of osteophytes that bulge into the neural foramen; hypertrophy of the facet joint further compromises its capacity. At the same time, partial subluxation of the posterior joint with upward and forward movement of the superior articular surface narrows the lateral recess of the spinal canal.[58] At first extension and rotation of the spine aggravate the process, so that dynamic stenosis (Figure 67-4) may produce intermittent compression and symptoms, although, as the condition advances, permanent compression occurs.

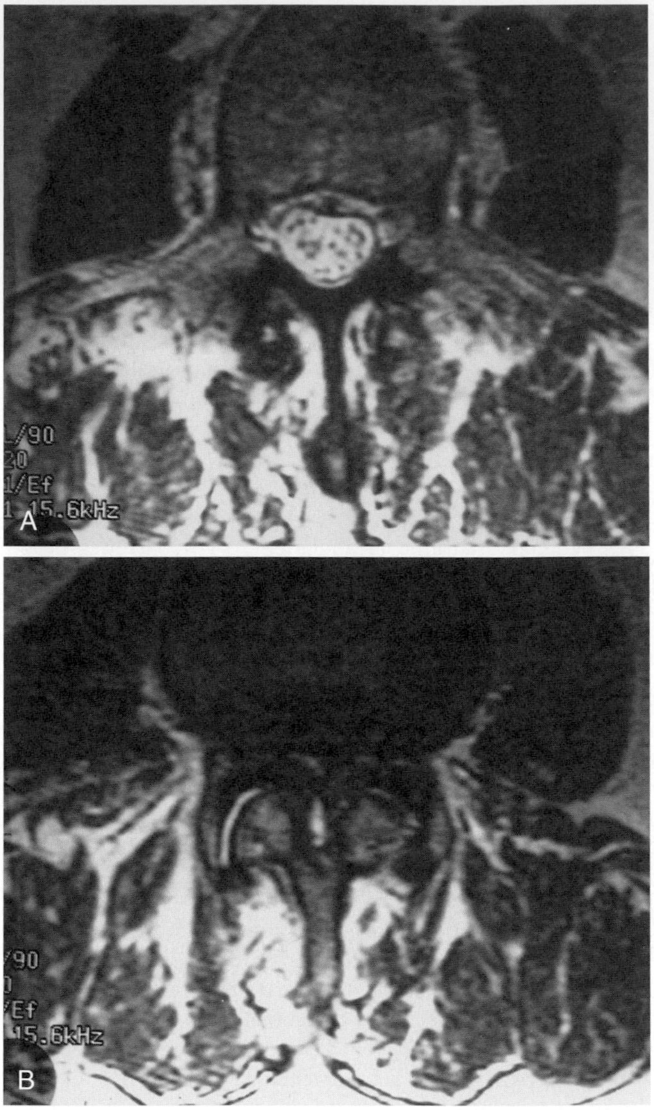

Figure 67-4. Magnetic resonance images of (A) normal lumbar spine and (B) severe spinal canal stenosis.

Typically, patients complain of pain and stiffness of the back, accompanied by the insidious onset of sciatic pain. These symptoms are generally aggravated by standing or walking and relieved by rest or lying, particularly when the spine is flexed. Patients complain of paresthesias in the legs, which are also precipitated by the same types of activity. In chronic nerve root entrapment caused by stenosis, coughing and straining aggravate the pain, and nerve root stretch tests are generally negative. Some patients show mild weakness of the legs, although objective sensory deficits are rare. The progression of symptoms and signs is generally much slower than for a herniated nucleus pulposus.[59–61]

Nerve root entrapment may complicate degenerative spondylolisthesis. This develops when degeneration of the facet joints and laxity of the disk annulus allow the upper vertebral body to slide forward on the lower. The L4–L5 intervertebral joint is most commonly affected, but other intervertebral levels can be involved and produce sciatic pain and symptoms of nerve root compression.

Neurogenic claudication

Narrowing of the central spinal canal can develop as a result of a combination of degenerative hypertrophy of the facet joints, hypertrophy and corrugation of the ligamentum flavum, and bulging of the disk and osteophytes. As the available space in the spinal canal narrows, there is compression of multiple nerve roots of the cauda equina and its circulation. The symptoms of claudication develop. Bilateral leg pain is precipitated by walking or standing and improved with rest, especially when the spine is flexed or when the patient sits or squats.[61]

Patients frequently develop a stooped posture. As the distance walked increases, a heavy leaden weakness builds up in intensity, accompanied by burning paresthesias and a fear of the limb giving way.[62] Sometimes neurologic signs are present only after an exercise provocation test on a treadmill.

In older adults, the clinical picture is often confused with the effects of peripheral vascular disease. Sharr et al[63] reported that urinary symptoms due to a neuropathic bladder often complicate central stenosis of the spinal canal.

Investigations

Plain radiographs reveal the extent and severity of degenerative changes of the disks and facet joints. Radiography has been superseded by CT and MRI of the lumbar spine, which reveal the cross-sectional anatomy of the spinal and neural canals and can reveal the degree of degeneration of the disk. However, only MRI can adequately display detail of the neural structures.

Radionuclide scanning is generally not helpful, as increased uptake is common in areas of osteoarthritis, but it can exclude spinal infection or neoplasm.

Management

The majority of elderly patients do not require surgical decompression, and their symptoms can be controlled by analgesic and anti-inflammatory medication and modification of their activities of daily living. Rest and physical treatment, combined with restriction of spinal movement, often produce satisfactory results. However, older adults can withstand surgery well, and age alone is rarely a contraindication to operation. Surgery is indicated when sciatic pain and other symptoms significantly reduce a patient's physical capacity or cannot be controlled by medical treatment. Signs of severe nerve root compression, such as weakness or sensory loss, neurogenic claudication, and cauda equina compression, are firm indications for surgical intervention. The aim of surgery is to decompress the spinal canal and neural foramina, thus freeing the nerve roots. Getty et al[64,65] obtained satisfactory results in 85% of patients after a partial undercutting facetectomy. However, low backache persists after surgery in many patients, owing to the background degenerative changes, and patients must be advised accordingly.[66,67] However, this effect may be in part related to the surgical approach, as persistent back pain is not reported as commonly following minimal access surgery in the elderly.[68] Approaches to the spine using minimal access surgical techniques (MAST) are becoming more commonplace and may have a particular role in the treatment of the older adult. MAST involves utilizing smaller skin incisions and working through small portals or "tubes" via a muscle splitting/sparing approach; in contrast to the traditional "open" surgical approaches, which involve stripping the paraspinal muscles off the spine to gain adequate access. MAST techniques have been shown to minimize surgical trauma and blood loss, reduce postoperative pain, and hasten mobilization/recovery. These advantages may be particularly important when treated a potentially frail population. Rosen et al[68] recently described their experience utilizing a MAST approach for lumbar decompression in a cohort of 50 patients with a mean age of 81 years. They observed no mortality or significant morbidity in their cohort and showed statistical improvement in multiple validated clinical outcome scales with a mean follow-up of 10 months. In addition to MAST, other novel approaches, such as dynamic stabilization, are promising adjuncts to decompressive procedures and are intended to address the issue of concomitant back pain without the need for a surgical arthrodesis.[69,70] However, all of these approaches still require the rigors of future randomized clinical trials to prove their potential merits.

KEY POINTS

Disorders of the Spinal Cord and Nerve Roots

- The majority of pathologies observed in the spines of older adults relate to degenerative processes.
- Spinal cord compression in the elderly population is most frequently caused by cervical spondylosis or metastatic vertebral body tumors.
- Less common causes of cord compression in the elderly population include intraspinal tumor and thoracic disk protrusion.
- The clinical presentation of cervical myelopathy is usually either insidious gait disturbance or numb, clumsy hands.
- In patients with advanced rheumatoid arthritis, subluxation at the craniocervical junction may require surgical treatment by internal decompression and fixation.
- The incidence of spinal cord injury in the elderly is rising, and the causes and sequelae are unique in this population.
- Claudicant leg pain needs to be differentiated between neurogenic and vascular etiologies.
- Given current operating room techniques, age alone should not deter surgical intervention when indicated.

For a complete list of references, please visit online only at www.expertconsult.com

CHAPTER 68

Infections of the Central Nervous System

Steven L. Berk
James W. Myers

Bacterial meningitis is a disease that presents particular challenges in the elderly patient. The mortality rate from bacterial meningitis is higher in elderly people than in younger adults. Bacterial meningitis has become a more common problem in elderly patients over the past 2 decades. In 1973, Fraser et al[1] reported that the mean age of death from meningitis in Olmsted County, Minn., had gone from 11.5 years in the period 1935 to 1946 to 64 years during the period 1959 to 1970. In the latter period more than one half of all deaths from meningitis occurred in those over 60 years of age. The incidence of bacterial meningitis rose from 5 cases per 100,000 to 15 cases per 100,000.[1] A Centers for Disease Control and Prevention survey performed between 1978 and 1981 showed an increasing incidence of meningitis in older patients[2] as did a survey on the incidence of meningitis conducted in Rhode Island.[3] In one review of 445 adults treated for bacterial meningitis at the Massachusetts General Hospital, 56% of community-acquired meningitis occurred in patients over 50 years of age.[4] In this study and all previous studies, the mortality rate was much higher in older patients. The mortality rate in the Massachusetts General Hospital study was 37 in those over 60 years of age compared with 17 in younger adults. In the Rhode Island study, 55% of elderly patients died compared with an overall mortality rate of 10%.[3]

The increased incidence of meningitis in this age group probably is explained, in part, by the more aggressive care given to elderly patients, including more rigorous evaluation of fever, change in mental status, and coma. Nosocomial meningitis particularly related to neurosurgical procedures is also a cause of the increasing incidence of meningitis in this age group. Durand et al[4] have shown that nosocomial meningitis has increased from 28% of all meningitis between 1962 and 1970 to 45% of all cases of meningitis from 1980 to 1988. Many of these cases occur in the chronically ill, frequently hospitalized elderly.

Bacteria may reach the subarachnoid space of the elderly patient by several different mechanisms.[5] Elderly patients with focal infections may develop bacteremia and seed the meninges. This occurs, for example, in the elderly patient with pneumococcal pneumonia, or less frequently in the patient with pyelonephritis and gram-negative meningitis. Meningitis develops by way of direct inoculation of bacteria into the meninges such as occurs in head trauma or after a neurosurgical procedure. Elderly patients are prone to frequent falls and head injuries. *Staphylococcus aureus*, coagulase-negative staphylococci, and gram-negative bacilli are responsible for most cases of meningitis secondary to head trauma or neurosurgery. Meningitis may occur from contiguous spread of infection to the meninges as in patients with otitis media, sinusitis, or mastoiditis. This mechanism of infection is probably somewhat less common in elderly people, compared with younger adults.

In the bacteremic, elderly patient, symptoms of fever, chills, and rigors will usually be present but afebrile bacteremia in elderly people is well described. Patients with contiguous spread of infection usually complain of localized findings, such as ear or facial pain. Bacteria in the subarachnoid space will cause an inflammatory reaction in the pia and arachnoid matter that will manifest itself as neck pain and stiffness with protective reflexes that cause the Kernig and Brudzinski signs. Structures that lie within the subarachnoid space are involved in the inflammatory reaction. Pial arteries and veins may become inflamed and cranial nerve roots damaged.

A diffuse encephalopathy may occur. Abnormal mental status results from cerebral ischemia, edema, or toxic encephalopathy. Confusion, headache, or lethargy is a manifestation of this diffuse, inflammatory process. Papilledema, hydrocephalus, and other focal findings may occur as a result of pus occluding the foramina of Luschka and Magendie, resulting in increased intracranial pressure.

The clinical features of meningitis in elderly patients are more subtle than in younger adults. This is a recurring theme in almost all studies that involve older patients with meningitis.[6,7] Most, but not all, studies have found that elderly patients with bacterial meningitis are less likely to have neck stiffness and meningeal signs. At the same time, older patients often have cervical spine disease and poor neck mobility, making interpretation of clinical signs more difficult. Berman et al[8] found meningismus present in only 58% of elderly patients with meningitis. Gorse et al[9] compared signs and symptoms of patients with meningitis over 50 years of age to those in patients under 50. Older patients had more mental status abnormalities and were more likely to have seizures, neurological deficits, and hydrocephalus. Berk,[6] Roos,[10] Massanari,[11] and others have noted that a delay in diagnosis is frequently associated with meningitis in the elderly and this delay may explain the high mortality rate noted in this group of patients.

Elderly patients with bacterial meningitis may not have as pronounced fever or may at times be afebrile. The change in mental status that occurs in elderly people may be attributed to senility, delirium, psychosis, transient ischemia, or stroke. In the elderly patient who has undergone neurosurgery, postoperative lethargy may be mistakenly attributed to an expected postoperative course. A stiff neck in an elderly patient may not arouse the same concern that it would in a young adult.

Physical examination is a critical part of the evaluation of an elderly patient with suspected meningitis. Nuchal rigidity is reported in between 56% and 92% of elderly patients depending on the series.[7] When neck stiffness is the result of meningeal irritation, the neck will resist flexion but can be rotated from side to side. A funduscopic and cranial nerve examination are mandatory to alert the clinician to associated increased intracranial pressure or brain abscess. Mental status should be carefully described and followed. Lethargy and coma are poor prognostic signs. Examination of the head should include a search for skull fracture, avulsion, or hematoma. Careful otoscopic examination is also a necessity as otitis media may be missed in the elderly patient, particularly when mental status is abnormal and a history cannot be obtained. The elderly patient may have pneumonia and concomitant meningitis. Gorse et al[9] found pneumonia to be much more common in older adults with meningitis. The elderly patient may not complain of respiratory symptoms so examination of the lung may be the first clue to pneumonia. Examination of the heart is necessary to detect underlying valvular heart disease that might predispose the elderly patient to endocarditis with seeding of the meninges. Examination for costovertebral tenderness, decubitus ulcers, and petechial lesions will also provide important information in determining the source and causal agent in meningitis.

Performance of a lumbar puncture without delay is the critical element in the diagnosis of bacterial meningitis in both young and old. About 35% of elderly patients with meningitis have focal neurologic findings.[9] Because lumbar puncture is contraindicated in patients with brain abscess, computed tomography (CT) or magnetic resonance imaging (MRI) will be necessary in some older patients. However, the high mortality rate from meningitis in the elderly makes time of the essence in the diagnosis and treatment of meningitis in this group. Many infectious disease experts now support the strategy of beginning empirical antibiotic therapy, pending lumbar puncture, particularly when a delay of hours is anticipated due to an imaging study.

There is very little in the literature to suggest that the cerebrospinal fluid (CSF) findings in elderly patients with meningitis differ from young adults with meningitis. Lumbar puncture will show purulent fluid with white blood cell counts between about 500 and 10,000 cu/mm. Polymorphonuclear leukocytes predominate, usually making up more than 90% of total cell count. Meningitis caused by *Listeria monocytogenes* sometimes has a mononuclear cell predominance. At least one study has shown that elderly patients with meningitis are more likely to have a lack of cellular response in CSF than younger adults.[12] Those elderly patients with meningitis who have few cells in CSF but many bacteria have a poor prognosis.[13] CSF glucose levels are usually low in bacterial meningitis. CSF to serum glucose ratios are usually less than 50%. Seventy percent of patients with meningitis will have a ratio less than 31%.[14] Spinal fluid protein is elevated above 50 mg/dL. Very high protein levels are associated with poor prognosis. Gram stain of CSF will be positive in 60% to 90% of all patients with meningitis.[14] In the study by Berman et al,[8] only 50% of elderly patients with meningitis had a positive Gram stain. The Gram stain is most likely to be negative in patients who have received prior antibiotic therapy. In those patients whose Gram stain is negative, a variety of methods to detect bacterial antigen are now in common use. These include latex fixation, coagglutination, and counterimmunoelectrophoresis. The limulus lysate assay has been used to detect gram-negative meningitis, an important cause of meningitis in elderly people. Other tests such as lactic acid levels and measurement of C-reactive protein have been recommended to help distinguish bacterial from viral meningitis, but clinical decisions are rarely based on them.

Blood cultures are recommended in all patients in whom bacterial meningitis is suspected. In the study by Berman et al,[8] almost one-half of all elderly patients with meningitis had concomitant bacteremia. In addition, other cultures—such as sputum, urine, and wound—may be extremely helpful in determining the causal agent and source of infection.

Streptococcus pneumoniae is the most common organism to cause meningitis in elderly patients.[5] *S. pneumoniae* was responsible for more than one half of all cases of meningitis in the elderly in several studies.[15–17] The organism caused 43% of all cases in the study of Berman et al[8] and 24% of cases in the study of Gorse et al.[9] Gram-negative bacilli cause meningitis in elderly patients both by bacteremic spread of infection, such as in urinary tract infection or pneumonia, and as a nosocomial infection after neurosurgery.[18,19] *Escherichia coli* is the most common organism to cause meningitis secondary to bacteremic spread. *E. coli* and *Klebsiella pneumoniae* are the more common gram-negative bacilli to cause meningitis after neurosurgery but more unusual organisms, particularly *Acinetobacter*[20–22] have been more commonly reported. In a review of 581 cases of bacterial meningitis in elderly patients between 1967 and 1980, about 8% of cases were caused by gram-negative bacilli[6] (Figure 68-1). However, more recent studies have shown gram-negative bacilli to be responsible for 20% to 25% of cases.[8,9] This increase is not unexpected in light of the reported increase in nosocomial meningitis in all age groups. Gram-negative meningitis occurs at the extremes of life: in the neonate and debilitated elderly people. In a study of 158 patients with gram-negative meningitis in New York City, more than one half of the patients were over 60 years of age. Almost all of these elderly patients died.[23] However, third-generation cephalosporins have replaced chloramphenicol for treatment of gram-negative meningitis with improvement in overall survival.

Listeria monocytogenes is also an organism more likely to cause meningitis in elderly people than the younger adult. Because this infection is T-cell mediated, it is possible that immunologic senescence of this system may explain the predisposition of elderly people to this infection. Although *Listeria* accounts for 4% to 8% of all cases of meningitis in elderly people, it is an extremely rare cause of meningitis in young healthy adults. Of 53 cases of *L. monocytogenes* meningitis in New York City, 77% of patients were older than 50 and 87% of these elderly patients died.[23]

Meningococcal meningitis is the most common cause of meningitis in young adults, but a less common cause of meningitis in elderly people. The incidence of meningococcal meningitis in the elderly patient population varies from one study to another, reflecting the epidemic nature of the disease. Outbreaks have occurred in nursing homes and institutional settings.[24] The infection should be considered in elderly patients who have meningeal signs and have a petechial or macular rash. No focus of infection will be noted.

S. aureus was the most common cause of meningitis in elderly people in a Mayo Clinic study between the years 1948 and 1958.[25] All cases were secondary to neurosurgery. Overall the organism is probably responsible for about 10% of cases of meningitis in older patients, either as a neurosurgical infection or part of a complicated staphylococcal sepsis secondary to pneumonia or endocarditis. Coagulase-negative staphylococci have become a more common cause of meningitis in elderly people, being associated with CSF shunts and other neurosurgical procedures.

β-Hemolytic streptococci are a relatively rare cause of meningitis in elderly people. However, this appears to be

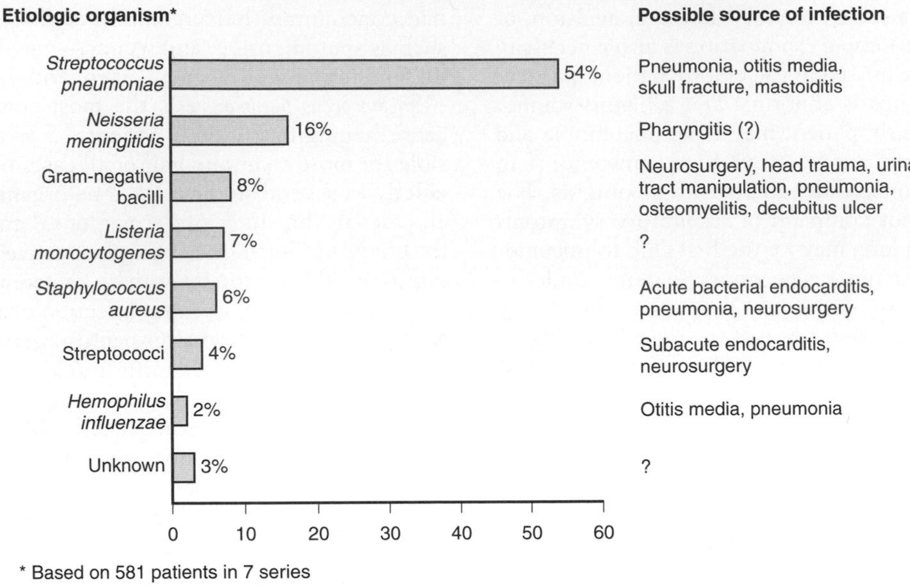

Figure 68-1. Bacterial meningitis in elderly patients. *(Modified from Berk SL, Smith JK. Infectious diseases in the elderly. Med Clin North Am 1983;67:273–93.)*

another organism that causes life-threatening infection and meningitis at the extremes of life.[26] *Hemophilus influenzae*, a cause of meningitis in children, is unusual in adults and elderly people. When *H. influenzae* does occur in older patients, it is usually a nonencapsulated organism.[27] This is in contrast to children, where the type B encapsulated organism is most likely to cause infection.

The treatment of bacterial meningitis requires prompt initiation of antibiotic therapy. The antibiotic chosen must have excellent activity against the causal agent. Information from the history and physical examination in combination with a careful review of the CSF Gram stain will be the foundation on which the causal agent will be determined and the optimal antibiotic chosen. An infectious disease specialist, when possible, should be involved in the case as the mortality rate from the disease is high and the margin of error is small. The antibiotic chosen should be bactericidal for the causal agent and must diffuse across the blood-brain barrier. Table 68-1 lists the causal agent and the antibiotic generally recommended.

However, the particular epidemiology of the hospital or community of the patient will take on increasing importance in determining the antibiotic of choice. The rapid emergence of penicillin-resistant pneumococci in the United States has created some uncertainty in regard to the initial treatment of pneumococcal meningitis. Given the rising incidence of high-level penicillin-resistant organisms, empirical therapy of pneumococcal meningitis should include vancomycin and a third-generation cephalosporin.[28] Pneumococci with an MIC of > 2 μg/mL are especially worrisome in that failures have been noted when these patients were treated with cephalosporin alone.[29] The role of dexamethasone, rifampin, and the new fluoroquinolones for pneumococcal meningitis is unclear at this time, and infectious disease consultation is advised. In the treatment of gram-negative meningitis, the antibiotic sensitivity pattern of gram-negative bacilli at a particular hospital is also critically important. If the infection has occurred after a neurosurgical procedure, the organisms responsible for prior neurosurgical infections should be noted. If *Pseudomonas aeruginosa* is suspected as the causal agent, ceftazidime is the antibiotic of choice. Cefotaxime or ceftriaxone is generally used for other gram-negative bacilli including *H. influenzae*. Ampicillin is the drug of choice for *L. monocytogenes*. Oxacillin or nafcillin are drugs of choice for methicillin-sensitive staphylococci; vancomycin is the antibiotic of choice for methicillin-resistant staphylococci and most coagulase-negative staphylococci. As previously noted, ampicillin plus a third-generation cephalosporin is recommended for treatment of meningitis in elderly people when the causal agent is unknown. Although corticosteroids are now recommended in the treatment of acute bacterial meningitis in children, there is no evidence at present to establish their use in the adult or elderly patient. Elderly patients with meningitis are generally admitted to an intensive care unit, where vital signs and neurologic status can be carefully monitored. Some patients will be severely dehydrated or volume depleted, and others will be in septic shock. Colloid or crystalloid may be necessary to improve blood pressure and urine output. Inappropriate antidiuretic hormone secretion may accompany central nervous system (CNS) infections but should be self-limited if hypotonic solutions are avoided.

Table 68-1. Antibiotic of Choice for Bacterial Meningitis

Streptococcus pneumoniae	Penicillin
Streptococcus pneumoniae (penicillin resistant)	Vancomycin + ceftriaxone
Staphylococcus aureus (methicillin sensitive)	Nafcillin
Staphylococcus aureus (methicillin resistant)	Vancomycin
Gram-negative bacilli	Third-generation cephalosporin (see text)
β-Hemolytic streptococci	Penicillin
Listeria monocytogenes	Ampicillin
Neisseria meningitidis	Penicillin
Hemophilus influenzae	Ceftriaxone or cefotaxime

The comatose, elderly patient requires specialized care. The patient may need frequent suctioning, particularly if pneumonia is present. The patient should be turned frequently to prevent decubiti. A condom catheter is preferable to a Foley, unless urinary retention develops. In patients who develop relapsing or prolonged fever, a repeat lumbar puncture is necessary. Drug fever, phlebitis, urinary tract infection, and pulmonary emboli are all possible explanations for prolonged fever.

The currently available pneumococcal vaccine is routinely recommended in all patients over 65 years of age. Although there are no specific data to support the prevention of pneumococcal meningitis in the elderly, it is clear that the vaccine does decrease the incidence of serious pneumococcal respiratory infection. Because most cases of pneumococcal meningitis in older patients are caused by pneumonia as the initial infection, it is likely that a vaccination program in elderly patients would be of benefit in preventing meningitis.

FOCAL LESIONS, ENCEPHALITIS, AND CHRONIC MENINGITIS

Brain abscess

A brain abscess often presents as a mass lesion with focal neurologic deficits. Since the advent of the CT scan, mortality has decreased from 30% to 50% to as low as 4% to 20%. The duration of symptoms before hospitalization usually has a mean of 15 days.[30] Risk factors for adverse outcomes include a severe change of mental status on admission, neurologic abnormalities on admission, and a short duration between the first symptoms and presentation suggesting a rapid progression. Fever may be absent in 40% to 50% of patients; common symptoms such as headache, change of mental status, and focal neurologic deficits may be misdiagnosed as cerebral tumors or cerebral vascular accidents, which are very common in elderly people.

The white blood cell count is ordinarily normal to slightly elevated. A lumbar puncture, which may be dangerous, particularly in patients with focal neurologic signs, reveals nonspecific findings. Seventeen percent of patients may have a white count greater than 500, suggesting a bacterial meningitis. Cultures of the spinal fluid, however, are usually negative.[30] Because 15% to 40% of patients with brain abscesses may die within 24 to 48 hours of a diagnostic lumbar puncture, this should be avoided in most cases.

The radiologic appearance of a "doughnut ring" lesion may be detectable in the majority of patients with brain abscesses. However, ring-enhanced lesions can also be seen with necrotic tumors and cerebral infarction. Surrounding edema may also be seen on CT scan and might be an indication for corticosteroids.[31,32] In cases of a single abscess, the most common location is generally that of the frontal lobe or parietal lobe rather than the occipital or temporal. Sites of brain abscesses are often independent from presumed origin of infection except for the possibility of ear and sinus infections more often leading to abscesses within the frontal brain.

Generalized seizures can prompt hospitalization of many patients including older adults. Often 50% of patients with a brain abscess may have a focal neurologic sign such as a hemiparesis or focal seizure. Patients may also present with a diffuse neurologic dysfunction such as a coma, generalized seizure, or neuropsychiatric manifestations. Funduscopic examination may also reveal papilledema. In Seydoux and Francioli's study[30] of 39 cases of brain abscesses, predisposing factors were not equally distributed in the different age groups in contrast to previous studies. They were more common in patients less than 50 years of age. Direct spread from a sinus or otologic focus appears to be more common with brain abscesses in younger adults, and was infrequently noted in patients older than 60 years of age. A short duration of symptoms before hospitalization also characterized patients between 20 and 60 years of age and was often associated with a poor outcome. The microbiology of brain abscesses does not appear to be significantly different between younger and older patients. Often viridans streptococcus and *Streptococcus milleri* are the most frequently isolated aerobes. *Fusobacterium* and other anaerobes were also common isolates.

Surgery is the only procedure that allows optimal microbiologic documentation. Several authors recommend medical therapy, particularly in cases in which the abscess is less than 2 cm in diameter and when the lesion is of high density, suggesting a cerebritis. Repeated aspiration and serial CT scans may be required to achieve a satisfactory response.[33–35]

A combination of a β-lactam agent with chloramphenicol or metronidazole generally has been recommended as standard therapy for brain abscesses. Microbiologic data obtained from a stereotaxic biopsy will be a further guide to therapy. The optimal duration of brain abscesses has been variable.[36] Usually most authors recommend approximately 4 to 6 weeks of antibiotics, including the combination of parenteral and oral agents. Neurologic sequelae can be quite high, occurring in as much as 46% of cases.[30]

Subdural empyema

Subdural empyema may arise as a complication of a sinusitis or otitis media. Presenting symptoms can often mimic a brain abscess. A contrasted study of the CNS is indicated and neurologic drainage is mandatory. Antibiotic therapy is targeted at many of the same organisms that cause brain abscess. Length of therapy is generally several weeks with intravenous antibiotics.

Tuberculous meningitis

Tuberculosis of elderly people is a serious disorder. Previously this was thought to be a diagnosis of the pediatric age group but recent reports indicate a rising incidence in elderly people.[37] Tuberculous meningitis is often an insidious disease and may be especially difficult to diagnose in elderly people. Nonspecific symptoms of fatigue, anorexia, nausea, and an altered mental status may suggest dementia in an elderly patient. A miliary picture on chest x-ray may be the only feature that is useful to distinguish tuberculous meningitis from cryptococcal meningitis. Duration of symptoms may range from 2 days to 6 months. Hospitalization is often precipitated by change in mental status, headache, or fever. Meningeal signs are present in less than one half of the cases. Ocular palsies, particularly due to involvement of nerve VI, are found in 30% to 70% of cases.

CSF findings often reveal a protein level above 50 and a low glucose below 40. Acid-fast positivity varies among the studies but can range anywhere from 10% to 80% depending on how many spinal taps were performed. A chest x-ray and purified protein derivative should be routinely obtained. Several attempts have been made to develop a rapid, common, and specific method for diagnosing tuberculous meningitis.

Adenosine deaminase activity has been detected in the spinal fluid. At levels greater than 9 units/L, the test was found to be sensitive and specific. Levels can also be increased in patients with sarcoid or lymphoma. Levels appear to perhaps correlate with disease activity. Radioimmunoassay has been used for detecting a *Mycobacterium tuberculosis* antigen. The assay becomes negative after therapy.

Tuberculostearic acid, a structural component of *M. tuberculosis*, can be identified by gas-liquid chromatography and may also be useful to diagnose tuberculosis.[38] Recent methodologies, such as polymerase chain reaction (PCR) testing and immunomagnetic enrichment, may also prove to be useful for cases of tuberculosis including tuberculous meningitis.[39–41]

Prognosis is influenced by age, duration of symptoms, and neurologic deficits. Mortality is greatest in patients younger than age 5 and older than 50 (60%). Clinical staging is often based on neurologic status: stage I—rational, no focal neurologic signs or hydrocephalus; stage II—confusion, depression, or focal neurologic deficits; stage III—stuporous or dense paraplegia or hemiplegia. Isoniazid (INH), pyrazinamide (PZA), and rifampin penetrate the blood-brain barrier to achieve adequate CSF concentrations. Multidrug-resistant tuberculosis may require several drugs.[42] Many authorities recommend the adjunctive use of corticosteroids for stage II and III patients, beginning with the dose of prednisone at 80 mg/day, which may be gradually tapered over 4 to 6 weeks as guided by the patient's symptoms. If hydrocephalus is present, ventricular shunting procedures may be beneficial.

Cryptococcal meningitis

Cryptococcal meningitis may present in a manner very similar to tuberculosis. Between 20% and 50% of patients with *Cryptococcus* may have no underlying disease such as human immunodeficiency virus (HIV). Spinal fluid findings are very similar to tuberculosis in that there is a lymphocyte predominance. The India ink test may be positive in 50% or more of cases. A cryptococcal antigen is often positive in 90% of cases using a rapid simple latex fixation test. A CT scan may be helpful to rule out hydrocephalus, which is not uncommon in cryptococcal meningitis.

Poor prognostic signs for cryptococcal meningitis may be related to a high CSF opening pressure, low CSF glucose, fewer than 20 white blood cells in the CSF, and high titers of cryptococcal antigen in a positive India ink, and the presence of HIV disease.

Amphotericin B is the traditional drug of choice for cryptococcal meningitis.[43,44] Flucytosine can serve as a useful adjunct, particularly when trying to lower the dose of amphotericin B to prevent renal insufficiency. However, flucytosine has bone marrow suppressive toxicities. Fluconazole is particularly useful for maintenance therapy but may also be useful as an acute therapy for patients with cryptococcal meningitis as well, particularly for those patients with less poor prognostic parameters.[45] Liposomal amphotericin B is also a new modality that may prove to be useful for treatment for cryptococcal meningitis. Combination therapy with fluconazole and flucytosine has also been investigated in patients with acquired immunodeficiency syndrome.

Coccidiomycosis is another common cause of chronic meningitis syndrome and a careful travel history may be an important clue to disease. Residents of the southwestern United States and Mexico appear to be at increased risk for this disease. Two thirds of the patients, however, may have no risk factors. Blacks, Filipinos, pregnant women, and patients with HIV disease appear more likely to have disseminated disease. CSF parameters are very similar to cryptococcal and tuberculous meningitis. Detection of complement fixation antibody in the CSF is specific and sensitive for the diagnosis. Amphotericin B has been the traditional drug of choice. Many experts often recommend the use of an Ommaya reservoir for intraventricular therapy. Newer data suggest that fluconazole may be helpful as an alternative to amphotericin B for long-term treatment of *Coccidioides* meningitis.[46]

Summary of Management Algorithm

Pneumococcal Meningitis

- Begin empirical therapy with vancomycin and a third-generation cephalosporin
- Dexamethasone administration is generally not recommended in adults
- Modify therapy based on the organism's MIC to penicillin

Herpes Simplex Encephalitis

- Begin therapy with high-dose acyclovir pending diagnostic tests
- An abnormal EEG can be suggestive of the diagnosis
- Temporal lobe enhancement on a cranial CT or MRI is highly suggestive of the diagnosis
- A positive CSF herpes simplex PCR test can eliminate the need for a brain biopsy

Herpes simplex encephalitis

Herpes simplex encephalitis is a serious infection of the CNS most commonly caused by herpes simplex virus type I. Mortality of untreated biopsy-proven cases is 60% to 80%, with fewer than 10% of the patients being left without any neurologic sequelae. This illness occurs in all age groups with an equal number of cases between the sexes. It has no seasonal association. Mortality may be higher in patients over 50 years of age.[47]

Patients may have an abrupt onset of personality change, altered mental status, fever, and headache. Localizing signs such as speech deficits, olfactory hallucinations, temporal lobe seizures, hemiparesis, and nasal field defects are common and may suggest the diagnosis. The spinal fluid findings are nonspecific with an elevated number of lymphocytes. An elevated number of polymorphonuclear leukocytes may be found early in the disease process. This will later change to a mononuclear site cell predominance as the disease progresses. An elevated red blood cell count can be suggestive of the diagnosis but is not required. The electroencephalogram pattern may consist of slow wave complexes at regular 2- to 3-second intervals, usually localized to the temporal lobe. CT scanning eventually becomes positive in more than 70% of the patients but MRI is more sensitive and results are abnormal earlier in the course of the disease.

The virus cannot usually be isolated from the spinal fluid but newer PCR-based methodology may be helpful in making the diagnosis.[48–51] The definitive diagnosis of herpes simplex encephalitis can be made by brain biopsy and appropriate culture and histology. Effective therapy usually consists of acyclovir at a dose of 10 mg/kg every 8 hours for

10 days, which must be adjusted for renal function in the elderly patient as acyclovir can cause nephrotoxicity, particularly in patients that are dehydrated. Survivals correlate with the patient's level of consciousness at the initiation of treatment. Neurologic sequelae are higher if treatment is delayed or the patient is comatose. A high index of suspicion is often required to make the diagnosis and to begin effective therapy for herpes simplex encephalitis. Rarely herpes encephalitis patients may relapse.[52,53]

Spirochetal infections

NEUROSYPHILIS

Several studies have suggested that neurosyphilis remains an important and frequently encountered entity. An estimated two symptomatic cases of neurosyphilis occur per 100,000 patients yearly. Syphilis is often the cause of reversible dementia in an elderly patient. Although neurosyphilis is often felt to be a late manifestation of syphilis, spirochetes invade the nervous system throughout the entire course of syphilis. Syphilitic meningitis may occur at the same time as the rash of the secondary syphilis. Most patients with cerebrovascular syphilis have had a duration of approximately 5 to 10 years. This can manifest as a stroke in a young person. Elderly patients typically have a presentation of paretic neurosyphilis or tabes dorsalis. The interval between infection and symptoms often ranges from 20 to 30 years for these syndromes. Both races appear easily susceptible. Men, however, have an increased risk as compared to women. The neurologic examination may be entirely normal with neurosyphilis, and the diagnosis may only be made by an abnormal CSF examination. As the disease progresses, intellectual function can decline and psychotic changes can occur. Symptoms include irritability, fatigability, personality changes, impaired judgment, depression, confusion, and delusions. Patients may have coarse, movement-induced facial, lingular, and labial tremors. Patients also may have difficulty with distorted handwriting, and abnormal reflexes and focal findings may also occur.[54] Untreated, the disorder is fatal within a few months to 3 or 4 years. Penicillin treatment can effectively reverse the CSF abnormalities and arrest the disease, but the neurologic outcome depends on the degree of structural CNS damage that had occurred at the time of therapy.[55] CSF findings in general paresis include an opening pressure between 50 and 300. The cell count is usually less than 100 in 90% of the cases. The glucose may be normal or moderately reduced. The protein is greater than 100 in 25% of cases. CSF and blood serology are generally positive in greater than 95% of cases.[54]

Tabes dorsalis continues to be a common form of CNS syphilis, although the percentage seems to be decreasing. This disease, again, is much more common in men than in women. It has the longest incubation period, being as high as 50 years in some patients. A triad of symptoms including lightning pains, dysuria, and ataxia may be seen in patients. A triad of signs including Argyll Robertson pupils, areflexia, and a loss of proprioception are characteristic of this disorder. Lightning pains last for a few seconds to minutes at a time and usually occur in the lower extremities. These can be separated by interval-free periods of a few months. Pain sensation is often strikingly impaired compared with that of hot and cold sensation.[55] Reduction or loss of ankle or knee jerks can occur in approximately 80% to 90% of patients. Pupillary abnormalities are noted in 79% of patients and consist of pupils that accommodate but do not react. In the elderly patient, diabetes can mimic tabes. Other rare causes mimicking tabes include Wernicke's encephalopathy and Charcot-Marie-Tooth disease. As the disease progresses, sensory ataxia becomes a problem. Many patients may have a positive Romberg sign. Less common abnormalities include syphilitic optic atrophy and gastric crises. Characteristic CSF findings of tabes usually include a normal opening pressure in 90% of the patients. Only 9% to 10% of patients have a cell count greater than 160. The protein is usually normal to moderately elevated. The majority of patients have an abnormal serum and CSF venereal disease research laboratory (VDRL) test. In the series by Merritt,[54] completely normal findings including an unreactive CSF and blood serology occurred in 2 of the 100 cases reported. In "burned-out" tabes, the fluid may be entirely normal. Penicillin treatment should clear the CSF and arrest progression of the disease; however, findings such as urinary incontinence, lightning pains, and gastric crises may not completely respond to penicillin therapy.

An unreactive peripheral blood FTA-ABS usually excludes the diagnosis of neurosyphilis, and in most cases a CSF examination would not be warranted. Any patient with a positive blood serology for syphilis and neurologic symptoms would warrant a lumbar puncture. An abnormal CSF VDRL test would constitute proof of neurosyphilis. Patients with only an abnormal protein or cell count might also be strongly considered for penicillin therapy. In patients with signs of neurosyphilis but with an unreactive CSF (normal cells and protein), such as in "burned out" neurosyphilis, the neurologic deficit is probably due to fixed structural damage and will probably not respond to additional penicillin.[55] A treponemicidal level has been assumed to be 0.3 IU/mL. Comparisons of serum and CSF penicillin levels after benzathine penicillin use suggest that benzathine penicillin may not reach adequate treponemicidal levels in the CSF. Adequate levels are achieved by adequate intravenous penicillin doses given for neurosyphilis. The present authors generally tend to treat patients with neurosyphilis with 18 to 24 million units/day for approximately 10 to 14 days. Adequate therapy is suggested by a normal spinal fluid cell count and a falling protein count at 6 months following treatment.[56–59] Repeat CSF examination should be performed every 6 months for the next 2 years during which time the protein count should fall and the cell count should remain normal. The VDRL will probably also disappear during this time period or reach a low-level "serofast" state. Any increase in the cell count or major deviation from this response would require retreatment with high-dose penicillin. Neurosyphilis is often an indication to consider desensitization if the patient has a penicillin allergy. Ceftriaxone may be a reasonable alternative in some patients. Penicillin allergy would be an indication for infectious diseases and allergy consultation. Many patients who have a positive serum test and no symptoms could potentially be treated with three injections of benzathine penicillin over a 3-week period. However, this would only be warranted if the physician is sure there is no symptoms of neurosyphilis. A negative CSF would be reassuring to the patient and physician before embarking on this treatment course. Hypothyroidism, cryptococcal, and tuberculous meningitis, or other causes of reversible dementia need to be considered in the differential diagnosis of neurosyphilis.

Lyme disease

The CNS effects of Lyme disease are receiving increasing attention in the literature. Lyme disease can cause a meningitis in the second stage weeks to months after the tick exposure. Bell's palsy and peripheral neuropathy syndromes are quite common. A CSF pleocytosis is often found with an elevated protein and a normal to low CSF sugar. Local CSF antibody production occurs. A positive enzyme-linked immunosorbent assay test for Lyme disease is usually recommended to be followed by a Western blot test. Ceftriaxone is generally considered the treatment of choice for the CNS manifestations of syphilis.[60] An exception might possibly be the use of doxycycline for facial nerve palsy.

KEY POINTS
Infections of the Central Nervous System

Fifty-six percent of community-acquired meningitis occurs in patients over 50 years of age.

Bacteria reach the subarachnoid space by three mechanisms:

1. Bacteremia
2. Head trauma and neurosurgery
3. Contiguous spread from sinusitis or otitis

Clinical features may be more subtle in elderly patients.

CSF findings in elderly patients resemble those of younger adults.

Streptococcus pneumoniae is the most common organism causing meningitis in elderly patients. *Listeria* is more likely to cause meningitis in older patients than in young adults.

Pneumococci may be resistant to β-lactam therapy. The addition of vancomycin to third-generation cephalosporins is recommended initially until culture results are available.

Focal Lesions

Brain abscess often presents as a mass lesion.

CSF findings are nonspecific.

Ring-enhancing lesions are detected by CT in the majority of patients.

Often viride streptococci and *Streptococcus milleri* are isolated.

A combination of metronidazole and a third-generation cephalosporin is usually recommended.

Subdural empyema arises as a complication of sinusitis and otitis media.

Tuberculous Meningitis

Tuberculosis

1. Meningeal signs are often absent.
2. CSF glucose levels are typically low.
3. Ocular palsies are common.
4. Acid-fast positivity varies.
5. Prognosis is related to clinical stage.

Cryptococcal Meningitis

India ink is positive about 50% of the time.

Poor prognostic signs include a high titer of antigen and fewer than 20 WBCs/hpf in the CSF.

Herpes Simplex Encephalitis

May present as an abrupt personality change, olfactory hallucinations, or temporal lobe epilepsy.

MRI is more sensitive than CT.

A CSF PCR test is usually positive.

Spirochetal Infections

Neurosyphilis

1. Often a cause of reversible dementia.
2. Elderly patients have tabes dorsalis or paretic syphilis more often than younger patients.
3. CSF serology is usually positive.
4. Patients who have a positive serum FTA-ABS and an abnormal cell or protein count should be considered for therapy.

Lyme Disease

Bell's palsy is common.

Ceftriaxone is the therapy of choice for all forms of CNS Lyme disease with the possible exception of facial nerve palsy.

For a complete list of references, please visit online only at www.expertconsult.com

CHAPTER 69

Metabolic Bone Disease

Roger M. Francis

INTRODUCTION

Bone is a living, dynamic tissue that undergoes constant remodeling throughout life. This is necessary to allow the skeleton to increase in size during growth, respond to the physical stresses placed on it, and repair structural damage due to structural fatigue or fracture. In addition to its mechanical properties, bone also plays an important role in calcium homeostasis, acting as a mineral reservoir that can be drawn on to maintain normocalcemia. The skeleton comprises two types of bone: cortical (or compact) and trabecular (or cancellous) bone. Cortical bone is predominantly found in the shafts of the long bones, whereas trabecular bone is mainly located in the vertebrae, pelvis, and the ends of long bones, where it forms a lattice-like structure within an outer shell of cortical bone. Trabecular bone has a larger surface area, undergoes greater remodeling, and is therefore more responsive to changes in calcium homeostasis than cortical bone. The respective proportion of cortical and trabecular bone varies with the anatomic site, but overall the skeleton is composed of 80% cortical and 20% trabecular bone.

The three major cell types involved in bone remodeling are osteoclasts, osteoblasts, and osteocytes. Osteoclasts are multinucleate cells derived from macrophage-monocyte precursors, which resorb bone, releasing mineral and removing degraded organic material. Osteoblasts are derived from fibroblast precursors and synthesize bone matrix or osteoid, which is subsequently mineralized around foci of crystal formation known as matrix vesicles. The matrix vesicles are extruded from osteoblasts by exocytosis and contain promoters of crystal formation such as alkaline phosphatase and pyrophosphatase. Osteocytes are mature osteoblasts that become trapped within calcified bone. These are interconnected by long dendritic processes, which may serve as mechanosensory receptors, leading to the production of paracrine factors that regulate bone resorption and formation.

Bone remodeling is initiated by a period of bone resorption lasting about 2 weeks, when osteoclasts erode an area of bone. Osteoblasts are then attracted to the resorption cavity, where over the subsequent 3 months new bone matrix is deposited and mineralized. The processes of bone resorption and bone formation are usually closely coupled, but bone formation exceeds resorption during skeletal growth, allowing the skeleton to increase in size and density. Later in life, resorption outstrips bone formation, leading to involutional bone loss. Bone remodeling may be influenced by mechanical forces applied to the skeleton, by paracrine factors, and by circulating hormones such as estrogen, testosterone, calcitonin, parathyroid hormone (PTH), and 1,25-dihydroxyvitamin D (1,25[OH]$_2$D).

One of the major regulators of bone remodeling is the receptor activator of nuclear factor kappa B (RANK) and RANK ligand (RANKL) system. RANKL, which is produced by osteoblasts, attaches to RANK on the cell surface of osteoclasts and osteoclast precursors, leading to stimulation of osteoclast differentiation and proliferation.[1] The interaction of RANKL and RANK is blocked by osteoprotegerin (OPG), a soluble decoy receptor produced by osteoblasts and marrow stromal cells.[1] Studies show relationships between circulating concentrations of OPG and bone mineral density (BMD), and it is now apparent that the beneficial effects of osteoporosis treatments may be mediated in part by changes in the RANK, RANKL, and OPG system.[2–4]

Bone mass changes throughout life in three major phases: growth, consolidation, and involution. Up to 90% of the ultimate bone mass is deposited during skeletal growth, which lasts until the closure of the epiphyses. There is then a phase of skeletal consolidation lasting for up to 15 years, when bone mass increases further until the peak bone mass is achieved in the mid-30s. Involutional bone loss then starts between the ages of 35 and 40 in both sexes, but in women there is an acceleration of bone loss in the decade after the menopause. Overall, women lose 35% to 50% of trabecular and 25% to 30% of cortical bone mass with advancing age, whereas men lose 15% to 45% of trabecular and 5% to 15% of cortical bone.

OSTEOPOROSIS

Osteoporosis is a skeletal disorder characterized by compromised bone strength, predisposing a person to an increased risk of low trauma or fragility fractures. The three major fragility fractures are those of the forearm, vertebral body, and femoral neck, but fractures of the humerus, tibia, pelvis, and ribs are also common. These fractures are a major cause of mortality, morbidity, and health and social service expenditure in older people, but this is particularly the case with hip fractures. The annual health and social service cost of fragility fractures in the United Kingdom has been estimated at £1.7 billion, of which almost 90% is attributable to hip fractures.[5]

There is a strong inverse relationship between bone density and fracture risk, with a two- to three-fold increase in fracture incidence for each standard deviation reduction in BMD. The risk of fracture is also determined by other skeletal risk factors, such as bone turnover, trabecular architecture, skeletal geometry, and previous fragility fracture. Nonskeletal risk factors for fracture include postural instability, physical and mental frailty, and conditions associated with falling.[5,6]

Prevalence of osteoporosis

The World Health Organization (WHO) has quantitatively defined osteoporosis as a BMD 2.5 standard deviations or more below the mean value for young adults (T score <-2.5).[7] The prevalence of osteoporosis, as defined by a T score <-2.5 at the hip, increases in white women in the United States from 8% in the seventh decade to 47.5% in the ninth decade, whereas the prevalence at the forearm, spine, or hip rises from 21.6% to 70%.[7] As regards the resulting probability of fragility fractures, the lifetime risk for a 50-year-old woman in the United Kingdom is 53.2%, compared with 20.7% for a 50-year-old man.[8] The risk of individual symptomatic fractures in a 50-year-old woman is

16.6% for the forearm, 3.1% for the vertebra, and 11.4% for the hip, whereas the corresponding figures for a 50-year-old man are 2.9%, 1.2%, and 3.1%.[8]

Pathogenesis of osteoporosis

Bone mass at any age and therefore the risk of fracture is determined by the peak bone mass, the age at which bone loss starts, and the rate at which it progresses.

PEAK BONE MASS

Genetic factors account for as much as 80% of the variance in peak bone mass. Other potential determinants of peak bone mass include exercise, dietary calcium, smoking, alcohol consumption, and hormonal factors.[6]

INVOLUTIONAL BONE LOSS

Bone loss starts between the ages of 35 and 40 in both sexes, possibly related to impaired new bone formation as a result of declining osteoblast function. The onset of bone loss is likely to be genetically determined, and the subsequent rate of bone loss may also be influenced by genetic factors. Recent studies suggest that a number of gene polymorphisms influence BMD and fracture risk.[6] The genes involved include those regulating RANKL, OPG, and the estrogen receptor gene.[9] Although the individual effect of variation in these genes is relatively small, the combined impact of these is similar to other major risk factors for fracture.[9,10]

Bone loss increases in the decade following the menopause in women, because of the marked reduction in the circulating estradiol concentrations. Other causes of age-related bone loss include low body weight, smoking, excess alcohol consumption, physical inactivity, declining vitamin D concentrations, and secondary hyperparathyroidism.[6]

Body weight is an important determinant of bone density and fracture risk, as bone loss is more rapid in postmenopausal women with low body weight and individuals with osteoporotic fractures are lighter than expected. The protective effects of high body weight on bone density and fracture risk may be due to the stimulation of bone formation by greater mechanical loading, increased conversion of adrenal androgens to estrogens in fat, and the shock-absorbing properties of subcutaneous fat.

Smoking may increase bone loss by reducing the age at menopause by several years, decreasing plasma estrogen levels by increasing their metabolism and possibly depressing osteoblast function. The deleterious effect of smoking on the skeleton may also be due in part to the association with low body weight. Although alcoholism is a recognized cause of osteoporosis, the effect of modest alcohol consumption on bone density remains unclear.

The decline in physical activity with advancing age is also likely to cause further bone loss. Physical activity is important to the skeleton because the associated weight-bearing and muscular activity stimulates bone formation and increases bone mass, whereas immobilization leads to rapid bone loss. The importance of physical activity is underlined by a number of studies, which show that physical inactivity is associated with an increased risk of hip fracture.

The role of dietary calcium intake in the pathogenesis of bone loss remains controversial. Although there is a relationship between dietary calcium and bone mass in adolescence, studies show little correlation between calcium intake and bone density or bone loss in postmenopausal women. Other nutrients that have been suggested as potential determinants of the rate of bone loss include fluoride, protein, and sodium, but their importance is still uncertain.

There is a reduction in circulating 25 hydroxyvitamin D (25OHD) and $1,25[OH]_2D$ concentrations with advancing age, because of decreased cutaneous production and impaired metabolism of vitamin D. This is likely to contribute to the observed increase in circulating PTH with age. There is a weak relationship between serum 25OHD and bone density in middle-aged women, with an inverse correlation between bone density and serum PTH, suggesting that vitamin D status may influence bone loss. Other studies show that vitamin D insufficiency and secondary hyperparathyroidism are common in older patients with osteoporosis and fractures.[11]

SECONDARY OSTEOPOROSIS

In addition to the factors influencing the attainment of peak bone mass and subsequent involutional bone loss, there are a number of conditions that may accelerate the development of osteoporosis. Secondary causes of osteoporosis may be found in up to 30% of women and 55% of men with symptomatic vertebral crush fractures.[6] The most frequently encountered are oral steroid therapy, male hypogonadism, hyperthyroidism, myeloma, skeletal metastases and the use of antiepileptic drugs.

Clinical features of osteoporosis

Osteoporosis is generally considered to be asymptomatic until fractures occur. Fractures of the forearm and hip are usually easy to diagnose, but vertebral crush fractures may be more difficult to detect clinically. Only 30% of patients come to medical attention after a vertebral fracture, and there are many other causes of acute back pain.[12] Classically, however, a vertebral fracture is associated with an acute episode of back pain lasting for 6 to 8 weeks before settling to a more chronic backache. The pain may radiate anteriorly but rarely radiates to the hips or legs. Individuals with vertebral fractures may also be aware of loss of height of several inches and notice the development of a kyphosis. Physical signs include a kyphosis, local tenderness over the spine, and horizontal skin creases and abdominal protrusion resulting from the loss of trunk height.

Diagnosis of osteoporosis

Before the development of techniques that accurately measure bone density, osteoporosis was usually only detected after a fracture had occurred. The term *osteoporosis* was therefore reserved for the fracture syndrome resulting from reduced bone density. With the advent of bone densitometry and the development of effective treatments that decrease fracture risk, the term *osteoporosis* is increasingly used to describe reduced BMD before fractures have occurred.

Although accurate measurements of lumbar spine and femoral BMD can be made using dual energy x-ray absorptiometry (DXA), a population-based bone density screening program cannot be justified, as there is little evidence that such as strategy is effective in the prevention of fragility fractures.[7] Nevertheless, an opportunistic case-finding strategy has been advocated in countries such as the United Kingdom, where a number of indications for BMD measurements are recognized.[13] These include previous fragility fracture, untreated hypogonadism, oral glucocorticoid therapy, other secondary causes of osteoporosis, and radiologic osteopenia.[13] Although spine BMD may be spuriously elevated in older people, because of degenerative changes and aortic calcification, femoral neck and total hip measurements are less affected by osteoarthritis.

BMD measurements may be of limited value in the investigation of frail elderly patients with hip and other fragility fractures, many of whom will have osteoporosis and should therefore benefit from treatment. Furthermore, U.K. guidelines recommend that all people over the age of 65 years who are likely to be on treatment with oral glucocorticoids for at least 3 months should be offered treatment for osteoporosis.[14]

BMD measurements may be expressed as standard deviation units above or below the mean value for normal young adults or relative to the mean value for control subjects of the same age, to give T and Z scores, respectively. Although the WHO definition of osteoporosis (T score <-2.5) may be useful in epidemiologic studies, it does not necessarily represent a threshold for treatment. This is important as 70% of women above the age of 80 years have a T score <-2.5, but only a proportion of these will sustain an osteoporotic fracture.[7] Furthermore, although more than half of patients with hip fractures have osteoporosis, fewer than 50% of those with other fragility fractures have a T score <-2.5 on DXA measurement.[15]

As the value of BMD in predicting fracture risk is relatively poor, there has been growing interest in using the combination of BMD and clinical risk factors for fracture to estimate the absolute risk of fracture. The WHO has developed a fracture risk assessment tool (FRAX), which estimates the 10-year risk of fractures of the major fragility fractures and of hip fracture in particular.[16,17] Country-specific algorithms use age, gender, and the presence or absence of appropriately weighted risk factors, with or without femoral neck BMD measurements, to estimate fracture risk.[18] The clinical risk factors for fracture used in FRAX, which are at least in part independent of bone density, are made up of low body mass index (BMI), prior fracture after age of 50 years, parental hip fracture, current smoking, oral steroid therapy, alcohol intake > 2 units/day, and chronic conditions associated with bone loss such as rheumatoid arthritis.[16–18] Guidelines are being developed that will guide clinicians on the absolute risk of fracture above which osteoporosis treatment should be considered.[19]

Investigation of osteoporosis

As vertebral fractures may not always be easy to diagnose, spine x-rays should be considered in patients with acute back pain, loss of height, or kyphosis, to look for evidence of vertebral deformation, degenerative arthritis, or other pathology. Although spine x-rays are useful in the diagnosis of vertebral fracture, they are unreliable in the assessment of bone density. Spine x-rays may also show lytic or sclerotic lesions, which raise the possibility of neoplastic disease. Further investigations are then required, which may include isotope bone scan and magnetic resonance imaging (MRI) scan.[12]

In patients with vertebral fractures, causes of secondary osteoporosis should be identified by careful history, physical examination, and appropriate investigation (Table 69-1), because specific treatment of underlying conditions such as hyperthyroidism, hypogonadism, and primary hyperparathyroidism increases bone density by up to 15%. Underlying causes of secondary osteoporosis should also be sought in older men and women presenting with hip and other nonvertebral fractures after minimal trauma. Serum 25OHD and PTH measurements may be used to confirm the diagnosis of vitamin D insufficiency and secondary hyperparathyroidism, but these are probably unnecessary if calcium and vitamin D supplementation is planned. Routine biochemical profile is worthwhile, as hypocalcemia and hypophosphatemia may indicate possible vitamin D deficiency osteomalacia, but these measurements lack diagnostic specificity or sensitivity. Serum 25OHD and PTH measurements are also useful in the further investigation of possible vitamin D deficiency osteomalacia, which is particularly likely in housebound patients or those with previous gastric resection, malabsorption, or the long-term use of antiepileptic drugs. Investigations for secondary osteoporosis should also be performed in patients found to have a BMD below the normal range for their age (Z score <-2.0), to identify underlying causes of bone loss, which may be modified.

Table 69-1. Investigations for Secondary Osteoporosis in Older People with Low Trauma Fractures or Low BMD

Full blood count
ESR or CRP
Biochemical profile
Thyroid function tests
Serum testosterone, sex hormone binding globulin, LH, FSH (men)
Serum and urine electrophoresis (vertebral fractures)
Serum 25OHD and PTH

Management of osteoporosis

All patients with fragility fractures should be given general advice on lifestyle measures to decrease further bone loss, including eating a balanced diet rich in calcium, moderating tobacco and alcohol consumption, and, if possible, maintaining regular physical activity and exposure to sunlight. As bone loss continues into old age in both men and women, the need for specific treatment should be considered in all patients with osteoporosis or fragility fractures. Although most studies of the treatment of osteoporosis have recruited few women above the age of 80 years, there is no evidence of an attenuated response to treatment with advancing age.

A number of treatments have been shown to increase BMD and decrease the risk of vertebral and hip fractures. The Royal College of Physicians has published guidelines on the management of osteoporosis,[13] grading its recommendations on the levels of evidence for each therapeutic intervention (Table 69-2). Grade A recommendations are based on randomized controlled trials, whereas grade B recommendations result from controlled studies without randomization, studies with a quasi-experimental design, and epidemiologic studies. Although the grading of the strength of the recommendations based on study design is useful, this takes no account of study size, the magnitude of the treatment effect, the patient groups studied, or the other potential risks and benefits of treatment.

Table 69-2. Effect of the Major Treatment Options on the Risk of Vertebral, Non-vertebral, and Hip Fractures

	Vertebral Fractures	Non-vertebral Fractures	Hip Fractures
Raloxifene	A	ND	ND
Alendronate	A	A	A
Risedronate	A	A	A
Zoledronate	A	A	A
Ibandronate	A	(A)	ND
Strontium ranelate	A	A	(A)
Teriparatide	A	A	ND
Calcium and vitamin D	ND	A	A

Grading of recommendations updated and adapted from the Royal College of Physicians Clinical Guidelines for Prevention and Treatment of Osteoporosis. Royal College of Physicians and Bone and Tooth Society of Great Britain. Osteoporosis clinical guidelines for prevention and treatment. Update on pharmacological interventions and an algorithm for management. London: Royal College of Physicians; 2000. (ND indicates that fracture reduction has not been demonstrated, whereas (A) reflects that a beneficial effect on fractures risk was only found in posthoc subgroup analysis.)

HORMONE REPLACEMENT THERAPY (HRT)

Although HRT was previously used in the prevention and treatment of osteoporosis in younger postmenopausal women, the situation changed with the publication of the results of the Women's Health Initiative Study.[20] This randomized controlled trial compared the effects of HRT with placebo in 16,608 postmenopausal women aged 50 to 79 years. Although this showed a reduction in colon cancer as well as vertebral, hip, and other factures, the benefits were outweighed by the increased risk of breast cancer, coronary heart disease, stroke, and thromboembolism.[20] As a result of this study, HRT is no longer recommended for the prevention of osteoporosis, but it may be useful in younger postmenopausal women with osteoporosis and severe climacteric symptoms and in those unable to tolerate other osteoporosis treatments.

RALOXIFENE

Raloxifene is a selective estrogen receptor modulator (SERM), which has estrogen agonist actions on the skeleton but acts as an estrogen antagonist on the breast and endometrium. The Multiple Outcomes of Raloxifene Evaluation (MORE) study in postmenopausal women with osteoporosis showed that raloxifene increased lumbar spine and femoral neck bone density by 2% to 3%, reduced the risk of vertebral fractures by 30% to 50%, and decreased the incidence of breast cancer by 76%.[21,22] There is no evidence that raloxifene decreases the risk of hip or other non-vertebral fractures. The main side effect of raloxifene is hot flashes, particularly when used shortly after menopause, but there is also an increased risk of venous thromboembolism. It is generally used in younger postmenopausal women with osteoporosis who are at high risk of vertebral fractures, but whose risk of non-vertebral fractures is low.

BISPHOSPHONATES

Bisphosphonates have become the treatment of choice for patients with osteoporosis, because of their proven antifracture efficacy and good safety profile. Intermittent cyclical etidronate therapy is now rarely used, because although it reduces the incidence of vertebral fractures, there are no interventional studies investigating the effect of treatment on hip fracture incidence.[13] Alendronate and risedronate have been shown in large studies to increase BMD and decrease the incidence of vertebral, hip, and other non-vertebral fractures.[13,23–25] These oral agents are available as daily or weekly preparations but need to be taken on an empty stomach, 30 minutes before food, to ensure that they are absorbed from the bowel. Ibandronate has also been shown to improve BMD and decrease the incidence of vertebral fractures, but although a posthoc subgroup analysis suggests that it prevents non-vertebral fractures, no reduction in hip fractures has been demonstrated.[26] Ibandronate is available as a monthly oral preparation and a three-monthly intravenous injection. Annual intravenous infusions of zoledronate in women with osteoporosis have been shown to decrease the risk of vertebral fractures by 70% and hip fractures by 41%.[27] A further study in patients with recent hip fracture demonstrates that annual intravenous zoledronate decreases the risk of vertebral and non-vertebral fractures but also reduces mortality by 28%.[28]

Although the antifracture studies with alendronate only recruited patients up to the age of 81 years, there was no evidence of any attenuation of the benefits with advancing age.[29] Risedronate has been shown to decrease vertebral fractures in women above the age of 80 years,[30] but although there is no definite evidence that it reduces the risk of hip fractures in women in this age group recruited on the basis of clinical risk factors for fracture,[25] there is no reason to suspect it will be ineffective in elderly women with osteoporosis. Over a third of the patients in the major study of zoledronate in osteoporosis were above the age of 75 years, suggesting that it is effective even in this older age group.[27]

Oral bisphosphonates are generally well tolerated, but upper gastrointestinal side effects are not uncommon. Esophagitis has been reported with oral bisphosphonates, but the risk of this complication may be reduced by following the manufacturers' advice that these agents should be taken with water and recumbency avoided for 30 minutes. Intravenous bisphosphonates may cause an acute phase response, with transient flulike symptoms lasting for a few days. The severity of these symptoms may be reduced by the administration of paracetamol for 3 days starting on the day of bisphosphonate administration. Intravenous zoledronate may also cause symptomatic hypocalcemia, so it is important ensure that the patient is vitamin D replete before administering this treatment. Increased bone pain has been reported with bisphosphonate treatment but appears to be an uncommon side effect. The major antifracture study of intravenous zoledronate showed an increase in serious atrial fibrillation,[27] but this was unrelated to the timing of infusion and was not found in other studies with zoledronate,[28] Osteonecrosis of the jaw has been reported in patients receiving high dose intravenous bisphosphonates in malignancy, but this appears to be uncommon in patients taking lower-dose bisphosphonates for osteoporosis.[31]

STRONTIUM RANELATE

Strontium ranelate is a dual action bone agent which reduces bone resorption and increases bone formation. A large randomized controlled trial of strontium ranelate in postmenopausal women with osteoporosis and at least one vertebral fracture showed increases in BMD of 12.7% in the lumbar spine and 8.6% in the hip after 3 years' treatment.[32]

About 50% of this apparent increase is spurious, because of the skeletal incorporation of strontium, which has a higher atomic number than calcium. This study also demonstrated a 41% reduction in the incidence of new vertebral fractures.[32] Another large study in women with osteoporosis showed a 16% reduction in the incidence of non-vertebral fractures with strontium ranelate, but in a posthoc subgroup analysis in women aged over 74 years with low BMD (T score < −3.0), there was a 36% reduction in hip fractures.[33] Recent data suggest that strontium ranelate decreases the incidence of vertebral and non-vertebral fractures in women above the age of 80 years.[34] Strontium ranelate is available in powder form in sachets, the contents of which are dissolved in water. Preferably it should be taken at bedtime, at least 2 hours after eating, to ensure adequate absorption from the bowel. Strontium has been generally well tolerated in clinical trials, but reported side effects include diarrhea and an increased risk of venous thromboembolism. A severe hypersensitivity reaction associated with drug rash, eosinophilia, and systemic symptoms (DRESS) has been reported, which occurs within 3 to 6 weeks of starting treatment with strontium ranelate, but this is fortunately very rare.

PARATHYROID HORMONE

The continuously high circulating concentrations of PTH found in primary and secondary hyperparathyroidism is associated with an increase in bone turnover, but bone resorption is stimulated more than bone formation, resulting in loss of bone from the skeleton. In contrast, intermittent administration of PTH stimulates bone formation more than resorption, resulting in an increase in bone mass and density. Recombinant human parathyroid hormone 1–34 (teriparatide) and parathyroid hormone 1–84 have anabolic actions on the skeleton when administered by daily subcutaneous injection. Studies show a larger increase in BMD than that observed with bisphosphonates.[35-37] Teriparatide decreases the incidence of vertebral and non-vertebral fractures, but no reduction in hip fractures has been demonstrated.[35] There also appears to be no attenuation of the effects of teriparatide on BMD or fracture reduction with advancing age.[36] Parathyroid hormone 1–84 has also been shown to reduce the incidence of vertebral fractures.[37] These agents are generally well tolerated but may cause transient mild hypercalcemia, nausea, dizziness, and headaches. As these preparations are 10-fold more expensive than bisphosphonates, their use is often restricted to patients with severe osteoporosis or those who fail to respond to bisphosphonates. There is evidence that concomitant administration of a bisphosphonate may attenuate the anabolic effect of PTH treatment,[38] but there is only transient attenuation after previous treatment.[39]

CALCIUM AND VITAMIN D

Calcium and vitamin D supplementation has been shown to reduce the incidence of hip and other non-vertebral fractures in older people living in care homes, where vitamin D deficiency and secondary hyperparathyroidism are common.[40] In contrast, recent large studies cast doubt on the role of calcium and vitamin D supplementation in the primary or secondary prevention of low-trauma fractures in community-dwelling older people.[11,41] Nevertheless, a recent meta-analysis shows a small reduction in hip fractures with calcium and vitamin D (relative risk 0·82, 95% confidence intervals 0·71 to 0·94), with no beneficial effect of vitamin D alone on fracture incidence.[42]

Calcium and vitamin D supplementation may cause abdominal bloating, other gastrointestinal symptoms, and change in bowel habit. These may account for the relatively poor compliance and persistence with supplementation, particularly with combined calcium and vitamin D preparations. Calcium and vitamin D supplementation is probably most appropriate in older people who are housebound or living in residential or nursing homes, where vitamin D insufficiency and secondary hyperparathyroidism are common.[11] The National Institute of Health and Clinical Excellence (NICE) in the United Kingdom recommends that patients receiving treatment for osteoporosis should also receive calcium and vitamin D supplementation, unless the clinician is confident that the patient has an adequate dietary calcium intake and is vitamin D replete.[43]

OTHER TREATMENTS

Calcitonin is a potent antiresorptive agent with a rapid but short-lived effect on osteoclast function. The Prevent Recurrence of Osteoporotic Fractures (PROOF) study of 1255 women with established osteoporosis showed only marginal improvements in BMD with intranasal calcitonin.[44] Although there was a 36% reduction in new vertebral fractures with doses of 200 IU calcitonin daily, no significant decrease in fractures was seen with 100 or 400 IU daily.[44] In view of the unconvincing data on the antifracture efficacy of calcitonin, it is generally only used when other treatments are contraindicated or not tolerated. Nevertheless, there is some evidence that the short-term use of calcitonin may be useful in the management of pain associated with acute vertebral fracture.[45]

Patients with established osteoporosis have lower calcium absorption than age-matched control subjects, which may be due to reduced serum $1,25[OH]_2D$ concentrations or to relative resistance to the action of vitamin D metabolites on the bowel.[46] Malabsorption of calcium in osteoporosis can be overcome by pharmacologic doses of parent vitamin D or by low doses of the active vitamin D metabolites, such as calcitriol and alfacalcidol. Studies of the effect of treatment with vitamin D metabolites on BMD and fracture incidence in established osteoporosis have produced conflicting results.[46] A study comparing calcitriol with calcium supplementation in women with vertebral fractures showed a significantly lower incidence of new vertebral fractures with calcitriol, but this was because of an increase in fracture rate with calcium rather than a reduction with calcitriol.[47] The inconsistent results of antifracture studies, potential risk of hypercalcemia, and the need for regular monitoring of serum calcium and renal function limit the use of vitamin D metabolites in the management of osteoporosis.

FUTURE TREATMENTS

Denosumab is a monoclocal antibody directed against RANKL, which it binds with high affinity and specificity. This inhibits the stimulatory action of RANKL on bone resorption. A randomized controlled trial in postmenopausal women with low BMD showed rapid suppression of bone resorption with twice yearly subcutaneous injections of denosumab, with significant increases in BMD.[48] Although the results of studies examining the effect of denosumab on fractures are still awaited, this appears to be a promising treatment for osteoporosis. Other potential antiresorptive treatments for osteoporosis include cathepsin K inhibitors[49] and new SERMs such as bazedoxifene.[50]

Novel anabolic treatments for osteoporosis include agents that inhibit the formation or action of sclerostin, a protein produced by osteocytes that is a potent inhibitor of bone formation.[51] Selective androgen receptor modulators (SARMs) are also being evaluated as potential treatments for osteoporosis.[52] Calcium-sensing receptor antagonists (calcilytics) stimulate the release of PTH, so they may also prove to be anabolic treatments for osteoporosis.[53]

FALLS ASSESSMENT

The risk of fragility fracture is determined not only by skeletal factors, but also by nonskeletal risk factors associated with a propensity for falling.[5,6] A study in older men and women presenting to hospital with a fragility fracture showed a higher prevalence of skeletal risk factors (53%) and falls-related risk factors (75%) than documented osteoporosis (35%) as defined by a BMD T score <−2.5.[54] All patients with fragility fractures should therefore undergo falls assessment. Risk factors for falling are divided into intrinsic factors, including poor vision, neurologic disease and medication, and extrinsic or environmental factors, such as trailing wires, loose carpets, and ill-fitting footwear. Intrinsic causes of falls should be sought by history, examination, and review of medication, whereas extrinsic or environmental causes may be identified from the history and home visit. In older patients with unexplained falls or syncope, tilt testing may also be useful.

A number of randomized controlled trials have assessed the effect of modifying risk factors for falling, but the results have not all been consistent. A recent meta-analysis concluded that there is only limited evidence that multifactorial falls prevention programs in primary care, community, or emergency care settings are effective in reducing the number of fallers or fall-related injuries.[55] Although it is logical that preventing falls will reduce the incidence of fractures, no randomized controlled trial of falls prevention has been adequately powered to examine the effect on fracture risk. Nevertheless, a recent controlled study suggests that a single visit by an occupational therapist reduces the risk of falling in older women after hip fracture.[56]

EXTERNAL HIP PROTECTORS

An alternative approach to fracture prevention is to decrease the impact of falls using external hip protectors, which are incorporated into specially designed underwear. A Danish study block randomized 665 elderly residents of nursing homes to receive external hip protectors or to serve as controls.[57] Over the 12-month study, there was a reduction in hip fracture risk of over 50% in those using the hip protectors. In the group randomized to receive hip protectors, the only patients who fractured were not using hip protectors at the time. A systematic review has examined the effect of external hip protectors in community-dwelling older people and in those living in residential or nursing home.[58] Pooled data from 11 studies in institutionalized older people, including six randomized controlled trials, showed some reduction in hip fractures (relative risk 0.77, 95% confidence intervals 0.62 to 0.97). In contrast, data from three individually randomized controlled trials in community-dwelling older people showed no reduction in hip fractures with hip protectors.[58]

CHOICE OF TREATMENT

In considering the choice of treatment in the individual patient, a number of factors are important. These include the underlying pathogenesis of bone loss, the evidence of efficacy in any particular situation, the cost effectiveness of treatment, tolerability, and patient preference. Although hormonal treatments are likely to be more effective in younger postmenopausal women with osteoporosis, where bone loss is largely due to estrogen deficiency, the risks of HRT outweigh the potential benefits in most cases.[20] Raloxifene may therefore be appropriate in younger postmenopausal women, who are at high risk for vertebral fractures. In contrast, calcium and vitamin D supplementation may be more appropriate in frail elderly people, who are likely to have vitamin D insufficiency and secondary hyperparathyroidism. Bisphosphonates are effective across a wide age range, but oral bisphosphonates may be inappropriate in individuals with cognitive impairment because of difficulties in coping with the complex instructions on administration. The use of alendronate may be precluded in older patients with hiatus hernia, esophageal disease, and peptic ulcers, because of concern about the risk of esophagitis. In patients with upper gastrointestinal disease and those with difficulty following the instructions for taking oral bisphosphonates, strontium ranelate or intravenous bisphosphonates provide alternative treatment options.

A number of factors may influence compliance and tolerability. Raloxifene is likely to aggravate hot flashes, particularly in women close to the menopause, so may be more appropriate in postmenopausal women between the ages of 55 and 70 years. Oral bisphosphonates have complex instructions for administration, which can preclude their use in unsupervised patients with cognitive impairment. Calcium and vitamin D supplements may be poorly tolerated in some individuals, because of gastrointestinal side effects and bowel symptoms.

A schematic representation of the management of osteoporosis is provided in Figure 69-1. All individuals should be given lifestyle advice on diet, exercise, tobacco and alcohol consumption, and exposure to sunlight. In younger postmenopausal women with osteoporosis at high risk of vertebral fractures, raloxifene may be useful, particularly if there is also a significant risk of breast cancer. In older women at high risk of vertebral and non-vertebral fractures, bisphosphonates are currently the treatment of choice, but strontium ranelate provides a useful alternative, particularly above the age of 80 years. In frail, housebound, or institutionalized older people, calcium and vitamin D supplementation should be considered, because of the high prevalence of vitamin D insufficiency and secondary hyperparathyroidism. In patients with a past history of recurrent falls, measures should be taken to reduce the incidence of falls. Consideration should also be given to the use of external hip protectors, especially where caregivers are available to encourage compliance with their use.

OSTEOMALACIA

Osteomalacia is a generalized bone disorder characterized by an impairment of mineralization leading to accumulation of unmineralized matrix or osteoid in the skeleton.[59,60] There

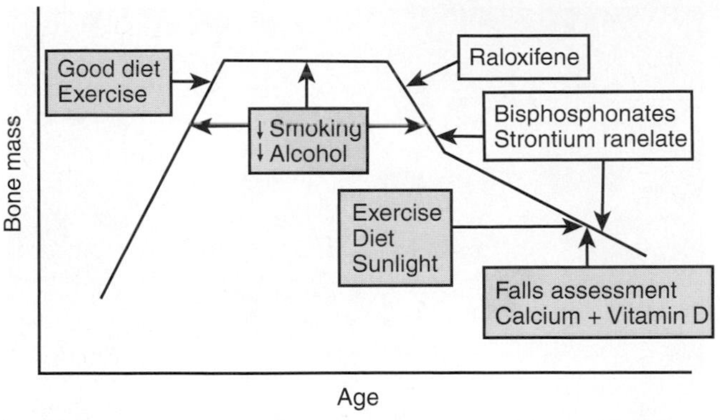

Figure 69-1. Schematic representation of the major therapeutic options in patients with osteoporosis of different ages, together with lifestyle measures in the shaded boxes.

Table 69-3. Classification of the Major Causes of Osteomalacia

Deficiency	Cause	Clinical Form
Vitamin D	↓ Sunlight exposure	Housebound elderly
	↓ Dietary vitamin D	Asian immigrants
	Malabsorption	Small bowel disease
25OHD	Abnormal vitamin D metabolism	Antiepileptic drugs
		Liver disease
$1,25[OH]_2D$	↓ 1α-hydroxylase activity	Renal failure
Phosphate	↓ Tubular reabsorption	Familial
		Tumoral
		Sporadic
	Phosphate depletion	Use of phosphate binders

are a number of causes of osteomalacia, but the majority of cases are due to vitamin D deficiency, abnormal vitamin D metabolism, or hypophosphatemia (Table 69-3).

Adequate amounts of calcium and phosphate are essential for mineralization of osteoid to proceed normally, and although vitamin D is important in the homeostasis of calcium and phosphate, the precise role of the vitamin D metabolites in mineralization remains uncertain. The major source of vitamin D is from cutaneous production, following the exposure of the precursor 7-dehydrocholesterol to ultraviolet irradiation.[61] The diet provides much smaller amounts of vitamin D, but this becomes essential when cutaneous production is limited. Vitamin D itself has little biologic activity and is metabolized in the liver to 25OHD, the major circulating form of vitamin D. This undergoes further hydroxylation in the kidneys to form $1,25[OH]_2D$, the hormonally active metabolite of vitamin D, which regulates calcium absorption from the bowel, influences bone remodeling, and affects muscle function.[61]

Vitamin D deficiency osteomalacia predominantly occurs because of reduced cutaneous production of vitamin D resulting from lack of exposure to sunlight, increased skin pigmentation, or adherence to strict religious dress codes where the skin is covered.[59,60] It is therefore particularly seen in the housebound elderly or Asian immigrants, particularly when the dietary intake of vitamin D is poor.[62,63] Vitamin D deficiency osteomalacia is also seen with malabsorption or after gastric surgery and is related to reduced sunlight exposure, decreased absorption of vitamin D, and malabsorption of calcium or phosphate.

Antiepileptic drugs and severe liver disease are also associated with low plasma 25OHD levels and the development of vitamin D deficiency osteomalacia.[59,60] Antiepileptic drugs induce liver enzymes, which metabolize vitamin D to biologically inactive polar metabolites, whereas liver disease may be associated with impaired 25 hydroxylation of vitamin D. In addition, patients with epilepsy or liver disease may be less exposed to sunlight and therefore have reduced cutaneous production of vitamin D.[59,60]

Renal impairment leads to the development of osteomalacia because of reduced production of $1,25[OH]_2D$, malabsorption of calcium, and low plasma calcium, though plasma 25OHD concentration may also be low because of reduced sunlight exposure. Hypophosphatemic osteomalacia may result from decreased renal tubular reabsorption of phosphate as in familial, tumor-associated, and sporadic cases, or from phosphate depletion associated with the use of phosphate binders.[59,60]

Osteomalacia in the elderly

Vitamin D deficiency is the commonest cause of osteomalacia in the elderly. Renal failure is a smaller but significant cause in this age group. There is a reduction in plasma 25OHD with advancing age, which is mainly due to reduced sunlight exposure, though decreased capacity for cutaneous production, low dietary intake, poor absorption, and impaired hepatic hydroxylation of vitamin D may also contribute to this condition.[61] Plasma 25OHD concentrations are lower in individuals living in residential care than in people living in the community, and they are lowest in residents of long-term geriatric wards.[62] The reduction in renal function with age is associated with decreased plasma $1,25[OH]_2D$ concentrations which may contribute to the development of osteomalacia in the elderly.[61]

Osteomalacia is essentially a histologic diagnosis, so there is little information on its overall prevalence in the elderly. Nevertheless, as mentioned previously, low 25OHD concentrations are common in older people, particularly in subjects who are housebound or institutionalized. As about 10% of elderly people are housebound, a significant proportion are at risk of developing osteomalacia because of absent cutaneous production of vitamin D, and several investigators have shown that osteomalacia occurs in about 4% of elderly people admitted to hospital.[64,65] An early histologic study from Leeds suggested that up to 40% of patients with hip fracture have evidence of osteomalacia, but the criteria used for this diagnosis were either excess osteoid or decreased calcification fronts.[66] Using the stricter diagnostic criteria of the combination of increased osteoid seam width and reduction in calcification fronts, a subsequent study from Cardiff showed osteomalacia in only 2% of patients with hip fracture.[67]

Clinical features of osteomalacia

The presentation of osteomalacia may be variable, and the diagnosis may be easily missed in the early stages of the disease because of the vague nature of the symptoms. The patient may complain of aches and pains, aggravated by muscular contraction, but tending to persist after rest. Although there is a propensity for fracture in osteomalacia, the soft

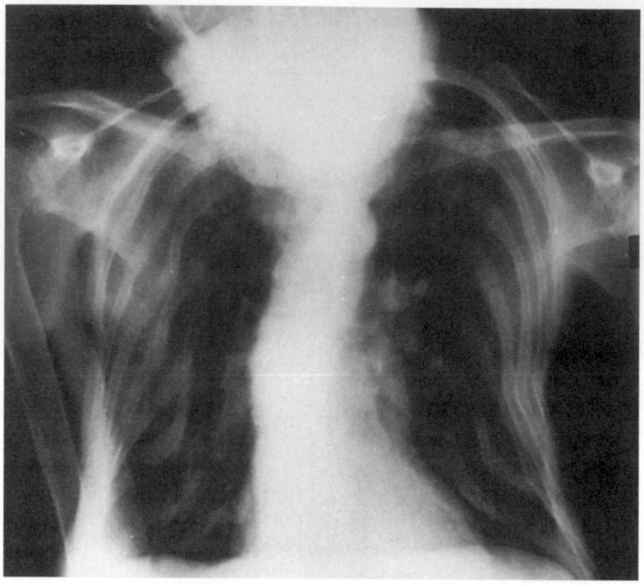

Figure 69-2. Chest x-ray of a woman with osteomalacia, showing deformity of rib cage as a result of bone softening.

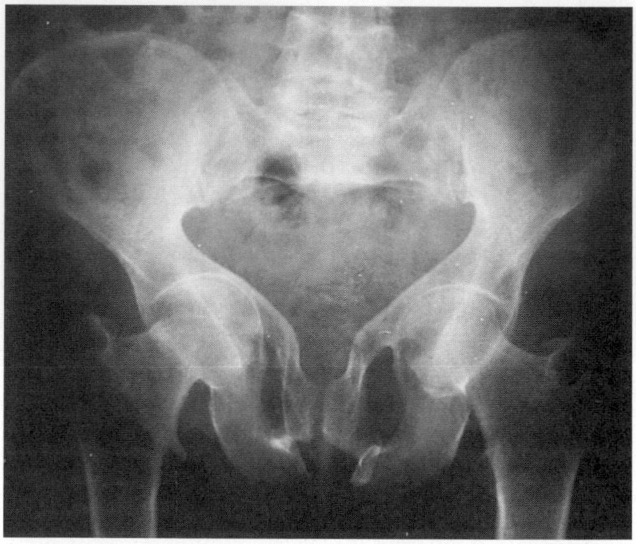

Figure 69-3. X-ray of the pelvis of a woman with osteomalacia, showing deformity of the pelvic bones as a result of bone softening.

elastic bone also deforms easily, leading to kyphosis, scoliosis, and deformity of the rib cage, pelvis, and long bones. The patient may also develop a proximal myopathy, causing a waddling gait and difficulties rising from a chair or climbing stairs. Occasionally, the hypocalcemia associated with osteomalacia leads to latent tetany, with paraesthesias of the hands and around the mouth, cramps, a main d'accoucheur appearance of the hands, and positive Chvostek's and Trousseau's signs.

Radiology in osteomalacia

The classic radiologic appearances of osteomalacia are relatively rare and may not be found in the early stages of the disease. Osteomalacic bone is softer than normal and so becomes easily deformed. The intervertebral discs balloon out and deform the adjacent vertebrae to give them a uniformly biconcave codfish appearance. Similar deformity may occur in osteoporosis, but the biconcavity is more regular in osteomalacia than with osteoporosis, where the extent of vertebral deformity is variable. There may be radiologic evidence of deformity of the rib cage, pelvis, and long bones (Figures 69-2 through 69-4). A characteristic finding in osteomalacia is Looser's zones or pseudofracture, which consist of a large area of osteoid. These appear as bands of decalcification surrounded by more dense bone, which occur perpendicular to the bone surface, often where nutrient arteries enter bone (see Figure 69-4). Looser's zones are seen particularly in the proximal femur, humeral neck, pubic rami, ribs, metatarsals, and the outer border of the scapula. There may also be radiologic evidence of secondary hyperparathyroidism, with subperiosteal erosions in the metacarpals or phalanges.

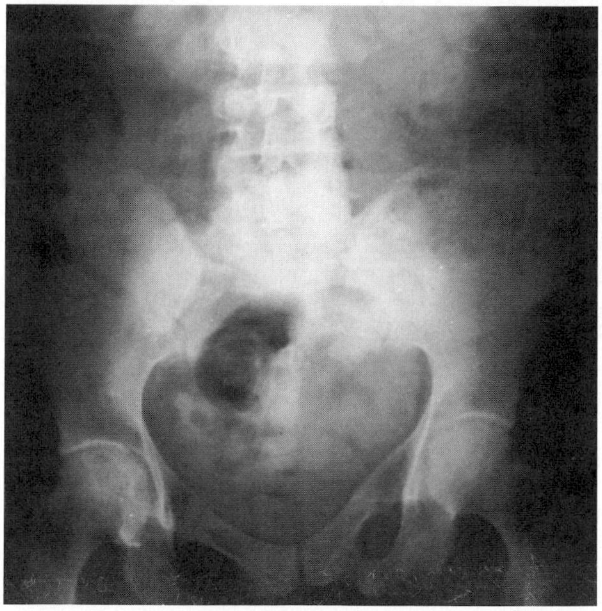

Figure 69-4. X-ray of the pelvis of a woman with osteomalacia, showing Looser's zones in the pubic rami.

Biochemical findings in osteomalacia

The biochemical findings in the major types of osteomalacia are shown in Table 69-4. In vitamin D deficiency osteomalacia, the plasma calcium tends to be low because of reduced calcium absorption resulting from low plasma 25OHD and $1,25[OH]_2D$ concentrations. The hypocalcemia leads to secondary hyperparathyroidism, which in turn stimulates the renal tubular reabsorption of calcium and reduces tubular reabsorption of phosphate. Plasma phosphate is therefore often low in osteomalacia because of reduced absorption from the bowel and decreased renal tubular reabsorption. The secondary hyperparathyroidism also increases bone remodeling, which is reflected in elevation of the plasma alkaline phosphatase and other biochemical markers of bone turnover. Not all patients with vitamin D deficiency osteomalacia will have hypocalcemia, hypophosphatemia, and raised alkaline phosphatase, and these abnormalities may occur individually in the elderly with intercurrent illness, so they lack specificity in the diagnosis of osteomalacia in the elderly.[68]

Table 69-4. Biochemical Abnormalities in Major Types of Osteomalacia

	Vitamin D Deficiency	Renal Failure	Hypophosphatemic
Hypocalcemia	59%	63%	9%
Hypophosphatemia	68%	0%	73%
↑ Alkaline phosphatase	88%	88%	27%
↓ 25OHD	80%	58%	0%
↓ $1,25[OH]_2D$	75%	81%	36%
↑ PTH	90%	100%	11%

Data derived from Peacock M. Osteomalacia. In: Nordin BEC, editor. Metabolic Bone and Stone Disease, 2nd ed. Edinburgh: Churchill Livingstone; 1984, pp. 72–111.

In osteomalacia associated with renal failure, hypocalcemia is seen in the majority of cases, although the plasma phosphate is normal or high because of reduced urinary excretion of phosphate. The plasma $1,25[OH]_2D$ is low because of impaired production by the kidneys, and the plasma 25OHD may also be reduced because of inadequate exposure to sunlight. Plasma alkaline phosphatase is raised in the vast majority of cases, whereas the serum PTH is invariably elevated.[59]

In hypophosphatemic osteomalacia, the major biochemical abnormality is a low plasma phosphate, though this may vary in severity. A few cases may also show hypocalcemia, low plasma $1,25[OH]_2D$, and elevation of serum PTH (see Table 69-4).

Diagnosis of osteomalacia in the elderly

The only definite way of diagnosing osteomalacia is by histologic examination of undecalcified bone and demonstrating excess osteoid and reduced calcification fronts or mineralization rate. Histologic confirmation of the diagnosis is required in the minority of cases, however. In patients with a typical history of bone pain and muscle weakness, with radiologic evidence of Looser's zones or typical biochemical changes there is little indication for bone biopsy. When the diagnosis is less clear-cut, measurement of plasma 25OHD and serum PTH may be useful, as the combination of low plasma 25OHD and elevated PTH is a strong indicator of the presence of osteomalacia. An alternative approach is to use a therapeutic trial of vitamin D in subjects likely to have osteomalacia and to monitor any subsequent clinical and biochemical improvement.

Treatment of osteomalacia

In cases of vitamin D deficiency osteomalacia, the condition will heal with ultraviolet irradiation or vitamin D treatment.[61] It has been suggested that vitamin D deficiency is treated with oral 50,000 IU vitamin D weekly for 8 weeks, followed by long-term vitamin D 800 to 1000 IU daily, to prevent recurrence of vitamin D deficiency.[61] Unfortunately, high-dose oral vitamin D is not always easy to obtain. Furthermore, although IM injections of 300,000 units vitamin D every 6 to 12 months provides an alternative approach to treatment, the absorption from the administered oily solution is relatively poor.[69] For these reasons, many clinicians treat patients with vitamin D deficiency osteomalacia with combined calcium and vitamin D supplements, providing 1000 to1200 mg calcium and 800 IU vitamin D daily. The addition of supplemental calcium ensures that sufficient mineral is available for mineralization of the osteoid to occur.

In patients with osteomalacia associated with malabsorption, the active metabolites of vitamin D may be required, which are usually given in a dose of 1 to 4 μg daily of either alfacalcidol or calcitriol. Calcium supplements may also be required, but the serum calcium should be monitored to avoid the development of hypercalcemia. Magnesium supplements may also be necessary if hypomagnesemia is present. If malabsorption is due to bacterial overgrowth, pancreatic insufficiency, or celiac disease, appropriate treatment of the underlying disorder with antibiotic therapy, pancreatic enzyme supplements, or gluten-free diet should be instituted.

In patients with osteomalacia and renal impairment, either alfacalcidol or calcitriol should be used in a dose of 1 μg daily, together with calcium supplements as required. Serum calcium and renal function should be monitored regularly on this treatment.

Treatment of osteomalacia leads to a resolution of the proximal myopathy and any symptoms of hypocalcemia within a few weeks, although the bone pain may take longer to improve. The biochemical abnormalities also persist for up to 6 months after treatment is started, and the bone remains histologically and structurally abnormal during this time. Care should therefore be taken to avoid falls during rehabilitation, as these may easily lead to fractures of the abnormal bone. The plasma calcium and phosphate returns to normal within a few weeks, whereas the plasma alkaline phosphatase rises further on treatment and may take many months to return to normal. Serum PTH also remains elevated for up to 6 months. Ultimately, radiologic abnormalities such as Looser's zones and changes of secondary hyperparathyroidism will resolve on treatment, though deformity will persist despite the remodeling of bone.

Paget's disease

Paget's disease of bone is a common condition characterized by increased bone turnover, which can involve one or more of the bones in the skeleton. Although the condition may be asymptomatic, it can cause significant morbidity in older people, including bone pain, skeletal deformity, pathologic fractures, deafness, and osteoarthritis.[70]

Prevalence of Paget's disease

The United Kingdom has the highest prevalence of Paget's disease in the world, but there is considerable regional variation in prevalence across the country.[71,72] By the eighth decade of life, up to 8% of men and 5% of women in the United Kingdom have evidence of the condition.[73] Studies suggest that Paget's disease is also common in the rest of Europe and in British migrants to Australia, New Zealand, and South Africa.[70,71] In contrast, the condition is rare in Scandinavia, Asia, and Africa.[71] There has been a decrease in the prevalence of Paget's disease in the United Kingdom and New Zealand over the past 25 years,[74,75] but this trend has not been observed in the United States or Italy.[71] The reason for the decrease in prevalence of Paget's disease is unclear, but may reflect environmental changes or the immigration of people from countries with a low prevalence.[71]

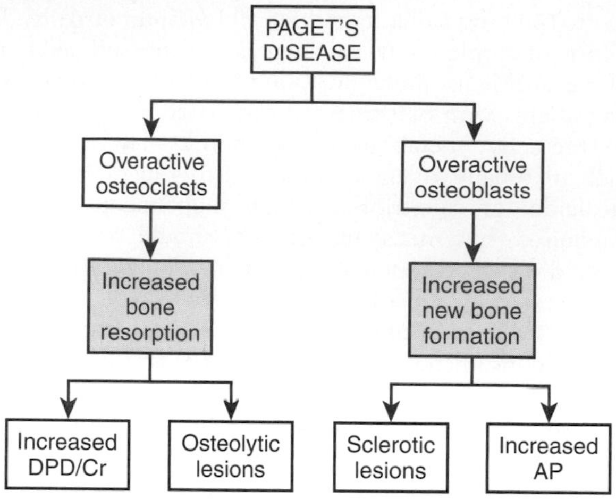

Figure 69-5. Pathophysiology of Paget's disease of bone, with the biochemical changes in the shaded boxes.

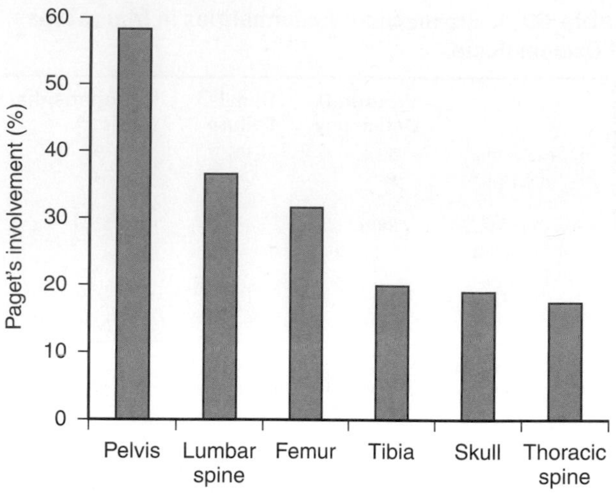

Figure 69-6. Skeletal involvement in 889 patients with Paget's disease. (*Data derived from Davie M, Davies M, Francis R, et al. Paget's disease of bone: A review of 889 patients. Bone 1999;24 (Supplement):11S–12S.*)

Pathophysiology of Paget's disease

Paget's disease is characterized by increased bone resorption mediated by enlarged, hyperactive osteoclasts.[71] There is also an increase in osteoblastic activity and new bone formation (Figure 69-5). This is associated with biochemical changes, including increased bone resorption markers, such as urine deoxypyridinoline/creatinine (DPD/Cr) and by an elevation of alkaline phosphatase (AP). The rapid bone turnover leads to the deposition of woven bone, which is more vascular, structurally weak and prone to deformity and fracture. Inclusion bodies resembling paramyxoviruses have also been seen in affected osteoclasts,[76] but their role in the pathogenesis of Paget's disease remains uncertain.[71] Osteoclast precursors from patients with Paget's disease appear to be particularly sensitive to factors that stimulate bone resorption, including $1,25[OH]_2D$ and RANKL.[77] Increased circulating concentrations of RANKL have also been reported in Paget's disease, but this requires confirmation in future studies.[78]

The etiology of Paget's disease remains uncertain. There is a significant genetic component to the condition, as about 15% of patients have a family history of the condition. The risk of developing the condition may be up to 10-fold higher in first-degree relatives of patients with Paget's disease.[71] Recent work has identified gene mutations that may contribute to the development of Paget's disease and related conditions. The most important of these is in the sequestosome 1 (*SQSTM1*) gene, which encodes for a protein involved in RANK/RANKL signaling.[79] Mutations in the *SQSTM1* gene are found in 20% to 50% of cases of familial disease and 5% to 20% of cases of sporadic disease.[71] A much more rare cause of Paget's disease is a mutation in the *VCP* gene, which is associated with hereditary inclusion-body myopathy and frontotemporal dementia.[80]

Although genetic factors may predispose to the development of Paget's disease, it is likely that other factors may influence its expression. The clustering of cases of Paget's disease within families includes spouses, so may reflect not only genetic factors but also shared environment. It has been suggested that Paget's disease may result from a slow virus infection, which either causes the disease or triggers it in a susceptible individual. As mentioned earlier, inclusion bodies resembling paramyxoviruses have been seen in affected osteoclasts, but their role in the pathogenesis of Paget's disease remains uncertain. Other factors that may influence the development of Paget's disease in susceptible individuals include mechanical forces, low dietary calcium intake or vitamin D deficiency during childhood, and occupational exposure to toxins.[71]

Clinical features of Paget's disease

Paget's disease may present at any age over 30, but is most often diagnosed in the sixth decade of life. The condition is more common in men than in women. The majority of people with radiologic evidence of Paget's disease are asymptomatic and do not come to medical attention. The condition is therefore often an incidental finding in patients having x-rays for an unrelated reason.

The bones most commonly involved in Paget's disease are the pelvis, spine, femur, tibia, and skull (Figure 69-6), although the distribution of the disease is usually asymmetrical. The extent of skeletal involvement is generally constant within an individual, with previously unaffected bones rarely becoming involved long after diagnosis. The most common presentation is with pain, which may be due to the Pagetic changes in the bone itself or to the effects of skeletal deformity on surrounding structures. The cause of bone pain in Paget's disease may be difficult to determine. It may be due to periosteal stretching, to microfractures, or to direct nerve stimulation by substances released by osteoclasts during bone resorption.

Paget's disease may also cause skeletal deformity, as the affected bones thicken, enlarge, and become more elastic. Classically, this causes frontal bossing of the skull, bowing of the long bones and deformity of the pelvis (protrusio acetabuli). Pagetic bone is more likely to fracture, and fissure fractures may also occur on the outer aspect of bowed long bones.

Thickening of the skull may cause compression of the cranial nerves, particularly the auditory nerves, resulting in deafness. Other cranial nerves are only rarely involved in Paget's disease. The increased vascularity of Pagetic bone may also result in neurologic deficit because of a "vascular steal" syndrome. Softening of the base of the skull may rarely lead to basilar invagination, causing brainstem compression. Vertebral involvement may result in crush fractures or more rarely spinal cord compression.

A major management problem is the development of secondary degenerative arthritis in joints adjacent to involved bone. This is frequently more disabling than the Paget's disease itself and will not respond to treatment of the underlying bone disease. Other complications of Paget's disease include high output cardiac failure, because of the increased vascularity of the affected bone, which although often described is rarely seen. Sarcomatous change also occurs only rarely but has a poor prognosis.[81]

Diagnosis and investigation of Paget's disease

The diagnosis of Paget's disease is reached through a combination of clinical assessment and selected investigations. Although the history rarely leads directly to a diagnosis of Paget's disease, it is important to seek clues to other conditions that may coexist with or masquerade as it. Examination may reveal skeletal deformity, especially of the skull or long bones, which may feel warm to the touch. There may also be signs of associated degenerative arthritis. A full neurologic assessment is advisable in symptomatic patients, though abnormalities other than deafness are not often found.

The diagnosis of Paget's disease is usually confirmed radiologically. x-rays may show an increase in size of affected bones, alteration of bone texture with areas of sclerosis and lucency (see Figure 69-5), skeletal deformity, and evidence of degenerative arthritis in adjacent joints. The radiologic appearances are often said to be pathognomonic, but skeletal metastases from occult carcinoma of the prostate or breast should be considered in the differential diagnosis. Prostate specific antigen should therefore be measured in all men with probable Paget's disease. Rarely, bone biopsy may be required if the diagnosis remains uncertain.

The extent of the bone disease can be assessed by isotope bone scan, although x-rays of areas with increased uptake may be advisable, if there is any doubt about the diagnosis. Serum alkaline phosphatase and biochemical markers of bone resorption are often markedly raised in Paget's disease, reflecting increased osteoblast and osteoclast activity respectively (see Figure 69-5), so they may be used to assess the activity of the condition and its response to treatment.

Treatment of Paget's disease

Treatment of Paget's disease is directed at suppressing the overactivity of osteoclasts, thereby decreasing bone turnover.[82] Although calcitonin was used for several decades in the management of Paget's disease, bisphosphonates have now become the treatment of choice. These agents are generally used in patients with symptomatic Paget's disease, but their role in asymptomatic individuals is unclear. The PRISM study showed no apparent benefit of intensive bisphosphonate treatment aimed at returning alkaline phosphatase to normal, compared with those given symptomatic treatment for bone pain.[71]

BISPHOSPHONATES

Oral antiresorptive therapy for Paget's disease became practical for the first time with the introduction of etidronate in the late 1970s. Disodium etidronate 400 mg daily decreases the biochemical markers of bone turnover by 40% to 60%.[82] Unfortunately, prolonged therapy with etidronate leads to impaired mineralization, so courses of treatment should not exceed 6 months. There is also evidence that previous treatment with etidronate decreases the efficacy of subsequent courses of treatment.[82]

Intravenous infusions of pamidronate decrease the biochemical markers of bone turnover by 50% to 80%, resulting in prolonged remission in many patients with Paget's disease.[82] Pamidronate may be given by weekly infusion of 30 mg for 6 weeks or by three fortnightly infusions of 60 mg. The intravenous route of administration avoids the potential problems of oral bisphosphonates, such as poor absorption from the bowel, the need to take medication in a fasting condition, and gastrointestinal side effects. These advantages are offset by the need for intravenous infusion and transient flulike symptoms that may follow treatment.

Oral tiludronate 400 mg daily for 3 months decreases the biochemical markers of bone turnover by at least 50% in 70% of patients.[83] This may avoid the need for further treatment for at least 18 months. A comparative study in 234 patients with Paget's disease showed that significantly more responded to 3- or 6-month treatments with tiludronate 400 mg daily (60.3% and 70.1%) than to 6-month treatments of etidronate at 400 mg daily (25.3%).[84] This study also showed an attenuated response to etidronate in patients who had previously received this bisphosphonate.

A North American study compared the effect of risedronate 30 mg daily for 2 months or etidronate 400 mg daily for 6 months in 123 men and women with documented Paget's disease.[85] At 12 months, alkaline phosphatase decreased into the normal range in 73% of patients who had taken risedronate, compared to 18% with etidronate. Previous treatment with etidronate had no significant effect on the subsequent response to risedronate but resulted in a blunted response to further etidronate. There was a significant reduction in pain with risedronate, whereas etidronate was associated with nonsignificant improvement.

Pooled data from two identical, randomized controlled trials compared a single intravenous infusion of 5 mg zoledronate with a 2-month course of oral risedronate 30 mg daily in 347 patients with Paget's disease.[86] After 6 months, alkaline phosphatase had returned into the normal range in 88.6% of patients receiving zoledronate, compared with 57.9% in the risedronate group. Although pain scores improved in both groups, there appeared to be greater improvement in quality of life with zoledronate than risedronate.[86] A subsequent study followed up 296 patients who had responded to treatment with either zoledronate or risedronate for a further 18 months.[87] In patients treated with zoledronate, the mean alkaline phosphatase remained in the middle of the reference range, whereas it increased in a linear fashion from 6 months with risedronate.

Although bisphosphonates decrease bone pain and reduce the activity of Paget's disease, there is currently no evidence that any treatment will prevent skeletal deformity, fractures, or other complications of the condition.[71] The choice of bisphosphonates for the management of Paget's disease depends on patient preference and tolerability. Despite its low cost, etidronate should no longer be used because it is much less effective than other bisphosphonates. The main choice lies between IV zoledronate or pamidronate infusions and oral risedronate.

CALCITONIN

Calcitonin has a direct, receptor-mediated action on osteoclast function. In vivo studies show that within 30 minutes of calcitonin administration, osteoclasts cease synthetic activity and begin to detach from bone. Recruitment of osteoclasts and fusion of precursor cells is also halted, resulting in a rapid reduction in bone resorption. Calcitonin has a short half-life, so osteoclast activation recommences as soon as local concentrations return to basal levels. Salmon and porcine preparations of calcitonin are also weakly antigenic, and neutralizing antibodies are formed during treatment by some patients, which may limit their long-term efficacy. Nevertheless, subcutaneous or intranasal calcitonin has proved to be useful in the management of Paget's disease, where it decreases bone pain and reduces the biochemical markers of bone turnover.[82] Calcitonin is now generally only used in patients unable to tolerate bisphosphonate treatment

FRACTURES IN THE ELDERLY

The mechanical properties of an individual bone are determined by the amount of bone present, skeletal architecture, and bone quality. Aging is associated with a reduction in bone mass, disruption of trabecular architecture, and an increased prevalence of disorders such as osteomalacia and Paget's disease, which adversely affect the quality of bone. Nevertheless, the risk of fracture is determined not only by skeletal factors but also by nonskeletal risk factors including postural instability, physical and mental frailty, and conditions associated with falling.[5,6] It is therefore not surprising that the incidence of fractures increases with advancing age. Whereas fractures in young adults usually occur after extensive trauma, fractures in the elderly may result from minimal trauma, such as falling from standing height. The major fractures occurring in older people are those of the forearm, vertebral body, humerus, pelvis, and hip.[8,88] The incidence of these fractures increases with advancing age and is higher in women than men because of their lower peak bone mass, different patterns of cortical and trabecular bone loss, smaller skeletal size, and greater risk of falls. Fractures are also more common in older residents of care homes and nursing homes than in community-dwelling people of the same age.[89] This probably reflects the higher risk of falls and lower BMD in institutionalized older people compared with those living in the community.[90]

There is considerable geographic variation in fracture incidence around the world,[91] which may reflect differences in bone mass due to race, smoking, alcohol consumption, and physical activity. The absolute number of fractures in the elderly is rising rapidly, partly because of the increasing numbers of elderly people and a rising age-specific incidence of fractures,[92] If present demographic trends continue in the United Kingdom, the number of young elderly will remain reasonably constant over the next few decades, whereas the number of people over the age of 85 will increase considerably. Many of these elderly people will be frail, and therefore at greater risk of falls and fractures. There has been an increase in the age-specific incidence of fractures of the forearm, vertebral body, humerus, and hip over the past few decades,[93,94] which has been attributed to the increased survival of frail individuals and secular changes in smoking, alcohol consumption, diet, and physical activity. Although the age-specific incidence of fracture may now be reaching a plateau or even declining,[95] the aging population means that an increase in the absolute number of fractures is inevitable, in both the developed and developing world.[96]

Forearm fractures

These are the most common fractures before the age of 75.[8,88] The incidence rises steeply at the menopause in women and then plateaus above the age of 65, whereas the incidence changes little with age in men.[97] It has been suggested that the rise in incidence at the menopause is due to an increase in postural instability and therefore falls in women at this age.[98,99] The absence of a further increase in incidence of forearm fractures after age of 65 may be due to the fact that the arm is less likely to be used to break a fall in the elderly. About 50% of postmenopausal women with Colles fracture have evidence of osteoporosis at the forearm, spine, or hip.[100] Forearm fractures are also associated with an increased risk of vertebral and hip fractures in both men and women.[101–103]

Vertebral fractures

The incidence and prevalence of vertebral fractures is difficult to quantify, as many patients with this fracture do not seek medical attention.[12] The European Vertebral Osteoporosis Study (EVOS) showed that the overall prevalence of vertebral deformity increased in women from 5% at the age of 50 years to 25% at 75 years, whereas the corresponding figures for men were 10% and 18%.[104] The higher prevalence of vertebral deformity in young men compared with women may be due to greater exposure to trauma. There was also a large variation in the prevalence of vertebral fractures across Europe, which may reflect differences in physical activity and other lifestyle factors.[105] Subsequently, the European Prospective Osteoporosis Study (EPOS) showed that the incidence of radiologically apparent vertebral fractures approximately doubles in women every 10 years, from less than 5/1000 person-years at the age of 50 years to about 25/1000 person-years by the late 1970s.[106] In men, the incidence also increases with age, but at a slower rate.[106]

In addition to back pain, loss of height, and kyphosis, vertebral fractures may also result in loss of energy, emotional problems, sleep disturbance, social isolation, and reduced mobility.[12,107] There is also an increased mortality associated with vertebral crush fractures, but this may be due to coexisting conditions associated with osteoporosis rather than the fracture itself.[108] Data from the Study of Osteoporotic Fractures in the United States show that mortality increases with the number of vertebral fractures.[109] It has been estimated that the acute cost of vertebral fractures in the United Kingdom is £12 million/year,[110] but the real cost may be substantially higher because of the associated long-term morbidity. Patients with symptomatic vertebral fracture consult their general practitioners 14 times more than control subjects in the year following fracture,[110] so they are likely to continue to use health and social service resources at an increased rate. Previous vertebral fracture increases the risk of further vertebral fractures and hip fracture.[111,112] An incident vertebral fracture is associated with a 20% risk of further vertebral fracture in the next year.[112]

KEY POINTS
Metabolic Bone Disease

- Fractures are a major cause of excess mortality, morbidity, and health and social service expenditure in older people.
- The risk of fracture is determined by skeletal and nonskeletal risk factors.
- The incidence of osteoporosis, osteomalacia, and Paget's disease increases with advancing age, contributing to the risk of fracture in older people.
- Treatments are available for osteoporosis, which improve bone density and reduce the risk of vertebral, hip, and other non-vertebral fractures.
- In addition to the increased risk of fracture, osteomalacia, and Paget's disease may also lead to bone pain and skeletal deformity.
- The most common cause of osteomalacia in older people is vitamin D deficiency, which can be corrected by appropriate supplementation.
- Bisphosphonate treatment in Paget's disease reduces bone turn-over and decreases bone pain.

Hip fractures

This is the most important fracture in the elderly because it causes greater mortality, higher morbidity, and more expenditure than all other fractures combined. The incidence of this fracture rises steeply with age in both sexes, though it is considerably higher in women than men.[8,88] The remaining lifetime risk of a hip fracture in a 50-year-old woman is 11.4% for the hip, whereas the corresponding figure for a 50-year-old man is 3.1%.[8]

The risk of hip fractures is determined not only by BMD but also by nonskeletal risk factors. Studies show an increased risk of hip fracture with causes of secondary osteoporosis, such as oral corticosteroid therapy, thyroid disease, and hypogonadism, and with conditions associated with falling, like previous stroke, Parkinson's disease, and dementia.[113–117] Hip fractures are associated with a considerable mortality, particularly in individuals with multiple comorbid conditions.[118] This excess mortality following femoral neck fractures has been reported to be about 17% over 5 years, though most deaths occur within 6 months of fracture.[119] In addition to the excess mortality, femoral fractures are associated with considerable morbidity, with many patients becoming more immobile and more dependent. Between 25% and 50% of individuals are more dependent after fracture, with deterioration occurring more often in women over the age of 75 years, those with a poor clinical result, and those who were already dependent before fracture.[120–122] It has been estimated that the average cost of hip fracture in the United Kingdom is £12,000, of which £4,800 is due to acute costs.[112]

For a complete list of references, please visit online only at www.expertconsult.com

CHAPTER 70

Arthritis in the Elderly

David L. Scott

Rheumatic diseases are common in elderly people and are often undiagnosed or undertreated. Elderly patients have similar types of musculoskeletal disorders as those from younger age groups, with some differences in pattern, severity, and effect. Some diseases, particularly osteoarthritis and polymyalgia rheumatica, are more common in elderly people. The main rheumatic diseases of the elderly, summarized in Table 70 1, include inflammatory arthritis, degenerative arthritis, connective tissue diseases, soft tissue rheumatism, and back pain.

Arthritis is the most common cause of disability in people over 75 years of age.[1] One hospital-based survey in London showed 76% of patients admitted to an acute elderly unit had peripheral arthritis, 48% had arthritis directly contributing to their functional disability, and 19% did not volunteer information about their joint disease.[2] The prevalence of disabling joint diseases increases as people age; osteoarthritis is the dominant problem. A survey from North America[3] showed that adults over age 65 years accounted for 37% of arthritis cases in 2005 will account for 50% by 2030. Arthritis in the elderly is a major and growing medical problem.

DISEASE MECHANISMS

Joint inflammation involves many pathologic mediators including T- and B-cell activation, cytokine release, and joint destruction. The key changes are summarized in Table 70-2. A key change is synovial lining cell proliferation, accompanied by increased vascularity in the subintimal layer. At the margins of the synovium the pannus forms overlying cartilage and bone and causes destructive changes.

The causes of rheumatoid arthritis (RA) and other forms of inflammatory arthritis are unknown. One concept is that, in genetically predisposed patients, an infective agent or other stimulus triggers innate immunity by binding to toll-like receptors on dendritic cells and macrophages.[4] Smoking has been strongly implicated in this process.[5] This results in a local immune response involving cytokines and other inflammatory mediators together with other components of the innate immune system like complement and neutrophils. Subsequent T-cell activation creates a multimolecular immune/inflammatory cascade. Finally, joint damage, associated with the development of locally invasive "pannus" tissue, occurs through the actions of proteases, growth factors, and activated osteoclasts.

Symptoms and signs of arthritis

Local symptoms include pain, tenderness, swelling, and stiffness in the joints, periarticular tissues, ligaments and tendons, and muscles. Pain is the predominant symptom in inflammatory arthritis as well as in degenerative arthritis.[6,7] Usually persistent and moderately severe, it is often worse on movement, and it invariably limits patients' lifestyles.

Stiffness is the most characteristic arthritic symptom. It comprises both early morning stiffness and postexercise stiffness. Morning stiffness points toward inflammatory arthritis or polymyalgia rheumatica. It usually lasts longer than 60 minutes and can be prolonged. Postexercise stiffness points more toward osteoarthritis. Tenderness and swelling of the joints or tendons usually go together and indicate an inflammatory synovitis or tendonitis. They vary from very subtle to gross symptoms. Some elderly patients minimize the extent of their joint swelling, even though it is extensive on examination. Bony swelling of the joints usually indicates osteoarthritis.

Systemic symptoms vary. In rheumatoid arthritis or polymyalgia rheumatica, they can be quite marked and include malaise, anorexia, weight loss, and depression. Low-grade fevers can occur, especially in connective tissue disorders.

Investigations

Investigations range from full blood counts and routine biochemistry to immunologic measures of rheumatoid factor and analysis of synovial fluid for crystals. The main tests are summarized in Table 70-3.

RHEUMATOID FACTOR

Rheumatoid factors are antibodies against the Fc fragment of IgG. Rheumatoid factors react against different species of IgG, including human and rabbit. Rheumatoid factors can involve different immunoglobulin classes, giving IgM, IgG, and IgA rheumatoid factors.[8] Different subclasses of antibody can also be involved, such as IgA_1 and IgA_2 rheumatoid factors. Most tests detect IgM rheumatoid factor. There is some evidence that IgA rheumatoid factor is more related to joint destruction. Rheumatoid factor positivity goes with worse disease and poorer outcome in rheumatoid arthritis and is associated with subcutaneous nodules, vasculitis, and other extraarticular features. Osteoarthritis, gout, and psoriatic arthritis should all be negative on tests for rheumatoid factor.

Table 70-1. The Main Musculoskeletal Disorders of the Elderly

Type of Disorder	Examples
Inflammatory synovitis	Rheumatoid arthritis Gout Pseudogout Septic arthritis
Degenerative arthritis	Osteoarthritis
Vasculitis and connective tissue diseases	Polymyalgia rheumatica Temporal arteritis Systemic lupus erythematosus
Soft tissue rheumatism	Rotator cuff shoulder lesions Frozen shoulder
Back pain	Mechanical back pain and disc disease Lumbar spondylosis and spondylolisthesis Spinal stenosis Osteoporotic vertebral fracture Spinal malignancy

ANTICYCLIC CITRULLINATED PEPTIDE ANTIBODIES (ANTI-CCP)

These were initially described as antibodies to keratin in buccal mucosal cells and keratinized esophageal cells. They were variously termed antiperinuclear factor, antikeratin antibodies, and antifilaggrin antibodies. They target citrullinated proteins. Citrulline is a nonstandard amino acid. It is formed from arginine by enzymic degradation. Citrullination occurs as part of the inflammatory reaction. A number of enzyme-linked immunosorbent assays can detect antibodies to citrullinated proteins. The second generation assays used cyclic epitopes selected from libraries of citrullinated peptides to provide the most sensitive assays. Anti-CCP assays are more sensitive and more specific for rheumatoid arthritis than rheumatoid factor assays.[9]

Table 70-2. Key Immunologic Mechanisms

Cytokines and immune regulation	Regulate inflammation and autoimmunity in the joints
Cytokines and bone	Also responsible for osteoclast maturation and activation; hierarchical role for receptor activator of nuclear factor-κ β ligand (RANKL) together with TNF, IL-17, and IL-1
T-cell activation	T-cell activation, particularly toward T helper 1 cells, is associated with the presence of many interleukins in the synovial tissue and drives inflammation
B cells	Critical roles in synovitis via antigen presentation and cytokine release
Macrophages	Macrophage-derived cytokines drive many of the proinflammatory pathways in synovial tissue

Table 70-3. Laboratory Investigations

Class of Test	Category	Example of Abnormality
Hematology	Hemoglobin	Anemia in rheumatoid arthritis
	White blood cell count	Leukocytosis in septic arthritis
	Platelet count	Thrombocytopenia in systemic lupus erythematosus
	ESR	Elevated in polymyalgia rheumatica
Biochemistry	Creatinine	High with involvement in systemic vasculitis
	Uric acid	Elevated in gout
	Creatine kinase	Elevated in polymyositis
Immunology	Rheumatoid factor	Positive in rheumatoid arthritis
	Anticyclic citrullinated peptide antibodies	Positive in rheumatoid arthritis
	Antinuclear antibody	Positive in systemic lupus erythematosus
	C-reactive protein	Elevated in rheumatoid arthritis
	Immunoglobulins	Elevated in Sjögren's syndrome
	Complements C3 and C4	Low in active systemic lupus erythematosus
Synovial fluid microscopy	Crystals	Present in gout and calcium pyrophosphate crystal deposition disease
Culture	Bacteria	Septic arthritis

OTHER IMMUNOLOGIC TESTS

Antinuclear antibodies are more important in connective tissue diseases, although rheumatoid arthritis is a common cause of low-titer positive antinuclear antibodies. There are many types of antinuclear antibodies, and the less specific IgM subclasses are more often seen in RA. Osteoarthritis, gout, and psoriatic arthritis should be negative for antinuclear antibodies.

The other main area of testing is for acute-phase changes. An elevated C-reactive protein level—together with a high erythrocyte sedimentation rate (ESR) and changes in several serum proteins—characterizes active RA. It is termed the acute-phase response. It is mediated by the cytokine network, especially IL-1 and IL-6. The levels of these cytokines can be measured directly, but they are labile and secreted in pulses and thus are poor measures of disease activity in many cases.

IMAGING IN ARTHRITIS

The modalities of imaging are summarized in Table 70-4. Currently plain joint radiographs remain the most widely used method for determining the extent and nature of structural changes in arthritis. The main radiologic changes include periarticular osteoporosis and sclerosis, loss of joint space (reflecting cartilage damage), juxta-articular erosions, marginal osteophytes, joint destruction, and ankylosis.[10] Although joint radiographs offer one of the most objective methods of assessing joint destruction, they are not ideal assessments of disease progression and overall status.

An important development has been the widespread introduction of high-resolution ultrasound.[11] This is better than clinical examination and conventional x-rays in diagnosing and assessing joint and bursal effusion and synovitis. It is the imaging modality of choice for tendon pathology. It is also more sensitive in detecting erosions. The main changes seen on ultrasound comprise effusions, synovial swelling indicating synovitis, tendonitis, and tendon rupture and erosions. Doppler ultrasound, particularly power Doppler or color Doppler imaging, allows an assessment of synovial vascularity. It can therefore help distinguish inflamed and nonvascular synovial swelling.

Magnetic resonance imaging (MRI) gives excellent images in arthritis and can show softtissue changes, cartilage changes, bony erosions, and inflammatory change in the synovium.[12] Gadolinium-based intravenous contrast agents

Table 70-4. Imaging Methods

Modality	Example
Plain radiology	X-rays of hands in rheumatoid arthritis
Magnetic resonance imaging	Imaging of knee joint to show internal derangement
Ultrasound	Imaging shoulder joint to identify rotator cuff tear
Computed tomography	Imaging of sacroiliac joint if infection suspected
Bone scan	Showing active joints in inflammatory synovitis
DEXA	Identifying osteoporosis with inflammatory synovitis

are useful for defining the extent and severity of synovitis. MRI is the most sensitive approach for identifying destructive changes in early arthritis and for defining the benefits of early treatments. It remains more of a research investigation at present.

Physiologic measurements and diagnostic assessments can both be achieved using nuclear medicine techniques and densitometry. Most experience comes from bone scintigraphy, which evaluated a combination of bone blood flow and osteoblastic activity. Its resolution is poor and this is a limiting factor. The three-phase bone scan looks at initial uptake, the blood pool interval, and subsequent localization within the bones.[13]

Densitometry has many advantages for assessing bone changes. It can be either whole-body densitometry or localized views of specific joints, particularly the hand and wrist.[14] Although patients with osteoarthritis often have generalized osteoporosis, they may also have localized bone loss at sites of inflammation.

Drug therapy in arthritis

ANTIINFLAMMATORY DRUGS

Nonsteroidal antiinflammatory drugs (NSAIDs) are a diverse group of drugs; their name distinguishes them from steroids and analgesics. They are one of the most frequently used groups of drugs. However, their benefits must be set against significant risks from gastrointestinal, renal, and cardiac toxicity, which cause a substantial number of deaths each year.[15–17] NSAIDs can be used locally; they are less effective used in this way but also less likely to cause adverse events. The central effect of NSAIDs is inhibiting cyclooxygenase (COX). Conventional NSAIDs inhibit COX-1, which is responsible for the production of "housekeeping" prostaglandins critical for normal renal, gastric, and vascular function and COX-2, which is responsible for driving inflammation. Newer NSAIDs focus on selectively inhibiting COX-2, with the intention of reducing unwanted adverse effects, particularly gastric ulcers.

Ibuprofen, the first nonaspirin NSAID, was identified in the early 1950s, and by the 1970s it was being widely prescribed for the treatment of arthritis. Subsequently a large number of NSAIDs were identified. NSAIDs such as diclofenac, ibuprofen, and naproxen are well established and have been available for many years. New COXIBs, or COX-2 (cyclooxygenase 2) specific inhibitors, such as celecoxib, have been introduced more recently. The main NSAIDs are summarized in Table 70-5.

NSAIDs reduce the signs and symptoms of acute synovitis and relieve pain and are widely used in RA, osteoarthritis, gout, back pain, and soft tissue rheumatism. They are highly effective in the short term. Their longer-term benefits are less certain.

Adverse effects are the major problem-limiting factor using NSAIDs. The risks increase markedly with age and NSAIDs must be used carefully in the elderly. Minor adverse effects such as dyspepsia and headache are commonplace. Central nervous system side effects, such as drowsiness and confusion, are often underestimated. Hematologic side effects are very unusual. NSAIDs can also exacerbate asthma and cause rashes, though these effects are usually mild. The main adverse effects are shown in Table 70-6.

Gastrointestinal adverse effects are the main problem with NSAIDs. They include dyspepsia, gastric erosions, peptic ulceration, bleeding, perforation, hematemesis or melena, small bowel inflammation, occult blood loss, and anemia. Between 10 and 20 out of every 1000 RA patients taking NSAIDs for 1 year will have serious gastrointestinal complications. The mortality risks attributable to NSAID-related gastrointestinal adverse effects are four times that for those not using NSAIDs. Many patients who have serious gastrointestinal complications do not have prior dyspepsia. In the absence of warning signs, there is no way to ascertain if a patient is at the point of developing serious problems. Therefore, if NSAID use is unavoidable, some protective strategy is needed, particularly in those patients at greatest risk. There are several potential options.

One approach is co-prescribing proton pump inhibitors like omeprazole. This is effective and acceptable to

Table 70-5. Main Nonsteroidal Anti-inflammatory Drugs

Class	Drug	Common Dose	Comments
Conventional NSAIDs	Diclofenac	75 mg slow release bid	Rapid onset of action but concerns about liver toxicity
	Ibuprofen	600 mg tid	Short half-life giving great flexibility means frequent dosing
	Naproxen	500 mg bid	Effective without major toxicity concerns
COXIBs	Celecoxib	200 mg bid	Reduced gastric toxicity but unresolved concerns about cardiac adverse events
	Etoricoxib	60 mg daily	Reduced gastric toxicity and once daily dosing, but fluid retention makes it unsuitable for patients with cardiac problems

Table 70-6. Adverse Effects of NSAIDs

Type of Adverse Reaction	Example
Gastrointestinal	Indigestion Erosions Peptic ulcer Hemorrhage and perforation Small bowel enteropathy
Hepatic	Hepatocellular damage Cholestasis
Renal	Acute renal failure Interstitial nephritis
Hematologic	Thrombocytopenia Neutropenia Hemolytic anemia
Skin	Photosensitivity Urticaria Erythema multiforme
Chest	Bronchospasm Pneumonitis
Central nervous system	Headache Dizziness Confusion
Cardiac	Increased risk of myocardial infarctions Cardiac failure Hypertension

patients. Another approach is to co-prescribe prostaglandin analogues, like misoprostol. This is also effective but causes added side effects such as diarrhea and is less well tolerated than proton pump inhibitors. The final approach is to use a safer NSAID—one of the newer COX-2 drugs. Although COXIBs increase the incidence of gastrointestinal adverse events compared to placebo, the magnitude is substantially less than with standard NSAID therapy.

There have been concerns that NSAIDs and COXIBs increase the risk of heart attacks and strokes. This is an area of controversy.[18,19] Some trials and some observational studies have found more cardiac problems; other trials have not done so. It is generally recommended that the lowest dose for the shortest period of time is a sensible policy. Patients at risk of cardiac disease should not receive NSAIDs and in particular should avoid COXIBs. As well as cardiac infarctions, some NSAIDs have an increased risk of fluid retention and can cause an increased propensity to cardiac failure.

DISEASE-MODIFYING DRUGS AND IMMUNOSUPPRESSION

Disease-modifying antirheumatic drugs (DMARDs) and immunosuppression are mainly used to treat inflammatory synovitis. The assessment of their effect includes clinical, laboratory, functional, and radiologic approaches. A central theme of therapy—disease control—is based on overcoming the inflammatory synovitis and thus reducing the progression of joint damage.[20] The effects of generalized inflammation indicated by the acute-phase response on the progression of RA are well known, as is the association between radiologic progression and acute-phase proteins such as C-reactive protein. However, normalizing an elevated acute-phase response may be insufficient, and only patients who consistently maintain low ESR and C-reactive protein levels have less radiologic progression.

A number of DMARDs are used and they are summarized in Table 70-7. Methotrexate is currently the dominant DMARD. Over half of all patients with rheumatoid arthritis treated with DMARDs who are seen in specialist units are receiving methotrexate. The only other DMARDs used to any appreciable extent are sulfasalazine and leflunomide. A systematic review comparing trials of the main DMARDs concluded that methotrexate, sulfasalazine, and leflunomide all showed similar efficacy.[21]

In patients with definite inflammatory arthritis, DMARDs are usually started as soon as the diagnosis has been made. They are then usually continued unless they have to be stopped for toxicity or loss of effect. In patients who are well controlled on DMARDs, stopping treatment leads to a high risk of flares. DMARD use is similar in all stages of arthritis. Patients need DMARDs in early disease and are equally likely to need them in later stages of the disease.

Table 70-7. Main Disease-Modifying Antirheumatic Drugs

Main Drugs	Minor Drugs	Rarely Used
Methotrexate	Hydroxychloroquine and chloroquine	Cyclosporine
Leflunomide	Injectable gold	Auranofin
Sulfasalazine	Azathioprine	Cyclophosphamide

Conventionally DMARDs were given singly. However, there is extensive evidence that they are also effective in combinations.[22] One approach is step-down treatment, which involves starting combinations together and then stopping one or more DMARD. The alternative is step-up treatment, which involves starting one DMARD and then adding another if needed. Combinations can involve two DMARDs, three DMARDs, or DMARDs and steroids. They are also often combined with biologics (discussed later).

DMARDs have a range of adverse events, and these vary between drugs. Gastrointestinal problems are common and include anorexia, nausea, vomiting, and diarrhea. Stomatitis with erythema, painful ulcers, and erosions is often seen. Alopecia is frequent with some drugs, particularly methotrexate, and causes particular concern in women. Skin reactions ranging from rashes to urticaria and cutaneous vasculitis affect many patients. Many DMARDs increase the risk of infections, including opportunistic infections, fungal infections, and viral problems like herpes zoster sometimes. The risks of blood and hepatic toxicity mean many DMARDs require monitoring with blood and liver function tests. Although with modern treatment the risks are minimized and the benefits of monitoring are less certain, it has become part of the standard approach to DMARD treatment. Chest problems are a particular concern with methotrexate and a pretreatment chest X-ray is needed; therapy should be paused or stopped if patients develop chest symptoms such as a cough.

Biologics

These agents have revolutionized the treatment of inflammatory arthritis. Conventional drugs such as DMARDs inhibit small molecules. However, as cytokines are large peptides, they can only be inhibited by large molecules. The biologics that inhibit cytokines are proteins, based on immunoglobulins. It may be possible to replace biologics with small molecules that inhibit intracellular cytokine targets, but so far this aspiration remains unfulfilled.

The dominant biologics are tumor necrosis factor (TNF) inhibitors. Three of these are now available, and these are summarized in Table 70-8. They are effective in rheumatoid arthritis and psoriatic arthritis and also in ankylosing spondylitis.[23–28] Depending on the biologic, they are either given by infusions or by self-injection every week or fortnight. They are usually given with methotrexate or an equivalent DMARD. They are rapidly effective and improve both synovitis and function. In addition, they reduce erosive damage.

Biologics are usually given only to patients in whom conventional DMARDs have proved ineffective and in whom there is evidence of ongoing synovitis. There is debate about their early use and currently this is not usually recommended.

When a TNF inhibitor is stopped for toxicity, another agent is usually started. There is less certainty when the TNF inhibitor is not effective. Many experts recommend starting an alternative biologic in this situation. It is an area of controversy.

The main alternative biologic is rituximab, which inhibits B cells.[29] It is mainly used in patients who have failed TNF inhibitors. A course of rituximab comprises two intravenous infusions 2 weeks apart. It is given with methotrexate. If there is evidence of continued disease activity, another course is given after 6 to 12 months. Some patients have had repeated

Table 70-8. Main Tumor Necrosis Factor Inhibitors

TNF-α Inhibitor	Site of Action	Dosing Schedule	Disease-Modifying Drugs
Adalimumab	Mainly binds soluble and transmembrane TNF-α	Subcutaneous fortnightly	Best to co-prescribe methotrexate
Etanercept	Binds TNF-α and competitive inhibitor of TNF receptor	Subcutaneous twice weekly	Best to co-prescribe methotrexate
Infliximab	Mainly binds soluble and transmembrane TNF-α	IV administration every 4 to 8 weeks	Needs co-prescribed methotrexate or equivalent

courses. Other biologics that inhibit T cells or interleukin-6 have either entered or are about to enter clinical practice. It is an area of rapid development.

Biologics cause local reactions at the injection sites. The main risk is serious and opportunistic infections. Biologics should not be started or should be discontinued when serious infections occur. Tuberculosis is a particular concern. There have been some reports of demyelinating-like disorders and a few cases of pancytopenia and aplastic anemia. Another potential problem is cardiac failure, and patients in whom this is a problem should not receive TNF inhibitors.

Finally there are concerns about the risk of lymphomas. The size of the risk is uncertain because the incidence of lymphoma increases in severe RA irrespective of treatment with immunotherapies. As a result, there is a preexisting increased risk of lymphoma in patients who are likely to receive TNF-α inhibitors.

Steroids

Glucocorticoids, which are invariably termed steroids in routine settings, have been used for more than 50 years to treat arthritis. Their efficacy and toxicity have been known since the 1950s.[30,31] Although their use extends well beyond rheumatoid arthritis, in other settings such as acute gout there is less evidence supporting their use.[32] The long-term side effects of steroids, particularly osteoporosis, remain a substantial obstacle limiting their routine use. Short courses of oral prednisolone or a depot intramuscular injection are often used in active disease when commencing therapy with a DMARD or to control flares of arthritis.

The more prolonged use of oral steroids is advantageous in early disease. There is strong evidence based on the work of Kirwan[33,34] that steroids reduce erosive progression, particularly when used in early rheumatoid arthritis. In this setting, the benefits of steroids outweigh their risks.

SUPPORTIVE NONDRUG THERAPY

Physiotherapy, occupational therapy, supplying aids, and appliances such as walking sticks, modifying footwear such as fitting insoles and providing surgical shoes, and chiropody all have important roles. Of equal importance is providing patient education and general advice about arthritis, together where possible with simple exercise programs.

RHEUMATOID ARTHRITIS

Epidemiology

Rheumatoid arthritis is a common disorder. We know the incidence of new cases of RA from prospective studies such as the Norfolk Arthritis Register; there will be in the region of 50 new cases of inflammatory synovitis each year per 100,000 population in the United Kingdom.[35] Most of these will be due to RA. There is marked geographic variation in the incidence of RA. Its cause is uncertain.

There is also a considerable amount of information about the prevalence of established RA. In Europe, this varies from 0.5% to 2% or more depending on the exact population studied.[36] Recent U.K. data suggests the prevalence of RA is relatively static at just under 1% of adults.[37] The prevalence of RA increases with age, and it is especially frequent in elderly women. A study in North America in the early 1960s showed that it was rare in men before the age of 45 years and in women before the age of 35 years. In the over-65 age group its prevalence increased to 1.8% in males and 4.9% in females.[38]

Clinical features of rheumatoid arthritis

Persistent joint inflammation is the central diagnostic feature of RA. The joints are swollen, tender, and stiff. Morning stiffness is prolonged and may last over an hour. The joint involvement is symmetrical and usually involves the hands (proximal interphalangeal and metacarpophalangeal joints), wrists, and feet (proximal interphalangeal and metatarsophalangeal joints). The elbows, knees, and ankles are often involved as well.

The synovitis is accompanied by systemic features of ill health with malaise, weight loss, occasional intermittent fever, and constitutional upset in many cases. As the arthritis progresses there are characteristic destructive changes—for example, ulnar deviation and the Swan neck and Boutonnière deformities of the fingers.

Subcutaneous nodules are a classic extra-articular feature. They are found on extensor surfaces such as the elbows or sites of pressure such as the lower back or in some parts of the hands. There are many other extra-articular features, which are summarized in Table 70-9. Extra-articular disease can occur at any time in the course of RA. Up to 40% of patients may have one or more extra-articular features.[39] The most common features are rheumatoid nodules (30-year cumulative incidence, 34%), secondary Sjögren's syndrome (30-year cumulative incidence, 11%), and pulmonary fibrosis (30-year cumulative incidence, 7%). About 10% of patients have severe extraarticular features; these patients have worse outcomes and higher mortality rates.[40]

Clinical assessment

The core dataset, which has been agreed on internationally,[41] is summarized in Table 70-10. The measures give a good overall picture of RA and permit assessment of progression and response to treatment. Disease activity can be assessed by counting the number of active joints. The best joint count has been an area of recent investigation. Prevoo et al[42] contrasted several available methods. The various

Table 70-9. Extraarticular Features of Rheumatoid Arthritis

Extraarticular Feature	Specific Example
Subcutaneous nodules	Pressure area at elbow
	In wall of olecranon bursa
	At sacrum
Pulmonary	Pleural effusion
	Interstitial fibrosis
Cardiac	Pericarditis
	Valvular disease
Ocular	Keratoconjunctivitis sicca
	Episcleritis
	Scleritis
Neurologic	Carpal tunnel syndrome
	Mononeuritis multiplex
	Peripheral neuropathy
	Cervical myelopathy
Renal	Amyloidosis
	Drug toxicity
Vasculitis	Nail-fold infarctions
	Leg ulcers
	Systemic vasculitis
Hematologic	Anemia
	Felty syndrome

Table 70-10. Clinical Measures in Rheumatoid Arthritis

Index	Measures
Core data set	Number of swollen joints
	Number of tender joints
	Pain assessed by the patient
	Patient's global assessments of disease activity
	Physician's global assessments of disease activity
	Laboratory evaluation of an acute-phase reactant (ESR, C-reactive protein, or equivalent)
	Disability measure
Disease activity score (DAS28)	Tender joint count
	Swollen joint count
	Patient global assessment
	ESR
Simple disease activity index (SDAI)	Tender joint count
	Swollen joint count
	Patient global assessment
	Physician global assessment
	C-reactive protein
Clinical disease activity index (CDAI)	Tender joint count
	Swollen joint count
	Patient global assessment
	Physician global assessment

indices had similar reliability and validity, and no joint index was superior for measuring disease activity. The implication is that the simplest index, the 28-joint count, is best. Other studies have also concluded that the 28-joint count gives all the necessary information. Disability is assessed using standard questionnaires. The most widely used is the Health Assessment Questionnaire (HAQ).[43]

Clinical outcomes

Studies of antirheumatic therapy tend to show that it is successful in the short term, whereas there are poor results in the longer term. Prospective long-term clinical studies show that most patients first seen as inpatients are moderately or severely impaired by 20 years, and the average outpatient has a 30% chance of severe disability.[44]

Rheumatoid arthritis leads to premature death. In hospitalized patients with RA, it is the direct cause of nearly 20% of deaths. Wolfe et al[45] reported results from a large study examining 922 deaths in 3501 patients with RA. The standardized mortality ratio was 2.3. The causes of death in RA do not differ much from those in the normal population, although there is an increase in infection and lymphatic malignancies as a cause of death. The average shortening of life is in the region of 4 to 5 years. Patients with severe RA are most likely to die early.

Specific problems in the elderly population

Rheumatoid arthritis is increasingly becoming a disease of later life. The most common time for developing the disease is the sixth decade, and as it lasts 10 to 20 years, many patients with RA are over 65 years old. One aspect, the impact of age on disease onset, has been studied in detail. Compared with young-onset RA, elderly-onset patients more frequently have an acute onset, commonly have polymyalgic and constitutional features, usually have higher levels of disease activity when first seen, and are more often male,[46–49] confirming a significant influence of age on disease expression at presentation.

When its onset is in old age, it is often overlooked or ignored by patients and physicians. It is difficult to manage complex RA in an elderly person, especially if he or she has other problems with mobility. RA is frequently associated with other diseases, and such comorbidity can be a serious clinical problem. Finally, elderly people have increased risks of adverse effects with antirheumatic drugs such as nonsteroidal antiinflammatory agents, and this makes management more complex.

SERONEGATIVE SPONDYLARTHRITIS

These diseases include ankylosing spondylitis, reactive arthritis, arthritis in Crohn's disease and ulcerative colitis, Reiter's syndrome, and psoriatic arthritis. They are characterized by sacroiliitis, inflammatory back disease, oligoarthritis of large joints, and an enthesopathy. Psoriatic arthritis is the most important seronegative arthritis in the elderly.

Epidemiology

As a group, these disorders are less common than RA.[50,51] Their prevalence varies across populations in relation to the frequency of HLA-B27; this gene is closely associated with the development of ankylosing spondylitis and, to a lesser extent, other members of this group. Estimates suggest that about 0.3% of adults have psoriatic arthritis, but estimates vary and there may be an underestimation of mild disease.

Clinical features

Most forms of seronegative arthritis involve a small number of large joints, particularly the knee and hip joints. Joint involvement is usually asymmetric. Psoriatic arthritis has a more complex pattern.[52] In some patients, there is a polyarthritis, which is similar to rheumatoid arthritis. In many patients, there is an oligoarthritis, with two or three joints involved. Some patients have a monoarthritis. A specific variant is a destructive arthritis mainly involving the distal joints. Occasional patients have arthritis mutilans, which is a progressive destructive form of arthritis. These different patterns change over time, and one form of psoriatic arthritis can merge with the other. The deformities of psoriatic arthritis lead to shortening of digits because of severe joint or bone lysis, with the most severe form being the telescoping of digits. Bony fusion of joints may also occur. Radiologic changes include "pencil in cup" and ankylosis, and there is periosteal reaction, enthesitis, and spinal involvement. Another feature is dactylitis, which is inflammation of an entire digit because of to inflammation affecting both joints and tendons.

The extraarticular features of psoriatic arthritis are very different from those seen in RA. Rheumatoid nodules are absent. Other findings include iritis, mucous membrane lesions, iritis, urethritis, diarrhea, and aortic root dilatation.

OSTEOARTHRITIS

Osteoarthritis (OA) is a heterogeneous condition with a variety of causes and patterns of expression. It is analogous to kidney or heart failure in which similar clinical and pathologic features develop irrespective of the underlying causes and could be considered as "joint failure." Older age is the most significant factor in its development in a general population.[53] The joint most commonly affected is the knee, and osteoarthritis of the knee is one of the most common causes of pain and disability in the community. There is a rise in the annual consultation rate for osteoarthritis,[54] and this may reflect not only an increased incidence of disease but also decreased tolerance of joint problems. Many patients who consult with osteoarthritis have other medical problems, and it is difficult to dissociate which was the main cause of seeking medical advice.[55]

Osteoarthritis can be considered as a synovial joint syndrome rather than a single disease. Pathologically it is characterized by a loss of, and change in, the composition of cartilage proteoglycans leading to failure of normal responses to stress. The results include cartilage fibrillation and loss, bone exposure, and a clinical syndrome of pain and disability. Rare forms of heritable chondrodysplasia lead to premature osteoarthritis but, in most instances, its cause is either excess, inappropriate, or insufficient mechanical demand or traumatic, infective, inflammatory, endocrine, or metabolic disease. There remain idiopathic ("primary") cases in which no cause is demonstrable.

Epidemiology

The prevalence of OA varies depending on how it is defined, which joints are studied, and the features of the population being studied.[56] All studies show OA prevalence increases steeply with age. Radiologic OA in people over 45 years varies from 20% to 37% in different studies.[57] Fewer patients have symptomatic OA.

In Europe and North America, there is a similar prevalence, rising from less than 1% of those aged under 35 years to over 30% of those aged over 75 years.[58,59] Both hand and knee forms of osteoarthritis are more common in women than in men. Hip osteoarthritis is less common, and its prevalence rates in men and women appear to be more similar. The incidence of symptomatic osteoarthritis has been studied less often. One study from North America showed the incidence of knee and hip osteoarthritis was 200 per 100,000 person-years.[60] Felson et al[61] evaluated 869 patients from the Framingham osteoarthritis study and found rates of incident disease were 1.7 times higher in women than in men, progressive disease occurred slightly more often in women, but rates did not vary by age. Among women, approximately 2% per year developed incident radiographic disease, 1% per year developed symptomatic knee osteoarthritis, and about 4% per year experienced progressive knee osteoarthritis.

Clinical features

Osteoarthritis is characterized by articular pain, bony enlargement, morning and inactivity stiffness, and associated functional disability and radiography changes. These features are summarized in Table 70-11.

Pain is the predominant symptom in osteoarthritis. It varies in severity and its exact nature both between patients and in individual cases over a period of time. Although pain is more marked in patients with severe joint destruction on x-rays, there is often no close relationship between pain and radiography abnormalities. Causes of pain in osteoarthritis include raised intraosseous pressure, inflammatory synovitis, periarticular problems, periosteal elevation, muscular changes, fibromyalgic amplification, and central neurogenic changes. There is often relatively little relationship between the severity and clinical importance of pain, stiffness, and physical function.[62]

Most patients with osteoarthritis experience stiffness. "Stiffness" may refer to difficulty initiating movement, problems in completing a full range of movement, or the ache or pain of a joint on movement. It is often present first thing in the morning, but lasts only 10 to 25 minutes in many cases. More characteristically it comes on after inactivity, when it is frequently termed "gelling" of a joint.

Many patients have loss of movement or instability of one or more joints. Sometimes patients note that a joint will suddenly "give way." In some joints, there is a sensation of inflammation due to an associated synovitis and the joint is swollen, tender, and warm.

On examination there is firm or bony swelling around the joint and crepitus on movement. The most characteristic bony swellings are the Heberden's and Bouchard's nodes of hand osteoarthritis. Coarse "crepitations" are usually felt on movement of the involved joint. In severe disease, they can be audible. Effusions occur in some cases, especially in knee osteoarthritis.

There are problems in diagnosing osteoarthritis. Although a set of clinical criteria has been developed,[63] these have been criticized for using rheumatoid patients who had not been age- and sex-matched as controls, using osteophytes as

Table 70-11. Clinical and Radiologic Features of Osteoarthritis

Clinical Features	Radiologic Features
Pain	Loss of joint space
Stiffness, including gelling after exercise	Marginal osteophytes
Bony tenderness	Subchondral sclerosis
Bony enlargement	Tibial spiking
Crepitus	Loss of alignment
Normal ESR and negative tests for rheumatoid factor	

a feature of osteoarthritis, for circularity, and for inadequate validation.[64] Loss of cartilage on x-rays has been reported as the one feature present in all attempted definitions, but these are based on pathologic changes that are not often available to the clinician making the diagnosis. Furthermore, the relationship between the incidence of symptoms and the degree of radiologic change is not clear. Almost all people over the age of 65 years have at least one joint with evidence of radiographic osteoarthritis, but the proportion with symptoms varies with joint, age, and sex.

Clinical subgroups

Osteoarthritis includes several different subgroups that may all have different natural histories, patterns of joints affected, and different rates of disease progression. These include knee/hand osteoarthritis (often known as "generalized osteoarthritis"), inflammatory/erosive osteoarthritis, rapidly progressive osteoarthritis, secondary osteoarthritis, hypertrophic and atrophic osteoarthritis, and destructive osteoarthritis of the elderly.

Set against the classification of osteoarthritis into such distinct subgroups are the findings of Cushnaghan and Dieppe,[65] who found a strong relationship between age and the number of involved sites. This was thought to be due to the slow addition of new joint sites with age. However, there was no evidence of well-defined clinical subsets of patients. Subsequent follow-up after 3 years[66] showed most patients reported an overall worsening of their condition, but pain severity did not change. There was an overall increase in disability. Although there were strong correlations between changes in x-ray appearances (joint space, osteophyte, and subchondral bone sclerosis), there were no relationships between radiographic and clinical changes.

Inflammatory osteoarthritis and destructive disease in the elderly deserve special consideration. Destructive osteoarthritis with radiographic findings of rapid severe joint destruction can be a diagnostic problem. The x-ray changes mimic septic arthritis, rheumatoid, and seronegative arthritis. Rapid progression of pain and disability are consistent clinical features. The condition mainly affects the shoulder, knee, and hip.[67] Progression to complete joint destruction takes only 1 to 2 years. Most patients are elderly women. This disease is a relative rarity.

POLYMYALGIA RHEUMATICA AND GIANT CELL ARTERITIS

Polymyalgia rheumatica and giant cell arteritis, which is also known as temporal arteritis, are related diseases that form two ends of a single spectrum. They are both diseases of the elderly population and their mean age of onset is 70 years, with a range from 50 to 90 years. Their onset is characteristically dramatic, and many patients can give the exact date and hour of their first symptoms. Occasionally the onset is insidious and the symptoms may have been present for months or longer before the diagnosis.

Paulley and Hughes,[68] in 1962, were the first to link these two conditions, suggesting polymyalgia has many of the manifestations of temporal arteritis. Since then, most authorities recognize the relationship between the two conditions.

Epidemiology

These diseases are relatively uncommon. One study from North America suggested the annual incidence of biopsy-proven giant cell arteritis between 1950 and 1985 in North America was up to 20 in 100,000 people over 50 years of age.[69,70] It was approximately three times more frequent in women. Studies from Europe suggest an incidence of 16.8 per 100,000.[71] In the United Kingdom, the prevalence of polymyalgic symptoms in people over 65 years of age is approximately 330 per 100,000.[72]

Clinical features

Both polymyalgia rheumatica and giant cell arteritis are associated with fever, fatigue, anorexia, weight loss, and depression. Occasionally patients present with a fever.

POLYMYALGIA RHEUMATICA

The onset usually involves pain and stiffness in the muscles of the shoulder and neck. There is eventual involvement of the pelvic girdles in some patients. The symptoms are bilateral and symmetric. Stiffness is a predominant feature, especially after rest or in the morning, and usually lasts for longer than an hour. Muscle pain is diffuse, movement accentuates the pain, and it can be worse at night. Muscle strength is usually unimpaired, although the pain makes testing difficult. There is often an associated synovitis especially of the knees, wrists, and small joints of the hands. It is usually transient and mild and erosive changes are unusual. The arthritis may overlap with rheumatoid disease in an elderly person.

GIANT CELL ARTERITIS

Headache is a predominant symptom and is present in a majority of cases. It often begins early in the course of the disease and may be a presenting symptom. Pain is severe and localized to the temple; there may be associated scalp tenderness. Visual disturbance is described in about 25% of cases; visual loss is less common and can involve 5% to 10% of cases, but blindness remains a significant risk owing to involvement of the ophthalmic artery, which is an end artery. Rare features of giant cell arteritis include hemiparesis, peripheral neuropathy, and deafness. Involvement of the coronary artery occasionally leads to myocardial infarction.

GOUT

Gout is one of the most common forms of arthritis affecting the elderly.[73] It is caused by an inflammatory response to the formation of urate crystals. These crystals develop secondary to hyperuricemia. Gout can occur in both acute and chronic forms. The hyperuricemia may be due to environmental or genetic factors. Although it most frequently affects middle-aged males, there is an increasing frequency in elderly females taking diuretic tablets. The acute form is usually relapsing and self-limiting. The chronic form is associated with tophus formation and bone and joint destruction.

Epidemiology

Hyperuricemia has been investigated in many populations. In males, the prevalence of hyperuricemia rises steeply after puberty; in females, the prevalence rises after the menopause, although levels in women are usually lower than in men. It is difficult to determine the precise incidence and prevalence of gout, as it is a remitting and relapsing disease and patients frequently are misdiagnosed. It is rare in children and premenopausal women. It is uncommon in men under the age of 30, and the peak onset in men is between 40 and 50 years. In women it occurs later.

The epidemiology of gout is changing, with an increasing number of females having the disease. This is probably because of changes in lifestyle, drug therapy, and increased longevity. Gout remains the most common inflammatory arthritis in males over 40 years of age.[74] The prevalence of gout is between 5 and 28 per 1000 males and between 1 and 6 per 1000 females. The plasma urate concentration is the most important determinant of the risk of developing gout.[75] An important identifiable cause is concomitant thiazide diuretic therapy.

Clinical features

Asymptomatic hyperuricemia is far more frequent than gout. The risk of gout increases with a rising level of serum uric acid. However, many years of hyperuricemia may precede the onset of acute gout, and many individuals with hyperuricemia do not develop the disease. When there is a severe acute overproduction of urate, as, for example, occurs with cytotoxic chemotherapy, there is a high risk of acute gout.

Acute gout is characterized by the rapid onset of pain, its exquisite nature, and the swelling and associated redness around the affected joint. The classic presentation is in the first metatarsophalangeal joint, and in time this is affected in over 80% of patients with gout—this is known as podagra. Many joints may be involved. The lower limbs are involved more frequently than the upper limbs. Redness over the affected joints is a feature that sets gout apart from most other noninfective causes of arthritis. The swelling can be very marked over the entire region. The natural history of acute gout varies: mild attacks may resolve within 1 or 2 days. More severe attacks may last 1 or 2 weeks. Approximately 90% of initial attacks of gout are monoarticular.

Sometimes gout presents early in its course with polyarticular involvement, and it can then be easily confused with other forms of arthritis. In the elderly population, gout is often more indolent and is frequently mistaken for osteoarthritis, which results in a delay in diagnosis. In elderly people, polyarticular gout can be the presenting feature of an attack, especially in elderly women. Acute gout can be precipitated by a variety of factors, including acute illness, trauma, surgery, and alcohol and drugs, which increase the uric acid concentration.

Incomplete resolution of acute gout normally indicates a concurrent arthropathy, especially osteoarthritis. However, a substantial proportion of patients with acute gout go on to develop a chronic phase of the disease. This is characterized by the formation of tophi. These are firm nodular or fusiform swellings that can occur at most sites of the body but are especially common on the hands and feet and around the ear. The inflammatory process in chronic gout is often mild although there can be supra-added acute episodes. Most of the disability is due to the presence of tophi that can become ulcerated and infected. Long-term problems with chronic gout are usually due to the deposition of tophi in the kidney.

Associated disorders

Gout is associated with obesity, hypertension with diuretic therapy and particularly thiazide diuretics, excess alcohol intake, hyperlipidemia, and other vascular disorders. There are also associations with renal impairment, psoriasis, myeloproliferative disorders, and treatment with cytotoxic drugs.

Treatment

Therapy is directed toward controlling the symptoms in acute episodes and preventing further attacks and complications in chronic gout.[76] Acute attacks of gout can be treated by oral NSAIDs, oral colchicine, or joint aspiration and injection of corticosteroid. Some patients respond to oral or IM steroids (Depo-Medrone). When NSAIDs are used, a conventional drug NSAID such as diclofenac or naproxen should be started as soon as possible, and the treatment should be continued until 48 hours after the attack has resolved. A proton pump inhibitor may be needed for gastric protection. Etoricoxib is an alternative COXIB. When NSAIDs are contraindicated, not tolerated, or have been ineffective in previous attacks, oral colchicine can be used at 500 μg, two to four times a day, until pain is relieved or diarrhea or vomiting occurs. Steroids may be preferable to colchicine.

In patients with recurrent acute attacks, tophi, or radiographic changes of gout, preventive treatment is required. This normally involves allopurinol, which inhibits the enzyme xanthine oxidase. The dosage varies from 100 to 600 mg daily; it is usual to start with a low dose and build up. The initiation of allopurinol may lead to an acute episode of gout, and it is conventional to start allopurinol at the same time as giving NSAID therapy. Allopurinol may make an acute attack of gout worse, so it is used subsequent to control of the joint inflammation with NSAIDs. If allopurinol toxicity occurs, options include other xanthine oxidase inhibitors, allopurinol desensitization, or a uricosuric. The uricosuric benzbromarone is more effective than allopurinol and can be used in patients with mild to moderate renal insufficiency, but it may be hepatotoxic. When gout is associated with the use of diuretics, the diuretic should be stopped if possible. For prophylaxis against acute attacks, either colchicine (0.5 to 1 mg daily) or an NSAID with gastroprotection, if indicated, is recommended.

CALCIUM PYROPHOSPHATE CRYSTAL DEPOSITION (CPCD)

This disease is associated with calcium pyrophosphate dihydrate crystal deposition. Although it is usually sporadic, there are familial forms and it can be associated with other metabolic disturbances. It is predominantly a disease of the elderly population, presenting with an acute self-limiting arthritis that is termed "pseudogout." There is a strong association and overlap with osteoarthritis. It mainly involves the large joints such as the knees and wrists. There is a spectrum of pathology. In some cases, there is only chondrocalcinosis, which is the deposition of calcium in articular cartilage and is usually asymptomatic. In other patients, there is more widespread deposition of pyrophosphate dihydrate, and an associated synovitis develops. Thus, although many patients with pseudogout have chondrocalcinosis, the latter can occur by itself and be asymptomatic or it may be seen against the background of osteoarthritis.

Epidemiology

Chondrocalcinosis has a female preponderance and is associated with aging. It is rare under the age of 50 years. In those aged between 65 to 75 years, it affects 10% to 15% of the population, and over the age of 85 years it affects up to 60% of the population.[77] The large population-based radiographic survey from Framingham,[78] which looked at a population ranging in age between 63 and 93 years, found an overall prevalence of 8%. No epidemiologic data exist for pyrophosphate arthropathy, although it is generally thought to occur in the elderly with a female preponderance. Most studies show that the mean age of presentation is between 65 and 75 years. It is rare in younger cases although occasionally seen. There are many associated conditions, including diabetes, anemia, Paget's disease, and hypothyroidism. The strongest association is with hemochromatosis.[79]

Clinical features of calcium pyrophosphate crystal deposition disease

Pyrophosphate crystal deposition disease can present as an acute synovitis, as chronic arthritis, or as an incidental finding. The classic presentation is the acute synovitis of pseudogout, which is the most common cause of an acute monoarthritis in the elderly population. The typical attack develops with severe pain, stiffness, and swelling maximal between 6 and 24 hours after the onset. The patient often describes the pain as very severe. There may be overlying erythema. Examination shows a tender joint with signs of marked synovitis such as warmth, a large intense effusion, joint line tenderness, and restriction of movement. Fever is common, and this can be marked. Elderly patients often appear unwell and mildly confused. The acute attacks are self-limiting and usually resolve within 1 to 3 weeks.

Chronic pyrophosphate arthropathy is also predominantly found in elderly and female patients. It mainly involves the knees, wrists, and shoulder joints. Presentation is with chronic pain, early morning and inactivity stiffness, reduced movement, and functional impairment. Acute attacks may be superimposed on this chronic history. Symptoms are often restricted to just a few joints, but occasionally multiple joint involvement is observed. Affected joints usually reveal signs of osteoarthritis, such as bony swelling, crepitus, and varying degrees of synovitis. Knee joints may be warm with some tenderness, effusion, and soft tissue thickening.

Examination may show more widespread evidence of osteoarthritis. There may also be occasionally more severe inflammatory features, and the presentation may develop into pseudo-RA, although the infrequency of tenosynovitis and the absence of extraarticular disease normally allows distinction.

Most patients present a benign course, and a majority of patients show stabilization of symptoms.[80] Occasionally, progressive severe destructive arthritis may occur, especially involving the knees, shoulders, or hips. This is almost entirely confined to elderly women, usually accompanied by severe night and rest pain and associated with a poor outcome.[81]

Atypical presentations are commonplace. A notable example is marked shoulder pain and stiffness that suggest polymyalgia rheumatica. A study from Spain[82] described 36 patients who met the diagnostic criteria for both polymyalgia and calcium pyrophosphate deposition disease. As a group, these patients were older and had peripheral arthritis more frequently.

Treatment

The aspiration of synovial fluid in acute synovitis associated with calcium pyrophosphate crystal deposition disease can markedly improve the initially severe symptoms. Analgesics and NSAIDs are usually given, and these also rapidly improve symptoms. Colchicine is effective but rarely warranted. For severe polyarticular attacks unresponsive to aspiration and injection, oral steroids may be considered although their efficacy is unproved. Once the synovitis is settling, active mobilization with attention to muscle training is worthwhile.

Unlike with gout, there is no specific therapy for chronic pyrophosphate arthropathy. Treatment of the underlying metabolic disease has little effect on outcome. The main objective is to reduce symptoms and maintain and improve function. Exercise programs, a reduction in obesity, and building up muscle strength are all immensely valuable. If osteoarthritic joint damage is a particular problem, surgical replacement must be considered.

APATITE DEPOSITION DISEASE

Periarticular deposits of calcific material that are predominantly carbonated apatites or intraarticular deposits of a variety of basic calcium phosphates, also predominantly apatites, are observed in a variety of disease settings. Calcific periarthritis and the acute synovitis associated with apatite deposition have different etiologies and clinical courses but are united by the presence of calcium deposits in bone.

The presence of calcific periarthritis has been recognized for many years. However, the relationship between apatite deposition and joint diseases is more recent and was not described in detail until 1976.[83]

Epidemiology

Calcific periarthritis is relatively common. In one large study of office workers, published in the 1940s, there was a prevalence of 2.7% of shoulder calcification.[84] Subsequent studies have found relatively similar high levels of shoulder calcification. There have been few studies of the epidemiology of articular apatite deposition, mainly because the relationship between pathologic and radiologic findings and symptoms of arthritis or the presence of an arthropathy or acute synovitis is uncertain. However, the finding of apatite particles in 30% to 60% of osteoarthritic synovial fluids may be of some pathologic relevance.[85]

Clinical features

Calcific deposits around the shoulder and elsewhere are often asymptomatic. They may be associated with a number of clinical syndromes. The most striking presentation is acute calcific periarthritis.[86] Over 70% of attacks occur around the shoulder, although other sites may be involved. The episode may be preceded by mild trauma or illness but is often spontaneous. Patients present with a sudden onset of severe pain described as "acute hyperalgia." Within hours there is often associated swelling that might be hot and red. There is extreme local tenderness. Movement around the shoulder is limited. The condition appears to be initiated by a rupture of the calcific deposit leading to crystals being shed into the adjacent periarticular tissues. Sites other than the shoulder that may be involved include the greater trochanter, the epicondyle, the wrist, and around the knee.[87]

In 1981, McCarty et al[88] described an important large-joint destructive arthropathy associated with apatite deposition. The shoulder is often involved, and the condition is often termed *Milwaukee shoulder.* Patients are usually over 70 years of age, and 90% are female. They present with a short history, over weeks and months, of pain, swelling, and loss of function of a shoulder. Aspiration shows a large quantity of synovial fluid, which may be blood-stained and contains apatite crystals.

Treatment

Acute calcific periarthritis requires high doses of NSAIDs; colchicine or local steroid injections are useful in some patients. Apatite deposition in osteoarthritis requires no specific treatments.

The destructive arthritis associated with Milwaukee shoulder is a difficult management problem. Antiinflammatory drugs, analgesics, and local steroids have all been used, but they are often ineffective. However, as symptoms do appear to be reduced in a majority of patients over a few months, conservative and simple symptomatic measures may eventually allow a resolution of the symptoms to occur as part of the natural history of the disease. Some centers recommend more intensive treatment such as tidal irrigation, which has been reported to result in considerable benefit.[89]

KEY POINTS
Arthritis in the Elderly

- Arthritis is common in the elderly.
- Over 30% of women over 75 years of age have clinical features of osteoarthritis.
- Over 5% of women over 75 years of age have rheumatoid arthritis.
- Arthritis causes substantial pain and disability and is a major factor in limiting quality of life.
- The treatment of arthritis is similar in elderly and younger people, although drug therapy requires greater caution in the elderly population.
- Intensive treatment of inflammatory arthritis is effective in elderly people, and there is no reason not to prescribe disease-modifying antirheumatic drugs or biologics for these patients.

For a complete list of references, please visit online only at www.expertconsult.com

CHAPTER 71

Connective Tissue Diseases

Anthony J. Freemont

INTRODUCTION

Connective tissue is found in all the organs of the body, usually forming a supporting scaffold for the cells or blood vessels within the tissue. In addition there are tissues that are composed exclusively of connective tissue. These fall into two major groups: those consisting of cells within an extracellular, collagen-rich matrix (bone, cartilage, fibrous tissue) and those with an internalized, specialized organic "matrix" (smooth, cardiac, and skeletal muscle and fat).

With age, connective tissues change their structure and function. The detailed mechanisms underlying this are dealt with in Chapter 12, but briefly, although there are diverse specific pathogenic mechanisms driving age-related tissue events, there are a number of generic processes that explain the changes seen in most tissues. At the whole body level these include a decrease in the amount of and receptiveness to circulating cytokines and growth factors or trophic hormones (e.g., the GH/IGF-1 axis). At the tissue level these include decreased amounts of tissue (e.g., bone in osteoporosis) and failure of normal responsiveness to load (an important homeostatic element in the biology of connective tissues). At the level of the cell these processes include reduced efficiency and number of stem cells and synthetic ability of increasingly senescent end cells.[1,2] And at the matrix level they are changes in the structure of matrix molecules (e.g., posttranslational cross-linking of collagen fibers by advanced glycation end products), bringing with it reduced functional efficiency.[3]

These changes can affect connective tissues anywhere,[4] not just in those tissues that consist primarily of connective tissue. However, in the latter group the effects can be profound, leading to poor mobility, altered ability to withstand cold, metabolic syndrome,[5] weakness, and an increased risk of falls, fractures, and age-associated "degenerative" diseases such as osteoarthritis and osteoporosis. As understanding of the causes of altered connective tissue function with age increases, it is becoming clearer that many of the predisposing factors are potential targets for improving quality of life in the elderly.

Diseases of three of the connective tissues—bone (Chapters 19 and 69), articular cartilage (Chapters 19 and 70), and skeletal muscle (Chapter 73)—together with some of the consequences of alterations in the connective tissue components of elements of the cardiovascular system (Chapter 14), blood (Chapters 21 and 93) and skin (Chapter 95), or disorders associated with the increasing prevalence of infection (Chapter 13) and cancer (Chapter 94) are described in detail elsewhere. This chapter concentrates on the common disorders of the connective tissues not already covered, and their associations with aging.

Once osteoporosis, osteomalacia, osteoarthritis, and sarcopenia are accounted for, the number of disorders of connective tissues that characteristically have an onset in the elderly age group (as opposed to those that accumulate throughout life but only present a significant disease burden in the elderly) is surprisingly small. The reasons why certain connective tissue diseases arise in the elderly population are not known. In this chapter, only those disorders characterized by a peak age of onset in the elderly population are discussed. Coverage cannot be exhaustive or comprehensive, but important issues and diseases affecting elderly people are highlighted.

NONMETABOLIC DISEASES OF BONE

The major nonmetabolic diseases of bone affecting the elderly are fracture, osteomyelitis, and Paget's disease.

Fracture

There is a higher incidence of both metastasizing epithelial neoplasms and osteoporosis in the elderly population. Both can weaken bone to a point where fracture is more likely to occur under "normal loading," predisposing the elderly to a higher incidence of pathologic fracture.

In addition, in the elderly there is impoverished fracture healing, probably as a consequence of a complex of diminished numbers of mesenchymal stem cells, poor stem cell maturation, and abnormalities in the humoral pathways that regulate osteoblast differentiation and function.[6] Poor fracture healing and an increase in the complication rate associated with fracture (e.g., thromboembolism) and illness/surgery/immobilization (e.g., confusion, infection) make even relatively trivial fractures serious events in the elderly, with a high incidence of significant morbidity, institutionalization, and death.[7]

Osteomyelitis

In the general population, osteomyelitis is a bacterial infection of bone marrow that usually reaches the bone by hematogenous spread from a primary site elsewhere. It is most commonly pyogenic, and the most common causal organism is *Staphylococcus aureus*. A second and increasingly common cause of osteomyelitis is consequent on orthopedic interventions such as joint replacement and internal fracture repair.[8] Joint replacement particularly is increasing in the elderly, and although the procedure is highly successful, a proportion (1% to 5%) of implant sites become infected, which is compounded in the elderly by comorbid conditions such as relative ischemia, diabetes, and reduced innate immunity. An appreciation that low-grade infection can underlie prosthesis failure in the elderly has led to a reassessment of diagnostic modalities[9] and improved detection of implant-associated osteomyelitis, but diagnosis and treatment remain the most significant problems in orthopedics, particularly in the aging population.

Paget's disease

Paget's disease is a disorder of poorly understood etiology that affects one or, rarely, more than one bone.[10] Paget's disease is believed to develop slowly, manifesting itself predominantly in the elderly population. Initially, perhaps in every case, there is a local decrease in bone mass, which is only later followed by the characteristic osteosclerosis. Usually, clinical features manifest themselves only in the later stages of the disease. The incidence varies widely across the world, being highest in northwest

England where at postmortem as many as 10% of individuals over 70 years of age show changes attributable to Paget's disease.

Histologically there is a generalized increase in bone cell activity that, in severe cases, leads to deposition of woven bone and uncoupling of osteoblastic and osteoclastic activity. Together these two factors lead to the laying down of excessive quantities of weak bone. The bone marrow is very vascular and the normal hematopoietic marrow is replaced by fibrous tissue. By electron microscopy, osteoclasts are seen to contain structures resembling viral particles (Figure 71-1), and modern research techniques, including immunohistochemistry and in situ hybridization, have demonstrated the presence of Morbillivirus within bone cells.[11] Causative links between the presence of the virus and altered osteoclast activity have given clues to the underlying biology of the disease and placed the osteoclast at the center of the disturbed bone cell biology.[12] There is, however, considerable controversy over the nature of this virus, or even its existence,[13] and increasingly opinion as to the cause of Paget's disease is moving toward it having a genetic basis.[14]

The abnormal bone matrix is weak leading to bone pain and fracture. Increased bone cell turnover predisposes to the development of primary bone malignancies, particularly osteosarcoma, fibrosarcoma, and malignant fibrous histiocytoma making Paget's disease the most common cause of primary bone malignancies in the elderly. Particularly in the elderly where there is a high incidence of impaired cardiac function, the increased vascularity within the affected bone or bones can lead to high-output cardiac failure.

Excessive bone cell activity causes an increase in the serum alkaline phosphatase and urinary collagen breakdown products. As the disease is driven by the osteoclast, symptomatic relief can be obtained by the use of drugs that suppress osteoclast function, notably bisphosphonates and calcitonin.

CARTILAGE DISORDERS

Chondroid tissues are characterized by the expression of the matrix molecules type II collagen and aggrecan and the transcription regulating gene Sox-9. The diversity of tissues expressing these genes is just beginning to be recognized with clear biologic distinctions being drawn between articular cartilage, growth plate, the cartilage of chondroid joints (e.g., costosternal joints), nonskeletal (e.g., nasal, auricular, bronchial) cartilage, structural fibrocartilage of synovial joints, the annulus fibrosus, and nucleus pulposus of the intervertebral disk and the vitreous humor of the eye.

By far the most common symptomatic disorder of cartilage in the elderly is osteoarthritis, which is covered in Chapter 70. Other common disorders include chondrocalcinosis (deposition of calcium pyrophosphate crystals) and degeneration of the intervertebral disk.

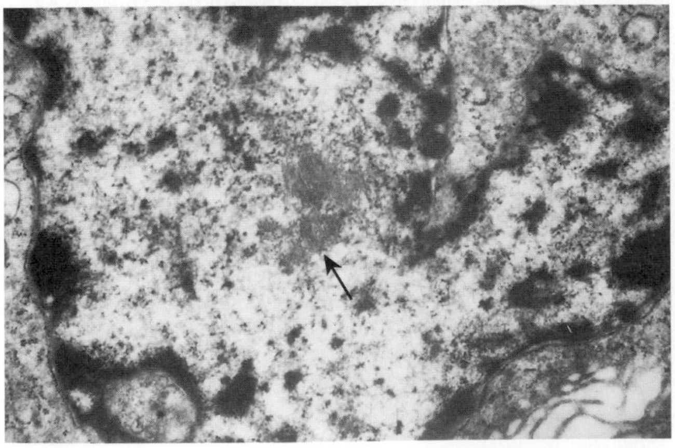

Figure 71-1. Osteoclast nucleus containing viral inclusions *(arrow)* in Pagetic bone (×27,000).

Degeneration of the intervertebral disk

Degeneration of the intervertebral disk (IVD) is attracting increasing interest as modern molecular pathology techniques allow the biology of this predominantly human disease to be studied; advances in biologic therapies, tissue engineering, and regenerative medicine offer potential therapeutic modalities; and diskogenic back pain makes an increasingly large impact on health and the economy.

In degeneration there are profound alterations in IVD cell and matrix biology, which include decreased synthesis of aggrecan, a switch in collagen subtype production from type II to type I, increased matrix breakdown by locally produced metalloproteinases, premature cellular senescence, and cell loss through apoptosis. The current view is that these changes are driven by altered cytokine regulation in the IVD, with interleukin 1 (IL-1) and tumor necrosis factor-α (TNF-α) having central roles in the processes leading to degeneration and diskogenic pain.[15] Currently, novel therapies are being developed to reverse the altered biology using cytokine modulators (such as IL-1 receptor antagonist and anti-TNF); replace the damaged tissues (particularly the nucleus pulposus, which is believed to be the seat of the altered cell biology) using disk replacements or biomaterials that have the same properties as the nucleus pulposus; or regenerate the IVD in vivo using a combination of stem cell therapy, smart biomaterials, and gene therapy.[16] Until such therapies are developed for widespread use, the treatment for diskogenic back pain in the elderly remains largely symptomatic.

DISORDERS OF FIBROUS TISSUE, LIGAMENTS, AND TENDONS

Disorders of fibrous tissue, particularly the organized fibrous tissues of ligaments and tendons, are common. They include proliferations such as keloid and the fibromatoses; trauma, either to the structure itself or to its insertion into bone (the enthesis); myxoid degeneration (e.g., ganglion formation); altered balance of connective tissue components; and metaplasia. Of these, two disorders, Dupuytren's disease and traumatic enthesopathy, are particularly common in the elderly.

Dupuytren's disease

Dupuytren's disease is a disorder in which there is a nodular proliferation of fibroblasts within the palmar fascia and its digital extensions, leading to dense collagen deposition, thickening and contracture within the fascia, and permanent deformity of the adjacent finger.

Many theories have been put forward to explain Dupuytren's disease.[17] They include changes induced by mast cell and epidermal chemical mediators, alterations in the vasculature, and paraneoplastic changes in DNA. None has been unequivocally accepted.

Within the palmar fascia, the fibroblastic proliferation is focal, leading to small nodules of very active fibroblasts (Figure 71-2). The nodular proliferation flits from area to area of the fascia, resulting in a generalized increase in collagen deposition. As the collagen "matures," internal fiber cross-linking leads to an overall reduction in fiber length and consequent contracture. The patient complains of a slowly progressive, painless nodule in the fascia that, as it worsens, shortens the affected area of tissue, causing further thickening and fascial contracture. Each fascial slip is attached to a finger, and the contracture leads to a permanent flexion deformity of the digit.

The clinical presentation is diagnostic, as are the biopsy appearances. Surgical excision is the treatment of choice, but the potential progression of the disease is not affected.[18]

Traumatic enthesopathy

Enthesopathy is the name given to a disparate group of disorders that occur at the entheses. The most striking of these are the inflammatory enthesopathies, seen in ankylosing spondylitis (AS) and rheumatoid arthritis (RA). Active enthesopathic AS is not specifically a disease of elderly people, and RA is discussed in Chapter 70.

There are two other major causes of enthesopathy: hyperparathyroidism and trauma.

Although the incidence of primary hyperparathyroidism peaks in elderly women (Chapter 91), it is usually a mild form of the disease and the abnormal activity of the parathyroid glands is often brought under control by an early resetting of the homeostatic mechanisms while the serum calcium is still within the normal range. There is therefore little of the bone erosion that is seen in classical advanced disease. In more severe disease, hyperosteoclasis at the enthesis can weaken the insertion, leading to pain and ligament failure.

Age-associated changes in collagen in the ligament/tendon and cartilage, weaken the structures in or around the entheses and lead to the increased incidence of partial or complete physical failure encountered during exercise in the increasingly fit elderly population. Trauma at the enthesis leads to a repair process, with development of painful bony outgrowths called "traction spurs," particularly at sites of maximum load—around the shoulder girdle, at the insertions of the plantar fascia and Achilles tendon into the calcaneum,[19] and the long ligaments of the spine into vertebral bodies.

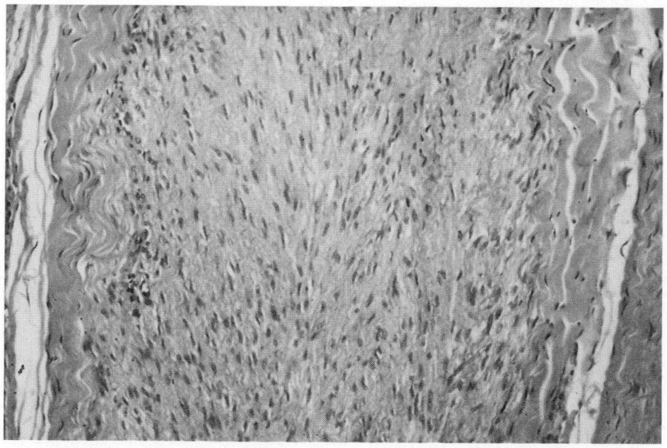

Figure 71-2. Cellular proliferation within a Dupuytren nodule (H&E ×200).

NEOPLASMS OF CONNECTIVE TISSUE

Although many benign and malignant connective tissue neoplasms are seen in the elderly population, only rare primary connective tissue neoplasms have their peak incidence in this age group. These are all rare and are either benign neoplasms of soft connective tissues or malignant neoplasms of soft connective tissues or bone. The group includes benign neoplasms of soft tissues (spindle cell/pleomorphic lipoma, atypical fibroxanthoma, elastofibroma, cellular angiofibroma), malignant neoplasms of soft tissues (pleomorphic sarcomas of the group that used to be known as malignant fibrous histiocytoma but is now recognized as a spectrum of pleomorphic malignancies that have a similar histologic pattern but different immunophenotype [Figure 71-3], pleomorphic liposarcoma, undifferentiated pleomorphic sarcoma with giant cells, myxofibrosarcoma, and fibrosarcoma), and malignant neoplasms of bone (Pagetic sarcoma, chondrosarcoma).

Elastofibroma

One of these, elastofibroma, is particularly interesting in view of the highly significant age-associated changes that occur in the connective tissue matrix molecule elastin.[20–22]

Elastofibroma is a benign, slow-growing tumor found mainly in the subscapular area in elderly women. It consists of fibrous tissue containing large numbers of elastin fibers. These can be recognized in conventionally stained sections (Figure 71-4), but stains for elastin are characteristic and show exactly how much elastin is present within the tumor.

The etiology is unknown. There is some evidence that it may be associated with trauma, but the evidence for this is far from convincing and a familial incidence could point

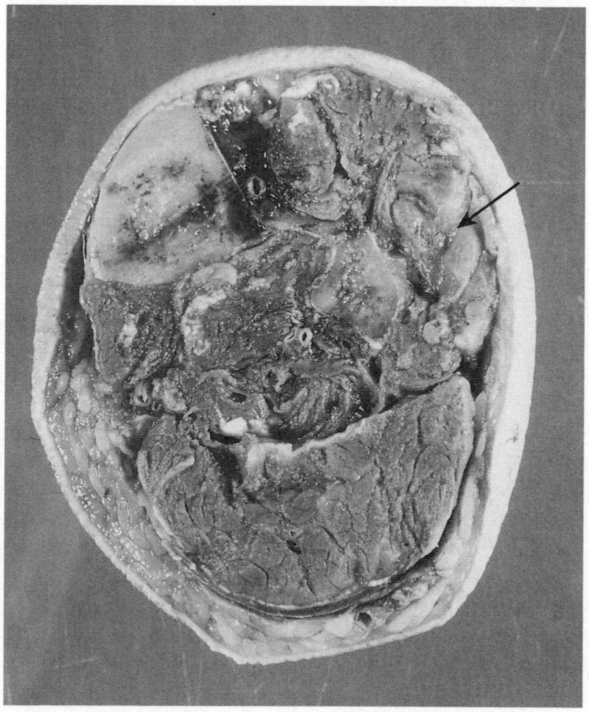

Figure 71-3. Macroscopic image of a pleomorphic sarcoma (*arrow*) in the lower leg. Diameter approximately 5 cm.

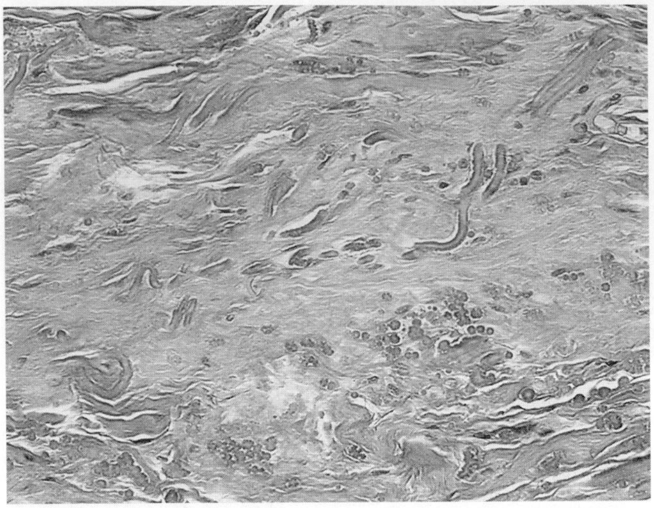

Figure 71-4. H&E stained section of an elastofibroma. Note the wormlike and somewhat ragged edged elastin fibers viewed from the side on in the upper part of the figure and from the end on in the lower part (×300).

toward a genetic predisposition. There have been studies showing recurrent DNA gains at bands Xq12-q22 and 19,[23] and clonal chromosomal changes have been reported.

Whatever else, the major feature of these tumors is the presence of abnormal elastin. Immunohistochemical, electron microscopic, and molecular studies have shown that the elastin fibers differ only slightly in amino acid composition from normal elastin.[24] The changes seem to have resulted from abnormal synthesis rather than some sort of abnormal degradation. The changed amino acid composition leads to morphologic changes in the elastin fibers such that under the electron microscope they appear as irregular, somewhat fern-shaped aggregates of electron-dense material surrounded by and incorporating microfibrils and collagen fibers. Whether this has any relationship to or bearing on the recognized age-associated abnormalities in elastin fiber structure, which have been described as being the one factor that will prevent extreme longevity in humans, is unknown,[25] but examination of these tumor cells that are actively overproducing abnormal elastin may be one route to gaining a better understanding of the altered biology of elastin in the elderly.

IMMUNE-MEDIATED CONNECTIVE TISSUE DISORDERS

This group of clinicopathologic entities is characterized by an immune response against "self-antigens," leading to damage to "connective tissues" and blood vessels in multiple organs, notably joints, skin, glomeruli, and large and small blood vessels. Pathogenetically, all of these disorders exhibit immune complex deposition, or formation, within affected organs (usually on basement membranes) and consequent tissue damage. The intriguing thing about these disorders is that the balance of the organs affected by the disease process varies from condition to condition, so that in rheumatoid arthritis the joints are most commonly and severely affected, whereas in polyarteritis nodosa it is the blood vessels, and in systemic lupus erythematosus it is the skin and kidney. Like all autoimmune diseases, they most commonly present in young adult women. Only giant cell arteritis and polymyalgia rheumatica stand out as being disorders predominantly of the elderly.

Giant cell arteritis and polymyalgia rheumatica

Giant cell arteritis is a relatively uncommon disorder (approximately 1:1000 over 60 years) manifesting as an arterial vasculitis with a predilection for the arteries of the head, particularly the external carotid and the retinal branch of the internal carotid arteries, of elderly women (F:M = 3:1).[26] The American College of Rheumatology has proposed diagnostic criteria.

Early in the disorder there is a leukocytoclastic vasculitis, so called because the vessel wall contains viable polymorphs and polymorph debris, evidence of complement activation, and generation of toxic polymorph products. Not only do polymorphs perish in this environment, but so too do the smooth muscle cells of the arterial wall, leading to segmental mural necrosis. Later the distinctive picture of chronic inflammation with giant cells within the wall of the vessel appears. The giant cells are of two types: immune-competent cells, primed to an unknown antigen; and foreign-body type cells that are phagocytosing the internal elastic lamina (Figure 71-5). Thrombus formation is commonly seen. The disease has a focal distribution within the vessel and, in any one location, a short time course. After the inflammation has spontaneously settled, the vessel wall undergoes fibrosis. Extensive fibrosis can be used to indicate earlier destructive inflammation, even in the absence of active inflammation. Care must be taken in interpreting this feature as fibrosis and segmental loss of the internal loss of the internal elastic lamina is a "normal" finding in the elderly population.

The etiology of the vasculitis is not known. There is familial aggregation and association with HLA-DR4. In the serum there are raised levels of IgG, total complement, C3, and C4. Circulating immune complexes have been demonstrated in up to 90% of patients. They have also been seen attached to the internal elastic lamina, perhaps by absorbance. Whether the key role of the elastic lamina in immune complex absorption and its recognition by multinucleate macrophages is another manifestation of the importance of abnormal elastin synthesis in age-associated disorders of connective tissues is not known, but it is certainly intriguing.[27]

POLYMYALGIA RHEUMATICA

The localized disorder giant cell arteritis is associated with a generalized condition known as polymyalgia rheumatica. It is characterized by low-grade fever, weight loss, ill-defined pain, malaise, fatigue, and stiffness in the shoulder girdle, upper arms, and neck. Movement accentuates the pain, which is at its worst at night. Affected joints, particularly the knees and sternoclavicular joints, are actively inflamed. There is an increase in the number of cells within the synovial fluid and a normochromic, normocytic anemia. The erythrocyte sedimentation rate (ESR) is very high but there is no leukocytosis. Tests for autoantibodies are negative. It responds to steroids.

METABOLIC DISORDERS

Prominent among the metabolic disorders affecting connective tissues in the elderly are disorders in which crystals and abnormal proteins accumulate in the tissues.

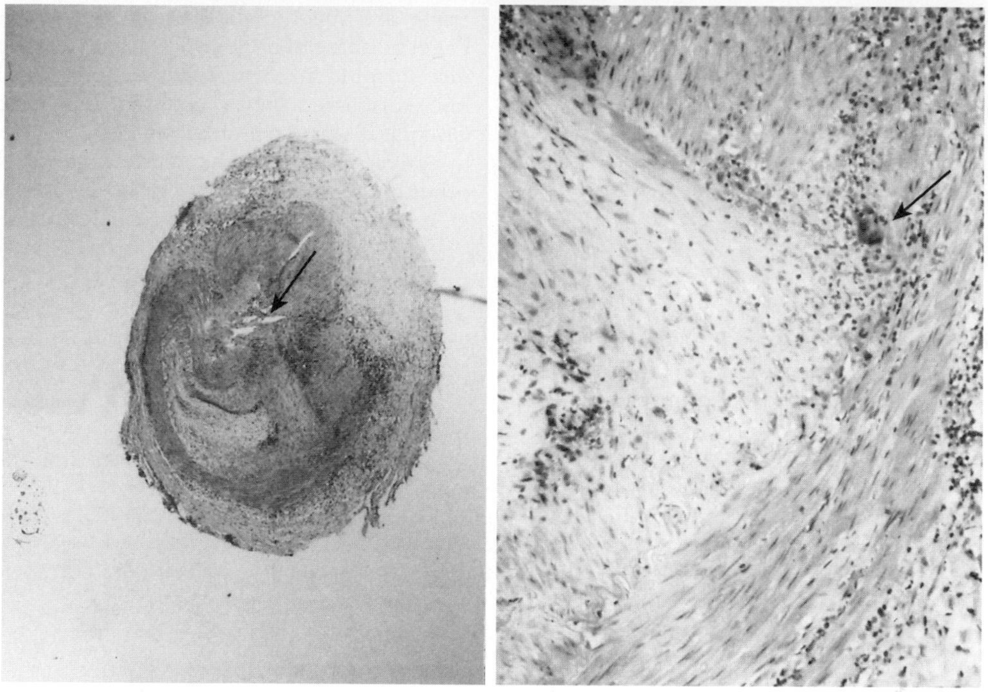

Figure 71-5. Artery from a patient with giant cell arteritis. The left panel shows virtual occlusion (*arrow*) of the lumen (H&E, ×10). The right panel shows inflammation including giant cells (*arrow*) in the wall (H&E, ×150).

Crystal deposition disease

The main symptomatic crystal deposition diseases affecting the elderly are gout and pseudogout.[28]

Gout is caused by the precipitation of crystals of monosodium urate in joints. Uric acid, from which urates are formed, is a breakdown product of purine metabolism. Most is excreted by the kidney. Alteration in uric acid excretion, either idiopathic or secondary to diuretic therapy, leads to an increase in monosodium urate in the blood and extracellular fluid and its precipitation in the tissues. Cartilage, particularly articular fibrocartilage and nonarticular hyaline cartilage, and subcutaneous connective tissue are the most common sites of its accumulation. Here aggregates of the crystals induce a macrophage response. These "tophi" may ulcerate. In elderly people, tophaceous or nontophaceous gout occur most commonly consequent upon an idiopathic decrease in urate excretion, generalized deterioration in renal function, or the use of certain diuretics. Therapy can be challenging in the elderly.[29]

Pseudogout is one of three manifestations of deposition of calcium pyrophosphate crystals in the elderly. The first is chondrocalcinosis, a disorder in which the crystals are deposited in articular tissues, mainly fibrocartilage. Despite being extremely common over the age of 70, it is generally not symptomatic. The second is in osteoarthritis in which calcium pyrophosphate crystals are a common finding in cartilage and synovial fluid and where they are believed to have some pathogenic role in disease progression. The third is pseudogout in which the presence of crystals in the synovial fluid leads to an acute crystal arthritis similar to gout.

Accumulation of abnormal proteins

Two conditions, diabetes and amyloidosis, cause abnormal proteins to accumulate in the elderly at least in part because the molecules are not as readily degraded as their normal counterparts. In terms of connective tissues, the most significant effects are alteration in structural proteins and thickening of vascular basement membranes leading to altered tissue nutrition. In diabetes a major cause of abnormal proteins to form is hyperglycemia, which leads to the production of advanced glycation end products (AGEs) that in turn induce cross-linking of collagens and other connective tissue matrix molecules.[30] In amyloidosis, tissue dysfunction is caused by deposition of molecules that have changed from their conventional structure of an α helix to a β pleated sheet. The greatest interest in amyloids in the elderly has focused on neurodegeneration-associated amyloid deposition in the brain, but amyloids are far more widely spread in the aging

KEY POINTS
Connective Tissue Diseases

- Age-associated disorders of connective tissues are among the most important for determining quality of life in the elderly.
- Connective tissue cells and matrices change structure or function markedly with increasing age. In particular AGE-induced cross-linking and cellular senescence affect tissue function.
- Connective tissue diseases restricted to the elderly population are rare as most connective tissue disorders are ones in which the incidence in the elderly is similar to that in other adults, or are present in the elderly following asymptomatic progression over many years.
- Most of the key connective tissue diseases affecting the elderly are among the most important diseases in the world.
- Elastin is a key matrix molecule for determining pathologic processes in the elderly.
- To fully understand connective tissue diseases in the elderly requires an understanding of the biology of the aging cell and matrix molecules.

population, with one estimate of the incidence of senile systemic amyloidosis (SSA) as 25% of those over 80.[31] In SSA the major component of the amyloid (AS amyloid) is derived from normal transthyretin (prealbumin). The most common site for age-associated amyloids to accumulate in connective tissues in the elderly is in and around joints and in the walls of arteries. In these sites it is generally benign, but there is an association with osteoarthritis.

SUMMARY

The connective tissues are the most abundant tissues in the body. Diseases of connective tissue can occur at any time of life and most present first during middle age. Some are specific to the elderly population, including Paget's disease of bone, Dupuytren's disease, elastofibroma, pleomorphic sarcoma, giant cell arteritis, and senile amyloid, discussed here; osteoporosis, osteoarthritis, and vascular disease, which are among the most common noninfective diseases in the Western world, are discussed in other chapters.

For a complete list of references, please visit online only at www.expertconsult.com

CHAPTER 72

Orthopedic Geriatrics

Robert Victor Cantu
Kenneth J. Koval

INTRODUCTION

Orthopedic care of geriatric patients presents unique challenges. Geriatric patients often have multiple medical comorbidities that affect decisions regarding timing and type of surgery. Bone quality is often substantially inferior to that of younger patients, and many older patients have preexisting arthropathies, making fixation more challenging and sometimes making arthroplasty the favored treatment. Coordination of care with an internal medicine or geriatric team is often helpful to provide the best outcome and to minimize complications. This chapter addresses many of the challenges the orthopedist must deal with when caring for geriatric patients.

Osteoporosis

The World Health Organization has defined osteoporosis as a bone mineral density (BMD) value of 2.5 standard deviations or more below the young adult mean.[1] Patients with known osteoporosis are at a substantial risk for fracture. The majority of patients with a fragility fracture involving the spine, hip, wrist, or proximal humerus, however, do not meet the BMD definition of osteoporosis.[2] This fact can make it difficult to know which patients should receive pharmacologic treatment to prevent the risk of fracture. This finding also suggests that patients who have had a single fragility fracture should receive treatment for osteoporosis, even if their BMD is not 2.5 standard deviations below the mean.

Despite improvements in pharmacologic treatment, osteoporosis continues to afflict millions of aging Americans and people worldwide. Fragility fractures result in pain, disability, and medical complications and affect as many as 1 in 3 women and 1 in 12 men during their lifetime. It is estimated that worldwide, 323 million people suffer from osteoporosis, and that number is projected to be 1.55 billion by the year 2050.[3] It has been predicted that the number of hip fractures in the year 2050 will be 6.3 million.[3] The medical expenses following fragility fractures are substantial.[4] The annual cost of osteoporosis and fragility fractures in Europe is estimated at 13 billion euros.[4] The majority of that cost results from hospitalization after fracture.

Patients who have sustained a single fragility fracture have a 1.5 to 9.5 times higher risk of sustaining a second fracture than do those who have never had a fracture.[5] One study found 20% of patients had a second fracture within 1 year.[6] Despite this risk, many patients who have had a fragility fracture are not started on preventive medication. In one study, only 7% of patients admitted with a fragility fracture were receiving osteoporosis treatment.[3] Surprisingly, this number only increased to 11% at the time of discharge. At a minimum, patients should be started on calcium and vitamin D after sustaining a fragility fracture. Antiresorptive medications should also be considered.

Osteoporosis has a dramatic effect on fracture fixation. Traditional nonlocked plates and screws may not achieve adequate purchase in osteoporotic bone. Intramedullary implants or locked plates should be considered to improve fracture fixation and maintain alignment.[7] Augmentation of bone with methylmethacrylate cement can enhance screw purchase, but care must be exercised to prevent extravasation into the soft tissues or into the fracture site. In elderly osteoporotic patients, certain fractures may be better treated with arthroplasty rather than open reduction internal fixation.

Several authors have looked at the costs of trying to screen for osteoporosis and institute antiresorptive treatment before the onset of a fragility fracture.[8–11] A study in Australia looked at 1224 women 50 years old and older and categorized them into age groups.[12] Dual-energy x-ray absorptiometry (DEXA) scanning was performed on all women, and the percentage with osteoporosis was 20% in the 50–59 age group, 46% in the 60–69 age group, 59% in the 70–79 age group, and 69% for those older than 80 years. It was estimated that if all women over 50 years of age were started on antiresorptive medication the risk of fracture would decrease by 50% in those with osteoporosis and by 20% in those without. They calculated the cost per fracture averted in the 50–59 age group at $156,400 and in the over-80 group at $28,500. It was concluded that treating all women over age 50 with antiresorptive medication was not financially feasible. The authors also concluded that for women over 60 years of age with osteoporosis, instituting antiresorptive therapy would decrease fragility fractures by 28% and was cost effective.[12]

GERIATRIC TRAUMA

Patients older than 65 years of age account for 28% of all fatal injuries in the United States, although they represent only 12% of the population.[13,14] Additionally, the population over 65 years of age is the fastest growing segment in the United States. Treatment of fractures in the elderly is often more complicated than in the young, healthy age group as elderly fracture patients often have preexisting medical problems that affect fracture management. One of the most common comorbidities in elderly patients is cardiopulmonary disease, which can limit their ability to tolerate surgery and participate in rehabilitation. Neurologic disorders, such as Alzheimer's disease and Parkinson's disease, are also common. Some patients have residual weakness or contractures from a previous cerebrovascular accident. Any of these disorders can affect gait and balance and limit weight-bearing restrictions that younger patients could comply with. Endocrine problems, particularly diabetes, are common in the elderly. Diabetic patients generally have vascular compromise secondary to small vessel disease and are immunosuppressed. Nonoperative treatment of select fractures may be preferred in these patients, particularly if there is a preexisting diabetic ulcer near the planned operative field.

For multiply injured elderly patients, the injury severity score (ISS) may underestimate the degree of injury. An elderly patient may present with a lower ISS than a young adult and still be unstable or even "in extremis," in the sense that minimal further insult can tip these patients past the point of recovery. At the same time, if their injuries are not rapidly stabilized, these patients may deteriorate beyond the point at which they can survive. It is this tightrope that

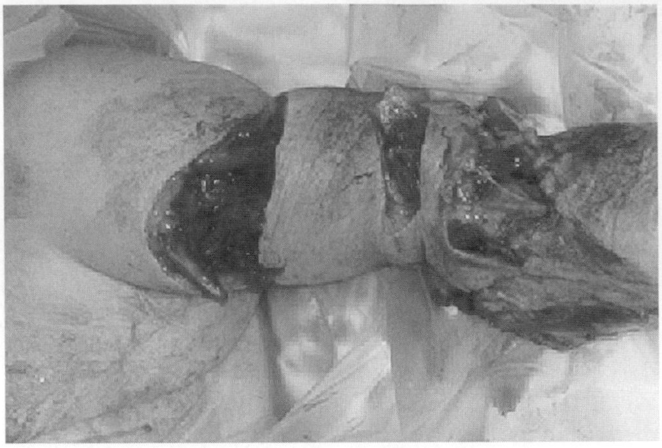

Figure 72-1. Grade IIIC humerus fracture in elderly trauma patient with multiple injuries. Treatment was immediate amputation.

the orthopedic trauma surgeon must walk when treating the elderly patient with multiple fractures. In such cases, simple splinting or external fixation of upper extremity fractures and external fixation of lower extremity fractures may represent the best initial treatment.

Few studies have focused specifically on the impact of orthopedic injuries in elderly trauma patients.[15–17] One retrospective, multicenter study attempted to define factors associated with increased morbidity and mortality rates in elderly patients who had sustained major trauma.[15] Of 326 patients with an average age of 72.2 years, there was an overall mortality rate of 18.1%. Of patients who required bony stabilization, 77% had this accomplished within 24 hours of admission. The mortality rate for patients who underwent fracture stabilization within 24 hours was 11%, and for those who were fixed after 24 hours it was 18%, but this difference was not statistically significant.[15] The three complications with the highest mortality rates were acute respiratory distress syndrome (ARDS) (81%), myocardial infarction (62%), and sepsis (39%).

For the elderly trauma patient with a mangled extremity, early amputation should be considered. Elderly patients may not be able to withstand the multiple surgeries required to salvage severe, open fractures, especially those with vascular insult. If a severely injured limb becomes infected, the cascade of sepsis and multiple system organ failure can proceed quickly. Although this is often a difficult decision, early amputation in the elderly patient can be a life-saving procedure (Figure 72-1).

ANESTHETIC CONSIDERATIONS

One aspect of orthopedic care in the elderly that should not be underemphasized is pain control. Early stabilization of fractures is one factor in pain control. Once fractures are stabilized, there is a minimization of narcotic use, which can improve respiratory function and mental status. Patients whose fractures are stabilized and have adequate pain control can be weaned from ventilators more easily, can obtain a more upright posture, and have reduced delirium; these are all critical for survival in the elderly. Selective use of nerve blocks or catheters for continuous infusion, such as a femoral nerve block catheter following a femur fracture, can greatly aid in pain relief and minimize narcotic requirements.

Periarticular fractures

Treatment of periarticular fractures in the elderly often differs from treatment in younger patients. Fractures involving the proximal humerus, elbow, hip, and occasionally the knee sometimes fare better with a joint arthroplasty rather than open reduction internal fixation (ORIF) in the elderly. Several studies have compared ORIF to joint arthroplasty for displaced femoral neck fractures in the elderly.[18–20] The complication rate following ORIF, including need for revision surgery, is substantially higher than it is for the arthroplasty group. Controversy exists as to whether hemiarthroplasty or total hip arthroplasty is the best treatment. Some studies seem to show improved results with total hip arthroplasty.[21,22] Dislocation rate is a concern with total hip arthroplasty, especially in patients with neurologic disorders such as Parkinson's disease or patients with hemiparesis after a stroke.

Distal humerus fractures are another example of a periarticular injury in the elderly that may have better outcomes with arthroplasty rather than ORIF. Frankle et al reported on a retrospective review of 12 patients who underwent ORIF and 12 who underwent total elbow arthroplasty for distal humerus fractures.[23] The total elbow group performed better on the Mayo Elbow Performance Score with 11 (excellent) and 1 (good) compared to 4 (excellent), 4 (good), 1 (fair), and 3 (poor) in the ORIF group. Muller et al reported on their results with 49 distal humerus fractures in patients older than 65 years treated acutely with total elbow arthroplasty.[24] Inclusion criteria included patients who were "high compliance" and "low demand." Average range of motion at follow-up (average, 7 years) was an arc from 24 to 131 degrees. A total of five revision arthroplasties were performed during the follow-up period. They concluded that the procedure is recommended when the appropriate inclusion criteria are met.

For periarticular fractures best treated with ORIF, the advent of locked plates has allowed for improved fixation, especially in patients with osteoporotic bone. Results so far have been encouraging. In one retrospective review of 123 distal femur fractures treated with the Less Invasive Surgical Stabilization (LISS) system, 93% healed without bone graft, the infection rate was 3%, and there was no loss of distal fixation.[25] In a prospective study of 38 complex proximal tibia fractures treated with the LISS system, 37 of 38 healed with satisfactory alignment, there were no infections, and the average lower extremity measure (LEM) score was 88.[26] Another review of 77 proximal tibial fractures treated with LISS showed 91% healed without complication.[27] The overall union rate was 97% with an average time to full weight bearing of 12.6 weeks; the infection rate was 4%.

Acetabular fractures are challenging to treat at any age. Helfet et al was one of the first research teams to report on open reduction and internal fixation of acetabular fractures in the elderly.[28] In their review of 18 patients age 60 or older followed for 2 years after ORIF, the mean Harris hip score was 90 points. All fractures healed, and only one patient had loss of reduction. Complications included two pulmonary emboli and one missed intra-articular fragment requiring reoperation. The authors concluded that "open reduction and internal fixation of selected displaced acetabular fractures in the elderly can yield good results and may obviate the need for early and often difficult total hip arthroplasty."[28]

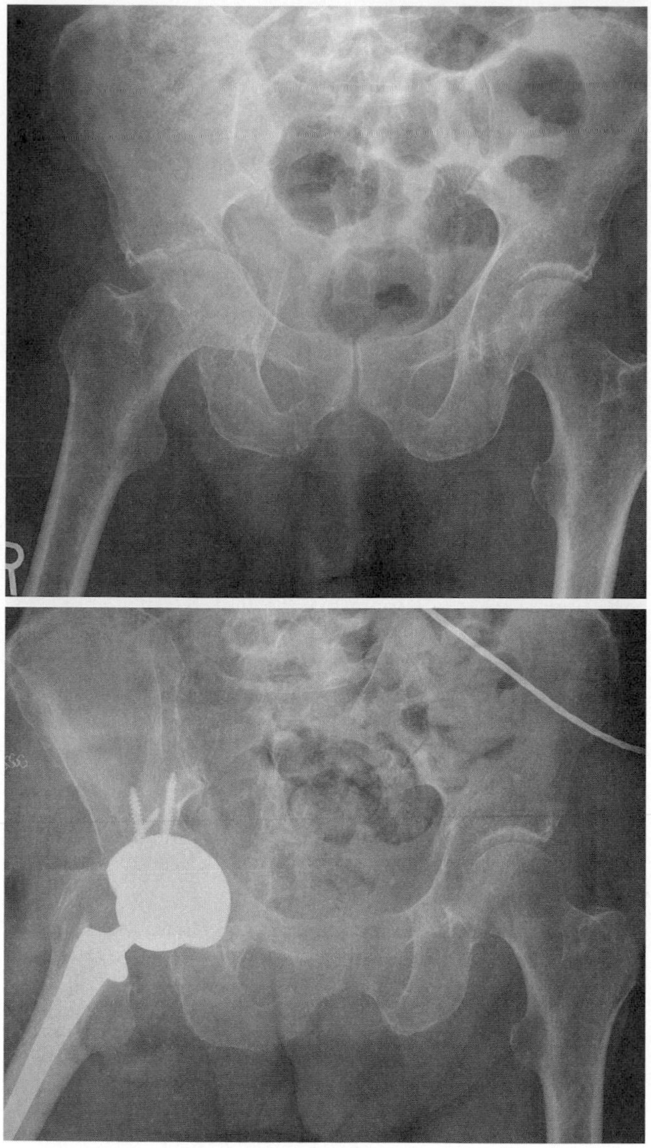

Figure 72-2. Displaced acetabular fracture in elderly male treated with acute primary total hip arthroplasty.

More recent work has suggested primary total hip arthroplasty may be a viable option for select acetabular fractures in the elderly (Figure 72-2). To perform arthroplasty in the acute setting is challenging and may require internal fixation of the fracture to provide enough stability to hold the arthroplasty. Mears has reported on his results with this approach in 57 patients with a mean follow-up of 8.1 years and mean age of 69 years.[29] The mean Harris hip score was 89, and 79% of patients had a good or excellent outcome. He concluded that this is a viable option for patients with a low likelihood of a favorable outcome with fracture treatment alone.

Periprosthetic fractures

As the number of patients with total joint replacements continues to rise, so do the number of patients sustaining periprosthetic fractures. These typically occur from low-energy falls, but the bone quality around the prior implant is often of poor quality making fixation of these fractures challenging. The first step in deciding on the best treatment is to assess the stability of the prior arthroplasty implants. If the implants are

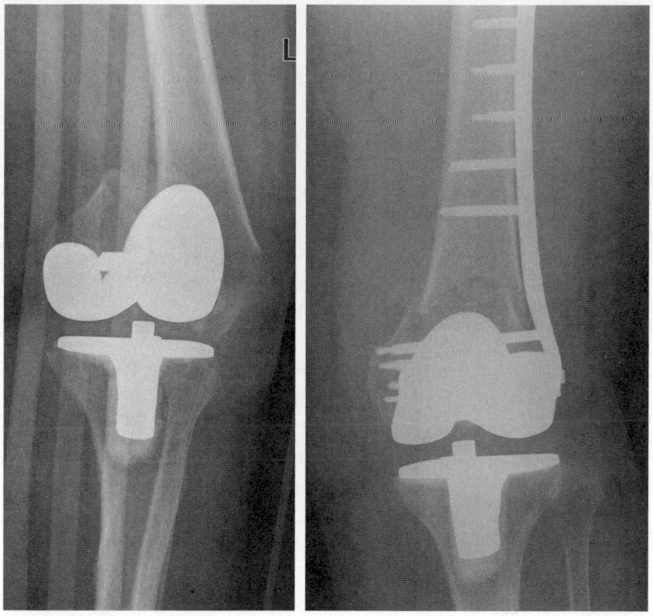

Figure 72-3. Periprosthetic distal femur fracture in osteoporotic bone treated with locking submuscular plate.

loose, then revision arthroplasty with long stem components is typically the best option. The goal is to use stems that extend beyond the fracture by at least two cortical diameters of the bone involved. If the implants are well fixed, then reducing and fixing the fracture is usually the preferred treatment. For certain fractures, such as a supracondylar periprosthetic femur fracture above a total knee replacement, intramedullary (IM) nailing may be employed, provided the knee replacement was cruciate sparing and the femoral component has an open slot for the nail. Other fractures may best be treated with plating. The techniques of plating have advanced to the point most fractures can be treated with indirect reduction to avoid devascularizing the fracture. Plates should overlap the arthroplasty implants to avoid stress risers. Locked plates have provided improved results for many periprosthetic fractures occurring in osteoporotic bone (Figure 72-3).

Prevention of fractures in the elderly

The first step in prevention of fragility fractures is identifying a patient's risk factors. Some risk factors cannot be changed, such as age, family history, rheumatoid arthritis, or a history of hyperthyroidism or hyperparathyroidism. Many risk factors can be modified, however, and include avoiding cigarette smoking, sedentary lifestyle, excessive alcohol use, low body mass index, and lack of dietary calcium vitamin D. Some medications can contribute to osteoporosis, such as glucocorticoids, cyclosporin, methotrexate, heparin, and anticonvulsants.

Multiple approaches to prevent osteoporosis and fragility fractures exist. They include nonpharmacologic means such as well-balanced diet and exercise, adequate sunlight exposure, not smoking, vitamin D and calcium supplementation, and selected use of hip protectors. Adequate exercise seems to be an important modifiable factor in the prevention of fragility fractures. Exercise not only helps prevent osteopenia and osteoporosis, but it also improves balance and aids in fall prevention in the elderly. A multicenter, randomized controlled trial found that group exercise programs were beneficial in preventing falls and improving physical performance in "prefrail" elderly patients.[30] Exercise does not have to be strenuous to achieve results as programs involving the principles of tai chi have been shown to be effective.

Medical treatments include the antiresorptive bisphosphonates such as alendronate, risedronate, and ibandronate. Nasal calcitonin and raloxifene have also been used to limit bone resorption. Teriparatide is an anabolic agent that improves bone density by increasing osteoblast activity. The FDA has withdrawn approval of hormone replacement with estrogen for osteoporosis prevention, except in selected postmenopausal women.[31]

Calcium and vitamin D are relatively inexpensive and do have benefit in the prevention of osteoporosis. The recommended doses for maximal benefit are 800 IU of vitamin D and 1000 to 1200 mg of elemental calcium. One review article recommended that three types of individuals should take vitamin D and calcium supplementation to prevent osteoporosis: (1) patients receiving glucocorticoid treatment, (2) patients with documented osteoporosis, and (3) patients at high risk for calcium or vitamin D deficiency, in particular older men and women.[32]

Adequate dietary protein seems to be another factor in the prevention of osteoporosis and fragility fractures. Diets deficient in protein can lead to loss of bone mass and decreased bone microarchitecture and strength.[33] Elderly patients who were given a diet with increased protein following a fragility fracture were found to have decreased postfracture bone loss, increased muscle strength, and reduced medical complications during their hospital stay. One author has stated that dietary protein is "as essential" as calcium and vitamin D for bone health and prevention of osteoporosis.[33] One prospective trial examined soy protein on bone health.[34] Soy protein contains phytoestrogens, which are also thought to be beneficial for bone health. Patients were placed on a diet that included 35 mg of soy protein per day. At the 12-week point, the levels of serum alkaline phosphatase had significantly increased and urinary deoxypyridinolone had decreased. It was concluded that soy protein "can be effective in protecting bone mass."[34]

Hip protectors have been proposed as a relatively inexpensive way to limit hip fractures. A meta-analysis of the Cochrane register of controlled trials concluded that hip protectors are an "ineffective intervention" in the home setting, whereas their utility in nursing or residential care settings is "uncertain."[35] The main reason for their ineffectiveness seems to be lack of compliance in using them.

FOLLOW-UP

The orthopedist may be the only physician a patient sees after a fragility fracture. Close communication between the orthopedist and the patient's internist is needed to implement osteoporosis treatment after a fragility fracture. In a 2006 survey of 140 orthopedists and internists in the United Kingdom, 45% of the internists believed the orthopedist would refer the patient for osteoporosis treatment if it was indicated.[36] When presented with the scenario of a 55-year-old female with a low-energy Colle's fracture, 56% of the orthopedists did not request further investigation for osteoporosis. Better awareness of patients at risk for osteoporosis and better communication between the orthopedist and internist as to who will initiate further evaluation and treatment are required to limit the growing burden of fragility fractures.

GERIATRIC-ORTHOPEDIC CO-CARE

Several studies have looked at the effectiveness of co-care between orthopedics and geriatrics regarding inpatient care of elderly patients with orthopedic injuries.[37–39] Most studies have focused on elderly patients with hip fractures. Previous studies have shown mixed results, but many do show some advantages. The keys to success seem to be careful targeting of the population, a proactive rather than a reactionary strategy, and attention to improving specific outcomes rather than just a general geriatric assessment.

A prospective, randomized trial was carried out on 126 patients 65 years and older admitted to a tertiary academic medical center following a hip fracture.[39] Patients were randomized to either a proactive geriatrics consultation or usual care. The group receiving the geriatrics consultation had a reduction in the incidence of delirium by one third and a reduction in severe delirium by one half.[39] Fisher et al conducted a study on 951 patients 60 years and older admitted with a hip fracture over a 7-year period to a single institution. For the first 3 years of the study, patients did not have routine geriatric medicine evaluation, whereas during the final 4 years, there was routine geriatrics consultation. During the second phase, significant reductions in mortality (4.7% vs. 7.7%, $p < 0.01$) and rehospitalization rates (7.6% vs. 28%) were seen.[38]

CONCLUSIONS

Orthopedic care of the elderly presents many challenges. Poor bone quality can make the goal of stable internal fixation difficult if not impossible in some patients. Comorbid medical conditions can dictate what types of treatment a patient can tolerate. Rehabilitation of injuries may be limited because of the patient's overall physical condition. For some periarticular fractures, performing a joint arthroplasty rather than trying to reconstruct the fracture may result in a more predictable and functional outcome. Shared care between the orthopedist and the internal medicine or geriatric team seems to improve overall outcomes for many elderly patients. Communication between the orthopedist and the patient's primary care physician is needed to ensure proper osteoporosis management. Each case requires an assessment of both patient and fracture characteristics to determine the most appropriate treatment.

KEY POINTS

Orthopedic Geriatrics

- Approximately 1 in 3 women and 1 in 12 men will sustain a fragility fracture.
- Injury severity scores may underestimate degree of injury for elderly patients.
- Joint replacement may provide the best treatment for some fractures in the elderly.
- Orthopedic and geriatric co-care may improve outcomes for hip fracture patients.

For a complete list of references, please visit online only at www.expertconsult.com

CHAPTER 73

Sarcopenia

Yves Rolland
Bruno Vellas

DEFINITION

Irwin Rosenberg defined sarcopenia in 1989 to describe a recognized age-related decline in muscle mass among the elderly.[1] This large and supposedly involuntary loss of muscle tissue in the elderly was considered responsible in part for the age-related decline in functional capacity. Since 1989, various definitions of sarcopenia have evolved as our understanding of the aging process and the changes that occur therein progress along with improved body composition measurement techniques and the availability of large representative data sets. Despite this increasing knowledge and improved technology, a worldwide operational definition of sarcopenia applicable across racial/ethnic groups and populations lacks consensus. One current definition of sarcopenia includes a loss of muscle strength and functional quality in addition to the loss of muscle protein mass.

EPIDEMIOLOGY

After 50 years of age, muscle mass is reported to decline at an annual rate of approximately 1% to 2%, but strength declines at 1.5% per year and accelerates to as much as 3% per year after age 60.[2] These rates are high in sedentary individuals and twice as high in men as compared to women.[3] However, men, on average, have larger amounts of muscle mass and shorter survival than women, which implies that sarcopenia is potentially a greater public health concern among women than men. The current prevalence of sarcopenia in populations varies depending on the definition used, the limitations of past epidemiologic and clinical data from small samples, and mixed information from the different measurement techniques employed. In the New Mexico Elder Health Survey, sarcopenia affects about 20% of men between age 70 and 75 years, about 50% of those over age 80 years, and between 25% and 40% of women have sarcopenia in the same age ranges.[4] However, Baumgartner later recognized that these estimates, which were based on a bioelectric impedance equation, might be biased and published revised prevalence estimates based on dual-energy x-ray absorptiometry (DEXA) ranging from 8.8% in women and 13.5% men aged 60 to 69 years, and up to 16% in women and 29% in men older than 80 years.[5] In a healthy elderly community-dwelling population 70 years of age and older in the French Epidemiologie de l'osteoporose (EPIDOS) study, only 10% of the women had sarcopenia[6] based on the Baumgartner's index, but cut points derived from a different reference group. Using a similar definition, Janssen reported, retrospectively, that 35% of the elderly in the population-based National Health and Nutritional Examination Survey III (NHANES III) had a moderate degree of sarcopenia and 10% a severe degree of sarcopenia.[7] Findings from a separate study by Melton et al using yet another definition suggests that sarcopenia affects 6% to 15% of persons over the age of 65 years.[8]

OPERATIONAL DEFINITION OF SARCOPENIA

Despite the recognition of the need for a consensus operational definition of sarcopenia since 1995[9] and the relative agreement among clinicians and epidemiologists on a theoretic definition of sarcopenia, development of a consensus operational definition useful across clinics, studies, and populations is still lacking.

The quantitative approach

Baumgartner et al[4] summed the muscle mass of the four limbs from a DEXA scan as appendicular skeletal muscle mass (ASM) and defined a skeletal muscle mass index (SMI) as ASM/height^2 (as kg/m^2). Individuals with a SMI two standard deviations below the mean SMI of a middle-age reference male and female population from the Rosetta study[3] were defined as gender-specific cut points for sarcopenia. Several authors have used this definition.[4,6,8] A limitation may be the ability of DEXA to distinguish water retention or fat tissue infiltration within muscle or soft tissue. There are few published data to date, however, for the impact of variation in these on sarcopenia prevalence estimates. Chen et al[10] and others[11] reported strong correlations (r > 0.94) between DEXA and magnetic resonance imaging (MRI) measures of skeletal muscle mass, indicating that this increasingly available method is useful for cross-sectional studies and screening. Another potential limitation is that this approach does not account for the joint effects of fat mass or body weight. Most obese adults have increased muscle mass in addition to a high fat mass but a low muscle mass in relation to their total body weight, whereas thin elderly have a high proportion of muscle mass in relation to their total body weight. Thus, the SMI potentially misclassifies the obese elderly with a high SMI and mobility and functional limitations and the thin elderly with a low SMI and none or a few mobility or functional limitations. Some investigators have taken a different approach and tried to build control for fat mass or body weight into the index, rather than adjusting statistically for these when analyzing associations with other variables.[5,12]

Recently, Janssen et al used data from the National Health and Nutrition Survey III to try to improve prevalence estimates in the United States. In addition, receiver operating curves were used to determine the sex-specific skeletal mass cut point below which the risk of physical disability significantly increased.[7] Women whose SMI was below 5.75 kg/m^2 muscle mass had an increased risk for physical disability (OR = 3.31, 95% CI; 1.91–5.73) and men whose SMI was below 8.50 kg/m^2 had an increased risk for physical disability (OR = 4.71, 95% CI; 2.28–9.74). As note earlier, a limitation of current methods of measuring muscle mass in defining sarcopenia is systematic errors introduced by the age-related increase in fatty infiltration of muscle tissue. Intramuscular adipose tissue infiltration, measured by MRI[13] and computed tomography (CT), improves our understanding of fat infiltration and muscle tissue impairment, but they are costly and often inaccessible. Ultrasound can accurately measure cross-sectional thicknesses and areas in subcutaneous adipose and muscles tissues,[14,15] and bioelectrical impedance can provide estimates of muscle mass, but these can have large errors and are sample and population specific.[16] Anthropometry has been used with limited success to detect sarcopenia in ambulatory settings. Changes in body weight loss are insufficient because an increase in fat mass can obscure a loss in muscle tissue leading to the condition referred to as *sarcopenic obesity*.[4]

The qualitative approach

The main effect from a loss of muscle mass is reduced muscle strength, which is an important factor to consider in defining sarcopenia. Muscle strength is measured with simple and complex equipment. Grip strength is a simple estimator of total muscle strength but is not useful in those with hand arthritis. Leg muscle strength, assessed as maximal lower extremity muscle strength or power, is a good measure of functional status, but it is properly measured with a dynamometer (e.g., Biodex or Kin Com) by a trained technician and is strongly associated with measures of mobility.[17] Including a measure of muscle strength in an operational definition is logical, as several authors have reported that muscle strength, more than muscle mass, is independently associated with physical performance.[18] Moreover, different factors, such as physical activity or hormones, can underlie and contribute in varying degree to the loss of muscle strength and loss of muscle mass. The loss of muscle quality, an important component of the definition of sarcopenia, supposes an assessment of both muscle strength and muscle mass.

Muscle power is strongly related to functional limitation more than muscle mass or muscle strength.[19] Muscle power is strength multiplied by speed, and it is defined as muscle work (muscle strength multiplied by a distance) divided by time. Muscle power declines considerably with aging and at a higher rate than muscle strength. A muscle power assessment is probably closer to a theoretic definition of sarcopenia than muscle strength alone, but muscle power does not include a quantitative measure. Using muscle power to define sarcopenia[20] could include muscle contraction speed and a measure of muscle quality in addition to muscle strength. Defining sarcopenia on muscle strength or muscle power only has several other limitations. Osteoarthritis and other comorbidities common with old age can induce underestimates of strength and power from pain affecting individual performance. Loss of muscle strength in the upper or lower limbs can have separate causes and be associated with different outcomes. Moreover, isokinetic, isometric, concentric, and eccentric muscle strength represent different aspects of muscle strength that are probably not affected at the same level during the process of sarcopenia.

Research is needed to validate the parameters (muscle mass, muscle strength, muscle quality) that could be used to define sarcopenia. An operational definition of sarcopenia should include components that contribute to physical function, but these components may be under different mechanisms or treated by different approaches. However, estimates of the prevalence of sarcopenia in populations with complex and variable combinations of muscle mass, strength, and power measurements have not yet been proved. Moreover, a clinical tool may not be useful in epidemiology, and vice versa.

ETIOLOGY OF SARCOPENIA

Multiple risk factors and mechanisms contribute to the development of sarcopenia. Lifestyle behaviors such as physical inactivity, poor diet, and age-related changes in hormones and cytokine levels are important risk factors. Postulated mechanisms include alterations in muscle protein turnover, muscle tissue remodeling, the loss of alpha-motor-neurons, and muscle cell recruitment and apoptosis.[21] Genetic susceptibility also plays a role and explains individual and group differences in rates of sarcopenia. The relative influences of these factors on sarcopenia components such as muscle mass, muscle strength, and muscle quality are not well understood,[22] Each factor in the etiology and pathogenesis of sarcopenia potentially contributes differently to the loss of muscle mass, strength, or quality.

Lack of physical activity

Inactivity is an important contributor to the loss of muscle mass and strength at any age.[23–25] Inactivity results from bed rest studies indicate that a decrease in muscle strength occurs before a decrease in muscle mass,[26] and low levels of physical activity result in muscle weakness that, in turn, results in reduced activity levels, loss of muscle mass, and loss of muscle strength. Thus, physical activity should be protective for sarcopenia, but some studies suggest that the amount of protection depends on the type of activity.

Loss of neuromuscular function

The neurologic contribution to sarcopenia occurs through a loss of alpha motor-neuron axons.[27] Decreased electrophysiologic nerve velocity, related to the dropout of the largest fibers, reduces internodal length and segmental demyelination occurs with the aging process,[2] but the role of demyelization in sarcopenia seems minor.[28] The central drive that contributes to a decrease in voluntary strength is supposed to be preserved. The progressive denervation and reinnervation process observed during aging and resulting in fiber type grouping is the potential primary mechanism involved during the development of sarcopenia. From cross-sectional findings, the decline in motor neurons starts after the seventh decade with a loss of alpha motor neurons in the order of 50%,[29] and this affects the lower extremities with their longer axons more than the upper limbs.[2] The reduction in alpha motor-neuron number and in motor unit numbers results in a decline in coordinated muscle action and a reduction in muscle strength. Reinnervation contributes to the final differentiation of nerve fibers and the repartition between the type I fibers (slow, oxidative fibers) and the type II fibers (fast, glycolytic fibers).

During aging, the number of satellite cells and their recruitment ability[30] decrease with a greater decrease in type II than type I fibers. Satellite cells are myogenic stem cells that can differentiate to new muscle fibers and new satellite cells if activated during the process of regeneration,[31] but this regeneration may lead to imbalance, and the number of type II muscle fibers may decline following damage.

Altered endocrine function

There is evidence linking age-related hormonal changes to the loss of muscle mass and muscle strength. However, controversy persists regarding their respective roles and effects on skeletal muscle in adulthood and old age.

INSULIN

Sarcopenia may be accompanied by a progressive increase in body and intramyocellular fat mass, which are associated with an increased risk of insulin resistance.[8] Insulin's role in the etiology and pathogenesis of sarcopenia could be important even if its effect on muscle synthesis remains controversial.[32–34] Insulin selectively stimulates skeletal muscle mitochondrial protein synthesis,[35] but it is unclear if the anabolic effect of insulin on muscle synthesis is impaired with advancing age.

ESTROGENS

There are conflicting data on the effects of estrogens on sarcopenia. Epidemiologic and interventional studies suggest that estrogens prevents the loss of muscle mass,[22,36] as their decline with age increase the levels of proinflammatory cytokines suspected to be involved in the sarcopenia process such as tumor necrosis factor alpha (TNF-α) and interleukin 6 (Il-6).[37] Estrogens also increase the level of sex hormone–binding globulin, which reduces the level of serum-free testosterone, thus hormone replacement therapy (HRT) should decrease rather than increase muscle mass,[38] Both these mechanisms may play a marginal role involving estrogen during the development of sarcopenia.

GROWTH HORMONE AND INSULIN-LIKE GROWTH FACTOR 1

Insulin-like growth factor-1 (IGF-1) and growth hormone (GH) decline with age[39] and are potential contributors to sarcopenia. GH replacement therapy lowers fat mass, increases lean body mass, and improves blood lipid profile. IGF-1 activates satellite cell proliferation and differentiation and increases protein synthesis in existing fibers.[40] There is also evidence that IGF-1 acts in muscle tissue by interacting with androgens,[41] but there are conflicting results on its effect on muscle strength despite the apparent increase in muscle mass.[42,43]

TESTOSTERONE

Testosterone levels gradually decrease in elderly men at a rate of 1% per year, and epidemiologic studies suggest a relationship between low levels of testosterone in elderly men and loss of muscle mass, strength, and function. The increase in sex hormone–binding globulin levels with age results in lower levels of free or bioavailable testosterone. Clinical and experimental studies support the hypothesis that low testosterone levels predict sarcopenia with low testosterone resulting in lower protein synthesis and a loss of muscle mass.[44] Testosterone induces in a dose-dependent manner an increase numbers of satellite cells, which is a major regulating factor of satellite muscle cell function.[41] When administered to hypogonadal subjects or elderly subjects with low levels, testosterone[45] increased muscle mass, muscle strength, and protein synthesis. Despite evidence that dehydroepiandrosterone (DHEA) supplementation results in an increase of blood testosterone levels in women and an increase of IGF-1 in men, few studies have reported an effect on muscle size, strength, or function.[46]

VITAMIN D AND PARATHYROID HORMONE (PTH)

With aging, 25-OH vitamin D levels decline. Several cross-sectional studies have reported the association between low 1,25-OH vitamin D and low muscle mass, low muscle strength, decreased balance, and increased risk of falls.[47,48] One recent longitudinal epidemiologic study reported an independent association between low serum vitamin D and sarcopenia.[49] Nuclear 1,25-OH vitamin D receptor has been described in muscle cells,[50] and low levels of vitamin D have been shown to decrease muscle anabolism. Low vitamin D may also influence muscle protein turnover through reduced insulin secretion. Low levels of vitamin D are associated with raised PTH, but previous studies suggest that high PTH is also independently associated with sarcopenia.[22,49]

High level of cytokines

Chronic medical conditions, such as chronic obstructive pulmonary disease (COPD), heart failure, and cancer, are highly prevalent in elderly and are associated with an increased serum level of proinflammatory cytokines and loss of body weight, including lean mass. This condition can occur in younger adults or elderly persons and is called cachexia. This acute hypercatabolism differs from the long-term age-related process that leads to sarcopenia. However, aging is also associated with a more gradual, chronic, increased production of proinflammatory cytokines, particularly IL-6 and IL-1, by peripheral blood mononuclear cells. There is some evidence that increased fat mass and reduced circulating levels of sex hormones with aging contribute to this age-related increase in proinflammatory cytokines that constituted catabolic stimuli.[51] Thus, the aging process itself is associated with increased catabolic stimuli, but there is still a lack of evidence for the hypothesis that cytokines predict sarcopenia in prospective studies.[22,52,53] Nevertheless, sarcopenia is one of the outcomes of cytokine-related aging process.[54]

Obesity is linked to inflammation[55] and may have an important role in the process leading to sarcopenia.[21] Being both obese and sarcopenic is a condition named *sarcopenic obesity*.[56] Sarcopenic obesity has been reported to predict the onset of disability more than sarcopenia or obesity alone. This condition occurs in about 6% of the community-dwelling elderly and to about 29% of men and 8.4% of women over 80 years of age. It has been hypothesized that sarcopenic obesity is associated with increased fatty infiltration of muscle, but confirmatory data are lacking. Fatty infiltration of skeletal muscle is associated with reduced strength[57,58] and functional status, and it is hypothesized that infiltration affects muscle function.[58] These findings suggest a role of fat mass in the etiology of sarcopenia.

Mitochondrial dysfunction

The role of mitochondrial dysfunction in sarcopenia is currently controversial.[59] Mitochondrial function may be affected by the cumulative damage to muscle mitochondrial DNA (mtDNA) observed with aging. This may result in a reduction of the metabolic rate of muscle cell protein synthesis, adenosine triphosphate synthesis[60] and finally to the death of the muscle fibers and the loss of muscle mass.[61,62] However, low physical activity could be the primary reason for mitochondrial dysfunction in the elderly. Some investigators report that the decline in mitochondrial functions with aging of can be attenuated by physical activity.[63] Others report that mitochondrial impairment is only partially reversed after physical training, but it does not reach the level of improvement observed in young.[62,64,65]

Apoptosis

Accumulated mutations in muscle tissue mitochondrial DNA are associated with accelerated apoptosis of myocytes, and apoptosis may also be the link between mitochondria dysfunction and loss of muscle mass. Evidence suggests that myocyte apoptosis is a basic mechanism underlying sarcopenia,[66] and muscle biopsies of older persons show differences associated with apoptosis[67] compared with younger subjects. Reports also suggest that type II fibers (those fibers preferentially affected by the sarcopenia phenomenon) may be more susceptible to death via the apoptotic pathway.[68]

Genetic influence

Genetic factors are major contributors to variability in muscle strength and likely contribute to susceptibility to sarcopenic agents. Genetic epidemiologic studies suggest that between 36% and 65% of an individual's muscle strength,[69] 57% of lower extremity performance[70] and 34% of the ability to perform the activities of daily living (ADL)[71] are explained by heredity. Sarcopenia and poor physical performance in elderly are also associated with birth weight in both men and women independent of adult weight and height, which suggests that exposures very early in life may additionally program risk for sarcopenia in old age in genetic susceptible individuals.[72,73]

Few studies have explored potential candidate genes determining muscle strength. In an analysis of the myostatin pathway, a possible muscle mass regulator, linkage was observed to several areas. Several genes were implicated as positional candidate genes for lower extremity muscle strength.[69,74–76] The actinin alpha 3 (ACTN3) R577X genotype is of interest, as it has been shown to influence knee extensor peak power in response to strength training as has a polymorphism in the angiotensin-converting enzyme (ACE) gene.[74,77] Also, polymorphisms in the vitamin D receptor (VDR) may be associated with muscle strength because of the relationship between vitamin D and its known effect on both smooth and striated muscle.[78] Polymorphisms in the VDR have been associated with sarcopenia in elderly men,[79] muscle strength and body composition in premenopausal women,[80] and muscle strength in older women.[81]

Low nutritional intake and low protein intake

Muscle protein synthesis rate is reported to be reduced 30% in the elderly, but there is controversy as to the extent to which this reduction is due to nutrition, disease, or physical inactivity rather than aging.[82,83] It is recognized by some that protein intake in elders should exceed the 0.8 g/kg per day recommend intake.[84] Muscle protein synthesis is also decreased in fasting elderly subjects, especially in specific muscle fractions like mitochondrial proteins,[85] and thus, the anorexia of aging and its underlying mechanisms contribute to sarcopenia by reducing protein intake.

Muscle protein synthesis is directly stimulated by amino acid and essential amino acids intake,[86] and protein supplementation has been explored in the prevention of sarcopenia. However, many interventional studies have not reported a significant increase muscle mass or protein synthesis with a high protein diet even when accompanied by resistance training.[87–89] The lack of effect of protein intake on protein synthesis stimulation may have several explanations.[38] A higher splanchnic extraction of dietary amino acids has been already reported.[90] This could limit the delivery of dietary amino acids to the peripheral skeletal muscle.

CONSEQUENCES OF SARCOPENIA

Increased clinical and epidemiologic interest in sarcopenia is related to the hypothesis that age-related loss of muscle mass and strength results in decreased functional limitation and mobility disability among the elderly (Figure 73-1). Sarcopenia also plays a predominant role in the etiology and pathogenesis of frailty, which is highly predictive of adverse events such as hospitalization, associated morbidity, and disability and death.[91] The annual health care cost attributable to sarcopenia is estimated at $18 billion in the United States alone.[92] Several epidemiologic cross-sectional studies have documented associations between low skeletal muscle mass and physical disability[7] or low physical performance,[58] with the level of disability two to five times higher in the sarcopenic groups. Sarcopenia also results in decrease in muscular strength and endurance.[93] Then, we can speculate that sarcopenia is a predictor of disability in the elderly, but very few longitudinal studies[7,94,95] have demonstrated that sarcopenia predicts disability and have reported little or no effect of sarcopenia on mobility disability.[94,95] This weak association between sarcopenia and the risk of disability suggests that disability can result in cases of sarcopenia (see Figure 73-1).

Relationship between sarcopenia and physical performance

Part of the theoretic model for sarcopenia potentially involves the positive association between muscle mass and strength and in improved functional performance and reduced disability. The relationship between muscle mass and strength is linear,[96] but the relationship between physical performance (such as walking speed) and muscle mass is curvilinear[97] (Figure 73-2). Thus, a threshold defining the amount of muscle mass under which muscle mass predicts poorer physical performance and physical disability should be detectable, but a specific threshold may exist for each physical task. The relationships among strength, muscle

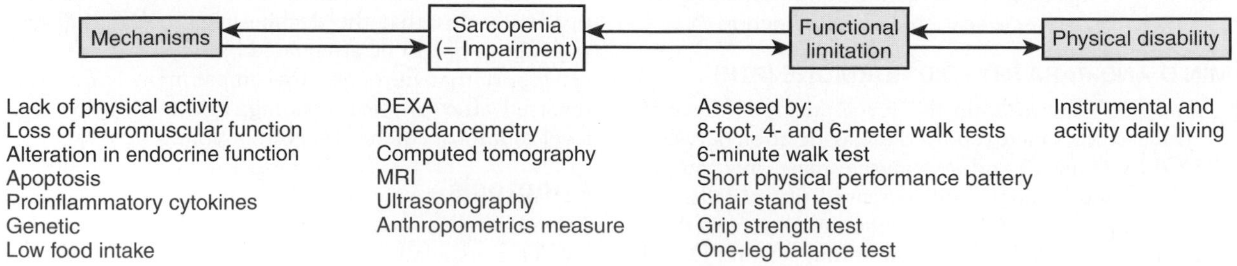

Figure 73-1. Sarcopenia and the disability process.

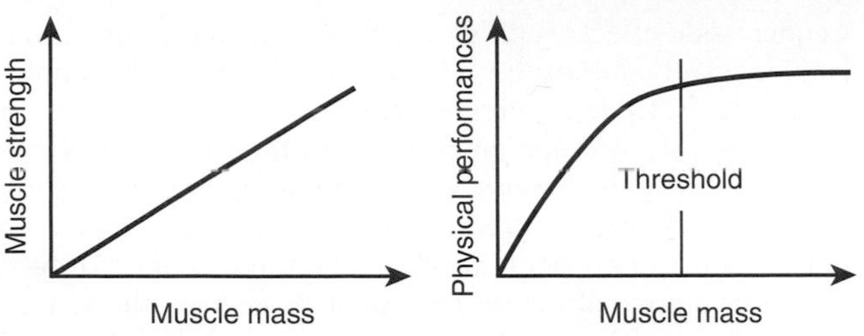

Figure 73-2. Relationship between muscle mass, muscle strength, and physical performances.

mass, and function have important implications regarding the selection of therapeutic approaches. An increase in muscle mass and strength in the healthy elderly could have little effect on a specific physical performance, but a small increase in muscle mass among sarcopenic elderly could result in a significant increase in physical performance despite a relatively small increase in muscle strength. An increase in muscle mass may have no effect on walking speed in the healthy elderly but a significant impact in very frail. However, differences in functional outcomes and population characteristics are major determinants in the success of interventional studies on sarcopenia, and these differences are attributable, in part, to these methodological considerations.

Treatment and future perspectives

Sarcopenia is treated currently with pharmacologic treatment and lifestyle interventions. Considerable evidence suggests that sarcopenia is a reversible cause of disability and could benefit from intervention, especially at the early stage of sarcopenia.[98–100] However, the effects and ability of these interventions to improve function and prevent disability and reduce the age-related skeletal muscle decline in elderly are unknown.

In treatment for sarcopenia, it could be argued that improving muscle strength or muscle power is more relevant clinically for the outcomes of disability or mobility than increasing muscle mass; however, increasing muscle mass is more important for other outcomes such as protein stores or thermogenesis. The notion that muscle strength and muscle mass are differentially affected by various treatment modalities is supported by experimental and clinical findings.[22] Although behavioral treatments, such as exercise, increase muscle mass and strength, pharmacologic treatments, such as growth hormone, increase mass without a significant change in strength.

Physical activity

No pharmacologic or behavioral intervention to reverse sarcopenia has proved to be as efficacious as resistance training. Muscle mass, strength, and muscle quality (strength adjusted for muscle mass) are reported to improve significantly with resistance training in older people.[101] Robust evidence in several studies indicates that resistance training such as weight lifting increases myofibrillar muscle protein synthesis,[102,103] muscle mass, and strength,[30,89,104–109] even in the frail elderly. Strength gains result from a combination of improved muscle mass and quality and neuronal adaptation (innervations, activation pattern). However, sarcopenia is observed in master athletes who maintain resistance training activities throughout their lifetimes.[110,111]

The American College of Sport Medicine (ACSM) and the American Heart Association (AHA) suggested that training at a 70% to 90% of 1-RM (maximal repetition) on two or more nonconsecutive days per week was the appropriate training intensity to produce gains in muscle size and strength, even in frail elderly.[112,113] Resistance training in elderly increases strength that is low in absolute terms but similar relative to muscle mass, but the increased muscle size is relatively moderate (between 5% and 10%) compared to the increase in muscle strength. Most of the increase in strength is in neural adaptation of the motor unit pathway,[2] but disuse results in a rapid detraining.[114] Several reports suggest that maintaining the benefits from resistance training is possible with as little as one exercise program per week.[115]

Whether aerobic training can reduce, prevent, or treat sarcopenia is an important practical question because resistance training is less appealing to many sedentary elders. Aerobic exercise does not contribute as much to muscle hypertrophy as resistive exercises, but it stimulates muscle protein synthesis,[116] satellite cell activation, and increased muscle fiber area.[117] A possible important aspect of aerobic exercises is that they reduce body fatness, including intramuscular fat, which is important for improving the functional role of muscle relative to body weight.

Leisure physical activity is not enough to prevent the decline in muscle mass,[118] but aerobic and resistance activities improve balance, lessen fatigue, increase pain release, reduce cardiovascular risk factors, and improve appetite. Thus, promoting an active lifestyle can prevent the functional effects of sarcopenia, but resistance training is the best approach to prevent and treat sarcopenia, although both training modalities contribute to the maintenance and improvement of muscle mass and strength in the elderly.

Nutrition

In malnourished elderly persons, poor protein intake is a barrier to gains in muscle tissue and strength from interventions such as resistance training. Increasing protein intake in elderly and especially in frail elderly can minimize the sarcopenic process.[119] However, it is not clear if protein supplementation in the absence of malnutrition enhances muscle mass and muscle strength, as protein supplementation alone or in association with physical training has proved unsuccessful.[113] New approaches, based on specific nutriments, including essential amino acids (leucine),[120] suggested an anabolic effect.[121] It has been reported that essential amino acids stimulate protein anabolism in elderly, whereas nonessential amino acids had no effect in association to essential amino acids.[86,122] The acute muscle protein synthesis in response to resistance training and essential amino acids ingestion is similar in old and young subjects but delayed in older subjects.[122] In supraphysiologic concentration, leucine stimulates muscle protein synthesis,[120] which may be related to a direct effect of leucine on the initiation of mRNA translation, and amino acid supplements are ineffective for muscle protein synthesis if they do not contain sufficient leucine.[123] The quantity and quality of amino acids in the diet are important factors for stimulating protein synthesis, and nutritional supplementation with whey proteins, a rich source of leucine, is a possible safe strategy to prevent sarcopenia.[124,125] However, caloric restriction can prevent the loss of muscle mass in animal and supposedly some human studies.[126,127]

The schedule of the protein supplementation is relevant to improve muscle protein synthesis. A large amount of amino acid supplementation in one meal per day is more efficient in increasing the anabolic effect than intermittent protein intake.[128] The anabolic effect of protein supplementation may be maximized with a large amount of a highly efficient nutritional supplement (such as essential amino acid and especially leucine) once a day. Another way to optimize postprandial protein anabolism is to administer "fast" protein (i.e., quickly digested protein by analogy with "fast" carbohydrate concept), which is an interesting nutritional strategy.[129,130] However, no randomized clinical trial actually supports the benefits of this specific approach on muscle mass synthesis.

Prevention of sarcopenia should occur throughout life. The possible influence of specific exposures at critical development periods may have a major impact on the risk of sarcopenia in old age.[72,131] An adequate diet in childhood and young adulthood affects bone development, and calcium maintenance is required throughout life, thus the same appears to be a reasonable lifestyle and treatment regime for sarcopenia.

Testosterone

About 20% of men older than 60 years and 50% of men older than 80 years are considered hypogonadic.[132] There are conflicting and inconclusive results of the effectiveness of testosterone therapy on muscle mass and muscle strength in elderly. Testosterone increases muscle mass and strength at supraphysiologic doses in young subjects under resistance training,[133] but such dose levels are not administered in the elderly. Some interventional studies report a modest increase in lean mass and most report no increase in strength.[113] For the few studies that report an increase in strength, the magnitude was lower than through resistance training. Moreover, the anabolic effect of testosterone on lean mass and strength seems weaker in the elderly than in young.[113] A recent meta-analysis indicated that there is a moderate increase in muscle strength among men participating in 11 randomized studies (with one study influencing the mean effect size).[134] Studies of DHEA have also reported no change in muscle strength.[113]

Testosterone is currently not recommended for the treatment of sarcopenia, and side effects associated with other androgens limit their use also. The potential risks associated with testosterone therapy (e.g., increased level of prostate-specific antigen, hematocrit, and cardiovascular risks) compared to the low level of evidence concerning the benefits on physical performances and function explain the actual recommendations.[135] High doses of testosterone have not be given in randomized controlled trial (RCT) for fear of prostate cancer,[136] and sense data from the Baltimore Longitudinal Study on Aging report a positive correlation between free testosterone blood level and prostate cancer.[137]

Growth hormone

GH increases muscle strength and mass in young subjects with hypopituitarism, but in the elderly, who are frequently GH-deficient, most studies report that GH supplementation does not increase muscle mass or strength,[113] even in association with resistance training.[113,138] GH increases mortality rate in ill and malnourished persons,[139] and potential serious and frequent side effects such as arthralgia, edema, cardiovascular side effect, and insulin resistance occur with GH supplementation.[43] To date, there is little clinical research support for the use of GH supplementation in the treatment of sarcopenia. Previous observations examining the association of IGF-1 with muscle strength and physical performance in older populations provide conflicting results.[140] Interestingly, in a study among obese postmenopausal women, the administration of GH alone or in combination with IGF-1 caused a greater increase in fat-free mass and a greater reduction in fat mass than those achieved by diet and exercise alone.[141] However, safety issues limit the clinical applications of these findings. Some studies have found that IGF-1 correlates with risk of prostate cancer in men, premenopausal breast cancer in women, and lung cancer and colorectal cancer in both men and women.[142]

Myostatin

Myostatin is a recently discovered natural inhibitor of muscle growth,[143] and mutations in the myostatin gene result in muscle hypertrophy in animals and in humans.[144,145] Antagonism of myostatin enhanced muscle tissue regeneration in aged mice[145] by increasing satellite cell proliferation. New approaches such as antagonist of myostatin drug may be relevant to the treatment of sarcopenia in the future.[146–148]

Estrogens and tibolone

A review on the effect of estrogen and tibolone on muscle strength and body composition[149] reports an increase in muscle strength, but only tibolone appears to increase lean body mass and decrease total fat mass. Tibolone is a synthetic steroid with estrogenic, androgenic, and progestogenic activity. HRT and tibolone may both react with the intranuclear receptor in the muscle fibers,[150,151] and tibolone may also act by binding androgen receptors in the muscle fibers and increasing free testosterone and GH. However, further research is needed to confirm these findings and the long-term safety of these drugs in the elderly population. In fact, no study has currently confirmed the positive findings in older persons.

Vitamin D

Vitamin D supplementation between 700 and 800 IU per day reduces the risk of hip fracture (and any nonvertebral fracture) in community-dwelling and nursing home elderly[152] and the risk of falls.[48] The underlying mechanism may be the increased muscle strength. Janssen et al reported an histologic muscle atrophy, predominantly type II fibers, in vitamin D deficiency.[153] Whether vitamin D prevents sarcopenia remains to be proved, but the relationship of vitamin D and calcium on muscle mass and function in the elderly is another important area for research.

Angiotensin II converting enzyme inhibitors (ACE inhibitors)

Growing evidence suggests that ACE inhibitors may prevent sarcopenia.[119,154,155] Activation of the renin-angiotensin-aldosterone system may be involved in the progress of sarcopenia. Angiotensin II infused in rats results in muscle atrophy,[146] and several mechanisms such as influences on oxidative stress, metabolic, and inflammation pathway have been suggested through epidemiologic and experimental studies. ACE inhibitor reduces the level of angiotensin II in vascular muscle cell, and angiotensin II may be a risk factor for sarcopenia through the related increase in proinflammatory cytokine production. ACE inhibitors may also improve exercise tolerance via changes in skeletal muscle myosin heavy chain composition.[156] The ACE gene polymorphism also affects the muscle anabolic response and muscular efficiency after physical training.[157]

Cytokine inhibitors

The age-related inflammation process is supposed to be an important factor in the development of sarcopenia, and anti-inflammatory drugs may delay its onset and progression. Cytokine inhibitors, such as thalidomide, increase weight and lean tissue anabolism in AIDS patients.[158] TNF-α produces muscle tissue atrophy in vitro. Anti-TNF-α antibodies, a treatment provided to rheumatoid arthritis patients, may also be an alternative therapeutic opportunity for sarcopenia.[159] However, the benefit/risk balance of these drugs is a major limitation that has not yet been tested in sarcopenic patients. Epidemiologic data also suggest that fatty fish consumption rich in the anti-inflammatory actions of omega-3 fatty acid may prevent sarcopenia.[160]

Genes

Many genetic factors contribute to muscle mass and strength.[161,162] Treatment based on the basic physiopathology of sarcopenia can be expected in the future.[163] Understanding the fundamental pathways leading to sarcopenia, such as the expression pattern of genes and proteomics, will probably determine future treatment strategies.

Apoptosis

Our understanding of the mechanisms of apoptosis suggests that caspase inhibitors may represent a possible future therapy.[164] Apoptosis may be reversible. For instance, exercise training reverses the skeletal muscle apoptosis and caloric restriction reduce apoptosis pathway stimulated by TNF-α.[127,165] Redox modulators such as carotenoids[166] seem to be important factors in influencing loss of muscle strength, functional limitation, and disability. Interest in all these molecules is actually suggested by basic research but may be studied in future clinical researches.

CONCLUSION

Improved understanding and treatment of sarcopenia would have a dramatic impact on improving the health and quality of life for the elderly, reducing the associated comorbidity and disability and stabilizing rising health care costs. However, continued research is needed to develop a consensus operational clinical definition of sarcopenia applicable in clinical management and clinical and epidemiologic research across populations. Sarcopenia is a complex multifactorial condition, the interrelated underpinnings and onset of which are difficult to detect and poorly understood. Thus, a comprehensive approach to sarcopenia requires a multimodal approach. Reducing the loss of muscle mass and muscle strength is relevant if the decrease in physical performances and increase in disability are affected. Defining target elderly populations for specific treatments in clinical trials is an important issue if the findings and their interpretation are to be inferred to other groups and populations of elderly individuals. An important clinical end point should be the prevention of mobility disability along with reducing, stopping, or reversing the loss of muscle mass, muscle strength, or muscle quality.

Currently, resistance strength training is the only treatment that affects the muscle aspects of sarcopenia. There are no pharmacologic approaches that provide definitive evidence in the ability to prevent the decline in physical function and sarcopenia. Current and future pharmacologic and clinical trials and epidemiologic studies could radically change our therapeutic approach to understanding and treating mobility disability in elderly.

KEY POINTS

Sarcopenia

- Definition of sarcopenia includes a loss of muscle strength and functional quality in addition to the loss of muscle protein mass.
- Sarcopenia affects about 20% of men between age 70 and 75 years, about 50% of those over age 80 years, and between 25% and 40% of women have sarcopenia in the same age ranges.
- A consensus operational definition of sarcopenia that is useful across clinics, studies, and populations is still lacking.
- Multiple risk factors and mechanisms contribute to the development of sarcopenia.
- Lifestyle behaviors, poor diet, and age-related changes in hormones and cytokine levels are important risk factors.
- The relationships among strength, muscle mass, and function have important implications in research and clinics.
- Evidence suggests that sarcopenia is a reversible cause of disability and could benefit from intervention.
- Muscle mass, strength, and muscle quality improve significantly in older people who participate in resistance training.
- No pharmacologic approaches provide definitive evidence in the ability to prevent sarcopenia.

For a complete list of references, please visit online only at www.expertconsult.com

CHAPTER 74

Podiatry

Katherine Ward
Mark A. Kosinski
Bryan Markinson

With population aging continuing to accelerate, particular attention must be paid to the multiple and complex disorders that impair functional independence and compromise quality of life of older adults. One of the most important and sometimes overlooked topics is that of proper foot health and function. Estimates of the prevalence of foot pain among community-dwelling older adults range between 36% and 70%, depending on definitions and populations studied.[1] Foot pain can easily jeopardize an individual's ability to perform many of the important instrumental activities of daily living, including cooking, shopping, housekeeping, doing laundry, and using transportation. Even so, as few as one third of older adults with disabling foot pain report receiving professional foot treatment.[2]

Foot pain in older adults may be caused by changes in gait, hereditary problems, or previous foot conditions that were not treated or treated inadequately. Changes in mental status, nutritional deficiencies, systemic and local disease, hospitalization and confinement to bed, polypharmacy, and other common elderly life situations may complicate the picture.

The myriad of changes associated with aging results in a diminished homeostatic reserve, commonly manifested with loss of ambulation. The ability of an individual to remain ambulatory may be the only dividing line between institutionalization and remaining an active and viable member of society.

Proper foot care must be provided for elderly patients in an attempt to promote pain-free ambulation. The consequences of immobility in this age group (bladder infections, pulmonary problems, and venous thrombosis) certainly underscores this point. Podiatric problems are often preventable or readily treatable. Podiatric care is just part of the comprehensive and interdisciplinary nature of geriatric medicine. Of note, it is coming under the same scrutiny as other areas, with a controlled trial of a multifaceted podiatry intervention now under way.[3]

In this chapter, the diagnosis, treatment, and prevention of common pedal problems are discussed.

ORTHOPEDIC/BIOMECHANICAL DISORDERS

Lower extremity joint impairment and painful foot disorders also represent major causes of treatable gait disturbances. Heel pain is a common complaint of older individuals, especially as the older population exercises more. Recent weight gain, increased walking or standing activities, hard floors or surfaces, and biomechanical abnormalities are the factors that predispose to the development of plantar calcaneal pain. Plantar calcaneal spurs (diagnosed by a lateral radiograph of the foot) are often aggravated by an atrophied fat pad. Conservative treatment includes rest, stretching exercises, nonsteroidal anti-inflammatory drugs (NSAIDs), and biomechanically sound footwear, such as a sneaker or running shoe, with a thick shock-absorbing insole. Viscoelastic heel cushions or heel cups (available commercially) can be inserted into existing shoes to provide cushioning. Prescription custom-made orthoses may be indicated to support the arch and to reduce traction of the plantar fascia from its origin on the calcaneus. Accordingly, shoe modification and orthoses are prescribed for the long term. Stretching of the Achilles tendon and plantar fascia may help diminish symptoms more rapidly. Recalcitrant cases may require a series of local injections (local anesthetic combined with a corticosteroid) into the area of maximum tenderness (usually the anteromedial tubercle of the calcaneus). Acute plantar heel pain can become a chronic condition, especially in patients who are overweight or have bilateral symptoms.[4] When appropriate therapy fails to achieve expected results (especially within 3 to 6 months), one should consider systemic disease as a possible cause of heel pain. Diseases such as rheumatoid arthritis, ankylosing spondylitis, psoriatic arthritis, and Reiter's syndrome can also cause heel pain.

Another common musculoskeletal problem in elderly people, which is often misdiagnosed, is posterior tibial tendon dysfunction. Suspect this problem in a presentation of sudden asymmetry in arch height. There may be swelling and tenderness on palpation of the tendon insertion around the medial and plantar aspect of the navicular, and these findings often extend along the course of the tendon proximally behind the medial malleolus. If not already present, an actual tear or even rupture of the tendon may result. Orthotics can control minor cases, but depending on the level of activity of the patient and the degree of discomfort, custom-made braces or surgical correction may be the best option.

The joints of the feet are also prone to osteoarthritis. Diagnosed by limited and painful range of motion with or without crepitation, this condition usually responds well to conservative measures. Joint space narrowing on radiographs is often a late finding. Shoe modifications such as balanced inlay orthoses and a forefoot rocker sole angled to follow the progression of gait provide good local treatment. Topical preparations such as capsaicin (Zostrix) cream have been shown to relieve pain caused by degenerative joint disease and may augment NSAID therapy, which is the mainstay of treatment.

Joint pains from hallux valgus, hammer toes, and mallet toes are also common lower extremity problems in elderly people (see Figure 74-1; see also Color Plate 74-1). The myth that these are caused by ill-fitting shoe gear is disproven by the studies of populations in the world who typically live their lives unshod. The same incidence of these deformities occur, pointing to a more biomechanical/genetic cause. Indeed, shoes aggravate these conditions and make them painful, with the development of corns and adventitious bursae. A hammer toe is one in which there is a flexion contracture at the proximal interphalangeal joint. An extensor contracture at the metatarsophalangeal joint may coexist. A mallet toe is contracted at the distal interphalangeal joint, and a claw toe is contracted at both. The most common problem associated with these deformities is the formation of corns dorsally over areas of prominence and medial and lateral, and interdigitally. If the above-mentioned conservative measures fail to alleviate the pain, surgical correction may be considered. Foot surgery can provide improvement of function and quality of life, even in the presence of chronic illnesses. Of course, a

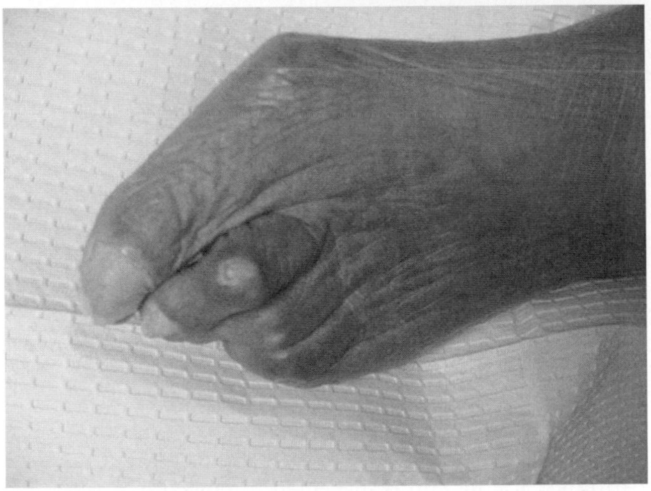

Figure 74-1. A bunion deformity with hammer toe of the second digit. Note preulcerative lesion over proximal phalangeal joint of second toe secondary to shoe pressure.

prudent comprehensive surgical work-up in conjunction with the primary care physician, and an anesthesiologist, would be obligatory. Fortunately, many forefoot procedures require only local anesthesia and are done on an ambulatory basis.

Your examination should always include watching the patient walk. Gait disturbances are a common sequela of age-related changes in the central and peripheral nervous systems (see Chapter 105). Features of pathologically induced gait disturbances are frequently nonspecific and overlap with those of senile ataxia, giving little clue as to the primary pathology. In Parkinson's disease and cerebellar atrophy, gait characteristics are specifically helpful in establishing the diagnosis. Shuffling and abducted gaits also produce increased stress and pressure on the soft tissues leading to dermal lesions (see Dermatology section below).

It is important to search for an underlying cause in the physical assessment because approximately 25% of gait disturbances in older adults have a treatable cause.[5] Serum studies may reveal vitamin B_{12} deficiency, hypothyroidism, osteomalacia, or drug toxicity. Radiographic studies assist in excluding bone disease. Remember that stress fractures may not be evident at the time of injury. If signs and symptoms are consistent with fracture, treat as such and repeat the radiograph in 10 to 14 days. Computed tomography, magnetic resonance imaging, myelography, and electrophysiologic studies may offer a definitive diagnosis in cases of primary central nervous system pathology. Common causes of gait disorders include neurologic (cerebrovascular accident, dementia, Parkinson's disease, etc.), musculoskeletal (arthritis, osteoporosis, myopathy, etc.), vascular, endocrine (hypothyroidism, diabetes), psychological (depression, fear of falling), and medications. Demonstration of poor gait, difficulty with chair transfer, and a loss of balance when standing on tiptoes suggests an underlying neurologic or musculoskeletal disorder.[6]

DERMATOLOGIC DISORDERS

Hyperkeratotic lesions (corns and calluses) are the most common podiatric complaints of elderly people. They frequently arise in areas of increased pressure or friction and over bony prominences. Although these conditions are common among all age groups, degenerative joint disease, atrophy of the plantar fat pad, and decreased pain threshold predispose elderly people to increased frequency of complaints. Depending on their depth and severity, there may be an associated adventitious bursa formation. Treatment consists of aseptic débridement and weight or pressure dispersion. Lesions on the plantar aspect of the foot should also be treated with a shock-absorbing insert to disperse the weight-bearing forces and augment an atrophic or displaced plantar fat pad.

It is especially important to débride chronic hyperkeratotic lesions in patients with vascular or neurologic impairment because untreated lesions may give rise to soft tissue breakdown, ulcerations, and bone infection. As noted earlier in this chapter, sneakers or running shoes are ideal footgear for biomechanical and dermatologic problems. A wide and high toe box is important for preventing pressure on the digits, and abundant cushioning on the sole of the foot is required to mitigate the excessive plantar pressures that cause the hyperkeratotic lesions.

Well-cushioned shoe gear is also required to mitigate the consequences of atrophied subcalcaneal or submetatarsal fat pads. When the natural fat found on the plantar aspect of the feet atrophies, the underlying bony structures become more prominent and cause pain. When such pain occurs under the plantar aspect of the metatarsal head, it is called metatarsalgia. The complaint is frequently a callus or inflammation of the area (bursitis). Diagnosis can be made by clinical examination, and radiographs may reveal underlying bone pathology. Treatment consists of débridement of hyperkeratotic lesions with padding to disperse the weight. Long-term treatment includes the use of soft tissue supplements such as plastizote, which can be added to foot orthotics or inserted directly into the shoe.

Expensive custom-molded shoes are often unnecessary for all but the most severe foot deformities. If they are indeed indicated, they should include a high, wide toe box, a bunion last, and an extra depth feature to accommodate weight-dispersive orthoses. Surgical correction should always be considered as the last resort, after all conservative measures have failed.

Maceration and fissuring of the interspaces is another common dermatologic finding in the elderly population. Vision and dexterity loss make it difficult to examine and care for the feet, and digital deformities precipitate moisture accumulation between the toes. The dark and moist environment between the toes predisposes the area to fungal and bacterial infection, which range from a mild annoyance to a severe debilitating infection. A Wood's light can be used to detect coral red fluorescence suggestive of *Corynebacterium minutissimum*, which is usually treated with topical erythromycin. Macerated toe web spaces may also be due to a fungal or yeast infection that can be treated with ciclopirox (Loprox) or clotrimazole solution (Lotrimin, Mycelex) applied interdigitally twice daily for 2 to 4 weeks. Of course, meticulous cleaning and drying of the area while bathing is also necessary. If lamb's wool or gauze is used to separate the toes, never encircle a digit; such dressings may become constrictive and severely compromise the circulation.

Interdigital tinea pedis (described previously), inflammatory tinea pedis, and chronic dry scaly tinea pedis are the three main categories of pedal dermatophyte infections.

Inflammatory tinea pedis, which is an acute vesicular eruption that has a particular predilection for the long arch, is caused by the dermatophyte *Trichophyton mentagrophytes*. It is usually severely pruritic, it may weep, and the severest of cases may require bed rest in addition to topical and/or oral antifungal therapy. The chronic form of tinea pedis, usually caused by *Trichophyton rubrum*, has a predilection for the arch as well, but is mainly confined to the lateral surfaces of the sole. Sometimes the entire plantar aspect is involved in what is classically described as a moccasin distribution. In contrast to the inflammatory type, these lesions are scaly and erythematous, and commonly display an arcuate shape.

There is also a decrease in skin hydration as aging progresses. Combined with diminished sebaceous and eccrine activity, dry, scaly, and hyperkeratotic skin often results. Peripheral heel hyperkeratosis is very common, but when fissures occur, severe pain and infection may ensue. This is a serious problem in the face of arterial insufficiency. Management includes débridement of the tissue, hydration of the skin, and avoidance of backless footwear. Chemical cautery with silver nitrate is often necessary to close a bleeding fissure. It is momentarily painful but works very effectively. Heel fissuring is more prevalent in the obese, and tends to be a chronic problem. In patients who have had total joint replacement, the presence of heel fissures should not be trivialized (see Figure 74-2).

Ulcerations of the leg, feet, and toes are also seen frequently in the geriatric population. The differential diagnosis of pedal ulcers includes arteriosclerosis obliterans, neurotrophic ulcers, chronic pernio, gout, mycobacterium tuberculosis, Raynaud's disease/phenomenon, scleroderma, and neoplasms, in addition to those caused by biomechanic, iatrogenic, or patient-induced diseases.[7]

Ischemic ulcers typically occur on the distal aspect of digits and over bony prominences. Symptoms include severe pain, often worse at night and relieved by dependency. They are characterized by poor granulation tissue, poor color of tissue (cyanotic, gray, or black), and poor bleeding upon débridement.

Neurotrophic ulcers commonly occur beneath pressure points or hyperkeratotic lesions. There is usually no pain because the patient is typically neuropathic. The ulcers are characterized by punched-out lesions with a red granular base and white fibrotic rim. Due to the high incidence of diabetic ulcers and their coexisting morbidity, this topic will be discussed thoroughly in a separate section within this chapter.

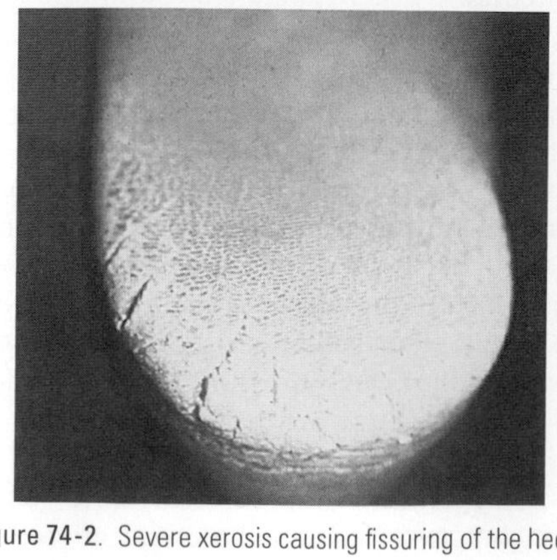

Figure 74-2. Severe xerosis causing fissuring of the heels.

Venous stasis ulcerations often follow chronic stasis dermatitis, which is secondary to incompetent venous circulation in the leg, as further described in Chapter 47. Poor arterial circulation is an added risk that will impair healing and increase the chance of infection.

Treatment of these ulcers must address their cause, and therefore requires a multidisciplinary approach. An ischemic ulcer requires a vascular consult as soon as possible, with possible revascularization. Neurotrophic ulcers require weight dispersion, débridement of devitalized tissue, and use of antibiotics when appropriate. Edema can be reduced with elevation of the foot (above heart level), and with compressive boots and stockings. Individuals with a history of venous stasis ulcers should wear elastic supports daily. Wound care must be performed regularly to ensure a clean, moist granular bed of the ulcer. Aerobic and anaerobic cultures must be performed if infection is suspected, followed by the appropriate antibiotic coverage.

It is important to keep in mind that a chronic ulceration, especially if it is not responding to appropriate therapy, has the potential for malignant degeneration. This is especially true for the common venous stasis ulcer. Any suspicious ulcer should be biopsied to include the most ominous border, along with normal skin for comparison.

NAIL DISORDERS

Identification of a fungal nail infection is easily performed with a KOH prep and fungal culture. The PAS (periodic acid-schiff stain) test is also used to detect the presence of viable or degenerating fungus organisms, and its sensitivity may be higher than that of the KOH test. Mycotic nail infections tend to respond poorly to topical therapy. The advent of safer oral agents such as Sporanox (itraconazole, Janssen Pharmaceutica) and Lamisil (terbinafine hydrochloride, Novartis) may help to achieve a cure in some patients, although the success of systemic agents is directly related to the vascular supply to the nail bed. A new topical antifungal, Penlac solution, 8% (ciclopirox, Dermik Laboratories), was approved by the U.S. Food and Drug Administration in 2000, and is indicated for mild to moderate onychomycosis due to *Trichophyton rubrum*. Older patients usually do well with serial nail débridement, which not only maintains comfort but decreases the chance of soft tissue infection, infected ingrown toenails, and subungual corns or ulceration.

It is important to differentiate mycotic nail infections from nail dystrophies secondary to systemic disease, vascular insufficiency, and trauma. For example, poor nutritional status can lead to toenails that are atrophic, thin, brittle, and lackluster, with possible longitudinal ridges. Other systemic diseases associated with common nail dystrophies include diabetes mellitus, syphilis, psoriasis, Reiter's syndrome, ischemia, gout, rheumatoid arthritis, and systemic lupus erythematosus.

Although patients invariably attribute periungual pain as being secondary to an ingrown or incurvated nail, it is important to rule out ischemia as the cause of the nail pain. Ischemic changes of the digit can often mimic nail pain and mislead both patient and physician.

Nail fold infections often exhibit adjacent chronic granulation tissue. In chronic infections, it may be prudent to biopsy such lesions. We are aware of patients in whom Kaposi's sarcoma, amelanotic melanoma, and squamous cell carcinoma of the nail groove have given the appearance of a pyogenic granuloma.

Subungual hematomas are not uncommon in older individuals, and usually result from microtrauma secondary to improperly fitting shoe gear. However, it is prudent to consider any subungual hyperpigmented lesion a melanoma until proved otherwise. In such cases, débride the nail plate as proximal as possible: many times part of the nail can be removed to reveal subungual debris consistent with previous hemorrhage or fungal infection. If a melanotic process is suspected, a biopsy must be performed.

FOOT PROBLEMS IN PATIENTS WITH DIABETES

Neuropathy, peripheral vascular disease, and immunopathy all play a role in the development of foot pathology in patients with diabetes. These three factors, combined with the reduced vision and mobility that impair the ability of older patients to inspect and care for their feet, can have disastrous consequences. When left unrecognized and therefore untreated, many minor foot problems (such as corns and calluses) progress to ulcerations and infections, producing the well-known morbidity associated with diabetes. Risk factors for diabetic foot ulcers include sensorimotor and autonomic neuropathy, peripheral vascular disease, limited joint mobility, high plantar pressures, bony deformities, history of previous ulceration, and visual or functional impairment.

Chronic sensory neuropathy is one of the most common long-term complications of diabetes mellitus. Symptoms frequently include numbness, dysesthesia, lancinating pain, burning, and hypersensitivity. Sensory loss is typically in a stocking-glove distribution and is often of insidious onset. In its early stages, patients may be unaware that a decrease in sensorium even exists. In those patients without diabetes, pedal neuropathy may be secondary to alcoholism, a herniated nucleus pulposus, heavy metals, vitamin deficiencies, and collagen diseases, among other systemic conditions.

Sensory neuropathy is often accompanied by a motor component. In the foot of a patient with diabetes, loss of motor fibers may lead to intrinsic muscle atrophy and imbalance between flexor and extensor muscles. Clawing of the toes, prominent metatarsal heads, and anterior displacement of an already atrophied plantar fat pad may increase the patient's risk for pressure-induced lesions.[8,9] Glycation of collagen leads to thickening and increased cross-linking of collagen bundles, resulting in thin, tight, and waxy skin and further restriction of joint movement.[10] Dry and atrophic skin is also caused by the autonomic neuropathy, which leads to denervation of the sweat glands. Cracks and fissures violate the skin defenses, leaving the patient vulnerable to bacterial infection.

Ulcerations may be caused by an acute event or repetitive minor trauma. It has been shown that constant pressure of 5 to 7 lb/square inch over a bony prominence can cause ischemic necrosis in less than 7 hours.[11] If an ulcer is indeed caused by pressure or a biomechanical problem, it will never resolve if weight is not dispersed from the affected area, regardless of how much débridement of local wound care is given.

Peripheral vascular disease is 20 times more common in patients with diabetes than in nondiabetic individuals.[12] Microvascular and macrovascular disease puts the patient at risk for gangrene and ulceration by reducing the perfusion pressure where tissue ischemia occurs. Diabetic occlusive disease has a predilection for the tibial and peroneal arteries, and tends to be bilateral and multisegmental. Ankle brachial pressure index (ABPI) and pulse volume recordings may be of questionable value in assessing peripheral circulation in patients with diabetes, but they are useful if they are low.[10] In general, be suspicious if the ABPI is greater than 1.0. A reading of less than 0.5 indicates serious arterial compromise and poor healing potential.

The best treatment for the foot of a patient with diabetes is patient education and thorough, frequent foot examinations. The foot examination should be a regular part of each office visit. Both shoes and socks should be removed and the feet should be checked for trophic and pretrophic skin changes, thickened or incurvated nails, and hyperkeratosis. Hemorrhage within a callus may be suggestive of ulcer formation. The interspaces should be carefully inspected for maceration or fissuring. Legs and feet should be evaluated for diabetic skin markers, such as bullous diabeticorum, diabetic dermopathy, and necrobiosis lipoidica, some of which may herald vasculopathy and retinopathy.

The neurologic examination should include evaluation of deep tendon reflexes, sharp/dull discrimination, light touch, proprioception, vibratory sensation using a 128 Hz tuning fork, and protective threshold using the Semmes-Weinstein monofilament. In fact, patients can do monofilament tests themselves. Vibratory sensation and proprioception, both carried by the posterior columns, are the first to be affected by diabetic neuropathy. Keep in mind that decreased vibratory sensation may also occur as part of normal aging. Diminished or absent knee and ankle jerk reflexes are also common with aging, and in the absence of other pathology do not require further evaluation. Autonomic neuropathy can be recognized clinically by the absence of sweating, a relatively fixed heart rate, and postural hypotension.

A palpable popliteal pulse may be an unreliable indicator of circulation in the lower extremity, as 40% of patients with diabetes having distal gangrene also have a popliteal pulse.[13] Similarly, a palpable dorsalis pedis or posterior tibial pulse is an unreliable indication of circulation in the toes. Twenty percent of patients with diabetes with palpable pedal pulses have significant small-vessel disease. Temperature gradient, capillary filling time, rubor on dependency, and pallor on elevation are useful adjunctive tests for assessing distal lower extremity circulation.

The pain of diabetic neuropathy is another common complaint of patients with diabetes. It is difficult to control, especially in patients with poor glucose control. Topical capsaicin (Zostrix) applied two or three times a day may provide some relief. Tricyclic antidepressants and nonsteroidal antiinflammatories may also prove advantageous, as are new drugs on the horizon.

Patients play an important role in preventing their foot problems. The following recommendations should be made at each office visit: stop smoking, inspect feet daily for cuts and blisters, inspect the inside and outside of shoes for foreign objects, do not walk barefooted, cut toenails straight across, avoid temperature extremes on the feet, and notify a physician of any problems immediately.

Summary of Management Algorithm

Diabetic Foot Ulcers

1. Evaluation
   a. Clinical appearance
   b. Depth of penetration
   c. X-rays to detect
      1) foreign body
      2) osteomyelitis
      3) subcutaneous gas
   d. Location
   e. Biopsy
   f. Blood supply (noninvasive vascular studies)
2. Débridement, radical
3. Bacterial cultures (aerobic and anaerobic)
4. Metabolic control
5. Antibiotics
   a. Oral
   b. Parenteral
6. Do not soak feet
7. Decrease edema
8. Non–weight-bearing
   a. Bed rest
   b. Crutches
   c. Wheelchair
   d. Special sandals
   e. Contact casting
9. Improve circulation (vascular surgery)

Source: Levin ME. The diabetic foot: pathophysiology, evaluation, and treatment. In Levin ME, O'Neal LW, Bowker J (eds). The Diabetic Foot, 5th Ed. St Louis, 1993, Mosby Year Book, pp 17–60. Reproduced with permission.

SUMMARY

Successful patient management must extend beyond diagnosis and disease treatment and include promotion of function and prevention of decline.[14] The podiatrist can be a valuable team member in the multidisciplinary approach of geriatric assessment; he or she can deliver proactive and preventive care that maintains or improves quality of life for older patients. The simple ability to ambulate comfortably is critical for our patient's feelings of overall well-being, self-esteem, and ability to interact in society. In addition, elderly people have become increasingly engaged in athletic activities, making them more prone to overuse, repetitive motion, and traumatic injuries. It is therefore necessary to prevent and treat the pedal manifestations of vascular, neurologic, musculoskeletal, and metabolic disorders to improve quality of life and ambulatory ability, while reducing pain and foot morbidity.

KEY POINTS
Podiatry

Orthopedic/biomechanical disorders:
- Heel pain
- Posterior tibial tendon dysfunction
- Osteoarthritis
- Digital deformities
- Pathologic gait

Dermatologic disorders:
- Hyperkeratotic lesions
- Bacterial infections
- Tinea pedis
- Xerosis/fissuring
- Ulcerations

Nail disorders:
- Fungal nail infections
- Nail dystrophies

Foot problems in patients with diabetes:
- Neuropathy
- Ulcerations
- Peripheral vascular disease

For a complete list of references, please visit online only at www.expertconsult.com

CHAPTER 75

Geriatric Dentistry: Maintaining Oral Health in the Geriatric Population

Andrea Schreiber
Robert Glickman

INTRODUCTION

Whereas dental textbooks address the management of medically compromised, older patients (generally including a review of the basic pathophysiology of a disease, the clinical signs and symptoms of the condition, common therapeutic interventions, and how either the disease itself or the medications for it might impact on planned dental care) in general, medical textbooks, even those on geriatric medicine, do not address the impact of oral health on the overall systemic health of a patient. The fact is that physicians are uniquely situated to screen elderly patients for common oral diseases.

Older adults tend to have low use rates of dental services, due perhaps to a lack of insurance coverage for these services or limited access to care secondary to infirmity. Although more than 90% of adults over the age of 75 seek medical care on a regular basis, only approximately a third of these individuals seek dental care.[1]

In a pilot study[2] investigating the physicians' role in the diagnosis and management of oral diseases in a geriatric population, four primary care physicians and four geriatricians were asked to identify oral conditions on 30 color slides. The rate of correct diagnosis was 55%, and appropriate treatment decisions were made 70% of the time.

In another study[3] performed to assess hospital physician knowledge and views concerning oral health in elderly patients, 70 respondents completed a survey and were asked to diagnose 12 different oral conditions demonstrated on clinical slides. Although 84% of respondents felt that it was important to examine the oral cavity, only 19% reported that they did so. Fifty-six percent of responding physicians did not feel confident in examining the oral cavity and 77% felt that that they had insufficient training to do so. Two of the 70 physicians (3%) were able to correctly identify all 12 oral conditions depicted in the slides.

The focus of this chapter will be on the maintenance of oral health for the geriatric patient and how physicians and dentists can ensure this goal. Topics to be covered include the definition of oral health, how oral health is measured, the changing dental needs of the geriatric population due to advances in medicine and dentistry, the impact of oral health on systemic health, recognition and management of common oral conditions in the elderly population and access to care issues for both community dwelling older adults and residents of long-term care facilities. Prevention and management of oral diseases will improve systemic along with oral health.[4]

Definition of oral health

Any discussion concerning the maintenance of oral health as a goal, must start with a definition of the term.[5] Mouradian[6] defined it as "...encompassing all of the immunologic, sensory, neuromuscular and structural functions of the mouth and craniofacial complex. Oral health influences and is related to nutrition and growth, pulmonary health, speech production, communication, self-image and societal functioning." Although the author was addressing the oral health needs of the pediatric population, this definition of oral health appears to apply to the population in general and to the geriatric population in particular. Conditions that adversely affect the oral and maxillofacial complex are common and pervasive in the elderly and can affect an individual's general health and quality of life.

Measures of oral health and function

Common measures of oral health include the number of teeth present in the mouth, the presence of caries (Figure 75-1, see also Color Plate 75-1) and restorations, and the presence or absence of periodontal disease (infection of the gingiva and tooth supporting structures) (Figure 75-2, see also Color Plate 75-2) and oral mucosal lesions (Figures 75-3 through 75-6, see also Color Plates 75-3 through 75-6). Many attempts have been made to quantify the effect of these parameters on oral function and the relationship of adequate oral function to an individual's quality of life. In a literature review[7] focused on determining the relationship between dentition and oral function, four specific areas were investigated: overall masticatory function, aesthetics/psychosocial ability, posterior dental occlusal stability and support, and other functions, including taste and phonetics. Eighty-three articles met inclusion criteria for review. Satisfactory masticatory function was linked to the total number of teeth present—specifically 20 teeth with 9 to 10 dental contacts (upper and lower teeth in occlusion). Patients with fewer teeth and/or fewer contacts demonstrated limited masticatory function. Dental aesthetics and psychosocial satisfaction was linked to the loss of anterior teeth with variations in satisfaction noted between age groups, cultures, and socioeconomic status. Occlusal stability

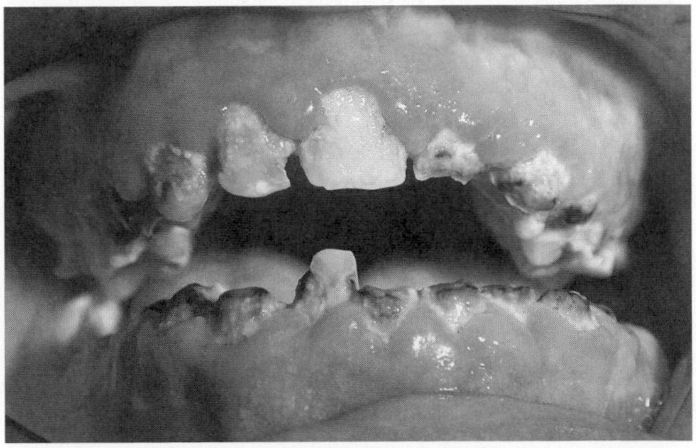

Figure 75-1. Rampant dental caries. *(Reprinted with the permission of Mirriam Robbins, DDS, New York University College of Dentistry.)*

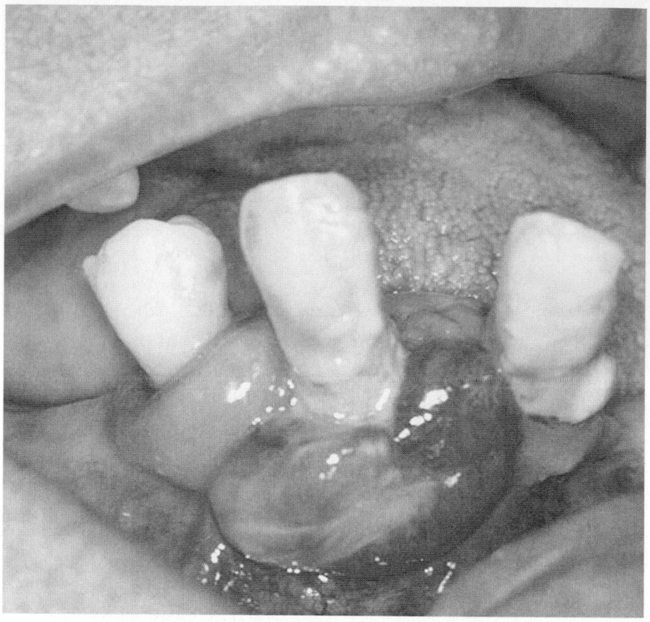

Figure 75-2. Periodontal abscess: associated with bone loss around root of tooth. *(Reprinted with the permission of Mirriam Robbins, DDS, New York University College of Dentistry.)*

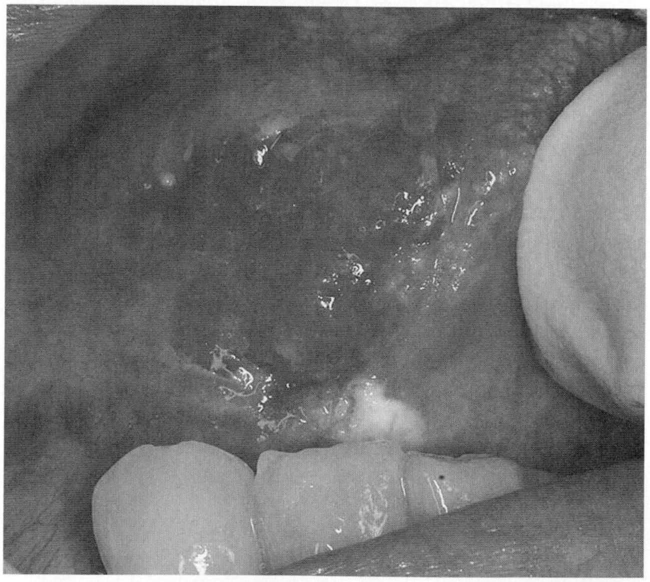

Figure 75-3. Oral dysplasias: right lateral border of tongue. *(Reprinted with the permission of Mirriam Robbins, DDS, New York University College of Dentistry.)*

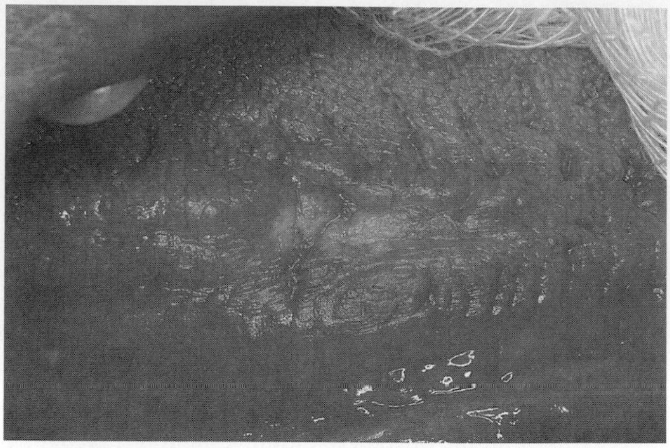

Figure 75-4. Leukoplakia or white lesion: left lateral border of tongue. *(Reprinted with the permission of Mirriam Robbins, DDS, New York University College of Dentistry.)*

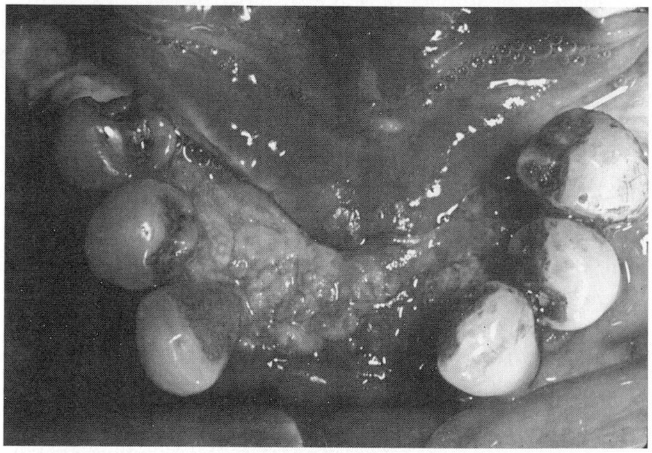

Figure 75-5. Squamous cell carcinoma: floor of mouth. *(Reprinted with the permission of Mirriam Robbins, DDS, New York University College of Dentistry.)*

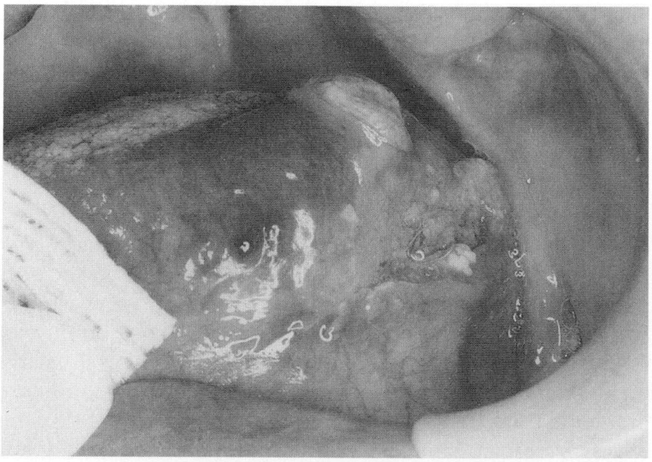

Figure 75-6. Squamous cell carcinoma: left lateral border of tongue. *(Reprinted with the permission of Mirriam Robbins, DDS, New York University College of Dentistry.)*

was noted with three to four posterior units in individuals with a symmetrical pattern of tooth loss and five to six posterior units in those with a nonsymmetrical pattern of bone loss. Patients did not attribute a high value to either phonetics or taste. The conclusion of the authors was that the World Health Organization goal of maintaining 20 natural teeth throughout life as a means of assuring an acceptable level of oral function is supported by current literature.

Measures of oral health-related quality of life (OH-QoL) assume functional and psychosocial impacts on the quality of life but exactly what is being measured by a variety of instruments designed for this purpose still remains to be clearly elucidated.[8]

Many efforts are underway to verify the validity of the quality of life assessment tools used to measure the impact of oral health on quality of life, or to add subscales to current tools to aid in quantifying a qualitative question.[9,10] In a survey study investigating the association between tooth loss, chewing ability, and association with oral and general health-related quality of life issues, two survey instruments were used (the Oral Health Impact Profile and the EuroQoL Visual Analogue Scale). In addition to the patient survey, functional tooth units were assessed by calibrated dentists on more than 700 Australians over the age of 50. The number of functional tooth units was positively related to chewing ability and general health, thereby reflecting the importance of oral health to general well-being.[11]

The aim of the Ontario Study of Oral Health of Older Adults (OSOHOA) was to document the natural history of oral diseases and disorders in older adults and to document the impact on physical, functional, and psychological well-being.[12] This was an observational cohort study of a random sample of adults who were over the age of 50 when recruited. The study consisted of a baseline phase and 3- and 7-year follow-ups. The ability to chew was assessed using an index of six different foods. Descriptive statistics were used to measure changes in chewing ability over time. The proportions of individuals experiencing increased chewing problems rose from 24% at baseline to 33.8% over the 7-year period. An increased prevalence and severity of chewing dysfunction was most noted for edentulous patients.

Other studies have noted that approximately one third of older adults have trouble biting some foods and that this percentage increases with advancing age and number of teeth missing.[13] Chewing ability or lack thereof can influence food choices and result in malnutrition in both community-dwelling and long-term care residents (Figure 75-7, see also Color Plate 75-7). Weight loss and poor nutrition in long-term care facilities have been linked to chewing problems.[14,15]

The changing need for dental care in geriatric patients

Advances in dental research have resulted in a lower incidence of tooth loss and caries in the general population as a result of the widespread use of fluoride, patient education, and dental hygiene programs.[16] Simply put, people are living longer with more teeth. The fully edentulous octogenarian is and will continue to be less frequently encountered in the twenty-first century. However, edentulous patients, despite the absence of teeth, may have a host of problems that can adversely affect oral and systemic health, including denture- or nondenture-related soft tissue lesions, oral candidiasis, malnutrition from ill-fitting dentures (Figure 75-8, see also Color Plate 75-8), or lack of thereof, resorption under existing dentures (Figure 75-9, see also Color Plate 75-9), gastrointestinal problems, masticatory insufficiency, swallowing disorders, and aspiration pneumonia. They are still susceptible to mucosal diseases (Figures 75-3 and 75-4, see also Color Plates 75-3 and 75-4) and oral cancers (Figures 75-5 and 75-6, see also Color Plates 75-5 and 75-6) despite the absence of teeth. The surgeon general's report on Oral Health in America in 2000 cited 30,000 new diagnoses of

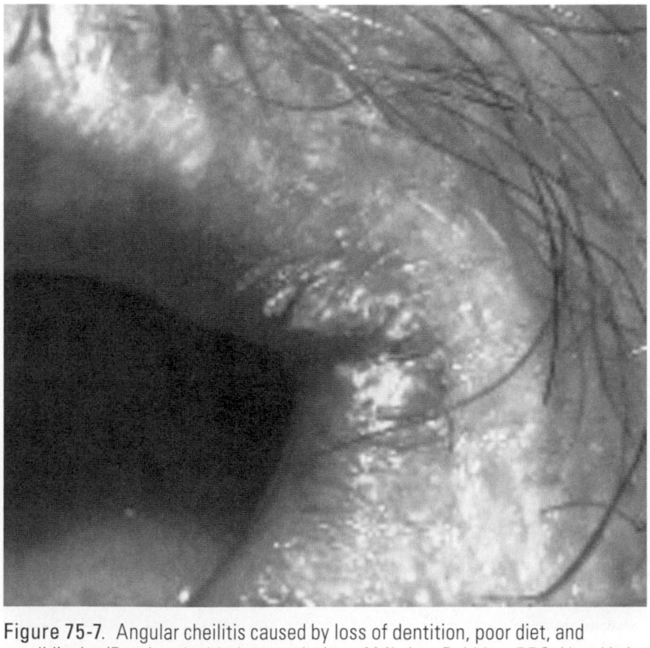

Figure 75-7. Angular cheilitis caused by loss of dentition, poor diet, and candidiasis. *(Reprinted with the permission of Mirriam Robbins, DDS, New York University College of Dentistry.)*

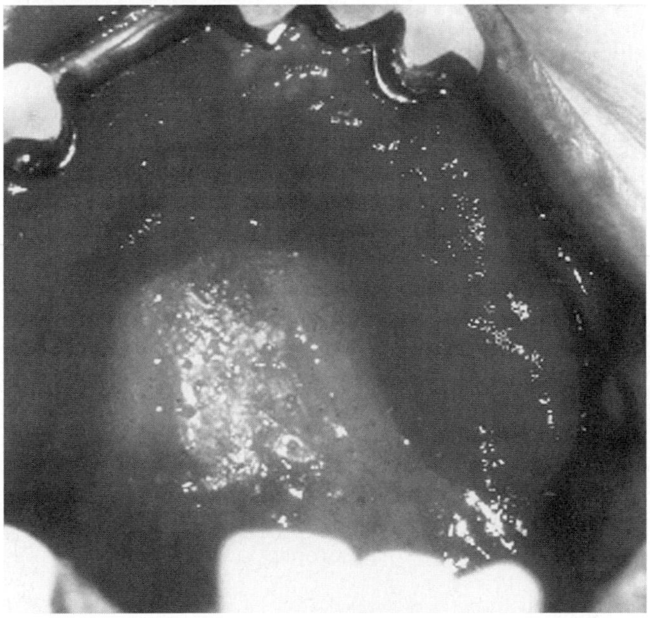

Figure 75-8. Denture stomatitis: ill-fitting denture and candidiasis. *(Reprinted with the permission of Mirriam Robbins, DDS, New York University College of Dentistry.)*

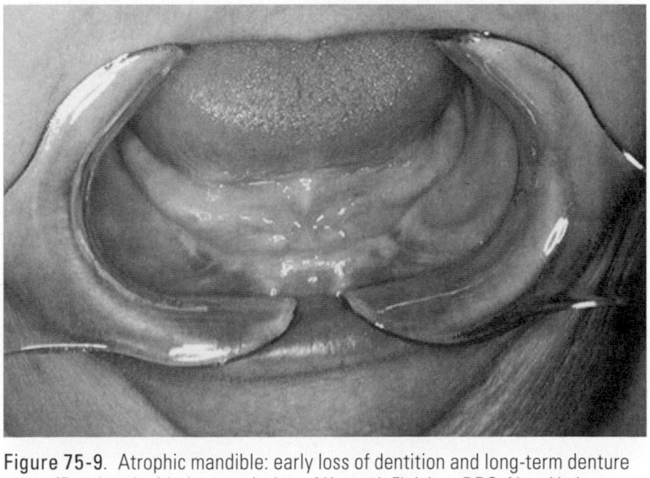

Figure 75-9. Atrophic mandible: early loss of dentition and long-term denture wear. *(Reprinted with the permission of Kenneth Fleisher, DDS, New York University College of Dentistry.)*

oral cancer each year, mainly in individuals with the median age in the sixth decade of life.[17]

The types of problems encountered by a dentate or partially edentulous geriatric patient may include dental caries, chronic facial pain and/or temporomandibular dysfunction, and benign or malignant lesions of the oral mucosa or jaws. Periodontal disease, an inflammatory disorder that results in alveolar bone loss and chronic tissue inflammation (Figure 75-10, see also Color Plate 75-10) is a primary cause of tooth loss in the elderly, which has been shown to have strong associations with the pathophysiology of certain systemic diseases including cardiovascular disease, cerebrovascular disease, and diabetes mellitus.[18] In fact, patients with periodontal disease are up to twice as likely to develop cardiovascular disease.[19] Medications taken for comorbid conditions may result in decreased salivary flow, which in turn impacts on the ability to chew, swallow, and cleanse the oral cavity. Additionally, xerostomia may be accompanied by painful or burning sensations. Finally, maxillofacial trauma as a result of gait disturbance, neuromuscular disease or in some cases elder abuse, is another factor affecting oral health in the geriatric population.[5]

As advances in medical research result in increasing patient life span, older adults have become the fastest growing portion of the population. In the United States, population projections indicate that by the year 2030 more than 20% of the population will be 65 years old or older.[20] Since concurrent advances in dental research have resulted in less tooth loss in older adults, these patients will require an increased need for dental care in the future, most especially with the advent of dental implants leading to less reliance on conventional dentures as a primary form of treatment. Although the trend is toward less tooth loss in older adults, there are still regional demographic variations, with higher levels of edentulism in areas of lower socioeconomic status. With increased tooth retention comes the continued risk of recurrent and cervical caries. The pattern of caries differs in the geriatric versus the general population in that coronal (chewing surface) caries are less frequent than root caries. Root or cervical caries (Figure 75-11, see also Color Plate 75-11) are characterized by rapid progression and increased difficulty in restoration, often necessitating extraction (Figure 75-1, see also Color Plate 75-1).[20,21]

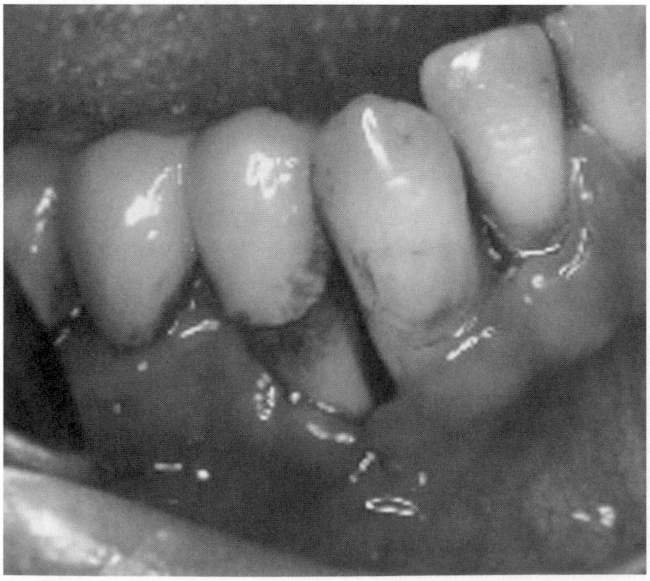

Figure 75-10. Severe periodontal bone loss. *(Reprinted with the permission of Mirriam Robbins, DDS, New York University College of Dentistry.)*

Dentists are now challenged with treating an increasing number of community dwelling older adults with chronic but stable systemic diseases, along with caring for the dental needs of the more debilitated and frail elderly with both physiologic and cognitive impairments. According to the surgeon general's report in 2000, more than 20% of homebound or institutionalized elderly require emergency dental care annually. As this population increases, so too will the need for care.[17]

Oral health impact on systemic health

The well established links between oral and systemic diseases have served as a "wake-up" call to improve oral hygiene and access to dental care for elderly patients in long-term care facilities.[22,23] One such risk is aspiration pneumonia, which has long been recognized as a common cause of death in infirm homebound and long-term care facility residents. Bacterial pneumonia is directly linked to aspiration as a result of dysphagia and/or poor oral hygiene and the elevated numbers of respiratory pathogens within oropharyngeal secretions. Attention to improved oral hygiene is a method or strategy to decrease the incidence of bacterial pneumonia in susceptible populations.[24]

The main causes of community-acquired pneumonia are *Streptococcus pneumoniae* and *Haemophilus influenzae*. The organisms more frequently associated with hospital-acquired pneumonia are *Staphylococcus aureus* and *Pseudomonas aeruginosa*. Hospital-acquired pneumonia commonly occurs in the frail elderly with compromised immune systems.

Aspiration is most likely to occur in patients with functional dependence on oral care and feeding.[25,26] Studies have demonstrated increased levels of bacteria in the oral secretions of institutionalized versus home-dwelling seniors.[27] Aspiration occurs most frequently with feeding or during sleep. The risk of developing an infection subsequent to aspiration depends on the state of the individual's host defenses—cough reflex, mucociliary adequacy, and cellular immunity—and on the type and volume of aspirate. The

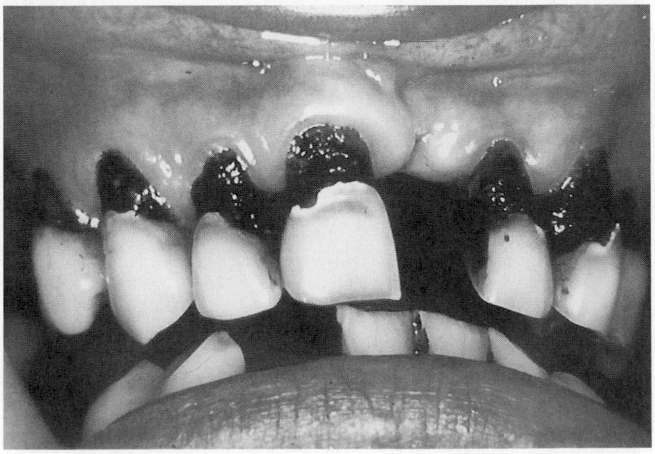

Figure 75-11. Severe cervical decay. *(Reprinted with the permission of Mirriam Robbins, DDS, New York University College of Dentistry.)*

higher the bacterial load of the aspirate and the lower the host defenses, the greater the risk.[28]

Oral care for functionally dependent elderly patients in long-term care facilities has been documented as being sorely lacking in numerous studies.[29,30] Poor oral hygiene leads to the proliferation of dental plaque, which is a biofilm responsible for dental and periodontal disease (Figure 75-2, see also Color Plate 75-2). As the biofilm matures, organism shedding is facilitated. Reduced salivary flow in the elderly as a consequence of medications, aging, or disease may also enhance microbial growth in the oral cavity. Similarly, long-term use of broad-spectrum antibiotics may contribute to the overgrowth of certain organisms in the oral cavity.

A study by Adachi et al[31] investigated the incidence of fevers greater than 37.8° C and aspiration pneumonia in the residents of two nursing homes for 2 years. Patients who received professional oral health care were compared with patients who did not. The prevalence of fevers and the rate of aspiration pneumonia was significantly lower in the patient group who received professional oral health care, than in the group who did not. It has been demonstrated that improved oral hygiene efforts in long-term care facilities has resulted in a decreased incidence of fevers and pneumonia deaths. Effects of improved oral health care on other systemic diseases, such as cerebrovascular accident, diabetes mellitus, and myocardial infarction have yet to be fully investigated.

Desvarieux et al[32] investigated the relationship between periodontal disease and tooth loss with subclinical atherosclerosis. Subjects received comprehensive periodontal examination, a carotid scan, and evaluation of cardiovascular disease risk factors. A significant association was noted between observed prevalence of carotid plaque formation and the number of teeth missing. Approximately 60% of individuals missing more than 10 teeth demonstrated carotid artery plaque, and this association was greatest among patients over the age of 65. The mechanisms underlying the relationship between periodontal disease and cardiovascular disease are not well understood but are likely due to chronic bacteremia and elevated inflammatory markers. Interestingly, in a follow-up study, gender variations were noted in the relationship between periodontal disease, tooth loss, and subclinical atherosclerosis, with men being affected more frequently than women.[33]

The relationship between cardiovascular disease/stroke and periodontal disease has been the object of numerous studies in the last decade, most focusing on the role of inflammatory markers, such as C-reactive protein (CRP), interleukin, and tumor necrosis factor. Periodontal disease results in elevations of CRP and interleukins, but a clear link between periodontal disease and the pathogenesis has yet to be elucidated. The therapeutic implications for such an association are significant given the prevalence of periodontal disease in the general population and the relative ease with which oral hygiene improvement can be accomplished. Other risk factors for the development of cardiovascular disease, such as gender, hypertension, obesity, hyperlipidemia, and smoking, are less readily addressed and modified. Animal studies indicate that chronic infections lead to increased systemic inflammation and the accelerated development of atherosclerotic plaque.[34]

The results of the meta-analysis of five prospective cohort studies involving more than 85,000 patients indicated that patients with periodontal disease had a 1.14 times higher risk of developing cardiovascular disease than those patients without periodontal disease. The highest risk (1.24) was assigned to individuals with less than 10 remaining teeth. The meta-analysis of five case control studies involving more than 1400 individuals demonstrated an even higher risk of individuals with periodontal disease developing cardiovascular disease.[35]

Issues facing community dwelling versus long-term care facility residents

Ohrui[36] studied more than 400 Japanese nursing home residents evaluating the relationship between dental status and mortality. Participants were divided into three groups: individuals with adequate dentition, edentulous individuals who wore full dentures, and individuals without adequate dentition and without dental prosthesis. All groups were followed for 5 years. The 2- and 5-year risks for mortality were greater for the functionally edentulous individuals than for the other groups. Ohrui concluded that the dental status of institutionalized elderly should be systematically evaluated and optimized.

Elderly patients with dementia may demonstrate difficulty with activities of daily life including oral care, and as such, they pose unique challenges to caregivers in the community and within institutions. Connell and McConnell[37] evaluated changes in the nursing home environment that could foster improved oral health care. The changes included modification of the physical environment to compensate for cognitive defects and physical incapacity and staff instruction on cues to overcome cognitive and noncognitive deficits. Improved visual cues, single step cues, and closing doors to decrease distractions all resulted in improved oral hygiene status. Improved wheelchair access to sinks, access to mirrors, and change from conventional toothbrushes to those designed with better grip handles also resulted in improved oral hygiene.

A study of 192 nursing home residents investigating oral health status, cognitive function, and the need for dental treatment as assessed by dental professionals and nursing staff was performed by Nordenram et al.[38] The results indicated that dentate status coupled with a loss of cognitive function was predictive for the need for oral treatment. The patients with the best cognitive function were found to have better chewing ability. Thirty percent of patients were found to have a functional chewing deficit based on lack of dentures, ill-fitting dentures, or poor dental status. Assessment of need by staff versus dental practitioners was compared, as clinical dental function and oral hygiene were assessed by both groups. The two groups varied widely in their assessment of the oral health status of the nursing home residents, as the dentists found that 93% of residents required oral hygiene assistance, whereas the nursing assessment was that only 11% of the population required such aid. Such disparity in findings between nursing home staff and dentists clearly indicates the need for improved training in the recognition of oral hygiene neglect and related oral health conditions.

Physical disability, cognitive impairment, or a combination of the two can result in making nursing home residents who are no longer functionally independent vulnerable to poor oral health. Numerous studies have documented the need for improved oral health care for both long-term care residents and homebound elderly. Reports of severe periodontal disease, untreated root caries, and poor oral hygiene on remaining teeth and on dentures abound in the literature. Frenkel et al[39] reported that more than 70% of nursing home residents had not seen a dentist in 5 years and that more than 20% reported untreated dental problems.

Murray et al[40] observed soft tissue lesions and dry mouth in 6% of their nursing home population. Oral hygiene, as measured by the amount of calculus on crowns of teeth or on dentures, increased with patient age and length of time of denture wear. Less than a quarter of nursing home patients demonstrated minimal or no calculus present.

In an article reviewing the prevalence and consequences of poor oral health care or lack of care in geriatric patients in long-term care facilities, Pino et al[41] concluded that the effects on the general health and well-being of these patients was far-reaching. Poor oral hygiene or oral health neglect may result in problems that range from socially embarrassing to life threatening. Systemic complications, including deep fascial space infections, endocarditis, cavernous sinus thrombosis, and brain abscesses, are well documented in both dental and medical literature. Nutritional status, conversing, smiling, and eating are all dependent on adequate oral health.

The institutionalized elderly are not the only individuals at risk. Studies of oral health status in the United States and Europe document the need for attention to oral health care in the elderly. Tooth loss results in masticatory insufficiency that can result in swallowing and digestive disorders, in addition to poor diet due to the need to alter food choices. Periodontal disease may present clinically with erythematous, edematous gingival tissue associated with bleeding, tooth mobility, and fetid oris locally (Figure 75-2, see also Color Plate 75-2), and aspiration pneumonia and local and distant spread of infection systemically.[41]

In a study evaluating functional tooth number (greater or less than 10) and overall mortality in more than 500 individuals aged over 40 who were followed for 15 years, Fukai et al[42] found that adults aged over 80 demonstrated increased mortality and decreased functional tooth number in comparison to the other groups. An increased risk of malnutrition was assessed on 130 community dwelling older adults in Japan using the Mini Nutritional Assessment tool (MNA). Factors affecting increasing risk of malnutrition were found to include cognitive impairment, physical disability, poor oral health status, and difficulty with meal preparation resulting in unbalanced diets. Twelve percent of participants were found to be at risk for malnutrition.[43]

Recognition and management of common oral conditions in the elderly population

CARIES AND PERIODONTAL DISEASE

Although the incidence of caries (tooth decay) is highest in children and young adults, dentate geriatric patients are not immune from the development of these lesions. To the contrary, cervical or root caries and recurrent caries under existing restorations are common in elderly dentate patients. Cervical caries tend to progress more rapidly than caries on occlusal surfaces, and restoration of teeth with cervical caries is often more difficult, leading ultimately to extraction. Partially edentulous elderly adults often alter their diets to softer consistency foods, which are high in carbohydrates and which increase the chance of caries formation, especially when coupled with inadequate home care. The CDC estimates that 30% of adults over the age of 65 have untreated caries and that 94% of adults with one or more natural teeth have experienced caries.[44]

Periodontal disease is a chronic inflammatory process involving the gingiva and alveolar bone, which ultimately results in gingival erythema, edema, bleeding, recession, and loss of alveolar bone resulting in tooth mobility and ultimately tooth loss.

In a study of more than 300 patients aged 65 to 95, Stabholz et al[45] found that caries accounted for 30% of extractions and periodontal disease accounted for 65% of extractions performed. In another study that followed 179 geriatric patients at three long-term care facilities over a period of 30 months, a logistic regression demonstrated that the relative risk of a worsening periodontal condition or loss of teeth was twice as high for those patients not enrolled in a preventive program than for those that were.[46] The benefit of an oral health preventive program in the severely frail elderly or terminal patient appears to demonstrate no significant improvement.[47]

EDENTULISM, PARTIAL EDENTULISM, DENTURES, AND IMPLANTS

Caries and periodontal disease, left untreated, are the primary causes of tooth loss.

Although the number of teeth present is a common tool used in evaluating oral health and masticatory function, evaluation of functional tooth units, which involves description of the arrangement and number of remaining teeth, is perhaps a more reliable tool to evaluate masticatory function in the elderly population. Hildebrandt et al[48] found that a low number of functional tooth units resulted in food avoidance patterns and swallowing of coarser boluses of incompletely chewed food.

The fabrication of full or partial dentures has long been the primary method of ensuring masticatory sufficiency in adults with missing teeth. Long-term use of these prostheses often leads to resorption of alveolar bone and associated soft tissue changes including ulcerations and hypertrophic areas. This ultimately results in the need for dentures to be continuously refitted. In some cases, resorption may be so severe as to obviate the fabrication of stable prostheses. The advent of dental implants (Figure 75-12, see also Color Plate 75-12) and the ability to provide implant supported bridges and dentures have improved the masticatory capabilities, diet, and nutrition of countless adults in the last 2 decades. The greatest benefit appears to be for patients with the most ridge resorption.[49] Implant supported prostheses may demonstrate secondary benefits, such as improvements in facial esthetics and lip support that complement improvements in masticatory function.[50]

In a survey of 125 patients, loss of function was the most common complaint of wearers of full dentures, whereas patients with fixed prostheses demonstrated fewer complaints.[51]

Before the advent of implants for treatment of full or partial edentulism, removable dental prostheses were the primary means of oral rehabilitative care. Full and partial dentures did and do provide for improvements in mastication, swallowing, speech, and facial aesthetics. Implant supported prostheses

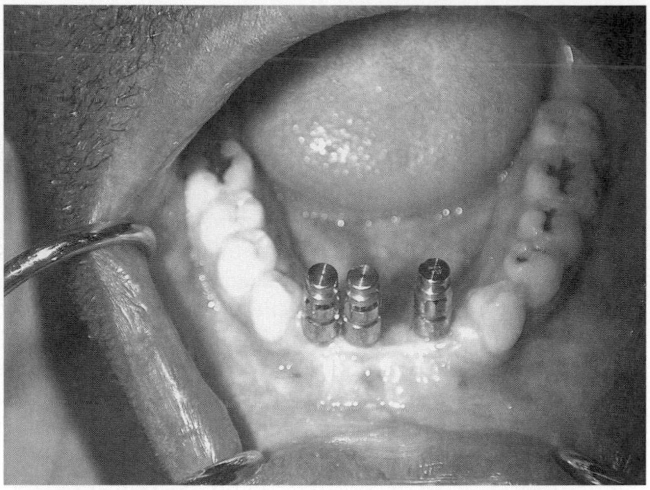

Figure 75-12. Dental implants: before fabrication of prosthesis/bridge. *(Reprinted with the permission of Mirriam Robbins, DDS, New York University College of Dentistry.)*

provide a more comfortable, functional, and stable alternative to conventional dentures. A study[52] was conducted of 15 patients over 60 years of age who were treated with implant supported lower dentures and then evaluated for impact of this treatment on their quality of life. The reported benefits of this treatment included improvements in eating, speaking, and social interactions.

Dental implants to treat either full or partially edentulous conditions have become a common treatment option, with more than 90% success rate reported at 10 years. Neither advanced age nor systemic disease are absolute contraindications to implant placement.[53] Some studies appear to have demonstrated an increased risk of implant failure associated with diabetes mellitus, smoking, oncologic treatments (including chemotherapy and head and neck radiation), and postmenopausal hormone therapy.[54] Patients should be evaluated as candidates for implants based on the level of control of their systemic diseases, their ability to withstand surgical stress, life expectancy, and quality of life.[55] Evidence of implant failure due to systemic disease is not prevalent.[56]

Grant and Kraut[57] placed 160 implants in the maxillas and mandibles of 47 patients all aged over 79 and with a median age of 89 years. All but one of the implants healed successfully. The authors concluded that geriatric patients in stable medical condition are suitable implant patients. It appears that concerns about the success of osseointegration in elderly patients as regards to bone remodeling and resorption and decreased soft tissue response may not be entirely warranted. There is no strong body of evidence to support an increased failure rate of implants based on advanced patient age. A review of the literature regarding the success of implants in elderly patients revealed that old age, in and of itself, is not a significant concern.[58] Al Jabbari[59] concluded that even limitation in oral hygiene capacity in old age is not a contraindication to implant placement. Treating dentists need to first consider if the patient is in optimal condition to withstand the procedure and be less concerned about whether osseointegration is likely to occur in the elderly patient.

SALIVA AND SALIVARY GLANDS

Xerostomia may occur with medication use, chemotherapy, radiation therapy for head and neck cancer, or as a symptom of Sjögren's syndrome. Common sequelae include an inability to tolerate a dental prosthesis, difficulty swallowing, alteration of nutritional status, and increased incidence of dental caries because of changes in the dental plaque biofilm. The decreased ability to chew comfortably can result in malnutrition, and decreased enjoyment of food and the social interaction of meals.[60] Dry mouth is a common complaint in the elderly, possibly secondary to polypharmacy for multiple comorbid conditions. It is more common among patients who take several medications, especially if antipsychotics are included.[61]

Dry mouth or xerostomia has a number of possible causes including smoking, use of alcohol or caffeinated beverages, mouth breathing, and a host of medications. Some drugs may cause the sensation of dry mouth, whereas others may result in measurable hyposalivation.[62] The drugs that are most commonly implicated in dry mouth are antipsychotics, tricyclic antidepressants, β-blockers, antihistamines, and atropine.[63] Advancing age and medication use were shown to be related to objective evidence of hyposalivation, whereas female gender and psychiatric issues were strongly correlated to subjective complaints of oral dryness.[64]

No specific medication has been singled out as being more xerogenic, but polypharmacy does increase the likelihood of dryness. Severity of dryness complaint appears to be increased with female gender and antianginal, antiasthma, and antidepressant medications.[65]

Drugs can affect salivary flow rate or composition by antagonizing or mimicking any of the regulatory aspects of salivation. The mechanism of action of xerogenic drugs may be due to an anticholinergic action mediated by parasympathetic (M3 muscarinic receptors) neurotransmission to the salivary glands.[60] Tricyclic antidepressants have been shown to reduce salivary flow whereas selective serotonin release inhibitors do not. This lower incidence of dry mouth complaint is thought to be related to the lower anticholinergic effects of this group of medications. Approximately one quarter of patients on tricyclics develop a complaint of dry mouth. Muscarinic receptor antagonists, such as oxybutynin, which are used to treat the overactive bladder symptoms of frequency and urgency with or without incontinence, are nonspecific for the bladder and also cause dry mouth. Tolterodine demonstrates in vivo selectivity for the bladder over the salivary glands and may be a good choice for elderly patients who are taking other xerogenic medications.

Anticholinesterase inhibitors such as donepezil, used in the treatment of Alzheimer's disease, may also induce dry mouth. Many antihypertensive agents including β-blockers, ACE inhibitors, and α-methyldopa have been associated with complaints of dry mouth.

A study of 175 home-dwelling elderly patients[61] who were hospitalized for an acute change in health status were compared with 252 outpatients. The parameters evaluated included medical diagnosis, prescribed medications, oral examinations, and analysis of saliva samples. Sixty-three percent of hospitalized and 57% of outpatients complained of dry mouth, whereas 13% of hospitalized and 18% of outpatients complained of burning mouth. There were no differences in the biochemical analysis of the saliva between the two groups. The complaint of dry mouth was associated with polypharmacy, whereas this was not the case for the complaint of burning mouth. Dry mouth and burning mouth were rarely reported simultaneously.

The management of dry mouth is challenging, and saliva substitutes have been the mainstay of treatment for many years along with alcohol-free mouth rinses, increased water intake, lubricating gels, and alteration of food consistency (blenderized diet). Since dentate patients diagnosed with xerostomia are prone to an increased incidence of caries, a comprehensive and aggressive caries monitoring protocol should be instituted including fluoride treatments, sealants, and use of sugar-free lubricating gum. Stimulation of salivary secretion with Yohimbine, an α_2-adrenoreceptor antagonist has been somewhat effective in patients being treated with psychotropic drugs. Another strategy, for patients on multiple medications, is for physicians to evaluate the xerogenic potential of each of the mediations prescribed for an individual and to alter the medication regimen if at all possible. A persistent dry mouth may necessitate alteration of drug dose or prescription.[61]

ORAL LESIONS

Oral mucosa possesses an essential protective function, which is presumed to diminish with age as the tissue becomes more permeable. This theory appears to be supported by the reported increased incidence of oral lesions with advancing age.[66] However, Wolff and Ship[67] found that the incidence of oral mucosal lesions in healthy adult seniors was not significantly higher than that of the general population. Other factors contributing to the development of oral mucosal lesions include general health and nutrition status, medication usage, and the presence of ill-fitting dentures.

Common oral mucosal conditions of elderly denture wearers include candidiasis (Figure 75-13, see also Color Plate 75-13), epulis fissuratum (soft tissue hyperplasia), traumatic ulcers, angular cheilitis (Figure 75-7, see also Color Plate 75-7), and coated tongue. Although the majority of oral mucosal lesions appear to be benign, premalignant and malignant lesions are also present, usually in the form of leukoplakias (Figure 75-4, see also Color Plate 75-4), erythroplakias, and squamous cell carcinomas (Figure 75-6, see also Color Plate 75-6).

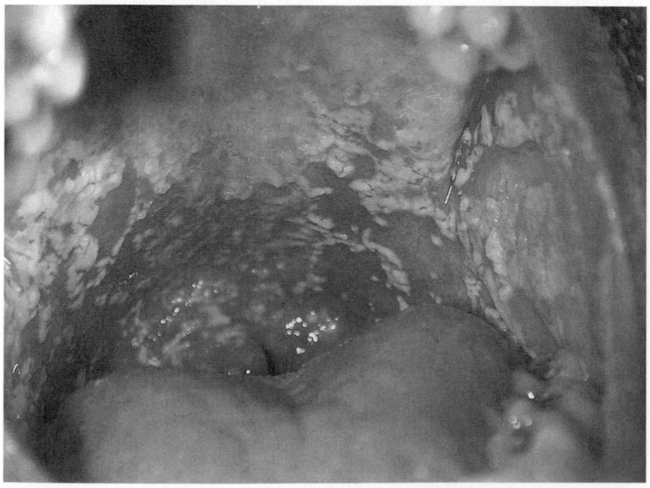

Figure 75-13. Oral candidiasis: note striae throughout indicative of fungal infection. *(Reprinted with the permission of Mirriam Robbins, DDS, New York University College of Dentistry.)*

Denture stomatitis is a generally asymptomatic, inflammatory process found on mucosal surfaces underlying full or partial removable dentures (Figure 75-8, see also Color Plate 75-8), with a commonly reported prevalence of 10% to 75% of denture wearers.[68] Causal factors for the development of denture-related stomatitis include trauma from ill-fitting dentures, poor oral hygiene, reduced vertical dimension (atrophy), continuous use of prosthesis, unstable occlusion, hyposalivation, and nutritional deficiency. The increased incidence of lesions was associated with a greater number of years of denture use. Interestingly, advanced age and high alcohol consumption did not correlate with incidence of these lesions.[69]

A retrospective study of 4098 adults, investigating the prevalence of oral lesions and association of those lesions with age, dentures, tobacco, or alcohol use, found that the overall prevalence of oral mucosal lesions appeared to be linked to risk behaviors and age. More than 27% of the male adults and 22% of the female subjects were noted to have a mucosal lesion. The use of alcohol and tobacco appeared to be linked to the incidence of leukoplakia, nicotinic stomatitis, and frictional lesions. Denture-related lesions, in the form of candidiasis and traumatic and frictional lesions, appeared to be the most prevalent.[70]

The incidence of oral mucosal lesions[71] in a Thai population of 500 adults over the age of 60 was investigated in relationship to type of lesion, age, sex, and presence or absence of dentures. The incidence of oral mucosal lesions in this study population was 83.6%, with no significant gender difference. The incidence of oral mucosal lesions appeared to increase with advancing age and denture use. The three most prevalent oral mucosal conditions were traumatic ulcers, fissured tongue, and lingual varices. Premalignant lesions were detected in 5% of subjects, and squamous cell carcinoma was detected in less than 1% of the subjects.

In one study,[72] older patients, especially females, appeared to be at increased risk of developing malignant lesions, and curiously, those who never smoked appeared to be at greater risk. Oral squamous cell carcinoma most commonly occurred on the ventral and lateral tongue, floor of the mouth, and retromolar regions.

Angular cheilitis is characterized by cracking fissures at the commissures of the lips, which may be caused by saliva accumulation in this region secondary to ill-fitting dentures, candida infections, or vitamin deficiencies (B) (Figure 75-7, see also Color Plate 75-7). Discomfort with eating and speaking are often attendant complaints. Treatment is aimed at the cause and may include topical antifungal ointments, vitamin supplements, dietary changes, and denture adjustments—or in some cases the fabrication of new dentures or implant supported prostheses.

Poor oral hygiene, immune compromise, or both can lead to an overgrowth of candida on dentures, resulting in denture stomatitis and oral-pharyngeal candidiasis (Figure 75-13, see also Color Plate 75-13). It is frequently asymptomatic and found on routine examination. On occasion, complaints of a painful or burning sensation may be elicited. Common clinical characteristics include erythema or pinpoint hyperemic areas in denture-bearing locations. Frank fungal colonies are also sometimes observed. If the affected region is limited to the denture-bearing areas, dentures should be routinely brushed and may be soaked in chlorhexidine or a dilute hypochlorite solution. In more extensive areas, oral antifungal troches are administered. Denture stomatitis may occur in up to one half of edentulous patients who wear full dentures.[39]

Oral cancer occurs most frequently in the older population, usually in or after the sixth decade of life, with more than 95% of cases occurring in individuals over the age of 45.[17,73] These cancers account for approximately 3% of all cancers in the United States. The National Institute of Dental and Craniofacial Research estimates that more than 28,000 Americans will be diagnosed and that 7000 individuals will succumb to oral cancer this year. Oral cancer affects men more frequently than women by a ratio of approximately 2:1. Tobacco and alcohol use remain primary risk factors for the development of oral cancers, the risks increasing with increased usage of either or both substances. The 5-year survival rate remains at 59%.[74]

Early detection remains the key to improved prognosis. Common clinical signs and symptoms include nonhealing ulcers and areas of leukoplakia, erythroplakia, or mixed lesions. Lesions that do not resolve upon removal of a suspected irritant or within a few weeks of detection should be biopsied because histologic evaluation is necessary to determine if any dysplastic or malignant changes are evident. If a malignancy is detected, treatment is then predicated on the staging of such lesions and may involve surgical ablation, chemotherapy, radiation therapy, reconstruction with vascularized grafts, and oral rehabilitation.

CONCLUSION

Compromised oral health may result in a variety of illnesses and conditions that can adversely impact an individual's quality of life or life span. Engaging in conversation, enjoying a good meal, kissing a loved one, smiling and laughing—many of life's "little pleasures"—require a functioning and esthetically acceptable dentition. The ability to engage in these activities improves socialization, self-esteem, and the quality of life of all but the most infirm and cognitively impaired individuals. Additional benefits of good oral health on an individual's systemic health include improved diet and nutrition and decreased frequency of aspiration pneumonia in the frail elderly population. The association between periodontal disease and cardiovascular disease, stroke, diabetes, and myocardial infarction may prove to have the most far-reaching health benefit.

The key to maintaining oral health in the geriatric population remains timely access to care. Community dwelling dependent seniors, homebound frail elderly, and long-term care facility residents face many more obstacles to receiving dental care than do healthy, independent seniors. Therefore, physicians play a primary and crucial role in ensuring adequate oral health of these individuals. Familiarity with common oral conditions afflicting both dentate and edentulous elderly adults is the first and most basic step in assuring improved oral health in these patients.

KEY POINTS

Maintaining Oral Health in the Geriatric Population

Definition of Oral Health:

- Conditions that adversely affect the oral and maxillofacial complex are common and pervasive in the elderly and can affect an individual's general health and quality of life. Physicians are in a unique position to screen elderly patients for common oral disorders. Impact on Quality of life.
- Poor oral health and loss of teeth adversely affect nutritional status and gastrointestinal health by limiting food choices secondary to masticatory insufficiency. In addition, socialization and psychologic well-being may also be affected. Oral Health Impact on Systemic Health.
- The link between oral and systemic disease has been reinforced in recent years, specifically in relationship to cardiovascular disease. The risk of aspiration pneumonia in nursing home residents has been demonstrated to be decreased with improvements in oral hygiene care. Recognition and management of common oral diseases of the elderly.
- Improvement of oral health hinges on recognition of common conditions, including caries, periodontal diseases, partial or complete edentulism, salivary gland dysfunction, benign and malignant lesions of the mucosa, and bony structures.

For a complete list of references, please visit online only at www.expertconsult.com

CHAPTER 76

The Upper Gastrointestinal Tract

David A. Greenwald
Lawrence J. Brandt

Symptoms of gastrointestinal disorders are frequently mentioned by older Americans during visits to the doctor, and the digestive diseases producing these symptoms are among the most common hospital discharge diagnoses for elderly patients in the United States.[1,2] As the elderly population expands and the demand by older individuals for medical care grows, it becomes increasingly important for physicians to be acquainted with the manifestations of diseases of the upper gastrointestinal tract in members of this age group.

THE ORAL CAVITY

The most proximal of the digestive organs traditionally is considered to be the esophagus; patients with complaints thought to originate within the oral cavity or pharynx are referred to a dentist or a specialist in disorders of the ear, nose, and throat. The oral cavity, however, is examined easily by the general practitioner and may reveal the cause of unexplained or apparently unrelated abnormalities; thus evaluation of the upper gastrointestinal tract should begin with the mouth.

The mouth and nutrition

Changes in the oral cavity occasionally limit the ability of elderly people to eat and enjoy a normal diet. Problems with eating sometimes are severe enough to cause malnutrition and prompt a search for a wasting illness.[3] The number of general oral health problems has been shown to be a strong predictor of involuntary weight loss in elderly people.[4]

A variety of abnormalities of oral structure and function may contribute to malnutrition. The muscles of mastication may become impaired during aging as the result of a decrease in (lean) body mass.[5] Eating occasionally becomes difficult because of tooth loss as a result of periodontal disease, poor dentition, or loosening of dentures caused by resorption of mandibular bone.[6]

A reduction in food intake by elderly individuals is sometimes related to a change in taste perception. The number of taste buds decreases after age 45, resulting in a decrease in taste sensation, especially the ability to appreciate salty and sweet foods.[7–9] Diminished perception of sour and bitter tastes is associated with palatal defects and typically occurs in patients who wear dentures. Taste sensation may also be altered directly by medications or indirectly affected by a drug's unpleasant flavor. Agents associated with abnormal taste perception (dysgeusia) include tricyclic antidepressants, sulfasalazine, clofibrate, L-dopa, gold salts, lithium, and metronidazole. Medications with anticholinergic properties interfere with taste by reducing salivary gland secretions and producing xerostomia. Age alone, however, is not associated with a reduction in stimulated saliva flow in nonmedicated subjects.[10]

Although abnormal perception may lead to deficient nutrition, some primary nutritional disorders may be responsible for dysgeusia and glossitis. For example, vitamin B_{12} and niacin deficiency are associated with a "bald" or magenta-colored tongue, respectively. Taste sensation and eating habits also are disturbed by processes that interfere with the sense of smell, which typically is diminished substantially by age 70.[11]

Vascular lesions

Diminutive vascular lesions of the upper gastrointestinal tract are poorly understood and rarely reported. The nomenclature for these lesions is confusing, and the terms *arteriovenous malformation, vascular ectasia, angiodysplasia*, and *telangiectasia* are usually used interchangeably with little regard as to their true meanings.

The lips are a frequent site of senescent vascular lesions resembling those of hereditary hemorrhagic telangiectasia (Osler-Weber-Rendu disease), and involvement often includes the upper gastrointestinal tract. In addition to this form of small vascular abnormality, patients often have sublingual varices, or "caviar lesions" (Figure 76-1). The walls of these dilated vessels are thick, but the endothelial lining is hypoplastic.[12] In males, sublingual varices may be associated with the occurrence of capillary phlebectasias, or Fordyce lesions, of the scrotal skin (Figure 76-2).

Because vascular abnormalities are often responsible for cryptogenic gastrointestinal bleeding, their presence in the mouth should suggest that similar lesions elsewhere in the gastrointestinal tract may be responsible for blood loss in such cases.[13] Not every individual, however, with bleeding vascular lesions of the gastrointestinal tract has involvement of oral structures, and the presence of oral lesions does not preclude existence of an unrelated distal bleeding lesion.

The oral mucosa

A number of abnormalities of the oral mucosa are encountered in elderly patients. These changes may be the result of medical therapy, signify the presence of a systemic disease, or represent premalignant changes.

Candidiasis

Candidiasis is usually caused by the fungus *Candida albicans*. This organism is part of the normal gastrointestinal flora, and its presence is not sufficient by itself to produce disease. Mucosal candidiasis occurs only after a change in other constituents of the normal flora or in the presence of an immunologic abnormality. In elderly patients, the widespread use of antibiotics and immunosuppressive chemotherapy for malignancies is most often responsible for the development of mucosal candidiasis.

The typical oral lesions of candidiasis are soft, white plaques that resemble cottage cheese. Characteristically, these plaques can be peeled from the mucosa, leaving the underlying surface raw and bleeding. This observation is important because most other white, plaquelike lesions, for example, leukoplakia, cannot be stripped off the mucosa.

A diagnosis of candidiasis is made by smearing scrapings of the lesion on a glass slide, macerating them with 20% potassium hydroxide, and examining this preparation under a microscope for the presence of typical hyphae. A definitive diagnosis can be made by culture on selected media.

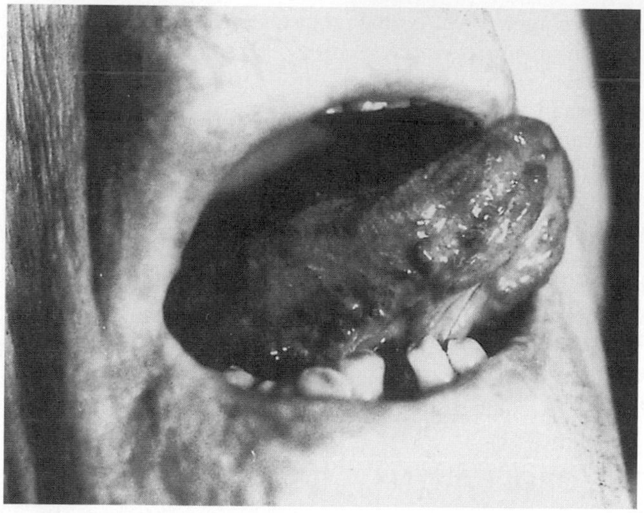

Figure 76-1. Caviar lesion (sublingual varices) in a patient with occult upper gastrointestinal bleeding. *(Reproduced from Brandt LJ. Gastrointestinal disorders of the elderly. Lippincott-Raven, 1986, New York.)*

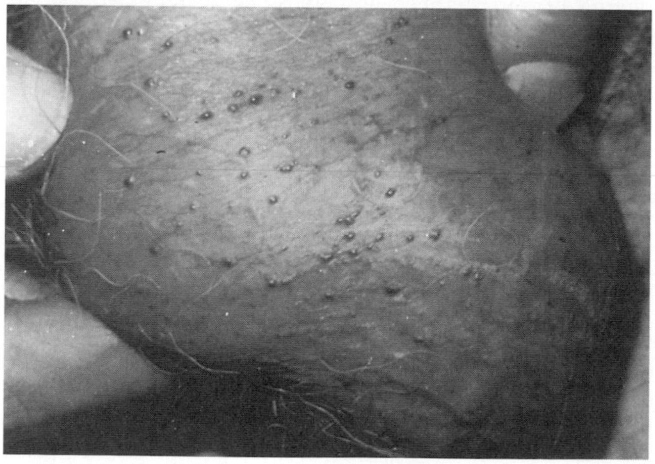

Figure 76-2. Phlebectasias in the scrotum of the same patient as in Figure 76-1. *(Reproduced from Brandt LJ. Gastrointestinal disorders of the elderly. Lippincott-Raven, 1986, New York.)*

Therapy usually consists of reestablishing the normal microbiologic flora by discontinuing antibiotics. In the immunocompromised host and the individual with significant morbidity, topical therapy with nystatin suspensions or troches is usually successful, although treatment with absorbable oral agents such as fluconazole may be required. Antifungal agents may be supplemented by the use of topical anesthetics to provide symptomatic relief (see later discussion).

Stomatitis

Cancer patients treated with radiation or chemotherapy frequently develop painful inflammation and erosions of the oropharyngeal mucosa. Stomatitis complicating cancer therapy is the direct consequence of drug and radiation toxicity to susceptible, rapidly dividing cell populations of the upper gastrointestinal tract and the indirect consequence of neutropenia, which impairs regeneration of injured tissues. Radiation to the head and neck also causes xerostomia secondary to fibrosis of the salivary glands. An absence of lubrication by saliva further aggravates mucosal damage, and a lack of salivary IgA permits overgrowth of bacteria and fungi. Oral lesions may become infected, contributing to persistent injury, discomfort, and poor nutrition and posing a risk of more widespread infection in immunocompromised individuals.

The initial therapy for stomatitis is promotion of good oral hygiene. Brushing and flossing are contraindicated in neutropenic patients because of the risk of disseminated infection. Instead, mouthwashes containing dilute hydrogen peroxide or a salt and soda solution are used to reduce mucosal bacterial and fungal colonization.

A number of therapeutic mouthwash "cocktails" have been recommended to relieve symptoms, promote healing, and treat superficial mucosal infection in patients with stomatitis.[14] Some of these cocktails have been tested in controlled trials, but the use of most is empirical, based on the known analgesic, antibiotic, and protective effects of widely available liquid medicines. Viscous lidocaine (2%) is frequently used as a topical anesthetic, as is diphenhydramine, which is often mixed with oral antacids or kaolin-pectin. Many recipes include sucralfate suspension because it coats damaged epithelium and promotes the production of mucus and protective prostaglandins. Antibiotics used alone or in combination in mouthwash cocktails to treat superficial infection include chlorhexidine gluconate, nystatin, tetracycline, neomycin, vancomycin, and clindamycin. Hydrocortisone and other glucocorticoids also have been added to reduce inflammation, but rapid absorption across the denuded oral mucosa into the systemic circulation may compromise the patient's immune defenses. Artificial saliva replacements (Salivart, Moi-Stir, Xero-Lube) are also available for patients with xerostomia.

Hairy tongue

"Hairy tongue" is characterized by hypertrophy of the filiform papillae of the tongue and a lack of normal desquamation. In this condition, the color of the tongue varies from yellow to brown or black, depending on staining by exogenous substances, such as tobacco or food, and on the presence of various chromogenic microorganisms.[15,16] Hairy tongue is frequently seen in patients who have had extensive radiotherapy to the head and neck. Although these individuals are usually asymptomatic, some complain of nausea, dysgeusia, and halitosis. On occasion, the lingual papillae reach such considerable length that they brush against the soft palate, gagging the patient.

Many organisms have been cultured from papillary scrapings from this entity; there is, however, no proof of a cause-and-effect relationship with any microorganism, and invasion of the lingual epithelium has not been demonstrated. Species of microorganisms that have been isolated are, in all probability, simply colonizing an already abnormal, excessively papillated tongue.

Therapy for this disorder consists of vigorous brushing of the tongue to promote desquamation and to remove accumulated debris. In extreme cases, topical treatment with podophyllin, an alcoholic extract of the mayapple, may result in a dramatic response.

Leukoplakia

The term *leukoplakia* was introduced by Schwimmer in 1877 to describe any white plaque. Today, some authors use this term to refer to histologic zones of hyperkeratosis, acanthosis, and chronic inflammation, whereas others reserve it to describe malignant dyskeratosis and epithelial atypia. Although leukoplakia is considered by many clinicians to be a premalignant condition, its natural history is uncertain because of a lack of uniform definition in case selection. The term should be abandoned because of its lack of specificity. Any persistent white lesion of the oral mucosa should be biopsied in an attempt to make a specific histologic diagnosis.

Leukoplakia is more common in men than in women, and most often occurs during the sixth and seventh decades.[17] It can be found anywhere in the oral cavity, although it is most common on the buccal mucosa, tongue, and floor of the mouth. Leukoplakia varies in appearance, partly depending on the age of the lesion. Some investigators consider verrucous patches to be of higher malignant potential than smooth plaques, whereas others believe that granular pinkishgray to red islands, also called erythroplakia, are most likely to be associated with carcinoma in situ or even invasive malignancy. Such controversy stresses the importance of taking a biopsy in the management of all such lesions. Approximately 10% of patients with leukoplakia have or will develop invasive carcinoma in the lesion.[17–19]

Once the diagnosis of leukoplakia has been substantiated by microscopic examination of a biopsy specimen, therapy is initiated. When dysplasia is present, or when the lesion fails to resolve after a source of physicochemical trauma has been eliminated, treatment consists of ablation.

Epidermoid carcinoma

Approximately 5% of human cancers arise in the mouth; 95% of oral malignancies are epidermoid carcinomas.[18,19] The lower lip is the most common site of malignancy in the area of the oral cavity. Epidermoid carcinoma of the lip occurs almost exclusively in elderly men; causal factors include actinic radiation, syphilis, and tobacco use, especially pipe smoking.

Carcinoma of the lip varies in clinical appearance and may be bulky or ulcerated. It metastasizes slowly, usually to the ipsilateral submental or submaxillary lymph nodes. Surgical resection or radiation therapy produces equally good results, with cures in approximately 80% of affected individuals. Successful treatment depends on the duration of symptoms, size of lesion, and presence of metastases.

Within the oral cavity, one half of epidermoid carcinomas originate in the tongue, and the rest arise with equal frequency in the palate, buccal mucosa, floor of the mouth, and gingiva. The disease is seen mainly in older individuals and occurs most often in males. Factors suspected of contributing to the development of oral cancer include tobacco, alcohol, nutritional deficiencies, syphilis, and miscellaneous forms of physicochemical trauma, such as irritation from pipe stems and dentures. Almost 90% of patients have a combination of predisposing factors.

Intraoral epidermoid carcinomas display a considerable amount of histologic variation, although lesions tend to be moderately well differentiated. Early carcinomas arising in the tongue typically are painless, even though they may ulcerate. Pain develops later, as the lesions grow, especially if they become secondarily infected. Tumors are usually located on the lateral or ventral surface of the tongue. The site of the primary lesion is of prognostic importance because cancers of the posterior aspect of the tongue tend to be more aggressive. Nodal metastases are located on either or both sides of the neck. Tumors also spread by direct invasion. Early detection is mandatory if patients are to survive more than a year after diagnosis.

Keratoacanthoma is a spontaneously resolving benign lesion often mistaken for epidermoid carcinoma.[20] It occurs most frequently in adults 50 to 70 years of age, involves the upper and lower lips equally, and usually presents as a painful umbilicated lesion seldom more than 1 to 1.5 cm in diameter. It initially appears as a small nodule, which reaches full size within 4 to 8 weeks. It persists as a static lesion for another 4 to 8 weeks, after which the keratin core is expelled and the mass resorbed over a period of 6 to 8 weeks. Recurrence is rare.

THE OROPHARYNX

The oropharyngeal phase of swallowing is exceedingly complex, requiring the participation of multiple distinct structures in the mouth, pharynx, and esophagus coordinated by six cranial nerves and orchestrated by the swallowing center of the central nervous system. After food has been masticated and moistened with saliva, the tongue initiates swallowing by thrusting the food bolus into the oropharynx. The soft palate prepares for the arrival of the bolus by elevating, so that material from the mouth cannot enter the nasal passages. The glottis also shuts, and the epiglottis tilts downward to prevent the bolus from entering the trachea. Relaxation of the upper esophageal sphincter in association with contraction of the pharyngeal muscles allows propulsion of food into the esophagus.[21]

Striated muscle involved in the oropharyngeal phase of swallowing, like the muscles of mastication, may be impaired during aging by a decrease in lean body mass. A radiographic study of 100 individuals beyond the age of 65 suggested that 22 had pharyngeal muscle weakness along with abnormal cricopharyngeal relaxation with pooling of barium in the valleculae and pyriform sinuses.[22] Several individuals also were noted to have tracheal aspiration of barium. All the subjects, however, were asymptomatic. Thus, although functional changes in the oropharyngeal phase of swallowing may occur with aging, these changes have not been identified as a cause of morbidity in elderly people.

Oropharyngeal dysphagia

Patients with oropharyngeal (cervical or "transfer") dysphagia complain of difficulty shifting food from the front of the mouth into the back of the throat, or of trouble initiating a swallow once the food bolus has been positioned in the oropharynx. Symptoms may be most severe when the patient attempts to swallow liquids. Signs of transfer dysphagia include nasal regurgitation or aspiration of oral contents during swallowing as a result of a failure to seal the nasopharynx or the trachea by appropriate muscle contraction. Inasmuch as oropharyngeal dysphagia may be due to a neuromuscular disorder, the patient may display other signs of neuromuscular dysfunction, including dysarthria, nasal speech, cranial nerve dysfunction, weakness, or sensory abnormalities.[23]

A variety of conditions interfere with the transfer of food from the mouth to the esophagus (Table 76-1).[24] Mechanical lesions, including tumors, abscesses, and strictures, may block passage of the food bolus or disrupt structures that

Table 76-1. Causes of Oropharyngeal Dysphagia in Elderly People

Malignancy—pharyngeal carcinoma
Central nervous system disease—tumor, Parkinson's disease, stroke
Peripheral nervous system disease—diabetes mellitus
Muscle disease—hypothyroidism
Mechanical—strictures, osteophytes, thyromegaly
Postoperative—laryngectomy
Medications
Motility disorders of the upper esophageal sphincter

directly mediate the oropharyngeal phase of swallowing. A neoplasm, infection, or cerebrovascular accident may damage the central nervous system, producing brain stem or pseudobulbar palsy and associated transfer dysphagia. The initiation of swallowing also may be impaired by degenerative diseases of the central or peripheral nervous system, the motor end plate, or the muscle itself. Finally, oropharyngeal dysphagia is often caused by a failure of upper esophageal sphincter function. Many of these problems are encountered in older individuals.

Cricopharyngeal achalasia

The term *cricopharyngeal achalasia*, partly derived from the Greek word meaning "absence of slackening," is a misnomer, as the cricopharyngeus muscle of patients with this disorder is capable of relaxing. The problem in cricopharyngeal achalasia is failure of the muscle to function in synchrony with other elements of the swallowing mechanism. As a result, the pharyngeal muscles propel all or part of the food bolus against a closed sphincter, producing symptoms of cervical dysphagia.

Cricopharyngeal achalasia is usually encountered in elderly individuals. Many disorders may cause this problem, but central nervous system diseases predominate. The clinical features are those of oropharyngeal dysphagia in general. Depending on the cause, the onset of symptoms may be sudden, as with a cerebrovascular accident, or intermittent, as with more insidious disorders such as diabetic neuropathy. The natural history of cricopharyngeal achalasia is also variable, again probably reflecting its many causes: dysphagia may diminish, remain unremitting, or follow a relapsing, remitting course. Most individuals with this disorder have more difficulty swallowing liquids than solids. Many patients have a pulmonary presentation with laryngitis, bronchitis, recurrent pneumonia, bronchiectasis, and pulmonary abscesses as the sequelae of otherwise quiet cricopharyngeal dysfunction.[25] In some patients, symptoms result in such a fear of eating that weight loss, malnutrition, and psychological problems overshadow the motility disorder.

Postintubation dysphagia

Special mention must be made of cervical dysphagia occurring as a sequela of endotracheal intubation. Unilateral vocal cord weakness is a common complication of endotracheal intubation and because the vocal cords are important to the formation of a tight laryngeal seal during the oropharyngeal phase of glutition, patients with vocal cord weakness may experience coughing and aspiration with swallowing. Individuals who have undergone a tracheostomy also may develop symptoms of oropharyngeal dysphagia. Scar formation from a tracheostomy occasionally prevents normal elevation and anterior rotation of the larynx, causing decreased pharyngeal contraction and incomplete upper esophageal sphincter relaxation during swallowing.

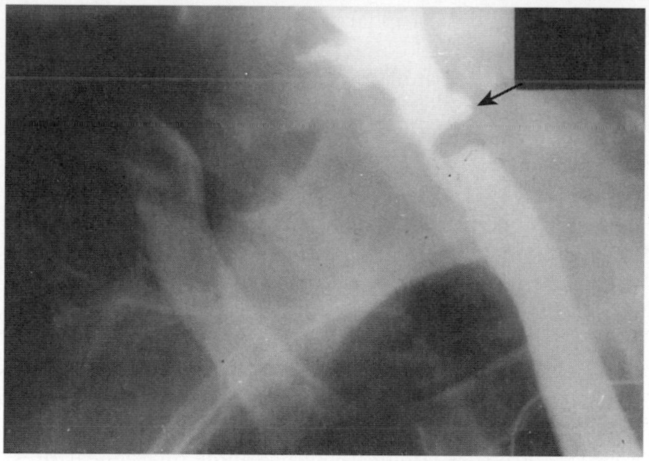

Figure 76-3. Oblique view of a barium-filled esophagus showing a small Zenker's diverticulum (*arrow*) proximal to a hypertrophied cricopharyngeus. *(Reproduced from Brandt LJ. Gastrointestinal disorders of the elderly. Lippincott-Raven, 1986, New York.)*

Management of oropharyngeal dysphagia depends only in part on its cause. Any underlying disorder, such as parkinsonism, should be treated. If dysphagia persists despite such therapy, or if significant complications result from impairment of the swallowing mechanism, treatment can be directed at the esophagus itself.

Bougienage of the upper esophageal sphincter with mercury-weighted rubber dilators is beneficial to some patients but often gives only temporary relief. This technique is contraindicated by the presence of a pharyngoesophageal diverticulum because of the high risk of perforation (see later discussion).

Many individuals with cricopharyngeal achalasia benefit from surgical interruption of the upper esophageal sphincter.[26] Failure to respond is observed most often in patients with central nervous system disease or peripheral neuropathy, although even these individuals are occasionally relieved of symptoms by this procedure. Serious complications following cervical myotomy are rare. Botulinum toxin injection and balloon dilation also have been employed. Gastroesophageal reflux or severe distal esophagitis indicating reflux is an absolute contraindication to cricopharyngeal myotomy unless the lower esophageal defect is corrected first.

Pharyngeal diverticula

ZENKER'S DIVERTICULUM

Zenker's diverticulum (Figure 76-3) is a posterior herniation of the hypopharynx through the triangular area just above the upper esophageal sphincter where the oblique and transverse fibers of the cricopharyngeus muscle join. It is seen once in every 1000 routine upper gastrointestinal series and is more frequent in males. Approximately 85% of cases occur in individuals over the age of 50.[27]

Symptoms of Zenker's diverticulum usually develop insidiously. An annoying irritation in the back of the throat is an early complaint, which may be followed later by the more classic symptoms of oropharyngeal dysphagia. Occasionally, an affected individual complains of a noise like the "roar of the ocean" or a "washing machine" during swallowing. Postcibal and nocturnal regurgitation of undigested food are common complaints. Obstructive symptoms may be caused by associated cricopharyngeal achalasia or, rarely, by compression of the esophagus by a large diverticulum.

Incoordination and incomplete relaxation of the upper esophageal sphincter during swallowing have been described in association with Zenker's diverticulum, lending support to the theory that cricopharyngeal dysfunction leads to high pharyngeal pressures, which result in the formation of hypopharyngeal diverticula. Many patients with a Zenker's diverticulum, however, have normal function of the upper esophageal sphincter or even reduced upper esophageal sphincter pressure, suggesting that high pharyngeal pressures may be due to stiffening of the pharyngeal muscles with loss of compliance.[28]

Zenker's diverticula most often are seen during x-ray examination but when small may be missed in the posteroanterior view because of superimposition over the main column of barium in the esophagus; this problem can be avoided by rotating the patient during the study (Figure 76-3). Endoscopic examination of the upper gastrointestinal tract in the presence of a hypopharyngeal diverticulum may be associated with an increased risk of perforation; however, this danger is minimized by passage of the instrument under direct vision.

Complications include compression and obstruction of the distal esophagus by a large diverticulum, respiratory difficulties caused by aspiration of diverticular contents, and diverticulitis with perforation. Rarely, carcinoma may develop in a Zenker's diverticulum.[29] Worsening of dysphagia, weight loss, and the appearance of blood in regurgitated material suggest the development of a malignant neoplasm.

The therapy for a symptomatic Zenker's diverticulum includes surgical excision alone or cricopharyngeal myotomy with or without removal of the diverticulum.[30] Endoscopic techniques for the treatment of Zenker's diverticulum also have been described.[31]

Lateral pharyngeal diverticula

Lateral pharyngeal diverticula, or pharyngoceles, occur with increased frequency in elderly people and are especially common in men.[32] They develop in the gap between the superior and middle pharyngeal constrictors. Symptoms are the same as those of a Zenker's diverticulum. In addition, patients may complain of a neck mass that enlarges with a Valsalva maneuver. Increased intrapharyngeal pressure may be an important causal factor, as exemplified by the frequency of this entity in muezzins and wind instrument players. Surgical repair is safe and effective.

THE ESOPHAGUS

The muscularis propria of the esophagus is composed of striated muscle fibers proximally and smooth muscle fibers distally. The central nervous system governs the activity of the striated muscle by means of sequential activation of extrinsic nerves. In humans, the dominant mechanism for control of the smooth muscle of the esophagus is unknown; both central and intramural neural pathways have been demonstrated. Orderly peristaltic contractions of esophageal muscle are necessary for normal esophageal function.

Although no information is available about the effects of aging on the regulation of esophageal muscle activity, alterations in esophageal muscle function have been identified manometrically in elderly individuals. These changes were described first in 1964 by Soergel et al,[33] who referred to motility disturbances in the elderly as "presbyesophagus." Soergel and his co-workers studied 15 subjects beyond the age of 90 and found a variety of abnormalities; 13 of their patients, however, had diseases known to affect esophageal motility. Subsequent studies have confirmed that, in the absence of other disorders, esophageal motility may be abnormal in elderly individuals, but the only manometric change identified in all the published work is a reduction in the amplitude of muscle contraction after a swallow.[34–36]

Elderly people also may be noted to have disordered motility, or "tertiary contractions," during a barium esophagogram, but this finding is rarely associated with symptoms.[37] Because motility changes that develop with aging do not appear to have clinical importance, the diagnosis of presbyesophagus should be abandoned. Elderly patients with dysphagia should be evaluated for the presence of disease processes involving the esophagus, and complaints should not be ascribed to motility changes occurring as a result of age alone.

Dysphagia and heartburn

Dysphagia and heartburn (pyrosis) are the principal symptoms of esophageal diseases; patients with esophageal disorders, especially elderly people, also may complain of respiratory difficulties, painful swallowing (odynophagia), chest pain resembling the pain of myocardial ischemia, regurgitation, and vomiting.[38–40]

Dysphagia is caused by impaired passage of food through the esophagus and is experienced immediately after the act of deglutition. Patients often complain that food "sticks on the way down." Since sensation in the esophagus is referred proximally, lesions at the gastroesophageal junction often appear as symptoms experienced at the level of the sternal notch. When a patient has symptoms apparently originating in the area of the proximal esophagus, evaluation of the entire esophagus, often with both esophagoscopy and barium radiography, is required.

The pattern of dysphagia frequently suggests the nature of the underlying disease.[41] Schatzki observed that a correct diagnosis can be made after taking a careful history in up to 85% of patients with this complaint.[42] Thus intermittent dysphagia connotes a motility disorder or a pliant mechanical obstruction such as an esophageal web. Progressive dysphagia often represents a neoplasm. Individuals who experience difficulty in swallowing liquids and solid food usually have a primary neuromuscular abnormality and disordered esophageal motility, whereas dysphagia produced only by solid foods is associated with mechanical obstruction of the esophagus.

Heartburn is a manifestation of the reflux of gastric contents into the esophagus and, as its name suggests, is described as being a hot sensation behind the sternum or in the left parasternal area. Pyrosis is relieved by antacids and intensified by bending at the waist or lying supine, especially when the stomach is full. Pyrosis also may be aggravated by some medications, smoking, and ingestion of alcohol, fruit juices, caffeine, chocolate, or peppermint. Discomfort is often accompanied by regurgitation of gastric contents, belching, vomiting, or secretion of saliva (water brash). The nature or extent of esophageal abnormalities associated with gastroesophageal reflux and heartburn cannot be predicted on the basis of the intensity of symptoms, especially in elderly people; severe reflux disease as evidenced by esophageal ulcers may be present in the absence of substantial symptoms.[43]

Esophageal motility disorders

After individuals with structural lesions have been excluded, more than 50% of adults of all ages with a complaint of dysphagia are found to have esophageal motility disorders.[44,45] These abnormalities may be primary or secondary and are classified according to their manometric signatures. Most often, adults with dysphagia have disordered motility with nonspecific and inconsistent manometric features.

NONSPECIFIC SECONDARY MOTILITY DISORDERS

In elderly people, nonspecific disorders of esophageal motility frequently are secondary to a systemic disease. Examples of generalized disorders sometimes responsible for esophageal dysmotility are myxedema, amyloidosis, connective tissue diseases, and diabetes mellitus.

Approximately 50% of patients with diabetic neuropathy have abnormal esophageal motility. Findings in these individuals include a decrease in the amplitude of muscle contraction, delayed esophageal emptying, esophageal dilation, and reduced lower esophageal emptying sphincter pressure. In patients with diabetes, the severity of motility changes correlates with the severity of other neuropathic complications; however, affected individuals usually do not have significant dysphagia. For this reason, esophageal symptoms in a diabetic must be fully evaluated and not simply attributed to diabetes.

PRIMARY AND SECONDARY ACHALASIA

Primary achalasia is the second most common motility disorder diagnosed in patients with nonstructural dysphagia, but it is rare in elderly people.[46] In persons beyond the age of 50, achalasia is most often secondary to gastric adenocarcinoma (Figure 76-4); pancreatic adenocarcinoma, oat cell carcinoma, reticulum cell sarcoma, and anaplastic lymphoma are responsible for isolated cases.[47,48] Manometric findings in secondary achalasia are identical to those in the primary disorder: absence of esophageal peristalsis, usually in association with elevation of resting lower esophageal sphincter pressure and failure of the lower esophageal sphincter to relax following an appropriate stimulus. The elevation of resting lower esophageal sphincter pressure typical of achalasia is less pronounced in elderly people, who also experience less chest pain in association with this disorder than do younger patients.[49] Pneumatic dilation typically is the treatment of choice for patients with primary achalasia.

Patients with both primary and secondary achalasia may experience progressive difficulty in swallowing. Food collects in the esophagus, which may become distended and tortuous even when the patient has an underlying carcinoma. In the absence of proximal dilation of the esophagus, a diagnosis of malignancy is favored. When the patient reclines, pooled food flows out of the esophagus back into

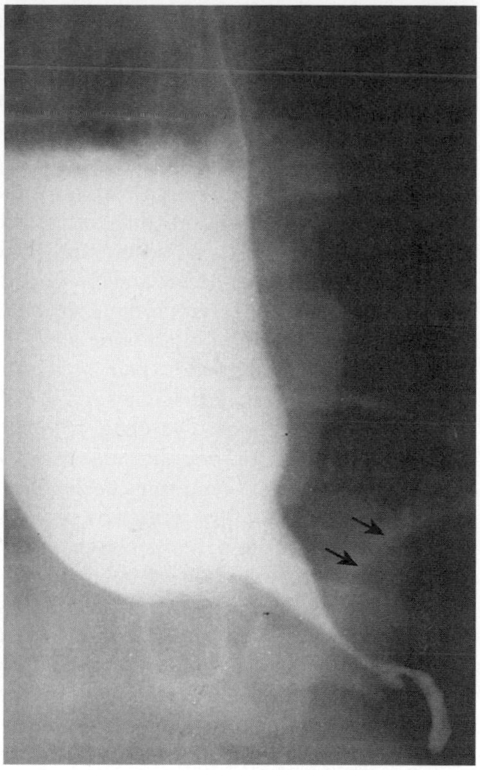

Figure 76-4. Barium esophagram showing tapering of the distal esophagus simulating achalasia. The subtle presence of a mass in the gastric fundus (*arrows*) suggested a diagnosis of carcinoma. *(Reproduced from Brandt LJ. Gastrointestinal disorders of the elderly. Lippincott-Raven, 1986, New York.)*

the pharynx, resulting in coughing and aspiration. Affected individuals, therefore, may have aspiration pneumonia. In addition to an infiltrate, a chest x-ray may reveal an air-fluid level in the esophagus and absence of the gastric air bubble. Because the presentations of primary and secondary achalasia may be identical, malignancy must be excluded in an elderly patient with this syndrome. Computed tomographic x-rays of the chest and upper abdomen, and endoscopy with biopsy of the distal esophagus, are recommended.[50] Endoscopic ultrasound may be helpful in differentiating primary from secondary achalasia.

The pathogenesis of secondary achalasia is unknown. Submucosal infiltration of the distal esophagus by tumor has been noted in some cases and normal histologic appearance in others.[51] It is possible that, in the absence of tumor infiltration, the motility disorder reflects a paraneoplastic neuropathy; manometric and roentgenographic abnormalities may disappear after resection of a gastric carcinoma or therapy for a lymphoma.[52,53]

DIFFUSE ESOPHAGEAL SPASM

Although primary esophageal motility disorders usually occur in middle-aged individuals, manometric recordings in elderly persons with intermittent dysphagia occasionally display the pattern of diffuse esophageal spasm.[38] *In this motility disturbance,* the patient has simultaneous, repetitive muscle contractions of prolonged duration occurring spontaneously or after a swallow. Normal peristalsis is present most of the time, explaining the intermittent nature of symptoms, which may be triggered by hot or cold food, pills, or carbonated beverages. The pathogenesis of diffuse esophageal spasm is obscure; on the basis of case reports, some have speculated that in some cases this disorder represents a stage in the development of achalasia.

"NUTCRACKER" ESOPHAGUS AND NONCARDIAC CHEST PAIN

It is usually assumed that in persons free of significant coronary artery disease with chest pain resembling the pain of myocardial ischemia, symptoms are due to an esophageal motility disorder. Such patients, however, rarely have chest pain during esophageal manometry, and provocative testing may be used to precipitate symptoms. Provocative testing with intravenous edrophonium chloride and infusion of acid into the esophagus causes chest pain in about 30% of subjects with a history of noncardiac chest pain.[54] A similar number of patients with noncardiac chest pain have been found to have an esophageal motility disorder, but only 25% of these individuals have symptoms during provocative testing.[44] It is often difficult, therefore, to prove that the esophagus is the source of the patient's complaints.

The most common motility disorder found in patients with noncardiac chest pain is "nutcracker" esophagus.[44] This abnormality is characterized by peristaltic muscle contractions of extremely high amplitude and long duration in the distal portion of the esophagus. A defect in esophageal transit can be demonstrated in many affected patients using a radionuclide marker. In one large series of individuals with noncardiac chest pain, 50% of patients with a motility disorder had nutcracker esophagus; other symptomatic individuals were found to have diffuse esophageal spasm.[44] A causal role for these motility defects in the production of chest pain has not been proved. In recent studies, many patients with noncardiac chest pain were found to have musculoskeletal disorders.

A number of medications have been used to treat primary esophageal motility disorders, especially diffuse esophageal spasm and nutcracker esophagus. Nitrates, anticholinergics, calcium channel blockers, or sedatives are occasionally effective in relieving symptoms of dysphagia and chest pain; their benefit in this setting, however, has never been evaluated in an appropriately designed trial. Some patients also obtain relief from dysphagia after bougienage.

Hiatus hernia

The incidence of hiatus hernia (Figure 76-5) increases with each decade of life from less than 10% of those under age 40 to approximately 40% in the sixth and seventh decades and 70% in patients beyond the age of 70. Symptoms such as pyrosis and regurgitation formerly attributed to the hernia are now known to be due to lower esophageal sphincter dysfunction. Sphincter dysfunction and gastrointestinal reflux are independent of the presence of a hiatus hernia, and the common "sliding" hiatus hernia is not considered by itself to be pathogenic.

One type of hiatus hernia that deserves special mention is the paraesophageal hernia (Figure 76-6), an uncommon hernia that occurs most often in persons between the ages of 60 and 70. Paraesophageal hernias often result in significant complications and therefore are of major importance. These hernias are frequently asymptomatic or cause only nagging discomfort until mechanical entrapment occurs. Such a catastrophe is associated with progressive distention of the incarcerated segment, vascular embarrassment, hemorrhage, gangrene, and perforation. In the absence of contraindications, a paraesophageal hernia demands surgical repair.

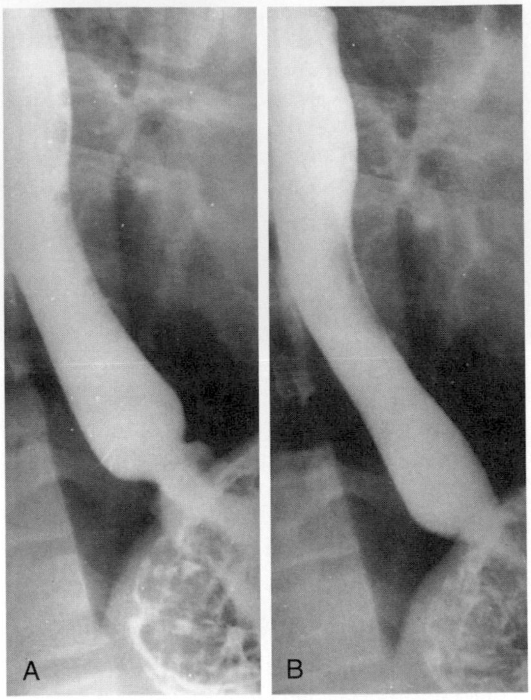

Figure 76-5. A small hiatus hernia sliding in (**A**) and out (**B**) of the thorax. The esophagogastric junction is seen above the diaphragm. *(Reproduced from Brandt LJ. Gastrointestinal disorders of the elderly. Lippincott-Raven, 1986, New York.)*

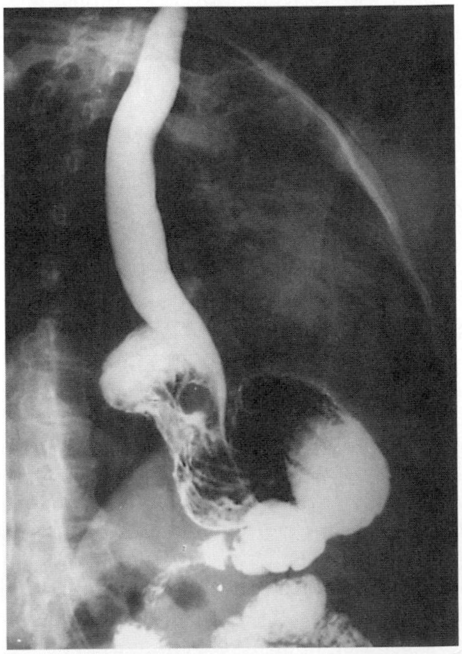

Figure 76-6. Barium esophagogram demonstrating a paraesophageal hernia with the gastric fundus above the diaphragm. The esophagogastric junction is at the level of the diaphragm. *(Reproduced from Brandt LJ. Gastrointestinal disorders of the elderly. Lippincott-Raven, 1986, New York.)*

Reflux esophagitis

The only notable change in the lower esophageal sphincter seen with aging is a reduction in the amplitude of postdeglutitive contraction or relaxation. Nevertheless, because the secretion of gastrin, which potentiates contraction of the lower esophageal sphincter, increases with age, and because gastric acid secretion declines with age in many individuals, it is unusual for reflux esophagitis to appear for the first time in elderly people.[55] The nature or extent of esophageal injury associated with gastroesophageal reflux cannot be predicted on the basis of the intensity of symptoms in older patients.[43] Complications of chronic, asymptomatic reflux such as stricture formation may be the initial clinical presentation of esophagitis in about 20% of affected elderly patients. When an aged individual complains of the recent onset of pyrosis, other causes of esophageal symptoms, such as candidiasis, must be considered. The therapy of reflux in elderly patients is the same as in younger patients, however, attention must be paid to the potential development of adverse effects of medications (see later discussion).[56]

Barrett's metaplasia

In patients with Barrett's metaplasia, the lower esophagus is lined for a variable distance by columnar, rather than the usual stratified squamous, epithelium.[57] The metaplastic columnar epithelium may be continuous with the columnar epithelium of the stomach and extend in tongues into the distal esophagus, or it may be present in islands surrounded by normal squamous epithelium. The importance of Barrett's metaplasia lies in its association with reflux esophagitis, (deep) esophageal ulcers, (high) esophageal strictures (Figure 76-7), and adenocarcinoma. The metaplastic columnar lining is believed to develop as a consequence of prolonged gastroesophageal reflux. Esophageal squamous epithelium damaged by exposure to gastric contents is replaced by a specialized columnar epithelium (intestinal metaplasia), a junctional type of epithelium, or a gastric fundic type of epithelium. Each of these three cell types may be seen alone or in combination with the others.

Most cases of Barrett's esophagus probably occur between the ages of 50 and 70; the exact incidence is unknown. The most common symptoms are those related to the reflux of stomach contents, and the entity is diagnosed best by esophagoscopy with multiple biopsies. The presence of specialized columnar epithelium establishes the diagnosis of Barrett's esophagus.[57] If the columnar epithelium in the biopsy specimen is one of the other two types, the biopsy must have been taken at least 3 cm above the gastroesophageal junction to make the diagnosis. Intestinal metaplasia can be recognized in situ by staining with Alcian blue.

Stricture and neoplasia are long-term complications of Barrett's esophagus. There is increasing evidence that cancer arises only in the specialized columnar epithelium. By careful screening using esophagoscopy with a directed biopsy every 1 to 2 years, premalignant dysplastic changes can usually be detected.[58,59] The development of severe dysplasia or carcinoma in situ requires resection of the involved esophagus. Thermal ablation of Barrett's epithelium with multipolar electrocoagulation, laser coagulation, or argon plasma coagulation has been investigated. Destruction of the Barrett's epithelium by these techniques is successful initially, but recurrence of the Barrett's tissue may occur. Therapy of reflux usually results in symptomatic improvement, but regression of the columnar epithelium does not occur without surgery.

Lower esophageal ring

A lower esophageal or Schatzki ring (Figure 76-8) is a thin, annular ridge of mucosa projecting perpendicularly into the esophageal lumen at or near the squamocolumnar

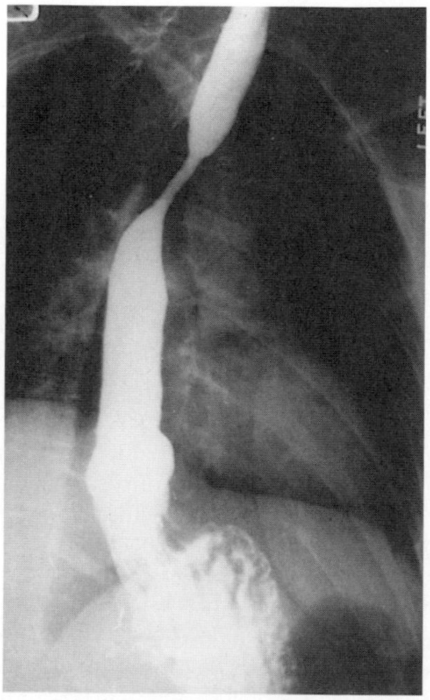

Figure 76-7. Barium esophagogram revealing a stricture of the esophagus at the level of the aortic arch in a patient with Barrett's esophagus. A hiatus hernia is also present. *(Reproduced from Brandt LJ. Gastrointestinal disorders of the elderly. Lippincott-Raven, 1986, New York.)*

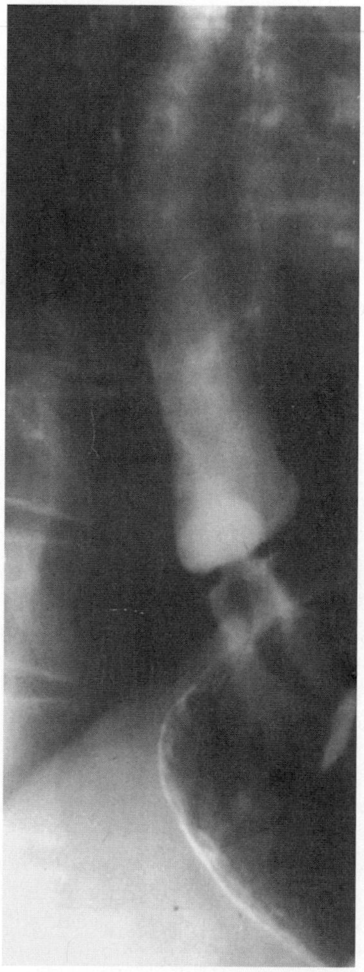

Figure 76-8. A Schatzki ring prevents passage of a barium pill in a patient with intermittent dysphagia. *(Reproduced from Brandt LJ. Gastrointestinal disorders of the elderly. Lippincott-Raven, 1986, New York.)*

junction.[60–62] A Schatzki ring may be asymptomatic, found incidentally during evaluation of the upper gastrointestinal tract for unrelated reasons, or it may cause intermittent episodes of dysphagia and an uncomfortable sticking or pressing sensation as a result of food lodging above the ring. Episodes commonly occur during hurried meals, meals requiring a great deal of mastication, or meals consumed with alcohol, hence the appellation "steakhouse syndrome." As the lumen of the ring diminishes to less than 12 mm (0.047 in.) in diameter, attacks become more frequent. Attacks usually last several minutes or more until the patient regurgitates the food bolus or flushes it into the stomach with a beverage.

Total obstruction of the esophagus secondary to food impaction frequently brings patients to the emergency department. Relaxation of the esophagus by administration of a small dose of intravenous benzodiazepine or 1 mg of glucagon is occasionally effective in relieving the impaction. Papain solution (meat tenderizer) should not be used to try to digest the meat because its use has been associated with esophageal perforation. If the impacted bolus does not pass, it must be removed by esophagoscopy. Alternatively, it may be gently nudged into the stomach if a patent lumen can be seen distally, the esophageal mucosa is intact, and there is no bone or other sharp object present. Multiple biopsies to disrupt the ring or dilation with bougies are techniques used to treat symptomatic rings.

Dysphagia aortica

Degenerative changes in the aorta may produce compression of the esophagus and dysphagia. Obstruction of the upper esophagus is occasionally caused by a thoracic aneurysm, while the distal esophagus may be squeezed between an atherosclerotic aorta posteriorly and the heart or esophageal hiatus anteriorly. Most patients are women beyond the age of 70.[63–65] Symptoms are usually prevented by having the patient thoroughly masticate solid food, but occasionally the obstruction is severe enough to warrant surgical mobilization of the esophagus at the hiatus.[66]

Medication-induced esophageal injury

Esophageal injury can occur as a result of the local caustic effects of medications.[67,68] The most frequent offenders are antibiotics, especially tetracyclines, potassium chloride, ferrous sulfate, nonsteroidal anti-inflammatory drugs, alendronate, and quinidine.

Most patients with medication-induced esophageal injury have no underlying esophageal disorder. Some individuals, however, have nonspecific, asymptomatic disorders of esophageal motility, peptic strictures, esophageal compression from left atrial enlargement, a prominent aortic knob, or mediastinal adhesions following thoracic surgery. Pills commonly lodge in the esophagus at the level of the aortic knob or the lower esophageal sphincter without the patient's knowledge. Many cases of pill-induced esophageal injury probably remain unrecognized with full recovery. The most frequent symptoms of medication-induced esophageal injury are odynophagia and retrosternal pain. Symptoms usually resolve within 6 weeks of stopping the medication or changing it to a liquid formulation; damage, however, may result in esophageal stricture formation or, occasionally, hemorrhage or perforation. Pills should always be taken with a generous amount of water, and elderly patients should not take pills immediately before bedtime because a decrease in salivation and esophageal motor activity accompanies sleeping.[69]

Esophageal diverticula

Diverticula of the esophagus are much less common than diverticula of other parts of the gastrointestinal tract. In a review of 20,000 barium studies on the upper gastrointestinal tract, Wheeler noted only six midesophageal (traction-type) and three epiphrenic (pulsion-type) diverticula, as compared with 1020 duodenal diverticula.[70] The terms *traction* and *pulsion* refer to commonly accepted theories regarding the pathogenesis of esophageal diverticula. Traction diverticula are thought to be caused by the effects of fibrotic disease in structures contiguous with the esophagus, whereas pulsion diverticula are hypothesized to result from increased intraluminal pressure. Pseudodiverticulosis of the esophagus also has been described.

MIDESOPHAGEAL DIVERTICULA (TRACTION DIVERTICULA)

Traction diverticula occur most commonly in the middle third of the esophagus, where a large group of lymph nodes lies in direct contact with the esophageal wall. Nodal inflammation of this area may lead to periesophagitis, fixation of the esophagus to the lymph nodes, and distortion of the esophageal wall. In the past, tuberculosis was the most common cause for this process; any infection with lymph node involvement, however, may lead to the formation of a traction diverticulum.

Traction diverticula usually occur in patients of middle age or older and are slightly more common in men. They rarely cause symptoms, perhaps because they are small, have a broad neck, and can contract and empty because they contain all the layers of the esophageal wall including muscle.

EPIPHRENIC DIVERTICULA (PULSION DIVERTICULA)

Pulsion diverticula are found in the lower 10 cm of the esophagus, usually on the right wall. Like traction diverticula, they contain all the layers of the esophageal wall; the muscular layer, however, may be quite attenuated.

Epiphrenic diverticula usually develop in males during middle age. Patients may complain of dysphagia or chest pain, but symptoms are probably due to an associated esophageal motor abnormality, such as achalasia or diffuse esophageal spasm.[71] The occurrence of an epiphrenic diverticulum without an underlying motility disorder or a hiatus hernia appears to be rare.

Many epiphrenic diverticula are asymptomatic, and in these instances no therapy is required.[72] Treatment of esophageal reflux or an underlying, motility disorder may afford the patient symptomatic relief.[73,74] In cases of larger diverticula, surgical resection may be necessary.[75]

INTRAMURAL PSEUDODIVERTICULOSIS

In esophageal pseudodiverticulosis, dilation of the excretory ducts of submucosal glands causes multiple small (1 to 3 mm) invaginations of the esophageal wall.[76,77] These defects involve all, or segments of, the esophagus in a circumferential fashion. Pseudodiverticula are best detected by barium contrast studies; their roentgenographic appearance is quite

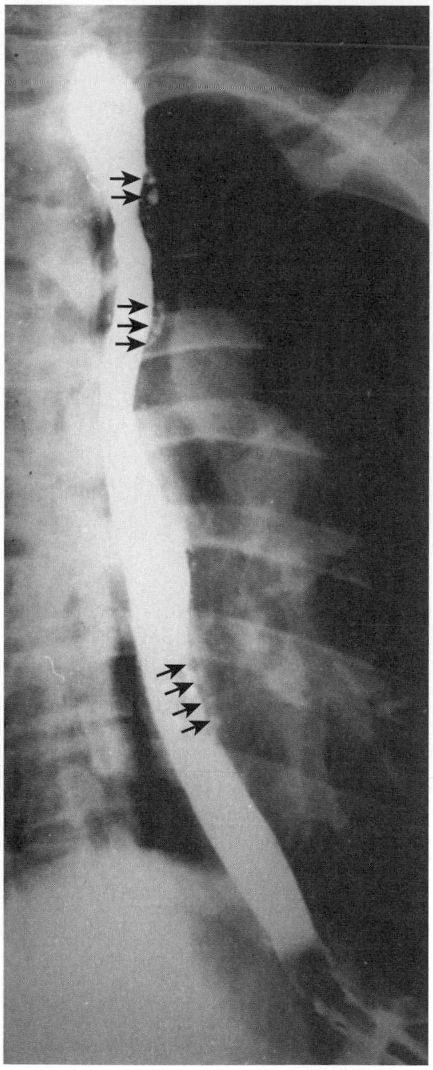

Figure 76-9. Intramural pseudodiverticulosis with multiple outpouchings (*arrows*) on a barium esophagogram. *(Reproduced from Brandt LJ. Gastrointestinal disorders of the elderly. Lippincott-Raven, 1986, New York.)*

characteristic (Figure 76-9). Pseudodiverticulosis is usually diagnosed during the seventh decade of life in patients with dysphagia. In at least 20% of cases, gastroesophageal reflux, a motility disorder, or a malignancy is found, and in approximately one half of patients, smears or cultures of the esophageal mucosa reveal *Candida albicans*. Stenoses, or areas of reduced distensibility, are found in up to 90% of cases of pseudodiverticulosis and preferentially seem to involve the upper esophagus. Surprisingly, there is no fixed relationship between the narrowed area and the segment involved with pseudodiverticula.

The cause of pseudodiverticulosis is unknown. The term *adenosis* has been used to refer to this entity because the number of deep esophageal mucous glands is markedly increased. Therapy consists of treatment of associated abnormalities. Coexisting strictures should be evaluated to ensure that they are benign.

Esophageal candidiasis

Infection of the esophagus is rare in patients without acquired immunodeficiency syndrome, with the exception of infection with *C. albicans*. *C. albicans* is a normal inhabitant of the alimentary tract; the yeast form is found in almost 50% of oral washings and 80% of stool samples.[78] The population of *C. albicans* is suppressed in healthy adults by other intestinal flora. Comparison of fecal specimens from subjects aged 70 to 100 with those of individuals aged 20 to 69 have revealed fungi to be more common in the elderly group. This finding may be explained by a diminution in esophageal peristalsis, a reduction in gastric acid secretion, and age-related alterations in cellular and humoral immunity.

In the absence of antibiotic therapy or an underlying immune disorder, esophageal candidiasis is a disease of elderly people. Most cases in this age group, however, occur in association with predisposing conditions, including malignancy, therapy with immunosuppressive or cytotoxic drugs, diabetes mellitus, malnutrition, and treatment with broad-spectrum antibiotics.[79,80]

In the proper clinical setting, dysphagia, odynophagia, substernal burning, or an awareness of food passing down the esophagus should suggest the possibility of candida infection, although even in the presence of infection with *C. albicans*, up to one half of patients may be asymptomatic. Esophageal candidiasis often results from the extension of oral lesions, and a careful examination of the oral cavity is important in any debilitated patient complaining of esophageal symptoms.

A diagnosis of candida esophagitis may be suggested by an abnormal barium esophagogram, although a normal study does not exclude the presence of this organism. Esophagoscopy is the best method for detecting candida infection; raised white plaque, hyperemia, ulceration, and friability are characteristic. The gross appearance of candida esophagitis may be confused with that of exudative esophagitis, and therefore the diagnosis must be confirmed by brushings and by taking biopsies. Typical hyphae are revealed under the microscope in scrapings placed on a glass slide and macerated with 20% potassium hydroxide.

In the appropriate setting, a trial therapy may be initiated without attempting an invasive diagnosis. As in oral and vaginal candidiasis, therapy usually consists of promoting the reestablishment of normal microbiologic flora by discontinuing antibiotics. In an immunocompromised host or in an individual with significant morbidity, fluconazole is considered the drug of choice. Odynophagia can be treated with viscous lidocaine or with a "swish-and-swallow" preparation of the type used to treat stomatitis (see previous discussion). Failure to respond to simple treatment necessitates endoscopic confirmation of the diagnosis and often systemic therapy with additional antifungal agents.

Esophageal neoplasms

Esophageal cancer (Figure 76-10) occurs most frequently after age 55 and is three times more common in males than in females in the United States, and two times more common in males than in females in the United Kingdom.[1] In the United States, it accounts for approximately 2% of all reported cancers. Factors associated with the development of esophageal cancer include alcohol and tobacco use, thermal irritation, poor oral hygiene, and esophageal stasis.[1,81,82] Furthermore, an association has been noted with certain esophageal diseases, notably achalasia, Barrett's esophagus, lye stricture, and Plummer-Vinson syndrome, and with previous gastric surgery.[83–85]

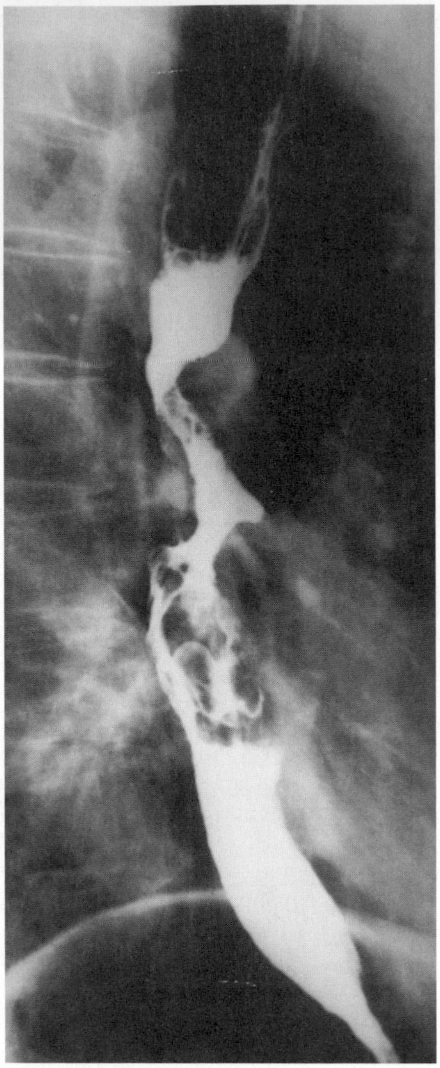

Figure 76-10. Barium esophagogram demonstrating an ulcerating esophageal carcinoma. *(Reproduced from Brandt LJ. Gastrointestinal disorders of the elderly. Lippincott-Raven, 1986, New York.)*

Surveillance, epidemiology, and end results (SEER) data show an increase in adenocarcinoma from 8% to 18% of all esophageal cancers during the years 1973–1984; it now represents the most rapidly increasing malignancy in the United States.[86] Esophageal adenocarcinoma is either cancer of the gastric fundus or a malignancy that has developed in a segment of Barrett's esophagus. Squamous cell carcinoma most commonly involves the middle third of the esophagus. Local spread occurs early and because the esophagus dilates so readily, dysphagia, the most common complaint at the time of diagnosis, is a late symptom.

In elderly people an important manifestation of esophageal cancer is an achalasia-like syndrome. Primary achalasia is uncommon in patients beyond the age of 50. Elderly individuals who have symptoms of achalasia of less than 1 year's duration associated with notable weight loss should be suspected of having a malignancy, most often gastric adenocarcinoma. The pathogenesis of secondary achalasia is unknown; in some cases the lower esophagus is infiltrated with tumor cells, but in other cases achalasia may reflect a paraneoplastic process.

The prognosis for esophageal cancer is dismal. Management is directed at relieving progressive obstruction.[87–89] Surgical resection and radiation are the accepted modes of treatment. Surgical resection offers the only chance for long-term survival, but fewer than half of all patients having esophageal cancer have a resectable lesion. If there is evidence of nodal or distant metastases, a thoracotomy should be avoided. Thoracic radiation, while useful, may be followed by the development of esophagitis, usually within 3 weeks of initiating therapy and continuing for several weeks after its completion. Chemotherapy may result in symptomatic improvement but does not substantially prolong survival. New chemotherapeutic agents should be administered under an investigational protocol. Combined modality therapy may offer advantages over more traditional approaches. Palliative therapy with endoscopically placed stents, lasers, or photodynamic therapy is often very useful and has improved the quality of life for many patients, albeit without prolonging survival.

THE STOMACH

Aging is associated with alterations in both the motor and secretory functions of the stomach but, as in other parts of the gastrointestinal tract, changes in gastric physiology attributable to age alone rarely are responsible for symptoms.

The motor activity of the stomach allows it to behave as two individual, albeit coordinated, organs: one that processes liquids and another that processes solids. The fundus and proximal body of the stomach serve as a reservoir for liquids. In contrast, the distal gastric body and the antrum grind solids into small particles and pump them into the duodenum. The activities of both the proximal and distal stomach are controlled by complex neural and hormonal mechanisms. Studies employing food labeled with radioactive isotopes suggest that gastric emptying of liquids is prolonged in elderly persons, whereas emptying of solids is unaffected by age.[90,91]

Changes in gastric secretion also occur in individuals as they grow older. In the past, almost every study on gastric acid production showed a decline in basal and stimulated acid output with advancing age.[92] Work by Goldschmiedt et al,[93] however, suggests that in the absence of *Helicobacter pylori* infection, aging is actually associated with an increase in gastric acid secretion. Previous confusion about the effect of aging on gastric acid secretion is probably related to the high incidence of *H. pylori* infection and chronic atrophic gastritis with secondary achlorhydria in older individuals (see later discussion).[94]

Gastric and duodenal mucosal injury

Advances in our understanding of the pathobiology of gastric and duodenal mucosal injury, and improvements in our ability to examine the upper gastrointestinal tract and detect diseases responsible for mucosal injury, make it important for physicians to use descriptive and diagnostic terminology carefully in clinical practice.[95,96] Unless diagnostic findings are reported with a precision that accurately reflects current understanding of mucosal injury, the benefits of medical advances made during the past few decades may be lost to patients.

In usual cases of gastric or duodenal mucosal injury, endoscopic inspection often reveals the presence of gross epithelial defects. Small epithelial defects, or erosions, do not penetrate the muscularis mucosae. Ulcers are defined as being larger than 3 mm in diameter and extend a variable distance through the muscularis mucosae, in some instances freely perforating into the peritoneal cavity or penetrating into an adjacent organ. A typical ulcer is composed of four layers or zones: a superficial layer of fibrinopurulent debris overlying a zone of inflammation, a layer of granulation tissue, and, at its base, a collagenous scar. Both erosions and ulcers may be sources of bleeding.

Diffuse mucosal erythema, a common finding at endoscopy, in most instances represents microvascular congestion and, although it is interpreted by many endoscopists as indicating the presence of "gastritis," this conclusion is unjustified. Mucosal erythema due to microvascular congestion is caused by a variety of factors and is without any specific causal significance or clinical association.[96] Conversely, patients often have histologic gastritis without the presence of mucosal erythema.

The term *gastritis* implies the presence of inflammation and should not be used unless examination of a biopsy specimen has revealed typical mucosal inflammatory changes, including infiltration of the lamina propria with polymorphonuclear leukocytes and mononuclear cells. Neutrophils are seen early in the course of inflammation (acute gastritis). With the passage of time, mononuclear cells, mainly plasma cells, and eosinophils appear in increasing numbers (chronic gastritis). Most patients with gastritis have a predominance of mononuclear cells in the lamina propria with a lesser number of neutrophils (chronic active gastritis).[97] The inflammatory changes of gastritis are accompanied by signs of cell injury and regeneration. Cell damage and death cause submucosal hemorrhage and edema and lead to development of epithelial defects. Hemorrhage and edema may be visible grossly at endoscopy and evident on microscopic examination of biopsy specimens, as are erosions and ulcers. In response to injury, the epithelium regenerates by proliferation and differentiation of mucous neck cells, a process that leads to elongation and tortuosity of the gastric pits (foveolar hyperplasia). The vast majority of cases of gastritis are caused by infection with *H. pylori* (type B gastritis). Gastritis also may be due to other less common bacterial infections, granulomatous disease, autoimmune disease (type A gastritis), and hypersensitivity reactions.

Other agents of gastric injury damage the mucosa without exciting an inflammatory response. This gastropathy is sometimes referred to as type C gastritis, an unfortunate misnomer given the noninflammatory nature of the process.[98] Microscopic examination of biopsy specimens from patients with gastropathy typically reveals vascular congestion and edema of the lamina propria, hypertrophy of the muscularis mucosae, and mucosal regenerative changes with foveolar hyperplasia.[99] As in gastritis, cell damage and death are accompanied by submucosal hemorrhage and edema and lead to the development of epithelial defects. The latter changes are all often grossly visible on endoscopy. The most common causes of gastropathy are ingestion of nonsteroidal anti-inflammatory drugs (NSAIDs) and ethanol.

Helicobacter pylori, gastritis, and peptic ulcer disease

Infection with *H. pylori*, a spiral gram-negative microaerophilic rod, is the most common chronic bacterial disease in humans. This organism attaches to receptors on the surface of gastric mucous neck cells and is also found on metaplastic gastric epithelium in the duodenum but not on the duodenal mucosa itself or on metaplastic duodenal mucosa in the stomach (Figure 76-11).[100] *H. pylori* causes alterations in cell structure and function, inflammation, metaplasia, and cell death.[101] A number of virulence factors, including urease, make it possible for the organism to colonize the stomach and produce disease.[102]

H. pylori infection is the most common cause of chronic gastritis (type B antral gastritis) and is one of the two principal causes of peptic ulcer disease, the other being ingestion of NSAIDs. More than 90% of patients with duodenal ulcer and more than 75% of patients with gastric ulcer also have *H. pylori* infection and chronic active gastritis.[102] The relationship between ulcer disease and gastritis was recognized long before the causal role of *H. pylori* in the pathogenesis of peptic ulcer disease was understood. *H. pylori* infection also has been linked to the development of gastric cancer, another gastritis-associated disease.[103]

Infection with *H. pylori* is usually acquired during childhood and occurs most often in persons living under conditions of poverty, crowding, and inadequate sanitation.[104] The prevalence of *H. pylori* infection in the United States and in the nations of western Europe increases with advancing age, a result of the poorer living conditions in these countries during the early years of the twentieth century.[105] Thus regardless of present socioeconomic status, infection is most prevalent in older individuals. The incidence of peptic ulcer disease also increases progressively with advancing age, reflecting the age-related increase in *H. pylori* infection.

Under experimental conditions, acute infection with *H. pylori* causes transient dyspeptic symptoms accompanied by the development of active antral gastritis.[106] Mucosal

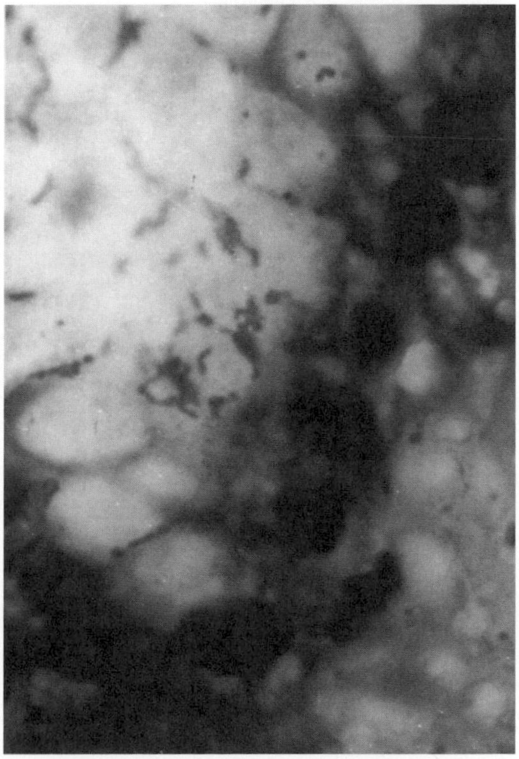

Figure 76-11. Gastric biopsy showing *H. pylori* in the surface mucous layer (Giemsa stain, 1000x). *(Courtesy of Sumi Mitsudo.)*

inflammation apparently may resolve spontaneously in the minority of patients or become chronic, gradually spreading proximally into the body and fundus of the stomach. As the disease progresses, inflammation extends into the deeper, glandular part of the epithelium containing the gastric secretory cells. These include parietal cells, which make hydrochloric acid and intrinsic factor; chief cells, which make pepsin; pylorocardiac gland cells, which make mucus; and endocrine G cells, which make gastrin. Normal glands are gradually destroyed and replaced by metaplastic glands (intestinal metaplasia) or by atrophic gastric mucosa (atrophic gastritis), a process that takes many years. Atrophic gastritis often is associated with low serum gastrin levels and antibodies to gastrin-secreting cells. Patients with chronic active gastritis frequently also have submucosal hemorrhage, edema, epithelial erosions (erosive gastritis), and peptic ulcers.

Individuals with active gastritis and gastric mucosal atrophy are usually asymptomatic but may complain of intermittent dyspepsia, abdominal pain, distention, nausea, and vomiting (nonulcer dyspepsia). The relationship, if any, between symptoms of nonulcer dyspepsia and gastritis is unclear (see later discussion); many persons with dyspepsia do not have gastritis, and many persons with gastritis do not have dyspepsia.[107] Dyspeptic symptoms may be due to the development of a gastric or duodenal ulcer, although at least 50% of patients with acute ulcers are asymptomatic.

H. pylori infection may be diagnosed by a transendoscopic pinch biopsy of the stomach. Microscopic examination of biopsy specimens from infected individuals reveals chronic active gastritis and typical spiral gram-negative rods in the mucus coating the surface epithelium (Figure 76-11). The absence of gastritis strongly argues against *H. pylori* infection, whereas its presence suggests that a failure to identify *H. pylori* is due to sampling error. Tissue also may be implanted in commercially available agar plates containing urea and a pH indicator. If *H. pylori* is present in the tissue specimen, bacterial urease will split the urea into bicarbonate and ammonia, raising the pH and producing a color change. Because infection may be patchy, testing several specimens obtained from different parts of the stomach improves the sensitivity of the assay.

Noninvasive diagnosis of *H. pylori* infection can be made by detecting serum antibody to bacterial antigens. This method of diagnosis is satisfactory, presuming there is no indication for endoscopy if the patient has not previously been treated with antibiotics to which *H. pylori* is sensitive. Antibody titers decrease gradually after eradication of infection, but qualitative serology remains positive for a number of years, leaving what has been referred to as an "immunologic scar." The presence of an immunologic scar makes it impossible to use antibody testing to assess the effectiveness of therapy or the occurrence of reinfection. This problem is avoided by using the urea breath test, which is positive only in a setting of active infection. In the urea breath test, the patient is given an oral dose of urea labeled with either a stable (^{13}C) or unstable (^{14}C) isotope of carbon. If the patient is infected with *H. pylori*, the urea will be metabolized by bacterial urease to ammonia and bicarbonate, and bicarbonate containing the isotopic tracer will be converted to CO_2 and expired. The presence of labeled CO_2 in samples of expired gas indicates active *H. pylori* infection. A stool assay for detection of *H. pylori* also is available commercially.

Simultaneous treatment with a combination of two antibiotics and a proton pump inhibitor is the most consistently effective means of curing *H. pylori* infection.[108] *H. pylori* is sensitive to a variety of antimicrobial agents, including metronidazole, tetracyclines, macrolides, some quinolones, β-lactams, bismuth preparations, and proton pump inhibitors. The most commonly used regimen is a combination of amoxicillin, clarithromycin, and a proton pump inhibitor. Regimens containing metronidazole are limited by the frequent occurrence of bacterial resistance to this agent. Because of the morbidity caused by *H. pylori* infection, the National Institutes of Health Consensus Development Panel has published guidelines mandating treatment of all *H. pylori*-infected ulcer patients, including those currently without an active ulcer crater or dyspeptic symptoms.[109] The significant treatment failure rate makes it desirable to document a cure by conducting a urea breath test 4 weeks after the completion of therapy. In addition to antibiotic therapy for *H. pylori* infection, patients with acute ulcers should be treated with an antisecretory agent to promote ulcer healing.

Nonsteroidal anti-inflammatory drugs, gastropathy, and peptic ulcer disease

Nonsteroidal anti-inflammatory drugs (NSAIDs) are among the most frequently prescribed medicines in the world. Approximately 3 million people in the United States, or 1.2% of the population, take at least one NSAID daily. Uncounted others regularly use over-the-counter NSAID preparations, including aspirin. As a result, NSAID-related morbidity is exceedingly common; each year 2% to 4% of chronic NSAID users have a serious drug-induced complication involving the gastrointestinal tract.[110] The use of NSAIDs and complications of NSAID use are most prevalent in elderly people.[111–113] In the United Kingdom, NSAID prescription rates for the entire population increased steadily from 1967 to 1985 and did so in direct proportion to the age of the recipient, with progressively more prescriptions being written for progressively older patients.[114] Thus in 1985, an astonishing 1400 NSAID prescriptions were written for every 1000 women in the United Kingdom aged 65 years or older. These chronic NSAID users are estimated to have a twofold to threefold greater mortality rate than nonusers because of drug-related gastrointestinal complications.

Each and every nonselective NSAID is capable of injuring the gastrointestinal mucosa and does so in a dose-dependent fashion roughly proportional to its anti-inflammatory effect. Virtually 100% of patients who take a NSAID preparation, including aspirin, develop acute gastropathy during the first 1 to 2 weeks of therapy.[115] This gastropathy has the typical histologic features described above and characteristically is associated with submucosal hemorrhage and some degree of edema, both of which are often grossly visible at endoscopy. Many NSAIDs, such as aspirin, are weak acids that remain nonionized as the tablets break up and are dispersed in low-pH gastric secretions. Because they are nonionized, NSAIDs move easily across the membranes of epithelial cells and then ionize at the neutral pH of the cytoplasm. In the ionic form, they interact with cell constituents and cause cell damage and death.[116] Dead epithelial cells leave shallow mucosal defects (erosions), which may bleed. Patients often have dyspeptic symptoms during this acute phase of injury.

In a significant minority of chronic NSAID users, mucosal defects enlarge and form true ulcers; approximately 12% to 30% of patients develop a gastric ulcer, and 2% to 19% of patients develop a duodenal ulcer.[117] Elderly people seem to be particularly vulnerable to the harmful effects of NSAIDs. In a study of peptic ulcer disease in persons aged 65 and older, Griffin et al[118] found that almost 30% of ulcers diagnosed in these individuals may have been caused by NSAIDs. The principal mechanism by which NSAID use leads to the development of peptic ulcers is dose-dependent systemic inhibition of prostaglandin synthesis. Prostaglandins protect the upper gastrointestinal mucosa by stimulating the secretion of bicarbonate and mucus, increasing mucosal blood flow, and promoting a number of cellular processes crucial to mucosal defense and repair. A decrease in prostaglandin synthesis tips the balance between defensive and aggressive factors in the upper gastrointestinal tract in favor of those that injure the mucosa, leading to the formation of ulcers and the possible development of complications, including hemorrhage, obstruction, perforation, and penetration into an adjacent organ.

The cyclooxygenase-2 (COX-2) specific agents have been shown to be equally efficacious as nonselective NSAIDs in the treatment of both osteoarthritis and rheumatoid arthritis, but with significantly fewer gastrointestinal side effects. These agents have a greater affinity for COX-2 as compared with COX-1; COX-2 is induced in response to inflammation, whereas COX-1 is a constitutive enzyme that functions in a variety of maintenance and housekeeping roles. Many studies have demonstrated a decreased incidence of both gastric and duodenal ulcers in patients taking COX-2 selective agents as compared with those using nonselective NSAIDs. The use of COX-2 selective agents is associated with ulceration rates in the gastrointestinal tract that are no different than a placebo.[119] Some COX-2 specific agents have been withdrawn from the market because of adverse side effect profiles; celecoxib remains available in the United States as of 2009.

A variety of treatment strategies for preventing the development of gastric and duodenal ulcers in patients on chronic NSAID therapy have been tested.[120] Many commonly used medicines are without any demonstrable prophylactic benefit in this setting. Ranitidine and omeprazole have been shown to prevent duodenal but not gastric ulcers in arthritis patients taking NSAIDs.[120–122] Similar results were obtained by Taha et al[123] in arthritis patients treated with prophylactic famotidine; however, in the same study, high-dose famotidine reduced the incidence of both duodenal and gastric ulcers.[123] An alternative approach to ulcer prevention in patients who require chronic NSAID therapy is prostaglandin replacement with an oral synthetic prostaglandin E analog. The prostaglandin E_1 analog, misoprostol, like famotidine, has been shown to prevent development of both duodenal and gastric ulcers.[124] This agent also reduces the incidence of bleeding, perforation, and gastric outlet obstruction in patients on chronic NSAID therapy.[112] The use of misoprostol has been limited by its tendency to cause loose stools, abdominal cramps, and flatulence in a significant minority of individuals during initiation of treatment.

The large number of eligible patients makes it impossible to prescribe prophylactic famotidine or misoprostol for every NSAID user, or to use COX-2 selective agents in all. Instead, an effort should be made to identify and treat those who both require chronic NSAID therapy and are at greatest risk for developing a significant NSAID-related complication. Included in this high-risk group are elderly people and persons with a history of peptic ulcer disease or previous upper gastrointestinal bleeding, individuals also taking steroids, and patients with cardiovascular disease.[112,113] Once an ulcer develops, a serious complication is often the first sign of its presence. Approximately 50% of persons with ulcers have no dyspeptic symptoms. Patients taking NSAIDs who have dyspeptic symptoms require evaluation for ulcer disease and possible *H. pylori* infection, and those with ulcers should be treated with an antisecretory agent and also antibiotics, if indicated.

Peptic ulcer disease in elderly people

Ulcer disease, whether due to *H. pylori* infection, NSAID use, or some other less common cause, frequently exhibits a virulent course in elderly people with more complications and higher mortality than in the young.[125–127] A duodenal ulcer occurs two to three times more frequently than a gastric ulcer, but the latter is responsible for two of every three deaths from peptic ulcer disease in older individuals, and the death rate increases with advancing age.

The presentation of ulcer disease in elderly people tends to be acute, often with bleeding or perforation, but symptoms may be subtle; this is particularly true of gastric ulcers. Gastric ulcers produce chronic blood loss more commonly than duodenal ulcers, and resultant anemia may lead to cardiac or neurologic symptoms. Weight loss and fatigue suggesting malignancy may be the only complaints, a presentation characteristic of giant ulcers. So-called geriatric ulcers (Figure 76-12) high in the cardia may cause misleading symptoms such as dysphagia mimicking esophageal neoplasm or

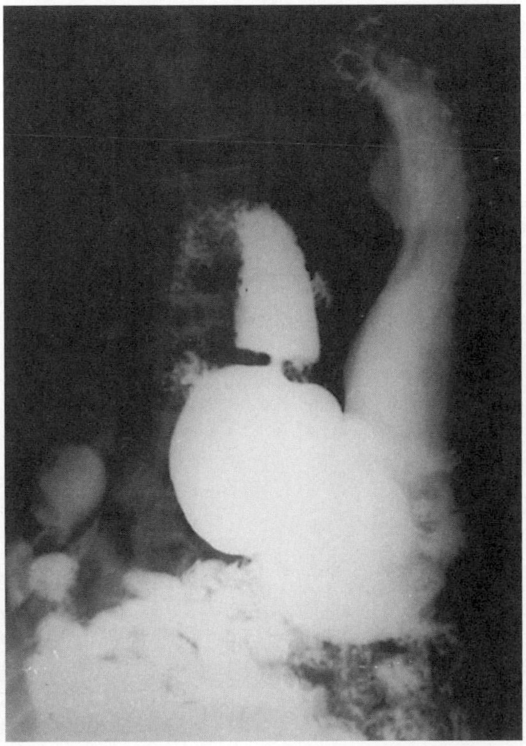

Figure 76-12. Upper gastrointestinal series revealing a large benign "geriatric ulcer" high on the lesser curvature. *(Reproduced from Brandt LJ. Gastrointestinal disorders of the elderly. Lippincott-Raven, 1986, New York.)*

chest pain suggesting angina. A history of NSAID use is commonly obtained from elderly patients with peptic ulcer disease.

The complication rate of peptic ulcer disease rises progressively from 31% in patients 60 to 64 years of age to 76% in those 75 to 79 years of age. Surgery should not be withheld or delayed solely because of advanced age because it is often life-saving in older patients. Bleeding, the most common complication, accounts for one half to two thirds of all fatalities (see later discussion). Perforation is the second most common complication of peptic ulcers in elderly people. The presentation of a perforated ulcer is subtle in this age group, delaying the correct diagnosis and contributing to the high mortality rate. Gastric outlet obstruction complicates ulcer disease in 10% to 15% of patients beyond 60 years of age, generally occurring in those with a long history of disease; an obstructing malignant lesion must be excluded in such patients.

Duodenal ulcers greater than 2 cm in diameter were once considered a distinct entity because of their poor prognosis, but it is probable that most of these "giant" duodenal ulcers are caused by either *H. pylori* infection or NSAID use, just like smaller lesions. Giant duodenal ulcers occur most often in men over 70 years of age who have no prior history of peptic ulcer disease. The most frequent complaint is of abdominal pain radiating to the back or right upper quadrant, suggesting pancreatic or biliary disease. Pain may be relieved by antacids, but aggravated by eating, and is often accompanied by significant weight loss. The ulcer crater is so large that it sometimes is mistaken for the duodenal bulb on an upper gastrointestinal series (Figure 76-13). Although giant duodenal ulcers were often fatal 30 years ago, today they usually respond to therapy with histamine antagonists or proton pump inhibitors and with antibiotics when indicated by the presence of *H. pylori* infection.

Giant gastric ulcers have a diameter of more than 3 cm.[128,129] They also are most likely caused by either *H. pylori* infection or NSAID use. Giant gastric ulcers are slightly more common in males and are usually seen in patients over 65 years of age. Pain is not a prominent complaint, but only about 10% of patients are completely free of pain. Pain may radiate to the chest, periumbilical region, or lower abdomen. Morbidity and mortality rates are high, with hemorrhage being the most common complication. These ulcers are usually benign and can be treated with histamine antagonists or proton pump inhibitors and with antibiotics when there is documented *H. pylori* infection. Patients should be followed carefully with endoscopy to demonstrate healing. Candidiasis of the ulcer crater may delay healing and requires adjunctive antifungal therapy.

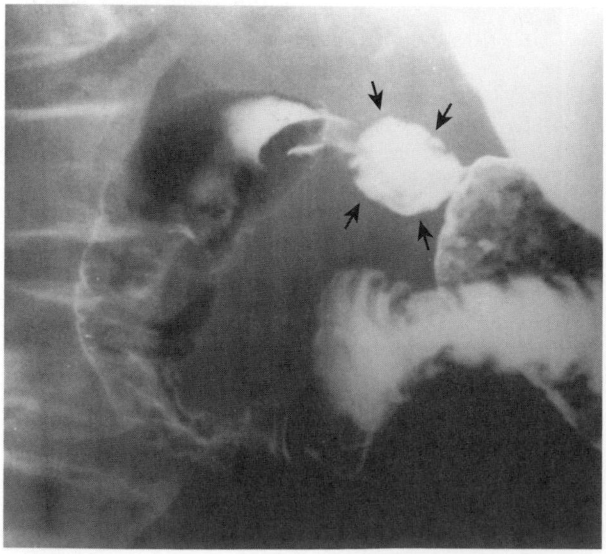

Figure 76-13. Upper gastrointestinal series demonstrates a giant duodenal ulcer resembling the duodenal bulb (*arrows*). *(Reproduced from Brandt LJ. Gastrointestinal disorders of the elderly. Lippincott-Raven, 1986, New York.)*

A number of potential problems must be considered in prescribing acid-suppressive therapy for elderly patients with peptic ulcer disease. Many antacid preparations contain large amounts of mineral salts, which may produce undesirable effects, such as fluid retention, diarrhea, or constipation. Aluminum hydroxide forms insoluble chelates with a number of drugs, including digoxin, quinidine, and tetracycline, interfering with their absorption. Histamine antagonists variably inhibit the oxidative metabolism of many drugs, prolonging their duration of action. Cimetidine impairs the elimination of lidocaine, nifedipine, phenytoin, propranolol, quinidine, theophylline, and warfarin, to mention a few. Ranitidine is a less potent inhibitor of mixed-function oxidases than cimetidine, and alterations in drug metabolism caused by ranitidine are usually not associated with pharmacologic effects. Famotidine has no effect on the oxidative metabolism of drugs. Intravenous administration of cimetidine in elderly patients with impaired renal function may produce mental confusion in a dose-related fashion. Cimetidine may also cause a mild elevation of serum creatinine levels unassociated with impairment of renal function. Ranitidine is a rare cause of hepatitis, and ranitidine and famotidine may cause headache. Sucralfate frequently causes constipation in elderly individuals. The National Institutes of Health Consensus Development Panel has published guidelines mandating antibiotic treatment of all ulcer patients infected with *H. pylori*, including those without an active ulcer crater or dyspeptic symptoms.[109]

Nonulcer dyspepsia

Patients with nonulcer dyspepsia suffer from chronic, recurrent upper abdominal pain and nausea, which may or may not be related to meals and which occurs in the absence of an ulcer crater.[130] Nonulcer dyspepsia is at least twice as common as true peptic ulcer disease. Most patients with this problem have no recognizable pathologic abnormality, although many have histologic gastritis.[107] Nonulcer dyspepsia is further defined by the absence of reflux esophagitis, disease of the biliary tract or pancreas, or most symptoms of irritable bowel syndrome. The criteria used to select patients for inclusion in clinical studies of nonulcer dyspepsia are very inconsistent, perpetuating confusion about this diagnosis among physicians and patients.[131]

The cause of nonulcer dyspepsia is unknown; numerous explanations have been proposed for this syndrome, including psychosocial factors, altered sensation, abnormal gastrointestinal motility and compliance, and *H. pylori* infection.[130,131] Gas washout studies show that individuals with nonulcer dyspepsia do not have increased gas in their digestive tracts, and therefore complaints of bloating are probably explained by sensitivity to normal volumes of gas; in some, the transit of infused gas is abnormal, suggesting a motility disorder. Gastric antral hypomotility and impaired gastric emptying of solids have been observed in 40% to 50% of patients with nonulcer dyspepsia, and treatment with drugs that affect upper gastrointestinal motility relieves symptoms in many patients.[132–134] Thirty to 50% of patients with symptoms of nonulcer dyspepsia have chronic active gastritis, even when the gastric mucosa appears grossly normal at endoscopy. It has been suggested that nonulcer dyspepsia is part of the spectrum of disease caused by *H. pylori*, which includes chronic active gastritis, duodenitis, and peptic ulcer disease. The successive development of nonulcer dyspepsia, duodenitis, and duodenal ulcer disease has been termed Moynihan's disease.[135] *H. pylori* infection, however, has not been shown to be the cause of nonulcer dyspepsia, nor has a definite relationship between nonulcer dyspepsia and peptic ulcer disease been proved.[136]

In practice, therapy for nonulcer dyspepsia is the same as for peptic ulcer disease, despite the fact that in double-blind, placebo-controlled trials, histamine antagonists, and proton pump inhibitors are only a little better than a placebo in treating this disorder, and the role of gastric acid hypersecretion in nonulcer dyspepsia is unproved by formal measurements of basal and peak acid outputs.[137,138] Peptic ulcer disease, NSAID use, *H. pylori* infection, and gastric cancer must be excluded in elderly patients who have dyspeptic complaints.

Upper gastrointestinal bleeding

Thirty-five percent to 45% of all cases of acute upper gastrointestinal hemorrhage occur in patients beyond age 60, and of these, half are caused by peptic ulcer disease.[139–141] Other important causes of gross upper gastrointestinal bleeding in elderly people are gastric erosions and esophagitis; these two entities in combination with peptic ulcer disease account for 70% to 80% of hospital admissions for upper gastrointestinal bleeding in older patients.

It is unclear whether elderly patients with upper gastrointestinal hemorrhage frequently have a long history of underlying acid-peptic disease, for example, chronic peptic ulcer disease, or whether they usually bleed from newly developed lesions. In one series, 36% of older individuals admitted to the hospital with acute upper gastrointestinal bleeding gave no history of preceding symptoms.[139] Alternatively, some patients complain of prior epigastric pain, pain in other parts of the abdomen, anorexia, dyspepsia, pyrosis or, simply, weight loss. Elderly patients with acute upper gastrointestinal bleeding usually have hematemesis, although 30% of patients have only melena.[139] Hemorrhage is often seen in persons with chronic medical illnesses, the most common being degenerative joint disease. Therapy with NSAIDs for rheumatologic and other problems has been found to be an important cause of upper gastrointestinal bleeding in elderly patients.[141,142] Other causes include disease found in younger patients, and entities seen almost exclusively in older individuals. Geriatric ulcers and giant duodenal ulcers are not associated with an unusually high incidence of hemorrhage, whereas giant gastric ulcers frequently do bleed.[129]

Aortoenteric fistula is an uncommon cause of gastrointestinal hemorrhage seen most often in men during the seventh and eighth decades of life. The most common cause is rupture of an arteriosclerotic abdominal aortic aneurysm. Other causes of aortoenteric fistulas include graft-enteric fistula, aortitis, mycotic aneurysm, carcinoma, trauma, foreign body, and peptic ulceration.[143,144] The overwhelming majority of fistulas between the aorta and the alimentary tract occur in the duodenum and, as a result, usually produce upper gastrointestinal bleeding. Other reported sites of communication include the esophagus, stomach, distal small bowel, and colon. Most patients experience an initial self-limited or "sentinel" bleed, followed hours to days later by massive hemorrhage. Mortality rate is very high but may be reduced by early endoscopic detection of the fistula during investigation of the cause of bleeding. An elderly patient with an aortic graft who has upper gastrointestinal bleeding, no matter how trivial, must undergo immediate endoscopy because of the possible presence of a graft-enteric fistula.

Another rare cause of massive upper gastrointestinal hemorrhage in elderly people is a dilated gastric artery with an overlying mucosal defect, typically located within 2 cm of the cardioesophageal junction. This lesion, called exulceratio simplex, or the ulcer of Dieulafoy, often requires surgical therapy, although it has been treated effectively with electrocautery, laser, argon plasma coagulation, and banding.[145,146]

Occasionally, vascular abnormalities of the type found in Osler-Weber-Rendu syndrome (hereditary hemorrhagic telangiectasia) may also be responsible for upper gastrointestinal bleeding in elderly people. There may be no history of childhood epistaxis and no family history of similar occurrences, although typical telangiectatic lesions are often found in the oral cavity, lips, nailbeds, and skin.

The hospital course of elderly patients with upper gastrointestinal bleeding is similar to that of younger patients with respect to duration, amount of blood transfused, and frequency of surgery.[147,148] Older patients, however, suffer significantly more morbidity than do younger patients; complications include cardiac, neurologic, and renal disease; sepsis; and reactions to medications and transfusions. Elderly patients are more likely than young patients to die during a hospital admission for gastrointestinal bleeding, especially if peptic ulcer is the cause.

The evaluation and treatment of upper gastrointestinal bleeding in elderly people are the same as in younger individuals. Age per se is not a contraindication for surgery; the decision to operate on an individual patient must be made in the context of the clinical setting. Early surgery should be contemplated for elderly patients who have bled from ulcers, who have signs of major hemorrhage (e.g., hypotension), and when endoscopic findings imply a significant risk of recurrent bleeding.

Volvulus of the stomach

Volvulus of the stomach is a relatively rare condition occurring most often after age 50 and requires relaxation of the gastric ligaments for its development.[149,150] Gastric volvulus may be responsible for chronic abdominal symptoms or may be manifested acutely with strangulation and gangrene.

Gastric volvulus is classified according to the axis around which the stomach rotates: torsion about a longitudinal axis formed by a line connecting the cardia and pylorus is known as organoaxial volvulus; rotation about a vertical axis passing through the middle of the lesser and greater curvatures is

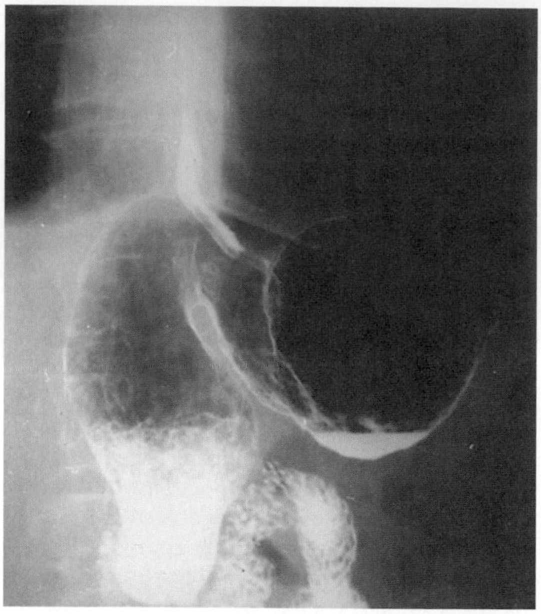

Figure 76-14. An organoaxial volvulus of the stomach identified on upper gastrointestinal series. *(Reproduced from Brandt LJ. Gastrointestinal disorders of the elderly. Lippincott-Raven, 1986, New York.)*

referred to as mesenteroaxial volvulus. Approximately 60% of affected patients have the organoaxial type, 30% have the mesenteroaxial type, and 10% have a combination form. Rotation may be partial or complete; complete twists often severely impair gastric blood flow and may cause gangrene, whereas partial twists may be asymptomatic or responsible for chronic symptoms.

Organoaxial volvulus usually has an acute presentation and often is associated with the presence of a large paraesophageal hiatus hernia or eventration of the diaphragm. Patients complain of the abrupt onset of upper abdominal or lower thoracic pain. Vomiting gives way to retching, and it is difficult to pass a nasogastric tube beyond the gastroesophageal junction. This group of symptoms and signs has been referred to as the Borchardt's triad. Roentgenograms may reveal a gas-filled viscus in the chest or an "upside-down stomach" in the upper abdomen (Figure 76-14). Gangrene ensues in approximately 5% of cases, mostly in individuals with a traumatic diaphragmatic hernia. Organoaxial volvulus usually requires surgical correction.

Mesenteroaxial volvulus is often intermittent and incomplete. Affected persons complain of chronic postprandial pain, belching, bloating, vomiting, and early satiety; strangulation is rare. Diagnosis is made by barium roentgenogram. Decompression with a nasogastric tube may return the stomach to its normal position. Surgery is indicated for persistent symptoms. Some patients have been successfully treated by fixation of the stomach with two percutaneous endoscopic gastrostomy tubes; these are removed after adhesions fix the stomach to the anterior abdominal wall.

Benign gastric tumors

The incidence of benign gastric tumors increases with age. A hyperplastic polyp accounts for 75% to 90% of such growths and typically is a small, solitary lesion at the junction of the gastric body and antrum.[151] Hyperplastic polyps are not considered true neoplasms and are not premalignant. They rarely produce symptoms and thus are found incidentally in an evaluation of the upper gastrointestinal tract. In contrast, adenomatous polyps are true neoplasms and account for 10% to 25% of gastric polyps. The mean incidence of malignant change in gastric adenomas is reported to be anywhere from 6% to 75%, probably reflecting their heterogeneity in size, age, and histology (tubular, villous, or mixed).

Gastric polyps may occur in some gastrointestinal polyposis syndromes, but the only one appearing in older individuals is the Cronkhite-Canada syndrome. This disorder is acquired, not inherited, and is characterized by diffuse gastrointestinal polyposis, protein-losing enteropathy, and ectodermal abnormalities, including hyperpigmentation, alopecia, and dystrophic nail changes. Polyps in this syndrome are hamartomas composed of tubules and mucus-filled cysts.

Mesenchymal tumors, including leiomyomas, fibromas, and tumors of neural origin, account for a significant percentage of benign gastric tumors. Symptoms of these tumors are usually related to their size and not their type. Pain and bleeding are the most common manifestations.

Malignant gastric tumors

GASTRIC ADENOCARCINOMA

Inexplicably, the incidence of gastric cancer is decreasing in elderly people, while relatively more cases are being diagnosed in younger patients.[152] Nevertheless, the vast majority of gastric cancers occur in patients beyond 60 years of age.[1] Carcinoma of the stomach is usually incurable by the time symptoms appear because symptoms often do not develop until the tumor is large. Initial symptoms are often mild and nonspecific. The tendency to treat dyspepsia in older patients without a diagnostic evaluation prompted Sir Heneage Ogilvie to say in the early 1900s, "in carcinoma of the stomach, alkalis are the undertaker's best friend."

Vague epigastric discomfort, anorexia, early satiety, and weight loss are the most frequent symptoms of gastric cancer. Physical examination may reveal enlarged left axillary and supraclavicular lymph nodes, an umbilical nodule, or a hard palpable left hepatic lobe. Rarely, the patient develops acanthosis nigricans, dermatomyositis, or an explosive outbreak of skin tags or keratotic lesions (sign of Leser-Trélat), raising the suspicion of a visceral neoplasm.

Laboratory abnormalities are nonspecific. Surgical excision is the only potentially curative treatment. Seventy percent to 90% of patients with gastric cancer are considered suitable for laparotomy, but only half are found to be eligible for potentially curative resections and death occurs in most of these individuals within 1 year. Five-year survival rates are 5% to 15%. Combined chemotherapy and irradiation may be of some benefit, but irradiation alone is ineffective except for palliation of bone pain from metastases.

GASTRIC LYMPHOMA

The stomach is the most frequent site of primary, extranodal lymphoma and accounts for one half to three fourths of patients with lymphoma of the gastrointestinal tract. Gastric lymphoma produces nonspecific symptoms, but epigastric pain with weight loss and a palpable mass in a

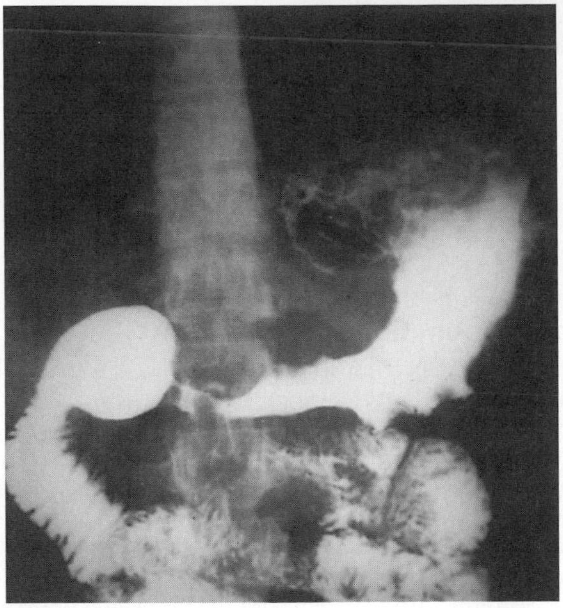

Figure 76-15. Upper gastrointestinal series showing a gastric lymphoma with antral narrowing mimicking an adenocarcinoma. *(Reproduced from Brandt LJ. Gastrointestinal disorders of the elderly. Lippincott-Raven, 1986, New York.)*

patient who is otherwise well is typical. Radiographically, lymphoma resembles carcinoma in up to two thirds of cases (Figure 76-15). Large, ulcerated masses, hyperrugosity, polypoid lesions, or antral narrowing suggests lymphoma. A definitive diagnosis cannot be made from gastroscopic brush cytology and biopsy, and laparotomy may be necessary. Therapy is wide excision followed by radiation and leads to a 5-year survival rate of about 40% to 50%.

SYSTEMIC DISEASES

Diabetes mellitus

Patients with long-standing diabetes mellitus often have profound abnormalities of gastrointestinal motility, including delayed gastric emptying of solids.[153] Such abnormalities are frequently without clinical manifestations, although difficulty controlling plasma glucose, due to an inconstant and unpredictable rate of gastric emptying, may be a subtle indication of gastroparesis. Gastric atony may be manifested by a gradual onset of upper abdominal fullness, satiety, and vomiting. Gastroparesis and accompanying hypochlorhydria probably underlie the development of gastric bezoars and bacterial and fungal overgrowth in this population.

Diabetic gastroparesis is caused by an abnormality of the autonomic nervous system almost always associated with peripheral or autonomic neuropathy. Metoclopramide has been used to improve gastric motility and relieve symptoms but causes intolerable central nervous system effects in many patients.

Amyloidosis

The gastrointestinal tract is involved in 50% to 75% of patients with amyloidosis, and in approximately one half of these cases the stomach is affected. It is unusual for signs and symptoms of gastrointestinal involvement to be directly attributable to the amyloidosis per se. Outlet obstruction may be caused by an obstructing mass of amyloid in the distal stomach. Amyloid may also diffusely infiltrate the gastric wall, making surgery difficult, and may be associated with giant gastric ulcers resistant to medical therapy. Prognosis is related to that of the primary disease.

KEY POINTS

The Upper Gastrointestinal Tract

- Evaluation of the upper gastrointestinal tract should begin with the mouth; changes in the oral cavity, such as candidiasis, stomatitis, leukoplakia, and vascular lesions, may limit the ability of elderly people to enjoy a normal diet.
- Oropharyngeal, or transfer, dysphagia is an important problem in the elderly, caused by uncoordinated muscular contractions that are the result of a wide spectrum of disorders including stroke and Parkinson's disease.
- Dysphagia, or difficulty swallowing, in the elderly should not be ascribed to aging alone and should prompt a search for the presence of disease processes involving the esophagus, such as gastroesophageal reflux disease, esophageal motility disorders, structural abnormalities including rings and webs, and neoplastic disorders.
- Aging is associated with alterations in both the motor and sensory functions of the stomach, but changes in physiology related only to aging rarely account for dyspeptic symptoms.
- Peptic ulcer disease in the elderly is very common, largely due to the frequent use of NSAIDs for arthritis and pain, and often is associated with severe complications including bleeding and perforation.

For a complete list of references, please visit online only at www.expertconsult.com

CHAPTER 77

The Pancreas

Ceri Beaton
Malcolm C. A. Puntis

BACKGROUND

The pancreas is a retroperitoneal organ located deep to the stomach and has both endocrine and exocrine functions. Some knowledge of its development and structure is necessary as a foundation on which to base an understanding of the diseases that affect it and its changes with age.

Development of the Pancreas

The pancreas begins to develop at day 26 as dorsal and ventral endodermal buds arising from their respective aspects of the primitive tubular foregut. The ventral bud arises together with the embryonic bile duct, and it then migrates posteriorly around the duodenum. Late in the sixth week, the two pancreatic buds fuse to form the definitive pancreas (Figure 77-1). The dorsal pancreatic bud gives rise to part of the head, the body, and the tail of the pancreas, whereas the ventral pancreatic bud gives rise to the uncinate process and the remainder of the head. The two ductal systems fuse, and the proximal end of the dorsal bud duct usually degenerates leaving the ventral pancreatic duct as the main duct opening at the ampulla. The opening of the dorsal duct, if it persists, forms the accessory duct. The pancreatic endoderm of each bud develops into an epithelial tree that will form the duct system draining the exocrine products manufactured in the acini. Endocrine cells arises separately from the ducts and aggregate into the islets.[1]

A failure of migration or fusion of the early pancreatic buds can result in pancreas divisum (this occurs in about 7% of people); alternatively, the pancreas can surround the duodenum resulting in an annular pancreas. Abnormal development of the ventral duct can result in a common channel whereby the junction of the biliary and pancreatic ducts is outside the wall of the duodenum allowing reflux and mixing of bile and pancreatic juice; this can result in damage to the bile duct in the fetus resulting in a choledochal cyst or damage to the pancreas causing acute pancreatitis.

Anatomic Relationships

The adult pancreas is a retroperitoneal structure 12 to 15 cm long extending from the duodenum to the hilum of the spleen. The neck of the pancreas lies anterior to the superior mesenteric vein and the uncinate process curls around the vein to lie on its right and the posterior border. Posterior to the head and uncinate process is the inferior vena cava. The splenic artery and vein pass deep to the upper border of the pancreas and provide much of its vascular supply. The right-hand border of the head is closely applied to the concavity of the duodenum, and its superior part is related to the portal vein.

Histology

The pancreas has a lobulated structure and there are intralobular ducts penetrating the secretory acini, which are flask-shaped structures consisting of typical zymogenic cells. The larger interlobular ducts contain some nonstriated smooth muscle.

The million or so islets of Langerhans are distributed throughout the adult pancreas and consist of endocrine cells. The alpha cells constitute 15% to 20% of the islet cells and produce glucagon. The insulin-secreting beta cells constitute about 65% to 80%; delta cells (3% to 10%) produce somatostatin. The PP cells (3% to 5%) produce pancreatic polypeptide, and the epsilon cells (<1%) produce ghrelin.

Exocrine function

The pancreas secretes 1400 mL per day of an alkaline, bicarbonate-rich solution containing proenzymes that are converted into active enzymes (proteases, lipases, and glycosidases such as amylase). In the gut, a proenzyme, like trypsinogen, is converted into trypsin by enterokinases; trypsin then, in turn, releases more trypsin from trypsinogen.

Enzyme secretion is stimulated by cholecystokinin released by the duodenum in response to the presence of food. Secretin, also released from the gut wall, controls the secretion of water and electrolytes, most of which is secreted from the ducts of the pancreas.[2]

Pancreatic exocrine function deteriorates with age; the secretion of bicarbonate and enzymes have been found to be reduced in a group of subjects with average age 72 years compared with a group with average age 36 years.[3] However, 80% to 90% of pancreatic function must be lost before malabsorption becomes apparent, and this happens only occasionally in the elderly where other causes of malabsorption are more common.[4]

Endocrine function

Synthesis and release of insulin from the beta cells of the pancreas is controlled by the level of glucose in the beta cells, which will reflect the plasma level. However, overall control of pancreatic function is the result of many complex interrelated feedback loops. Somatostatin, for example, secreted from the delta cells in response to an increasing blood sugar level, inhibits enzyme release and decreases gut motility. The full complexity of the hormonal control of glucose in the body is as yet not fully elucidated; however, it is clear that there are some functional changes with age.[5]

Age changes

Besides the age-related changes in pancreatic function, there are morphologic changes; after the age of 60 the pancreas shrinks and can become more fatty.[6] Patchy fibrosis can also occur in the pancreas from the seventh decade onward, but without the other changes of chronic pancreatitis this age-related focal lobular fibrosis is associated with ductal papillary hyperplasia, which can be premalignant.[7]

TUMORS OF THE PANCREAS

Adenocarcinoma is the most common pancreatic tumor, accounting for 90% of all tumors in the pancreas; it is a malignant tumor with a poor prognosis. Many of the remaining 10% are cystic, often with a more benign behavior but malignant change cannot be ruled out. Truly benign tumors such as fibromas, lipomas, and hemangiomas do occur but are exceedingly rare.

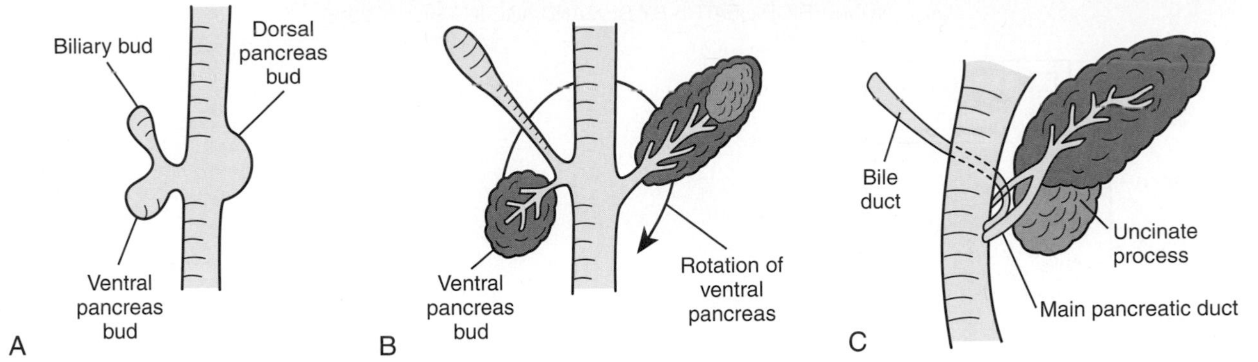

Figure 77-1. Embryology of the pancreas. A, The two pancreatic buds form at 26 days of development. B, Rotation of the ventral pancreas. C, At 45 days, the final position is reached and the ventral and dorsal pancreases have fused.

CYSTIC TUMORS

These tumors are often an incidental finding on imaging, but once they have been detected, determining the exact nature of a cystic lesion in the pancreas is difficult in spite of modern computed tomography (CT), magnetic resonance imaging (MRI), and ultrasound (US) by both transcutaneous and endoscopic techniques. It is often difficult to distinguish an inflammatory lesion from a neoplasm.[8,9] Biopsy is often difficult or inconclusive, and the general advice is to err on the side of resection.[10] Although these tumors tend to occur more commonly in the young or middle aged, they also occur up to the seventh and eighth decades and they are more likely to be malignant in patients older than 70 years, when resection should be considered.[11]

Solid-pseudopapillary neoplasm

These occur most commonly in young women and are generally benign but can undergo malignant change. They should be treated by resection, which results in an excellent prognosis.[12]

Serous cystadenoma

This is sometimes known as a serous microcystic tumor. The mean age of presentation is in the sixth decade, and 70% occur in females. The vast majority are benign; only a handful of cases of malignant serous cystic tumor of the pancreas have been reported.[13]

Mucinous cystic neoplasm

This neoplasm accounts for 50% of cystic tumors and is either malignant or potentially so. It is most common in middle-aged women and it should be treated by resection of the affected part of the pancreas.[14]

Intraductal papillary mucinous neoplasm (IPMN)

This tumor is twice as common in males as in females and has a mean age at presentation in the seventh decade. It is characterized by copious mucous draining at a patulous ampulla from a dilated duct. It has a favorable prognosis following appropriate resection.[15,16]

Lymphoepithelial cyst of the pancreas

This is a rare epithelium-lined cystic lesion similar histologically to a branchial cyst.[17]

Cystic islet cell tumors

This tumor results from cystic degeneration of a solid endocrine tumor. Although it is rare, it is important to consider this diagnosis when evaluating a cystic lesion in the pancreas and test for endocrine activity in order to exclude a functioning tumor, although the majority of these tumors are in fact nonfunctioning.

Von Hippel–Lindau syndrome

This is rare genetic condition with autosomal dominant inheritance. Several types of pancreatic tumor can occur in this condition including serous cystadenoma, multiple cysts, and endocrine tumors.[18]

SOLID TUMORS

Adenocarcinoma

EPIDEMIOLOGY AND AGE INCIDENCE

Pancreatic cancer is the sixth most common cause of cancer death in the United Kingdom and the fourth most common in the United States. In 2005, the number of deaths from pancreatic cancer in the United Kingdom was 7238, with a rate of 12.1 per 100,000 population; for the United States in 2004, the death rate was 9.24 per 100,000 population.[19,20]

The incidence of pancreatic cancer in the United Kingdom increases sharply with age and the average age at presentation is 69 years.[19,21] (See Figure 77-2.)

Pancreatic ductal adenocarcinoma has the lowest 5-year survival rate for all cancers for both men and women at 2% in the United Kingdom and 5% in the United States. The mortality rate is 94% of the incidence rate.[20,22] The mortality rate for pancreatic cancer remained static across most of the world from 1992 to 2002.[23]

Risk factors for pancreatic adenocarcinoma include chronic pancreatitis, diabetes mellitus, smoking, possible relation to increased body mass index (BMI), and genetic (BRCA2, Peutz-Jeghers, von Hippel-Lindau and hereditary nonpolyposis colorectal cancer).[24,25]

PRESENTATION

Approximately 85% of patients present with disseminated or locally advanced disease, and symptoms frequently include epigastric or back pain, anorexia, weight loss, and obstructive jaundice.[26]

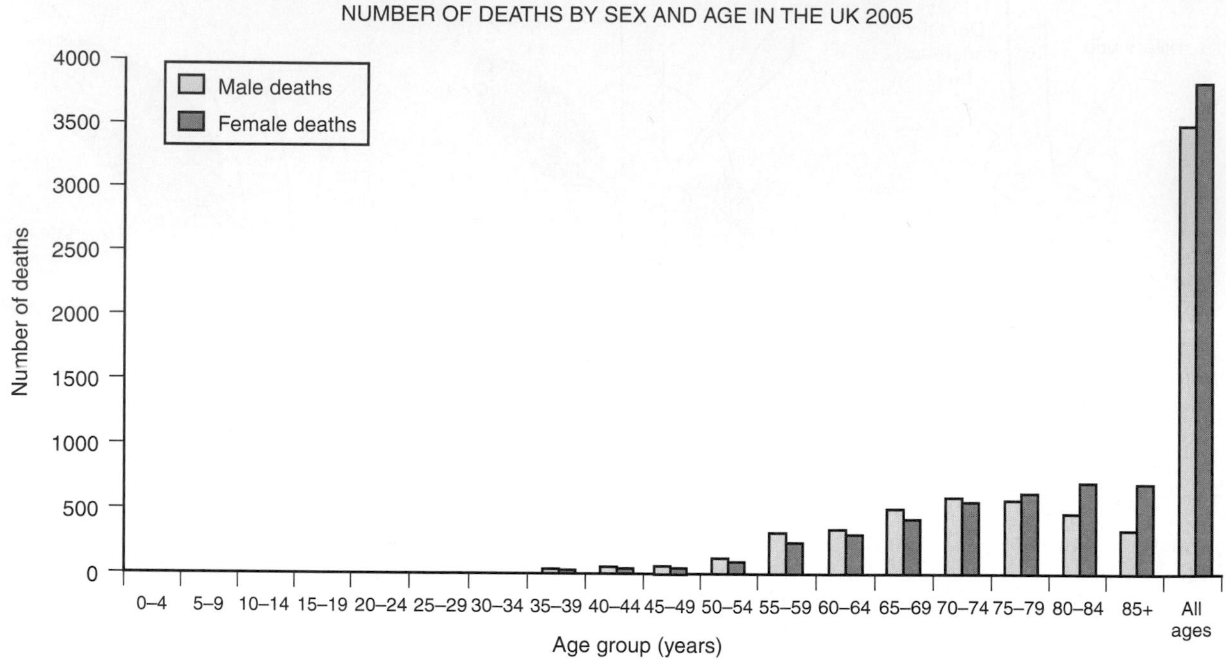

Figure 77-2. Death rate from pancreatic cancer in the United Kingdom in 2005. *(Derived from Cancer Research UK 2008 data.)*

PAIN Pain can be caused by tumor compression of surrounding structures, tumor size, invasion of pancreatic nerves, and invasion of the anterior pancreatic capsule. Pain intensity at presentation has been found to correlate with survival (29 months for patients without pain, 9 months for those with severe pain).[27] Back pain may predict unresectability and shortened survival after resection.[28]

WEIGHT LOSS Weight loss is a common presenting symptom and can be due to anorexia, catabolic metabolism, or malabsorption; however, weight loss is also a common symptom in the elderly and can be nonspecific.

JAUNDICE Sixty percent to 70% of pancreatic adenocarcinomata affect the head of the pancreas, and these patients often present with obstructive jaundice resulting from compression of the biliary tract.[21]

OTHER Tumors of the body and tail of the pancreas are frequently associated with late presentation and inoperability. When an older patient presents with a new diagnosis of diabetes mellitus, then the presence of an underlying pancreatic cancer should be borne in mind especially if the patient has other suggestive symptoms. Tumor has been found to be the underlying cause in 1% of patients over 50 years old diagnosed with diabetes.[29] Other presentations may include acute pancreatitis and acute upper gastrointestinal or retroperitoneal hemorrhage.[21]

DIAGNOSIS

The investigations performed in suspected pancreatic cancer are undertaken with the following aims:

- Establishing the diagnosis
- Locating the tumor
- Staging the tumor
- Assessing resectability
- Obtaining a tissue diagnosis

Blood Tests

SERUM ANTIGENS

Carbohydrate antigen 19-9 (CA 19-9) is a glycoprotein synthesized by pancreatic cancer cells as well as being produced by normal epithelial cells of the pancreas, bile ducts, stomach, and colon.[30] It has been found to have a sensitivity of 70% to 90% and specificity of 75% to 90% for pancreatic cancer, but it is also elevated in obstructive jaundice, chronic pancreatitis, and biliary and gastrointestinal cancers.[30,31] Other tumor markers such as carcinoembryonic antigen (CEA) and carbohydrate antigen 125 (CA 125) have limited use because of lower sensitivity and specificity.[31] Although tumor markers cannot actually confirm a diagnosis, they are particularly useful later in the patient's management when a rise in CA19-9, especially if it originally decreased after treatment, may indicate a recurrence. It is of no use as a screening test.[32]

Imaging

TRANSABDOMINAL ULTRASOUND

Transabdominal ultrasound (US) is frequently the first-line imaging investigation performed in the elderly patient presenting with upper abdominal symptoms. The results are variable and dependent on the operator, the patient's body habitus, and the presence of overlying gas-filled bowel loops. The sensitivity of diagnosing pancreatic cancer with ultrasound ranges from 44% to 95%,[30,33,34] with the very high sensitivities in groups where patients were not scanned on an intention to treat basis and difficult scans were excluded from the analysis.

COMPUTED TOMOGRAPHY

Computed tomography (CT) is considered the imaging modality of choice in pancreatic cancer as it can give additional staging information by imaging the chest, abdomen, and pelvis, and more detailed information regarding the resectability of pancreatic tumors. Helical CT has been found to be effective in detecting and staging adenocarcinoma, with sensitivity of up to 97% for detection and up to 100% accuracy in predicting unresectability, although it is not as good at predicting resectability.[35] When directly compared with endoscopic ultrasound (EUS) and MRI in a cohort of patients deemed fit for surgery, CT had the highest accuracy in assessing the extent of the primary tumor (73%), locoregional extension (74%), vascular invasion (83%), and tumor resectability (83%).[36] Multidetector CT used with an appropriate protocol for timing the injection of contrast agent can provide images in both venous and arterial phases, and the data can then be reformatted in transverse, coronal, and sagittal planes allowing for improved precision in assessing any vascular involvement.[21] The value of CT in predicting resectability, however, can be as low as 38%, with patients predicted to have resectable disease on CT found to be unresectable at laparotomy, with the most common causes of unresectability including small peritoneal or liver metastases and vascular involvement of the tumor.[35] The contrast material used for CT is potentially nephrotoxic, and patients must be well hydrated and serum creatinine checked; this may be a problem in the elderly, in whom renal impairment is more common.

MAGNETIC RESONANCE IMAGING

MRI has the advantage of demonstrating the anatomy of the biliary tree better than CT, but in comparison to multidetector CT, MRI is not thought to offer any diagnostic advantage with respect to the pancreas.[37] Magnetic resonance cholangiopancreatography (MRCP) has been shown to be as diagnostically effective as endoscopic retrograde cholangiopancreatography (ERCP) in patients with symptoms suggestive of pancreatic cancer (84% sensitivity and 97% specificity).[38] MRCP has the added advantage of fewer complications, compared with ERCP, although a number of elderly patients are unable to tolerate the confined space in an MRI scanner.

ENDOSCOPIC RETROGRADE CHOLANGIOPANCREATOGRAPHY

In the diagnosis of cancer of the pancreas, ERCP has a sensitivity and specificity of 70% and 94%[38] and offers the opportunity to obtain a cytologic diagnosis by sampling bile or taking brushings. The value of such sampling can be questionable, however, as a sensitivity of only 60% has been reported with a specificity of 98%.[39] ERCP carries a significant rate for serious complication such as pancreatitis, cholangitis, hemorrhage, and death.

ENDOSCOPIC ULTRASOUND

Endoscopic ultrasound (EUS) is rapidly growing in importance. The high-frequency ultrasound probe positioned in the stomach and duodenum allows high-resolution imaging of the pancreas and surrounding tissue. The accuracy of EUS in evaluating tumor and nodal status was found to be 69% and 54%, respectively,[40] and EUS has been found to be at least as valuable as CT[41] and equal if not superior to CT in evaluating vascular invasion.[42] EUS also offers the opportunity of performing fine needle aspiration of the tumor to aid diagnosis, but in potentially resectable patients this should generally only be performed via the duodenum rather than the stomach as the duodenum will be removed during resection and there have been concerns regarding seeding malignant cells in the needle track.

POSITRON EMISSION TOMOGRAPHY

Positron emission tomography (PET) exploits the increased glucose metabolism observed in malignant tumors by administering a radioactive glucose analogue and scanning for increased uptake by tumor cells. PET images may be captured with coincident CT images to aid in localizing any accumulation of tracer. There is still uncertainty about the ability of PET scans to distinguish between inflammatory and malignant lesions.[43] PET is useful in diagnosing small (<2 cm) tumors and has sensitivity and specificity as good as EUS, ERCP, and US and is particularly useful in detecting distant metastasis—for example, cervical nodes.[44]

Management

RESECTABLE DISEASE

The only curative treatment for pancreatic cancer is surgical resection; however, only 15% of patients presenting with pancreatic cancer are considered to be resectable.[26] Preoperative imaging is useful for determining clearly inoperable tumors, but at operation a further proportion will be found to be inoperable because of local or distant involvement of other tissue.

To be considered as resectable on imaging, there should be no involvement of the superior mesenteric artery or celiac axis, a patent superior mesenteric vein (SMV) and portal venous confluence and no evidence of distant metastasis. At the time of surgery, findings including previously unidentified metastasis or a tumor that cannot be dissected of the SMV would preclude progression to resection.

Surgical options for resecting cancer of the head of the pancreas include the traditional Whipple pancreaticoduodenectomy or a pylorus-preserving pancreaticoduodenectomy (PPPD). PPPD involves dividing the bile duct close to the liver hilum, dividing the duodenum 2 cm beyond the pylorus, dissecting the pancreas off the superior mesenteric vein, and dividing the pancreas between the head and neck and dividing the small bowel at the duodenal-jejunal flexure. The reconstruction then involves three anastomosis: restoring gut continuity by a pylorus-jejunal anastomosis, connecting the stump of the bile duct to the jejunum just distal to the pylorus-jejunal anastomosis, and finally a pancreatic anastomosis. This last anastomosis is the Achilles' heel of the operation and there is much debate about the technique.[45] The authors prefer a pancreaticogastric anastomosis rather than the alternative pancreaticojejunal anastomosis. Most surgeons use the technique that in their hands gives them good results; however, the published leakage rate is up to 10% in some series.[46]

The Whipple procedure differs in that a distal gastrectomy is also performed, although it would be expected to cause possible long-term morbidity because of gastric dumping, marginal ulceration, and bile reflux gastritis when compared to the PPPD. There have been questions regarding adequacy of resection in a PPPD, but a Cochrane review in 2008 has demonstrated no significant difference between a Whipple and PPPD in terms of in-hospital mortality, overall survival, and morbidity rates.[47]

The overall complication rate for PPPD is around 39% with a mortality rate ranging from 0 to 7%.[47–49] Early complications including postoperative bleeding and bile leak are quoted at rates of 4.8% and 1.2%, respectively, in a meta-analysis.[47] Other significant early complications that are of particular importance in the elderly because of preexisting comorbidities include cardiac and respiratory complications, and the elderly have been shown to be treated for significantly more cardiac events following PPPD (13% versus 0.5%).[50] The overall mortality for pancreatic cancer resections in octogenarians is over twice that for younger patients (15.5% vs. 6.7%).[51] Late complications related to the nature of the operation include delayed gastric emptying, which occurs in 21% of PPPD patients, and pancreatic fistula in 11%.[49] Pancreatic endocrine function is generally maintained,[52] and pancreatic exocrine function should be assessed by measuring fecal elastase, as malabsorption will result in malnutrition postoperatively.[53]

Surgery for cancer of the body and tail of the pancreas is less frequently performed, as patients usually have only nonspecific symptoms and a diagnosis is often only made when the tumor is inoperable. However, when a distal pancreatectomy is possible, it involves dissecting the pancreas off the SMV, dividing the pancreas, and then oversewing the cut end. A splenectomy is also performed in cancer operations to ensure as much clearance as possible.

The question of the appropriateness of performing surgery of such magnitude in an elderly patient is an important one. The patient should be evaluated on an individual basis with regard to comorbidities and fitness for anesthetic, possibly using assessments such as Physiological and Operative Severity Score for the enUmeration of Mortality and Morbidity (POSSUM), a multifactorial scoring system[54] and cardiopulmonary exercise testing (CPX) (which defines the physiologic stress level at which the patient becomes anaerobic).[55] Patients must be made fully aware that their short-term function, and nutritional condition may be compromised after a major pancreatic resection.[50]

It has been demonstrated that patients older than 75 years of age, when compared with patients younger than 75 years of age, undergoing pancreatic surgery for cancer have increased mortality rates (10% compared with 7%), are more frequently admitted to the intensive care unit unplanned (47% compared with 20%), are treated for more cardiac events (13% compared with 0.5%), are more likely to have a compromised nutritional and feeding status, and are more likely to be transferred for further nursing care before the discharge home.[50] The operative mortality rate for pancreatic cancer surgery has been shown to increase with advancing age: 7% at 65 to 69 years, 9% at 70 to 79 years, and 16% at 80+ years.[51] However, when looking at significant predictors of survival, some studies have not found age to be an independent variable.[56,57]

UNRESECTABLE DISEASE For patients with unresectable disease, the three most important symptoms for palliation are pain, jaundice, and gastric outlet obstruction. A multidisciplinary team consisting of representatives from surgery, medical oncology, gastroenterology, radiology, and palliative care medicine is essential for the optimal palliation of symptoms.[58]

PAIN

The World Health Organization approach to pain management in patients with advanced cancer is still recommended,[59] and analgesics should be titrated according to the three-step analgesic ladder: (1) nonopioids, including nonsteroidal anti-inflammatory agents, (2) weak opioids, and (3) strong opioids. Attention should be paid to the route of administration in pancreatic cancer patients, as gastric outlet obstruction may be present and absorption of oral analgesics may be unpredictable.

In patients with severe pain, a celiac plexus block (CPB) with neurolytic solutions may provide analgesia by interrupting visceral afferent pain transmission from the upper abdomen. This can be performed percutaneously, surgically (at the time of laparotomy or bypass), or under EUS guidance. In a prospective, randomized, double-blinded, placebo-controlled trial percutaneous CPB with absolute alcohol has been shown to significantly improve pain relief in patients with unresectable pancreatic cancer, compared with opioids although CPB did not affect quality of life or survival.[60] The major complications from percutaneous CPB include lower extremity weakness, paresthesia, lumbar puncture, and pneumothorax, and they have been quoted at a rate of 1%. The technique of EUS-guided CPB has therefore developed in popularity recently and has been found to be safe and effective in pancreatic cancer.[61,62]

JAUNDICE

Jaundice can have severe consequences, including intolerable itching, liver dysfunction, and eventually hepatic failure caused by bile stasis and cholangitis;[63] relief of the jaundice has been shown to result in a dramatic increase in quality of life.[64] Biliary drainage can be achieved by endoscopic or percutaneous placement of a biliary stent or by a surgical biliary-enteric anastomosis. Biliary stents are plastic (Teflon and polyethylene) or made of an expandable metal meshwork. Plastic stents are associated with a higher complication rate including migration, blockage, and infection, although they can be replaced and are cheaper, whereas metal stents have a significantly longer time to first blockage but cannot be removed and are not recommended for patients with a prognosis greater than 2 years because of metal fatigue.[63,65]

Percutaneous stenting is often performed if endoscopic stent placement was difficult or impossible in patients with hilar obstruction, bilateral or multiple strictures, or previous upper gastrointestinal tract surgery. In the case of metal percutaneous stenting, it provides good palliation with a procedure-related morbidity rate of 9%.[66] The choice of an endoscopic or percutaneous approach may depend on local expertise.

A Cochrane review of palliative biliary stents for obstructing pancreatic carcinoma concluded that based on meta-analysis, endoscopic stenting with plastic stents appears to be associated with a reduced risk of complications but with a higher risk of recurrent biliary obstruction before death when compared with surgery. No trials comparing endoscopic metal stents to surgery were identified.[67]

GASTRIC OUTLET OBSTRUCTION

A number of patients with unresectable pancreatic cancer will develop functional or mechanical gastric outlet obstruction (GOO); this can be caused by a dysfunction of gastric or duodenal motility as a result of celiac nerve plexus infiltration by tumor or duodenal blockage caused by tumor infiltration of the wall and lumen. These cases should be fully assessed radiologically with a video contrast meal to assess both motility and the existence of tumor blockage before planning management. For mechanical blockage, surgical gastrojejunostomy can be performed either laparoscopically or at open operation. It should, however, be performed at the time of laparotomy if the intended resection of a pancreatic cancer is found to be not possible and it may be combined with a biliary bypass. This method of preempting GOO was studied by comparing two groups that underwent either single bypass (hepaticojejunostomy) or double bypass (hepaticojejunostomy and retrocolic gastrojejunostomy) and researchers found that there was a significantly higher incidence of GOO in the single bypass group (41% as compared to 5%) with no significant difference in length of stay, survival, or quality of life.[68]

It is, however, pointless to trying to drain a stomach that is paralyzed. Pharmacologic agents such as metoclopramide or erythromycin may occasionally be helpful in this situation.

Endoscopic palliation with a self-expanding metal duodenal stent is an option in GOO. It has been found to be simple and effective with no complications related to the insertion or the stent, and a 93% reported improvement in symptoms.[69] Subsequent stent obstruction was observed, however, in 11% of patients.

CHEMORADIOTHERAPY Chemotherapy with or without radiotherapy can be used as an adjuvant treatment in patients following attempted curative resection for pancreatic cancer or as a primary treatment in advanced or metastatic pancreatic cancer. The decision to recommend chemotherapy or chemoradiotherapy for an elderly patient with pancreatic cancer should be made after careful evaluation of the patient's health status, comorbidities, and quality of life, and consideration that physiologic decline and alterations in pharmacodynamics may make the older patient more susceptible to cytotoxic medication.[70]

The role of adjuvant chemotherapy following curative resection for carcinoma of the pancreas still remains controversial. A recently published meta-analysis of randomized controlled trials estimated a prolongation of median survival time of 3 months for patients in the chemotherapy group, but there was no difference in the 5-year survival.[71] A randomized controlled trial specifically looking at the impact of gemcitabine in patients following gross complete resection of pancreatic cancer demonstrated an improved disease-free survival of 7.5 months with no difference in overall survival or quality of life.[72]

A Cochrane review evaluated various chemotherapeutic regimens used in advanced inoperable pancreatic cancer and concluded that chemotherapy (5-fluorouracil [5-FU] combination regimens), when compared with best supportive care, resulted in improved mortality at 1 year.[73] There was no significant difference in outcomes when chemotherapeutic regimens (mostly including 5-FU and gemcitabine) were compared with each other, although current trends seem to favor gemcitabine as it is clinically more acceptable.[73] The evidence for the use of chemoradiotherapy was less convincing, and the authors suggest that although there may be benefit from using chemoradiotherapy over supportive care or radiotherapy alone, the potentially greater toxicity needs further review.[73]

The evidence for chemo- and chemoradiotherapy specifically in an elderly population with advanced pancreatic cancer is limited to retrospective evaluations of patients who had been considered suitable for therapy. Chemotherapy with gemcitabine-based regimens was found to be as acceptable in patients over 70 as in those under 70 with no difference in overall survival, but more elderly patients required dose reduction and experienced increased toxicity.[74] Chemoradiotherapy (5-FU and radiotherapy) was also found to be acceptable in the over-70s, with no difference in toxicity and an actual increase in median survival for elderly patients (11.3 months versus. 9.5 months).

NEUROENDOCRINE TUMORS

Pancreatic neuroendocrine tumors (pNET) are rare with an incidence of 1 to 2 per 1 million population.[75] They have a median age of presentation of 57 years.[76] pNETs are a heterogeneous group of tumors that can be classified according to functionality, tumor localization, rate of proliferation, and metastatic disease.[77] The World Health Organization (WHO) classification defines three types of pNET: well-differentiated neuroendocrine tumor (WDT), well-differentiated neuroendocrine carcinoma (WD-Ca), and poorly differentiated neuroendocrine carcinoma (PD-Ca).[76] This classification is useful in estimating prognosis with 5-year survival rates quoted as WDT, 95%; WD-Ca, 44%; and PD-Ca, 0%.[76]

Management is controversial involving surgery, chemotherapy, octreotide therapy, interferon-α, and peptide receptor radionuclide therapy. The main goal of surgery is curative resection of tumor, but other indications include relief of symptoms from hormone-secreting tumors or obstruction.[77]

ACUTE PANCREATITIS

Acute pancreatitis is an acute inflammatory process of the pancreas with variable involvement of the other regional tissues or remote organs.[78] It is a potentially fatal disease, and the incidence in the United Kingdom is increasing although the mortality has decreased. The incidence and mortality increase with age.[79] (See Figure 77-3.)

Etiology

Acute pancreatitis has multiple causes. Gallstone disease (44% to 54%) and alcohol (3% to 19%) are the predominant causes in the United Kingdom, although in the elderly population gallstones is the most common cause.[79] Drugs are responsible for a small proportion (about 5%) of cases of acute pancreatitis, and as the elderly are more likely to

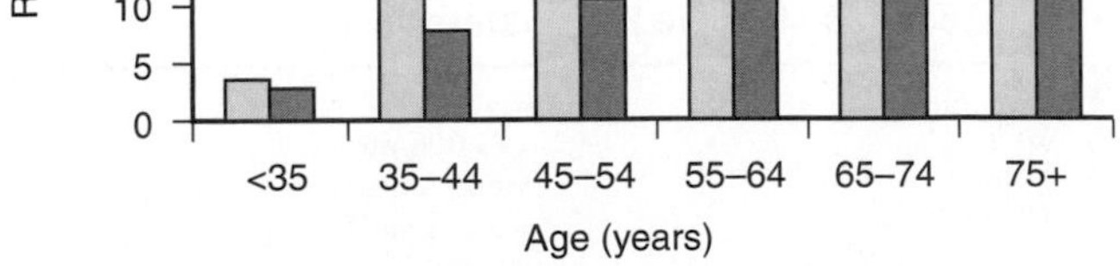

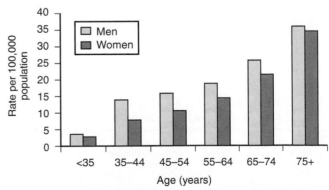

Figure 77-3. Rate of acute pancreatitis by age group in the United Kingdom, 1987–1998. *(Data derived from Goldacre MJ, Roberts SE. Hospital admission for acute pancreatitis in an English population, 1963–98: database study of incidence and mortality. BMJ 2008;328:1466–9.)*

be prescribed medications such as furosemide, nonsteroidal anti-inflammatory drugs, steroids, some antibiotics, and cancer drugs, this should be considered as a possible etiologic factor. Other causes include hypertriglyceridemia, hyperparathyroidism, trauma, and infection. There is accumulating evidence that the underlying cause of acute pancreatitis is premature intracellular activation of trypsin.[80]

Presentation

Abdominal pain and vomiting are the most common presenting symptoms of acute pancreatitis, and an elevation of plasma amylase (to four times normal) will often confirm the diagnosis. The serum amylase level peaks early and then declines over 3 to 4 days; in a patient presenting late, this peak may be missed. A raised serum lipase is more specific for pancreatitis and persists for slightly longer. The amylase level may be increased for other reasons, such as acute gastrointestinal ischemia, gastrointestinal perforation, or a leaking abdominal aortic aneurysm; it should be noted that these conditions are also more common in the elderly.[81]

Assessment

Immediate assessment should include clinical evaluation, blood tests (including complete blood count; liver, bone, and renal profiles; blood glucose), a chest x-ray, and any other tests necessary because of comorbidities present in an elderly patient. It is important to determine the severity of an attack of acute pancreatitis in order to help predict outcome and manage the patient in a suitable setting; care in a high-dependency unit is recommended for patients with severe acute pancreatitis.[82] There are several methods for assessing severity: Ranson[83] and Imrie or Glasgow[84] are specific acute pancreatitis scoring systems based an a range of factors; a score of 3 or more predicts a severe attack (Table 77-1). APACHE II is based on an assessment of Acute Physiology and Chronic Health. It is more complicated to calculate than Imrie or Ranson scores but can give an accurate initial prediction of severity; a score greater than 8 predicts a severe attack.[82] Additionally, it may be used repeatedly to assess the progress of a patient.[85] Trypsinogen activation peptide (TAP)[86] and C-reactive peptide (CRP).[87] are based on the assay of a single marker and are useful adjuncts to assessing severity. The British Society of Gastroenterology (BSG) guidelines recommend that APACHE II is performed on admission and the Glasgow score be calculated at 48 hours.[82]

Abdominal ultrasound is useful in acute pancreatitis to confirm the presence of gallstones or bile duct dilatation. Gas-filled loops of bowel overlying the pancreas will often diminish the value of these images; contrast-enhanced ultrasound may, however, be more helpful.[88] Early CT is occasionally indicated for diagnosis if clinical or biochemical findings are inconclusive and alternative diagnoses need to be excluded. Abdominal contrast-enhanced CT is most useful in acute pancreatitis between 6 and 10 days after admission to look for pancreatic necrosis in patients with persisting organ failure, signs of sepsis, or clinical deterioration.[82]

Table 77-1. The Glasgow Scoring System Includes a Point for Each of These Parameters

Albumin	< 32 g/l
WCC	>15,000/mm³
LDH	> 600 units/L
AST/ALT	> 200 units/L
Glucose	10 mmol/L
Calcium	< 2 mmol/L
Urea	> 16 mmol/L
Po_2	<8 KPa

Management

Approximately 75% of acute pancreatitis is *mild* and is usually self-limiting, requiring simple supportive management.[89] *Severe* acute pancreatitis, however, can produce a systemic inflammatory response syndrome (SIRS) and subsequent multiorgan dysfunction syndrome (MODS). The principles of management in severe acute pancreatitis (SAP) are, therefore, to support each organ system and establish appropriate monitoring to detect deterioration or the onset of complications, which may need some form of intervention. Elderly or obese patients should also be managed in a high-dependency unit.[90]

RENAL

Adequate and timely intravenous fluid (IV) replacement lowers the risk of developing renal insufficiency and failure. Rapid or aggressive fluid resuscitation can be difficult in the elderly patient who may well have underlying cardiac or respiratory compromise.[91] Hemofiltration or hemodialysis can be necessary if renal failure develops.

RESPIRATORY

Respiratory failure is the most frequently encountered single organ malfunction in SAP, and all patients should receive oxygen therapy and monitoring with oxygen saturation, arterial blood gas sampling, clinical evaluation, and radiologic investigation. Intervention with positive pressure ventilation may be required, and in severe cases high-frequency ventilation may be indicated.

CARDIAC

Cardiac failure is more commonly seen in those with preexisting cardiac problems including hypertension, myocardial infarction, and atrial fibrillation and is therefore more common in elderly patients. Inotropic support is often needed in these patients.

GUT

Gut anoxia and the inflammatory syndrome can result in intestinal barrier failure and subsequent bacterial translocation, which has been suggested as a factor in the development of infected pancreatic necrosis. Enteral nutrition is recommended by the BSG guidelines (2005) as it may help preserve gut mucosal barrier function.[82] Enteral feeding may be nasojejunal or, if the stomach is emptying, nasogastric. If the stomach is, however, not draining, nasogastric aspiration should be used to manage the gastric stasis.[92]

GENERAL

The inflammatory response alters capillary permeability and results in edema and hypovolemia.[93] As already mentioned, aggressive IV fluid replacement should be initiated in the patient with SAP,[94] and cardiovascular response should be monitored with, for example, central venous pressure measurement, Swan-Ganz catheter or the pulse contour computer (PiCCO),[95] and urinary output measurement. There is no consensus as to whether prophylactic antibiotics should be administered.[96]

The elderly patient is more likely to have pre-existing organ dysfunction and so the capacity to tolerate an insult such as SAP is limited; this is reflected by the higher incidence in development of organ failure in the elderly (64% compared with 48%).[97]

MANAGEMENT OF PANCREATIC NECROSIS

Nonperfusion of the pancreas on contrast-enhanced CT implies pancreatic necrosis and indicates a poor prognosis.[98] The Atlanta Classification provided a definition of necrosis, but it has not been strictly adhered to and a more recent classification has been suggested.[78,99] It is important to determine if the necrosis is infected, as sterile necrosis can be left to resolve.[100] Infection may be confirmed by CT-guided needle aspiration. Untreated, infected necrosis is almost always fatal and the necrosis must be débrided and drained at open operation or by a minimally invasive technique.[89,90]

MANAGEMENT OF FLUID COLLECTIONS

Fluid collection can occur within or adjacent to the inflamed pancreas (i.e., within the lesser sac) or elsewhere in the abdomen, remote from the pancreas. There is much controversy in the literature concerning the nomenclature and management of these collections.[78,99] In essence, sterile collections will often resolve, whereas an infected collection (a pancreatic abscess) will need drainage by open operation, endoscopy, or a minimally invasive technique; the choice often depends on local expertise and preference.[82]

CONCLUSIONS

Pancreatitis is more likely to be severe in the elderly, and this contributes to the higher mortality rates observed in elderly patients: 2.7 deaths per 100 patients in the 45- to 54-year-old age group compared with 18.9% in those 75 years or older.[101] Patients with SAP, especially the elderly in whom there may be complicating comorbidities, should me managed in a specialist unit by experienced intensivists and pancreatic surgeons. Those patients who survive long-term management of complications such as diabetes and malabsorption caused by destruction of the pancreas will require specialist management. Attempts must be made to determine the cause of the pancreatitis to try to prevent further attacks. Patients with gallstone pancreatitis will require either cholecystectomy or ERCP and duct clearance.

CHRONIC PANCREATITIS

Chronic pancreatitis is an inflammatory disease resulting in progressive, irreversible destruction of the pancreatic parenchyma affecting exocrine and endocrine function. Onset is typically in the fourth decade with a strong male predominance, and presentation in those over 65 years is rare.[102] Chronic pancreatitis shortens life expectancy by 10 to 20 years and is therefore not typically a disease of the elderly.[102]

In up to 80% of cases of chronic pancreatitis (CP), the etiology is alcohol related,[103] and long-term alcohol consumption (>35 years) increases the risk of developing CP.[104] The remaining 20% of cases of chronic pancreatitis can be attributed to tropical CP, hereditary CP, pancreatic strictures, pancreas divisum, pancreatic trauma, or idiopathic CP. Idiopathic senile chronic pancreatitis is a subtype of idiopathic CP that presents after the age of 50 and is more prevalent in the elderly.[105] Various theories have been proposed as to the mechanism of cell destruction, inflammation, fibrosis, and atrophy seen in CP, but this is still controversial.

The predominant symptoms of CP include pain, typically remitting and relapsing; exocrine dysfunction characterized by weight loss and malabsorption secondary to steatorrhea; and endocrine dysfunction manifesting as diabetes mellitus. Patients often present with symptoms related to the complications of chronic pancreatitis, which include pseudocysts, ductal calculi, distal bile duct strictures, pancreatic duct strictures, and duodenal stenosis.

The diagnosis of chronic pancreatitis can be difficult, but clinical history and examination, biochemical investigations, and radiologic investigations should be used in combination. Fecal elastase is a useful test to confirm pancreatic exocrine failure and has increasing sensitivity with increasing severity of disease. Other pancreatic exocrine function tests are possible but are more unreliable and generally not used.

The role of imaging in CP is both diagnostic and therapeutic. Ultrasound can be used to demonstrate changes in pancreatic tissue and the ductal system; however, CT has greater sensitivity in identifying pancreatic atrophy, pancreatic calcification, dilatation of the pancreatic duct, and pseudocysts, which are typically seen in chronic pancreatitis. MRCP is a useful, noninvasive method of imaging the biliary and pancreatic ductal system, especially if the pancreatic duct is dilated, and the administration of secretin can improve duct visualization. ERCP can provide similar images and has the advantage of offering therapeutic interventions such as sphincterotomy, dilatation of strictures, extraction of calculi, and stenting, although these procedures do carry a complication rate of 5% to 10%.[106] EUS has become a useful tool in the diagnosis of CP, particularly in the early stages,[107] and is useful therapeutically in celiac

KEY POINTS

The Pancreas

Pancreatic Adenocarcinoma

- The incidence increases with age.
- It has the lowest 5-year survival for all cancers.
- Most patients present with advanced disease.
- It is managed with surgery, chemotherapy, or palliation.

Acute Pancreatitis

- It is most commonly caused by gallstones in the elderly.
- Severity scoring is important to indicate prognosis and guide management.
- Management is supportive according to BSG guidelines with input from intensivists.
- It results in a higher incidence of organ failure and death in elderly.

Chronic Pancreatitis

- It is not typically a disease of the elderly.
- It is often caused by alcohol.
- It is characterized by pain and pancreatic insufficiency.

plexus blockade, drainage of pseudocysts, and obtaining a tissue diagnosis. The incidence of pancreatic cancer is increased in chronic pancreatitis. Radiologic imaging may be utilized to distinguish between the two diseases; although this can be difficult and the conclusion is often equivocal,[108] many patients will be found to be inoperable when they are diagnosed.

Management of patients with CP initially involves symptom control and the goal should be to improve quality of life. Pain should be initially treated with analgesics according to the analgesic ladder, but if this becomes intractable, then celiac plexus block can be considered—operatively, percutaneously, or endoscopically.

The main indications for surgery in CP are intractable pain, suspicion of malignancy, and involvement of adjacent organs. It is recommended that surgery should be individualized according to pancreatic anatomy (small or large duct), pain characteristics, exocrine and endocrine function, and medical comorbidity.[109] In an elderly patient, careful consideration should be given to the risks and benefits of what is potentially major and complicated surgery. Options include gastrojejunostomy, feeding jejunostomy, PPPD, Whipple procedure, total pancreatectomy, lateral pancreaticojejunostomy (Puestow procedure), duodenum-preserving pancreatic head resection (the Beger's procedure), and local resection of the pancreatic head with longitudinal pancreaticojejunostomy (the Frey's procedure).

The nutritional status of a patient with CP should be carefully assessed and addressed with appropriate feeding and supplements, and exocrine insufficiency should be managed with enzyme supplements. Endocrine dysfunction may require referral to a specialist diabetologist.

The prognosis for patients with CP is poor, with a 20-year survival rate of 45% and a significantly worse survival for older patients and those with alcoholic CP.[110]

For a complete list of references, please visit online only at www.expertconsult.com

CHAPTER 78

The Liver

Joanna Hurley
John Trevor Green

STRUCTURE

Decline in liver mass and a reduction in hepatic blood flow are commonly cited features associated with increasing age. A reduction in liver volume both in absolute terms and in relation to total body mass is known to occur after the age of 50,[1] and studies using ultrasound have estimated that total hepatic volume declines somewhere between 20% and 40% across the lifespan in humans.[2] Postmortem data suggest that livers of subjects older than 60 years exhibit increased hepatocyte volume despite decline in total liver size.[3] However, other studies using liver scintigraphy have suggested that total hepatic mass in elderly subjects is not diminished, but that the mass of functional hepatocytes is decreased.[4] Aging in the liver is also associated with reduction in hepatic blood flow of the order of 30% to 50%. Both total and functional hepatic flow decrease with age, and this reduction is particularly evident after the age of 75.[5] The effects of aging on hepatocyte structure are less clear. There is an increase in the binuclear hepatocyte index and polyploidy, and decreased hepatic concentration of smooth endoplasmic reticulum.[6] Within hepatocytes, mitochondrial volume increases, yet the number of mitochondria per hepatocyte is decreased with age.[7] There are reports of thickening of the endothelial lining by 60% and an 80% decline in the number of endothelial cell fenestrations with increasing age.[8] The resultant implications of these changes are impairment of sinusoidal blood flow and hepatic perfusion, as well as reduced uptake of macromolecules such as lipoproteins from the blood,[2] which may contribute to hyperlipidemia and vascular disease.[9] The term *brown atrophy* is used to describe the macroscopic change seen in the liver with advancing age. This is due to age-related accumulation of the brown pigment lipofuscin within the lysosomes of hepatocytes. Studies in rodents have demonstrated that this may contribute to hepatocyte dysfunction by impairing metabolism, secretion, or excretion.[9]

FUNCTION

The structural changes with increasing age observed in human and animal studies do not appear to directly reflect any functional degeneration of the elderly liver. Certainly, there are no liver diseases specific to advancing age, and compared to other systems such as the musculoskeletal and cardiovascular systems, the liver appears to be less affected by aging.[10] Elderly patients with abnormal liver biochemical tests should be investigated in the same way as younger patients as these changes cannot be attributed to an aging liver. Serum concentrations of liver enzymes remain unaltered, with albumin concentrations and synthesis rates remaining stable in old age.[11] The exception is alkaline phosphatase (ALP), which has been reported to increase by approximately 20% between the ages of 20 and 80,[12] probably as a result of bone ALP leakage into blood. Values for serum bilirubin in some reports have been shown to be slightly decreased with increasing age, perhaps explained by an effect of reduced cellular muscle mass and decreased hemoglobin concentration.[13] Hepatic secretion of cholesterol has been shown to increase with age, whereas bile flow and bile salt formation are reduced by 50%.[14] The hepatic clearance of high-density lipoprotein has also been found to be reduced with increasing age in humans.[2] The increased incidence of cholesterol gallstones in elderly patients may be explained by some of these changes. Kupffer cells—macrophages with a major role in the removal of endotoxins—have impaired phagocytic activity with increasing age and could explain the susceptibility of elderly patients to sepsis because of intra-abdominal infection.[10] It has also been reported that there is a 50% age-related decline in DNA base excision repair in mouse hepatocytes.[15] The DNA damaged by free radicals or other insults therefore undergoes repair at a slower rate in older animals, increasing the likelihood of cell dysfunction. In animal studies, it has been extensively reported that the liver has a decreased capacity to recover from severe hepatic injury with increasing age. Although the rate of regeneration is slower, the overall capacity for regeneration seems to be preserved.[2] These changes appear to demonstrate that hepatic function declines with age; however, the significance of this in relation to clinical practice remains unclear.

DRUG AND ALCOHOL METABOLISM

The effect of age on hepatic drug metabolism, unlike renal drug excretion, remains controversial although it is widely perceived that there is a decline in the rate of clearance of drugs undergoing liver metabolism with increasing age. Reduction in liver blood flow and mass with increasing age has been consistently shown to correlate with the reduction of metabolism of rapidly cleared drugs such as propranolol, amitriptyline, verapamil, and morphine.[16] Total hepatic enzyme activity is adversely influenced by changes in liver size, enzyme mass, and activity, yet metabolism of drugs such as phenytoin and warfarin, cleared in this manner, are unchanged with age.[17] Animal studies have demonstrated impaired enzyme activity with a reduction in microsomal content of cytochrome P-450 during aging in mice; however, this has not been reproduced in most human studies.[16] The clearance of drugs that undergo phase I metabolism appears to be unchanged in older people.[18] However, drugs that undergo phase II metabolism are affected by age. Clearance of drugs such as ibuprofen, many benzodiazepines, imipramine, and more recently ropinirole and citalopram have been shown to be reduced by 10% to 50% with increasing age.[19] Differentiation between frail and healthy elderly must be considered when interpreting data on drug metabolism. It has been demonstrated that clearance of paracetamol per unit body weight is significantly reduced in the frail elderly when compared with age matched fit subjects.[20] In addition, a reduction in the clearance of metoclopramide has also been described in frail but not in healthy subjects older than 65 years.[21] Influence of disease states, environmental factors, and co-administration of other drugs have been postulated as important factors affecting variance of hepatic drug metabolism with aging.[19] The physiologic effect of alcohol on the aging body differs to that in the young.[22] Reduced hepatic blood flow and fewer hepatocytes result in a prolonged effect of alcohol and comparably higher serum levels in the elderly despite a similar or reduced alcohol intake to that of younger subjects.[23] Ethanol is distributed almost completely in the body's water space, which is reduced with advancing age thus partially explaining increased blood alcohol concentration after intravenous administration in the elderly.[24] Animal experiments on older rats have revealed decreased alcohol elimination rates and reduced alcohol dehydrogenase activity within the liver.[22] In addition, animal studies have demonstrated an age-dependent reduced activity of cytochrome P4502E1, an important enzyme in the metabolism of alcohol, but to date, this has not been reported in humans.[25]

INVESTIGATIONS

Liver function tests (LFTs) refer to measurements of serum bilirubin, alkaline phosphatase (ALP), aspartate aminotransferase (AST), alanine aminotransferase (ALT), gamma glutamyl transpeptidase (GGT), and albumin, but they should also include the prothrombin time (PT). In general, conditions affecting the liver cell (hepatitis) cause a rise in AST and ALT, whereas biliary tree disorders (cholestasis) cause raised ALP and GGT. It is important to recognize that these enzymes are also present in other sites of the body, and when interpreting isolated elevation extrahepatic sources should be considered (Table 78-1). Raised liver enzymes often overlap between hepatitis and cholestatic patterns in clinical practice. Aminotransferases (AST, ALT) can also be elevated in both intra- and extrahepatic cholestasis.[26] Extrahepatic biliary obstruction causing irritation and secondary inflammation of hepatocytes results in mildly raised serum transaminases, and hepatitis can lead to a degree of cholestasis with consequent rise in ALP and GGT. In practice, when faced with this situation, it is helpful to recognize the pattern of the so-called dominant distribution of raised enzymes.[27] If the serum bilirubin is elevated to greater than twice the upper limit of the normal reference range, then the patient will be clinically jaundiced. Bilirubin can be raised in most types of hepatobiliary pathology,[27] often with an associated rise in liver enzymes. Initial evaluations should determine whether the hyperbilirubinemia is conjugated (direct) as seen in most types of liver disease, or unconjugated (indirect).[28] A low-serum albumin level and prolonged prothrombin time (PT) are sensitive indicators of impaired hepatic synthetic function, occurring in both acute and chronic liver disease, and are important prognostic indicators. When interpreting the serum albumin in elderly patients it must be taken into account that other factors may result in low levels of albumin. A prolonged PT may also arise from a deficiency of vitamin K, which is required for synthesis of clotting factors II, VII, IX, and X in the liver. This may be of particular significance in the elderly as dietary insufficiency can exhaust hepatic stores of vitamin K after just 4 weeks. Vitamin K deficiency can be excluded by giving intravenous replacement of 10 mg of vitamin K and then repeating the PT.

In chronic liver disease, blood loss from gastrointestinal bleeding as a result of upper gastrointestinal pathologies such as bleeding varices, can lead to iron deficiency anemia. This may be exacerbated by coagulopathy and thrombocytopenia secondary to the splenic enlargement seen in portal hypertension. Hypersplenism can also result in leukopenia and a mild anemia. A raised mean corpuscular volume (MCV) suggests excessive alcohol intake because of its direct toxic effect on the bone marrow. In addition, macrocytosis is also seen in patients with chronic liver disease due to failure of bone marrow to produce erythrocytes and reduced erythrocyte survival. In elderly patients, poor nutrition, particularly lack of dietary folic acid, can lead to hematinic deficiencies and may contribute to difficulties interpreting hematologic tests when there is underlying liver disease.

The true prevalence of abnormal LFTs in the elderly has yet to been clarified. However, research from the early 1980s showed 17% of elderly hospitalized patients had abnormal LFTs when screened without clinical indication.[32] In the United Kingdom, there is evidence that liver disease may be missed in all age groups as abnormal LFTs are often not investigated.[33] A thorough history is a mandatory part of a "liver screen" and should include the patient's

Table 78-1. Interpreting LFTs in the Elderly

Abnormality in Liver Enzymes	Consider
Elevated ALT and AST	Hepatitis A, B, C, and E Alcoholic liver disease Nonalcoholic fatty liver disease Autoimmune hepatitis Hereditary hemochromatosis Medications (e.g., NSAIDs, herbal drugs) Congestive cardiac failure and ischemic hepatitis Celiac disease
Elevation of AST only (normal ALT)	Nonhepatic source Cardiac, skeletal muscle, kidneys, brain, pancreas, lungs, leukocytes, and red blood cells[29]
Elevated ALP and GGT	Intrahepatic cholestasis (e.g., primary biliary cirrhosis); drugs (e.g., co-amoxiclav, erythromycin); sepsis Extrahepatic cholestasis (e.g., biliary obstruction), stones, strictures, malignancy Hepatic infiltration (e.g., malignancy)
Elevated GGT only (normal ALP)	Excess alcohol consumption Enzyme-inducing drugs (e.g., barbiturates, phenytoin)[26] Fatty liver, obesity, type II diabetes, hypercholesterolemia Renal failure Chronic obstructive pulmonary disease Pancreatic disease Myocardial infarction[30]
Elevated ALP only (normal GGT)	Extrahepatic source—bone Malignancy without liver or bone involvement (e.g., lung)[31] Amyloid, leukemias, granulomas
Isolated raised bilirubin (normal LFTs)	Unconjugated—hemolysis Inherited disorders (e.g., Gilbert syndrome)
Elevated PT only (normal LFTs)	Warfarin Vitamin K deficiency Malabsorption
Low albumin only (normal LFTs)	Malabsorption Malnutrition Urinary and gastrointestinal losses Acute illness[31]

alcohol consumption, current or recent drug use (prescribed or otherwise), risk factors for viral hepatitis, the presence of autoimmune diseases, family history of chronic liver disease, and factors such as diabetes, obesity, and hyperlipidemia. Elderly patients with elevated LFTs should be investigated initially with noninvasive serologic tests[28] (Table 78-2). It excludes Wilson's disease, which is rarely diagnosed over the age of 40. Liver disease in those with homozygote α_1-antitrypsin deficiency tends to become apparent in the age group of 50 to 60 years but is probably worth including as part of the screen. Serologic screening tests for celiac disease could also be included as this condition is recognized as causing asymptomatic elevation of transaminases, which subsequently normalize on a gluten-free diet.[34] There are several causes of LFT derangement in patients with a negative liver screen including drugs, sepsis, and other comorbidities. Many of the medications used in elderly patients can cause abnormal LFTs.[35] This should be borne in mind when reviewing a patient's drug history. In a district general hospital study of hospitalized patients with jaundice, the second commonest cause after cancer was found to be sepsis/shock.[36] A study of liver function tests in bacteriemia not of hepatobiliary origin demonstrated significant elevations in levels of GGT and ALP, and reduced albumin levels.[37] Other possible causes to consider include alcohol excess, fatty liver, obesity, diabetes, thyroid disease, and Addison's disease, which may also cause mild derangement of LFTs. Some expert reviews suggest that where there is a negative screen to treat the most likely cause of the abnormal LFTs—that is, alcohol (by abstinence), hepatotoxic drugs (by drug cessation), and nonalcoholic fatty liver disease (by weight reduction and diabetes control)—before more detailed investigation if LFTs remain abnormal after a period of observation.[28]

Table 78-2. Initial Serologic Tests in Elderly Patients with Abnormal LFTs

Screening Test	Disease	Other Clues
Hepatitis A IgM	Hepatitis A	Travel to endemic areas
Hepatitis B surface antigen (HBsAg)	Hepatitis B	Intravenous drug usage Blood transfusion
Hepatitis C virus antibody (HCV antibody)	Hepatitis C	Intravenous drug usage Blood transfusion
Hepatitis E IgM	Hepatitis E	Travel to endemic areas
Antimitochondrial antibody (AMA)	Primary biliary cirrhosis	Pruritus Female sex Presence of other autoimmune disorders
Smooth muscle antibody (SMA) Liver kidney microsomal antibody (LKM)	Autoimmune hepatitis	Presence of other autoimmune disorders Female sex
Transferrin saturation Ferritin	Hemachromatosis	Diabetes Joint symptoms
Serum Alpha-fetoprotein	Hepatocellular carcinoma	Known chronic liver disease
α_1-Antitrypsin level	α_1-Antitrypsin deficiency	Coexisting lung disease
Anti-TTG antibody	Celiac disease	Gastrointestinal symptoms of malabsorption
Lipid profile Serum glucose	Nonalcoholic fatty liver disease	Comorbidities (e.g., diabetes)

RADIOLOGY

The role of *abdominal ultrasound* is well established in the evaluation of the liver and biliary tree. It should be the first-line investigation in patients with any abnormality in liver function tests or where there is a suspicion of liver disease. It is safe and noninvasive and therefore an ideal investigation for use in elderly patients. The images require no adaption in interpretation compared to younger patients; the only change seen in the liver in increasing age is reduction in liver volume. It is particularly useful in the detection of focal liver lesions, when performed by an experienced operator.[27] The advent of contrast-enhanced ultrasound has been shown to improve the detection and differentiation of these focal lesions.[38] Detection of fatty liver is also possible, although ultrasound is unable to accurately quantify the amount of fat present.[26] Ultrasound is also useful in chronic liver disease, particularly evaluation of liver texture and size, and for assessing other upper abdominal organs including the spleen. Doppler facilities to detect blood flow provide useful information about vascular structures and in portal hypertension, reversed portal vein flow, and development of collateral vessels can be demonstrated. *Spiral computed tomography (CT)* can provide extra detail and is particularly effective in further characterization of focal liver lesions. It can also be used to detect diffuse liver disease because of fat, iron deposition, and cirrhosis as well as providing further information about other abdominal organs. There are no protocol adaptations that need to be specifically undertaken in elderly patients when undergoing CT scans of the liver; however, the intravenous contrast agent can cause renal failure in patients with underlying reduced creatinine clearance. Even elderly patients with a degree of cognitive impairment may be able to cooperate well with CT scanning, as examinations are now quicker; for example, the entire liver and pancreas can be imaged in one single breath hold.[39] Unenhanced *magnetic resonance imaging (MRI)* of the liver is comparable to enhanced spiral CT in the detection of focal liver lesions, while avoiding the disadvantage of radiation exposure and the potential nephrotoxic effect of iodinated contrast agent.[40] It has improved the characterization of underlying nodules and fibrotic changes in patients with cirrhosis, particularly when there is sideroblastic nodular regeneration.[41] MRI is also particularly useful in quantifying hepatic iron concentration and has a positive and negative predictive value of 100% in the detection of hemachromatosis.[40] Magnetic resonance cholangiopancreatography (MRCP) is the modality of choice for noninvasive assessment of the pancreatic duct,[42] giving further views of the biliary tree. It may even demonstrate common bile duct (CBD) stones not seen on endoscopic retrograde pancreatography (ERCP).[42]

LIVER BIOPSY

The need for further investigation of persistently abnormal LFTs in the elderly must depend on clinical context, considering the risks and benefits of the procedure and whether the findings will dictate further management. Liver biopsy is not specifically contraindicated in elderly patients, but a

25-year audit from Australia found that increasing age was a risk factor for major complications following the procedure, particularly in those age over 50.[43] The patient should be able to understand and cooperate with instructions given by the person performing the liver biopsy and be able to give informed consent.[44] Midazolam can be used as sedation in the very anxious, but this must be used with caution in elderly patients. It is important to correct clotting abnormalities prior to biopsy to minimize the potential risk.[44] The indications for liver biopsy can be broadly subdivided into the diagnosis of parenchymal disease and focal lesions. In parenchymal liver disease, biopsy is indicated in the diagnosis and classification of chronic viral hepatitis and is useful for planning treatment decisions. In hemochromatosis, it is recommended that liver biopsy is undertaken to define or exclude the presence of cirrhosis.[44] In autoimmune hepatitis, where 25% of patients are diagnosed over the age of 65,[45] liver biopsy is indicated in both diagnosis and follow-up.[46] It is not usually indicted for primary biliary cirrhosis or routinely in alcoholic liver disease, and its role in nonalcoholic fatty liver disease has not yet been clearly established. Liver biopsy may be useful in the investigation of acute liver dysfunction where routine serologic tests are unhelpful or there is an unusual course or severity of illness. It may also be of use in suspected drug reactions, especially herbal medicines. For the assessment of focal liver lesions, the indications for liver biopsy depend largely on the clinical picture.[44]

LIVER DISEASES

Liver disease in clinical practice can be classified into acute liver failure (ALF) and chronic liver disease. ALF is the term used to describe a clinical syndrome of sudden loss of hepatic function in a patient with no prior history of liver disease.[47] Chronic liver disease is caused by long-standing liver damage and commonly presents with the complications of cirrhosis. There are a number of recognized etiologies of acute and chronic liver disease as summarized in Table 78-3. As chronic liver disease is more commonly seen in the elderly population, this will be discussed first.

Liver injury caused by *chronic liver disease* of any etiology can result in cirrhosis, defined histologically as a diffuse process with fibrosis and nodule formation. As there are no diseases specific to liver aging itself, older patients are affected by the same conditions and have similar clinical manifestations as younger age groups.[48] However, older patients may present with more advanced disease and prognosis is poorer with increasing age.[49] It is important to recognize that there is a greater mortality rate from other diseases unrelated to the liver, especially pneumonia, in those age 80 or over with underlying cirrhosis.[49] Cirrhosis has a varied clinical presentation from an asymptomatic individual with abnormal LFTs to advanced decompensated liver disease indicated by the presence of complications such as jaundice, ascites, and portal hypertension with variceal bleeding. There are several recognized stigmata of chronic liver disease which include palmar erythema, Dupuytren's contracture, clubbing, spider nevi, and gynecomastia.

Table 78-3. Common Causes of Acute and Chronic Liver Disease Presenting in the Elderly

Causes of Acute Liver Failure	Causes of Chronic Liver Disease
Acute viral hepatitis A,B, C, and E	Chronic hepatitis B and C
Drug induced	Alcoholic liver disease
Ischemic hepatitis	Nonalcoholic fatty liver disease
Autoimmune hepatitis	Autoimmune liver disease—autoimmune hepatitis, primary biliary cirrhosis, primary sclerosing cholangitis
Portal or hepatic vein thrombosis	Hemochromatosis

The prevalence of *chronic hepatitis B (HBV) infection* is declining worldwide, but it is still high in elderly people of Asian origin. Although acute cases are rare, the natural history of HBV infection appears to be altered in the elderly with a higher risk of progression to chronic infection.[50] HBV in the elderly can present as chronic hepatitis, but more often as cirrhosis with older patients more likely to have advanced liver disease compared to younger ones.[51] HBV causes liver injury via an immune response against virus-infected hepatocytes. The aim of treatment is to reduce inflammation and fibrosis by preventing replication of the virus. Antiviral treatments (e.g., interferon-α, lamivudine) are available and indicated in patients of all ages with chronic HBV who also have markers of active viral replication (i.e., detectable HBV DNA), elevated aminotransferase levels, and chronic hepatitis on liver biopsy. The decision to treat must consider the presence of other comorbidities and the patient's overall general health, as the advantages of treatment of HBV in the elderly remain unspecified. That said, most elderly patients with chronic HBV infection even with advanced liver disease have no evidence of ongoing viral replication and therefore are not candidates for antiviral treatment.[51] The increased rate of adverse effects seen with interferon in older patients may render lamivudine as the treatment of choice, but these decisions should always be led by a specialist center. Screening for hepatocellular carcinoma is of importance where there is long duration of viral infection as it develops mainly in patients over age 50 with cirrhosis, although development may occur in those with either chronic hepatitis or simple HBsAg carriage.[51]

Chronic hepatitis C (HCV) can cause liver disease in the elderly, and in some southern European countries it is estimated that as many as one in two or three people over age 80 are infected.[52] It is anticipated as the population ages over the next few decades, so will the prevalence of HCV in older patients. Most of the elderly with HCV infection have previously acquired it from blood transfusions. The American Association for the Study of Liver Diseases (AASLD) recommends that anyone who received blood transfusion or blood products before 1992 be screened for HCV infection.[53] Chronic HCV develops in 55% to 85% of individuals initially infected with HCV,[54] and the progression of fibrosis is more rapid in those who acquire the infection at an older age.[55] The mechanism of this rapid progression in elderly patients has not been fully established, although factors such as a higher prevalence of the more aggressive genotype 1 and impaired immunity have been suggested.[56] Among HCV-infected individuals, cirrhosis becomes more prevalent with age,[56] with studies showing a mean age of 65.4 years for those with cirrhosis.[57] Accordingly elderly patients are more likely to present with a complication of cirrhosis or hepatocellular carcinoma (HCC).[58] HCC develops in 1% to

2% of patients with cirrhosis because of chronic HCV and the interval between infection and diagnosis of HCC may be shorter when the infection is acquired at an older age.[59] The current treatment of choice for active HCV infection is pegylated interferon-α and oral ribavirin.[53] The goals of treatment are to clear the virus and to prevent complications, such as cirrhosis and HCC. Only patients who have at least moderate inflammation and necrosis on liver biopsy and a significant risk of cirrhosis during their estimated life expectancy should be considered as candidates for therapy.[56] Treatment in elderly patients is controversial as they are more likely to experience adverse effects including lethargy, confusion and behavioral change,[60] but guidelines do not stipulate an upper age limit for antiviral therapy. Therapy is contraindicated for patients with reduced life expectancy from severe hypertension, heart failure, coronary artery disease, poorly controlled diabetes, or obstructive lung disease.[53] Adherence to therapy, which is essential to achieving a virologic response, may be suboptimal in older patients.[61] Studies have also shown that increasing age is an independent predictor of poor response to treatment, although sustained response rates of 45% have been observed in patients above 65 years.[62] Whether this benefits overall survival in the elderly population remains to be seen and the decision to treat must therefore encompass an individual's risks and benefits.

Alcoholic liver disease (ALD) is becoming an increasing problem among elderly individuals. Alcohol consumption is common in the elderly, and the prevalence of alcohol abuse probably underestimated.[63] Reasons for increased alcohol consumption may be explained by associated psychosocial problems, such as loss of spouses, loneliness, and mental health problems that occur with increasing frequency.[22] Although data suggest that most patients with severe ALD present in the fifth or sixth decade of life, a study from the United States reported the peak incidence of alcoholic cirrhosis in the seventh decade among white men.[64] An increased rate of complications and severity of disease at presentation is one important difference in the elderly population and the presence of other comorbidities may result in the increased capability of alcohol to cause a harmful effect.[65] This has implications for overall prognosis, which is dependent on the severity of disease at presentation. Those over the age of 70 years with alcoholic cirrhosis have been shown to have a mortality rate of 75% at 1 year.[66] Patients are living longer because of better therapeutic strategies, and therefore HCC is emerging as a major complication in later life.[23] In the elderly, the spectrum of symptoms and signs of ALD do not differ from those seen in younger adults and include jaundice, acute liver failure, and decompensated liver disease with portal hypertension. Nonspecific symptoms of ALD including general malaise and anorexia are more common.[67] Chronic alcohol ingestion can result in alcoholic fatty liver, which can be reversible even in the elderly with abstinence.[22] Patients are usually asymptomatic but may have hepatomegaly on examination. Alcoholic hepatitis may result from continued or increased alcohol intake, as well as recommencing drinking after a period of abstinence. Severe alcoholic hepatitis results in a potentially life-threatening illness, with deep jaundice, encephalopathy, ascites, and coagulopathy. Underlying cirrhosis may coexist, and signs of decompensated liver disease are common. The prognosis of alcoholic hepatitis is variable; however, ongoing alcohol abuse, the presence of cirrhosis, and severe malnutrition are important factors.[22]

A raised GGT supports a diagnosis of alcohol-related liver disease when serum AST:ALT levels are elevated at a ratio of 2:1, particularly in the presence of a raised MCV.[29] Bilirubin is a useful prognostic indicator and correlates well with the degree of histologic change in alcoholic steatohepatitis.[22] A careful alcohol history should be taken in all elderly patients and the opportunity for advice and counseling utilized, as alcohol abstinence is beneficial at any stage of ALD. Studies suggest that these brief interventions reduce hazardous alcohol consumption in the elderly similar to younger populations.[68] Withdrawal from alcohol in elderly subjects should be supervised by a health care professional.[69] Few clinical studies directly support or refute the hypothesis that withdrawal symptom severity, delirium, and seizures increase with advancing age, but several observational studies suggest that adverse functional and cognitive complications during alcohol withdrawal do occur more frequently in elderly patients.[23] Benzodiazepines such as chlordiazepoxide and diazepam are used, based on validated alcohol withdrawal protocols with dose and frequency individualized. Older hospital in-patients with concurrent serious illness may have increased sensitivity to adverse effects.[70] β-Blockers, clonidine, carbamazepine, and haloperidol may be used to treat withdrawal symptoms not controlled by benzodiazepines in the elderly. Attention to nutrition and replacement of B vitamins via an intravenous route are of great importance to prevent Wernicke's and Korsakoff's syndromes. For acute alcoholic hepatitis, intensive care management may be indicated. Selected patients may gain benefit from steroid therapy or pentoxifylline, an inhibitor of TNF-α.[71] Management of complications and continued encouragement of abstinence is the mainstay of treatment in alcoholic cirrhosis with liver transplant the ultimate therapy.

Nonalcoholic fatty liver disease (NAFLD) represents a spectrum of disorders characterized by predominantly macrovesicular hepatic steatosis that occur in individuals in the absence of consumption of alcohol in amounts considered harmful to the liver.[72] This spectrum includes fatty liver and nonalcoholic steatohepatitis (NASH) with inflammation and fibrosis, which can lead to cirrhosis. It is the probable cause of "cryptogenic cirrhosis" in many elderly individuals.[73] Risk factors for underlying NAFLD include obesity (particularly abdominal adiposity), diabetes and insulin resistance, rapid weight loss, drugs including amiodarone, and elevated triglycerides. Older age (>40 years) is an independent risk factor for more advanced liver disease in NAFLD.[74] For patients with the metabolic syndrome and NASH-associated cirrhosis, liver failure is the main cause of morbidity and mortality rather than cardiovascular disease.[75] It is estimated that 20% to 30% of the U.S. population is affected by NAFLD,[76] with 3.5% to 5% prevalence of NASH.[77] NAFLD commonly presents between the ages of 46 and 57 years,[10] and one study from Israel has reported a prevalence of NAFLD, as determined by ultrasound criteria, as high as 46% in a group of patients older than 80 years.[78] Prospective studies are few, but it is thought 10% to 15% of patients will progress to advanced fibrosis and cirrhosis.[79] The overall progression to cirrhosis is slow, but once developed, complications will occur in 45% within 10 years.[76] Elderly patients are therefore likely to constitute a considerable proportion of this cohort. Many patients are asymptomatic; however, initial symptoms can include fatigue, malaise, and right upper quadrant pain. The diagnosis can usually be made on the basis of a negative "liver screen," mild elevation of transaminases (ALT:AST ratio < 1), evidence of fat on abdominal ultrasound, or features of the metabolic syndrome.[74] Excess alcohol consumption must be excluded. A liver biopsy is the only way to determine the stage of NAFLD. No therapy has yet been proved to be of benefit although initial management should focus on lifestyle modification and the reversal of conditions associated with NAFLD.[80] There is a growing consensus that only patients with NASH require pharmacologic treatment.[81] Slow weight loss by dietary modifications and exercise are recommended to achieve weight loss and improve insulin sensitivity,[72] although this may prove to be challenging in the elderly with reduced mobility. Drug treatments for weight loss appear promising, but there may be issues with long-term tolerability relevant to elderly patients. Improvement of insulin resistance with metformin and thiazolidinediones have shown potential, but further randomized placebo-controlled trials are needed to assess efficacy and safety of these drugs.[80] Lipid-lowering drugs, antioxidants, angiotensin-converting enzyme inhibitors, and angiotensin receptor blockers are also the subject of ongoing studies.

Autoimmune hepatitis (AIH) is a chronic necro-inflammatory disease of the liver which can silently progress to cirrhosis.[45] It is characterized by hypergammaglobulinemia (usually IgG) circulating autoantibodies and morphologic changes of interface hepatitis.[7] Although it was initially thought to affect young women, it is now known to have a bimodal distribution with another peak between 50 and 70 years of age.[82] Studies have agreed that approximately 25% of cases of AIH present in those over 65 years of age.[45] It may present acutely, but commonly in the elderly presents in a more indolent form. However, patients over the age of 60 have been observed to have a higher rate of cirrhosis at presentation. Symptoms can be subtle and may include fatigue, upper abdominal pain, anorexia, and polymyalgia, but a lower rate of arthralgia when compared to younger patients.[45] Autoantibodies such as antinuclear (ANA), anti-smooth muscle (SMA), antiliver kidney microsomal (LKM) and antisoluble liver/pancreas (SLA/LP) antigens may be positive but are nonspecific. AIH in the elderly is almost always characterized by ANA and SMA antibodies, classified as type 1 (classic) disease; other pathologic autoantibodies occasionally seen in this population are anti-SLA/LP and antiactin.[83] The outcomes for elderly people with AIH appear to be no worse than they are for younger ones,[50] including those who are untreated.[84] It was traditionally believed that elderly patients had a milder disease course and controversy existed as to whether treatment was beneficial; however, it is now widely thought that these patients have an excellent prognosis if remission is induced. Treatment failure occurs less commonly in patients older than 60 years compared to younger adults, but it must be recognized by careful monitoring. The preferred initial treatment for severe AIH in the elderly is prednisolone in combination with azathioprine.[85] If there is relapse after remission, low-dose prednisolone or azathioprine as maintenance is used although sustained long-term remission free from medication is still possible after relapse and retreatment.[84] However, in the elderly, azathioprine is less well tolerated and use of prednisolone alone in a higher dose is associated with greater frequency of adverse effects. Bone protection must be instituted early. A recent study from Japan suggested ursodeoxycholic acid may be an effective drug for management of older patients with AIH.[86]

Primary biliary cirrhosis (PBC) is an autoimmune disease classically affecting middle-aged women, but it may be present in patients older than 65 years in 30% to 40% of cases.[50] Data from the 1990s revealed that in England, more than one third of patients with PBC were older than 65, with a median age at diagnosis of 62 to 63 years.[87] Symptom severity at first presentation does not differ in older subjects, although age is known to be an independent adverse prognostic risk factor in PBC when symptoms and complications of liver disease arise.[88] Diagnosis can be made in the presymptomatic stage, where antimitochondrial antibody (AMA) is detected in the serum but LFTs are normal. In the asymptomatic phase, patients have detectable AMA and abnormal LFTs (elevated ALP and GGT) but no clinical features of disease. However, up to 50% have established cirrhosis at diagnosis. When symptoms arise, lethargy and pruritus are characteristic. In late presentation, symptoms and signs of decompensated liver disease can dominate the clinical picture. Jaundice does not become apparent until late in the disease, and serum bilirubin is an important prognostic indicator. Other autoimmune diseases, especially Sjögren's syndrome, Raynaud's syndrome, or rheumatoid arthritis, may be present. Helpful investigations include raised immunoglobulins, particularly IgM and raised serum cholesterol. In the presence of investigations highly suggestive of the disease, some hepatologists believe a liver biopsy to be unnecessary, especially in elderly and frail patients, where management will not be affected.[44] Liver transplantation is the only effective treatment for patients with end-stage disease.[89] Immunosuppressants such as steroids are of no benefit. Ursodeoxycholic acid (UCDA) can improve LFTs and symptoms; however, it does not improve overall survival.[90] For pruritus, cholestyramine is the most commonly used agent, but other drugs such as rifampicin, naltrexone, and sertraline can be of benefit. Patients who have marked cholestasis are at risk of malabsorption of fat-soluble vitamins A, D, E, and K and should receive replacement where this occurs. Bone disease such as osteopenia, osteomalacia, and osteoporosis can complicate PBC, and prophylaxis is indicated.[91]

Hemochromatosis is an inherited disorder of iron metabolism. Liver damage results from progressive iron deposition, which also affects the pancreas, heart, endocrine organs (pituitary, occasionally thyroid, and adrenals), and joint synovia.[27] The gene for hemochromatosis (HFE) is located on chromosome 6, with 90% of cases associated with homozygous substitution of tyrosine for cysteine—the C282Y mutation.[92] It is characteristically diagnosed in men between 40 and 50 years, but in women, because of the protective effect of menstruation, presentation is classically a decade later. Raised serum ferritin and raised transferrin saturation (>60%) are suggestive of the diagnosis. Genetic testing for the HFE gene is now widely available, and, as already mentioned, MRI can be useful. Liver biopsy is recommended to define or exclude the presence of cirrhosis, in cases where biochemical and genetic testing do not give a clear diagnosis and where other causes of liver disease need to be excluded.[44] Presentation can be with symptoms and signs of the complications of chronic liver failure, especially if HCC has developed. The risk of HCC is particularly high in hemochromatosis, estimated at 30%.[26] Venesection should be performed once or twice weekly to remove 500 mL of blood (200 to 250 mg of iron) until serum ferritin is less than 50 mg/L. However, elderly patients with underlying heart failure may need smaller volumes of blood removed or less frequent phlebotomy. The aim of treatment is to prevent the onset of cirrhosis, and thus HCC. Life expectancy is similar to that of the healthy population if treatment can be achieved before the onset of cirrhosis or diabetes.[92] Transplantation for liver failure remains a viable option, although survival in this group is lower than in those transplanted for other indications.[93] Genetic screening of all first-degree relatives of any age is recommended given the effectiveness of early treatment in preventing complications that significantly reduce life expectancy.

Primary sclerosing cholangitis (PSC) can be diagnosed at any age but is commonly a disease of young males. There is a close association with inflammatory bowel disease, particularly ulcerative colitis. There is also increased risk of developing cholangiocarcinoma. LFTs usually show cholestasis, and AMA is negative. Other autoimmune markers including ANCA are nonspecific. Endoscopic Retrograde and Magnetic Resonance Cholangio-Pancreatography demonstrate multiple irregular strictures and dilatation of the biliary tree. Management involves symptomatic relief of cholestasis, bone disease prophylaxis, and replacement of fat-soluble vitamins. Where there are acute episodes of cholangitis, antibiotic treatment is indicated. Balloon dilatation or stenting may be undertaken if there is a focal obstructive biliary stricture. Liver transplantation remains the only effective treatment, although there is a high risk of subsequently developing colon cancer in those with ulcerative colitis.

COMPLICATIONS OF CIRRHOSIS

Portal hypertension results from cirrhosis of any cause but can occur acutely following portal vein thrombosis or occlusion of the hepatic vein *(Budd-Chiari syndrome)*. Although rare in the elderly, Budd-Chiari syndrome is a recognized complication of myeloproliferative diseases resulting in a hypercoagulable state. The development of *varices* in cirrhosis has important prognostic implications for the patient, as 30% will bleed from their varices, irrespective of age, within 2 years of diagnosis. The mortality rate for each bleeding episode is 30% to 50%.[94] Immediate survival rate after variceal bleeding is similar in elderly and younger cirrhotic patients, although midterm and long-term survival rates appear to be worse for the older group.[50] Initial management of a significant bleed requires stabilization of the patient, with care not to precipitate congestive cardiac failure in older individuals. Terlipressin (a vasopressin analogue) to reduce portal blood flow should be used with caution in the elderly as it may precipitate an ischemic event, which can either be cardiac, mesenteric, or peripheral[95] and is contraindicated in documented ischemic heart disease. Upper gastrointestinal endoscopy should be arranged urgently; endoscopic treatment using sclerotherapy, or preferably band ligation, has a high success rate of approximately 90% across all age groups.[95] If bleeding cannot be controlled endoscopically, balloon tamponade with either a Sengstaken–Blakemore tube or Minnesota tube can be undertaken. If there is continued bleeding despite endoscopic intervention, transjugular intrahepatic portal systemic shunt (TIPSS) can be employed. Following TIPSS there is a greater risk of encephalopathy in elderly patients, and it is recommended that careful assessment be undertaken so the risk of encephalopathy does not outweigh the benefit.[96] It also increases cardiac preload and may precipitate cardiac failure in those with heart disease.[97] Propranolol, a nonselective β-blocker for primary and secondary prevention, has been shown to be effective in lessening rebleeding and mortality by reducing portal pressure.[95] It should be used with caution in the elderly, as they are less tolerant to β-blockers and coexisting heart failure may increase the likelihood of adverse effects.

Ascites and peripheral edema are often the first signs of decompensated liver disease,[95] occurring in over half of all patients with cirrhosis over a 10-year period.[98] In a patient with known liver disease, it should not be presumed that the underlying cause of the ascites is cirrhosis. Patients should undergo an ascitic tap, and fluid should be sent for albumin and protein levels, culture and sensitivity, neutrophil count, and, if there is clinical suspicion, amylase and cytology. Patients with cirrhosis generally have low levels of protein or albumin in the ascites. Treatment is aimed at addressing the key underlying factors in the pathogenesis of ascites in cirrhosis formation—portal hypertension and sodium retention. Bed rest is no longer recommended for the treatment of uncomplicated ascites.[98] The risk of muscle atrophy, particularly in the elderly, and other complications can result in prolonged in-patient stays. However, salt restriction is important, and dietary salt should not exceed 90 mmol per day. Food with very low salt content in a hospital setting can be unpalatable[95] and reduces patient compliance; therefore, recognition and avoidance of malnutrition is important. There is controversy over the role of fluid restriction. Despite sodium retention, some patients have hyponatremia because of impaired free water clearance. Recently updated guidelines[98] recommend that water restriction be reserved for those who are clinically euvolemic with severe hyponatremia, who are not taking diuretics and only where there is a normal serum creatinine. In situations where the sodium is <120, diuretics should be stopped. Diuretic therapy remains the mainstay of treatment in ascites. Spironolactone, an aldosterone antagonist, is the first-line drug of choice, but amiloride or eplenorone are alternatives. If spironolactone alone does not achieve adequate diuresis, a loop diuretic such as furosemide may be added. Careful monitoring of fluid loss by recording body weight, together with serum urea and electrolytes should be undertaken particularly in the elderly.[95] Large volume paracentesis is reserved for patients who initially present with tense ascites. To prevent circulatory dysfunction, volume expansion with intravenous salt-poor human albumin is given. Although there are no data on the hemodynamic changes seen during paracentesis specific to elderly patients, it is reasonable to suggest that they should be carefully monitored. TIPSS is a highly effective treatment for refractory ascites; however, it may precipitate encephalopathy, and whether it has a positive impact on overall survival remains to be clarified.

Even with early diagnosis and prompt treatment, *spontaneous bacterial peritonitis (SBP)* carries a mortality rate of 20%.[99] It is diagnosed when the ascitic fluid neutrophil count is

>250 in the absence of a precipitating cause, such as an intra-abdominal and surgically treatable source of sepsis.[98] It is commonly caused by coliforms; however, culture can be negative. The symptoms are usually nonspecific, especially in the elderly where there may be a poor systemic and laboratory response to infection.[95] It should be suspected if there is abdominal pain, fever, or encephalopathy in a patient with ascites or deterioration in blood tests. Intravenous cefotaxime is the antibiotic of choice and will attain high ascitic fluid concentrations.[100] In a third of patients, renal impairment develops and this is a significant cause of mortality. Treatment with intravenous albumin has been shown to be associated with improvement in circulatory function compared with equivalent doses of fluid as colloid.[101] Continuous prophylactic antibiotics with oral norfloxacin or ciprofloxacin is recommended after an episode of SBP because of the cumulative recurrence rate of 70% at 1 year.[98] SBP is an indicator of poor prognosis and referral for liver transplantation should be considered.

Hepatorenal syndrome (HRS) is a serious complication in patients with advanced cirrhosis either alone or in association with SBP. Intense vasodilatation of the splanchnic circulation causes a relatively low and insufficient cardiac output with effective hypovolemia.[102] Marked vasoconstriction of the renal circulation results in "functional" renal failure with no structural damage to the kidneys.[103] Vasoconstrictors such as terlipressin together with albumin infusions are recommended as first-line treatment of HRS. Treatment should continue until there is reversal of HRS, defined as reduction in serum creatinine below 1.5 mg/dL, commonly seen in week 2,[104] although the optimum duration of treatment is unknown. In most studies of HRS, the incidence of ischemic side effects with terlipressin is approximately 13%,[102] although many studies exclude high-risk patients with ischemic heart disease or arterial disease and also the elderly.[105] TIPSS is an alternative treatment in HRS; however, the long-term survival benefits remain unknown.[103] Overall survival in HRS is poor, and liver transplantation again remains the treatment of choice.[106]

The exact underlying pathophysiology of *hepatic encephalopathy (HE)* remains poorly understood, but it is believed that failure to detoxify gut-derived toxins that are normally cleared by the liver is one of the main factors. Elevated circulating levels of ammonia, alteration in neurotransmitter systems, including increased levels of the neuroinhibitor GABA, decreased neuroexcitation, and an altered blood-brain barrier are all thought play an important role.[107] HE is characterized by the development of mental slowing, memory loss, disorientation, worsening somnolence, and occasionally coma in advanced stages.[95] Clinical examination findings include asterixis (liver flap), fetor hepaticus, increased reflexes, or muscular rigidity. Chronic persistent encephalopathy may result where there have been recurrent episodes of acute encephalopathy. Dysarthria, ataxia, dementia, and extrapyramidal signs in this context may be difficult to assess in elderly patients with underlying neurologic disorders. In its subclinical form, estimated to affect over 60% of patients with compensated cirrhosis,[95] diagnosis is challenging—in particular in elderly patients where it may be confused with cognitive impairment or early dementia. In addition, elderly patients with subdural hematoma, meningitis, or sepsis from urinary tract infections, cellulitis, or pneumonia may appear to be encephalopathic. It has also been described that a significant proportion of elderly patients with documented liver disease and a presumptive diagnosis of HE had coexisting treatable extrahepatic conditions.[48] When appropriate treatment was administered, including standard therapy for HE, 67% of these patients showed improvement in their encephalopathy. There are also a number of factors that can precipitate HE, and careful identification and treatment of these are important. They include gastrointestinal bleeding, electrolyte disturbance, dehydration, drugs including diuretics, infection, and constipation—especially if elderly patients are noncompliant with laxatives. There is no laboratory test to confirm the diagnosis, ammonia levels may be raised but do not correspond to the severity of symptoms, and electrophysiologic tests are rarely used outside of research. The drawing of a five-pointed star is often useful as constructional apraxia is a common feature of HE and should be assessed at the bedside. General treatment measures include short-term protein restriction to reduce the gut protein load, although in the elderly this should be instituted with caution as many have borderline nutrition to begin with.[95] Lactulose is the mainstay of drug therapy. It lowers colonic pH, dissuading replication of ammonia-producing bacteria and reducing absorption of ammonia, and increasing fecal nitrogen elimination by producing osmotic diarrhea.[108] Adverse effects such as diarrhea and abdominal cramps may make it difficult to tolerate in elderly, especially outside the hospital setting. Antibiotics such as neomycin can also be effective; however, long-term risks such as ototoxicity and nephrotoxicity limit their use. Chronic persistent HE is also an indication for liver transplantation.

Hepatocellular carcinoma (HCC) is a common complication of liver cirrhosis affecting the elderly,[109] with 35% to 40% of patients diagnosed over the age of 70 years.[110] An aging society and increased survival because of better treatments of the complications of cirrhosis are the likely explanations. HCV infection contributes to a greater risk of HCC in the elderly, because of its long natural history,[111] and is responsible for the rise in incidence of HCC seen in Western countries.[112] Five-year survival is poor in all age groups. HCC typically presents on a background of known cirrhosis, and it should be suspected in any patient with sudden decompensation. An elevated serum Alpha-fetoprotein (AFP) with characteristic radiologic imaging especially in the presence of cirrhosis is widely recognized as diagnostic. The potential risk of needle track spread should contraindicate biopsy when surgical resection is a viable option. Six-monthly assessment of AFP and imaging such as ultrasound or CT is indicated in patients with cirrhosis to screen for HCC,[113] as early diagnosis is vital in determining a favorable outcome, especially in older patients. Options in the treatment of HCC in cirrhotic patients include liver transplantation, surgical resection, and local ablation techniques. Previously, the role of resection surgery in HCC in elderly patients was uncertain because of the high operative mortality and high tumor recurrence rate. However, one paper[114] reported a low mortality rate for major hepatic resection in elderly cirrhotic patients and early surgical outcomes comparable to those of younger patients. Data on HCC in patients greater than 80 years[115] have shown that it is the advanced stage of HCC and not the patient's age or comorbidities that has the greatest impact on survival rate.

ACUTE LIVER FAILURE

As *acute liver failure (ALF)* is rare in the elderly, little is known specifically about the underlying causes, clinical course, and outcomes.[116] Despite extensive medical investigation, in some cases the etiology remains undiscovered. It often results in multiorgan failure, with cerebral edema and sepsis being the leading causes of death.[117] ALF commonly presents initially in a nonspecific manner with malaise or nausea. Jaundice then develops, followed by features of hepatic encephalopathy, and many patients evolve to coma within 1 week or less.[47] Elderly patients with ALF have been described as having a more protracted disease course,[116] and increasing age has been identified as an independent risk factor of mortality from all causes.[118] The presence of other coexisting diseases and smaller functioning liver mass is believed to render them more easily susceptible to succumbing to a lesser degree of hepatic necrosis.[116] Impaired regeneration, as described previously, can result in prolonged hepatocyte damage. The spontaneous survival rate for ALF is poor and has been reported as less than 50% for adults of any age.[119] In one study from Japan, incidence of ALF in autopsy cases of those more than 65 years of age was 0.2%.[116] The mortality rate of ALF in the elderly patients in this study was found to be 85%.

A variety of viral agents can cause acute liver disease. *Acute hepatitis A (HAV)* infection usually begins with a prodromal illness, before the appearance of jaundice. It is typically a self-limiting disease that resolves in the majority of patients within 6 weeks. Although rare in this age group, patients over 65 years are more susceptible to severe infections and are more likely to have serious complications.[50] ALF occurs in less than 0.35% of younger adults with HAV; however, in elderly patients this figure is higher. In addition, the mortality rate is increased, with the U.K. census data for 1979 through to 1985 demonstrating a mortality rate approaching 15% in those older than 75.[120] *Acute hepatitis B (HBV) and C (HCV)* infection is also rare over the age of 65 in the Western world, due in part to the lack of risk factors such as intravenous drug use and high-risk sexual behavior and the routine screening of donated blood for these viruses. However, sporadic cases and rare outbreaks may still occur.[50] Data from the United States have shown acute HBV still accounts for 3% of all adult ALF cases.[121] *Hepatitis E (HEV)* has emerged as an important cause of acute hepatitis in the elderly throughout the world. It has an overall mortality rate of between 0.5% and 4%. In a U.K. study of sporadic HEV, the majority of cases affected elderly males,[122] and data from Hong Kong suggest that older patients affected by HEV have a more severe illness leading to a higher mortality rate than patients with hepatitis A.[123] In a recent French study of patients with severe ALF resulting from acute HEV, the mortality rate for those older than 70 years was 71%.[124] It is possible that underlying liver disease from other etiologies may be a factor in the poor prognosis observed in these patients. Other viruses such as cytomegalovirus, Epstein-Barr virus, and yellow fever are rare but recognized causes of ALF.

Drug-induced ALF occurs with increased frequency in the elderly, because of either increased drug use and polypharmacy, but also accidental or intentional overdose. Worldwide, the major causative drugs include antituberculous drugs, antibiotics, nonsteroidal medication, and paracetamol (acetaminophen).[125] Anesthetic drugs of the halothane family cause hepatic failure and death more commonly in older compared to younger patients.[126] Although paracetamol poisoning is predominantly seen in adolescents and young adults, the majority of paracetamol-related deaths occur in the older population,[118] and it is widely held that older age is an independent risk factor for both development of ALF and subsequent death. In addition, accidental overdose and late presentation are seen more commonly in the elderly and are individual risk factors associated with poor prognosis.[118] *N*-acetylcysteine (NAC) is an effective therapy in the treatment of paracetamol overdoses, and when given within 24 hours of overdose it has been shown to decrease the risk of liver injury.[127] It can be used safely in elderly patients.

Ischemic hepatitis is thought to be more likely with older age. One U.K. study demonstrated the condition occurring in 1% of elderly patients acutely admitted to hospital with a variety of other conditions.[128] It is often difficult to recognize, as the classical signs of liver failure are not prominent. It is thought to be associated with an episode of hypotensive liver anoxia, which is usually the result of a significant drop in blood pressure.[129] In the absence of any other causes, a striking and reversible rise in serum transaminases (in the order of 10- to 20-fold) is generally accepted as diagnostic in the appropriate clinical setting.[130] A retrospective analysis has indicated that all patients with a clinical diagnosis of ischemic hepatitis had evidence of cardiac disease, usually right sided, suggesting underlying hepatic congestion may be an important part of the pathophysiologic process.[130] Prognosis in ischemic hepatitis is influenced by the underlying condition; in one U.K. study, the mortality rate was found to be one third in the elderly.[129]

Autoimmune hepatitis (AIH) can present as an acute severe hepatitis. Belgian data have demonstrated an acute presentation with pronounced jaundice and a biopsy showing severe necrotizing hepatitis present in 19% of the elderly population studied (4% of the total study group).[45] AIH should be considered in all elderly patients with acute liver failure as it typically responds favorably to corticosteroid treatment.[47]

If the liver has been severely damaged by any of the preceding conditions, emergency transplantation can be considered. Artificial liver-assist systems have not yet been proven to affect survival in ALF,[131] but the next generation of systems are being developed using hepatocyte cell-based therapy. These are promising developments for the future. At present, the mainstay of treatment is supportive, to allow time for the liver to recover from the acute insult and eventually regenerate.

LIVER TRANSPLANTATION

There is growing evidence to suggest that in end-stage chronic liver disease, advanced age should not be considered a contraindication to liver transplantation. More than 10% of patients undergoing liver transplantation in the United States in 2000 were over the age of 65 years.[132] Recently published data from the United Kingdom[133] demonstrated no significant difference in survival between age groups within the first 5 years after liver transplant. In addition, patients over 65 years were found to have lower rejection rates, probably because of reduced immune function, and have excellent graft survival. After 5 years, survival is significantly worse in older recipients. At this time point, one study showed a survival rate of 52% in those over 60 years compared to 75% in younger patients, with more deaths from malignancy in the older group.[134] In particular, good survival rates have been observed in those over 65 years who received transplants for PBC as their primary indication.[133] Chronologic age alone should not form the basis of refusal for liver transplantation; it is the overall general health of the patient that appears to be of greater importance.

FOCAL LIVER LESIONS

Pyogenic liver abscess is a disease of elderly patients, most often diagnosed after the sixth to seventh decades.[135] Untreated it is invariably fatal. Biliary tract disorders, such as cholangitis and portal pyemia from intra-abdominal sepsis, are common sources of liver abscess; however, few papers have remarked on etiologies in relation to age. Data suggest there are no age-related differences with regard to symptoms or laboratory data at presentation.[135] Classical presentation includes abdominal pain, fever, nausea, and vomiting. Examination findings may include a tender liver. Laboratory investigations may reveal an elevated white blood cell count, elevated liver enzymes (especially ALP), raised inflammatory markers, and a low serum albumin. Centrally necrotic liver metastases may sometimes be indistinguishable from abscess on conventional as well as contrast-enhanced ultrasound.[38] Blood cultures can be negative; abscess cultures are often of greater yield, with *E. coli* the most frequently isolated organism across all age groups. Treatment of pyogenic liver abscess is by complete percutaneous drainage of the abscess, either by needle or indwelling catheter. This is in combination with intravenous antibiotics, which should be continued for 14 days, followed by oral treatment for a minimum of 4 weeks depending on clinical response. A broad-spectrum cephalosporin with metronidazole is usually adequate, but advice from a microbiologist is useful. Surgery is rarely indicated. Progress can be monitored by serial ultrasound, and the search for the underlying cause should be attempted and treated if possible. Active management is well tolerated in the elderly, and there appears to be no appreciable difference in mortality rates compared with younger patients.[135]

Liver metastases are common in elderly patients, particularly of gastrointestinal origin; for example, 35% of those with colorectal carcinoma have liver metastases at presentation.[136] Weight loss, general malaise, and nonspecific abdominal discomfort are common presenting features. However, the finding of metastatic disease can be incidental. Liver biopsy may be indicated where the nature of the primary neoplasm is unknown, and with new immunohistochemistry techniques it may help to indicate the likely primary site and guide further treatment. Lymphoma, for example, resembles hypervascular metastases on ultrasound scanning[38] but has good prognosis if treated. However, if there is a history of a known primary malignancy, liver biopsy is often not required. Where surgical resection of the metastasis is under consideration, liver biopsy should not be undertaken. Colorectal metastases have the potential to be cured by liver resection, and increasing numbers of elderly patients are being referred for surgery. A recent U.K. study[137] has confirmed that low perioperative morbidity and mortality rates as well as good long-term outcomes can be achieved with an aggressive strategy in elderly patients with colorectal liver metastases.

Benign liver lesions include simple cysts, hemangiomas, and focal nodular hyperplasia (FNH), which can present in all age groups. There is no potential for malignant transformation, and patients can be reassured that no treatment is required. The majority of patients are asymptomatic, and these lesions are found incidentally on abdominal imaging. In cysts and hemangiomas, rupture or hemorrhage can occur, causing right upper quadrant discomfort. Mass effect from large lesions can also result in pain, but other causes of pain should be excluded first.[14]

KEY POINTS
The Liver

- There are no liver diseases specific to old age.
- Abnormal liver function tests in the elderly should be fully investigated, in the first instance with serologic tests.
- Alcoholic liver disease and chronic hepatitis C infection are becoming more prevalent in the aging population worldwide.
- No treatment of liver disease is contraindicated by age alone, only by the individual's frailty and comorbidity.
- Liver transplantation for chronic liver disease in selected elderly patients is achieving improved outcomes.

For a complete list of references, please visit online only at www.expertconsult.com

CHAPTER 79

Biliary Tract Diseases

Elias Xirouchakis
Andrew K. Burroughs

Jaundice, or icterus, is the yellow discoloration of sclerae, mucous membranes, and skin caused by accumulation of bilirubin: clinically, it is not obvious until the bilirubin concentration in the blood exceeds 51 μmol/L (3 mg/dL).

The appearance of jaundice is also related to the circulatory status and any accompanying edema. Particularly in elderly people, paralytic and edematose limbs tend not to have the typical pigmentation and it is possible to observe a one-sided icterus in patients with hemiplegia.

Jaundice can be classified in different ways, depending on the following:

- Prevalent form of bilirubin detectable in serum: it is divided into unconjugated, mixed, or conjugated hyperbilirubinemia.
- Site of impairment in bilirubin production or excretion pathway: it is classically divided into prehepatic, hepatocellular, and obstructive.

From a practical point of view, it is useful clinically to consider conditions that lead to icterus under the following categories:

- Isolated disorders of bilirubin metabolism
- Liver disease
- Obstruction of the bile ducts

ISOLATED DISORDERS OF BILIRUBIN METABOLISM

In these conditions, there is an increase in bilirubin production (hemolysis, ineffective erythropoiesis, blood transfusion, resorption of hematomas) or decreased hepatocellular uptake or conjugation (congenital hyperbilirubinemias). Liver function is otherwise normal and hyperbilirubinemia is often characterized by a predominant elevation in unconjugated bilirubin.

Jaundice resulting from hemolysis is usually mild with a serum bilirubin of 68 to 102 μmol/L (or 4 to 6 mg/dL), as normal liver function can easily handle the increased bilirubin derived from excessive breakdown of red blood cells. Unconjugated bilirubin is not water soluble and therefore will not pass into the urine, hence the term *acholuric jaundice*. Urinary urobilinogen is increased. Causes of hemolytic jaundice are those of hemolytic anemia. Investigations show raised unconjugated bilirubin but normal serum alkaline phosphatase, transferase, and albumin, and serum haptoglobins are low.

Most of the congenital and inherited defects are diagnosed in young people; the only condition that could incidentally be found in older patients is Gilbert's syndrome, the most common familial hyperbilirubinemia. It is asymptomatic and is usually detected as an incidental finding of a slightly raised bilirubin 17 to 102 μmol/L (or 1 to 6 mg/dL) on a routine check. No signs of liver disease are present. There is a family history of jaundice in 5% to 15% of patients.

Hepatic glucuronidation is approximately 30% of normal, resulting in an increased proportion of bilirubin monoglucuronide in bile. Most patients have reduced levels of UDP-glucuronosyl transferase activity, the enzyme that conjugates bilirubin with glucuronic acid. Evidence[1–3] has shown mutations in the gene encoding this enzyme with an expanded nucleotide repeat consisting of two extra bases in upstream 5′ promoter element. The abnormality appears to be necessary but is not in itself sufficient for the phenotypic expression of the syndrome.[4] Among the most relevant drugs that undergo glucuronidation are morphine, acetaminophen, chloramphenicol, and transplant immunosuppressants such as cyclosporine A and tacrolimus, but also the widely used antitumor drug metabolite of irinotecan SN-38.

The major importance of establishing this diagnosis is to inform the patient that it is not a serious disease and to prevent unnecessary investigations. Tests show only a raised unconjugated bilirubin, which is further raised on fasting, during mild illnesses or infections, after surgery, or during consumption of large amounts of alcohol; the reticulocyte count is normal. No treatment is necessary.

LIVER DISEASE

Primary sclerosing cholangitis (PSC) is a rare (8 to 13 cases per 100,000 persons) chronic cholestatic disease characterized by chronic inflammation and progressive obliterating fibrosis of the intra- or extrahepatic biliary ducts. It affects primarily caucasian men during their fourth or fifth decade of life.[5] Etiology is unknown: both immune (genetic) and nonimmune (infections, toxins, ischemic damage) mechanisms have been postulated. A genetic predisposition to PSC has been described, and there is a strong association between PSC and inflammatory bowel diseases (IBD). Coexisting IBD is seen in 50% to 80% of PSC patients, more commonly ulcerative colitis (UC) than Crohn's disease; in 2% to 10% of IBD patients, PSC is also present.[6] However, there is no correlation between severity of PSC and IBD, nor a temporal relation between the onset of the diseases. Furthermore, therapy of IBD has little effect on the course of PSC and vice versa. Other less common disease associations are thyroiditis, ankylosing spondylitis, and celiac disease.

Typical symptoms on presentation are pruritus and fatigue, but asymptomatic cases are being diagnosed more frequently because of routine testing monitoring of liver function tests particularly in IBD patients. One third of patients have episodes of acute cholangitis, with recurrent attacks; in advanced disease, jaundice is constantly present.

Liver enzymes and especially serum alkaline phosphatase levels are raised in the majority of patients; perinuclear antineutrophil cytoplasmic antibodies (pANCA) may be detected in 26% to 85% of PSC cases, but they lack specificity for diagnosis. Overlap syndromes with other forms of liver diseases have been described. PSC with autoimmune hepatitis-like features has been referred to as autoimmune cholangitis. These patients usually present with high serum alanine aminotransferase (ALT) levels, modest or no elevations in serum alkaline phosphatase, high titers of antinuclear (ANA) and anti–smooth muscle antibodies (SMA), and liver histologic findings typical of autoimmune hepatitis. Corticosteroid therapy may lead to improvements in symptoms and liver enzyme abnormalities.

The differential diagnosis for a patient with chronic cholestatic symptoms includes all the secondary causes of bile duct abnormalities, particularly biliary obstruction resulting from pancreatic, biliary, or metastatic malignant obstruction; strictures resulting from previous surgery; and malignant transformation and lymphomas. Rare causes are cryptosporidiosis and cytomegalovirus in patients with immunodeficiency.

Although endoscopic retrograde cholangiopancreatography (ERCP) has been the gold standard diagnostic technique in diagnosing PSC for many years, magnetic resonance cholangiopancreatography (MRCP) has replaced ERCP for diagnosis of PSC.[7,8] Typical findings are multifocal strictures of the biliary tree alternating with normal segments and ectatic ducts; liver biopsy shows fibro-obliterative ductal lesions in one third of cases. There is no correlation between histologic severity and radiologic findings.

The estimated median survival for PSC is about 12 years: for symptomatic patients; there is a significant reduction in life expectancy with a mean survival just under 10 years.[9] Cholangiocarcinoma develops in 6% to 20% of patients at a rate of 1% to 5% per year and can occur before the onset of cirrhosis, especially in patients with coexisting UC[10] as these patients have a higher risk of developing colorectal cancer. Hepatocellular carcinoma can develop in those with cirrhosis.

Different drugs including antifibrotic agents such as methotrexate or colchicine, penicillamine, and ursodeoxycholic acid (UDCA) have been used, but none of them has been shown to improve histology, liver function tests, symptoms, or survival. However, a few studies have emerged reporting improved liver enzymes and a possible survival benefit with high doses of UDCA (30 mg/kg/day).[11–13] Bone density and liposoluble vitamin deficiency should be monitored and treated appropriately, particularly in patients with advanced disease.[14] Preliminary reports suggest that UDCA therapy decreases the risk of colon cancer,[15,16] but further investigation is needed. Currently liver transplantation is the only life-extending treatment available, with 5-year survival rates of 75% to 85%. However, disease recurrence has been reported in up to 47% of cases, with the presence of IBD being the most important independent predicting factor.[17]

OBSTRUCTION OF BILE DUCTS

Obstruction can be mechanical or anatomic and is commonly due to stones, intrinsic disorders of the biliary tree (e.g., cholangiocarcinoma), or extrinsic compression, usually by pancreatic carcinoma.

Clinically, there is a considerable rise of serum conjugated bilirubin, alkaline phosphatase (ALP), and cholesterol. In contrast to what happens in cirrhosis, serum bilirubin levels rarely exceed 600 μmol/L, with a trend to a plateau, as, when conjugated bilirubin concentration increases, glomerular filtration and excretion also increase. In complex cases with prolonged partial obstruction, hepatocyte function is also affected, thus producing a mixed biochemical picture, with elevation of circulating unconjugated bilirubin. Patients do not usually have signs of chronic liver disease but may have signs indicating malignancy, and pruritus is usual.

On examination, in the presence of obstructive jaundice a palpable gallbladder may be found; this is due to malignant obstruction of the biliary tree, usually pancreatic head carcinoma (Courvoisier's sign) or to a stone impacted in Hartman's pouch, leading to a mucocele or an empyema (Mirizzi's syndrome).

Signs of infection such as fever, abdominal pain, and chills are common. Steatorrhea is responsible for weight loss and malabsorption of fat-soluble vitamins A, D, E, and K and calcium.

Gallstones

Diseases affecting the gallbladder and bile ducts occur commonly in elderly people. By the age of 70, cholelithiasis and choledocholithiasis are found in 13% to 50% of the population, and the figures rise to 38% to 53% in persons above the age of 80. There is geographic variation: gallstones are rare in the Far East and Africa and very common in native North Americans and in Chile and Sweden. They occur twice as frequently in women as in men, but this difference decreases with increasing age.

Gallstones can be distinguished in three types, depending on the major constituents: pure cholesterol, pure pigment (which can be black or brown), and mixed. Cholesterol stones are by far the most frequent, accounting for 80% to 90% of all gallstones in the West. They contain more than 70% cholesterol, often with some bile pigment and calcium. Cholesterol is slightly soluble in aqueous media and is transported in bile mixed with bile salts and phospholipids in the form of micelles and vesicles. These later become saturated when cholesterol cannot be solubilized any further. Therefore cholesterol supersaturation could result from (1) hepatic hypersecretion of biliary cholesterol (often observed in obese patients with gallstones), (2) decreased rates of bile salt or phospholipid secretion into bile (nonobese patients with gallstones, ileectomy, diseases of the ileum such as Crohn's disease, or surgical bypass of the ileum), or (3) a combination of cholesterol hypersecretion with hyposecretion of the solubilizing lipids (found in both American Indians and whites with gallstones, which could be the result of diminished 7-hydroxylation of cholesterol).[18]

With the passage of time and in the presence of a heterogeneous pronucleating agent, usually mucin gel in gallbladder bile, cholesterol supersaturation leads to precipitation of cholesterol monohydrate crystals from a phase of separated liquid to a crystalline phase, followed by agglomeration and growth of the crystals into mature and macroscopic stones.

Several factors have been reported to influence gallstone formation. More rapid crystallization of cholesterol in bile of patients with gallstones suggests that lithogenic bile may contain components (i.e., pronucleating agents) that accelerate crystallization or alternatively that normal bile may contain components (i.e., antinucleating agents) that inhibit crystallization. Mucin was the first biliary protein shown to promote cholesterol crystallization. Subsequently, it was shown that many glycoproteins that bind reversibly to concanavalin A-Sepharose also speed up cholesterol crystallization.[19] Two roles in the formation of gallstones have been proposed for mucins: (1) as a pronucleating/crystallizing agent for the nucleation/crystallization of cholesterol from saturated bile and (2) as a scaffolding for the deposition of crystals during growth of stones. Despite evidence that mucin overproduction is critical in the pathogenesis of gallstones, the mechanisms triggering mucin production during gallstone formation are still unclear. Furthermore, mucin secretion and accumulation in the gallbladder are determined by multiple mucin genes. Although the regulation of gallbladder mucin secretion and accumulation and its role in gallstone pathogenesis have been intensively studied in vivo and in vitro, no information is available on how individual mucin genes contribute to cholesterol gallstone formation and whether the epithelial mucins influence susceptibility to cholesterol gallstone formation.[19] Other nucleating factors such as nonprotein components of bile also expedite cholesterol crystallization. A low-density particle composed principally of lipids is a potent promoter of crystallization. Calcium bound to micelles and vesicles in bile may accelerate cholesterol crystallization by promoting fusion of cholesterol-rich vesicles.

Antinucleating factors include apolipoproteins AI and AII, and secretory immunoglobulin A and its heavy and light chains.[19]

Impaired gallbladder motility could precede gallstone formation. The stasis induced by the hypofunctioning gallbladder would provide the time necessary to accommodate nucleation of crystals and growth of gallstones within the mucin gel in the gallbladder.

Intestinal factors including decreased large bowel transit time, increased colonic gram-positive anaerobic bacteria, increased bile acid metabolizing enzymes, and higher intracolonic pH values compared to stone-free controls have also been documented. Together, these changes lead to increased deoxycholic acid formation, solubilization, and absorption.

Black pigment stones contain calcium salts of bilirubin, phosphate, and carbonate in addition to bilirubin polymers and mucin glycoproteins. The biliary lipids are normal. These stones form in the gallbladder and are seen in patients with chronic hemolysis (e.g., hereditary spherocytosis and sickle cell disease) where there is an increase in bilirubin, and also in cirrhosis.

Brown pigment stones have layers of cholesterol, calcium salts of fatty acids (mainly palmitate), and calcium bilirubinate. They form in the common bile duct as a result of stasis and infection, usually in the presence of *E. coli* and *Klebsiella* spp., which produce β-glucuronidase that converts soluble conjugated bilirubin back to the insoluble unconjugated state, which is prone to precipitation with calcium. They are also found with biliary strictures, sclerosing cholangitis, and Caroli's syndrome.

The most common presentation of gallstone disease is biliary pain. This occurs in the epigastrium and right hypochondrium, and it does not fluctuate but persists from 15 minutes up to 24 hours, subsiding spontaneously or with opioid analgesics; it may radiate round to the back in the interscapular region.

Complications of gallstones

ACUTE CHOLECYSTITIS, COMMON DUCT STONES, AND CHOLANGITIS

Acute cholecystitis occurs when a gallstone impacts in the neck of the gallbladder or in the cystic duct, leading to distension and inflammation. The inflammation is usually sterile, but within 24 hours gut organisms can be cultured from the gallbladder. Infections are polymicrobial in 30% to 80% of the episodes. Occasionally inflammation may be mild and quickly subside, sometimes leaving a gallbladder distended by mucus (mucocele). More commonly, the inflammation is severe, involving the whole wall and giving rise to localized peritonitis and acute pain. The gallbladder can become distended by pus (empyema) and, rarely, an acute gangrenous cholecystitis occurs with perforation and a more generalized peritonitis.

The patient is usually ill with fever and shallow respirations. Right hypochondrial tenderness is present, being worse on inspiration (Murphy's sign). There is guarding and rebound tenderness.

The presentation of biliary colic in the elderly patient with diabetes and diabetic neuropathy is obfuscated and atypical. In such patients, a condition as serious as gangrenous cholecystitis can present with minimal temperature increases, without significant leukocytosis and few, if any, abdominal complaints. Consequently, clinically significant cholecystitis can be interpreted as an episode of mild biliary colic.

At ultrasound (US) examination, with the detection of gallstones alone is insufficient for a diagnosis of acute cholecystitis. Additional criteria are as follows:

- Sonographic Murphy's sign (focal tenderness directly over the visualized gallbladder)
- Distention of gallbladder
- Presence of biliary sludge
- Pericholecystic fluid
- Gallbladder wall thickening (but not specific for acute disease)

Common bile duct stones are frequently found in elderly patients who present with concomitant cholecystitis. In the general population, 5% of patients presenting with cholecystitis have coexisting bile duct stones, but this figure rises to 10% to 20% in elderly people. Presentation can be with one or all of the triad of abdominal pain, jaundice, and fever. The pain is usually severe and situated in the epigastrium and right hypochondrium, and it may be accompanied by vomiting; it usually lasts for a few hours and then clears up, only to return days, weeks, or even months later. Between attacks the patient is well.

The jaundice is variable in degree, depending on the amount of obstruction. Urine is dark and the stools are pale. High fever and rigors indicate cholangitis. The liver is enlarged if the obstruction lasts for more than a few hours. Prolonged biliary obstruction or repeated attacks lead to secondary biliary cirrhosis, but this is now rare.

US examination reveals a dilated common bile duct, but stones are detected in only about 75% of cases. MRCP is very useful as an additional diagnostic test, particularly if the bowel hinders good visualization of the common bile duct, and is better than ultrasound in detecting stones in the lowest part of the common bile duct. Endoscopic ultrasound, when available, is a more accurate method of detecting a stone with a sensitivity and a specificity of more than 80% and 95%.

Acute cholangitis is due to bacterial infection of the bile ducts and is always secondary to bile duct abnormalities. The most frequent causes are common duct stones, biliary strictures, neoplasms, or following ERCP in the presence of large duct obstruction.

Symptoms are fever, often with a rigor, upper abdominal pain, and jaundice. Older patients can present with collapse and gram-negative septicemia and renal failure.

Initial therapy of acute cholecystitis and cholangitis is directed toward general support of the patient, including fluid and electrolyte replacement, correction of metabolic imbalances, and antibacterial therapy. In all but mild cases, pain relief with an opiate is required. In the absence of vomiting, the patient can soon tolerate oral fluids, and nasogastric aspiration is not often required.

Antimicrobial therapy is usually empirical. Initial therapy should cover the Enterobacteriaceae, in particular *E. coli*, and anaerobes, especially in elderly people and in patients with previous bile-duct–bowel anastomosis. In patients with moderate clinical severity, monotherapy with a ureidopenicillin—mezlocillin or piperacillin—is more effective than the combination of ampicillin with aminoglycoside. Additionally, in the most recent years quinolones have proved their efficacy and as they can also be administered orally, many clinicians use them as the first choice of therapy in biliary tract infections. Patients who are septic or who have a previous biliary stent in place may benefit from the addition of ampicillin as further coverage against *Enterococcus*. Therapy with aminoglycosides when necessary, mostly for *Pseudomonas aeruginosa*–related infections, should not exceed a few days because the risk of nephrotoxicity increases during cholestasis.[20] Relief of biliary obstruction is mandatory,[21] even if there is clinical improvement with conservative therapy, because cholangitis is most likely to recur with continued obstruction.

Endoscopic techniques are effective for removing bile duct stones by sphincterotomy and stone extraction and should be the first therapeutic approach because it is safer than surgery in elderly people[22] as the associated morbidity and mortality of endoscopic therapy is unchanged regardless of age. Stent insertion with bypass of common bile stones may be needed if stones cannot be removed or sphincterotomy is unsafe or as part of a two-stage procedure with delayed sphincterotomy. Sometimes endoscopic nasobiliary drainage may be required as a first step to relieve obstruction in the presence of sepsis, again followed by a second therapeutic endoscopy to remove stones.

Cholecystectomy[23,24] is the treatment of choice for virtually all patients with gallbladder stones and symptoms. Since the late 1990s, laparoscopic cholecystectomy has been the operation of choice.[25] In patients aged 65 to 69 years, mortality rates are comparable with those reported in the younger patients (0.3%), and patients can leave hospital in 24 to 48 hours. Accordingly, the complication rate is low and includes wound sepsis, bile duct injury (0.2%), and retained gallstones in the common bile duct.[26] In patients older than 70 years, complications can increase up to 13%, mostly represented by chest infections, whereas the mortality rate can increase up to 2%, especially when concomitant cholangitis or other comorbidities coexist. In addition, postoperative stay is significantly higher.[27] Laparoscopic cholecystectomy is not superior to the small incision cholecystectomy, and some surgeons prefer this "mini-laparotomy" approach, with a small surgical incision, because the length of stay in hospital and return to full activity is similar to that of laparoscopic surgery.[28–32]

Malignant obstruction

Obstructive jaundice can result from neoplasms of the gastrointestinal tract, arising from the biliary tree or most frequently from the pancreas. The usual presentation of this syndrome in the elderly consists of the insidious development of cholestasis and jaundice.

PANCREATIC CARCINOMA

Pancreatic carcinoma is the most common cause of malignant biliary obstruction. In the United States, pancreas cancer develops in approximately 30,000 patients per year, with about the same number in Europe and about 20,000 annual cases in Japan. Although it represents a rare form of cancer with age-adjusted rates in most countries, ranging from about 5 to 10 new cases per 100,000 persons per year, it is so lethal that it ranks fourth as a cause of death from cancer.[33] Usual presentation is in the sixth and subsequent decades of life.

PRIMARY ADENOCARCINOMA OF THE GALLBLADDER

Primary adenocarcinoma of the gallbladder represents less than 1% of all cancers; it occurs chiefly in patients over 70 years of age, more commonly in women, and has striking genetic, racial, and geographic characteristics, with an extremely high prevalence in Native Americans and Chileans. Gallstones are usually present, but a definite relationship is uncertain. Polyps that are larger than 1 cm, single, sessile, and echogenic are associated with a higher risk of malignancy. Anomalous junction of pancreaticobiliary ducts, chronic bacterial infections, certain occupational and environmental carcinogens, hormonal changes, and possibly a porcelain gallbladder are additional factors that predispose to cancer. Occasionally a mass can be palpable in the right hypochondrium.

The majority of cases are discovered during exploration for presumed gallstone disease, and cholecystectomy is performed if possible. The overall 5-year survival is 5%, and the 1-year mortality is 88%.

CHOLANGIOCARCINOMA

Cholangiocarcinoma is the most common primary tumor of the biliary tree; it is less common than hepatocellular carcinoma, representing less than 3% of gastrointestinal cancers, but is rapidly increasing in incidence in several countries.[34,35] There is no association with cirrhosis or viral hepatitis, whereas in the Far East it may be associated with infestation with *Clonorchis sinensis* or *Opisthorchis viverrini*. Primary sclerosing cholangitis, as described earlier, is an important risk factor.[36]

It usually develops at the hepatic hilum, from the junction between right and left hepatic ducts; more rarely the tumor arises from the common bile duct or intrahepatic ducts. Despite the central site of obstruction, the two hepatic lobes can present different degrees of dilatation of the biliary ductal system, with the left lobe usually more involved. Local invasion and proximity of vital structures within the porta hepatis contribute to the difficulty in achieving complete resectability, so that curative surgical resection is rarely possible: only one third of cases are suitable after staging.

Patients usually die within 6 months.[37–39] Even for resectable disease, 5-year survival rate is between 20% to 40%.

Liver transplantation alone is not a current option because of an almost universal likelihood of recurrence.[40] A protocol for treatment of unresectable disease combining external beam radiation therapy (EBRT) with brachytherapy, 5-fluorouracil chemosensitization, then liver transplantation has been used.[41] The most recent published survival following this regime, published in 2006, of 65 patients with a mean follow-up of 32 months was 91% at 1 year and 76% at 5 years.[42]

AMPULLARY TUMORS

Malignant tumors of the ampulla present with cholestatic jaundice, which may occasionally be intermittent. They may ulcerate and produce gastrointestinal hemorrhage or chronic anemia. The diagnosis is usually made at ERCP. Carcinoma of the ampulla can sometimes be resected, with a 5-year survival rate of 40%.

MANAGEMENT OF PANCREATICOBILIARY MALIGNANCY

The main goal in treating patients with malignant biliary diseases, presumed to be unresectable, is to provide palliation of jaundice, to avoid early liver failure caused by chronic obstruction, and improve the patient's nutritional and immunologic status. Surgical therapy consists of either attempting a curative resection of the tumor or performing a palliative operation. Unfortunately, the surgical cure rate of these tumors is less than 5%.

Staging techniques should be used in elderly people in order to select carefully those patients who are likely to have resectable disease. Multislice computed tomography scanning should be routine. Endoscopic ultrasound (EUS) is the most sensitive diagnostic modality currently available for predicting resectability.[43,44]

Palliative surgery is directed toward relieving jaundice by creating a biliary-enteric anastomosis. However, given the morbidity and 30-day mortality (up to 20%) for bypass procedure, nonoperative techniques of palliation are preferred in aged populations unless there is a concomitant or impending duodenal obstruction. Alternatively, stenting of duodenal obstruction with self-expanding metal stents that can be deployed endoscopically or placed radiologically can obviate the need for surgery. These stents do not preclude endoscopic management of pancreatic or biliary problems.

Endoscopic relief of jaundice has been used successfully for over 20 years, and endoscopic techniques have a high rate of success (up to 90% to 95% of cases). Greater success is achieved when treating distal bile duct obstruction, as complications occur less frequently. With tumors affecting the bifurcation of the hepatic ducts (Klatskin tumors), several stents can be placed into both the right and left intrahepatic ducts to provide decompression.

Plastic stents placed endoscopically have a propensity to clog or occlude within 6 months of placement, thus requiring exchange. Expandable metal stents seem to delay stent occlusion, but they are not removable and are more expensive than plastic stents. However, with a limited life span in many patients, metallic stents offer a one-step procedure with excellent palliation. A recent meta-analysis of seven randomized controlled trials confirmed a significantly reduced relative risk of stent occlusion at 4 months for metal compared to plastic stents[45] but reported no significant difference between the two stent types in terms of technical success, therapeutic success, 30-day mortality, or complications. Covered metallic stents that can be removed are now available, and these may offer a further advantage in patients with malignant obstruction and in those with benign strictures for whom surgery carries too high a risk.

INVESTIGATIONS OF THE BILIARY TRACT

Liver ultrasound

This is the imaging technique of choice in the evaluation of jaundice. In acute jaundice, if the clinical history and laboratory tests suggest an obstructive etiology, liver ultrasound should be the first imaging modality and can be considered as the "stethoscope" of the hepatologist. It can demonstrate changes in size and shape of the liver. Fatty changes and fibrosis produce a diffuse increased echogenicity. In established cirrhosis, there may be marginal nodularity of the liver surface and distortion of the arterial vascular architecture. The patency and diameter of the portal and patency of hepatic veins can be evaluated. The sensitivity of abdominal ultrasonography for the detection of biliary obstruction in jaundiced patients ranges from 55% to 91% and the specificity from 82% to 95%. US can demonstrate cholelithiasis and space-occupying lesions in the parenchyma greater than 1 cm in diameter, as well as enlargement of pancreatic head suggestive of carcinoma. The Achilles' heel of the visualization is the very low common bile duct. Ampullary carcinomas are usually too small to be directly visualized, but they can be suspected when a simultaneous dilatation of pancreatic and biliary duct is found without any other abnormality ("double duct sign"). Dilatation of the common biliary duct, which usually indicates biliary tract obstruction, is also common in patients who have undergone previous cholecystectomy. The major advantages of ultrasound are that it is noninvasive, portable, and relatively inexpensive. The major disadvantages are that it is operator dependent, and the images may be difficult to interpret in obese patients or patients with overlying bowel gas.

Computed tomography of the abdomen

This is useful in all hepatobiliary problems and is complementary to US. Pancreatic disease, enlargement of regional lymph nodes, and lesions in the porta hepatis can be visualized. Abdominal computed tomography (CT) permits accurate measurements of the caliber of the biliary tree. Using spiral (helical) CT and the multidetector channel row (MDCT) scanner technology, with a single breath-hold multiple thin slices can be obtained and reconstructed by a computer analysis program, giving very high quality images. Recently for the detection of choledocholithiasis, sensitivities of 88% to 96% and specificities of 92% to 96% have been reported.[46] Moreover helical CT improves diagnostic accuracy in relation to space-occupying lesions of the liver: it involves rapid acquisition of a volume of data during or immediately after intravenous contrast injection. Data can thus be acquired in both arterial and portal phases of enhancement, enabling more precise characterization of a lesion and its vascular supply. It remains the main imaging technique for the study of the liver, including screening for focal lesions, as it can detect nodules as small as 5 mm, differentiating benign masses from malignant and helping in staging hepatocellular carcinoma (HCC) in patients undergoing hepatic resection. In the case of cholangiocarcinoma, accuracies for arterial, portal, and biliary involvement of 92.7%, 85.5%, and 84% have been reported.[47]

CT is not as operator dependent as US and provides technically superior images in obese patients in whom the biliary tree is obscured by bowel gas. CT is not as accurate as US in detecting cholelithiasis, because only calcified stones can be seen clearly. Other considerations in the use of abdominal CT in patients with jaundice are its lack of portability, requirement for intravenous contrast, and expense.

Magnetic resonance imaging

MRI is a very useful investigation of hepatobiliary disease, especially in diagnosing and staging malignant disease. Alteration in weighting of the image leads to prominence of the ductal system in the biliary tree and pancreas, known as magnetic resonance cholangiopancreatography (MRCP). The basic principle of MRCP is to utilize T2-weighted images in which stationary or slowly moving fluid, including bile, has high signal intensity and all surrounding tissues including retroperitoneal fat and solid visceral organs are lower in signal. MRCP provides detail of the liver parenchyma and biliary tree; it can be employed when there are contraindications to percutaneous cholangiography (PTC) or ERCP, if therapeutic intervention is unlikely to be required, or as a first imaging test when there is a previous biliary-enteric or Billroth II anastomosis. MRCP has 95% sensitivity for detecting biliary obstruction, though it is inaccurate in assessing the grade of obstruction. Similarly, strictures cannot be well characterized due to a signal dropout. Its accuracy is equal to ERCP in determining the level of obstruction and whether it is due to a neoplastic process. Unlike PTC or ERCP, MRCP enables the biliary tract to be visualized above and below a complete obstruction. MRCP has an advantage over ERCP in being noninterventional and nonoperator dependent, and it does not require contrast injection, although unlike ERCP it is purely diagnostic. MRCP has already replaced direct diagnostic cholangiography in many clinical circumstances, but PTC and ERCP remain the tests of choice when a therapeutic intervention is necessary. MRCP has proved to be a useful tool for diagnosis of primary sclerosing cholangitis (PSC), with reported sensitivity of 83% and specificity of 98%,[8] and it can also provide information about the periductal tissue, allowing for a single modality to provide both diagnosis of PSC and screening for cholangiocarcinoma. Because of its lack of complications compared to ERCP, MRCP is the diagnostic treatment of choice, particularly for older patients who may have relative contraindications to ERCP.

Endoscopic ultrasound

Endoscopic ultrasonography (EUS) combines endoscopy with real-time, high-resolution ultrasound. Unlike transabdominal ultrasonography (US), it provides excellent sonographic visualization of the extrahepatic biliary tree without interference of bowel gas. After conscious sedation, the echoendoscope is placed in the duodenum and the extrahepatic biliary tract is scanned from the duodenum upon instrument withdrawal.

EUS is superior to US and CT for diagnosing bile duct stones.[48] Prospective studies have supported the accuracy of EUS compared to ERCP in the diagnosis of pancreatic and biliary conditions. In highly experienced hands, EUS has been found to be more sensitive than ERCP for choledocholithiasis.[49] The principal limitations of EUS are that it is an invasive procedure, its results are highly operator dependent, and procedure is not widely available in clinical practice. In addition, pathology identified at the time of EUS may require a subsequent therapeutic ERCP. Compared to high-resolution MRCP (using slice thickness <5 mm) in detecting bile duct stones, good-quality studies report that sensitivity of MRCP and EUS were 87% and 90%, respectively, and specificity was 95% and 99%, respectively (i.e., no significant difference).[50] Thus, MRCP should be the first-line investigation for common bile duct calculi because it is a noninvasive technique that does not require sedation nor admission to hospitals, and EUS should be performed when MRCP is negative in patients with moderate or high pretest probability. These would be patients with previous episodes of cholangitis and increased cholestatic tests.

Evidence comparing MRCP to EUS in the diagnosis of malignant strictures showed a lower sensitivity but a higher specificity for EUS being 80% and 90% and 80% and 65%, respectively.[44]

The failure rate of EUS (2.3%) is lower than that of ERCP (8.3%).[51] Morbidity rate of EUS is between 0 to 8% including complications like hypoxia resulting from sedation, transient abdominal pain, acute pancreatitis, and delayed bleeding; the mortality rate is zero.[52–54]

Endoscopic retrograde cholangiopancreatography

Previously (before MRCP) this was the gold standard investigation for the visualization of the biliary tree as well as the pancreatic ducts. The technique involves the passage of an endoscope into the second part of the duodenum and cannulation of the ampulla; contrast material is then injected into both systems, and the patient is screened radiologically. In experienced hands, this procedure is successful in demonstrating the intra- and extrahepatic biliary tree in 95% of cases. In comparison with abdominal US, CT, and MRCP, ERCP is more invasive and requires conscious sedation.

It is highly accurate for the diagnosis of biliary obstruction, with a sensitivity of 89% to 98% and specificity of 89% to 100%. In addition to providing radiographic images, other diagnostic and therapeutic procedures can be carried out in the same session:

- Common bile duct stones can be removed after balloon dilatation (if small) or after a diathermy cut to the sphincter has been performed to facilitate their withdrawal. Sphincterotomy has a complication rate of 8% to 12%: acute pancreatitis in 5% of cases, severe hemorrhage in 2%, with an overall mortality of 0.5% to 1%.[55] These complications are reduced in experienced hands and with the initial use of biliary stents or nasobiliary stents, particularly in septic patients. Endoscopic balloon dilatation preserves biliary sphincter function and is safer in terms of bleeding.
- The biliary system can be drained by passing a tube (stent) through an obstruction or placement of a nasobiliary drain.
- Biopsy specimens and brushing for cytologic study can be obtained.

Percutaneous cholangiography

This is a procedure that complements ERCP. Contraindications are as for liver biopsy. Under a local anesthetic, a fine flexible needle is passed into the liver. Contrast is injected slowly until a biliary radicle is identified and then further contrast agent is injected to outline the whole of the biliary tree. In the presence of obstruction, bile can be aspirated and a guidewire can be passed to allow stenting.

Its sensitivity (98% to 100%) and specificity (89% to 100%) are comparable with those of ERCP. In difficult cases, the two techniques are sometimes combined, with PTC showing the biliary anatomy above the obstruction and ERCP showing the more distal anatomy. It is the procedure of choice if there is a high obstruction proximal to the common hepatic duct when interventional procedures are needed, such as balloon dilatation and stent placement to relieve obstruction of the biliary tree, and also when altered anatomy precludes ERCP. PTC may be technically difficult in the absence of dilatation of the intrahepatic bile ducts. The rates of morbidity (3%) and mortality (0.2%) are similar to those for ERCP and are due to major complications: biliary leakage, sepsis, perforation, and bleeding.

KEY POINTS

Biliary Tract Diseases

- Jaundice is clinically evident when the bilirubin concentration exceeds 50 mol/L.
- A careful history, physical examination, and review of the standard laboratory tests should allow a physician to make an accurate diagnosis in 85% of cases.
- In acute jaundice, liver ultrasound should be the first imaging modality, particularly in elderly people.
- If there is any evidence of biliary obstruction and a therapeutic intervention is planned, ERCP or PTC are the investigations of choice.
- MRCP should follow ultrasound if this has been technically difficult, obstruction has not been ruled out, or therapeutic intervention is not needed.
- Liver biopsy is needed to confirm the presence, cause, and severity of chronic liver disease.

For a complete list of references, please visit online only at www.expertconsult.com

CHAPTER 80

The Small Bowel

Christopher A. Rodrigues

Diseases of the small bowel can be divided into two categories for clinical purposes. Diffuse processes such as celiac disease result in the malabsorption syndrome, whereas discrete diseases like small bowel tumors produce focal manifestations. Some conditions like Crohn's disease and radiation enteritis can cause a combination of malabsorption and focal features. Malabsorption in elderly people is not due to aging alone, as the absorption of most nutrients is unaffected with a few exceptions. Lactose malabsorption is common in otherwise healthy elderly individuals[1,2] and can coexist with other diffuse small bowel diseases. Calcium absorption declines with age because of a higher prevalence of vitamin D deficiency[3] Lastly, atrophic gastritis is more common in elderly people and can adversely affect the absorption of vitamin B_{12} and folic acid. Food-cobalamin malabsorption, the impaired release of the vitamin B_{12} from food, is due to reduced or absent gastric acid secretion or to the use of acid-suppressing drugs. This is the most common cause of B_{12} deficiency in elderly people,[4] pernicious anemica and terminal ileal disease/resection being much rarer. Folic acid absorption in the proximal jejunum is also pH dependent and declines with achlorhydria. However, jejunal bacterial overgrowth, another consequence of achlorhydria, can compensate for reduced absorption of the vitamin because of bacterial folate synthesis[5] Three conditions account for most cases of malabsorption in older individuals: bacterial overgrowth syndrome, celiac disease, and chronic pancreatitis (the latter is actually maldigestion resulting in malabsorption).

Steatorrhea, the typical symptom of fat malabsorption, is much less likely to occur in elderly patients who may even be constipated despite an increased stool volume. Carbohydrate malabsorption can cause watery diarrhea, abdominal distention, borborygmi, and flatulence. These symptoms are due to the action of bacteria on carbohydrate residues in the colon. The clinical presentation of malabsorption in elderly people is nonspecific. It consists of a variable combination of the following: fatigue, poor mobility, anorexia, nausea, diarrhea, anemia, weight loss, depression, and confusion.[6,7] Peripheral edema may result from hypoproteinemia. Vague generalized body ache and muscle weakness can be early clinical indicators of osteomalacia. Vitamin K deficiency may cause bruising, petechiae, and bleeding manifestations. Abdominal discomfort and distention are common, but abdominal pain is relatively rare. Recurrent abdominal pain occurs with chronic pancreatitis, inflammation as in Crohn's disease, subacute obstruction as a result of strictures, or chronic mesenteric ischemia.

The diagnosis of malabsorption should therefore be considered in elderly patients with clinical and anthropometric evidence of undernutrition, even in the absence of gastrointestinal symptoms. A dietary assessment is important in determining whether the malnutrition can reasonably be attributed to inadequate nutrient intake. The details of previous surgical procedures should be ascertained: gastric surgery or intestinal bypass procedures can result in the bacterial overgrowth syndrome, and extensive small bowel resection can cause malabsorption because of a critical reduction in the mucosal absorptive surface area.

INVESTIGATION OF SMALL BOWEL DISORDERS

Screening tests

Routine blood tests are often helpful in the diagnosis of small bowel disease. The full blood count and blood film may show anemia with macrocytosis, an iron deficient picture, or a dimorphic film. Macrocytosis, leukopenia, and thrombocytopenia suggest megaloblastic anemia. Ferritin, vitamin B_{12}, and red cell folate levels should be measured in patients with suspected malabsorption, even with a normal blood film, as typical changes may not be present in early deficiency. B_{12} deficiency should be further investigated with serologic tests for pernicious anemia (gastric parietal cell and intrinsic factor antibodies), celiac disease (discussed later, a rare cause of isolated B_{12} deficiency), and, if necessary, radiologic or endoscopic evaluation of the terminal ileum. A low B_{12} with a normal or increased red cell folate raises the possibility of small bowel bacterial overgrowth. Howell–Jolly bodies in the blood film indicate splenic atrophy, which occurs in association with celiac disease. Osteomalacia results in a raised alkaline phosphatase with low calcium and phosphate levels and is confirmed by a low serum 25-hydroxycholecaliferol. Vitamin K deficiency prolongs the international normalized ratio (INR). Hypoalbuminemia is a common though nonspecific finding, as it also occurs with poor dietary intake, injury, sepsis, and malignancy. Malabsorption is unlikely if these screening tests are completely normal.

Tests of absorption

Tests of nutrient absorption such as fecal fat estimation and xylose absorption are no longer used in clinical practice: they are cumbersome to perform, unpopular with patients and professionals, and relatively insensitive, often giving equivocal results. Furthermore, these tests provide no information about the underlying disease process. Lactose absorption is the only nutrient absorption test that is widely used.[8] In the standard lactose tolerance test, blood glucose levels are measured before, and 30 and 60 minutes after the ingestion of 50 g of lactose. A rise of less than 1.1 mmol/L indicates lactose malabsorption, and accompanying (transient) symptoms of abdominal bloating, discomfort, diarrhea, and wind are indicative of intolerance. Alternatively, a lactose hydrogen breath test can be used: after an oral dose of 25 to 50 g lactose, end-expiratory breath samples are collected every 30 minutes for 3 hours. Malabsorption of lactose results in fermentation of the sugar by colonic flora, producing a rise in breath hydrogen. This rise can also occur in patients with small bowel bacterial overgrowth, though usually much earlier than in patients with lactose malabsorption. Approximately 25% of patients will have a false negative test, and hence a trial of a lactose-free diet is reasonable if the diagnosis is suspected clinically.

Radiology and endoscopy

Double-contrast barium follow-through examination and enteroclysis (small bowel enema) have been used for many years to investigate the small bowel. Enteroclysis is probably more accurate but is more invasive. The role of abdominal ultrasound, computed tomography (CT) scanning, and magnetic resonance imaging (MRI) is described in the relevant sections.

Esophagogastroduodenoscopy (EGD) is the usual method for collecting fluid for culture and for obtaining biopsies from the distal duodenum. The detection of villous atrophy at endoscopy can be improved by viewing the duodenal mucosal surface at high magnification after spraying with indigo carmine.[9] Wireless capsule endoscopy was introduced in 2000[10] and can provide endoscopic images of the entire small bowel.[11] It consists of a capsule endoscopy system, which is swallowed and propelled by peristalsis, transmitting two images per second to a data recorder worn on a belt. Approximately 50,000 images are recorded over an 8-hour period, by which time the capsule will have reached the cecum in most patients. The images are then downloaded onto a computer workstation and are viewed as a video. Capsule endoscopy is currently used for the investigation of obscure gastrointestinal (GI) bleeding (discussed later), small bowel Crohn's disease, in suspected or refractory malabsorption syndromes (e.g., celiac disease), and in suspected small bowel tumors, including screening in familial polyposis syndromes.[12] The major drawbacks of capsule endoscopy are the inability to take biopsies, incomplete visualization of the mucosal surface, and capsule retention requiring surgical or endoscopic removal (1% to 7%).

Double-balloon enteroscopy (DBE), a technique that can traverse the whole of the small bowel using an enteroscope with an overtube, was first described in 2001. The enteroscope is inserted by either the oral or anal routes, and therapeutic procedures can be carried out.[11,13] General anesthesia is often required for this complex and prolonged technique. The overall diagnostic yield is between 43% and 83% with a subsequent change in management for 57% to 84% of patients. Complications include postprocedural abdominal pain, pancreatitis, bleeding, and small bowel perforation. Push enteroscopy is currently the most widely available technique for endoscopic examination of the small bowel. The instrument can be inserted 30 to 160 cm beyond the ligament of Treitz and has a channel for biopsies and therapeutic procedures including thermocoagulation of bleeding lesions, polypectomy, and placement of feeding jejunostomy tubes. Lastly, intraoperative enteroscopy, in which the small bowel is "pleated" over an endoscope at laparotomy or laparoscopy, is the most accurate technique but has a significant complication rate.

SMALL BOWEL DISEASES

Celiac disease

In celiac disease, sensitivity to dietary gluten in cereals like wheat, barley, and rye leads to a characteristic small bowel mucosal lesion, hyperplastic villous atrophy. The disease affects the proximal small bowel, decreases in severity distally, and may spare the distal jejunum and ileum. The wider use of serologic screening tests has altered our understanding of the epidemiology of the disease. It appears to be much more common than previously appreciated with current prevalence rates of approximately 1%.[14,15] Only 30% to 40% of patients are symptomatic, the rest have clinically silent disease. This variable clinical picture is probably related to the extent of affected bowel. Currently 60% of newly diagnosed patients are adults[16] with a peak incidence in the third decade and a second smaller peak in the fifth and sixth decades.[17] In a recent multicenter Italian study, only 60 (4.4%) of 1353 patients with celiac disease were over 65 years at diagnosis.[18] However, the seroprevalence of celiac disease in an English population of 7257 people aged 45 to 76 years was 1.2% with no significant difference between those under and over 65 years of age.[19] In a Finnish population-based study of 2815 individuals, the prevalence of celiac disease in those aged 52 to 74 years was 2.13%, double that in younger adults.[20] The female to male ratio in adults is approximately 2:1, and this is no different in elderly patients.[18,19]

Many elderly patients, like adults with celiac disease, are either asymptomatic or have trivial or nonspecific symptoms. However, in the Italian study referred to previously, 77% of patients over the age of 65 years presented with diarrhea and approximately 60% had weight loss and anemia.[18] Despite these typical features, the diagnosis was only made after a mean interval of 17 years in this group. Celiac disease should be considered in patients with unexplained anemia, macrocytosis, or evidence of splenic atrophy on the blood film even in the absence of diarrhea or steatorrhea. Folate deficiency is the most common cause of anemia, but malabsorption of iron or vitamin B_{12} can occur. Osteoporosis[21] and osteomalacia are common in untreated celiac disease, particularly in elderly patients.

Celiac disease is associated with a number of autoimmune conditions, the most important being insulin-dependent diabetes mellitus, autoimmune thyroid disease, Sjögren's syndrome, autoimmune hepatitis, primary biliary cirrhosis, and Addison's disease.[14,15,17,22] Dermatitis herpetiformis can be regarded as an extraintestinal manifestation of celiac disease as virtually all patients have an enteropathy with characteristic histologic changes. Neurologic disorders such as epilepsy, cerebellar syndrome, dementia, peripheral neuropathy, myopathy, and hyporeflexia have been reported in celiac disease.[23] IgA deficiency affects 2% to 3% of patients with celiac disease and can result in false-negative serologic tests. From 90% to 95% of celiac patients have the HLA class 2 molecule DQ2, and most of the remainder have DQ8. At least 1 in 10 first-degree relatives are affected.[15]

DIAGNOSIS

Serologic markers are now used routinely for screening patients and high-risk groups with associated disorders or a positive family history. IgA endomysial antibody (EMA) has a specificity of over 98% but antibody to IgA tissue transglutaminase (tTGA) is also very accurate and is a simpler and cheaper test.[14,22,24] Patients with an absent tTGA or those in whom there is a strong clinical suspicion of celiac disease should have an IgA level to exclude deficiency—this is routinely carried out by some laboratories. If IgA deficiency is present, tests for IgG tTGA or EMA should be carried out. Patients with positive serology should undergo an EGD in order to take three to four distal duodenal biopsies.[25] The typical histologic features of celiac disease are villous atrophy, crypt hyperplasia, intraepithelial lymphocytosis, and a lymphoplasmacytic infiltrate in the lamina propria. These changes, accompanied by a clinical response to a gluten-free diet, are adequate to establish the diagnosis.[22,26] Antibody titers can decrease or disappear with treatment, but this is not a reliable marker of histologic remission.[27,28] A repeat biopsy to confirm histologic remission is required only in asymptomatic patients or in those with an equivocal clinical response. Rebiopsy after a gluten challenge is rarely carried out now but may be required in cases where there is diagnostic difficulty, such as when the original biopsy was taken on a gluten-free diet. The absence of HLA DQ2 and DQ8 virtually excludes the diagnosis and is useful when the patient does not wish to undergo a gluten challenge. Lastly, 5% to 10% of patients have serology-negative disease, and thus histologic confirmation should be undertaken if the likelihood of celiac disease is high (e.g., in symptomatic patients with a positive family history).

MANAGEMENT

Most elderly patients respond to a well-balanced gluten-free diet and cope well with the change in lifelong eating habits. It is now generally accepted that patients can take a moderate amount of oats provided it is not contaminated with wheat gluten. Lactose intolerance can cause apparently resistant disease in some patients. However, milk and milk products are an important source of calcium and should be restricted only if they exacerbate symptoms—ideally after confirming the diagnosis with an objective test. Patients should receive supplements to correct nutrient deficiencies, as complete recovery of mucosal function can take months. Elderly patients with celiac disease should be given multivitamins and a calcium supplement initially. All patients with celiac disease should see a dietician, should be encouraged to join a patient support organization, and should have regular clinical follow-up.[14,15] Bone mineral densitometry should be carried out at diagnosis in all elderly patients with celiac disease. Bone mass improves, but does not normalize, in adult and elderly patients on a gluten-free diet, and other therapeutic measures are often required.[21] Approximately 5% of patients fail to respond to gluten withdrawal or relapse after an initial remission.[14,29,30] Some patients with refractory disease respond to corticosteroids or immunosuppressive agents. Others (a proportion of whom have small intestinal ulcers and strictures: ulcerative enteritis) have a cryptic T-cell lymphoma of the intraepithelial lymphocytes[31] with 5-year survival rates of less than 50%.[14] Patients with ulcerative enteritis often require surgery for complications such as perforation or obstruction.

NEOPLASMS

The two-fold increase in mortality in the first year after diagnosis is largely due to the development of malignant complications.[32] The overall risk of malignancy is less than previously reported[33] and is approximately 30% greater than that of the general population.[32] T-cell lymphoma of the small intestine is the most common tumor,[34–36] but there is an increased risk of developing squamous cell carcinomas of the esophagus, mouth, pharynx, adenocarcinoma of the small bowel, and colorectal carcinoma. The incidence of breast[32,35] and lung cancer[32] is decreased. Lymphoma may be the first manifestation of celiac disease, but the diagnosis should also be considered in established patients whose condition is either resistant to, or relapses on, a strict gluten-free diet. Weight loss is the most common symptom, and patients also experience profound lethargy, muscle weakness, abdominal pain, and diarrhea. The prognosis is poor: less than a fifth of patients survive for 30 months.[37] A gluten-free diet has a protective effect against the development of malignancy in celiac disease.[33,35,36]

Bacterial overgrowth syndrome

Intestinal bacterial counts normally increase abnormally and bacterial populations vary in different sections of the gastrointestinal tract: the jejunum is colonized by gram-positive aerobes and facultative anaerobes, ileal flora contain some strict anaerobes as well, and the colon is heavily populated by predominantly anaerobic bacteria.[38] Malabsorption can occur when the small bowel population increases and becomes more anaerobic. This is partly the result of direct injury to the intestinal mucosa, but uptake or binding of major nutrients and vitamin B_{12} by the proliferating bacteria also play a part.[39] In addition, fat absorption is affected by deconjugation of bile salts by anaerobic bacteria, resulting in impaired micelle formation. Folic acid and vitamin K are synthesized by bacteria, and folate levels are often normal or raised when bacterial overgrowth is present. Two factors are largely responsible for regulating bacterial growth: gastric acid and intestinal motility.[38,39] Gastric acid destroys microorganisms ingested with food and saliva. The interdigestive migrating motor complex, a cyclic fasting motility pattern, regularly propels luminal contents toward the colon, thus preventing stagnation and bacterial overgrowth.[40]

PATHOGENESIS

The classic disorders associated with bacterial overgrowth are those in which disordered intestinal motility, abnormal reservoirs, or abnormal communications between the proximal and distal intestine result in proliferation of bacteria. Examples of the former are diabetic autonomic neuropathy, late radiation enteropathy, collagen diseases such as scleroderma, and the numerous causes of chronic intestinal pseudo-obstruction. Partial small bowel obstruction due to strictures or adhesions has a similar effect. Abnormal reservoirs that permit stagnation of luminal contents may arise de novo—for example, small bowel diverticula—or as a result of surgery (e.g., the afferent limb of a Billroth II gastrectomy). Abnormal communications between the proximal and distal intestine result in contamination of the former by denser, more anaerobic bacterial populations. Examples of this group include gastrocolic and jejunocolic fistulas, right hemicolectomy with resection of the ileocecal valve, and surgical bypass of obstructed or diseased intestinal segments. Small bowel bacterial overgrowth in elderly people also occurs under conditions that impair gastric acid secretion, such as atrophic gastritis,[39,41] treatment with acid-reducing drugs,[42–44] or after surgery for peptic ulcer disease. Gut immune defenses may be impaired in elderly people and thus contribute to their susceptibility to overgrowth.[45]

CLINICAL PICTURE

Elderly patients who have bacterial overgrowth with malabsorption typically present with diarrhea, weight loss, and abdominal bloating associated with hypoalbuminemia and low B_{12} levels. Some anatomic abnormalities associated with bacterial overgrowth (e.g., small bowel diverticula) are more common with increasing age. Most patients who had surgery for peptic ulcer disease before the widespread use of proton pump inhibitors are now elderly. Bacterial overgrowth is thus more common in elderly people and is found in 52.5% to 70.8% of patients with symptoms of malabsorption.[6,44,46] It also affects 14.5% to 25.6% of elderly people with no gastrointestinal symptoms.[43,47–49] Some of these individuals are on acid-suppressing medication,[43] others have factors that are associated with slower small bowel transit: reduced intake of dietary fiber[43] and physical disability.[49] Subclinical malabsorption is probably present in a proportion who have low albumin and B_{12} levels, and this may also adversely affect bone mineral density.[50]

DIAGNOSIS

The literature on bacterial overgrowth is plagued by the absence of a reliable diagnostic test. Historically, culture of proximal small bowel aspirate (currently usually obtained during EGD) was the gold standard for establishing the diagnosis: proximal jejunal counts greater than 10^5 colony-forming units (cfu)/mL were accepted as abnormal.[38] Although this is probably true for postsurgical patients with blind loops, jejunal bacterial counts in healthy individuals are much lower, in the range of 0 to 10^3 cfu/mL, and a recent systematic review has found no evidence to support culture as a gold standard test.[51] Furthermore, this technique only samples a limited region of the small bowel and may miss overgrowth in the more distal segments. Breath tests were developed as an alternative to the invasive procedure and cumbersome culture techniques were involved.[51,52] However, these tests were largely validated against culture, which raises serious doubts about their reliability.

In the [^{14}C] glycocholate breath test, 5 to 10 μCi of glycocholic acid, a conjugated bile acid radiolabeled with ^{14}C is administered with a test meal. Bacterial deconjugation results in separation of [^{14}C]glycine from cholic acid, and $^{14}CO_2$ produced from the former is measured in breath samples collected over the next 4 to 8 hours. Terminal ileal disease or resection also results in a positive test because the bile acid is not reabsorbed and is then metabolized by colonic flora. The test has largely been abandoned because of its poor sensitivity with a false negative rate of 30% to 40%.

Breath hydrogen measurement after ingestion of 50 to 80 g of glucose or 10 to 12 g of lactulose is an alternative technique that avoids the use of a radioisotope. Metabolism of either carbohydrate by the abnormal bacterial population produces hydrogen, which can be detected by breath testing. The timing of the hydrogen rise is crucial for the lactulose test, as this sugar is not absorbed in the small bowel and produces a second, higher "colonic" hydrogen peak. It is not possible to reliably distinguish the peak produced by small bowel bacterial overgrowth from that due to normal colonic flora without using an oral contrast medium as well. Glucose is thus a better substrate as it is absorbed completely in the proximal small bowel. Furthermore, a small study in healthy volunteers has shown that even a 10-g quantity of lactulose accelerates small bowel transit,[53] and hence the glucose–hydrogen breath test is probably more reliable. Approximately 15% of individuals are colonized by colonic flora, which produce methane, not hydrogen, and false negative tests will occur unless breath methane and hydrogen are both measured.[52] In the [^{14}C]xylose breath test, elevated $^{14}CO_2$ levels appear in breath samples within 60 minutes of taking 10 μCi of [^{14}C]xylose with 1 g of unlabeled xylose by mouth. Although the sensitivities and specificities of breath tests are variable, even when compared against culture, they are simple to perform and are probably useful if positive. Until a better test for bacterial overgrowth becomes available the most practical strategy would be to test, treat, and then retest, in addition to evaluating the clinical response.[51] Patients with confirmed overgrowth should have a small bowel x-ray series to look for abnormal communications or reservoirs.

MANAGEMENT

The conditions underlying bacterial overgrowth (with the exception of strictures and some enteroenteric fistulas) are rarely amenable to surgical correction, and hence antibiotics are the mainstay of treatment.[39] Tetracycline was traditionally used to reduce bacterial flora, but about two thirds of patients do not benefit from this drug. Chloromycetin and clindamycin are rarely used now because of their toxicity. Co-amoxiclav and norfloxacin are effective in standard doses given for 7 to 10 days, as is metronidazole in combination with one of the cephalosporins.[54,55] Rifamixin is also effective and systemic toxicity does not occur, as the drug is not absorbed.[56] In some patients, a single antibiotic course produces a satisfactory response lasting for months, but many patients need cyclic courses given at monthly intervals for 4 to 6 months. Octreotide, a long-acting analogue of somatostatin, has been tested in small numbers of patients with connective tissue diseases and chronic intestinal pseudo-obstruction. It improves motility and appears to be highly effective on its own[57] or in combination with erythromycin.[58]

Prokinetic agents (including erythromycin) may play a role in the management of bacterial overgrowth, particularly in elderly patients with prolonged small bowel transit. Probiotics may also be helpful, but further work is required to define their role. Clinicians should avoid using acid-suppressing agents in elderly people without a clear indication: apart from their possible role in promoting clinically significant bacterial overgrowth, these drugs can cause food-cobalamin malabsorption and are implicated in an increased susceptibility to *Clostridium difficile* infection.

Crohn's disease

Crohn's disease is an idiopathic chronic relapsing disorder, characterized by transmural inflammation and ulceration, occurring in a segmental distribution. Intestinal ulceration ranges from aphthoid erosions to deep fissures, and the course is often complicated by the formation of strictures, abscesses, and fistulas. The disease has a predilection for the terminal ileum, but any region of the GI tract can be affected. The Vienna classification groups patients according to clinical phenotype including disease behavior and location.[59] The majority of patients (70%) initially have nonstricturing and nonpenetrating disease, approximately 17% have strictures, and 13% present with penetrating disease (i.e., fistulas or abscesses).[60] At diagnosis approximately 28% of patients have terminal ileal involvement only, 50% have ileocolic disease, and 25% colonic disease alone.[61] Small bowel disease is less common in older people.[62] In a recent series from northern France, 34% of patients over the age of 60 years had small bowel involvement compared to 64% of younger patients.[63]

Crohn's disease predominantly affects teenagers and young adults with a second smaller peak from the sixth to the eighth decades. Recent studies, however, have not described this bimodal pattern consistently.[64,65] Nevertheless, a substantial minority of patients with Crohn's disease first present in later life, and the numbers of affected elderly people will also increase because of longer life expectancy. In the French study quoted earlier, 24% of patients were diagnosed with Crohn's disease at or above the age of 60 years.[63] In another population-based study from Belgium, 23 of 137 patients (17%) were over the age of 60 years at diagnosis with an annual incidence of 3.5 per 100,000 (4.8 per 100,000 in patients under 60 years).[66] Smoking, a family history of inflammatory bowel disease, and (in most studies) previous appendicectomy are risk factors for Crohn's disease.[65]

CLINICAL PICTURE AND INVESTIGATIONS

The clinical features of Crohn's disease, including the extraintestinal manifestations, are no different in elderly patients. Diarrhea is the main symptom, but right iliac fossa pain, fever, and an abdominal mass are typical features. Stricture formation can lead to subacute or acute bolus obstruction, and fistulas to a wide variety of manifestations. Ileocecal Crohn's disease can mimic acute appendicitis or an appendiceal abscess; the differential diagnosis in older patients includes cecal diverticulitis, colonic carcinoma, and small bowel ischemia. Gastrointestinal infections, smoking, and nonsteroidal anti-inflammatory drugs can all precipitate relapse. There is no single definitive test for Crohn's disease.[67] The diagnosis is established (and disease activity assessed) by clinical features, inflammatory markers, endoscopic, or radiologic imaging and histology. Standard activity indices, incorporating some of these features (Crohn's disease activity index [CDAI], Harvey-Bradshaw Index) are used in trials but can also be helpful in clinical practice (e.g., in assessing patients for therapy with antitumor necrosis factor [TNF] agents).[68] For example, a CDAI of <150 is used to define remission, and severe disease is characterized by a score of >450.[68,69]

A discussion of investigative techniques used in small bowel Crohn's disease inevitably overlaps with the investigation of colonic disease. In practice, ileocolonoscopy will probably be the initial investigation of choice. Only a short segment of terminal ileum is examined at colonoscopy, and hence either a double-contrast barium follow-through or enteroclysis is traditionally used to define the extent and severity of small bowel disease. Advances in magnetic resonance imaging (MRI) (including MR enteroclysis) have resulted in improved small bowel visualization,[61,70,71] including the ability to distinguish between inflammatory and fibrotic strictures. MRI has the advantage of not using ionizing radiation and is likely to replace barium studies. CT and ultrasound imaging have been used for many years in Crohn's disease to outline phlegmons (inflammatory masses) and abscess cavities and to drain the latter percutaneously. Technical advances have extended the range of both these modalities. Ultrasound is now also employed to image the bowel wall and detect strictures. Contrast-enhanced examinations with multislice helical CT scanners have high sensitivity (71% to 83%) and specificity (90% to 98%) in the evaluation of small bowel inflammation.[71] As stated previously, wireless capsule endoscopy can provide endoscopic images of the entire small bowel.[11,61,71] In a meta-analysis of its use in nonstricturing small bowel Crohn's disease, the diagnostic yield was significantly better than other modalities for recurrent disease but not in a suspected initial presentation.[72] Push enteroscopy is rarely used in Crohn's disease, as the terminal ileum is not visualized with this technique. Double balloon enteroscopy can be used to take biopsies and do therapeutic procedures such as dilation of strictures.[1,13,61,71]

MANAGEMENT

Detailed guidelines (including a series of Cochrane reviews) usually discuss management under two headings: the induction of remission and the maintenance of remission.[6,73–75] The medical management of elderly patients with Crohn's disease is essentially the same as that in younger patients.[64] However, particular caution is required when using corticosteroids, immunosuppressive agents, and biologic drugs in this age group.

Sulfasalazine is not effective in small bowel Crohn's disease without colonic involvement. Mesalamine preparations coated with a pH-sensitive resin or in ethylcellulose-coated granules start releasing the drug in the small bowel. However, recent meta-analyses have shown that mesalamine is little better than placebo for induction of remission,[76] and the drug is ineffective for maintenance of medically induced remission.[77] Mesalamine only has a role in reducing the relapse rate after surgical resection.[78] Budesonide (9 mg daily), a topically active steroid with extensive first-pass metabolism in the liver, is recommended for mild/moderate localized ileocecal disease. Budesonide has a better side-effect profile compared to other corticosteroids and does not result in osteoporosis. Prednisolone (40 to 60 mg/day up to 1 mg/kg body weight) is used for severe ileocecal disease and for extensive small bowel disease: over 80% of patients go into remission or have a partial response by 4 weeks. However, corticosteroids cause many side effects. At 1 year only 32% of patients will have had a prolonged response, 28% become steroid-dependent (i.e., require at least 10 mg/day of prednisolone or budesonide 3 mg/day to prevent recurrence), and 38% require surgery.[79] Steroids have no role in maintaining remission in Crohn's disease, although budesonide may delay relapse.

Immunosuppressive agents such as azathioprine (2 to 2.5 mg/kg), 6-mercaptopurine (1 to 1.5 mg/kg), and methotrexate (15 to 25 mg im/sc weekly with folic acid) are used as steroid-sparing agents. They are effective in maintaining remission and may need to be taken long term. They should be used cautiously in elderly patients given their potential for serious toxicity, although, in clinical trials, 6-mercaptopurine has been tolerated by patients in the seventh decade as well as their younger counterparts.[80] Antibiotics, including antimycobacterial agents, are not effective as primary therapy for small bowel Crohn's disease although the former will be required for septic complications associated with penetrating disease. Monoclonal antibodies against TNF alpha (infliximab, adalimumab, certolizumab) are used in refractory disease, in patients who are intolerant to conventional treatment, for maintenance of remission, for fistulating disease, and for some extraintestinal manifestations.[81] These drugs are expensive and significant adverse effects have been reported including reactivation of tuberculosis, serious infections, optic neuritis, infusion reactions, and a possible increased risk of developing lymphoma. They increase mortality, in patients with class 3 to 4 congestive cardiac failure and are therefore contraindicated in this group.

Malnutrition is common in small bowel Crohn's disease and is due to a variable combination of reduced nutrient intake, malabsorption, and increased energy requirements resulting from inflammation, sepsis, or surgery. In most patients, nutrient intake can be increased by using small, frequent, low-fiber meals and supplementary polymeric sip feeds. Some patients benefit from tube feeding, and a few need parenteral nutrition. Enteral nutrition, with either elemental or polymeric diets, can also be used as a primary treatment for Crohn's disease but is less effective than corticosteroid treatment[82] and is also less acceptable to patients, despite the absence of side effects.

Patients with Crohn's disease are prone to osteopenia and osteoporosis. Bone loss occurs with corticosteroid use, as a direct result of the inflammatory process and also because of malabsorption of calcium and vitamin D in patients with extensive small bowel disease. Reduced bone mineral density is associated with low body mass index, male sex, long-standing disease, ileal resection, and active disease. Comprehensive guidelines for the prevention and management of osteoporosis in inflammatory bowel disease have been published.[21]

Surgery is required for obstruction as a result of strictures, for suppurative complications, and for disease that is refractory to medical treatment. Elderly patients usually tolerate surgery well. Although postoperative hospital stays are longer because of comorbidity, rates of mortality and of surgical complications are similar to those in younger patients.[83] Adenocarcinoma of the small bowel can complicate small bowel Crohn's disease. The risk of malignancy is higher in patients with disease confined to the small bowel than in ileocolic disease.[84] Patients with Crohn's disease also have a higher relative risk of developing colorectal cancer, lymphoma, and some extraintestinal malignancies.[84]

Small bowel ischemia

Small bowel ischemia can be acute or chronic and of arterial or venous origin. Arterial ischemia predominantly affects middle-aged and elderly people. Mesenteric vein thrombosis accounts for 5% to 10% of patients with acute mesenteric ischemia. It affects a younger cohort of patients (mean age 48 to 60 years) and will therefore not be discussed further.

Acute arterial mesenteric ischemia[85–87]

Acute arterial mesenteric ischemia is due to embolism, thrombus formation, or nonocclusive ischemia of the superior mesenteric artery (SMA) or its territory. Complete occlusion of the SMA, which supplies the jejunum, the ileum, and the right half of the colon, has catastrophic effects. Patients who survive frequently require long-term nutritional support and may need parenteral nutrition depending on the length of residual jejunum. Embolism accounts for 40% to 50% of cases and usually occurs in elderly people with predisposing causes such as atrial fibrillation, left-sided cardiac chamber enlargement, or myocardial infarction. Nonocclusive mesenteric ischemia occurs in 20% to 30% of cases and is due to vasoconstriction of the mesenteric circulation following a low-output state or circulatory collapse, for example, severe congestive cardiac failure (CCF), hypotension, cardiac arrhythmias or following cardiac arrest. Thrombosis (20% to 30%) occurs in the setting of widespread vascular disease, and 20% to 50% of patients have a history of abdominal angina in the preceding weeks to months.

DIAGNOSIS

Patients present with severe abdominal pain, but physical examination is initially either normal or reveals only tenderness. This disparity between symptoms and physical signs in an elderly patient with cardiovascular disease or a hypercoagulable state should alert the clinician to the possibility of mesenteric ischemia. Signs of peritonitis, hypotension, vomiting, fever, dark or bright red rectal bleeding, increasing distention, leukocytosis, and metabolic acidosis are features of intestinal infarction. Up to 25% of patients have abdominal distention or gastrointestinal bleeding without pain, and about a third of elderly patients may present with an acute confusional state.[88] Leukocytosis and raised serum levels of lactate, amylase, alkaline phosphatase, and phosphate are not reliable markers. Fluid levels, dilated loops of bowel, and "thumbprinting" on plain abdominal films occur in up to a third of patients, but specific radiologic features of infarction such as gas in the intestinal wall or portal vessels are rare. CT scanning is more accurate in delineating these changes, can also demonstrate thrombus in the mesenteric vessels, and is useful in excluding other causes of abdominal pain.[89] Duplex ultrasonography has a limited role, but CT and MR angiography are promising approaches that have a high sensitivity and specificity for pathology in the SMA.[90,91] Patients with abnormal films have a poor prognosis as even nonspecific changes usually signify intestinal necrosis. Mesenteric angiography is the gold standard for establishing the diagnosis and should ideally be performed before signs of infarction appear. It can, however, be difficult to differentiate between acute and long-standing vascular changes on an angiogram, particularly in patients with nonocclusive mesenteric ischemia.

MANAGEMENT

Management warrants aggressive measures in the appropriate patients, and initial resuscitation includes monitoring of central pressures, correction of hypovolemia, and inotropic support. Splanchnic vasoconstrictors, mainly norepinephrine (noradrenaline) and digitalis preparations, should be avoided. Broad-spectrum antibiotics are given empirically to treat the septicemia resulting from bacterial translocation across infarcted bowel. Early angiography is the cornerstone of management, even when the decision to operate has been made. The angiographic catheter is left in situ for two reasons: repeat angiography may be required, and the catheter can be used for intra-arterial infusion of the vasodilator papaverine. This relieves the associated mesenteric arterial spasm and improves perfusion perioperatively. Patients with established signs of infarction need emergency surgery with resection of infarcted bowel and embolectomy, thrombectomy, or arterial reconstruction. A second-look operation is often indicated 12 to 24 hours later to differentiate between viable and nonviable intestine. Full anticoagulation with heparin is controversial but is generally started 48 hours after embolectomy, thrombectomy, and arterial reconstruction. There are many case reports and small case series of successful thrombolytic[87] and endovascular therapy including angioplasty, stenting, and mechanical thrombus fragmentation in patients with SMA embolism or thrombosis.[92,93] These forms of therapy are generally only successful if carried out within 12 hours of presentation. The mortality rate of acute arterial mesenteric ischemia is 70% to 90% if the diagnosis is not made before irreversible infarction occurs. The overall mortality has improved since the late 1960s, probably because of earlier diagnosis and aggressive management with intensive care support. In one systematic review, mortality rates for arterial embolism, arterial thrombosis, and nonocclusive ischemia were 54.1%, 77.4%, and 72.7%, respectively.[94] Focal segmental ischemia causes localized infarction, often at multiple sites, and can be due to vasculitis, cholesterol, or atheromatous emboli and various nonvascular diseases. Management consists of surgical resection of the infarcted segment.

Chronic mesenteric ischemia

The syndrome of abdominal or intestinal angina is a rare condition that develops as a result of atherosclerosis of the splanchnic circulation.[85–87] Mesenteric blood flow fails to meet the increased metabolic demand that occurs after meals, resulting in pain with or without malabsorption and disordered motility. The pain begins within 30 minutes of a meal and gradually increases to a plateau, which lasts for up to 3 hours. It is located in the upper abdomen, can radiate to the back, and is gnawing or cramping in character. It is sometimes relieved by lying prone or squatting. Constipation, diarrhea, steatorrhea, abdominal bloating, and flatulence may also occur. Patients may miss or restrict meals in order to avoid provoking symptoms (sitophobia), and hence lose weight.

DIAGNOSIS

Clinical assessment often reveals evidence of widespread vascular disease. An abdominal systolic bruit may be present but is not a specific finding. Individuals with advanced atherosclerotic disease can have severe stenosis or occlusion of two or even all three main mesenteric arterial trunks and remain asymptomatic. Diagnosis therefore depends on the history as well as on angiographic findings of proximal stenoses in at least two of the main mesenteric trunks, with a collateral circulation indicating chronic ischemia. Occlusion of two vessels is found in over 90%, and three-vessel occlusion in over 50% of patients with chronic mesenteric ischemia.[87] It is important to exclude atypical angina pectoris and other causes of recurrent abdominal pain such as biliary pain due to gallstones and peptic ulcer disease. Duplex ultrasonography, CT, and MR angiography are used to evaluate symptomatic patients before angiography.[95]

MANAGEMENT

Surgical revascularization and percutaneous angioplasty with stenting are the two main therapeutic alternatives, both of which relieve symptoms in most patients. Surgery has higher revascularization rates and lower rates of restenosis or occlusion but also has a higher perioperative morbidity and mortality associated with longer hospital stays. Endovascular therapy is not feasible in all patients but is particularly suitable for those with short segments of disease. The choice of therapy will therefore be made on an individual basis, as many patients will have widespread vascular disease and other comorbidities.[95–97]

Small intestinal neoplasms

Primary small bowel tumors are relatively rare, accounting for only 1% to 2.4% of all gastrointestinal neoplasms.[98] Approximately two thirds of these tumors are malignant, and the small bowel is frequently involved by metastatic disease, particularly metastatic melanoma.

BENIGN TUMORS

Adenomas, leiomyomas, and lipomas are the most common benign tumors. Adenomas have a slight preponderance for the duodenum and ileum; lipomas are more frequent in the ileum. Leiomyomas are distributed more evenly in the small bowel but are more common in the jejunum. More than 50% of benign tumors are asymptomatic; the rest manifest with obstruction, intussusception, or occult bleeding. Adenomas and leiomyomas can undergo malignant transformation and should be removed by surgical resection or, in the case of adenomas, by endoscopic resection. Asymptomatic lipomas discovered incidentally can be left in situ, as malignant transformation is unknown.

MALIGNANT TUMORS

Data from the Surveillance, Epidemiology and End-Results (SEER) program estimated that 6110 American men and women would be diagnosed with small intestinal cancer in 2008, representing a progressive increase since the 1970s. The age-adjusted incidence for 2001–2005 was 2.2 per 100,000 for men and 1.6 per 100,000 for women with a median age of diagnosis of 67 years. The overall 5-year relative survival rate (RSS) for 1996–2004 was 57.8%; 31% of patients had localized disease at diagnosis with a 5-year RSS of 77%, 33% had regional spread (5-year RSS 62.2%), and 29% presented with metastases (5 year RSS 36%).[99] Adenocarcinomas (35% to 50% of tumors), carcinoid tumors (20% to 40%), lymphomas (14% to 18%), and sarcomas (10% to 13%) are the four major histologic types encountered.[98,100]

PRESENTATION AND DIAGNOSIS

Abdominal pain, bleeding, intestinal obstruction, and weight loss are the major manifestations, a palpable abdominal mass being less frequent. Perforation occurs in about 10% of cases, periampullary tumors can present with obstructive jaundice, and diarrhea is more common in patients with lymphoma. With small bowel carcinoids, the carcinoid syndrome, due to the release of serotonin and other vasoactive compounds, causes flushing, telangiectasias, diarrhea, bronchospasm, and, less commonly, right heart failure, but it only occurs when hepatic metastases are present[101,102]; 24-hour urinary 5-hydroxyindoleacetic acid and plasma chromogranin A are appropriate screening tests for carcinoid tumors.

The diagnosis of small bowel malignancy is often delayed because of the nonspecific history and the absence of clinical signs. Enteroclysis is more sensitive than barium follow-through in detecting tumors.[103] Modern multidetector-row CT scanning techniques have significantly improved the detection and staging of these relatively rare tumors.[104] CT scans and barium studies may be normal in patients with small bowel carcinoids, but larger lesions are characterized by fixation, separation, thickening, and angulation with a starburst appearance because of the desmoplastic reaction produced by the tumor. Somatostatin receptor scintigraphy has a sensitivity of up to 90% for detection of the primary tumor and of 61% to 96% for metastases.[101] Wireless capsule endoscopy, push enteroscopy, and DBE have transformed the investigation of small bowel tumors. The proportion of patients in whom the diagnosis is established only at laparotomy has correspondingly decreased.

Adenocarcinoma

The majority (52% to 55%) of adenocarcinomas arise in the duodenum, 18% to 25% in the jejunum, and 13% in the ileum.[105,106] The mean age of presentation is 55 to 65 years. These tumors have a poor prognosis, largely because of late presentation and delayed diagnosis: the overall 5-year survival rate is 26% to 31% with a median survival time of 20 months.[105,106] Surgical resection is curative in the appropriate patients without disseminated disease—usually a Whipple's pancreatoduodenectomy for lesions of the first and second parts of the duodenum and segmental resection for tumors at other sites. Chemotherapy and radiotherapy are not effective.

Carcinoid tumor

The small bowel is the most common site for carcinoid tumors, which are predominantly located in the ileum.[107,108] Duodenal tumors are rare. The mean age of presentation is 64 years, and 40% to 70% of patients will have regional or distant (most commonly hepatic) metastases at diagnosis.[101,108] However, carcinoid tumors grow slowly and are compatible with prolonged survival even with incurable disease. The overall 5-year survival rate is 61%, approximately double that of small bowel adenocarcinoma.[108] Surgical resection is the only curative treatment. When liver metastases are confined to one lobe, curative hepatic resection can also be carried out in patients with the appropriate functional reserve. The postoperative mortality of patients who undergo resection of the primary tumor or hepatic metastases is 6% with a 5-year survival of up to 87%.[101] Resection of the primary tumor and regional lymph nodes is even appropriate in some patients with unresectable hepatic secondaries, as nodal metastases are associated with intense fibrosis and can compromise the vascular supply of the involved small bowel.[101] The 5-year survival rate of patients with hepatic metastases is 18% to 32%.[102] Treatment options for patients with unresectable disease also include the somatostatin analogues octreotide and lanreotide, interferon, hepatic artery embolization, and chemotherapy. The serotonin receptor antagonists, cyproheptadine, and ondansetron are used for symptomatic control of the carcinoid syndrome.

Sarcoma

Gastrointestinal stromal tumors (GISTs) are rare soft tissue sarcomas of mesenchymal origin arising from the gastrointestinal tract.[109,110] These tumors were previously thought to originate from smooth muscle. However, only a minority exhibit the histologic characteristics of true smooth muscle tumors, and most GISTs express the tyrosine kinase growth factor receptor c-KIT, which is detectable by immunostaining for the CD 117 cell surface receptor. They are therefore now usually clearly distinguishable from leiomyomas and leiomyosarcomas. All GISTs have malignant potential, but tumors smaller than 2 cm in diameter can be regarded as essentially benign. The annual incidence is approximately 10 to 15 per million, and 20% to 30% arise from the small bowel. Most GISTs are diagnosed between the ages of 50 and 70 years. The primary treatment is surgical resection. Conventional chemoradiotherapy is not effective but imatinib, a tyrosine kinase inhibitor, can result in a complete or partial long-term response in up to two thirds of patients with unresectable or metastatic disease.[111,112] Leiomyosarcomas are slightly more common in the jejunum compared to the ileum and less than one fifth involve the duodenum. Surgical resection does not usually entail lymph node resection as these tumors rarely metastasize to the regional lymph nodes.[98]

Lymphoma

Most B-cell lymphomas occur in the ileum, whereas the majority of T-cell lymphomas are jejunal.[113,114] One-quarter of B-cell and 50% of T-cell tumors are multifocal with up to 10 lesions. Two thirds of primary small bowel lymphomas are of the B-cell type, the remainder being T-cell in origin.[1] Approximately 50% of T-cell lymphomas are associated with enteropathy, mainly celiac disease. Twenty percent of B-cell lymphomas are low-grade tumors of mucosa-associated lymphoid tissue (MALT lymphomas). Treatment is primarily by surgical resection, but the optimal treatment strategy with adjuvant chemoradiotherapy has not yet been established.[114,115] T-cell tumors have a worse prognosis, with 5-year survival rates of 25% compared to 50% for high-grade and 75% for low-grade B-cell lymphomas, respectively.[113] The overall 5-year survival in a population-based study of 328 primary small bowel tumors over a 25-year period was 54%.[116]

Obscure gastrointestinal bleeding

Obscure gastrointestinal bleeding is said to occur when bleeding from the gastrointestinal (GI) tract continues despite a normal EGD, colonoscopy, and barium follow-through or enteroclysis.[11,117,118] It accounts for approximately 5% of cases of GI blood loss and can be classified into overt and occult subtypes, depending on whether or not bleeding is clinically evident. Some patients, initially

KEY POINTS
The Small Bowel

- Celiac disease, small bowel bacterial overgrowth, and chronic pancreatitis are the main causes of malabsorption in older patients.
- Celiac disease has a prevalence of 1%, and 60% to 70% of patients are asymptomatic.
- Small bowel bacterial overgrowth occurs in 52% to 70% of symptomatic and 14% to 25% of asymptomatic elderly individuals.
- Crohn's disease has a bimodal distribution with a second peak in the elderly population.
- The mortality rate in acute mesenteric ischemia is still very high at 54% to 77%.
- Small bowel tumors are rare and account for only 1% to 2.4% of all gastrointestinal neoplasms.
- Wireless capsule endoscopy and double-balloon enteroscopy have transformed the investigation of small bowel disease.

thought to have obscure bleeding, actually have pathology that is within the reach of conventional endoscopes but that has been overlooked. Cameron's ulcers (ulcers within a hiatus hernia), Dieulafoy lesions, collapsed esophageal or fundal varices, angioectasias, and gastric antral vascular ectasias can be missed at EGD. Even experienced colonoscopists fail to detect small neoplasms or angioectasias on occasion. Hence, a second-look EGD (and less commonly a colonoscopy) is recommended before assuming that the small bowel is the source of blood loss. Technologic advances that permit endoscopic evaluation of the whole of the small bowel have altered the management of these patients since the early 2000s. The use of radionuclide studies and mesenteric angiography has correspondingly declined. The classification of GI bleeding has also changed and the conventional terms *upper* and *lower GI bleeding* to denote a source above and below the ligament of Treitz have been replaced. Bleeding above the ampulla of Vater, which is within the reach of an EGD, is termed *upper GI bleeding*. *Mid-GI bleeding* defines a bleeding source in the small bowel from the ampulla of Vater to the terminal ileum and is currently best investigated by wireless capsule endoscopy and enteroscopy. *Lower GI* or *colonic bleeding* is assessed by colonoscopy.

Vascular ectasias are probably the most common reason for mid-GI obscure blood loss in elderly people. Nonsteroidal induced small intestinal ulcers, small bowel tumors, small bowel varices, Crohn's disease, and aortoenteric fistulas are the other causes encountered. Radionuclide scans and mesenteric angiography are being replaced by the new modalities. Patients with obscure bleeding should first undergo wireless capsule endoscopy that has a diagnostic yield of 40% to 80%. If negative, a repeat examination should be considered or, depending on availability, DBE should be carried out (diagnostic yield 75%). Intraoperative enteroscopy, the most accurate (diagnostic yield 70% to 93%) but also the most invasive technique, is usually reserved for critically ill patients with persistent bleeding or when other modalities have failed to reveal the bleeding source. A bleeding vascular lesion in the proximal jejunum may be amenable to therapy via a push enteroscope, but a more distal source (hitherto usually dealt with by surgery) is now accessible via the double balloon technique.

For a complete list of references, please visit online only at www.expertconsult.com

CHAPTER 81

The Large Bowel

Arnold Wald

ANATOMY

The colon is a large, hollow organ that is derived embryologically from the primitive midguts and hindguts.[1] The appendix and transverse and sigmoid colons have mesenteries, whereas the ascending and descending colons do not. Like the stomach and small intestine, the colon has both circular and longitudinal smooth muscle layers, but uniquely, the longitudinal muscle of the colon is separated into three bundles known as taenia. The configuration of the taenia causes the colon to be divided into haustral folds, which presumably help to slow the passage of fecal material and thus facilitate absorption.

The superior mesenteric artery supplies the right colon to the midtransverse colon, whereas the inferior mesenteric artery supplies the left colon.[2] The anorectum derives its blood supply from branches of the internal iliac arteries.[3] In the distal transverse to mid-descending colon, the superior and inferior mesenteric arteries are linked by a series of anastomoses known as the marginal artery of Drummond. This anatomic arrangement increases the vulnerability of this area to ischemic damage.

Innervation of the colon is via the autonomic nervous system and the enteric neurons.[4] Parasympathetic innervation is by the vagus nerve in the right colon and by sacral parasympathetics from the second, third, and fourth sacral nerves. Sympathetic innervation is derived from the lowest cervical to the third lumbar nerves via the splanchnic nerves. However, colon function may persist even after vagal or splanchnic interruption because of the presence of a well-developed enteric nervous system, which can function in the absence of extrinsic innervation.

FUNCTIONS AND SYMPTOMS

The principal functions of the colon and rectum are to store fecal wastes for prolonged periods of time and to expel them in a socially appropriate manner. Storage is facilitated by adaptive compliance of the bowel and by muscular contractions of colonic smooth muscle, which retard the forward movement of stool, thereby promoting electrolyte and water absorption and reducing stool volume. Forward movement occurs principally by relatively infrequent peristaltic contractions, which move intraluminal contents over long distances. Continence is maintained by recognition of rectal filling and coordinated function of the anal sphincters and pelvic floor muscles to defer defecation until socially appropriate. Colonic motility and transit in healthy elderly people are similar to that in younger individuals,[5] whereas aging is associated with diminished anal sphincter tone and strength and a less compliant rectum.[6,7] The latter changes may lead to greater susceptibility to fecal incontinence in elderly people (see Chapter 103).

The major symptoms of colonic and rectal disorders are constipation, diarrhea, pain, and rectal bleeding. The conditions that produce these symptoms are not unique to the elderly population; those occurring with increased frequency in elderly people include diverticulosis, neoplasms, ischemic colitis, vascular ectasias, fecal incontinence, constipation, and antibiotic-associated diarrhea and colitis. Inflammatory bowel diseases occur in all age groups, but onset of these diseases is less likely in the elderly population. In short, a challenge of evaluating older people with bowel symptoms is that these not uncommon complaints can arise from disorders that range from the minimally disruptive to the likely fatal, with a higher probability of worse illness as age increases. As with any other illness, disease in the colon can present in elderly people who are frail as delirium, falls, or immobility.

DIAGNOSTIC TESTING

Radiology

CONTRAST STUDIES

Contrast examination of the large intestine has traditionally been done by using barium sulfate in either a single- or a double-contrast technique in which a thickened barium suspension is used to coat the mucosa followed by insufflation to expand the viscus. Alternatively, water-soluble contrast agents can be used if perforation is suspected.

The single-contrast technique is preferred when studying patients with suspected obstruction, diverticulitis, or fistula, whereas the double-contrast technique is preferred for demonstrating fine mucosal lesions and neoplasms. Although there continues to be some controversy concerning the choice of barium contrast or colonoscopy when investigating colonic diseases, most clinicians favor colonoscopy for its greater sensitivity and opportunity for biopsy and therapy. Contrast studies may be indicated in cases where severe stricturing disease or adhesions make colonoscopy hazardous, where conditions such as diverticulitis are suspected, if the location and nature of a colonic obstruction requires assessment, and if functional and structural information is required. A barium enema should not be attempted when increases in colon pressure may worsen the patient's condition, for example, in patients with suspected toxic megacolon or those with peritoneal signs that suggest ischemic colitis.

When patients complain of constipation or a recent change in bowel habit, barium radiographs complement sigmoidoscopy in detecting organic causes and are also useful in diagnosing functional megacolon and megarectum. Complete filling of the colon with barium is neither necessary nor desirable in patients with megacolon. However, conventional barium studies provide limited information about colonic motor function in most patients with chronic constipation.[8] Moreover, they are frequently inadequate in frail or hospitalized elderly patients.[9,10]

IMAGING TECHNIQUES

Abdominal computed tomography

This procedure allows visualization of the thickness of the bowel wall, the solid viscera within the abdomen, the mesenteries, and soft tissues adjacent to the bowel. It offers a modest advance in the diagnosis of diverticulitis by demonstrating inflammation of pericolic fat, abscesses that may contain collections of fluid and gas, and intramural sinus tracts. Fistulas to other organs can be identified when gas is found within the bladder or vagina. It also can identify extension of disease at a distance from the colon, including unsuspected intra-abdominal abscesses.

Computed tomography (CT) is also valuable when evaluating and managing complications of Crohn's disease, including abscesses, fistulas, and involvement of psoas muscles and ureters, and occasionally for percutaneous drainage of collections. Other complications, including sacral osteomyelitis, cholelithiasis, nephrolithiasis, and vascular necrosis of the femoral head associated with corticosteroid therapy, can also be diagnosed.

In appendicitis (and cecal diverticulitis, which is usually misdiagnosed as appendicitis), computed tomography may augment the clinical diagnosis by showing the periappendicular inflammatory process and differentiating phlegmon from abscess.[11] Occasionally, appendicoliths are identified, which are considered pathognomonic of appendicitis when associated with periappendicular inflammatory signs.

CT colonography is a new technique devised to detect colon polyps for screening purposes. Detection rates for colonic polyps of greater than 6 mm are similar to colonoscopy, but the test has low sensitivity for smaller polyps.[12] The use of 3-dimensional evaluation in addition to 2-dimensional evaluation may reduce perceptual errors.[13] CT colonography is now recommended as an alternative for colon polyp screening in the United States.

Anal and rectal endosonography

Endoscopic anal and rectal ultrasonography accurately delineates the layers of the rectal wall, the internal and external anal sphincters, and the levator muscles.[14] It can be used to evaluate pelvic floor structures in patients with fecal incontinence to detect occult sphincter injuries arising from childbirth or other conditions associated with potential injury to continence mechanisms.[15,16]

Endoscopic ultrasonography is a rapid, minimally invasive technique used to image rectal polyps, focal malignancy within polyps, tumor masses penetrating into the bowel wall, and extramural lesions such as prostatic tumors and ovarian lesions. Perirectal fistulas and abscesses can also be evaluated (including determining whether there is destruction of pelvic muscles). It is considered the reference standard for the preoperative staging of rectal and anal cancers with relatively high accuracy in categorizing tumors and lymph nodes.[17]

Colonoscopy and flexible sigmoidoscopy

These procedures are usually performed in the prepared colon except when evaluating diarrheal illnesses. Colonoscopic examinations provide unparalleled evaluation of the mucosal surfaces and opportunities for biopsy and therapy. These include diagnosis and determining extent of inflammatory bowel disease, evaluation of patients with overt or occult gastrointestinal bleeding, evaluation of chronic watery diarrhea, endoscopic sampling and removal of polyps, decompression of sigmoid volvulus or functional megacolon, and ablation of vascular lesions. Colonoscopy is generally done under conscious sedation, whereas flexible sigmoidoscopy usually is not.[18] In many elderly patients, the physician must be aware of their increased sensitivity to sedatives and analgesic medications. As elderly people are susceptible to hypotension and respiratory depression, careful monitoring of the patient during the procedure is especially important. Even so, such procedures are generally safe in experienced hands and when done in units that monitor blood gases and cardiorespiratory functions. Major complications include bleeding and perforation, which should not occur more than 2 or 3 times in 1000 routine diagnostic procedures.

Histopathology

Mucosal biopsies are often indicated when evaluating undiagnosed diarrhea, in longstanding ulcerative colitis during surveillance for precancerous dysplasia, in obtaining tissue for viral culture, and in evaluating polypoid or ulcerated lesions. In inflammatory disorders of the colon and rectum, biopsies serve to establish the presence, extent, and distribution of colitis and to differentiate ulcerative from Crohn's colitis and these disorders from other inflammatory conditions such as infectious colitis. Biopsies should be obtained from endoscopically normal and abnormal areas, as characteristic changes may be patchy and therefore missed if too few biopsies are obtained. This is especially true in pseudomembranous, collagenous, and lymphocytic colitis in which the distal colon may be spared. As hypertonic phosphate enemas and purgative laxatives may induce mucosal changes that can be mistaken for mild colitis, they should be avoided when evaluating suspected inflammation of the colon.

Fecal occult blood testing

Fecal occult blood tests (FOBTs) identify hemoglobin or altered hemoglobin compounds in the stool. Food containing peroxidases, such as melon and uncooked broccoli, horseradish, cauliflower, and turnips, may produce false positive results, whereas reducing agents such as ascorbic acid may decrease sensitivity.[19] Tests that extract the protoporphyrin from hemoglobin, such as Hemo Quant, are more specific and are quantitative but are also more time-consuming and expensive. Rehydration of Hemoccult slides increases sensitivity but decreases specificity and is not recommended. A weakly positive slide may become negative after 2 to 4 days of storage. Oral iron supplements do not interfere with any of these tests.

COLONIC DIVERTICULOSIS

Colonic diverticula are herniations of colonic mucosa through the smooth muscle layers. Diverticula occur in areas of anatomic weakness of the circular smooth muscle created by penetration of blood vessels to the submucosa. They are most commonly found in the sigmoid and descending colons and rarely, if ever, in the rectum.[20]

This disorder has been recognized with increasing frequency in modern Western countries.[21] Colonic diverticula are present in about one third of persons by age 50 and about two thirds by age 80. Dietary fiber insufficiency and the increased longevity of modern Western populations have been hypothesized to explain the increased prevalence of diverticulosis. Dietary factors may promote increased colonic motor activity and intraluminal pressures, whereas aging may lead to structural weakness of the colonic muscle.[20] As diverticula are asymptomatic in most individuals, caution must be taken before attributing nonspecific gastrointestinal symptoms to them.[22]

Painful diverticular disease

Painful diverticular disease is characterized by crampy discomfort in the left lower abdomen. Symptoms are often associated with constipation or diarrhea and with tenderness over the affected areas. These symptoms are similar to those of irritable bowel syndrome and partial bowel obstruction due to tumors or ischemia. Studies have shown that these patients have altered motor activity in the segments containing diverticula, which are associated with reporting of abdominal pain.[23] In contrast to diverticulitis, there is no fever, leukocytosis, or rebound tenderness.

Diverticulitis

Diverticulitis develops in approximately 10% to 25% of individuals with diverticulosis who are followed for 10 years or more; however, less than 20% of these patients require hospitalization. Inflammation begins at the apex of the diverticulum when the opening of a diverticulum becomes obstructed (e.g., with stool), leading to microperforation or macroperforation of a diverticulum.[24] The presence of a palpable mass, fever, leukocytosis, and/or rebound tenderness indicates an inflammatory process, which often remains localized in the adjacent pericolic tissues but may progress to a peridiverticular abscess.[25] Other complications include fibrosis and bowel obstruction, fistula formation to the bladder, vagina, or adjacent small intestine, and free perforation with peritonitis. The frequency of complications rises to about 60% with recurrent attacks of diverticulitis.

Making a clinical distinction between painful diverticular disease and diverticulitis carries a sizable rate of error.[24] In an elderly or debilitated patient, the absence of fever, leukocytosis, or rebound tenderness does not exclude diverticulitis.[25]

Recently, a disorder characterized by localized inflammation associated with diverticulosis (SCAD syndrome) has been described in older symptomatic patients.[26] Symptoms appear after the age of 40 years and are most often characterized by rectal bleeding, diarrhea, and abdominal pain.

Other disorders such as carcinoma, inflammatory bowel disease, and ischemia may mimic symptomatic diverticular disease. Diagnostic studies include barium enema, CT, ultrasonography, and colonoscopy. In most cases of suspected diverticulitis, barium enema should be delayed for about a week to allow some resolution of the inflammatory process. A single-contrast study should be performed cautiously to minimize the risk of perforation. Radiographic findings suggesting diverticulitis include longitudinal fistulas connecting diverticula over segments of colon, fistula into adjacent organs, a fixed eccentric defect in the colon wall, contrast outside the lumen of the colon or diverticulum, and intraluminal defects representing abscesses.[20] CT and ultrasonic imaging of the abdomen provide superior definition of colonic wall thickness and extraluminal structures and are the procedures of choice at the time of initial evaluation. Colonoscopy is a less attractive option during an acute episode and is best employed to exclude tumors or other conditions if other diagnostic tests are inconclusive.

The treatment of painful diverticular disease is designed to reduce symptoms based on smooth muscle spasm, in contrast to the treatment of diverticulitis, which is designed to treat bacterial infection (Table 81-1). Patients with severe pain, nausea and vomiting, or complications should be hospitalized and given intravenous antibiotics until clinical improvement occurs.

Surgery is recommended for patients with diverticulitis who fail to respond to medical therapy within 72 hours, for immunocompromised patients, and those who have fistula to the bladder with pneumaturia and urinary infection or fistula to the vagina with discharge of stool into the vagina. Although some surgeons recommend elective sigmoid resection after two episodes of diverticulitis, others favor a more conservative approach.[27] A one-stage operation, in which the diseased segment of bowel is resected and continuity restored by a primary anastomosis, is preferred.[28] In cases of generalized peritonitis or emergent surgery for perforation with abscess or high-grade obstruction, a two-stage procedure requiring a diverting colostomy should be used.[29] Large abscesses can often be drained percutaneously by an interventional radiologist using CT or ultrasonography as a guide.[30,31] Elective surgery can then be performed after 2 to 3 weeks of antibiotic therapy, often allowing for a single-stage resection.

Emergent surgery is required for generalized peritonitis or persistent high-grade bowel obstruction. Most patients with complicated diverticular disease require surgery, even if clinical recovery occurs, since there is a high risk of recurrent attacks.

Table 81-1. Medical Treatment of Diverticular Disease

Measure	Painful Diverticulosis	Diverticulitis
Diet	Increase fiber	Reduce fiber (or NPO)
Bulk laxatives	Sometimes effective	Not indicated
Analgesics	Avoid narcotics	Avoid morphine; meperidine is best
Antispasmodics	Propantheline bromide (15 mg tid); Dicyclomine hydrochloride (20 mg tid); Hyoscyamine sulfate (0.125 mg–0.250 mg q 4 h)	Not indicated
Antibiotics	Not indicated	**Oral:** Amoxicillin/clavulanate K^+ (875/125 mg bid) Ciprofloxacin (500 mg bid) and metronidazole 500 mg tid) Parenteral 1. Gentamicin or tobramycin (5 mg/kg/day) plus clindamycin (1.2–2.4 g/day) or 2. Levofloxacin 500 mg/day and metronidazole (500 mg q 8 h) 3. Piperacillin-tazobactam (3.375–4.5 gm q 6 h)

Updated and modified from Wald[20] with permission.

Most patients with localized inflammation associated with diverticulosis respond with long-term resolution of the disease to 5-aminosalicylate therapy. On occasion, spontaneous remissions may occur or persistent chronically active disease may require resective surgery.[26]

Bleeding

Bleeding associated with diverticula is typically brisk and painless and often arises from the proximal colon. Bleeding is thought to occur when a fecalith erodes into a vessel in the neck of the diverticulum or there is rupture of the penetrating arteriole in its course around the diverticular sac.[20]

An important indication for emergent colonoscopy is to identify the source of bleeding in patients with diverticula, as other lesions not seen by contrast studies may be the actual source. If bleeding is brisk, a bleeding scan or selective mesenteric angiography can often locate the site of bleeding; superselective embolization of distal arterial branches has been demonstrated to be highly effective and relatively safe (<20% ischemia rates)[32] (see Lower Gastrointestinal Bleeding).

APPENDICITIS

Elderly patients with appendicitis are at increased risk (about 60%) for perforation. They have a higher mortality and often do not exhibit a fever or elevated white blood cell count.[33]

Classically, the onset of abdominal pain is abrupt, begins in the midabdomen, relocates to the right lower quadrant, and is often associated with nausea, vomiting, and fever. Physical examination characteristically reveals signs of local peritonitis in the right lower quadrant, and the white blood cell count is frequently elevated. The differential diagnosis includes pyelonephritis, Crohn's disease, gastroenteritis, pelvic inflammatory disease, ovarian cyst, and cecal diverticulitis. In elderly patients, appendicitis may occur in association with colon cancer in which low-grade obstruction results in distention of the appendix and mimics true appendicitis.

If the diagnosis is uncertain, ultrasonography has been shown to have positive and negative predictive values of about 90% for appendicitis and is also useful in identifying another cause of symptoms in patients with right lower quadrant pain.[34] One sonographic criterion for acute appendicitis is visualization of a noncompressible appendix with a diameter of greater than 6 mm.

INFECTIOUS DISEASES

Clostridium difficile

Clostridium difficile is responsible for approximately 3 million cases of diarrhea and colitis each year and is the most common cause of nosocomial diarrhea in the United States.[35]

The vast majority of cases are associated with two protein exotoxins (A and B) produced by *C. difficile*. Toxin A is an enterotoxin that triggers diarrhea, epithelial necrosis, and a characteristic inflammatory process in animals, whereas toxin B is a cytotoxin in tissue culture but does not by itself cause toxicity in animals.[36] The disease spectrum ranges from mild diarrhea, with little or no inflammation, to severe colitis often associated with pseudomembranes, which are adherent to necrotic colonic epithelium. Acquisition of *C. difficile* occurs most frequently in elderly persons in hospitals or nursing homes, potentially because of environmental contamination with *C. difficile* and spores carried on the hands of hospital or institutional personnel.[37] Acquisition is often asymptomatic but may have clinical consequences if elderly patients receive certain antibiotics or chemotherapeutic agents. Other possible risk factors include surgery, intensive care, nasogastric intubation, and length of hospital stay. A smaller number of patients have antibiotic-associated diarrhea but no evidence of *C. difficile* infection.

Although virtually all antibiotics have been implicated, the most common are cephalosporins, ampicillin or amoxicillin, and clindamycin.[38] Less commonly mentioned antibiotics include other penicillins, erythromycin, and fluoroquinolones.

Currently, the United States, Canada, and Europe are experiencing an outbreak of a new virulent strain of *C. difficile* designated as ribotype 027.[39] This strain has been shown to be resistant to the newer fluoroquinolones, as is the case of other existing strains of *C. difficile*.[35]

The typical clinical picture of *C. difficile*–associated colitis includes nonbloody diarrhea, lower abdominal cramps, fever, and leukocytosis. Fever is usually low grade although, on occasion, it can be quite high. In severe cases, dehydration, hypotension, hypoproteinemia, toxic megacolon, or even colonic perforation may occur.

In severely ill patients, the diagnostic test of choice is flexible sigmoidoscopy or colonoscopy. As the distal colon is involved in the majority of cases, flexible sigmoidoscopy is usually satisfactory; however, changes may be confined to the right colon in up to one third of cases, making colonoscopy necessary if less extensive procedures do not confirm a suspected diagnosis. The yellowish-gray pseudomembranes are densely adherent to the underlying colonic mucosa, interspersed with mucosa that appears normal. Mucosal biopsies may exhibit characteristic findings of epithelial necrosis and micropseudomembranes ("volcano lesions") even when pseudomembranes are not grossly visible. Endoscopy particularly has a role in severely ill patients who present atypically and therefore require a rapid diagnosis.[40]

Several tests identify *C. difficile* or its toxin. The enzyme immunoassay (EIA) for toxin A and/or B is the preferred test to detect toxin. On average, EIA tests range in sensitivity from 87% to 96% in confirmed cases of *C. difficile* diarrhea.[41] Thus it should be emphasized that a negative EIA test does not exclude a diagnosis of *C. difficile* colitis.

The offending drug should be discontinued if possible. If symptoms persist, patients who are not seriously ill should receive oral metronidazole 500 mg tid for 7 to 10 days. Patients who are seriously ill and those with complicated or fulminant infections should receive oral vancomycin 125 mg PO qid for 7 to 10 days.[42] If oral intake is not possible, metronidazole 500 mg IV q6h is given until oral administration can be accomplished. Metronidazole and vancomycin appear to be therapeutically comparable in nonseriously ill patients, but metronidazole costs less and there are current concerns about vancomycin-resistant enterococcus.[43] In general, fever resolves within 24 hours and diarrhea decreases within 4 to 5 days.

Relapses average about 20% to 25% following successful treatment with either agent,[44] often involving sporulation,

Table 81-2. Practice Guidelines for Prevention of *Clostridium difficile* Diarrhea

1. Limit the use of antimicrobial drugs.
2. Wash hands between contact with all patients.
3. Use enteric (stool) isolation precautions for patients with *C. difficile* diarrhea.
4. Wear gloves when contacting patients with *C. difficile* diarrhea/colitis or their environment.
5. Disinfect objects contaminated with *C. difficile* with sodium hypochlorite, alkaline glutaraldehyde, or ethylene oxide.
6. Educate the medical, nursing, and other appropriate staff members about the disease and its epidemiology.

From Fekety,[40] with permission.

which leads to relapse within 4 weeks after completion of successful treatment. These episodes invariably respond to another course of antibiotic therapy. About 5% to 10% of patients have multiple relapses. In such individuals, vancomycin in conventional doses should be followed by a 3-week course of cholestyramine 4 g tid and/or Lactinex 500 mg PO qid, or vancomycin 125 mg PO every other day. Others advocate a 6-week schedule consisting of a 2-week course of vancomycin given daily in the standard dose, a 2-week course in the same dose given every other day, followed by a 2-week course at the same dose given every third day. *Saccharomyces boulardii* is a nonpathogenic yeast which inhibits the binding of toxin A to rat ileum, with consequent prevention of enterotoxicity.[45]

Guidelines for prevention of *C. difficile* diarrhea and colitis are based upon a few simple practices and attitudes and are shown in Table 81-2.[40]

Shigella

These organisms consist of four groups: (1) *Shigella dysenteriae*, (2) *S. flexneri*, (3) *S. boydii*, and (4) *S. sonnei*, the last of which accounts for most clinical infections in Western countries. In contrast to other enteric pathogens, very few organisms are needed to produce infection, which is spread by fecal-oral transmission between humans and which continues to occur despite high standards of water purification and sewage disposal. At least 30 gene products are involved in *Shigella* invasion and its intercellular spread. Disease is caused by invasion of colonic epithelial cells, perhaps in part mediated by cytotoxins produced by *S. dysenteriae* and *S. flexneri*, but enterotoxins may also contribute to early symptoms of nondysenteric diarrhea.[46] Enterotoxins similar to Shigalike toxins secreted by enterohemorrhagic *Escherichia coli* are believed to mediate the hemolytic-uremic syndrome associated with severe colitis caused by *S. dysenteriae* type I.

SYMPTOMS

Colitis is heralded by the passage of bloody mucoid stools associated with urgency, tenesmus, abdominal cramping, fever, and malaise. The frequency of stools is highest during the first 24 hours of illness and gradually diminishes thereafter.

DIAGNOSIS

Stool examination reveals numerous polymorphonuclear cells, and leukocytosis is common. Stool culture grown on selective media is the definitive diagnostic study. Sigmoidoscopy is usually not necessary, but if done, will demonstrate a friable hyperemic mucosa. Barium contrast studies are not indicated.

TREATMENT

If the illness is mild and self-limited, antibiotics can be withheld. As resistance to sulfonamides, ampicillin, tetracycline, and even trimethoprim-sulfamethoxazole is now common, treatment with a fluoroquinolone (e.g., ciprofloxacin 500 mg twice daily for 5 days) is indicated in frail or otherwise debilitated patients with acute disease to shorten the illness and the period of fecal excretion of the organism.[47] Antidiarrheal agents prolong the clinical illness and carrying of the organism and should not be administered.[48] The development of a chronic carrier state is rare and difficult to treat.

Pathogenic *Escherichia coli* that cause colitis

These organisms commonly cause disease in developed countries and are a major cause of diarrhea in tourists visiting underdeveloped countries. As older individuals increasingly engage in overseas travel, these organisms can be a major impediment to a successful trip.

Of the five major classes of pathogenic *E. coli*, only enteroinvasive (EIEC) and Shiga toxin–producing *E. coli* (STEC) primarily involve the colon. Both produce a clinical illness similar to that of shigellosis. Once thought to be a pathogen restricted to developing countries, STEC has been shown to produce diarrhea in the United States and is a relatively uncommon cause of traveler's diarrhea. It is more difficult to identify in stool cultures and is not a reportable illness. The clinical illness is generally milder than with shigellosis. A reasonable approach is to treat with a fluoroquinolone similar to treatment for shigellosis.[35]

Preventive measures include eating cooked food only while it is still hot and avoiding local water, including fruits and vegetables washed with local water. In elderly tourists, the disease can be shortened by prompt use of a fluoroquinolone.[46]

Shiga toxin–producing *E. coli* 0157:H7

This organism has been identified as a major pathogen in the United States and Canada, causing approximately 70,000 cases in the United States annually.[35] In addition to sporadic infections, epidemics have been traced to consumption of undercooked and raw ground beef, as healthy cattle serve as the primary reservoir for Shiga toxin–producing strains. Infections have also been associated with exposure to patients with bloody diarrhea, contaminated water supplies, and nonpreserved apple cider. Clinical manifestations include nonbloody diarrhea, hemorrhagic colitis, and hemolytic-uremic syndrome (HUS).[49] Unlike most bacterial enteric diseases, *E. coli* 0157:H7 is often characterized by low-grade fever or the absence of a fever.[50] The pathogenesis of colitis has been linked to Shigalike toxins (verocytotoxins 1 and 2), which bind to a glycolipid on the surface of colonocytes, but adherence factors may also play a role. Older age is both a risk factor for this infection and increases the risk of HUS and death. It is generally believed that antibiotics are not indicated for active infections and appear to predispose to hemolytic-uremic syndrome.[49]

An important emerging group of related pathogens are the non-0157 toxin–producing *E. coli*, which can produce an illness similar to 0157:H7 strains.[51] Indeed, in Europe, a majority of STEC strains belong to the non-0157 serogroup.

Campylobacter species

Campylobacter jejuni and *C. coli* are among the most common bacterial causes of diarrhea and can be manifested by gastroenteritis, pseudoappendicitis, or colitis. These organisms are usually transmitted from animals to humans through contaminated food and water and sometimes by direct contact with pets. Constitutional symptoms usually precede diarrhea and abdominal cramps by up to 24 hours, and colitis may be characterized by fever and dysentery lasting for a week or more. Diagnosis is made by stool culture. Convalescent carriage up to a mean of 5 weeks is common after the onset of illness and is significantly reduced by antimicrobial treatment.

Although the infection is usually self-limited, antibiotics may be given if the illness is severe or in patients who are immunosuppressed.[52] Treatment consists of erythromycin or fluoroquinolones; macrolides such as azithromycin and clarithromycin show excellent in vitro activity. Resistance rates to fluoroquinolones of up to 88% have been reported in Europe and Asia. In areas of high resistance, azithromycin 500 mg daily for 3 days is an effective alternative.

Entamoeba histolytica

This organism remains a primary cause of dysentery, which may be complicated by fulminant colitis, toxic megacolon, bleeding, stricture, and perforation. Severe disease is more common in elderly people and in patients who are immunosuppressed or debilitated.[53] The disease is typically acquired by ingesting cysts from contaminated water or fresh vegetables but can also be transmitted venereally through sexual practices that promote fecal-oral transmission. Studies on germ-free animals suggest that intestinal disease does not develop unless bacteria are present. This may partly account for the effectiveness of metronidazole, which is also active against anaerobic bacteria.

Three separate stool specimens should be examined if the diagnosis is suspected. A wet preparation should be performed within 30 minutes of passage to look for motile trophozoites, which may contain ingested red blood cells. A formalin-ethyl acetate concentration preparation should be examined for cysts. Barium, bismuth, kaolin compounds, magnesium hydroxide, castor oil, and hypertonic enemas all interfere with the ability to detect the parasite in stools.[53]

Colonoscopy may reveal erythema, edema, friability of the mucosa, and scattered ulcers 5 to 15 mm in diameter, covered with a yellow exudate. These ulcers may occur anywhere in the colon but are most common in the cecum and ascending colon. Biopsies from the edge of these ulcers may reveal typical "hour-glass" ulcers containing trophozoites. Cathartics and enemas should not be used because they interfere with identification of the parasite.

As these techniques may miss identifying the parasite, serologic tests for antiamebic antibodies should also be obtained in suspected cases. The indirect hemagglutination assay (IHA) is positive in 75% to 90% of patients with amebic dysentery and in virtually all patients with amebic liver abscesses. The IHA remains positive for years after treatment of invasive amebiasis.[53]

Treatment of acute amebic dysentery consists of metronidazole 750 mg three times daily for 5 to 10 days or, if not tolerated orally, 500 mg q 6 h by the intravenous route.[54] This should be followed by luminal acting oral drugs such as paromomycin 25 to 35 mg/kg in 3 doses daily for 7 days or iodoquinol 650 mg three times daily for 20 days to eliminate all cysts and prevent possible relapse.

Cytomegalovirus

Cytomegalovirus (CMV) is a member of the herpes virus family, which enters a lifelong latent phase after primary infection in immunocompetent persons. In patients who are immunocompromised with diminished T-cell function, reactivation may occur and may become persistent, with reappearance of IgM anti-CMV antibodies in the serum. Among the gastrointestinal syndromes associated with CMV are focal and diffuse colitis.

CMV colitis is associated with severe small-volume diarrhea, abdominal pain, and fever. Colonoscopy may reveal variable degrees of focal erythema, petechial hemorrhage, erosions, and in advanced cases, scattered ulcers. Mucosal biopsy may reveal characteristic intranuclear inclusions ("owl-eye" lesions) or cytoplasmic inclusions in vascular endothelial cells. In cases in which a biopsy is not diagnostic, polymerase chain reaction assay or in situ hybridization techniques may be helpful, together with serum IgM CMV-specific antibodies.

The treatment of choice is ganciclovir (5 mg/kg IV q 12 h for 21 days) to achieve remission.[55] For patients who relapse after discontinuation of the drug, chronic maintenance therapy (6 mg/kg five times per week) may be instituted. Valganciclovir is as effective as IV ganciclovir because of improved bioavailability over previous oral agents. As the drug has hematologic side effects such as neutropenia, regular blood counts should be obtained. Human immunodeficiency virus (HIV)-infected patients with CMV colitis should be placed on maintenance therapy indefinitely. Foscarnet is used in patients who do not respond to ganciclovir or who cannot tolerate its toxicity.

INFLAMMATORY BOWEL DISEASE

Both ulcerative colitis and Crohn's disease are more common in early adulthood but are found with increased frequency in older adults. In part, this is because increasing numbers of patients with inflammatory bowel disease (IBD) now live into old age. In addition, both ulcerative colitis and Crohn's disease exhibit a bimodal age of onset,[56,57] the peak incidence occurring in the third decade and a minor later peak between the ages of 50 and 80 years; more than 10% of cases have their onset after the age of 60. This pattern persists even when other diseases that mimic inflammatory bowel disease, such as ischemic colitis and infectious causes, have been excluded. The reasons for this bimodal pattern are unknown.

ULCERATIVE COLITIS

Ulcerative colitis is a chronic inflammatory process of unknown cause that affects the mucosa and submucosa of the colon in a continuous distribution. Enhanced humoral immunity is more evident in ulcerative colitis than Crohn's disease and probably reflects disturbed immunoregulation leading to unrestrained T-cell activation and cytokine release.[58]

HISTOPATHOLOGY

Histologically, there are diffuse ulcerations and epithelial necrosis, depletion of mucin from goblet cells, and a polymorphonuclear and lymphocytic infiltration involving the superficial layers of the colon to the muscularis mucosa. The finding of crypt microabscesses is characteristic but not pathognomonic. The inflammatory process invariably involves the rectum and extends proximally for variable distances but does not involve the gastrointestinal tract proximal to the colon. Involvement of the rectum only is designated ulcerative proctitis, whereas disease extending no further than the splenic flexure is designated as left-sided disease.

SYMPTOMS AND SIGNS

Symptoms commonly are similar to those seen in younger persons.[59] The severity of ulcerative colitis may be classified as mild, moderate, and severe and is generally proportional to the extent of colonic inflammation (Table 81-3). Most patients exhibit diarrhea, with or without blood in the stools, although older patients with proctitis only occasionally have constipation or hematochezia. Systemic manifestations occur during more severe attacks and carry a poorer prognosis. Indeed, despite the occurrence of less extensive disease in older patients, they more often have a severe initial attack and have higher mortality and morbidity than do younger patients.[60]

Toxic megacolon is a feared complication of ulcerative colitis, which occurs more frequently in elderly patients. Abdominal radiographs show colonic dilation, often to impressive proportions, and patients may exhibit mental confusion, high fever, abdominal distention, and overall deterioration.[61]

Extraintestinal manifestations may occur in ulcerative colitis, including arthralgias, erythema nodosum, pyoderma gangrenosum, uveitis, and migratory polyarthritis. These disorders occur less frequently than in Crohn's disease and are generally associated with increased disease activity.

DIAGNOSIS

The diagnosis is made by sigmoidoscopy and rectal mucosal biopsies since the disorder invariably involves the rectum. The extent of the disease is determined by colonoscopy or barium radiography, both of which should be avoided in patients who are severely ill because of the danger of inducing perforation or toxic megacolon. The characteristic findings are diffuse erythema, granularity, and friability of the mucosa without intervening areas of normal mucosa. Inflammatory pseudopolyps indicate more severe erosion of the mucosa and must be distinguished from true polyps.

Particularly in elderly people, it is important to exclude other diseases that may mimic ulcerative colitis, including Crohn's colitis (see later discussion), ischemic colitis, radiation proctocolitis, and diverticulitis. In acute presentations, infectious agents should be excluded with appropriate stool cultures, including *Salmonella, Campylobacter, Shigella*, amebiasis, *Yersinia*, and *E. coli* 0157:H7. Finally, *C. difficile*–associated diarrhea and pseudomembranous colitis should be considered in elderly persons, particularly those who have recently been treated with antibiotics, reside in institutions, or have recently been hospitalized.

TREATMENT

The treatment of ulcerative colitis is based on the extent and the severity of the disease (Table 81-4). Medical therapy consists of a number of effective drugs, which are administered intravenously, orally, or rectally. The major classes of drugs are corticosteroids, 5-aminosalicylate (5-ASA) products, immunomodulators, and anti-TNF-α agents.[62] In elderly people, some drugs must be used more carefully than in younger patients. For example, corticosteroids have higher risk complications, such as hypertension, hypokalemia, and confusion, whereas sulfasalazine, 5-ASA products, and immunomodulators are generally tolerated well.[60]

SEVERE DISEASE

Patients with severe or fulminant disease, including toxic megacolon, should be hospitalized for intravenous therapy. This treatment consists of hydrocortisone or

Table 81-3. Proposed Criteria for Assessment of Disease Activity in Ulcerative Colitis*

Factor	Severe	Mild
Bowel frequency	>6 daily	<4 daily
Blood in stool	++	+
Temperature	>37.5° C on 2 of 4 days	Normal
Pulse rate (beats/min)	>90	Normal
Hemoglobin (allow for transfusion)	<75%	Normal or near normal
Erythrocyte sedimentation rate (mm in 1 hr)	>30	<30

*Moderate disease is intermediate between severe and mild classifications.
(Data from Truelove and Witts: Br Med J 1955;2:4941-8, with permission.)

Table 81-4. Medical Treatment of Ulcerative Colitis

Indication	Drug	Dosage
Mild to moderate distal disease	Hydrocortisone enemas	hs
	5-ASA enemas	hs
	Sulfasalazine	2–4 g/day PO
	Mesalamine	2.4–4.8 g/day PO
Mild to moderate disease extensive disease	Sulfasalazine	2.4 g/day PO
	Mesalamine*	2.4–4.8 g/day PO
	Balsalazide*	6.75 g/day PO
	Prednisone	40–60 mg/day PO
Severe disease (recently receiving steroids)	Prednisolone	60–80 mg/day IV
	Hydrocortisone	300 mg/day IV
Severe disease (not recently receiving steroids)	Corticotropin (ACTH)	120 units d/IV
	Infliximab	5 mg/kg IV at 0.2 and 6 wk; then every 4–8 wk
Maintenance of remission	5-ASA (mesalamine) enemas	o.n. or q 3rd night
Distal disease	Sulfasalazine	2 g/day PO
Pancolonic	Mesalamine*	1.2–2.4/day PO
	Balsalazide*	3 g/day PO
	Azathioprine	2–2.5 mg/kgBW/day PO
	6-Mercaptopurine	1.5 mg/kgBW/day PO
	Infliximab	5 mg/kg/BW q 4–8 wk IV

Abbreviations: *ASA*, aminosalicylate; *ACTH*, adrenocorticotrophic hormone.
*If patient is intolerant of sulfasalazine.

adrenocorticotrophic hormone (ACTH) infused in fluids containing sufficient amounts of potassium to prevent hypokalemia. One study suggests that ACTH is superior for treating patients who have not previously received corticosteroids, whereas hydrocortisone tends to be more effective in those who have.[63] If ACTH or hydrocortisone does not produce significant improvement within 2 to 3 days, IV cyclosporine may be attempted with close monitoring of renal function, an especially important consideration in an elderly patient.

Once improvement is noted, the patient should be converted to oral maintenance therapy (see later discussion). However, in some cases, surgery is preferred unless the patient is an extremely poor operative risk.

Infliximab is a chimeric monoclonal antibody of the IgG subclass directed against human TNF-α, an important proinflammatory cytokine that is elevated in ulcerative colitis and Crohn's disease. Several large multicenter studies have showed efficacy in patients with moderately to severely active ulcerative colitis who fail conventional therapy. The dose of infliximab is 5 mg/kg body weight IV at 0, 2, and 6 weeks followed by infusions every 8 weeks[64] and is now accepted as part of the standard treatment options in patients with ulcerative colitis.

MODERATELY SEVERE DISEASE

Oral corticosteroids are used to achieve remission or to sustain remission after intravenous therapy. Initial therapy should be 40 to 60 mg/day in divided doses, followed by conversion to a single morning dose. Corticosteroids should be viewed as acute phase drugs and should not be used as long-term maintenance therapy because of significant side effects related to both the dose and duration of therapy. Diabetes, congestive heart failure, osteoporosis, cataracts, and hypertension are common in elderly people and may be exacerbated by corticosteroids.[60] Corticosteroid reduction should be accomplished in stepwise fashion while monitoring clinical activity and appropriate laboratory studies.

5-ASAs may be started together with oral corticosteroids. Sulfasalazine is quite effective and inexpensive but is somewhat limited by side effects, which are often dose-dependent and occur in as many as 30% of patients. Side effects include nausea, anorexia, headache, and, less commonly, a generalized rash; in most cases, these conditions are due to the inactive sulfapyridine carrier rather than the 5-ASA moiety. If side effects occur, patients should be switched to the more expensive 5-ASA products such as mesalamine. Diarrhea is a potential side effect of all 5-ASA drugs.

If patients fail to respond to 5-ASA drugs and cannot be weaned from oral corticosteroids, a trial of azathioprine or 6-mercaptopurine should be considered as an alternative to surgery.[65] These drugs act slowly and have a response time ranging from 3 to 6 months. Complete blood counts should be monitored frequently when these agents are used.

An alternative approach is to use infliximab in an induction dose similar to those with severe disease. Before starting this therapy, a skin test for tuberculosis should be placed, as infliximab has been associated with reactivation of latent *Mycobacterium tuberculosis*.

MILD DISEASE

Patients with mild disease can be treated effectively with 5-ASA drugs, which can be administered orally, by enema in cases of left-sided disease, or by suppositories in patients with proctitis. Corticosteroid enemas are also effective in left-sided disease but in general are not more effective than 5-ASA products. As up to 60% of the rectal corticosteroid may be absorbed, they also are less suitable for maintenance therapy. Budesonide is a nonsystemic steroid with a significant first-pass hepatic metabolism, which does not affect the adrenal-pituitary-hypothalamic axis. It is available in both foam and enema for mild to moderate proctosigmoiditis or left-sided disease.[66]

MAINTENANCE THERAPY

For patients in remission, long-term maintenance with a 5-ASA product reduces the frequency of relapses.[67] The usual maintenance dose of sulfasalazine is 1 g bid with little or no long-term adverse effects. For patients who are intolerant to sulfasalazine, mesalamine 1.2 mg/day is also effective. For those with ulcerative proctitis or left-sided colitis, 5-ASA suppositories and enemas, respectively, are very effective when given every night to every third night. Nonsteroidal anti-inflammatory drugs have been reported to activate quiescent inflammatory bowel disease and should be avoided if possible.[68]

SURGERY

Indications for surgery include failure of medical therapy for acute fulminant disease, inability to wean patients from long-term corticosteroid therapy, development of precancerous colonic lesions identified during surveillance studies, and suboptimal response to medical therapy in chronic ulcerative colitis.

The surgical procedure most commonly performed for acute fulminant colitis in all age groups is subtotal colectomy and ileostomy. In the elderly patient, proctocolectomy and ileostomy also remains the most popular choice for chronic failure of medical treatment or because of the development of premalignant changes. Although procedures that avoid ileostomy, such as the ileoanal reservoir, are a viable choice for many younger patients, the increased morbidity of the treatment makes its use less attractive in elderly patients who also are at greater risk for fecal incontinence because of age-associated changes in anal sphincter function.

RISK OF COLON CANCER

The risk of developing colorectal cancer in elderly patients with ulcerative colitis is approximately nine times that of the general population of that age group.[69] The risk in all age groups increases about 8 years after the onset of the disease and is greatest in those with universal colitis. Carcinoma almost always develops many years after quiescent disease has been present and occurs at an earlier age than in the general population. For this reason, yearly colonoscopy has been recommended to detect mucosal dysplasia, which is considered a premalignant lesion in ulcerative colitis. Biopsies are obtained randomly throughout the colon and in areas that appear suspicious. Despite some shortcomings in the interpretation of biopsies and in the outcome of surveillance programs, all patients with longstanding ulcerative colitis should receive periodic colonoscopy and biopsy to look for evidence of mucosal dysplasia. The presence of low-grade dysplasia in the absence of active inflammation is an indication for proctocolectomy.[69]

CROHN'S DISEASE

Crohn's disease is a chronic inflammatory process of unknown cause that most often affects the terminal ileum and/or colon and is characterized by transmural inflammation of the bowel wall, often with linear ulcerations and granulomas.

HISTOPATHOLOGY

Histologically there is transmural inflammation affecting all layers of the bowel and often associated with submucosal fibrosis. Other features that serve to distinguish this disease from ulcerative colitis are linear ulcerations, fissures, fistulas, discrete mucosal ulcers, granulomas, skip areas, and frequent rectal sparing.[70] The disease can involve all areas of the gastrointestinal tract, from the mouth to the anus, but most frequently involves the ileum and colon. According to most published series, Crohn's disease confined to the colon (Crohn's colitis) occurs more frequently in elderly than in younger persons, and left-sided colitis appears to be prevalent in elderly women.[60]

SYMPTOMS AND SIGNS

As with ulcerative colitis, the clinical picture in elderly patients is similar to that in younger individuals and includes rectal bleeding, diarrhea, fever, abdominal pain, and weight loss. In patients with colorectal involvement, perianal disease, including fistulas, may be an early manifestation. The prevalence of extraintestinal manifestations such as migratory arthritis, pyoderma gangrenosum, iritis, and erythema nodosum is similar to that in younger patients. Common laboratory abnormalities such as anemia, leukocytosis, hypoalbuminemia, and elevated sedimentation rate vary with the severity of the illness. Rarely, the disease may be manifested by peritonitis due to bowel perforation, but this occurs more commonly with ileal disease. In elderly patients, peritonitis may occur atypically with mild abdominal pain, often minimal abdominal findings, and mental confusion. Uncommonly, Crohn's colitis is characterized by massive lower gastrointestinal bleeding or bowel obstruction.

DIAGNOSIS

Prolonged delays in diagnosis probably occur more frequently in elderly patients. It has been speculated that there is a tendency for Crohn's colitis to appear in a more indolent fashion than does ileal or ileocolonic involvement.[60]

As the disease may often not involve the rectum and the distribution in the colon is often not confluent, colonoscopy and barium radiography are the diagnostic tests of choice. Both procedures can identify the characteristic ulcerations, skip lesions, and areas of colonic narrowing. Barium studies are superior for identifying fistulas from the intestine to adjacent visceral organs, whereas colonoscopy provides superior examination of the mucosa and allows mucosal biopsies to be obtained. Biopsies should also be obtained from grossly normal-appearing mucosa to help distinguish Crohn's colitis from other diseases that may mimic it. This is particularly important because of the increased frequency with which diverticula occur in elderly people and because of the tendency for ischemic colitis to occur in a discontinuous distribution.

Computed tomography provides superior definition of the wall of the colon and can identify extraintestinal abdominal pathology, such as abscesses in patients with fever or palpable masses. Computed tomography and ultrasonography can also identify renal lithiasis or ureteral obstruction, which often occur silently.

Perianal involvement is a well-recognized manifestation of Crohn's disease and may be characterized by rectal or anal strictures, fissures, fistulas, abscesses, prominent skin tags, and ulcers. Venereal disease (uncommon in elderly people) and carcinoma should be excluded, particularly as the latter may complicate long-standing Crohn's proctitis. Infectious agents should be excluded by appropriate studies.

Small bowel follow-through remains a frequently used radiologic examination to assess the extent of small bowel involvement and to detect fistulas and strictures.[70] Increasingly, capsule endoscopy is being used in patients without strictures because it appears to be more sensitive than radiology in the small bowel.[71] Assessment of the small intestine should be done at least once in every patient, usually at the time of diagnosis, to stage the disease.[70]

TREATMENT

As with ulcerative colitis, treatment of Crohn's disease is based on its extent and severity and its distribution. Medical therapy encompasses all the drugs used in treating ulcerative colitis[62]; in addition, selected antibiotics and methotrexate are helpful in some patients (Table 81-5).

Table 81-5. Medical Treatment of Crohn's Disease

Indications	Drug	Dosage
Ileocolitis or colitis	Mesalamine	2.4–4.8 g/day PO
	Metronidazole	10–20 mg/kg/day PO
	Prednisone	40–60 mg/day PO
	Budesonide	9 mg/day PO
Perineal disease	6-Mercaptopurine or	50 mg/day up to 1.5 mg/kg/day
	Azathioprine or	50 mg/day up to 2.5 mg/kg/day PO
	Metronidazone or	1–2 g/day PO
	Ciprofloxacin	500 mg bid PO
	Infliximab	5 mg/kg/IV q 4–8 wk
Refractory disease	6-Mercaptopurine or	50 mg/day to 1.5 mg/kg/day PO
	Azathioprine or	50 mg/day up to 2.5 mg/kg/day PO
	Infliximab or	5 mg/kg/IV q at 0, 2, and 6 wk
	Adalimumab	40 mg SC q 2 wk after loading dose of 160 mg SC followed by 80 mg SC in 2 wk
	Certolizumab	400 mg SC at 0, 2 and 4 wk
	Methotrexate	25 mg SQ/wk
Maintenance of remission	Sulfasalazine or	2 g/day PO
	Mesalamine	800–1200 mg/day PO
	6-Mercaptopurine or Azathioprine	50 mg/day up to 1.5 or 2.5 mg/kg/day, respectively
	Methotrexate	15 mg SQ/week
	Infliximab	5 mg/kg BW q 4–8 wk IV
	Adalimumab	40 mg SC q 2 wk
	Certolizumab	400 mg SC q 4 wk

ILEOCOLITIS AND COLITIS

Patients with mild to moderate disease often respond to 5-ASA products in doses similar to those used for ulcerative colitis. If the disease remains mild or only moderate in severity but responds inadequately to 5-ASA drugs, metronidazole 125 to 250 mg three times daily or ciprofloxacin 500 mg once or twice daily can be tried before using immunomodulating agents.[72] Alternatively, budesonide 9 mg daily, a steroid with fewer side effects than prednisone, can be tried.

If the disease worsens despite conservative therapy or if the patient has moderate to severe symptoms, corticosteroids are begun in doses similar to those used in ulcerative colitis. After remission is induced, prednisone is tapered at a rate of 5 to 10 mg/wk until a dose of 20 mg/day is achieved. Subsequently, prednisone should be reduced by 5 mg/day every 3 weeks while monitoring clinical activity and laboratory studies.

Approximately 60% of patients who cannot be weaned from oral corticosteroids respond to azathioprine (up to 2.5 mg/kg per day) or 6-mercaptopurine (up to 1.5 mg/kg per day). Response may not occur for 6 to 9 months.[73] These drugs can be continued indefinitely, but at least one attempt should be made to discontinue them after 1 year of therapy to see if quiescence can be maintained. The folate antagonist methotrexate 25 mg IM once weekly appears to be effective in many patients who are resistant or intolerant to azathioprine or 6-mecaptopurine and has been used successfully to maintain remission.[74]

Infliximab is now often used for the treatment of active Crohn's disease, which is resistant to immunomodulating agents[75,76] and also for active fistulizing disease.[77] At all ages, a skin PPD and chest radiograph should be obtained before therapy because of reports of reactivation of latent tuberculosis. In the elderly, infliximab is contraindicated in patients with moderate to severe heart failure and should be used cautiously in patients with mild heart failure.[70] Infliximab-treated patients should not receive concomitant immunosuppression with azathioprine, 6-MP, methotrexate, or corticosteroids chronically, as side effects may be increased with no demonstrable benefits.

To avoid the problem of the development of antibodies to infliximab, fully humanized anti-TNF agent have been approved for treating Crohn's disease. Their advantage is that they are administered subcutaneously every 2 weeks, thus obviating the need for infusions and lessening the risk of reactions to infliximab.[78,79]

PERIANAL DISEASE

Perianal fistulas and abscesses can be terribly debilitating and frustrating to treat. Although perianal disease often improves with standard therapy for bowel inflammation and control of diarrhea, some patients continue to have persistent symptoms. Short-term success has been reported with metronidazole in doses of 1.5 to 2 g/day, but side effects at these doses are not uncommon and relapses occur when the drug is discontinued or tapered. Ciprofloxacin 500 mg twice daily is a more expensive alternative, albeit one with fewer side effects, but again there is a high relapse rate when the drug is discontinued. If an abscess develops, incision and drainage should be performed.

If perianal disease remains unresponsive to therapy, surgical diversion of the colon may be performed in an attempt to allow healing, but this too may be unsuccessful. Azathioprine or 6-mercaptopurine may be helpful in some patients with refractory disease.[80] Infliximab, a monoclonal antibody directed at human tumor necrosis factor, has been reported to be effective in severe Crohn's disease and those with resistant fistula.[77]

SURGERY

Unlike ulcerative colitis, Crohn's disease cannot be cured by surgery. Therefore surgical procedures should be reserved for patients who do not respond to medical therapy.

Proctocolectomy with ileostomy is the best surgical option for patients with extensive Crohn's colitis. In elderly patients who are debilitated or malnourished, an initial subtotal colectomy with ileostomy is less debilitating and permits weight gain and improved physical well-being. If proctectomy is subsequently required, it can be done with a low complication rate but may not be necessary if rectal disease is mild or absent. More limited colonic resections may be appropriate if severe disease is localized or obstructive symptoms are caused by relatively circumscribed bowel involvement.

LYMPHOCYTIC AND COLLAGENOUS COLITIS (MICROSCOPIC COLITIS)

Lymphocytic and collagenous colitis are uncommon disorders characterized by chronic watery diarrhea and histologic evidence of chronic mucosal inflammation in the absence of endoscopic or radiologic abnormalities of the large bowel. They comprise two histologically distinct disorders, which have been grouped under the term "microscopic colitis" and which differ principally by the presence or absence of a thickened collagen band located in the colonic subepithelium.[81,82] Both lymphocytic and collagenous colitis occur most commonly between ages 50 and 70 years, with a strong female predominance and a frequent association with arthritis, celiac disease, and autoimmune disorders.

In both lymphocytic and collagenous colitis, there is a modest increase in mononuclear cells within the lamina propria and between crypt epithelial cells, primarily consisting of $CD8^{+}$T lymphocytes, plasma cells, and macrophages.[83] In collagenous colitis, there is a thickened subepithelial collagen layer, which may be continuous or patchy. Although inflammatory changes occur diffusely throughout the colon, the characteristic collagen band thickening is highly variable, occurring in the cecum and transverse colon in more than 80% of cases and less than 30% of the time in the rectum. Although involvement of the left colon appears to be less intense, multiple biopsies of the left colon above the rectosigmoid during flexible sigmoidoscopy is sufficient to make the diagnosis in about 90% of cases.

Patients with collagenous and lymphocytic colitis usually have chronic watery diarrhea, with an average of eight stools each day, often with nocturnal stools, ranging from 300 to

1700 g per 24 hours, occasional fecal incontinence, abdominal cramps, and decreased symptoms when fasting.[84] Nausea, weight loss, and fecal urgency have also been reported but are variable. Diarrhea is generally longstanding, ranging from months to years, with a fluctuating course of remissions and exacerbations. In one series of 172 patients, the median time from onset of symptoms to diagnosis was 11 months, whereas in another of 31 patients, it was 5.4 years. Physical examinations are usually unremarkable and blood in the stool is absent. Routine laboratory studies are also normal.

Examination of fresh stools showed fecal leukocytes in 55% of 116 patients with collagenous colitis. Mild steatorrhea, mild anemia, low serum vitamin B_{12} levels, hypoalbuminemia, and mild steatorrhea have been reported in variable numbers of patients but are not characteristic. Autoimmune markers that have been identified in patients with collagenous colitis include antinuclear antibodies (up to 50%), pANCA in 14%, rheumatoid factor, and increased C_3 and C_4 complement components.

Colonoscopic examinations are usually normal. Infectious agents should be excluded by testing for stool ova and parasites, standard stool cultures, and *C. difficile* toxin assays. Many patients have been diagnosed to have irritable bowel syndrome, a disorder that can be excluded by abnormal colonic biopsies and the finding of increased stool volume, both of which are not characteristic of irritable bowel syndrome.

There have been very few controlled trials for either collagenous or lymphocytic colitis and therapy is largely empirical. NSAIDs and other colitis-inducing medications should be stopped.[82] About one third of patients respond to antidiarrheal agents, such as loperamide or diphenoxylate with atropine and bulk agents such as psyllium or methylcellulose; however, they do not exhibit improvement in inflammation or collagen thickness. In an open-label trial of bismuth subsalicylate in 12 patients,[85] eight chewable tablets per day for 8 weeks resulted in resolution of diarrhea and reduction of stool weight within 2 weeks, and in nine patients, colitis resolved, including disappearance of collagen band thickening. Although the basis for its efficacy is unknown, bismuth subsalicylate possesses antidiarrheal, antibacterial, and anti-inflammatory properties.

The majority of other treatment trials for collagenous colitis and lymphocytic colitis have studied 5-ASA compounds and bile acid resins. Alone or in combination, these agents appear to improve diarrhea and inflammation in some but certainly not all treated patients. Although corticosteroids given in either the oral or enema route provide symptomatic improvement and decreased inflammation in more than 80% of cases, relapse usually occurs quickly after stopping the drug.[84] Moreover, long-term corticosteroids have undesirable effects, especially in older patients.

Budesonide is a topical steroid with both a high receptor-binding affinity and a high first-pass effect in the liver. It has similar efficacy to prednisone but fewer significant side effects. The recommended dose is 9 mg once daily with tapering by 3 mg daily for 2 to 4 weeks.[86,87] Recurrences may occur and maintenance with 3 mg once daily may be necessary in some patients.

Azathioprine and methotrexate may be considered in steroid-refractory patients.[88] Some studies suggest that older patients are more likely to be controlled with antidiarrheal agents or require no medication, in contrast to younger patients.[89]

COLONIC ISCHEMIA

The blood supply to the colon is derived mainly from branches of the superior and inferior mesenteric arteries and is characterized by a rich collateral circulation, except for the potentially susceptible marginal artery of Drummond and the arc of Riolan located at the peripheral junction of the two mesenteric arteries.[90] Occlusion of a major artery results in immediate opening of collateral vessels to maintain an adequate blood supply to the bowel. Intestinal ischemia may occur as a result of generalized reduction of blood flow (nonocclusive ischemia), redistribution of blood flow (e.g., vessel obstruction with poor collateral circulation), or a combination of the two. Colonic ischemia is the most common vascular disorder of the intestines in the elderly population and one that is often misdiagnosed unless there is a high index of suspicion and an aggressive diagnostic approach is used in patients suspected of having this disorder.[91]

The clinical spectrum of colonic ischemia includes a vast array of presentations and may be associated with a number of potentiating factors. Ischemia may be classified as reversible and irreversible; the former may have submucosal or intramural hemorrhage or transient ischemic colitis, which completely resolves within weeks to months, depending on the severity of the process. Irreversible ischemia may be characterized by chronic ulcerations, strictures of varying lengths, colonic gangrene, or fulminant transmural colitis.[92]

In most cases, the cause of colonic ischemia cannot be established with certainty and no vascular occlusions can be identified. A significant minority of patients are found to have a potentially obstructing process in the colon, such as a benign stricture, diverticulitis, or carcinoma. Other contributing factors include hypotension, dehydration, congestive heart failure, use of digitalis, polycythemia, volvulus, and cardiac arrhythmias.

Symptoms and signs

The most common manifestation is the sudden onset of mild to moderately severe left lower abdominal cramping pain; this is often accompanied by bloody diarrhea or hematochezia, which may not appear until 24 hours later. Frank hemorrhage is not characteristic of ischemia. Physical examination reveals tenderness at the site of the involved bowel; these sites encompass the distal transverse, splenic flexure, and/or descending colons in about two thirds of patients. Peritoneal signs may last for several hours, but persistence beyond that time suggests a transmural process. Fever, leukocytosis, absence of bowel sounds, and abdominal distention also suggest the possibility of bowel infarction.

Diagnosis

If the diagnosis is suspected on clinical grounds, colonoscopy with minimal insufflation with air is the preferred diagnostic test. When an ischemic segment is encountered, biopsies should be taken from the edge of the ulcerated area and of noninvolved tissue, and the procedure aborted. Barium studies may reveal "thumbprinting" in the affected areas of the colon, which represents submucosal or mucosal hemorrhages and edema during the early phase of the process. This corresponds to the hemorrhagic nodules noted on colonoscopic examination. There is no meaningful role for mesenteric angiography in patients with colon ischemia, unless there is involvement of the right colon with suspected mesenteric ischemia of the small intestine.

Treatment

Patients should be managed with bowel rest, intravenous fluids, or plasma expanders, and in severe cases, systemic antibiotics such as gentamicin and clindamycin.[93] Corticosteroids are of no benefit and should not be administered. In mild disease, symptoms resolve within several days, and radiologic healing occurs within several weeks, although some patients may not heal for up to 6 months.

If the patient continues to have diarrhea, bleeding, or significant obstructive symptoms for more than several weeks, surgical resection is usually indicated. If colonic infarction is suspected, emergency laparotomy with resection of nonviable bowel is needed.[94] With colonic infarction and gangrene, the mortality rate in the elderly with multiple co-morbid conditions approaches 50% to 75% with surgery and is universally fatal with nonsurgical treatment.

Prognosis

Recurrent episodes of colonic ischemia occur in less than 10% of patients. Attempts should be made to correct or remove underlying conditions that predispose to this disorder. Peripheral vasculopathy and right colonic involvement are associated with more severe disease.

COLONIC PSEUDO-OBSTRUCTION

Acute colonic pseudo-obstruction, sometimes termed Ogilvie's syndrome, is characterized by nonobstructive, nontoxic dilation of the colon.[95] This condition may develop after surgical procedures, especially orthopedic ones, and also occurs in a setting of serious coexisting illness, including sepsis, pneumonia, acute pancreatitis, spinal cord injury, or administration of anticholinergic, narcotic, or psychotropic drugs. This disorder can compromise respiratory status and cause cecal perforation. The risk of cecal perforation is said to rise when the diameter of the cecum increases beyond 10 cm. A variant of this disorder is "megasigmoid syndrome," often described in psychotic patients but not exclusively seen within this group.

After obstruction has been excluded, treatment includes correction of electrolyte imbalances, discontinuation of offending drugs, treatment of underlying infection or inflammation, nasogastric suction, a rectal or colonic decompression tube with positioning of the patient on the right and left sides at intervals of several hours, or medical treatment with intravenous neostigmine.[96] Decompression with colonoscopy may be attempted if there is severe dilation and no response to medical therapy.[97] Surgical decompression under local anesthesia using a stab-wound cecostomy can be performed if other measures fail. Postdecompression x-ray films should be obtained for several days to document continued resolution.

Relapses are common after successful decompression of acute colonic pseudo-obstruction, being as high as 33%. The administration of 29.5 g PEG daily in two divided doses after successful treatment resulted in no relapses versus a 33% relapse rate for patients receiving a placebo.[98]

Chronic colonic pseudo-obstruction, with or without colonic dilation (megacolon), may be associated with amyloidosis, muscular dystrophy, myxedema, dementia, multiple sclerosis, Parkinson's disease, quadriplegia, schizophrenia, and idiopathic visceral neuropathy and myopathy. There may be esophageal, gastric, small intestinal, and genitourinary dysfunction. Although most patients have constipation, diarrhea occurs if there is small bowel bacterial overgrowth or overflow around a fecal impaction.

Subtotal colectomy may be necessary in some patients with refractory symptoms and if anorectal function is normal. If anorectal dysfunction is present, proctocolectomy with ileostomy is indicated. Sigmoid resection may be all that is necessary in patients with megasigmoid syndrome. Most patients can be treated conservatively.

VOLVULUS

Factors thought to contribute to colonic volvulus include increasing age, chronic constipation, fecal retention, poor peritoneal fixation during embryologic rotation of the hindgut, and, in some areas of the world, diets very high in fiber.[99] The clinical setting typical of a sigmoid volvulus is an elderly institutionalized individual with a history of chronic constipation or laxative abuse.[99]

The sigmoid colon, with its copious mesentery, is most commonly involved, but cecal volvulus can occur when fixation to the posterior parietal wall is incomplete. Volvulus of the transverse colon is by far the least common. Patients have a sudden onset of severe abdominal pain, followed by rapid and marked abdominal distention. Compromise of blood flow occurs as a result of twisting of the mesentery and marked distention of the loop.

Abdominal x-rays reveal massive distention of a single loop of bowel; the obstructed loop frequently is shaped like a coffee bean, with the concavity marking the point of torsion. The concavity points to the left lower quadrant in patients with sigmoid volvulus, and to the right lower quadrant when cecal volvulus is present. Administering contrast through the rectum confirms the diagnosis by the appearance of the pointed twist of the contrast column.

Closely related to a cecal volvulus is a cecal bascule in which malfixation allows the cecum to fold anteriorly and in a cephalad direction, which can result in a flap-valve obstruction with cecal distention. Abdominal x-rays reveal distention of the cecum, but no "bird beak" is seen on a barium enema, as in volvulus. However, treatment is identical to that for conventional cecal volvulus.

Attempts to untwist a sigmoid volvulus may be made by gently inserting an endoscope as far as the twisted segment.[100] Successful detorsion must be followed by careful observation should the bowel continue to be ischemic. Nonoperative decompression is more successful with a sigmoid than with a cecal volvulus; indeed, attempts to treat a cecal volvulus by nonoperative means can be dangerous, and even if successful, recurrence rates are high. Opinion is divided as to whether the first episode of sigmoid volvulus should be treated with resection. Fixation without resection is not considered a useful option. Certainly, patients with more than one episode of sigmoid volvulus should have resection.

In elderly and frail patients with cecal volvulus, early surgical intervention to untwist the volvulus followed by cecal fixation (cecopexy) is frequently all that is necessary unless bowel necrosis is present. If the latter is present, resection with ileostomy is indicated. In healthy elderly patients, cecal resection with reanastomosis is the preferred option.

NEOPLASTIC LESIONS

Colonic polyps may be classified into: (1) neoplastic polyps, which include adenomatous polyps and carcinomas; (2) non-neoplastic polyps, which include hyperplastic, inflammatory, and hamartomatous types; and (3) submucosal tumors, such as lipomas, leiomyomas, hemangiomas, fibromas, lymphoid polyps, and carcinoids.[101]

Most (80%–90%) colonic polyps are either adenomatous or hyperplastic, and of these about 75% are adenomas. However, when only polyps less than 5 mm are considered, half are hyperplastic and most are found in the rectosigmoid colon. Current evidence has suggested that hyperplastic polyps are not of clinical importance.[102] However, this view may be too simplistic. There are serrated polyps that appear to be hyperplastic but with important histologic differences, which do have malignant potential. In contrast, it is widely accepted that most carcinomas arise from adenomas.

Adenomatous polyps

These polyps arise from mucosal glandular epithelium and can be described based on the following characteristics:

1. Size: Approximately 25% of adenomas are larger than 1 cm, and more than 80% of large adenomas occur in the left colon and rectum.
2. Architecture: More than 80% of adenomas are tubular, 5% to 15% are villous, and the rest are tubulovillous. Those with a higher proportion of villous elements tend to be larger and carry a higher risk of malignant transformation.
3. Dysplasia: All adenomas are dysplastic, but high-grade dysplasia is strongly associated with malignancy.

In the United States, prevalence rates in men and women are similar. Except in familial syndromes, colonic adenomas are rare before the age of 40, increase steadily, and reach a peak after the age of 60. Population studies suggest that the environment strongly contributes to adenoma prevalence and probably to the frequency of colon cancer as well. For example, obesity may be a risk factor whereas nonsteroidal anti-inflammatory drugs (including aspirin) are associated with decreased risk.[103]

It is logical to identify and remove all benign adenomas at an early stage to prevent progression to carcinoma. In one study, screening and polyp removal by rigid sigmoidoscopy during the previous 10 years resulted in a 70% reduction in the risk of fatal cancer of the rectum and distal colon compared with the outcome in nonscreened subjects.[104] In the National Polyp Study, colonoscopic polypectomy reduced the incidence of colorectal cancer by 76% to 90% during a follow-up of almost 6 years.[105] These findings form the basis for current screening recommendations.

There is epidemiologic evidence that aspirin and other, nonsteroidal anti-inflammatory drugs (NSAIDs) may reduce the risk of colorectal cancer.[106] Several large studies, although not all, have found a significant reduction in death rates from colon cancer among both men and women who use NSAIDs on a regular basis. Such observations are supported by laboratory studies demonstrating that aspirin and other cyclooxygenase inhibitors demonstrate chemopreventive effects in animal models of colon carcinogenesis. There currently are insufficient data supporting the use of NSAIDs as colorectal cancer chemopreventive agents outside appropriately designed trials.

Management of polyps

Criteria for the adequacy of colonoscopic polypectomy are well established for pedunculated malignant polyps.[107,108] In patients having favorable criteria, the risk of residual tumor is 0.3% for pedunculated lesions and 1.5% for sessile lesions, whereas the risk is 8.5% for those having unfavorable criteria. Surgery is therefore strongly considered in the latter situation, although recommendations should be individualized based on patient age and comorbid conditions.

The following recommendations for treatment after polypectomy are based on recent information.[109]

1. Patients should undergo complete colonoscopy at the time of polypectomy and removal of all synchronous polyps.
2. In 3 years the first follow-up colonoscopy should be performed to check for missed synchronous and/or metachronous adenomas. If the results are negative, subsequent surveillance intervals may be increased to 5 years.
3. Selected patients with multiple adenomas or those with large sessile polyps (>3 cm) or those with suboptimal initial clearing examinations require colonoscopy at 1 year or sooner and again 3 years later if the colon is clear.

Screening strategies

It is generally accepted that colorectal cancer largely can be prevented by the detection and removal of adenomatous polyps. Screening tests may be divided into those that primarily detect cancer early, and those that can detect cancer early and also detect adenomatous polyps that can be removed.[110] Although a yearly FOBT for all patients 50 years and older has been suggested, controversy exists regarding the cost and benefits of such a policy. The sensitivity of Hemoccult II tests for detecting asymptomatic colorectal cancer ranges from 45% to 80% in mass-screened populations and is less than 25% for detecting polyps 1 cm or larger in diameter.[111,112] Thus a FOBT is a relatively effective way to screen for asymptomatic cancers but is ineffective in detecting even sizable premalignant polyps. Moreover, at least 50% of screened individuals over the age of 40 are false-positive or have an upper gastrointestinal source of bleeding. However, the specificity of an unrehydrated FOBT is about 98% to 99%.

A recent systematic review of colorectal cancer screening using the fecal occult blood test indicated that screening had a 16% to 25% reduction in the relative risk of CRC mortality for studies that used biennial screening.[113]

A recently published consensus document expressed the strong opinion that colon cancer prevention should be the goal of screening and indicated a preference for tests designed to detect both early cancer and adenomatous polyps if resources are available and patients are willing to undergo an invasive procedure.[110] Testing options under this scenario include flexible sigmoidoscopy or double contrast barium enema every 5 years, full colonoscopy every 10 years, and computed tomographic colonography every 5 years for asymptomatic adults aged 50 years or older. The finding of adenomatous polyps on flexible sigmoidoscopy should be followed by colonoscopy to remove all polyps followed by a repeat colonoscopy in 3 to 5 years depending upon number of polyps and histology. Although somewhat controversial, many believe that finding polyps on imaging studies should be confirmed by colonoscopy with removal of any polyps. Others believe that polyps less than 1 cm may be watched with repeat studies every 2 years.[12]

Colorectal cancer

Colorectal cancer is the third most commonly diagnosed cancer and the second most common cause of cancer death in the United States and the United Kingdom.[113] Epidemiologic evidence strongly suggests that colon cancer is an acquired genetic disease produced by chronic exposure to environmental carcinogens. Thus deaths from colon cancer increase slowly by middle age and rise steeply thereafter. Moreover, immigrants from areas of low incidence acquire, within a single generation, the increased risks of the indigenous population in areas of higher incidence.[114] Except for the increased risk for colorectal cancer among individuals with ulcerative colitis and those with a family history of colorectal cancer, no high-risk exposures have consistently been identified in the United States. However, epidemiologic evidence implicates both decreased dietary fiber and increased consumption of animal protein and fat. That colorectal cancer is caused by cumulative alterations in the cellular genome, and not by a single genetic alteration, may explain the long latency period between initial exposure to carcinogen(s) and the appearance of cancer.[115]

In about 80% of cases, somatic mutations in the APC gene on chromosome 5 are the earliest recognized genetic alterations in sporadic colonic carcinogenesis and are found in the smallest adenomas. These mutations permit unregulated proliferation at the base of the colonic crypt. A multistep genetic model for sporadic colorectal tumorigenesis involves sequential mutations in cellular oncogenes and tumor suppressor genes.[115,116] Two cellular proteins associated with the APC gene have been identified and appear to be involved in cell adhesion, which may provide an important clue to the mechanism of tumor initiation.

In about 15% of sporadic cases, a colon cancer "susceptibility gene" on the short arm of chromosome 2 has been identified in patients with families with hereditary nonpolyposis colon cancer (HNPCC) and in sporadic colon cancers as well. Widespread mutations in short, repeated DNA sequences due to defective or mutant DNA mismatch repair enzymes have been identified on chromosome 2p. At least six such repair genes have now been identified in the pathogenesis of colon cancer.[117] These tumors appear to have a genetic pathogenesis different from that of the hereditary polyposis syndromes that result in different clinical features and less aggressive behavior.

Colonic cancers can be classified by gross appearance, histology (well to poorly differentiated, mucinous, signet-ring type) or by DNA content.[114] In general, poorly differentiated carcinomas have a somewhat worse prognosis than well-differentiated tumors. More helpful is staging, for example, by the Astler and Coller modified Dukes (Dukes-Turnbull) classifications: A, tumor limited to the muscularis mucosa; B1, tumor extends into the muscularis propria or, B2, penetrates through serosa with no lymph node involvement; C1, four or fewer regional lymph node metastases or, C2, greater than four nodes involved; and D, distant metastases. Actuarial 5-year survival rates diminish from 85% to 95% for Dukes A lesions to less than 5% for Dukes D lesions. As expected, prognosis is much poorer when there is vascular or neural invasion.

In an attempt to provide a uniform classification, the American Joint Committee on Cancer introduced the tumor-node metastases (TNM) classification for CRC.[118] This system classifies the extent of the primary tumor (T), the status of regional lymph nodes (N), and the presence or absence of distant metastases (M). Cases are assigned to one of five stages (O through IV); it has in most cases replaced the Dukes classification in therapeutic trials.

The primary treatment for colorectal cancer is surgical resection. Preoperative studies include a complete evaluation of the colon, preferably by colonoscopy and a chest x-ray. Routine measurement of carcinoembryonic antigen (CEA) is often done. Although serial measurements of CEA have been advocated to detect early recurrences after surgery, cancer cures attributable to CEA monitoring appear to be infrequent[119] and it must be questioned whether such a practice is justified in view of the substantial cost or the emotional stress that CEA testing may cause patients. Abdominal imaging studies are most useful for detecting advanced disease (i.e., hepatic metastases) but are less useful in finding localized extracolonic spread. Moreover, such information can be obtained directly at the time of surgery, and the presence of metastases does not influence the need for surgery or the type of surgery that is performed. In contrast, rectal endosonography is superior to computed tomography and magnetic resonance imaging in staging rectal cancers.[17]

There is no benefit from adjunctive radiation therapy for colon cancer outside the rectum. However, adjuvant chemotherapy with fluorouracil (and levamisole)[120] or fluorouracil and leucovorin has been associated with a significant reduction in tumor recurrence and enhanced survival in patients with stage III colon cancer.[121] These data support the use of postoperative adjuvant chemotherapy in stage III colon cancers. In contrast, the benefit of adjuvant fluorouracil-based therapy in stage II colon cancer is less clear.[122] Adjuvant combined radiotherapy and chemotherapy improve postsurgical survival in patients with rectal carcinoma, albeit with increased and often severe toxicity.[123] Some patients with unresectable rectal cancer may become surgical candidates following radiation therapy.

LOWER GASTROINTESTINAL BLEEDING

The two most frequent causes of acute lower gastrointestinal bleeding in elderly patients, defined as originating below the ligament of Treitz, are diverticulosis and vascular ectasias (angiodysplasia).[124] These two entities account for two

Table 81-6. Clinical Presentation of Common Causes of Lower Gastrointestinal Bleeding

Symptom	Young Adult	Middle Age	Elderly
Abdominal pain	IBD	IBD	Ischemia, IBD
Painless bleeding	Meckel's diverticulum, polyp	Diverticulosis, polyp, cancer	Angiodysplasia, diverticulosis, polyp, cancer
Diarrhea	IBD, infection	IBD, infection	Ischemia, infection, IBD
Constipation	Hemorrhoids, fissure, rectal ulcer	Hemorrhoids, fissure	Cancer, hemorrhoids, fissure

Abbreviation: *IBD*, inflammatory bowel disease.

thirds of hemodynamically significant lower gastrointestinal bleeding (Table 81-6). The most common causes of chronic lower gastrointestinal bleeding are hemorrhoids, angiodysplasia, and colonic neoplasms. Known causes of acute lower gastrointestinal bleeding other than angiodysplasia and diverticulosis make up perhaps 25% of all bleeding episodes. These include neoplasm; radiation enterocolitis; ischemic, ulcerative, and Crohn's colitis; solitary rectal ulcer syndrome; and internal hemorrhoids. Less frequently reported causes of bleeding include small intestinal and Meckel's diverticula, vasculitis, and Dieulafoy lesions of the small intestine and colon.

Angiodysplasia

Angiodysplasia are small clusters of dilated and tortuous veins, which appear in the mucosa of the colon and in the small intestine.[125] They are thought to result from age-associated degeneration of colonic submucosal veins, are often multiple, and are an important cause of lower gastrointestinal bleeding in the elderly population; two thirds of patients with angiodysplasia are over 70 years of age. The principal theory concerning their development is that repeated episodes of low-grade partial obstruction of submucosal veins occur during muscular contraction or from increased intraluminal pressure, resulting in dilation and tortuosity of the vein.[126] This process may extend to the mucosal veins, which are drained by the submucosal vein. Finally the precapillary sphincter becomes incompetent, and a small arteriovenous communication with an ectatic tuft of vessels develops. The tendency of vascular ectasias to occur in the right colon is best explained by the greater tension on the bowel wall, as expressed by Laplace's law relating tension to the diameter of the bowel lumen. A review of the literature casts doubt on a causal association between vascular ectasias and aortic stenosis.[127] Nevertheless, it has been reported that recurrent bleeding from these lesions decreases after replacement of a stenotic aortic valve.[128]

Vascular ectasias remain asymptomatic in most individuals. The usual manifestation is that of painless subacute or recurrent bleeding, which stops spontaneously in most cases. Bleeding may consist of bright red blood, maroon stools or (rarely) melena, or may be occult.[124] About 10% to 15% of patients have episodes of brisk blood loss, and up to half exhibit iron deficiency anemia.

Diagnosis may be made by colonoscopy or angiography; of the two, colonoscopy is preferred, since it can exclude other causes of bleeding and can be used for therapeutic interventions.[129,130] Because lesions are small, often multiple, and difficult to see, thorough cleansing of the colon is necessary to provide adequate visualization of the mucosa. Colonoscopy is usually performed after bleeding has stopped and within 48 hours to permit identification of other bleeding sources.

Mesenteric angiography is the diagnostic procedure of choice when acute bleeding is brisk. The finding of tortuous, densely opacified clusters of small veins that empty slowly represents the advanced ectatic process. Early filling of the vein, indicative of the presence of an arteriovenous communication, is found in most patients who are studied for bleeding. Extravasation of contrast into the bowel lumen is seen when there is active bleeding at a rate of at least 0.5 mL/min; because bleeding is often intermittent, a bleeding site is identified by angiography in only a minority of patients.

Bleeding can be controlled acutely by intra-arterial administration of vasopressin in doses ranging from 0.2 to 0.6 units/min. This often permits stabilization of the patient and appears to be more effective when bleeding is from the right colon. When bleeding cannot be controlled, surgery is required. Colonoscopic therapeutic modalities generally involve thermal ablation techniques, but rebleeding remains a significant problem.[131] A right hemicolectomy is performed if bleeding from the right colon has been identified by angiography or colonoscopy and if other sources of bleeding have not been identified. The extent of resection should not be influenced by the presence of left colonic diverticulosis. Recurrent bleeding, probably due to undetected ectasias, occurs in up to 20% of patients who may require either more extensive colonic resection or exploratory laparotomy.

Treatment should be conservative whenever possible and consists of blood or iron replacement as appropriate. For recurrent bleeding, transcolonoscopic electrocoagulation or laser coagulation may be attempted; difficulties include identifying the ectatic lesion(s) and excluding other causes of blood loss if bleeding has stopped. Perforation of the right colon with coagulation therapy is a hazard.[132]

The development of capsule endoscopy may reduce the need for diagnostic laparotomy in patients with recurrent bleeding from obscure sites.[133]

Vasculitis

Inflammation and necrosis of blood vessels may lead to ischemia and ulceration, resulting in pain and/or bleeding. Polyarteritis nodosa, Churg-Strauss syndrome, Henoch-Schönlein purpura, systemic lupus erythematosus, rheumatoid vasculitis, Behçet's disease, and essential mixed cryoglobulinemia have all been reported to produce gastrointestinal bleeding and are best diagnosed with endoscopic procedures in the appropriate clinical setting.

Dieulafoy lesions

These lesions have been reported to cause bleeding, in several cases massive, in the small intestine and colon.[134] They are characterized by a small mucosal defect with minimal inflammation and a congenitally large, tortuous, thick-walled arteriole at the base which ruptures into the bowel lumen. The histology of these vessels is normal, and their abnormality is their size relative to their superficial location. Bleeding can be localized with angiography, although occasionally colonoscopy can identify the lesion if bleeding has stopped and the colon is well prepared. Surgical resection, embolization therapy, or thermal coagulation therapy are the treatments of choice.

Evaluation and management of lower gastrointestinal bleeding

The first goal of management is to rapidly assess the severity of bleeding and cardiovascular status of the patient and to resuscitate those with major blood loss (Figure 81-1). Vital signs reflecting orthostatic changes and other signs of hypovolemia should be checked immediately and at frequent intervals thereafter. If signs of shock or hypovolemia are present, one or two large-bore intravenous catheters should be placed to facilitate fluid resuscitation. Initial blood work, including hemogram, platelet count, coagulation profiles, routine blood chemistries, and type and cross-match should be obtained immediately. Only after these critical tasks are completed should a more detailed history and physical examination be performed to help determine the site of bleeding and potential causes. Another important step is to distinguish acute bleeding from active bleeding superimposed on chronic blood loss. This is best done with the hematocrit and mean corpuscular volume; if the latter is low, chronic bleeding should be suspected.

The third step is to consider the location of the gastrointestinal bleed based on characteristics of the bleeding and a BUN/creatinine ratio.[135] Although hematochezia, defined as the passage of red blood through the rectum, suggests a lower gastrointestinal source, up to 20% of patients with upper gastrointestinal bleeding may have hematochezia because of the rapid passage of large amounts of blood through the small and large intestines.[136]

Such patients always show evidence of severe hemodynamic compromise, and most have a BUN/creatinine ratio greater than 25 on initial evaluation.[135] On the other hand, melena is often characteristic of upper gastrointestinal bleeding but can also be seen in patients with bleeding from the small intestine or right colon when colonic transit is slow. Fresh unclotted blood dripping into the toilet after

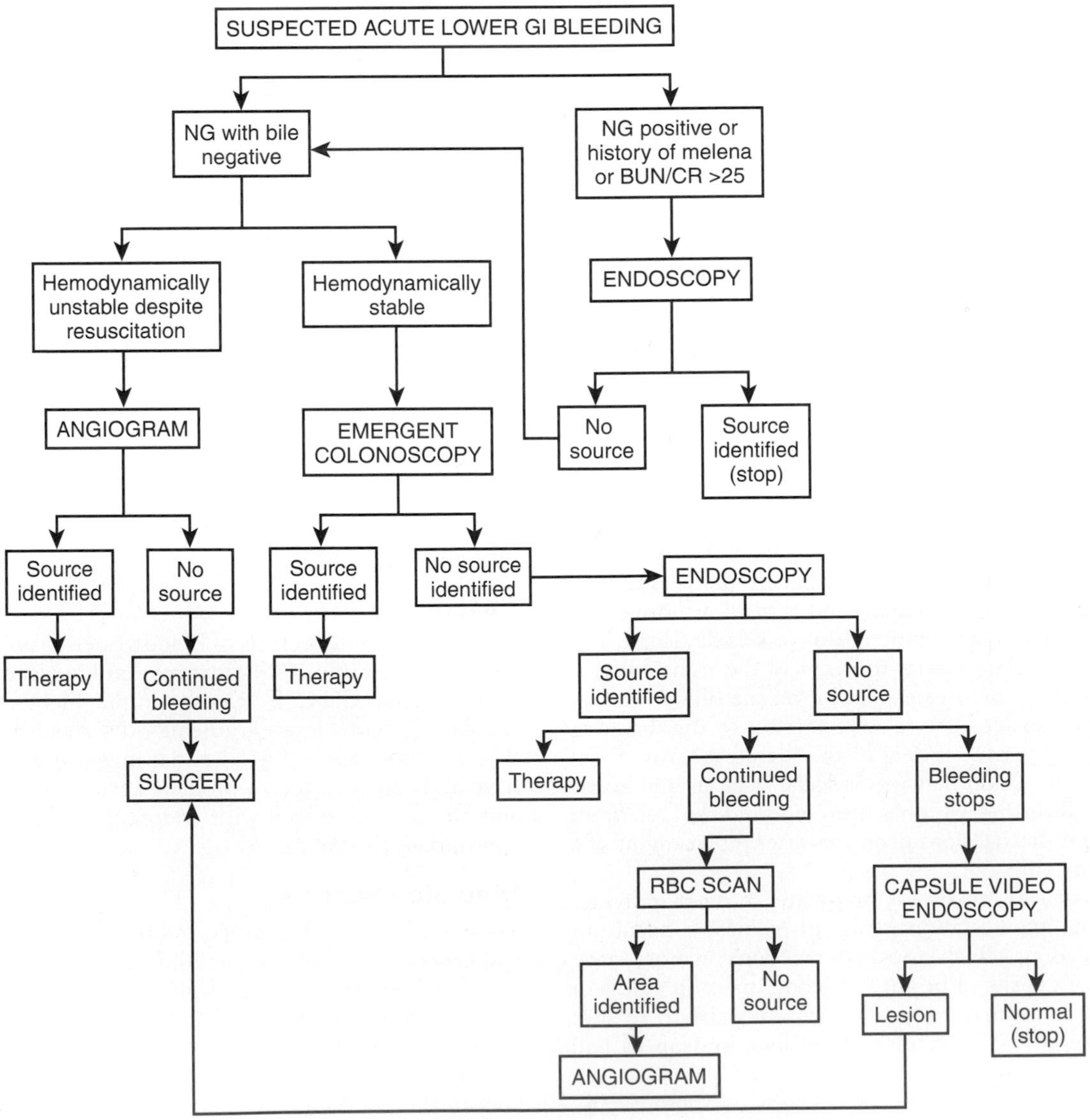

Figure 81-1. Suspected acute lower gastrointestinal bleeding.

defecation suggests a very distal anorectal source, whereas blood streaking the stool suggests origin in the left colon.

Exclusion of an upper gastrointestinal site begins with passage of a nasogastric tube and examination of gastric contents for red blood, coffee ground materials, and bile. The presence of bile and an absence of blood or coffee ground materials significantly diminishes but does not exclude bleeding proximal to the duodenojejunal junction; thus, an upper endoscopy should be performed in a setting compatible with an upper gastrointestinal source. There is no role for occult blood testing of a nasogastric aspirate in the absence of coffee grounds or bloody material. Finally, hemorrhoidal and low rectal bleeding should be excluded by sigmoidoscopy in patients thought to have lower gastrointestinal hemorrhage.

When evaluating stable patients with acute lower gastrointestinal hemorrhage, colonoscopy preceded by oral bowel preparation is preferred in identifying and potentially treating a colonic bleeding source. If an emergency colonoscopy is to be considered, the nasogastric tube should be left in place to permit rapid administration of a polyethylene glycol electrolyte solution to cleanse the colon.

If bleeding is active and bowel preparation cannot be done, scintigraphy with ^{129}Tc-labeled red blood cells can be used in an attempt to locate a bleeding site. This technique detects active bleeding at rates of approximately 0.1 mL/min, and the patient can be serially scanned for up to 36 hours if bleeding is intermittent. Site localization may be impaired if delayed films are taken too infrequently and, of course, the patient must be actively bleeding at the time of the study. Although there were initial enthusiastic reports of an approximately 90% rate of detection of active bleeding, subsequent studies have yielded conflicting results.[137,138] These latter reports have raised serious concerns regarding a rigid policy of routinely performing nuclear scintigraphy before mesenteric angiography, particularly in high-risk patients for whom rapid diagnosis is preferred. It may be more accurate if upper gastrointestinal bleeding has been excluded.[138] If bleeding is active and severe and/or scintigraphy is not diagnostic, selective mesenteric angiography can be used to detect extravasated contrast into the bowel when bleeding rates are 0.5 to 1.0 mL/min, or to demonstrate vascular lesions, neovascularity, or tumors in the absence of extravasation.[139] Sensitivity declines when bleeding is recurrent or chronic. Attempts have been made to increase diagnostic sensitivity and accuracy by using systemic heparinization, intra-arterial vasodilators, or thrombolytic agents during angiography if the initial study is negative.[140] More extensive experience is needed to determine whether the increased yield justifies the increased risk of bleeding complications.

Angiography also offers the potential for local therapy, provided selective catheterization can be achieved. These modalities include infusion of vasopressin to control acute arterial bleeding in colonic diverticular disease or angiodysplasia, and selective embolization of an identified bleeding site with a gelatin sponge, vascular coils, or polyvinyl alcohol particles.[141] Complications include electrolyte disturbances, cardiovascular complications, and bowel ischemia with vasopressin infusion and bowel infarction following embolization. The latter should be attempted only at centers that have the expertise to perform superselective catheterization. Some investigators report that urgent colonoscopy is superior to selective mesenteric angiography in identifying the source of severe lower gastrointestinal bleeding. If bleeding is massive, emergent surgery with or without intraoperative endoscopy may be the best option. There is little or no place in modern surgical practice for blind colonic resection.

If no source of bleeding is detected by colonoscopy and no further bleeding occurs, a small bowel enteroscopy or capsule endoscopy should be performed. Enteroscopes can often be advanced to 60 to 100 cm past the ligament of Treitz if the procedure is done by experienced personnel.[142] The diagnostic yield has varied from 30% to 60%, with arteriovascular malformations accounting for most of the causes of bleeding. Video capsules allow visualization of most or all of the small intestine.

Barium radiographic procedures have no role in the evaluation of patients with acute lower gastrointestinal bleeding. They are unable to demonstrate active bleeding and interfere with attempts to perform colonoscopy or mesenteric angiography. Even if a lesion is detected, there is no proof that it is the source of the bleeding.

KEY POINTS
The Large Bowel

- Principal functions of the colon are to store fecal wastes and to expel them in an appropriate manner. Colonic dysfunction may result in constipation, diarrhea, or fecal incontinence.
- Making a clinical distinction between painful diverticular disease and diverticulitis carries a sizable rate of error in elderly people. Computed tomography and ultrasonography often help in this process, which is important as treatment approaches.
- Both ulcerative colitis and Crohn's disease are found with increased frequency in elderly people. There are more and better drugs to treat these patients, both acutely and to maintain remissions.
- Colonic ischemia is often underdiagnosed in elderly people, is characterized by the sudden onset of abdominal pain and bleeding, and often is benign and reversible. Colonoscopy is the diagnostic procedure of choice.
- Colon cancers are a frequent but often preventable cause of death in both men and women. The aggressive use of colonoscopy to detect premalignant polyps is the gold standard for prevention and should begin at age 50 in persons of normal risk.
- Lower gastrointestinal bleeding in elderly people is most often associated with angiodysplasias and diverticulosis. Colonoscopy is the preferred diagnostic test, whereas scintigraphy and angiography are helpful if no source of bleeding is seen or if bleeding is so brisk as to exclude colonoscopy.

For a complete list of references, please visit online only at www.expertconsult.com

CHAPTER 82

Nutrition in Aging

C. Shanthi Johnson
Gordon Sacks

NUTRITION IN AGING

The nutrition goals in caring for older adults are to maintain or even improve their overall health and quality of life as well as to prevent or treat age- and nutrition-related problems by improving the nutritional status of individuals and population groups. Whether defined as "the condition of a population's or individual's health as affected by the intake and utilization of nutrients and non-nutrients"[1] or as the degree of balance between nutrient intake and nutrient requirements, nutritional status is extremely important to overall health and to maintaining optimal nutritional status. Optimal nutritional status also has been shown to influence the aging process, various physiologic systems and functions, body composition, and the onset and management of various chronic conditions. The process of aging also affects nutritional status. Specifically, aging directly contributes to the changes in nutritional needs, although requirements for specific nutrients can decrease, increase, or remain the same.[2] With aging, changes in economic and social status arise that contribute to decreased access to food, poor food choices, nutrient deficiencies, and poor nutritional status, which in turn lead to increased risk of illness, poor health, and limited mobility and independence, as illustrated in Figure 82-1.[3]

Like overall health, nutrition is influenced by social determinants such as income, educational level, social support, gender, culture, and other factors outlined in the population health framework.[4,5] Such factors partly account for the wide and stubbornly resistant disparities in nutritional and health status that exists in populations. For example, research in the area of food costing shows that seniors living alone are not able to afford nutritious diets.[6] The consumption of vitamin and mineral supplement is higher among those older adults with higher levels of education.[7] Furthermore, seniors who live alone and lack social support tend to have poorer nutritional status compared to elderly individuals with social support.

NUTRITION SCREENING AND ASSESSMENT

Many physiologic factors impact the nutritional status and well-being of older adults. An inadequate or excess intake of nutrients is the result of ingestion and utilization of nutrients from a variety of dietary sources, as well as other various elements (e.g., age-related changes, medication intake, socioeconomic factors, and functional and cognitive capacity). These factors facilitate the depletion or storage of tissue stores, change in plasma nutrient levels, enzymatic activity, and other physiologic functions, which affect anthropometric indicators (e.g., weight, body composition). As a result, anthropometric measures, as well as biochemical, clinical, and dietary factors, are critical and must be considered in the assessment of an individual's nutritional status.

Anthropometric measures are used to assess nutritional status through the examination of body proportions and composition, as well as the fluctuations in these indicators over time, and include body weight, weight history, height or other estimates of stature, body mass index (BMI), skin-fold thickness, and circumference measurements.[8,9] Self-reported measures are often inaccurate, and trained technicians should adopt standardized measurement protocols to reduce measurement error.[10,11] Body weight is a key indicator in nutritional status, and one's weight history serves as an indicator of nutritional risk. Periods of excessive or significant weight loss include 2% body weight in a week, 5% in a month, 7.5% in 3 months, or 10% in 6 months. In addition to weight changes, height changes, which are largely due to the shortening of the spine, are reliable indicators of an at-risk individual. If an individual is unable to stand or stand straight, estimates of stature can be estimated via arm span, demispan, or knee height. Arm span measurements can determine the maximal height in adulthood rather than one's actual height, whereas age-, gender-, and race-specific equations are used to estimate stature from knee height measures[12] with supine knee height valued as more reliable than seated knee height. Once height and weight measures are obtained, body mass index (BMI) can be calculated. Body weight (kg) is divided by height squared (m), which evaluates weight independent of height but does not directly measure body fat. For older adults, a BMI of less than 24 is associated with poor nutritional health, a BMI between 24 and 29 is believed to be a healthy weight, and a BMI of over 29 is seen as overweight and may lead to health problems.[13] Skinfold thickness measurements are used to determine body fatness. However, with aging, skin changes in thickness, elasticity, and compressibility, and skinfold thickness is not a reliable measurement for older adults as a result. Body fat stores can be assessed through circumference measurements (e.g., waist, waist-to-hip ratio, and upper arm circumference), much like measures that are used to estimate skeletal muscle mass (somatic protein stores). Body fat measurement can be used as a quick screening tool to pinpoint high-risk individuals who may be susceptible to under- or overnutrition and are useful alone or combined with height and weight measurements.

Another useful measure for individuals at risk for nutritional problems is *biochemical data*, which can be used to find subclinical deficiencies (e.g., through blood or urine specimens). Through such tests, biochemical indicators of visceral protein status, which include serum albumin, thyroxine binding prealbumin, serum transferrin, and retinol binding protein as well as total lymphocyte counts, can be substantiated. Although serum albumin is a commonly used screening tool, it is not always a reliable measure in older adults. Values can be elevated because of dehydration, or values can decline because of age-related degeneration of muscle mass. Other biochemical measures such as total cholesterol, high-density lipoprotein, low-density lipoprotein, and triglycerides are used to assess lipid status and are also used to measure micronutrient status (e.g., iron status). Biochemical measures of iron status can include hemoglobin, hematocrit, mean cell volume, mean cell hemoglobin concentration, and total iron binding capacity. A combination of these measures is used for a proper clinical diagnosis

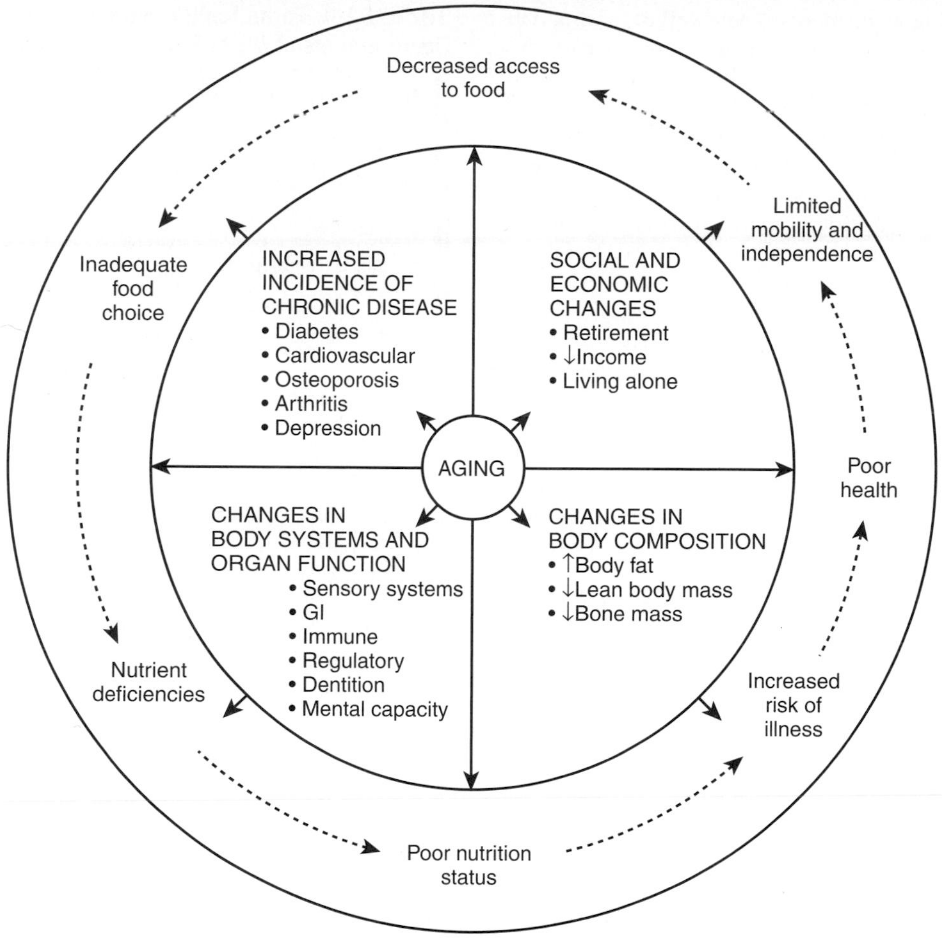

Figure 82-1. Changes in economic and social status contribute to decreased access to food, poor food choices, nutrient deficiencies, and poor nutritional status, which lead to increased risk of illness, poor health, and limited mobility and independence.

and can be compared to normative age and gender group values.

Clinical indicators are also used to assess nutritional status, and the components of clinical assessment can include medical history and physical signs and symptoms associated with nutritional deficiencies, functional status, and cognitive status. Some clinical signs and symptoms are nonspecific and attributed to the aging process rather than to a particular nutritional deficiency. Functional status can be assessed in several different ways, usually with a focus on the person's abilities to perform basic activities of daily living (ADL), which include basic self-care such as bathing, feeding, and toileting and instrumental activities of daily living (IADL), which includes activities such as cooking, shopping, and managing one's own affairs. These can serve as clinical indicators useful in the assessment of nutritional status. The inability to execute such tasks may indicate a higher risk of poor nutrition, although some clinical signs may be nonspecific and attributed to aging rather than to a specific deficiency. Clinical assessment can include physical signs and symptoms affiliated, not only with nutritional deficits, but also functional and cognitive status. Both functional and cognitive status can be assessed in multiple ways.

Dietary assessment is an integral component in the measurement of nutritional status and can be categorized as retrospective or prospective. A retrospective assessment involves the recall of all foods and fluids consumed in a particular time frame (often 24 hours). Retrospective assessment can be unreliable if the individual has problems with cognition status. In this case, a prospective assessment may be favored, as this involves keeping a written record of all foods and fluids consumed in a given period of time (e.g., 3 days including 2 weekdays and a weekend day or 7 days). Although this aids those with cognitive challenges, it does pose a problem for those individuals who suffer from a particular functional disability such as arthritis of the hand or poor vision. A 3-day food record with intakes of 2 weekdays and one weekend day recorded is considered to be one of the better dietary assessment methods as it does not depend on memory and can provide detailed intake data, although no single best method exists.

Given that a comprehensive assessment of nutritional status is complex and time-consuming, rapid screening is beneficial to identify those who might be at risk for poor nutrition and individuals who might need in-depth assessment. Several screening tools exist. The DETERMINE checklist determine your nutritional health checklist developed as part of the Nutrition Screening Initiative provides public awareness about basic nutrition information and can help identify individuals at risk for poor nutrition in community settings. The checklist is widely used in the United States[14] and is executed in two stages or levels. Level I can include the following assessments: body weight, eating habits, living environment, and functional status—particularly ADLs and IADLs—and is usually filled out by the individual's primary caregiver.[15] The level II screen can include anthropometric measurements, laboratory data, polypharmacy, and cognitive status assessments. Based on the assessment, specific nutritional care plan or support is provided. In Canada, a screening tool titled Seniors in the Community: A Risk Evaluation Tool for Eating and Nutrition Version II (SCREEN II) has been developed for assessing nutritional risk among community-dwelling seniors.[16] The Mini Nutritional Assessment (MNA) is also widely used for initial screening and assessment for individuals in the community as well as in the long-term care settings.[17,18]

In addition to these commonly used screening tools, several others exist. These include the Payette Nutrition Screening Scale, the Nutritional Risk Index (NRI), the Nutritional Risk Score (NRS), the Nutritional Risk Assessment Scale (NuRAS), the Prognostic Nutritional Index (PNI), the Sadness-Cholesterol-Albumin-Loss of weight-Eating-Shopping (SCALES) measurement, and the Subjective Global Assessment (SGA). Screening tools are beneficial for identifying individuals at risk or as an educational tool as they can provide simple, rapid, and reliable assessments.[19] Even so, screening tools may have limited value in apparently healthy elderly people.[20] It is therefore important to select and use appropriate screening tools based on the target group (e.g., home care, long-term care), ease of use, and psychometric properties (validity/reliability).

Although researchers and clinicians have traditionally relied on the nutritional assessment and screening based on anthropometric, biochemical, clinical, and dietary considerations as well as the presence of various risk factors that could predispose one to have less than optimal nutritional intake, we need to consider what the appropriate indicators of nutritional health are in the context of the aging population. Is it the nutrient intake of macro- and micronutrients or body mass index (an indicator of weight status based on the proportion of weight for height) as we have traditionally measured, or should we pay attention to the variety, moderation, and balance in food group consumption, or should we include indicators of food security such as availability, access, and affordability of nutritious diet? How do we measure availability and access to traditional diet and the quality and safety of traditional foods or cultural foods for the minority populations? There is a considerable need for identifying appropriate indicators of nutritional health among the aging population.

NUTRITIONAL REQUIREMENTS

Determination of a person's nutritional requirements is critical to ensure optimal nutrient intake. Reduction in energy requirements is one notable difference between individuals over 65 years of age and their younger counterparts.[21] For example, energy needs for individuals 51 to 75 years of age typically decrease by approximately 200 kcal/day. After age 75, energy needs decrease on average by an estimated 500 kcal/day for men, whereas women's energy needs decrease an estimated 400 kcal/day.[22,23] The decrease in energy needs is largely attributed to the age-related reduction in resting metabolic rate and activity-related energy expenditure.[24–26] Historically, decreases in energy expenditure have been attributed to less physical activity, reduced mean muscle mass, and lower metabolic rate with advancing age. Yet other problems, including chewing difficulties, living alone, and low income, contribute to a decline of intake in the elderly. The third National Health and Nutrition Examination Survey (NHANES III, 1976–1980) reported that women and men aged 60 to 69 years and 70 to 79 years consumed an average of 550 kcal/day and 745 cal/day less than women and men aged 30 to 39 years, respectively.[27]

Table 82-1. Formulas for Estimating the Energy Requirements of Older Persons (kcal/day)

Harris-Benedict Equations	
Males:	BEE = 66.4730 + 13.7516 (Wt) + 5.003 (Ht) − 6.7550 (A)
Females:	BEE = 655.0955 + 9.5634 (Wt) + 1.8496 (Ht) − 4.6756 (A)
World Health Organization Equations	
Males:	BEE = 8.8 (Wt) + 1128 (Ht) − 1071
Females:	BEE = 9.2 (Wt) + 637 (Ht) − 302
Weight-Based Method	
20–25 (Wt)	

Wt = weight (kg); Ht = height (cm); A = age (yr).

Different methods exist for estimating the energy requirements of older individuals, and knowledge of patient-specific information is required such as height, weight, and age. One simple method, only requiring a patient's weight, estimates energy expenditure in the range of 20 to 25 total kcal/kg/day. Thus, the energy requirements of an elderly 70-kg individual could be met with the provision of 1400 to 1750 total kcal/day. These estimates appear to be appropriate because indirect measurements of energy expenditure in critically ill older adults were found to be 22 to 25 kcal/kg/day.[28] If weight gain is the desired objective, an increase in calories up to 30 kcal/kg/day may be warranted.

Although widely used to predict energy expenditures, the Harris-Benedict equations (Table 82-1),[29] which are based on the measurement of oxygen consumption and carbon dioxide production using direct calorimeter, are likely not accurate for older adults. They were developed in 1919, and although subjects ranged in age from 15 to 74 years, only 9 of the 239 healthy male and female subjects studied were greater than 60 years of age. In consequence, some authorities favor more recent equations established by the World Health Organization (see Table 82-1). Recommendations from the National Research Council include multiplying the calculated energy expenditure by coefficients accounting for various levels of physical activity.[30] An activity coefficient 1 to 1.12 times the energy expenditure is used for older adults who are sedentary or fairly inactive. Activity coefficients of 1.27 to 1.45 should be used to account for energy expended by the elderly with highly active lifestyles.

In contrast to declining energy requirements, protein requirements actually increase with advanced age because of the loss of skeletal muscle mass. Because of changes in metabolism, changes in body composition, and protein utilization efficiency, the age-related increase in protein needs is necessary for the repletion of body protein. In addition, infections, surgery, trauma, and pressure ulcers may also increase protein needs as a person ages. Sarcopenia is used to describe the age-associated loss in skeletal muscle and its functional consequences.[31] The etiology of sarcopenia is currently unknown. However, loss of muscle mass has been linked to neurogenic processes, dietary protein deficiencies, and sedentary lifestyles. There is no consensus on the recommended daily protein intake to enhance muscle protein anabolism and minimize the loss of muscle mass with age. Studies show that the average adult needs 0.8 gm of protein/kg of body weight in order to maintain protein equilibrium, whereas older adults require as much as 1.0 to 1.2 gm of protein/kg of body weight.[32–35] This level of protein intake is generally recognized as safe and appropriate for maintaining nitrogen equilibrium in free-living, healthy elderly persons. Increasing protein intake to dosages of 1.2 to 1.5 g/kg/day may be required in older individuals with pressure ulcers who are undernourished or those with burns or gastrointestinal diseases that exhibit extraordinary nitrogen losses.[36] Elderly patients generally tolerate moderately high protein intakes without deterioration in renal function. However, subjects with existing renal disease should avoid high-protein diets as they may hasten a greater decline in renal function.[37]

Another key factor in maintaining healthy nutritional status is an appropriate intake of dietary fat. Fats contain twice as many calories per gram as carbohydrates or proteins, and given the fact that higher intakes of dietary fat are associated with an increased risk of developing diabetes, heart disease, and other chronic ailments, lower-fat choices, such as skim milk rather than whole milk, are recommended. However, for older adults who are unable to consume enough of their daily energy requirement, the risks associated with a higher fat intake may be overlooked in favor of meeting the necessary daily energy requirement.

To maintain a healthy nutritional diet and nutritional status, one must maintain an opportune intake of vitamins and minerals as one ages. Because energy needs decrease while vitamin and mineral needs increase, the challenge of creating an optimal intake for the elderly is vital. According to the dietary reference intakes (DRI), calcium, vitamin D, and vitamin B_6 needs increase with age. For example, 1200 mg/day of calcium is essential to protect against bone loss. Similarly, the DRI indicates that vitamin D needs increase from 5 μg to 10 μg for individuals aged 51 to 60, and 5 μg to 15 μg for those over age 70. Hypovitaminosis D is currently a significant problem among elderly individuals. An age-related decline in vitamin D intake is correlated with lower dietary intakes, less sun exposure, less efficient skin synthesis of vitamin D, and impaired kidney function, which in turn impairs the conversion of vitamin D from its inactive to active form. Also, insufficient levels of folate and vitamins B_6 and B_{12} are known to contribute higher than normal levels of serum homocysteine, a known risk factor in the development of coronary artery disease, stroke, and depression, as well as a decrease in cognitive function. Individuals over age 50 need to consume more vitamin B_{12} or rely on supplements to avoid the malabsorption of food-bound B_{12}, because as many as 30% of older adults are deficient in vitamin B_{12} daily.

Water is often overlooked as an essential nutrient, and inadequate hydration poses an additional risk for increased morbidity and mortality in the elderly. Age-related decline in intracellular water and fluid reserves, paired with changes in renal function (causing an inability to concentrate urine), can result in difficulty maintaining appropriate fluid levels in older adults. Not only do these physiologic factors impair fluid levels, but altered thirst perception resulting in reduced fluid intake also becomes an obstacle. Furthermore, external factors provide the elderly with more impediments to balanced fluid intakes. Residents of long-term care facilities (LTCF) are especially at risk for dehydration because of their limited access to oral fluids or underlying conditions (vomiting, diarrhea, colostomy/ileostomy) that increase fluid losses. Institutional issues including inadequate staffing and a subsequent need for better supervision places the frail elderly at greater risk.[38] Untreated dehydration in hospitalized elderly can result in mortality exceeding 50%.[39] As a result, LTCF staff members use specific triggers to detect inadequate hydration (Table 82-2). As such, older adults should make a conscious effort to increase fluid intake and not just rely on thirst perceptions. A water intake of 1 mL per calorie ingested or 30 mL/kg per day is generally recommended to meet dietary water requirements and achieve adequate fluid intake in older adults.[40]

Table 82-2. Risk Factors for Dehydration Among Residents of Long-Term Care Facilities

Deterioration in cognitive status in the past 90 days
Failure to eat or take medication
Diarrhea
Fever
Swallowing problems
Communication problems

Adapted from Weinberg AD, Minaker KL. Council on Scientific Affairs, American Medical Association. Dehydration: evaluation and management in older adults. JAMA 1995;274:1552–6.

In accordance with Canada's Food Guide to Healthy Eating, dietary guidelines have been created to help avoid energy and vitamin deficiencies in the older population, by encouraging the elderly to meet their needs from healthy dietary sources. The DRI encourages older adults to acquire 45% to 65% of their daily energy intake from complex carbohydrates in order to obtain enough dietary fiber (25 to 30 gm/day). Dietary recommendations from the 2005 Dietary guidelines for Americans include the consumption of nutrient-dense beverages from the food groups that limit saturated and trans fats, cholesterol, added sugar, salt, and alcohol; a diet rich in fiber found in natural sources such as fruit, vegetables, and whole grains; and limiting sodium intake to 1500 mg per day. Other recommendations such as the consumption of calcium and vitamin D through foods or supplements and the maintenance of a healthy body weight through a balanced diet and exercise also play a key role in helping older adults meet their daily nutritional needs.

COMMON NUTRITIONAL PROBLEMS AND DEFICIENCIES

Imbalance between nutrient intake and nutrient requirements or less than optimal nutritional status can result from less than optimal dietary intake, age-related changes, disease conditions and their treatment, or other contextual factors such as cultural and religious beliefs, practices, and socioeconomic conditions. This imbalance can result in nutrition-related problems and deficiencies among older adults. The most common nutritional deficiencies include malnutrition, which encompasses both under- and overnutrition, micronutrient deficiencies, and dehydration. Malnutrition is common in elderly adults and can be divided into protein energy malnutrition and micronutrient deficiency. Whether the imbalance is a result of poor dietary intake, age-related changes, disease conditions/treatments, or other factors such as cultural or religious beliefs, practices, or socioeconomic issues, malnutrition varies in its prevalence. Protein energy undernutrition varies from 1% to 15% in the community to 25% to 85% in long-term care facilities.[41] It is important to recognize that undernutrition is not simply a result of poor dietary intake but is the combination of many factors that interrupt the balance between intake and need. The presence of cognitive decline or dementia, depression, chronic disease, or functional deficits are also factors in undernutrition, which are common in individuals suffering from sarcopenia (loss in skeletal muscle and its functional consequences as one ages) and geriatric failure to thrive (GFTT), a syndrome where individuals suffer involuntary weight loss and cannot maintain functional capacity or social and cognitive skills with no visible cause. Although the exact prevalence is unknown, the incidences increase with age and are more common in men and those living in LTCF. In both cases, nutritional interventions and the use of an interdisciplinary team approach have been successful through an increase of energy and protein intake through both dietary sources and oral supplements.[42] Other interventions such as exercise programs have also been beneficial to prevent sarcopenia.

Micronutrient deficiencies among older adults occur when calcium, vitamin D, iron, vitamin B_{12}, and other minerals or vitamins are lacking. Such deficiencies are common and can be easily remedied through the use of supplements. Vitamin D deficiency is widespread among all age groups but is especially prevalent among the elderly.[43] Adequate vitamin D nutrition is important for maintaining healthy bone status and reducing the risk of fractures and osteoporosis. The Institute of Medicine (IOM) recommendations for vitamin D daily intake are 400 IU for adults 51 to 70 years old and 600 IU for adults > 71 years old.[44] Calcium also plays an important role in maintaining bone health in the elderly. The IOM-recommended calcium intake for adults 51 years and older is 1200 mg/day, with the maximal dose of elemental calcium not to exceed 500 mg at any one time.[44] Calcium carbonate is the most cost-effective form of calcium, well absorbed, and tolerated by most individuals when consumed with a meal. Of note, calcium citrate is the preferred form to be used in elderly with intestinal absorption problems, such as achlorhydria or inflammatory bowel disease.[45] Noteworthy changes in B vitamin status occur with advancing age. Observational studies suggest that low plasma concentrations of B vitamins folate, cyanocobalamin (B_{12}), and pyridoxine (B_6) in elders may be linked to greater bone loss.[46] Concern for toxicity of fat-soluble vitamins, such as vitamin A, exist in older adults because of increased liver stores and declining renal function associated with increasing age. Osteoporosis and hip fracture are associated with vitamin A intakes that are only twice the current recommended daily intake of 1000 μg retinol equivalents (RE)/day in males and 800 μg RE/day in females.[47] Thus, caregivers of elders who take vitamin supplements should understand the risks and effects that chronic high intakes of vitamin A may have on bone loss.

The prevalence of obesity has steadily increased since the late 1980s. Obesity is generally defined as an unhealthy excess of body fat characterized as a body mass index (BMI ≥ 30 kg/m^2). In 1991, approximately 15% of individuals aged 60 to 69 years old and 11% of those over 70 years old were obese.[48] The prevalence of obesity in these same age groups increased to approximately 23% and 16%, respectively, 9 years later.[49] Higher risks of mortality and other serious medical complications, including hypertension, arthritis, obstructive sleep apnea, urinary incontinence, and cancer, are associated with older men and women who have a BMI over 30 kg/m^2. The current treatment guidelines for weight management in older persons are lifestyle intervention involving diet, behavior modification with physical activity, and pharmacotherapy.[50] A reduction in calorie intake by 500 to 750 kcal/d with an intake of 1 g protein/kg/d of high-quality protein is recommended. Regular physical activity in the form of stretching and aerobic and resistance activity is important to increase flexibility and endurance while preventing frailty. Experience with weight-loss medications is limited, however, orlistat appears to be the safest for older individuals. Bariatric surgery is reserved for selected individuals who fail diet and medication therapy and continue to suffer from disabling obesity. The perceived benefits of the procedure in terms of quality of life must be weighed against the postoperative morbidity and risk of potential complications.

NUTRITIONAL STRATEGIES

Several strategies can be used to increase dietary intake of the frail elderly person. High nutrient-dense feeds can be incorporated into the diet if the individual tolerates traditional solid foods. Peanut butter spread on whole-wheat bread, enriched cereal, or powdered instant breakfast products can be substituted at breakfast to increase caloric intake. High-protein and high-calorie snacks, in the form of crackers and cheese, milkshakes, or sandwiches, can be given throughout the day to supplement oral intake.[36] Dietary adjustments and special utensils are often beneficial when physical or neurologic disorders contribute to poor oral consumption. Institutionalized residents often require assistance from staff for eating and drinking.[51] Use of semicircular tables is a simple method to assist understaffed caregivers in feeding several residents at a time in an LCTF. Modified spoons have been used to decrease spillage by elders afflicted with hand tremors. Changes in food texture, such as pureed vegetables or puddings, can avoid intake problems in subjects with poor dentition. Patients with swallowing dysfunction should be taught appropriate eating positions and safe swallowing techniques to minimize dysphagia.

Enteral nutrition (EN) delivered through a feeding tube can be initiated when older subjects are unable to maintain adequate nutrient and fluid intake by oral ingestion. Small-bore gastric or duodenal tubes may be placed through the nose to provide short-term (i.e., a few weeks) enteral access to treat elderly patients admitted for rehabilitation after hip or knee surgery, patients with pressure ulcers, or those with temporary swallowing disorders. Chronic disorders such as head/neck cancer, stroke, head injuries, or neuromuscular disorders impairing the ability to swallow would necessitate placement of a long-term (months to years) enteral access device. Long-term enteral access is achieved with gastric tubes that are inserted directly into the stomach by a surgeon in an operating room or by a gastroenterologist at the bedside. Percutaneous endoscopic gastrostomy (PEG) tubes placed with an endoscope are becoming more common than open surgical gastrostomy tubes because the expense and risks associated with an invasive surgical procedure can be avoided. If gastroparesis or an anatomic defect is present that prevents normal gastric emptying, a feeding tube placed in the jejunum is most appropriate to reduce the risk of aspirating EN into the lungs.

Complications of EN include pulmonary aspiration, diarrhea, and mechanical obstruction of the feeding tube. Aspiration of EN remains one of the most dangerous complications of EN administration. Mortality rates from aspiration of gastric contents range from 40% to 90%.[52] Recommendations for reducing the risk of aspiration in older individuals receiving gastric feedings include elevating the head of the bed over 30° and frequent exams for abdominal distention. EN is often identified as a cause of diarrhea, despite numerous other factors such as medications, hyperosmolar EN formulations, hypoalbuminemia, and infection. Sorbitol is used as a vehicle for many liquid formulations of pharmacologic agents and has been associated with diarrhea. Antibiotics or prokinetic agents like metoclopramide are examples of concurrent therapies more likely to cause diarrhea than the EN formulation. *Clostridium difficile* is a well-known cause of diarrhea in patients receiving EN and should be ruled out before antidiarrheal agents are initiated.

Elderly patients who require nutrition support but do not have functional or accessible gastrointestinal tracts are candidates for parenteral nutrition (PN). This may include patients with severe inflammatory bowel disease (e.g., Crohn's disease or ulcerative colitis), malabsorption (e.g., celiac sprue), bowel obstruction, a history of extensive bowel surgery (e.g., short bowel syndrome), and severe acute pancreatitis when enteral nutrition has failed. The primary goal of PN should be to prevent undernutrition from inadequate energy and nutrient intake or to treat undernutrition and its complications. Guidelines published by the American Society for Parenteral and Enteral Nutrition exist for appropriate use of PN.[53] Table 82-3 lists some monitoring guidelines for fluid, electrolyte, and micronutrient abnormalities that should be performed in geriatric patients during PN administration.

NUTRITION PROGRAMS AND SERVICES

Many services are available to support the nutritional and health needs of the elderly. Examples include meal-delivery programs, community meals, grocery-delivery services, food banks and food stamps, and nutrition screening and education initiatives. In-home programs such as the Elderly Nutrition Program (ENP) in the United States, mandated through the Older Americans Act, provides in-home and community-based nutrition services to individuals over 60 years of age and targets those at highest economic and social need.[54] ENP offers meal-delivery services and congregate meals, as well as nutrition screening and assessment. Although a program such as ENP is not available in Canada, for-profit and not-for-profit organizations provide a similar array of services.

Many *meal-delivery services* in Canada, such as the Meals on Wheels program, offer meals for elderly Canadians for a nominal fee, and many church groups, for-profit, and not-for-profit organizations offer similar programs for those who have difficulty preparing meals for themselves, thereby placing them in a high-risk category. These meal-delivery services provide one hot meal, usually lunch, to people's homes at least 5 days a week. Frozen meals are also available to the elderly on request. The delivered meal is required to meet one third of the daily nutritional requirement. However, for the frail, largely homebound elderly, one meal is insufficient to meet nutritional needs and avoid nutritional deficiencies. This type of meal-delivery service has shown benefit to seniors who have difficulty preparing meals for themselves and are at risk for poor nutrition. A recent study examining the impact of home-delivered breakfast and lunch showed significant improvement in nutritional intake and quality of life among frail, homebound older adults.[55]

Congregate and community meals offered by churches and other community-based organizations not only assist the

Table 82-3. Complications of Parenteral Nutrition and Management Techniques

Complication	Management
Mechanical	
Pneumothorax	Possible chest tube placement; minimize number of catheter insertions; placement by experienced personnel
Air embolism	Placement by experienced personnel
Catheter occlusion	Anticoagulation locally with urokinase or streptokinase; routine line flushing
Venous thrombosis	Anticoagulation; catheter removal
Metabolic	
Hyperglycemia	Slowly initiate PN; check blood glucose frequently before advancing nutrition; administer insulin if needed
Hypoglycemia	Decrease amount of insulin administered; avoid abrupt discontinuation of PN by tapering rate of infusion; administer 10% dextrose if PN is abruptly discontinued
Hypertriglyceridemia	Decrease lipid volume administered; increase length of infusion time; avoid lipid administration >60% of total calories; assess risk factors for hypertriglyceridemia
Electrolyte disturbance	Monitor fluid intake and output and serum chemistries; replace electrolytes as necessary
Essential fatty acid deficiency	Provide 8% to 10% of total calories as lipid
Prerenal azotemia	Increase fluid intake; decrease protein administered; increase nonprotein calories; analyze nitrogen balance
Gastrointestinal	
Cholestasis	Avoid over-feeding; use gastrointestinal tract as soon as clinically able
Gastrointestinal atrophy	Use gastrointestinal tract as soon as clinically able
Infectious	
Catheter-related sepsis	Remove catheter and place at alternate site; adequately care for catheter site; possible treatment with intravenous antibiotics

elderly by providing them with balanced meals, but they also function as social events that many seniors would otherwise not experience. The community meals can be served as breakfast, lunch, or dinner, and their frequency ranges from once a week to once a month. Economic need can be offset through the use of *food stamps* or *food banks* on a short-term basis. The selection of foods offered in food banks primarily includes dry goods and nonperishable food items. Some food banks in Canada have facilities for refrigeration and offer selected perishable foods. For accessing these services, a rent receipt, identification, and proof of income may be required. *Community kitchens* allow small groups of individuals to pool resources and cook meals together that are later taken home, thus saving money and creating social time for elderly individuals. If mobility is an issue, *grocery-delivery services* are available for a fee and can be accessed via telephone or the Internet. Lastly, *nutrition screening* and *education programs* are offered through government agencies such as the ENP who utilize the DETERMINE checklist to aid seniors with nutritional risk assessments. Other lectures and community nutrition education programs are also offered to elderly individuals.

ETHICAL CONSIDERATIONS

A common but controversial issue is the withdrawal of nutrition when death is imminent (i.e., within 6 months). Although families may decide to discontinue life-sustaining medical treatment such as mechanical ventilation or dialysis, nutrition and hydration are often considered a basic human right. Most health care professionals agree that the wishes of the individual constitute the most important factor to consider in the development of a nutritional care plan.[56] Thus, most health care teams consider it ethical and acceptable for a competent individual to refuse or halt administration of artificial nutrition, although cultural differences are notable.[57,58] If an individual is considered incompetent, caregivers should provide family members the support needed to facilitate a thoughtful decision with the individual's quality of life taken into consideration. Communication among all parties involved (health care personnel, patients, family, friends, guardian) is paramount in making informed decisions concerning the delivery of artificial nutrition and end-of-life issues. Providing hydration solely without EN or PN is an appropriate alternative, as patients do not suffer from signs of dehydration. Additional information concerning the ethics of forgoing life-sustaining treatments may be found at www.partnershipforcaring.org/homepage/index.html.

KEY POINTS
Nutrition in Aging

- Nutrition affects aging and aging affects nutrition; each amplifies the impact of the other on health status.
- Nutrition assessment combines anthropomorphic, biochemical and clinical/dietary evaluation. Several screening tools exist, but appear to have their greatest impact when screening targeted populations, such as people receiving home care.
- Average energy requirements decrease with age; typically men >75 years require 500 fewer kcal/day, and women 400 fewer kcal/day. Protein requirements, however, increase due to the loss of skeletal muscle mass. The minimum requirement for muscle anabolism has not been established, but absent renal impairment, most older adults can tolerate moderately high protein intakes.
- Individuals over age 50 need to consume more vitamin B_{12} or rely on supplements to avoid the malabsorption of food-bound B_{12}, since as many as 30% of older adults are deficient in vitamin B_{12} daily.
- Water is often overlooked as an essential nutrient.
- Protein energy undernutrition varies from 1% to 15% in the community to 25% to 85% in long-term care facilities.
- Vitamin D deficiency is widespread among all age groups, but is especially high in older adults.

For a complete list of references, please visit online only at www.expertconsult.com

CHAPTER 83

Obesity

Krupa Shah
Dennis T. Villareal

INTRODUCTION

Obesity is defined as an unhealthy excess of body fat, which enhances the risk of morbidity and untimely mortality. Obesity is a growing epidemic in developed countries and is also becoming increasingly problematic in our aging population. Obesity in older adults is accompanied by an untoward burden of chronic disease, metabolic complications, and a worsening in quality of life. More important, obesity in older adults exacerbates the age-related decline in physical function, which leads to frailty and disability. The current treatment designed for weight loss in older persons includes lifestyle intervention (diet, exercise, and behavior modifications), pharmacotherapy, and surgery. Existing evidence indicates that weight-loss therapy in obese older adults prevents or delays functional decline and medical complications, as well as improves quality of life. However, weight-loss therapy in the older adult population is controversial because it can potentially lead to adverse effects on a person's muscle and bone mass. This chapter describes the clinical importance of obesity in older adults and provides medical professionals with evidence-based treatment guidelines for obesity in the elderly.

MEASUREMENT

Body mass index (BMI) and waist circumference are widely used and accepted as simple methods to classify overweight and obesity. BMI is calculated as weight (kg)/height squared (m^2). However, the measurement of height is often unreliable and impractical in older adults in nursing homes. In this situation, it seems that using alternative measurements such as arm span may be more reliable.[1] Central obesity, as measured by waist circumference, is the excessive accumulation of fat in the abdomen. It is an independent predictor of comorbidities like diabetes, hypertension, and cardiovascular disease.[2] Table 83-1 incorporates both BMI and waist circumference in the classification of overweight and obesity and estimates relative disease risk.[3]

OBESITY PREVALENCE

The prevalence of obese older adults is rising sharply. According to National Health and Nutrition Examination Survey (NHANES) data from the period 1991-2000, the prevalence of obesity has increased dramatically for those in the age range of 60 to 69 and 70 to 79 years,[2,3] by 56% and 36%, respectively.[4] Only the very old, such as individuals older than 85 years of age, remain relatively constant in body fat percentage. The prevalence of obesity in older adults is likely to continue to increase and challenge our health care systems.[5] Moreover, obesity poses an increasing dilemma for long-term care facilities and raises concerns about nursing home preparedness and access.[6] The global growth rate for age-related obesity in developed counties is predicted to be 15% to 20%, and the same trends are now being observed even in developing countries as they gain more economic affluence.[7]

THE RELATIONSHIP BETWEEN BODY COMPOSITION AND AGING

Aging is associated with significant changes in body composition. After the age of 30 years, individuals tend to show a progressive decrease in fat-free mass (FFM), such as muscle and bone, and an increase in fat mass. Moreover, in women after the age of 60 years, data from some studies suggest an accelerated loss of FFM.[8,9] FFM attains its peak during the third decade of life, whereas fat mass reaches its peak during the seventh decade followed by a subsequent decline thereafter.[9] In addition, aging is associated with the redistribution of body fat. The intra-abdominal fat (central adiposity) increases with aging, whereas the subcutaneous fat and total body fat decrease with aging.[10]

The hormonal changes with aging may explain some of the age-related shifts in proportion of fat and FFM. These age-related changes include a reduced production of the anabolic hormones, growth hormone, insulin-like growth factor-1 (IGF-1), testosterone, and dehydroepiandrosterone (DHEA), without a concomitant decline in the catabolic hormone, cortisol.[11,12]

CAUSES OF OBESITY IN THE ELDERLY

Obesity results when total energy intake exceeds the energy output. Energy intake neither changes nor declines with advancing age. Hence, the decrease in total energy output (EO) is an important contributor in the gradual accumulation of body fat with aging. Aging is associated with a decrease in all major components of EO. These components are basal metabolic rate (which explains 70% of EO), thermal effect of food (10%), and physical activity (20%). The resting metabolic rate decreases with age largely because of an age-related decline in FFM.[13] The thermic effect of food also declines with aging. The decline in physical activity with aging contributes ~50% of the reduction in EO that occurs with aging.[14]

ADVERSE EFFECTS OF OBESITY

Obesity is associated with several complications that are commonly known to increase mortality and morbidity[15] (Table 83-2). In addition, obesity has a detrimental effect on physical function and quality of life in the elderly. These adverse effects of obesity are discussed in this chapter.

Mortality

Obesity is associated with increased cardiovascular and overall mortality in both younger and older adults.[16] Even though obesity is associated with a higher relative risk of death for younger adults than for older ones, an elevated BMI increases absolute mortality and health risks linearly up to 75 years of age.[17] The relationship of obesity in individuals 75 years or

Table 83-1. Classification of Overweight and Obesity by BMI, Waist Circumference, and Associated Disease Risk[18]

	BMI (kg/m^2)	Obesity Class	DISEASE RISK* (RELATIVE TO NORMAL WEIGHT AND WAIST CIRCUMFERENCE)	
			Men <40 in; Women <35 in	Men >40 in; Women >35 in
Underweight	<18.5		—	—
Normal†	18.5–24.9			—
Overweight	25.0–29.9	I	Increased	High
Obesity	30.0–34.9	II	High	Very high
	35.0–39.9		Very high	Very high
Extreme obesity	>40	III	Extremely high	Extremely high

*Disease risk for type 2 diabetes, hypertension, and CVD.
†Increased waist circumference can also be a marker for increased risk even in persons of normal weight.

Table 83-2. Adverse Effects of Obesity in the Elderly

Disorders Directly Caused by Obesity	Disorders Aggravated by Obesity
Metabolic syndrome	Osteoarthritis
Hypertension	Urinary incontinence
Dyslipidemia	All cardiopulmonary abnormalities
Coronary artery disease	Postoperative complications
Diabetes mellitus	Cataracts
Neoplasia	
Obstructive sleep apnea	

older with total mortality is equivocal. In very old persons, the prevalence of obesity could actually be lower. One explanation for this demographic shift is selective mortality. The underlying diseases can themselves increase the risk of early mortality in obese adults, thus causing an underestimation of the relation between obesity and mortality in older adults. Although those who are vulnerable to the adverse effects of obesity die at a younger age, the remaining surviving group of obese older adults are called the "resistant" survivors.

Comorbid disease

Obesity and increased abdominal fat are associated with increased morbidity (see Table 83-1), mortality, and poor quality of life.[15] The prevalence of medical conditions commonly associated with obesity—such as hypertension, diabetes, dyslipidemia, and cardiovascular disease—increases with age.[18] Therefore, obesity and weight gain during middle age may contribute to medical complications and the increasing health care expenditures that occur during old age.[19]

The age-related glucose intolerance increases with abdominal obesity and lack of physical activity. Older people who are physically active and do not have increased abdominal girth are much less likely to develop insulin resistance and type 2 diabetes mellitus.[20] In addition, obese older adults have higher prevalence of dyslipidemia (high triglyceride and low high-density lipoprotein [HDL])[21] and hypertension.[22] In a 15-year longitudinal study, increased BMI in older men was associated with an increase in new cases of coronary heart disease and cardiovascular disease mortality.[23]

Functional impairment and quality of life

Advancing age causes physical dysfunction because of both a progressive decline in muscle mass and strength and an increase in joint immobility and arthritis.[24] These functional limitations adversely affect the activities of daily living (ADL) and quality of life. Obesity exacerbates this age-related decline in physical function. In addition, medical comorbidities like diabetes, heart disease, and pulmonary disorders frequently coexist with obesity and contribute to functional decline. Moreover, older adults who are obese (BMI greater than 30) have a greater rate of nursing home admissions than those who are nonobese (BMI between 18.5 and 24.9).[25] Both cross-sectional studies[26,27] and longitudinal studies[28] have consistently demonstrated a strong link between a decline in physical function of older persons and an increase in BMI.

Obesity is also associated with frailty syndrome in older adults. In one study, 96% of community-living obese (BMI greater than 30) older subjects (65 to 80 years old) were frail, as determined by physical performance test scores, peak oxygen consumption, and self-reported ability to perform ADL.[29] In another study, which was conducted in older women (70 to 79 years old), obesity was linked with a marked increased risk of frailty, determined by weakness, slowness, weight loss, low physical activity, and exhaustion.[30]

Despite having higher absolute muscle mass, obese older adults are particularly susceptible to the adverse effects of obesity because not only do they have smaller muscle mass relative to their body weight (relative sarcopenia)[31] but they also have age-related decline in muscle mass leading to sarcopenic obesity.[32] With higher fat mass and lower muscle mass, physical activity becomes progressively more difficult. Hence, sarcopenic obesity acts synergistically with aging to augment disability. This leads to functional dependence, inactivity, and poor quality of life.

BENEFICIAL EFFECTS OF OBESITY

It should be noted that a potential benefit of obesity with aging is the protection from osteoporosis-related fractures. Higher body weight is associated with greater bone mineral density.[33] This is explained by the bone-stimulating effects of carrying extra body weight as well as hormonal changes (e.g., increased adipose tissue conversion of androstenedione to estrone). Heavier individuals have been found to have higher bone densities even in their non-weight-bearing bones. Furthermore, in the event of a fall, the extra cushioning provided by body fat can serve as protection against fractures, particularly of the hip.

MECHANISMS BY WHICH OBESITY INCREASES MORTALITY AND MORBIDITY

Adipose tissue is recognized as a source of inflammatory mediators by producing cytokines such as tumor necrosis factor-alpha (TNF-alpha) and interleukin-6.[34] It appears that the relationship between obesity, insulin resistance, and atherosclerosis may depend partially on the increased production and the release of these inflammatory mediators from adipose tissue. It is postulated that the visceral fat (intra-abdominal fat) is most responsible for producing these deleterious cytokines, which in turn leads to diabetes, coronary artery disease, and malignant disease more commonly seen in older adults. Similarly, cytokines and inflammatory mediators produced by adipose tissue may play an important role in the pathophysiology of sarcopenic obesity.[35] A better understanding of the mechanisms that lead from gain in fat mass to muscle loss or vice versa seems to be crucial. Thus, more research is needed to better characterize this new area.

EFFECTS OF INTENTIONAL WEIGHT LOSS IN OLDER ADULTS

Body composition

Because weight loss results in a decrease in both fat mass (75%) and FFM (25%),[36] it is possible that weight loss in obese older persons could worsen the age-related loss of muscle mass. Nevertheless, adding regular exercise to a weight loss program can attenuate the loss of FFM. This effect was observed in a randomized controlled trial conducted on obese older subjects. There was no significant difference in the loss of FFM after regular exercise was added to a diet-induced weight loss program compared to a control group that did not lose weight.[31]

Medical complications

It is well known that weight loss improves or normalizes metabolic abnormalities associated with obesity in young and middle-aged persons.[37] Clinical trials conducted in obese older adults have shown similar results. It was observed that a decrease in multiple coronary artery disease risk factors (including the prevalence of the metabolic syndrome) and insulin resistance, as well as an increase in insulin secretion, resulted from weight-loss therapy in obese older adults.[38,39]

Physical function and quality of life

Data from studies conducted in overweight and obese older persons with or without joint disease have shown that the combination of moderate diet-induced weight loss and exercise therapy improves both subjective and objective measures of physical function and health-related quality of life.[31,40,41] Weight loss in combination with exercise training has also been shown to have beneficial effects on muscle strength and muscle quality (muscle strength/cross-sectional area).[31,42]

Most of the weight loss studies that analyzed physical function as an outcome have included an exercise component. Therefore, data on the effect of weight loss alone on physical function are limited. Nevertheless, one study demonstrated that diet-induced weight loss programs can indeed improve both endurance capacity and exercise tolerance in obese older adults despite the loss of FFM.[43] These findings indicate that obesity is a remediable cause of frailty.

Mortality

In epidemiologic studies, it has been observed that older adults who lost weight, or who experienced weight recycling, had an increased relative mortality risk compared to those who were weight-stable.[23,44] However, it was not described whether the observed weight changes were intentional or unintentional. Self-reported weight change was used, and in addition, unintentional weight loss is a frequent complication of underlying serious illnesses, which can confound the explanation of weight-loss effects on mortality. Furthermore, there have not been any randomized controlled trials of weight loss that examined mortality as an outcome.

Bone mineral density

Weight loss can have adverse effects on bone mass. Prospective interventional studies conducted in young and middle-aged adults report that weight loss causes bone loss that may be proportional to the amount of weight loss.[45–47] A clinical trial conducted in young and middle-aged persons showed that diet-induced weight loss, but not exercise-induced weight loss, is associated with reductions in bone mineral density (BMD) at weight-bearing sites. This suggests that exercise is an important component of a weight loss program designed to offset the adverse effects of diet-induced weight loss on bone.[48] Regular exercise can potentially attenuate weight loss–induced bone loss. Therefore, including exercise as part of a weight-loss program is particularly important in older persons to reduce bone loss. However, one study showed that moderate weight loss, even when combined with a multicomponent exercise, decreases hip BMD in obese older adults.[49] It is unclear whether the beneficial effects of weight loss and exercise on physical function lower the overall risk of falls and fractures, despite the decline in hip BMD. Additionally, it is unknown whether the bone loss associated with intentional weight loss increases the risk of osteoporotic fractures in obese persons.

TREATMENT

Weight loss in obese persons, regardless of age, can improve obesity-related medical complications, physical function, and quality of life.[15] In older adults, improving physical function and quality of life may be the most important goals of therapy. The current therapeutic options available for weight management in older persons are (1) lifestyle intervention involving diet and exercise therapy, (2) pharmacotherapy, and (3) surgery.

Lifestyle intervention

Lifestyle intervention is just as effective in older subjects as in younger subjects.[31] The combination of an energy-deficit diet, increased physical activity, and behavior therapy results in moderate weight loss and is associated with a lower risk of treatment-induced complications. Weight-loss therapy that reduces muscle and bone losses is recommended for older adults who are obese and who have functional limitations or metabolic complications.

DIET THERAPY

A successful diet-induced weight-loss program should help patients set realistic, yet clinically meaningful weight loss goal of an 8% to 10% reduction in initial body weight by 6 months. Following a calorie-reduced (calorie deficit ~500 to 1000 kcal/d) but balanced diet that provides for as little as 1 or 2 pounds of weight loss a week is recommended for a safe

Summary of Management Algorithm

Initial Evaluation

- A comprehensive medical history, physical examination, relevant laboratory tests, and medication review should be performed to evaluate the patient's current health status and comorbidity risks.
- Further information such as the patient's willingness to lose weight, prior attempts at weight loss, and current lifestyle should be gathered before starting weight loss therapy.
- Health professionals should facilitate in setting personal goals for the patient and welcome family members and care providers to participate in the management.
- Health professionals should personalize the weight loss plan after taking into considerations the special needs of this population.
- Advocate a combination of energy-deficit diet, exercise, and behavior modification.

Weight Loss Therapy

- Recommend a moderate energy intake (calorie deficit ~750 kcal/day) containing 1.0 g/kg high-quality protein/day, multivitamin, and mineral supplements (1500 mg Ca and 1000 IU vitamin D/day).
- Recommend referral to a registered dietitian trained in behavior therapy for nutritional education, counseling, and behavior modification techniques.
- Advocate a combination of energy-deficit diet, exercise, and behavior modification.
- Bariatric surgery may be an alternative for patients who have failed multiple weight loss attempts.
- Weight maintenance efforts should be implemented once weight loss goals have been achieved.

Exercise Therapy

- Evaluate the need for stress test before starting an exercise regimen.
- Recommend an exercise regimen that is gradual, personalized, and monitored.
- Recommend a multicomponent exercise program including stretching, aerobic activity, and strength exercises.

and effective weight-loss program.[15] Because of the increased risk of medical complications, a very-low-calorie diet (<800 kcal/d) should be avoided. The diet should contain 1.0 g/kg high-quality protein/d,[50] a multivitamin, and mineral supplements to ensure that all daily recommended requirements are met. This includes 1500 mg Ca/d and 1000 IU vitamin D/d to prevent bone loss. It is important that health professionals help older adults set personal goals, closely monitor their progress, and use encouragement strategies to improve adherence to the weight-loss program. The diet therapy should be consistent with the National Cholesterol Education Program Expert Panel (Adult Treatment Panel III)'s Therapeutic Lifestyle Changes Diet (Table 83-3).[51]

Referral to a registered dietitian with experience in weight management is often necessary to ensure that appropriate nutritional counseling is provided. Patients should be educated on food composition, portion control, food preparation, and preferences. Counseling from an exercise specialist or a behavioral therapist who has weight-management experience can also facilitate behavior modification. A specific behavioral therapy strategy includes self-monitoring, goal setting, social support, and stimulus control.[52] These techniques can be utilized to improve compliance.

Table 83-3. Nutrient Composition of the Therapeutic Lifestyle Changes Diet[51]

Nutrient	Recommended Intake
Saturated fat*	<7% of total calories
Polyunsaturated fat	Up to 10% of total calories
Monounsaturated fat	Up to 20% of total calories
Total fat	25% to 35% of total calories
Carbohydrates†	50% to 60% of total calories
Fiber	20 to 30 g per day
Protein	Approximately 15% of total calories
Cholesterol	<200 mg per day
Total calories‡	Balance energy intake and expenditure to maintain desirable body weight

*Avoid trans fatty acids as well because they increase low-density lipoprotein (LDL) and lower high-density lipoprotein (HDL) cholesterol levels.

†Carbohydrates should be derived from foods rich in complex carbohydrates, including whole grains, fruits, and vegetables.

‡Daily energy expenditure should include at least moderate physical activity.

It is important to realize that changes in the diet and activity habits of older adults may present special challenges because older adults have an increased burden of comorbid conditions, depression, hearing and visual difficulties, and cognitive dysfunction. This increase in chronic disabilities with aging reduces physical activity and functional capacity. Older adults are more likely to have unique psychosocial situations such as dependency on others, cognitive impairment, institutionalization, widowhood, loneliness, isolation, and depression. These situations should be addressed because such factors pose a challenge to weight loss. Because dependency in older age is common, lifestyle-change programs must include participation by family members and caregivers. A successful weight loss and maintenance program should be based on sound scientific rationale. The program must not only be safe and nutritionally adequate, but it must also be practical and applicable to the patient's ethnic and cultural background.

EXERCISE THERAPY

The introduction of an exercise component early in the treatment course can improve physical function and ameliorate frailty in older adults.[31] In addition, exercise is a key component in maintaining weight loss. The exercise program should be started gradually and must be customized individually with consideration of diseases and disability. It should be started at a low to moderate intensity, duration, and frequency to prevent injuries and promote adherence. Subsequently, the exercise program should gradually intensify over time with longer duration and with more frequency, if feasible. The goals of regular exercise in obese older persons are to increase flexibility, endurance, and strength. Therefore, a multicomponent exercise program that includes stretching, aerobic activity, and strength exercises is the most appropriate. Very old and frail persons should not be excluded from these activities.

PHARMACOTHERAPY

Clinical trials that studied the role of pharmacotherapy in obesity treatment have enrolled very few older individuals. Therefore, limited data are available to determine the efficacy and safety of pharmacotherapy for obesity treatment in older adults.

The use of pharmacologic agents to treat obesity can further burden older patients. Most obese older patients are on a host of other medications for concomitant illnesses, which would increase the likelihood of noncompliance or errors with obesity pharmacotherapy. In addition, the potential side effects could have serious implications in older adults. Moreover, health insurance and Medicare often do not cover weight-loss drugs. This can cause an additional financial burden in older patients because they tend to live on a fixed income. All medications should be carefully reviewed because some medications can cause weight gain (e.g., antipsychotics, anticonvulsants, steroids, and antidepressants). Furthermore, weight loss–induced clinical improvements may require changes in medications in order to prevent iatrogenic complications.

BARIATRIC SURGERY

The available evidence concerning the effectiveness and safety of bariatric surgery in older adults is insufficient because only a handful of studies include older adults. Consequently, bariatric surgery should be considered in select older adults—those who have disabling obesity that can be ameliorated with weight loss and have failed multiple weight loss attempts in the past. The specific bariatric surgical procedure that is performed depends on the skill and experience of the surgeon. A multidisciplinary team should carefully evaluate the potential surgical candidates to make certain that the risk of postoperative morbidity and mortality is acceptable and that the perceived benefits of the procedure outweigh the risk of potential complications. A preoperative evaluation should include an assessment for depression, which is common in older adults and could influence outcome. Postoperative care should include monitoring for nutrition-related abnormalities, particularly osteoporosis and deficiencies in iron and vitamin B_{12}.

CONCLUSION

There has been a dramatic increase in the prevalence of obesity in older adults. Obesity exacerbates the age-related decline in physical dysfunction and the increase in metabolic abnormalities, which leads to frailty, disability, and poor quality of life. It is particularly important to consider weight-loss therapy in order to improve physical function in obese older persons and prevent or improve medical complications associated with obesity. Therapeutic approaches must consider the potential undesirable effects of weight loss on muscle and bone masses.

KEY POINTS

Obesity

- The increase in prevalence of obesity in older adults is a major public health issue.
- Obesity causes frailty in older adults by exacerbating the age-related decline in physical function.
- Lifestyle intervention such as weight loss, behavior modification, and exercise therapy should be considered in older adults to improve physical function, quality of life, and medical complications associated with obesity.
- The treatment must consider the potential adverse effects of weight loss on bone and muscle mass.

For a complete list of references, please visit online only at www.expertconsult.com

CHAPTER 84

Diseases of the Aging Kidney

Latana A. Munang
John M. Starr

INTRODUCTION

Older adults are particularly vulnerable to renal diseases as changes in the aging kidney diminish the capacity to respond to various physiologic and pathologic stresses. The diagnosis of renal disease in older people remains challenging, and the causes are seldom as straightforward as in younger people. The etiology is often multifactorial, and other concomitant nonrenal conditions such as diabetes and vascular disease commonly complicate the clinical picture.

DIAGNOSTIC PROBLEMS IN OLDER ADULTS

Atypical presentation of disease

As with any illness, the presentation of renal disease is often different in older adults compared to younger people. They may present with nonspecific symptoms that could be associated with a decline in their cognition or function or decreased mobility and falls, or they may be completely asymptomatic. Clinical examination findings can be hard to interpret. Typical signs of renal disease in younger people such as decreased skin turgor and postural hypotension are common in older adults without necessarily signifying hypovolemia and dehydration. Leg edema is also common, particularly in those with reduced mobility without necessarily indicating volume overload.

Measuring renal function

Although serum creatinine is most commonly used to detect renal dysfunction, it is an insensitive measure in older people because levels depend on age, sex, muscle mass, and diet. Renal disease is often undetected in older adults as their muscle mass is relatively lower and their serum creatinine levels may fall within the normal range even when renal function is severely diminished.[1] Nevertheless, in the context of acute renal failure, changes in serum creatinine remain the best marker of kidney function. In chronic kidney disease however, the glomerular filtration rate (GFR) is the preferred indicator and can be estimated by creatinine clearance, through a timed urine collection or formulae such as the Cockcroft-Gault[2] or Modification of Diet in Renal Disease[3] (MDRD). The four-variable MDRD formula (Table 84-1) is the current method of choice in older people[4,5] and is recommended by current guidelines.[6] Cystatin C, a cysteine protease inhibitor freely filtered by the kidney, is an alternative serum marker of kidney function that is unaffected by age, sex, and muscle mass and approximates direct measurements of GFR more precisely. It is more sensitive in detecting early kidney dysfunction in older people and has been shown to be a strong prognostic indicator of death and cardiovascular disease,[7] but it has yet to come into routine clinical use.

Collecting urine specimens

Obtaining a clean urine sample for analysis can be challenging, particularly in bed-bound female patients or incontinent patients, but not impossible with good nursing care. An early morning urine sample is preferable to exclude postural proteinuria. Occasionally, catheterization may be necessary, but it should only be performed as a last resort as the procedure itself can cause infections.

Interpretation of urine examinations

In older people, urinalysis often shows increased leukocytes and epithelial cells, which are not necessarily pathologic. Mixed growth of organisms on culture is frequently a result of contamination, although mixed infections may occur in those with indwelling urinary catheters. Urinalysis may also reveal red cell casts, hematuria, or proteinuria as a result of intrinsic renal disease and should prompt further investigations and specialist input.

INFECTIONS OF THE URINARY TRACT

Up to 25% of women and 10% of men aged over 65 years have asymptomatic bacteriuria, which is defined as ≥100,000 colony-forming units per mL urine on two or more consecutive tests in the absence of any clinical symptoms. This figure rises to >50% in women and >35% in men aged over 80 years.[8] The prevalence is higher in people in institutionalized care, people with urinary catheters, and people with diabetes. Routine screening and treatment is not recommended, as unnecessary antibiotics result in more adverse effects and antimicrobial resistance without any clear benefits in mortality and morbidity.[9] The only exceptions are those who are symptomatic or those about to undergo invasive urologic procedures such as transurethral resection of prostate or cystoscopy.

Urinary tract infections (UTI) occur when bacteria which colonize the superficial epithelium of the urinary tract breach this mucosal barrier. Once this barrier is breached, bacteria are able to invade bladder epithelial cells[10]—hence, the recommendation for treating asymptomatic bacteriuria in patients undergoing invasive urologic procedures. Recurrent UTI may occur because of susceptibility of the mucosal barrier, for example, in trauma secondary to urinary catheters, stones, or neoplasia or in people with problems clearing bacteria from bladder epithelial cells because of impaired immune response.

The diagnosis of UTI is based on clinical evaluation of symptoms and signs indicating breach of the mucosal barrier. The usual features of dysuria, urinary frequency, and urgency may be absent in older patients. Other typical symptoms and signs that significantly increase the likelihood that a UTI is present are hematuria, back pain, and costovertebral angle tenderness, whereas a history of vaginal discharge, vaginal irritation, or presence of vaginal discharge on examination significantly reduces the probability.[11] UTI is also associated with urinary incontinence in women[12] and should be excluded in people presenting with this symptom. Distinguishing asymptomatic bacteriuria from a clinically significant UTI may be difficult, particularly in those with cognitive impairment. A systematic review of the use of dipstick tests to diagnose or rule in UTI indicates that a positive result for either the leukocyte esterase or nitrite test showed the highest sensitivity and the lowest negative

Table 84-1. Estimation of GFR Using the Four-Variable MDRD Equation

$$GFR(mL/min/1.73\ m^2) = 186 \times \{[\text{serum creatinine } (\mu mol/L)/88.4]^{-1.154}\} \times \text{age (years)}^{-0.203} \times 0.742 \text{ if female, and} \times 1.21 \text{ if African American}$$

Reprinted with permission from the American Society of Nephrology. Levey AS, Greene T, Kusek J, Beck G. A simplified equation to predict glomerular filtration rate from serum creatinine. J Am Soc Nephrol 2000;11:155A.

likelihood ratio.[13] However, a study in younger women aged 16 to 50 years found that a 3-day course of trimethoprim reduced dysuria equally in those with and without positive nitrite tests on urinary dipstick even though the dipstick test reliably predicted who did and who did not have a UTI.[14] It is unclear whether this is generalizable to older adults, but it raises the question of balancing symptomatic relief against potential promotion of antibiotic resistance. The problem of promoting antibiotic resistance also occurs with regard to management of recurrent UTI. In women aged 21 to 72 years, both cranberry juice and cranberry tablets reduced the risk of UTI by around 20%,[15] and this may be a useful first-line approach, though benefit in older age groups is less certain. There is a paucity of evidence to support long-term antibiotic prophylaxis in older adults, and attention to risk factors such as local hygiene, diabetic control, and catheter use is more important.

Although mild uncomplicated lower UTI can be managed safely in the community, bacteremic urinary sepsis carries a significant mortality rate of 25% to 60%.[16] The most common causative organisms are *Escherichia coli*, *Klebsiella*, *Pseudomonas,* and *Proteus*. Several guidelines have been published with treatment recommendations.[17–18] Uncomplicated lower UTI in women should be treated empirically with three days of trimethoprim or trimethoprim-sulfamethoxazole (cotrimoxazole). Longer courses of antibiotics have not been found to be better than short courses in older women.[19] A 3-day course of ciprofloxacin is equally effective,[20] but this antibiotic should not be used as a first-line approach in older people, especially in hospitals, because of its association with increased risk of the hypervirulent ribotype 027 *Clostridium difficile*–associated diarrhea.[21]

The evidence for treating UTI in men is less robust. Most infections are associated with prostatitis or instrumentation of the urinary tract, and a 2-week course of quinolone therapy may be needed, though this has to be balanced against *C. difficile* risk as noted previously. Catheter-associated UTI is a major problem in older people, causing symptoms in 30% of patients, bacteremia in 4%, and a three-fold increase in the risk of death in the hospital.[22] Symptomatic infections require broad-spectrum antibiotics based on local susceptibility patterns, then adjusted to culture results. A catheter change should be considered in those with long-term indwelling catheters before commencing antibiotics. There is some evidence to support the use of antimicrobial urinary catheters to prevent catheter-associated UTI in hospitalized patients,[23] which thus may be a useful adjunct to the general measures of avoiding catheter use when possible and careful catheter care.

Pyelonephritis refers to infection of the upper urinary tract. This mostly occurs through ascending infection from the urethra and urinary bladder. Prostatic hypertrophy in men causes urinary obstruction, increasing susceptibility to infection. Immunocompromised and chronically ill patients, as well as those with renal calculi or any abnormality of the renal tract, are at a higher risk of complicated pyelonephritis. Clinical presentation ranges from mild illness to septic shock, often associated with fever, flank pain, and costovertebral tenderness as well as lower-urinary tract symptoms. Older people may be completely asymptomatic and only diagnosed with chronic pyelonephritis when they are found to have renal failure. Prompt antibiotic treatment is important in acute pyelonephritis because of the high risk of bacteremia as well as complications such as intrarenal and perinephric abscess. Most cases require hospital admission and parenteral antibiotics, although outpatient oral treatment is effective in selected uncomplicated cases.[24]

ACUTE RENAL FAILURE

Acute renal failure (ARF) refers to the sudden reduction in the capacity of the kidney to excrete nitrogenous waste products and maintain adequate fluid and electrolyte homeostasis. Despite the lack of a universal definition of ARF,[25] commonly accepted criteria are a substantial rise in serum creatinine from baseline or beyond a set limit, with or without a reduction in urine output. The RIFLE classification scheme[26] (Table 84-2) attempts to further stratify ARF into severity categories with clinical outcomes, and it has been validated in several studies.[27]

ARF is more common in older people with an incidence of 949 to 1129 per million population (pmp) in those aged over 80 years.[28] It is also more common in hospital inpatients, particularly within the intensive care unit. The causes of ARF have traditionally been divided into three categories: prerenal, intrinsic, and postrenal. There is substantial overlap between these categories, particularly the first two, and causes are often multifactorial in older adults.

Prerenal ARF

This is an appropriate physiologic response to renal hypoperfusion, which may occur as a result of true hypovolemia from dehydration, blood loss, vomiting or diarrhea, or functional hypovolemia in sepsis, cardiac failure, or decompensated liver cirrhosis. Drugs such as nonsteroidal anti-inflammatory drugs (NSAIDs), angiotensin-converting enzyme (ACE) inhibitors, or angiotensin II receptor blockers (ARBs) interfere with autoregulation of renal blood flow and can cause ARF in preexisting renal disease or hypoperfused kidneys. ACE inhibitors and ARBs can also cause hemodynamically mediated ARF in patients with renal artery stenosis in a solitary kidney or bilateral renal artery stenosis.[29] The integrity and function of the kidney is usually preserved after these insults, and prerenal ARF is reversible if perfusion and oxygenation is normalized by correcting the underlying cause promptly.

Intrinsic renal failure

Intrinsic ARF involves structural injury to renal cells, most commonly acute tubular injury. Unfortunately, many causes of acute tubular injury are iatrogenic in nature, through diagnostic procedures, therapeutic interventions, or nephrotoxic medications. The most common drugs causing hospital-acquired renal failure are aminoglycoside antibiotics.[30] They

Table 84-2. RIFLE Classification of ARF[29]

	GFR Criteria	Urine Output Criteria
Risk of renal dysfunction	Serum creatinine increased 1.5 times or GFR decrease >25%	<0.5 mL/kg/hour for 6 hours
Injury to the kidney	Serum creatinine increased 2 times or GFR decrease >50%	<0.5 mL/kg/hour for 12 hours
Failure of kidney function	Serum creatinine increased three times or GFR decrease 75% or serum creatinine >350 μmol/L (with an acute increase of > 44 μmol/L)	<0.3 mL/kg/hour for 24 hours or anuria for 12 hours
Loss of kidney function	Persistent ARF, complete loss of kidney function > 4 weeks	
End-stage renal disease	End-stage renal disease > 3 months	

Reproduced with permission of BioMed Central. Bellomo R, Ronco C, Kellum JA, Mehta RL, Palevsky P, and the ADQI workgroup. Acute renal failure—definition, outcome measures, animal models, fluid therapy and information technology needs: the Second International Consensus Conference of the Acute Dialysis Quality Initiative (ADQI) group. Critical Care 2004;8:R204–R212.

are directly toxic to renal tubules; therefore, serum levels should be closely monitored.

Drugs can also cause acute tubulointerstitial nephritis, a pertinent problem considering the prevalence of polypharmacy among older people. A thorough drug history of current and recent medications is therefore crucial, including any over-the-counter preparations. Common culprits include NSAIDs, diuretics, allopurinol, proton-pump inhibitors, and antimicrobials such as penicillin, ciprofloxacin, and acyclovir. A rash, fever, and arthralgia may also suggest acute interstitial nephritis. Stopping the offending drug should improve renal function, but corticosteroids are often used to help recovery by diminishing the inflammatory process.

Radiocontrast nephropathy is a growing problem accounting for 11% of ARF cases in hospitals.[30] The rise in serum creatinine generally occurs 2 to 5 days after exposure to contrast medium. The risk is four-fold higher in patients with preexisting renal disease and diabetes, whereas contrast osmolality and volume are also directly correlated to nephrotoxicity.[31] Regional hypoperfusion causing hypoxia and direct tubular toxicity are mechanisms thought to be involved but the underlying pathophysiologic process is still poorly understood. There is some evidence supporting the use of periprocedural hydration as prophylaxis, but the optimal type, route, volume, and timing require further studies to determine this. Other prophylactic measures using antioxidants such as *N*-acetylcysteine or ascorbic acid may be beneficial, but current evidence is still inconclusive. Contrast media should therefore be avoided if at all possible, but if used, it should involve the lowest volume of iso-osmolar contrast, and other potentially nephrotoxic medications should be temporarily stopped.

Cholesterol embolism can occur following vascular procedures such as cardiac surgery, angiography, angioplasty, and stenting. It can also occur following thrombolysis and anticoagulation. Showers of small cholesterol crystals break off from atherosclerotic plaques and occlude arterioles or larger vessels. It can affect almost any organ in the body including the kidney, and it can be difficult to recognize. Malignant hypertension, mesenteric, and cutaneous ischemia as well as encephalopathy may be more prominent than the associated ARF. Symptoms and signs usually manifest weeks to months after the procedure. One study found the incidence of cholesterol embolism to be 4%,[32] but true incidence is difficult to determine because of the lack of large epidemiologic studies.

Acute tubular necrosis may also be caused by endogenous renal insults. In rhabdomyolysis, skeletal muscle breaks down, releasing its contents and causing myoglobinuria, accounting for 7% to 10% of cases of ARF.[33] This is caused by muscle injury resulting from direct trauma, metabolic disorders, prolonged exercise or seizures as well as medications such as statins and neuroleptics. Up to a third of rhabdomyolysis patients will develop ARF,[33] and this is important to exclude in older people sustaining a stroke or a fall with a prolonged lie.

Multiple myeloma is another condition mostly affecting older adults, of whom approximately 50% will develop renal failure.[34,35] This is mediated through the direct toxic effects of light chains to renal tubules or intratubular obstruction by their casts. The associated hypercalcemia and hyperuricemia may also give rise to intratubular crystals. Renal failure is reversible in approximately half of these cases, and this is associated with better long-term survival.[34]

Acute tubular necrosis can also be caused by renal ischemia, making prerenal ARF and ischemic acute tubular necrosis part of the same continuum. The most common cause is sepsis, particularly with multiple organ failure. Postoperative acute tubular necrosis may also occur, again often with prerenal causes.

Glomerulonephritis refers to immune-mediated conditions causing inflammation in the kidney, usually classified according to their histologic appearances. Previously thought to be rare in older people, it is now recognized to be a frequent finding as increasing numbers of renal biopsies are performed in this patient group. Rapidly progressive or crescentic glomerulonephritis is more common in older than younger patients.[36] The clinical features depend on the underlying causes, which include antibodies to the glomerular basement membrane, connective tissue diseases, infections, and systemic vasculitides (Table 84-3). Prompt diagnosis and treatment is essential to prevent irreversible loss of renal function. The presence of blood, protein, or red cell casts on urinalysis are useful clues. A full history and examination will often narrow down the differential diagnosis.

Postrenal ARF

An obstructive cause must be ruled out in all patients with ARF as prompt relief of the obstruction should result in improvement and recovery of their renal function. The longer this is delayed, the higher the risk of irreversible damage. Prostatic disease is a common cause and a history of hesitancy, poor stream, dribbling, and nocturia is usually present. Other causes include renal calculi, urethral strictures, retroperitoneal fibrosis, renal papillary necrosis, and pelvic malignancies. Examination may reveal a palpable bladder and a large residual volume following catheterization, unless

Table 84-3. Common Causes of Crescentic Glomerulonephritis and Associated Clinical Features

Causes	Clinical Features
Antiglomerular basement membrane (GBM) antibody	Goodpasture's syndrome—hemoptysis and pulmonary hemorrhage Anti-GBM disease—renal involvement only
Immune complex–mediated disease	Connective tissue diseases • Systemic lupus erythematosus—fever, malaise, myalgia, Raynaud's phenomenon, hypertension, edema, frothy urine • Essential mixed cryoglobulinemia—peripheral neuropathy, arthralgia, skin purpura • Henoch-Schönlein purpura—skin purpura, arthritis, abdominal pain, gastrointestinal hemorrhage Infection-associated causes • Poststreptococcal infection—edema, hypertension, hematuria • Endocarditis—fever, sweats, weight loss Glomerular disease • IgA nephropathy—frank hematuria, hypertension • Membranoproliferative nephropathy—hypertension, edema
Antineutrophil cytoplasmic antibodies (ANCA)-associated systemic vasculitis	• Wegener's granulomatosis—nasal and upper airway symptoms, pulmonary nodules and infiltrates, c-ANCA positive • Microscopic polyangiitis—general malaise, weight loss, cutaneous lesions, p-ANCA positive • Churg-Strauss syndrome—late-onset asthma, eosinophilia, gastrointestinal upset, peripheral neuropathy, p-ANCA positive
Others	• Malignancies: solid organ carcinomas and lymphoma • Drugs: penicillamine, hydralazine

the obstruction is more proximal. Ultrasound scan of the renal tract should show hydronephrosis. However, the sensitivity of renal ultrasonography is only 80% to 85%,[37] and serial ultrasound scans or other radiologic imaging methods such as computed tomography or pyelography may be indicated.

Immediate Management

The principal aim is to treat any life-threatening features promptly and stop the decline in renal function before it becomes irreversible. Hypotension, shock, and respiratory failure will be obvious clinically and sepsis should be treated immediately with appropriate antibiotics and fluid resuscitation, preferably in a high-dependency or intensive care unit. Other life-threatening features associated with ARF are hyperkalemia, pulmonary edema, and severe metabolic acidosis.

Hyperkalemia is dangerous because it precipitates fatal cardiac arrhythmias. ECG changes include absent or flattened P waves, broadening of the QRS complex, tall-tented T waves, and eventually ventricular fibrillation or asystole. If any of these Electrocardiogram (ECG) changes is present or if the serum potassium is >6.5 mmol/l, treatment should be started immediately. The myocardium should be stabilized with intravenous calcium, followed by an infusion of insulin and dextrose to increase cellular potassium uptake. Salbutamol has a similar effect to insulin. These measures simply redistribute potassium within the body, and the excess potassium still needs to be excreted, either through restoration of renal function with increased renal potassium excretion or renal replacement therapy (RRT) if the patient remains oliguric or anuric.

Pulmonary edema resulting from volume overload in oliguric or anuric patients is difficult to treat. Respiratory support with oxygen is mandatory, and ventilation may be considered depending on the clinical situation. Opiates and a nitrate infusion may reduce cardiac workload. Large doses of diuretics may be needed to induce diuresis. However, if unsuccessful, then fluid can be removed by RRT.

Severe metabolic acidosis can be treated with intravenous sodium bicarbonate, but there is little evidence that this is beneficial. The acidosis will improve as renal function recovers, but severe acidosis in patients who remain oliguric or anuric will require RRT.

Subsequent Management

The cause of ARF needs to be determined so treatment is targeted appropriately. Thorough history-taking and examination should enable the clinician to establish a differential diagnosis. Several blood tests and radiologic investigations may be helpful (Table 84-4). A renal biopsy may be necessary for accurate histopathologic diagnosis, and although there is a risk of bleeding, it is reasonably safe in older people.[38]

Crucial to the management of ARF is accurate assessment of the patient's volume status and hydration. The majority of patients will be volume deplete and require intravenous fluids. However, bearing in mind the high prevalence of cardiac disease among older people, in particular diastolic dysfunction, this needs to be done cautiously to avoid acute pulmonary edema caused by overzealous fluid resuscitation. Assessment of fluid balance can be difficult in older adults, so a central venous pressure monitor may be useful but is not without its risks.

A urinary catheter should be inserted early, not just because it may relieve obstruction, but to allow accurate measurement of urine output. Relief of upper urinary tract obstruction will require either percutaneous nephrostomy or retrograde cystoscopy with urethral catheterization. Postobstructive diuresis may be up to 20 liters a day,[29] requiring careful management to prevent prerenal ARF resulting from the subsequent volume depletion. Hyperkalemic renal tubular acidosis may also occur but generally resolves spontaneously.

All nephrotoxic medications should be stopped as soon as renal failure is identified. Some drugs are removed by dialysis, and this should be considered when elimination is slowed down because of the associated ARF—for example, in toxicity resulting from lithium, salicylates, barbiturates, and inorganic acids. Special considerations and dose adjustments

Table 84-4. Useful Investigations in ARF

Investigation	Comments
Urea and electrolytes	Identifies renal failure, hyperkalemia, and acidosis
Full blood count	Identifies anemia, infection
Clotting	Coagulopathy may occur
Group and save or cross-match	If acute bleeding suspected
Calcium, phosphate	Hypercalcemia may occur in multiple myeloma
Creatinine kinase, myoglobin	If rhabdomyolysis suspected
Blood cultures, as well as cultures of sputum, urine, wound sites	To identify causative organism in septicemia
Immunoglobulins, protein electrophoresis	If multiple myeloma suspected
Autoantibodies • Antinuclear (ANA) • ANCA • Anti-GBM • Antiextractable nuclear antigen (ENA)	If glomerulonephritis suspected
Complement	
Cryoglobulins	
Rheumatoid factor	
Antistreptolysin O (ASO) titer, throat swab	If poststreptococcal glomerulonephritis possible
Hepatitis and HIV serology	If urgent hemodialysis considered
Other serology • Cytomegalovirus (CMV) • Epstein-Barr virus (EBV) • Varicella-zoster virus (VZV)	If immunosuppressive treatment considered
Urinalysis	Identifies blood, protein, red cell casts
Spot urine protein:creatinine ratio	To quantify proteinuria
Midstream urine	Microscopy, culture, and sensitivities in infection Bence-Jones protein in multiple myeloma
Renal ultrasound scan or other radiologic imaging	Identifies urinary obstruction, size of kidneys, renal calculi, other structural abnormalities of renal tract
Electrocardiogram	Changes may occur with hyperkalemia
Renal biopsy	May be required for histopathologic diagnosis

are also necessary when prescribing drugs such as antibiotics and analgesia, as their pharmacokinetics may be altered in renal failure.

Once the cause of ARF is identified, definitive treatment should be commenced as soon as possible. Hypovolemia caused by bleeding may need endoscopic or surgical intervention. Uremia itself induces platelet dysfunction and coagulopathies requiring correction with vitamin K and blood products. Glomerulonephritis as suggested by the history, urinalysis, and autoimmune serology requires early involvement of nephrologists. Immunosuppression with corticosteroids or other agents, and occasionally plasma exchange, are necessary treatment measures once the diagnosis is clear.

RENAL REPLACEMENT THERAPY

Life-threatening conditions such as severe metabolic acidosis, pulmonary edema, and hyperkalemia refractory to medical therapy may require urgent RRT in the form of peritoneal dialysis, hemodialysis, or continuous RRT. Other indications for initiation of RRT include poisoning with a dialyzable toxin and severe uremia with its complications of pericarditis, encephalopathy, and neuropathy.

Peritoneal dialysis uses the peritoneum as the semipermeable membrane for dialyzing. Solutes pass from blood into the dialysate along their concentration gradient, and water by an osmotic gradient created by adding glucose or a polymer to the dialysate. This method is less efficient at solute and fluid removal compared to hemodialysis and is rarely used in the acute setting in developed countries. It is still useful where hemodialysis resources are limited and when anticoagulation or vascular access is not possible.

Hemodialysis involves passing blood into a dialyzer, where it interfaces with dialysate across a semipermeable membrane. Molecules diffuse across this membrane and large volumes of fluid can be removed by ultrafiltration. Good vascular access and anticoagulation with heparin is required. Intermittent hemodialysis is more suitable in severe hyperkalemia, has a lower risk of bleeding, and costs less, but adequacy and hemodynamic control are more difficult. Continuous RRT—for example, continuous venovenous hemofiltration (CVVH) or continuous venovenous hemodiafiltration (CVVHD)—is preferred for patients with cerebral edema and multiple organ failure as it offers better hemodynamic stability and biochemical and fluid volume control. Slowly extended daily dialysis (SLEDD) combines the advantages of both intermittent hemodialysis and continuous RRT by removing fluid more slowly with greater hemodynamic and metabolic control and may be preferable in the elderly. No particular modality has been proven to have better outcomes.[28]

Age alone should not preclude a patient from receiving RRT. However, each patient should be assessed individually, taking into account his or her premorbid functional level and other nonrenal comorbidities, as well as the patient's wishes and that of his or her family. Even so, at the moment we lack an evidence base that would suggest when, if ever, a patient might be too frail to withstand hemodialysis.

Outcome

Mortality in ARF has been estimated at 40% to 70%.[39] Prognosis is worse with increasing age and comorbidity and those with hospital-acquired ARF.[40] Fifteen percent to 30% of ARF survivors remain dependent on long-term RRT,[41] and many more never fully recover renal function and continue to have chronic kidney disease with its associated risks and complications. Prevention of ARF is therefore vital, with good clinical care and judicious use of potentially nephrotoxic drugs and procedures. Once present, ARF needs to be identified and treated promptly to maximize chances of full renal recovery.

CHRONIC KIDNEY DISEASE

Chronic kidney disease (CKD) is defined as at least 3 months of either decreased GFR of <60 mL/min/1.73m^2 or kidney damage, which may be indicated by persistent microalbuminuria, proteinuria, or hematuria; radiologically demonstrable structural abnormalities; or biopsy-proven chronic glomerulonephritis. The stage of CKD is determined by the level of kidney function, regardless of the underlying cause of renal failure (Table 84-5).[6,42]

Table 84-5. Classification of CKD

Stage	GFR (mL/min/1.73m²)	Description
1	>90	Normal kidney function, but with evidence of kidney damage
2	60–89	Mildly reduced kidney function with evidence of kidney damage
3	30–59	Moderately reduced kidney function
4	15–29	Severely reduced kidney function
5	<15 or on dialysis	Established renal failure

Reprinted with permission from the National Kidney Foundation. National Kidney Foundation. KDOQI Clinical Practice Guidelines for Chronic Kidney Disease: Evaluation, Classification and Stratification. Am J Kidney Dis 2002;39(suppl 1):S1–S000.

CKD mainly affects older people. The prevalence in the United States is estimated to be 13%, with 37% of those aged over 70 years having CKD stage 3 and above.[43] An English study found the prevalence of significant CKD to be 5554 pmp, with almost 90% of those not referred to nephrologists being aged over 70 years.[44]

Causes of CKD

The most common cause of CKD is diabetes mellitus, accounting for 22% of people commencing RRT in the United Kingdom.[45] In older adults, renovascular disease and hypertension are also important causes, but in the majority of cases the primary renal diagnosis remains unconfirmed. Other causes more common in older patients include obstructive uropathy, myeloma, and systemic vasculitis. Glomerulonephritis, pyelonephritis, and polycystic kidney disease predominantly affect younger patients.

Clinical manifestations and complications

CKD is often asymptomatic, even in advanced stages. A large proportion of CKD is found incidentally on blood tests done for other reasons. Clinical features include poor appetite, nausea and vomiting, tiredness, breathlessness, peripheral edema, itch, cramps, and restless legs.

CKD is associated with increased mortality and morbidity, particularly from cardiovascular disease. The cardiovascular risk increases exponentially as CKD progresses, so the risk is increased 2-fold to 4-fold in stage 3 and 10-fold to 50-fold in stage 5.[46] Hypertension is common in CKD because of sodium retention and activation of the renin-angiotensin system. Most CKD patients also have other traditional cardiovascular risk factors such as age, diabetes, dyslipidemia, and smoking. Renal dysfunction itself causes oxidative stress, vascular calcification, increased circulating cytokines as a result of chronic inflammation, and elevated asymmetrical dimethylarginine (ADMA) levels that inhibit nitric oxide synthesis contributing to endothelial dysfunction and accelerated atherosclerosis. All of these mechanisms lead to a higher prevalence of myocardial infarction and ischemic heart disease, cardiac failure, stroke, and peripheral vascular disease.

Other complications of CKD involve the bones, anemia, acidosis, and malnutrition. Renal bone disease and anemia start at stage 3. The production of active 1,25-dihydroxyvitamin D is impaired, and secondary hyperparathyroidism occurs because of hypocalcemia and hyperphosphatemia. This is particularly significant in older people because of the high incidence of osteoporosis. Anemia is due to erythropoietin deficiency, decreased erythrocyte life span, and blood loss. If left untreated, it may contribute to cardiac failure, cognitive impairment, and poor quality of life. Metabolic acidosis and malnutrition occur mainly at stages 4 and 5. Acidosis accelerates bone loss, muscle wasting, and hypoalbuminemia, as well as decline in renal function. Anorexia, dietary restrictions, increased catabolism, and chronic inflammation all contribute to malnutrition in CKD, causing muscle weakness, poor exercise tolerance, and increased susceptibility to infection.

Management

The rate of deterioration in renal function can be assessed by reviewing previous biochemistry results. Serum creatinine should always be rechecked so that any rapid decline can be identified and treated promptly. Any potentially reversible causes of renal failure should be considered, such as medications and infections. Urinalysis is important to check for hematuria and proteinuria. A urologic malignancy should always be excluded in macroscopic hematuria with a normal GFR. Proteinuria requires confirmation by laboratory testing, but 24-hour protein quantification is cumbersome and unnecessary. This can be estimated by multiplying the urine protein:creatinine ratio (P/Cr) measured from a spot urine sample by a factor of 10. P/Cr ≥45mg/mmol is considered positive for proteinuria.

Clinical guidelines have been published outlining the management of CKD and indications for referral to nephrologists.[6,47] Most patients up to stage 3 can be managed safely in the community, but disease progression should be monitored with regular kidney function tests. The rate of GFR decline can be estimated by graphing 1/creatinine over time and can be as high as 7 to 8 mL/min/year.[48] Changes in the gradient of the curve indicating a faster rate of decline should prompt investigations for potentially reversible causes. CKD progression is accelerated with proteinuria and uncontrolled hypertension.

The mainstay of treatment in CKD is optimal management of cardiovascular risk factors. Not only does this reduce mortality and morbidity, it also slows the progression of early CKD to established renal failure (ERF). Smoking, weight loss, exercise, alcohol, and sodium consumption are important issues to address. Aspirin and lipid lowering agents should be considered in all patients, and diabetics should aim for target glycated hemoglobin (HbA1c) of 6.6% to 7.5%. Hypertension should be carefully controlled, aiming for a target blood pressure of 130/80, and 125/75 if P/Cr >100mg/mmol. All patients with proteinuria and diabetics with microalbuminuria should be on ACE inhibitors or ARBs. Serum creatinine and potassium should be rechecked 2 weeks after commencing or increasing the dose of these drugs, withdrawal should be considered if creatinine increases by >20% or GFR falls by >15%, and investigations for renal artery stenosis may be warranted.

All CKD patients should have their hemoglobin (Hb), potassium, calcium, and phosphate monitored at least annually. Treatment with erythropoiesis-stimulating agents and intravenous iron should be considered in anemic patients with Hb <11g/dL, aiming to maintain a stable Hb between 10.5 and 12.5g/dL, depending on their functional needs.[49] If the parathyroid hormone concentration is raised and serum

25-hydroxyvitamin D is low, treatment with ergocalciferol or cholecalciferol with calcium supplement should be commenced. Phosphate binders are also useful in hyperphosphatemia, aiming for a phosphate level ≤1.8 mmol/L. Renal ultrasonography or other radiologic imaging may be indicated, especially in patients with lower urinary tract symptoms, intractable hypertension, and unexpected deterioration in GFR.

As CKD progresses to stages 4 and 5, patients should have blood tests mentioned earlier checked every 3 months. They should also receive dietetic input regarding appropriate sodium, fluid, potassium, and phosphate restrictions. Supplementary sodium bicarbonate can be used to correct acidosis, aiming to maintain plasma bicarbonate ≥20 mmol/L. All patients with stages 4 or 5 of CKD should discuss their condition with a nephrologist, unless there are other mitigating factors—for example, terminal illness. This is to ensure that patients are adequately informed about their treatment options as they approach ERF. Most patients need a minimum of 1 year to prepare themselves and their caregivers for RRT,[50] but late referral is significantly more frequent in older patients, contributing to excess mortality.[51]

ESTABLISHED RENAL FAILURE

The number of older patients on RRT continues to grow, and the median age of patients starting dialysis in the United Kingdom is 65 years.[45] Guidelines recommend starting RRT when GFR falls below 15 mL/min/1.73m^2 with symptomatic uremia, difficult fluid balance, or blood pressure control and progressive malnutrition. RRT should be started when GFR falls below 6 mL/min/1.73m,^{2} even when the patient is asymptomatic.[52]

The most common form of RRT in older adults is hemodialysis. Subcutaneous arteriovenous fistula is the preferred vascular access and should be formed at least 6 months before commencing dialysis. In the short to intermediate term, synthetic grafts, central venous catheters, and semipermanent tunneled central catheters may also be used. Most patients undergo three hemodialysis sessions per week, each lasting 3 to 5 hours, usually in hospital units. Access to home hemodialysis is limited but may be considered for appropriate patients and is associated with good outcomes.[53]

Peritoneal dialysis allows greater independence as it can be carried out in the patient's own home and tailored to the patient's daily routine. However, it is contraindicated in patients with a history of major abdominal surgery or peritoneal adhesions, unrepaired inguinal hernias, or compromised respiratory function, which unfortunately excludes many older people. Common problems include infection and fluid overload resulting from inadequate ultrafiltration, and conversion to hemodialysis may be necessary.

Transplantation can restore renal function completely and is clearly preferable to dialysis. Scarce donor organs, however, means that many older patients are not considered for transplantation because of their comorbidity and shorter life expectancy. Only 14% of renal transplant recipients in the United Kingdom are aged over 60,[54] despite no age limit to transplantation. Renal transplantation has been shown to be worthwhile in older patients with good graft survival rates, provided they are carefully selected and their immunosuppression tailored sensibly.[55,56] Main complications are graft rejection, infection, and malignancy, but cardiovascular disease remains the leading cause of death.

RRT may not always be in the best interest of all older patients. In heavily dependent patients with more comorbidity, survival on RRT is not significantly longer than those treated palliatively.[57] Many older patients on RRT spend a considerable proportion of their time in the hospital with a higher risk of developing multiple complications.[58] Conservative management aims to relieve the symptoms of ERF and maximize health for the remainder of patients' lives. This includes treating anemia with erythropoiesis-stimulating agents and controlling nausea and pruritus with appropriate drugs. Many renal units now have conservative care specialist nurses to facilitate this treatment option for patients. End-of-life care is equally important, not just in patients who choose not to dialyze but also for those who choose to withdraw from dialysis. Close collaboration with palliative services and primary care is essential.

Outcome

Mortality increases exponentially with declining GFR, by 17% for stage 3 and nearly 600% for stage 5.[59] Most patients are more likely to die of cardiovascular disease before reaching ERF. In a 5-year observational study in the United States, 3% of patients with CKD stages 2 through 4 eventually required RRT, whereas 24% died.[60] Our efforts should therefore concentrate on early identification and good management of cardiovascular risk factors, which will also delay progression to ERF.

CONCLUSION

The number of people with renal disease will continue to increase as our population ages and the diabetes epidemic grows. Early recognition of risk factors is essential as the disease is often asymptomatic in older people. Age per se should not be a contraindication to good treatment, and appropriate patients should be referred to nephrologists promptly. Bearing in mind the great heterogeneity of older people, each patient should be considered individually. Patients need to be adequately informed about the likely course and prognosis of their disease to guide them in making choices about treatment options.

KEY POINTS

Diseases of the Aging Kidney

- Renal disease is frequently underdiagnosed and undertreated in older people because they present with nonspecific or no symptoms and their serum creatinine may be normal.
- Asymptomatic bacteriuria does not require treatment.
- Iatrogenic renal failure is a growing problem because of nephrotoxic drugs and radiocontrast agents.
- Good management of cardiovascular risk factors is important in chronic kidney disease to reduce mortality and morbidity and delay progression to established renal failure.
- Appropriate referral to nephrologists improves outcomes.

For a complete list of references, please visit online only at www.expertconsult.com

CHAPTER 85

Disorders of Water, Electrolyte, and Mineral Ion Metabolism

M. Shawkat Razzaque

INTRODUCTION

Water is the main component of living cells and tissues. Water balance is important for the proper physiologic function of various organ systems. An imbalance of water homeostasis, in the form of either dehydration or overhydration, can lead to severe health problems. Even mild alteration of the water balance can significantly affect the homeostasis of electrolyte and mineral ions, including sodium, potassium, calcium, and phosphorus; in addition, the body requires adequate amounts of magnesium, chloride, copper, fluoride, iodine, iron, selenium, and zinc. To maintain adequate functionality of the organ systems, the body needs to continuously recycle and replace water, electrolyte, and mineral ions. A unique coordination among the neural, endocrine, gastrointestinal, and renal systems maintains the necessary balance of water, electrolytes, and mineral ions in the body. As people age, this system becomes more prone to disruptions that can have clinical consequences.

WATER BALANCE

The mechanisms underlying the regulation of water balance are not yet clearly understood; however, increased knowledge of the effects of water channels in the kidney, namely aquaporins, as well as the functions of antidiuretic hormone (ADH) has provided molecular insights. ADH, also known as vasopressin, is a peptide hormone secreted by the hypothalamus. ADH secretion is influenced by several factors, including increased plasma osmolarity that activates receptors in the hypothalamus to release ADH. In normal physiologic conditions, water intake and water output are tightly regulated. If water output exceeds intake, a thirst sensation is stimulated to facilitate fluid intake. Higher serum osmolality, hypotension, and hypovolemia can stimulate thirst. In mild water disturbances, the kidneys conserve water according to the needs of the body. In conditions of severe volume depletion or hypertonicity, secretion of ADH is stimulated to reabsorb more water in the kidneys, resulting in the excretion of concentrated urine. In contrast, in conditions of hypotonicity, ADH is suppressed, and diluted urine is excreted. Similarly, when the blood pressure falls, stretch receptors in the aorta and carotid arteries are activated to stimulate ADH secretion so that the body can retain enough fluid to restore blood pressure. In addition, stretch receptors in the atria of the heart are activated when a larger than normal volume of blood returns to the heart from the veins; this activation of atrial stretch receptors inhibits ADH secretion, resulting in excretion of excessive fluid.

Maintaining water, electrolyte, and mineral ion balance becomes difficult in elderly individuals, as older people tend to retain less water than younger individuals. A healthy 30- to 40-year-old person usually has a total-body water content of 55% to 60%; however, by the age of 75 to 80 years, the total-body water content declines to 50%, which is even more marked in elderly women.[1] In aged individuals, the urine-concentrating ability of the kidneys is reduced, and this may lead to more water loss through the urine.[2] Impairment of water homeostasis in elderly individuals is also associated with decreased renal mass,[3] reduced cortical blood flow,[4] and a decreased glomerular filtration rate,[5] as well as altered responsiveness to sodium balance.[4] Moreover, elderly individuals with urinary incontinence tend to drink less to avoid frequent micturition. Diarrhea, vomiting, or gastrointestinal bleeding can also contribute to water dysequilibrium in elderly individuals. Common neurologic disorders, including dementia, anorexia, or depression, can affect water intake and water balance in older individuals. Similarly, poorly controlled diabetes, strokes, draining wounds, fever, rapid breathing, infection, or burns can destabilize not only water balance but also electrolyte balance in the elderly.

ELECTROLYTE BALANCE

The serum concentration of sodium usually reflects the status of water homeostasis in the body. The elderly show impairments in thirst sensation, renal function, and factors that regulate salt and water balance, and they are thus more vulnerable to age-associated diseases and iatrogenic events involving water and electrolytes disturbances. A comprehensive review of all the aspects of the regulation of electrolytes is beyond the scope of this chapter. Rather, emphasis will be given to the conditions that are associated with abnormal regulation of sodium and potassium, the two most extensively studied electrolytes.

Sodium is one of the major cations in the extracellular fluid, and it mostly determines serum osmolality. Systemic electrolyte disturbances, either in the form of hyponatremia or hypernatremia, are common in older adults and most evident in hospitalized patients or individuals living in long-term care facilities. Cross-sectional studies have found that hyponatremia may be present in as many as 15% to 18% of the individuals living in chronic care facilities.[4] In contrast, about 30% of nursing home residents who required acute hospitalization have hypernatremia.[6] Impaired water metabolism can be attributed to electrolyte imbalance in the form of hyponatremia or hypernatremia. For instance, elderly individuals have a reduced ability to excrete a water load,[7] which may contribute to hyponatremia and be aggravated by receiving intravenous fluids.[4] When hyponatremia is accompanied by central nervous system manifestations (hyponatremic encephalopathy), the morbidity is quite high. Hyponatremia can cause confusion, drowsiness, muscle weakness, and seizures, and a rapid fall in the sodium level can intensify these symptoms.

Dysequilibrium of salt and water input and output can lead to hypernatremia. In a hypernatremic microenvironment, cells become dehydrated, as increased extracellular sodium extracts water out of the cells. Dehydrated cells start to shrink, and to protect cells from such shrinkage, the resting potentials of electrically active membranes are altered. Within an hour of hypernatremia, intracellular organic solutes are formed and they try to restore cell volume to minimize structural damage. It is important to note that the effects of cellular dehydration are marked in the components of the central nervous system, where stretching of shrunken neurons and alteration of membrane potentials from electrolyte flux may result in loss of cellular functions. In extreme cellular shrinkage, subsequent stretching may lead to rupture of the bridging or overlaying veins in the brain, resulting in intracranial hemorrhage. The available evidence supports the fact that a hyperosmolar microenvironment resulting from water loss can induce neuronal cell shrinkage and brain injury, while uncontrolled water replacement can lead to the development of cerebral edema.

The prevalence of high plasma tonicity is significantly higher in adults older than 50 years of age, an indicator of cell dehydration.[8] Among adults aged 70 years or older, the prevalence of plasma hypertonicity can be as high as 30%.[8] Hypertonicity is positively associated with older age, Hispanic and African-American race, impaired glucose tolerance, diabetes, and hemoconcentration. In a community-based longitudinal observational study with more than 500 adults aged 70 years or older, plasma hypertonicity (≥300 mOsm/L) was suggested to be associated with early frailty.[9] Taken together, plasma hypertonicity is an important determining factor for ill health in elderly individuals.

Potassium likewise needs to be adequately balanced to help maintain normal function of the organ systems. Hypokalemia is often caused by the use of a diuretic and may also result from prolonged diarrhea or vomiting. It is important to note that in prolonged hypokalemia, the body tends to produce less insulin, which may lead to increased blood sugar levels. Moreover, hypokalemia is also associated with fatigue, confusion, muscle weakness, and cramps. In patients consuming digoxin to treat heart failure, even a moderately low level of potassium can cause abnormal heart rhythms. Hyperkalemia, however, poses much more health risks than hypokalemia. The most common cause of hyperkalemia is kidney failure or the use of drugs that impair potassium excretion by the kidneys (Table 85-1). These drugs include the diuretics spironolactone, triamterene, and amiloride, and angiotensin-converting enzyme (ACE) inhibitors, or angiotensin receptor blockers. Moreover, the use of nonsteroidal anti-inflammatory drugs (NSAIDs), cyclosporine or tacrolimus, trimethoprim or sulfamethoxazole, heparin, ketoconazole, and metyrapone can also lead to the development of hyperkalemia. One of the severe complications of hyperkalemia is severe cardiac arrhythmias.

As will be apparent, maintenance of an adequate electrolyte and mineral ion balance is essential for normal functionality of the vital organ systems, and this balance is often disrupted because of water imbalance in elderly individuals.

Table 85-1. Causes of Hyperkalemia

Excessive Potassium Load
- Excess in diet
- Hemolysis
- Internal hemorrhage
- Parenteral administration
- Potassium supplements

Reduced Potassium Excretion
- Acute or chronic kidney disease
- Decreased mineral corticoid activity
- Drugs
    - ACE inhibitors
    - Angiotensin II blockers
    - Cyclosporine
    - NSAIDs
    - Potassium-sparing diuretics
- Hyporeninemic hypoaldosteronism
- Renal tubular disease (e.g., tubular acidosis)

Redistribution of Potassium
- Acute tubular necrosis
- Cell depolarization
- Congenital adrenal hyperplasia
- Digitalis toxicity
- Electrical or thermal burns
- Head trauma
- Insulin deficiency
- Metabolic acidosis
- Rhabdomyolysis
- Succinylcholine

MINERAL ION BALANCE

Here we emphasize calcium and phosphate homeostasis and the disorders associated with their dysregulation. Maintaining normal calcium and phosphate balance is crucial for various essential biologic activities that include, but are not limited to, energy metabolism, signaling activities, and normal skeletal growth, development, and function. Abnormal mineral ion metabolism can affect the functionality of almost all the tissues or organ systems. In spite of the wide biologic importance and clinical significance of maintaining normal calcium and phosphate homeostasis, it is not yet clearly elucidated how homeostasis of these mineral ions is regulated.

A healthy adult usually contains ~25,000 mmol (~1 kg) of calcium. More than 99% of this is in the bone and less than 1% (~20 mmol) is in the extracellular fluid. In healthy individuals, the extracellular calcium concentration is remarkably stable, and a balance exists between the extracellular calcium concentration and the body calcium content. The extracellular calcium concentration depends on the balance between the amount of calcium entering the extracellular fluid (mainly from bone) and the amount of calcium leaving the extracellular fluid (in urine). Any functional impairment can lead to an abnormal extracellular calcium concentration. For instance, septicemia and sepsis can lead to the development of hypocalcemia. Reduced activities of parathyroid hormone or vitamin D deficiency are also associated with hypocalcemia. In addition, pancreatitis and a low dietary intake of calcium can facilitate development of hypocalcemia. Generalized weakness, numbness of the extremities, confusion, and seizures are a few commonly encountered complications of hypocalcemia. In contrast, hypercalcemia is found in skeletal diseases that are associated with abnormal release of calcium from the bone into the circulation. Skeletal metastasis of tumor cells and hyperparathyroidism can cause hypercalcemia. Mild hypercalcemia may not produce visible symptoms; however, more severe forms may cause dehydration, loss of appetite, nausea, vomiting, confusion, and even coma. Severe hypercalcemia needs immediate medical attention.

The total phosphorus content in the adult human body is about 12 g/kg, and most of it is present in mineralized tissue. The serum phosphate level is held relatively stable by the regulated excretion of phosphate through the kidney. This control is primarily mediated by the action of parathyroid hormone and fibroblast growth factor 23 (FGF-23). Identification of FGF-23 as a "phosphatonin" has significantly enhanced our understanding of phosphate homeostasis.[10] FGF-23 is a 30 kDa-secreted protein that is mainly produced in the bone by osteocytes.[11] It is presumed that bone-derived FGF-23 exerts its influence in the proximal tubules to induce urinary phosphate excretion to maintain phosphate homeostasis, but it is not yet clear how it interacts with or influences molecules that are also involved in regulating mineral ion homeostasis, including the transient receptor potential cation channel, subfamily V, member 5 (TRPV5), sodium–phosphate cotransporter 2a (NaPi2a), Calbindin$_{28k}$, the Na^+/Ca^{2+} exchanger, and plasma membrane ATPase in the kidney.

Altered regulation of FGF-23 has direct relevance to human diseases, as gain-of-function mutations of FGF-23 have been shown to be associated with autosomal dominant hypophosphatemic rickets (ADHR).[12] These mutations are believed to prevent the proteolytic cleavage of the FGF-23 protein, with the net effect being phosphate wasting and skeletal defects, perhaps because of the enhanced biologic activities of FGF-23. Similarly, the increased serum level of FGF-23 in patients with oncogenic osteomalacia (OOM) is the causative factor for tumor-induced phosphate wasting.[13] Likewise, X-linked hypophosphatemia (XLH) is caused by inactivating mutations of the gene encoding the phosphate-regulating gene with homologies to endopeptidases on the X chromosome, resulting in increased FGF-23 serum levels that lead to phosphate wasting and osteomalacia.[14] Moreover, the presence of inactivating mutations in the dentin matrix protein 1 (*DMP1*) gene has been described in patients affected with autosomal recessive hypophosphatemia (ARHP),[15] a rare genetic disorder with similar clinical features to those seen in patients with OOM, XLH, and ADHR. The clinical similarities of these diseases are thought to be due to increased activity of circulating FGF-23 protein. In contrast, patients with familial tumoral calcinosis (FTC) are characterized by the presence of ectopic calcifications and elevated serum levels of phosphate resulting from loss-of-function mutations in the FGF-23 gene.[16] A list of the diseases caused by abnormal regulation of FGF-23 can be found in Table 85-2.

Table 85-2. Serum Parameters in Human Phosphate Wasting Diseases*

Normal Range†	XLH	ADHR	OOM	ARHR
Phosphorus (2.4–4.1 mg/dL)	Low	Low	Low	Low
Calcium (8.5–10.2 mg/dL)	Normal	Normal	Normal	Normal
PTH (10–55 pg/mL)	Normal	Normal	Normal	Normal
$1,25(OH)_2D$ (39–102 pmol/L)	Low/normal	Low	Low/normal	Normal
FGF23 (220–540 RU/mL)	High	High	High	High

*Note that a low serum phosphate level is always accompanied by a high fibroblast growth factor (FGF)-23 level, irrespective of the disease type.[10] XLH: X-linked hypophosphatemia; ADHR: autosomal dominant hypophosphatemic rickets; OOM: oncogenic osteomalacia; ARHR: autosomal recessive hypophosphatemic rickets.
†Normal value ranges may vary among different laboratories.

In general, hypophosphatemia can produce a wide range of complications including rickets and osteomalacia, cardiac contractility defects, skeletal muscle weakness, anorexia, irritability, confusion, and seizures (Table 85-3), whereas hyperphosphatemia can cause nephrocalcinosis, nephrolithiasis, and band keratopathy. The main causes of hyperphosphatemia are listed in Table 85-4. Moreover, dysregulation of calcium, phosphate and vitamin D metabolism in chronic kidney diseases play an important role in the development of secondary hyperparathyroidism. Such imbalance is associated with renal osteodystrophy and high cardiovascular mortality caused by coronary artery calcification and myocardial fibrosis of the uremic hearts.[17] Animal studies have shown that increased vitamin D activity and hyperphosphatemia are associated with development of features of premature aging,[18–20] although the human application of such observations requires additional examination. It is, however, clear that the elderly population is particularly at risk of developing clinical complications related to low vitamin D levels, as their ability to generate the precursor of vitamin D in the skin is reduced with the advancement of age, changes in lifestyle that reduce outdoor physical activities, and immobility.[21,22] Moreover, the public health messages and widely spread information of the adverse effect of chronic unprotected sunlight exposure, at times, may lead to overprotection. Older individuals may either avoid sunlight

Table 85-3. Clinical Symptoms/Diseases Arising Because of Hypophosphatemia

Anorexia
Cardiac arrhythmias
Coma
Confusion
Congestive heart failure
Encephalopathy
Hemolysis
Irritability
Leukocyte dysfunction
Metabolic acidosis
Muscle weakness
Myalgias
Osteopenia/osteomalacia
Platelet dysfunction
Respiratory failure
Rhabdomyolysis
Seizures

Table 85-4. Causes of Hyperphosphatemia

Acromegaly
Berylliosis
Chronic kidney disease
Diabetic ketoacidosis
Diphosphonate therapy
Excessive intravenous administration
Hypoparathyroidism
Metabolic acidosis
Multiple myeloma
Pseudohypoparathyroidism
Respiratory acidosis
Rhabdomyolysis
Sarcoidosis
Tumor lysis syndrome
Tumoral calcinosis
Vitamin D toxicity

or use protective agents to reduce sun exposure, which would further contribute to inadequate vitamin D levels, leading to osteoporosis and a higher incidence of fracture.[23]

CONCLUSION

Older adults tend to have a reduced reserve of water because of their impaired ability to restore water balance. The hormonal mediators of water, electrolyte, and mineral balance are less responsive with age, making older adults more susceptible to age-related diseases. Moreover, the thirst sensation diminishes with age, along with the urine-concentrating abilities; this all leads to a significantly reduced ability to maintain water, electrolyte, and mineral ion balance, which confers increased risks of disease in elderly individuals.[24] Dehydration is often linked to infection, and is associated with mortality in elderly individuals. As such, health care professionals should monitor the risk factors and signs of dehydration in elderly patients to reduce the disease burden related to water, electrolyte, and mineral imbalance.

For a complete list of references, please visit online only at www.expertconsult.com

CHAPTER 86

The Prostate

Nicholas J. R. George

The prostate gland lies between the bladder base and pelvic floor and is intimately associated with each structure. Secretions of the seminal vesicle and vas deferens are conducted through its substance to the ejaculatory duct, which terminates in the urethra at the verumontanum. Exocrine secretion products, largely under androgenic control, are discharged into prostatic acini and include zinc, citric acid, and numerous enzymes—acid phosphatase, coagulases, fibrinolysins, and proteolytic enzymes—that form a significant part of the seminal plasma acting to support the physiologic changes required for transport of spermatozoa.

DEVELOPMENT

The embryonic prostate differentiates in response to androgen secretion by the fetal testis commencing about the eighth week of intrauterine life.[1] Androgenic activity at the time of puberty results in rapid growth to a weight of approximately 20 g by the age of 20 years. Thereafter, weight remains reasonably constant until 40 to 50 years of age when growth of benign adenomatous (prostatic) hyperplasia (BPH) becomes increasingly common with advancing years. Autopsy studies reveal BPH in more than 40% of men in their 50s and almost 90% of men in their 80s;[2] figures are confirmed by community-based studies involving transrectal ultrasound estimation of prostatic volume.[3]

Castration before puberty prevents prostatic development as well as the later emergence of both BPH and prostate cancer. Removal of testes in the adult leads to involution of the gland,[4] but replacement reactivates growth though only to and not beyond the normal adult size.

The action of androgen on the prostate cell is highly complex and only partially understood. Within the prostate, testosterone is converted to its active metabolite, 5α-dihydrotestosterone (DHT), by the 5α-reductase enzyme located on the nuclear membrane. Most evidence suggests that prostatic epithelial cells per se are unresponsive to DHT, which acts via signaling between stromal and epithelial components of the tissue; epidermal growth factor (Figure 86-1) and transforming growth factor-α (TGFα) provide the most potent mitogenic stimulus.[5] The importance of DHT to prostatic growth has been illustrated by the studies of Imperato-McGinley and colleagues into males from the Dominican Republic with an autosomal recessive form of male pseudohermaphroditism caused by deficiency of the 5α-reductase enzyme. These children develop phenotypically into men at puberty with normal serum testosterone, but with prostates that remain impalpable.[6] These observations form the basis of the development of the 5α-reductase inhibitors presently widely prescribed for men with early symptomatic BPH.

Morphology

Early work by Lowsley[7] concerning the anatomy of the prostate has been superseded in recent years by the extensive studies of McNeal and associates.[8,9] They described peripheral and central zones of the gland (Figure 86-2) as distinct from earlier lobe terminology; the central zone, approximately one third of the gland mass, completely surrounds the ejaculatory ducts, whereas the peripheral zone extends to the apex and wraps around the central zone like an eggcup. The benign prostatic hypertrophy mass arises from the periurethral zone (within the transitional zone) and this extends from the bladder neck to the region of the verumontanum, but never caudal to that structure. By contrast, prostate cancer usually arises from the peripheral zone, explaining the difficulties in identifying early disease endoscopically via the urethra (discussed later).

Much confusion has been created by this conflicting prostatic terminology over the years. Surgeons refer to "lateral" and "middle" lobes at operation, but clearly these are all contained within the periuretheral transitional zones. The true exocrine prostate is not removed in operations for BPH, although patients frequently assume—not unnaturally—that "prostatectomy" means removal of the entire gland. The operation of radical prostatectomy for cancer does, however, involve extirpation of all prostatic tissue—each zone and contained BPH tissue en bloc.

The substance of the prostate consists of glandular tissue, stroma, and smooth muscle. The preprostatic sphincter lies at the bladder neck (Figure 86-3) and is responsible for preventing retrograde ejaculation during intercourse. This α-adrenergic muscle is inevitably removed during the operation of transurethral resection (TUR) for BPH, but lack of leakage following the procedure shows, however, that this sphincter is not normally responsible for urinary continence. α-Adrenergic fibers are present throughout the gland and

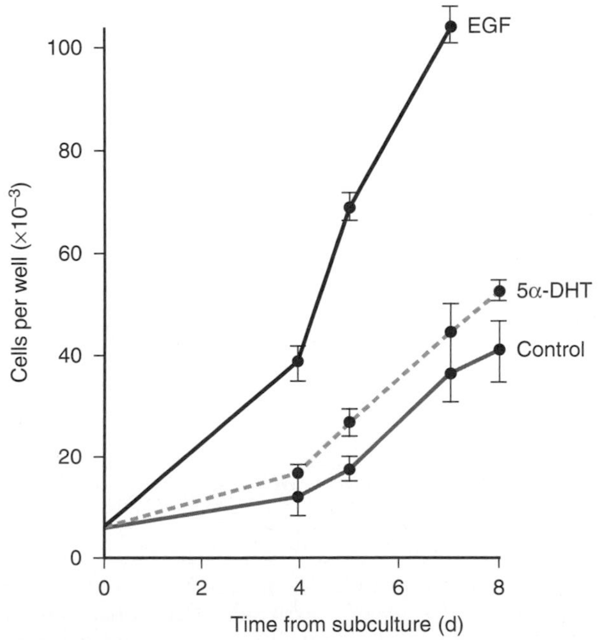

Figure 86-1. Prostate epithelial cells (CAPE-1) in culture. 5-α-DHT stimulation is no greater than control, whereas EGF stimulation leads to significantly enhanced stimulation.

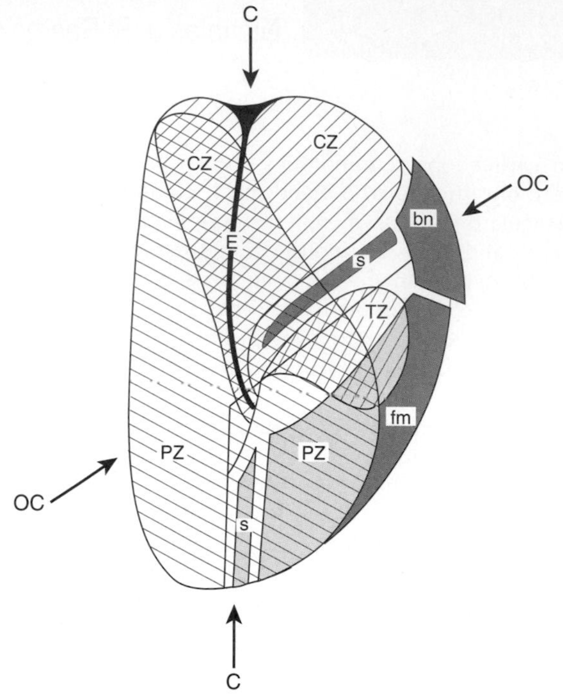

Figure 86-2. Sagittal section through prostate, showing zonal architecture relative to urethra. PZ, peripheral zone; CZ, central zone; TZ, transitional zone; bn, bladder neck; fm, fibromuscular stroma; s, preprostatic, and distal striated sphincter; E, ejaculatory ducts; C, true coronal plane; OC, oblique coronal plane. *(Data from McNeal JE. Origin and evolution of benign prostatic hypertrophy. Invest Urol 1978;15:340.)*

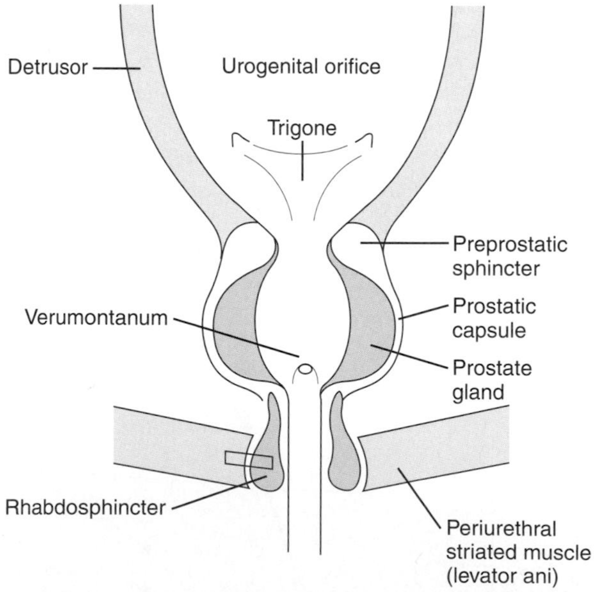

Figure 86-3. Distal sphincter and bladder neck mechanism in the male. P, periurethral striated muscle (levator ani); R, rhabdosphincter; V, verumontanum; PG, prostate gland; PC, prostatic capsule; PPS, preprostatic sphincter; T, trigone; UO, ureteric orifice; D, detrusor. *(Adapted with permission from George NJR. Bladder and urethra: function and dysfunction. In: Weiss RM, George NJR, O'Reilly PH, editors. Comprehensive urology, London: Mosby; 2001, pp. 67–79.)*

may be implicated in the etiology of chronic inflammatory conditions of the gland (discussed later); pharmacologic manipulation by α-adrenergic blocking agents provides a useful therapeutic approach to patients with mild prostatic obstruction.

The continence mechanism lies intimately related to the apex of the prostate at the level of the pelvic floor. Studies by Gosling[10] and coworkers clearly show that the true external urethral sphincter lies within a sleeve of connective tissue, which separates it from the periurethral striated (levator ani) pelvic floor muscle (see Figure 86-3). This latter muscle is innervated via the pudendal nerve and is responsible for emergency continence requiring extra voluntary effort such as occurs during laughing, coughing, or sneezing. The nerve supply to the (slow twitch) specialized external urethral sphincter remains debatable; horseradish peroxidase techniques have suggested it travels via the pelvic nerve to terminate in the ventral horn of S2-S3 on Onuf's Nucleus X.[11] Damage to this sphincter, which by anatomic definition must be distal the verumontanum, during TUR by inexperienced surgeons will inevitably lead to postoperative genuine stress incontinence.

ASSESSMENT OF THE PROSTATE

The prostate is relatively accessible to a number of techniques that may confirm normal or abnormal morphologic features. In a broader sense, prostatic investigations may also encompass assessment of vesicourethral dysfunction, the gland being intimately involved in the storage and voiding disorders of the lower urinary tract.

Rectal examination

Digital rectal examination can by definition only assess the posterior aspect of the peripheral zone of the prostate. The periphery of the gland and the midline sulcus, as well as the texture of the gland may be recorded, but inevitably the experience of the examiner is crucial for accuracy of diagnosis. Rectal examination gives a poor indication of prostatic size; glands may protrude variably into the rectal lumen and other factors, such as a full bladder in acute or chronic retention of urine, may displace the bladder base and prostate downward leading to an erroneous assessment of volume. Additionally, prostatic size is not related to the presence or absence of outflow tract obstruction,[12] but nevertheless the examination remains an essential technique of assessment, particularly with regard to the detection of neoplastic change.

Plain X-ray of abdomen

A single film showing kidneys, ureter, and bladder (KUB) may frequently be performed before prostatic surgery, chiefly to exclude bladder stone. Although the size of the gland cannot be assessed on these films, abnormalities such as calcification may be seen within the gland substance, perhaps indicating past inflammatory disease within the prostatic ducts.

Intravenous urogram

For many years, urography was routinely performed before prostatectomy,[13] and although it is now accepted that this is unnecessary in the majority of cases,[14] radiologists continue to report on the size of the prostate as judged by shadows on bladder films (Figure 86-4). Clinical experience suggests that such assessment can be very misleading, not only because of other causes of intravesical impressions

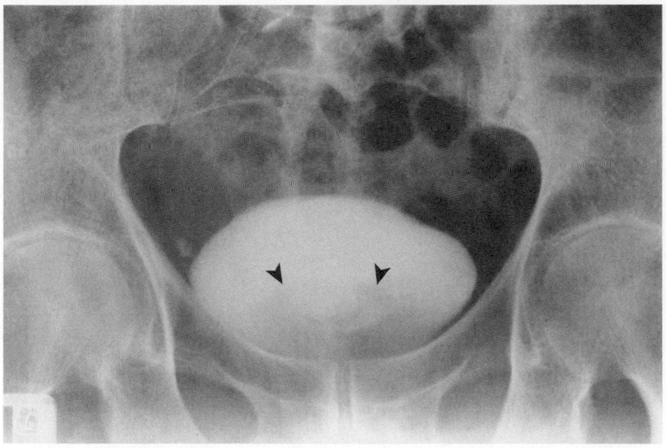

Figure 86-4. Bladder film from intravenous urogram series. Shadows at base of bladder (arrows) are a poor indicator of prostatic size and may represent bladder tumor or other intravesical pathology.

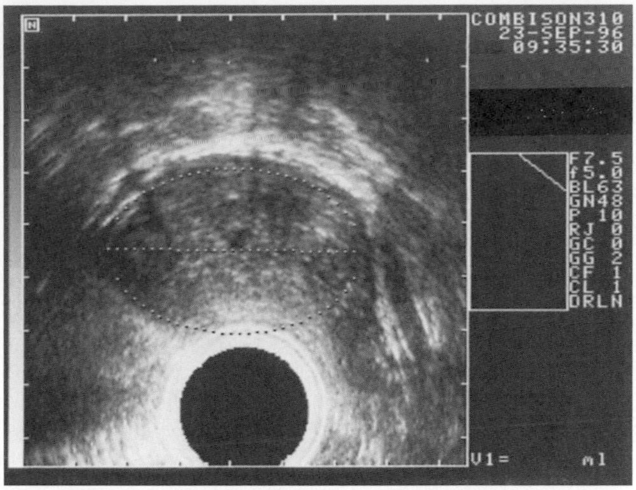

Figure 86-5. Transrectal ultrasound scan of prostate, showing relatively homogeneous pattern within, but with loss of capsular definition on the left. Biopsy from this area showed well-differentiated prostatic cancer.

(i.e., bladder tumor) but because of technical factors such as the variable angle of incidence of the X-rays through the pelvis.

Transrectal ultrasound

Transrectal ultrasound (TRUS) imaging of a prostate is now accepted as the principal methodology by which accurate anatomic detail of the gland may be obtained. Modern machines linked to sophisticated software packages may give high resolution in both multiple transverse and sagittal planes. Additionally, computer-assisted guided needle biopsies may retrieve tissue from exactly specified areas of the gland to distinguish between benign and malignant disease.

In practice, TRUS technology is rarely applied unless it is necessary to exclude or confirm the presence of carcinoma. Patients with straightforward symptom complexes thought on the basis of tests including prostate-specific antigen (PSA) to be due to BPH are likely to be offered therapy without the need further to image the gland and its appendices.

By contrast, despite insensitivity as a "screening tool," TRUS with biopsy as indicated is an essential preoperative investigation in patients with a suspicious prostate on rectal examination and in those—often younger—patients in whom PSA tests indicate the possibility of cancer. It has been suggested that the cancer detection rate obtained by the traditional sextant biopsy technique could be significantly improved by an extended core protocol,[15] though sensitivity for capsular bulge/spread (Figure 86-5) and seminal vesical spread (stage T3b) remains relatively poor.[16]

It will be appreciated that the large literature that has amassed relating to TRUS and TRUS biopsies relates to the enormous effort to detect prostate cancer in PSA "screened" younger men; for older men (taking into account age adjusted PSA ranges, discussed later), the search for neoplasm becomes more measured as age advances. *Nevertheless, the identification of biologically significant prostate cancer that may adversely affect quality of life is important at any age.*

Computed tomography

Computed tomography (CT) scanning is not commonly employed in the diagnosis of prostatic disorders. Although good resolution may be obtained with modern multislice machines, the technique is not routinely utilized in the treatment algorithm of BPH (see the benign prostatic hyperplasia algorithm). Cross-sectional imaging may occasionally be of advantage in those few older men being considered for radical therapy to a neoplastic gland; however, radiopathologic insensitivity relating to patients with low PSA values (< 20 ng/mL), micrometastatic spread, and detectable nodes (<8 mm) ensure that CT is not routinely utilized for "early" disease,[17] even in younger men. It may be of help in clinical management of T3/T4 disease or radiotherapy planning.[16]

Magnetic resonance imaging

Magnetic resonance imaging (MRI) is not routinely used for the diagnosis of prostate cancer. However, the technique is increasingly utilized in the staging of patients in whom the diagnosis has been established but in whom the curative possibility of radical corrective treatments remains uncertain (Figure 86-6). A number of factors may confuse interpretation of scans; in particular postbiopsy hemorrhage within the gland may cause difficulty. Biologically youthful older men may also choose active treatment and in this group with an increased statistical chance of higher staged disease MRI may identify those unsuited for radical intervention.

Despite variable data regarding sensitivity and specificity,[18] good images of capsular distortion and seminal vesical infiltration may be obtained, particularly when the technique employs endorectal (er-MRI) coils. Mullerad and coworkers[19] found er-MRI to offer significantly more diagnostic information in 106 patients before radical prostatectomy when compared to digital rectal examination (DRE) or TRUS biopsy findings.

MRI spectroscopy is a relatively novel technique presently under active evaluation in which the pretreatment ratio of intraprostatic elements (e.g., choline and citrate) is correlated to subsequent observations such as Gleason score.[20]

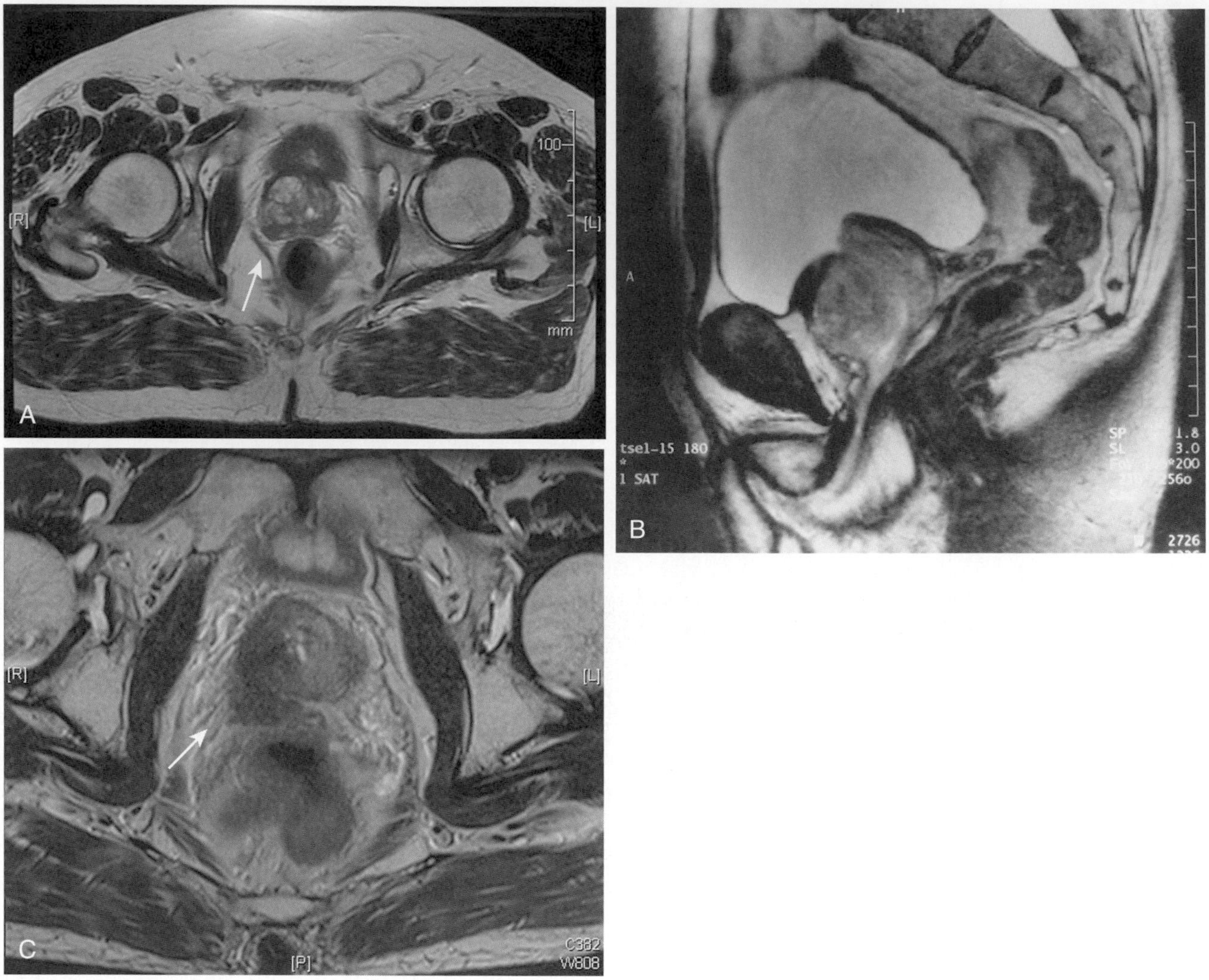

Figure 86-6. MRI scans. **A**, Transverse (axial) section through prostate. Posterio-laterally on the left a distortion of the capsule is clearly seen but penetration has probably not occurred. **B**, Sagittal section through the prostate. The relationship of bladder, prostate and other pelvic structures is clearly seen. **C**, Transverse section showing invasion of right seminal vesicle (T3b). Left SV normal.

Magnetic resonance (MR) scans are commonly employed to detect sites of anatomic treatment failure (PSA elevation) after radical retropubic prostatectomy before salvage therapy; recent studies utilize similar imaging following treatment failure of new therapeutic modalities such as high-intensity frequency ultrasound (HIFU).[21]

Overall it is accepted that the acquisition and interpretation of MR scans requires highly trained personnel. Most uroradiologists agree that under such circumstances there is a marginal advantage to MRI as compared to transrectal ultrasound even when performed by an experienced operator in terms of practical staging diagnostics in patients with localized prostate cancer.[22]

SERUM MARKERS OF PROSTATIC DISEASE

Acid phosphatase

Since the report of Gutman and Gutman[23] noting high acid phosphatase levels in men with metastatic prostate disease, acid phosphatase estimations were widely used in the staging of prostate cancer. Unfortunately, lack of sensitivity with regard to localized disease precluded its use for cancer detection, and the test has now effectively been replaced by PSA, although some authorities still employ it to monitor results of therapy in patients with proven bony metastatic disease.

Prostate-specific antigen

This serum protease was isolated from prostatic tissue in 1979 by Wang and associates[24] and has rapidly emerged as the most important marker of prostatic epithelial activity. Contrary to widespread public opinion, this marker is not cancer specific (Figure 86-7) but may be elevated in other pathologies such as inflammation or benign hyperplasia. Prostate-specific antigen (PSA) varies with the proportion of ductal epithelial cells, so it is not surprising that higher values are found in patients with larger glands and that age-adjusted ranges have been proposed.[25] Damage to epithelial cells either by inflammation or other means such as elective prostate biopsy may elevate levels markedly, often for some weeks, making interpretation difficult in an already

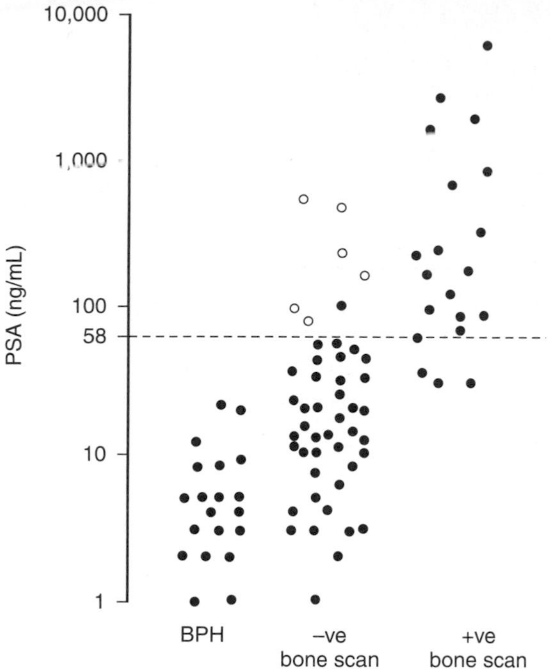

Figure 86-7. Prostate-specific antigen levels in patients with benign prostatic hyperplasia, localized prostate cancer (bone scan negative), and metastatic prostate cancer. Open circles represent seven patients with raised acid phosphatase suggesting metastatic disease despite apparently negative scans. The degree of overlap between the values can be clearly seen, illustrating that PSA is a marker of prostate epithelium and not a specific indicator of prostate cancer. Dotted line: discriminant analysis identifies 58 ng/mL as optimum cutoff distinguishing between skeletal and nonskeletal disease. See text for details. *(Data with permission from Pantelides ML, Bowman SP, George NJR. Levels of PSA that predicts skeletal spread in prostate cancer. Br J Urol 1992;17:299–303.)*

cancer-anxious patient. To avoid unnecessary interventions, *no diagnostic pathway should be entered without at least two confirmatory PSA records.*

In general, cancer may be found on biopsy in 25% to 30% of men with PSA between 4 and 10 ng/mL and an ever-increasing proportion in those with greater values. Most patients with PSA above 50 ng/mL will have skeletal metastases (see Figure 86-7). Despite age-adjusted ranges cutoff values remain problematic,[26] and even below 4 mg approximately 15% of men may have positive biopsies.[27]

The level of PSA at presentation guides therapeutic choices available to those later found to have cancer confirmed on biopsy. For patients with PSAs >20 ng/mL, high surgical margin positivity following radical prostatectomy determines that this modality is rarely (discussed later) offered under these circumstances; this option is usually offered to patients with a PSA under 10 ng/mL. Naturally, surgery is usually reserved for patients with cancer discovered at an early age (<70 years), but extended life expectancy has led many surgeons, particularly in the United States, to offer this modality to otherwise fit men between 70 and 80 years of age.

Although such radical treatment options may not be appropriate to the majority of elderly men, increased life span and regular medical checkups determine that active management of elevated PSA levels in this group is of increasing clinical importance. *No patient, whatever his age, should be allowed to develop by default the morbidity associated with skeletal metastases.* Annual PSA checks are a minimum standard for care of the elderly with subsequent management (discussed later) based on PSA risk stratification.

PSA CHARACTERISTICS AND PSA ISOFORMS

Various aspects of PSA characteristics have been studied to improve its performance in relation to clinical risk including PSA velocity (doubling time) and aged-specific reference ranges,[25] which, though very helpful in younger men, are of limited value in the older age group where larger volumes of benign tissue serve to confuse the picture.

Studies have extended the utility of PSA by showing that it may exist in the serum in two modes: free and bound or complexed forms.[28] Determination of these fractions has added new impetus to the search for a test that can distinguish between BPH and cancer; tumor cells may stimulate production of α-chymotrypsin (ACT), with which binding may occur, leading to higher levels of complexed PSA-ACT than is detected in patients with simple BPH.[29] The determination of the free or complex forms in practical terms is usually limited to the most difficult diagnostic group of patients—those with a presenting PSA between 4 to 10 ng/mL. Free levels below 15% have been associated with the increased chance of a positive biopsy (30% to 50%), but a prospective multicenter study showed only a moderate increase in specificity when compared to total PSA values.[30] Other isoforms such as proPSA and benign PSA have failed significantly to improve on the free PSA performance.[31] PCA3, a marker over expressed in 95% of patients with prostate cancer, is measured in urine after rectal examination.[32] It shows diagnostic promise particularly in the problematic 4 to 10 ng group but is not yet widely accepted in clinical practice.[33]

CLINICAL ASPECTS OF PROSTATIC DISEASE

Prostatitis

Inflammation of the prostatic ducts and acini may occur at any age, although it is more common in its typical form in the third, fourth, and fifth decades. The infection, commonly by coliform organisms, may lead to severe systemic illness with high fever, rigors, and acute perineal discomfort. More chronic forms of the disorder may be difficult to eradicate, and it is suggested that spasm of α-adrenergic smooth muscle as well as general pelvic floor tension may contribute to poor duct drainage and, hence, persisting symptoms. Combination therapy using both antibiotics and smooth/striated muscle relaxants has been advocated in such cases.[34]

In older men, prostatic infection is usually related to the presence of residual urine and outflow tract obstruction. Infection commonly spreads distally down the vas deferens leading to epididymo-orchitis; in earlier times, bilateral vasectomy was commonly performed at the time of (open) prostatic surgery to prevent this almost inevitable consequence of the infected residual. In general, the presence of lower urinary tract infection associated with poor bladder emptying will demand surgical intervention after a period of suitable antibiotic treatment so as to reduce the residual volume. In patients for whom surgery is inappropriate or contraindicated, direct installation of antibiotics into the bladder by a self-catheterization has been described[35] and tried in the elderly with some success.

Benign prostatic hyperplasia

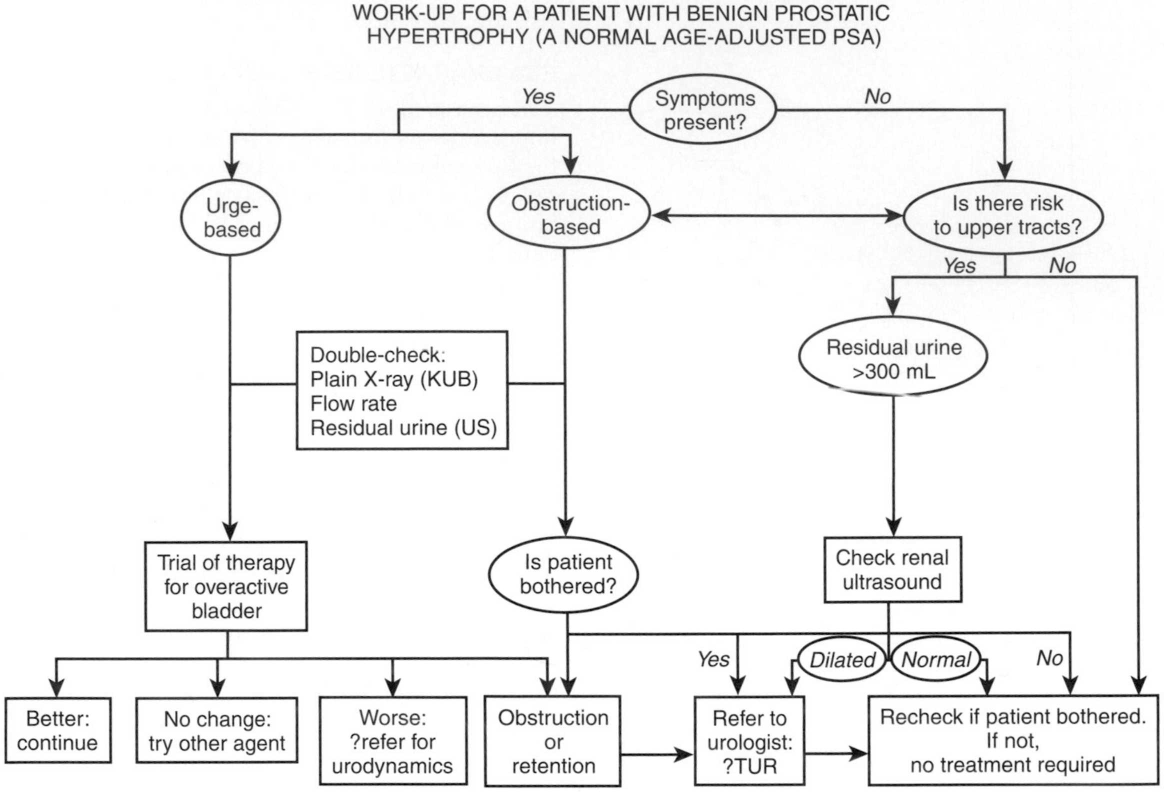

SYMPTOM COMPLEXES AND TERMINOLOGY

It has already been noted that BPH arises chiefly in the periurethral zone and affects a high proportion of men as part of the aging process. It is essential to appreciate, however, that the presence of hyperplasia per se does not imply either significant obstruction to the lower urinary tract or association with particular clinical symptom complexes that may be related to vesicourethral dysfunction rather than the enlarged prostate gland.

These three components—hyperplasia, symptoms, and obstruction—have been brought together in a classic diagram by Hald[36] (Figure 86-8) demonstrating that although all three may be found in a minority of cases, each may exist alone or with one other in a random association.

Urologists have argued for many years against the usage of the common phrase *prostatism* employed to describe a wide range of symptoms relating to the male lower urinary tract. Not only does this imply, often wrongly, that the symptoms may be due to the hyperplasia, but it also suggests that therapeutic attention to the gland will cure the patient. *Obstruction* should be reserved for those patients proven to be obstructed by urodynamic tests—lower urinary tract symptoms (LUTS) more exactly describe the symptom complex that may or may not be associated with the gland.[37]

Associated detrusor dysfunction

The reaction of the bladder to the presence of emergent BPH is responsible for the symptom complexes that are associated with the condition. These changes are best understood if the filling and voiding segments of the micturition cycle are considered independently.

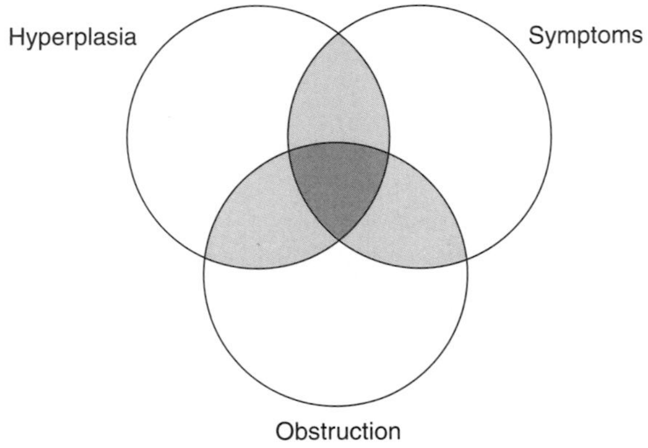

Figure 86-8. Interlocking diagram demonstrating the interdependence of lower urinary tract symptoms, outflow tract obstruction, and hyperplastic tissue when considering symptoms of patients with "prostatism." Significant volumes of hyperplasia may not necessarily be associated either with obstruction or symptoms, whereas all three may be present in some cases. *(Adapted with permission from Hald T. Urodynamics in benign prostatic hypertrophy: A survey. The Prostate 1989; (suppl 2):69–77.)*

FILLING PHASE

The bladder, receiving urine at 1 mL/min from the kidneys under normal circumstances in temperate climates, normally responds by accommodating the physiologic volume (400/500 mL) at low (less than 5 cm H_2O) intrinsic detrusor pressure. This normal reaction to filling may be observed even in the presence of significant outflow obstruction.

More commonly, however, the growth of the emerging gland may give rise to *bladder overactivity*—abnormal intrinsic detrusor pressure waves during filling that lead the patient to experience frequency, nocturia, urgency, and possibly urge incontinence. Unfortunately, not all bladder overactivity is related to prostatic obstruction, there being a significant association with old age and neurologic disorder (when overactivity is correctly called detrusor hyperreflexia). Careful studies have shown that approximately two thirds of older men being investigated for "prostatic" symptoms have bladder overactivity, and of these only two thirds will lose their overactivity following prostatectomy.[38] Unfortunately, there is no test at present that can detect preoperatively which patients will not lose their bladder overactivity postoperatively. Persistence of the disorder following surgery leaves a very unhappy patient with significantly worse urge symptoms that may take many months to settle (Figure 86-9).

VOIDING PHASE

As with the filling phase, significant prostatic hyperplasia may not necessarily affect vesicourethral function. This observation presumably explains in part the large number of elderly men who have apparently enlarged glands on rectal examination but who deny any impairment to micturition performance. More typically, however, two types of bladder dysfunction are found in association with BPH—typical high-pressure obstructed voiding or relatively low-pressure underactive detrusor function.

High-pressure/low-flow voiding is the classic reaction to mechanical blockage of the urethra by BPH leading to typical symptoms of hesitancy, poor stream, and gradually increasing frequency by day and night. Additionally (discussed earlier) symptoms of bladder overactivity may superimpose problems related to urgency and urge incontinence.

Low-pressure/low-flow underactive bladders have been recognized only relatively recently but may account for 20% to 25% of patients with outflow tract symptomatology. The reason for the abnormal detrusor function remains unknown, although the condition has been likened to a nonobstructive myopathy.[39] Men with low-flow voiding also complain

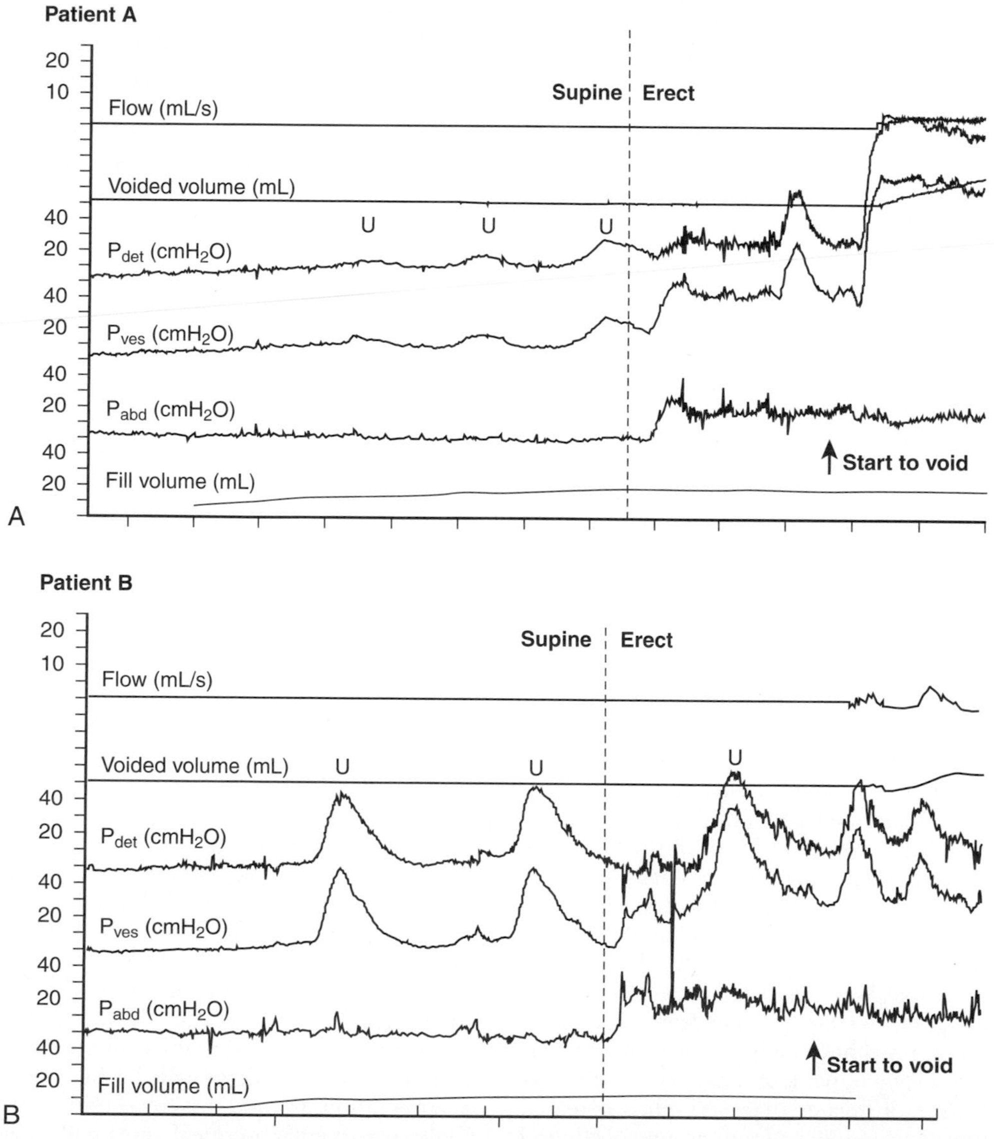

Figure 86-9. Urodynamic (cystometry) traces from patients with (A) bladder overactivity probably associated with obstruction, and (B) bladder overactivity probably not associated with obstruction. In both cases the patient presented with urgency, frequency, and a poor flow. It remains extremely difficult to determine which patient might benefit from outflow tract surgery without urodynamic investigation. In the cases illustrated, patient A would probably benefit significantly from surgery, whereas patient B would probably become significantly worse. P_{det}, intrinsic detrusor pressure; P_{ves}, pressure within bladder; P_{abd}, pressure within abdomen (rectal line). U: patient experienced urgency sufficient to mention to the investigator. Vertical dotted line: commencement of move from supine to erect investigation position.

of frequency and poor stream (often prolonged and interrupted), which is impossible to separate from high-pressure/low-flow voiding except by invasive urodynamic tests (Figure 86-10). It has been recognized increasingly that inclusion of such low-pressure/low-flow patients in prostatectomy series leads to reportedly "poor outcomes" from the procedure.[40,41] In this group, an otherwise satisfactory outcome from TURP will not include a "fire hose" postoperative flow rate, but patients may be well satisfied with such outcomes if counseled appropriately in the preoperative period.

Bladder dysfunction and retention

Sudden increase in prostate size, such as may occur during hemorrhage or infarction, may cause acute (painful) retention of urine, but these conditions are unusual. It is a common observation that patients on urologic waiting lists for outflow tract obstruction rarely present in acute retention; by contrast men admitted with this condition have usually not seen their general practitioner previously, and the precipitating factor seems often to relate to acute fluid loading and subsequent overstretching of the unrelieved bladder—as happens, for example, during a long coach trip.

Chronic (painless) retention of urine is broadly divided into two forms: the relatively common low-pressure "floppy" bladder, which may become complicated by infection but which has normal upper tracts; and the unusual high-pressure "tense" bladder, which frequently is seen in patients with few if any lower tract symptoms but which usually is associated with bilateral upper tract dilatation and obstructive uropathy.[42]

High-pressure chronic retention (HPCR) is specifically associated with sterile urine, late onset enuresis (discussed later), and renal impairment in its later stages. However, elevated creatinine levels may occur for many reasons in the elderly, and this has led to a misdiagnosis of HPCR in many patients with other forms of retention, the true incidence of the condition only being approximately 1 in 20 men with significant retention of urine.[42]

Investigation in benign adenomatous hyperplasia

Audit studies have lead to rationalization of investigations required to assess the patient with BPH. Frequency/volume charts filled in by the patient at home are helpful in revealing nonprostatic causes of urinary tract disorders such as fluid excretion patterns related to cardiovascular disease or excessive tea drinking. Following urine microscopy and culture, rectal examination, and palpation of the abdomen for chronic retention of urine, plain X-ray of the abdomen (KUB) will detect potential operative problems such as bladder calculus. An independent flow rate test, correctly performed (greater than 150 mL voided, no Valsalva pushes permitted) is mandatory (see Figure 86-10). Intravenous urography is no longer advised unless the patient complains of, or is found on urine testing to suffer from, significant hematuria.[43] As noted previously, only 5% of men with significant residual urine have upper tract changes; for this reason, if a residual urine of greater than 300 mL is detected by suprapubic ultrasound, upper tract ultrasound is advised to assess renal anatomy. In summary, audit studies suggest that patients without blood in their urine or residual urine < 300 mL do not require any form of upper tract studies before consideration for surgery.

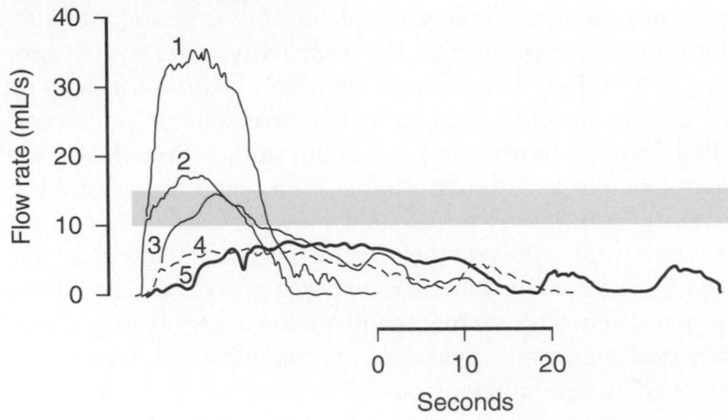

Figure 86-10. Independent flow rate traces. 1: Normal flow rate, younger male. 2,3: Normal flow rates, older male (>70 years). 4,5: Poor flow rate. It is not possible to determine whether the reduced rate is related to outflow tract obstruction or underactive detrusor function—see text for details. Stippled line: lower limit of normality.

Management of patients with benign adenomatous hyperplasia

Many patients come to their doctor because a friend has recently been admitted in acute painful retention or they have seen a television program about prostate cancer. A negative workup followed by reassurance permits these patients to return to their normal lifestyle without the need for any intervention.

PATIENTS WITH INCONTINENCE

Stress incontinence is rare in neurologically normal males and when observed is usually the result of prostatic surgery where the sphincter mechanism has been damaged during the procedure. By contrast, urge incontinence is common, particularly in the older age group, and is chiefly related, in the presence of sterile urine, to bladder overactivity. The therapeutic approach to overactivity is mentioned later and is discussed more fully in Chapter 109. "Late onset" enuresis, mentioned earlier, refers to the loss of a small amount of urine (damp nightwear or underclothes) when the patient is asleep at night or dozing by day. Direct enquiry is usually required for this highly specific symptom of HPCR to be elicited.

PATIENTS WITH HIGH PRESSURE/LOW-FLOW VOIDING

Advice for patients with uncomplicated obstructive symptoms—hesitancy, poor stream, and moderate frequency/nocturia (no urge or urge incontinence)—will depend to a large extent on the patient's own circumstances and preferences. Frequency may not trouble a retired man as much as a clerical officer at his desk. Reassurance, particularly concerning prostate cancer, may be all that is required, and it is tempting to propose that the reduction in α-adrenergic periprostatic tone might be responsible for the noted improvement.

More usually, however, active intervention will be required, and typically the choice will be between medical therapy and operation (transurethral resection of the prostate, TUR). Only in particularly critical cases will (irreversible) surgery be considered before a trial of (reversible) medical treatment, which typically will involve the use of $alpha_1$ blocking agents, alpha reductase inhibitors (ARI), or a combination of both (Table 86-1).

Table 86-1. α-Blockers

Nonselective α-Blockers
Phenoxybenzamine
Selective α-Blockers
Prazosin
Alfusozin
Indoramin
Selective Long-Acting α-Blockers
Terazosin
Doxazosin
Tamsulosin
Type II 5α Reductase Inhibitor
Finasteride
Dual 5α Reductase Inhibitor
Dutasteride

α-Blockers are reasonably fast acting, producing symptomatic relief greater than the observed increment in flow rate might suggest.[44] Modified release preparations permitting a long-acting single daily dose may be of benefit to elderly patients. α-Blockers are the accepted first-line therapy for most men with obstructive BPH symptoms and are always indicated for those patients undergoing trial removal of urethral catheter such as maybe required, for example, after routine orthopedic surgery.

The slow ARI onset of action has long been recorded.[45] Finasteride, a type 2 ARI, was initially considered no better than placebo when treating symptomatic BPH in the veterans' group study,[46] but despite its very slow onset of action, the Medical Therapy of Prostate Symptoms (MTOPS) Study later suggested a benefit for Finasteride in symptom scores and risks of subsequent painful retention in patients with relatively small glands (a mean of 36.3 mL).[47] The socioeconomic cost-effectiveness of the reduced acute retention rate had been questioned in a widely quoted editorial comment[48] on an earlier study, which observed that treatment with Finasteride for 4 years reduced the probability of surgery and acute painful retention.[49] Nevertheless, a recent analysis of MTOPS follow-up data demonstrated that Finasteride led to a significant reduction in prostate volume (25%) over a 4½-year period;[50] whether such dual therapy remains economically viable continues as a matter of debate.

Further combination studies have examined men with larger (a mean of 55 mL) prostates, perhaps more appropriate for an elderly population, and found symptomatic improvement using an alpha blocker and the dual 5ARI dutasteride, which was greater than either drug taken alone.[51] Importantly, it is advisable that any Finasteride cancer–related anxieties aroused by the Prostate Cancer Prevention Trial (PCPT) should be discussed carefully with the patient before ARI treatment.[52] Finally, it is noteworthy that, despite the relatively slow onset of action, Finasteride has been found to be effective in reducing bleeding from the prostate surface, which can be persistent and troublesome in some elderly patients.[53]

For patients with severe "simple" obstruction, TUR offers the unquestioned gold standard in terms of measured outcomes. Despite the significant comorbidity of the elderly treatment population, a rapid resolution of symptoms ensures that the great majority of patients submitted with the correct indications are delighted with the results of treatment.

PATIENTS WITH UNDERACTIVE DETRUSOR FUNCTION

It has already been emphasized that it is not possible to separate patients with underactive function from those with true obstruction unless full preoperative urodynamic tests are performed;[40] hence, overall, it is not surprising that in the absence of such tests, some patients are not satisfied with their postoperative micturition performance.[41] Nevertheless, some improvement is seen and the disappointment is a relative measure of the difference in postoperative flow rates between obstructive and underactive groups. The reversibility of medical therapy makes it ideal for a trial of treatment in this group, and transurethral resection may be reserved for those who are dissatisfied or who cannot tolerate blockade therapy.

PATIENTS WITH IRRITATIVE SYMPTOMS

As previously noted, overactive bladder (OAB) is common in men with both obstructed and unobstructed bladders. Although a complete diagnostic picture may be obtained by urodynamic tests on each patient, few units can afford the academic luxury of this purist approach; hence, trials of therapy are commonly practiced in elderly patients with the frequency urge syndrome (see Figure 86-9A).

Physiologic bladder contraction is mediated by a stimulation of postganglionic parasympathetic cholinergic receptors on detrusor smooth muscle, and of the forms of muscarinic receptor, the M3 subtype is thought to be the most important for bladder contraction.[54] Hence, atropine and atropine-like agents will induce a lessening of the contraction wave with corresponding decrease in detected urgency by the patient.

Early descriptions of such pharmacologic agents[55,56] and subsequent variations in release rate[57] were precursors of a plethora of publications comparing efficacy, safety, and side-effect profiles.[58–60] New-generation extended release (ER) preparations such as tolterodine ER and solifenacin have been studied, although only a minority of the patients were elderly men.[61] Similar constraints applied to a systematic review of antimuscarinic therapy, and it is acknowledged that more studies are required to address urge problems in the elderly population.[62]

Despite these laudable efforts, many will be familiar with the statement about any treatment for overactive bladder: "one is always surprised when it works."

New modalities for treatment of benign prostatic hyperplasia

Although it is accepted that transurethral resection remains the gold standard for treatment of patients with obstructive BPH,[63] a number of new modalities have been introduced, including prostate incision, laser therapy, stent therapy, and varieties of thermotherapy. All these techniques have their vociferous supporters, but all agree that for the patient with a significant volume of hyperplastic tissue obstructing the bladder outlet, endoscopic transurethral resection remains the treatment of choice. The need for critical evaluation of the new technology in terms of outcome measures continues to be debated in urologic circles.

Prostatic surgery in the elderly

Advances in anesthetic techniques and in some cases introduction of preoperative cardiopulmonary testing[64] have allowed a complete reappraisal of treatment options in the elderly, and it is now rare for a patient to be refused prostatectomy on anesthetic grounds alone. Although many patients over 100 years of age have been treated satisfactorily—an unnecessary urethral catheter is undesirable at any age—the chief contraindication to operation is presently the inability of the patient mentally to appreciate what is being offered to alleviate his symptoms. Hence, apart from a few seriously compromised patients, modern anesthesia permits straightforward decisions to be made about the elderly patient, and "lesser" operative techniques such as urethral stent insertion[65] no longer require consideration under these circumstances.

Prostate cancer

Since the 1980s, prostate cancer has increasingly been recognized as a major health problem for both younger and older male patients.[66,67] It is now the most common cancer diagnosis in U.K. men, accounting for 24% of new cases,[68] 35,000 of which were diagnosed in 2004.

However, the increasing age of the population and the very slow growth of some tumors mean that, unlike many other neoplasms, not every cancer is a life-threatening event for the patient. Many older men die *with* rather than *of* their prostate cancer, but the prediction as to whether the disease as identified in any one individual patient carries a good prognosis remains extremely difficult. This overall problem is illustrated by the wide difference between the *incidence* and *mortality* of the disease in many Western countries.

In the United States in 2002, the incidence/mortality ratio was 8:1, whereas in Holland it was 2.6:1,[67] demonstrating that the diagnostic tests were detecting many more cancer cases than were later dying of the disease. The essential question relates to which of the detected cancers

Prostate cancer

WORK-UP FOR A PATIENT WITH PROSTATE CANCER
CONCENTRATING ON PATIENTS OVER 70 YEARS OF AGE

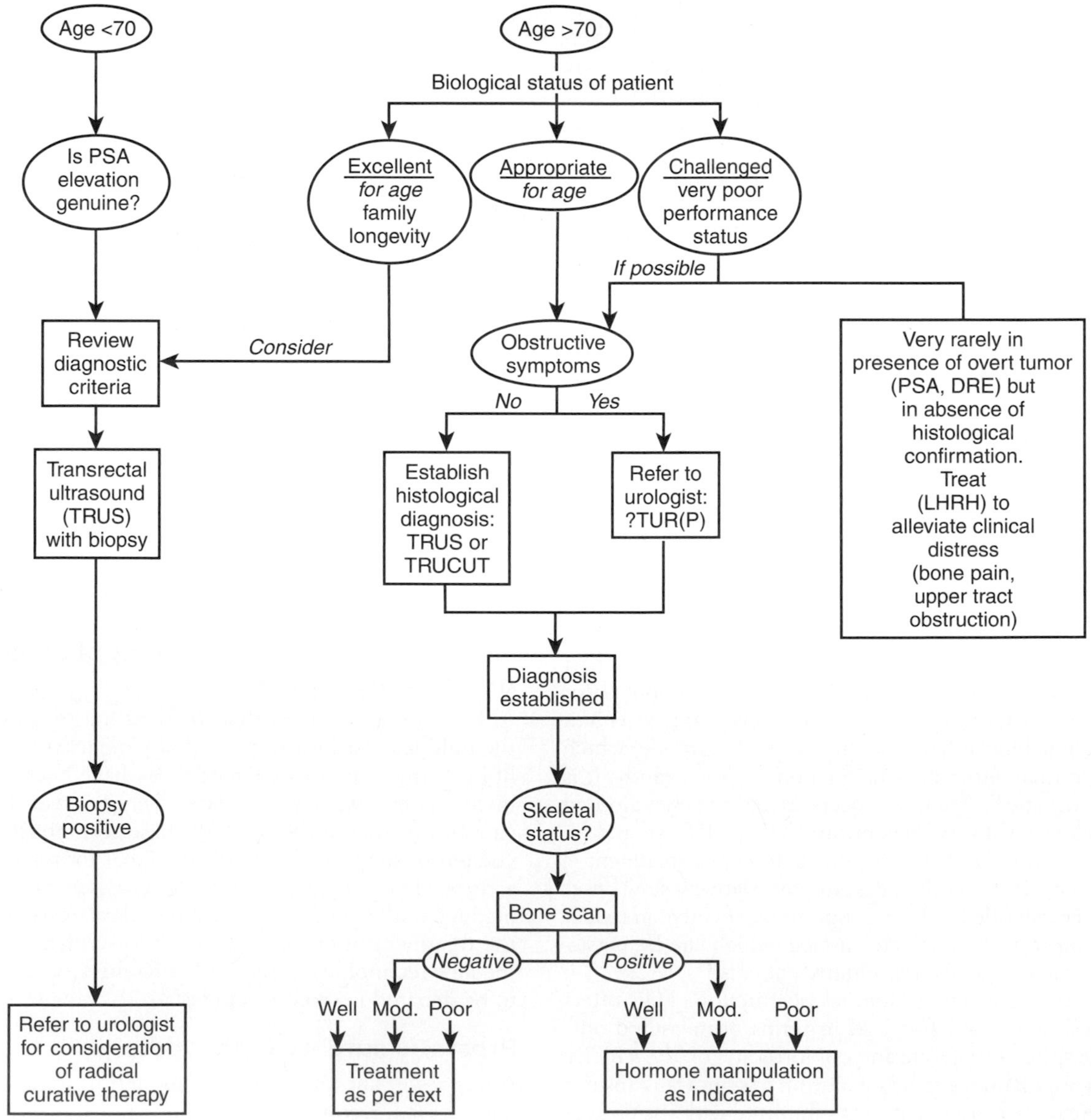

Well, Gleason ≤6; Moderate, Gleason 7; Poor, Gleason ≥8

are capable of progressing and leading eventually to the patient's death.

SITE OF DISEASE

Anatomically, most cancers (70% to 75%) are found in the peripheral zone of the gland (see Figure 86-2). Approximately 20% of lesions are thought to originate in the transitional zone, whereas the remainder are located in the central zone. As such, the educated finger on rectal examination should detect most nodules or palpable lesions; in a minority, the transurethral resection of the transitional zone (i.e., for an obstructive lesion thought to be BPH) may occasionally eradicate unsuspected tumor in that area.

EPIDEMIOLOGIC STUDIES

Prostatic disease is rare in the Far East, Japan, and China. Classical migratory studies have clearly shown, however, that the incidence of the disease increases as males move to a more Western lifestyle. Significant racial differences also exist; within the San Francisco Bay area, Japanese Americans are eight times less likely to suffer from the disease than African Americans.[69]

PROSTATE CANCER AND THE ELDERLY

It has already been mentioned that the disease is being diagnosed at an earlier stage in younger men. At the present time, the question of whether to screen for prostate cancer and which treatment to offer for the cases so detected remains at the forefront of medical debate.[70] Views are strongly expressed because a tumor discovered at age 53, however indolent its growth pattern, is likely to carry a significant risk of death within the patient's natural life span. For the older person, however, the decision criteria are different, and it is in this context that the following variants of disease presentation are discussed.

Localized prostate cancer

Localized prostate cancer may be detected incidentally or it may be discovered as part of the investigation of a man with developing lower urinary tract symptoms. Prostate-specific, antigen-led ultrasound biopsy may reveal carcinoma (stage T1C, Table 86-2) in a patient who merely presented with anxiety, no symptoms, and a normal rectal examination (i.e., BPH in texture). However, for the elderly patient, lower urinary tract symptoms—irritation or obstruction—are more often the reason for a first visit to his doctor.

PSA ELEVATION IN OLDER MEN

Although elevation above the age-related cutoffs will almost invariably lead to TRUS-led biopsy in younger men, the same interventional stance may not be appropriate in all older men. Biologically fit septuagenarians *may* follow the protocol pathway of their younger counterparts (discussed later), but increasingly as age progresses management will be more conservative bearing in mind the high incidence of microscopic prostate cancer found in postmortem studies of urologically asymptomatic men. Hence, the common referral of an elevated PSA in an older man (e.g., PSA 18, age 80) will demand an exquisite level of judgment from both doctor and patient, who, after full informed consent, will have to decide between biopsy and an expectant policy. The answer of course will depend on the individuals concerned, but there must be a strong argument for a careful watchful waiting approach and diagnostic/intervention only if a slowly rising (minimal doubling time) PSA enters the range (35 to 40 ng/mL) statistically associated with impending bony metastatic disease, which, as mentioned previously, must be avoided at all costs. This argument is driven by the scientific literature identifying therapy-related problems such as bone fracture associated with long-term androgen deprivation.[71]

Table 86-2. TNM Staging of Prostate Cancer: 1997 Revision

Primary Tumor, Clinical (T)		Primary Tumor, Pathologic (pT)		Regional Lymph Nodes (N)		Distant Metastasis (M)	
TX	Primary tumor cannot be assessed	pT2	Organ confined	NX	Regional lymph nodes cannot be assessed	MX	Distant metastasis cannot be assessed
T0	No evidence of primary tumor	pT2a	Unilateral	N0	No regional lymph node metastasis	M0	No distant metastasis
T1	Clinically inapparent tumor not palpable or visible by imaging	pT2b	Bilateral	N1	Metastasis in regional lymph node or nodes	M1	Distant metastasis
T1a	Tumor incidental histologic finding in 5% or less of tissue resected	pT3	Extraprostatic extension			M1a	Nonregional lymph nodes
T1b	Tumor incidental histologic finding in more than 5% of tissue resected	pT3a	Extraprostatic extension			M1b	Bone(s)
T1c	Tumor identified by needle biopsy (e.g., because of elevated PSA)	pT3b	Seminal vesicle invasion			M1c	Other site(s)
T2	Palpable tumor confined within prostate	pT4	Invasion of bladder, rectum				
T2a	Tumor involves one lobe						
T2b	Tumor involves both lobes						
T3	Tumor extends through the prostatic capsule						
T3a	Extracapsular extension (unilateral or bilateral)						
T3b	Tumor invades seminal vesicles						
T4	Tumor is fixed or invades adjacent structures other than seminal vesicles: bladder neck, external sphincter, rectum, levator muscles, or pelvic wall						

Following histologic confirmation, bony metastatic disease may be confirmed by isotope bone scan, but it has been suggested that PSA is a superior predictor of a negative scan if levels are less than 20 ng/mL, and thus the time-consuming and expensive scan may be avoided.[72] Regardless of the economic arguments, however, the demonstration of a negative bone scan may be a great comfort to an older man who is likely to have widespread osteoarthritic changes in his skeleton.

TREATMENT OF LOCALIZED DISEASE

Four options are available for the treatment of older men with apparently localized disease: watchful waiting, radical radiotherapy, brachytherapy, or radical prostatectomy. The therapeutic choice will depend *inter alia* on the histologic grade of the tumor, the PSA level at diagnosis, and the biologic age of the patient.

WATCHFUL WAITING OR ACTIVE SURVEILLANCE. Since early studies from Scandinavia[73] and England,[74] there has been a general admission that overtreatment is common in older men who may never experience a clinical problem following discovery of the disease,[75] and hence major efforts have been made to establish safe and expectant treatment protocols for patients, particularly those with low-risk disease.[76,77] Moderate and particularly poor-grade levels of disease have always been associated with poor survival.[74]

Watchful waiting implies a low-key but persistent observation of an often elderly man who may have either histologically proven disease or nonbiopsied PSA elevation (discussed earlier); by contrast, active surveillance implies an interventional management protocol that will include rebiopsy of the gland at specified intervals to detect silent (non-PSA-detected) upgrading of histologic pattern.[78] The ideal protocol for such regimes has yet to be agreed,[79] but increasing (Internet) awareness of the overtreatment dilemma has led even younger patients (e.g., age 60 to 70) to explore the safety aspects of expectant treatment with their physicians.[80] The personal and economic importance of this debate, particularly in North America, is emphasized by the remarkable incidence/mortality data already mentioned.

CONVENTIONAL RADIOTHERAPY. Local tumor control is dependent on clinical T stage and tumor bulk. In the United Kingdom, radiotherapy was traditionally the mode of treatment for those patients with nonmetastatic (i.e., bone scan negative) disease in whom markers, grade or stage (as judged by rectal examination), pointed to the need for local primary control rather than an attempt to "cure" localized disease. In general, at that time, results of comparative trials with surgery were unfavorable, but it is generally agreed that patients entered to the radiotherapy arm of such studies were poorly staged when compared to those submitted ("selected") to radical surgery. However, centers in the United States in particular have reported more favorable outcomes when patients, accurately staged (including PSA) for localized disease, were submitted either to radical radiotherapy or radical surgery.[81,82] Hence, for the many older men in whom watchful waiting or radical surgery is either contraindicated or not the patient's choice, radiotherapy remains an entirely acceptable method of treatment with minimal short- or long-term complications.

BRACHYTHERAPY. Brachytherapy—the implantation of an interstitial radiation source within the prostate—has gained rapid popularity in both younger and older men with localized prostate cancer. Relative simplicity, short (if any) in-patient stay, and rapid return to normal activity constitute the unarguable attractions of the technique. Within the United States it is estimated that brachytherapy, chosen by only 4% of men with localized prostate cancer in 1996, will soon be the treatment of choice for the majority, particularly elderly patients.[83]

Selection criteria for men suitable for brachytherapy are strict. Large prostates (>60 mL), prominent median lobes, previous transurethral resection of the prostate (risk of incontinence), and significant comorbidity (previous pelvic irradiation, diabetes) are contraindications. The treatment morbidity includes irritative voiding symptoms (80%), urinary retention (13%), and late complications of radiation proctitis, stricture, and incontinence.[84]

Along with external beam and surgery, brachytherapy has established itself as a safe, reliable treatment for correctly staged localized prostate cancer and is a popular choice for elderly patients in particular who wish to consider active treatment options. As always, technical expertise allied to up-to-date hard and software will be necessary to deliver optimum results.[84]

RADICAL SURGERY. Radical prostatectomy has always been the first choice in the United States for the treatment of localized prostate cancer, particularly in younger men. However, enthusiasm has been taken to levels where > 90% of patients with low or moderate risk cancers elect for active therapies.[75] Such observations have confirmed the trend to overtreatment,[85] particularly in the elderly; to emphasize this point it has been noted that, in the this age group, more than 300 men would have to undergo surgery to prevent one prostate cancer death at 10 years.[76]

Nevertheless, the treatment preference of biologically fit elderly men with 10-year life expectancy should be respected. Although the majority of the surgical workload will naturally involve younger men, good results can be expected with carefully selected older patients. These comments and caveats apply equally to patients choosing either open or the newly fashionable robotic assisted surgery.[86]

TREATMENT SUMMARY

Observational studies, while making due allowance for pathologic stage and grade, have shown that the biologic age of the patient is the most important factor in making a decision between the treatment options. Whereas there is little doubt that the man of 55 years of age should be offered radical therapy on the basis of the 10- to 15-year predicted survival data, for men over 70 the choice widens to include more conservative approaches such as watchful waiting/active surveillance. Patient preference remains an important part of the therapeutic decision process.

Local-regional disease

The first problem with local-regional disease is to define its boundaries. Disease metastatic to bone, described later, is self-evident; more problematic is the boundary between truly localized (theoretically curable) prostate cancer and disease that has spread away from the gland so as to render it, in all probability, an eventual candidate for palliative treatment only. Certainly in the United Kingdom, where the "PSA screening effect" has generally had a lesser impact than in the United States, patients with locoregional disease constitute the majority of new patients attending the prostate cancer clinic at the present time.

Before the PSA era, anatomic findings on DRE essentially defined "locally advanced" disease—T3 or T4 prostates with a negative bone scan. Subsequently, Partin (and others) added preoperative PSA and Gleason biopsy data to clinical stage data to produce tables capable of predicting the pathologic stage.[87,88] Naturally, these tables were primarily designed to indicate whether curative therapy was possible for an individual patient, but the reverse and probably more important observation was to predict and define the group with locoregional disease.

Subsequently D'Amico further refined the chances of disease spread by risk stratification; "high risk" being defined as stage T2c, PSA >20 ng/mL and biopsy Gleason score ≥ 8.[89] Such disease, even in the presence of apparently negative cross-sectional imaging, will have a high chance of micrometastatic locoregional spread.

Clearly, spread away from the prostate will demand treatment strategies able to contain the threat of micrometastatic disease; combinations of radiation therapy, androgen deprivation therapy (ADT), or chemotherapy remain under active investigation.

Two important randomized prospective studies have addressed the role of ADT in this patient group. In these trials Neo adjuvant[90] and adjuvant[91] luteinising hormone (LHRH) therapy was found significantly to improve local control in patients treated with external beam radiotherapy. Although it might be expected that patients randomized to early hormone therapy might show an initial treatment advantage, updated reports[92,93] have confirmed an ongoing benefit, at least in certain patient subgroups. It seems likely that these and other studies[94] will impact positively on the large number of patients presenting with nonlocalized non-(bony) metastatic disease.

Metastatic disease

Until relatively recently, a majority of patients with prostate cancer presented with bony metastases.[74] Increased public awareness and PSA "screening" since the mid-1990s have reduced this figure to 10% to 12% at presentation,[95] although great geographic variation continues to exist. Worldwide it is accepted that even with immediate treatment, the survival of such patients is approximately 50% at 2 to 2½ years and 10% to 14% at 5 years.

TREATMENT OF METASTATIC DISEASE

HORMONAL MANIPULATION. Androgen deprivation treatment (ADT) has, since 1940 when Huggins discovered the hormone-dependent nature of the tumor, been the mainstay of treatment for metastatic prostate cancer. Remission occurs for a variable period—usually 9 to 12 months—before prostate markers, which usually fall following treatment, start to rise again. Approximately 10% to 15% of patients fail to respond significantly to the hormonal manipulation, which may be achieved by either medical or surgical means. Bilateral subcapusular orchidectomy was the traditional approach to androgen deprivation, and the serum testosterone rapidly falls into the "castrate" range. Medical therapy by LHRH analogue[96] has, however, become widely established, although the injections are expensive and the serum testosterone does not fall for 8 to 10 days, which may be of clinical importance. It has to be emphasized to the patients that the side-effect profile of these two treatments—impotence and hot flushes—is identical, a point not always well made by the manufacturers.

Diethylstilboestriol (DES) 5 mg was for many years used to achieve the required hormonal manipulation. Well-publicized cardiac toxicity, however, has led many to avoid this medication even at the lower 1 mg dose, although some continue to advocate the approach in combination with daily aspirin.

NONSTEROIDAL ANTIANDROGENS. Nonsteroidal antiandrogens have the attraction of blocking the action of testosterone peripherally without the major side effect problems associated with traditional hormonal manipulations. Each compound, however, has particular drawbacks. Flutamide leads to significant gastrointestinal upset and diarrhea, whereas bicalutamide, which has the attraction of once daily dosage,[97] also causes some breast tenderness and leads to elevation of serum testosterone because of a central agonist action effecting a rise in luteinizing hormone. Bicalutamide is licensed for the treatment of metastatic disease in conjunction with LHRH analogues.

Androgen withdrawal syndromes whereby altered expression of the androgen receptor permits an agonist response to antiandrogenic agents, particularly Flutamide, have been described.[98] Predictive factors for such a response are high baseline alkaline phosphatase and prolonged drug exposure. The literature suggests that significant PSA reductions might occur in one third of patients with a time to onward progression of 3 to 6 months, and a trial withdrawal of nonsteroidals should always be undertaken in those patients on dual therapy with PSA progression.

Maximum androgen blockade (MAB), the addition of an antiandrogen to (usually) LHRH therapy, has been intensively investigated. Although emotive arguments are frequently put forward, particularly for younger, fit patients with metastases, no significant benefit has been found to accrue from dual therapy.[99,100] Despite this scientific conclusion, it is difficult to avoid offering dual therapy in some patients.

THE TIMING OF TREATMENT

Unusually for a neoplastic condition, the timing of treatment for androgen sensitive prostatic disease is a matter for debate; different approaches can be taken under differing circumstances. Intermittent deprivation therapy and the maintenance of the androgenous environment for cases with low-risk nonmetastatic disease are examples of this dilemma.

Intermittent androgen suppression (IAS) is a technique advanced on the Darwinian basis that the emergence of androgen independent cells might be restricted by the return of the androgenous environment; an improved quality of life (especially sexual activity) might accompany such restoration. Implicit also is the assumption that immediate is preferable to deferred treatment (discussed later). Inclusion criteria, treatment regimens, and timing protocols for IAS vary considerably;[101] most investigators exclude patients who fail to achieve a nadir of 4 ng/mL PSA after 6 months initial (usually combined) therapy and patients with metastatic disease in bone (TxNxM1b) at diagnosis. Ideal cases are patients with biochemical failure after surgery or radiotherapy and some men with TxN1-3 M0 disease, although it is realized that this latter group is associated with enhanced survival on conventional treatment.[102]

The debate on early or delayed treatment was reignited when the Medical Research Council (MRC) initiated a trial of less than ideal construction, which was widely quoted on publication in 1997.[103] The trial showed clearly that delayed therapy in patients with metastatic disease to bone was associated with significantly worse morbidity—but not inferior prostate cancer–specific survival—and there seems little doubt that treatment should be commenced immediately in such patients even if no symptoms are present; this applies particularly to patients at risk from spinal collapse. (It had been argued previously that patients with asymptomatic bone metastases [a relatively small group] should not receive immediate ADT as they would suffer the side effects of treatment with no possibility of symptomatic improvement.)

Conclusions relating to patients with nonmetastatic disease were more controversial. Early work by the veterans research (VACURG) group when corrected for cardiovascular (estrogen associated) mortality as well as later studies involving node positive postprostatectomy patients[104] seemed to suggest that early ADT would be beneficial for overall survival. The MRC Mo subanalysis also supported this conclusion,[103] but later analysis of long-term follow-up data reversed this finding. EORTC 30891 subsequently reported a "modest" advantage for early ADT in terms of survival but no difference in prostate cancer mortality between the treatment arms. The reason for the reduction in non-cancer deaths, which led to the survival advantage in the immediate group, remains unexplained.[105]

It may be concluded that, bearing in mind the prevalence of CaP in the elderly population, the case for early ADT, particularly in newly diagnosed low-risk disease in elderly patients, has yet to be made with conviction. Meticulous watchful waiting protocols would appear to be the prudent way forward for these patients.

ROLE OF ESTROGENS AND CHEMOTHERAPY

The great majority of prostate cancers eventually achieve hormone refractory status and regrowth commences. This point probably marks the most difficult therapeutic decision point for the physician and, particularly, the older patient. Estrogens (DES) may directly inhibit growth factors and may produce a PSA response for up to 6 to 9 months in some cases.[106] Naturally, such patients will be carefully monitored for thromboembolic events, and the estrogen will typically be prescribed with low-dose (75 mg) soluble aspirin to counter such side effects. At the time of writing, diethylstilboestrol (1 to 3 mg daily) is probably the first treatment choice for patients with newly emerging hormone-resistant prostate cancer.

Chemotherapy, certainly in the United Kingdom, has not previously been routinely associated with older men suffering from prostate cancer. Nevertheless, therapeutic advances and reduced toxicity are gradually opening the door to a treatment modality that intuitively should be the rational answer to a disease with a widespread micrometastatic profile. Modest survival advantage from Docetaxel-based therapy in patients with bone metastases[107] has encouraged further work to identify ideal patient groups to undergo further trials; common and distressing side effects include fatigue, diarrhea, Alopecia, and neuropathy.

Theoretically, chemotherapeutic options with lesser toxicity should be of great interest in the nonmetastatic (e.g., postprostatectomy) setting. Slow trial recruitment, however, underscores the reluctance to submit patients—particularly older more frail patients—to chemotoxicity. Active debate continues on this question, which centers on quality of life for the elderly.

BONE PAIN

Bone pain remains the most troublesome aspect of the disease for the patient and it is often difficult to manage. Radiotherapy remains the basis of local control. Radiation should not be used in hormone—naïve disease as ADT will usually provide rapid and lengthy relief from pain. Focal treatment to local reemergent lesions ("spot welding") is effective for pain relief and may (significantly) prevent fracture and improve quality of life. Metabolically guided therapies such as diphosphonate treatment may reduce skeletal related events, although the natural history of microfracture associated with the metastatic skeleton has always made objective assessment of benefit difficult.[108] Radionuclide-based therapy (Strontium[89]) and hemibody radiation[109] are infrequently used today.

MANAGEMENT OF BONE PAIN. The management of a patient in the early stages of prostate cancer is relatively simple. Given that satisfactory exchange of information has occurred, first-line therapy is usually effective, and the patient may be seen and reassured on an infrequent basis. The emergence of resistant disease and bone morbidity in particular heralds the need for multidisciplinary team support. Apart from any medical and surgical intervention that may be required, close cooperation with a radiation – oncologist will be essential. Perhaps most important will be the integrated team of support nurses with analgesic expertise who will be crucial to the administration of palliative care at the end of the disease process.

PROSTATE CANCER IN THE ELDERLY: A PATIENT SYNOPSIS

Despite every endeavor, those patients who are destined to progress do so relentlessly, albeit at a slow, drawn-out pace. This poses particular problems as age advances.

Figure 86-11 illustrates a typical episode in an 82-year-old patient presenting with LUTS and subsequently diagnosed with well-differentiated Gleason 3+3 adenocarcinoma following TUR in 1996. PSA was stable between 20 and 25 in the years before the transurethral resection. Bone scan was negative at diagnosis, remaining so during four further tests (red dots) but converting in December 2005.

A watchful waiting policy was instituted, but slow progression led to hormonal manipulation by subcapsular orchidectomy in 1997 (a). Following a long period of remission, hormone-resistant disease gradually emerged, and bicalutamide was added in 2004 (b) but stopped 10 months later because of further progression (c). Stilbestrol was then commenced in 2005, and this was effective

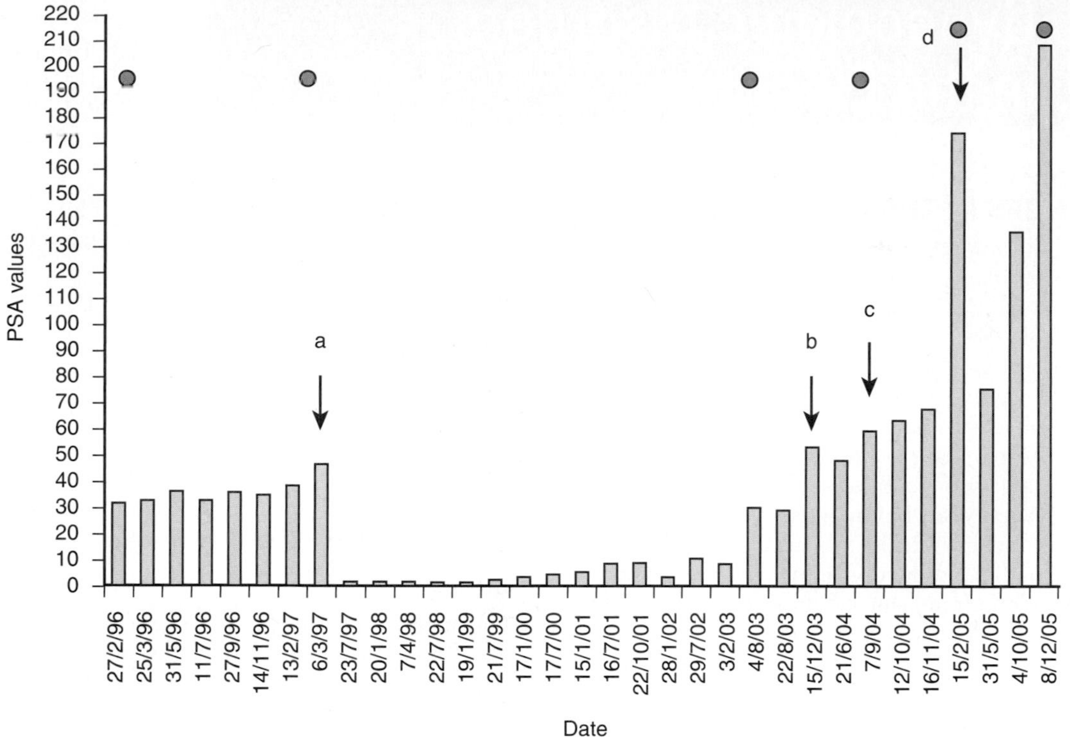

Figure 86-11. Sequential PSA records in man diagnosed with low-grade prostate cancer at age 82. See text for details.

KEY POINTS
The Prostate

- Anatomic knowledge of the sphincter apparatus assists understanding of continence mechanisms.
- Physicians offering prostate-specific antigen (PSA) tests to patients should fully understand the implications of an abnormal result.
- "Prostatic" symptoms may not be related to disease of the prostate gland.
- Elderly patients with localized prostate cancer have a wide range of therapeutic options.
- Elderly patients with metastatic prostate cancer should be treated, even if no symptoms are present.

for 12 months (d). Despite the final PSA rise and eventual development of bony metastases, chemotherapy was declined and the patient died on the palliative care pathway in 2006 aged 92.

Quality of life was excellent for the great majority of the patient's final years. It is to be regretted, as noted earlier, that a low-toxicity chemotherapy regime is not available to arrest disease before M1 conversion.

For a complete list of references, please visit online only at www.expertconsult.com

CHAPTER 87

Gynecologic Disorders in the Elderly

Tara K. Cooper
Oliver Milling Smith

AGE CHANGES IN THE GENITAL TRACT

The female physiologic aging process accelerates after menopause, particularly in the genital tract.

Hormone changes

In perimenopausal women the ovary becomes less responsive to gonadotrophins, which results in a gradual increase in the circulating levels of follicular stimulating hormone (FSH) and later luteinizing hormone (LH) and a subsequent decrease in estradiol concentrations. FSH levels can fluctuate markedly several years before menses cease, so is a poor diagnostic test, but eventually follicular development fails completely, estradiol production is no longer sufficient to stimulate the endometrium, amenorrhea ensues and FSH and LH levels are persistently elevated, reaching peaks 3 to 5 years after menopause. Thereafter there is a gradual decline to premenopausal levels 20 years later.[1] In the reproductive years, the ovary has three components for steroid biosynthesis: the maturing follicle, the functioning corpus luteum, and the stroma. After menopause, the stroma is the only source of estrogen.

Estrone is the major postmenopausal estrogen and it is derived from the conversion of androgens, mainly androstenedione, produced by the ovaries and adrenal glands. The efficiency of this process increases with age and estrone levels rise to four times that found in young women. This conversion also correlates with weight as fat has the ability to aromatize androstenedione to estrone.[2]

The other postmenopausal estrogens include estriol, which is weak and does not seem to have a significant role, and estradiol, which although secretion is minimal with blood levels being reduced by 90%, has 10 times greater biologic activity than estrone so still has an important role to play in maintaining hormone dependent tissues.[3]

Progesterone in the postmenopausal woman is derived mainly from the adrenal glands and levels fall steadily. Production of testosterone remains relatively unchanged and surgical oophorectomy will, therefore, result in a decrease of serum testosterone levels of up to 50%.[4]

Anatomic changes

The major change is atrophy, which results in smaller and smoother structures, flattened epithelial surfaces, and fibrous stroma with much reduced vascularization and fat content.

OVARY

The postmenopausal ovary is small and sclerotic with absence of follicular activity. The cortex involutes and germinal inclusion cysts are found. Lipid droplets may be seen in the stroma as evidence of continuing steroidogenesis.

UTERUS

There is a marked reduction in uterine size so that the uterine body to cervix ratio reverts from the 4:1 of reproductive life to the 2:1 of childhood. In the myometrium, there is interstitial fibrosis and thickened blood vessels due to obliterative, subintimal sclerosis. The endometrium becomes a single layer of cuboidal cells with a few inactive glands, which may be dilated because of blocked ducts.

CERVIX AND VAGINA

The cervix becomes more flush with the vaginal vault and the squamocolumnar junction recedes into the endocervical canal; this can cause stenosis of the external os.

The vagina becomes thinner, atrophic, and less elastic which can make it more vulnerable to trauma. Reduction in estrogen also reduces natural defenses against infection.

VULVA

Postmenopausal changes are characterized by skin shrinkage, loss of prominent landmarks, and sparse, graying hair. The epidermis is thinner although there is increased keratinization. These features may coincide with a vulvar epithelial disorder (discussed later).

PELVIC FLOOR

Aging produces pelvic floor weakness. Damage to the nerve supply starts with parturition[5] and progressive denervation is found in association with prolapse[6] (discussed later). An important element of pelvic floor support is collagen, which diminishes after the climacteric.

MENOPAUSE

The cessation of ovarian function at menopause has many short- and long-term consequences. Early menopause symptoms (e.g., mood swings, hot flashes, and night sweats) affect most women to varying degrees and those who have problems may be treated effectively by hormone replacement therapy (HRT).

More relevant is the prolonged effect of estrogen deficiency postmenopausally. The average age of menopause has remained around 51 years for centuries. With female life expectancy now reaching over 80 years, there has been a massive increase in the number of postmenopausal women, and the morbidity/mortality secondary to the effects of ovarian failure becomes increasingly important. At present there is poor correlation between early symptoms and late consequences; therefore, it is not possible to select women for prophylactic HRT to obtain the most beneficial outcome.

Osteoporosis

In postmenopausal women there is accelerated bone loss so that by age 70 years 50% of bone mass is lost, whereas men lose only 25% by 80 years.[7] This is due to increased bone resorption by osteoclasts and reduced new bone formation, leading to increased turnover. Altered calcium metabolism may be a contributory factor, but the primary defect is generalized connective tissue loss with reduced bone mineral content following breakdown of the organic collagen matrix.[8]

The resultant osteoporosis dramatically increases the elderly female fracture rate: 50% of women aged 75 years will have sustained one or more fractures at the most common sites of wrists, vertebral bodies (resulting in the classic "Dowager's hump"), and neck of femur. The latter is the most significant consequence of osteoporosis because of its high morbidity and mortality: there is a 20% death rate within the first year, and half of survivors will fail to regain their independence.[9]

Older people are also at increased risk of falls: 35% to 40% of over 65s living at home fall at least once a year, rising to 50% for the over 80s.[10] Ten percent to 15% of falls lead to serious injuries, with up to 10% resulting in fracture, 1% to 2% of these being hip fractures.[11]

Two years of HRT results in a 66% reduction in hip fracture in the subsequent 2 years,[12] and taken for 10 years produces a 60% reduction in the overall mortality rate related to osteoporotic fractures.[13] However, recent studies have highlighted the potential risks of HRT and it is no longer recommended as first-line prophylaxis or treatment for osteoporosis (see section on HRT).

Cardiovascular disease

Cardiovascular disease (CVD; includes coronary heart disease and stroke) is five times more common in men than in premenopausal women but by 70 years the sex difference is lost. Overall, CVD is the most common cause of death in women. In younger women, estrogen exerts cardioprotective effects through a vasodilatory effect and an alteration in lipid metabolism. Ovarian failure causes increased levels of cholesterol, triglyceride, and low-density lipoprotein (LDL), and a reduction in high-density lipoprotein (HDL). These changes contribute to an increased predisposition to ischemic heart disease.[14]

Theoretically therefore, estrogen therapy should reverse these effects, and previous observational data suggested a cardioprotective effect of HRT,[15] but a wide variety of randomized clinical trials have observed that HRT does not reduce and indeed may slightly increase the risk of cardiac events after menopause.[16]

Skin and dentition

Skin changes have been attributed to the aging process, but estrogen deficiency and light exposure are significant factors. Skin thickness declines after menopause by 30% in the first 10 years, which is comparable to bone loss over the same time.[17] When HRT is started early, there is maintenance of skin collagen and thickness.

Estrogen deficiency also affects teeth—one third of women over 65 in the United States are edentulous. HRT may be protective.

Hormone replacement therapy

Estrogen therapy has been widely regarded as the appropriate treatment for the consequences of ovarian failure, either for symptom relief or prevention of long-term effects. However, publication of the Women's Health Initiative (WHI) study and Million Women Study (MWS) has led to considerable uncertainties among health professionals and women about the role of HRT.[18,19]

Recent recommendations suggest that treatment choice should be based on up-to-date information and targeted to individual women's needs. Currently, most women who request HRT do so for symptom relief, and duration of use is usually less than 5 years. The merits of long-term use need to be assessed for each individual at regular intervals (e.g., annually).[20]

HRT should currently not be prescribed solely for possible prevention of CVD and dementia, and it is no longer recommended as first line therapy for osteoporosis prevention.

If HRT is to be used, it should be in the lowest dose required to relieve symptoms. It may be given orally or parenterally (i.e., transvaginally, transdermally, or subcutaneously). There is an additional need for progesterone in nonhysterectomized women because unopposed estrogen therapy causes endometrial hyperplasia, which may lead to adenocarcinoma. Twelve to 14 days of progesterone each month reduces these risks[21] and may be administered orally or transdermally. When HRT is given in this cyclical sequential regime, there is a withdrawal bleed at the end of each course. In women at least 1 year postmenopausal, progesterone can be given continuously which prevents endometrial proliferation, so there is no bleeding. The levonorgestrel intrauterine system (Mirena, Schering) can fulfill this role. Women who start on cyclical HRT can be changed to a continuous combined product when they reach the age of 55.

Oral estrogen

Oral administration is the most widely used route and is convenient, relatively inexpensive, and generally well tolerated. Many combinations are available commercially, both cyclical and continuous. In perimenopausal women who do not wish frequent withdrawal bleeds, a three-monthly bleed preparation can be tried. Tibolone is a synthetic steroid with estrogenic, progestogenic, and androgenic properties and acts as a continuous combined product. It also improves libido and may have less effects on breast tissue.[22]

The main disadvantage of the oral route is that estrogen passes directly to the liver, where it is inactivated and partially metabolized to the less effective estrone—this is called the "first pass" effect and means that higher doses are required than with parenteral therapy. It may also result in altered hepatic metabolism with changes in clotting factors and increased renin substrate, which predisposes to hypertension.

Transdermal estrogen

Transdermal patches may be matrix or reservoir in type and require changing once or twice weekly. Combination patches with progesterone are also available. Estradiol is delivered at a controlled rate depending on surface area. The first pass effect is avoided and hepatic metabolism not affected, thus reducing the risk of thrombosis. The main problems are with adhesion, and transient skin reactions can occur in up to 30% of women; the frequency is less with matrix patches. A transdermal gel may be used instead.

Topical estrogen

Vaginal creams and pessaries are used primarily for treating atrophic vaginitis. Systemic absorption is minimal, but if use is prolonged, progesterone therapy should be considered. In general, a short course is adequate: a 14-day course should be followed by 2 nights' application each week for up to 6 weeks. A problem with this route in the elderly is reduced acceptability and impaired manual dexterity for self-administration. A district nurse may help or a slow-release soft vaginal ring provides 3 months' therapy. Other alternatives include a low-dose hydrophilic vaginal tablet, which has a fine, prelubricated, and preloaded applicator (Vagifem)—because of its low dose and lack of systemic absorption, this product is acceptable for use in patients with a history of breast cancer.

Subcutaneous implants

Estradiol implants can be inserted in the lower abdominal wall under local anesthesia, and serum levels are sustained for several months depending on the dose. Levels tend to be higher, and symptoms tend to return more quickly despite therapeutic serum levels, requiring more frequent implants (tachyphylaxis). This method is now rarely used.

Contraindications and risks with hormone replacement therapy

There are few contraindications to HRT, which provides estrogen replacement at below the normal premenopausal plasma concentrations and those achieved with the high-dose synthetic steroids used in the combined oral contraceptive pill. The main contraindications are estrogen-dependent breast or endometrial cancers, although women with treated breast cancer and debilitating menopausal symptoms may be given HRT under specialist supervision, and there is no evidence of increased recurrence rates.[23]

More recent reports have suggested a small increase in the risk of venous thromboembolism with HRT, which was not thought previously to exist.[24] Patients with other risk factors should therefore be treated with caution and preferably with transdermal HRT. It is not necessary to stop HRT before surgery as most patients will fall into a moderate risk category (in view of age) and receive antithrombosis prophylaxis.

HRT may be given where there are preexisting gynecologic conditions (e.g., endometriosis and fibroids), but the latter may fail to shrink and cause heavier withdrawal bleeds.

The benefits of HRT are considerable, but there are increasing concerns with the safety of long-term therapy particularly in relation to breast cancer and CVD (discussed previously). Also, although initially protective against endometrial cancer, use greater than 10 years causes a modest increase in this cancer too.[25] Changing to continuous combined HRT as soon as appropriate reduces the endometrial risk.[26]

Despite extensive educational products and improved therapies such as "no bleed" continuous HRT, compliance is poor and 50% of patients do not remain on HRT 12 months after starting treatment, even when at risk of osteoporosis.[27]

Alternatives to hormone replacement therapy

Symptomatic relief from hot flashes can be achieved with clonidine, venlafaxine (not yet licensed) and progesterone. There is also a growing trend toward "natural" products such as black cohosh, red clover, and natural progesterone cream. There are some data on the safety and efficacy of red clover[28] but less so with other products, and one study shows no pharmacologic activity for progesterone cream[29] and any benefits are likely to be a placebo effect.

VULVAR DISORDERS

Vulvar epithelial disorders are important because of the severity and chronicity of symptoms (most commonly itching, soreness, and irritation), and their association with carcinoma. Management is often difficult especially as patients may present to a variety of specialists including gynecologists, dermatologists, geriatricians, or general practitioners. Treatment may therefore be improved by utilization of a dedicated vulvar skin clinic if available.

To accurately diagnose vulvar pathology, full examination is required because of the significant overlap of vulvar disease symptoms. Other skin and mucosal membranes should be examined and swabs taken to screen for infection. Importantly, if lesions do not respond to initial treatment or doubt exists as to their etiology, they should be biopsied to assist diagnosis and subsequent management.

There have been conflicting views about pathogenesis, diagnosis, and terminology of vulvar disorders. Lesions may be infective, inflammatory, localized variants of generalized dermatoses, premalignant, and malignant. Extensive classifications are available, but this review will focus on the general management and some specific common conditions.

Symptoms

Vulvar skin is more sensitive than other epithelium because it is subjected to increased heat, friction, and occlusion. Aging is also a factor and some chronic vulvar disorders represent an advanced stage of atrophic change. Patients with any of the myriad of diseases of the vulva may complain of symptoms such as dryness, itch, ulceration, and pain.

GENERAL MEASURES FOR VULVAR CARE

1. Avoidance of tight, restrictive, or occlusive clothing
2. Avoidance of irritants such as soaps, fragrances, or urine (if incontinent)
3. Use of emollients and soap substitutes
4. Treatment of any detected infection

Dermatologic conditions

The vulvar skin may be affected by a variety of dermatologic conditions including psoriasis, urticaria, and the bullous diseases such as pemphigus. The more common inflammatory conditions found in the elderly patient include contact dermatitis and lichen planus, which are described next.

ECZEMA/DERMATITIS

Eczema is a term used synonymously with dermatitis. This inflammatory condition affects many skin sites, classically on the flexural site of the body. Vulvar itch may, however, be attributed to eczema. The condition may be endogenous (atopic) or exogenous (contact) in nature. In the elderly population, urine is a common irritant but a history indicating a change in soap, fragrances, underwear, and so on should be sought. Management of dermatitis starts with identifying and avoiding the causative irritant and general measures of vulvar care as illustrated above. Topical steroids may relieve the itch and can be of value to try and break the "itch-scratch" cycle, which can lead to thickening with accentuated skin margins (lichenification), termed *lichen simplex*. Secondary infection may complicate dermatitis, and swabs should be taken to identify treatable infection.

LICHEN PLANUS

This inflammatory condition may also affect hair, nails, and mucosal membranes. The classic lesions are purple papules, sometimes with a lacy white surface pattern (Wickham's striae). The usual complaint is of soreness, but

Table 87-1. Classification of VIN (International Society for the Study of Vulvar Disease, 2004)

Usual type
Warty type
Basaloid type
Mixed
Differentiated type

itch, dyspareunia, and discharge may be present. If the patient is sexually active and concern exists over vaginal narrowing, then vaginal dilators may be of benefit. A more severe presentation of lichen planus may involve an erosive vulvar lesion leading to profuse discharge and scarring. Treatment involves general vulvar care including the use of emollients and high-potency topical steroids.

Premalignant vulvar disorders

Premalignant conditions of the vulva are rare but include a spectrum of disorders such as vulvar intraepithelial neoplasia, lichen sclerosus, and Paget's disease of the vulva.

VULVAR INTRAEPITHELIAL NEOPLASIA

Although the incidence of this condition is rising in the younger population, 80% of cases occur in women over the age of 50. Vulvar intraepithelial neoplasia (VIN) represents an abnormal proliferation of epithelial cells and is almost certainly associated with exposure of the human papilloma virus (HPV), in particular subtypes 16 and 18. Smoking represents an additional strong risk factor.

Clinically the complaint may be of itch, pain or a burning sensation but around half of cases will be asymptomatic. There are no typical appearances of VIN and the lesions may be unifocal or multifocal. Assessment of malignant transformation potential is difficult, but it is generally agreed that "differentiated type" has the greatest potential for malignant change of around 30% with "usual type" around a 2% to 5% chance of transformation.[30] Differentiated type is often found in the elderly population and may be associated with lichen sclerosus. VIN may also be described as VIN 1, 2, or 3. The International Society for the Study of Vulvar Disease revised this classification in 2004 because of a lack of evidence of disease continuum from VIN 1 to VIN 3 (Table 87-1).

DIFFERENTIATED TYPE

Surgical treatment involves wide local excision and is often mutilating, creates anxiety, affects sexual function, and unfortunately suffers from relapse rates. For this reason, a prudent management plan may often involve watching with repeated biopsies to exclude change. No single ideal therapy for VIN exists. Surgery may be destructive and medical treatments troubled by side effects. Treatment is recognized to be difficult and referral to a specialist vulvar skin clinic is advised.

LICHEN SCLEROSUS

Lichen sclerosus (LS) is a common problem affecting the aging vulva. The etiology is uncertain, but there is an association with genetic and hormonal factors and autoimmune disease.[31] The vulvar appearance varies but the characteristic lesions are a "figure of eight" configuration around the vulva and anus of white plaques together with atrophy. The condition does not extend to the vagina. Loss of tissue architecture is common with fusion of tissue occurring, which may lead to introital stenosis. Chronic scratching complicates the picture, so the skin may be thickened (i.e., lichenified). Although the clinical appearance varies, there are characteristic histologic features, including an atrophic epidermis with hyalinization and areas of thickening (hyperkeratosis), and inflammation.

In the elderly, management may include investigating for the presence of autoimmune disorders such as pernicious anemia, thyroid disease, and diabetes. General vulvar care advice should be given. However, the mainstay of treatment should include topical use of a potent steroid such as dermovate. This should be applied daily at first, reducing as symptoms improve (a 30-g tube is expected to last 3 to 6 months).

Malignant change has been quoted at between 2% to 9%,[32] and punch biopsies under local anesthetic should be taken of any suspicious areas to exclude atypical change. Squamous carcinoma is more likely when there is a failure to respond to topical steroid use or with the presence of ulceration, raised lesions, or lymph node involvement. These patients should report alteration in symptoms and be checked every 6 months to yearly, again ideally at a dedicated vulvar skin clinic if available.

Although the condition is associated with atrophy, topical estrogen is ineffective and should be considered only for vaginal use.

EXTRAMEDULLARY PAGET'S DISEASE

This rare condition is a neoplasm of apocrine bearing skin. It has a peak incidence at 65 years of age. Clinically it has similar symptoms to other skin conditions of the vulva. Lesions will often appear as "white islands" with bridges of hyperkeratinization. A biopsy is required to make diagnosis. Treatment is specialized and may involve surgery or radiotherapy after appropriate discussion by a multidisciplinary team. Prognosis is good if confined to epidermis, and the challenge is therefore early detection.

Vulvar discomfort

A complaint of severe pain or discomfort in the vulva for over 3 months is termed *vulvodynia*. Localized pain to light touch at the vaginal vestibule (where vaginal meets vulva) is known as localized vulvodynia (previously known as vestibulitis).

In the elderly population, vulvar pain is more commonly generalized and characterized by pain, burning, stinging, irritation, and rawness. This is often termed *dysesthetic vulvodynia* or *generalized vulvodynia*. Unlike vestibulitis, which is provoked by touch, women with dysesthetic vulvodynia have a more constant neuropathic pain. The complaint of itch is uncommon and examination is usually normal. Etiology is uncertain, but it is now recognized that both psychological and physical factors are involved.[33] Depression is a possible factor, as these patients often live alone. Assessment includes neurologic and local examinations with urethral, vaginal, and endocervical swabs to exclude infections. Pathology is rarely found.

Initial treatment should involve explanation of the condition, emphasizing this is a real condition although often no physical findings are present. General vulvar care as previously described should be given, and in some cases use of low strength topical corticosteroids or anesthetics (e.g., 5% lidocaine) may benefit. The use of pelvic floor exercises to improve muscle tone and blood supply and vaginal retraining dilators can also be used. Some symptoms will respond to low-dose tricyclic antidepressants such as 10 mg of amitriptyline at night, increasing the dose as side effects permit to a usual dose of between 60 to 150 mg per day. The use of the neuroleptic gabapentin has also been reported as a second-line therapy.[34]

UTEROVAGINAL PROLAPSE

Urogenital prolapse occurs when there is a weakness in the supporting structures of the pelvic floor allowing pelvic viscera to descend and ultimately fall through this anatomic defect. An increase in life expectancy has meant that prolapse has become an increasingly important problem. Although a benign condition, quality of life can be severely affected with bladder, bowel, and sexual dysfunction described. The lifetime risk for having surgery for prolapse is 11%,[35] and approximately 60% of elderly women have some degree of prolapse. Prolapse of the anterior and posterior vaginal walls occurs independently or together, resulting in any combination of urethrocele, cystocele, rectocele, and enterocele, which are displacements of the underlying urethra, bladder, rectum, and pouch of Douglas (and any contents), respectively. Classification of prolapse has traditionally been described as first-, second-, or third-degree prolapse depending on the relationship of the lowest part of the prolapse to the introitus.

Prolapse is most commonly related to childbirth—50% of patients with prolapse are parous[36]—and postmenopausal hormone deficiency when lack of estrogen causes collagen loss and ligament atrophy.[37] Congenital weakness of sustaining structures and the natural aging process are other factors. Additionally, factors leading to increased abdominal pressure such as obesity, constipation, and chronic cough will exacerbate prolapse symptoms.

The main supports of the uterus and upper vagina are the transverse cervical, or cardinal, ligaments, the pubocervical fascia, and the uterosacral ligaments. The middle third of the vagina is supported by fascia, and the lower third of the vagina is buttressed by fibers of the pelvic floor. In the erect posture, the anterior vagina rests on the posterior wall, which is strengthened by the rectovaginal fascia and perineal body.

The patient commonly presents with a dragging or bearing down sensation of gradual onset that is worse with activity and settles with rest. A lump may be seen or felt. Urinary symptoms such as frequency, urgency, incontinence, and incomplete/slow emptying result from distortion of the prolapsed bladder and urethra, but they may also be due to atrophy, infection, or detrusor overactivity.[38] Digital replacement of the anterior or posterior vaginal wall is sometimes necessary before micturition or defecation may proceed.

With prolonged uterine descent, edema occurs because of the interference with venous and lymphatic drainage, leading to epithelial hyperkeratinization and decubital ulceration. Bleeding may result but carcinoma rarely develops. With severe prolapse, it is possible to cause ureteric obstruction with subsequent hydronephrosis. In the elderly patient with complete procidentia, a degree of ureteric obstruction is likely and ultrasound investigation should be organized. Further investigation should include pelvic abdominal assessment to exclude a mass. Prolapse is assessed with the patient in the left lateral position if possible, although standing up may provide good assessment of the degree of prolapse. The practitioner may ask the patient to cough repeatedly and look for signs of stress incontinence, as this may assess urinary signs. Occult stress incontinence may occur in the elderly patient after correction of prolapse by either conservative or surgical methods. It may therefore be advisable to arrange cystometry and uroflowmetry to evaluate potential stress incontinence. If stress incontinence is discovered, then this may be addressed at the time of managing the prolapse.

Physiotherapy may have a role in the treatment of prolapse, although the evidence supporting its effectiveness is weak and in the elderly patient is less likely to benefit. Surgery offers definitive treatment. but suitability of the patient depends on the severity of symptoms, the degree of incapacity, and the patient's operative fitness. It includes, as appropriate, anterior or posterior pelvic floor repair, vaginal hysterectomy, or vault suspension if hysterectomy has already occurred. It is now standard practice to give subcutaneous heparin pre- and post operatively to reduce venous thromboembolism risk and antibiotics for surgical prophylaxis. Most patients tolerate surgery well because of improved anesthetics and minimal postoperative morbidity. The procedures lead to greater mobility and return to an independent life. Evidence suggests that surgical procedures for prolapse in the elderly do not carry any increased morbidity as compared to the younger patient.[39]

Recurrence of prolapse will trouble about a third of patients who undergo a surgical corrective procedure.[40] The use of synthetic mesh is becoming increasingly more common in the treatment of patients with recurrent defects.[41] Complications associated with the use of synthetic material may include dyspareunia or troublesome infection. The use of such procedures should therefore be reserved for specialists in this surgical field rather than the general gynecologist.

When surgery is contraindicated or declined, conservative measures may be used. It is useful to remember that it is common for women to tolerate a procidentia for years without complaint, and in general prolapse is a benign condition. However, if symptoms are troublesome, then a polyvinyl ring pessary can be inserted. The pessary should be inspected and cleaned or renewed every 4 to 6 months to prevent vaginal ulceration occurring. In this event, the ring should be removed for a few weeks to allow epithelial healing. The use of local estrogen may help healing if hypoestrogenic atrophy is present. If the ring pessary is not effective, usually because of expulsion, a shelf pessary exists to reduce prolapse. Shelf pessaries lead to a higher degree of vaginal trauma, including the possibility of rectovaginal or vesicovaginal fistulae. However, in the elderly population, because of comorbidities preventing surgery or the large degree of prolapse, they may be more suitable than the more common ring pessary. They should be inspected in the same way but are more difficult to remove and replace. Varieties of other support or space-occupying pessaries exist[40] but are less commonly used in routine practice. An awareness of their existence is useful for the elderly patient with troublesome prolapse who is difficult to treat by nonsurgical procedures.

URINARY INCONTINENCE

Lower urinary tract symptoms are common and are due to a wide variety of underlying mechanisms. Diagnosis based on history and examination alone may be correct in only 65% of women complaining of urinary tract symptoms.[42]

Urinary incontinence is particularly disabling and distressing in the elderly, but, with modern investigation and treatment, symptoms may be alleviated if not cured. Causes of urinary incontinence can be broadly divided into overactive bladder, stress incontinence, and other causes of leakage. Continuous leakage is more likely to be associated with neurologic disorders, overflow, urethral diverticulum, or a vesicovaginal fistula.

Overactive bladder (OAB)

Detrusor overactivity is classically associated with frequency, urgency, urge incontinence, and nocturia. Uninhibited detrusor muscle contractions are usually the cause of incontinence in geriatric patients. Urodynamic investigations have shown detrusor overactivity in 80% of the elderly population. Most cases of OAB are idiopathic, but the condition is amplified in the presence of neurologic conditions such as stroke, Parkinson's disease, or multiple sclerosis.[43] The pathophysiology is uncertain but may occur by a reduction of functional innervation of the bladder wall.

Investigation should include a midstream urine sample to exclude infection. Simple and noninvasive tests such as daily urinary frequency/volume and incontinence charts are important. The diagnosis of detrusor overactivity is, strictly speaking, a diagnosis made at the time of urodynamic investigation. However, it is not practical for all elderly patients with symptoms of OAB to undergo this test, and often a clinical diagnosis can be made; however, if doubt exists as to the cause of urinary incontinence or if there is poor response to treatment, urodynamics are required. Ultrasonography is a useful method to check postvoid residual volumes and to exclude incontinence secondary to overflow.

Conservative treatment of OAB should include monitoring and reducing fluid intake to around 1.5 to 2 liters per day. Bladder irritants such as caffeine and alcohol should be avoided. In the elderly, the patient's medications should be reviewed to ensure there are no unnecessary diuretics or other medications. Constipation may aggravate the problem and should be treated. The use of a specialist nurse to help with behavioral therapies such as bladder retraining can improve symptoms. Many professionals advise combining this with pelvic floor exercises if the patient is capable.

Pharmacologic agents can be used when conservative measures fail. There is a large placebo effect with these agents and the difficulty is to find the right drug for the right patient. The side effects are often poorly tolerated, and this is particularly evident in the elderly patient. Anticholinergic/antimuscarinic drugs inhibit the parasympathetic action upon the bladder and hence reduce detrusor muscle contractions. They unfortunately may cause constipation, dry mouth, and dry eyes. In the older patient, reduced drug metabolism and elimination must be considered together with potential drug interactions. Oxybutynin, tolterodine, solifenacin, trospium, darifenacin, and propiverine all have level 1 evidence for their effectiveness. Trospium is made from a compound that does not cross the blood-brain barrier and may be useful in older patients on polypharmacy. The tricyclic antidepressant, imipramine at 25 to 50 mg twice daily, can be useful in treating symptoms of nocturia and nocturnal enuresis. There is limited value in estrogen therapy for either urge or stress incontinence,[44] but it has a place when urinary symptoms are associated with significant estrogen deficiency.

Surgical options such as cystoplasty or urinary diversion for the treatment of OAB should be reserved for patients in whom all other methods of treatment have failed, and they are rarely undertaken.

Stress incontinence

Urodynamic stress incontinence is diagnosed by filling cystometry and is defined by involuntary leakage on exertion, coughing, or sneezing in the absence of detrusor activity. It is the most common cause of incontinence in women in reproductive or early postmenopausal years and is often suffered in silence despite good available treatments. It is associated with damage to the pelvic floor (usually as a result of childbirth) and causes of increased abdominal pressure such as constipation, cough, and obesity.

The treatment of genuine stress incontinence should be nonoperative initially as good results for mild/moderate leakage can be achieved with conservative measures without compromising further surgical procedures.[45] Conservative measures involve pelvic floor exercises with or without the use of biofeedback or electrical stimulation. The use of vaginal cones and weights is less common, as their effectiveness has been difficult to prove.

Surgical procedures, however, offer effective treatment. Colposuspension has traditionally been the gold standard of treatment. It is major abdominal surgery and is associated with voiding difficulties in 12% to 25% of cases and de novo overactive bladder symptoms in around 15% of cases.[46] The use of this procedure has largely been superseded by the use of tension-free vaginal tapes. A large number of variations are available for these midurethral tape procedures; however, the best body of evidence exists for the Gynecare tension free vaginal tape (TVT), which is a synthetic polypropylene, monofilamentous mesh that is inserted vaginally at the level of the midurethra into the retropubic space to provide tension-free support under the urethra. The procedure may be performed under local anesthetic and carries a low morbidity with de novo overactive bladder symptoms occurring in around 6%. The reported 2-year cure rate for the TVT is 84%, and it has been shown to be equally efficacious as colposuspension.[47] Evidence suggests that surgical procedures for incontinence in the elderly do not carry any increased morbidity as compared to the younger patient[48] and should therefore be considered to improve quality of life.

GYNECOLOGIC CANCER IN THE ELDERLY

An association has been noted between aging and cancer development, and there is a tendency for cancers to be at a more advanced stage at presentation. The management of gynecologic cancer patients is now mostly centralized in units staffed by experienced gynecologic oncologists where the care and outcome is improved. Decisions for care should be undertaken by a multidisciplinary team (MDM) involving, among others, the gynecologist, medical and radiologic oncologists, pathologists, and the patients themselves.

Female genital cancer affects five main sites.

Vulva

Vulvar carcinoma is seen most frequently in the 60-to-70-year-old age group and accounts for about 5% of genital neoplasia. Early symptoms are pruritus or an asymptomatic lump, but late presentation is more common because of embarrassment and is usually in the form of bleeding or an offensive discharge. Ninety-five percent of tumors are squamous in type, but occasionally malignant melanoma can occur. The lesion commonly arises in the labium majorum and spreads directly to the urethra, anus, and vagina and by regional lymph glands—the superficial inguinal and prefemoral nodes. Lateral tumors tend to spread to the ipsilateral nodes, but centrally placed tumors may involve the contralateral nodes. Hematologic spread is rare and a late phenomenon leading to metastases to lungs, liver, or bone. The most significant prognostic indicator is nodal status. Overall groin negative patients have a 90% 5-year survival rate.

The aim of management is to carry out the most conservative procedure likely to lead to cure. Radical vulvectomy with bilateral groin node dissections is no longer the treatment of choice, as morbidity is high. Early stage disease is often treated with wide local excision with ipsilateral nodal dissection if the tumor is greater than 1.5 cm from the midline.[49] Central tumors merit bilateral nodal dissection. Full groin node dissection is often performed if tumor is greater than 4 cm and superficial nodes are negative. Thirty percent to 70% of patients who have undergone a full node dissection will have long-term lymphedema and recurrent cellulitis.[50]

Advanced disease may be treated by radical surgery sometimes necessitating exenteration. Five-year survival rates are less than 50%, and the postoperative morbidity very high.[50] Preoperative radiotherapy may be used to reduce tumor bulk and the risk of recurrence. Radiotherapy is additionally used to treat recurrence (if not previously used), and it is also helpful in the palliative setting.

If a large vulvar defect results from surgery, repair may be possible using a myocutaneous flap with rectus abdominis or gracilis muscle. Nursing management may be difficult because of increasing problems with catheterization, poor healing, and discharge, which may be infective or lymphatic in origin.

Vagina

Primary vaginal squamous cancer is rare and virtually confined to the elderly. Usually vaginal malignancy is metastatic adenocarcinoma with blood or lymphatic spread from the uterus and, rarely, kidney, breast, or colon. Direct invasion may occur from bladder, cervical or vulvar lesions. Presenting symptoms are postmenopausal bleeding, offensive discharge, and eventually fistula formation. Diagnosis is by biopsy and the treatment is usually radiotherapy, although vaginectomy can be considered for primary lesions. Other surgical measures include urinary diversion for a fistula or palliative vaginal closure (colpocleisis). Endometrial metastases show some response to high-dose progesterone.

Cervix

Worldwide, cervical carcinoma is still the most common gynecologic malignancy over all age groups. In developed countries, the incidence is falling significantly as a result of screening programs. In the United Kingdom, screening programs stop at 60 years, but if an abnormal smear is found in a woman over this age it is 16 times more likely to lead to a diagnosis of invasive cancer compared with women younger than 30 years.[51] Types 16 and 18 of the human papillomavirus (HPV) have been incriminated in the pathogenesis of invasive squamous carcinoma and are detectable in more than 90% of cases. The recent introduction of a vaccine against the high-risk HPV subtypes[52] may change the face of cervical cancer in future generations, but vigilance is still required.

Elderly patients will present with such symptoms as offensive vaginal discharge and postmenopausal or postcoital bleeding. Pain is experienced late and related usually to diffuse pelvic infiltration or bony metastases. The first sign of this cancer may be obstructive renal failure from hydronephrosis because of advanced disease.

Diagnosis is by biopsy of suspicious areas preferably under general anesthesia so that clinical staging and evaluation of histologic tumor grade is achieved. Squamous cell cancer accounts for more than 80% of cases. Lymphatic metastases occur quickly; hence, up to 50% of early lesions have pelvic spread at presentation. Tumors confined to the cervix may be treated by radical hysterectomy and pelvic node dissection, or radiotherapy. Both treatments carry similar 5-year survival rates[53] in early stages. In the elderly, radiotherapy may be more commonly used because of the fear of radical surgery complications or because of the more advanced presentation of disease. However, a fit elderly patient with early stage disease will tolerate the procedure well and should not be denied it on the basis of age alone. In advanced disease, the tumor may infiltrate locally causing fistula formation to the bladder or rectum. As in other squamous carcinomas, the success of chemotherapy is limited.

Corpus uteri

Endometrial carcinoma is the most common gynecologic malignancy in the elderly. Postmenopausal bleeding is the most frequent symptom and occurs early; hence, prognosis tends to be good with an overall 5-year survival rate for all stages of around 70%.[54] There are significant associations with nulliparity, late menopause; obesity, diabetes, and hypertension (Saint triad); unopposed estrogen replacement therapy and tamoxifen use. The incidence of uterine cancer is increasing in the United Kingdom, and this has much to do with the increasing obesity rates. Eighty percent of primary endometrial cancers are adenocarcinomas arising from the glandular endothelium often on a background of atypical hyperplasia. Hyperplasia is associated with unopposed estrogen action, and when described as atypical, surgical hysterectomy is warranted as undiagnosed carcinoma may be present. Serous, clear cell, squamous, and undifferentiated carcinomas are less common but more aggressive malignancies. More rarely, sarcomatous and mixed mesodermal tumors occur, and they have a poorer prognosis.

Approximately 90% of women present with postmenopausal bleeding (PMB), and patients with this complaint have around a 10% chance of being diagnosed with endometrial cancer. The recommended initial assessment of PMB should involve a transvaginal ultrasound scan to measure endometrial thickness. A thin endometrium on ultrasound has a high negative predictive value and is reassuring.

Where a thickening is detected, an endometrial biopsy is required. Thresholds for endometrial thickness will vary between regions but commonly are between 3 and 5 mm (or greater if currently on HRT). Ultrasound assessment is of little value where tamoxifen use is present due to subendometrial cystic changes. In this situation, first-line investigation should involve hysteroscopy with endometrial biopsy.[55] However, most cases of PMB are due to benign conditions including atrophic vaginitis and simple endometrial or cervical polyps.

Endometrial tumors spread directly to cervix, vagina, and peritoneal cavity via fallopian tubes. Myometrial invasion is common and may lead to serosal involvement. Lymphatic spread involves external iliac, internal iliac, obturator, and para-aortic nodes. Hematologic spread may lead to lung metastases. The staging of endometrial cancer relies on surgical assessment of intra-abdominal disease combined with pathologic assessment of hysterectomy specimen. If tumor extends to less than 50% of myometrial depth, lymph node spread exists in fewer than 5% of cases. If endometrial biopsy suggests high-grade disease or high malignant histology or if imaging suggests deep myometrial involvement, then it is recommended that care should be provided via a dedicated gynecologic oncologist via a multidisciplinary team.

Treatment should involve as a minimum, total hysterectomy, bilateral salpingo-oophorectomy, peritoneal cytology, and upper abdominal inspection. The debate regarding the necessity of lymphadenectomy in these patients led to the Medical Research Council funded ASTEC trial. One of the study's primary aims was to assess the benefit, or otherwise, of pelvic lymphadenectomy in patients where disease is thought to be confined to the corpus. Recruitment for this trial has now closed, and the preliminary results were presented at the European Society of Gynaecological Oncology in 2005. The society suggested that there was no benefit for survival or prevention of recurrence in performing lymphadenectomy for early stage endometrial cancer.

Radiotherapy may be given when the women cannot undergo surgery for medical reasons. Postoperative radiotherapy for stage 1 disease will reduce local recurrence from 14% to 10% but has no effect on overall survival.[56] Radiotherapy is therefore given based on individual risk stratification—myometrium invasion beyond 50%, tumor grade, and age all influencing this decision. Usually radiotherapy is a combination of vaginal radiotherapy to reduce vault recurrence and external beam radiotherapy. Side effects are common, occurring in 25% of women, and include frequent bowel movements, urinary frequency, pain, and scarring. Patients with advanced disease may be suitable for surgery with adjuvant chemoradiotherapy. Treatment for advanced disease is usually palliative, involving chemotherapy to treat systemic disease and radiotherapy for problems such as vaginal bleeding or bony metastases.

Progestational agents may be used for palliation or when the patient is unfit for other treatment. Tumor deposits may regress for a time; however, high-grade tumors often lack progesterone receptors.

Vaginal vault recurrence can be successfully salvaged with either surgery or radiotherapy with 3-year survival rates of approximately 70%.

Ovary

Ovarian cancer remains the most lethal gynecologic malignancy and is currently the fifth leading cause of female cancer deaths. It affects those aged 65 years and older more frequently than younger women, with almost 50% of ovarian tumors occurring in this age group. More of the older women are likely to present with advanced disease and are less likely to be offered radical surgery and chemotherapy. The onset and progress is often insidious, so a high index of suspicion is necessary in postmenopausal women with nonspecific symptoms such as abdominal discomfort and swelling, malaise, and weight loss. In a postmenopausal woman with ascites, ovarian cancer should be the diagnosis until proven otherwise. Hereditary ovarian cancers are unlikely to represent more than 10% of all ovarian cancers. Currently there is no satisfactory screening method for ovarian neoplasia that has been shown to reduce morbidity. Screening should only be offered to high-risk individuals, with enrollment into a screening trial encouraged. Screening is therefore not advisable for the elderly population. The tumor marker CA125 is an indicator of ovarian malignancy, but it may not be elevated in all ovarian carcinomas and is often not elevated in early stage disease. However, inclusion of CA125 levels with menopausal status and ultrasound findings provides a useful algorithm termed Risk of Malignancy Index (RMI) (Table 87-2). Using RMI provides an 87% sensitivity, 89% specificity, and 75% positive predictive value.[57] The RMI's greatest value is in allowing triaging of patients to the care of a gynecologic oncologist or general gynecologists. Many postmenopausal ovarian cysts are an incidental finding, and if the RMI is low, no action is required.

All high-risk patients should be managed by a multidisciplinary team and have any surgery performed by a trained gynecologic oncologist. In advanced stage disease, operative mortality is around 1% and major morbidity about 5%.

Ninety percent of ovarian malignancies in older women are epithelial adenocarcinomas, but other ovarian components may become malignant and give rise to such histologic types as sex cord and germ cell tumors. Up to 10% of ovarian masses are metastases from elsewhere, particularly colon and breast. Granulosa cell tumor is the most common sex cord malignancy and may occur after menopause. Hormone

Table 87-2. Risk of Malignancy Index (RMI = Ultrasound Score × Menopausal Status × CA125)

Ultrasound score	0	No suspicious features
	1	One suspicious feature
	3	Two to five suspicious features
Menopausal score	1	Premenopausal
	3	Postmenopausal
CA125		

Suspicious ultrasound features are multiloculated cyst, solid areas, metastases, bilateral lesions, and ascites.

Triaging According to RMI

	RMI	Percentage of Women	Risk of Malignancy
Low risk	<25	40%	<3%
Moderate risk	25–250	30%	20%
High risk	>250	30%	75%

production can cause vaginal bleeding because of endometrial hyperplasia.

A complete history is essential to make diagnosis and assess fitness for surgical and nonsurgical management. Investigation includes hematologic and biochemical profiles, chest x-ray, and ultrasound screening of the pelvis, liver, and kidneys. Magnetic resonance imaging (MRI) or computed tomography (CT) scans are not routinely indicated but may assist in surgical planning and assessment of the upper abdomen.

Laparotomy establishes the diagnosis, and examination of abdominal contents provides accurate staging, which will influence treatment and prognosis. Debulking of the tumor with bilateral salpingo-oophorectomy, total hysterectomy, and infracolic omentectomy is the mainstay of treatment. Peritoneal washings and upper abdominal/diaphragmatic assessment is carried out at the time of laparotomy. Complete tumor removal may be difficult, but the greater the reduction of tumor bulk, the more effective is adjuvant therapy and ascites is better controlled. Although cytoreductive surgery is still the gold standard of care for advanced disease, results from trials of primary surgery versus neoadjuvant chemotherapy with interval surgery have suggested a benefit in advanced disease.[58] Larger trials on this question are awaited. Postoperative chemotherapy is used in all but stage 1 disease, and indeed many patients will have residual disease after surgery.

The platinum compounds, cisplatin and carboplatin, remain the agents of choice; they are toxic and side effects include myelosuppression, nephro- and neurotoxicity, and severe emetogenesis. Combination therapy of platinum drugs with paclitaxel has been shown to provide some survival benefit over cyclophosphamide/cisplatin (the previous standard of care).[59] However, this has not been demonstrated in other large trials.[60] Forty percent to 50% of patients with extensive disease will have complete remission with platinum, but the majority relapse within 2 years. A less aggressive option is the oral alkylating agent, chlorambucil, which is sometimes used in the elderly.

Failure of first-line treatment is ominous, as recurrent disease is often resistant to further therapy, but taxanes are tried in these patients with some success. Retreatment with platinum-based drugs is appropriate if the tumor was originally sensitive and a disease-free interval of greater than 1 year has occurred. Recurrent ascites is a major problem and requires repeated paracentesis; spironolactone may reduce the fluid and limit recurrence. Radiotherapy is limited to unresectable tumors and patients with symptomatic recurrence and is used only for palliation. The most common indication for palliative surgery is bowel obstruction, and referral to surgeons should be considered despite poor prognosis in order to ensure an optimized quality of life.

In knowing that most patients with ovarian cancer present late and die of the disease, although cure is the ultimate goal, it is not often achieved. Surgery and chemotherapy will have a significant impact on a patient's quality of life. Therefore, the informed patient's wishes should always be listened to in planning his or her care.

SEXUALITY AND AGING

There is a view that sexuality in the elderly is irrelevant and sexual activity unnecessary. The facts are, however, that sexual drive is not exhausted with aging, and as life expectancy increases it is necessary to recognize that continued sexual activity is an important component of increasing age to promote satisfactory relationships, personal well-being, and quality of life. There will be an increasing demand from this age group for advice and expert help on sexual matters.[61] Many older people have problems because they grew up in sexually restricted times, so that ignorance is widespread.[62] Society has an obsession with youth and its sexuality while largely stereotyping the elderly and ignoring their difficulties in this area. In addition, as is generally the case with disabled people, the organization of institutions for the elderly does not recognize their sexuality, so their needs—for example opportunities for privacy—are ignored.[63]

A longitudinal study[64] has shown that sexual activity remains relatively constant within a stable relationship and only declines following a negative event, particularly for the male partner—for example, the death of the spouse. Many factors contribute to changing sexuality such as age, physical appearance, self-image, culture, education, and social attitudes.

Sexual behavior and age

A steady reduction in male sexuality from early and middle years has been observed.[65] A common phenomenon in older men is erectile dysfunction due to penile arterial insufficiency, the effect of such drugs as antihypertensives, and illnesses like diabetes.[66] Brecher[67] noted that 75% of 70-year-old men continued to have some sexual activity.

Waning sexuality with age is also related to previous experience.[68] In both sexes, low activity levels in youth are associated with a greater decrease in later life.

An early study observed little change in women's capacity for sexual activity until later life.[69] However, questionnaires[70,71] from both sexes between ages 45 and 71 were analyzed. A greater reduction was noted in sexual interest and activity in women, the most significant change being between 50 and 60 years. At 66 to 71 years, 50% and 10% of women and men, respectively, had no sexual interest.

Sexual interest also depends on the availability of a partner. Women, who tend to marry older men who die before them, are often left alone and may experience difficulty finding a new partner.[62] Thus, masturbation may become a more regular activity. It has been found that female sexual activity was highest in those currently married and it progressively reduced in the divorced, widowed, and never married.[72] Resumption of interest a year after widowhood is more likely when death of the partner was expected, there had been extramarital experience, and, in younger women, activity diminished when the marriage had been sexually satisfying and there was still a strong attachment to the lost partner.[73]

A common problem following postmenopausal lack of estrogen is vaginal atrophy and dryness causing dyspareunia,[69] which leads to a loss of interest and activity. It has been observed[74] that the more sexually active women (with coitus and masturbation) had less vaginal atrophy, suggesting that activity protects the vagina by stretching and possibly stimulating hormone production. The use of HRT has been studied.[75] Estrogen, androgen, and a combination of both and placebo were compared in oophorectomized women. The results indicated a beneficial effect of androgen alone or with estrogen on sexual motivation and coital frequency. Thus, the evidence suggests that female sexuality is affected by aging but initially less so than by menopause, and the hormones involved are estrogen and androgen. Testosterone treatment has been recommended in women where other therapeutic and counseling techniques have not helped.[76] Tibolone is an oral HRT preparation that contains androgen and has been shown to improve sexual problems including reduced libido.[77] Alternatively, a 6-week trial of testosterone undecenoate, 40 mg daily, may be used; if there is no beneficial effect, the drug should be stopped. A subcutaneous implant of 50 mg testosterone is also effective. With either treatment there is little risk of masculinizing effects, for example, hirsutism or deepening of the voice; however, if these symptoms occur, treatment should be discontinued.

Sexual response and aging

It has been noted[76] that with age, vasocongestive changes following sexual stimulation develop more slowly in both sexes; these alterations are gradual so that the couple adjusts to activity that is less intense but may be as enjoyable. Older men will develop erections more slowly and maintenance of the erection is not as good and if lost is more difficult to regain.

In women, vaginal lubrication diminishes and takes longer; there is less vaginal elasticity so that there is shrinkage in the absence of coitus. There are changes elsewhere; for example, nipple erection and breast engorgement are less marked and orgasmic capacity may be reduced[78]; also the sense of touch in the genital area may be reduced or experienced as unpleasant or painful, which can further inhibit orgasm.

Management of couples with sexual problems

The management of these disorders should be guided by the same principles irrespective of age and condition of the patient, although the emphasis may vary. Both partners should take part in therapy, because although one usually presents a problem the other invariably contributes to it, and the treatment is obviously facilitated by cooperation. After an initial discussion, the couple should be seen separately so that confidential interviews are obtained including information not to be disclosed to the partner. A preliminary medical and social history may suggest contributing factor(s) and helps rapport to be established before turning to more sensitive questions.

Ignorance about sexuality is common, so there is a need for basic education and permission to experiment, for example, with different methods of stimulation and coital positions. Couples, particularly older ones, frequently have difficulty talking to each other about sexual anxieties or needs, and discussion with the therapist increases their mutual understanding and ability to communicate.

For men with psychogenic, organic, or mixed erectile dysfunction (ED), various treatments have become available in recent years. A concise account of these is available.[79] Following a full assessment to screen for conditions associated with ED, systemic treatment can be with type 5 phosphodiesterase inhibitors such as Sildafenil and Tadalafil or local intercavernosal or intraurethral prostaglandin therapy (Alprostadil).

There are currently limitations to the prescription of ED drugs in the National Health Service; they are allowed only in men who have had, for example, prostate surgery, renal failure, spinal cord injury, diabetes mellitus, multiple sclerosis, or some other specific medical condition. Those suffering severe emotional stress resulting from ED are entitled to a prescription, but many health authorities have not provided funding, so the men have to rely on a private script from their hospital clinic or general practitioner.

Mechanical devices have been tried for ED, such as vacuum cylinders and penile prostheses. The latter technique involves referral to a specialist urologist for detailed counseling and management.

KEY POINTS
Gynecologic Disorders in the Elderly

- The female aging process accelerates after menopause, particularly in the genital tract, as a consequence of cessation of ovarian estrogen production.
- Hormone replacement therapy is now only advocated for symptomatic relief, but patients should be assessed on an individual basis and fully informed of the risks and benefits.
- Diagnosis of vulvar disorders requires detailed history and examination and biopsy when indicated. Management should be by a dedicated vulvar skin clinic where available.
- Newer surgical mesh treatments for urinary stress incontinence and uterovaginal prolapse are suitable for the elderly, and some can be performed under local anesthesia.
- An elderly patient with gynecologic cancer should be offered the same surgical treatment recommended to younger women. Management should be by a multidisciplinary team.
- There is no age limit to the expression of sexuality, and the elderly should be offered a full range of counseling and treatment where appropriate.

For a complete list of references, please visit online only at www.expertconsult.com

CHAPTER 88

Cancer of the Breast in the Elderly

Lodovico Balducci

INTRODUCTION

The management of breast cancer in the older woman is an increasingly common problem. The incidence and prevalence of this neoplasm increase with age, and the options available for its management have become more numerous.[1,2] This is the consequence of the aging of the population, more wide utilization of breast cancer screening in the older woman, and the prolonged survival of breast cancer patients.

The geriatrician or the primary care provider may be involved in a number of decisions and interventions related to the management of breast cancer, including screening, referral for treatment, and management of short- and long-term treatment complications.

BREAST CANCER PRESENTATION: DIAGNOSIS AND STAGING

Diagnosis

More and more women 70 and older are undergoing mammographic screening.[3] The indirect evidence of benefits supports this practice. The Surveillance Epidemiology and End Results (SEER) data indicate that women 70 to 79 who had at least two mammograms were less likely to die of breast cancer than those who were not screened, and this benefit was present even in subjects with moderate degrees of comorbidity.[4,5] For these individuals, the most common presentation of breast cancer is an asymptomatic abnormality in the radiograph.

Other forms of presentation include an asymptomatic breast nodule, nipple discharge, and, more rarely, symptoms related to metastatic disease such as bone pain or edema of an upper extremity.[6] Occasionally, breast cancer may manifest with metastases to the axillary lymph nodes without any sign of neoplasm in the corresponding breast.[6]

When the breast cancer is suspected because of nipple discharge or enlarged lymph nodes, radiographic examinations necessary to confirm the suspicion include simple mammography, digital mammography, ultrasound, and magnetic resonance imaging (MRI) of the breast.[7,8,9] Although there is general agreement that digital mammography and MRI are more sensitive than regular mammography, controversy persists over the technique that is preferable in individual situations.

The cancerous nature of any abnormality found by imaging or by physical exam needs to be established by a biopsy. This may include a fine needle aspiration of a palpable mass or a core biopsy of a radiographic abnormality. Occasionally the biopsy may be avoided in women with very limited life expectancy, for whom the cancer does not appear life threatening and further management is impractical.[10]

Staging

The management of breast cancer is determined primarily by the stage of the disease—that is, by its extension. A discussion of the current staging systems is beyond the scope of this chapter. As a general rule, breast cancer can present as localized, locally advanced, and metastatic disease. The tests utilized for staging include positron emission tomography (PET) scan; computed tomography (CT) (or MRI) of chest, abdomen, and brain; and radionuclide bone scan.

There is general agreement that in the presence of small tumors, without microscopic involvement of the axillary lymph nodes, these tests are unnecessary, unless the patient has specific symptoms, such as bone pain or headaches, suggesting bone and brain metastases, respectively. Likewise the majority of oncologists would perform a full staging of patients with locally advanced disease or of those in whom one or more metastases have been documented. An area of controversy is whether the staging tests are necessary for patients with local tumor and microscopically involved lymph nodes. The National Comprehensive Cancer Center (NCCC) guidelines recommend that full staging be performed in patients who are asymptomatic but have three or more microscopically involved lymph nodes.[10]

A number of circulating tumor markers may be useful in the management of breast cancer, including carcinoembryonic antigen (CEA), Ca15-3, and 27–29. The value of these assays is controversial.[11] In older patients with metastatic disease, tumor markers may be followed in lieu of imaging tests, which are more risky and expensive, to follow the disease response to treatment.

The location of metastases has important clinical implications. If untreated, brain metastases, lymphangitic lung metastases, and widespread liver metastases may be associated with a survival shorter than 1 year, whereas patients with bone and skin metastases may survive several years. Patients with metastases to long bones are at high risk of pathologic fractures and may need surgical fixation; those with metastases to the spinal cord are at risk of spinal cord compression that may lead to paraplegia and sphincter dysfunction in a period of a few hours. In the presence of vertebral metastases, the practitioner should have a high grade of suspicion for this complication. Upon diagnosis of vertebral metastases, an MRI of the spine is indicated, and this should be repeated in the presence of worsening pain or the appearance of neurologic signs, including weakness, sensory levels, and sphincter dysfunction.[12]

PATHOLOGY OF BREAST CANCER AND MOLECULAR MARKERS OF CLINICAL INTEREST

In an increasing number of cases breast cancer presents at diagnosis as "carcinoma in situ," as a result of more widespread use of mammography. The distinction between "ductal carcinoma in situ" (DCIS) and "lobular carcinoma in situ" (LCIS) is clinically relevant, as LCIS has a high probability of recurrence both in the same and in the contralateral breast.[13]

Table 88-1. Pathologic and Molecular Markers of Breast Cancer

Marker	Prognostic Value	Predictive Value
Tumor size	Prognosis worsens with increasing tumor size	Unestablished
Tumor grade (degree of tumor differentiation)	The more undifferentiated the tumor, the poorer the prognosis	
Number of microscopically involved axillary lymph nodes	Prognosis worsens with increasing number of lymph node involvement	Unestablished
Hormone receptors	Prognosis improves with the richness in hormone receptors	Response to endocrine therapy
Ki67	Measurement of cell proliferation; the highest the value the highest the risk of recurrence	Unestablished
HER2neu	Increases risk of recurrence	Predicts response to trastuzumab and lapatinib and poor response to hormonal therapy
Genetic profile	Predicts risk of recurrence in the case of hormone receptor—rich breast cancer with uninvolved lymph nodes	May predict response to chemotherapy

A number of pathologic and molecular prognostic factors have been identified for invasive carcinoma of the breast in the early stages (Table 88-1).[14,15] Estrogen and progesterone receptors are a harbinger of more indolent disease and predict the benefits of hormonal treatment. The overexpression of epidermal growth factor receptor II (HER2 neu) is a harbinger of very aggressive disease but, more important, predicts response to the monoclonal antibody trastuzumab[16] and to the small molecule tyrosine kinase inhibitor lapatinib,[16] two agents that have substantially improved the survival of patients with this aggressive form of breast cancer. The development of microarray techniques has allowed researchers to study the genetic profile of many cancers and their prognostic and predictive values. A 21-gene assay (oncotype) is now available for clinical use: it predicts those patients with hormone receptor–rich tumors and uninvolved axillary lymph nodes who are at risk of systemic recurrence and may benefit from adjuvant chemotherapy in addition to hormonal therapy.

MANAGEMENT OF BREAST CANCER

Common forms of treatment for breast cancer are listed in Table 88-2.

For the purpose of this chapter, it is useful to define some terms that will recur frequently: adjuvant and neoadjuvant therapy, breast preservation surgery, and sentinel lymph node. *Adjuvant therapy* is treatment given in addition to definitive treatment in patients with no evidence of disease with the goal of preventing tumor recurrence. *Neoadjuvant therapy* is treatment administered before definitive treatment with the goals of preventing later recurrences and of reducing tumor size making it amenable to surgery or to lesser surgery (breast preservation). *Breast preservation surgery* consists of partial mastectomy followed by radiation therapy to the breast. Although it has been in high favor since the late 1980s, the use of breast preservation has recently declined because of the discovery by MRI that a large number of patients with breast cancer harbor in the same breast small, unsuspected focuses of DCIS.[17] The need of postoperative irradiation of the breast in women 70 and older has been questioned, as the risk of local recurrences decreases with age[18] and postoperative radiation does not appear to improve survival. External beam irradiation is particularly inconvenient for older women as it requires daily visits to the treatment center for 5 weeks. New forms of postoperative irradiation, such as brachytherapy or hypofractionation treatment, are administered over a shorter period of time and may be more compatible with the needs of older individuals.

Sentinel lymph node is the first lymph node draining the tumor and it may be identified at surgery in the majority of cases. If the tumor does not involve the sentinel lymph node, a full axillary dissection and the consequent complications (lymphedema) may be avoided.[18] A disadvantage of the sentinel lymph node sampling is that it requires a two-stage surgery—that is, if the lymph node is positive for cancer, the patient needs another operation for lymph node dissection.

We will discuss treatment now by stage.

Carcinoma in situ

Surgery is still the mainstay of treatment of DCIS and LCIS. DCIS may be managed with total mastectomy or partial mastectomy, followed by radiation therapy.[14] Postoperative radiation therapy after partial mastectomy reduces by half the risk of local recurrences that are further reduced by systemic treatment with the estrogen antagonist tamoxifen. Risks and benefits of tamoxifen need to be carefully assessed, as the drug does not prolong the patient's survival and the risk of local recurrence is minimal. LCIS may be treated with local excision or with bilateral mastectomy (given the risk of bilateral recurrence).

Localized diseases

Mastectomy or breast preservation surgery with sentinel lymph node sampling is the commonly used procedure. Patients with positive sentinel lymph nodes undergo axillary dissection at a later time. The choice of adjuvant treatment depends on the hormonal status and risk of systemic recurrence. In patients with cancer rich in hormone receptors, adjuvant hormonal therapy for at least 5 years reduces by 50% the risk of recurrence and by 30% the risk of mortality.[20] Nowadays most oncologists prefer aromatase inhibitors to estrogen antagonists. Aromatase inhibitors appear to be more effective, do not cause endometrial cancer, and have a lesser risk of deep vein thrombosis, but they may cause osteopenia and osteoporosis and have higher risk of disabling arthralgias.[21] Current investigations explore the benefits of continuing the treatment beyond 5 years. The benefits of adjuvant chemotherapy decline with the patient's age[19] and have not been conclusively demonstrated in

Table 88-2. Forms of Cancer Treatment

Form of Treatment	Specific Treatment	Clinical Considerations	Complications
Local treatment	Surgery	The most common form of treatment of localized breast cancer. Both partial and total mastectomy may be performed under local anesthesia. It may be used occasionally in the management of metastatic disease, including fixation of bones at risk for fractures and resection of brain metastases.	
	Radiation therapy	Used in combination with surgery for breast preservation. In addition it may be used for palliation of painful bony metastases and for treatment of brain metastases after total mastectomy is indicated for large tumors (more than 5cm in diameter).	
Systemic treatment	Hormonal therapy: Estrogen antagonists Aromatase inhibitors Progestins Estrogens Androgens	Used in the management of breast cancer whose tumor is positive for hormone receptors. It may be used both in the metastatic and in the adjuvant and neoadjuvant setting.	Estrogen antagonists may cause uterine cancer and deep vein thrombosis. Aromatase inhibitors cause severe arthralgias and osteopenia.
	Cytotoxic chemotherapy	Used in the management of breast cancer whose tumor is poor in hormone receptors and occasionally in those who are rich in hormone receptors. It may be utilized in the metastatic and in the adjuvant and neoadjuvant setting.	Older patients are at increased risk of neutropenia and cardiotoxicity and mucositis.
	Targeted treatment Bevacizumab Trastuzumab Lapatinib	It enhances the activity of some chemotherapy agents. Very effective in the management of tumors who have an overexpression of HER2neu.	Complications include hypertension, clotting, bleeding, and visceral perforation (postsurgical). Trastuzumab may cause reversible cardiomyopathy. Lapatinib can cause diarrhea and interactions with drugs metabolized by the CyP450 system.
	Bisphosphonates	Utilized in patients with bony metastases to delay the development of pain, fractures, and other bone complications.	

women 70 and older.[19] In addition to acute complications, including alopecia, nausea and vomiting, neutropenic infections, adjuvant chemotherapy may be associated with two late complications: myelodysplasia/acute myelogenous leukemia[22] and chronic cardiomyopathy (in patients treated with anthracyclines).[23] A user-friendly computer system (found at www.adjuvantonline.com) allows a fairly precise estimate of the risk of recurrence and the benefit of chemotherapy in individual situations.[24] In patients whose tumor overexpresses HER2neu, the addition of trastuzumab for 1 year to adjuvant treatment has further reduced the risk of recurrences by 50%.[25] The benefits of this compound greatly overwhelm the risks, which include reversible cardiomyopathy in older patients.

Locally advanced disease

The management of locally advanced but unresectable disease includes neoadjuvant therapy, aimed to make the tumor smaller, followed by a local form of treatment: radiation therapy, surgery, or both.[26] This presentation of breast is dramatic and requires aggressive treatment to prevent local complications. Fortunately, it is rare, but in older women it may result from inadequate screening and ineffective self-examination.[27]

Metastatic disease

The management of metastatic disease is determined by the nature of the metastases, by the concentration of hormone receptors, and by the presence of HER2neu overexpression. Some general points may be made:

- Life-threatening metastases (lymphangitic lung spread or extensive liver metastases) should be treated with chemotherapy, irrespective of hormone receptor status, to achieve a rapid response and save the patient's life. These are rare in older individuals.
- Patients with hormone receptor–rich tumors should be treated with three lines of hormonal therapy, including aromatase inhibitors, estrogen antagonists, and progestins, before starting chemotherapy. The use of estrogen in high doses and androgens has become limited because of their toxicity.
- Patients whose tumors overexpress HER2neu should receive trastuzumab as part of their treatment. If this agent is contraindicated, then oral lapatinib is the treatment of choice.
- Patients who have hormone receptor–poor tumors and those whose cancer has failed three lines of hormonal treatment may receive chemotherapy. The majority of oncologists would use single agent chemotherapy

sequentially to reduce the toxicity. Particularly indicated in older individuals, because of minimal toxicity are the oral prodrug capecitabine, pegylated liposomal doxorubicin, and gemcitabine.
- Patients with bony metastases should receive a bisphosphonate in combination with other systemic treatments to delay pain and fractures.
- Patients with a single brain metastasis may benefit from surgical removal or radiosurgery. Multiple metastases require total brain irradiation.

CONCLUSIONS

The management of breast cancer in older women is predicated on individual life expectancy and disease aggressiveness. The basic treatment principles are the same as for younger women with the following considerations:

- Postoperative radiation therapy may not be indicated for breast preservation at age 70 and over.
- The risk of complications resulting from hormonal therapy and chemotherapy increases after age 70. Of particular concern are endometrial cancer and deep vein thrombosis with tamoxifen; disabling arthritis and osteoporosis with aromatase inhibitors; and neutropenic infections, mucositis, and anthracycline cardiomyopathy with cytotoxic chemotherapy.
- Long-term complications of chemotherapy in older women include myelodysplasia/acute leukemia and congestive cardiomyopathy.
- A number of chemotherapy agents are particularly suitable for the management of older women with metastatic breast cancer resistant to hormonal therapy.

KEY POINTS

Cancer of the Breast in the Elderly

- Breast cancer is in general more indolent in older than in younger women. However, the disease is lethal in women of all ages. The management should be guided by the aggressiveness of the individual cancer and the life expectancy and functional reserve of individual patients.
- Screening mammography reduces breast cancer—related mortality in women with a life expectancy of 5 years or longer. Life expectancy rather than chronologic age should direct the implementation of cancer prevention.
- Therapeutic principles are the same in women of all ages. Controversy persists about the benefits of adjuvant chemotherapy in women 70 and older with hormone receptor–positive tumors. Genomic and proteomics may help identify older women who definitely benefit from adjuvant chemotherapy.

For a complete list of references, please visit online only at www.expertconsult.com

CHAPTER 89

Adrenal and Pituitary Disorders

Paul E. Belchetz
Peter Hammond

DISORDERS OF THE ADRENAL CORTEX

The need for normal adrenal functioning continues into old age. After decades of speculation, there is now firm evidence that the patterns of basal and stimulated levels of cortisol secretion are substantially unchanged in the healthy aging population. Subtle age-related changes have been described related to the metabolism of adrenal hormones, and morphologic features such as nodules appear quite commonly in the aging adrenal glands. Their importance arises from much readier and often serendipitous recognition as advanced imaging techniques are more widely used. It is therefore relevant to open this chapter with a résumé of the physiologic and biochemical actions of adrenal steroids, mechanisms controlling their secretion, and techniques available for assessing the function and anatomy of the adrenal glands.

Physiologic responses to adrenocortical steroids

Of the multitude of steroids found in the adrenal cortex, only the secretions of cortisol and aldosterone have undisputed and vital endocrine roles. The distinction between glucocorticoid and mineralocorticoid hormone actions is based on physiologic observations, backed by differential effects on critical enzyme systems in target tissues.

Glucocorticoids. Cortisol (hydrocortisone) is the natural glucocorticoid of humans and most other mammals (but not the rat, which is unable to synthesize cortisol and uses corticosterone instead). It has long been recognized that cortisol, especially in high doses, has mineralocorticoid properties and this has led to the widespread use of dexamethasone, a synthetic glucocorticoid, effectively without mineralocorticoid properties as the benchmark glucocorticoid.[1]

This practice has passed from laboratory experiments to clinical investigation, as will be discussed later. There are growing reasons to question the validity of such assumptions, although the pragmatic clinical tests have proven value. There has previously been a tendency to subdivide the actions of glucocorticoids into those seen at low doses and termed physiologic, and those seen with high doses, classically causing cushingoid side effects, as pharmacologic. There is no sound scientific basis for this differentiation as new effects are not seen with high doses, although the clinical sequelae are, of course, striking.

The term *glucocorticoid* derives from the effects on carbohydrate metabolism: antagonism of insulin action, promotion of hepatic glycogen synthesis, and participation in the defenses against hypoglycemia. It may affect resource use by virtue of tissue differences in response of the key glycolytic enzyme, phosphoenolpyruvate carboxykinase.[2] Glucocorticoids have many other actions, often permissive in nature. These include vascular and renal responses affecting control of blood pressure and extracellular water content. Other critical roles include actions on protein and lipid synthesis and complex interactions with the immune system. In addition there is the well-recognized but poorly characterized function that enhanced glucocorticoid secretion plays in combating stress. The stimuli recognized as stressful and capable of evoking enhanced cortisol secretion are numerous, including: fever, trauma, hemorrhage, and plasma-volume depletion, hypoglycemia, and even psychological disturbance. A unifying hypothesis is thus hard to achieve; but with regard to inflammatory processes, it is now widely believed that the role of glucocorticoids is to curtail the effects of the rapidly responding cytokine and acute-phase protein production, which if protracted could be potentially damaging.[3]

Mineralocorticoids. The action of aldosterone is ostensibly simpler, operating primarily via renal mechanisms to control extracellular sodium and potassium levels with secondary consequences on fluid balance and blood pressure. The effects of mineralocorticoids on other tissues such as the colon, brain, and pituitary are documented, but their significance is much less certain. The secretion of aldosterone and its circadian rhythm are maintained in the elderly despite a decrease in tonic levels of renin, its principal regulator.[4]

Adrenal androgens. The adrenal cortex also synthesizes androgens. These include androstenedione and dehydroepiandrosterone; much of the latter is conjugated and secreted as the sulfate. The function of adrenal androgens remains obscure, although much has been made of the phenomenon in childhood of the so-called "adrenarche," when enhanced amounts are made from about the age of 7 years. By contrast with cortisol production, there is a well-documented fall in adrenal androgen production in old age, to as little as 5% of young adult levels, with decreased ACTH responsiveness, which has been termed the "adrenopause."[5]

Apart from effects on body hair, it is not at all clear what function the secretion of adrenal androgens serves in normal adults. It has been postulated that the decline in dehydroepiandrosterone levels is, in part, responsible for the increased atherogenesis and, hence, cardiovascular disease in old age, but recent evidence does not support this hypothesis.[6] It appears more likely that dehydroepiandrosterone has an immunomodulatory, and possibly antioncogenic, action. Dehydroepiandrosterone replacement in an elderly person increases natural killer (NK) cell cytotoxicity and is claimed to dramatically improve the sense of physical and psychological well-being.[7]

Biochemical actions of steroid hormones

The effects of hormones on tissues depend on the distribution of specific receptors. Recent advances in knowledge have simultaneously clarified aspects of steroid hormone action and raised paradoxes that await definitive resolution. Steroids are lipophilic and readily enter cells: steroid receptors are intracellular. The classic model of steroid action is that steroid hormones bind to cytoplasmic receptors, forming activated complexes that are translocated to the nucleus where specific genes are activated, leading eventually to protein products as the end point of hormone influence.[8] A similar pattern was proposed for the structurally dissimilar thyroid hormones. Molecular cloning techniques have not only revealed that all steroid hormone receptors show strong homologies to each other and the proto-oncogene c-*erb*-A, but that the latter actually appears to be a thyroid-hormone receptor. All these receptors share homologies, both in the hormone and the DNA-binding domains, and can be regarded as constituting a superfamily of genes, whose products are transcriptional regulatory proteins evolved from a common ancestor gene.[9] The steroid-hormone receptor is bound to a protein complex containing the heat-shock proteins hsp 90, hsp 70, and hsp 65. Exposure to steroid hormone leads to dissociation of the receptor from the complex so that the receptor is able to bind the hormone.[10] Along with the classic genomic mechanisms, the cortisol-glucocorticoid receptor complex can interact with other transcription factors such as nuclear factor-κB and also nongenomic pathways via membrane-associated receptors and second messengers.[11]

The new complex of hormone-plus receptor adopts a different molecular conformation, exposing the DNA-binding domain of the receptor. Thus far, the generalized scheme for steroid hormones applies to glucocorticoids. When it comes to identifying the molecular basis for mineralocorticoid and glucocorticoid actions, difficulties arise. The type-1 receptor—originally considered to bind mineralocorticoids with higher affinity than glucocorticoids—shows no such distinction with more modern techniques. Indeed there is a marked kinship shown at the molecular level as well.[12,13] A possible explanation for the failure of the great molar excess of cortisol to swamp the type-1 receptor with regard to aldosterone binding has been suggested for tissues such as kidney, gut, and salivary glands. These tissues possess a potent 11-hydroxysteroid dehydrogenase enzyme system, which rapidly converts cortisol to cortisone, and cortisone does not bind measurably to the receptor.[14]

Acting through the genome, glucocorticoids enhance several key metabolic enzymes, such as hepatic tyrosine aminotransferase[15] and tryptophan oxygenase.[16] In addition to this classic mode of action, it has also been suggested that many of the actions of glucocorticoids on the immune system are mediated by a specific protein product termed *lipocortin* (now known as *annexin A1*), which acts as a second messenger.[17] This has multiple sites of action especially, inhibiting polymorphonuclear leukocyte trafficking, reduction of pro-inflammatory cytokines and stimulation of anti-inflammatory cytokines.

Regulation of adrenal function

Regulation of glucocorticoid production. Cortisol secretion is under the immediate control of pituitary ACTH secretion acting to promote the conversion of cholesterol to pregnenolone by the removal of the six-carbon fragment from the cholesterol side chain. These steps occur within the mitochondrion. A complex cascade of cytochrome-P450 variants has been implicated as steroidogenesis proceeds, shuttling from mitochondrion to endoplasmic reticulum and back. The chronic effects of ACTH affect many more steps in steroidogenesis than just cholesterol side-chain cleavage.[18]

Physiologic control of ACTH secretion involves three major areas: circadian rhythms, stress, and negative-feedback inhibition by cortisol. ACTH is synthesized as part of a large 31-kDa precursor polypeptide pro-opiomelanocortin.[19] This is cleaved and the major fragments, including ACTH and β-endorphin, are usually cosecreted in equimolar proportions. The stimulus to ACTH release is from the hypothalamus by way of the hypothalamopituitary portal vessels conveying corticotrophin-releasing factors.[20]

These are a complex of polypeptides, the major constituent of which is a 41-residue moiety, corticotrophin-releasing hormone (CRH). However, this alone has less potent ACTH-releasing properties than crude hypothalamic extracts. It has been shown that vasopressin (AVP) and probably other, as yet unidentified, compounds act synergistically with CRH.[21] The secretion of these corticotrophin-releasing factors appears to be pulsatile-driving pulses of ACTH and cortisol in turn. The circadian rhythm is composed of pulses of varying amplitudes and frequency, with a nadir reached at midnight, but the onset of activity at about 3 AM to 4 AM reaching a peak at 8 AM to 9 AM. The pulses of ACTH and cortisol decline in size and frequency thereafter, although there is often a secondary rise at about lunchtime, which seems to be related to food ingestion.[22]

As mentioned earlier, there is a formidable array of apparently unrelated stressors that can stimulate the release of ACTH and cortisol. There is preliminary evidence that the relative importance of CRH, AVP, and oxytocin varies according to the stimulus.[23] Where inflammation is involved, there is growing evidence for interleukin-1, interleukin-6, and tumor necrosis factor (TNF) having the capacity to stimulate the hypothalamic-pituitary-adrenal axis, thus providing a loop to suppress their own production.[24]

Reports suggesting extrahypothalamic production of ACTH secretagogues lack confirmation of authenticity or physiologic significance.

Negative feedback of cortisol on ACTH production constitutes a sensitive homeostatic regulatory mechanism. The sites of negative feedback include not only the ACTH-producing cells of the anterior pituitary itself, but also higher centers including the hypothalamus and CA3 field of the hippocampus.[25]

Regulation of aldosterone production. Aldosterone is produced by the distinct outer part of the adrenal cortex, the zona glomerulosa. In humans this is found in cell clusters rather than in a distinct zone. The main regulation of aldosterone is by the renin-angiotensin system. The stimuli to renin release from the juxtaglomerular cells of the kidney are low-renal perfusion pressure, sodium depletion, and hypokalemia, although hyperkalemia acting directly on the zona glomerulosa is a more potent stimulus to aldosterone release than hypokalemia. Renin acts on renin substrate or angiotensinogen, released into the circulation from the liver, to form angiotensin-I. This decapeptide is converted to the octapeptide angiotensin-II by angiotensin-converting enzyme (ACE), which is of widespread distribution, but most importantly found in the pulmonary bed.[26]

Angiotensin-II, apart from being a powerful arteriolar vasoconstrictor, stimulates aldosterone secretion from the adrenal cortex. Aldosterone, as mentioned earlier, acts powerfully to retain salt (and obligatorily water), but promotes kaliuresis, hence closing the homeostatic feedback loop. There are other minor influences recognized as acting on aldosterone secretion, including ACTH, dopamine, and serotonin.

Adrenocortical function in normal aging

Numerous studies indicate that basal, circadian, and stimulated cortisol secretion remains intact well into old age.[27–33] This is particularly important with regard to the ability to withstand stress, and the cortisol response to exogenous ACTH has been shown to be normal in elderly patients following myocardial infarction.[34] There are well-documented changes in the metabolism of corticosteroids with age-related decrease in the catabolism of cortisol.[35,36] Because of the intact negative feedback mechanisms there is a commensurate reduction in cortisol production rate. Aldosterone secretion is also normally well preserved in the healthy geriatric population.[37] The recognized decline in adrenal androgen production[30,38–41] has been referred to earlier.

Tests of adrenal function

Tests of adrenal function in elderly people are for the foregoing reasons largely those established for the younger adult population. The diminishing reliance on urinary collections is beneficial for practical reasons, and also means that some of the physiologically irrelevant changes alluded to earlier will not prove distracting. The key to successful and safe investigation is careful selection.

Adrenal insufficiency. To investigate possible adrenal insufficiency, the basal measurement of greatest value is the plasma cortisol, measured at the circadian peak at 8 AM to 9 AM. Measurement of midnight cortisol is uninformative. If the 9 AM cortisol is less than 150 nmol/L, the diagnosis of adrenal insufficiency is made, and if greater than 450 nmol/L, the patient is normal. For values in between, adrenal reserve should be assessed by measuring plasma cortisol before the intramuscular administration of 250 μg tetracosactrin (synthetic $ACTH_{1-24}$) and then 30 minutes after. If secondary adrenal insufficiency is suspected, central mechanisms need assessing. Although the insulin-induced hypoglycemia test is still the gold standard for younger patients, and indeed, has been used successfully in the elderly,[42] there are serious hazards attending its use. If the 9 AM plasma cortisol is not greater than 180 nmol/L, if there is a history of epilepsy, or if there is a significant risk of ischemic heart disease (surely present in all elderly patients), the test is contraindicated.

Alternative tests have been suggested, including several varieties of the metyrapone (Metopirone) test. This drug blocks the 11-hydroxylase enzyme, which is a crucial step in cortisol biosynthesis. If negative-feedback mechanisms are intact, metyrapone provokes enhanced ACTH secretion, which drives adrenal synthesis of 11-desoxycortisol. In the classic version, the adrenal response is measured by urinary 17-oxogenic steroid excretion,[43,44] but altered production of urinary metabolites in old age plus the nonstandardized assays used for the measurements diminish the value of this approach. Other investigators have proposed measurement of the plasma 11-desoxycortisol response, but this, too, has not been fully validated, especially in the elderly age group.[45–47] Finally, it has been proposed that the ACTH level should be directly monitored, and this has been evaluated in a geriatric population.[48] The difficulties of ACTH measurements are many, standardization nonexistent, and the assay is costly and not widely available; thus as a practical test this version does not bear further consideration. Most importantly, it does not assess what one needs to know: the capacity to secrete cortisol adequately in the face of stress. It is popular in North America, but for reasons of tradition rather than sound science.

A test by which contrast has much to recommend is the glucagon stimulation test. In the most widely used version, 1 mg of glucagon is injected subcutaneously and blood samples then taken basally at 90 minutes and thereafter at 30-minute intervals up to 240 minutes. As with the insulin test, the patient fasts overnight. There is no correlation between the cortisol response (or growth hormone response, because it is a reliable test of reserve of this hormone) and blood glucose changes. The diagnostic power of the test closely approaches the insulin stress test.[49] Glucagon is, however, safe to use even in the presence of heart disease and in epilepsy. The length of sampling period is dictated by the variable time taken to reach peak cortisol secretion—this adds inconvenience and expense. The use of intramuscular glucagon has been a simpler, more reliable version requiring samples only at 0, 150, and 180 minutes.[50] It is a more reliable test than the short synacthen test when compared with the insulin tolerance test as the reference.[51] As with the insulin tolerance test, a peak plasma cortisol of 550 nmol/L or higher is regarded as a satisfactory response to glucagon.

Another useful aid in distinguishing primary and secondary hypoadrenalism is the long ACTH-stimulation test using depot tetracosactrin 1 mg intramuscularly and sampling at 0, 30, and 60 minutes as with the short test, but taking further samples at 4, 8, 16, and 24 hours.[52] The atrophied adrenals following ACTH deficiency can usually be stimulated, albeit subnormally, over this time span—in contrast to the flat response in Addison's disease.

Glucocorticoid excess. Adrenal hyperfunction usually means cortisol excess or Cushing's syndrome. Conventional methods of investigation are employed first to establish the presence of the syndrome. The 24-hour urine-free cortisol is a simple and reliable test.[53,54] Its value derives from the fact that at normal levels of plasma, cortisol is much bound to a high-affinity cortisol-binding globulin (CBG). The free cortisol level (though thought to be the biologically active fraction) is generally small, and is readily excreted in the urine. Because the capacity of CBG is limited, and saturated with even minor degrees of cortisol hypersecretion, there tends to be a nonlinear and marked rise in urinary-free cortisol. The overnight dexamethasone suppression test is much used, but also much criticized for unacceptable error rates.[55] If a patient is genuinely thought to have Cushing's syndrome, inpatient investigation is usually required. The low-dose dexamethasone test (0.5 mg orally taken strictly every 6 hours for 48 hours) and high-dose dexamethasone test (2 mg every 6 hours for 48 hours) were originally described in terms of suppression of urinary cortisol metabolites and proved useful in the differential diagnosis of pituitary-dependent Cushing's syndrome from other causes of the syndrome, namely adrenal tumors (benign and carcinoma) and ectopic ACTH secretion from a wide variety of neoplasms.[56] More commonly, the plasma cortisol response is relied upon these days.[57] The basis of this test is that in Cushing's syndrome the pituitary lesion, most commonly a microadenoma only a few millimeters in diameter, is not truly autonomous, but shows blunted suppression of ACTH secretion, especially with high-dose dexamethasone. The plasma cortisol is an accurate index of ACTH secretion because its measurement is not affected by the concomitant presence of dexamethasone. (This useful property of dexamethasone can be used to assess adrenal reserve in seriously ill patients with suspected Addison's disease in whom glucocorticoid therapy may need to be given empirically, and the cortisol response to tetracosactrin assessed at the same time to establish diagnosis.) There is increasing use of synthetic CRH, either of ovine or human composition.[58,59] Though many investigators find this a helpful and safe test, as with all tests used in Cushing's syndrome it is not infallible.[60] Nevertheless, it is useful to know that there is a preservation of response in the healthy elderly population.[33]

In cases of adrenal carcinoma it is not unusual to have mixed patterns of steroid excess. Virilization in women is not uncommon, and plasma testosterone is raised. A striking rise in dehydroepiandrosterone sulfate is characteristic of adrenal carcinoma,[61] and this large production of a weak androgen may greatly raise the urinary 17-oxosteroid excretion.[62]

Mineralocorticoids. The mineralocorticoid status can be monitored by measurement of plasma aldosterone and also plasma renin activity both lying and standing (if clinically possible). The latter measurement of renin requires prior consultation with the laboratory so that rapid handling can be arranged to prevent artefactual results. Primary hyperaldosteronism is very uncommon in the elderly population and is diagnosed by raised aldosterone and suppressed plasma renin activity in hypertensive patients who usually exhibit hypokalemic alkalosis. The much more frequent occurrence of secondary hyperaldosteronism is indicative of disease outside the adrenals, such as renal artery stenosis, cardiac failure, or hepatic cirrhosis leading to raised renin, driving the normal zona glomerulosa to secrete high levels of aldosterone.

Hyporeninemic hypoaldosteronism occurs predominantly in the elderly population and is characterized by hyperkalemia, a hyperchloremic metabolic acidosis, and moderate hyponatremia. It is more common in men, and is often associated with diabetes mellitus, particularly in the presence of autonomic failure or renal impairment. It is aggravated by potassium-sparing diuretics, β-blockers, and nonsteroidal anti-inflammatory drugs.[63]

Imaging techniques in adrenal disease. The adrenal glands are readily visualized using CT scanning, especially if the patient is at all obese. Ultrasound can be useful, but is much less valuable than CT.[65] There is growing experience with magnetic resonance imaging (MRI), which may provide an indication of the likely functional status of any lesion. However, potential pitfalls arise with the exquisite sensitivity but nonspecificity of this and advanced CT scanning techniques.[64]

There remains a small role for isotopic scintigraphy in the diagnosis of adrenal hyperfunction, perhaps more for extra-adrenal or bilateral pheochromocytomas using metaiodobenzylguanidine than the use of selenocholesterol or its variants in Cushing's and Conn's syndromes.[66] Angiography is invasive, but much less so with the advent of digital venous imaging (DVI), which can be useful in adrenal disease. The pituitary may require imaging in Cushing's disease—often the tiny size of the tumor defies even the latest generation CT scanners,[67] but it does seem that MRI with gadolinium enhancement offers a slight edge.[68] In cases of hypopituitarism, CT scanning may be valuable.

As a final resort, venous sampling under radiographic control may be useful in the diagnosis of adrenal, pituitary, or ectopic sites of hormone production.[69] This approach in the elderly patient should be undertaken only if, after the most careful consideration, a balance of cost-benefit factors points inescapably in this direction. In practice this will rarely be the case.

CLINICAL PATTERNS OF ADRENAL DISORDERS

The patterns of adrenal disease do not differ greatly in the elderly population from those in younger adults. Because these are well-described in standard textbooks of clinical medicine and endocrinology, full descriptions will not be given here in all cases. Instead, emphasis will be placed on points particularly relevant to an elderly person.

Adrenal insufficiency

Primary adrenal failure (Addison's disease) characteristically begins insidiously with nonspecific symptoms, although gastrointestinal features, including weight loss, are often prominent, and in the elderly person functional status may be diminished.[70] Though the characteristic ACTH-mediated pigmentation is a useful feature if present, it is occasionally absent.[71] A large survey suggested that in elderly patients Addison's disease was not only more likely to be tuberculous than in younger patients, but likely to prove fatal and the diagnosis be made at post mortem.[72] Other rarer causes of adrenal failure, such as hemorrhage and amyloid, should be borne in mind.[73]

Though metastases are commonly found in the adrenal glands, they only exceptionally compromise cortisol secretion.[74] The therapeutic dividend from diagnosing Addison's disease is so great that the cortisol response to tetracosactrin should be assessed at the slightest suspicion. It is emphatically not necessary for the electrolytes to be disturbed or random cortisol to be "subnormal" for the significant adrenal insufficiency to be present. Secondary adrenal insufficiency is considered later.

Cushing's syndrome and adrenal carcinomas

Cushing's syndrome is rare in elderly people. It is most frequently due to ectopic ACTH production, usually by small-cell carcinoma of the lung, but these patients typically have cachexia and profound hypokalemia, rather than the characteristic cushingoid appearance. If due to pituitary-dependent disease, transsphenoidal surgery may be considered because it causes little constitutional disturbance. Nevertheless, in mild cases medical treatment with metyrapone alone may suffice and be more appropriate. This mode of treatment is certainly appropriate with other forms of Cushing's syndrome, such as ectopic ACTH secretion. The mixed picture of Cushing's syndrome and virilization in adrenal carcinoma may be difficult to recognize: the hirsuties and thinning of capital hair may be much more prominent than the features of cortisol excess (Figure 89-1). Indeed, the main features of Cushing's syndrome may be skin atrophy and fragility with spontaneous bruising. Obesity and plethora may be conspicuously absent. In the elderly person certain features are more marked, particularly impaired cognitive function, myopathy, osteoporosis, and diabetes. Hypokalemia is common in all forms of Cushing's syndrome other than pituitary-dependent, although a patient with the nodular hyperplasia variety of Cushing's disease was diagnosed following an admission precipitated by an acute diarrheal illness in which the plasma potassium fell to 1.2 mmol/L. Subclinical Cushing's syndrome is increasingly being

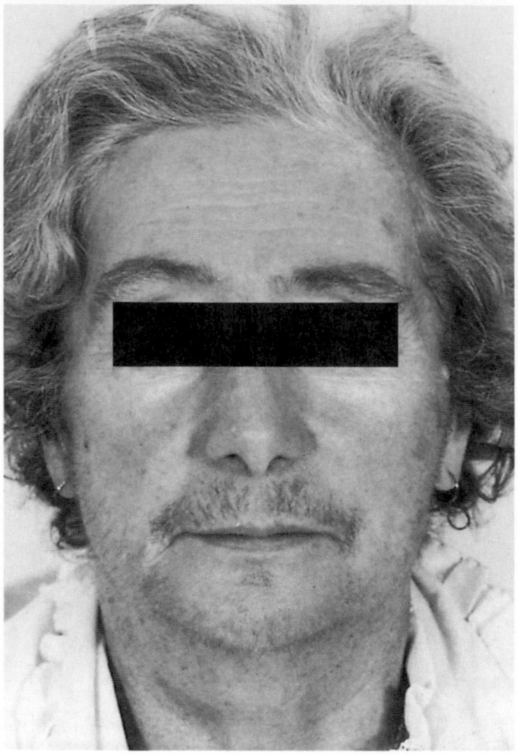

Figure 89-1. Patient with a metastasizing adrenal carcinoma causing virilization and Cushing's syndrome. Note hirsuties, slight scalp recession, but absence of cushingoid facies.

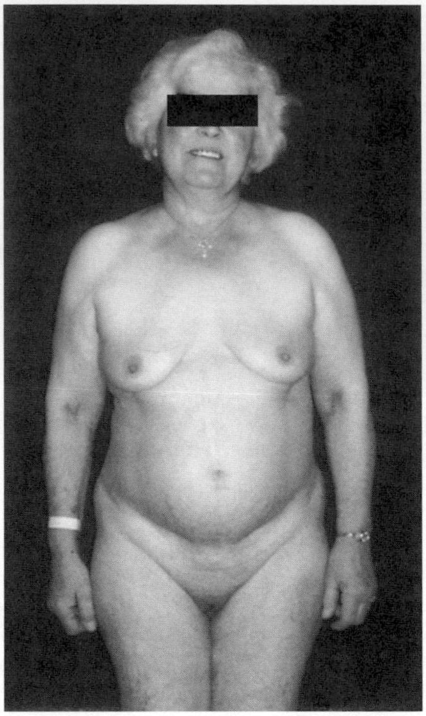

Figure 89-2. Patient with adrenal carcinoma causing Cushing's syndrome and feminization.

recognized in cases of adrenal incidentaloma (see later discussion) and is associated with increased cardiovascular risk.[75,76]

Adrenal carcinomas may occasionally secrete estrogen. This was retrospectively recognized in a youthful looking elderly woman with Cushing's syndrome (Figure 89-2) following removal of her large adrenal tumor (Figure 89-3) when she had a brisk vaginal blood loss. Rescue of preoperative urine specimens revealed high estrogen levels. Treatment is primarily surgical unless there are widespread metastases. The use of opDDD is probably helpful, but may be associated with severe side effects, in which case it should not be persevered with.[77]

Iatrogenic glucocorticoid excess

The most common cause of Cushing's syndrome in an elderly person is the exogenous administration of steroids for a variety of medical disorders. The side effects of steroid therapy, often aggravating preexisting problems, are usually more marked in the elderly group. Particular problems include decreased cognitive function, emotional lability, and dysphoria; osteoporotic fractures; myopathy and muscle wasting with limitation of mobility; skin fragility; and impaired glucose tolerance. Furthermore, patients on maintenance steroids (>10 mg prednisolone daily or equivalent for more than 2 weeks) are at risk of adrenal insufficiency in the event of intercurrent illness, and the daily steroid dose should be doubled for at least 3 days in these circumstances.

Incidentalomas

Last, but very far from least, is the vexed problem of what to do with a patient who for usually quite unrelated reasons has an abdominal ultrasound or CT scan that reveals an

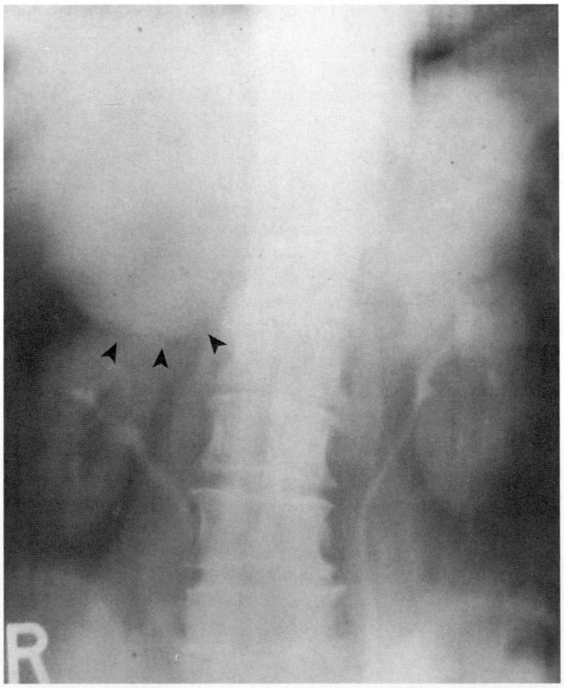

Figure 89-3. Intravenous pyelogram, showing large right-sided adrenal mass depressing the right kidney.

unsuspected adrenal mass.[78,79] Because about 20% of adrenocortical carcinomas are nonfunctioning in the absence of any clinical endocrine syndrome, it is probably prudent to repeat the scans at intervals, particularly for lesions greater than 3 cm diameter, since lesions progressing to greater than 6 cm diameter are almost always malignant. However, the problem must be kept in proportion. Adrenal cancer is rare, with an annual incidence approximately two per million.[80] Autopsy studies show that benign nodules are extremely common, especially with advancing age, and particularly in hypertensives.[81] Most are microscopic, but lesions of greater than 1 cm are found in approximately 1% of patients undergoing abdominal CT.[82] Clearly, there is a need for biochemical screening to exclude pheochromocytoma, Conn's, and also Cushing's syndrome. Hypertension and hypokalemia are particularly good indicators of functioning lesions. It has been estimated that the frequency of these conditions in 100,000 patients with an adrenal incidentaloma would be 6500 pheochromocytomas, 7000 Conn's syndrome, and only 35 Cushing's syndrome. However, subclinical cortisol hypersecretion has been reported in up to 25% of patients with adrenal tumors incidentally discovered on CT in a number of studies.[83,84] Cumulative worldwide experience indicates that most adrenal incidentalomas are benign, but a significant number are malignant, especially large lesions, and in patients with a history of malignancy.[85,86] Late diagnosis of genetic disorders can occur in the elderly including pheochromocytoma in the proband of a family with MEN2a, a woman aged 73;[87] and an 88-year-old woman with congenital adrenal hyperplasia, due to 21-hydroxylase deficiency, presenting with adrenal insufficiency.[88]

PITUITARY DISORDERS

Pituitary tumors

Pituitary tumors are increasingly uncommon in the elderly population, with the exception of nonfunctioning (null-cell) adenomas, which increase in incidence over the age of 50. These tumors have local complications—usually due to compression of the optic chiasm causing bitemporal hemianopia, or more rarely due to invasion into surrounding structures, such as the cavernous sinus—or features of hypopituitarism (see later discussion). Functioning pituitary tumors are associated with the characteristic syndromes of hormone excess, notably, acromegaly and Cushing's disease, and behave in a similar fashion to tumors in younger patients, although it has been suggested that the somatotroph adenomas causing acromegaly are more benign in the elderly person, and thus medical therapy could be considered as a first-line option.[89] However, advances in neurosurgical techniques mean that almost all tumors can be at least debulked by the transsphenoidal approach; the relative simplicity and low morbidity and mortality of this procedure make it the treatment of choice for even the very elderly patient, especially one having visual field defects.[90–95]

Other sellar lesions are very rare, although two occur more commonly in the elderly. Pituitary metastases may present like nonfunctioning tumors. Pituitary incidentalomas-adenomas, usually less than 1 cm in diameter, without clinical sequelae, may be identified on a CT or MRI scan performed for other indications in the same way as adrenal incidentalomas and have a prevalence of up to 10% in the over-80 age group, but intervention is not required in such cases.

Hypopituitarism

Hypopituitarism may be caused by pituitary adenoma as in younger age groups. A valuable clue in postmenopausal women is finding inappropriately low gonadotrophin levels, although it has been reported that these can be depressed in nonspecific illness in the extremely elderly.[48] More important, because subtler and more difficult to diagnose, is idiopathic hypopituitarism, in which the pituitary fossa is normal in size. Key features may be orthostatic hypotension, hyponatremia (reflecting adrenal and thyroid insufficiency causing water overload, possibly from inappropriate ADH secretion), or hypothyroidism with inappropriately low TSH.[96–99] Computed tomography scanning may indicate a number of abnormalities ranging from a thickened pituitary stalk to empty sella.[97] Replacement therapy with hydrocortisone and thyroxine is gratifyingly effective. As with patients on steroid therapy, those patients needing replacement hydrocortisone should be advised to double the dose of hydrocortisone for 3 days with intercurrent illnesses, and they need parenteral steroids if they cannot tolerate oral medication while unwell.

Growth hormone deficiency. Growth hormone secretion declines by about 15% per decade from a peak at about 30 years of age,[100] and stimulated growth hormone secretion, using both pharmacologic agents and physiologic stimuli, such as exercise, is diminished in elderly people. This fall in growth hormone secretion is due to a decline in the frequency[101] and amplitude[102] of growth hormone pulses, probably the result of an increase in somatostatinergic tone. Furthermore, there is a decrease in circulating levels of insulin-like growth factor-I (IGF-I), the peripheral mediator of the somatic effects of growth hormone—although, in contrast to young adults, the IGF-I levels do not show as strong a correlation with 24-hour growth hormone secretion.

Some of the features of aging are similar to the characteristics of adult growth hormone deficiency, such as the decrease in lean body mass and bone mineral density, the increase in fat mass,[103] and possibly, neuropsychological sequelae and increased cardiovascular mortality.[104] The availability of recombinant growth hormone has made the treatment of adult growth hormone deficiency possible, and recently there has been interest in its effects on the healthy elderly individual. In those with low IGF-I levels, administration of growth hormone increases lean body mass, skin thickness, lumbar spine bone density, and nitrogen retention, and decreases adipose tissue. No effect was seen on bone density at other sites or on serum cholesterol, and nonsignificant increases in blood pressure and fasting glucose have been reported. Side effects of fluid retention, in some cases causing bloating or carpal tunnel syndrome, arthralgia, headaches, lethargy, and gynecomastia may occur.[105]

KEY POINTS

Adrenal and Pituitary Disorders

- Adrenal cortex produces cortisol, aldosterone, and adrenal androgens.
- Steroids act by genomic and membrane-mediated effects plus intracellular conversions.
- Clinical consequences of disordered steroid production/exposure
- Incidentally diagnosed adrenal nodules in old age
- Age-related decline in adrenal androgen and growth hormone secretion
- Diagnosis and management of pituitary disease in the elderly

At present, the only group for whom growth hormone therapy can be recommended are those with pituitary disease, requiring at least one form of pituitary hormone replacement therapy, in whom growth hormone deficiency has been demonstrated using a pharmacologic stimulation test and who have symptoms of growth hormone deficiency. Elderly patients with hypothalamic-pituitary disease and growth deficiency are distinguishable from elderly controls with respect to lipid profiles, body composition, and quality of life.[106] They respond as positively to growth hormone replacement as do younger patients.[107–110]

Isolated ACTH deficiency. Less frequent is the development of isolated ACTH deficiency. This has been seen in an octogenarian who developed frequent hypoglycemic comas associated with raised insulin levels. The clue that this was not due to an insulinoma came from the equimolar secretion of insulin and C-peptide. Replacement therapy with hydrocortisone completely abolished the hypoglycemic episodes.[111]

For a complete list of references, please visit online only at www.expertconsult.com

CHAPTER 90

Disorders of the Thyroid

Myron Miller

Although thyroid disorders occur over the entire age range, many appear to be increasingly common with advancing age. It is important to recognize that the clinical features of thyroid disease may be significantly altered in the aged individual, so that symptoms and physical findings typical in young persons may be modified, different, or absent in the elderly population.

The diagnosis of a thyroid disorder may be further influenced by the age of the patient as a consequence of normal aging-associated changes in thyroid physiology. Of great importance is the impact of nonthyroidal illnesses that frequently occur in the elderly person on many of the tests used to assess thyroid function.[1] Management may be influenced by the presence of the many coexistent medical disorders common in an aging population.

MORPHOLOGY

The normal aging process is accompanied by changes in the gross and microscopic appearance of the thyroid gland. Early studies based on autopsy data indicated that overall mass declines from the normal range of 15 to 25 g so that with increasing age a progressively larger proportion of individuals will have glands weighing less than 20 g.[2] In contrast, data obtained in recent years by ultrasound in healthy subjects reveal that aging results in little change in size of the thyroid.[3]

With advancing age, there is progressive fibrosis, the appearance of lymphocytes, a decrease in follicle size, and a reduction in the amount of colloid.[4] Although these changes are common in the elderly population, they are by no means characteristic of all aged persons. More important, there does not appear to be a decline in thyroid function concomitant to the morphologic changes, and neither weight nor histologic appearance correlate with common measures of thyroid function.[5]

Hypothalamic–pituitary–thyroid regulation

The production of thyroid hormones is regulated by the hypothalamic–pituitary–thyroid axis. Thyrotropin-releasing hormone (TRH) is synthesized in the hypothalamus and functions to stimulate release of thyroid-stimulating hormone (TSH) from the anterior pituitary by binding to receptors on the cell membrane of TSH-producing thyrotropes. Thyroid-stimulating hormone is regulated by the negative feedback of the thyroid hormones thyroxine (T4) and triiodothyronine (T3) acting on the pituitary gland.

The neuroendocrine mechanisms controlling TSH release may be altered during the normal aging process. Thus, serum TSH concentration, which undergoes circadian variation, exhibits smaller fluctuations in elderly than in young men.[6] The ability of TRH to stimulate TSH release may be affected by both the age and gender of the individual. Several studies have documented that elderly men have an impaired TSH response to TRH stimulation, with peak serum TSH values in men over the age of 60 showing approximately a 40% reduction compared with young men.[7–12] In women, however, there does not appear to be an effect of age on TSH responsiveness.[13]

The ability of the pituitary gland to synthesize TSH does not appear to be diminished by the aging process, as reflected by the observation that pituitary TSH content undergoes no significant change over the life span.[14] The 24-hour TSH secretion has been reported to be decreased in healthy elderly men,[10] but the secretion rate of TSH has also been reported to be higher in elderly subjects than in young individuals.[15] However, circulating levels of TSH remain constant with advancing age, and the elevations that are commonly seen in elderly persons must be considered as evidence for failing thyroid function.[16]

Thyroid-stimulating hormone exerts its effects by binding to the membrane of thyroid follicular cells. The response of these cells to TSH stimulation is not impaired by aging, as reflected by T4 and T3 release into the circulation following either TRH or TSH administration.[17]

Within the thyroid gland, T4 and T3 synthesis results from the trapping of iodide by follicular cells, subsequent oxidation of iodide leading to iodination of tyrosine, and coupling of two iodinated tyrosines. In the normal adult, approximately 80 μg of T4 and 30 μg of T3 are produced daily.[18] In elderly individuals, T4 and T3 production declines to approximately 60 and 20 μg per day, respectively. These changes may be related to the decrease in thyroidal iodide accumulation, which has been observed with aging.[19]

Thyroid hormone secretion and metabolism

In response to TSH stimulation, T4 and T3 stored in thyroid follicles are hydrolyzed from thyroglobulin and released into the circulation where they are bound to albumin, thyroid- binding prealbumin (TBPA), and thyroid-binding globulin (TBG), with less than 0.1% of the hormones circulating in the free form. Thyroid-binding globulin is the primary thyroid hormone transport protein, carrying about 70% of bound hormone, and its levels do not appear to differ between healthy young and old individuals.[9] A greater T4-binding capacity of TBG has been observed in the elderly population but appears to be without clinical significance.[20,21]

The small proportion of T4 and T3 in the free state (FT4 and FT3) is composed of the biologically active forms of the hormones and is responsible for peripheral thyroid hormone action and metabolism. Circulating levels of both FT4 and FT3 remain constant over the age span, and a decrease in concentration, especially FT3, should be considered a consequence of illness rather than as a result of normal aging.[9,16,17,20,22] Approximately 20% to 30% of circulating T3 is directly secreted by the thyroid gland, with the remaining 70% to 80% resulting from 5′-monodeiodination of the outer ring of T4 in peripheral tissues.[18] T4 degradation is decreased with advancing age so that, by age 90, the degradation rate is approximately 50% that of young subjects.[17,23,24] This change appears to be due to an age-related reduction in the activity of monodeiodinase enzymes in peripheral tissue.[25] T3 degradation is less affected by aging.[17,25] A consequence of these changes is a decline in T4 metabolic clearance rate and an increase in the half-life of circulating T4 from approximately 6 days in young persons to over 9 days in individuals who have reached their ninth decade.[23,24,26] Because serum T4 concentration is not affected by aging, the prolongation of T4 half-life implies that there is an aging-related decline in T4 production by the thyroid gland.

Part of T4 degradation involves 5-monodeiodination of the inner ring of the molecule and results in the generation of the biologically inactive reverse T3 (rT3).[18,27] The outer-ring 5′-monodeiodinase is sensitive to a variety of influences including starvation, febrile illness, elevation of glucocorticoid concentration, and drugs such as propranolol, amiodarone, and iodinated contrast materials.[18,28] As a result of inhibition of the enzyme activity, there is impaired T4 conversion to T3, with a decline in serum T3 concentration and a parallel rise in rT3 concentration. Serum rT3 is not affected by normal aging, and an increase must be considered to be a consequence of illness or drug-induced alteration in T4 degradation.[22,25,29]

Thyroid hormone action

The primary thyroid hormone acting on peripheral tissue and responsible for the broad range of thyroid actions is FT3. FT3 and, to a lesser amount, FT4 act on peripheral tissue cells by binding to specific nuclear receptors and subsequently affect DNA transcription, RNA formation, and new protein synthesis.[30–32] There are two T3 receptor genes, located on chromosomes 17 and 3, whose product is a group of T3 receptors.[32] Protein products coded for by the c-*erb*-A gene family, the cellular counterpart of the viral oncogene v-*erb*-A, have been demonstrated to be nuclear receptors for thyroid hormone.[33,34] At the level of the pituitary, thyroid hormone action results in inhibition of synthesis and release of TSH.[35,36]

Thyroid hormone action appears to be diminished as part of the aging process. Oxygen consumption is decreased and is reflected clinically by a decline in basal metabolic rate.[37] In aging animals, there is decreased ability to stimulate hepatic enzyme synthesis following exposure to thyroid hormone.[38] Clinical support for diminished thyroid hormone action is provided by the observation that typical features of hyperthyroidism are often absent in the elderly population of patients.

Thyroid function in advanced aging

Studies in healthy centenarians ranging in age from 100 to 110 years provide further information regarding the extent to which aging alone contributes to change in measures of thyroid function. There was no difference in serum FT4 of the centenarians as compared to both healthy elderly (aged 65 to 80 years) and healthy younger adults (aged 20 to 64 years), but serum FT3 was reduced in the centenarians. Serum TSH was also lower in the centenarians, and for the older groups as a whole there was an inverse relationship between serum TSH and age. Serum rT3 was increased in the centenarians, suggesting that there was reduced outer-ring deiodination of T4. Thus, in healthy aging persons, thyroid function was preserved into the eighth decade, whereas advanced old age was associated with reduced thyroid activity that was likely to be due to a decrease in TSH secretion and impairment of peripheral 5′-deiodination.[1,39]

ASSESSMENT OF THYROID FUNCTION

Circulating thyroid hormones

Screening of the secretory status of the thyroid gland can be accomplished by measurement in the blood of TSH, total circulating T4 and T3 concentrations, and FT4 and FT3 concentrations through use of radioimmunoassay or immunometric assays.[12] The development of "super sensitive" immunoassays for TSH have allowed differentiation of normal from suppressed levels of the hormone so that this single measurement can provide evidence supporting a diagnosis of primary hypothyroidism, secondary hypothyroidism, or hyperthyroidism.[40–42] It now appears that this assay may be the best initial test of thyroid function in evaluating patients for suspected under- or overactivity of the thyroid gland.[40] Although it has been suggested that the generally accepted value of 5 mU/L as the upper limit of normal for the adult population may actually be as high as 10 mU/L in individuals who have reached their eighth decade, it is more likely that TSH values between 5 and 10 mU/L indicate mild thyroid dysfunction.[42]

Total and free concentrations of T4 and T3 are commonly used to document the status of thyroid secretory activity. It appears to be well supported that the normal range for these hormones is unaffected by aging and that deviations from normal must be considered as evidence for thyroid disease or for other illness or states that may affect hormone measurement.[16,17,20,22,25,43]

Serum-free T4 is best measured by equilibrium dialysis[44,45] or more easily by the use of T4-specific antibodies.[46,47] Less reliable estimates of FT4 concentration can be obtained from the FT4 index, which involves measurement of both total T4 and a measure of thyroid hormone-binding protein capacity such as the T3 resin uptake.

Low T4 states

In addition to the expected reduction in total T4 seen in primary or secondary hypothyroidism, total T4 may be low because of a variety of other causes. Levels of TBPA may be acutely lowered in the presence of infectious disease, protein-wasting states, surgery, and malnutrition with accompanying decline in total T4. More important, TBG levels can be depressed as a result of X-linked congenital deficiency, severe catabolic illness, chronic hepatic disease, glucocorticoids, and androgen administration.[48] Binding of T4 to TBG can be inhibited by drugs such as furosemide and high-dose salicylates.[49] The anticonvulsants carbamazepine and phenytoin can reduce serum T4 by stimulating an increase in hepatic enzyme metabolizing activity.[49] In from 20% to 74% of patients with nonthyroidal illness, an inhibitor of T4 binding to TBG has been detected, which may contribute to the measurement of a low T4 in these patients.[48,50]

The finding of a low T4 concentration in the presence of nonthyroidal illness has been termed the *euthyroid sick syndrome*.[51] In mild to moderate forms, measurement of FT4 will be normal even though total T4 concentration is reduced.[45,48] However, severe illness can result in marked reduction of both total and free T4 concentrations. When this circumstance occurs, the prognosis of the patient is poor with a mortality rate of approximately 80% having been reported.[52] The ability to differentiate these patients from those with hypothyroidism can be difficult.[53] Although serum TSH is usually in the normal range, occasionally mild to moderately elevated concentrations are found. This is especially true in the recovery phase of the illness when values can rise to as high as 20 mU/L. Within 4 to 20 weeks after clinical recovery, all measures of thyroid function usually will have returned to normal.[54]

Low T3 states

The serum concentration of total T3 is easily affected by many nonthyroidal illnesses, and low values are often seen in elderly ill patients, giving rise to the "low T3 syndrome." This consequence of systemic illness is the earliest and most common of the alterations in thyroid hormone levels.[16,17,28,43,48,53,55,56] In response to many acute illnesses, there is decreased peripheral 5′-monodeiodination of T4 to T3 with consequent reduction in serum T3 concentration and increase in serum rT3. Lowering of TBPA and TBG in the presence of acute and chronic illness further contributes to the marked fall in serum T3 characteristic of the sick elderly person. Often, the possibility of a diagnosis of hypothyroidism is raised and can usually be excluded by the absence of an increase in TSH and by the demonstration of normal or increased serum levels of rT3.

Cytokines such as interleukin-1, interleukin-6, and tumor necrosis factor (TNF) could be involved as intermediaries in the development of low T4 and T3 states. Many patients with nonthyroidal illnesses and low T4 or T3 also have elevated serum concentrations of cytokines.[57,58] Experimental increase of TNF-α has been observed to induce low serum concentrations of T4, T3, and TSH.[59]

High T4 states

Although less common than low thyroid hormone states, nonthyroidal factors can result in elevation of serum T4 concentration.[53,60] A euthyroid increase in total T4 can occur as a result of overproduction of TBG, a disorder that may be familial.[61] More commonly, TBG increases because of therapy with estrogen or tamoxifen or as a transient acute-phase reactant during acute hepatocellular injury. In these circumstances, serum-free T4 will be normal. On occasion, mild to moderate levels of illness can increase FT4 in the patient with euthyroid sick syndrome as a result of impaired T4 monodeiodination by peripheral tissues.[48,51]

Thyrotropin-releasing hormone test

The response of serum TSH to exogenously administered TRH is a useful method of assessing the dynamics of the pituitary–thyroid axis. In the normal individual, the bolus intravenous administration of 500 μg TRH results in a prompt rise in serum TSH, with peak values achieved in 30 minutes.[7,8] The minimal normal response should be an increase of greater than 2 mU/L over the basal value, with many normal subjects reaching peak concentrations up to 30 mU/L.[12] As previously stated, many elderly males respond less well to TRH stimulation than do younger subjects or women at all ages.[7–13] Failure to respond to TRH supports a diagnosis of hyperthyroidism, whereas a normal response excludes the diagnosis. Subnormal responses may be seen in patients with severe illness, depression, or hypercortisolism as well as in euthyroid patients with thyroid adenomas or multinodular goiter. An exaggerated response of serum TSH is characteristic of primary hypothyroidism.[42]

Measures of iodine uptake

The ability of the thyroid gland to trap iodide and other ions such as technetium (Tc) has been the basis for assessment of both thyroid gland function and morphology. The oral administration of ^{131}I to normal individuals results in an accumulation of 5% to 25% of the dose in the gland by 24 hours.[62,63] Because of considerable overlap between normal and hypothyroid subjects, low values for 24-hour ^{131}I uptake are of lesser diagnostic usefulness in establishing a diagnosis of hypothyroidism. Further, exposure to increased amounts of iodide in the diet or to iodine-containing drugs or radiographic contrast media result in a marked reduction of ^{131}I uptake. Elevated values are useful in supporting a diagnosis of hyperthyroidism, although some elderly patients with toxic nodules may have 24-hour ^{131}I uptake values within the normal range. The 24-hour ^{131}I uptake is usually obtained in a patient with an established diagnosis of hyperthyroidism in order to calculate the dose of ^{131}I to be given for ablation therapy.

Thyroid scanning with ^{99m}Tc, or now more commonly with ^{123}I, is useful in the evaluation of the patient with a palpable single thyroid nodule where demonstration of activity within the nodule markedly reduces the likelihood of the nodule representing an area of malignancy. In the elderly hyperthyroid patient, scanning can be used to differentiate a diffusely overactive thyroid from the gland with single or multiple toxic nodules.[64]

Other thyroid imaging procedures

Currently available imaging techniques can provide high-quality anatomic detailing of thyroid structure, including real-time ultrasonography, computed tomography (CT), and magnetic resonance imaging (MRI). These procedures can be useful in evaluating patients with single and multiple nodules by identifying cysts, areas of hemorrhage, and tissue calcification. Ultrasonography may be of value in determining which regions of the thyroid are most appropriate for fine-needle aspiration. Both CT and MRI are expensive and have few clinical indications at present, but they may be of occasional value in assessing the extent of tracheal compression by a thyroid mass, in determining the extent of substernal goiters, and in determining the extent of local invasion or metastasis by thyroid cancers.[65]

Antithyroid antibodies

Many thyroid disorders, including hyperthyroidism of the Graves' disease type[66] and hypothyroidism of the Hashimoto type, are believed to be the result of autoimmune disease.[12,67] As a consequence, high levels of serum antibodies to both thyroglobin and to microsomes are commonly found in patients with thyroid disease. Low levels of antithyroglobulin antibody (titer less than 1:100) may be present in patients without clinical signs of a thyroid disorder. Moderate to high titers (1:1600 to 1:25,600) can be found in patients with nonthyroid autoimmune disorders.[12]

Thyroid antibodies in the serum increase in incidence progressively with increasing age, reaching a peak incidence of 20% to 25% in women above the age of 50 years and 5% to 10% in similarly aged men.[68,69] However, in a highly selected population of healthy elderly individuals ranging from 65 to 110 years, the prevalence of antithyroid antibodies was low and did not differ from the prevalence in healthy young persons.[1] This finding suggests that the high incidence of antithyroid antibodies in aging populations is a reflection of disease and is not a consequence of normal aging. In many patients, the findings of high-serum antithyroglobulin or antimicrosomal antibody titers are accompanied by an elevation of basal serum TSH concentration and reduced levels of serum T4, suggesting the presence of an autoimmune thyroiditis and a failing thyroid gland.[70]

From a diagnostic standpoint, high titers of antithyroid antibodies are commonly found in patients with documented hypothyroidism and suggest a diagnosis of chronic lymphocytic or Hashimoto's thyroiditis. In patients with hyperthyroidism, elevated antithyroglobulin and antimicrosomal antibody titers are more characteristic of patients with Graves' disease than of those with toxic nodules.

Thyroid-stimulating immunoglobulins

Thyroid-stimulating activity similar to that of TSH can be found in the IgG portion of serum obtained from many patients with hyperthyroidism resulting from Graves' disease. These immunoglobulins have been demonstrated to be antibodies directed against the TSH receptor.[66] Thyroid-stimulating immunoglobulins can be detected by both radioreceptor assays utilizing radiolabeled TSH and by bioassay based on stimulation of cyclic AMP release from isolated thyroid cell cultures.[71–75] Both methods reveal positive tests for TSH receptor antibodies in over 85% of patients with untreated Graves' disease and in essentially 100% of patients with severe Graves' ophthalmopathy. Positive tests are infrequent in Hashimoto's disease and rare in nodular thyroid disease, including toxic nodular goiter. Monitoring of antibody levels may be useful in predicting the likelihood of sustained remission in patients with Graves' disease who are treated with antithyroid drugs.[76]

Serum thyroglobulin

Thyroglobulin involved in intrathyroidal synthesis of T4 and T3 can gain entry to the circulation where it can be detected in normal individuals at low levels by means of immunometric assays.[77] Many elderly people have circulating antithyroglobulin antibodies, which can interfere with accurate estimation of thyroglobulin concentration. Normal individuals have been found to have serum concentrations of thyroglobulin of less than 5 μg/L and levels appear to be unaffected by age. Concentrations can be increased in patients with hyperthyroidism, benign nodules, and inflammatory disorders, such as subacute thyroiditis. High levels are found in the majority of patients with thyroid cancer.

In patients with thyroid cancer previously treated by surgical or radioiodine ablation, measurement of serum thyroglobulin appears to be a sensitive indicator of tumor recurrence, either locally or by metastases. However, caution must be observed in interpreting blood levels because elevations above normal can be found in patients whose ablation has not been complete and have been left with small remnants of nonmalignant thyroid tissue.[77]

SCREENING FOR THYROID DYSFUNCTION

Disorders of thyroid function become increasingly common with advancing age and include both overt and subclinical hyperthyroidism and hypothyroidism (discussed later). As a consequence, a number of organizations have recommended that screening for thyroid dysfunction be initiated in the general population as a means of early detection of altered thyroid function. The American College of Physicians has recommended that women over the age of 50 should have serum TSH testing followed by measurement of free thyroxine if the TSH level is undetectable or greater than 10 mU/L.[78,79] The American Academy of Family Physicians recommends that thyroid function be measured periodically in all older women. The American Thyroid Association has published guidelines for the detection of thyroid dysfunction, which recommend that all adults, both men and women, be screened with measurement of serum TSH starting at age 35 and then repeated every 5 years thereafter, with more frequent screening for individuals who may be at higher risk of developing thyroid dysfunction.[80] Other organizations have not recommended routine screening of asymptomatic persons.

HYPERTHYROIDISM

Overproduction of thyroid hormone leads to the clinical condition of hyperthyroidism. This disorder, also referred to as thyrotoxicosis, is accompanied by a broad array of symptoms and signs that can differ markedly between young and old patients.

Demography

In the past, hyperthyroidism was regarded as a disorder with preferential expression in young to middle-aged individuals, especially women. It is now clear that this disorder is also common in the elderly population.[78] The proportion of patients with hyperthyroidism who are over 60 years of age is estimated to be 15% to 20%.[81,82–85] Many studies confirm that hyperthyroidism is far more common in women than men, with estimates of female preponderance ranging from 4:1 to as high as 10:1.[81,84,86]

Etiology

In young persons, Graves' disease remains the most common cause of hyperthyroidism and is the consequence of thyroid receptor antibodies, which have stimulatory effects on the thyroid gland.[66,72,74,75] With increasing age, there is a change in etiology so that more cases are due to multinodular toxic goiter and fewer to Graves' disease.[81,87] It is estimated that more than 50% of hyperthyroid patients over the age of 60 years have thyroxicosis resulting from multinodular toxic goiters. Multinodular goiters are common in the elderly population and may not be clinically apparent.[5] Many clinical observations support the concept that long-standing euthyroid multinodular goiters may undergo change to become overproductive of thyroid hormones[81] (Table 90-1).

Another less common cause of hyperthyroidism in the elderly population is toxic adenoma (Plummer's disease), usually identifiable on thyroid scanning by the demonstration

Table 90-1. Etiology of Hyperthyroidism and Hypothyroidism in the Elderly Population

Hyperthyroidism	Hypothyroidism
Toxic multinodular goiter	Autoimmune disease
Graves' disease	Radioiodine or surgical thyroid ablation
Toxic adenoma	Hypothalamic/pituitary disease
Exogenous thyroid hormone	Iodine-induced
Subacute thyroiditis (early)	Iodine deficiency
Iodine-induced	Subacute thyroiditis (late)
	Inborn disorder of thyroid hormone synthesis

of a solitary hyperfunctioning nodule with suppression of activity in the remainder of the thyroid gland.[88,89] Hyperthyroidism can occur in a previously euthyroid person following ingestion of iodide or iodine-containing substances (the Jod Basedow phenomenon). This is usually a self-limiting disorder lasting several weeks to several months.[90] Most commonly, this occurs following exposure to iodinated radiocontrast agents and to amiodarone.[91] Up to 40% of persons taking amiodarone will have serum T4 levels above the normal range, but only about 5% will develop clinical hyperthyroidism.[92] Amiodarone is fat-soluble and has a long half-life, so drug-induced hyperthyroidism can be prolonged and difficult to treat.[93,94]

The possibility of hyperthyroidism must always be considered in the elderly person who is receiving thyroid hormone, especially if the dose is greater than 0.15 mg of L-thyroxine daily. Patients who have received such doses for many years without evidence for hyperthyroidism may insidiously develop features of hyperthyroidism as they age past 60 years because of age-associated slowing in thyroid hormone metabolism.[95]

Rare causes of hyperthyroidism in the elderly population include TSH-producing pituitary tumors[96,97] and ectopic TSH production by nonpituitary tumors. These can be recognized by the finding of unsuppressed levels of serum TSH in the presence of increased amounts of circulating thyroid hormone. An additional uncommon cause of hyperthyroidism is overproduction of thyroid hormone by metastatic follicular carcinoma.

Transient hyperthyroidism may occur in patients with subacute thyroiditis as a result of increased discharge of thyroid hormone into the circulation during the inflammatory phase of the illness.[98] In a similar fashion, radiation injury to the thyroid can be accompanied by transient increase in circulating thyroid hormone levels with associated symptoms.

T3 TOXICOSIS

In a small proportion of cases of hyperthyroidism, measurement of serum thyroid hormone concentrations result in the expected increase in serum T3, but with the finding that serum T4 is within the normal range, although often at the upper end. This circumstance has been designated as *T3 toxicosis* and can occur with any type of hyperthyroidism, but it is found more commonly in patients with toxic multinodular goiter or solitary toxic adenoma.[89] The diagnosis will not be missed if T3 is measured in patients with clinically suspected hyperthyroidism who do not demonstrate elevated levels of serum T4 or free T4.

Clinical presentation of hyperthyroidism

As with other disorders occurring in the elderly person, the clinical presentation of hyperthyroidism often differs from the classic description of the disease in younger individuals[81,82,99–101] (Table 90-2). Presenting features may be progressive functional decline, including weakness, fatigue, changes in mental status, loss of appetite, weight loss, cardiac arrhythmia, and congestive heart failure. A symptom complex peculiar to the geriatric hyperthyroid patient is "apathetic hyperthyroidism," in which the patient lacks the hyperactivity, irritability, and restlessness common to the young patient with thyrotoxicosis and presents instead with weakness, lethargy, listlessness, depression, weight loss, and the appearance of a chronic, wasting illness. Often, the initial impression in such patients is that of depression, malignancy, or cardiovascular disease.[102,103]

The elderly patient with Graves' disease often differs from younger patients in the nature and severity of expected classic symptoms and in physical findings. Clinically detectable thyroid enlargement, present in almost all younger patients, is absent in as many as 37% of elderly patients.[81] Infiltrative ophthalmopathy with severe proptosis and exophthalmos occur infrequently in the elderly group. Thus, none of the elements of the classic triad of Graves' disease (clinical hyperthyroidism, diffuse goiter, and infiltrative ophthalmopathy) may be recognizable in the elderly patient in whom the diagnosis may be suspected only on the basis of laboratory studies.[81,99,100]

Several reports have attempted to compare symptoms and objective physical findings in young and elderly patients with hyperthyroidism. Symptoms less commonly present in the elderly group include nervousness, increased sweating, tremor, increased appetite, and increased frequency of bowel movements. Symptoms more common include marked weight loss (present in over 80% of patients), poor appetite, worsening angina, edema, agitation, and confusion. Similarly, physical findings differ in elderly patients. In addition to absence of palpable goiter and eye signs of exophthalmos, pulse rate is slower, and reflexes are often not hyperreflexic. Cardiac arrhythmias, especially atrial fibrillation and ventricular premature beats, are more common. Lid lag and lid retraction are frequently seen.[81,99–104]

The spectrum of symptoms and findings that result from thyroid hormone excess is broad and can involve almost all body systems. Of special concern in the elderly are the impacts of hyperthyroidism on the cardiovascular system. Thyroid hormones act on the myocardium to sensitize the heart to β-adrenergic stimulation with resultant increase in heart rate, stroke volume, cardiac output, left ventricular mass, ejection fraction and shortened left ventricular ejection time.[104–106] These changes underlie the clinical consequences of increased systolic blood pressure, widened pulse pressure, palpitations, tachycardia, increased risk of atrial fibrillation, often with a slow ventricular response, exacerbation of angina in patients with preexisting coronary artery disease, and precipitation of congestive heart failure, which responds less readily to digoxin treatment owing to increased renal clearance of the drug.

Echocardiographic data further define the cardiac changes in hyperthyroidism. Specifically, it has been demonstrated that diastolic function is enhanced as evidenced by increased

Table 90-2. Frequency of Symptoms and Signs of Hyperthyroidism

	Kawabe et al[99] (%)	Davis and Davis[81] (%)	
	Young Elderly	Elderly	
Symptom/sign	($n = 48$)	($n = 45$)	($n = 85$)
Palpitation	100	60	63
Goiter	98	58	64
Tremor	96	71	55
Excessive perspiration	92	66	38
Weight loss	73	85	69
Eye signs	71	28	57
Arrhythmias (atrial fibrillation and ventricular premature contractions [VPC])	4.6	16.4	62

From Griffin MA, Solomon DH. Hyperthyroidism in the elderly. J Am Geriatr Soc 1986;34:887–92.

isovolumic relaxation and left ventricular filling in hyperthyroid patients.[107] These alterations in hemodynamic parameters may explain many of the cardiovascular signs and symptoms of hyperthyroidism and many of the cardiac complications associated with hyperthyroidism, including decreased exercise tolerance and increased risk of congestive heart failure.

Gastrointestinal consequences of hyperthyroidism in an elderly person include weight loss, poor appetite, and occasionally abdominal pain, nausea, and vomiting.[81,82] Diarrhea and increased frequency of bowel movements resulting from thyroid hormone action on intestinal motility can occur but are often absent in the elderly in whom constipation is likely to be present. Hepatic actions of thyroid hormone can lead to alterations in liver enzymes, including elevation of alkaline phosphatase and γ-glutamyl transpeptidase levels, which return to normal following restoration of thyroid function to normal.

Weakness, especially of the proximal muscles, is a major feature of hyperthyroidism in elderly patients and is often accompanied by muscle wasting.[81,103] As a consequence, disorders of gait, postural instability, and falls can be significant symptoms. Tremor occurs in more than 70% of elderly thyrotoxic patients, but this sign must be distinguished from other causes of tremor common in the elderly which are usually more coarse or primarily present at rest.[99,100] A rapid relaxation phase of the deep tendon reflexes is common in young patients but is often difficult to assess in the older patient. Central nervous system manifestations may be a prominent component of the symptom complex of the elderly patient and include confusion, depression, forgetfulness, irritability, and a shortened concentration span.[87,108] These cognitive impairments may point to a diagnosis of dementia and failure to consider the presence of hyperthyroidism.

Other clinical manifestations of hyperthyroidism in the elderly population may include glucose intolerance and, occasionally, the unmasking of latent diabetes mellitus. Mild elevations of serum calcium can occur and hyperthyroidism can contribute to the development of osteoporosis, especially when other risk factors for osteoporosis are present. Men with Graves' disease may present with gynecomastia, decreased libido, and erectile dysfunction.[109]

Diagnosis of hyperthyroidism

Because of the altered clinical presentation of hyperthyroidism in an elderly person, suspicion must always be high and the laboratory should be used for any patient with possible symptoms. It is not uneconomical to employ screening tests for thyroid status in all geriatric patients undergoing initial clinical evaluation.[78,104]

Serum T4 or free T4 and measurement of serum TSH by modern ultrasensitive methods are the preferable screening procedures for thyroid dysfunction.[42,111] The findings of a normal serum T4 with suppressed serum TSH raises the possibility of T3 toxicosis and calls for measurement of serum T3.[47,48,87] Determination of FT4 concentration by one of the direct measurement techniques may be useful when there is reason to suspect an alteration in thyroid-binding proteins.[44,47] Demonstration of anti-TSH receptor antibodies can be helpful in making a diagnosis of Graves' disease.[66,72,75]

The TRH stimulation test, although useful in evaluating the patient with borderline laboratory tests, is rarely performed in contemporary times.[8,12] A significant rise in serum TSH will exclude the likelihood of hyperthyroidism, but an inadequate rise of TSH can only be considered as supportive of the diagnosis.

Thyroid scanning with ^{99m}Tc or radioiodine and measurement of ^{123}I uptake can be useful in distinguishing Graves' disease from toxic multinodular goiter.[62,63] Scanning may demonstrate the presence of a small diffusely active goiter that could not be detected on physical examination. Very low ^{123}I uptake in a patient with elevated circulating thyroid hormone levels suggests exogenous thyroid hormone ingestion (factitious hyperthyroidism), the hyperthyroid phase of subacute thyroiditis, or iodine-induced hyperthyroidism.

Management of hyperthyroidism

The first step in management of the patient with hyperthyroidism is to determine the underlying etiology and to exclude the possibility of one of the transient forms that may require supportive therapy directed toward the primary process (hormone ingestion, iodine exposure, subacute thyroiditis). Although the vast majority of patients with either Graves' disease or toxic multinodular goiter can be treated using antithyroid drugs, radioactive iodine, or surgery, radioactive iodine ablation is the preferred treatment in the elderly patient.[112–114]

In the patient with suspected hyperthyroidism who is still undergoing investigation, a useful initial step in treatment is the administration of β-adrenergic blocking agents such as propranolol, metoprolol, or atenolol. These agents are especially indicated in patients who have palpitations, tachycardia, angina, or agitation as symptoms since use of the β-blockers can lead to quick symptom control. These drugs act by interfering with some peripheral actions of thyroid hormone but do not correct the hypermetabolic state. The drugs, however, do not interfere with laboratory assessment of thyroid function and can allow control of symptoms until definitive treatment can be undertaken.

Once a diagnosis of Graves' disease or a toxic nodular goiter is established, treatment should be started with one of the antithyroid drugs, propylthiouracil or methimazole.[115] Methimazole has the advantage of often being effective when given once daily, whereas propylthiouracil is usually given in three divided doses. These agents impair biosynthesis of thyroid hormone and lead to depletion of intrathyroidal hormone stores and consequently to decreased hormone secretion. A decline in serum T4 concentration is usually seen by 2 to 4 weeks after initiation of antithyroid drug therapy, and the dose can be tapered once thyroid hormone levels reach the normal range in order to avoid development of hypothyroidism. In 1% to 5% of patients, the antithyroid drugs may cause fever, rash, and arthralgia. Drug-induced agranulocytosis occurs in 0.1% to 0.3% of treated persons and is seen more commonly in the elderly population. It is most likely to occur within the first 3 months of treatment, especially in patients who receive more than 30 mg/day of methimazole.[115] Routine periodic monitoring of the white blood cell count is not recommended, but measurement is called for if the patient experiences the onset of fever, sore throat, or oral ulcerations, and the drug must be discontinued if there is evidence of neutropenia. Long-term antithyroid drug administration can be used as a primary therapy in patients over the age of 60 with Graves' disease, who appear to respond more rapidly and have a greater likelihood of long-lasting remission than younger persons.[116,117] Long-term antithyroid drugs are rarely successful in inducing sustained remission in elderly patients with toxic multinodular goiter.

The recommended definitive treatment in the elderly group is thyroid ablation through use of ^{131}I.[112–114] Once the patient has been rendered euthyroid by antithyroid drugs, these agents should be stopped for 3 to 5 days, following which ^{131}I is given orally. Therapy with β-blockers can be maintained and antithyroid agents can be restarted 5 days after radiotherapy and continued for 4 to 10 weeks until the effect of radioiodine is achieved. Many therapists attempt to calculate a dose that will render the patient euthyroid without subsequent development of hypothyroidism. These calculations are based on a clinical estimate of thyroid gland size, 24-hour ^{131}I uptake, and whether the gland is diffusely overactive or contains toxic nodules. In spite of this approach, many patients will still develop permanent hypothyroidism following ^{131}I therapy.[118] It is not unreasonable to treat all elderly patients with a large dose of ^{131}I to assure ablation of thyroid tissue and avoid the possibility of recurrence of hyperthyroidism. Using this approach, patients are monitored following treatment until their serum thyroid hormone levels reach the hypothyroid range and are then put on permanent replacement therapy with exogenous thyroid hormone. Hypothyroidism may be evident as early as 4 weeks after treatment and can occur at any time after treatment. With all dosing regimens, by 12 months posttherapy 40% to 50% of patients are hypothyroid and hypothyroidism continues to occur thereafter at the rate of 2% to 3% per year.[119] Periodic monitoring of thyroid status is a necessity for any patient treated with ^{131}I who has not yet become hypothyroid.

Surgery is not recommended as a primary choice for treatment of hyperthyroidism in the elderly patient. The frequent accompaniment of hyperthyroidism by many coexisting disorders, including cardiac, pulmonary, and central nervous system disease, puts the patient at increased operative risk. In addition, postoperative complications of hypoparathyroidism and recurrent laryngeal nerve damage represent significant problems, especially when surgeons not highly experienced in thyroidectomy perform the surgery.[120] Surgery may be of value for the rare patient with tracheal compression secondary to a large hyperfunctioning goiter.

ATRIAL FIBRILLATION

This condition occurs in 10% to 15% of hyperthyroid patients, most of whom are elderly.[106,121] In a retrospective study of 163 hyperthyroid patients with atrial fibrillation, approximately 60% had spontaneous reversion to sinus rhythm after becoming euthyroid. Most of these reversions occurred with 3 weeks of becoming euthyroid, whereas no patient reverted if atrial fibrillation was still present after 4 months of euthyroidism or if atrial fibrillation had been present for more than 13 months before becoming euthyroid.[122] Thus, the patient who remains in atrial fibrillation beyond 16 weeks of return to the euthyroid state is a candidate for cardioversion.

While in the hyperthyroid state, the patient with atrial fibrillation is more sensitive to the anticoagulant effect of warfarin, resulting in a greater lowering of activity of coagulation factors II and VII and greater increase in the prothrombin ratio and partial thromboplastin time.[123] Many older persons with hyperthyroidism and atrial fibrillation are at increased risk for thromboembolic events, especially those with a prior history of thromboembolism, hypertension, or congestive heart failure or who have evidence of left atrial enlargement or left ventricular dysfunction.[106] In the absence of contraindications, anticoagulant therapy should be given with warfarin in a dose that will increase the international normalization ratio (INR) to 2.0 to 3.0. Careful monitoring of the dose of warfarin is necessary, and warfarin should be continued until euthyroidism has been achieved and a normal sinus rhythm has returned.[105,124]

ACUTE HYPERTHYROIDISM

Acute hyperthyroidism or *thyroid storm* can occur in the patient with either known or undiagnosed hyperthyroidism who is subjected to acute stress such as an operative procedure, trauma, or infection or who is exposed to iodine-containing drugs. It can also occur in the elderly patient treated with ^{131}I who did not receive adequate antithyroid medication before therapy.[125] In these patients, features of severe hyperthyroidism may develop over several hours and include fever, tachycardia, vomiting, diarrhea, dehydration, severe restlessness, and disorientation. Patients with cardiac disease are at especially high risk for acute heart failure or acute myocardial ischemia.

Thyroid storm is a life-threatening condition and must be treated vigorously and promptly.[126,127] Immediate treatment involves administration of antithyroid drugs and iodide to interfere with thyroid hormone production. Propylthiouracil is given in an initial dose of 900 to 1200 mg followed in several hours with sodium iodide or oral Lugol's solution. High-dose β-blockers such as propranolol and high-dose corticosteroids are also given to blunt peripheral action of thyroid hormones and to inhibit T4 to T3 conversion in peripheral tissues. Supportive measures include sedation, fluids, antipyretics, and cooling blankets, plus antibiotics if infection is present.[126]

SUBCLINICAL HYPERTHYROIDISM

The finding of suppressed or nondetectable serum TSH along with normal total and free serum T4 or T3, often in the upper end of the normal range, is defined as subclinical hyperthyroidism. Etiology ranges from excessive thyroid hormone replacement therapy to thyroid disease, with the most common cause in the elderly person being long-standing multinodular goiter.

Demography

The finding of subnormal TSH concentrations in the elderly is not infrequent. The prevalence of subclinical hyperthyroidism appears to vary with geographic area and dietary iodine intake.[128] Individuals with low iodine intake are more commonly affected because of compensatory growth of the thyroid gland in response to low iodine and thus the tendency to develop hyperplastic nodules that may become autonomously functioning thyroid tissue. One study in Italy reported that individuals living in iodine-deficient areas had an age-related increase in subclinical hyperthyroidism from a prevalence of 0.7% in children to a prevalence of 15.4% in individuals over the age of 75.[129] Similarly, in a U.S. population of 2575 persons over the age of 60 years, 101 were found to have low TSH and, of these, 30 had no history of past or present thyroid disease. Over a 4-year follow-up period, most had normal TSH on subsequent testing, but two became overtly hyperthyroid with an increase in serum T4 to above normal values.[130] In a prospective study, persons age 85 years were followed with serum TSH and free T4 until age 89. Of 12 with subclinical hyperthyroidism at baseline, 1 became overtly hyperthyroid, 5 had persistent subclinical hyperthyroidism, 5 became euthyroid, and 1 developed subclinical hypothyroidism.[131] In a study of 1210 persons in England, low TSH was found in 6.3% of women and 5.5% of men.[132] However, repeat measurements of serum TSH 1 year later showed a return of TSH to the normal range in the majority of cases. Several studies suggest that the conversion rate to overt hyperthyroidism ranges from 1.5% to 13% within 1 year.[130,132–135] Thus, the natural history of subclinical hyperthyroidism is variable, sometimes disappearing over time.[136]

Clinical presentation

Individuals with thyroid function values indicating the presence of subclinical hyperthyroidism generally have no or only mild clinical features suggestive of hyperthyroidism.[133] However, persons with subclinical hyperthyroidism are at increased risk of developing atrial fibrillation as reflected by a cumulative incidence of 28% over a 10-year period in individuals over the age of 60 years, representing a 3-fold increase in risk.[121,134] There may be other cardiac consequences of persistent subclinical hyperthyroidism including increased prevalence of atrial premature beats, increased heart rate, increased left ventricular mass, enhanced systolic function, impaired diastolic function, and reduced exercise performance (Table 90-3).[137,138]

Many studies suggest that apparently asymptomatic individuals with subclinical hyperthyroidism have accelerated loss of bone mineral, which is benefited by treatment.[139–141] Postmenopausal women with subclinical hyperthyroidism and nodular goiter who were treated with ^{131}I with subsequent normalization of serum TSH had an increase in bone mineral density at the spine and hip after 2 years of follow-up, whereas a similar group of women who were not treated showed progressive bone loss.[142] Therefore, the finding of suppressed TSH and normal T4 in an asymptomatic elderly person calls for periodic retesting of thyroid function, including measurement of FT4. In the presence of significant osteopenia or if there is subsequent development of clinical features of hyperthyroidism, atrial fibrillation, or increased thyroid hormone production, restoration of thyroid function to normal should be undertaken.

Table 90-3. Findings and Potential Adverse Effects of Subclinical Hyperthyroidism

Functional Cardiovascular Alterations
Increased cardiac contractility
Impaired left ventricular diastolic filling
Impaired systolic function during exercise
Increased left ventricular mass index
Increased intraventricular septal thickness
Increased left ventricular posterior wall thickness
Decreased large and small artery elasticity
Prolonged QTc interval
Clinical Cardiovascular Consequences
Increased heart rate and frequency of atrial premature beats
Increased incidence of atrial fibrillation
Lower serum total and low-density lipoprotein (LDL) cholesterol concentrations
Reduced exercise capacity
Increased mortality due to cardiovascular disease
Bone Loss
Osteopenia
Osteoporosis
Diminished Quality of Life

Impaired quality of life as assessed by questionnaire has been reported in subclinical hyperthyroidism.[131] In individuals over the age of 55 years with subclinical hyperthyroidism, an increased incidence of dementia and Alzheimer's disease has been reported, especially in those who have circulating antithyroid antibodies detected.[143] Long-term studies of patients with untreated subclinical hyperthyroidism have demonstrated an increase in both cardiovascular and all-cause mortality.[132,144]

Treatment

Treatment of subclinical hyperthyroidism is controversial because of the low rate of progression to overt hyperthyroidism. A long-term study of patients with untreated subclinical hyperthyroidism demonstrated an increase in both cardiovascular and all-cause mortality.[145] When these data are coupled with the findings of diminished self-reported ratings of quality of life and a higher rate of osteopenia in persons with subclinical hyperthyroidism, it is reasonable to consider earlier, more aggressive treatment, especially in individuals who already manifest these changes.[146–148]

Although there have been no randomized prospective trials evaluating the treatment of subclinical hyperthyroidism, there is a consensus that therapy should be initiated in elderly individuals with heart disease or evidence of other problems, such as bone loss, that may be impacted by this entity and who have serum TSH levels less than 0.1 mU/L. A consensus panel of endocrinologists has recommended treatment for those with TSH suppression of <0.1 mU/L but recommends periodic retesting of thyroid function in patients with partial TSH suppression of 0.1 to 0.4 mU/L.[149,150] It has been suggested that all postmenopausal women, individuals over age 60, and those with a history of heart disease, osteoporosis, or symptoms be treated if the TSH is less than

0.1 mU/L and that a similar approach be considered if the TSH is between 0.1 and 4 mU/L in this same population.[151,152] Treatment leading to the return of serum TSH to normal has been associated with significant improvement in cardiovascular function including a decrease in the heart rate, total number of beats during 24 hours, number of atrial and ventricular premature beats, and reduction in left ventricular mass index, interventricular septum thickness, and left ventricular posterior wall thickness at diastole.[153]

HYPOTHYROIDISM

Hypothyroidism is the clinical state that results from inadequate peripheral tissue response to thyroid hormone action. Most commonly, this occurs as a consequence of decreased thyroid hormone production from the thyroid gland,[154,155] but in rare instances can result from tissue unresponsiveness to the presence of adequate amounts of thyroid hormone in the circulation.[156,157] Deficient thyroid hormone release most commonly is the result of disease or dysfunction of the thyroid gland itself and is referred to as "primary hypothyroidism." In some patients, pituitary TSH release is inadequate, leading to failure of the thyroid gland and "secondary hypothyroidism." Rare cases of "tertiary hypothyroidism" have been identified in which the underlying mechanism is failure of synthesis or release of hypothalamic TRH.

Demography

Hypothyroidism is relatively common in the general population and shows a clear sex and age relationship.[78,83] The Whickham, England, study identified hypothyroidism, based on measurement of serum TSH, in 19 per 1000 women with a mean age at diagnosis of 57 years and a prevalence 10-fold more common in women than in men. The incidence rate of elevated serum TSH showed a direct relationship to age in women, increasing from 4% to 5.7% of women under age 45 to 17.4% of women over the age of 75 years. In men, elevated serum TSH was present in 1.6% to 3.5% of those under age 65 and increased to 3.5% to 6.9% in persons over the age of 65 years.[84] Similarly, study of the Framingham population in the United States revealed clear elevation of serum TSH in 5.9% of women between the ages of 60 and 89 years and borderline elevation in an additional 7.7%. Men of the same age had elevated serum TSH in 2.4% of subjects, with another 3.3% showing borderline levels.[158]

Many population studies carried out in Great Britain, Sweden, Switzerland, West Germany, Japan, and the United States confirm the high frequency of hypothyroidism in the population, its predominance in women, and its progressive increase with advancing age.[78,85,110,159–165] Based on the clear influence of age on the risk of development of hypothyroidism, it is reasonable to screen all elderly individuals for the possible presence of the disorder through measurement of serum TSH.[78]

Etiology

Hypothyroidism can arise as a consequence of inborn or acquired disorders/diseases of the thyroid gland, from exposure to agents affecting thyroid-hormone synthesis, and from disease or disturbance of hypothalamic–pituitary production of TRH and TSH (see Table 90-1). In the elderly population, the most common cause of thyroid failure is Hashimoto's disease.[155] This autoimmune disorder is characterized histologically by continuous replacement of normal thyroid tissue with lymphocytic and fibrous tissue, ultimately leading to a reduced mass of functional thyroid elements and decline in hormone production.[4] Many patients can be identified by demonstrating the presence of antithyroglobulin and antimicrosomal antibodies in their serum.[67,68,71] Much evidence has accumulated for the presence of another family of immunoglobulins that are capable of blocking the action of TSH on thyroid cells either by interfering with TSH binding to its receptor or by blocking both pre- and postreceptor processes.[67,166]

There is a question over whether or not the presence of antithyroid antibodies in the serum can predict the subsequent development of hypothyroidism.[167] In a study of subjects with demonstrated thyroid antibodies, hypothyroidism developed at a rate of 5% per year. Other reports do not support the predictive value of antithyroid antibodies, although they document the strong association of the antibodies with the presence of increased serum TSH and clinical hypothyroidism.[168]

Some patients with previously diagnosed Graves' disease may go on to develop an autoimmune hypothyroidism.[169] This consequence may be related to the presence of TSH-blocking antibodies. Other forms of thyroiditis, such as subacute and silent thyroiditis, may progress from a transient hyperthyroid state to euthyroidism, and finally, to permanent hypothyroidism.

A major cause of hypothyroidism is the prior treatment of hyperthyroidism, especially Graves' disease, by either radioiodine[118,119] or subtotal thyroidectomy.[170] Both treatments have been demonstrated to be followed by a continuous, life-long risk of developing hypothyroidism, with a rate 1 year after initial treatment of 20% to 40% and an annual incidence of 2% to 4% each year thereafter. Any patient with a prior history of surgical or radioiodine treatment of hyperthyroidism should have yearly monitoring of thyroid status with serum TSH and/or T4.

Iodide and iodine-containing drugs can result in inhibition of thyroid-hormone synthesis (Wolff-Chaikoff effect) with ensuing hypothyroidism, which is usually reversible when the source of exogenous iodine or iodide is removed.[171] Common sources of iodine ingestion are expectorants (potassium iodide), topical antifungal or antiseptic agents (betadine), iodine-containing radiographic contrast agents, and the antiarrhythmic agent, amiodarone.[172] Long-term lithium therapy can also lead to impaired thyroid hormone synthesis and to inhibition of thyroid hormone release. As many as 20% of patients taking lithium may develop hypothyroidism.[49]

Impairment of production or release of TSH from the anterior pituitary or of TRH from the hypothalamus leads to secondary and tertiary hypothyroidism, respectively. These alterations can be the consequence of pituitary or hypothalamic tumors, surgical or traumatic injury, radiotherapy, or infiltrative diseases such as histiocytosis, sarcoidosis, tuberculosis, or amyloidosis. These patients may have isolated abnormalities of the TRH–TSH–thyroid axis or, more commonly, other associated disorders of hypothalamic, anterior, and posterior pituitary function.

Iodine deficiency in the past accounted for many cases of hypothyroidism, usually with an accompanying goiter. With the routine use of iodized salt and common exposure to many iodine-containing agents in the diet, this is now a rare cause of hypothyroidism in the United States. However, in many underdeveloped parts of the world, iodine deficiency remains as a common cause of failure of thyroid hormone production.

Clinical presentation of hypothyroidism

Hypothyroidism, particularly in the elderly population, is a disorder with insidious onset characterized by the emergence of symptoms and signs over many years, so that neither the patient nor close associates may be aware of the process.[173,174] Consequently, the manifestations of hypothyroidism are often attributed to "old age" or to other disorders common in the elderly person. Depending on recognition of the "classic" clinical features of hypothyroidism will invariably result in failure to make the diagnosis in many symptomatic patients.[175] In one study, only 10% of patients with a laboratory-confirmed diagnosis were recognized as being hypothyroid on clinical examination.[176] Similar results have been found in other investigations.[158,159,161,177]

Central nervous system manifestations are a significant consequence of hypothyroidism in the elderly population. Mental slowing is common, along with complaints of fatigue and excessive sleepiness. The possibility of psychiatric disorder is raised by patients who present with depression, delirium, or paranoid ideation.[159,178,179] So-called myxedema madness with psychotic behavior is infrequent. Alterations in level of consciousness can occur with confusion and coma. An acute decline in mental status may be precipitated by the stress of infection or trauma, exposure to the cold, or exposure to drugs such as sedatives and narcotics.[180] Seizures can occasionally be due to severe hypothyroidism. The possibility that hypothyroidism may be a cause of reversible dementia has led to much study of patients undergoing dementia evaluation. Most reports confirm that whereas hypothyroidism is common in patients with dementia, only rarely is the dementia truly reversible with thyroid hormone therapy, although there may be overall improvement in the patients' functional state.[159]

Classic cold intolerance and diminished sweating are often present in the elderly hypothyroid patient, but these symptoms are also common in euthyroid elderly. Hypothermia may be found. Dry skin, puffiness of the face, periorbital edema, coarsened and thinned hair, thinning of the outer parts of the eyebrows, brittle nails, and yellowing of the skin are common features of the patient, but these also occur with great frequency in patients of advanced age whose thyroid function appears normal.

Coarsening of the voice with slow and sometimes slurred speech should increase the awareness of possible hypothyroidism. Hearing impairment may be due to thyroid insufficiency, or, more commonly, hypothyroidism may aggravate a hearing disorder of other cause.

An important feature of thyroid deficiency in the elderly group is physical slowing with accompanying symptoms of fatigue, weakness, and occasionally muscle stiffness. Arthralgia can also lead to physical slowing. Entrapment neuropathy with paresthesias can occur, especially involving the carpal tunnel.[181] Other aspects of neurologic involvement in hypothyroidism include impairment of reflex function, leading to the classic delayed or "hung-up" relaxation phase of the reflex. Not infrequently, there may be hyporeflexia or complete loss of reflexes, especially of the Achilles tendon.

In the elderly patient, assessment of changes in weight may give little insight into a possible diagnosis of hypothyroidism. Weight gain may occur, but decrease in appetite may be sufficient to result in weight loss. Bowel motility may be slowed with resultant constipation, but here again, this is a common complaint of the nonhypothyroid elderly.

The myocardium is affected by thyroid-hormone deficiency, with the most common changes being bradycardia and narrowed pulse pressure. Reduced cardiac output is the consequence of slowed heart rate, decreased ventricular filling, and a decrease in ventricular contractility.[106,182] The myocardium may undergo myxedematous infiltration with resultant cardiac enlargement, symptoms of ischemic heart disease, and development of pericardial effusion.[183] Reduced cardiac output results in decrease of glomerular filtration rate and consequent renal retention of sodium and water, so that peripheral edema may develop even in the absence of overt congestive heart failure.

Alterations in peripheral vascular resistance can lead to hypertension. Pulse wave analysis from recordings at the radial artery in patients with hypothyroidism demonstrates increased augmentation of central aortic pressures and central arterial stiffness. These changes, along with increased cardiac afterload and with hypothyroid-associated endothelial dysfunction, contribute to increased cardiovascular risk. These abnormalities are reversed by appropriate thyroid hormone replacement.[184] Other cardiovascular risk factors for patients with hypothyroidism include smoking, elevated levels of homocysteine, elevated C-reactive protein, coagulation abnormalities, and insulin resistance.[185]

Electrocardiographic abnormalities may be seen including slow heart rate, low voltage of the QRS complex, flattening or inversion of T waves, prolonged QT interval, and ventricular arrhythmias.[106] The echocardiogram often demonstrates features of decreased left ventricular contractility with increased systolic time interval and prolongation of isovolumic relaxation time. Small pericardial effusions may be present in as many as 50% of hypothyroid patients but usually do not affect cardiac function.[186,187]

Hematologic, metabolic, and other systemic impacts of hypothyroidism are more likely to be detected by laboratory evaluation than by clinical examination.[188] Anemia of the normocytic or macrocytic type can be found in about one third of patients,[159] appears to be mediated by insufficient production of erythropoietin, and is directly attributable to the lack of thyroid hormone. Serum iron may be low in some patients, but serum levels of folic acid and B_{12} are usually normal. Pernicious anemia occurs frequently in association with autoimmune forms of hypothyroidism and should be looked for in hypothyroid patients with persistent anemia after hormonal treatment or in patients with macrocytosis and low serum B_{12}.

Changes in blood lipoprotein composition are common in hypothyroidism and have implications for atherogenesis. Short-term hypothyroidism is associated with an increase in plasma lipoprotein (a) and T3 therapy rapidly lowers lipoprotein (a) together with apolipoprotein B and low-density lipoprotein (LDL) cholesterol, supporting the hypothesis that thyroid hormone is capable of regulating plasma lipoprotein (a) and apolipoprotein B in a parallel manner. Elevated concentrations of lipoprotein (a) in combination with LDL cholesterol may be involved in the increased risk of cardiovascular disease, which is associated with hypothyroidism.[189] Changes in LDL receptor activity are significantly correlated with changes in LDL cholesterol, but not changes in lipoprotein (a). The LDL receptor pathway appears to be involved in the catabolism of lipoprotein (a) to a limited extent.[190] Hypothyroidism has been associated with elevated levels of total and high-density lipoprotein (HDL) cholesterol, total/HDL cholesterol ratio, apolipoprotein AI, and apolipoprotein E. The increase in apolipoprotein AI without a concomitant increase in apolipoprotein AII suggests a selective elevation of HDL2. These effects were found to be reversible with treatment of the hypothyroidism.[191]

Hyponatremia may be found in elderly patients with hypothyroidism. The clinical picture is that of the syndrome of inappropriate antidiuretic hormone secretion—that is, dilutional hyponatremia, concentrated urine, normal or expanded intravascular volume, and sodium excretion in the urine. The mechanism appears to be an increased release of antidiuretic hormone as well as altered renal blood flow with increased tubular reabsorption of sodium and water.

Evidence suggestive of myopathy is provided by elevated levels of serum creatine phosphokinase (CPK), which may be very high. Decreased renal clearance of the enzyme largely contributes to these increased levels.

MYXEDEMA COMA

This condition is an extreme, life-threatening form of hypothyroidism that occurs almost exclusively in the elderly population. Presentation is that of an elderly person with rapid development of stupor, seizures, or coma, often in association with infection, stress, exposure to the cold, or following administration of sedatives, tranquilizers, or narcotics.[180] History or symptoms of hypothyroidism may have been present for a long time. Hypothermia of profound degree is often present along with more common signs of hypothyroidism. Respiratory depression with hypoxia and carbon dioxide retention is commonly present and may necessitate intubation and ventilatory assistance. Blood pressure may be low, along with bradycardia and features of shock. Laboratory data will reveal, in addition to marked hypothyroxinemia, hyponatremia, hypoglycemia, elevation of serum CPK, anemia, and evidence of respiratory acidosis with increase in P_{CO_2}. Chest X-ray often reveals cardiomegaly, because of either dilated myocardium or pericardial effusion. Electrocardiogram typically shows low voltage. Recognition of the syndrome and prompt initiation of therapy is essential, because the mortality rate is probably in excess of 50%.

Laboratory diagnosis of hypothyroidism

The findings of low total and free serum T4 concentration along with elevation of serum TSH clearly establish a diagnosis of primary hypothyroidism, and these two findings require no further investigation.[42] Measurement of serum T3 in an elderly patient is of little diagnostic value because many disorders or drugs common in this age group lead to reduced concentrations of T3.[28] Conversely, in some patients with hypothyroidism, serum T3 levels may remain in the normal range.

The failure to find elevation of serum TSH in a patient with reduced serum T4 or T3 concentrations and clinical features suspicious for hypothyroidism requires that more extensive laboratory evaluation be carried out. The differentiation between secondary or tertiary hypothyroidism and the various "sick euthyroid" syndromes may be difficult. Normal values of FT4 point against hypothyroidism, but low FT4 may be seen in both conditions. Measurement of rT3 may be useful because its concentration will be low in true hypothyroidism and is generally normal or increased in nonthyroidal illness.[28]

The TRH test may occasionally be of value because patients with secondary hypothyroidism will show blunted or absent rise in TSH, whereas sick euthyroid individuals usually will respond to TRH with a rise. The measurement of antithyroid antibodies may indirectly support a diagnosis of hypothyroidism if the titers are high, but the levels themselves cannot indicate the functional state of the thyroid gland.

Therapy for hypothyroidism

The establishment of a diagnosis of hypothyroidism generally calls for initiation of thyroid hormone replacement. In the vast majority of patients, the preferred form of treatment is with synthetic L-thyroxine. There is little role for treatment with T3 because peripheral conversion of T4 to T3 is capable of providing adequate amounts of T3.

It is now well established that the usual replacement dose of T4 is lower in the elderly than in the young patient, largely as a result of an age-related reduction in the rate of T4 clearance.[192–196] The mean daily dose of T4 for patients over the age of 65 years has been estimated to be 0.110 mg (1.6 μg/kg), but it varies in individual patients from 0.05 to 0.2 mg. Determination of the optimum T4 dose is based on monitoring of serum TSH and is defined as the dose of T4 that will reduce serum TSH into the normal range.[197] There is a suggestion that the magnitude of initial serum TSH elevation correlates with the final T4 replacement dose.[196]

Excessive thyroid hormone replacement should be avoided. Elderly patients treated with L-thyroxine in standard doses and with serum T4 in the normal range have often been found to have suppressed serum TSH. Even though clinically evident features of hyperthyroidism are not detectable, metabolic effects of increased thyroid hormone can occur and include increased nocturnal heart rate, shortened systolic time interval, increased urinary sodium excretion, and increased hepatic and muscle enzyme activity.[198,199] Of even greater consequence is the observation that patients on thyroid hormone replacement who have suppressed serum TSH also have evidence for increased bone resorption with consequent risk of accelerated rate of osteoporosis and, possibly, increased risk of fracture.[199–201]

In the elderly patient, initiation of hormone replacement should be with small doses, which are then slowly increased until full replacement has been achieved.[192,193] For most older patients, a dose of 0.025 mg daily of L-thyroxine is an appropriate starting amount. Subsequent increases can be in increments of 0.025 mg daily at 4- to 8-week intervals until the serum TSH has been normalized. It is not usual for the decline in TSH to lag behind the attainment of normal values for serum T4. This approach to treatment minimizes the risk of possible adverse effects of thyroid therapy, which include provocation of anginal pain, myocardial infarction, congestive heart failure, and arrhythmias.

Special attention must be given to the patient who, in addition to hypothyroidism, has an established diagnosis of ischemic heart disease. In this circumstance, it may be difficult to achieve full hormone replacement without provoking cardiac symptoms. An attempt should be made to maximize the antianginal regimen, including administration of β-blockers, vasodilator agents, and calcium-channel blockers.[202,203] Should this approach fail, the patient should undergo evaluation for the possibility of angioplasty or coronary artery bypass surgery.[204]

In the patient who is thought to have secondary or tertiary hypothyroidism, consideration must be given to the possibility that there may be coexistent ACTH deficiency with resultant hypoadrenalism. Because the increased metabolic state resulting from thyroid replacement can precipitate the clinical picture of adrenal insufficiency, glucocorticoid replacement should be started concomitantly with thyroid hormone if there is any likelihood that ACTH deficiency is present. Some patients with long-standing, severe primary hypothyroidism may also develop signs of adrenal insufficiency following the initiation of thyroid hormone, owing to metabolic impairment of adrenal hormone production from the hypothyroidism itself. Should any features of hypoadrenalism be suspected, prompt treatment with physiologic doses of glucocorticoids should begin. After a euthyroid state has been achieved, the steroid dose may be tapered and discontinued. In some patients, it may be prudent to start treatment with both thyroid and glucocorticoid hormones and discontinue the latter as the patient approaches euthyroidism.

The treatment of myxedema coma warrants special consideration. The patient should be cared for in an intensive-care setting.[126,205–207] If the diagnosis is suspected, therapy must be started at once, even though laboratory confirmation has not yet been obtained.[126,205–207] Treatment with thyroxine is necessary to correct the hypothyroid state with an initial dose of 300 to 500 μg given intravenously, because both intestinal and intramuscular absorption are likely to be unreliable.[205,206] In a review of 87 patients with myxedema coma, initial thyroxine doses greater than 500 μg were associated with a mortality rate of 53%, whereas the mortality rate in patients treated with an initial dose less than 500 μg was 9%. Mortality was highest in patients over the age of 65 years.[208] Once there is evidence of a clinical response such as rise in body temperature and heart rate, the daily dose of thyroxine should be reduced to 50 to 100 μg, given orally as soon as possible, and adjusted further as necessary by monitoring of serum TSH.[206] T3 or combinations of T4 and T3 are not recommended in an elderly patient because the acute metabolic impact of T3 can lead to cardiac arrhythmia or myocardial infarction.

Adrenal insufficiency can be present in patients with myxedema coma. In life-threatening situations, blood for measurement of cortisol should be drawn and intravenous stress doses of glucocorticoids should be given and continued until there is laboratory confirmation of status of adrenal function. A decision can then be made to either continue treatment for adrenal insufficiency or to taper and discontinue the glucocorticoid.

Supportive therapy must be promptly initiated and may include ventilatory support for respiratory failure, antibiotics for infection, external rewarming for hypothermia, and correction of hypotension by fluid replacement or dopamine. Hyponatremia, if severe, should be treated.

SUBCLINICAL HYPOTHYROIDISM

As a result of a number of large laboratory survey studies, a significant population of individuals has been identified who have serum levels of TSH above the accepted upper limits of normal, but in whom serum concentrations of total and free T4 and T3 are normal, and symptoms of hypothyroidism are usually mild or lacking.[78,83,177,209,210] This syndrome has been termed *subclinical hypothyroidism* and is most commonly found in women above the age of 60 years.[211–214] It is thought that the failing thyroid gland responds with an increase in TSH secretion, which, in turn, is capable of further driving the thyroid to maintain normal levels of T4 and T3 until true thyroid failure ensues. Antithyroid antibodies are often present, suggesting an autoimmune etiology.

Demography

In the Framingham study, 5.9% of subjects over the age of 60 years had clearly elevated serum-TSH concentrations (>10 mU/L) with normal serum T4 levels, and an additional 14.4% had slightly elevated serum TSH (5 to 10 mU/L) with normal serum T4.[158] A thyroid screening survey of 1149 community-residing women with mean age of 69 ± 7.5 years identified 10.8% as having subclinical hypothyroidism.[214] Other studies have established a prevalence rate of between 25 and 104 per 1000 persons with the highest rate occurring in women over age 55 years. The incidence in women between 40 and 60 years of age may be as high as 10%. Data from the Whickham study indicate that 60% of subjects with serum TSH values greater than 6 mU/L and 80% of those with TSH values greater than 10 mU/L had demonstrable antithyroid antibodies in their serum. Of the entire population of women, 5% had both elevated TSH levels and antithyroid antibodies.[84]

Of clinical importance is the question of what is the likelihood that the person with laboratory criteria for subclinical hypothyroidism will go on to develop clinical hypothyroidism. In a long-term follow-up study, women who initially had antithyroglobulin and antimicrosomal antibodies along with a serum TSH of greater than 6 mU/L developed overt hypothyroidism at the rate of 5% per year. No cases developed in women with borderline elevation of TSH only (6 to 10 mU/L), and only one case developed in the 67 women who had antithyroid antibodies with normal TSH levels.[212] Other studies support progression to overt hypothyroidism at the rate of 7% per year in women with elevated serum TSH and high titers of antithyroid antibodies with ranges from 1% to 20% per year.[76,215,216] There is a relationship between the degree of elevation of TSH and the long-term risk of progression to overt hypothyroidism. An initial TSH greater than 12 mU/L resulted in a 77% incidence of overt hypothyroidism by 10 years of follow-up.[217,218] It is clear that the presence of antithyroid antibodies, which indicate the presence of chronic autoimmune thyroiditis, constitutes a significant risk factor for the development of clinically apparent hypothyroidism in women who are found to have isolated elevated values of serum TSH.[84,166]

Clinical manifestations

Subclinical hypothyroidism has been associated with a number of potentially adverse clinical findings, particularly those affecting the cardiovascular system (Table 90-4). There is evidence that systolic contractility on effort and left ventricular diastolic contractility at rest are decreased in patients with subclinical hypothyroidism.[219] These changes may have little functional significance in the resting state, but symptoms can develop during cardiopulmonary exercise. The altered contractility and clinical response to exercise are corrected with thyroid hormone treatment.[220–222] Although subclinical hypothyroidism has been associated with a prolongation of the QT interval, little has been reported regarding its clinical consequences.

The relationship between subclinical hypothyroidism and cardiovascular disease has been the subject of many clinical studies, which have yielded conflicting results. A study of 1922 patients indicated that subclinical hypothyroidism was not associated with an adverse cardiovascular risk profile.[223] This observation was further supported by data from several large longitudinal studies of community-residing persons.[121,224]

Contrarily, a number of studies suggest that subclinical hypothyroidism is a risk factor for cardiovascular disease. The relationship between subclinical hypothyroidism or autoimmune thyroid disease and coronary heart disease (CHD) was evaluated in a Japanese study of patients diagnosed as having CHD by coronary angiogram (the CHD group) and healthy subjects matched for age, sex, and body mass index (the control group). Thyroid function, thyroid autoantibodies, and serum lipid concentrations were measured in the CHD and control groups. The CHD group exhibited significantly decreased levels of serum free T3 and free T4 and significantly increased serum TSH levels as compared with the control group, indicating a significant decrease in thyroid function in the CHD patients. Serum HDL cholesterol levels were significantly decreased in the CHD group.[225] Another Japanese study of men and women of mean age 58.5 years found 10.2% to have subclinical hypothyroidism. Men with subclinical hypothyroidism had a prevalence of ischemic heart disease four times greater than euthyroid men but no increase in intracranial hemorrhage or cerebral infarction. Over 12 years of follow-up, there was a significant increase in all-cause mortality in the subclinical hypothyroid men but not in women.[226] Another longitudinal study of men and women with a mean age of 50 years found a significant increase in prevalence of coronary heart disease in both men and women with subclinical hypothyroidism who had a TSH level greater than 10 mU/L.[227] Similarly, a study of 2730 men and women age 70 to 79 years who were followed for a period of 4 years revealed an increased risk for congestive heart failure in persons with subclinical hypothyroidism who had TSH levels of 7 mU/L or greater.[228] In this population, subclinical hypothyroidism was not associated with an increased risk for coronary heart disease, stroke, peripheral arterial disease, or cardiovascular-related or total mortality.

Among elderly residents of a nursing home, 6% were found to have subclinical hypothyroidism, and of these, 83% had dyslipidemia and 56% had evidence of coronary artery disease in contrast to a 16% incidence of coronary artery disease in euthyroid residents.[229] A possible contributing factor for the increased risk of vascular occlusive disease is the finding of an increase in factor VII activity, which may result in a hypercoagulable state with increased risk of thromboembolism.[230]

Table 90-4. Findings and Potential Adverse Effects of Subclinical Hypothyroidism

Ventricular Function
Impaired systolic function on effort
Impaired left ventricular diastolic function at rest/delayed relaxation time
Right ventricular systolic and diastolic dysfunction
Increased risk of congestive heart failure
Peripheral Vasculature
Increased systemic vascular resistance
Impaired vasodilatation
Increased carotid artery intima-media thickness
Increased arterial stiffness
Increased pulse wave velocity
Increased diastolic blood pressure
Increased peripheral vascular disease
Dyslipidemia
Increased total cholesterol
Increased low-density lipoprotein (LDL) cholesterol
Increased apolipoprotein B
Increased lipoprotein A
Atherosclerosis
Increased ischemic/coronary heart disease
Increased risk of myocardial infarction
Increased aortic atherosclerosis
Coagulation
Increased factor VII activity
Central Nervous System
Depressed mood, fatigue, decreased energy
Memory impairment
Dementia
Mortality
Increased cardiac mortality
Increased all-cause mortality

There have been many reports indicating that subclinical hypothyroidism is associated with alterations in circulating concentrations of lipids that may enhance the risk for development of vascular disease.[222,231–237] A study of 2108 community-residing persons demonstrated that in the 119 person subgroup (5.6%) with subclinical hypothyroidism, there was a significant increase in total serum cholesterol and in LDL cholesterol with no change in HDL cholesterol.[227] In other studies, decreased HDL and increased lipoprotein (a) and apolipoprotein B have been described, along with an accompanying higher prevalence of ischemic heart disease.[236,238,239]

Women with hypercholesterolemia have an increased likelihood of having coexisting subclinical hypothyroidism.[240] Patients with subclinical hypothyroidism have been noted to have a relative increase in low-density lipoprotein and decrease in high-density lipoprotein with a higher prevalence of ischemic heart disease.[241] In a large group of elderly women with evidence of aortic atherosclerosis, 13.9% were found to have subclinical hypothyroidism; and in those women with a history of myocardial infarction, 21.5% had subclinical hypothyroidism.[214] Similarly, the presence of subclinical hypothyroidism was accompanied by a high prevalence of both aortic atherosclerosis and myocardial infarction, with an even higher prevalence in those who also had detectable antimicrosomal antibodies.

As in patients with overt hypothyroidism, those with subclinical hypothyroidism have been shown to have alterations in peripheral vasculature. Both diastolic blood pressure and pulse wave velocity were significantly increased in patients with subclinical hypothyroidism as compared to euthyroid persons.[231] Pulse wave analysis has also demonstrated increased arterial stiffness in patients with subclinical hypothyroidism, which improved after thyroid hormone treatment.[232] Carotid intima-media thickness, a recognized risk factor for cardiovascular disease, has been found by high-resolution ultrasonography to be increased and positively related to age, TSH, and LDL cholesterol levels.[239] In a nursing home population with mean age 79 years, 78% of persons identified with subclinical hypothyroidism were found to have symptomatic peripheral vascular disease.[242]

Subclinical hypothyroidism also can affect central nervous system function with patients reporting memory impairment, depressed mood, anxiety, and a variety of somatic complaints. Thyroxine treatment has been reported to improve these symptoms as well as to improve sense of well-being and performance on psychometric testing.[222,243–245]

Treatment

Thus, attention must be given to the question of whether or not the detection of subclinical hypothyroidism warrants treatment—a topic of considerable controversy. Treatment with L-thyroxine has resulted in improved systolic and diastolic functioning, improvement in left ventricular ejection fraction with exercise, and a decrease in systemic vascular resistance.[235,246,247] Several studies have reported that treatment with L-thyroxine results in a decrease in total and LDL cholesterol, an increase in serum high-density lipoproteins, and a decrease in low-density lipoproteins and apolipoprotein B.[236–238,241,248–251] There are no substantive data as yet to indicate that early treatment of subclinical hypothyroidism with thyroid hormone replacement is effective in reducing the risk for subsequent development of atherosclerosis or coronary artery disease.

Several publications have dealt with the divergent opinions on treatment for subclinical thyroid dysfunction.[149,150,152,252,253] Two reports on subclinical thyroid disease were prepared by a panel of experts appointed by the American Association of Clinical Endocrinologists, the American Thyroid Association, and the Endocrine Society, who carried out an exhaustive review of the literature using principles of evidence-based medicine. These reports addressed issues of screening, evaluation, and management of patients with subclinical thyroid disease and culminated in a consensus statement of conclusions and recommendations prepared by the panel members, which was published in 2004.[149,152] Subsequently, a response document from representatives of three organizations was prepared and published in 2005, pointing out areas where there was disagreement with the consensus conference recommendations.[150]

The consensus panel concluded that routine treatment of patients with subclinical hypothyroidism with serum TSH levels of 4.5 to 10 mU/L was not warranted but indicated that treatment is reasonable for patients with TSH levels greater than 10 mU/L. This recommendation was based on data from patients with a TSH level above 10 mU/L regarding the projected rate of progression from subclinical to overt hypothyroidism and the effects of thyroxine treatment on symptoms, depression, lipid profiles, and cardiac function.[149]

The three sponsoring societies disagreed with some of the consensus panel's conclusions. Thus, the three societies recommend routine screening for subclinical thyroid disease according to previously published guidelines. Further, they recommend routine treatment of patients with subclinical hypothyroidism who have TSH levels between 4.5 to 10 mU/L.[150]

At present, a conservative approach is to monitor patients identified with the syndrome with serum TSH and T4 at 6- to 12-month intervals. Replacement therapy with thyroxine should be given to those patients with serum TSH greater than 10 mU/L and to those with TSH between 4.5 and 10 mU/L who have either high levels of antimicrosomal antibodies or symptoms consistent with mild hypothyroidism.

NODULAR THYROID DISEASE AND NEOPLASIA

The development of thyroid nodules is an age-related process that occurs more commonly in women than in men.[84,254–256] Autopsy studies have demonstrated that thyroid nodules are frequently found in the elderly population, even when clinical examination of the neck has failed to reveal abnormality.[254,256] Autopsy data reveal that an increase in frequency of nodules is evident in women and men over age 30 with a progressive increase to a frequency of 90% in women and 50% in men aged over 70 years. These observations are supported by ultrasound data, which have found thyroid nodules in approximately 50% of women over the age of 50 years.[257]

Clinical presentations

Thyroid nodules most commonly are asymptomatic; the patient may discover them accidentally, or the physician may find them during the course of a physical examination or as an incidental finding on CT or MRI of the head, neck, or chest. Of greatest concern is the finding of a single palpable nodule, which raises the possibility of thyroid malignancy. In many such patients, further evaluation will reveal the presence of multiple nodules. Although a single nodule is more likely to harbor a malignancy than a multinodular thyroid, only approximately 10% of clinical single nodules will, in fact, be malignant.

Patients with thyroid nodules should be questioned for the history of external radiation exposure of the head, neck, and upper thorax. It is well established that radiation of the thyroid results in a marked increase in risk of developing thyroid malignancy. In the United States, it was common practice for many years, up to the 1950s, to treat facial acne, tonsillar enlargement, cervical adenitis, and thymic enlargement with external radiation. It is estimated that several million people were irradiated, many of whom are now in the over-60 age group. Although a history of irradiation in a patient with nodular thyroid increases the likelihood of malignancy, it is important to note that irradiation also increases the development of benign nodules. Of individuals who as children received low-dose head and neck irradiation, 87%

Table 90-5. Risk Factors for Malignancy in a Thyroid Nodule

- Male
- Age greater than 60
- History of irradiation of head or neck area
- Family history of thyroid cancer
- Solitary on clinical examination
- Increase in size
- Hard on palpation
- Hoarse voice
- Suspicious ultrasound characteristics
  - Size greater than 1 cm
  - Solid rather than cystic
  - Hypoechogenicity
  - Central hypervascularity
  - Presence of microcalcifications
  - Irregular borders

have ultrasound-detectable nodules, from 16% to 29% will develop palpable thyroid nodules, and of these, approximately one third will be malignant.[258,259] Nodules are apparent after a latency of 10 to 20 years, and the incidence of malignant nodules reaches a peak 20 to 30 years after exposure.[255,258]

Occasionally, a thyroid nodule will be associated with acute onset of neck pain and tenderness. This circumstance may be the result of acute or subacute thyroiditis or hemorrhage into a preexisting nodule.

The finding of multinodular thyroid increases in areas of iodine deficiency. Often there is a history of goiter dating back to childhood or young adult years. Very large multinodular goiter, particularly those with a sizable substernal component, may compress the trachea and lead to complaints of dyspnea. Disturbances of swallowing may also occur. This presentation is most common in older women. A large substernal goiter sometimes is first recognized when the patient has had a chest radiogram and is noted to have compression or deviation of the trachea or a superior mediastinal mass.[260]

Differential diagnosis

The entities that present as thyroid nodules are many. Most are the result of benign thyroid lesions and include follicular and colloid adenomas, acute and subacute thyroiditis, Hashimoto's thyroiditis, and thyroid cysts. Malignant thyroid neoplasms include papillary, follicular, medullary, and anaplastic carcinomas, as well as thyroid lymphoma and metastases to the thyroid. Nonthyroid lesions may also present as apparent thyroid nodules and include lymph nodes, aneurysms, parathyroid adenomas and cysts, and thyroglossal duct cysts.[261]

The likelihood that a single nodule is malignant increases if there is a history of radiation exposure, if it occurs in a man, has been observed to undergo increase in size, is accompanied by hoarseness of the voice suggestive of impingement on the recurrent laryngeal nerve, and is stony hard on palpation (Table 90-5).

Age appears to be a risk factor for the development of thyroid cancer. The National Cancer Data Base of 53,856 patients with thyroid cancer indicates that approximately 25% of all thyroid cancers are first diagnosed in individuals who are older than 60 years.[262,263] The overall

Table 90-6. Occurrence of Thyroid Malignancy in the Older Patient, and 10-Year Survival

	Percentage of Cancer Patients		Percentage
Cancer Type	>Age 40	>Age 64	10-Year Survival*
Papillary/mixed	79	60–67	<65
Follicular	13	20–25	<57
Medullary	3	5	<63
Anaplastic	2	6	0
Lymphoma	3	5	≤100

*Age at diagnosis >60 years.

histologic distribution of thyroid cancer is 79% papillary, 13% follicular, 3% Hurthle cell, 3.5% medullary, and 1.7% anaplastic.[262] Age is a factor in predicting histologic type of malignancy[262,264] (Table 90-6). In patients over the age of 60 years, papillary carcinoma accounts for approximately 67% of thyroid cancers. Follicular carcinoma, the next most common histologic type, has a peak frequency in both the fourth and sixth decades of life with a mean age at diagnosis of 44 years. It, along with Hurthle-cell carcinoma, makes up approximately 23% of the thyroid malignancies in the over-60 age group. Medullary carcinoma has a peak incidence in the fifth and sixth decades and accounts for 5% of thyroid cancers in the elderly population.[262,265]

Anaplastic carcinoma of the thyroid is almost exclusively a disease of older persons and accounts for approximately 6% of thyroid cancers in this age group. It is invariably fatal in a short period of time from its first diagnosis, especially when greater than 5 cm in diameter.[266] Clinically, it often arises in an area of previous thyroid disease and is recognized by its rapid growth, rocklike consistency, and local invasiveness with recurrent laryngeal nerve involvement and tracheal compression.

Lymphoma and metastatic cancers make up the remaining thyroid malignancies in elderly people. Lymphoma is characterized by a rapidly enlarging painless neck mass, which may cause compressive symptoms and initially may be difficult to differentiate from anaplastic carcinoma on clinical appearance alone. Hashimoto's thyroiditis is commonly present in patients with lymphoma.[276]

The rapid onset of a painful, tender thyroid mass with an accompanying fever and leukocytosis is highly suggestive of acute suppurative thyroiditis. Similarly, the development of a painful, tender, firm thyroid mass without fever and leukocytosis points toward a diagnosis of subacute or granulomatous thyroiditis. A history of an antecedent upper-respiratory tract infection with a sore throat further supports the diagnosis. This disorder may be accompanied in its acute phase by transient hyperthyroidism as a result of leakage of thyroid hormones from damaged follicular cells. Another consideration in the patient with acute onset of a painful, tender neck mass is hemorrhage into a previously asymptomatic thyroid cyst or adenoma.

Evaluation of a thyroid nodule

The major objective of evaluation in the patient who is found to have a thyroid nodule, especially an apparently single nodule, is to determine if the nodule is benign or malignant. A number of diagnostic modalities are available.

Blood tests of thyroid function will usually give normal results, with the exception of the patient with a hyperfunctioning adenoma or toxic multinodular goiter. In some patients with nodular disease secondary to Hashimoto's thyroiditis, serum TSH may be increased. Several reports have shown that serum TSH may be an independent predictor of thyroid malignancy with the risk of malignancy in a thyroid nodule increasing with higher levels of TSH, even within the normal range, so that the likelihood of malignancy was 52% when TSH was 5 mU/L or greater.[268,269] Measurement of serum thyroglobulin is often elevated in patients with thyroid cancer but cannot reliably differentiate malignancy from benign adenoma or thyroiditis.[77] Its major usefulness is in the early recognition of recurrence or metastasis in patients with papillary or follicular carcinoma who had previously undergone total thyroidectomy. Elevation of serum calcitonin concentration greatly supports a diagnosis of medullary carcinoma.[270]

Determination of functional status of a nodule by isotope imaging is useful. Malignant tissue rarely is able to take up iodine, so that identification of a nodule as "warm" or "hot" by ^{123}I or technetium scanning makes the likelihood of malignancy in the nodule remote. In addition, scanning may reveal that an apparent single nodule is, in fact, part of a multinodular thyroid, again decreasing the risk of malignancy. The finding of a nonfunctioning or "cold" nodule does not establish a diagnosis of malignancy because 95% of thyroid nodules are cold, and of these, the incidence of malignancy is 5%.[271] For this reason, isotopic scanning is no longer considered as an initial diagnostic test.

High-resolution ultrasonography can detect lesions as small as 2 mm and can permit classification of a nodule as solid, cystic, or mixed solid–cystic.[272] The technique often demonstrates multinodularity in a gland with a single palpable nodule. The value of ultrasonography in establishing a diagnosis of malignancy is limited because there is considerable overlap in the ultrasound characteristics of benign and malignant nodules. The following ultrasound features increase the probability of malignancy: (1) size greater than 1 cm, (2) solid rather than cystic, (3) hypoechogenicity, (4) central hypervascularity, (5) presence of microcalcifications, and (6) irregular borders (see Table 90-5).[273] The procedure may be useful for detecting recurrent or residual thyroid cancer and for screening individuals who have had a history of irradiation exposure. It may also be of value in the patient suspected of having thyroid lymphoma, because this malignancy often produces a characteristic asymmetrical pseudocystic pattern.[274]

Computed tomography and MRI can provide detailed information on thyroid anatomy. These procedures are expensive and appear to add little to initial clinical assessment for malignancy.[65] However, they may be useful in determining the extent of disease in patients with anaplastic carcinoma or lymphoma of the thyroid. Additionally, CT and MRI can provide information about the size and substernal extent of large goiters and compression of neck structures.

In patients with nontoxic nodular goiter, thyroid hormone has been used to suppress TSH on the assumption that benign lesions were more likely to be TSH-dependent and, therefore, likely to decrease in size. The procedure involves giving L-thyroxine in a dose sufficient to suppress serum TSH and monitoring the size of the thyroid nodule for a period of 3 to 6 months. Because of the subjective nature of assessment of thyroid nodular size and the demonstration that suppressive therapy had little significant effect on goiter or nodule size during several well-controlled trials of L-thyroxine, there does not appear to be justification for future use of this procedure.[275,276] In addition, the administration of suppressive doses of L-thyroxine to elderly patients carries substantial risk for precipitation or aggravation of ischemic heart disease and for acceleration of bone loss.

Fine-needle aspiration (FNA) of the thyroid to obtain tissue for cytologic or histologic examination appears to be the most reliable and accurate method of separating benign from malignant disease.[277–279] FNA is indicated in any patient with a solitary nodule and when there is suspicion of thyroid malignancy from clinical, ultrasound, or scanning findings. In skilled hands, the procedure is safe, inexpensive, and capable of determining the presence or absence of malignancy with 95% accuracy. The reliability of FNA can be further increased if done in conjunction with real-time sonographic guidance. The cytopathologic findings from FNA are assigned to four categories: positive for malignancy, suspicious for malignancy, negative for malignancy, and nondiagnostic. In the case of a nondiagnostic aspirate, repeat FNA is recommended. Surgery is recommended for all patients with a malignant cytologic diagnosis. For patients with a suspicious interpretation of the FNA, thyroid scanning is recommended with surgical excision to follow if the lesion is hypofunctioning. The patient with benign cytology can be managed subsequently by observation. The patient with clinical or FNA features suggestive of lymphoma should have a large-needle or surgical biopsy done to confirm the diagnosis.[274]

Management of thyroid nodules

The management of thyroid nodules largely depends on the results of the diagnostic evaluation, especially the determination as to whether the nodule has a high risk of being malignant based on ultrasound characteristics and FNA results.[280] Nodules identified as being "warm" and with associated normal thyroid hormone production and no compressive symptoms warrant only observation with examination at intervals of 6 to 12 months. "Hot" nodules are managed similarly as long as thyroid function is normal. If evidence for hyperthyroidism is found, then appropriate treatment for this condition should be initiated.

Management of the "cold" nodule is more complex.[281] When possible, FNA biopsy should be performed.[277–279] Demonstration of benign cytology in either a solid or a cystic nodule indicates that the patient can be managed subsequently by observation. The combination of suspicious cytology by FNA and cold appearance on scanning should lead to a recommendation of surgical excision. If FNA reveals malignant cells, operation is recommended with little need for further study.

Only a surgeon experienced in the procedure should perform surgery for thyroid carcinoma. If a diagnosis of malignancy has not been firmly established preoperatively, the nodule should be removed with a wide margin of uninvolved tissue and examined by frozen section. If a diagnosis of papillary or follicular carcinoma is confirmed or has been made before surgery, near-total thyroidectomy should be carried out because of the high frequency of multicentricity of malignancy and the need to remove functional thyroid tissue in order to monitor the patient with whole-body radioiodine scanning in the future.[263,280,282–284] Regional lymph nodes should be explored and removed if there is evidence of metastatic involvement. Postoperatively, attention must be paid to the possible complications of recurrent laryngeal nerve injury and hypoparathyroidism, which may be transient or permanent. Almost certainly, patients will become hypothyroid following surgery and will require hormone replacement, which should be in a dose sufficient to suppress serum TSH to levels below normal, if clinically tolerated.

Postoperatively, and at 6- to 12-month intervals thereafter, it will be necessary to discontinue thyroid replacement for a period of up to 6 weeks to allow endogenous serum TSH levels to rise sufficiently high (>30 mU/L) to promote tissue uptake of ^{131}I. Alternatively, replacement thyroid hormone can be continued and recombinant human TSH (rhTSH) can be given intramuscularly at 24-hour intervals for two doses.[285] Twenty-four hours after the second dose of rhTSH or after the period of thyroid hormone withdrawal, blood is obtained for measurement of thyroglobulin and then large scanning doses of ^{123}I are administered and neck and total-body scans are performed at 24, 48, and 72 hours. If serum thyroglobulin is elevated or if areas of uptake are found, large ablative doses of ^{131}I are then administered and replacement therapy reinstituted 48 hours later. This approach reduces the recurrence rate of both papillary and follicular carcinoma and prolongs survival.[263,283,284,286] In the patient whose initial surveillance thyroid scan shows no areas of uptake and in whom the serum thyroglobulin levels are below 0.1 ng/mL, subsequent monitoring can be done by periodic measurement of serum thyroglobulin while continuing on thyroid hormone replacement without the need for thyroid hormone withdrawal.[287] As long as the serum thyroglobulin remains below 0.1 ng/mL, the risk of thyroid cancer recurrence is very low. Patients followed in this way should also have periodic neck ultrasonography performed.

The 10-year survival rate when initial diagnosis is made over the age of 60 years is estimated to be less than 65% for patients with papillary carcinoma, whereas 10-year survival falls to less than 57% in older patients with follicular carcinoma and is lower yet for patients with medullary carcinoma.[264,288] In patients with follicular carcinoma, increased size (greater than 3 cm) was associated with increased recurrence, and distant metastases at time of diagnosis predicted a high risk of subsequent death.[265] Patients with radioiodine-resistant differentiated thyroid cancer have shown a positive response to treatment with motesanib diphosphate, an orally active inhibitor of vascular endothelial growth factor receptors.[289] For medullary carcinoma, the operative procedure of choice is total thyroidectomy because the disease is often multicentric. Routine dissection of the lymph modes is also recommended. The majority of medullary carcinomas do not respond to ^{131}I therapy so that patients with inoperable residual or recurrent disease are treated palliatively with external irradiation. The survival declines with increase in age at time of initial diagnosis, being substantially lower in patients over age 60 years. Approximately two thirds of patients in their seventh decade will have persistent disease after surgery.[290] The efficacy of surgery can be monitored postoperatively by measurement of blood calcitonin concentration, both in the basal state and after stimulation.[270] Survival rates for thyroid malignancy initially diagnosed in patients over the age of 60 years are given in Table 90-6.

The management of anaplastic carcinoma of the thyroid remains unsatisfactory.[286] Relief of symptoms of compression can sometimes be achieved by surgery followed by high-dose (45 to 60 Gy) external irradiation.[291] Chemotherapy with doxorubicin may be beneficial in combination with surgery and external irradiation.[266,292]

Patients with thyroid lymphoma should have clinical staging carried out by means of CT or MRI. The survival rate can approach 100% in response to aggressive external irradiation in combination with CHOP (cytoxan, Adriamycin, vincristine, prednisone) chemotherapy.[274]

Subtotal thyroidectomy has been the traditional therapy for compressive goiter.[293] However, large compressive goiters can respond to ablation doses of ^{131}I (25 to 125 mCi) with significant shrinkage of the thyroid and accompanying relief of compressive symptoms such as stridor, dyspnea, and dysphagia.[260,276,294,295] Improvement in the response to ^{131}I has been observed when patients were given rhTSH before radioiodine administration.[296] In these patients, replacement doses of L-thyroxine sufficient to keep serum TSH within the normal range should be given following either surgery or radioiodine treatment to maintain suppression of thyroid tissue and to avoid the late development of hypothyroidism.

If acute, suppurative thyroiditis is suspected, treatment with antibiotics is called for. The microorganisms most commonly responsible are *Staphylococcus aureus*, *Streptococcus hemolyticus*, *Escherichia coli*, *Pneumococcus*, and *Salmonella*. Rarely, surgical drainage of a fluctuant mass will be necessary. Nodules found in association with subacute thyroiditis require no special care and may diminish in size as the disease resolves.

Summary of Management Algorithm

Hyperthyroidism

- Use β-blockers for rate control of tachyarrhythmias.
- ^{131}I ablation is preferred treatment.
- If atrial fibrillation is present:
  - Use anticoagulants
  - Use cardioversion if normal sinus rhythm has not occurred by 16 weeks after normalization of thyroid function
- Use high-dose antithyroid drugs plus iodide for thyroid storm.

Subclinical Hyperthyroidism[297]

- Normalize thyroid function with antithyroid drugs or ^{131}I if:
  - There are clinical features of hyperthyroidism
  - Atrial fibrillation occurs
  - There is evidence for osteopenia or osteoporosis
  - TSH is suppressed <0.1 mU/L
  - There is an increase in T4, free T4, T3, or free T3 during follow-up
- Monitor TSH/free T4 at 6- to 12-month intervals in asymptomatic patients with TSH 0.1 to 0.4 mU/L.

Hypothyroidism

- Treat with L-thyroxine:
  - Start with low-dose 12.5 to 25 μg daily
  - Increase by 12.5 to 25 μg at 2- to 4-week intervals
- Monitor treatment response with serum TSH.
- If coronary artery disease and angina are present, start β-blocker along with L-thyroxine.
- For myxedema coma:
  - Provide supportive care in intensive-care setting
  - Treat immediately with IV L-thyroxine 300 to 500 μg
  - Give IV glucocorticoids until adrenal status is determined

Subclinical Hypothyroidism[297]

- Initiate treatment with L-thyroxine if:
  - TSH is >10 mU/L
  - TSH is 4.5–10 mU/L and
    - Antithyroid antibody titers are >1:1600.
    - Dyslipidemia is present.
    - Coronary artery disease is present.
    - Symptoms suggestive of mild hypothyroidism are present.
- Monitor TSH/free T4 at 6- to 12-month intervals in patients with TSH 4.5 to10 mU/L, negative antithyroid antibodies, and no evident symptoms of hypothyroidism.

Thyroid Nodules/Malignancy

- If suspicious nodule is present, do FNA biopsy.
- If positive diagnosis is made of differentiated thyroid cancer:
  - Treat with near-total thyroidectomy
  - Follow with ^{131}I ablation of any thyroid remnant
  - Subsequent yearly follow-up with ^{123}I scans and serum thyroglobulin

KEY POINTS
Disorders of the Thyroid

- Both disease states and drugs commonly used in the elderly can affect measures of thyroid function.
- Disorders of thyroid function increase in prevalence with increasing age.
- Because aging can alter the clinical presentation of both hyperthyroidism and hypothyroidism, screening for thyroid dysfunction is warranted for all persons over the age of 50 years.
- Treatment of both subclinical hyperthyroidism and subclinical hypothyroidism may prevent the later occurrence of significant adverse clinical events.
- Treatment of both hyperthyroidism and hypothyroidism in elderly people differs from the approach to treatment in younger persons.
- Thyroid malignancy increases in prevalence with increasing age, and initial diagnosis in the older person carries higher risk of subsequent recurrence or decreased survival.

For a complete list of references, please visit online only at www.expertconsult.com

CHAPTER 91

Disorders of the Parathyroid Glands

Jane Turton
Michael Stone
David E. C. Cole

INTRODUCTION

Most individuals have only four parathyroid glands, which are usually located at the superior and inferior poles of the thyroid gland and which arise from the second and fourth branchial arches during fetal development[1] (Figure 91-1).

A parathyroid gland is oval, yellow in color, measures about 5 mm across, and usually weighs less than 35 mg. Within a gland, there are four cell types: chief cells, clear cells, oxyphil cells, and adipose cells.[2]

PHYSIOLOGY OF PARATHYROID HORMONE

Parathyroid hormone (PTH) is produced by the chief cells and is an 84 amino acid polypeptide with biologic activity in the N-terminal portion of the molecule. It is synthesized as pre-pro-PTH and is then sequentially processed to pro-PTH and finally to intact PTH (1-84). PTH is secreted as intact PTH and also in the cleaved C-terminal PTH form (C-PTH). The proportion of C-PTH secreted relative to intact PTH changes in response to circulating free calcium concentration.

Intact PTH has a half-life of less than 5 minutes. It is metabolized by Kupfer cells in the liver, resulting in cleavage of its N-terminal portion and the intracellular degradation of the N-terminal fragment. C-terminal fragments are released back into the circulation from the liver. These fragments are cleared by the kidneys and may be elevated in renal failure. C-terminal fragments have a longer half-life than the intact hormone and constitute the majority of circulating PTH forms.

PTH secretion exhibits both a circadian rhythm, with a peak in the early hours of the morning and nadir in late morning/early afternoon,[3] and a seasonal variation that is highest in the winter and lowest in the summer.[4]

The secretion of PTH occurs predominantly in response to a fall in extracellular free calcium concentration, which is sensed by the calcium sensing receptor (CaSR) on parathyroid chief cells. The CaSR is a G-protein coupled receptor found in the intestine, kidney, thyroid C-cells, brain, and bone, where it is involved in local calcium homeostatic processes.[5] The gene mutation of the CaSR in familial benign hypocalciuric hypercalcemia results in an alteration of the calcium homeostatic set point.[6]

The secretion of PTH is also influenced by circulating levels of 1,25-dihydroxyvitamin D ($1,25(OH)_2D_3$) phosphate and magnesium. $1,25(OH)_2D_3$ suppresses PTH secretion by inhibiting gene transcription. Hyperphosphatasemia increases PTH synthesis and secretion; the converse holds for hypophosphatemia. In states of significant chronic magnesium deficiency, PTH secretion is impaired. An acute magnesium deficiency may, however, increase PTH secretion.

In the kidney, PTH stimulates 1α-hydroxylation of 25-hydroxyvitamin D_3 ($25(OH)D_3$) to produce the biologically active $1,25(OH)_2D_3$, promotes calcium reabsorption in the distal convoluted tubule, and inhibits the reabsorption of phosphate from the proximal tubule.

In the small intestine, PTH has a small direct local effect, and circulating $1,25(OH)_2D_3$ produced in the kidney promotes gastrointestinal absorption of calcium and phosphate.[7]

PTH increases osteoclastic resorption of bone at cortical surfaces and causes the release of calcium into the extracellular fluid. The net result of PTH action is an increase in extracellular calcium levels and a reduction in phosphate levels.

CALCIUM HOMEOSTASIS AND CHANGES WITH AGE

In the elderly, average PTH levels can be up to 35% higher than those measured in a young adult population.[8,9] The cause of this is multifactorial and is the result of the following conditions:

- A fall in $1,25(OH)_2D_3$ production by the aging kidney as the glomerulofiltration rate falls from 125 mL/min at age 20 years to 60 mL/min at age 80.[10]
- A reduction in the responsiveness of renal 1α-hydroxylase to circulating PTH.[11]
- A reduction in dietary intake and absorption of calcium and vitamin D.[12]
- A reduction in vitamin D production in the skin as a result of less frequent and efficient sunlight exposure. Individuals who are housebound or living in nursing

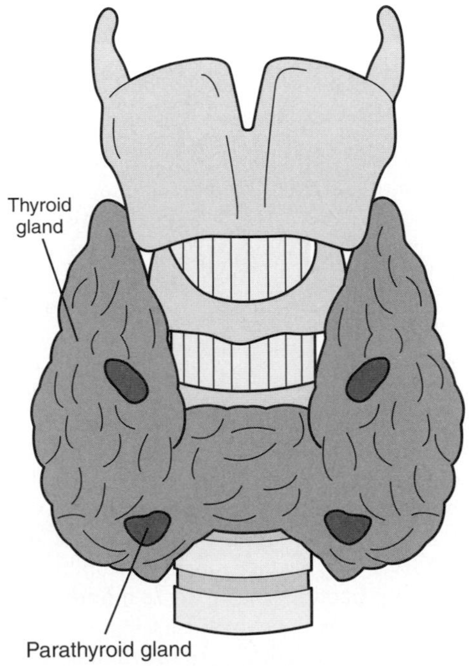

Figure 91-1. Anatomic drawing of parathyroid glands.

Table 91-1. Clinical Investigation of Parathyroid Disorders

Measurement of
Bone profile: calcium, phosphate, albumin, alkaline phosphatase
Renal profile: sodium, potassium, urea, creatinine
Plasma PTH
Serum 25(OH) vitamin D
Magnesium
(Lithium)
24-hour urinary calcium, phosphate, sodium and creatinine
Bone density measurement: dual x-ray absorptiometry
X-rays and isotope bone scan
Sestamibi and ultrasound scan for preoperative assessment of primary hyperparathyroidism

Table 91-2. PTH Assay, Calcium, and Vitamin D Assays

PTH Assay

Blood for PTH assay should be collected into tubes containing EDTA, as PTH is more stable in EDTA.[14] Intact PTH is measured by noncompetitive immunoassay, which recognizes the C-terminal region. Specificity for the intact PTH is achieved by using a signal antibody that binds to the N-terminal (1-34) region.

Calcium and Vitamin D Assay

Total calcium is usually measured using dye-binding spectrophotometric techniques. Forty percent of calcium in blood is bound to albumin, so changes in serum albumin may alter the total calcium result. Laboratories correct for this by reporting an "adjusted calcium" result.

The more physiologically relevant ionized calcium fraction (by direct ion-specific electrode) may be measured using electrochemical methods.

Nutritional vitamin D status is assessed using an assay for serum 25-hydroxyvitamin D (25(OH)D), which has a physiological half-life of 3 weeks.

homes are at particular risk of developing abnormal PTH secretion secondary to vitamin D deficiency[13] (Tables 91-1 and 91-2).[14–16]

SECONDARY HYPERPARATHYROIDISM

Secondary hyperparathyroidism is the most common disorder of calcium homeostasis in the elderly and has a prevalence of 20% to 60% in the population aged over 75 years.[17] It occurs when there is vitamin D deficiency or insufficiency, and the resultant decrease in serum calcium causes parathyroid gland hyperplasia, which in turn causes a physiologic increase in PTH production.

The combination of vitamin D deficiency and secondary hyperparathyroidism is associated with an increased risk of fracture.[17,18] There is an associated increase in mortality from cardiovascular disease[19] independent of bone mass, serum 25(OH)D, and renal function.[20–22]

The first-line treatment for secondary hyperparathyroidism is a combined preparation of elemental calcium 1000 to 1200 mg and vitamin D3 20 micrograms (800 IU) daily. Chapuy et al showed that reducing PTH levels and improving serum 25(OH)D_3 levels using this combination could reduce risk of hip fracture by 30% at 18 months and that this efficacy was maintained out to 3 years.[23]

If for any reason a patient cannot or will not adhere to this regime, vitamin D_2 or D_3 alone, 1α-hydroxycolecalciferol, or 1,25-dihydroxycolecalciferol can be used. 1,25-dihydroxycolecalciferol is particularly useful for patients with renal failure although careful monitoring of serum calcium is required.

Case Report: Secondary Hyperparathyroidism

A female Caucasian nonsmoker age 81 years presented to our clinic with a history of falls and a past history of wrist fracture, osteoarthritis, hypertension and hypercholesterolaemia. She was independent in her activities of daily living and mobile with a walking stick but lacked confidence to go outside alone. Her diet was low in calcium. She was referred for a bone density scan and diagnosed osteoporotic (Neck of Femur T score –3.0). She was taking a statin and mild opiate analgesia for arthritic pain. A biochemical screen for secondary causes of osteoporosis was performed, which revealed a profound vitamin D deficiency, secondary hyperparathyroidism, and mild hypocalcaemia. She was treated with a combined preparation of calcium 1000 mg and 800 IU ergocalciferol daily, which normalized her biochemistry (see below).

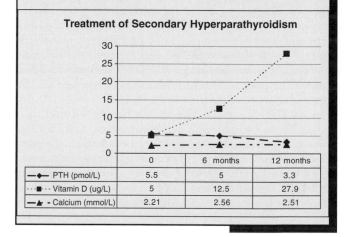

Treatment of Secondary Hyperparathyroidism

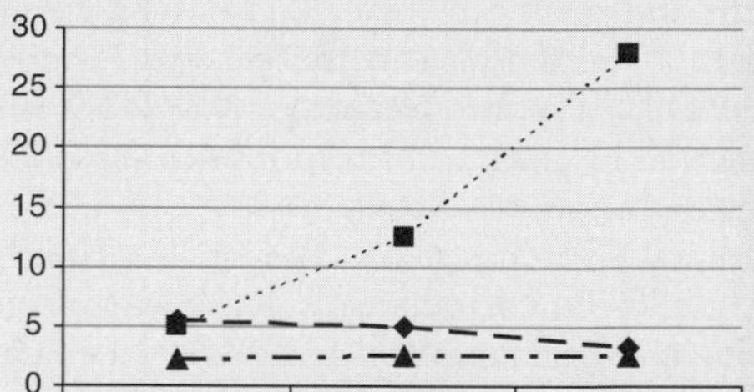

	0	6 months	12 months
PTH (pmol/L)	5.5	5	3.3
Vitamin D (ug/L)	5	12.5	27.9
Calcium (mmol/L)	2.21	2.56	2.51

PRIMARY HYPERPARATHYROIDISM

The biochemical presentation of primary hyperparathyroidism (HPT) is a raised plasma PTH and hypercalcemia. The peak incidence occurs between ages 55 to 64 years at 1:1000. The prevalence is 2% in persons aged over 75 years, and it is three times as common in women as in men.[24] Primary HPT is caused by a single adenoma in 80% of cases, four-gland hyperplasia in 15% of cases, and carcinoma in fewer than 1% of cases.[25] A rare but notable form of hypercalcemia, which can mimic primary hyperparathyroidism, is benign familial hypocalciuric hypercalcemia.

Changes in the levels of circulating PTH have been shown to have an effect in the bone and in the brain. There is an increase in the bone remodeling space, and in trabecular bone, high levels of PTH increase bone formation. However, in cortical bone, high levels of PTH increase bone loss, cause a fall in bone mineral density (BMD), and increase the risk of fracture independent of 25(OH)D_3 levels.[26,27]

In the brain, high levels of PTH can cause mood disturbance and memory loss secondary to the action of PTH on the PTH_2 receptor.[28]

Case Report: Primary Hyperparathyroidism

A female Caucasian age 75 years presented with a history of bone and muscle pain, low mood, indigestion, and a BMI of 18.5 She was referred for bone densitometry, which confirmed severe osteoporosis. Screening for secondary causes of osteoporosis revealed hypercalcemia (corrected calcium 2.68 mmol/L), normal 25(OH)D_3, a raised PTH of 6.8 pmol/L, and raised urinary calcium excretion. She had no vertebral fractures. She was prescribed regular vitamin D_2 and an oral bisphosphonate. She was referred for parathyroidectomy. At surgery, she had a solitary right lower parathyroid adenoma measuring 20 × 3 × 2 mm removed. Since her surgery, her PTH and calcium have remained in the normal range. Her mood has improved, and the muscle and bone pains have eased. Bone mineral densities have increased by 7.5% in the 12 months since her surgery.

A common presentation of primary hyperparathyroidism follows measurement of serum calcium and the identification of individuals with asymptomatic hypercalcemia. The very elderly can present with an acute disequilibrium hypercalcemia as their renal function progressively declines or if they become acutely dehydrated[29] (Table 91-3).

Although most patients are now identified while asymptomatic, they can present with symptoms of lassitude, fatigue, mood swings, muscle pain, generalized weakness, and memory loss.[25] The classical presentation of primary hyperparathyroidism comprising bone cysts, pathologic fractures, and renal calculi as described by Von Reckinghausen in 1891 is very rare.[30]

The treatment of primary hyperparathyroidism can be conservative or surgical. The conservative management involves regular monitoring (serum calcium, BMD, and PTH) and the use of oral or intravenous bisphosphonates. Although the effects on serum calcium are limited and transient,[31] they are effective in treating the associated loss of bone.[32] The use of calcium and vitamin D supplements with bisphosphonates is accepted practice in postmenopausal osteoporosis; however, in primary hyperparathyroidism, calcium supplementation should not be used. It is, however, safe to prescribe regular vitamin D_3 alone to these individuals to ensure that serum vitamin D levels remain normal.

The use of surgery as treatment is becoming more acceptable, even for very elderly patients, because improvements in imaging have led to successful minimally invasive surgical techniques.[33] The indications for surgery are detailed in Table 91-4. The usual imaging and localization techniques are sestamibi and ultrasound scanning (Figures 91-2 and 91-3), and during surgery intraoperative sampling of parathyroid hormone[34] is performed, which confirms when the hyperfunctioning tissue has been removed (Figure 91-4).

After parathyroidectomy, patients can have increases of up to 12% in bone mineral density in the first year, even without further treatment,[35] and the dilemma regarding the use of calcium and vitamin D supplementation is removed. The mood disturbance and memory loss associated with hyperparathyroidism has also been shown to improve after surgery.[36,37]

Table 91-3. Symptoms and Signs of Acute Hypercalcemia

Differential Diagnosis of Hypercalcemia in the Elderly
Primary hyperparathyroidism
Malignancy
Renal failure
Addison's disease
Hyperthyroidism
Immobilization
Medications: thiazide diuretics, calcium supplements, lithium
Milk alkali syndrome
Paget's disease (when immobilized)
Sarcoidosis
Tuberculosis
Vitamin D or vitamin A intoxication
Symptoms of Acute Hypercalcemia
Neurological: drowsiness, confusion, irritability hypotonia, coma
Gastrointestinal: anorexia, nausea, vomiting, acute pancreatitis
Cardiovascular: arrhythmias
Renal: polyuria, polydipsia, dehydration

Table 91-4. Indications for Parathyroidectomy: National Institutes of Health Consensus Conference on Primary Hyperparathyroidism 1991 and 2002 Recommendations for Surgery[33]

1991 Recommendations
Typical bone, renal, gastrointestinal, or neuromuscular symptoms
Life-threatening hypercalcemia
Calcium level 11.4–12.0 mg/dL (2.9–3.0 mmol/L)
Urine calcium level >400 mg/day (10 mmol/day)
Renal stones
BMD 2 SDs <age, sex-matched controls (z score)
Reduced creatinine clearance <30%
Age <50 y
Patient request;
Adequate follow-up unlikely
2002 Additional Recommendations
Calcium level >1 mg/dL (0.25 mmol/L) above normal for each laboratory
BMD T score < −2.5 at any site (WHO definition of osteoporosis)

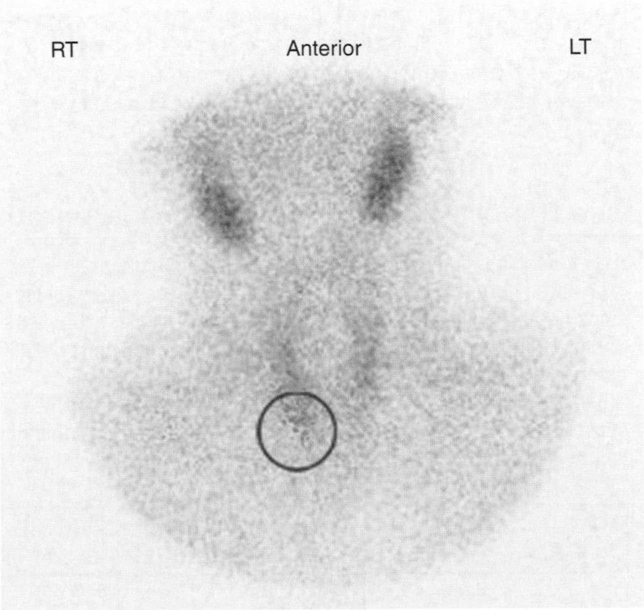

Figure 91-2. Sestamibi scan showing increased uptake at lower right lobe of thyroid.

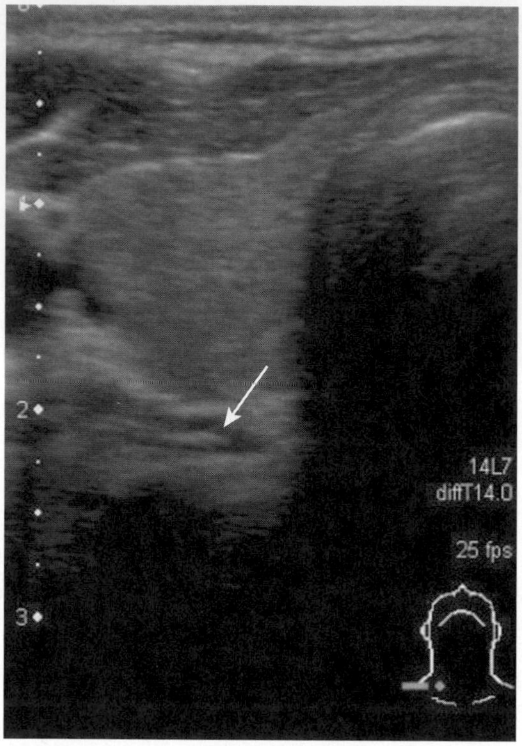

Figure 91-3. Ultrasound showing a hyperechoic region behind right lower lobe of thyroid.

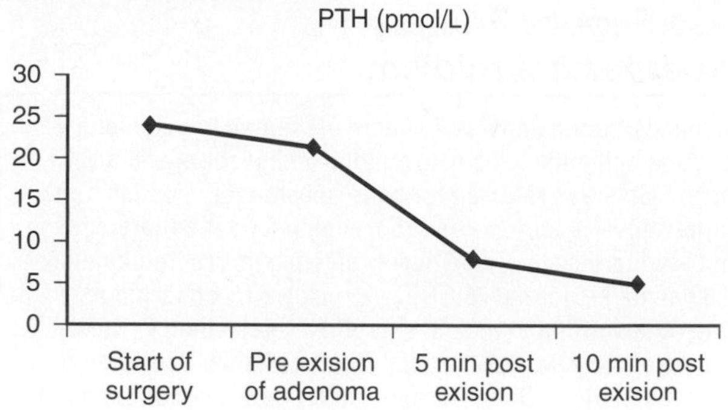

Figure 91-4. Graph of changes in PTH when hyperfunctioning parathyroid tissue is removed. Intraoperative PTH assay is carried out rapidly during the operation and takes 10 to 12 minutes. A drop in PTH of >50% indicates complete removal of the hyperfunctioning tissue.

Calcimimetic medications initially developed for the treatment of hyperparathyroidism related to renal disease and for the treatment of hypercalcemia of malignancy may now be used to treat primary hyperparathyroidism. These medications alter the sensitivity of the calcium sensing receptor in the parathyroid glands, thus reducing the levels of circulating PTH and calcium.[38]

LITHIUM

Hypercalcemia and hyperparathyroidism is common in patients treated with lithium. It has an incidence of 6.3% to 50%, and it can mimic primary hyperparathyroidism.[39,40] However, there are subtle differences between primary HPT and lithium-induced HPT. In lithium-induced disease, there is usually a normal serum phosphate, severe hypercalcemia is rare, 24-hour urinary calcium excretion is low or normal, and there is no adenoma. However, there is a hyperplasia of the parathyroid glands, and the condition is reversible on withdrawing lithium.[41]

Hypercalcemia can occur many years after initiation of lithium therapy, but it is also a recognized effect of a single dosing with lithium, which causes an acute elevation of serum PTH by direct stimulation of the parathyroid gland.[42] Surgical treatment of hypercalcemia with subtotal parathyroidectomy is usually unsuccessful when it is a result of lithium administration, and the hypercalcemia can recur if lithium therapy is continued.[43]

TERTIARY HYPERPARATHYROIDISM

In individuals who have prolonged secondary hyperparathyroidism as a result of renal failure, there is severe hyperplasia of the parathyroid glands, and the set point for normal inhibition of PTH secretion by calcium is altered. The hyperplastic parathyroid glands show a reduction in CaSR expression, and unlike secondary hyperparathyroidism, patients have high serum calcium and high PTH.

There are indications for parathyroid surgery in this condition, including severe bone pain, fractures, hypercalcemia,

Case Report: Lithium-Induced Hyperparathyroidism

A 65-year-old female presented to clinic with hypercalcemia and osteoporosis identified by screening in a gastroenterology clinic (corrected serum calcium 2.78, total spine T score −4.4, total hip T score −1.9). She had clinical risk factors for osteoporosis, namely smoking, a history of thyrotoxicosis, and celiac disease. She was being treated for bipolar disorder with oral lithium. She was adherent to a gluten-free diet and was taking 1000-mg calcium with 400 IU ergocalciferol and oral bisphosphonates as treatment for her osteoporosis at the time of presentation. Her PTH was raised; vitamin D was normal, and her 24-hour urinary calcium was low (see table). She had preoperative imaging for primary hyperparathyroidism, which did not identify an adenoma and she was not offered surgery. Her calcium and ergocalciferol were replaced with calciferol, and since then serum calcium has remained within normal limits. She continues to be treated with oral bisphosphonate for her osteoporosis.

PTH (0.9–5.4 pmol/L)	Calcium (2.20–2.60 mmol/L)	25(OH)D (8–50 ng/ml)	Phosphate (0.8–1.45 mmol/L)	24-Hour Urinary Calcium (<7.0 mmol)
6.6	2.78	25.8	1.34	0.7

Case Report: Tertiary Hyperparathyroidism

A 74-year-old male, who had received a renal transplant at age 58 years presented with osteoporosis (total spine T score −2.2, NOF T score −2.8, total hip T score −2.2), gross heterotopic calcification with chalky discharge, cardiovascular disease, and multiple falls.

Biochemically he had a vitamin D deficiency (25(OH)D 12.5 mcg/L), hyperparathyroidism (PTH 29.0 pmol/L), and a raised calcium x phosphate product (calcium 2.57, phosphate 1.81). He had CKD stage 4 disease with a creatinine of 350 micromol/L. He was managed conservatively with intermittent oral etidronate, phosphate binders, and low-dose alfacalcidol as he was unfit for parathyroid surgery. He subsequently died after suffering a hip fracture.

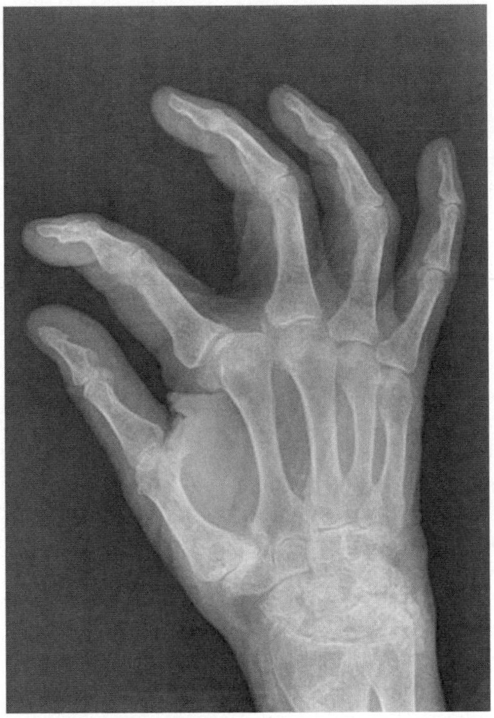

Figure 91-5. Heterotopic tissue calcification in a periarticular distribution.

heterotopic calcification, and bone cysts; however, if this condition is treated surgically, there is a risk that some patients will subsequently develop adynamic bone disease (Figure 91-5).

HYPOPARATHYROIDISM

Hypoparathyroidism is much less common than hyperparathyroidism. It is unusual for it to present for the first time in the elderly. It presents clinically as hypocalcaemia and is a result of insufficiency or resistance to PTH. It can occur after surgery for thyroid or parathyroid disease or reflect autoimmune disease. The reduction in PTH leads to an increase in renal calcium loss and reduced absorption of calcium in the gut because of a fall in 1,25(OH)D_3 production. Treatment is with hydroxylated products of vitamin D, Ca supplementation, and thiazide diuretics to reduce renal calcium loss.

KEY POINTS

Disorders of the Parathyroid Glands

- Vitamin D deficiency and secondary hyperparathyroidism is common in the elderly.
- Treatment of frail elderly people with simple calcium and vitamin D supplementation significantly reduces the risk of fractures.
- Acute disequilibrium hypercalcemia is an important, life-threatening cause of confusion in the elderly.
- The differential diagnosis of raised serum calcium and raised parathyroid hormone includes primary hyperparathyroidism, lithium-induced hyperparathyroidism, familial hypocalciuric hypercalcemia, and tertiary hyperparathyroidism.
- More elderly patients are now being considered for parathyroid surgery because of improvements in preoperative imaging and the use of minimally invasive surgical techniques.

For a complete list of references, please visit online only at www.expertconsult.com

CHAPTER 92

Diabetes Mellitus

Alan J. Sinclair
Simon C. M. Croxson

Diabetes mellitus remains a significant personal and public health burden with unmeasured socioeconomic implications.[1–4] Although detailed and focused studies in older people need to be planned, there is the recognition that as a common disabling disorder, diabetes requires interventional strategies at an early stage and the involvement of both patients and caregivers in defining goals of care and treatment plans.[5,6]

During the last decade, a number of factors suggest that care delivery has been enhanced and attitudes have changed.[7] In particular, there is more recognition that older patients with diabetes may be different from younger counterparts[8]; for example, they have a high degree of comorbidity, an age-related impairment of functional ability, and an increased vulnerability to hypoglycemia and its consequences. They may also require a different approach to care, which involves a greater focus on managing disability and functional impairment.[9] This chapter provides an account of the scientific and clinical basis of managing older people with diabetes, which should be a basis for enhancing the quality of diabetes care delivered. Although this is a large topic, the chapter should be read in conjunction with the European guidelines on diabetes in older people, which are currently being updated.[10] Modern aims of care have been identified and should form the basis of any care package (Table 92-1).

DIABETES DEFINITION, CLASSIFICATION, AND DIAGNOSIS

Diabetes is defined by hyperglycemia and the tendency to develop specific complications, particularly retinopathy; indeed, the gold standard test for diabetes would be to leave the subject untreated for several years after which the presence of retinopathy is diagnostic.[11–13] The diagnostic criteria were developed to diagnose type 2 diabetes mellitus (previously known as non–insulin-dependent diabetes mellitus), since type 1 diabetes (previously known as insulin-dependent diabetes mellitus) is generally obvious clinically. A venous plasma glucose level equal to or exceeding 11.1 mmol/L (200 mg/dL)[14,15] following glucose challenge identifies those subjects who have a dramatically increased risk of retinopathy.[11–13,16] The cutoff value of 11.1 mmol/L does actually separate normoglycemic and diabetic populations (each with a gaussian distribution of 2-hour values) in different age groups, suggesting that the World Health Organization (WHO) criteria (see later discussion) apply in both elderly and young people.

Table 92-1. Aims in Managing the Elderly Diabetic Person

- Maintain an optimal level of well-being and quality of life
- Avoid hyperglycemic malaise and optimize nutritional status
- Assess comorbidity state
- Avoid adverse drug events, particularly hypoglycemia
- Maintain lower limb strength
- Recognize disability and limit handicap

The majority of elderly diabetic people have type 2 diabetes, but type 1 does occur[17] and the age-specific incidence of type 1 is the same from 30 to 80 years of age.[18] Type 1 diabetes in the elderly population may have a very insidious onset, when it is termed "latent autoimmune diabetes of the aged" (LADA). LADA has been shown to be quite common in some series (e.g., 10% to 15% of diabetic adults and 50% of the nonobese type 2 diabetic subjects[19]); the autoantibody screen is not used in routine clinical practice in elderly people because it is not particularly predictive. Diabetes may also be secondary to or exacerbated by other conditions such as pancreatic disease, endocrine disease such as Cushing's syndrome, acromegaly, or thyrotoxicosis, and (most commonly) drug therapy with high-dose thiazide diuretics, oral glucocorticosteroids, and oral β-blockers. A comprehensive list of diabetogenic drugs is given in the National Diabetes Data Group criteria.[14] The majority of subjects with secondary diabetes are elderly.[20] A simple classification of diabetes mellitus in the elderly population is given in Table 92-2.

Recently, the diagnostic criteria were revised by both the American Diabetes Association (ADA)[21] and the WHO[22]—see Table 92-3 and www.diabetes.org.uk/info/carerec/newdiagnotic.html. These revisions have attempted to make screening for diabetes easier, but the ADA criteria have created pitfalls for the unwary. Both sets of criteria lower the threshold for an abnormal fasting plasma glucose (FPG) from 7.8 to 7.0 mmol/L, which addresses the low sensitivity of the fasting plasma glucose to detect an elevated 2-hour postchallenge glucose. Many studies have shown that this decrease in FPG increases the sensitivity of the FPG (e.g., from 65% to 81% in Bristol, U.K.), but the test still misses diabetic subjects with elevated 2-hour plasma glucose levels.[23] Isolated postchallenge hyperglycemia is not a benign mild condition; it carries increased risk of death.[24] Finally, the ADA reintroduced the concept of impaired fasting glucose (IFG) for subjects with a fasting glucose of 6.0 to 6.9 mmol/L. It is true that the risk of macrovascular disease increases once the FPG exceeds 6.0 mmol/L, but these IFG subjects have 2-hour postchallenge glucose levels, putting them clearly into normal, IFG, or diabetic categories, which require different management. In the predominantly European population of Bristol,[23] one third of IFG subjects have each category of glucose tolerance, whereas in the high-risk Gujerati population of Leicester, U.K., all IFG subjects have either diabetes

Table 92-2. Classification of Diabetes in Elderly People

Primary
Type 1
Type 2
Obese
Nonobese
Maturity-onset diabetes of the young

Secondary
Pancreatic disease
Drugs (e.g., steroids)
Other endocrine conditions (e.g., Cushing's syndrome, acromegaly, thyrotoxicosis)

Table 92-3. WHO Values for Diagnosis of Diabetes Mellitus and Other Categories of Hyperglycemia[22]

	GLUCOSE CONCENTRATION (mmol/L)		
	WHOLE BLOOD		
	Venous	**Capillary**	**Plasma (Venous)***
Diabetes mellitus:			
Fasting *or*	≥ 6.1	≥ 6.1	≥ 7.0
2 hours after glucose load	≥ 10.0	≥ 11.1	≥ 11.1
Impaired glucose tolerance (IGT):			
Fasting (if measured) *and*	<6.1 *and*	<6.1 *and*	<7.0 *and*
2 hours after glucose load	6.7–9.9	7.8–11.0	7.8–11.0
Impaired fasting glycemia (IFG):			
Fasting *and* (if measured)	5.6 *and* <6.1	5.6 *and* <6.1	6.1 *and* <7.0
2 hours after glucose load	<6.7	<7.8	<7.8

*Corresponding values for capillary plasma are:
For diabetes mellitus: fasting, 7.0; 2 hr, 12.2.
For impaired glucose tolerance: fasting, <7.0; and 2 hr, 8.9 and <12.2.
For impaired fasting glycemia: 6.1 and <7.0, and if measured, 2 hr, <8.9.
For clinical purposes, the diagnosis of diabetes should always be confirmed by repeating the test on another day unless there is unequivocal hyperglycemia with acute metabolic decompensation or obvious symptoms.

or IGT on the 2-hour PG.[25] These facts are important if the FPG is used for diagnosing diabetes.

The latest WHO and International Diabetes Federation (IDF) criteria simplify matters greatly by introducing the term *intermediate hyperglycemia* as somewhere between normal glucose tolerance (fasting venous plasma glucose <6.1 mmol/L and 2-hours postchallenge of <7.8) and diabetes (fasting venous plasma glucose = 7.0 mmol/L and 2-hour postchallenge of 11.1 mmol/L).[26]

IMPAIRMENT OF GLUCOSE TOLERANCE WITH AGING

The prevalence of diabetes mellitus increases with advancing age and is predominantly type 2. This age-related impairment has been confirmed by more recent studies indicating that glucose intolerance begins in the third decade and continues throughout adulthood.[27–30] The magnitude of the rise has been estimated to be 0.33 to 0.72 mmol/L (5.9 to 13.0 mg/dL) per decade in 1- and 2-hour postglucose ingestion samples. The rise is more pronounced in women (about 0.55 mmol/L [9.9 mg/dL] higher than in men).[30] The National Health and Nutrition Examination Survey (NHANES III) of U.S. residents found a rise in prevalence of impaired glucose tolerance (IGT) of 11.9% in those aged 40 to 49 years to 20.7% in those aged 60 to 74 years;[31] this survey also demonstrated increasing prevalence rates of diabetes with age from 3.4% to 24.4% (Figure 92-1).

Several possible mechanisms may contribute to glucose intolerance during aging and these are listed in Table 92-4. The impairment is clearly multifactorial, being characterized by delays in glucose-mediated insulin secretion, insulin-induced suppression of hepatic glucose output, and a rise in insulin-mediated glucose uptake.

EPIDEMIOLOGY OF DIABETES MELLITUS IN THE ELDERLY POPULATION

To promote rational health care planning involving an accurate assessment of the public health burden of diabetes and a needs assessment, we require better ways of identifying

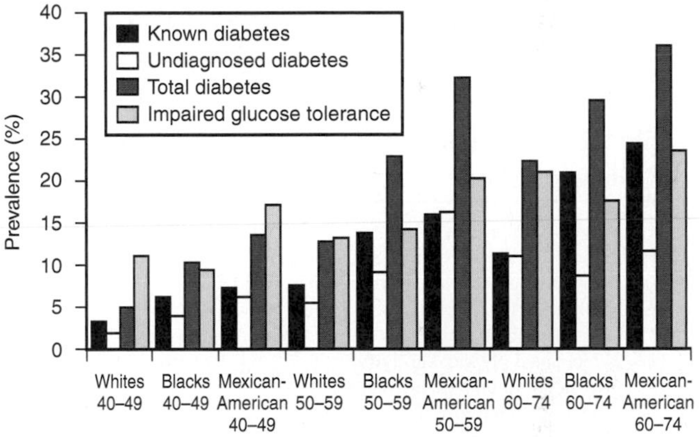

Figure 92-1. Data from NHANES III: rising abnormalities of glucose tolerance with age. *(From Harris MI, Flegal KM, Cowie CC et al. Prevalence of diabetes, impaired fasting glucose, and impaired glucose tolerance in U.S. adults: the Third National Health and Nutrition Examination Survey, 1988–1994. Diabetes Care 1998;21:518–24.)*

individuals with the disease since approximately 50% may be undiagnosed.[32] However, even studies of subjects with previously diagnosed diabetes can provide useful information. For instance, the surveys of Poole, Oxford, and Southall (U.K.) of European subjects with diagnosed diabetes[33] reveals that 60% of known diabetic subjects are aged 60 years or more.

The prevalence of diabetes rises from youth to old age (Figure 92-1). However, the Melton (U.K.) screening survey,[34] the East and West Finland screening survey,[35] and a survey of Pima Indians[36] found static prevalences from age 65 to 85, suggesting that the age-related increase in diabetes prevalence levels off after age 65. Most developed countries have a prevalence of approximately 17% in their elderly white population and around 25% in nonwhite populations.[15,31,35–47] The prevalence in white British elderly people is only around 9%,[34,48] although the prevalence in nonwhite British elderly people is still approximately 25%,[49] and the prevalence in care-home residents is 25%.[50]

The prevalence of previously diagnosed diabetes in the United Kingdom elderly population has increased over the last few decades and one could argue that this is because of a higher rate of ascertainment, rather than a true increase. Evidence from screening in Glostrup, Denmark, shows an increased true prevalence in the Danes because of increased obesity and decreased exercise,[51] and NHANES III has shown a true increase in prevalence[31] from NHANES II[32] (Table 92-5).

The risk of developing type 2 diabetes is increased by parental history,[32,47,52] obesity,[32,45,47,51,52] hypertension,[45,52] lack of exercise,[45,52] and nonwhite race.[31,32] In subjects with these risk factors, exercise seems to protect against the development of diabetes.[52] This is important when advising the offspring of patients who are told to stay slim, avoid refined carbohydrates, exercise more (climb 15 flights of stairs per day), and be aware of their risk of diabetes and hypertension.[52] Targeted screening of at-risk individuals is now also advised (e.g., fasting venous plasma glucose every 3 years for offspring of diabetic patients, after the age of 40 years),[21] remembering to advise the subjects to buy life insurance before the test rather than after.

Table 92-4. Mechanisms of Decreased Glucose Tolerance in Old Age

- Delayed/decreased glucose-induced insulin secretion
- Impaired insulin-mediated glucose uptake in skeletal muscle and adipose tissue because of predominantly postreceptor defect
- Other factors:
  - Increased body fat
  - Decreased physical activity
  - Reduced dietary carbohydrate
  - Impaired renal function
  - Hypokalemia
  - Increased sympathetic nervous system activity
  - Diabetogenic drugs

IMPACT OF DIABETES MELLITUS IN THE ELDERLY POPULATION

Overview

Diabetes places a significant vascular burden on older patients with diabetes, which is partly explained by the traditional risk factors present and also by the effect of aging, itself. Older patients appear to have 2 to 3 times more need for hospital care than the general population[53] for various conditions such as heart failure, stroke, and coronary heart disease. This increase occurs from middle age onwards.[54] Older people with diabetes also use primary care services 2 to 3 times more than nondiabetic controls.[54,55]

Several studies have defined the prevalence of elderly patients in hospital diabetic populations. In a study from the Edinburgh Royal Infirmary, elderly patients aged 65 years and over with diabetes accounted for 60% of the overall bed-occupancy because of diabetes, giving a mean hospital prevalence of 4.6%.[2] A Cardiff-based study of three district general hospitals found a hospital prevalence (pooled data) of 8.4% with a mean age of 65 years.[58]

Diabetes in older subjects is associated with considerable morbidity, mainly because of the long-term complications.[48–51] A population-based study from Oxford[59] measured the incidence of complications over a median period of 6 years in 188 patients aged 60 years and over by using a structured questionnaire and clinical examination. Incidence rates of ischemic heart disease, stroke, and peripheral vascular disease were 56, 22, and 146 per 1000 person-years, which are slightly higher than found in the Framingham study,[63] since the Oxford study involved an older age group. Retinopathy occurred at a rate of 60 and cataract at 29 per 1000 person-years, whereas proteinuria (albumin concentration greater than 300 mg/L) was 19 per 1000 person-years. Incidence rates appeared to be unrelated to sex or duration of diabetes, but stroke and peripheral vascular disease rose significantly with age.

Table 92-5. Prevalence of Diabetes in Different Screened Elderly Populations

Study	Year	Ref.	Age	Sex	Ethnic Origin	DIABETES rate (%)	IGT RATE (%)
Melton, U.K.	1991	44	65–85	MF	White	9.1	7.1
Coventry, U.K.	1988	59	60–79	MF	White	7.0	—
Coventry, U.K.	1988	59	60–79	MF	South Asian	27.8	—
NHANES II, U.S.	1976–1980	42	65–74	MF	White	17.9	23.0
NHANES II, U.S.	1976–1980	42	65–74	MF	Nonwhite	26.4	14.5
NHANES III, U.S.	1988–1994	37	60–74	MF	White	22.3	20.9
NHANES III, U.S.	1988–1994	37	60–74	MF	Black	29.5	17.6
NHANES III, U.S.	1988–1994	37	60–74	MF	Hispanic	36	23.5
California, U.S.	1972–1974	47	60–89	MF	White	16.1	—
Tampere, Finland (F)	1977	48	85	MF	White	17.0	—
Fredericia, Denmark (F)	1981–1982	53	60–74	M	White	7.2	—
Glostrup, Denmark (U)	1967	54	70	MF	White	10.0	25
Glostrup, Denmark (U)	1977	54	80	MF	White	12.0	36
Glostrup, Denmark	1996–1997	63	60	M	White	12.3	15.9
Glostrup, Denmark	1996–1997	63	60	F	White	6.8	13.1
East/west Finland (pm gtts)	1984	45	65–84	M	White	29.8	31.8
Gothenburg, Sweden	1980	55	67	M	White	10.8	14.2
Amsterdam, Holland (D)	1985	56	65	MF	White	23.6	—
Kuopio, Finland	1986–1988	57	65–74	MF	White	17.8	20.8

Abbreviations: *F*, FBG–based survey; *D*, recruitment details scanty; *pm gtts*, testing performed in afternoon, which may increase diabetes prevalence; *U*, previously undiagnosed diabetic subjects only recorded.

In Poole, a coastal town in southern England, the prevalence of diabetic neuropathy, an important cause of foot ulceration and amputation, was determined in 1077 diabetic subjects,[60] who comprised 94% of the known diabetic population. Neuropathy was diagnosed by the presence of neuropathic symptoms plus one or more physical findings, such as loss of light touch or impairment of pain sensation. The overall prevalence of neuropathy was 16.3% (compared with 2.9% in nondiabetic controls) with similar values in both type 1 and type 2 diabetes patients.

A community survey from Nottingham, U.K.,[61] of 98 elderly diabetic patients (mean age 73 years) registered with two inner-city general practices, studied the impact of diabetes in terms of complications and frequency of hospital and general practice contacts. Figure 92-2 shows that diabetic subjects had significantly higher prevalences of stroke, cognitive impairment, diminished leg pulses, visual impairment, and absent vibration senses (vibration perception threshold greater than 50 V at one or more sites, as a marker of neuropathy) compared with nondiabetic controls. Disability was present in four out of five patients. Cataract was the most common cause of disability associated with visual impairment.

Visual loss

Diabetic retinopathy was the third main cause of blindness and partial sight registration in one epidemiologic study in Avon, U.K.[64] However, the diabetic person also has a greater risk of cataract, glaucoma, retinal artery thrombosis, and retinal vein thrombosis. Thus it is no surprise that blind registrations for diabetic subjects in Nottingham, U.K., are eight times higher than the subjects not known to have diabetes,[60] with 16% of elderly diabetic subjects having blind or partial-sight registrations. The diabetic blind registration is predominantly due to maculopathy, which is treatable, unlike most forms of age-related macular degeneration, the main cause of blind registration in the elderly population.

Many cross-sectional studies show that good glycemic control is associated with less chance of developing retinopathy.[80,81] The U.K. Prospective Diabetes Study has now shown, in a prospective randomized controlled trial of aggressive versus conventional (when the trial was started) treatments, that both blood glucose lowering and blood pressure lowering decrease the risk of retinopathy.[67–70] Duration of disease is also associated with increased risk of retinopathy. Because the elderly diabetic subject has often had type 2 diabetes for at least 5 to 7 years before diagnosis,[71] it is not surprising that diabetic retinopathy is already present at diagnosis in 10.5% of elderly subjects in whom only one pupil was dilated[72]; 23.8% of subjects of all ages in the U.K. Prospective Diabetes Study had retinopathy at presentation.[73]

Laser photocoagulation can preserve vision in edematous and exudative maculopathies if visual acuity is 6/9 or better,[74,75] and it has been calculated that screening and treating diabetic retinopathy would prevent 56% of blind registrations that are caused by the retinopathy.[76] Interestingly, the EURODIAB controlled trial of lisinopril in insulin-dependent diabetes (EUCLID) showed a 50% reduction in progression of retinopathy in type 1 diabetic subjects randomized to ACE inhibitor.[77]

Cataract has been shown to be more common in diabetic subjects[78,79] even at the time of diagnosis,[80] and its presence predicts increased mortality.[81] However, The U.K. Prospective Diabetes Study showed that aggressive blood glucose reduction decreased the rate of cataract extraction.[67]

Although some studies show an association of diabetes with open-angle glaucoma,[82] other studies do not.[83–85] There is some evidence that glaucoma is associated with worse retinopathy[86] and neovascularization is associated with glaucoma,[87] particularly if there is rubeosis iridis. It is well accepted that retinal venous thrombosis is a complication of diabetes,[88] and there is some evidence that retinal artery thrombosis is associated with diabetes.[80,89]

Age-related macular degeneration seems very common in diabetic patients; the theoretical reasons for this are discussed in the paper by Klein et al.[90] However, most studies show no such association,[91–93] and only one study has shown such an association in men aged 75 or more.[90]

The gold standard ophthalmologic assessment is slit-lamp examination by an experienced user,[94] but this is often not practicable. Mydriatic retinal photography has a sensitivity of detection of eye disease of 89%, which is significantly better than the sensitivity of direct ophthalmoscopy of 65%.[94] If photography is not available, subjects need measurements of visual acuity and dilated fundoscopy by experienced observers each year; this is probably worth doing opportunistically anyway because even photography misses 11% of retinopathy. Although exudative maculopathy is easy to spot in the dilated eye (exudates around or within one disk's diameter of the macula), macular edema is practically impossible to distinguish from a normal eye by ophthalmoscopy; hence, the importance of measuring the corrected visual acuity. Reasons for referral to an ophthalmologist are set out in Table 92-6.

Foot disease

Limb amputation remains an important health problem in the diabetic population, with the rate of lower limb amputation being 15 times higher than for nondiabetic patients.[95]

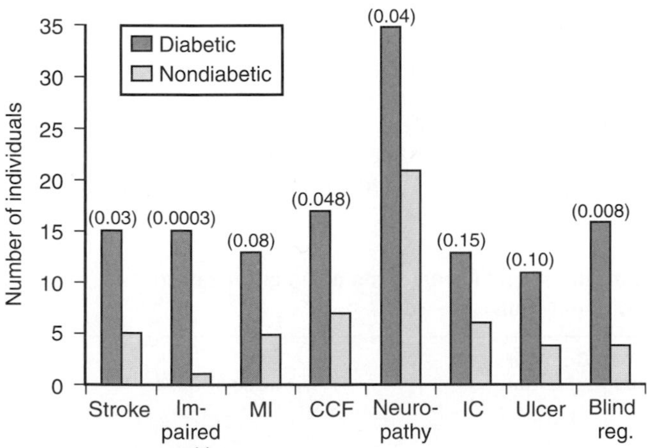

Figure 92-2. Comparison of morbidity between diabetic and nondiabetic individuals. *P* values are shown in parentheses. *(From Dornan TL, Peck GM, Dow JDC, et al. A community survey of diabetes in the elderly. Diab Med 1992;9:860–5.)*

It is three times higher in diabetic men than in women.[96] Elderly people are particularly affected.[97]

In 1986 the total annual cost of major leg amputations in diabetic patients in the United Kingdom was estimated to be in excess of £13 million[98]; in the United States, the direct medical care costs for all amputations in the diabetic populations, not including rehabilitation, exceeded $500 million.[99] A recent study from the Netherlands[100] estimated the direct costs associated with diabetes-related lower limb amputations and found it to be more than £10,000 per hospitalization, with a mean inpatient stay of 42 days. This study identified increasing age and a higher level of amputation as important factors leading to increases in both the period of hospitalization and the associated costs (Table 92-7).

The mortality rate for amputees is high. Recent evidence indicates that the 3-year survival following lower extremity amputation is about 50%,[101] with a median life expectancy after amputation of less than 2 years.[96] Only 5% of elderly amputees become fully independent postoperatively.[102]

In about 70% of cases, amputation is precipitated by foot ulceration[103,104] whose principal antecedents include peripheral vascular disease and peripheral neuropathy, both of which increase with age. Other at-risk groups include those with limited joint mobility, bony abnormalities, diabetic nephropathy, excess alcohol intake, visual impairment, and patients living alone.[97]

Various risk factors that increase the likelihood of foot ulceration have been identified (Table 92-8). Peripheral sensorimotor neuropathy is the primary cause or contributory factor in 90% of cases.[105,106] Both small (often unmyelinated) and large (usually myelinated) nerve fibers are affected, which leads to the common symptoms of numbness, lancinating and burning pain, "pins and needles," and hyperesthesia, which is typically worse at night.[97] Physical examination reveals a glove and stocking loss of pain, fine touch, and thermal sensation (small fibers), with coexisting vibration and proprioceptive loss (large fibers). Small muscle atrophy in the foot can also occur because of motor fiber loss, which can cause flexor/extensor muscle imbalance resulting in clawed toes, prominent metatarsal heads, and forward displacement of the metatarsal foot pads.[107] This can lead to abnormally high foot pressures developing, which can increase the risk of foot ulceration and lead to gait disturbances. In elderly patients with peripheral neuropathy, this may give rise to further foot injuries and falls. The presence of visual loss may exacerbate the situation.[108] A trivial foot injury in a patient with severe neuropathy can eventually lead to the development of a Charcot joint, which is a chronic neuroarthropathy whose prevalence varies from 0.15% to 7% depending on the study population.[97] The majority of subjects have had diabetes for at least 10 years, and most are elderly people.

Peripheral blood flow in patients with diabetes is disturbed, with loss of blood flow autoregulation, increased arteriovenous shunting, and changes in capillary blood flow. Some of these abnormalities may be reversible or ameliorated by improved glycemic control.[109] Risk factors for peripheral vascular disease include smoking, hypertension, and hypercholesterolemia, with prevalence increasing with both advancing age and duration of diabetes. Symptoms include intermittent claudication and/or rest pain with lower limb ulceration or gangrene being important clinical outcomes. Radiologic investigation may show medial arterial calcification, which has been reported to be associated with both diabetic peripheral somatosensory and autonomic neuropathy.[110] Objective assessment of limb blood flow by Doppler ultrasound can be affected by extensive medial calcification, giving rise to a misleadingly high ankle-pressure index.[111]

It seems logical that interventions designed to prevent diabetic foot disease and amputations in patients with diabetes should be directed to the prevention of peripheral neuropathy and peripheral vascular disease and the prevention, early detection, and treatment of foot lesions. Several studies using staff and patient education and a multidisciplinary approach to foot care have demonstrated a reduction in diabetes-related amputations.[112,113] However, elderly people require more assistance than the young because they have difficulty perceiving foot problems and touching their feet.[114] By incorporating an intensive multidisciplinary approach in a diabetes foot clinic,[112] a London-based study demonstrated a 44% decline in amputation rate after 2 years. By use of suitable-fitting shoes, the recurrence rate of foot ulcers was reduced from 83% to 26%. At the University Hospital of Geneva, an 85% reduction in the rate of below-knee

Table 92-6. Reasons for Referral to an Ophthalmologist

- Cataract either obscuring examiner's view of fundus or impairing patient's vision
- Diabetic maculopathy as evidenced by exudates within 1 disk diameter of macula or any unexplained loss of visual acuity
- Preproliferative changes, such as intraretinal microvascular abnormalities, venous changes (beading, loops, dilation), six cotton wool spots in one quadrant, large blot hemorrhages, arteries replaced by white lines
- Proliferative changes, such as new vessels visible or vitreous hemorrhage
- To complete blind registration

Table 92-7. Duration of Hospitalization for Lower-Extremity Amputations, and Mean Costs of Hospitalization (Including Hospital Stay and Surgery) by Age Group in the Diabetic Population

Age Group	Duration of Hospitalization*	Mean Costs of Hospitalization (£)	Number of Cases
<45	25.5 ± 20.5	6516	53
45–64	38.7 ± 36.0	9734	521
75	43.3 ± 42.9	10,928	655
Total	41.8 ± 39.1	10,531	1575

*Results expressed as mean ± SD in days.

Table 92-8. Risk Factors for Foot Ulceration in the Elderly Population

- Peripheral sensorimotor neuropathy
- Autonomic neuropathy
- Peripheral vascular disease
- Limited joint mobility
- Foot pressure abnormalities
- Previous foot ulcer
- Smoking and alcohol

amputations was seen over a 4-year observation period by a combination of education and training in foot care in patients with diabetes.

With many elderly patients having great difficulty in performing the most routine foot care,[114] often as a result of poor vision and reduced mobility, it becomes very important to design strategies that enable partners and other caregivers to have a role in prevention and treatment of foot lesions. Educational material needs to be concise and repeated regularly,[97] and video presentations may also be helpful. The accompanying box on foot care education provides general principles of foot care reflecting a positive approach that can be adapted to many patients in clinical settings.

General Principles of Foot Care Education

- Target the level of information to the needs of the patient. Those not at risk may require only general advice about foot hygiene and shoes.
- Assess the ability of the patient to understand and perform the necessary components of foot care. If this is limited, then the spouse or caregiver should be involved at the beginning of the process.
- Suggest a positive approach to foot care with "do's" rather than "don'ts"—the principle of active rather than passive foot care is more likely to be successful and acceptable to the patient.
    - Do inspect the feet daily.
    - Do report any problems immediately.
    - Do have your feet measured every time new shoes are bought.
    - Do buy shoes with a square toe box and laces.
    - Do inspect the inside of shoes for foreign objects every day before putting them on.
    - Do attend a fully trained chiropodist regularly.
    - Do cut your nails straight across and not rounded.
    - Do keep your feet away from heat (fires, radiators, and hot water bottles) and check the bath water before stepping into it.
    - Do wear something on your feet to protect them at all times and never walk barefoot.
- Repeat the advice at regular intervals and check that it is being followed.
- Disseminate advice to other family members and other health care professionals involved in the care of a patient.

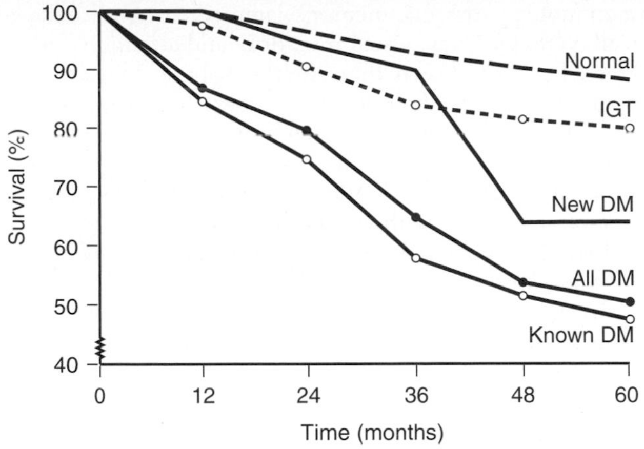

Figure 92-3. Mortality of elderly subjects in Melton Mowbray, according to glucose tolerance status. *(From Croxson SCM, Price D, Burden M et al. Mortality of elderly people with diabetes. Diab Med 1994;11:250–2.)*

Mortality

It is a widely held belief that diabetes mellitus confers little or no excess mortality risk in older patients, with life expectancy being similar to nondiabetic risk after age 70 to 75 years.[115–117] This apparent finding was explained by a shorter life in elderly subjects with other competing causes of death minimizing the effect of diabetes.[118] In line with this, most early reports indicated that the ratio of death rates in diabetics to rates in the general population falls progressively with age, especially in those aged 65 years and over, though it remains above unity up to age 80 years.[118] More recently, one study actually found a significantly lower mortality in patients aged 75 years and over (mortality ratio 0.88) compared with the general population,[119] and these contradictory findings have created uncertainty about the true impact of this metabolic disorder on the older diabetic population.

It is important to determine whether premature death because of diabetes is observable in elderly patients because this evidence would provide guidance to those responsible for providing health services on how best to focus their resources. An unequivocal finding of increased mortality would argue for a more sustained commitment to diabetic health care provision and research. Alternatively, the absence of excess mortality could redirect care strategies toward reducing morbidity and disability only.

A recent literature review by the authors has confirmed that diabetes in later life imposes an excess mortality risk[121] associated with a reduction in life expectancy in both sexes, even in patients aged 75 years and over. The pattern of excess mortality is relatively consistent, even though the duration of follow-up varied between studies. In the Melton study by Croxson et al[120] a substantial increase in excess mortality was seen in diabetic subjects aged 65 years and over (Figure 92-3), and impaired glucose tolerance was found to be associated with a relative risk of death of 1.7 (95% confidence interval 0.8 to 3.5). Most studies report a higher mortality in female diabetics and in both sexes; excess mortality is predominantly because of macrovascular disease.

Dementia

There is now better evidence that diabetes may be associated with decreases in psychomotor speed, frontal lobe/executive function, verbal memory, processing speed, complex motor functioning, working memory, immediate and delayed recall, verbal fluency, visual retention, and attention.[122] Earlier studies had shown that elderly diabetic subjects have impaired cognitive function,[123–126] but these studies were generally not population-based, excluded subjects with dementia,[123–126] and generally used a large battery of tests to show the deficit.[124–126] Worse cognitive function in these tests was associated with worse glycemic control.[123–126]

There are several possible explanations for the lower cognitive function in the known diabetic subjects, apart from abnormal plasma glucose levels. First, depression has been found to be associated with known diabetes.[129,130] Second, hypertension is associated with diabetes and insulin resistance[131] and is itself associated with decreased cognitive function;[132] there is even evidence to suggest that among hypertensive subjects, hyperinsulinemia is associated with worse cognitive function.[133] Third, cerebrovascular disease is 2 to 3 times more common in people with known diabetes,[61,134] which again might be associated with cognitive impairment. Fourth, there is evidence that cortical atrophy is associated with diabetes. Some studies suggest that the excess dementia is because of vascular disease,[128] whereas others suggest an excess of Alzheimer type of dementia.[127] It is likely that the current diagnosis and classification of dementia in diabetic subjects is inaccurate owing to the multiple risk factors present.[135] However, it is vitally important to exclude iatrogenic hypoglycemia (e.g., from long-acting sulfonylureas) as a cause of confusion because it is eminently treatable, although the authors have seen patients rendered permanently confused by a single episode of profound hypoglycemia.

Glycemic control appears to play a role in altering cognitive function. In one study, patients with a HbA_1c of greater than 7.0% had a fourfold increase in developing cognitive impairment.[136] A study in type 1 diabetes has shown that cognitive impairment is worsened by increasing duration of diabetes and may also be associated with recurrent hypoglycemia.[137]

Whatever the reason, known diabetic subjects appear to have poorer cognitive function than subjects not known to have diabetes. It is interesting to note the two studies that suggest that improving glycemic control improves cognitive function.[138–140] Impaired cognitive function should be borne in mind when treating elderly diabetic subjects because it has implications for their safe treatment. It may cause difficulty with glycemic control as a result of erratic taking of diet and medication. This may occur with hypoglycemia where patients forget that they have taken medication and repeat the dose. One should enlist the help of family and services to optimize glycemic control to see if this makes any difference; if it does not, accept that one has to change glycemic targets to less strict, but safer control.[141] It is important to consider screening for other treatable causes of cognitive impairment.

Several recommendations relating to best practice in this area are derived from the European guidelines[10]:

- Each functional assessment must include a measure of the three domains of function: global/physical, cognitive and affective (grade of recommendation A). *Specific assessment of cognitive dysfunction and depressive illness by screening methods are an essential part of this process and can be undertaken by either medical and/or nursing and therapy staff.*
- Optimal glucose regulation may help to maintain cognitive performance and improve learning and memory. Evidence level 2+; grade of recommendation C.

RESIDENTIAL CARE AND THE HOUSEBOUND

Greater numbers of older people are now living within care homes and other forms of residential care. Several studies have shown that diabetes is an independent risk factor for admission to a care home.[142,143] Again, the number of diabetic residents identified is just the tip of the iceberg. These were prevalences of 12% diagnosed and 15% undiagnosed diabetes in a study of Birmingham residential care homes,[50] and in Canada a routine screening program led to 30% of residents being diagnosed as diabetic.[144] Residence of nursing home is a risk factor for hyperosmolar nonketotic coma and carries increased mortality.[145] Compared with nondiabetic residents, diabetic residents have increased rates of stroke, peripheral vascular disease, amputation, urinary catheter, foot ulcer, renal impairment, and dementia.[50,146] They suffer poor nutrition, with 20% of residents being at least 20% underweight[147] but recent trends in obesity in the West suggest that the proportion of obese residents being admitted to nursing homes in the United States has risen from 15% to 25% over a decade.[148] Diabetes is a risk factor for pressure sores, although this is less of a problem in rural American nursing homes,[149] so it may be preventable.

It is very clear that the residents of care homes receive inadequate diabetes care compared with their noninstitutionalized peers[146,150,151]; (Table 92-9). Various common problems make diabetes management more complex in these patients.[152] The following are some of the problems:

- There may be irregular oral intake owing to: (1) confusion and/or a poor appetite because of concurrent illness; or (2) dysphagia because of stroke or other neurologic or gastroenterologic disorders. Lack of regular calorific intake can be particularly troublesome for insulin-treated patients.
- Recurrent urinary, chest, and other infections can render the diabetic person liable to hyperglycemia, and possibly ketosis with poor metabolic control.
- Leg ulcers and pressure sores may deteriorate rapidly.
- There can be an increased vulnerability to hypoglycemia (especially in those taking sulfonylureas or insulin) owing to poor appetite and difficulties in ensuring sufficient and regular caloric intake.
- There may be inadequate facilities to cater for the dietary needs of residents with diabetes, and inadequate knowledge on the part of catering staff—including the need for snacks outside main meals.
- Adequate arrangements for regular diabetes review may be lacking, particularly for those discharged from hospital clinics and who are unable to visit their primary care physician.
- There may be insufficient provision of health professional input, particularly of specialist nurses, dietitians, dental surgeons, opticians, and state-registered chiropodists and doctors, including hospital specialists.

Table 92-9. Care Received by Diabetic Subjects in Care Home or Free Living[151]

	Care Home (%)	Free Living (%)
Annual review	44*	84
Chiropody	60*	96
Optician	36*	76
Dietitian	48	60†

*$P < 0.05$ care home resident versus free living elder.
†Not significant.

Some time ago, the British Geriatrics Society (Special Interest Group in Diabetes)[153] and the British Diabetic Association[154] published guidelines. In particular the BDA monograph is an excellent reference work on the subject and an incentive to improve care, and this document is being updated by Diabetes UK and is available in 2009. The European guidelines have a section devoted to Care Home diabetes and several of their recommendations are given below:

- At the time of admission to a care home, each resident requires screening for the presence of diabetes. Level of evidence 2++, grade of recommendation B.
- Each resident should have an annual screen for diabetes. Level of evidence 2+, grade of recommendation C.
- Each resident with diabetes should have an individualized diabetes care plan with the following minimum details: dietary plan, medication list, glycemic targets, weight, and nursing plan. Level of evidence 2+, grade of recommendation C.

See the accompanying box on improving care.

Improving Care Within Residential Nursing Home Settings

- Each resident should have an individual diabetes care plan agreed between patient (or relative), doctor (who is responsible for diabetic care), and home care staff.
- There should be increased community support from experienced health professionals, such as diabetes specialist nurses and dietitians.
- Diabetic patients living in residential and nursing homes should have ready access to other specialist health professionals.
- Each resident with diabetes should be reviewed by either the family doctor or a hospital consultant physician/geriatrician at least once a year.
- Patients in residential and nursing homes should be included in any local audit of diabetic care.

GLUCOSE CONTROL IN DIABETES MELLITUS

Overview

A major trial to guide the clinician is the U.K. Prospective Diabetes Study (UKPDS). The initial outcomes of intensive blood glucose control[68] were disappointing, with sulfonylurea or insulin use reducing microvascular end points from 11.4% to 8.6% (i.e., by approximately one quarter) at 10 years. A 1% decrease in HbA_1c,[67] was associated with a significant reduction in any diabetes end point (21% decrease), diabetes related death (21% decrease), all-cause mortality (14% decrease), any myocardial infarction (MI) (14% decrease), any stroke (12% decrease), microvascular end points (37% decrease), cataract extraction (19% decrease), amputation or peripheral vascular disease death (43% decrease), and heart failure (16% decrease). The U.K. study looked at intensive control from time of diagnosis; however, the recent Kumamoto intervention study in middle-aged Japanese subjects with type 2 diabetes for 6 to 10 years found that intensive insulin treatment with good control delayed the onset and progression of specific diabetic complications[155]; that study suggests that the thresholds for developing specific complications are: HbA_1c 7%, fasting plasma glucose 6.7 mmol/L, and postprandial plasma glucose 10 mmol/L.

The main concern is that striving for normoglycemia using insulin or sulfonylurea drugs might result in hypoglycemia. Compared with younger subjects, aging individuals perceive fewer symptoms of hypoglycemia, need a lower plasma glucose level to elicit symptoms, exhibit a reduced counter-regulatory response to hypoglycemia, and recover more slowly from the hypoglycemic insult.[157–160] Thus the elderly person may have few symptoms of hypoglycemia until developing neuroglycopenia,[161] when nothing can be done about it. Hypoglycemia may be missed entirely or misdiagnosed, especially as one third of hypoglycemic events in the elderly have nonspecific symptoms.[162] Although age is an independent risk factor for drug-induced hypoglycemia,[163] elderly people are taught very little about it.[164] In the Diabetes Control and Complications Trial and Kumamoto studies,[155,165] the risk of hypoglycemia increased dramatically, as the HbA_1c decreased below the upper normal limit. However, the usual control of the elderly diabetic person's glycemia is poor.[61]

Sensible and appropriate diabetic care requires a considered judgment of the risks and benefits of treatment. A framework for this management is assisted by the aims of care, which are:

- Achieve metabolic targets at lowest daily doses of therapeutic agents
- Prevent hypoglycemia
- Reduce and limit other associated adverse drug reactions
- Limit weight gain on sulfonylureas and insulin therapy
- Ameliorate microvascular complications
- Attend to macrovascular risk factors and disease

Unless there are other reasons to treat the elderly diabetic individual differently from the younger diabetic person, aim for an HbA_1c level less than 7%, fasting plasma glucose 5.0 to 7.0 mmol/L, and random plasma glucose less than 11.1 mmol/L. See the accompanying box on "Treatments to Improve Glucose Control."

Pathologic basis for the treatment of type 2 diabetes

Type 2 diabetes mellitus accounts for more than 90% of cases of diabetes in old age,[166] with the remainder being predominantly type 1. Type 2 diabetes has been characterized

Treatments to Improve Glucose Control

Improve β-cell dysfunction by:

- Stimulating pancreatic β-cells to secrete more insulin; for example, by the use of sulfonylureas or other insulin secretagogues
- Lowering circulating levels of glucose, for example, by dietary modification
- Introducing exogenous insulin to replace the function of the failing β-cell

Decrease insulin resistance by:

- Using drugs that decrease insulin resistance (e.g., metformin, peroxisome proliferator-activated receptor γ agonists, and probably a minor effect of some sulfonylureas)
- Directly reducing hyperglycemia, for example, by dietary modification
- Limit the dietary intake of monosaccharides, for example, by:
  - Diet
  - Drugs that delay the absorption of monosaccharides by inhibiting breakdown of polysaccharides (e.g., α-glucosidase inhibitors such as acarbose)

Initial Care Plan for the Older Adult With Diabetes

- Set realistic glycemic goals.
- Agree upon the frequency of diabetic follow-up by primary or secondary health care team.
- Organize monitoring of glycemic control by the patient and/or caregiver; for example, by home urine or blood glucose monitoring or, if the patient cannot manage this, by regular review.
- Advise on stopping smoking, on exercise (ideally a minimum of 3 weekly brisk walks of 30–45 min duration), and on alcohol intake.
- Refer to social or community services as appropriate.

by a combination of insulin resistance (at both hepatic and peripheral tissue levels) because of a potentially decreased number of insulin receptors and a postreceptor defect, and β-cell dysfunction characterized by defective insulin secretion.[167] Other disturbances are often associated with hyperglycemia, including hypertension, dyslipidemia, and obesity; this is referred to as Syndrome X, Reaven's syndrome, or the Deadly Quartet.[168] Syndrome X is associated with increased risk of large vessel disease, and further abnormalities associated with this syndrome and increased vascular risk are being described (e.g., microalbuminuria, abnormal plasminogen activator inhibitor-1 levels).

Treatments for glucose control

Specific treatments aim to reverse or ameliorate the previously discussed defects of glucose control in one or more of the following ways: improvement of β-cell dysfunction; decrease of insulin resistance; and limitation of dietary intake of monosaccharides (see box on "Treatments to Improve Glucose Control").

Table 92-10. Risk Factors for Hypoglycemia[174,175]

- Choice of sulfonylurea/insulin
- Tight glycemic control
- Increasing age
- Male gender
- Recent discharge from hospital
- Polypharmacy
- Change of or new hypoglycemic treatment
- Impaired renal function
- Excess alcohol
- Hepatic impairment
- Cardiac failure

DIETARY TREATMENT

The foundation of any treatment in diabetes is diet.[169] Complex carbohydrates should comprise 50% to 55% of the energy intake, and come from food high in fiber (bread, pasta, rice, and potatoes). Up to 25 to 50 g of added sucrose is allowed, but one would generally not advertise this since refined carbohydrate is very prevalent in the Western diet. The diet should contain as much fiber as possible, but realistically one is looking at a maximum of 30 g per day. Fat intake should be limited to 30% to 35% of energy intake.

Although diet is vitally important, it is unlikely to achieve glycemic targets when used alone. In the U.K. Prospective Diabetes Study, only 6% of subjects were controlled on diet at the end of the second year.[170]

In most cases, diet alone will fail, and most patients will need oral hypoglycemic drugs. Although there are many hypoglycemic drugs available, the mainstays are metformin and sulfonylureas as these are relatively cheap.

SULFONYLUREAS

Sulfonylureas bind to a specific sulfonylurea receptor on the pancreatic β-islet cell, which blocks ATP-sensitive potassium channels and hence stimulates insulin release.[171]

Hypoglycemia is the main side-effect of note, and risk factors for hypoglycemia are given in Table 92-10.

Glibenclamide appears particularly likely to cause hypoglycemia and death, more so than other sulfonylureas[174–177] including chlorpropamide[68,177] and metformin.[178] The deaths of elderly patients from hypoglycemia in a Swedish study,[179] and the finding that some elderly subjects experience a prolonged hypoglycemic effect from it,[180] has placed a question mark over glipizide. Gliclazide has a low (but not zero) risk of hypoglycemia[181–186]; it may be less likely to cause weight gain, the other common problem with sulfonylureas,[181,183–186] and achieves glycemic targets with low rates of secondary failure.[184] If hypoglycemia is a major worry, then tolbutamide has the lowest risk[175,176] and can be used if the patient's creatinine is over 200 μmol/L.[172] Several longer-acting or slow-release preparations are now on the market, including gliclazide MR, and these may aid compliance.

METFORMIN

Metformin reduces insulin resistance particularly in the liver, and so decreases hepatic glucose output by decreasing gluconeogenesis.[187] Metformin decreases gluconeogenesis from lactate, but plasma lactate levels stay stable since metformin increases oxidation of lactate.[187] However, older biguanides

Table 92-11. Contraindications to Metformin

- Renal impairment (creatinine >120 μmol/L)
- Hepatic impairment (including alcohol abuse) as indicated by abnormal liver function tests
- Cardiac failure, even if treated
- Critical limb ischemia
- Any acute illness
- Use of intravenous radiologic contrast media

decreased oxidation of lactate, hence the unpredictable high risk of lactic acidosis. Lactic acidosis is a condition of the elderly group.[188] Metformin is predictable and safe if used correctly.[178] The contraindications[172,173] are given in Table 92-11 and they must be observed. Advantages of metformin are that it does not cause hypoglycemia on its own, it does not cause weight gain, and it is inexpensive. It probably decreases HbA_1c by about 1% to 1.5%, and fasting plasma glucose by 4 to 5 mmol/L,[189–192] which is similar to sulfonylureas. In the U.K. Prospective Diabetes Study, metformin was used in obese subjects; all-cause mortality, and any diabetes-related end points were significantly lower on intensive treatment with metformin than with insulin or a sulfonylurea.[191] Metformin is now available as a slow-release preparation and in combination with either pioglitazone or rosiglitazone.

Apart from lactic acidosis, other side effects include gastrointestinal disturbance, which may be minimized by gradual introduction of the agent. Metformin may also cause vitamin B_{12} malabsorption, so it is wise to check B_{12} levels every 5 years, and particularly if the subject has neuropathy.

ACARBOSE

This is an α-glucosidase inhibitor that inhibits the breakdown of polysaccharides in the small bowel, which are then digested or fermented more distally. This leads to lower but more sustained postprandial glucose levels and flatulence, which is the main limiting factor in the use of acarbose. Its advantages are low risk of hypoglycemia on its own (though if the patient is rendered hypoglycemic by co-prescription of a sulfonylurea, polysaccharides will be slower to correct this) and little weight gain.

Although acarbose can be successfully combined with metformin, sulfonylureas, or insulin, its use in many older people with diabetes may be limited because of gastrointestinal side effects and the need for frequent dosing.

THIAZOLIDINEDIONES (TZDS)

These agents are generally well tolerated in older people and can produce a lowering of HbA_{1c} of up to 1.5%. Their use in patients with diabetes has recently come under scrutiny because of evidence that suggests an increased risk of cardiovascular events in patients on thiazolidinediones with the risk apparently confined to rosiglitazone.[193] Further analysis of data from ongoing studies is taking place but inevitably there has been restricted use by some clinicians.

Thiazolidinediones reduce insulin resistance by activating the peroxisome proliferator-activated receptor γ (PPAR γ).[193] They do not cause hypoglycemia but because they cause fluid retention and may increase the risk of heart failure, they are contraindicated in this latter condition and in those with a history of heart failure. Rosiglitazone should also not be used in those with acute coronary syndrome or in those with ischemic heart disease or peripheral arterial disease. There has also been recent concern that TZDs are associated with an increased risk of bony fractures due to bone loss. This needs further investigation but may warrant clinicians considering the overall fracture risk of patients with diabetes before they decide on treatment with a TZD.

They are safe in mild-to-moderate renal impairment, and pioglitazone is safe even with creatinine clearance as low as 2 mL/min. They can be used as monotherapy (although not all countries have a monotherapy license),[194] combined with metformin[195,196] or a sulfonylurea,[197] or combined with insulin (pioglitazone only) but treatment must be stopped if significant fluid retention develops. A TZD can be added (triple license) to existing treatment with metformin and a sulfonylurea, if human insulin is likely to be unacceptable. It takes 6 weeks at least to achieve the full effect on plasma glucose levels. Both drugs are available in combination with metformin.

Prandial glucose regulators, the meglitinides, and amino acid derivatives

Repaglinide acts on the β-cell for a short time to rapidly and potently stimulate insulin release. Therefore it is taken just before each meal. It is predominantly metabolized to inactive metabolites by the liver, and is safe in mild-to-moderate renal impairment. In a comprehensive review,[198] it appears that repaglinide is as effective as sulfonylureas at reducing HbA_{1c}, but with better postprandial glucose levels, and slightly less risk of symptomatic hypoglycemia. It cannot be used with sulfonylureas. However, its use with metformin has been studied in a crossover study with three arms, which found that metformin plus repaglinide (mean HbA_{1c} decrease 1.41%) exerted a greater hypoglycemic effect than monotherapy with metformin (0.33%) or repaglinide (0.38%) without significant hypoglycemia.[199] Similarly, it can be used effectively in combination with a thiazolidinedione.

Nateglinide is safe in mild-to-moderate renal impairment, and very usefully safe in mild-to-moderate hepatic impairment.[200] It has a modest hypoglycemic effect as monotherapy, but is licensed only in the United Kingdom for use with metformin, with which it works well.[201]

Newer therapies are becoming available that offer greater choice in the management of type diabetes. These are represented by incretin-based treatments. Exenatide that is a GLP-1 (glucagon-like peptide-1) is an effective glucose-lowering agent and is often considered when oral agents fail to achieve glycaemic targets and the patient is unwilling to accept a thiazolidinedione or insulin. It lowers HbA_{1c} by about 0.9% when used at a dose of 10 μg twice daily given subcutaneously. It also lowers weight by an average of 1.4 kg. Treatment may be complicated by nausea. A once-daily analogue, liraglutide, is also now available. The combination of reduced risk of hypoglycaemia (unless used with a sulphonylurea) and weight loss may be advantageous in older patients unless they are very frail where the impact of nausea and weight loss would not be desirable.

Other new treatments are stagliptin and vildagliptin which are oral DPP-IV inhibitors that can decrease HbA_{1c} by 0.7–1.0% as monotherapy but can be used with other oral agents. These are weight neutral compounds and have a low risk of hypoglycaemia unless used with a sulphonylurea.

Table 92-12. Indications for Insulin

- Type 1 diabetes
- Type 2 diabetes, inadequately controlled by oral means
- Type 2 diabetes, with an intercurrent illness and associated hyperglycemia
- Type 2 diabetes, with other illnesses contraindicating oral therapy (e.g., liver disease)
- Type 2 diabetes during prolonged surgery
- Hyperglycemic coma

INSULIN

This is the required therapy for type 1 diabetes, and in view of the progressive deterioration of glucose homeostasis it is commonly needed in type 2 diabetic individuals.

There is often a reluctance to start an elderly diabetic patient on insulin, but given the wide range of insulin and injection devices available, and the benefits of improved glycemic control discussed previously, this attitude is generally inappropriate. Indications for insulin treatment are given in Table 92-12.

There are several advantages to short-acting insulin analogues. They are more convenient for the patient, being given as the meal arrives. They cause fewer hypoglycemic reactions, particularly overnight, and because patients need fewer snacks between meals to prevent hypoglycemia, weight gain may be less problematic.[202] They can also be given after a meal,[203] which is very useful if one does not know whether the patient is going to eat until he or she has eaten, as in subjects with dementia or where there is intermittent vomiting as in diabetic gastroparesis.

A twice-daily (bid) regimen is the most common. For the older type 1 diabetic subjects, twice-daily premixed insulins seem to work well. For the older type 2 diabetic person going on to insulin, one would generally use a twice-daily isophane regimen[204] since it gives good control with low risk of hypoglycemia[156,205]; one can add soluble insulin later if required.

The more intensive "basal bolus" regimen uses a daily intermediate- or long-acting insulin (isophane- or zinc-based) given before bed or before an evening meal, and a bolus quick-acting insulin (either soluble or quick-acting analogue) given before each meal.

One combines insulin with an oral agent in a regimen of daytime oral agent plus bedtime insulin regime, or when trying to limit weight gain on the insulin. Limiting the weight gain associated with insulin has been noted with sulfonylureas,[206,207] but is particularly effective with metformin co-prescription.[208,209] The main side effect of insulin is hypoglycemia, and one should be aware that 3 AM hypoglycemia is quite common. If this occurs on a regime with the isophane before teatime, moving the isophane to bedtime generally helps. Patients who are frail or who have poor vision may still be able to dial the dose by counting audible clicks, or using the preset preloaded Optiset pen (Aventis), or have someone else prepare the pen for them to use at the correct time. However, sometimes it is necessary to have caregivers or district nurses give the insulin, in which case a once-daily regime is generally necessary. The diabetes specialist nurses are vital for high-quality, safe insulin treatment, particularly initiation.

Choice of treatment strategy

The first step is to identify the rare elderly-onset type 1 diabetic individuals who need insulin treatment. For the other subjects, the initial treatment is a trial of diet for 6 to 12 weeks with instruction by a trained dietitian. Patients and caregivers should be educated about the indications for referral to hospital as an outpatient and when admission is likely to be required. Oral agents are likely to be needed to get to target HbA_1c and we would recommend the following:

For normal weight (body mass index 20 to 25 kg/m^2) and overweight patients (body mass index >26 kg/m^2), metformin should be considered first and titrated to 1.5 to 3 g per day according to gastrointestinal tolerability if there are no contraindications (see Table 92-11). If there are contraindications, or if metformin fails, then a sulfonylurea should be considered as monotherapy or combination therapy, respectively. A thiazolidinedione should be used if the patient is on either metformin or a sulfonylurea and cannot take the alternative agent; commonly this will be an individual on a sulfonylurea who cannot take metformin owing to renal impairment, when a thiazolidinedione will probably be suitable.

For underweight patients (body mass index <20 kg/m^2), one should question the diagnosis of type 2 diabetes. Does this patient have type 1 diabetes needing insulin, or diabetes secondary to chronic pancreatic disease (also probably needing insulin), thyrotoxicosis, or coexistent underlying malignancy? In thin type 2 diabetic subjects, sulfonylureas should be taken as first-line therapy; unless there is a dramatic long-lasting effect, insulin treatment should be used if the sulfonylurea fails to achieve control quickly.

For demented patients or people with a chaotic lifestyle who cannot be relied upon to eat regularly, hypoglycemia is a major worry. Metformin is the first choice, particularly if the once-daily long-acting formulation is available to allow supervision of once-daily medication. If the person is still poorly controlled, and cannot be adequately supervised, a thiazolidinedione is a safe next agent. If the problem is just a chaotic lifestyle, then one of the prandial glucose regulators is sensible.

For people with diabetes secondary to steroid use, the plasma glucose is raised over the afternoon and evening. Intermediate-acting sulfonylureas cause hypoglycemia before breakfast.[210] A short-acting insulin secretagogue, such as tolbutamide or repaglinide, before midday and evening meals works quite well or, if insulin is needed, a rapid-acting analogue before midday and evening meals is a good start—although it may need converting to a complete basal bolus regimen. Hypoglycemic medication must be decreased as the steroid dose is decreased.

The European guidelines have provided a series of glycemic targets to guide treatment and these are as follows[10]:

For older patients with type 2 diabetes, with single system involvement (free of other major comorbidities), a target HbA1c (DCCT aligned) range of greater than 7% should be aimed for. Evidence level 2++; grade of recommendation B. The precise target agreed upon will depend on existing cardiovascular risk, presence of microvascular complications, and ability of individual to self-manage.

For older patients with type 2 diabetes, with single system involvement (free of other major comorbidities), a target HbA_{1c} (DCCT aligned) with a range of 6.5–7% should be aimed for. Evidence level 2++; grade of recommendation B. The precise target agreed will depend on existing cardiovascular risk, presence of microvascular complications, and ability of individual to self-manage.

HOME MONITORING OF DIABETIC CONTROL

Blood glucose monitoring is recommended for insulin-treated patients on at least two occasions per day for those who are in poor metabolic control, but for stable patients a four-point profile once per week is adequate. Blood glucose estimations should be done before meals and at bedtime. Blood glucose monitoring is also valuable for patients with poor metabolic control (e.g., if considering insulin treatment) or who are at risk of hypoglycemia.

For patients with type 2 diabetes who are taking oral agents, home blood glucose monitoring should be offered, although it is not essential. Monitoring is only of value when a patient or caregiver or doctor is able to interpret and act upon the results.

HYPOGLYCEMIA IN THE ELDERLY PATIENT

Sulfonylurea-induced hypoglycemia is a problem, if severe, owing to the prolonged nature of the event. It is frequently misdiagnosed as a cerebrovascular event, or classified as "confusion query cause." Glibenclamide and chlorpropamide are very long-acting, but other sulfonylureas can have a prolonged effect in the setting of renal or hepatic impairment. Diazoxide, which has a direct inhibitory effect on insulin secretion, may be used as an adjunct to treatment. In the unconscious patient, diazoxide can be given as a slow intravenous infusion of 300 mg over 30 minutes, and can be repeated every 4 hours if necessary. Glucagon can be used in insulin-treated patients to good effect and is valuable since one does not need venous access. However, it should not be used in sulfonylurea-induced hypoglycemia since it stimulates the remaining β-cell activity (upon which the sulfonylureas depend for their efficacy) to release further insulin.

Insulin-induced hypoglycemia is more common, and nocturnal hypoglycemia may present as morning headaches or disturbed sleep. Any subject taking more than 1 unit of insulin per kilogram bodyweight should be closely questioned for unrecognized hypoglycemia.

HYPERGLYCEMIC COMA

Immediate Management of Hyerglycemic Comas

- Be aware of hyperglycemic coma as a possibility.
- Test for hyperglycemia, ketosis, and acidosis.
- Screen for any precipitating illness (e.g., infection, cerebral or myocardial infarction, inadequate treatment).
- Institute a slow insulin infusion guided by frequent bedside blood glucose monitoring to halve glucose level over 4 hours.
- Arrange prompt, adequate fluid replacement with 0.9% saline (if Na less than 155 mmol/L) or 0.45% saline (if Na greater than 155 mmol/L) at 500 mL/hr over first 4 hours.

Diabetic ketoacidosis (DKA) may occur at any age, whereas hyperglycemic hyperosmolar nonketotic (HONK) coma occurs predominantly in subjects aged over 50 years.[212] The tendency to hyperosmolality in HONK coma may be worse in elderly people who may not appreciate thirst well, may have difficulty drinking enough to compensate for their osmotic diuresis,[212,214] and may also be on diuretics.[215] It also appears that hyperosmolality not only worsens insulin resistance, but may also inhibit lipolysis.[214]

Diabetic ketoacidosis may be defined as hyperglycemia occurring in conjunction with ketoacidosis as evidenced by significant ketosis (3+ Ketostix in urine or plasma) and significant acidosis (venous plasma bicarbonate less than 15 mmol/L or arterial pH below 7.2). HONK comas may be defined as hyperglycemia occurring in conjunction with raised plasma osmolality (greater than 350 mmol/L) with no evidence of ketoacidosis. The osmolality may be measured directly in the laboratory using a freezing-point depression technique, or can be estimated approximately by calculating the sum of $2 \infty (Na^+ + K^+)$ + urea + glucose, concentrations in mmol/L.

All studies of hyperglycemic comas show a progressive increase in mortality with age.[213,216,217] In Birmingham, the mortality due to DKA rose from 5% in the age range 60 to 69 to 100% at age 90,[213] although the number of 90-year-olds was small. Most studies suggest that death is primarily because of acute illnesses, such as pneumonia and myocardial infarction.[213,216,217] There has been no apparent decrease in mortality over the past 20 years.[213,216]

The cause of the hyperglycemia may be infection, myocardial infarction, inadequate hypoglycemic treatment, or inappropriate drug treatment. Often, a particular cause cannot be identified[213,216]; for instance, there was no apparent cause in 354 out of 929 admissions with DKA in Birmingham.[213] Thiazide diuretics and steroids are known to increase blood glucose levels and may precipitate DKA; thiazide diuretics and furosemide may be particularly likely to precipitate HONK coma.[215]

Management of hyperglycemic coma

This is covered in greater detail elsewhere.[211] The history and examination should pay special attention to previous diabetic symptoms and treatment, any precipitating infection, infarction or medication, evidence of heart failure, and the degree of dehydration (see box on "Immediate Management of Hyperglycemic Comas"). Blood should be tested for glucose, urea, electrolytes, creatinine, cardiac enzymes, and cultures. Urine and sputum should also be cultured and an electrocardiogram and chest x-ray obtained.

Acidosis should be identified by measurement of either venous bicarbonate or arterial blood gas pH. Urine (or plasma from blood in a lithium heparin tube left to stand) should be dipstick-tested for ketone bodies. Intravenous (IV) fluid replacement should be at a rate of 500 mL/hr over the initial 4 hours, reducing to 250 mL/hr. The patient needs more rapid infusion where there is shock due to hypovolemia, and here a central line is invaluable to monitor aggressive infusions, particularly in the presence of cardiac failure or recent MI. There is a wide choice of IV fluid depending on the condition of the patient. In DKA or a HONK coma with plasma sodium level less than 155 mmol/L, use 0.9% saline. If the plasma sodium level rises above 155 mmol/L, then use 0.45% saline,[211,212,214] although if the plasma glucose level is less than 15 mmol/L, 5% dextrose could be used. If the patient is shocked because of hypovolemia, then a plasma volume expander may be needed.

An insulin pump (50 units human soluble insulin in 50 mL of 0.9% saline) is undoubtedly the easiest way to deliver the required insulin, and syringe pumps are now very reliable. The dose of insulin infused is varied according to the result of blood glucose testing, which is initially performed hourly, and then less frequently as the readings stabilize.

Subjects with a HONK coma may need very small doses of insulin to reduce plasma glucose levels; however, if the patient is in hypercatabolic state or has marked insulin resistance, as in obesity or in some subjects with type 2 diabetes, larger doses of insulin may be required. The plasma glucose should halve over 4 hours; if it does not, check that the insulin is actually being given, and increase the insulin infusion rate as necessary—for example, initially by 25%, aiming to reduce the plasma glucose level by 5 to 10 mmol/L per hour.

The potassium level needs to be checked 2 hours after starting treatment, and then 4-hourly until stable; if the level is 4.0 to 5.0 mmol/L, add 20 mmol/L of KCl to each liter of IV fluid, and add 40 mmol/L if the potassium level is below 4.0 mmol/L.

Thrombotic complications may occur or may well have occurred before hospitalization in subjects with a HONK coma. Most authors recommend prophylaxis against deep venous thrombosis with heparin 5000 units tds subcutaneously.[211,212,214] If there is decreased consciousness, pay particular attention to pressure areas and use pressure-relieving mattresses and bootees because heels in particular are very prone to ulceration. Unconscious diabetic subjects with hyperglycemia should have a nasogastric tube passed. As the subject improves and the plasma glucose falls below 15 mmol/L, one can either change to 5% dextrose, or feed the patient, to further reduce ketone bodies in DKA. The immediate management of these comas is summarized in the accompanying box on "Immediate Management of Hyperglycemic Comas." Please note that lactic acidosis will not be covered in this chapter.

BLOOD PRESSURE CONTROL IN DIABETES MELLITUS

Hypertension is very common in elderly people with type 2 diabetes (up to 50% prevalence in some studies, and becoming more prevalent as the target blood pressure decreases). The U.K. Prospective Diabetes Study[69] showed that a 10 mm Hg systolic BP reduction led to significant reductions in any diabetes end point (12% reduction), diabetes-related death (17%), all-cause mortality (12%), MI (12%), stroke (19%), microvascular end points (13%), amputation or death from peripheral vascular disease (16%), and heart failure (12%). The U.K. study used either ACE–inhibitor-based or β-blocker–based regimens to similar effect, although the ACE inhibitor was better tolerated.

Which agent should be used? Given the HOPE, United Kingdom, Syst-Eur, and SHEP studies, one could make a case for ACE inhibitor, long-acting dihydropyridine calcium channel blocker or thiazide diuretic as first-line agents of choice, or a combination if necessary [218] (e.g., use of an ACE inhibitor plus either a diuretic or a generic calcium channel antagonist in subjects of African-Caribbean descent). If the systolic pressure is more than 10 mm Hg from target, then 98% of patients will need at least two agents to control their blood pressure, so the question is academic: patients will be taking as many as they can tolerate. One worry is the diabetogenic effect of thiazide diuretics; in SHEP the whole thiazide group's mean glucose rose 1 mmol/L, but we do not know how many needed an escalation of their hypoglycemic medication. If glycemic control is borderline, we generally use indapamide instead of a thiazide since indapamide is said to be metabolically inactive. The main worry about ACE inhibitors (and sartans) is atheromatous renal artery stenosis, which is common in diabetic people with peripheral vascular disease.[219] In practice we look at the peripheral circulation and creatinine and, if worried, request Doppler ultrasound of renal arteries.[220]

The European guidelines offer a series of recommendations relating to blood pressure lowering in older patients with diabetes[10]:

- The threshold for treatment of high blood pressure in older subjects with type 2 diabetes should be 140/80 mm Hg or higher for more than 3 months and measured on at least three separate occasions during a period of lifestyle management advice (behavioral: exercise, weight reduction, smoking advice, nutrition/dietary advice). Level of evidence 2++; grade of recommendation B.

  This decision is based on the likelihood of reducing cardiovascular risk in older subjects balanced with issues relating to tolerability, clinical factors and disease severity, and targets likely to be achievable with monotherapy and/or combination therapy, and with agreement with primary care colleagues.

  As most subjects aged 70 years and over with type 2 diabetes and hypertension will already by definition have a high CV risk, no additional weighting for extent of CV risk has been applied. A lower value of blood pressure should be aimed for in those who are able to tolerate the therapy and self-manage, and/or those with concomitant renal disease.
- Optimal blood pressure regulation should be aimed for to help to maintain cognitive performance and improve learning and memory. Evidence base 2++, grade of recommendation B.

LIPID CONTROL IN DIABETES MELLITUS

Coronary heart disease (CHD) is the most common cause of mortality in type 2 diabetes and remains the principal challenge for older people with this metabolic disorder. Elevated levels of blood lipids is an independent risk factor for CHD and there is published evidence of cardiovascular benefit using a lipid lowering regimen, although this is limited in older subjects. As part of a multifaceted approach to the metabolic consequences of diabetes, effective management of blood lipids is essential to optimize vascular outcomes. Attention to risk factors such as smoking and other metabolic derangements such as blood pressure are also of paramount importance.

Diabetic dyslipidemia is characterized by high triglycerides, low HDL-cholesterol, and an LDL-cholesterol that is rich in highly atherogenic, small, dense LDL particles, which contribute to cardiovascular risk.[221] Can we alter this? The Scandinavian Simvastatin Survival Study (4S)[222] included 2282 subjects with angina or previous myocardial infarction aged 60 to 70 years with hypercholesterolemia (total cholesterol >5.5 mmol/L) randomized to a placebo or simvastatin to achieve total cholesterol below 5.2 mmol/L; this resulted in a 27% lowering of risk of death and a 29% lowering of risk of a coronary end point (nonfatal MI or CHD death). Subgroup analysis examined the diabetic subjects of all ages, and showed a much greater absolute risk reduction in diabetic than in nondiabetic people,[223] with very similar relative risk reductions—emphasizing the much greater benefit of addressing vascular risk in the diabetic than the nondiabetic subject.

The Cholesterol And Recurrent Events (CARE) study[224] took subjects with an acute myocardial infarction in the preceding 3 to 20 months with total cholesterol below 6.2 mmol/L (mean 5.4 mmol/L) who were randomized to placebo or pravastatin 40 mg per day. In 2129 subjects aged 60 to 75 years, pravastatin resulted in a 27% relative risk reduction of major coronary events over the 5-year follow-up. The elderly subgroup benefited more than average from the pravastatin.

Thus it appears that lipid reduction benefits the elderly diabetic person. In secondary prevention, a total cholesterol level more than 5.0 mmol/L indicates the need for treatment. In primary prevention, risk assessment is based on age, gender, blood pressure, and microalbuminuria using the color charts.[225]

We would not measure lipids in subjects aged more than 80 years because there is at present no evidence that dyslipidemia has an adverse effect at that age. However, a more recent study provides convincing evidence of benefit irrespective of age. The Heart Protection Study[226] included adults with diabetes aged 40 to 80 years treated with simvastatin 40 mg or a placebo over a 5-year period. Treatment led to an average fall in LDL-cholesterol of 1.0 mmol/L and resulted in a highly significant reduction of 27% in the incidence in first nonfatal myocardial infarction or coronary death and a 25% reduction in first nonfatal stroke or fatal stroke. Evidence of benefit was observed after as early as 12 months of treatment.

One should also attend to other cardiovascular risk factors and consider whether the dyslipidemia is secondary to thyroid, hepatic, or renal disease.

VASCULAR PROPHYLAXIS

Diabetic patients have a twofold to threefold increase in the rate of cerebrovascular accidents or myocardial infarctions, and have a worse outcome than nondiabetic people from either myocardial infarction or stroke.[227]

Aspirin should be used as secondary prophylaxis in all diabetic people with evidence of macrovascular disease, and it should be strongly considered as primary prevention in diabetic subjects with other risk factors for macrovascular disease, such as hypertension, cigarette smoking, dyslipidemia, obesity, and albuminuria (macro or micro).[228] Because of the platelet defects associated with diabetes, it is recommended that the dose of aspirin should be 300 mg per day,[228–230] although the American Diabetes Association's position statement (http://www.diabetes.org/DiabetesCare/supplement198/s45.htm) advocates a dose of 81 to 325 mg enteric-coated aspirin per day. If the patient cannot tolerate aspirin, then clopidogrel[231] can be used.

The elderly diabetic person is at increased risk of atrial fibrillation (odds ratio: 1.4 for men and 1.6 for women)[232] and at twofold increased risk of thromboembolism from atrial fibrillation.[233,234] We can find no subgroup analysis of the major atrial fibrillation trials to examine the benefits of warfarin specifically in older diabetic subjects. It appears that the adverse event rate in diabetic people drops from 8.6 events per 100 patients per year to 2.8 events with warfarin use.[234] It is important to check for retinal new vessels when diabetic subjects are placed on warfarin, although the Early Treatment Diabetic Retinopathy Study[235] showed no excess vitreous or preretinal hemorrhages in subjects given aspirin for vascular prophylaxis.

Despite our efforts, patients are still likely to suffer myocardial infarction. The Diabetes mellitus, Insulin Glucose infusion in Acute Myocardial Infarction (DIGAMI) study[236,237] reported on treating subjects with acute myocardial infarction and either diabetes or raised random plasma glucose (i.e., not necessarily diabetic) with either an intensive insulin infusion and then a four-times daily insulin regimen or conventional treatment. Over a mean follow-up of 3.4 years, there was a 33% death rate in the treatment group compared with a 44% death rate in the control group, an absolute reduction in mortality of 11%. The effect was greatest among the subgroup without previous insulin treatment and at a low cardiovascular risk. Evidence is continuing to accumulate that the diabetic person should have a glucose/insulin infusion after a myocardial infarction.

CARE ISSUES AND FUTURE INITIATIVES

Diabetes mellitus in old age is increasingly recognized to be a specialist area. It demands skills and commitment often not available to hard-pressed general physicians attempting to cope with the dramatic increase in scientific knowledge and the escalation of clinical involvement required by most employers, whether in hospital or primary care settings. This final section explores several topical themes within the emerging discipline of "geriatric diabetology," which focuses on service delivery.[238]

Models of care

Four models of care are usually defined in relation to managing older adults with diabetes.[239] In the first, where there is effectively a breakdown in patient and doctor education and communication, the patient is essentially self-caring. This model should be avoided. A primary care-based approach is a common and often an acceptable model as long as there is an enthusiastic and informed commitment to diabetes care. It has several advantages, including increased convenience for both patients and relatives, familiarity with practice staff, and continuity of care. Disadvantages such as lack of on-site specialist input and unstructured follow-up practices may lead to suboptimal care.

Hospital service-based care is a third model and has the advantage of regular specialist input, but has two main disadvantages. These are the lack of clinic time to deal with the vast numbers of patients needed to be seen, and the fact that junior medical staff are often expected to provide this "expert" opinion. The extra inconvenience for patients traveling large distances and the excessive waiting times discourage many patients from being involved in this practice. Primary care physicians should always be involved.

The fourth model is the favored one and consists of a "shared care" approach between the hospital (diabetologist or geriatrician) and primary care. Joint management policies are essential for this to be a worthwhile and effective partnership, with an emphasis on early referral to secondary care when problems develop. Good communication is important and a common diabetes record card is mandatory. Clear boundaries of responsibility need to be established, and educational strategies should form the basis of a common approach to management.

Diabetes specialist nurses for elderly people

Diabetes specialist nurses are an invaluable addition to a diabetes service and can act as a link between primary and secondary care sectors.[240] They have many other roles (see box on "Roles of the Diabetic Specialist Nurse for Elderly People") and we feel strongly that some of these specialist nurses should be appointed specifically to manage older diabetic patients. In conjunction with the primary care physician, community dietitian, social worker, chiropodist, geriatric liaison sister, and geriatrician (or diabetologist), they should constitute a "Community Diabetes Team" that will provide multiprofessional diabetes health care.

Special considerations

Providing specialist care for older patients with diabetes requires an up-to-date approach to implementing research findings or at least questioning them and deciding if they are applicable. Recent evidence suggests that examining older patients admitted to the hospital with diabetes for the presence of depression may be a valuable aid to improving outcomes.[241]

The recent introduction of amylin analogues (e.g., pramlintide) and dipeptidyl peptidase-IV inhibitors (sitagliptin and vildagliptin) create new opportunities for treatment in aging subjects but their use needs to be defined from both an efficacy approach but also from a safety standpoint. The emergence of an increased risk of fractures (especially of the hip and wrist) in subjects treated with TZDs[242] has more recently been of concern prompting clinicians to consider fracture risk generally in patients before starting a TZD. There remains a great deal to achieve in enhancing diabetes care for older inpatients but recent work by the National Diabetes Support Team (U.K.) has provided a series of recommendations, some of which deal specifically with older people which may bring about an improvement in outcomes.[243] (See box on "Roles of the Geriatrician in Elderly Diabetic Care.")

Diabetes mellitus remains an exciting challenge for all health professionals involved in clinical geriatrics, and progress is being made in improving all aspects of the care of this common and serious condition.

Roles of the Diabetic Specialist Nurse for Elderly People

- To teach, advise, and counsel patients and caregivers both in the clinic and in the patient's home.
- Where possible, to educate patients to achieve self-care.
- To teach self-monitoring of blood glucose (or urinalysis, if appropriate) and instruct in the use of special monitoring techniques for patients with physical problems, partial-sightedness, or blindness.
- Teaching and advising on insulin administration.
- To liaise with and refer to other health professionals, chiropodists, community nurses, general practitioners, etc.
- To commence insulin treatment in the patient's home.
- To advise and guide residential and nursing home staff to manage patients with diabetes.
- To provide continuing support and advice to patients and health care providers when specific problems arise relating to diabetes.

Roles of the Geriatrician in Elderly Diabetic Care

- To assess coexisting disease that impacts on diabetes management
- To manage increasing dependency and disability
- To recognize and manage cognitive impairment
- To assess and treat urinary incontinence
- To liaise between hospital and community support services
- To provide respite programs for spouses and caregivers
- To be a member of a hospital diabetic clinic team

KEY POINTS
Diabetes Mellitus

- Diabetes is very common in elderly people, and is frequently undiagnosed.
- Type 2 predominates, but type 1 and secondary diabetes also occur.
- Diabetes has considerable associated morbidity (predominantly macrovascular disease and conditions with mixed etiology, such as dementia and foot ulcers) and increased mortality.
- Glycemic targets are a compromise between improved cognition and quality of life with a lower plasma glucose level, and risks of drug side effects with still lower target levels.
- Control of vascular risk factors using hypotensive and lipid-lowering drugs and antiplatelet and anticoagulant drugs is vitally important.
- There must be secondary amelioration of complications, such as eye and foot disease.

For a complete list of references, please visit online only at www.expertconsult.com

CHAPTER 93

Blood Disorders in the Elderly

Bindu Kanapuru
William B. Ershler

There is the old maxim "Hematology is the study of blood, and the organs it perfuses." With such perspective it would seem impossible to adequately provide a comprehensive review in a single chapter. Instead, we provide broad strokes of the key topics of modern hematology with particular focus on geriatric issues of clinical relevance.

Most circulating cells are derived from a single hematopoietic stem cell. The life span of blood cells is genetically predetermined. Therefore, hematopoiesis is a lifelong continuous process. Stem cells lack the surface molecules, which are associated with differentiation (maturation), but they do express the CD34 molecule on their surface, a feature that has important clinical implications. Hematopoietic stem cells give rise to unipotent progenitor cells, which then divide and differentiate into recognizable cells of a specific lineage. This differentiation process is considered to be random. Once a specific cell line is determined (leukocyte, erythrocyte, etc.), the progenitor cells go through further differentiation to manifest their ultimate predestined phenotype. This is accomplished by upregulation of specific receptors under the influence of multiple cytokines and growth factors. Certain of these cytokines, for example erythropoietin and granulocyte-colony stimulating factor, have, in recent years, become important clinical tools.

With aging, there is a notable reduction in the capacity to produce new blood cells. Yet unless there is substantial physiologic stress, the number of circulating cells remains fairly constant. Quantitative deficiencies are only apparent when stress produces a demand that exceeds reserve proliferative capacity. Such might occur during an acute infection or after cytotoxic chemotherapy. Significant qualitative deficiencies in blood cell function are not thought to be a consequence of aging but may be associated with age-associated chronic diseases.

Acknowledging that the discipline of hematology extends way beyond what is presented, we attempt in the pages that follow to provide an overview of blood disorders of particular relevance to older people. We focus primarily on the hematologic problems that will be encountered by the practicing geriatrician. These include anemia, myelodysplasia, myeloproliferative disorders, hematologic malignancies, and disorders of hemostasis.

ANEMIA

Anemia is a significant health problem in the elderly because of both a high prevalence and significant associated morbidity (Table 93-1).[1] Although there is a long-established perspective that anemia in the elderly is of little consequence, studies have shown that even mild decreases in hemoglobin levels are associated with reduced quality of life, clinical depression, falls, functional impairment, slower walking speed, reduced grip strength, loss of mobility, worsening comorbidities, and mortality and have called for a greater focus on this problem.[2] Currently, screening for anemia is not generally practiced, and thus it is typically discovered during a workup for other conditions, at a time when many of its deleterious effects may have already occurred.

The World Health Organization (WHO) defines anemia as a hemoglobin level of less than 13g/dL in adult males and less than 12g/dL in adult females.[3] In older men and women, anemia by this definition is associated with an increase in mortality.[4–9] It has been pointed out the WHO criteria do not take into account inherent racial variations, particularly with respect to African Americans who may have lower levels of hemoglobin without significant adverse outcomes.[10,11] In a study that analyzed 1018 black and 1583 white adults aged 71 to 82 years, anemia was associated with increased mortality in whites but not blacks.[10,11] The issue of defining criteria for the diagnosis of anemia is quite relevant in the context of age as well. Older women, for example, have better physical performance and function at hemoglobin values between 13 and 15 g/dL than between 12 and 12.9 g/dL,[12] suggesting perhaps that a cutoff level of 12 g/dL is too low. Nevertheless, the WHO definition remains the current standard utilized in most current epidemiologic surveys and many clinical laboratories.

Prevalence of Anemia

Guralnik and colleagues examined the third National Health and Nutrition Examination Survey (NHANES III) database, a nationally representative sample of community-dwelling persons and determined age- and sex-specific prevalence rates of anemia in the total U.S. population.[13] For those over the age of 65 years, by WHO criteria, approximately 11% were anemic (see Table 93-1). The prevalence of anemia was lowest (1.5%) among males between 17 and 49 years of age and highest (26.1%) in males over 85 years. Among those 65 years and older, the prevalence rate was notably higher in African Americans as compared to whites and Hispanics. Prevalence rates of anemia in the elderly vary in community-dwelling and institutionalized populations. It is also quite clear that anemia is more common among frail elderly. In the

Table 93-1. Anemia Prevalence in the Elderly Using the WHO Criteria

Study (ref)	Age	Population	Prevalence
Gurlanik (13)	≥65 years	Community-dwelling elderly Americans	10.6%
Ferruci (256)	>70 years	Community-dwelling elderly Italians	11%
Denny (257)	≥71	Community-dwelling	24%
Joosten (258)	≥65 years	Hospitalized	24% (defined as Hb < 11.5 g/dL)
Artz (43)	Most ≥65 years	Nursing-home	48%
Robinson (17)	Most >65 years	Nursing home	53%

nursing home, for example, anemia prevalence approaches 50% or higher.[14–17]

Pathogenesis

In younger adults with anemia, the cause is usually readily apparent. In older patients, however, discerning the cause of anemia can oftentimes be challenging (Table 93-2). Inflammation, nutritional deficiencies, and renal insufficiency are commonly observed, but for as many as one third of elderly anemic individuals (and almost 50% for those residing in nursing homes), the anemia cannot be attributed to conventional causes, a condition now termed *unexplained anemia*.[18]

ANEMIA OF INFLAMMATION

Chronic diseases, such as atherosclerosis, diabetes, arthritis, infection, and malignancy, increase in prevalence with age and each is characterized by inflammatory processes. Although there are several ways in which inflammation can negatively influence erythropoiesis, disordered iron kinetics is a common feature.[19] During inflammation, there is reduced iron absorption from the gastrointestinal tract and defective reutilization of iron sequestered in reticuloendothelial cells. Hepcidin, a 25 amino acid polypeptide produced in the liver in response to inflammatory stimuli, down-regulates intestinal iron absorption as well as macrophage and monocyte iron release, thereby creating functional iron deficiency and resultant hypoproliferative anemia.[20–24] Reduced secretion of erythropoietin due to the action of inflammatory cytokines is also known to play a role in the anemia of chronic inflammation.[25]

IRON DEFICIENCY ANEMIA

The prevalence of iron deficiency in the elderly may range from 2.5% to as high as 30% in some studies. Iron deficiency is usually secondary to iron loss rather than inadequate intake and is important to identify because it may be a manifestation of an occult malignancy. For example, in one study, of 114 outpatients referred to a gastroenterologist for investigation of iron deficiency, 45 had upper gastrointestinal and 18 had colonic sources of bleeding.[26] In an older study of 100 patients in whom the site of bleeding could not be established by any means other than laparotomy, a malignancy was found to be the cause in 10%.[27] In a survey of 1388 patients over 65 years of age, 25% were anemic and approximately one third were iron deficient. Of those with iron deficiency, gastrointestinal endoscopy found 57% to have an upper gastrointestinal lesion and 27% to have colonic lesions. In total, gastrointestinal malignancy was found in 15% of those with iron deficiency anemia.[28]

Iron deficiency may be the result of gastrointestinal malabsorption, particularly in patients who have had bowel resection, inflammatory bowel disease, or who are on chronic antacid therapy. Furthermore, malabsorption of iron may be an early manifestation of celiac disease.[29,30]

For patients who present with anemia and microcytic red blood cell indices, serum levels of iron, ferritin, and transferrin saturation are typically low and total iron-binding capacity is elevated. The coexistence of chronic inflammatory disease may complicate analysis. To determine whether patients with chronic inflammation and anemia are iron deficient, measurement of the soluble transferrin receptor is frequently useful. Under conditions of iron deficiency, transferrin receptor is upregulated and increased levels are found in the serum. An index, derived by dividing the serum level of soluble transferrin receptor by the log of the ferritin level, has been shown to be helpful.[31] A ratio of less than 2 denotes anemia of chronic inflammation, whereas values greater than 2 identify patients with either uncomplicated iron deficiency anemia or a combination of both iron deficiency and inflammation.

B_{12} AND FOLATE

Since the implementation of the Food and Drug Administration's policy of folic acid fortification of cereal grain products *in 1998*, there has been a dramatic reduction in measurable folate deficiency. Just 2 years after implementation, examination of the NHANES cohort IV (1999–2000) compared with cohort III (1988–1994) revealed the prevalence of low-serum folate concentrations (<6.8 nmol/L) decreased from 16% before to 0.5% after fortification.[32] Thus, folic acid deficiency is currently an uncommon cause of anemia. Vitamin B_{12} deficiency, however, remains a problem, particularly in geriatric populations.[33] The great majority of B_{12} deficiency in the elderly is due to food cobalamin malabsorption with true dietary deficiency or pernicious anemia being significantly less common. An age-associated atrophic gastritis with or without antacid therapy is a frequent antecedent. Macrocytic indices, the hallmark of B_{12} deficiency, may not be apparent because of concomitant inflammatory disease or iron deficiency. In addition to red cell changes, patients with B_{12} deficiency may also present with a myriad of hematologic abnormalities including leukcopenia, thrombocytopenia, and pancytopenia,

Table 93-2. Features of Anemia by Classification

	MCV	Iron/TIBC	Ferritin	ESR/CRP	EPO	CrCl	Misc
IDA	Small	Low/hi	Low	wnl	High	wnl	
ACI	Small	Low/low	Low to High	High	High	wnl	
CKD	wnl	wnl	wnl	wnl	Low	<30 cc/min	
B_{12}/ Folate	Large	wnl	wnl	wnl	High	wnl	levels
Hypo-thyroid	Large	wnl	wnl	wnl	High	wnl	TSH up
MDS	wnl - Large	wnl	wnl	wnl	High	wnl	marrow
UA	wnl	wnl	wnl	wnl	Low	>30 cc/min	

Abbreviations: IDA, iron deficiency anemia; ACI, anemia of chronic inflammation; CKD, chronic kidney disease; B_{12}, vitamin B_{12}; MDS, myelodysplastic syndrome; UA, unexplained anemia; TIBC, total iron binding capacity; ESR, erythrocyte sedimentation rate; CRP, c-reactive protein; EPO, serum erythropoietin, CrCl, creatinine clearance.

occasionally requiring the diagnosis of myelodysplasia or aplastic anemia. B_{12} deficiency is usually suspected by the finding of an elevated mean corpuscular volume (MCV) either on routine screening or for evaluation of the cause for anemia. However, other causes for macrocytosis are more common, and these include excessive alcohol intake, drug intake (particularly antineoplastic agents), reticulocytosis, myelodysplasia, and hypothyroidism. Levels of B_{12} below 200 pg/mL quite reliably indicate vitamin B_{12} deficiency; however, measurement of *methylmalonic acid levels and homocysteine (which are elevated)* may be necessary to establish the diagnosis for those with higher serum B_{12} levels. Treatment with both intramuscular B_{12} and crystalline oral B_{12} are effective in the elderly, even in patients with cobalamin food malabsorption.

RENAL INSUFFICIENCY

Chronic kidney disease (CKD) is an important cause of anemia in the elderly.[34,35] Reduced renal erythropoietin (EPO) production is the primary factor leading to anemia in CKD. Serum EPO levels have been shown to be inappropriately low at a creatinine clearance of < 40 mL/min.[36] The precise degree of renal dysfunction sufficient to cause anemia remains controversial. Mild hemoglobin decreases in adults may be detected at a creatinine clearance of 40 to 60 mL/min.[37,38]

A study among community-dwelling elderly suggested anemia and low EPO levels independent of age and other factors at a creatinine clearance < 30 mL/min.[39] In a nursing home of 6200 residents, 59% were found to be anemic and 43% had calculated creatinine clearances of < 60 mL/min. Their analysis indicated that renal impairment, even at mild levels increased the risk of anemia.[17]

UNEXPLAINED ANEMIA

Increasingly, it has become recognized that approximately *one third of older adults* with anemia do not have an obviously discernible cause upon routine evaluation (Table 93-3). Typically, this anemia is generally mild (hemoglobin concentration in the 10 to 12 g/dL range), normocytic, and hypoproliferative (low reticulocyte count). It has been postulated that the cause relates to a number of factors including testosterone,[40] occult inflammation,[41] reduced hematopoietic reserve with advancing age,[42] inappropriately low-serum erythropoietin level,[43] and myelodysplastic syndromes (discussed later). It is clear that this anemia is associated with a low-serum erythropoietin level for the degree of anemia. The EPO level usually falls within the normal reference range. However, this is abnormal because serum EPO should rise with falling hemoglobin concentration. The diagnosis of "unexplained anemia" assumes the clinician has excluded serious causes. The threshold to pursue a bone marrow examination to exclude myelodysplastic syndromes remains unknown. However, we advocate considering a bone marrow examination in all patients requiring red cell transfusion who otherwise have an unexplained anemia. Macrocytosis, thrombocytopenia, neutropenia, splenomegaly or unexplained constitutional symptoms of fever, chills, early satiety, bone pain, or weight loss should prompt consideration of a bone marrow examination.

Table 93-3. Features of Unexplained Anemia

Hemoglobin	10.5 to 12 g/dL
Reticulocyte index	Low
MCV	80 to 95 fL
Serum iron	Mildly low normal
TIBC	Normal
% Iron saturation	Mildly low normal
B_{12}, folate, ESR, TSH	Normal
Platelet and white blood counts	Normal
Creatinine clearance	<90 to >30 mL/min

MYELODYSPLASIA

Myelodysplastic syndromes (MDS) include a heterogeneous group of disorders characterized by dysplastic changes within the bone marrow and impaired proliferation in one or more cell lines (erythroid, myeloid, or megakaryocytic).[44] As such, peripheral cytopenias and symptoms related to anemia, leukopenia, or thrombocytopenia are common manifestations of the disease. MDS occurs primarily in older males with a median age of 76 years. Each year approximately 15,000 patients will be diagnosed with this disorder, although this might be an underestimate.[45]

Classification

The long-established French-American-British (FAB) classification[46] defined five distinct types of MDS: refractory anemia (RA), refractory anemia with ringed sideroblasts (RARS), refractory anemia with excess blasts (RAEB), refractory anemia with excess blasts in transformation (RAEB-T), and chronic myelomonocytic leukemia (CMML). The WHO has modified this general classification based on salient bone marrow cytogenetic features (e.g., deletion of the short arm of the fifth chromosome [5q-]) and other histopathologic or clinical features (Table 93-4).[47] Thus, RAEB is divided into two groups based on the number of blasts and the RA and RARS into those with only anemia or those with multilineage involvement. These modifications have enabled a more accurate estimation of prognosis.[48]

Pathogenesis

Although in a majority of cases, no distinct cause for MDS can be identified, in many there is an association with prior chemotherapy, particularly with alkylating agents or topoisomerase inhibitors, and with prior radiation therapy.[49,50] Treatment-related MDS patients are usually younger and have a worse prognosis than de novo MDS patients.[49] Prolonged exposure to high concentrations of benzene and pesticides appear to increase the risk of MDS possibly by inducing chromosomal abnormalities.[51] Carcinogens present in cigarette smoke appear to have a similar effect in increasing the risk of MDS, especially of the type associated with deletions of chromosome 5 and 7.[52] A familial etiology for MDS has also been postulated.[51] Chromosomal abnormalities are frequently seen in MDS, and they are very similar to those in acute myelogenous leukemia (AML) including complex karyotypes.[49] Several mechanisms may be involved in the pathogenesis of MDS, including alteration in apoptotic pathways, cytokine regulation, bone marrow microenvironment, mitochondrial enzymes, and immune regulation.[53] Furthermore, there is evolving evidence that some MDS cases have an autoimmune basis because clinically MDS may be associated with other autoimmune disorders and

Table 93-4. WHO Classification and Criteria for the Myelodysplastic Syndromes

Disease	Blood Findings	Bone Marrow Findings
Refractory anemia (RA)	Anemia	Erythroid dysplasia only < 5% blasts < 15% ringed sideroblasts
Refractory anemia with ringed sideroblasts (RARS)	Anemia	Erythroid dysplasia only < 5% blasts ≥ 15% ringed sideroblasts
Refractory cytopenia with multilineage dysplasia (RCMD)	Cytopenias (bicytopenia or pancytopenia) No or rare blasts No Auer rods $<1 \times 10^9$/L monocytes	Dysplasia in ≥10% of cells in two or more myeloid cell lines < 5% blasts in marrow No Auer rods < 15% ringed sideroblasts
Refractory cytopenia with multilineage dysplasia and ringed sideroblasts (RCMD-RS)	Cytopenias (bicytopenia or pancytopenia) No or rare blasts No Auer rods $<1 \times 10^9$/L monocytes	Dysplasia in ≥10% of cells in two or more myeloid cell lines ≥ 15% ringed sideroblasts < 5% blasts No Auer rods
Refractory anemia with excess blasts-1 (RAEB-1)	Cytopenias < 5% blasts No Auer rods $<1 \times 10^9$/L monocytes	Unilineage or multilineage dysplasia 5% to 9% blasts No Auer rods
Refractory anemia with excess blasts-2 (RAEB-2)	Cytopenias 5% to 19% blasts Auer rods ± $<1 \times 10^9$/L monocytes	Unilineage or multilineage dysplasia 10% to 19% blasts Auer rods ±
Myelodysplastic syndrome, unclassified (MDS-U)	Cytopenias No or rare blasts No Auer rods	Unilineage dysplasia in granulocytes or megakaryocytes < 5% blasts No Auer rods
MDS associated with isolated del(5q)	Anemia < 5% blasts Platelets normal or increased	Normal to increased megakaryocytes with hypolobated nuclei < 5% blasts No Auer rods Isolated del(5q)

laboratory evidence has documented oligoclonal T-cell patterns in up to 50% of cases.[54]

Clinical and laboratory features

Patients with MDS may be asymptomatic or present with symptoms and signs related to qualitative or quantitative defects of erythrocytes, leukocytes, and platelets.[55] Fatigue, which significantly affects quality of life,[56] exertional dyspnea, fever, and infections are some of the reasons for consulting a physician. Complete blood count usually reveals anemia with normocytic or macrocytic indices. Moderate leukopoenia and thrombocytopenia or thrombocytosis may be present. Bone marrow examination may reveal a normal or hypercellular pattern with dysplastic features identified in erythroid, myeloid, and megakaryocytic cell lines, or in all three (trilinear). Commonly seen changes in peripheral blood and bone marrow include anisocytosis, macrocytosis, basophilic stippling, ringed sideroblasts, pseudo-Pelger Huët abnormality, blast cells, and hypersegmented neutrophils, micromegakaryocytes, and large platelets.[55]

PROGNOSIS

The International Prognostic Scoring System (IPSS)[57] divides patients into low, intermediate-1 (INT-1), intermediate-2 (INT-2), and high categories (Table 93-5). It is based on the number of cytopenias (hemoglobin level of less than 10 g/dL, an absolute neutrophil count of less than 1500/μL, and a platelet count of less than 100,000/μL), chromosomal abnormalities, and percentage of bone marrow blasts and is used to estimate overall survival and predict progression to AML. Median survival ranges from less than 3 months regardless of age in the high-risk groups to almost 12 years in those less than 60 years in the low-risk group. In the low-risk group, patients over 70 years seem to have a worse prognosis than younger patients, but age does not seem to significantly change prognosis in the high-risk category. Other factors found to be of prognostic importance include WHO subtypes[58] and transfusion dependence. Older age did not influence prognosis in the refractory anemia group, which is usually associated with good prognosis.[58] Also, MDS associated with 5q deletion is associated with a good prognosis.[59]

Treatment

Supportive care in the form of transfusions, iron chelating therapy, and adequate treatment of infections is the backbone of treatment in MDS. In the low and INT-1 groups, treatment is deferred unless significant cytopenias are present. Patients with deletion 5q have a relatively good prognosis and experience an excellent response to the thalidomide analog lenalidomide. In one series, 67% of patients became transfusion independent after treatment with 10 mg of daily lenalidomide and continued to remain so for more than 2 years.[60] Recombinant erythropoietin with or without granulocyte-stimulating factor is used to treat symptomatic anemia in those with low-serum erythropoietin levels and symptomatic anemia.[61] Older patients in the low INT-1 category but with neutropenia or thrombocytopenia and inpatients in the INT-2 and high-risk group who are ineligible

Table 93-5. Myelodysplastic Syndrome (MDS) International Prognostic Scoring System (IPSS): Prognostic Variables

IPPS Score	0	0.5	1.0	1.5	2.0
Marrow blasts %	<5	5–10	—	11–20	21–30
Karyotype	Good*	Intermediate*	Poor*	—	—
Cytopenias	0/1	2/3	—	—	—

*Good = normal, -y, del(5q), del(20q); poor = complex (>3 abnormalities) or chromosome 7 anomalies; intermediate = any other abnormalities.

for transplantation are best treated with DNA methyltransferase inhibitors, such as decitabine[62] or azacytidine,[63] as both have been shown to improve quality of life. Although intensive therapy with allogeneic stem cell transplantation has been traditionally reserved for younger patients, reduced intensity conditioning regimens have extended this therapy to selected older patients with favorable results. Assessment with the Hematopoietic Cell Transplantation Comorbidity Index (HCT-CI) has been used in elderly MDS patients and may help select patients for whom the risk-benefit ratio is favorable for this form of aggressive therapy.[64]

MYELOPROLIFERATIVE DISORDERS

Myeloproliferative disorders (MPDs) are characterized by clonal proliferation of hematopoietic stem cells. They include polycythemia vera (PV), essential thrombocythemia (ET), chronic idiopathic myelofibrosis (CIF), and chronic myelogenous leukemia (CML). CML is identified by the presence of the translocated *bcr-abl* gene and typically has three phases: a chronic phase, seen in more than 80% of patients, a blastic phase, and an intermediate, accelerated phase.

The 2008 WHO classification has replaced the term *disease* in MPD with *neoplasm* to indicate the possibly malignant nature of these disorders.[47,65] The myeloproliferative neoplasm (MPN) group includes mast cell disease, chronic eosinophilic and neutrophilic leukemia, hypereosinophilic syndrome, and other previously unclassified bone marrow disorders in addition to CML, PV, CIF, and ET. The common feature of these disorders is evident clonal proliferation without dysplasia.

Epidemiology

PV and CIF are more often diagnosed in the elderly[45] and equally in both genders, with a median age of 70 years. Incidence rates for all age groups have ranged between 0.7 to 2.6/100,000 for PV and 0.3 to 1.5/100,000 in CIF, but rates as high as 23.5/100,000 have been reported for those between 70 and 79 years for age in PV. An increased incidence among Ashkenazi Jews has been reported. Incidence for ET ranged between 0.59 and 2.53/100,000 with almost twofold higher rates seen among females than males. Unlike PV, ET is diagnosed at a younger age and is often seen in association with pregnancy. A significant trend toward an increase in ET incidence has been observed, especially among men, although the trends for PV and CIF do not show any change.[45] Familial studies have shown an almost fivefold increased risk for PV and sevenfold risk for ET in first-degree relatives with myeloproliferative disorders.[66]

Etiology

Identification of a specific (V617F) mutation in the Janus Kinase-2 (*JAK2*) gene improved our understanding of the pathogenesis of myeloproliferative disease.[67] *JAK2* V617F can be identified in almost 95% of PV patients[68] and in more than 50% of ET and CIF patients.[69] Increased activity of this gene enhances the sensitivity of the mutated stem cells to hematopoietic growth factors like erythropoietin, thrombopoietin, stem cell factor, and granulocyte-stimulating factor, causing clonal trilinear proliferation of myeloid precursors. Additionally a mutation in the *mpl* gene, which involves the thrombopoietin receptor, is also thought to play a minor role in the pathogenesis.[70] The *bcr-abl* fusion gene formed as a result of translocation of the *abl* gene from chromosome 9 to the *bcr* region on chromosome 22 causes transcription of proteins with abnormal tyrosine kinase activity resulting in clonal proliferation recognized most commonly in CML.[71] Clonal evolution with additional chromosomal abnormalities frequently involving the 17th are seen in more than 50% of patients in accelerated phases of the disease.[72]

Production of growth factors by cytokines secreted from megakaryocytes and monocytes are hypothesized to play a role in proliferation of fibroblasts, changes in extracellular matrix, and angiogenesis seen in CIF.[73] Abnormal homing of stem cells and endothelial progenitor cells CD34+ to peripheral hematopoietic organs are also known to play a role in the extramedullary hematopoiesis of myelofibrosis.[74] Secondary myelofibrosis can result as progression of PV and ET, although progression of true ET has been highly debated.

Clinical features and diagnosis

The characteristic clinical features vary by specific myeloproliferative disorder. In ET, they are related to abnormalities in platelet number and function, and this is manifest predominantly as thrombotic episodes, although hemorrhagic episodes are also encountered.[75] Thrombotic events can precede the diagnosis of the disease and can involve both microvascular and large vessel arterial circulation causing ischemic strokes, peripheral vascular disease, and myocardial infarction in addition to venous thrombosis.[76] Erythromelalgia, a specific microvascular condition seen in ET, typically presents with erythremic, burning sensation of the extremities and ulceration of the toes.[77] The risk of thrombosis increases with age in both PV and ET.[78] Higher incidence of cardiovascular complications is also seen in those older than 65 years who had history of thrombosis.[79] It appears that the presence of *JAK2* mutation[80] and leukocytosis[81] may be additional risk factors for thrombosis in MPN patients. Hemorrhagic complications usually occur in patients with very high platelet counts ($>1500 \times 10^9$/L), and clinical presentation can vary from minor bruising or epistaxis to life-threatening gastrointestinal bleeding.[78] CIF may be asymptomatic in more than 30% of the patients, and diagnosis may be suspected on the basis of a leukoerythroblastic blood picture, presence of classic tear drop cells, or an enlarged spleen usually in the prefibrotic stage.[82] Presentation in CML is similar to that seen in other MPNs with constitutional symptoms and hemorrhagic manifestations. A finding of low leukocyte alkaline phosphatase (LAP) scores characterizes CML as compared to PV, ET, and CIF, which typically have normal LAP scores.

General signs and symptoms in patients with myeloproliferative disorders include splenomegaly, which can run the spectrum of mild and of little concern to uncomfortable and even life threatening if rupture occurs. Pruritus may be present in more than 50% of the patients. Patients with MPD also have a high incidence of fatigue, which may substantially decrease the quality of life.[83] Weight loss, night sweats, fever, and bone pain are also seen.

Diagnosis

The diagnosis of MPN has undergone a radical change with the identification of the JAK2 mutation. Previously standard criteria included physical signs and parameters based on peripheral blood counts, oxygen saturation, bone marrow findings, red cell mass, and the presence of splenomegaly. The new WHO criteria, an update of the previous 2001 criteria, include detection of JAK2 mutation along with bone marrow biopsy in the diagnosis of *bcr-abl* negative MPNs. Important changes also include lowering the platelet threshold number for diagnosis of ET from 600 to 450 × 10^9/L and establishing a 2g/dL increase of hemoglobin from normal levels as criteria for PV.[84] Different algorithms using serum EPO levels, morphology of bone marrow megakaryocytes, bone marrow reticulin staining, and use of fluorescence in situ hybridization (FISH) for *bcr-abl* have been proposed to enable differentiation of MPNs from one another.[84] It is especially important to differentiate the cause of isolated thrombocytosis because the prognosis of ET is very different from thrombocytosis seen in early prefibrotic CIF and that resulting from CML. The diagnosis of ET also may require exclusion of reactive thrombocytoses like cancer, iron deficiency anemia, and inflammatory conditions.[85] The diagnosis of CML is straightforward by identification of the Philadelphia chromosome by cytogenetics or *bcr-abl* gene by FISH technique.

Prognosis

As mentioned previously, survival times vary markedly in each of the described myeloproliferative diseases. One study shows 3-year survivals as high as 92% for ET and 88% for PV. However, older age was associated with lower overall survival for myeloproliferative diseases as a group[90] in <50 years and 66% in those >80 years of age).[45] ET and PV are associated with reduction in life expectancy, significant morbidity related to thrombosis, hemorrhage, and a small but definite risk for either leukemogenic transformation or marrow fibrosis, especially in the elderly.[86] Fatigue present in more than 80% of these patients has significant negative effect on quality of life.[83] It is now recognized that those with JAK2 mutation,[80] especially those with higher allelic burden and higher leukocyte counts, have a tendency to higher rates of thrombosis. Age >60 years, a previous history of thrombosis,[79] and a high platelet count (>1,500 × 10^9/L) have been previously identified as important prognostic factors for thrombosis in these patients. Patients in the prefibrotic stage of CIF have relatively good prognosis, with survival of almost 12 years. However, for those with high-risk CIF, life expectancy is significantly reduced.[87] The median length of survival can be as short as 1 year for those at highest risk. AML occurring in patients with primary myelofibrosis carries the worst prognosis with a dismal median survival of less than 3 months. Numerous scoring systems in CIF using hemoglobin levels, age, and white blood cell count have been described to predict prognosis,[88] and older age[9] appears to be a common negative prognostic factor.[89]

Treatment

Treatment in PV and ET is generally recommended to reduce morbidity associated with qualitative and quantitative changes in blood cells. Phlebotomy to reduce hematocrit to less than 45% is the mainstay of treatment in PV, as this has reduced the incidence of thrombosis.[75] Low-dose aspirin has been shown to reduce the risk of micro- and macrovascular complications and is recommended for treatment in all patients with PV.[90] In the European Collaboration on Low-dose Aspirin in Polycythemia vera (ECLAP) study, which randomized predominantly asymptomatic low-risk PV patients, cardiovascular death, nonfatal myocardial infarction, nonfatal stroke, and major venous thromboembolism were fewer among those treated with 100 mg aspirin daily as compared to placebo-treated controls (relative risk = 0.4 [95% CI 0.18 – 0.91], p = 0.0277).[91] Total and cardiovascular mortality were also reduced by 46% and 59%, respectively. There was no significant increase in the risk of bleeding. In younger, low-risk ET patients, treatment is generally not required although low-dose aspirin can be used to reduce microvascular symptoms.[92] However, in elderly patients, aspirin may be recommended based on the ECLAP study, especially if other traditional risk factors for vascular disease are also present.[92]

The evidence for benefit with treatment with hydroxyurea (HU) in high-risk ET patients has been clearly demonstrated, particularly with reference to reduced thrombosis (1.6%) compared to no treatment (10.6%).[93,94] Superior benefit was also seen when HU was compared to other cytoreductive agents including anagrelide.[93] Studies with HU in PV have not been as consistent, and a higher risk of leukemic transformation has been observed in treated patients. However, in high-risk PV and ET patients, HU is considered the standard of care.[75]

Primary myelofibrosis is a potentially fatal disease, and allogeneic hematopoietic stem cell transplantation is the only potentially curative therapy currently available. However, age and increasing comorbidity are strong negative prognostic factors for survival, even in these patients, and only 14% of myelofibrosis transplant patients older than 45 years survived 5 years after an allogeneic hematopoietic stem cell transplant (HSCT), as compared to 62% of younger patients.[95] In that same series, those with a Charlson comorbidity index of 4 to 6 had a greater than twofold risk of mortality. Reduced-intensity conditioning (RIC) regimens have increased response rates and event-free survival (EFS) in older patients, but in most of these studies, patients are considered old at age 60. It can be said that for patients younger than 70 years of age with low comorbidity, RIC regimen and allogeneic transplantation is a reasonable option worthy of clinical investigation.[96] Optimum treatment for those 70 years and older remains investigational and outside of a clinical trial may be supportive management alone. Control of symptomatic anemia, elevated leukocytes, or platelets may require pharmacologic intervention, but treatment is primarily palliative.

Erythropoietin and danazol were commonly employed to correct anemia, but a recent retrospective study[97] found an increase in risk of transformation to leukemia with the use of these agents in myelofibrosis, and thus enthusiasm for this approach has been tempered. High response rates for patients with anemia and splenomegaly with lenalidomide have been observed in those with the del (5q) group of myelofibrosis.[98]

The management of CML has changed dramatically since the late 1990s. Survival in CML patients depends on the phase of the disease, with median survival ranging from 5 years in those who present with chronic phase to less than 3 months for the blastic phase.[99] Prognostic classification developed by Social and Hasford incorporating variables like percent blasts, spleen size, platelet count, basophil and eosinophil counts, and age distinguishes three groups: low, intermediate, and high risk with good correlation with survival.[100] With the introduction of the oral tyrosine kinase inhibitor, imatinib, treatment of CML has improved considerably, and it appears that response rates and overall survival for older patients is comparable to that observed for younger patients.[101] Although no prognostic models are currently available for imatinib, complete cytogenetic response to treatment (i.e., disappearance of the Philadelphia chromosome on samples from bone marrow) identifies patients with favorable prognosis.

Current projections are for those treated in chronic phase with imatinib 400 mg daily,[102] overall survival rates exceed 75% at 6 years. Resistance to imatinib may occur and is usually associated with the presence of mutation in the kinase domain of *abl*. Newer drugs that bind to both active and inactive domains, such as dasatinib and nilotinib,[103] have enhanced survival in patients with imatinib refractory patients. Unless under investigational circumstances, the current role for hematopoietic stem cell transplantation is currently restricted to patients who are refractory to imatinib treatment.[104] The tyrosine kinase inhibitor drugs as a whole are well tolerated, and even the initial grade III and IV adverse effects of myelosuppression and liver toxicity experienced with imatinib are reduced to less than 2% at 5 years. Because these drugs are metabolized by CYP3A4 enzymes, which also are involved in the metabolism of drugs commonly used in the elderly, care to minimize drug-drug interactions are important, and attention to the potential for cardiac conduction delays (prolonged QTc) is of particular concern for those with preexisting cardiac disease.[104]

OTHER HEMATOLOGIC MALIGNANCIES COMMON TO OLDER PATIENTS

Multiple myeloma

Multiple myeloma (MM), the second most common hematologic malignancy diagnosed in the United States, is a disorder characterized by monoclonal proliferation of plasma cells (>10%) within the bone marrow. Typically, in MM, abnormal amounts of monoclonal immunoglobin or light chains (kappa or lambda) are present in the serum or urine. Manifestations related to involvement of the bone predominate, but symptoms resulting from the extramedullary effects of the circulating abnormal protein or hypercalcemia are also frequently observed. The median age of myeloma diagnosis is 70 years, and it occurs more frequently in African Americans and in males. The annual incidence in the United States is 4.4/100,000. Curiously, MM incidence and mortality rates are decreasing. However, the 5-year relative survival rates continue to be less than 20% for patients 65 years and older.

ETIOLOGY

Lower socioeconomic status, education, and dietary habits seem to account for the difference in incidence between African Americans and whites in the United States.[105,106] Familial studies have shown the risk of myeloma is higher in patients with a family history of hematologic malignancy, possibly implicating genetic predisposition.[107] Risk is also known to be higher after radiation or exposure to pesticides, certain chemicals, and asbestos[108] and also in those with a history of inflammatory disease[109] or allergies.[110] High levels of human herpes virus-8 (HHV-8) virus have been reported in bone marrow stromal cells of myeloma patients, indicating a possible viral etiology for the disease in selected cases.[111]

PATHOGENESIS

Bone pain is the primary symptom in approximately 70% of patients. Radiographs reveal either localized punched-out lytic bone lesions or diffuse osteoporosis, usually in bones with active hematopoietic tissue. The discrete lytic lesions are characterized by large and numerous osteoclasts on the bone-reabsorbing surface. Excess of osteoclast activating factors like RANKL, MIP-1α, and IL-6 coupled with a decrease in osteoblast activity caused by the presence of inhibitors such as Dickkopf-1 (DKK-1) contribute to the characteristic osteolytic bone lesions. With bone demineralization and with decreased activity because of pain, hypercalcemia may be expected. The symptoms of hypercalcemia (drowsiness, confusion, nausea, and thirst) are nonspecific, but their occurrence should alert the physician to investigate this possibility. Cardiac arrhythmias, renal insufficiency, and profound central nervous system (CNS) depression can develop as hypercalcemia progresses.

The circulating monoclonal protein at high levels can cause increased whole blood viscosity. This occurs most frequently with IgM (see Waldenstrom's disease, discussed later in the chapter) but may also occur with IgA, or even IgG myeloma. Increased viscosity compromises circulation including that to the brain, kidney and heart, and thus symptoms of confusion, light-headedness, or chest pain may result. The myeloma protein itself may cause tubular damage within the kidney, and renal insufficiency is a major consequence of uncontrolled myeloma.

CLINICAL FEATURES

It is important to differentiate myeloma from other plasma cell dyscrasias that occur with increasing frequency with age. Monoclonal gammopathy of undetermined significance (MGUS) is considered a benign disorder secondary to age-associated immune dysregulation.[112] The features of MGUS (Table 93-6) include a marrow with less than 10% plasma cells (and without dysplastic features characteristic of myeloma plasma cells), less than 3 g/dL monoclonal protein in the serum, and no end organ damage. Patients with MGUS will have stable, not increasing, levels of paraprotein. It is important to recognize MGUS and to follow closely, as some patients with early MM will present with features of MGUS only to progress to the more aggressive myeloma. About 1% of patients considered to have MGUS progress to MM per year.[113,114] MGUS patients who have >1.5 g/dL of

Table 93-6. Early Myeloma versus MGUS

	Early Multiple Myeloma	Monoclonal Gammopathy of Undetermined Significance (MGUS)
Pathogenesis	Neoplastic plasma cell disorder (malignant)	Disordered immunoregulation or possibly benign B cell neoplasm
Bone marrow	Frequently >10% plasma cells with many dysplastic features (myeloma cells)	Usually, 10% normal appearing plasma cells
Bone	Lytic bone lesions or diffuse osteoporosis	Usually no bone disease
Symptoms	Bone pain, constitutional symptoms (fatigue, weight loss), or those associated with kidney failure or hyperviscosity	Usually no symptoms
Serum spike	Progressively rising	Stable

monoclonal protein other than IgG and an abnormal urinary light chain ratio are at a greater risk of progression to MM. Follow-up every 3 months is recommended for patients with two or more of these conditions present, as opposed to less frequent intervals in those patients without.[115]

Smoldering myeloma has the same laboratory features as MM but without end organ damage. Solitary plasmacytoma is an isolated tumor consisting of plasma cells either in bones (solitary myeloma of bone) or soft tissue (extramedullary plasmacytoma) without systemic involvement.[116] In 1% to 2% of patients, MM can progress to plasma cell leukemia, which is more common in younger patients, has more than 20% plasma cells, and is more aggressive than MM.

Renal dysfunction is seen in more than 20% of myeloma patients at the time of diagnosis.[117] The pathogenesis of the renal disease is frequently multifactorial with contributions from paraproteins, tubular damage, tissue deposition of light chains, amyloidosis, hyperuricemia, or infection.[118–120]

Pathologic fractures are also common. Fatigue related to anemia occurs in 30% to 60% and usually occurs in patients with hemoglobin levels less than 10g/dL.[121] Signs of amyloidosis (present in up to 30% of myeloma patients) like macroglossia may also be present. Although constitutional symptoms can occur because of anemia, hyperviscosity, hypercalcemia, renal insufficiency, or infection, it should be remembered that in the elderly these symptoms might be less pronounced. The clinical presentation of MM has changed over the years with a lower percentage of patients presenting with end organ damage.[122] Especially in the elderly, MM is usually suspected by the presence of normocytic normochromic anemia and mild renal failure or hypergammaglobulinemia. Because of the catabolic effects of myeloma-associated cytokines, older patients may present with normocytic anemia and a drop in serum cholesterol, even before other signs or symptoms of the disease appear.

LABORATORY DATA AND DIAGNOSIS

Complete blood count, metabolic profile with liver function tests, serum LDH level, serum beta-2 microglobulin, serum-free light chain assay, serum and 24-hour urine protein, electrophoresis and immunofixation, a skeletal survey, and bone marrow are all important in the initial workup of MM patients.[123] Hypercalcemia, renal insufficiency, anemia, and bony abnormalities, which are the hallmarks of end organ damage in MM, are usually identified with the preceding evaluation. Other laboratory abnormalities include hypoalbuminemia, elevated LDH and beta-2 microglobulin, and platelet and coagulation abnormalities as well as rouleaux formation (stacking of red cells) apparent on the peripheral blood smear.[121]

Protein electrophoresis detects a monoclonal protein in approximately 80% of the patients in the serum and in 75% in the urine. Immunofixation (or immunoelectrophoresis) allows identification of the isotype, and this is usually IgG (60%) or IgA (20%). Of the 20% without detectable monoclonal protein by serum protein electrophoresis, most will have either kappa or lambda light chains detected in the urine (light chain myeloma). Only about 1% of myeloma will be truly "nonsecretors".[121] In the absence of monoclonal protein, the diagnosis of MM is established by finding of >30% plasma cells in the marrow.

PROGNOSIS

Traditionally the Durie-Salmon staging (predominantly clinical features and amount of paraprotein) has been used to identify patients at higher risk of death, as it is a good indicator of tumor burden in MM. However, the international staging system (ISS) has been shown to more accurately provide prognostic information. This staging system is based on the levels of serum beta-2 microglobulin and albumin, as well as other measures. In one survey, in stage I or low-risk MM (serum beta-2 microglobulin <3.5 g/dL and serum albumin >3.5 g/dL), median survival was 62 months. In contrast, for stage III (serum beta-2 microglobulin >5.5 g/dL), median survival was 29 months, and for the intermediate stage (stage II), the median survival was 44 months.[124] Certain cytogenetic abnormalities including those detected by fluorescence in situ hybridization (FISH) such as deletion of chromosome 13, hypoploidy, t(4;14), t(4;16), 17p-, when combined with a plasma cell labeling index >3% and selected laboratory data (LDH and CRP) have been shown to improve prognostic accuracy.[125]

Although most prior studies have not distinguished significant differences in clinical features of myeloma in young versus older patients, two reports are notable. The first compared those above and below the age of 70 years, and the second compared those above and below 50 years. Both showed that older patients presented with more advanced stage, poorer performance, and more adverse clinical features including lower hemoglobin, and higher creatinine, and in both reports the response rates and survival were less for the older group.[126,127]

TREATMENT

Older patients with MGUS and smoldering or asymptomatic myeloma need careful follow-up in an effort to detect and intervene if evidence for progression to more aggressive disease occurs. In patients with symptomatic myeloma, treatment includes two components, one to manage the disease and the second to provide supportive treatment to control complications or end organ damage. In older patients, treatment is especially difficult as improvements in progression-free survival and overall survival may come at an expense of increased toxicity and poor quality of life. Proper selection of patients using geriatric assessment may reduce the possibility of these adverse outcomes.

Previously, vincristine, doxorubicin, and dexamethasone were used as initial aggressive therapy, although it was difficult to prove that this was more effective than oral melphalan and prednisone (MP) in terms of overall survival. Recently, thalidomide and dexamethasone have become the agents of first-line therapy and are even used as induction therapy before transplantation. Bortezomib (a reversible inhibitor of 26S proteosome) alone or in combination has also been used for myeloma with excellent results.[128] Retrospective studies have shown similar toxicity profiles and survival outcomes in both younger and older patients despite the elderly receiving reduced chemotherapy doses.[129]

Currently the standard of care in elderly myeloma patients is treatment with melphalan, prednisone, and thalidomide (MPT). In patients between 65 and 75 years of age, median overall survival was 51.6 months for MPT compared to 33.2 months for MP and 38.3 months for autologous transplantation with reduced intensity melphalan conditioning regimen.[130] The complications from MPT include an increased risk of venous thromboembolism, especially when administered with high-dose dexamethasone and erythropoietic stimulating agents as well as peripheral neuropathy, infection, and constipation. Other combinations, which have shown benefit in older patients, include bortezomib or lenalidomide in combination with dexamethasone. Objective response rates as high as 90% have been seen with both these regimens.[131,132] The efficacy of maintenance therapy is not currently established and should not be offered outside of a clinical trial.

Treatment with bisphosphonates has benefit with regard to lytic bone disease, bone pain, and osteopenia.[133,134] Radiation is used as a palliative measure to reduce bone pain and along with dexamethasone to stabilize tumors of the spine to prevent spinal cord compression and compression fractures. Newer surgical techniques like vertebroplasty and kyphoplasty have improved the care of patients with bony complications in MM. Appropriate use of erythropoietic agents for management of anemia, aggressive management of infections including prophylactic antibiotics, immunoglobulin use, and management of hyperviscosity and hypercalcemia are all important for reducing morbidity in MM patients.

Lymphoma

Lymphomas are neoplastic disorders of B and T lymphocytes, which predominantly involve lymphoid organs. They are made up of a heterogeneous group of disorders, each with distinct etiology, histology, and clinical and prognostic features. Broadly, they can be classified as Hodgkin's, which make up less than 10% of the lymphoid neoplasm and non-Hodgkin's lymphoma.[135] Hodgkin's lymphoma, characterized by an owl eye–like inclusion in the nucleus referred to as Reed Sternberg cells on histology, usually has a predictable pattern of spread and predominantly involves lymphoid organs (lymph nodes, spleen, and liver), whereas non-Hodgkin's lymphoma (NHL) may involve extranodal tissues and can have widespread systemic involvement at presentation.

Classification of lymphoma has undergone numerous changes. The World Health Organization classification is the current accepted and widely used classification. B lymphomas, as the name implies, primarily arise from lymphocyte of B cell lineage and constitute more than 90% of NHL as compared to T-cell lymphomas.[135] B-cell and T-cell lymphoma subtypes are further subclassified based on the maturation level of the cells. Categories under mature B- and T-cell lymphomas include distinct morphologic, immunophenotypic, and clinical subtypes.[136]

EPIDEMIOLOGY

NHL is a disease that affects all age groups with almost 50% of incident cases occurring in those over 65 years of age. Age-adjusted incidence in those over 65 years of age for 2001–2005 was as high as 88.4/100,000 compared to 9.4/100,000 in those younger than 65 years. Diffuse B-cell lymphoma is the most common B-cell subtype in all ages including those above 75 years. Anaplastic large cell lymphoma, lymphoblastic cell, and Burkitt's lymphoma are less frequently encountered in the elderly.[125] White males have the greatest incidence of all lymphomas with the exception of peripheral T-cell lymphoma and mycosis fungoides, which are more common in African Americans. Asians have the lowest incidence of lymphoma.[135] There is an equal distribution of lymphoma subtypes between sexes, although a lower incidence of follicular lymphoma and higher incidence of mycosis fungoides lymphomas have been observed among black females.[135] A decreasing trend in the incidence of lymphomas has been seen in younger but not older age groups. The incidence of mantle cell and Burkett's lymphoma has increased in those over 75 years of age.[135] The reason for these trends in the elderly, particularly among certain NHL subtypes, is not known, although age-related changes in immune function may be contributing.

ETIOLOGY

Environmental, infectious, genetic factors, and certain diseases are all known to play a role in the genesis of NHL, mostly by altering or activating immune processes.[137] Immunodeficiency is associated with a greatly increased risk of NHL. It is estimated that human immunodeficiency virus (HIV) patients have an almost 100-fold increased risk for NHL. An increase in NHL has also been reported in association with transplantation, rheumatoid arthritis, Sjögren's syndrome, and systemic lupus erythematosus, especially for diffuse follicular lymphoma and marginal cell lymphomas. NHL has been associated with the use of pesticides, especially in those with t(14;18) subtype, and with use of permanent dark hair dyes in women.[138] Obesity and a diet high in animal fat and protein are also known to increase the risk of NHL.[139] Hepatitis C, Epstein-Barr virus, *Heliobacter pylori*, *Campylobacter jejuni*, and *Plasmodium falciparum* are all known to be associated with specific subtypes of lymphoma.[140] Chromosomal translocations, for example, t(14;18) involving the *bcl-2* proto-oncogene in 85% to 90% of follicular lymphoma[141] and the t(8;14) and other translocations involving the c-*myc* proto-oncogene in 100% of Burkett's lymphoma, can promote lymphoma development.

DIAGNOSIS AND WORKUP

The diagnosis hinges on a tissue diagnosis, usually obtained by lymph node biopsy. A comprehensive evaluation starts with a complete physical examination to document all involved areas as well as pattern of spread. Further diagnostic procedures include imaging studies to determine occult areas of involvement. These would include computed tomography, magnetic resonance imaging, and positron emission tomography (PET), either alone or in combination. Bone marrow biopsy is often recommended to rule out extranodal involvement.

CLINICAL FEATURES, PROGNOSIS, AND MANAGEMENT

AGGRESSIVE LYMPHOMAS. Diffuse large B-cell lymphoma (DLBCL) is the most common lymphoma subtype seen in the elderly.[142] Although characterized by an aggressive course without treatment, DLBCL has a high chance of cure with therapy. DLBCL may present as localized disease, but this is very unusual. More commonly, the disease manifests in an advanced stage and with extranodal involvement (e.g., the gastrointestinal tract or bone marrow).[143] Patients may also present with severe systemic systems and sometimes with rapidly progressive organ failure. Immunophenotyping reveals subtypes based on their derivation from germinal center or activated B cells. *bcl-2*, *bcl-6*, *p53*, CD10, and *mum1* expression also may recognize distinct clinical types of diseases with different presentation and prognosis. Cytogenetic analysis reveals a deletion of 18q as the most frequent abnormality (20% of cases) as well as a number of other nonrandom alterations. Mantle cell lymphoma—identified by the presence of B-cell markers (CD19, CD20, and CD22), the T-cell marker CD5, and the lack of CD23 and CD10[144] antigens—is an aggressive type of lymphoma that presents in more than 75% of the cases at an advanced stage.[143] It is a disease of elderly males with a median age at presentation of 68 years and a 2:1 male-to-female ratio.[143] Despite intensive treatment, the 5-year survival is less than 40%. Lymphadenopathy and bone marrow involvement are common, and splenomegaly is present in more than 60% at diagnosis. Leukemic expression (peripheral blood involvement) is also common in mantle cell lymphoma. Cytogenetic analysis typically reveals t (11;14)(q13;q32) in more than 85% of patients involving the *bcl-1* oncogene and the overexpression of cyclin D1.[144]

The International Prognostic Index (IPI), which risk-stratifies patients based on age, tumor stage, LDH level, number of extranodal sites, and performance status, is useful in determining treatment.[145]

TREATMENT

Although many studies have shown no definite age difference in clinical presentation,[125] treatment of lymphomas in the elderly is associated with significant bias, which may account for some of the observed poorer outcomes.[142,146] More than 60% of elderly lymphoma patients have at least one comorbidity,[125] and physiologic changes in the key organ reserve may render an older patient more vulnerable to chemotherapy toxicity. As mentioned earlier, a careful comprehensive assessment of comorbidities, functional status, and social factors are likely to improve outcomes.

Randomized studies have shown that the standard regimen of cyclophosphamide, doxorubicin, vincristine, and prednisone (CHOP) is safe, well tolerated, and comparably effective in young and old patients.[147] However, complete response is still seen in only 40% of elderly patients. The introduction of rituximab, a monoclonal antibody to the lymphocyte cell surface antigen CD20, has greatly improved response rates and survival for patients of all ages with NHL. In previously untreated 60- to 80-year-old patients with DLBCL, Rituximab-CHOP (R-CHOP) resulted in a 76% complete remission rates with relapse-free survival of 70% at 2 years—a considerable improvement from CHOP alone and without any increase in toxicity.[148] Thus, R-CHOP is currently the standard of care for elderly patients with DLBCL. The use of Granulocyte-Colony Stimulating Factor (G-CSF) has also been recommended in the elderly if neutropenia is the only limiting factor to treat patients with CHOP regimens.[149] Standard treatment for mantle cell lymphoma, such as R-CHOP, results in better remission rates and time to treatment failure but does not significantly improve survival, and for this histology, more aggressive treatment might be required.[150] In the elderly, hyper-fractionated cyclophosphamide, vincristine, doxorubicin, dexamethasone (hyper-CVAD) regimens alternating with high-dose methotrexate and cytarabine have shown response rates as high as 90%.[151] Yet when rituximab was added to this regimen, a high rate of toxicity and shorter failure-free survival was seen in those over 65 years of age (50% vs. 73%).[151] However, rituximab used alone for 2 years as maintenance therapy after a modified hyper-CVAD regimen without methotrexate and cytarabine showed a complete remission rate of 64% with acceptable toxicity and has been recommended in patients over 65 years of age.[152] Rituximab in combination with fludarabine, cyclophosphamide, and mitoxantrone in relapsed patients is associated with improved survival in relapsed or recurrent mantle cell lymphoma as compared to standard chemotherapy.[153]

INDOLENT LYMPHOMAS. Follicular lymphoma (FL) accounts for 20% of lymphomas in the elderly population. Small painless lymphadenopathy without other symptoms may be the most common presentation.[154] Bone marrow involvement may be present in up to 60% of patients but usually does not signify poor prognosis unless infiltration is extensive and associated with peripheral cytopenias.[143] Sometimes fever and weight loss may be present with lymphadenopathy and warrant immediate investigation. Translocation t(14;18) juxtaposing the *bcl-2* oncogene with the Ig heavy chain promoter may be detected in more than 90% of follicular lymphomas.[155] Follicular lymphomas are graded from I to III based on the number of large cells in the malignant nodules. Initially, grade III FL was thought to be associated with worse clinical outcomes, but subsequent studies have shown this not to be the case.[156] Historically, FL has been considered an indolent lymphoma with a median survival of 8 to 10 years but generally not curable with standard chemotherapy. The follicular lymphoma International Prognostic Index (FLIPI) was established, which is a modification of the IPI[157]; five adverse prognostic factors were selected: age >60 years, advanced stage, hemoglobin level (<120 g/L), number of nodal areas (more than four vs. four or fewer), and serum LDH level (above normal vs. normal or below). Three risk groups were defined: low risk (zero to one adverse factor), intermediate risk (two factors), and poor risk (three or more adverse factors), and this system effectively predicts prognosis. Transformation to an aggressive type of lymphoma may occur, especially in those with high-risk FLIPI, and portends poor prognosis.[157,158]

In older patients where maintaining quality of life is an important end point, treatment is commonly deferred unless symptoms or signs of progressive disease develop. Under carefully monitored circumstances, this delay in treatment initiation has been shown to not significantly influence survival.[159] The decision to start radiotherapy, a potentially curative treatment in early stage disease, is highly individualized, and age >60 years is found to be an adverse factor with regard to the effectiveness of localized approaches such as these.[160] No standard chemotherapy regimens are currently available for treatment of FL. Rituximab-based therapy combined with traditional chemotherapy regimens including CHOP[161] and fludarabine[162] have shown durable response rates as high as 90%.[163] For elderly patients with comorbidities or functional impairment, rituximab as a single agent is both well tolerated and an effective treatment.[164]

Marginal cell lymphoma includes three categories: mucosa-associated lymphoid tissue (MALT) lymphoma (typically located in the gastrointestinal tract), splenic marginal zone lymphoma (SZL), and nodal zone lymphoma (NZL).[165] Gastrointestinal MALT is the most common extranodal presentation of MALT lymphoma, and the stomach is the most common organ involved.[166] Pathogenesis is mainly related to the presence of infection with *Helicobacter pylori*,[167] which is seen in almost all cases and investigations to identify this organism is mandatory in MALT lymphomas.[168] Other commonly involved regions include salivary gland, ocular adnexa, lung, skin, and Waldeyer's ring.[166] Patients with gastric MALT typically present with symptoms of dyspepsia or abdominal pain, and upper endoscopy and biopsy will reveal a tumor with the characteristic histology.[168] Although prognosis of low-grade MALT (86%, 5-year survival) is excellent,[169] those who present with advanced disease and poor IPI scores do not fare well. Eradication of *H. pylori* with antibiotics has been very effective in treatment of localized gastric MALT and is the standard treatment when *H. pylori* is identified. Initial treatment in those who have *H. pylori* negative disease or t(11;18) translocation (associated with resistance to *H. pylori* treatment),[170] radiotherapy, or rituximab is usually employed.[171] Treatment of MALT in other sites involves locoregional radiotherapy or surgery, although individualized treatment taking into consideration the patient's functional status and preferences is the preferred approach. Splenic marginal zone lymphoma and nodal zone lymphoma are primarily seen in women. An association with hepatitis C infection is seen in some SZL and NZL. The spleen is commonly involved in SZL as is the bone marrow.[172] M-protein (paraprotein) and immunologic abnormalities may be seen in a high percentage of patients and are associated with a poor prognosis.[173] As with indolent lymphomas, asymptomatic or elderly patients may be frequently followed for development of symptoms or progression to aggressive lymphoma. Hepatitis C patients may be successfully treated with appropriate therapy,[166] but splenectomy is the preferred treatment for hepatitis C–negative patients.[173] Nodal zone lymphoma primarily presents with extensive peripheral and central lymphadenopathy. Survival is lower than the other NZLs and treatment is not defined, but rituximab-based therapies have been used with varying success.[166]

Waldenström macroglobulinemia (WM) (lymphoplasmacytic lymphoma) is a low-grade lymphoma identified by IgM monoclonal protein in serum and presence of characteristic intertrabecular infiltration of bone marrow with plasmacytoid lymphocytes. Immunophenotyping reveals surface IgM+, CD10–, CD19+, CD20+, CD22+, CD23–, CD25+, CD27+, FMC7+, CD103–, and CD138 cells.[174] The median age of diagnosis is 63 years, and the disease occurs more commonly in the white population. Symptoms in WM are primarily related to direct tumor infiltration or with the effects of IgM protein. Infiltration can occur within any organ causing hepatomegaly, splenomegaly, and lymphadenopathy, and the bone marrow is almost always involved.[175] Hypercalcemia secondary to lytic bone lesions may be seen. Hyperviscosity due to presence of pentameric IgM molecules can give rise to headaches, ocular symptoms epistaxis and even altered consciousness.[175] Primary amyloidosis can occur in WM and typically involves the heart and peripheral nerves leading to cardiac failure and severe peripheral neuropathy. The lung may also be involved. Cardiomyopathy is more common in the elderly and is a primary cause of death in WM.[176] Renal dysfunction can be related to glomerulonephritis secondary to tissue infiltration with tumor, cryoglobulin deposition, or the result of IgM antibody against glomerular basement membrane. Cold agglutinin disease resulting from IgM antibody directed at the red cell antigens can lead to chronic immune hemolytic anemia. Cytopenias may also occur because of bone marrow infiltration of the tumor. Twenty percent of patients may have no symptoms at diagnosis.

Asymptomatic WM patients usually do not require treatment and may be followed by observation alone.[177] A close watch, especially to monitor symptoms of hyperviscosity, is imperative, especially in those with serum monoclonal levels greater than 5 g/L.[178] Measurement of serum viscosity is usually not helpful although symptoms rarely occur at levels less than 4 cp. Plasmapheresis is the treatment of choice in reducing hyperviscosity in these patients.[179] Treatment is usually recommended for symptomatic patients and those with a hemoglobin level less than 10g/dL and platelet count less than 100×10^9/L.[177] Median survival is about 5 to 10 years in WM[178] and older age; high serum β2 microglobulin, poor performance status, and cytopenias predict a poor prognosis.[180] Especially in older people, survival may be affected by concomitant comorbidities, as only 50% of deaths in WM patients have been attributable to the disease. Options when cytoreductive treatment is required include single-agent therapy with chlorambucil, fludarabine, or rituximab with reported median response duration as high as 60 months[181] and combination therapy with CHOP and cyclophosphamide and prednisone (CP),[181] although their specific activity in people over 65 years is not known.

T-CELL LYMPHOMAS. Peripheral T-cell lymphoma and angioimmunoblastic lymphoma (AIBL) are the two most common T-cell lymphomas encountered in the elderly. Derived from post-thymic lymphocytes, they can identify by expression of T-cell receptor αβ or γδ chains and CD3+, CD4+, or CD8+ cells. Median age of presentation is generally greater than 60 years with a male preponderance. Clinically they present in advanced stages with higher rate of "B" symptoms, worse performance scores and a higher IPI.[182] Involvement of the skin is common in peripheral T-cell lymphoma

(PTCL), and allergic manifestations and symptoms related to proteinuria are typically seen in AIBL as well as a high seropositivity for Epstein-Barr virus.[183] Molecular cytogenetics reveal a high rate of chromosomal abnormalities and T-cell receptor (TCR) clonality in β or γ genes. Peripheral T-cell lymphoma and AIBL generally have a poor prognosis when compared with B-cell lymphomas.[184] IPI is useful in predicting prognosis, with survival less than 1.5 years in the high-risk group and longer than 10 years in the low-risk group,[185] although other molecular findings like *p53* expression[186] have also been shown to correlate with poor survival. Treatment with six to eight cycles of standard CHOP or more aggressive regimens for patients with AIBL are all reasonable approaches but should be individualized based on acceptable toxicity and a goal to maintain quality of life in the elderly.

HODGKIN'S LYMPHOMA

Hodgkin's lymphoma (HL) constitutes about 8%[135] of total lymphomas in the population. Incidence of HL at 2.5% is relatively low and typically demonstrates a bimodal pattern of distribution with highest rates seen between 20 to 30 years of age (4.3%) and between 70 to 84 years of age (4.4%). In the younger age groups, HL is more often diagnosed in females than males, whereas the reverse is true in the elderly.

The characteristic feature of HL is the presence of lymphadenopathy, which develops in a contiguous fashion, and the presence or absence of systemic symptoms, which provide useful prognostic information. Of the histologic variants of HL, the nodular sclerosing variety is most common, but the mixed cellularity type appears more frequently in older patients than in younger patients. Elderly patients with Hodgkin's present in more advanced stages and with more constitutional ("B") symptoms (fever, weight loss, night sweats) but with less bulky disease than younger patients.[187] Accurate staging is imperative such that curative therapy can be effectively prescribed. Positron emission tomography/computed tomography (PET/CT) has become an excellent method to assist in staging.

Traditionally, stage I and II in the absence of B symptoms have been considered to have a good outcomes. Additional prognostic factors have come to light in both early stage and advanced disease, which further define survival and necessitate treatment modification. In early stage disease, bulky disease (mediastinal mass on chest x-ray greater than one third of the intrathoracic diameter, or mass greater than 35% of the thoracic diameter at T5-6, or any other mass greater than 10 cm) identifies a subset of patients with less favorable disease especially associated with resistance to radiation. The international prognostic score,[188] which awards one point each for albumin <4 g/dL, hemoglobin <10.5 g/dL, male, age >45 years, stage IV disease, leukocytosis (white blood cell count at least 15,000/mm^3), lymphocytopenia (lymphocyte count less than 8% of white blood cell count or lymphocyte count less than 600/mm^3), can predict freedom from disease progression (FFP) and overall survival and has proven a useful adjunct to staging in assessing the type of therapy to be undertaken. Those who had none of the above had 84% rate of FFP compared to 42% for the presence of five or more.

A treatment of doxorubicin, bleomycin, vinblastine, and dacarbazine (ABVD) has become the standard of care for HL. In early stage disease, four to six cycles are administered depending on the presence of bulky disease. In the presence of favorable factors, two cycles may be sufficient. Involved field radiation after completion of chemotherapy and complete response may reduce relapse rate in these patients,[189] but the long-term risk of second malignancy is of concern for younger patients. Reports have been inconsistent regarding outcomes of elderly patients following chemotherapy. Doxorubicin-based regimens and involved field radiation have been shown to be equally effective in the elderly[190] who have been selected appropriately. Nonetheless, treatment regimens should be chosen with an eye on potential toxicity in older patients. A retrospective analysis of elderly patients from the German Hodgkin's group[191] showed that with the exception of minor reactions like nausea and pain, frequency of adverse effects were greater in elderly (>60 years) than younger patients. This excessive toxicity resulted in a reduction of the treatment dose and number of cycles, and early termination of treatment. As a result, lower response rates and overall survival were observed. Although Hodgkin's disease was still the most common cause of death in the elderly and younger patients, mortality resulting from treatment-related toxicity and second malignancies was more common in older patients. Appropriate assessment in the elderly to individualize treatment programs based on a comprehensive pretreatment evaluation may minimize toxicity, treatment reductions, and less favorable outcomes. Currently, elderly Hodgkin's lymphoma patients are more likely to experience treatment-related cardiovascular disease, second malignancy, and death.[192,193] Age-appropriate cancer screening, annual chest imaging, thyroid function tests, and tests to detect cardiovascular risk factors are essential in all treated patients to identify and prevent late toxicities associated with therapy for HL.

Chronic lymphocytic leukemia

Chronic lymphocytic leukemia (CLL)/small lymphocytic leukemia is a disorder classified as a mature (peripheral) B cell neoplasm according to the WHO classification.[194] There are almost no reported cases under the age of 30 years and only about 10% of the cases occur in those below 55 years of age. Although not significant, there has been a trend toward a slight decrease in the incidence rates of CLL, including in those aged 75 years and above.[135] It is a disease predominantly seen in the white population occurring slightly more frequently in males and the incidence is very low among Asians and Pacific Islanders.[135] An increased risk of CLL has been observed in patients with pernicious anemia,[195] chronic sinusitis, recurrent pneumonia, and herpes simplex and zoster viral infections.[196,197] Interestingly, there is a decreased incidence of CLL in patients with chronic rheumatic as well as nonrheumatic valvular heart disease. Population and family studies have highlighted the importance of genetic factors in the etiology of B-cell CLL (B-CLL). The relative risk of CLL in first-degree family members can be eightfold higher than in controls.[198,199] Some have suggested the risk increases with the degree of relationship between the affected member and the family members,[198] and it is apparent that the age at onset of disease occurs earlier in successive generations—a phenomenon termed *anticipation*.[200]

CLINICAL FEATURES AND DIAGNOSIS

A rapid proliferation in the use of automated meters to evaluate peripheral blood counts have caused an increase in diagnosis of asymptomatic individuals with elevated lymphocyte counts and those in early stage CLL.[201,202] The median age of patients diagnosed in early stage also is increasing. Lymphadenopathy is the most common feature in symptomatic patients, and the lymph nodes are usually painless and mobile on examination.[203] Inguinal lymphadenopathy is uncommon. Nonspecific symptoms such as malaise, fatigue, and weight loss also predominate in symptomatic CLL patients. Other findings include anemia, hepatomegaly, and splenomegaly.[204] Bruising secondary to thrombocytopenia may also occur in these patients. Cytopenia seen in CLL may result from bone marrow failure (more common) or secondary to autoimmune disease.[205] Clinical features are similar in younger and older patients,[206] except that younger patients (<50 years) usually present with a higher hemoglobin level.[207] Autoimmune hemolytic anemia can occur in CLL as a presenting feature or during the course of the disease with a prevalence of approximately 4%. Older males appear to have a higher rate of autoimmune hemolytic anemia.[208] Treatment with steroids for this condition is frequently successful[208] but can significantly increase the morbidity and mortality if prolonged treatment is required by elderly patients. Other autoimmune disorders like immune thrombocytopenic purpura and pure red cell aplasia occur but are uncommon. Infections secondary to hypogammaglobulinemia may precede the diagnosis of CLL but more commonly occur during the course of the disease especially following CLL treatment. Although bacterial infections with encapsulated organisms are the most common, fungal and viral infections are also fairly frequent.[209] Transformation to diffuse B-cell lymphoma (Richter's) also occurs in CLL patients with a 10-year incidence of 16.5%,[210] and older people appear to be at an increased risk.[211] This can occur even in early stage disease and is heralded by the development of systemic symptoms and rapidly growing lymphadenopathy.

CLL cells contain either unmutated or mutated immunoglobin heavy chain variable (IGHV) genes. ZAP-(zeta chain associated protein) 70 is a 70 kDa intracellular tyrosine kinase involved in T-cell receptor signaling.[212] By gene expression analyses, it was discovered that CLL cells with unmutated IGHV differed from CLL cells with mutated IGHV in the expression levels of a small subset of genes, one of which encodes ZAP-70. It has been established that patients with CLL cells that have unmutated IGHV have more aggressive disease, and that measurement of ZAP-70 may be used as a surrogate marker for the expression of unmutated IGHV.[213] Furthermore, the expression of the cell surface marker CD38 on CLL cells also defines those with more aggressive disease,[214] but the two markers (ZAP-70 and CD38) do not always coincide.[215] Using both markers, clinicians are now better prepared to determine which patients at presentation are likely to be best served by aggressive treatment (those positive for ZAP-70 or CD38) and those for whom specific therapy can be delayed.

DIAGNOSIS AND MANAGEMENT

The international working group recently updated CLL guidelines[216] for diagnosis and management. CLL is usually diagnosed by the presence of lymphocytosis in the peripheral blood $>5 \times 10^9/L$ present at least for 3 months, with <55% of atypical cells (prolymphocytes or lymphoblasts). Flow cytometry is essential in the diagnosis of CLL and reveals the characteristic immunophenotype with CD5+, CD23+, FMC7−, weak expression of surface Ig (sIg), and weak or absent expression of membrane CD22 and CD79b.[217] Bone marrow usually has ≥30% lymphocytes, although bone marrow examination is not required for diagnosis.

Clinical staging using Rai[218] or Binet[219,220] classification is used both to provide prognosis and guide therapy. It is well known that CLL is a heterogeneous disease with survival for some only 2 years and for others, 2 decades. However, it is also appreciated that more than 30% of the patients show progression from an early to more advanced stages within 3 years of diagnosis.[221] Numerous prognostic indicators have been identified that can detect these individuals at high risk of progression and that also correlate with survival.

Features associated with poor prognosis include older age,[222] absolute lymphocyte count $> 50 \times 10^9/L$, diffuse bone marrow involvement, low platelet count, lymphadenopathy, low hemoglobin, and the presence of fever.[223,224] A diagnosis of CLL has significant effects on psychological quality of life (more so in the elderly), and this aspect should be considered in decision making.[225]

Currently the guidelines do not recommend treatment for early asymptomatic disease (Stage 0 Rai and Stage A Binet),[216] as more than 50% of these patients are alive at 10 years, and treatment for indolent disease did not improve outcome. For all stages, more than 65% of patients >80 years old did not receive treatment at the time of initial diagnosis as compared to <45% in those less than 40 years. However, analysis of relative survival from the National Cancer Database[226] revealed that elderly patients do succumb to CLL more often than from existing comorbid diseases.

TREATMENT OF CLL

Treatment in the early and intermediate stages is offered only for those with CLL-attributable symptoms. Chlorambucil with or without prednisone was initially the drug of choice, but this has been largely replaced by fludarabine, either alone or in combination with cyclophosphamide or rituximab.[227] However, the incidence of autoimmune hemolytic anemias is increased in patients treated with fludarabine, and hematologic toxicity does appear to increase in those over 70 years of age. Pentostatin, cyclophosphamide, and rituximab has also been found to be effective treatment of CLL with no significant differences in overall response (83% vs. 93%) or complete response rate (39% vs. 41%) when older (70 years) were compared with younger patients (<70 years).[228] In patients with 17p deletion (associated with p53 mutations and poor prognosis), alemtuzumab, a humanized anti-CD52 monoclonal antibody, achieved objective response rates as high as 40%.[229] Curiously, older patients appeared to do better than younger patients, and currently this agent is recommended as frontline therapy for those over 70 years with 17p deletion or refractory CLL. There is an increased risk of infections with alemtuzumab, and appropriate prophylaxis should be administered. Reduced intensity allogeneic stem cell transplantation may be considered for younger patients (<65 years) with good performance status after first remission or refractory disease, but supportive care and observation may be best for older patients in that setting.

ACUTE MYELOGENOUS LEUKEMIA

Acute myelogenous leukemia (AML) is primarily a disease of the elderly. The median age at diagnosis is 67 years and according to the National Cancer Institute's Surveillance,

Epidemiology and End Results (SEER) registry, the age-adjusted incidence rates for people aged 65 years and older is 16.4/100,000 as compared to 1.7/100,000 for those under 65 years.[230] Furthermore, there is a progressive increase in the incidence of AML with age up to 85 years with the highest incidence and mortality in those 74 to 85 years old. Although in the earlier years incidence of AML has shown to increase with each year, the annual percentage change in the age groups 65 to 74 years and >75 years has shown a significant downward trend for the years 2001–2005. However, the mortality rates continue to increase in those over 75 years. There is a slight gender difference, with males being more affected, and this difference becomes more pronounced with age.

AML diagnosis is made by the demonstration by a minimum of 20% myeloblasts in a bone marrow sample. Environmental, genetic, and iatrogenic factors have been implicated in its etiology.[231] AML may arise *de novo* or, as commonly the case with older patients, as a progression of MDS or after treatment for a primary malignancy (secondary, or treatment-related AML).[232] In people over 60 years of age, cigarette smoking (number of cigarettes and duration of smoking) is associated with an increased risk, particularly of the M2 subtype of FAB AML classification.[233] A higher carrier rate of Human T-cell lymphotropic virus-1 (HTLV-1) type virus has been observed in patients with acute promyelocytic (FAB M3) leukemia.[234]

As with most of the hematologic malignancies, classification schemes have recently been revised in consideration of new molecular and genetic understandings of disease pathogenesis. Thus, the classic French American British (FAB) system has been replaced by the WHO classification of acute leukemia (Table 93-7).

Clinical features in AML are related to uncontrolled proliferation of leukemic blasts in the bone marrow and infiltration into body tissues. Anemia and thrombocytopenia are frequently seen. CNS infiltration, which is more often seen in those with initial white blood counts >100,000/mm³ and in those with monocytic leukemia, may manifest as meningeal involvement, bleeding, or as distinct mass (chloromas). Lumbar puncture should be considered in patients with neurologic features if imaging studies do not reveal pathology. Chloromas may also present as a space-occupying mass when present on the spine. In the elderly, more subtle symptoms like weakness, fatigue, or generalized malaise may be initial presenting features. Acute promyelocytic leukemia may manifest with disseminated intravascular coagulation (DIC) and bleeding manifestations. Elderly patients with AML typically present with a worse performance status and a greater percentage of complex and high-risk karyotypic abnormalities but lower numbers of peripheral and bone marrow blasts.[235] Cytogenetic evaluation and immunophenotyping are absolutely essential in the initial workup of leukemia to classify subtypes and determine prognosis.[236] Although age itself is a poor prognostic factor in AML, the demonstration of high-risk karyotypes or immunophenotypes might portend an even greater risk of standard therapy failure.[237]

Table 93-7. WHO and FAB AML Classifications

WHO		FAB
I	AMLwith recurrent genetic abnormalities	
	t(8;21)(q22;q22);(AML1/ETO	
	inv(16)(p13;q22) or *t*(16;16)(p13;q22); (CBFβ/MYH11)	
	t(15;17)(q22;q12)(PML/RARα)	
	11q23(MLL) abnormalities	
II	AML and MDS, therapy related	
	Alkylating agent related	
	Topoisomerase type II inhibitor related	
III	AML with multilineage dysplasia	
	Following MDS	
	Without antecedent MDS	
IV	AML not otherwise categorized	
	AML without maturation	M1
	AML, minimally differentiated	M2
	AML with maturation	M3
	Acute monocytic leukemia	M4
	Acute myelomonocytic leukemia (AMMoL)	M5
	Acute monoblastic leukemia AMMoL with eosinophilia	M5e
	Acute erythroid leukemia	M6
	Acute megakaryoblastic leukemia	M7
V	Acute leukemia of ambiguous lineage	

Acute promyelocytic leukemia (FAB M3) is usually associated with favorable cytogenetic alterations and is also effectively treated by the use of all-trans retinoic acid and daunorubicin or arsenic trioxide.[238] Studies have shown that standard induction therapy is associated with better outcomes in those over 60 years with low-risk features compared to best supportive care.[239] Although the rate of hospitalization is greater in these patients, treatment is often quite gratifying with a return to a baseline level of functioning after discharge. For those younger than 75 years with good performance status and favorable cytogenetics,[240] cytosine arabinoside combined with an anthracycline followed by consolidation therapy is still considered the standard of care. Reduced intensity conditioning regimens followed by stem cell transplantation can be effective curative therapy for older patients with excellent performance status once in remission. However, this approach is still considered investigational and should be performed in the setting of a clinical trial. New treatment approaches may also be relevant for older patients. For example, treatment with gemtuzumab, an ozogamicin calicheamicin conjugated to monoclonal antibody specific for the CD33 receptor, was associated with improved median survival in older patients with relapsed disease.[241] For patients with significant comorbidities or over the age of 75 years and with unfavorable cytogenetics or other high-risk factors, the standard induction therapy (cytosine arabinoside and an anthracycline, such as daunorubicin) often results in poor outcomes, and these patients may best be managed by low-intensity therapy or supportive care. However, involvement of the patient in decision making and consideration of available psychosocial support are important in all decisions regarding AML management. Support with granulocyte colony-stimulating factor (G-CSF) after chemotherapy may be considered in older patients, as it has been shown to improve remission rates and reduce hospitalizations.[242]

The elderly are susceptible to tumor lysis syndrome, which should be considered in all patients, particularly those who present with very high white counts. Also, the elderly are particularly susceptible to the cerebellar toxicity of certain drugs, most notably cytosine arabinoside. When this drug is used in higher doses, such as during remission consolidation, careful neurologic checks should be performed before each dose of drug.

DISORDERS OF HEMOSTASIS

Hemostasis is maintained by intricate and complex interactions involving vascular, platelet, and coagulation components. With advancing age, alterations in function of at least one of these components is likely, and there is a tendency for either bleeding or clotting to result. This may be a consequence of aging, but it is equally likely to be associated with use of one or many prescription drugs that can influence coagulation or platelet function. However, as a general rule, coagulation defects in elderly people may be treated just as they are in other age groups.

Senile purpura

Senile purpura occurs mainly on the extensor surfaces of the forearms and hands and may be seen in many otherwise normal older people. Loss of subcutaneous fat and changes in aging connective tissue permit undue mobility of older skin, and shearing forces result in rupture of small vessels. Platelets are typically normal both qualitatively and quantitatively in patients with senile purpura, and no correlation has been shown with ascorbic acid deficiency.

Purpura resulting from platelet defects

Thrombocytopenia may occur as a primary (idiopathic) disorder or a secondary phenomenon (drug-induced or associated with other blood diseases, infections, neoplasia, or various other conditions). Occasionally thrombocythemia, thrombasthenia, or combined defects may be present.

AUTOIMMUNE (IDIOPATHIC) THROMBOCYTOPENIC PURPURA

Autoimmune (idiopathic) thrombocytopenic purpura (ITP) is usually secondary to IgG auto antibodies against platelets that sensitizes the platelets for destruction[243] and has a higher incidence in the elderly as compared to the younger population.[244] Antibody to platelet antigens may be observed in a number of medical conditions including in the setting of systemic lupus erythematosus, HIV, immunodeficiency disorders, or B-cell lymphoproliferative syndromes (e.g., CLL). In older people, the onset is usually insidious and is not clearly related to another illness. More than two thirds may present with signs of mucosal or visceral bleed (e.g., hematuria). The course is usually chronic and intermittent. An association of chronic ITP with current or past infection with *H. pylori* infection suggests an association that might be very relevant in older patients.[245]

Few platelets are seen in the peripheral blood smear, and those present are large ("megathrombocytes"). The bone marrow typically reveals an increase in megakaryocytes. There is usually no splenomegaly. Diagnosis is primarily clinical; testing for the presence of antibodies on platelet surfaces is, however, associated with many false positive results, and the assay has not proven of great value under most circumstances.[246] Treatment is usually initiated if bleeding occurs or prophylactically in the setting of a very low platelet count (usually less than 10,000/μL) or before surgery. Therapy usually involves corticosteroids (prednisone 1 to 2 mg/kg per day), which results in improvement in about 80%, but sometimes only after 2 or more weeks of treatment.[247] Other approved treatment options include intravenous immunoglobin and danazol. Anti-CD20 antibody (rituximab)[248] and the new thrombopoietin (TPO) receptor agonist eltrombopag[249] are currently being evaluated. Splenectomy is usually considered only for refractory cases but provides excellent cure rates with complete remission in more than 60% of the cases.[250]

Secondary thrombocytopenia

Drugs are an important cause of thrombocytopenia. They may be direct marrow toxins or cause idiosyncratic, hypersensitivity reactions or immune-mediated platelet destruction. Some drugs are known to cause selective thrombocytopenia only by decreasing megakaryocytes. Commonly used drugs associated with thrombocytopenia include sulfonamides, penicillin, tetracycline, desipramine, chlorothiazide, digitoxin, insulin, cimetidine, and myelosuppressive drugs used as chemotherapeutic agents.[251] Secondary thrombocytopenia is seen with acute and chronic leukemia, lymphoma, infection, myelodysplastic syndromes and myeloproliferative disorders, chemotherapy treatment, collagen vascular diseases, splenomegaly, paraproteinemia, cirrhosis of the liver, and hypersensitivity reactions.

Heparin-induced thrombocytopenia results from antibodies against heparin, which bind to and activate platelet Fc receptors.[252] Patients are at risk of severe bleeding from the thrombocytopenia, as well as arterial thrombosis, and one or the other can be lethal. Management includes immediate discontinuation all heparin-related products including low-molecular weight heparin and warfarin and use of alternative antithrombotics like argatroban and hirudin before restarting warfarin.[252] Although the incidence of this complication is low, the widespread use of heparin in clinical practice makes it a familiar problem.

Thrombotic thrombocytopenic purpura

Thrombotic thrombocytopenia purpura (TTP) is a disseminated thrombotic microangiopathy that can be triggered by infection, drugs (e.g., clopidogrel), autoimmune disease, or without a known risk factor. The syndrome is due to deficiency of the ADAMTS-13 protein. ADAMTS-13 is a protease discovered in normal plasma that cleaves von Willebrand factor and prevents platelet aggregation and clot formation.[253] TTP has a rapid onset, with widespread manifestations appearing over the course of 1 or 2 days. In the classic case, fever, thrombocytopenia with bleeding, microvascular hemolytic anemia, acute renal failure, and CNS disturbances are seen. Elevated LDH, bilirubin, and low haptoglobin are often present, and schistocytes or fragmented red blood cells may be seen on the peripheral blood smear. Other clotting studies are usually normal, fibrinogen levels are normal or increased, and split products are usually absent.

TTP is usually treated by large-volume plasma exchanges. Cryodepleted (vWF poor) plasma can be used in combination with steroids. This form of therapy has decreased the mortality rate of TTP from 90% to less than 50%. In patients with TTP who do not respond to plasma exchange, a combination of steroids, antiplatelet agents, and emergency splenectomy has been used with some success.

Coagulation defects in the elderly

Survival with congenital coagulation disorders in later life is possible, especially in von Willebrand's disease. Acquired disorders include vitamin K deficiency, which leads to a reduction in prothrombin (factor II) and in factors VII, IX, and X. This condition may occur in malabsorption syndromes, liver disease, prolonged obstructive jaundice, and biliary fistula and with oral broad-spectrum antibiotic therapy. Renal failure, extracorporeal circuits, and acquired inhibitors may result in significant blood coagulation defects.

Anticoagulant therapy with warfarin reduces hepatic synthesis of the same four factors. Although warfarin has been associated with increased risk of hemorrhagic complications, particularly intracranial hemorrhage,[254] maintaining INR values between 2.0 to 3.0 remains appropriate in the elderly[254] to derive adequate benefit. Levels of D-dimer, fibrinogen, factor VIII, and thrombin are known to increase with age and may explain the high incidence of vascular disorders in the elderly. These have also been shown to predict adverse outcomes including hospitalization, mortality, and poor functional outcomes.

Disseminated intravascular coagulation

A syndrome of diffuse intravascular coagulation (DIC) may be seen in elderly people in an acute, subacute, or chronic form. There is typically a serious underlying disease process leading to thromboplastic substances entering the circulation or directly injuring endothelial cells. Liver disease, acute pancreatitis, incompatible transfusions, cancer, and nonbacterial thrombotic endocarditis have also been associated with the occurrence of DIC.[255] DIC may also complicate the clinical course in acute promyelocytic leukemia in the elderly. Criteria for diagnosis are not well defined; the most useful are a low platelet count, prolonged prothrombin time, positive plasma protamine test for fibrin, monomer–fibrinogen complexes, D dimers, and levels of fibrinogen and fibrin degradation products related to the clinical condition. Primary treatment should include control of underlying disease.

Therapy may include restoration of depleted blood components with platelet and fresh frozen plasma infusions in bleeding patients. The use of heparin in the treatment of DIC remains controversial. Most studies have found heparin to be of little or no value and may, in fact, result in exaggerated thrombocytopenia or thrombosis. Even in complex situations such as promyelocytic leukemia, the routine use of heparin remains controversial.

ACKNOWLEDGMENT

This work was supported in full by the Intramural Research Program, National Institute on Aging, National Institutes of Health.

KEY POINTS

Blood Disorders in the Elderly

- Aging without disease is associated with minor changes in hematologic functions.
- Anemia in older persons is of clinical importance. It is important to find the cause and treat it when possible.
- Older patients with lymphoma, myeloma, chronic leukemia, or myelodysplasia can be effectively managed with standard or new agents, but a pretreatment comprehensive assessment is needed to tailor treatment and avoid toxicity.

For a complete list of references, please visit online only at www.expertconsult.com

CHAPTER 94

Geriatric Oncology

Margot A. Gosney

Cancer is a major cause of death and morbidity in elderly patients. Within England and Wales, there were 138,454 cancer deaths in 2005; of these, 51% (70647) were 75 years or older.[1] Although total U.K. death rates fell between 1999 and 2005, the total number of older people dying from cancer has increased. In the United States, cancer incidence rates increased from the mid-1970s through to 1992 and then decreased from 1992 to 1995, although since then the incidence rates have been essentially stable. The rates of breast cancer in women and prostate cancer in men have increased, but a compensatory fall in lung cancer in men has resulted in a stable total population.[2] As the incidence and prevalence of cancer increases, coupled with improved diagnostic certainty and life expectancy, many doctors will be faced with caring for elderly patients with cancer. It is estimated that over 5% of National Health Service (NHS) expenditure is used in cancer care, with elderly patients responsible for a large proportion of this expenditure. A European study found that Britain ranked 10th for men and 11th for women, when considering 5-year cancer survival. This is despite the fact that Britain spends more on cancer than other major European countries.

Although cancer was chosen as a key area in the "Health of the Nation"[3] document, elderly people were not specifically targeted, and in the Department of Health document, "A Policy Framework for Commissioning Cancer Services,"[4] which provides guidance for purchasers and providers of cancer services, there is no mention of involvement of geriatricians in the acute care or rehabilitation of elderly patients with cancer. The Cancer Reform Strategy launched on December 3, 2007, although setting a clear direction for development of cancer services in England over the following 5 years, does little to focus on the needs of older cancer patients.[5] The National Service Framework for older people and Living Well in Later Life (March 2006) do not highlight cancer as a particular problem in old age.[6,7]

The true impact of cancer in older people is unknown because of poor histologic verification; often the first registration of cancer is at death certification. In the United States, in an attempt to focus attention on geriatric oncology, the American Cancer Society, the American Society of Clinical Oncology, and other research groups have formed subgroups specifically to deal with the problem of geriatric oncology. In the Netherlands, age-specific cancer mortality rates have increased with increasing age for both males and females during 1991–1995,[8] and this may reflect better identification of cases, worse survival, or a combination of both.

It is clear from work by Grulich et al that there is a change in cancer mortality with age.[9] Between 1970 and 1990 for males and females aged 75 to 84, there was a 16% and 18% respective increase in cancer mortality. This is in contrast to males and females aged 45 to 54 who have had a 19% and 17% decrease in cancer mortality.

It should, however, be remembered that cancer mortality is influenced by a variety of factors that are closely associated with age. In the United States between 1980 and 1988, there was a large increase in breast cancer incidence as a result of an increase in uptake of mammography. However, despite this substantially higher incidence rate, particularly for women age 50 and older, the mortality rate fell as a result of improved treatment and early detection.[10]

CANCER AND AGING

There is no doubt that older people are more likely to develop cancer and differences in tumor growth and spread occur as a result of aging. The relationship between cancer and aging is complex, and various factors, including changes in host tumor defenses and exposure to carcinogens, have roles to play in the etiology of tumors. Although there are several distinct theories of cancer causation in older people, including decreased ability to repair DNA, oncogene activation or amplification, tumor suppressor gene loss, decreased immune surveillance, prolonged duration of carcinogenic exposure, or increased susceptibility of aged cells to carcinogens, no one theory has universal backing.[11]

There is debate as to whether carcinogenesis and aging are related phenomena. Many believe such a relationship exists,[12,13] with some postulating that cancer develops because of normal processes occurring during aging[14] and others favoring a common etiologic origin for both cancer and aging.[15] There is a relationship between chromosomal alterations and malignancy.[16] Several inherited disorders, featuring both chromosomal breakage and an increased frequency of malignant disease, show abnormalities of DNA repair or recombination,[17] and many genetically determined syndromes have both an accelerated progression of biologic aging and a high frequency of malignant disease.[18]

The increased incidence of cancer with age can be interpreted by the two major theories of aging.[11,19] The first, the damage or error theory, holds that over time there is an accumulation of damage to vital areas of cellular or organ function, which culminates in the manifestations of the aging process. Mutations may occur in certain key genes or in many individual genes on a random basis. The multistep model of carcinogenesis fits with this theory as successive cancer-causing mutations accumulate during the aging process.[20] The alternative or program theory considers aging as a latter stage of a program that proceeds through embryogenesis to growth development and maturation. During aging, certain genes become expressed and others are shut down.

In 1858, Virchow[21] stated that each tissue present in the body has a limited response to injury. Since then, further work has described how various tissues of the body respond to damage. Those tissues having continuously mitotic cells, such as the gut and marrow, develop tumors, whereas those with intermittently mitotic cells, such as endothelial or smooth muscle, develop degenerative diseases such as atherosclerosis, but only rarely malignant change. Nonmitotic cells such as the neurone virtually never develop tumors but are associated with disorders such as Alzheimer's or Parkinson's disease, illustrating that frequent cell turnover is required for tumor development.[22]

Alterations in DNA methylation in some genes is more common in older subjects and results in an increase in cancer.[23] The formation of DNA adducts in a variety of tissues is seen in chemical carcinogenesis,[24] and, in certain animal models, adduct-like compounds (L-compounds) accumulate with age.[25] These compounds do have the capability to carry mutations, DNA chain breaks, and gene rearrangements.[25] Further evidence for the role of altered DNA repair in cancer causation is provided by the increased susceptibility of cells from older persons to chromosomal damage by ^{3}H-thymidine and to the toxic consequences of irradiation.[26]

When comparing young and aged rats, the activity of DNA repair and metabolic activation enzymes was found to decline in the aged group, and the accumulation of spontaneous DNA damage may affect vital functions.[27]

In considering cancer in elderly people, the role of factors that increase life span (geroprotectors) and their effects on tumor development must be noted. Geroprotectors are of three types. First are those that decrease the mortality of a long-living subpopulation, are effective in inhibiting carcinogenesis, prolong tumor latency, and decrease the incidence of cancers (e.g., calorie-restricted diet). Second are those that increase the survival in a short-living subpopulation without a change in the maximum life span and may increase tumor incidence in an exposed population (e.g., tocopherol). Finally, there are geroprotectors that prolong the life span equally in all members of the population, postpone the beginning of population aging, and in general do not influence the incidence of tumors but do prolong tumor latency (e.g., β-mercaptoethylamine).[28]

A large body of literature describes the gradual alteration of immune function that occurs with advancing age and that may contribute to the increase in malignancy. Many of these changes occur with the onset of thymic involution, which begins at puberty and results in only 10% of thymic function remaining by the age of 45. Although the total population of T lymphocytes does not decline, the number of suppressor and killer cells decreases, the helper-suppressor ratio reverses, and there is an increase in the number of immature lymphocytes in the peripheral blood. Immune surveillance depends on the integrity of lymphocytes, and thymic function is critical for monitoring and disposing of cells that harbor replicative aggregations. Thymic hormones decline with age and have also been shown to be significantly lower in age-matched patients with malignant disease.[29] The role of thymic factors in the improvement of immunocompetence, in both viral infections and cancer, is still developing.[30] Although reduction in immune surveillance may play a role in the development of cancer in older people, if it were to result in tumor development as seen in immunosuppressed patients, a lack of tumor diversity would be expected, which is not the case.[31]

Administration of L-arginine acts directly on the pituitary to increase thymulin levels and, thus, the number of lymphocyte peripheral subsets.[29] However, there are no data on the use of L-arginine in immune activation in elderly patients with cancer.

There is conflicting opinion regarding the growth and spread of cancer in older patients, and although some evidence shows death to be earlier in older subjects, coexisting diseases have obvious effects on morbidity and mortality. Some experimental work has demonstrated slower tumor growth, fewer metastases, and longer survival in older rodents and others have shown decreased tumor growth associated with impaired T-cell function.[32] Cultures from melanoma cell lines have demonstrated that T cells from young, but not old, donors stimulate the growth of tumor cells, and T cells from young, but not old, mice produce angiogenic factors resulting in a richer vascular supply that may be responsible for increased growth and metastases. The therapeutic implications of angiogenic factors produced by T cells have yet to be explored. Additionally, a relationship between anergy and cancer mortality, although not statistically significant, has been noted in older patients.[33]

Many elderly subjects have been exposed to carcinogenic agents as a result of their occupation (asbestos; inorganic chemicals such as arsenic or nickel; and plant products such as aflatoxin, polycyclic hydrocarbons, and dyes). Lifestyle and diet are dominated in older subjects by tobacco consumption and atmospheric pollution, and although studies have shown an increased incidence of cancer of the endometrium and breast associated with diet, other dietary factors such as fiber does protect against the development of carcinoma of the bowel.

The relationship between cancer and aging is clearly complex and various factors, including exposure to carcinogens and changes in the host defense, have roles to play in the etiology of tumors. With further understanding of normal aging, its relationship to carcinogenesis should be further understood.[34]

CANCER PREVENTION

There are two main approaches to cancer prevention: *primary prevention*, which may be less applicable to older people, relates to changes in lifestyle, exercise, and diet to preclude the development of cancer; and *secondary prevention*, which involves screening tests and examinations to aid early detection of tumors, thereby decreasing morbidity and mortality, increasing the chance of cure, and prolonging the disease-free interval following therapy.

Cancer becomes 100 times more common in men and 30 times more common in women between the ages of 25 and 75 years.[35] Therefore, secondary prevention should perhaps be targeted at older people rather than the young.[36]

PREVENTION STRATEGIES

Prevention has been classified into three types.[37] Primary prevention aims to prevent the onset of a disease, and secondary prevention aims to halt progression of a disease once it has been established. By identifying the disease early, often while the patient is still asymptomatic, prompt and effective treatment may be given to stop the disease. Tertiary prevention aims to rehabilitate people with an established disease to minimize residual disabilities and complications.

The focus of many cancer studies is in both primary and secondary prevention. Approximately 80% of all cancers are potentially preventable, and many public health strategies have been aimed at behavior modification such as smoking cessation, healthy diet, and protection from sunlight.[38]

Primary prevention and health promotion for older people are important issues not only for cancer but other common causes of morbidity and mortality, such as stroke and cardiovascular disease. With regard to cancer, primary prevention may include elimination of environmental carcinogens through chemoprevention (i.e., estrogen antagonists for breast cancer).[39] Primary prevention, even at extreme old age, may result in a decreased incidence of heart disease, colon cancer, and hypertension.[40]

For screening to be applicable, a disease must be common, curable if diagnosed early, and the test involved must be highly sensitive. Screening in the United Kingdom is almost exclusively for tumors of the breast, cervix, and colon and is more commonly performed in younger people. Older subjects are less likely than those from younger age groups to participate in screening and cancer detection behaviors,[41] and this may be due to inadequate knowledge about cancer,[42–44] lower educational level,[45] perceived susceptibility,[46] and ethnic background.[47] Other factors such as fear of cancer[48] and its treatment, difficulty differentiating between normal physiologic changes and early symptoms or signs of cancer[49,50] and fatalism[51,52] have also been implicated. Men participate less than women in screening procedures,[53,54] although the role of ethnicity, marital status, availability of screening test, and physician attitude are all known to have effects on this gender inequality. It has been found that elderly people who scored highly in a health perception questionnaire which measured current health, prior health, health outlook, health worry/concern, resistance or susceptibility to illness, and rejection of the sick role, were also more likely to have participated in cancer screening programs.[53] This perception of health by older people playing an important role in cancer prevention has been reported by others.[55–57]

Older subjects involved in health promotion have significant improvement in their quality of life, and therefore this should be advocated.[58]

If screening of older subjects is to increase, the involvement of health care providers will be important.[59,60] Many exploratory studies have found that individuals failing to undertake cancer screening tests have cited lack of involvement with the health care providers in the previous year, as well as in some countries the financial implications of undertaking such screening. Ageist attitudes must not prevent physicians from recommending screening, nurses must not remove patient's autonomy, and screening services must not exclude those most at risk.[61] Education of health care practitioners, instilling confidence in their ability to teach certain self-examination techniques to patients and increasing the education of patients, is essential.[62]

To improve the early detection of cancer, several questions, including the attitudes of older people toward screening and the barriers perceived by the patient, especially for skin, breast, and cervical cancer, need to be explored.[63–65] Elderly people must be encouraged to take all "red flag" symptoms seriously and not delay seeking a medical opinion. In addition, they should be educated about self-examination, access to screening, and the good outlook of a cancer diagnosis, if treated early.

Breast cancer studies have shown a positive relationship between stage of disease and age at diagnosis,[66] which has not improved with time.[67] However, older women are less likely to participate in screening programs for breast cancer than are younger women.[68] In the United Kingdom in 1988, screening by mammography of women aged 50 to 64 on a triennial basis was recommended by the Forrest Report, and national coverage was achieved by the mid-1990s.[69] Evidence from Hendry and Entwistle,[70] in a study involving 1500 women aged 65 to 69 years, which achieved a screening uptake of 74.6% and a cancer detection rate of 9.3/1000, suggests that the extension of screening to women aged 70 years would be both beneficial and cost-effective. The extension of screening to this age group appears to have been well received. On March 31, 2007, 76% of women aged 53 to 64 years resident in England had been screened at least once in the previous 3 years. In addition, at that point the overall screening of women aged 65 to 70 years had achieved a rate of 67.7%, which was an 8.7% increase from March 2006.[71]

Mammography reveals more tumors in older patients than in younger subjects,[72] increases the proportion of early cancers detected,[73] and thereby reduces mortality.[74–78] Only 16% of all mammographies performed in the 1980s were on women aged over 60 years.[79] Factors that previously reduced the number of elderly women attending for mammography; considering themselves less at risk for developing breast cancer[80] and considering self-examination to be adequate are still seen but less commonly. Haigney et al assessed the views of both older women and hospital doctors on the performance of clinical breast examination.[81] Despite older women stating they would accept clinical breast examination if it was offered by their doctor, only 7% of doctors said that they would routinely perform such an examination on women over 50 years of age. Previous assumptions that older women will not attend for routine screening have been inaccurate. An overall predicted uptake of previous non-attendees was found to be 50%, and when studied by age group, 67% of patients aged 65 to 69 years, 53% of patients aged 70 to 99 years, and 27% of patients aged ≥85 years attended for mammographic screening.[82] This, however, is now reflected in the age groups included within screening but is difficult to extrapolate to those who are not invited by letter.

The American Cancer Society (ACS) recommends that women begin monthly breast self-examination at the age of 20 and between 20 and 39 years have a clinical breast examination every 3 years. The society then recommends that from age 40 onward women should have an annual mammogram and a clinical breast examination. Unlike the United Kingdom's National Screening Programme, there was no upper age limit to the 1997 ACS recommendations as long as the women are in good health.[83]

In 2003, the ACS reviewed its recommendations in a number of key clinical groups. A group of experts considered the screening of older women and women with comorbid conditions. They recommended that screening decisions should be individualized, and as long as the woman was in reasonably good health and fit enough to be a candidate for treatment, she should continue to be screened with mammography. However, if the individual had a life expectancy of less than 3 to 5 years, severe functional limitations, or multiple or severe comorbidities likely to limit life expectancy, it may be appropriate to consider cessation of screening.[84] The argument for the extension of screening to older women focused on the aging population, the finding that 45% of all new breast cancer cases were in women aged 65 and older,[85] and that 45% of all cancer deaths occur in women aged 65 years or older.[86] Data obtained from the Surveillance, Epidemiology and End Results (SEER) program showed a life extension of 178 days for those over 85 years and 617 days for those aged 65 to 69 years old[87] if screening was extended. Hughes and colleagues studied individuals below or above the age of 70 years diagnosed with breast cancer between the years 1980 and 2000. When considering two 10-year cohorts and after adjustment for clinical stage, there was no significant improvement in survival in any age group. However, when compared with an age-matched group in the general population, the elderly breast cancer patients had a 62% increased risk of death.[88]

Unfortunately, despite well-documented evidence of the benefits of screening for colorectal cancer (CRC), there is a relatively low participation rate, particularly when comparing the screening programs that exist for breast or cervical cancer.[89] Colorectal screening uses fecal occult blood, digital rectal examination, and either sigmoidoscopy or colonoscopy. Although well accepted in the United States, until recently it was not commonly performed in the United Kingdom.[90,91] Colon cancer is related to the presence of premalignant adenomas, which are more common in elderly people.[92,93] There is controversy about some of the earlier studies, which showed no increased survival following screening.[94] More recent studies have sufficient evidence to suggest that population screening of people aged over 50 years can reduce mortality rates from bowel cancer.[95,96]

The U.K. NHS Bowel Screening Programme currently offers screening every 2 years to all men and women aged 60 to 69 years. Although individuals aged over 70 years can request a kit, they are not sent one automatically. Controversy exists about the upper age limit of 69 years, as Hardcastle et al[95] and Kronborg et al[96] suggested an upper age limit of 74 years. It is expected that for every 100 patients screened, 98% will get a normal result and be returned to routine screening and the remaining 2% will be offered a colonoscopy. For every 20 individuals offered colonoscopy, 16 will accept the invitation and of them, half are likely to have nothing abnormal detected, 38% are likely to have one or more polyps detected, and 12% are likely to have colorectal cancer detected.[97] The third arm of the U.K. Bowel Cancer Screening pilot study concluded in 2008. Goodyear et al reported a 49% reduction in presentation with a symptomatic cancer and a proportionate rise in the number of asymptomatic colorectal cancers that were detected by screening. In the screened population, there was a significant increase in early Dukes A tumors and an odds ratio of 0.27 for Dukes D cancers.[98] However, there is no evidence yet that colorectal cancer screening will be recommended routinely in individuals 70 years or above.

Despite good screening methodologies, nonattenders will always give a variety of reasons for nonparticipation, including time-related or priority-related, not noticing a test in the mailbox, or forgetting. Much work is required to ensure that individual decision making is not hampered by poor communication or failing to address specific concerns.[99]

In 1997, the U.K. government accepted the advice of the National Screening Committee not to introduce a population screening program for prostate cancer because it would be neither cost-effective nor acceptable.[100] The main reasons against such an introduction were that prostate specific antigen (PSA) has a low specificity and that it cannot reliably distinguish males with prostate cancer from males without the disease. It must, however, be remembered that despite its dubious role in screening, both PSA and C-reactive protein (CRP) are significant predictors of cancer-specific survival in prostate cancer.[101] A U.S. study that followed a representative sample of 7889 men found evidence of 32% undergoing PSA screening. The authors found that this was higher than the number who were undertaking fecal occult blood screening (22.8%) and comparable with the numbers of women aged 75 years or older (29%) undergoing cervical cancer screening. In this population, the majority reported that their doctor first suggested screening and within these, at least two thirds reported that the risks and benefits of screening were fully discussed with them before commencement.[102] The role of screening may become more important, as further evidence becomes available around the efficacy of specific treatments for colorectal cancer.

Although PSA testing is widespread in the United States, the impact of screening remains controversial and may also result in treatment costs in largely asymptomatic patients who will die from unrelated causes.[103]

Although lung cancer is common, it is generally considered that survival is not improved by screening programs. Despite physicians considering that older subjects have little or no benefit from smoking cessation, there is evidence that elderly smokers have no less ability to stop smoking with increasing age[104] and innovative clinics may increase the rate of smoking cessation in an elderly population.[105] It has been known for some time that immediately after cessation of smoking, a decline in the risk of developing lung cancer is seen and by 15 years the risk is that of a lifelong nonsmoker.[106] Using modeling data from a meta-analysis of epidemiologic studies, it has been predicted that 18 million deaths from lung cancer will occur in China before 2033. If, however, there were a complete but gradual cessation of both smoking and solid-fuel use by 2033, there would be 6.5 million fewer deaths from lung cancer (i.e., a reduction of 8% to 26% would occur).[107] The absolute reduction in the number of smoking-related cancers in some studies has been less significant, however.[108]

The role of spiral computed tomography and positron emission tomography in the detection of early stage lung cancer in individuals considered to be at higher risk has been well described. In an Italian study with patients (mean age 58 years) of whom a number were up to the age of 84 years, there was little evidence for the routine use of screening.[109] In 2008, there was a U.K. call for a randomized trial initiated by the Health Technology Assessment to address this question in a systematic way.

The screening for cervical cancer has been aimed particularly at young women. Data from the late 1980s suggested that fewer than one half of all women aged 65 years or older had had a Papanicolaou screen in the previous 3 years.[110] It is known that individuals assessed by their postcode of residence show that the most deprived patients are at increased risk of cervical cancer. In the United Kingdom, the regional differences in the socioeconomic gradients are greatest for lung and cervical cancer in the north of England.[111] Although there is some evidence that cancer screening behavior with regard to breast and cervical cancer is not affected by disability status, the quality of the experience during cancer screening does increase the likelihood of the individual undertaking future routine screening.[112] Fahs et al,[113] using a Markov computer model, found that the early detection of cervical cancer through screening programs may improve survival rates regardless of the patient's age. In addition, screening older women for cervical cancer remained cost-effective although for women aged over 64 years with a history of regular negative smears, regular screening becomes inefficient and the cost increases. Most studies of the cost benefit of screening women for cervical cancer using a Papanicolaou test only recruit women up to the age of 64 years, and this coupled with the increasing use of human papillomavirus DNA testing as well as vaccination of younger individuals should reduce the incidence of cervical cancer in older women in the future.[114] Various methods of improving participation in cervical screening, including the availability of testing in older persons accommodation[115] and creating educational interventions, have been recommended.[116]

INCIDENCE

Overall cancer incidence rates are higher for males than for females, and males have a greater probability of dying from cancer compared with females.[117–119]

Malignant disease has a rising incidence with age, particularly for tumors of the prostate, stomach, colorectum, pancreas, and esophagus.[120–123] The most common cancer site for adult males (aged 25 years or older) is the lung, and for adult females it is the breast.[124,125] In the case of primary lung and breast tumors, although there is a similar rise in incidence with age, this reduces in the very old group, which may be due to poorer standards of diagnosis and certification or due to an increase in deaths from other causes. In 1996, Smith[126] found that although mortality rates increase with age, the relative frequency of cancer deaths declined. Almost 40% of all deaths between the ages of 50 and 69 years, but only 4% of deaths in those aged 100 years or older, were due to malignant disease. Of the 524 patients aged 100 years or older who died from malignant disease in the United States in 1990, the most common single site was the breast in 70 women, with 45 men dying of carcinoma of the prostate.[126] Similar studies in England and Wales looking at patients aged over 100 at the time of death showed a decreased mortality rate for males but a slow nonexponential increasing mortality rate in females.[127] This, however, has not been a consistent finding, since de Rijke and colleagues found in a Netherlands study that the total cancer incidence rates in both men and women were highest in the age group 85 to 94 years. Within middle-aged groups, there was a stable rate of the most common tumors, but increasing rates in the oldest age groups. Although they speculated that it might be due to a real increase as a result of changes in mortality from other diseases, they also suggested that it was caused by an artifactual increase resulting from increased cancer detection rates in the very elderly group.[122] With increasing interest in older patients with malignant disease, the latter rather than the former seems more likely.

DIAGNOSIS

For many patients, early diagnosis is the key to improved survival. There is evidence that stage of disease varies in older subjects at presentation. In breast cancer, it has been found to be earlier in these subjects when screening is utilized and the number of cancer cases diagnosed, and confirmed by mammography in older women appears to be increasing.[128] However, many older patients delay seeking medical advice, and this may result in cancer being diagnosed at an advanced stage. The delay in diagnosis may have the same cause as the failure to participate in screening, namely a general lack of awareness of possible signs and symptoms of malignancy. Older people may still view cancer to be untreatable and to be invariably fatal. Some studies have found that elderly patients may have difficulty accessing diagnostic interventions.[129] It must be realized that this factor is now being superseded by factors such as race, poverty, and, in some countries, insurance status.[130] Older people are significantly less likely to have their cancer verified histologically compared with younger patients.[131–133] Death certificate only diagnosis in older patients with cancer may occur, although with better cancer registry data, this trend should reduce in all age groups.[134]

The diagnostic tests offered to older patients are influenced by the medical specialty to which they are referred. Fleming and Fleming found that geriatricians were less likely to recommend mammography when compared to general physicians,[135] and older people with suspected lung cancer are less likely to be investigated by geriatricians than by chest physicians.[136] There is controversy as to whether the patient's age alone influences the method and the thoroughness of diagnostic investigations. Mulcahy et al concluded that the patient's age did not influence the method of detecting colorectal cancer.[137] However, they did find that significantly more older patients with colorectal cancer were likely to present as emergency cases with advanced disease when compared with younger patients. These emergency cases are often referred to medicine or geriatric medicine rather than surgical units, and this may be partly explained by atypical presentation and the general frailty of the patient.[138] The relative lack of investigations that are undertaken in an elderly person may be partly due to the oncologist's lack of understanding about normal aging. Geriatricians are experienced in assessing preexisting disability and concurrent disease and in understanding functional status, level of dependency, and psychological adjustment. This enables joint decisions with regard to further therapy before the rehabilitation and, it is hoped, recovery of the elderly patient with cancer.[139]

With improved screening and diagnostic tests, older patients should present with an earlier stage cancer. The knowledge of and ability to treat comorbidity should ensure that older patients are just as likely to be investigated as their younger counterparts. This should be particularly encouraged in patients with tumors, where low-risk elective surgery can be undertaken and found to have similar morbidity and mortality in all age groups.[140]

STAGE OF DISEASE

Cancer staging is an important component of management. There is little doubt that both histology and stage of the cancer are independent predictors of survival.[141] There is a clear relationship between age and stage at diagnosis and between age at diagnosis and treatment received by the patient with cancer.[142,143] In general, older patients are more likely to have advanced or unstaged disease when compared to younger patients,[144] although other factors, including greater material deprivation, also affect the age at diagnosis.[145] It must therefore be remembered that those older patients living in increased poverty may present later with their tumors. Although data from the 1990s[146] found that patients over 74 years of age were more likely to have unstaged tumors, the discrepancy between unstaged stomach cancer (26.9%) and breast cancer (2.4%) is more likely to be due to the diagnostic techniques available at this time, rather than chronologic age alone. Older patients are also more likely to have "unknown" stage at diagnosis. Bergman et al[147] and Martin et al[148] found that older women with breast cancer were more likely to be diagnosed as stage unknown or stage 3 when compared with younger women. In contrast, Busch et al found a lower proportion of older women (≥ 75 years) with breast cancer stage 2 or unknown when compared to younger women (13.7% vs. 8.3%),[149] although for stages 1, 3, and 4 there were comparable proportions for both age groups.

Older women with ovarian cancer have a higher proportion of advanced disease (stages 3 and 4) than younger women, and age remains a prognostic indicator.[150,151] As with breast cancer, there are reports that older women have the highest proportion of unstaged ovarian cancer.[152]

Although there have been some conflicting data regarding colorectal cancer stage at presentation, in a study of more than 172,000 patients with colorectal cancer, unstaged tumors were more likely to be found in the older group. Ironically, survival was significantly higher in the unstaged group, except for patients who were aged 65 years or older.[153]

TREATMENT

Elderly patients should receive therapy comparable to their younger counterparts, although this may not always have been the case. In the 1980s and 1990s, older people with cancer were less likely to receive definitive treatment than younger patients.[154] With the increasing inclusion of older individuals (although often not over 70 years of age) in cancer screening, there are few patients who should not, following assessment of comorbidity, be considered for active curative treatment. There is, however, an issue regarding the inclusion of older individuals in clinical trials. When a comparison of the 1990 incidence data from the National Cancer Institute (NCI) Surveillance, Epidemiology and End Results (SEER) program[155] was made to the NCI Treatment Trials, which included more than 8000 elderly patients, a significant discrepancy between the incidence of cancer and participation in cancer treatment protocols was found. Only 39% of males and 25.9% of the women involved in the trials were 65 years or older; as a result, the United States, under the auspices of the NCI, has sponsored a number of trials specifically targeting older patients. Unfortunately, cancer data from the United States including years 1995–2002 suggested that cancer treatment is not always consistent with evidence-based guidelines and pointed out that there are economic, racial, geographic, and age-related disparities in cancer treatment.[156] U.S. data comparing 1996–1998 with 2000–2002, showed an increase in the total number of trial participants, with only 1.3% of 65-to-74-year-old patients and 0.5% of patients aged over 75 years being represented. With increasing age participation becomes reduced.[157] During the 1980s and 1990s, there was evidence that age affected decision making regarding curative cancer therapy,[158] and many of the older drugs caused a number of adverse drug reactions, particularly in older individuals. However, when side effects of chemotherapeutic agents are considered, there is some evidence that younger patients report more nausea, fatigue, and vomiting than do their older counterparts.

The reasons behind the underrepresentation of older subjects in treatment figures are complex. The patient may not have full investigation and staging and therefore not be eligible to enter into a trial. Some argue that older patients are more likely to suffer from toxicity with chemotherapy, although newer drugs have reduced toxicity and allow good palliation for most cancers.[159]

As noted earlier, when side effects of chemotherapeutic agents are considered, studies have documented that younger patients report more nausea, fatigue, and vomiting than do their older counterparts.[160] However, Dibble et al found that vomiting immediately after chemotherapy for breast cancer was equally prevalent in younger and older age groups and delayed vomiting occurred more frequently in younger women with a larger body mass index.[161] One possible explanation for the reduction in nausea and vomiting in older people is that younger patients have higher anxiety levels and a greater expectation of being sick.[162] Other studies have confirmed that nausea expectation and younger age are risk factors for chemotherapy-induced nausea and vomiting.[163]

Putative problems with compliance in older people has been cited as a reason for their nontreatment, and elderly women with breast cancer have been found not to follow the prescribed adjuvant chemotherapy, although the reasons for this were not clear.[164] Further planning with regard to patient education is required as more elderly people undergo complex oral chemotherapeutic regimes at home. Other studies have shown, in contrast, that older patients are more compliant with therapeutic regimens than are younger patients.[165]

Other reasons given for the nontreatment of elderly subjects with cancer have included advanced disease at presentation, and although there is some evidence that patients over 55 years of age have more advanced disease, at presentation this is not universal.[66,142,143,166–168]

Some doctors caring for elderly patients with cancer consider that they are less likely to wish to receive treatment than their younger counterparts. This was not the finding of Yellen and colleagues,[169] who used structured scenarios to assess patients' willingness to accept toxic chemotherapy to enhance survival and found that older patients were as willing to choose chemotherapy as were younger patients, though the former required a greater survival advantage before they would choose a toxic regime over a less toxic alternative.

Myths about cancer may affect treatment. If older patients believe that cancer treatments are worse than the disease itself[170] or they have a greater fear of cancer than younger patients do,[171] they may decline treatment. If adequate information is given to older patients, they are likely to accept treatment in a similar fashion to younger patients[172,173] and indeed may experience less emotional distress following the diagnosis of cancer.[174]

Poor life expectancy in elderly subjects has been cited as a further reason for nontreatment; however, life expectancy tables should not be used to gauge who should receive therapy.

Unfortunately, many patients with cancer, irrespective of their age, consider that they have not fully participated during the treatment decision-making process. There is evidence that if patients perceive that they have been poorly involved, they have increased anxiety, which impacts on their quality of life.[175] However, Bilodeau and Degner found that older women with breast cancer preferred to assume a passive role in treatment decision making.[176] Whereas most younger women felt that stage of disease, likelihood of cure, and treatment options were the most important aspects of the information they received, older women considered that self-care issues were more important.[176,177] The attitudes of physicians with regard to informing older people about a cancer diagnosis may also influence the treatment that they receive. Although anecdotal evidence suggests that older people do not wish to receive a diagnosis of cancer, 80% of respondents aged 65 to 94 years wanted to be informed of a cancer diagnosis, with 70% of the respondents wanting their relatives also to be informed when the diagnosis was made.[178] This is in contrast to the feelings of relatives of patients with cancer, when 66% did not want the diagnosis to be disclosed.[179] It must, however, be remembered that collusion and nondisclosure to patients have a negative effect on those caring for the patient.[180]

The presence of comorbidity is associated with less treatment for cancer. Following an interview of 800 patients aged 65 years or older with newly diagnosed cancer of the breast, prostate, colon, or rectum, logistic regression was used to assess factors potentially influencing the receipt of definitive treatment by each individual. The study showed that for breast and prostate cancer, there was a clear increase in the percentage of patients not receiving definitive treatment with increasing age,[181] and in colorectal cancer, men were more likely to receive definitive therapy than women.[181] Other studies have found factors determining nontreatment with chemotherapy to include impaired ability to perform activities of daily living, access to transportation, being unmarried, low income, and low educational achievement.[181] Surprisingly, the presence of other medical disorders, although reducing definitive treatment, was not statistically significant in the analysis. In contrast, advanced age, impaired access to transportation, and poor functional and cognitive status showed little influence on receipt of surgical therapy.

Coexisting diseases are well documented in older patients with cancer. Approximately 25% of patients over the age of 75 years with cancer have vascular disease, and almost 10% have coexisting chronic obstructive pulmonary disease or diabetes mellitus.[182] Unfortunately, patients with some coexisting diseases, irrespective of age, are less likely to receive curative treatment for their cancer.[183] It is important that such patients are included in clinical trials to determine the effect of comorbidity on treatment tolerance and survival,[184,185] although many exclusion criteria are derived from a desire to study "pure" patients rather than the pragmatic approach, which often characterizes the specialty of geriatric medicine.

SURGERY

Surgery is considered to be the treatment of choice for most cancers, and patients should not be denied surgery on the basis of chronologic age.[186] Nonetheless, mortality and morbidity rates are often increased in older patients who undergo surgery for a variety of difficult cancers. Consultation and teamwork can, however, minimize mortality and morbidity.[187] In a review of 105 patients aged 75 years or older with a variety of recurrent solid tumors, postoperative mortality was 3.8% with a 5-year survival rate of over 40% for selected patients.[188] This figure is continuing to improve, and it is essential that a full assessment of patient suitability for surgery is undertaken.[189]

Advanced age per se is often used by either the patient's family or the physician to justify not proceeding with surgery. This ageist attitude is, however, fortunately declining. Surgery for octogenarians now obtains better clinical outcomes in both cancer and noncancer patients.[190]

In older women with breast cancer, age is often independently negatively associated with the surgery being performed.[191] Unfortunately, primary surgical therapy varies significantly with age.[192] Elderly women are less likely to receive breast reconstruction surgery than are younger women, and ageist attitudes do unfortunately continue to prevail.[192]

Surgery is the treatment of choice for patients with colorectal cancer. Chronologic age should not be a reason to withhold surgery from such patients.[187,193–195] Although postoperative morbidity may be similar in young and older patients, mortality may be up to three times higher and both cancer-specific survival and disease-free survival significantly worse in older groups, after rectal cancer surgery. The role of additional comorbidity in individuals aged over 65 may have been the cause of the long-term cancer-related survival being worse in contrast to the short-term prognosis.[196] Unfortunately, older patients with colorectal cancer are more likely to present with advanced disease, twice as likely to have emergency surgery, and less likely to undergo curative surgery.[197] Although the proportion of older patients undergoing curative surgery for colorectal cancer has increased,[198] this may be because surgery is performed on most patients regardless of age.[199]

Some patients with colorectal cancer will have solitary hepatic metastases, which are usually resected in younger individuals. When analyzing data from the resection of metastases in individuals aged 75 years or older, the overall survival at 1, 3, and 5 years was 90%, 64%, and 33%, respectively, and the disease-free survival was much lower at 1 and 3 years (74% and 42%). Although the authors suggest that this may affect those selected for liver resection, many older individuals would consider a 42%, 3-year, disease-free survival as being an adequate benefit, when compared to a hospital morbidity and mortality of 10% and 3%, respectively. Older individuals wish to be actively involved in such difficult decision making and may at times surprise medical practitioners in the risks that they are prepared to take.[200]

DRUG THERAPY

The normal physiologic changes of aging affect drug absorption, distribution, metabolism, and elimination; thus, when prescribing any drug for an elderly person, drug pharmacokinetics must be considered. Elderly patients with cancer may receive a wide range of drugs including chemotherapeutic agents, analgesics, antiemetics, antibiotics, and others, in addition to drug therapy that was previously prescribed for coexisting medical disorders.[201]

Although absorption is not significantly altered by age per se, some normal changes of aging do affect drug absorption. Oral drugs are modified by gastric motility and emptying time, whereas the absorption of parenterally administered drugs is dependent on local blood flow in muscles and fatty tissue. Drug distribution is affected by the decrease in total body water and albumin and the change in the ratio of lean body weight to fat. The reduction in albumin results in a greater concentration of unbound highly lipophilic drugs in the circulation able to exert their effects.

Drug metabolism is affected by decreased liver mass and hepatic blood flow as well as decreased microsomal enzymatic activity in the liver.[202] Elimination is affected by the reduction in glomerular filtration rate, decreased renal blood flow, and renal tubular function, and it is particularly important with cyclophosphamide and methotrexate, which are both excreted renally.

Unfortunately, as with younger patients with cancer, many older individuals will have multiple medications, which will increase the risk of adverse drug reactions, drug-to-drug interactions, and nonadherence. Many clinical trials do little to select "typical" geriatric medicine type patients; as a result, our progress in the understanding of many of the pharmacologic issues in treating older individuals with cancer are yet to be addressed.[203]

CHEMOTHERAPY

Chemotherapy, often a primary systemic form of treatment for cancer, possesses either cytotoxic or cytocidal activity.[204] McKenna found that adverse drug reactions from chemotherapy increased sevenfold for patients over 69 years of age when compared with younger patients.[205]

Older patients are less likely to receive chemotherapy, and if treated, it is more likely to be outside a clinical trial, although this continues to improve with time. This is due partly to age restrictions on trial entry and partly to clinicians, without clinical evidence, feeling the need to reduce drug dosages in such patients. All drug therapy in elderly people is affected by altered pharmacokinetics and pharmacodynamics, and some chemotherapeutic agents pose special problems.[39,206,207] Reduction of chemotherapeutic drug dosages may reduce toxicity at the expense of response rates, or lower response rates without any effect on toxicity, or result in better tolerance, but provide no survival advantage. Many researchers now consider that reducing doses on the basis of age alone is not justified, but data are lacking.

Other researchers have found that elderly subjects, when receiving drug dosages similar to their younger counterparts, have similar toxicity rates, although some trials do not clearly define how the patients over age 70 years were selected.[208]

A prospective pilot study by Chen et al found that although older patients undergoing chemotherapy did experience some toxicity, they could generally tolerate it with limited impact on their independence, other comorbidities, and quality of life levels.[209] This, however, is in contrast to the views of Repetto,[210] who considered that age was such a clear risk factor for chemotherapy-induced neutropenia and its complications, particularly in the treatment of lymphoma or solid tumors that without the use of colony-stimulating factors better outcomes would not be achieved.[210] Controversy still exists as to the prevalence of hematologic toxicity in older cancer patients, with some authors finding that increasing age alone does not increase the risk of hematologic toxicity during the treatment of some common malignancies, with chemotherapeutic agents known to cause neutropenia.[211] However, their paper evaluated all elderly patients of whom only about 50% of the individuals aged over 70 years received relatively full-dose chemotherapy.

To avoid unnecessary toxicity, a decision regarding dose reduction should be made on the onset of treatment, because if dose reductions vary from cycle to cycle of therapy, although tailored for individual patients, little evidence is accrued with regard to toxicity and efficacy. Although it is difficult to establish general rules regarding the administration of chemotherapy,[212] physicians must be aware of the diversity of levels of health among older people and tailor chemotherapy according to individual needs.[206]

Balducci and Beghe set out guidelines on the administration of chemotherapeutic drugs for older people,[207] which include the following:

- Age 75 years defines older age for chemotherapeutic agents.
- Chemotherapeutic agents that are excreted renally should be dose-adjusted according to the patient's glomerular filtration rate.
- Hematopoietic growth factors should be used in people receiving moderately toxic chemotherapy in order to reduce the duration and severity of neutropenia.
- High-dose chemotherapeutic regimens should be avoided because the functional reserve of many older people (≥75 years) is decreased, and this population is more susceptible to complications of chemotherapy.
- Palliation for frail patients may include some mild form of chemotherapy.

Although Balducci and other colleagues have been keen to point out that only a minority of elderly patients should be excluded from treatment because of reduced tolerance, there is little concrete advice on who to treat and at what doses, and in those who developed toxicity, what method of assessment should be undertaken before deciding on their next dosage of chemotherapeutic agent.[213,214] What is quite clear is that additional studies need to be undertaken to address both pharmacokinetic and pharmacodynamic changes that are present in older patients with cancer, and the need for these studies to be undertaken in not only in a systematic way but across multiple centers, to ensure that adequate numbers guide future therapy, is indisputable.[215]

There is an age-dependent decrease in bone marrow stem cells, which results in increased liability to neutropenic episodes. Hematopoietic factors reduce the duration of severe neutropenia and accelerate neutrophil recovery following chemotherapy. There is no evidence that older people respond differently from younger patients to such agents.[207]

HORMONAL THERAPIES

Hormonal therapies may provide a benefit to elderly patients with advanced cancer of the breast, prostate, and endometrium. In the management of metastatic breast cancer, the beneficial effects of estrogen therapy increase steadily with age in all postmenopausal women, probably because of the increased incidence of receptor-receptor positive tumors in older women that result in an increased response rate to such therapy.

Tamoxifen (an anti-estrogen drug) prolongs survival of patients with breast cancer and also reduces recurrence rates. It is particularly useful if the tumor is estrogen-receptor positive as seen in many postmenopausal women. Tamoxifen, however, should not be used as an alternative to surgery in all but the frailest elderly patients who would not survive such treatment.[216–218] Some researchers have found that tamoxifen alone appears to delay definitive treatment, and this should not be encouraged.[219–223] Although there is evidence that preoperative tamoxifen may be an appropriate approach before breast-conserving surgery,[173,224] its main role is in the prevention of recurrence of breast cancer in postmenopausal women. It should be administered daily for a maximum of 5 years, as there is yet no evidence for a longer duration of therapy.[225]

Martelli and colleagues found that elderly patients with early breast cancer and no palpable axillary lymph nodes could be safely treated with conservative surgery and adjuvant tamoxifen without the need for either axillary dissection or postoperative radiotherapy. They found during prolonged follow-up (median 15 years), 83% of the deaths were unrelated to breast cancer. This provides data that may enable some older women to choose more limited surgery and adjuvant tamoxifen over extensive surgery and postoperative radiotherapy.[226] In 2008, the results of two large trials that had investigated extending tamoxifen treatment beyond 5 years were both reported. It is now suggested that following 5 years of adjuvant tamoxifen, an aromatase inhibitor is used for a further 4 years in postmenopausal women.[227–229]

RADIOTHERAPY

If a tumor is radiosensitive, radiotherapy may be appropriate and have positive results for older patients in good health.[199,205,230]

Organ-specific tolerance to radiation is related to aging. Lymphocytes from both elderly experimental animals and humans are more susceptible to damage induced by ionizing radiation. When radiotherapy in elderly patients is palliative in intent, it is important that minimal toxicity is experienced. However, radiotherapy can be highly effective, with many older patients completing the treatment with no serious complications. Radiotherapy may be used at times with curative intent, particularly in early stage non-small-cell lung cancer which is inoperable. In such cases, a large fraction size can be given safely, even in older individuals.[231] Zachariah et al found that 94% of patients aged 80 years or older diagnosed with cancer of the head and neck, lung, pelvis, or breast tolerated and completed the planned course of radiotherapy, be it either curative or palliative, without serious complications.[232] Palliative radiotherapy is particularly good in patients with lung cancer, whose symptoms include hemoptysis, although it is less effective for the more common symptoms of dyspnea and cough. In such groups, side effects are often few and usually mild, with the majority of older patients tolerating delivery of their radiotherapy over 1 week.[233] Unless the patient is severely debilitated, there is no reason to modify a potentially curative approach.[234] When radiotherapy is being used for the treatment of cancer pain, there is no evidence that age influences the efficacy of such treatment, and factors such as the pain score before the onset of radiotherapy, or the presence of radiating pain, are much better predictors of who will benefit from the treatment.[235] Follow-up of such patients is often difficult, and the use of an Edmonton Symptom Assessment System (ESAS) by telephone follow-up may be more appropriate for older individuals.[236]

With regard to breast cancer, age unfortunately remains an independent factor that determines those patients who will receive postoperative radiotherapy, even after adjusting for other variables, including stage.[237] In breast cancer, patients who received adjuvant radiotherapy are generally younger, have fewer comorbidities, and are more likely to be white, married, and from an urban area. However, they are also more likely to have a surgeon who is female and who has a higher medical degree.[238] In the future, other factors may influence which older women undergo radiotherapy, and age may become less of an issue. Even in the twenty-first century, older women continue to be less well represented when considering postoperative radiotherapy following breast cancer.[39,239]

Myelosuppression may be problematic as elderly patients have less functional bone marrow and a slowed recovery of normal tissue. Fatigue may result in compliance problems, and radiation may result in dry skin that is more susceptible to infection.[240] The normal aging of the gastrointestinal tract may result in increased susceptibility to anorexia and stomatitis following radiotherapy.[241]

The more commonly seen radiation side effects that occur in elderly subjects are predicated on preexisting conditions; thus, radiation to emphysematous lungs will increase dyspnea, and irradiation of the mediastinum will impair declining left ventricular function. Compliance with radiotherapy in elderly subjects is additionally hampered by multiple visits and traveling. The use of split fractions does, however, reduce toxicity and is essential in the treatment of many tumors in older patients.

Patients with Non Small Cell Lung Cancer (NSCLC) who are unfit or refuse surgery may receive radiotherapy as an alternative treatment. Patients who accept radiotherapy, tolerate it well and consider it an acceptable treatment.[233]

Radiotherapy is a well-established and potentially curative treatment for small volume prostate tumors. It is often the preferred treatment because it carries fewer complications than surgery, and in some series 15-year disease-free survival rates of up to 85% have been achieved.[242,243] The median age of patients with prostate cancer treated with radiotherapy is increasing,[244] and more sophisticated single-session radiotherapy is now being used in younger men to provide curative treatment. It must be hoped that such methodologies can in the future be implemented in older men, as data suggest that morbidity may be considerably reduced compared to surgery.[245]

NURSING CARE

Unfortunately, elderly patients with cancer often have comorbidity, and this together with their socioeconomic status will influence the treatment that they receive.[246] Patients with cancer will have a variety of symptoms, and many report fatigue, which may be particularly difficult to treat in elderly patients with comorbidity.[247] Quality of life has become a more important outcome measure for cancer patients. This coupled with disease-free and overall survival time must be carefully considered in older individuals and should be an outcome measure that nurses caring for such patients should note.[248]

Ageism is an important adverse influence on the prevention and diagnosis of cancer, but also in the nursing care of elderly patients with cancer, and nurses are just as likely as others to be biased by ageism.[249] This may be due to the inadequate preparation of nurses[250] or to a perceived lack of attractiveness of a gerontologic career.[251] The nurse may view cancer prevention to be unnecessary, may promote dependency and learned helplessness, and may minimize the need for referral to clinicians or community resources.[250] Nurses caring for elderly patients on general medical wards will see the three symptoms—pain, fatigue. and insomnia—as being particularly prevalent in everyday geriatric medicine. These are the most prevalent, distressing, and often undermanaged symptoms that cancer patients experience.[252] When they occur together, they are associated with adverse outcomes and are often first detected by nurses.[252]

The experience of cancer for both the patient and family is stressful, and although many treatments for cancer can be given on an outpatient basis, many require prolonged hospitalization. Upon discharge to the community, much of the physical and psychological care of the patient is placed on the family. This puts an enormous stress on elderly patients and their caregivers. Not surprisingly, there is a high correlation between severity of symptoms and impact on activities of daily living.[253] Although younger cancer patients are more likely than older patients to need help with relieving distressing symptoms, elderly patients do report distressing symptoms and therefore should not be excluded from specialist palliative care services on the basis of their age. Somewhat surprisingly, Addington-Hall and colleagues found that cancer patients did not show increased independence with age, thus stressing the importance of access to both social services and community health services for cancer patients of all ages.[254] Many patients with cancer have depressive symptoms,[255] and there is a positive correlation between patients' self-care needs and mood.[256] Age is an important determinant in decision making when patients present with advanced stage cancer, although, surprisingly, whereas older patients have more comorbidities, they often have lower levels of depression, anxiety, and symptom distress. Their views about treatment goals focus on pain relief and comfort, but they receive fewer prescriptions for opioids.[257] This finding was confirmed by Kurtz et al,[258] who assessed the mental health of patients and family members and found that of the 208 patients in the study, 83 of whom were aged 65 years or older, the most common five symptoms were fatigue, pain, nausea, poor appetite, and constipation. In this study there was no relationship between age and level of symptoms, although older people tend to underreport and this may counteract a genuine age-related increase in symptoms.

Caregivers are more likely to be wives than husbands and to care single-handedly. Wives provide twice the hours of care that husbands provide, although this is compensated by female patients having more outside care than males.[259] Unfortunately, when illness or treatment results in restricted activity, when finance is limited, or when caregivers are not spouses, patients with cancer are more likely to report unmet needs.[260] Using data from noninstitutionalized elderly people without cancer, there is further evidence of married, disabled women receiving fewer hours per week of informal home care than do married, disabled men, again stressing the need to target resources, particularly to married, disabled women who without the input of their children may be deficient in necessary care.[261] When the patient was younger, the caregivers tended to be more depressed, and caring had a greater impact on the caregiver's schedule; friends did provide more support to the caregiver. In 82% of cases, the caregivers were spouses of the patients, and it is likely, therefore, that elderly spouses will be solitary caregivers and have little support from other friends and relatives.[256] Elderly caregivers require counseling, but this may present logistic difficulties. The use of telephone counseling is of potential value and removes the need for transport and alternative care arrangements.[262]

REHABILITATION

Where data are available on elderly patients following treatment for cancer, functional status assessment is usually via the Karnofsky performance status. This, however, is not specific to older subjects and ignores many of the more important activities of daily living that are included in the well-validated rating schemes that geriatric frequently use. Without accurate clinical assessment of older people with cancer, rehabilitation cannot be targeted. The role of comorbidity scores is limited, and therefore there is a need for an overarching comprehensive assessment.[263]

SURVIVAL

Relative survival is lower among older people with cancer than among their younger counterparts. There are many possible explanations for these differences, and these include the tendency for cancer to be diagnosed at a later stage in older subjects and differences in the treatments received by elderly patients. Other age-related factors, such as comorbidity, obviously alter outcome.[264,265]

With better diagnosis through screening methodologies, early evidence-based interventions, and good post-therapy care including rehabilitation, older patients will continue to benefit. The development of specialized shortened questionnaires for cancer patients will additionally facilitate the identification of symptoms that require palliation.[266] All clinicians caring for older people must consider that it is often much worse for patients not to understand some of the areas that clinicians find difficult to deal with. Patients wish to know the mode of disease progression, the mode of death, and the prognosis and are more content with realistic versus unrealistic timescales. In addition, a prognosis does not in itself cause depression, and therefore collusion and physician anxiety must not detract from information-giving, particularly with older patients.[267] Novel delivery of specialized care may be more appropriate to older patients, many of whom wish to remain at home. This not only improves quality of life, but there is evidence that it also improves survival.[268] In addition, near-death patients are often prepared to undergo chemotherapy even for very small gains, and this may be particularly so in older cancer patients.[269]

KEY POINTS
Geriatric Oncology

- Older people commonly develop cancer, which is poorly investigated and treated.
- The incidence and prevalence of cancer is increasing in those over 70 years of age.
- There is evidence for screening for certain tumors even in old age.
- Progress has been made in various therapy modalities, although older people need careful pretreatment assessment.
- Caregivers of people with cancer are also often elderly and may need particular support to enable them to fulfill a caring role.
- Although the links between aging and cancer are well documented, it is important to promote primary prevention in this age group.
- Validation of palliative care protocols in this elderly age group will support end-of-life care.

For a complete list of references, please visit online only at www.expertconsult.com

CHAPTER 95

Skin Disease and Old Age

Gopal A. Patel
Gangaram Ragi
W. Clark Lambert
Robert A. Schwartz

INTRODUCTION

Aging affects all organ systems, including the integument. Cell replacement, sensory perception, thermal regulatory function, and immune defense systems are among the many components compromised. The skin appearance changes, depending on environmental and genetic factors. The psychosocial impact, including cosmetic disfigurement and social stigma, in addition to vulnerability to skin disease, must be addressed in elderly patients. The role of the physician is to diagnose, treat, and guide patients through this visible component of aging, while preventing avoidable disease.

EPIDEMIOLOGY

The U.S. population that is older than 65 is greatly expanding. Skin complaints constitute a significant and growing portion of geriatric ambulatory patient visits. A 2005 study in the United States demonstrated that 21% of all patients seen by family practitioners had a skin problem. Seventy two percent of the time it was their primary complaint.[1] Also in 2005, the National Ambulatory Medical Care Survey showed that the number of outpatient visits was highest in the 45-to-64-year-old age group, a shift up from the 1995 survey, suggesting increasing medical use by the baby-boomer population, which is now entering the 65-and-older bracket.[2] Among all patient age groups, 1 in 20 visits to an outpatient office are of skin, hair, or nail concern.[2] Diseases such as cutaneous melanoma are on the rise, with lifetime risks shifting from 1/250 in 1980 to 1/65 in 2002 based on a U.S. population study.[3] These data emphasize the importance of skin disease recognition in the elderly.[4] Skin cancer, for example, is often preventable and with early diagnosis can be 100% curable. Also, the role of cosmetic services and the impact on psychosocial well-being that can be traced to skin disease is of added concern.

APPROACH TO THE PATIENT

A complete medical history is desirable for the skin disease patient, regardless of age. One should pay attention to medicines or chemicals used, including topical, systemic, cosmetic, or complementary and alternative ones. The duration of a complaint, previous therapy, close contacts, and patient opinions on etiology may assist or obfuscate diagnosis and treatment. Hygiene, including bathing and laundering habits, should be assessed. Geriatric patients should undergo a thorough skin evaluation under good lighting.

Older patients often have trouble with medication compliance. Dermatologic treatments are further challenging because of their frequent topical nature. Patients may need to apply creams on difficult-to-reach areas (e.g., feet, back) or may be immobilized. Shampooing, showering, or complicated treatment regimens can confuse and challenge geriatric patients. The clinician needs to be aware of all these barriers and accommodate accordingly.

SELECTED SKIN CONDITIONS

KEY POINTS
Skin Disease and Old Age

- Skin diseases are common in the elderly, and though rarely deadly, may degrade quality of life.
- Skin cancer is increasing in incidence in light-skinned Americans and is curable if diagnosed early.
- Xerosis and pruritus are the most common complaints of the elderly and may be manifestations of many systemic diseases.
- Early treatment, within 3 days of onset, is most effective for herpes zoster patients.
- Tobacco use and unregulated sun exposure are major preventable factors in skin cancer predisposition and skin aging.

Eczematous disorders

The geriatric patient population's chief complaint is often of a pruritic (itchy) rash or lesion that turns out to be an eczematous disease. The prevalence of eczema is between 2.4% and 4.1% in the U.S. population.[5] In the elderly, natural aging of the skin predisposes patients to eczematous diseases. In a Turkish study of more than 4000 patients, eczematous disorders constituted nearly 22% of diagnoses in the 65-to-74-year-old age group.[6]

XEROSIS (ECZEMA CRAQUELÉ, ASTEATOTIC ECZEMA)

Xerosis describes rough or dry skin, which is seen in almost all elderly persons. Conditions of low humidity, such as artificially heated rooms, especially forced hot air heating, exacerbate this condition. Xerosis is actually a misnomer, as water is not absent throughout the entire thickness of the skin. There is only diminished hydration in the superficial corneum.[7,8] Xerosis has also been misclassified as a sebaceous gland disorder. Though sebaceous gland activity decreases with age and thus depletes the skin's moisture, it only plays a partial role in xerosis development.[9] Other factors include an irregular epidermal surface caused by maturation abnormalities. Deficits in skin hydration and lipid content impair normal desquamation, leading to formation of the skin scales that characterize xerosis. Furthermore, old age results in altered lipid profiles and in decreased production of filaggrin, which are filament associated proteins that bind keratinocytes. Both features contribute to xerosis.[8]

Xerosis may appear scaly with accentuated skin lines, often occurring on the anterior legs, back, arms, abdomen, and waist. The scales are a result of epidermal water loss, and focal dryness may be deep enough to cause bleeding fissures.

Superimposed pruritus is possible, leading to secondary excoriations, inflammation, and lichen simplex chronicus.[8] Allergic and irritant contact dermatitis may also complicate xerosis. Secondary infection may follow a break in the skin barrier.[10] Xerosis is also a secondary feature of many of the selected conditions in this chapter.

Untreated xerosis progresses to flaking, fissuring, inflammation, dermatitis, and infection. Topical emollients make dry skin more comfortable and avoid such complications. Alpha-hydroxy acids (e.g., 12% ammonium lactate) are helpful because of their keratolytic nature, though some patients report stinging and irritation.[11] Formulations containing ammonium lactate or other alpha-hydroxy acids help to restore barrier function and improve xerosis.[12] Liberal use of moisturizers throughout the day is recommended. Topical steroids (classes III and VI) are recommended in moderate to severe cases, along with antipruritics for symptomatic itching. Further recommendations include decreasing hot water baths, reducing use of soap or harsh skin cleansers, avoiding rough clothes on the skin, utilizing humidifiers in dry environments, or adding emollient substances, such as oatmeal, to bathwater.

Simple xerosis is a common cause of pruritus in the elderly. Asteatotic eczema is a dermatitis superimposed on xerosis that often flares in the winter. It is dry, scaly skin, sometimes resembling, in extreme cases, cracked porcelain with bleeding from damaged dermal capillaries. The cracked porcelain, or "crazy paving," pattern is best termed eczema craquelé.[13] Asteatotic eczema is a common condition on the shins of geriatric patients, though it is also seen on other regions of the body. Several associations of asteatotic eczema exist: one related to hard soaps, one to corticosteroid therapy, one to neurologic disorders, and an idiopathic one often located on the shins of elderly patients. Prevention is the key to controlling this entity. Contributing factors include cleansers used, frequency of showers, diet, medications, and temperature exposure. Specifically, patients should reduce hot showers and irritant detergents. Creams, humidifiers, and topical steroids can improve the effects of asteatotic dermatitis.[13] Alcohol-based lotions feel good just after application but eventually cause increased dryness and should be avoided.

SEBORRHEIC DERMATITIS

Seborrheic dermatitis typically manifests as an erythematous and greasy-like scaling eruption, usually affecting areas with abundant sebaceous glands, including the scalp, ears, central face, central chest, and intertriginous spaces.[14] When present in the scalp, it tends to cause flaking known as dandruff. It may also appear as marked erythema over the nasolabial fold during times of stress or sleep deprivation. Seborrheic dermatitis is found in greater frequency with neurologic conditions such as Parkinson's disease, a concern in the geriatric population.[15] Facial nerve injury, spinal cord injury, syringomyelia, and neuroleptic treatment are also associated with seborrheic dermatitis.

The pathogenesis of seborrheic dermatitis, though controversial, has been attributed to the yeast *Malassezia* species (*Malassezia furfur, Malassezia ovalis*), formerly known as *Pityrosporum*.[16] This yeast is a normal inhabitant in more than 90% of healthy adults, but when overgrown it can be proportionally related to the severity of seborrheic dermatitis. Treatment options against *Malassezia* species have been effective for seborrheic dermatitis, supporting a causal relationship. Antifungals along with topical steroids are utilized, such as ketoconazole cream or shampoo and hydrocortisone valerate cream.[14] Furthermore, topical ketoconazole has inherent anti-inflammatory properties. One classic study comparing these two agents determined that 2% ketoconazole cream was 80.5% effective in resolving seborrheic dermatitis, as opposed to 94.4% efficacy with 1% hydrocortisone cream.[17] Though not as good as hydrocortisone, ketoconazole serves as an effective steroid sparing agent. The calcineurin inhibitors tacrolimus and pimecrolimus are macrolide immunosuppressants that are alternative agents for use on the face, to again reduce the use of steroids in this sensitive area. A 2008 randomized prospective controlled study comparing 1% pimecrolimus cream and 2% ketoconazole cream showed equal efficacy between the two, but there were greater side effects with pimecrolimus.[18] Side effects included burning, itching, and redness. Both tacrolimus and pimecrolimus have a black box label by the U.S. Food and Drug Administration (FDA) warning of skin cancer or lymphoma formation in some patients using this drug, though an established link remains controversial.[19] Shampoos with ketoconazole, selenium sulfide, salicylic acid, zinc pyrithione, or tar are also effective for seborrheic dermatitis in hair-bearing regions.[20]

Pruritus

Elderly patients often experience localized or generalized pruritus, which can be severe. The cause of itching in elderly patients is often difficult to determine. Renal, hematologic, endocrine, cholestatic, allergic, infectious, and malignant causes all potentially contribute to the elderly patient's itch.[21,22] Some of these are addressed here (Table 95-1).

Physiologically, specific C-fiber neurons that terminate at the dermoepidermal junction transmit the itch sensation to the brain. These fibers possess receptors sensitive to histamine, neuropeptide substance P, serotonin, bradykinin, proteases, and endothelin. Rubbing or scratching further stimulates these receptors.[23] As the itch and scratch cycle progresses; the skin is driven to a point of barrier function compromise, which is worrisome in elderly patients with limited means of self-care.

Table 95-1. Systemic Diseases Causing Pruritus

Uremia
Cholestasis
Pregnancy
Cancers (including lymphoma, leukemia, and multiple myeloma)
Polycythemia vera
Thyroid disease
Iron deficiency anemia
Diabetes mellitus
HIV infection
Multiple sclerosis
Drug hypersensitivity
Psychogenic causes
Senile pruritus
Sjögren's syndrome
Carcinoid syndrome
Dumping syndrome

Pruritus is one of the most distressing concerns of a patient suffering from cholestasis. The exact cause of pruritus in this disease is unknown, though an altered role of opioid receptor function has been suggested.[24] Treatment of the underlying disease process often resolves itching. However, some diseases, such as primary biliary cirrhosis (PBC), cannot easily be cured. Ursodeoxycholic acid (UDCA) treatment for PBC often does not resolve the patient's pruritus.[25] Cholestyramine, rifampin, naloxone, and phenobarbital are other agents utilized for pruritus, all of which have substantial side effects in the elderly.[26]

Generalized pruritus is recognized as a key marker of underlying malignancy, particularly lymphomas and leukemias.[27] Generalized pruritus is noted in up to 30% of patients with Hodgkin's disease and may be the only presenting symptom.[28,29] Pruritus is also a noted feature of multiple myeloma, polycythemia rubra vera, Waldenström's macroglobulinemia, and malignant carcinoid.[30]

Pruritus is best resolved by identifying and treating the underlying systemic etiology. Unfortunately, nonspecific therapies must often be employed for elderly patients with atypical disease presentation. Emollients are valuable interventions regardless of suspected etiology, as some level of pruritus exacerbating xerosis is present in most elderly patients. Topical use of alcohol, hot water, or harsh soaps and scrubbing must be discouraged. Proper humidity, cool compresses, nail trimming, and behavior therapy may all improve the itch and scratch cycle.[23] Topical anesthetics such as benzocaine and dibucaine have been utilized for relief. A trial of oilated soap and antihistamines may also be helpful before an invasive workup, including hematologic studies, imaging for malignancy, skin biopsy, skin scrapings, skin culture, and HIV tests.[30] Antihistamines should be used with caution as they are not universally effective and may cause sedation in the vulnerable and often highly medicated elderly patient.

Vascular-related disease

STASIS DERMATITIS

Stasis dermatitis is a common condition affecting 15 to 20 million patients over age 50 in the United States.[31] It often presents as a circumscribing dermatitis around the calf and ankle in patients with chronic venous insufficiency and venous hypertension. However, any body area constantly under pressure against a hard surface may be impacted. Pitting edema may be present in addition to loss of hair, waxy appearance and yellow-brown pigmentation.[32] If untreated, stasis dermatitis may progress to a chronic nonhealing wound with erythema and oozing. Stasis dermatitis results from poor function of the deep venous system in the legs, which leads to backflow and hypertension in the superficial venous system.[33] Often both lower legs show stasis dermatitis. An associated self-perpetuating cutaneous inflammatory response follows.[33] Workup includes venous Doppler studies to identify flow in the involved venous plexus.

Several treatment approaches are useful in resolving stasis dermatitis. Compression of the legs to control superficial venous hypertension is critical. This can be achieved by the use of Unna boots, compression stockings, or elastic wraps. In one study of more than 3000 patients, those with stasis dermatitis had a compliance of 46% for the use of compression stockings.[34] Leg elevation 6 inches above the level of the heart during sleep also improves blood flow. Topical treatments include corticosteroids and the calcineurin inhibitors, pimecrolimus and tacrolimus. Corticosteroids have an associated risk of tachyphylaxis and must be used carefully because of the high risk of infection in these patients.[35,36] Topical antibiotics such as bacitracin, neomycin, or polymyxin B may be added if there is evidence of skin barrier compromise and infection.

For more information on stasis ulcers please refer to Chapter 38.

CHERRY ANGIOMAS (CHERRY HEMANGIOMAS, CAMPBELL DE MORGAN SPOTS)

Cherry angiomas are the most common vascular proliferations of the skin and are nearly ubiquitous after age 30. They appear as firm, smooth, and red colored papules ranging in size from 0.5 mm to 5 mm. They may also appear as a myriad of tiny spots resembling petechiae. Though patients may be concerned with a new cherry angioma, the condition is benign. Cosmetic concern may merit electrocautery or laser coagulation treatment.[37]

VENOUS LAKES

Venous lakes are dark blue to violet colored papules that occur on sun-exposed areas of elderly patients. They are compressible lesions common on the face, lips, and ears. The differential diagnosis includes blue nevus and malignant melanoma. Venous lakes are benign lesions and treatment is for cosmetic purposes or bleeding. Electrodesiccation, excision, or lasers may be used to remove venous lakes.[38]

Infectious diseases

HERPES ZOSTER (SHINGLES)

Herpes zoster (shingles) is a reactivation of the varicella-zoster virus, the causative agent of varicella. It is a significant ailment of the geriatric population, constituting 690 to 1600 cases per 100,000 person-years in the 60-and-older age group.[39–41] The varicella zoster virus remains latent in the dorsal root ganglia of the nervous system after its initial infection usually resolves in childhood.[42,43] A weakening or impaired immune system is thought to precede reactivation, so underlying conditions such as lymphoma, leukemia, and possible HIV disease should be considered. Local steroid injection has also been associated with a herpes zoster flare.[44] Herpes zoster begins as a prodromal sharp pain localized to a dermatomal region, followed by a rash and vesicular eruption. Itching, burning, and weakness of muscles associated with the involved nerve may be noted. More than 20 vesicles outside of the primary dermatome suggest disseminated zoster, as may be seen in immunocompromised patients[45] or patients with granulocytic lesions. The long-lasting pain of zoster may be mistaken for gallbladder, kidney, or cardiac pain depending on location. Chronic pain or chronic pruritus localized to the dermatome may follow. These are known as postherpetic neuralgia (PHN) or postherpetic itch, respectively.[46]

Herpes zoster is diagnosed by a Tzanck smear of a sample scraped from the base of an intact vesicle. Appearance of multinucleated giant cells may indicate a herpetic infection. Treatment of herpes zoster includes early antiviral therapy, within 72 hours of onset. Acyclovir is a safe but variably efficacious agent, though famciclovir is also used. In one double-blind, randomized group study of 55 patients, it was found that famciclovir was well tolerated and had a more favorable adverse event profile than acyclovir.[47] Valacyclovir is an L-valanine ester form of acyclovir and is converted to acyclovir in vivo. It provides three to five times the oral bioavailability of acyclovir and has been shown in clinical trials to better reduce pain severity.[48] In 2006, the FDA approved the use of zoster vaccine live (Zostavax) for the prevention of shingles in immunocompetent patients over 60 years of age. According to the multicenter Shingles Prevention Study, vaccine administration reduces incidence, burden, and PHN complications in elderly patients.[49] Oral antibiotics covering staphylococci and streptococci are used to control secondary infection.[42]

PHN is most evident in the elderly, and 10% to 18% of zoster patients develop this neuralgia according to a community-based study in the United States.[50] Treatment is more challenging for PHN and requires concomitant use of pain medication, such as topical capsaicin. Prompt prescription of analgesia, recommended when zoster is still active, often reduces long-term negative outcomes for PHN.[51]

SCABIES

Scabies is among the oldest recognized infections to occur in humans, with more than 300 million yearly cases detected worldwide.[52,53] A U.K.-based study showed an incidence of 788 per 100,000 person-years of scabies.[54] Risk factors include nursing home residence, especially older (>30 years) and poorly staffed (>10:1 bed to health care provider) institutions.

The causative agent for scabies is the mite, *Sarcoptes scabiei*, whose life span is about 1 month. Transmission requires direct skin contact or indirect contact with bedding or clothing. Once the pregnant female mite is on a new host, she digs into the skin to lay eggs. The eggs, saliva, feces, and the mites themselves lead to a delayed type IV hypersensitivity reaction from 2 to 6 weeks after contact so that, at onset, multiple lesions are typically seen. These immune reactions lead to intense pruritus. In previously infected patients, the immune system response may present in 1 to 4 days after contact.[55]

Scabies manifests as papules, pustules, burrows, nodules, and also urticarial plaques. Severe pruritus impacts most patients unless they are immunocompromised.[56] In the latter case, scabies may resemble psoriasis or a hyperkeratotic dermatosis. The infection is not life-threatening but is often debilitating and depressing. Common areas infected include the finger webs, wrists, waistline, axillary folds, genitalia, buttocks, and nipples.[57] An area of concern should be scraped and microscopically examined for mites. Early confirmation is imperative to avoid secondary infection and rapid spread in the susceptible nursing home environment.[58] Treatment includes permethrin cream or rinse, which should be applied to all areas of the body for an 8- to 14-hour period. Mild burning, stinging, and rash may develop. Lindane cream, crotamiton, and sulfur have been utilized previously but with less efficacy. Ivermectin is an alternative agent with the benefit of oral administration, but the FDA has not officially approved its use for scabetic infection.[56] It is particularly helpful in cases of scabetic resistance to permethrin, though cases of ivermectin resistance are also documented.[59,60] Pruritus and inflammation may be handled with steroids and antihistamines.[61]

PEDICULOSIS

Parasitic lice are known to infest hair-bearing areas of the human body. Louse infection, or pediculosis, affects up to 12 million Americans each year. The offending human agents include *Pediculosis humanus humanus*, *Pediculosis humanus capitis* (larger body louse), and *Phthirus pubis* (pubic louse).[62] Similar to scabies, transmission may be direct or indirect through brushes, clothing, or bedding. Higher levels of crowding increase transmission rates, as seen in some nursing homes. Pathogenesis involves deposition of eggs (nits) on hair shafts and subsequent hatching under conditions of 70% humidity and temperatures of 28°C or higher.[61]

The main symptom of lice infestation is pruritus.[21] Bite reactions, excoriations, lymphadenopathy, and conjunctivitis are other possible manifestations. Hair combing may be associated with a "singing" sound because of the interaction of the tines with the nits. Red bumps on the scalp that progress to crusting and oozing are noted in *Pediculosis humanus capitis*. Pediculosis is further complicated by the potential of co-transported infections. Diagnosis is established by visualization of the lice or nits. This often requires a good light source and use of a comb to expose the hair. The difficult-to-remove nits on the hair shafts appear as white specks on examination.[62] Prevention is the best way to address lice infestations, such as avoiding continued contact with an infested individual. Chemical pediculicides—including permethrin, malathion, lindane, pyrethrin—are the main treatment modalities. These treatments should be repeated every 7 to 10 days and, because of increasing resistance, must often be rotated.[63] "Bug busting" with a wet comb and conditioner has limited efficacy. Dimethicone has recently been shown to treat pediculosis in a randomized controlled study where 69% of patients were cured, and only 2% had irritant reactions.[64] More studies are necessary for widespread recommendation of this treatment. All family members and contact persons should be included in therapy and prevention during patient treatment.

ONYCHOMYCOSIS

Fungal infections are among the most prevalent integumentary concerns in the elderly, and onychomycosis is a leading entity. Defined as a fungal infection involving the nail and nail plate, over 90% of onychomycosis is attributable to dermatophytes, known as *tinea unguium*, and 10% to nondermatophytic molds or *Candida*. The prevalence of onychomycosis has been estimated at almost 6.5% in the overall Canadian population.[65] Studies have shown that onychomycosis increases with age, possibly because of poor circulation, diabetes, trauma, weakened immunity, poor hygiene, and inactivity.[66] Some studies have shown the prevalence of onychomycosis in patients over 60 years of age to be 20%.[67]

Several classifications of onychomycosis exist, including distal-lateral subungual, superficial white, candidal, and proximal subungual. Distal-lateral subungual onychomycosis is the clinically most common type, often caused by *Trichophyton rubrum* invasion of the hyponychium, the white area at the distal edge of the nail plate. The nails become yellow and thick with parakeratosis and hyperkeratosis leading to subungual thickening and onycholysis. Superficial white onychomycosis is often associated with HIV infection and appears as a chalklike white plaque on the dorsum of the nail.[68] The proximal subungual type is also relatively uncommon and may present in either immunocompetent or immunocompromised patients. In this case, the infection penetrates near the cuticle and migrates distally resulting in hyperkeratosis, leukonychia, and onycholysis. *Trichophyton rubrum* is again the most causative agent. Candidal onychomycosis is seen in patients with chronic mucocutaneous candidiasis.[66]

A patient history, physical examination, microscopy, and culture are all critical to diagnosis. Onychomycosis is best diagnosed by clipping the toenail very proximally and scraping the newly exposed subungual debris for laboratory evaluation. Toenails are 25 times more likely to be infected than fingernails.[66] Typical presentation involves two feet and one hand (the dominant hand of a patient).

Treatment options include topical and systemic medications along with surgical approaches. A surgical trimming and debridement may be effective initially. Systemic therapy includes griseofulvin, fluconazole, itraconazole, or terbinafine.[69] Multiple double-blind controlled studies have shown terbinafine to be more effective than fluconazole or itraconazole for dermatophyte infections.[70–75] Systemic antifungals may have significant contraindications in patients on other medications. Topical treatments have poorer penetration and thus are less effective. Newer treatments are being investigated, such as AN-2690 by Anacor Pharmaceuticals, which allows for deeper penetration of topical therapy.[76]

Cutaneous cancer

KEY POINTS
Skin Cancer

- Current rates suggest that one in five people in the United States will develop skin cancer in his or her lifetime.
- Basal cell carcinoma is the most common type of skin cancer and the one least likely to metastasize.
- Melanoma comprises 4% of skin cancers, and suspicion is guided by ABCDE criteria (asymmetry, border irregularity, color variegation, depth, and evolution of lesion).
- Actinic keratosis is considered to be a precancerous form of squamous cell carcinoma, though its classification as malignant neoplasm is debated.
- All patients would use a dermatologist-recommended sunscreen appropriate for their skin type and should avoid sun exposure during the peak hours of sunlight.

Skin cancer is an increasingly important public health issue for the geriatric population. Current rates demonstrate that one in five people in the United States develop skin cancer at some point in their lifetime, with melanoma incidence increasing faster than any other cancer worldwide.[77] The economic burden of skin cancer is substantial in the United States.[77] The risk of skin cancer has been related to ultraviolet exposure, which has varying roles in basal cell carcinoma, squamous cell carcinoma, and melanoma pathogenesis. The use of sunblock, avoidance of peak hours of sunlight, and proper clothing are simple preventive measures all patients, young and old, can follow. Early detection is critical in the elderly patient, as a 100% cure rate is possible.[78]

ACTINIC KERATOSIS

Actinic keratosis (AK), or solar keratosis, may be defined as a premalignant precursor of squamous cell carcinoma or an incipient cutaneous squamous cell carcinoma.[79] There are about 5.2 million physician visits annually for AKs in the United States, 60% by the Medicare population.[80] These precancers are most common in light-skinned populations with year-round sun exposure who have not used appropriate sunscreens. Areas most affected include the forehead, scalp, ears, lower lip, forearms, and dorsal aspect of the hands.[81]

AK development is attributable to ultraviolet (UV) radiation-induced DNA mutation in select keratinocyte genes. With time, AKs may develop into invasive squamous cell carcinomas. They appear as small, skin-colored to yellowish-brown macules or papules, often with a dry adherent scale. They may feel rough to palpation, reminiscent of sandpaper, though are asymptomatic in most patients.[82] If an AK becomes painful, indurated, eroded, or greatly erythematous, squamous cell carcinoma transformation must be highly suspect. AKs may also proliferate and become exophytic so as to constitute a "cutaneous horn." This is particularly evident on the ear.[83] Treatment for few and discrete AKs is best performed with cryosurgery (liquid nitrogen), which approaches near 100% effectiveness and is convenient and economical. Topical treatment includes 5-fluorouracil, imiquimod, diclofenac, and photodynamic therapy with a light-sensitizing compound.[81] Sun safety practice is helpful for prevention, such as proper coverage and limited outdoor activity between 10 AM and 4 PM.

SQUAMOUS CELL CARCINOMA

Squamous cell carcinoma (SCC) is a cancer arising from the epithelium, with an estimated 200,000 cases diagnosed each year.[84] SCC is often separated into two groups based on malignant potential. The more common type develops from sun-damaged skin and AKs and is less likely to metastasize. For people in this group, the lifetime risk of having SCC after developing a single AK is between 6% and 10%.[85] The more aggressive type arises from areas of prior radiation or thermal exposure, chronic drains, chronic ulcers (Marjolin's ulcer), and mucosal surfaces. In general, prolonged UV radiation exposure induces DNA damage and subsequent carcinogenesis in select keratinocytes leading to SCC formation.[81]

SCCs arising from AKs often appear with a thick adherent scale. The tumor is soft to hard, locally movable, and has an erythematous, inflamed base. SCCs are frequently found on the same areas noted for AKs. If a SCC is diagnosed on a mucous membrane or on non-sun-damaged skin, it may be aggressive and can rapidly metastasize to regional lymph nodes. An SCC described as firm, movable, and elevated with minimal scale and a sharp border is usually derived from actinically damaged skin but not typically from a precursor AK. The differential diagnosis for SCC is wide, including seborrheic keratosis, melanocytic nevus, AK, and chromomycosis. Diagnosis is established by skin biopsy. When SCC is in situ, it is commonly known as Bowen's disease.[81] However, what Bowen originally described is slightly different and includes the presence of large atypical cells ("Bowen's cells") within the lesion.[86] Smaller SCCs are treated with electrodesiccation and curettage, whereas larger tumors in sensitive locations such as the face are often best handled with Mohs micrographic surgery. Other treatment options include radiation therapy, carbon dioxide laser, and oral 5-fluorouracil for refractory lesions.[87]

KERATOACANTHOMA

Keratoacanthomas (KAs) are a common and distinct neoplasm with a histologic pattern resembling SCC, thus challenging the diagnosis. They are often found in sun-exposed areas of light-skinned elderly patients, peaking at ages 50 to 70 years and increasing in incidence with advancing age.[88,89] The face, forearms, and hands are frequently afflicted sites, though any area is possible. The etiology of KAs is unknown, though they are likely derived from hair follicles, with UV light, chemical carcinogens, immunocompromised status, and viruses contributory to incidence and progression. KAs are usually solitary and appear as firm, round, skin-colored or erythematous dome-shaped papules. They often have a central umbilication with a keratin plug. Diagnosis is best established by incorporating affected tissue with normal lateral tissue in a biopsy specimen so as to help distinguish SCC from KA. KAs grow rapidly in a period of 2 weeks but may slowly involute over a period as long as 1 year if no intervention is implemented.[90] The primary therapy for KA remains surgical excision.

BASAL CELL CARCINOMA

Basal cell carcinomas (BCCs) are the most common type of cancer in pale-skinned individuals. It is estimated that more than 1 million new diagnoses are made each year in the United States, comprising 25% of all cancers diagnosed.[91] People who burn easily and severely in the sun without tanning are those at greatest risk for BCC. Fortunately, BCC only rarely metastasizes and is better described as a local infiltrator, with the potential of destroying underlying structures if unattended. However, our group and others have described a rare variant of facial BCC that is extremely aggressive and rapidly involves deep tissue, especially bone. Ultraviolet light exposure is the main etiologic agent, but x-rays, thermal injury, and scars may all contribute to BCC formation.[92]

There are five major subtypes of BCC. Noduloulcerative BCC is the most common with a pearly dome-shaped nodule, central umbilication, and telangiectatic border. This type enlarges slowly, with a 4-mm-sized tumor taking years to develop. Pigmented BCCs may display a uniform dark pigment and can resemble melanoma. Cystic BCCs are uncommon and are described as bluish gray cystic nodules. Superficial BCCs are flat plaques with pearly translucency and thin borders. This subtype is most common on the trunk, unlike the high occurrence on the face of other subtypes. Sclerosing BCCs appear as fibrosing and infiltrating plaques. When these resemble a scar, it is often an ominous sign of deep invasiveness.[92] Such "morpheiform" BCC must be excised with wide margins.

After biopsy-proven diagnosis, several treatment options are available. These include cryotherapy, curettage and electrodesiccation, radiotherapy, and excisional or Mohs micrographic surgery. For carefully selected thin and small BCCs, topical treatment options include imiquimod and 5-fluorouracil. A 2004 study of 5% imiquimod cream for superficial BCCs showed clearance rates near 75% based on clinical and histologic examination.[93]

MELANOMA

Melanoma, a malignancy of melanocytes, comprises 4% of all skin cancers but is the leading cause of skin cancer deaths worldwide.[94] According to the American Cancer Society, cutaneous melanoma accounts for 60,000 cases but about 9,000 deaths annually. Melanoma incidence per year peaks at 30 to 50 years of age. The median age of diagnosis is 59 years, with 19.5% of cases diagnosed between 55 and 64 years of age; 17.8% diagnosed between 65 and 74 years of age; 16.4% diagnosed between 75 and 84 years of age; and 5.5% diagnosed at older than 85 years of age. The median age for death is 68 years, with 15% dying between 45 and 54 years of age; 18.8% dying between 55 and 64 years of age; 21.3% dying between 65 and 74 years of age; 23.6% dying between 75 and 84 years of age; and 11.0% dying when older than 85 years of age. Incidence is 18.5 to 28.5 per 100,000 for white persons and 0.9 to 1.1 per 100,000 for black persons for all types of melanoma.[95] Malignant melanoma formation is a multistep process of mutations with risk factors including blistering tendencies in the sun, high number of dysplastic moles, actively changing mole, family history of melanoma, previous history of melanoma, and older age.[96]

There are several subtypes of melanoma. Superficial spreading melanoma is characterized as a flat or slightly elevated dark brown lesion with variegate colors. Nodular melanoma manifests as a rapidly growing dark brown or black papule or nodule that is at risk for ulceration and bleeding. Both are common on the trunk and legs.[96] Lentigo maligna is a slower-growing subtype on the rise in the United States, which when invasive is called lentigo maligna melanoma.[97] It is found on chronically sun-damaged areas of the head, also on the neck and arms with a peak incidence at 65 years of age. It is characterized as a brown to tan colored macule with possible areas of hypopigmentation and later raised blue-black nodules with dermal invasion. The last major subtype, acral melanoma, is the least common, comprising 2% to 8% of all melanomas in lightly pigmented people and 29% to 72% in darkly pigmented people. Although the proportion is higher in dark-skinned individuals, the incidence is similar across all skin types.[98] Acral melanomas are noted on the palms, soles, and subungual areas and thus are more difficult to identify with late diagnosis leading to poor outcome. They most often appear dark brown to black with irregular borders. The subungual type may show Hutchinson's sign, or proximal nail fold dark pigmentation.[99] Two percent to 8% of all melanomas are amelanotic, showing no pigmentation.[96]

Diagnosis involves a proper history and physical examination, along with lymph node evaluation. The ABCDE criteria frequently mentioned is a useful tool during the initial examination, and all components must be used in concert to establish a level of suspicion. The mnemonic stands for asymmetry, border irregularity, color variegation, diameter and evolution or change over time. A biopsy with pathologic confirmation is essential to rule out mimicking lesions such as pyogenic granuloma and pigmented basal cell carcinoma. After biopsy-confirmed diagnosis and evaluation for metastasis, the primary mode of treatment is surgery.[96]

ANGIOSARCOMA

Angiosarcomas are rare and malignant neoplasms of endothelial origin. The age-adjusted incidence for soft tissue sarcoma was 3.1 per 100,000 men and women per year in the 2000–2004 period, with angiosarcomas constituting 4.1% of such sarcomas.[100,101] Angiosarcomas have a peak incidence in the seventh decade, though any age group may be affected. Cutaneous angiosarcoma of the scalp and face is the most common form and appears as an enlarging bruise, dark blue to black nodule, or unhealed ulceration. After biopsy and staging, treatment remains challenging with a combination of surgery and radiation therapy most successful. Studies have demonstrated beneficial activity of paclitaxel and liposomal doxorubicin against angiosarcoma of the scalp and face.[102]

KAPOSI'S SARCOMA

Kaposi's sarcoma (KS) is a tumor of endothelial origin in which the classic form is usually found in men in their 60s. Human herpesvirus-8 is linked to the pathogenesis of all types of KS, including the classic form. Classic KS is found as a rare and indolent lesion in elderly men of Jewish and Mediterranean descent. Specifically, it represents about 0.2% of cancer in older American men of Mediterranean and Central-Eastern European (Ashkenazi) Jewish lineage in the United States.[103] In Israel, rates of classic KS of 2.07 in men and 0.75 in women per 100,000 persons were calculated.[104] Clinically, it is often apparent on the distal extremities as a bluish-red hematoma resembling a macule. It can develop into plaques and nodules and may become hyperkeratotic and ulcerate. The disease progresses slowly, and patients may live for decades with the tumor. Therefore, death in these patients may well be from other causes of aging.[104] In localized disease, treatment can be handled with radiotherapy and intralesional chemotherapy. System-wide chemotherapy, including agents such as doxorubicin, vincristine, and etoposide, are helpful in metastasized or aggressive KS. Immunotherapy including imiquimod, interferon-α and sirolimus have been utilized, but specific health concerns of each elderly patient need to be carefully addressed.[105,106] Other types of KS, including those in immunocompromised and AIDS patients, do not occur preferentially in the elderly.

Bullous pemphigoid

Bullous pemphigoid is an autoimmune blistering disease primarily of the elderly. The average age of affected patients is 65 years, and incidence reports vary by region.[107,108] Rates of 0.7 cases per 100,000 have been reported in Germany in 1995 and up to 4.3 cases per 100,000 in the United Kingdom in 2008.[108,109] The disease is characterized by large tense bullae on an erythematous base on flexor areas of the extremities, axillae, groin, and abdomen. Clear or sanguineous exudates exist in these bullae. The size can range from half a centimeter to 7 centimeters. Postinflammatory pigmentary changes may follow rupture of these bullae. Mucosal lesions are rare but heal quickly if present. There have been associations of bullous pemphigoid with other autoimmune conditions such as psoriasis, diabetes mellitus, and rheumatoid arthritis.[110]

Consistent with its autoimmune etiology, IgG and C3 have been demonstrated in the epidermal basement membrane of bullous pemphigoid. IgG autoantibodies specifically bind to hemidesmosome adhesion complexes (components BP180 and BP230) of the basement membrane.[111] A subepidermal blister forms with eosinophils, and possible lymphocytes, histiocytes, and neutrophils. Diagnosis is established with clinical and histologic contribution. A fresh blister biopsy shows eosinophils in a subepidermal cleft, whereas direct immunofluorescence demonstrates IgG or C3 linearly deposited at the basement membrane zone.[110]

Topical or systemic corticosteroids are used for treatment, with systemic therapy most effective for multiple lesion disease.[112] Before the start of systemic corticosteroids, tetracyclines, with possible niacinamide, may be explored for mild to moderate disease.[112]

The use of steroids in elderly patients should be coupled with calcium and vitamin D to help prevent osteoporosis complications. Supplemental anti-inflammatory agents such as dapsone are useful for tapering steroid doses. Dapsone therapy requires close evaluation of liver and bone marrow function as well as ruling out glucose-6-phosphate dehydrogenase deficiency, and the adverse effect profile is severe. Other ancillary treatments include azathioprine, methotrexate,[113] chlorambucil, cyclosporine, cyclophosphamide, plasmapheresis, and mycophenolate mofetil.[112,114] The effectiveness of plasma exchange or azathioprine as adjuncts has not been concluded.[112] Methotrexate is an excellent option in patients according to a 2008 Swedish study of 138 patients comparing methotrexate, prednisone, methotrexate plus prednisone, and topical steroid groups.[115]

Bullous pemphigoid may be fatal if appropriate treatment is not administered. The main predictors of poor prognosis include old age, female gender, associated chronic morbidities, and poor hygiene.[116,117] Mortality rates from 19% to 43% have been reported in some studies, and death may be related to chronic high-dose steroid use.[116,118–120]

Systemic concerns of the elderly with cutaneous complications

DIABETES MELLITUS

Diabetes mellitus (DM) is an endocrine disease of epidemic proportions in the United States. The Centers for Disease Control in a 2005 study showed that individuals over 60 years had a diabetes prevalence of 20.9%.[121] Diabetes manifests in many organ systems including the nervous, renal, ocular, integumentary, and cardiovascular. Elderly patients suffer greatly from complications such as functional disability, depression, cognitive impairment, injury, and urinary incontinence.

Diabetic dermopathy, also known as shin spots, is found in 9% to 55% of diabetics.[121–125] It appears as round slightly indented patches of brown to purplish skin. Diabetic dermopathy is the most common cutaneous complication of DM and suggests advanced internal disease of the heart, liver, or kidney.[122]

Diabetes mellitus is the cause of the greatest number of nontraumatic amputations in the United States. This is a result of nonhealing ulcers in diabetics with long-standing neuropathy and reduced pain sensation. Up to 25% of diabetics suffer from leg ulcers in their lifetime.[126] Proper and frequent examination of the feet and immediate treatment of ulcers is a critical component of diabetic patient care.

Perforating dermatosis is a condition found in diabetics who suffer from severe renal disease or in patients with chronic renal failure alone. This condition presents as hyperkeratotic, pruritic, and umbilicated papules and nodules on the extensor surfaces of the legs, trunk, and face.[127]

Acanthosis nigricans is probably the most recognized dermatologic sign of diabetes. It reflects insulin resistance and is common among the obese. This is a diffuse, darkened, and velvet-like thickening seen on the skin of the neck, axilla, groin, umbilicus, hands, submammary area, and areola. In exuberant form, this condition can also be a signal of internal malignancy; thus, thorough examination is critical.[27]

Necrobiosis lipoidica diabeticorum presents as a red papule that grows peripherally, becomes atrophic in the center, assuming an "apple-jelly"–like coloration, and eventually appears telangiectatic and porcelain like. Though rare, a striking 75% of patients with necrobiosis lipoidica have or will be diagnosed with diabetes.[128] Patients may respond to topical or intralesional corticosteroids among other medications, but strict diabetes management does not improve the papules of necrobiosis lipoidica.

THYROID DISEASE

Thyroid diseases, including hypo- and hyperthyroidism, impact up to 20% of elderly patients[129] Cutaneous manifestations of thyroid disease also depend on over- or underproduction of thyroid hormones. There is an increased incidence of alopecia areata and vitiligo associated with autoimmune thyroid disease.

Characteristic features of hyperthyroidism include palmar erythema, warm and moist skin, and fragile scalp hair or alopecia. These signs are often useful for diagnosis. Pretibial myxedema is a specific dermopathy of hyperthyroidism in Grave's disease (an antibody-mediated autoimmune thyroid reaction). Firm, nonpitting, nodules or plaques form on both legs in an asymmetric pattern. The color may be pink, purple, or fleshlike.[130] An accumulation of mucopolysaccharides in the dermis is suspected to lead to this appearance. These signature features of hyperthyroidism should trigger appropriate diagnosis and treatment of the underlying disease process. Hypothyroidism is a condition occurring in about 10% of females and 2% of males over 60 years of age.[131] It manifests with a cutaneous feature of myxedema that is more prolonged and diffuse. In advanced cases, the overall appearance of the skin becomes dry, scaly, and yellowish with sparse hair.[131] With progressing myxedema, the face may also appear flat and expressionless. Palmoplantar keratoderma, or hyperkeratosis on the palms and soles, is possible in severe cases. Hair and fingernails are prone to break as well.[129] Onycholysis, or separation of the nail plate from the nail bed, is found in patients with thyrotoxicosis and hypothyroidism but decreases in incidence in patients over 60 years of age.[130]

RENAL/ADRENAL DISEASE

Cushing's syndrome and Addison's disease are two conditions of the adrenal gland with cutaneous manifestations. In Cushing's disease, the main cause of Cushing's syndrome, there is hypersecretion of adrenocorticotropic hormone (ACTH).[132] ACTH levels may rise from neoplasms of the pituitary gland or from ectopic neoplasms such as oat cell lung cancer.[133] The primary clinical features include hypertension and weight gain. A "buffalo hump" or redistribution of fat to the upper back is evident, along with purple striae on the torso. Hypertrichosis, excessive bruising, poor wound healing, and hirsutism are additional complications.[132] In Addison's disease, autoimmune destruction of the adrenals leads to adrenocortical insufficiency. The main dermatologic feature is hyperpigmentation of skin creases, new scars, the vermilion border, nipple, and areas of constant pressure.[133] The mechanism is attributable to the stimulation of melanocytes by ACTH or the closely related melanocyte-stimulating hormone (MSH). This darkening of the skin may be the presenting feature.[134]

Chronic kidney disease (CKD) is a life-threatening condition affecting more than a third of patients 70 years of age and older according to the National Health and Nutrition Examination Survey.[135] Cutaneous examination of patients has shown that 50% to 100% have at least one dermatologic symptom.[136] The list of cutaneous sequelae is extensive, including pruritus, xerosis, ischemic ulcerations, prurigo nodularis, calcinosis cutis, calciphylaxis, Kyrle disease, bullous disease of dialysis, and nephrogenic fibrosing dermopathy. The majority of these improve with appropriate renal management.

Pruritus and xerosis have been attributed to uremia in CKD patients.[137–139] Pruritus may be local or generalized, mild or severe, or episodic or constant. Evidently, it is highly patient specific with no demographic biases.[136] Both xerosis and pruritus may improve with kidney disease management, with xerosis specifically responding to emollients.[139] Calcinosis cutis is the result of insoluble calcium deposition in the skin, appearing as multiple, firm, whitish papules, plaques, or nodules. They may ulcerate extruding a chalky white substance.[140] Calciphylaxis refers to vascular calcification with skin necrosis. Patients have firm painful lesions with central necrosis along a vascular track. These may begin initially as violaceous mottling.[141] Kyrle disease is the occurrence of widespread papules with central keratin and cellular debris plugs. It usually begins as a silvery scaled papule.[142] Bullous disease of dialysis resembles porphyria cutanea tarda with blistering and mechanical fragility of the skin in sun-exposed areas. The incidence is 1.2% to 9% in patients with CKD on hemodialysis.[143–146]

Nephrogenic fibrosing dermopathy is a condition with fibrosis of the skin and internal organs that is distinct but reminiscent of scleroderma. Large areas of indurated skin, brawny discoloration, and tightening occur. Nephrogenic fibrosing dermopathy occurs almost exclusively in patients with end-stage renal disease who have had imaging studies with gadolinium.[147]

NUTRITION

Proper nutrition, including daily recommended levels of essential vitamins and minerals, is critical in the elderly to prevent diseases with cutaneous manifestations such as scurvy and pellagra. Please find more information on these topics in Chapter 74.

MENOPAUSE

Menopause leads to significant changes in skin biology. On physical examination, the skin is thinner and less lubricated than premenopausal skin. The risk of infection is higher, and atrophy, pruritus, stiffness, alopecia, and dryness result.[148] Topical estrogen-based creams have shown some improvement in elasticity and moisturization. Specifically, collagen content and dermal thickness are improved with estrogen use after menopause.[149,150] The risks and benefits for each individual patient must be assessed before initiating therapy for moderate improvement.

TOBACCO USE

Tobacco use is a leading cause of preventable morbidity and mortality in the United States. In addition to risks of lung cancer, chronic obstructive pulmonary disease, and cardiac disease, the skin suffers significant damage from smoking. Early skin aging, SCC, melanoma, oral cancer, acne, and hair loss are some problems faced by long-term smokers. One study of 63 volunteers noted that a 35 pack-years smoking history led to a significantly greater skin furrow depth of the volar forearm when compared to non-smokers ($p < 0.05$).[151] A few specific signs of tobacco smoking include harlequin nail, which is a demarcation between the yellow and pink on the nail of a recent quitter. Smoker's face refers to a constellation of deep lines and furrows at right angles from the lips and corners of the eye, prominence of bony structures, and general graying of the skin. In vitro and epidemiologic evidence strongly support premature aging of skin from tobacco smoke.[152]

For a complete list of references, please visit online only at www.expertconsult.com

CHAPTER 96

Aging and Disorders of the Eye

Scott E. Brodie

Loss of vision, one of the most feared forms of medical disability, falls disproportionately on the elderly. Unfortunately, the damage to the delicate tissues of the eye from the various metabolic insults that may occur throughout life is generally cumulative. Consequently, most forms of ocular pathology occur ever more frequently, and in more debilitating forms, with increasing age.

Estimates of the prevalence of blindness from all causes vary by perhaps a factor of 13 between industrialized and Third World societies.[1] Nevertheless, regardless of the degree of economic development, the prevalence rate for blindness in any society is typically 100-fold greater among individuals over 65 years of age than among children in the same society.[2] In developed countries, the major causes of blindness are primarily cataract, glaucoma, and retinal disease (mostly macular degeneration and diabetic retinopathy), all of which are strongly related to advancing age.[3] In the Third World, the major causes of blindness are cataract, corneal scarring, glaucoma, and retinal disease.[4]

Delivery of adequate eye care to elderly individuals remains an unsolved problem, even in wealthy countries. Recent surveys in the United States have identified significant rates of untreated eye disease among the elderly. The nursing home population appears to be notably underserved.[5,6]

Discussion of age-related ocular problems is conveniently organized by considering the visual apparatus in anatomic order from anterior to posterior.

EYELIDS

The eyelids are vital for the proper circulation of tears and maintenance of the smooth ocular surface necessary for clear image formation by the eye. With increasing age, the skin of the eyelids, as elsewhere, loses elasticity, and the lids become more loosely apposed to the globe. Atrophy of the fascial planes within the eyelids may lead to herniation of the orbital fat into the lid tissue, producing the "bags under the eyes" frequently seen in the elderly (Figure 96-1). Atrophy or disinsertion of the aponeurosis of the levator palpebrae muscle, which ordinarily supports the upper eyelid, may cause the opened lid to fail to uncover the pupil, as seen in senile ptosis, despite normal levator muscle function (Figure 96-2; see also Plate 96-1). Senile ptosis must be differentiated from ptosis due to mechanical and neuromuscular causes, such as oculomotor nerve palsies and myasthenia gravis.[7]

Laxity of the lower lid may allow the free lid margin to rotate away from the eyeball, a condition known as ectropion (Figure 96-3). If severe, the lacrimal punctum may fail to make contact with the pool of tears adjacent to the lower lid. This prevents the normal conduction of tears into the lacrimal sac, which may result in persistent tearing (epiphora) even in the absence of lacrimal duct obstruction. More dangerous is entropion, in which a loosening of the adhesions between tissue planes in the lid allows the muscle tone of the orbicularis oculi to rotate the lid margin inward (Figure 96-4).[8] Frequently, the lashes come to rub directly against the cornea or conjunctiva, producing irritation or scarring.

The treatment of eyelid malpositions is generally surgical. For senile ptosis, resection of the levator aponeurosis is generally performed.[9] Ectropion and entropion are generally treated by resection of redundant lid tissue.[10]

Of the tumors of the eyelid skin, basal cell carcinomas are the most common. These tumors are frequently a consequence of lifetime exposure to sunlight. If the lesions are detected early, a curative local resection is often possible. In advanced cases, the tumor may cause massive destruction of facial structures by local extension. Metastases are very rare.[11]

LACRIMAL APPARATUS

The lacrimal apparatus consists of the lacrimal glands, which secrete the tears, and the lacrimal sac and ducts, which convey the tears into the nasal cavity. Secretory function of the lacrimal glands declines with age, and many elderly individuals develop "dry eye" syndrome. (This nonspecific reduction in tear production is much more common than the full-fledged Sjögren syndrome, which is an autoimmune disease process affecting both salivary and lacrimal secretion.[12]) Paradoxically, many tear-deficient patients complain of excess tearing, because the chronically irritated eyes may stimulate reflex tear production. Dry eyes are treated with artificial tear eyedrops, as often as needed. Some patients respond well to topical treatment with cyclosporin A.[13] In patients whose eyes dry out overnight, lubricant ointment at bedtime may be helpful. In severe cases, small silicone plugs may be placed to obstruct the lacrimal puncta,[14] or surgical

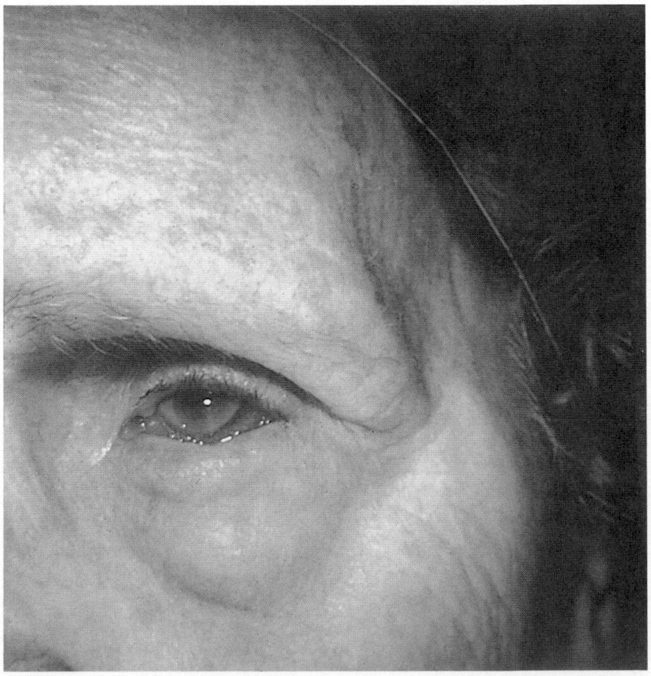

Figure 96-1. Prolapse of orbital fat through atrophic fascial planes in the eyelid produces "bags" under the eyes. *(Courtesy of Murray Meltzer, MD.)*

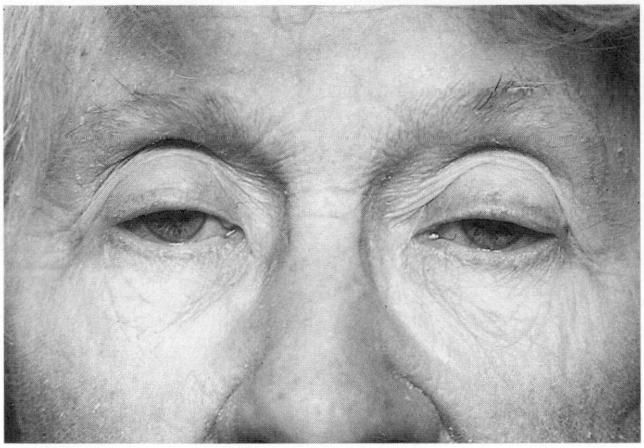

Figure 96-2. Senile ptosis. Note the low lid level and the loss of the normal lid folds. *(Courtesy of Murray Meltzer, MD.)*

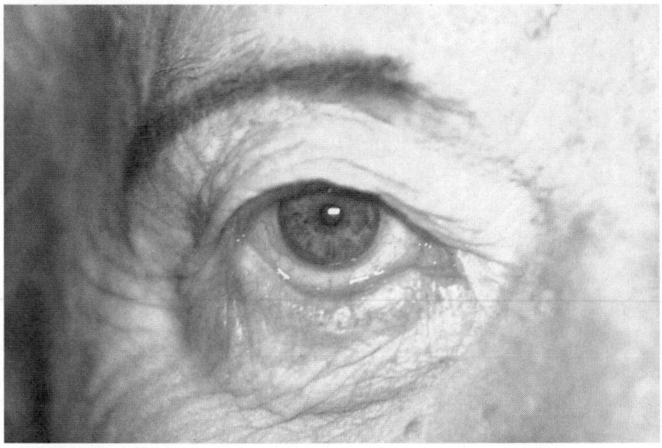

Figure 96-3. Ectropion. Laxity of the lower eyelid allows the lid margin to rotate away from the eyeball. *(Courtesy of Murray Meltzer, MD.)*

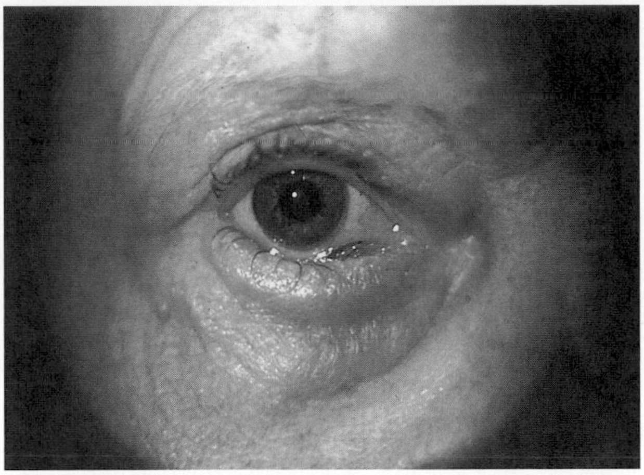

Figure 96-4. Entropion. Breakdown of the adhesion between the tissue planes in the eyelid allows the muscle tone of the orbicularis oculi muscle to rotate the lid margin inward. The eyelashes may chronically irritate the surface of the eyeball. *(Courtesy of Murray Meltzer, MD.)*

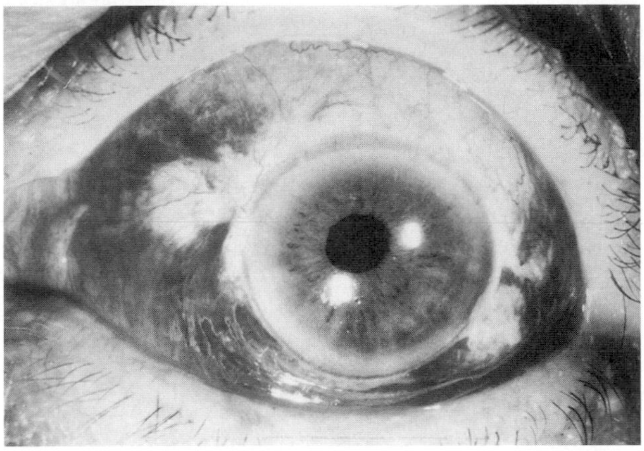

Figure 96-5. Subconjunctival hemorrhage. This small hematoma, seen through the transparent conjunctiva, is benign unless recurrent.

occlusion of the lacrimal puncta may be performed, in order to conserve the available tears.

Obstruction of the lacrimal ducts also leads to epiphora. Uncomplicated mechanical stenosis may occasionally be relieved with simple probing, but severe cases (often following bacterial infection of the lacrimal sac) are treated surgically: a dacryocystorhinostomy is performed to anastomose the mucosa of the nasal cavity to the lacrimal sac through an osteotomy made in the lacrimal bone.[15]

CONJUNCTIVA

Subconjunctival hemorrhage, a localized accumulation of blood seen between the conjunctiva and the globe, is frequently encountered in the elderly, either following minor trauma or occurring spontaneously (Figure 96-5; see also Plate 96-2). Such hemorrhages are rarely of any consequence, but they are often alarming in appearance. They resolve spontaneously without treatment over a period of several days. Occasionally, recurrent hemorrhages may suggest an underlying disease such as hypertension or a coagulation disorder.

Chronic exposure to sunlight, particularly at tropical latitudes, may cause a degeneration of the connective tissue in the exposed sector of the conjunctiva between the eyelids, leading to thickening of the conjunctiva (pingueculum), which may grow over the cornea from the periphery toward the pupil (pterygium). If the growth threatens to cover the visual axis, surgical excision may be indicated. Recurrence after surgery is, unfortunately, not uncommon.[16]

Tumors such as squamous cell carcinoma and melanoma may arise from the conjunctiva. Local excision and cryoablation may be adequate in early cases, but advanced cases may require orbital exenteration.[17]

CORNEA

The eye is unique in its requirement for transparent tissues, including the cornea and crystalline lens. The need for transparency places many constraints on the architecture and metabolism of these ocular structures. In particular, the eye must nourish these tissues with a cell-free fluid, as red blood cells preclude transparency. Similarly, the transparent tissues must rely primarily on anaerobic glycolytic metabolism, as the enzyme systems required for oxidative phosphorylation (aptly named cytochromes) strongly absorb visible light. Even in the absence of these absorbent components, the tissues must be constructed in a highly compact and regular manner, so that light scattering from tissue organelles does

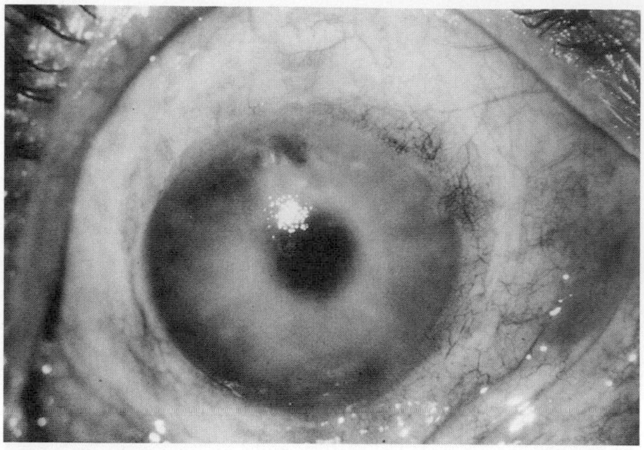

Figure 96-6. Corneal edema. The cornea is thickened and cloudy because of failure of the corneal endothelium to adequately dehydrate the tissue. *(Courtesy of Calvin Roberts, MD.)*

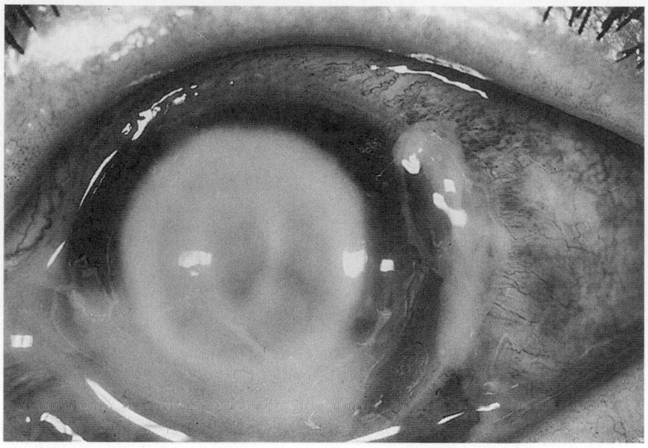

Figure 96-7. Corneal ulcer. A localized infection causes an epithelial defect and attracts an infiltrate of white blood cells. *(Courtesy of Michael Newton, MD.)*

not cause a white, opaque appearance. This requirement is met in the case of the cornea by a highly regular arrangement of collagen fibrils and an active metabolic pump in the corneal endothelial cell layer, which dehydrates the corneal stroma. (Absence of these tissue features explains why the sclera, which is otherwise histologically similar to the cornea, is opaque.[18])

The corneal endothelial cells, on which the dehydration critical for corneal transparency depends, do not divide during adulthood. Indeed, the endothelial cell density declines slowly with age.[19] If the number of endothelial cells falls below a critical level, the cornea imbibes fluid, swells, and becomes cloudy (Figure 96-6; see also Plate 96-3). Edema fluid percolates to the epithelial surface and may coalesce into subepithelial bullae. Mild cases may be managed with the use of hypertonic saline eyedrops and ointment to withdraw fluid from the cornea osmotically. If these measures fail, a corneal graft, which replaces the deficient endothelium, is necessary to restore vision.[20]

Bacterial ulcers of the cornea (Figure 96-7; see also Plate 96-4) seem to occur with greater frequency in the elderly, perhaps reflecting impairments of tear secretion, epithelial integrity, and cellular and humoral immunity, and are associated in the elderly with a poorer prognosis.[21] Intensive antibiotic therapy is generally required.[22]

The ring-shaped deposition of lipid in the far periphery of the cornea, referred to as *arcus senilis*, is completely benign.

UVEAL TRACT

The uveal tract (*uvea*) comprises the iris, ciliary body, and choroid, which form a continuous, highly vascular layer inside the sclera. Inflammation of the uvea occurs frequently: as a primary disease process, in response to infections, in many patients with rheumatic disease, and as a sequela to accidental or surgical trauma. Clinically, inflammatory cells are seen in the aqueous or vitreous humor. These inflammatory reactions can cause ocular injury by many mechanisms. They may occlude the trabecular meshwork, causing glaucoma. They may accumulate on the inner surface of the cornea as keratic precipitates, where they may injure or destroy the corneal endothelial cells and cause corneal edema. Inflamed tissues often develop pathologic adhesions, which may derange normal ocular function. Adhesions between the anterior surface of the peripheral iris and the anterior chamber angle (peripheral anterior synechiae) may occlude the trabecular meshwork, leading to chronic angle-closure glaucoma. Adhesions between the posterior surface of the iris and the anterior surface of the crystalline lens can seal off access of the aqueous humor to the anterior chamber (pupillary block), forcing the iris to bow forward (iris bombé). In cases where the peripheral iris becomes apposed to the trabecular meshwork, the egress of aqueous humor from the eye is blocked, resulting in angle-closure glaucoma. In the posterior segment, inflammatory cells in the vitreous humor may obscure vision and lead to fibrovascular proliferation that may distort the retina, or even cause a retinal detachment.

Treatment in most cases of uveitis is generally empirical. Dilation of the pupil with cycloplegic eyedrops is generally advisable to prevent posterior synechiae and pupillary block and to relieve the discomfort (photophobia) caused by light-induced miosis of the inflamed iris. If the inflammation is confined to the anterior segment, topical corticosteroid eyedrops are usually sufficient. In cases involving the posterior segment, periocular corticosteroid injections or systemic administration of corticosteroids are frequently required. Typically, workup for associated systemic disease is appropriate. If a treatable condition is discovered, such as syphilis or tuberculosis, specific treatment for the underlying condition may simultaneously cure the uveitis. In refractory cases, success may often be achieved with systemic administration of immunosuppressive drugs.[23]

Intraocular tumors in the elderly occur most frequently within the uveal tract. Melanomas are the most common primary tumor. Though prompt enucleation (surgical removal of the eyeball) was long the traditional management, many authorities now recommend that eyes containing small uveal melanomas be followed closely, rather than enucleated, as they have only a low propensity for metastasis.[24] Medium-sized tumors have been successfully treated in many cases with irradiation, either by temporary implantation of a radioactive plaque applied to the overlying sclera[25] or administered by external beam.[26] A large, prospective, clinical trial found no difference in 5-year survival between groups of patients randomized to treatment by radioactive plaque or by enucleation.[27] Primary enucleation is often

Major Causes of Blindness in the Elderly

In Developed Countries
- Cataract
- Glaucoma
- Diabetic retinopathy
- Macular degeneration

In Developing Countries
- Cataract
- Corneal scarring
- Glaucoma
- Diabetic retinopathy
- Macular degeneration

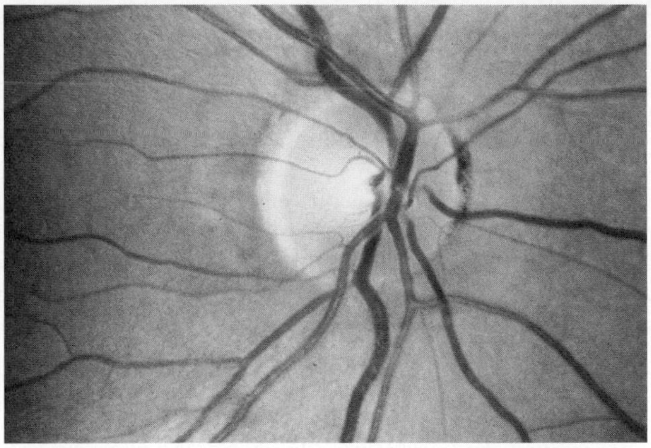

Figure 96-8. Normal optic nerve head. Cup-to-disc ratio is about 0.3.

recommended for large tumors. Metastatic melanoma is usually detected initially in the liver. Regular physical examinations and monitoring of hepatic enzyme activity in the serum are advisable for patients at risk.

Tumors metastatic to the choroid are actually more frequent than primary intraocular tumors. Lung primaries predominate in men, breast primaries in women.[28] As the eye is seldom the sole site of metastasis, these patients generally require systemic chemotherapy.

GLAUCOMA

Glaucoma is a form of progressive atrophy of the optic nerve, frequently associated with increased intraocular pressure (Figures 96-8 and 96-9; see also Plates 96-5 and 95-6).

Open-Angle Glaucoma

In many cases, the primary pathology is presumed to lie in the trabecular meshwork, the ring of porous tissue located in the anterior chamber angle through which aqueous humor drains from the eye. Impaired facility of aqueous outflow through the trabecular meshwork is generally idiopathic (so-called primary open-angle glaucoma). This condition is generally reported to increase in prevalence with increasing age, at least in most Western populations.[29] Loss of outflow facility may also arise from various insults to the trabecular meshwork, including trauma, uveitis, hemorrhage, and dispersion of intraocular pigment.

Visual impairment from open-angle glaucoma is generally insidious and chronic, with visual field damage occurring initially in the far periphery, where it is rarely noticeable except by formal testing. Our ability to diagnose this condition in its early stages is quite imperfect. The actual risk of visual field loss in untreated individuals with modestly elevated intraocular pressure is only 1% to 2% per year;[30] conversely, histologic studies have shown that as many as 40% of the optic nerve fibers must be destroyed before any abnormality of the visual field is detectable by standard techniques.[31]

Initial treatment is usually medical. The goal of therapy is to lower the intraocular pressure, with topical (or rarely, systemic) medications, to a level that is tolerated by the optic nerve, as demonstrated by the arrest of progressive visual field loss. Available medications include parasympathomimetic miotics (rarely used), anticholinesterase miotics

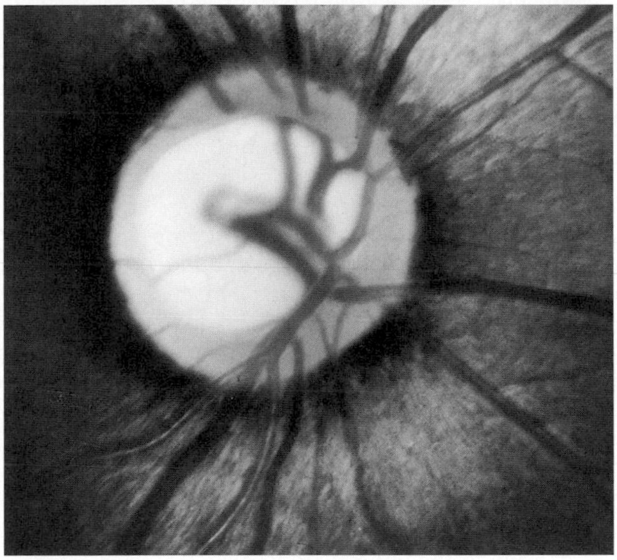

Figure 96-9. Glaucomatous optic nerve head cupping. Loss of neural tissue is seen as narrowing of the neural rim of the optic disc and enlargement of the central cup. (Compare with Figure 96-8.)

(rarely used), sympathomimetics, β-adrenergic blockers, carbonic anhydrase inhibitors, and prostaglandin analogs. The potential side effects of the various topical and systemic pressure-lowering drugs are occasionally serious, particularly in elderly patients (see Systemic Complications of Ophthalmic Medications, presented later). If medical treatment is unsuccessful or poorly tolerated, intraocular pressure may be further lowered by laser treatments to the trabecular meshwork or by "filtering surgery," which creates a fistula between the anterior chamber and the subconjunctival space, allowing easier egress of aqueous humor. Complications of filtering surgery may include hypotony, choroidal effusion, and cataract. Supplementary medical treatment after filtering surgery is may also be required. The optimal stage in the disease process for surgical intervention is unclear. Some authors have reported better long-term visual results with earlier surgery.[32] One large study suggests that laser treatment to the trabecular meshwork may also be suitable as initial therapy.[33]

Angle-Closure Glaucoma

Occasionally, alterations in intraocular anatomy may predispose the iris to cover the trabecular meshwork, suddenly preventing aqueous outflow and causing an acute elevation of the intraocular pressure. Common scenarios include adhesions between iris and lens (pupillary block), which may cause the iris to bow forward so as to occlude the trabecular meshwork, and dilation of the pupil, such as may occur spontaneously in the dark or following pharmacologic mydriasis. Gradual enlargement of the lens with increasing age or cataract formation is an important factor that predisposes the eye to this process in the elderly. Acute angle-closure glaucoma is generally a dramatic event, with symptoms including severe pain, blurring of vision, perception of colored haloes around lights, nausea, and vomiting. Diagnosis of acute angle closure is easy once attention is directed to the eye, but it may be missed if attention is diverted to the gastrointestinal symptoms. Cases have been reported from the emergency departments of general hospitals where concentration on the nausea and vomiting of a patient with acute angle closure has led to exploratory laparotomy!

The massive elevation of intraocular pressure following acute angle closure (often to triple the normal upper limit of 21 mmHg) may cause permanent optic nerve damage within a matter of weeks. Acute angle closure is initially treated by lowering the intraocular pressure with systemic and topical medications, including miotic eyedrops and systemic osmotic agents. In cases of pupillary block, a small hole (peripheral iridotomy) is made in the iris by laser or invasive surgery to bypass the pupillary block and allow passage of aqueous humor from the posterior segment into the anterior chamber. This prevents subsequent angle-closure attacks. Because the anatomic factors that predispose an eye to acute angle closure are generally found bilaterally, it is usually considered prudent to perform a peripheral iridotomy prophylactically in the fellow eye after an attack of angle closure.

Prolonged episodes of angle closure may result in permanent damage to the trabecular meshwork or even adhesions between the iris and sectors of the trabecular meshwork, leading to chronic angle-closure glaucoma. If the angle is sufficiently compromised, filtering surgery may be necessary.

Normal-Tension Glaucoma

Although elevated intraocular pressure has historically been the hallmark of the diagnosis of glaucoma, it has become clear in recent decades that many patients with otherwise typical glaucomatous optic atrophy and visual field loss seldom if ever are found to have elevated intraocular pressure. Identification and treatment of this so-called low-tension glaucoma (more accurately termed normal-tension glaucoma) remains problematic, although even in this cohort, reduction of intraocular pressure is thought to convey some benefit. This entity is probably more common than previously thought, as population-based surveys have demonstrated a substantial incidence of otherwise typical glaucomatous field loss in patients with normal intraocular pressures.[34]

CRYSTALLINE LENS

The crystalline lens of the eye is a unique ectodermal structure that develops entirely within the primordial lens vesicle. Only the cells on the extreme periphery of the lens divide, adding cells to the outer surface of the growing lens. Thus, the center of the adult lens represents the earliest tissue laid down during embryonic development. There is no mechanism by which these cells can turn over, unlike the situation in typical ectodermal structures, such as the skin. The metabolism of the lens is largely confined to anaerobic glycolysis, as neither hemoglobin-mediated oxygen transport nor cytochrome-mediated oxidative phosphorylation is available owing to the need for transparency. The lens is at a further metabolic disadvantage because of the need to maintain a state of great disequilibrium with its surroundings, as the lens must maintain the highest protein concentration and one of the lowest water concentrations of any tissue in the body. Thus, relatively modest metabolic insults or osmotic stresses may overwhelm the lens metabolism, resulting in protein denaturation and cataract formation.[35]

The lens of the eye continues to grow and mature throughout life. As the lens ages, it becomes more rigid and responds less effectively to changes in ciliary muscle tone, decreasing the effectiveness of accommodation, the eye's mechanism for focusing from distant to near objects. This loss of accommodation (presbyopia) is managed with reading glasses, bifocals, or other refractive strategies.

The lens responds to virtually any mechanical or metabolic insult by loss of optical clarity, resulting in the formation of a cataract (Figure 96-10; see also Plate 96-7). Several patterns of opacities are commonly encountered:

Oxidation ("browning reactions") of lens proteins, particularly in the older, central portions of the lens, is referred to as *nuclear sclerosis*, which may result in alterations in the refractive index of the lens as well as frank opacity. The most common refractive change is in the direction of an increase in myopia or decrease in hyperopia. In some instances, this refractive shift will allow the patient to read without reading glasses (so-called second sight). This improvement in visual performance is usually only temporary and often heralds the development of a more debilitating lens opacity. Refractive changes in the lens need not be uniform. Patients will occasionally report monocular diplopia resulting from inhomogeneous refraction by distinct portions of the lens resulting in two distinct images being formed on the retina.

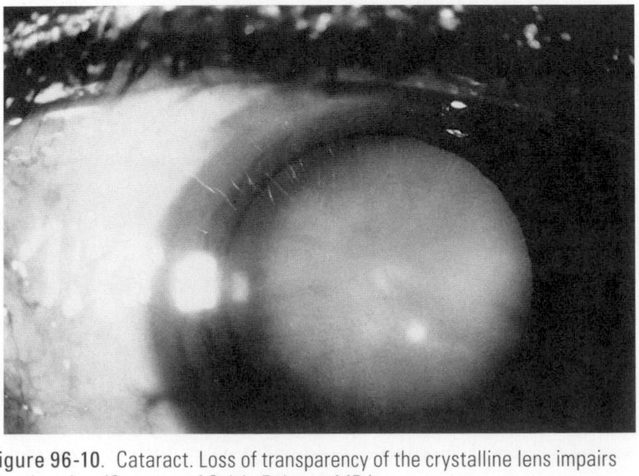

Figure 96-10. Cataract. Loss of transparency of the crystalline lens impairs visual acuity. *(Courtesy of Calvin Roberts, MD.)*

(The notion that monocular diplopia is generally indicative of hysteria is incorrect.)

Denaturation of lens proteins in a sector of adjacent cortical lens fibers results in a wedge-shaped or cuneiform cortical opacity. These are often found in the far periphery of the lens but frequently spare the optical zone near the center.

Aberrant proliferation of lens fibers on the posterior lens capsule produces a posterior subcapsular cataract. These are often induced by topical or systemic corticosteroid treatment and are frequently seen in other disease states, such as retinitis pigmentosa.

Treatment of cataract is generally surgical. With rare exceptions, the lens proteins that constitute the opacity are irreversibly denatured, precluding medical treatment.[36] Surgical strategies for removal of the lens material have evolved greatly. In all cases, an incision must be made in the eyeball. A cataract cannot be removed—even with a laser—without an ocular incision. The simplest operation is to remove the entire lens intact within its lens capsule, a so-called intracapsular procedure. At present, the extracapsular procedure, in which the opaque lens tissue is carefully aspirated from within the lens capsule, has become standard, as retention of the capsule to serve as a barrier between the anterior and posterior segments of the eye appears to reduce the rate of complications. Recently, greater emphasis has been placed on the development of minimally invasive surgical methods for cataract extraction. Often, the cataract can be liquefied by the mechanical action of a rapidly vibrating needle (phacoemulsification) and aspirated from the eye through an incision only 3 to 4 mm in length.[37] Frequently, such wounds can be constructed to be self-sealing, eliminating the need for sutures.[38]

Indications for cataract surgery should be determined in relation to the visual needs of each individual patient. Occasionally, cataract extraction is recommended for technical reasons, such as those rare cases when the lens is itself causing injury to the eye (as in phacolytic glaucoma, when lens proteins leak from a cataractous lens and occlude the trabecular meshwork) or when a cataractous lens prevents adequate visualization or treatment of disease of the posterior segment of the eye, such as diabetic retinopathy. Otherwise, cataract surgery is appropriate whenever the anticipated improvement in visual function would be of benefit to the patient. In general, a visual result of 6/12 (20/40) or better may be anticipated in 90% to 95% of cases without other known concurrent ocular disease; thus, surgery is generally recommended only when the acuity has fallen to the level of 6/15 (20/50) or worse. In some patients, difficulties with glare, contrast sensitivity, diplopia, or specific occupational demands may justify cataract extraction even with less severe loss of visual acuity.

Optical rehabilitation of the aphakic eye requires replacement of the focusing power of the cataractous lens that was removed. Where economic conditions permit, this is usually provided by means of a plastic intraocular lens prosthesis, which is generally implanted at the time of the primary cataract operation. Recent intraocular lens designs are even able to restore a degree of accommodation, reducing the need for reading glasses or bifocals in many cases.[39] Alternatives include contact lenses (often worn on an extended-wear basis) and thick "aphakic" spectacles, which subject the patient to substantial optical distortions and (if the aphakia is unilateral) may cause substantial difficulties because of unequal perceived image size in the two eyes. (Indeed, the difficulties with spectacle correction of unilateral aphakes are sufficiently severe that, if spectacle correction is the only modality of optical rehabilitation available, most surgeons recommend deferral of surgery until visual acuity in the *better* eye falls to 6/18 [20/60] or worse.) In some Third World countries, local custom may discourage the use of spectacles after cataract surgery. In these situations, the attitudes of the patient must be taken into account in the decision as to whether or not to perform a cataract extraction.

Some yellowing of the lens proteins is nearly universal with aging. Sufficient opacity to impair visual acuity results in more than 1.5 million cataract extractions each year in the United States, the vast majority in individuals over 65 years of age. In developing countries, the rate of cataract formation appears to be even higher, so that untreated cataract typically forms the largest single cause of acquired blindness.[3] In India, for example, even at the present rate of millions of cataract procedures each year, present surgical efforts continue to fall behind the rate of new cataract formation in the general population.[40]

Cataract formation may occasionally reflect an underlying metabolic abnormality, such as galactosemia or renal failure. Cataract onset is accelerated in diabetic patients and may be triggered by various drugs (particularly topical or systemic corticosteroids). In addition to these specific associations, several studies have shown a nonspecific excess mortality among cataract patients compared with age-matched control patients undergoing other elective surgical procedures.[41,42]

RETINA AND VITREOUS

Diseases of the retina, particularly diabetic retinopathy and so-called age-related macular degeneration (formerly referred to as "senile macular degeneration") constitute the most frequent cause of acquired blindness, at least in developed countries.

Diabetic Retinopathy

Diabetic retinopathy shows a steady increase in incidence and severity with increasing duration of diabetes mellitus, with significant visual complications rarely occurring before 10 to 15 years after the onset of the disease.[43] Thus, while juvenile-onset (type I) patients may develop severe retinopathy as early as the third decade, the retinal burden of adult-onset (type II) patients is borne largely by the elderly. The disease seems to attack primarily the retinal capillary circulation. Initially, small, innocuous microaneurysms are noted ophthalmoscopically. With time, the retinal capillaries begin to leak fluid into the surrounding tissue, causing retinal edema and precipitation of exudates into the retina, with a concomitant reduction in visual acuity (Figure 96-11; see also Plate 96-8) At this stage of the disease, loss of visual acuity may be reduced through the use of laser treatments, either directed at leaking microaneurysms or, if the leakage is diffuse, placed in a grid pattern over the leaky sectors of the retinal capillary bed.[44]

In later stages, perfusion of small regions of the retinal capillary bed fails (capillary dropout), leading to localized retinal infarctions, which may be seen ophthalmoscopically

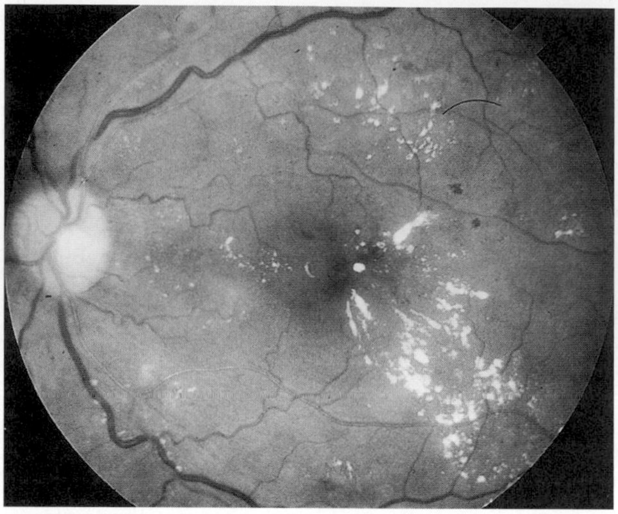

Figure 96-11. Background diabetic retinopathy. Microaneurysms ("dot hemorrhages"), intraretinal hemorrhages ("blot hemorrhages"), and "hard" exudates indicate deterioration of the retinal microcirculation.

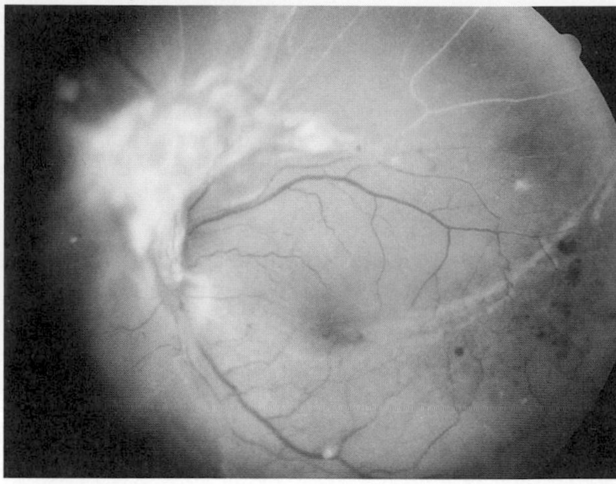

Figure 96-12. Proliferative diabetic retinopathy. A membrane of fibrovascular tissue has sprouted from the optic disc in response to prolonged retinal ischemia.

as cotton-wool spots. The remaining capillaries are often seen to become dilated, irregular, and leaky. Ultimately, in many patients, the ischemic retina develops a neovascular proliferative response, sprouting new blood vessels that may grow along the retinal surface or along the posterior surface of the vitreous body. These aberrant blood vessels are prone to leaking and hemorrhages. Vision may also be lost through traction exerted on the retina by fibroblastic membranes that accompany the neovascular proliferation (Figure 96-12; see also Plate 96-9). In severe cases, the neovascular response may extend to the anterior segment, producing neovascularization on the surface of the iris (rubeosis iridis). If the fibrovascular membrane extends over the anterior chamber angle, it obstructs filtration of aqueous humor through the trabecular meshwork, producing a refractory neovascular glaucoma.

Proliferative retinopathy may often be arrested through the ablation of a large fraction of the peripheral retina with laser photocoagulation.[45] In severe cases, blood in the vitreous cavity and fibrovascular membranes may be removed surgically by introducing mechanized suction-cutter instruments through small scleral incisions over the ciliary body (pars plana vitrectomy).

The benefit of tight control of blood glucose in the management of diabetic retinopathy depends on the stage of the disease. Many attempts to retard the progression of established retinopathy by improving the degree of glucose control have been disappointing.[46] Indeed, in some studies, tight control has been associated with a worsening of retinopathy. Similarly, in one study, successful pancreatic transplantation, with near-perfect normalization of blood glucose levels, failed to improve diabetic retinopathy, compared to the retinal disease in fellow pancreatic transplant patients whose allografts failed, requiring resumption of daily insulin injections, with the usual deficiencies in control of blood glucose.[47] However, it has been demonstrated (in both type I and type II patients) that better glucose control in recent-onset diabetic patients helps retard the onset of diabetic retinal disease.[48,49]

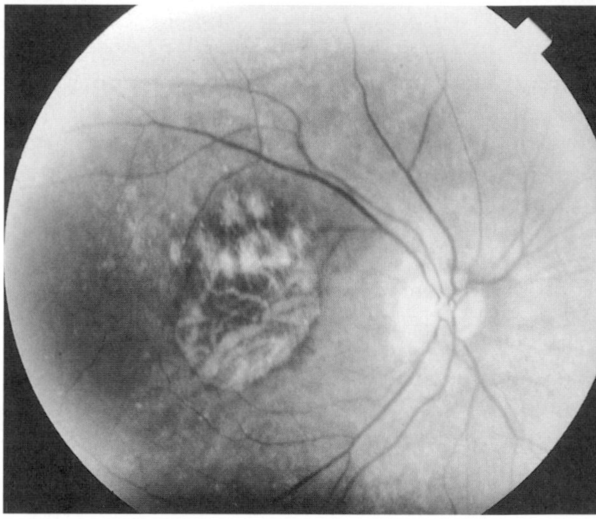

Figure 96-13. Atrophic ("dry") age-related macular degeneration. Geographic atrophy of the retinal pigment epithelium causes loss of central vision.

Age-Related Macular Degeneration

Age-related macular degeneration is a common cause of impaired vision, although not of total blindness, in the elderly population. In the "atrophic" form, the retinal pigment epithelium and choriocapillaris underlying the macula appear to degenerate, resulting in dysfunction of the overlying photoreceptors (Figure 96-13; see also Plate 96-10). There is no known treatment. In the "exudative" form, a neovascular net emanates under the macular region of the central retina from the choroidal circulation, proliferating between the retina and the underlying retinal pigment epithelium or underneath the pigment epithelium.[50] Leakage of plasma components and frank subretinal hemorrhage or scarring cause loss of vision (Figure 96-14; see also Plate 96-11).

Treatment of exudative macular degeneration has been revolutionized with the introduction of injectable drugs directed against the tissue factor, vascular endothelial growth factor (VEGF), which is elaborated by ischemic retina, stimulating increased vascular permeability and the sprouting and growth of new retinal blood vessels from adjacent vascular beds.[51] The initial anti-VEGF agent Pegaptanib sodium (Macugen, an aptamer directed against VEGF) significantly reduced the likelihood of progression of visual loss in patients with exudative macular degeneration, though improvement of visual acuity with treatment was unlikely.[52] The subsequent introduction of ranibizumab (Lucentis, a monoclonal antibody fragment directed against VEGF) has yielded even better results, preventing progression of visual loss in up to 90% of patients and actually inducing significant improvement of visual acuity in up to 40% of patients [53] (Figure 96-15; see also Plate 96-12). Bevacizumab, a similar monoclonal antibody directed against VEGF, has been used extensively to treat exudative macular degeneration on an off-label basis (often at considerable savings compared to ranibizumab) and appears to be equally safe and effective in numerous small case series and large cumulative series.[54] A formal head-to-head trial comparing these two drugs is now in progress.

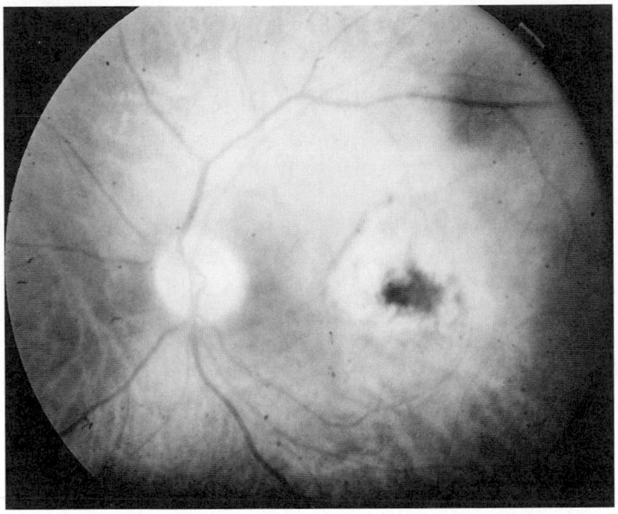

Figure 96-14. Exudative ("wet") age-related macular degeneration. Leakage and scarring from a subretinal neovascular membrane destroys central retinal function.

These anti-VEGF treatments are quite demanding of patient and physician. The drugs are administered under operating-room conditions (iodophore skin preparation, sterile drape and lid speculum, sterile gloves) by injection into the vitreous compartment of the eye through the sclera and pars plana of the ciliary body. After injection, the eye must be checked for elevation of intraocular pressure. Injections must be repeated every 4 to 6 weeks, potentially indefinitely. Each eye must be treated separately. Complications are rare, with an infection rate below one per thousand injections in competent hands, and rare incidents of cataract and retinal detachment. Close monitoring of patients in clinical trials of ranibizumab has suggested a possible small excess of thromboembolic events, but this has not been borne out by subsequent clinical experience.

Where available, anti-VEGF treatment has largely supplanted other treatment modalities for exudative macular degeneration. The role of combination treatment with anti-VEGF agents and other modalities (such as photodynamic therapy or corticosteroid medication) continues to be

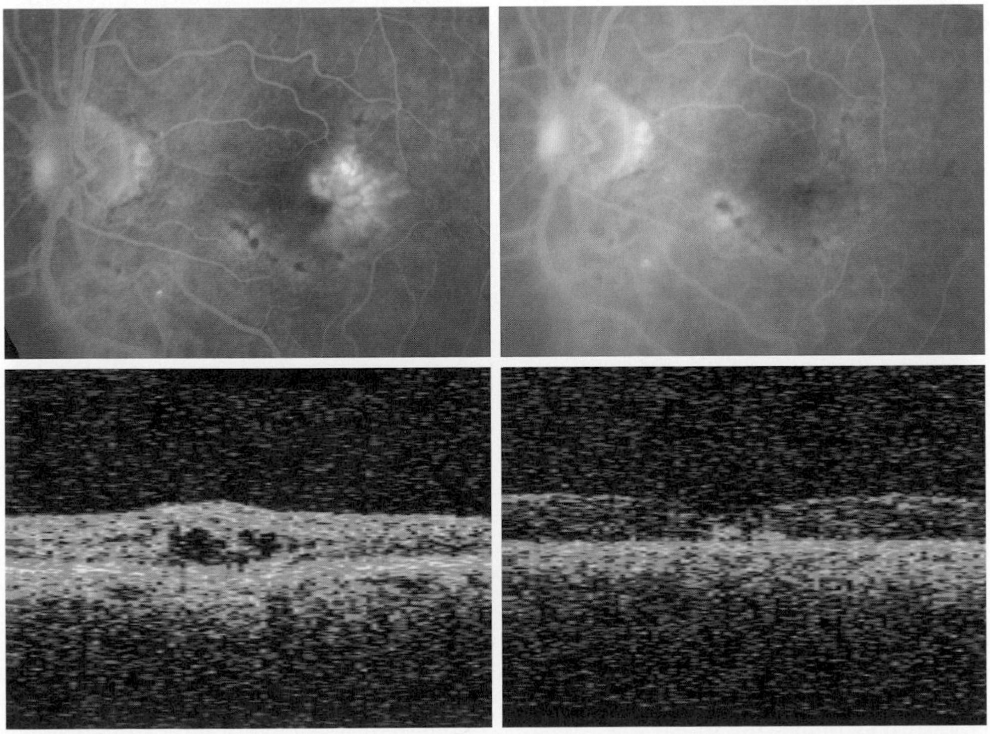

Figure 96-15. Treatment of wet age-related macular degeneration in a 90 year-old woman with intravitreal ranibizumab. Baseline images *(left)* show macular edema in fluorescein angiogram *(top – note patch of white fluorescence at temporal edge of fovea)* and in retinal cross-section as seen in OCT scan image *(bottom – extracellular fluid appears as dark clefts within retinal layers)*. After three injections of ranibizumab, edema has resolved *(right, top and bottom.* Note absence of white fluorescence in angiogram, and resolution of intraretinal clefts in OCT image, with restoration of normal foveal contour). Visual acuity improved from 20/100 (6/30) to 20/40 (6/12).

investigated, but additional benefits beyond those of anti-VEGF treatment have been difficult to demonstrate.[55]

Previous treatment modalities for exudative macular degeneration have included thermal laser[56] and photodynamic treatment using nonthermal laser.[57] In favorable cases, laser treatment of neovascular membranes outside of the foveal region may arrest the growth of these membranes before they undermine the central macula, thus helping to preserve central vision. Laser treatment of subfoveal membranes may ultimately limit the size of the central scotoma (blind spot) caused by macular degeneration[58] but is seldom recommended if anti-VEGF treatment is available.

Photodynamic therapy is an alternative modality of ablation treatment for subretinal neovascularization. Patients undergo intravenous infusion of a sensitizing agent that binds selectively to neovascular tissue. The involved retinal sector is then treated with a low-power (nonthermal) ultraviolet laser, which interacts with the sensitizing agent to create highly reactive singlet oxygen species in the target tissue. These molecules exert a cytotoxic effect sufficient in many cases to block perfusion of the subretinal neovascularization.[57] The treatment effect is often only transient, and retreatments are frequently required. Photodynamic therapy has the potential to ablate subretinal neovascular tissue with considerably less destruction of adjacent, healthy retinal tissue than is typically caused by traditional, thermal, laser treatments. In practice, photodynamic therapy appears to be a modest advance over previous ablation techniques, at least in selected patients,[57] but is not as effective as injection of anti-VEGF agents.[55]

It should be emphasized that these various modalities of treatment for age-related macular degeneration have significant limitations. Anti-VEGF agents are expensive and require frequent injection—in principle, indefinitely. Many patients fail to recover visual acuity. Few patients with advanced visual loss are restored to normal or near-normal visual function.

In both atrophic and exudative types of macular degeneration, the pathologic process appears to be confined to the posterior pole. These diseases thus spare the peripheral retina in nearly all cases, so that most affected patients indefinitely retain sufficient vision for independent ambulation and may be reassured that they are not going to go completely blind.

The pale white dots known as *drusen*, frequently seen in the retinas of older patients, are usually benign. They correspond to small deposits of amorphous hyaline material seen histologically between the Bruch's membrane and the retinal pigment epithelium. However, these lesions appear to serve as a predisposing factor in the evolution of exudative macular degeneration.[59] Elderly patients with drusen or who have lost vision in one eye to age-related macular degeneration may be advised to check their vision every day by examination of an Amsler grid, a 10-cm square of ruled graph paper. Any abnormality or distortion of the central vision should prompt an immediate examination of the retina. This will maximize the chance that a subretinal neovascular net will be discovered before it undermines the fovea, when treatment is most effective.

Studies suggest that nutrition may play a role in the development of macular degeneration. In one large prospective randomized study, patients at risk for age-related macular degeneration were randomized to dietary supplementation with a combination of antioxidant vitamins (C, E, β-carotene, and zinc) or to placebo. Treated patients at high risk for exudative macular degeneration (as indicated by the presence of large or confluent drusen, extensive geographic atrophy or advanced macular degeneration in the fellow eye) experienced a 27% reduction in risk compared with controls.[60] There was no benefit to patients at lesser risk. (The antioxidant plus zinc regimen was also of no value in preventing the development of cataracts.) Studies are now in progress to assess the benefit, if any, of additional nutrient supplements, including lutein, zeaxanthin, and omega-3 fatty acids.

Retinovascular Occlusive Disease

Both retinal arteries and retinal veins are subject to sudden occlusive events, particularly in the elderly. Retinal artery occlusions are usually either embolic or arteritic in nature. Embolic occlusions are due to the occlusion of a retinal artery by a small particle derived from the more proximal circulation, most commonly a cholesterol fragment from an ulcerated atherosclerotic plaque. A small refractile cholesterol crystal may often be visualized within a retinal artery (Hollenhorst plaque). Acutely, the affected sector of the retina appears pale and cloudy. Various measures to encourage migration of the occlusive plaque toward the retinal periphery have been recommended, including lowering of intraocular pressure by medical means or by withdrawal of a small amount of fluid from the anterior chamber with a fine needle and dilation of the retinal arterial tree by breathing an elevated concentration of carbon dioxide. No convincing benefit of these maneuvers has been demonstrated.[61]

Transient obscurations of vision, typically lasting less than 10 minutes (amaurosis fugax), are generally believed to represent embolic arterial occlusions that are quickly dislodged into the far retinal periphery.[62] These attacks indicate an elevated risk of occlusive stroke.[63]

Arteritic disease (e.g., temporal arteritis) may also cause occlusion of the arteries of the retina or optic nerve head. An elevated erythrocyte sedimentation rate is commonly, but not invariably, observed. The diagnosis is usually confirmed by temporal artery biopsy. Prompt treatment with systemic corticosteroids is indicated and may prevent visual loss in the fellow eye.[64] If the diagnosis of temporal arteritis is suspected, most authorities recommend immediate initiation of systemic corticosteroid treatment; it is unwise to wait until the erythrocyte sedimentation rate and the results of a temporal artery biopsy can be obtained, as the fellow eye may lose vision in the interim. If the tests are negative, the steroid treatment can usually be stopped promptly without a period of tapering doses.

Retinal vein occlusions result in a pattern of vascular tortuosity and intraretinal hemorrhage in the affected sector of the retina. Most retinal vein occlusions seem to be due to compression of a retinal vein by an adjacent retinal artery, frequently exacerbated by hypertension, arteriosclerosis, or glaucoma. Although there is no treatment for the occlusion itself, retinal vein occlusion carries a significant risk of subsequent neovascular complications, particularly glaucoma. In cases where retinal ischemia can be demonstrated (typically by fluorescein angiography or electroretinography), retinal ablation by laser photocoagulation can substantially reduce the risk of subsequent neovascularization.[65] Attempts to reduce retinal edema with injection of anti-VEGF agents have yielded promising results.[66]

OPTIC NERVE

The elderly are particularly susceptible to ischemic injury to the optic nerve. Infarctions of the entire optic nerve head cause sudden obscuration of vision in one eye and present ophthalmoscopically with optic nerve head swelling and hemorrhages. Many patients present with infarction of only a portion of the optic nerve head, resulting in sudden onset of a monocular visual field defect. As with retinal artery occlusions, it is important to distinguish between arteritic and nonarteritic occlusions,[67] as only the former respond well to systemic corticosteroids.

Ischemic optic neuropathy is also occasionally seen in the period following otherwise uncomplicated cataract extraction. Visual recovery is rare, and the benefit of corticosteroids in this setting is unproved.[68]

The term *papilledema* is reserved in ophthalmic usage for optic disc swelling as a result of increased intracranial pressure. In these patients, visual acuity is rarely impaired (at least initially); the only visual field abnormality is typically an enlarged blind spot. In chronic papilledema, optic atrophy may ensue, with progressive visual impairment. Treatment is directed at the underlying intracranial cause of the increased pressure. In occasional cases of idiopathic intracranial pressure elevations (pseudotumor cerebri), medical treatment with carbonic anhydrase inhibitors or surgical decompression of the central nervous system via a shunt or fenestration of the optic nerve sheath may be of value.[69] Other causes of optic disc swelling that must be distinguished from papilledema include ischemic optic neuropathy, malignant hypertension, and severe uveitis.

NEURO-OPHTHALMOLOGY

The oculomotor nerves and the posterior visual pathways are targets in the elderly for ischemic injury and for compressive injuries caused by intracranial mass lesions (typically tumors or aneurysms) and shifts of the intracranial contents. Sudden loss of function of a *single*, isolated cranial nerve is quite common. An isolated trochlear or abducens nerve palsy in a patient otherwise susceptible to atherosclerotic disease is usually a benign event, and spontaneous recovery is frequently seen.[70] Ischemic insults to the oculomotor nerve typically spare the pupillary fibers.[71] Patients with *multiple* cranial nerve deficits or in whom pupillary dilation has occurred require a thorough neurologic evaluation, preferably including computed tomography or magnetic resonance imaging, if available.

Abnormalities of the visual field should be thoroughly investigated. Scotomas that affect only one eye or that respect the horizontal meridian are generally the result of injury to the retina, optic disc, optic nerve, or to glaucoma. Injuries at or posterior to the level of the optic chiasm will impair vision in both eyes. Of particular importance are bitemporal hemianopsias, which suggest compression of the optic chiasm, typically by a pituitary tumor, and highly congruous homonymous field defects, which suggest an injury of the occipital cerebral cortex.

ORBIT

Tumors of the orbit generally present with horizontal, vertical, or anterior displacement of the globe (proptosis). In the elderly, the most frequently diagnosed entities include orbital pseudotumor (idiopathic inflammation of one or more orbital tissues, typically the extraocular muscles, lacrimal gland, or infiltration of the orbital fat), hemangiomas and lymphangiomas, lymphomas, and primary tumors of the lacrimal gland. Management frequently requires orbital exploration for histopathologic diagnosis, as well as for anatomic correction.[72]

Thyroid ophthalmopathy (Graves disease) is a well-known orbital problem. The impairment of ocular motility, lid retraction, and exophthalmos are largely due to the infiltration of the extraocular muscles. The orbital fat is rarely, if ever, involved.[73] Progression of the orbital disease is poorly correlated with the actual thyroid hormone levels, and restoration of the euthyroid state, although desirable for many reasons, is not particularly effective as a tool in the management of the ocular complications. Early cases respond well to systemic corticosteroids, but the benefits are often only temporary. In long-standing cases, patients should be monitored closely for signs of optic nerve compression and should be promptly offered surgical decompression (generally achieved by fracturing the orbital bones to provide greater room for the swollen orbital contents) if the optic nerve is at risk.[74]

OPHTHALMIC COMPLICATIONS OF SYSTEMIC DISEASES

The vision of elderly patients is at risk, not only from primary ocular diseases, but from the effects of systemic diseases as well. In addition to the effects of diabetes mellitus and thyroid disease mentioned earlier, a few of the more prominent disease entities with serious ophthalmic sequelae include hematologic disorders (such as leukemia and polycythemia), rheumatic diseases (including rheumatoid arthritis, ankylosing spondylitis, and systemic lupus erythematosus), Marfan syndrome, and renal failure. Treatment is usually directed at the primary disease process, but topical or systemic corticosteroids may be needed to control ocular inflammation.

In addition to the local, mechanical effects of metastasis to the eye or orbit, systemic malignancy may also exert a deleterious remote effect on retinal function, greatly impairing vision.[75] Chemotherapy directed at the primary malignancy has occasionally led to visual improvement.

OPHTHALMIC COMPLICATIONS OF SYSTEMIC MEDICATIONS

Many elderly patients receive several concurrent medications, some of which may frequently cause ocular symptoms. A few of the more common problems are described here.[76]

Tricyclic antidepressants have a mild parasympatholytic action, which may cause mydriasis and paralysis of accommodation. Major tranquilizers, such as chlorpromazine, may also cause mydriasis and interfere with accommodation and may cause a pigmentary retinopathy. Significant visual impairment has generally been reported only with protracted, chronic use. Chloroquine may also cause a "bull's-eye" maculopathy with impairment of central vision, particularly after prolonged use with a total dosage exceeding 100 g of the chloroquine base. Hydroxychloroquine appears to be less retinotoxic than chloroquine.

Systemic corticosteroids may precipitate an open-angle glaucoma (which frequently does not abate until several weeks after cessation of the drug), as well as accelerate the formation of cataracts. Digitalis derivatives may produce various visual disturbances, in addition to the classic "yellow vision" (xanthopsia). Ethambutol is also reported to produce dyschromatopsia, as well as optic atrophy and visual field defects. The antiimpotence drugs such as sildenafil may cross-react slightly with the retinal isoform of phosphodiesterase and may cause transient perception of a bluish haze or increased light sensitivity.[77]

Precipitation of an acute angle-closure attack by the mydriatic action of systemic medications is extremely rare.

SYSTEMIC COMPLICATIONS OF OPHTHALMIC MEDICATIONS

Because the dosages of topical eye medications are generally much smaller than the dosages used in systemic treatment, systemic complications from use of eyedrops are rare. However, these drugs are rapidly absorbed across the conjunctiva and nasal mucous membranes and occasionally cause systemic complications. Of course, it is also sometimes necessary to treat localized eye disease with systemic medications, which may cause further systemic problems.[76]

The topical anticholinergics used as mydriatic/cycloplegics may occasionally cause the full spectrum of systemic atropinic toxicity. Of the drugs in common use, cyclopentolate appears to cause these problems most frequently. Conversely, the parasympathomimetics, such as pilocarpine and carbachol, and the anticholinesterases, such as echothiophate, may cause side effects such as abdominal cramps, diarrhea, and nausea.

Topical adrenergic agents, such as Neo-Synephrine, may cause tachycardia, hypertension, and even frank arrhythmias. Conversely, topical β-blockers, such as timolol maleate, may cause the full spectrum of side effects of β-blockade, including bradycardia, asthma, and hypotension. The use of "cardioselective" β-blockers, such as betaxolol, has not completely eliminated these problems.

Topical use of chloramphenicol has resulted in a few reported cases of aplastic anemia, generally after prolonged treatment. There have also been rare reports of Stevens-Johnson syndrome following topical administration of sulfa antibiotics. Otherwise, there are few reports of serious systemic toxicity from topical antibiotics, other than local ocular hypersensitivity reactions.

Mannitol and glycerin are administered as osmotic agents to lower intraocular pressure in acute glaucoma. The fluid shifts that result may also cause congestive heart failure, renal shutdown, and altered mentation. Patients undergoing repeated treatments should be closely monitored for electrolyte imbalances and signs of renal decompensation.

Systemic carbonic anhydrase inhibitors, such as acetazolamide and methazolamide, are occasionally used to treat glaucoma. These are difficult drugs for many patients, frequently causing anorexia, depression, impotence, and paresthesias, in addition to such rare complications as bone marrow depression, gout, and acidosis. Carbonic anhydrase inhibitors are now available in topical formulations, which have largely eliminated many of these complications. Patients whose quality of life is intolerable on these medications should be offered medical or surgical alternatives.

LOW-VISION REHABILITATION

The rehabilitation of individuals who have sustained an irremediable loss of vision is an important component of effective medical care, particularly among the elderly. In the United States, more than two-thirds of individuals with acuity less than 6/18 are over 65 years of age. Conversely, of individuals over 65 years of age, 7.8% are reported to have acuity worse than 6/18, a fraction that increases to 25% among individuals over 85 years old. Loss of vision has been ranked as the third most common chronic condition (after arthritis and heart disease) for which individuals over the age of 70 require assistance with the activities of daily living.[78]

Low-vision rehabilitation attempts to allow vision-impaired individuals to make the most effective use of whatever vision they retain, so as to facilitate activities of daily living, prolong independence, and enhance self-confidence. Successful rehabilitation frequently requires the coordinated efforts of a team of care providers, including the ophthalmologist, optometrist, and occupational therapist, as well as the assistance and understanding of the patient's family and friends or caretakers. Rehabilitation is generally most successful if it begins as soon as permanent visual disability has been diagnosed. Critical to the functional outcome is the acceptance by the patient of the need to adopt compensatory visual strategies to cope with the loss of vision, rather than to continue vain attempts to reverse the visual loss.

Rehabilitation programs should center on the needs of the patient. A thorough functional history should be obtained. Emphasis should include the patient's perceptions of the impact of the visual disability on accustomed activities and on goals for the future. Every attempt should be made to identify specific tasks that the patient's visual limitations have curtailed and whose recovery would be particularly valued. Typical problems include inability to read, mend, or pay bills; loss of independent mobility; and difficulty with distance vision, such as watching television or reading signs.

The severity of the visual deficit should be determined, including measurements of visual acuity, visual fields, and contrast sensitivity. It is often helpful to be more specific in identifying the level of visual acuity than is typical in general ophthalmic practice. Placement of eye charts as close as 1 m may be used to expand the range of acuity testing. It is frequently essential to allow a substantially greater amount of time than usual for visual assessment in low-vision patients, especially the elderly.

Rehabilitation may then proceed.[79] A comprehensive program frequently entails the dispensing and instruction in the use of optical aids (such as spectacles, telescopes, and magnifiers) and nonoptical aids (such as improved lighting, large-print reading materials, high-contrast guides for reading and writing, and closed-circuit television magnifiers). Training in the use of residual vision, such as eccentric viewing for individuals who have lost central macular function, may be attempted but may require many hours of practice over many months in order to obtain optimal performance. Training in

KEY POINTS
Treatments for Major Causes of Blindness

Cataract
- Surgical extraction, ideally with intraocular lens implant

Glaucoma
- Initial: lower intraocular pressure with topical, systemic medications
- Additional options: laser treatment to trabecular meshwork; filtering surgery

Diabetic Retinopathy
- Tight control prevents or delays retinopathy in early stages
- Focal or grid laser treatment for macular edema
- Pan-retinal laser treatment for proliferative retinopathy
- Pars-plana vitrectomy for persistent vitreous hemorrhage or traction retinal detachment

Macular Degeneration
- Atrophic ("Dry")
  - No treatment available
- Exudative ("Wet")
  - Injection of anti-VEGF agents
  - Photodynamic therapy
  - (Thermal) laser ablation of neovascular membranes
- Dietary supplement with antioxidant vitamins and zinc may reduce risk of progression from "dry" to "wet" macular degeneration.

adaptations for activities of daily living and the introduction of suitable equipment, such as needle threaders or large-print playing cards, can help recapture self-confidence and facilitate independence. Professional counseling, often in a group setting, can play an important role in helping patients deal with the emotional impact of visual disabilities.

It is important that the patient adopt reasonable goals for low-vision rehabilitation. In nearly every case, it is impossible to recover the efficiency enjoyed before the loss of visual function. Each patient must individually decide whether the results achieved are worth the extra effort that will remain necessary to perform most visual tasks. The best results are achieved when specific tasks are targeted.

For a complete list of references, please visit online only at www.expertconsult.com

CHAPTER 97

Disorders of Hearing

Barbara E. Weinstein

DEMOGRAPHICS OF AGING AND HEARING LOSS

Americans are living longer and are healthier and wealthier than ever before. Life expectancies at ages 65 and 85 have increased dramatically. Under current mortality conditions, people who survive to age 65 can expect to live an average of nearly 18.7 more years, almost 7 years longer than persons aged 65 in 1900. The life expectancy of persons who survive to age 85 today is about 7.2 years for women and 6.1 years for men. Hence, in the United States half of all people who have ever lived to age 65 are currently alive. The increase in longevity brings with it an increase in the amount of time spent in all major activities including work and retirement. A significant proportion of older adults are gainfully employed. Labor force participation rates have risen dramatically for older men and women over the past few decades. Baby boomers are expecting to work longer; in 2004, a substantially larger proportion of people in their early to mid-50s work after 65 years of age as compared to 1992. Of interest is that in 2006, 15% of people over 65 were in the labor force. Because of the increase in life expectancy, older adults are spending a good deal of life in retirement. In fact, the average man aged 20 today can expect to spend a third of his life in retirement. The ability to communicate effectively takes on even greater importance as we move through the twenty-first century because of the lifestyle trends characterizing older adults, the increase in average income projected for older adults over the next 40 years, and declining disability rates.

As people age, the likelihood of experiencing one or more chronic conditions increases. Approximately 88% of adults over age 65 suffer from at least one chronic medical condition that requires ongoing care and management. Interestingly, 75% of U.S. health care expenditures are for the treatment of chronic conditions. Currently, 65% of Medicare beneficiaries have two or more chronic conditions, 43% have three or more, and 24% have four or more types of chronic conditions.[1] Hearing impairment is a major chronic condition recently recognized as a major public health problem. Currently, approximately 30% of the population over 65 years of age is hearing-impaired, rising to 40% to 50% among persons older 75 years and to more than 80% in persons over 85 years of age. The risk of experiencing a hearing loss increases dramatically with each additional decade. Nearly half of the 76 million baby boomers in the United States experience some degree of hearing loss. Self-reported hearing problems are less prevalent among persons of Asian and African decent than among whites or Native Americans. In addition to ethnicity and race, gender and baseline hearing thresholds and frequency play a role in hearing loss progression and severity.[2] The high prevalence of hearing impairment among persons over 85 years has implications for nursing home staff, as the majority of residents of nursing homes are in their ninth decade of life. That is to say, hearing loss will be the rule rather than the exception among nursing home residents and homebound older adults. It is projected that by the year 2030, at least 21 million Americans beyond age 65 will have a hearing impairment. Approximately 11% of adults suffering from age-related hearing loss experience permanent tinnitus, most commonly described as ringing in the ear. The prevalence of tinnitus rises with age, and age-related hearing loss is a major predictive factor. The sensation of dizziness is highly prevalent among people over the age of 65, accounting for 8 million primary care physician visits in the United States. Dual sensory impairments are prevalent among older adults, as well. Of persons over 70 years of age, 18% are reportedly blind in one or both eyes, 33% reportedly experience hearing problems, and approximately 10% report concurrent hearing and visual problems.[2] Despite the likelihood of experiencing either a sensory, physical, or mental disability, the majority (39%) of older adults assessed their health as excellent or very good in 2006.

Given the high prevalence of hearing loss among persons aged 65 years and older, it is no surprise that the majority of persons purchasing hearing instruments are in this age bracket. Hearing aid adoption rates are higher for older adults than for younger adults with comparable hearing loss.[3] Adults over 55 years of age make up 81% of all hearing aid users; yet the majority of older adults with hearing loss do not use hearing aids. The latter is consistent with the tendency of older adults to rate their health as good even in the presence of disability. The stigma associated with hearing aid use coupled with persistent complaints from experienced users about continued difficulty understanding speech in noisy environments have kept penetration rates stable over time.[3] Evidence of neural plasticity associated with auditory input from hearing aids and resulting improvements in sound perception should serve as inducement for physicians to understand hearing loss in older adults and the value of available medical and nonmedical interventions, depending on the type and degree of hearing impairment. Physicians play a pivotal role in the early identification of older adults with hearing and balance problems that require attention.

AGE-RELATED CHANGES WITHIN THE AUDITORY SYSTEM

The inner ear is composed of several functional components that are responsible for both hearing and balance. The sensory, neural, vascular, supporting, synaptic, or mechanical structures within the peripheral or central auditory systems are especially vulnerable to the effects of aging.[4] The organ of Corti, which extends from the basal convolution to the cupula or apex of the cochlea, houses the sense organ of hearing. It is the structure within the auditory system most susceptible to age-related histopathologic changes. The cochlea rests atop the basilar membrane and is composed of sensory cells (outer and inner hair cells along with their stereocilia), supporting cells, Reissner's membrane, the tectorial membrane, and stria vascularis, among other structures. The fact that various frequencies are registered in different parts of the cochlea is the basis for the tonotopic organization of the auditory system. The organ of Corti is the site of transduction of mechanical to neural energy, and age-related atrophy interferes with the transduction process integral to the reception of sound.

The most critical risk factor for the auditory sense organ is age.[5] The term *presbycusis* refers to hearing impairment associated with auditory system changes within the peripheral and central systems that cannot be accounted for by ototraumatic, ototoxic, genetic, or pathologic conditions.[4] The peripheral auditory system serves as the interface between the acoustic signals in the external environment and the brain. It is responsible for detecting and coding acoustic stimuli. In combination with the cognitive system, the central auditory system is responsible for perception—that is, modifying and analyzing the code it receives from the periphery. The changes the aging ear undergoes have been studied most extensively by Schuknecht and more recently by Willott, Chisolm, and Lister.[4,6,7] In general, hair cell loss is the rule rather than the exception in older adults. Loss of both types of hair cells is most severe in the basal region of the cochlea, with apical and midcochlear involvement of the outer hair cells as well. Although both outer and inner hair cells tend to degenerate with age, the outer hair cells are more vulnerable than inner hair cells, and their degeneration accounts in large part for the "normal" decline in hearing with age.[4] It is noteworthy that outer hair cells are most susceptible to the effects of noise and are vulnerable to ototoxic effects especially associated with ingestion of aminoglycosides.

Research clearly demonstrates a relation between age and loss of ganglion cells.[8] As would be expected, neural histopathologic studies suggest that age-related loss in ganglion cells is greatest near the base of the cochlea. Similarly, age is associated with a decrease in the average number of fibers in the cochlear nerve, with nerve fiber loss greatest within the basal 10 mm of the cochlea.[9] Neural degeneration can occur before or independently of sensory cell loss.[10] That is, loss of nerve fibers in one turn of the cochlea or in all turns has been noted without severe hair cell loss.[3] Stated differently, loss of inner or outer hair cells is not a condition for age-related pathology of ganglion cells.[3] In conclusion, two major age-related structural changes have been observed histologically in the inner ear and auditory nerve. These include extensive atrophy and degeneration of the hair cells, numerous supporting cells, and the stria vascularis, as well as a reduction in the number of functional spiral ganglia and nerve fibers that constitute the auditory portion of the eighth nerve.[10]

Histologic studies of the central auditory nervous system suggest that portions undergo age-related changes as well.[11] These apparent changes, which predominate in the auditory brain stem pathways and the auditory cortex, are not universal across individuals, nor are they universal across the nuclei or tracts within the auditory brain stem. These changes within the central auditory nervous system have profound implications for speech understanding in less than optimal listening conditions and interfere with hearing aid benefit. In short, the locus of the degenerative changes determines the functional effects of the physiologic changes.

Although within the peripheral auditory system the inner ear and central auditory pathways are most vulnerable to aging effects, the outer and middle ear do undergo changes with age. For the most part the changes do not have a dramatic effect on the transmission of sound energy, yet the changes are of relevance because of their functional implications. The glandular structure within the ear canal, most notably the sebaceous and cerumen glands, loses some of its secretory ability. There is also a decrease in the fat present in the ear canal and an increase in the thickness and length of hair follicles in the fibrocartilaginous portion of the canal. Additionally, failure of the self-cleaning mechanism that automatically expels cerumen/earwax, a naturally occurring substance that cleans, protects, and lubricates the external auditory canal, is common in older adults and accounts in part for its high prevalence. Interestingly, cerumen impaction is also more common in those with cognitive impairment and in individuals in nursing homes.[12] As a result, the skin in the external ear canal becomes dry, prone to trauma and breakdown, and cerumen tends to become more concentrated, hard, and impacted. One of the functional implications of an excessive buildup of cerumen and a common cause of hearing aid malfunction is physical obstruction of sound emanating from hearing aids. An additional consequence of gradual cerumen buildup is constriction of the ear canal leading to a blockage of the sound-conducting mechanism resulting in a conductive type hearing loss. More than 33% (estimates range from 19% to 65%) of adults over 65 years of age present with excessive or impacted cerumen, which is associated with close to 12 million people seeking medical care for cerumen removal.[12]

Moving medially beyond the ear canal is the middle ear including the tympanic membrane and tympanic cavity wherein the ossicles lie. The three middle ear ossicles (i.e., malleus, incus, stapes) are connected by joints, similar to joints in the body, and the cartilage within the incudostapedial and incudomalleolar joints undergoes degenerative changes consistent with osteoarthritis. According to a recent study, individuals with osteoarthritis and a negative family history of hearing loss, noise exposure, or chronic middle ear effusion had a higher prevalence of middle ear abnormalities and of sensorineural hearing loss (associated with degenerative changes in the inner ear) than the age-matched control group without arthritis.[13] As arthritis is a prevalent chronic condition for which potentially ototoxic medications are prescribed, individuals with osteoarthritis should undergo routine hearing and balance screening after age 65. A question about the presence or absence of tinnitus should be included in the screening given the high association between tinnitus and ototoxic medications.

Age-related morphologic changes also take place in the vestibular system. Most notably there is a significant loss of hair cells in the sensory receptors in the semicircular canals, the saccule and the utricle. Further, there is a decrease in primary vestibular neurons, and a significant loss of neurons in the cerebellum. Finally, the vestibulo-ocular reflex time decreases with age and the vasculature of the vestibular system all undergo changes with age. These changes in combination with changes in the ocular system with age increase the susceptibility of older adults to falls and dizziness. The rate of falls increases with age and falls, and the experience of dizziness accounts for a high proportion of primary care physician visits, emergency department visits and hospitalizations among older adults.[14] Despite the high prevalence and consequences of hearing and balance problems among persons of Medicare age, primary care physicians rarely screen for these conditions. Since the United States Preventive Services Task Force has given a "B" recommendation for office-based periodic screening for hearing loss this chapter will conclude with a recommended protocol for screening for these prevalent chronic conditions.

In addition to age-related degeneration, a number of other factors can lead to hearing loss in older adults. These include excessive exposure to occupational or recreational noise; genetic factors; diabetes; acoustic neuroma; trauma; cardiovascular disease; metabolic disease such as kidney problems and Ménière's syndrome; vascular disease; infections; and ingestion of ototoxic agents, most notably aminoglycosides, ethacrynic acid, and salicylates. Data suggest that type II diabetics experience significant impairments in hearing sensitivity and speech understanding relative to an age-matched and gender-matched group of adults without diabetes. Further, hearing impairment is more prevalent among adults with diabetes, and the association is independent of such risk factors for hearing loss as noise exposure, ototoxic medication use, and smoking.[15] Finally, older adults with hypothyroidism experience impaired speech understanding and reductions in audibility for pure tone signals.

Adverse drug reactions (ADRs) in the form of auditory or vestibular symptoms are prevalent and are known to be more severe among older adults.[16] ADRs in older adults occur for a variety of reasons including lack of compliance resulting from a compromised understanding of the prescription because of hearing or visual problems or possibly because of confusion between two medications that might sound alike (e.g., Plavix or Paxil) to a hearing-impaired person or may look alike to a visually impaired older adult. Some of the auditory or vestibular side effects of medications frequently prescribed for older adults include dizziness, ear discomfort, ear congestion, lightheadedness, vertigo, and tinnitus. Similarly, performance on selected electrophysiologic tests conducted by audiologists are affected by selected medications, so audiologists do instruct patients to suspend taking selected medications before performing vestibular studies.

In light of the variety of medical conditions associated with hearing loss and prevalent among older adults, individuals presenting with any of these conditions should be screened for hearing impairment and associated tinnitus. Impacted cerumen, otitis media, glossopharyngeal tumors, and otosclerosis are not uncommon. The latter conditions are associated with conductive hearing loss, yet they can occur in the presence of cochlear involvement. Finally, affective disorders such as depression and cognitive disorders such as senile dementia of the Alzheimer's type are also associated with sensorineural hearing loss. In fact, the prevalence of hearing loss is higher among persons with dementia than among those without it. In addition, inattention or confusion related to depression or dementia may give the impression of significant hearing loss and should be considered in a systematic geriatric assessment. Complete audiometric studies can help identify the existence and etiology of hearing loss in older adults. Hearing loss should be ruled out in individuals being worked up for cognitive or affective disorder.

BEHAVIORAL IMPLICATIONS OF ANATOMIC AND PHYSIOLOGIC CHANGES

The aforementioned age-related degenerative changes are associated with decrements in hearing for pure-tone and speech stimuli, poor word recognition, and decrements in comprehension of connected speech. In addition to loss of audibility for tonal stimuli, compromised frequency resolution and temporal processing, deterioration in central auditory processing, visual deficits, and age-related changes in cognitive abilities ensue and compromise communication.

Most studies on hearing loss characterizing noninstitutionalized older adults confirm that age-related hearing loss commonly referred to as *presbycusis* has several distinct features. First, pure-tone hearing sensitivity tends to decline with increasing age, and the hearing loss tends to be greatest in the frequencies above 1000 Hz. Further, the hearing loss tends to be bilateral, symmetrical, and sensorineural in origin, associated with damage to the sensory structures within the cochlea. The decline in high-frequency sensitivity appears to be greatest in males, whereas the decline in low-frequency thresholds tends to be greatest in females of comparable age.[5] The average hearing loss in males can be described as mild to moderately severe, bilateral, and sensorineural with a sharply sloping configuration, whereas women tend to present with a mild to moderate gradually sloping bilaterally symmetrical sensorineural hearing loss. The odds of hearing loss are higher in men versus women, and the probability of hearing loss is lower in black than in white individuals.[17] Additionally, age, gender, and frequency effects emerge in most cross-sectional and longitudinal studies of hearing loss, such that air conduction thresholds became poorer as age or frequency increase.[4,17,18,19] It is important to note that a large proportion of subjects in many of the cross-sectional and longitudinal studies had history of noise exposure and ototoxicity, so it is often difficult to tease out the hearing loss associated exclusively with aging. Interestingly, the rate of change in hearing varies with frequency and initial hearing threshold levels.[18] Further, hearing loss seems to be setting in at younger ages or prevalence of hearing loss is increasing among individuals younger than 65 years of age.[17] There is a subset of older adults including octogenarian men who do not present with clinically significant hearing loss.

Among residents of nursing facilities, the sensorineural hearing loss tends to be more significant, moderately severe sloping to severe, and more prevalent, affecting approximately 70% to 80% of residents. The fact that nursing home residents are older accounts for the high prevalence of more severe hearing loss among residents. Similarly, by the year 2011 when the first group of baby boomers will turn 65, there will be an increase in older adults with significant hearing loss who are homebound and are receiving palliative care who will have an increased need to communicate with health care professionals, caregivers, and family members.

The pure-tone hearing loss, site of involvement within the cochlea, eighth nerve, auditory brain stem pathways, auditory cortex, and cognitive factors including memory loss determine in large part the nature of the speech understanding problems experienced by older adults. The classic complaint of older adults with presbycusis, namely "I can hear people talking but cannot understand what they are saying, especially in noisy situations," aptly describes the problems that derive from the reduction in transmission, reception, and perception of the speech signal attributable to sensorineural hearing loss.

The speech recognition difficulties can in part be predicted from an understanding of the interaction between speech acoustics and the compromised audibility of selected frequencies associated with presbycusis. Ordinary conversation takes place over a frequency band that ranges from 250 to 6000 Hz and within a decibel range of about 35 dB. Consonant sounds and diphthongs such as s, sh, th, z, k, t, p, and g are relatively high in frequency or pitch and low in intensity (dB) or loudness. Conversely, vowel sounds such as a, i, o, and u are concentrated in the lower frequencies and are somewhat higher in intensity. Environmental noise is high in intensity and low in frequency as well. Audibility for consonant sounds is critical to the understanding of speech. Hearing loss afflicting most older adults with age-related hearing loss renders consonant sounds (e.g., s, th, t, z) with energy in the high frequencies inaudible, yet low-frequency vowel sounds and environmental noise can be heard normally. As a result of the configuration of hearing loss, older adults claim that they can hear people talking (vowels audible) but they cannot make out the words (consonants inaudible) especially in noise (audible).

A number of variables beyond the audiogram have a dramatic effect on speech understanding in older adults. Speech understanding difficulties are exacerbated in challenging acoustic environments such as a noisy room, as background noise tends to be audible given good low-frequency hearing, yet consonant sounds important to understanding are inaudible. Speech understanding in reverberant environments (e.g., large rooms with high ceilings and walls with windows or mirrors) is also compromised for older adults. Distance between the speaker and listener can erode speech understanding. Characteristics of the speaker's voice, complexity of the message, listener's knowledge of the language, use of gestures, and availability of contextual information influence speech understanding as well. Older adults have difficulty understanding fast speech and accented speech used by non-native speakers of English and understanding speakers with dialects.[20] Speech understanding is compromised when presented without the benefit of contextual information, when multiple speakers are talking, and when the speaker is not nearby. Age-related changes in cognitive processing, declines in rapid information processing, decrements in auditory temporal processing because of central auditory effects of peripheral pathology vary across older adults, but those individuals experiencing such changes have dramatic speech understanding difficulties.[20] Table 97-1 includes a list of tips for helping to ensure that your patients understand most of what is being communicated to them.

Table 97-1. Tips for Effective Communication With Patients with Hearing Loss

- Make sure your face and mouth are visible when speaking.
- If hearing difficulties are observed and no hearing aid or other hearing assist device is functioning, all communication with your patient should be conducted with the use of a commercially available personal sound amplifier.
- Speak when you are at most 3 to 6 feet from your patient.
- Repeat or rephrase what you have said if your patient doesn't understand you.
- Make sure your patient is paying attention to you when you speak.
- Raise the level of your voice to be understood, but never shout.
- Use gestures to enhance your spoken message.
- Be patient when repeating instructions to your patient.
- Make sure your lips and face are visible to your patient.
- Do not have anything in your mouth while conversing with your patient.
- Make sure your face is on the same level as your patient's when you are speaking.
- Make sure there is no glare on your face when speaking to your patient.
- Speak in an area with little noise.
- Turn off radio, close the door, and remove any other sound sources when speaking.
- Inform your patient when you change topics.
- Slightly decrease the rate of your speech.
- Write information down that is important, as multiple modalities are helpful.
- Make sure to provide a context for what you are trying to communicate.
- Make sure the receptionists and billing people in your offices look at your patient and not at the computer when they are checking them in or processing papers and make sure they speak slowly on the telephone or use an amplified telephone when contacting patients with hearing loss to ensure that the patients understand the message.

PSYCHOSOCIAL CONSEQUENCES OF DECREMENTS IN PURE-TONE SENSITIVITY AND SPEECH UNDERSTANDING

The behavioral implications of the hearing and speech understanding difficulties characterizing older adults are considerable. Untreated hearing loss impacts daily communication function; restricts one or more dimensions of quality of life including physical functional status and cognitive and emotional function; and interferes with one's capacity to meet personal and occupational demands.[21–25] Dalton and her colleagues reported that older adults with moderate to severe hearing loss were more likely than individuals without hearing loss to have impaired instrumental activities of daily living (IADLs) and activities of daily living (ADLs).[24] They also reported that severe hearing loss had a significant association with decreased function on the mental and physical component scores of the SF-36.

Moreover, the myth that hearing loss is harmless has been debunked, and it is becoming increasingly clear that, if untreated, hearing loss can be costly to the individual and family members. Untreated hearing loss is costly from an economic vantage point; it is associated with lost wages and lower income in retirement.[25] Kochkin's data revealed a link between household income and hearing loss severity, with individuals with mild hearing loss reporting a household income of $36,400 and persons with severe loss reporting an income of $33,600.

The adverse effects of untreated hearing impairment presents a global problem. A study conducted in a geriatric medicine clinic in Singapore attempted to quantify the psychosocial consequences of self-perceived handicap in a sample of 63 older adults ranging in age from 62 to 90.[26] They reported that of subjects with self-reported hearing difficulty and a fail on the pure-tone screen, 70% indicated that they would be happier if their hearing were normal, 40% indicated that difficulty hearing made them feel frustrated, and 43% admitted to feeling sad because of their hearing handicap.[26] Interestingly, the federal government in Australia is designing a comprehensive approach to managing age-related hearing loss because hearing impairment is the second highest cause of disability for every Australian man.[27]

In general, unaddressed hearing loss undermines familial relationships and impacts nearly every aspect of daily life, ultimately eroding the patient's quality of life. Specifically, hearing loss does the following:

- Negatively impacts communicative behavior
- Compromises efficiency at work
- Alters psychosocial behavior
- Strains family relations
- Limits the enjoyment of daily activities and leads to activity limitations and participation restrictions
- Jeopardizes physical well-being
- Interferes with the ability to live independently and safely
- Interferes with long-distance contacts on the telephone, potentially jeopardizing safety and security
- Interferes with medical diagnosis, treatment, management, and interventions in emergency rooms
- Compromises compliance with pharmacologic regimens
- Interferes with therapeutic interventions, compromising quality of care

HEARING TECHNOLOGIES

Once hearing loss is documented, the etiology determined, medical treatment ruled in or out, and the activity limitations and participation restrictions quantified, an older adult should undergo some form of audiologic rehabilitation. Audiologic rehabilitation (AR) is a patient management process designed to reduce activity limitations, decrease participation restrictions, improve communication efficiency, and improve quality of life. The goal is to help the individual overcome challenges posed by hearing impairment and sensory management in the form of hearing aids, hearing assistive technologies, or hearing implants. Approximately three quarters (74%) of the people fitted with hearing aids in 2006 were at retirement age or older.[3] Hearing aid adoption rates for people ages 85+ and 75 to 84 were 61% and 44%, respectively. Interestingly, hearing aid adoption rates decline precipitously among individuals in the younger age groups. It is notable that the average hearing aid purchaser is 70 years old, yet it is important to emphasize that most older adults with hearing loss *do not* use hearing aids.[3] The significant communicative and psychosocial effects of hearing loss, coupled with the fact that a high percentage of older adults suffer from hearing loss that affects ordinary daily life, and the efficacy of hearing aids in reducing the functional consequences of hearing impairment would indicate that older adults should be encouraged to purchase hearing aids before hearing loss becomes an intolerable burden and less responsive to intervention.

A number of variables are at play, which determine whether an older adult will consider hearing aid use, including the self-perception of the severity of hearing impairment and the perception that one can get along without hearing aids. The high cost of hearing aids, especially digital devices, is a deterrent to older adults on fixed incomes, as are reports from friends that hearing aids are of no value. Unfortunately, third-party reimbursement for hearing aids is limited, and economics dictates that nonmedical intervention for hearing loss may not be a priority.

Although a host of factors influence nonadoption rates, many variables are predictive of hearing aid candidacy, hearing aid satisfaction, and hearing aid success. These include but are not limited to the following: auditory, physical, sociologic, psychological, cognitive, and environmental factors. With regard to auditory variables, sensorineural hearing loss of nearly any degree can be remediated via a hearing aid, assuming the client is interested in pursuing amplification. Clinical experience suggests that motivation is one of the most important, yet least well understood, psychological factors that affects rehabilitation potential in general and hearing aid candidacy in particular.[22] It explains why behavior is initiated, why it persists, and why it is attenuated. Motivation to pursue intervention is optimal when an individual (1) knows what he or she wants, (2) expects it can be attained, (3) believes that the rewards are meaningful, and (4) considers that intervention takes place at a reasonable cost.[28] It is incumbent on the audiologist to understand the patient's motivations for pursuing a hearing aid so as to ensure that their needs and expectations are fulfilled. The audiologist can optimize the patient's motivation to purchase amplification by emphasizing the positive consequences associated with a hearing aid purchase and instilling realistic expectations regarding the advantages and disadvantages associated with hearing aid use.[28]

The new generation of hearing aids has impacted use and acceptance patterns, and an understanding of the technology can assure that physicians will partner with audiologists to encourage those with impaired hearing to seek assistance to overcome communication deficits. Present-day hearing aids improve audibility, tend to be more comfortable in the ear, can be manipulated to provide appropriate gain at selective frequencies, differentially compress high-intensity sounds, filter out background noise, and many have directional microphone technology, which picks up speech coming in front of the speaker and eliminates unwanted noise from behind the speaker. Hence, they are designed to meet the needs of individuals with varying auditory and nonauditory needs.

Hearing aids are basically miniature public address systems with several key components. They can be broken down into several categories ranging from traditional devices that are considered analog signal processing devices to digital signal processing systems, which can be described as low end, middle level, and high end. Table 97-2 contrasts the style unit, the signal processing technology, and the level of sophistication of available hearing aids.

The majority of hearing aids sold in 2008 were digital; approximately 8–10 different companies manufacture the large variety of hearing aids available to consumers. Hearing aid styles range from traditional behind the ear (BTE) to open fit mini BTE units, to custom in-the-ear (ITE), to in the canal (ITC), and completely in the canal (CIC). Mini-BTEs are a new category of hearing aid that utilizes transparent tubing and a variety of open earmold options. They are small BTE units with receivers in different locations and an earmold, which varies in terms of the amount of the ear canal that remains open. Many BTE units are ergonomically shaped,

Table 97-2. Hearing Aid Classification System

Style of Unit	Signal Processing Technology	Level of Sophistication
Traditional behind the ear (BTE)	Analog,* digital signal processing†	Low end
Mini-BTE (mBTE)	Analog, digital signal processing	Low end, middle level, high end
In the ear (ITE)	Analog, digital signal processing	Low end, middle level, high-end
In the canal (ITC)	Analog, digital signal processing	Low end, middle level, high end
Completely in the canal (CIC)	Analog, digital signal processing	Low end, middle level, high end

*Most basic and least expensive circuitry.
†Greater sound precision, less internal.

most are currently available in a variety of colors, many are water-resistant, and more and more do not include volume controls. Newer and smaller BTE units are attached to thin clear tubing or thin preformed tubing and are referred to as open fittings (i.e., open fitting, BTE). Similarly in-the-ear hearing aids are referred to as open canal devices. Open fittings simply refer to the fact that the ear canal remains relatively "open" or "unoccluded." When there is no occlusion, people with good low-frequency hearing and significant high-frequency hearing loss can be comfortably fitted with hearing aids that take advantage of their good low-frequency residual hearing and that are no longer susceptible to feedback (sound leakage), which traditionally was a problem. The basic components of all hearing aids include the amplifier, microphone, receiver, earmold, and battery. An important function of the amplifier, in combination with the receiver and earmold/molded piece, which delivers sound to the ear, is to control the maximum amount of amplification the user receives. This function is critical, as the appropriate amount of gain/amplification minimizes the possibility of hearing aid rejection because sound is amplified to an uncomfortably loud level. Open canal fittings in combination with digital signal processing have revolutionized the hearing aid industry by allowing special features to be included in hearing aids that lead to dramatic performance improvements. Present-day hearing aids include features that have increased their comfort, cosmetic appeal, ease of use with the telephone, and noise suppression capabilities.

Common product features include noise suppression circuitry, feedback reduction, automatic telecoils, directional microphones, low-battery indicators, power on delay, wind noise protection, Bluetooth technology, and data logging. The size, style, and amplifier type determine which battery powers the hearing aid. All hearing aids use 1.4-volt batteries, and at the time the hearing aid is dispensed, the audiologist will advise consumers on the correct battery type for the particular unit. Battery types range from the smallest (number 10 battery) to midsized batteries (312, 13), to the largest size battery (number 675). Approximately 40% of BTE hearing aids dispensed during the first part of 2008 used the smallest battery sizes (10 or 312) and were open canal fittings, which when appropriate to the hearing loss allow for considerable user comfort. The American Association of Retired Persons is one of the least expensive sources for purchasing batteries, but they are available at most drugstores, through Costco, battery clubs sponsored by dispensers, and at military bases for veterans. The size battery that a hearing aid accommodates depends in large part on the style and size of the hearing aid. Some hearing aids come with rechargeable batteries, which have advantages and disadvantages.

Various hearing aid styles are available to the hearing-impaired older adult once it is mutually decided that hearing aids are the appropriate intervention. According to a recent survey of hearing instrument dispensers, more than 95 percent of all hearing aids sold in 2008 used digital signal processing. Sixty-three percent of all hearing aids sold in the first half of 2009 were BTE devices, of which 42% used the smaller size ten batteries. Figures 97-1 and 97-2 display a BTE and mini-BTE. Approximately 49% of all hearing aids sold in the Untied States in 2007 were ITE units; of these, 9.8% were CIC units, 12.4% were ITC units, and the remainder full-shell/half-shell ITE units.[29]

Custom ITE hearing aids range in size and are identified according to their physical location and their dimensions within the concha of the outer ear or pinna. Custom in-the-ear hearing aids (ITEs, ITCs, and CICs) take full advantage of the size and shape of an individual user's ear (that is, it completely occupies the concha portion of the pinna). Typically the hearing aid for the right ear is red and the one for the left ear is blue, but other color options are available. ITC hearing aids are smaller than ITE units, having most of their components within the cartilaginous portion of the ear canal. For the most part, ITCs use small 312 batteries or even smaller size cells (i.e., 10), making the battery difficult to insert and remove for older adults with manual dexterity problems and reduced tactile sensitivity.

The electronic components of CIC hearing aids are deep within the external auditory canal, terminating close to the tympanic membrane. Figure 97-3 displays CIC hearing aids with the tiny components relative to a coin. The only piece visible is the thin piece of plastic extending outward from the faceplate of the hearing aid, which is used to remove the unit. The microphone of CIC hearing aids is located deep in the ear canal providing for a natural high-frequency boost, less wind noise, and theoretically better speech understanding because of the acoustic advantage provided by the outer ear. CICs use very small batteries, and some companies make devices to assist in battery insertion and removal.

Most of the hearing aid styles discussed thus far incorporate advanced features. The majority of units sold in 2009 included feedback reduction technology, noise reduction technology, directional microphone technology, and data logging technology. The bulk of behind-the-ear hearing aids sold in 2009 were of the receiver in the canal or receiver in the ear variety furthering the fitting candidacy for the hearing impaired. Availability of these "high-tech features" is no longer limited to low-end hearing aids, providing hearing aid dispensers with the ability to custom-tailor the response of the hearing instrument to the consumer's lifestyle, listening needs, and financial situation. Similarly, the dispenser can adjust the low frequencies independent of the high frequencies depending on the hearing configuration and the nature of the input sound, providing for improved

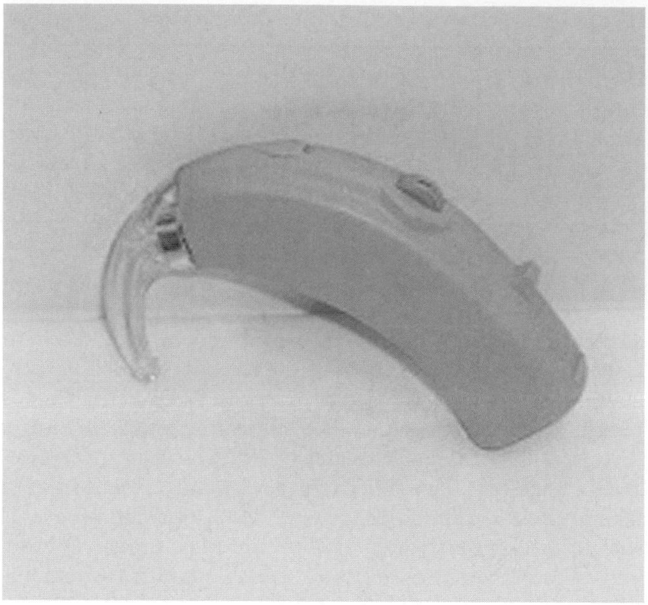

Figure 97-1. Traditional behind-the-ear hearing aid.

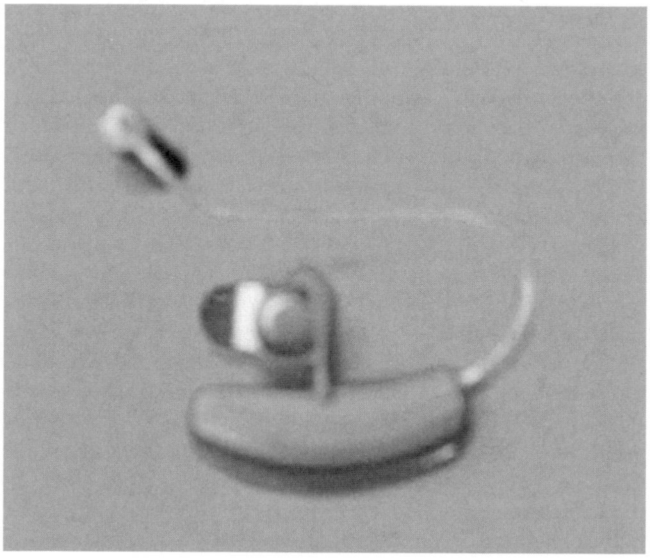

Figure 97-2. Mini-behind-the-ear hearing aid.

speech understanding in favorable and unfavorable listening environments. The availability of Bluetooth and automatic telephone settings, hearing aids without volume controls, and rechargeable batteries further increases the flexibility of hearing aids and appeals to people with varying technologic skills. Finally, the majority of hearing aid fittings are binaural given the listening and speech understanding advantages of two ears, especially in noisy situations. It is worth noting that because of cognitive or central auditory processing problems, some older adults are not candidates for binaural fittings, and the audiologist should explore the appropriateness of a binaural fitting before proceeding.

The average price of hearing aids in 2007 varied according to the style, the circuitry, the level of sophistication, programming flexibility, and the number of special features. The cost differs dramatically by qualifications of the dispenser and with geography as well. The average overall

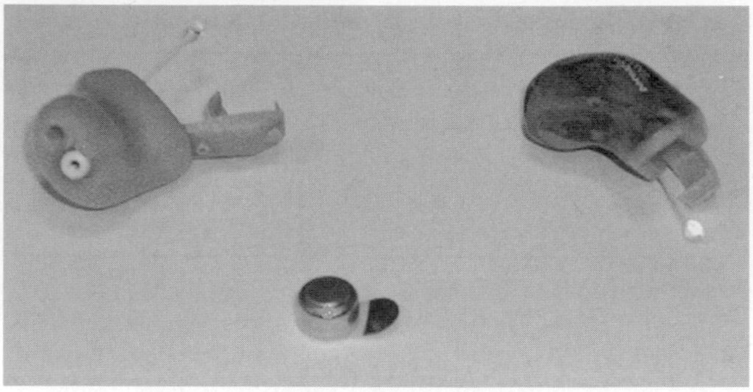

Figure 97-3. Completely in-the-canal hearing aids.

price in 2007 for an analog hearing aid was $857 as compared to $948 in 2006.[30] The average price for a low-end digital signal processing unit was $1269, the average price of a midlevel digital signal processing unit was $1943, and that of a high-end digital signal processing unit was $2714. The average price of a high-end DSP CIC unit was $2860, as compared to $2609 for a high-end DSP BTE unit and $1209 for a low-end DSP ITC unit.[30] The price typically includes a minimum 1-year warranty with an option to extend the warranty; but this too varies by manufacturer. Service connected veterans are eligible for hearing aids through the Department of veterans Affairs and the service and technology is consistently superb. The considerable financial investment associated with the purchase of hearing aids underlines the importance of referring the consumer to a qualified professional who spends time dispensing the product, orients the individual and family members to the hearing aid in an effort to optimize the fit, and has hours daily, as problems do arise on a relatively frequent basis. Finally, with the exception of cochlear implant surgery for severely and profoundly impaired individuals, support for hearing care is modest or unavailable in most health plans. However, recently selected managed care plans and more and more corporate plans for retirees have introduced some, albeit minimal, coverage toward the purchase of a hearing instrument.

The value of hearing aids lies in their ability to restore the reduced audibility and frequency resolution accompanying hearing loss and to increase loudness of the speech signal relative to background noise so that speech understanding is more comfortable and intelligibility improved in suboptimal situations. Older adults are enjoying improved speech understanding in noisy situations, and consumer satisfaction with hearing aids that include advanced features is growing. A task force convened by the American Academy of Audiology completed a systematic review of studies on the relationship between hearing aids and health-related quality of life in adults with hearing loss.[23] The task force was charged with reviewing and summarizing the evidence regarding the nonacoustic benefits of hearing aids in light of the rise in prevalence of adult onset hearing loss, the increase in sophistication of hearing aids, and the low proportion of adults using hearing aids. The task force concluded that hearing aids are in fact beneficial in several health and social domains over the short and long term, which should serve as an inducement for health professionals to refer the hearing impaired for an evaluation to consider candidacy for intervention. It is important to emphasize that their positive impact on quality of life and on brain plasticity is maximized when hearing aids are delivered close to the onset of the hearing loss, when two hearing aids are worn in the case of bilateral hearing loss, when hearing aids are worn on a regular basis, and, most important, when hearing-aids are delivered in the context of a holistic rehabilitation program. Brain plasticity occurs when functional representation of the brain is altered when the hearing-impaired are taught to effectively relearn and use the new speech input provided by hearing aids through some form of listening training designed to enhance auditory system.[31] It is also important to note that lack of amplification is associated with sensory deprivation, wherein speech understanding ability declines over time in unaided ears of adults with sensorineural hearing loss, whereas hearing for pure-tones and speech understanding ability either improves or remains stable over time with hearing aid use.[32]

The improved communication and reduction in social and emotional dysfunction perceived by older adults is sustainable over a period of 1 year of hearing aid use. Compared with the waiting list group, those older adults with mild to moderately severe sensorineural hearing loss who received hearing aids demonstrated an 85% improvement in social and emotional function, a 68% improvement in communication function, and a 26% improvement in depressive symptoms as assessed by the Geriatric Depression Scale. Improvements in psychosocial well-being and communication function associated with short-term hearing aid use are comparable for older and younger adults.[33] This finding is an important step toward dispelling the myth that older adults cannot derive significant benefits from hearing aids. Data from a 1999 study completed by the National Council on Aging (NCOA) revealed that hearing aid users are less depressed and more socially engaged than are older adults with comparable hearing loss who do not use hearing aids. Further, the NCOA study revealed that non–hearing aid users report more negative social effects of hearing loss than users, and non–hearing aid users reported higher levels of anger and frustration than hearing aid users.[34]

Hearing aids + audiologic rehabilitation = improved function

The benefits derived from hearing aids are enhanced when delivered in the context of a holistic audiologic rehabilitation (AR) program.[35] AR is an integral part of the solution to hearing loss and its negative consequence.[22,35,36] It is a highly variable process with several components, and current thinking suggests that AR and hearing aid fitting have a complementary relationship.[22,37] AR consists of (1) sensory management to optimize auditory function using hearing aids, assistive listening devices, or implantable devices; (2) instruction in the use of technology and control of the listening environment; (3) perceptual training to improve speech perception and communication; and (4) counseling to enhance participation and address emotional and practical limitations.[35,38]

Available cost utility analyses confirm that the most favorable outcomes are achieved when hearing aids are dispensed in the context of a comprehensive rehabilitation program.[32] Further, of the various approaches to AR, group programs that focus on counseling, communication strategies training, and computer-assisted techniques to enhance perceptual learning are of proven cost utility and effectiveness.[34,37] The systematic review recently completed by Hawkins concluded that that there is reasonably good evidence that hearing-related quality of life improves when adults participate in counseling-based group AR programs.[37] Table 97-3 summarizes the value of delivering hearing aids along with adjunctive counseling-oriented AR.

Table 97-3. The Value of Audiologic Rehabilitation + Hearing Aid Use

Features of Integrated Audiologic Rehabilitation Programs
• Provide an understanding of hearing aids, their care, maintenance, and use of the data logging feature.
• Promote realistic expectations regarding the value and capabilities of hearing aids.
• Maximize sensory input by providing the best possible visual and auditory signal.
• Help the patient understand the psychological and social problems resulting from hearing impairment.
• Maximize sensory integration by making the best use of the amplified auditory signal and the visible signal.
• Promote the use of cognitive processes necessary to derive meaning from incomplete sensory messages.
• Promote an understanding of how to create a positive communication environment.
• Develop within the individual assertive and interactive ways of communicating and repairing breakdowns.
• Empower the hearing impaired and help them to become proactive.
• Engage members of the individual's support system so that they partner with the hearing-impaired person.
• Help ensure understanding of compensatory communication strategies.
• Facilitate neural plasticity.
• Promote personal adjustment to hearing loss.

Device-related and personal adjustment counseling, perceptual and listening retraining, and familiarity with effective communication strategies will help debunk many of the myths surrounding hearing aid use and will provide realistic expectations critical to success. To ensure maximal benefit from hearing aids, older adults must have realistic expectations, patience, and the understanding that hearing aids are not very smart in that they do not automatically do a good job of helping the user to discriminate between the sounds the person wants to hear (i.e., speech) and those sounds the person wants to ignore (i.e., background noise).[32] New hearing aid users should not expect to suddenly hear normally. Users must understand that it takes time to realize the potential benefit from hearing aids, and thus they should not become discouraged early. Their ears and brains must become reeducated to hear selected patterns of sounds that have been made louder by the hearing aid. In a sense, new hearing aid users are suddenly being exposed to or bombarded with a world of sounds they have forgotten existed, such as the blare of street noises in the city, and they must become reoriented to or acquainted with the location and source of these "new" sounds. Table 97-4 summarizes what the elderly can realistically expect from hearing aids.

To better adapt to the hearing aid, new hearing aid users should wear the hearing aids for as many hours during the day as they feel comfortable with the units in their ears. Ideally they should wear their hearing aids in restricted situations at first, such as while at home with family members, while watching the television, or while eating dinner. Once the individual feels comfortable with amplified sound at home, he or she should venture into new hearing situations, at all times experimenting with the volume control to

Table 97-4. Realistic Expectations Regarding Capabilities of Hearing Instruments

Hearing aids will do the following:
- Enable the hearing impaired to hear many sounds they were unable to hear previously
- Enhance high-frequency sounds with reduced feedback
- Enable the hearing impaired to understand speech more clearly in noise, but not in all environments
- Improve sound quality
- Improve the ability of the hearing impaired to hear environmental sounds
- Require some time for adjustment
- Improve job performance
- Ease communication difficulties
- Stabilize speech understanding in the ear fitted with hearing aids
- Provide high value relative to cost

maintain speech input at a comfortable level and noise at a minimum. Although full-time use should be the goal, there are some exceptions. Persons with mild hearing loss may find their hearing aids useful in business meetings but burdensome in noisy situations such as restaurants or parties.

If patients complain that some intense sounds produce an uncomfortably loud hearing sensation, they should alert the dispensing audiologist at the follow-up visit, because a simple adjustment can usually be made. Many hearing aid users report that although at first they prefer "natural sounding" louder sounds as their ears and mind adjust, they tend to prefer a boost in the high-frequency response of the hearing aid that makes the consonants of speech crisper and easier to understand. It is of utmost importance that new hearing aid users schedule and keep all follow-up appointments (a minimum of 2 to 4 weeks following receipt of the hearing aid) so that the audiologist can make the necessary adjustments to ensure that sounds are comfortable, audible, tolerable, and understandable. At these visits, the audiologist and new hearing aid user work together to modify the response of the hearing aid for optimal speech understanding and user comfort. Finally, new hearing aid users should accept their hearing loss and not continue to consider it a disgrace or a stigma. They should not cover their hearing aids as a way of hiding the hearing loss, as hearing aids signal others that a hearing loss exists and that they should speak clearly. If the hearing aid users accept their hearing loss and hearing aids, so will persons to whom they are speaking. In short, acceptance of hearing loss and motivation to overcome its consequences are conditions for hearing aid satisfaction and success.

Implantable devices and hearing assistive technologies

Of the components of audiologic rehabilitation, sensory management, or the provision of some form of amplification ranging from hearing aids and hearing assistive technologies (HATs) to medical technologies such as a cochlear implant or bone-anchored hearing aid, is the treatment of choice. Since the late 1980s, there have been considerable improvements in speech-processing strategies used with cochlear implants; they are now a realistic option for healthy, older adults with severe to profound hearing loss for whom hearing aids are not conferring enhanced quality of life in important social environments. There are approximately 300,000 older adults suffering from non-age-related profound hearing loss for whom cochlear implants are a viable option.[39] Cochlear implantation is a cost-effective option for those older adults who qualify audiometrically and are considered good surgical candidates. The surgical procedure requires general aesthesia and can be completed within 3 hours.

Cochlear implants are small commercially available electronic devices surgically implanted into the inner ear. The array of electrodes bypasses the damaged hair cells and is inserted into the auditory nerve, directly stimulating it. It is noteworthy that age and duration of deafness have a negligible effect on postsurgical outcomes among subjects 65 years and older.[39] Available evidence suggests that cochlear implants improve the user's access to verbal communication and environmental sounds, and they enhance telephone communication and the user's enjoyment of music.[39] Interestingly, residual speech recognition carried higher predictive value for success than the age at which an individual received an implant.

In contrast to a cochlear implant, a bone-anchored hearing aid (BAHA) is surgically implanted into the skull behind the ear. Some consider it a surgically implantable bone-conduction hearing aid, as it works on a principle similar to that of bone-conduction hearing aids worn by individuals with chronic middle ear disease or external and middle ear deformities, which preclude use of traditional air conduction hearing aids. The BAHA delivers sound into the skull by means of sound vibration. These vibrations transfer sound from the bad ear side to the good ear side through the skull. The BAHA can be used in persons with conductive hearing loss, particularly those with chronically discharging ears, or in persons with complete or near complete single-sided deafness (SSD) or deafness in one ear.

The BAHA has three components: a titanium implant that is surgically implanted into the skull just behind the affected ear, which over time naturally integrates into the cranium; an external abutment that serves as a link between the titanium implant and the sound processor; and a sound processor, which picks up the sound, shapes it, and changes it into a vibratory stimulus that is passed through the abutment and titanium implant to vibrate the cochlea in both ears. The sound processor is either worn on the head or is worn on the body like a body hearing aid with a cord and receiver that snap onto the abutment. Older adults with SSD who have not experienced much success with hearing aids should consider speaking with an otolaryngologist to determine candidacy. Before proceeding with the surgical procedure, individuals can try the BAHA to gain a feel for the experience of hearing via bone conduction. Reports suggest that BAHAs have successfully reduced the emotional and social handicap experienced by persons with SSD from a variety of etiologies.

Surgical implants are appropriate for a select group of older adults with hearing impairment. Hearing aids in combination with AR are the primary nonmedical intervention for hearing impairment. However, for selected individuals, hearing aids do not provide for the easy clear listening in all communication environments. Their disadvantage lies in the fact that well-fit hearing aids can provide a favorable signal-to-noise (S/N) ratio if the environment is free of distractions and if the speaker is close to the person with the hearing impairment. However, in many listening situations, the hearing aid microphone at the listener's ear is typically some distance from the sound source, making speech difficult to understand especially in a noisy room. In essence, the farther away from the sound source one is, the softer the sound pressure and the less clear the speech signal.[40]

For the most part, the listening environments we live in are demanding, and hearing aids alone are insufficient to access auditory events that are not close to the person who is hearing impaired. HATS have proven invaluable in overcoming some of the environmental barriers to successful communication. They include auditory and nonauditory devices available to help individuals in a variety of listening situations.[40] Collectively, these devices rely on auditory, visual, or tactile information to augment speech understanding or to help the user to monitor environmental sounds. HATS are recommended based on an individual's communication needs including small group face-to-face communication, electronic media, telephone use and environmental alerting needs, large group communication, and noisy environments. HATS are designed to be used as a complement to or in lieu of hearing aids or cochlear implants. Their value, in part, lies in their simplicity and low cost. They enhance or help to maintain the functional communication capacities of the hearing impaired.

Divided into four distinct categories, these devices use alternate modes of sound transmission and different types of signal delivery modalities. The four categories include (1) sound-enhancement technologies, (2) television/media devices (television reception), (3) telecommunications technologies (telephone reception), and (4) signal-alerting technologies (reception of environmental warning sounds). Sound enhancement technologies enable a person with hearing impairment to understand speech clearly when the speaker is at a considerable distance away. This is accomplished by transmitting the signal directly to the listener's ear, thereby overcoming the barriers posed by distance and environmental noise. In short, the intensity of the signal relative to the noise (signal-to-noise ratio) becomes more favorable. Sound enhancement technologies include a microphone placed close to the sound source (within 6 inches), which picks up the signal, and via one of several modes of transmission, sends the signal to the listener's ear(s). Signals can be transmitted to the listener via a hard-wired connection between the microphone/amplifier/receiver and the headphones, via wireless radio transmission of signals (i.e., frequency modulated [FM] unit), via an induction loop system, or via infrared light.

Figure 97-4 shows an inexpensive, hard-wired system, available online and at audio stores, that health professionals can use when communicating one-on-one with patients who have difficulty understanding in the clinical setting. These personal amplifiers are ideal for use during an intake, when communicating at bedside with persons with hearing impairment, and when providing important recommendations to patients for whom compliance is key.

Personal FM systems are wireless communication systems that pick up the signal directly from the source and transmit it via radio waves to the hearing-impaired receiver. FM systems can be used with or without a hearing aid. They are more costly than hardwired systems, yet can facilitate listening in noisy environments, in large rooms with poor acoustics, or when the speaker is at a distance such as in a boardroom or at a conference. With this arrangement, the FM microphone transmitter is worn close to the source of speech (speaker), and the signal is delivered via FM signals to the listener's ears free of environmental noise. FM systems can be used outdoors and when the speaker and listener are in different rooms. FM systems benefit individuals with moderately severe to severe sensorineural hearing loss whose personal or professional lives demand adequate speech understanding to function effectively. When using FM systems in a large auditorium, the speaker talks into a microphone, and the signal is transmitted wirelessly to those in the audience wearing a stand-alone FM receiver, a BTE-FM system, a hearing aid with a telecoil system, or a cochlear implant equipped with a telecoil. If the hearing aid does not include a telecoil, the individual can link the hearing aid to an FM system using a small adapter known as a boot. Many companies manufacture behind-the-ear hearing aids that include an integrated BTE-FM system, whereas others manufacture hearing aids that can be coupled to an FM system. Present-day hearing aids that are equipped to receive FM signals also incorporate multimicrophone technology. Older hearing-impaired adults with moderately severe to severe sensorineural hearing loss or auditory processing problems should consider a BTE that incorporates an FM receiver as an option. When coupling an FM system to a hearing aid, older adults do experience improvements in communication performance in a variety of situations.[40] Further, BTE-FM systems are beneficial in restaurants, at lectures, in cars, and at noisy receptions.

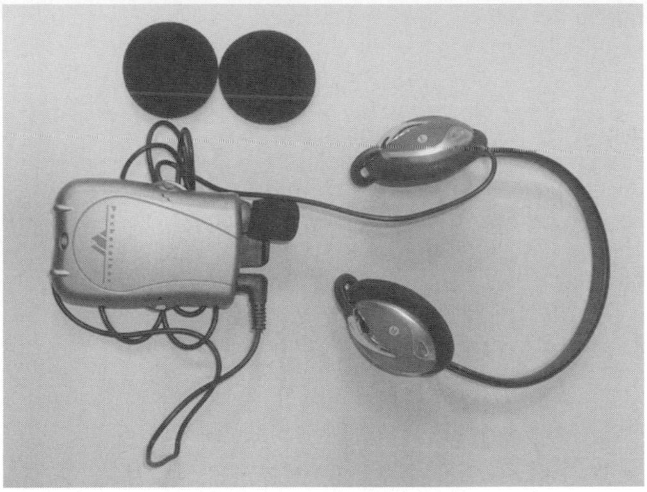

Figure 97-4. Personal amplifier.

In contrast to FM systems, which use radio waves to carry sound, infrared systems use invisible light, the wavelength of which is outside the range of human visibility, to transmit signals indoors in a single room.[41] Infrared systems can be used with different forms of media including television, stereo systems, and in large rooms where people congregate such as theaters or houses of worship. Infrared systems provide the best quality sound for radio and television and are widely used in theaters and in concert and lecture halls. Essentially the remote microphone of the system is placed within 6 inches of the media speaker to provide a favorable S/N ratio.

Telecommunication technology facilitates communication over the telephone. A variety of options are available ranging from portable amplifiers, speakerphones, amplified telephones, text messaging, and telecommunication relay services, such as text to voice, Internet protocol (IP) relay services, video relay services (VRSs), or text telephone services known as telecommunication systems for the deaf (TDDs).[41] TDDs are invaluable to persons with severe to profound hearing loss for whom it is impossible to discriminate speech that is transmitted by telephone. TDDs are approximately the size of a typewriter. Individuals communicating over the telephone merely type in their message, or use a relay operator who types in a message, which is displayed across the listener's TDD. The telephone company provides relay service free of charge for a person wishing to speak with a TDD user. E-mail is also an excellent form of telecommunication technology for a person with hearing impairment who is unable to communicate comfortably over the telephone. Bluetooth technology, open canal hearing aids, and hearing aid compatible cellular phones allow hearing aid users to comfortably speak on the phone while wearing hearing aids. Finally, signal-alerting technology includes any system that warns, signals, or alerts a person with a hearing loss. These systems use loud sounds, visual signals, or tactile signals to alert the hearing impaired to sounds in the environment. For example, a vibrator placed under the pillow can awaken the person with hearing loss in the morning, a strobe light attached to a smoke alarm can alert the hearing-impaired person to a fire, and vibrating pagers or wristwatches can alert the hearing impaired as well.[41] Signal-alerting devices are commercially available and are invaluable for hearing-impaired persons who are homebound, for persons with cognitive impairments, and for residents of nursing facilities who cannot hear external events because of hearing loss.

Audiologists are well equipped to guide persons and institutions about the system(s) that will best meet their needs and to arrange for them to purchase the necessary assistive listening devices. Hearing-impaired individuals have to be proactive about assistive technologies, as audiologists sometimes underestimate their value. A number of Web sites describe the alerting technologies available to the consumer.

SCREENING PROTOCOLS

Mounting evidence exists suggesting that at least 25% of persons between 65 and 75 years of age have undiagnosed hearing loss that may be detectable via routine, inexpensive hearing screening activities.[42] Further, fall-related injuries are among the most common, morbid, and expensive health conditions involving older adults. Falls account for 10% of emergency department visits and 6% of hospitalizations among persons over the age of 65 years and are major determinants of functional decline. Despite the high prevalence of hearing and balance problems among persons of Medicare age, the majority of physicians do not screen older adults because of reimbursement obstacles and a limited understanding of approaches to cost-effectively screen this population.[45]

In light of the functional consequences of unidentified hearing loss and balance problems, the variety of technologies available to overcome communication difficulties, and the proven value of physician referral screening programs, it is imperative that physicians periodically screen older adults for hearing loss and balance problems. Recognizing the detrimental effects of unidentified sensory loss, the U.S. Preventive Services Task Force recommends that persons over 65 years of age undergo periodic hearing evaluations and counseling regarding the availability of hearing aids.[44,45] Further, the national Medicare system will reimburse primary care physicians (PCPs) a fixed amount of money for completing the entire Welcome to Medicare examination, which includes hearing and balance screening using inexpensive, brief, reliable, and valid questionnaires.[44,45] In fact, it is now acknowledged that the health-related quality of life of older adults is improved when PCPs screen for hearing and balance problems.[43]

Self-report measures of high sensitivity and specificity, which are easy and inexpensive to use, have been recommended for use by PCPs to identify older adults at risk for hearing and balance problems. Audiologists and physicians alike have advocated the screening version of the Hearing Handicap Inventory for the Elderly (HHIE-S), which has the advantage of identifying patients who perceive hearing loss to be a problem and who are motivated to use hearing aids.[45–47] The Dizziness Handicap Inventory (DHI) is widely used for screening for dizziness, a condition for which there is considerable under-referral despite the morbidity and mortality associated with falls in older adults.[49]

A simple, reliable, and valid hearing screening protocol with good diagnostic accuracy has been advocated and validated by a number of investigators.[45–49] The procedure entails a pure-tone screen and administration of the 10-item screening version of the Hearing Handicap Inventory for the Elderly (HHIE-S). The purpose of the screen is to identify older persons with handicapping hearing impairment who require audiologic testing and intervention. The pure-tone screen involves use of the audioscope, a hand-held otoscope combined with a screening audiometer that delivers pure tones at 40 dBHL at four frequencies: 500, 1000, 2000, and 4000 Hz. The audioscope is shown in Figure 97-5. A patient fails the screen if he or she does not hear the tones at 1000 or 2000 Hz in one or both ears. The patient is instructed to raise his or her finger or hand when the tone is heard. The patient's response should be time-locked to the presentation of the stimulus signaled by a red indicator light on the audioscope. If otoscopic examination indicates the presence of cerumen impaction, this necessitates a failure and a referral. Further, patients complaining of tinnitus should be referred, as tinnitus could be a symptom of a significant medical condition for which efficacious treatments are now available.

Before or following the pure-tone screen, the patient should complete the HHIE-S using a face-to-face, paper-and-pencil, or computer-assisted presentation. A score of 10 or greater signifies the necessity of a referral. More specifically, scores of 0 to 8 signify no handicap, scores of 10 to 22 signify a mild to moderate handicap, and scores of 24 to 40 suggest significant self-perceived handicap. Scores on the HHIE-S are directly correlated to hearing aid uptake and have been shown to improve after the initiation of hearing aid use. Primary care physicians with firsthand experience with this screening protocol consider it to be simple, cost-effective, quick, and easy to administer.[46] Table 97-5 lists the items that make up the 10-item screening version (HHIE-S).[47] Scores on the questionnaire are highly predictive of hearing aid use such that individuals obtaining a score

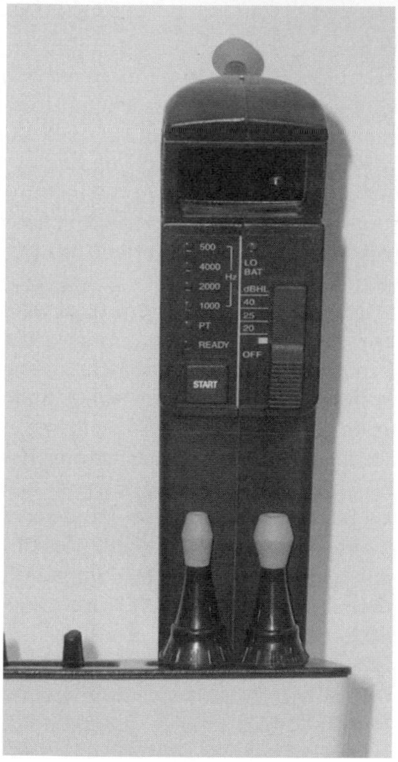

Figure 97-5. Audioscope.

Table 97-5. Screening Version of the Hearing Handicap Inventory for the Elderly (HHIE-S)

Instructions: Answer yes (4 points), sometimes (2 points), or no (0 points) for each question. If you are a hearing aid user, answer questions according to how you hear with the hearing aid. If the question does not apply, merely enter no as your response.

E-1. Does a hearing problem cause you to feel embarrassed when meeting new people?
E-2. Does a hearing problem cause you to feel frustrated when talking to members of your family?
S-1. Do you have difficulty hearing when someone speaks in a whisper?
E-3. Do you feel handicapped by a hearing problem?
S-2. Does a hearing problem cause you difficulty when visiting friends, relatives, or neighbors?
S-3. Does a hearing problem cause you to attend religious services less often than you would like?
E-4. Does a hearing problem cause you to have arguments with family members?
S-4. Does a hearing problem cause you difficulty when listening to TV or radio?
E-5. Do you feel that any difficulty with your hearing limits or hampers your personal or social life?
S-5. Does a hearing problem cause you difficulty when in a restaurant with relatives or friends?

Abbreviations: "S" items probe social/situational consequences of hearing loss; "E" items probe emotional consequences of hearing loss.

of 18 or greater on the HHIE-S are considered likely to purchase and benefit from hearing aid use, irrespective of hearing loss severity. Further, veterans with a high score on the HHIE-S who report perceiving a hearing handicap (question E-3) have a high likelihood of being fitted with hearing aids. Weinstein devotes an entire chapter of her textbook to strategies for identifying older adults with hearing loss including the use of multimedia and Web-based techniques.[28] Web sites containing the HHIE-S can easily be accessed, and several of these have links to audiology services nationwide.

WHEN AND TO WHOM TO REFER

Audiologists and otolaryngologists are hearing health care specialists who provide assistance to persons with hearing problems. The otolaryngologist is a medical doctor who diagnoses and treats medical diseases of the ear that may be causing a hearing problem. If medical treatment in the form of antibiotic therapy or surgical intervention is not indicated, persons with hearing loss should be seen by an audiologist. An audiologist is a professional with a doctoral degree who works with people who exhibit hearing, balance, and ear-related problems. Audiologists provide evaluative, rehabilitative, and preventive services. They work in a wide variety of settings, including private practice, hospitals, otolaryngology offices, government health facilities, and rehabilitation centers. Although audiologists can represent the point of entry into the hearing health care system, older

KEY POINTS
Disorders of Hearing

- Hearing loss prevalence increases with age such that over 50% of persons over 80 years of age have a hearing impairment.
- The majority of residents of nursing facilities have a hearing impairment.
- The hearing impairment and speech understanding difficulties that are a hallmark of presbycusis are associated with significant functional effects, including depression and isolation.
- Presbycusis arises because of atrophic age-related changes in the cochlea, auditory nerve fibers, auditory brain stem pathways, and the temporal lobe of the brain.
- Cerumen impaction is prevalent in older adults and can interfere with the proper functioning of hearing aids.
- The sensorineural hearing loss affecting a high proportion of older adults is typically not amenable to medical intervention.
- The most effective treatment for sensorineural hearing loss is hearing aids.
- Hearing aids are efficacious in ameliorating the functional, social, and emotional effects of hearing loss in older adults.
- The most favorable outcomes with hearing aids take place when a hearing aid is delivered in the context of a counseling-oriented rehabilitation program
- Counseling should assist the hearing impaired to do the following:
  - Understand hearing loss
  - Accept the handicapping effects of hearing loss
  - Overcome obstacles posed by hearing loss
  - Manipulate hearing aids and hearing assistive technologies independently
  - Understand principles of care and maintenance of hearing aids
  - Incorporate communication strategies into daily life

Sources of information about hearing loss and hearing aids are the American Academy of Audiology, the American Speech-Language-Hearing Association, and the Better Hearing Institute (BHI).

adults referred to audiologists by a physician are most likely to purchase audiologic services in the form of hearing tests, hearing aids, and AR. In the current health care delivery system, PCPs tend to be too busy to screen patients for hearing and balance problems. It behooves audiologists to partner with PCPs to develop an efficient, easily administered protocol to identify older adults with hearing/balance problems requiring evaluation and treatment.[43]

CONCLUDING REMARKS

Approximately 30% to 50% of older adults suffer from a handicapping hearing impairment that can interfere with the quality of their lives. Adults over 55 years of age make up 81% of all hearing aid users, yet the majority of older adults with hearing loss do not use hearing aids. The stigma associated with hearing aid use coupled with persistent complaints from experienced users about difficulty understanding in public places, especially noisy environments, has kept penetration rates stable but low over time.

Technologically sophisticated hearing aids in combination with some form of audiologic rehabilitation are more effective than ever before and are a boon to older adults who are living longer and retiring early yet continue to be confronted by difficulty understanding the speech of others, especially in noisy environments. Sound evidence is available demonstrating the improved audibility and enhanced speech understanding in noisy and reverberant environments afforded by today's digital hearing instruments, which reduce feedback, lessen the perception of extraneous noise, and include directional microphone technology that automatically picks up speech while suppressing unwanted noise emanating from behind the speaker. This improved communication translates into beneficial effects on the individual's health-related quality of life.

The availability of assistive listening devices that compensate for the shortcomings remaining with hearing aids is another avenue for persons with hearing impairment to pursue. The physician has reliable, valid, and inexpensive tools at his or her disposal to identify persons with hearing problems who require and can benefit from the expertise of audiologists. Working together, physicians and audiologists can reduce the burden of hearing loss and can promote the quality of life of the increasing population of older adults suffering from a handicapping hearing impairment.

For a complete list of references, please visit online only at www.expertconsult.com

CHAPTER 98

Health Promotion for the Community-Living Older Adult

Maureen F. Markle-Reid
Heather H. Keller
Gina Browne

INTRODUCTION

Older adults (>65 years of age) are growing in proportion and number in both developed and less-developed nations[1] as a result of economic prosperity, health care, improved sanitation, and improved education. In Canada, as in many other developed countries, there will be an aging of the population as the "baby boom" generation reaches the age of 65. The fastest-growing segment is those who are ≥80 years; currently 1 in 30 Canadians is over the age of 80, and this proportion is projected to increase to 1 in 10 by 2056.[2]

Increasingly, Canada's older citizens are aging in place, attributable to the aging of the population, technologic advances, budget constraints, and preferences of older adults, their families, and society, as well as changes in options for care. Over 90% of those aged 65 and over live in the community.[3] Rates of institutionalization for older people have decreased, and formal community-based care has expanded, such that the proportion of older people receiving community care now substantially outweighs the proportion receiving formal services through an institution.[4] Since the late 1980s in Canada, hospital beds have been reduced by 30% and nursing home beds by 11%, and ambulatory care has increased. The result is increasing pressure on community-based services to maintain accessible, high-quality, and comprehensive health care within the confines of economic constraints.[4–6]

The benefits associated with aging in place are well documented. Residing at home optimizes an older person's health,[7,8] independence, control, and sense of well-being,[9] as well as social connectedness, which positively influences health.[8,10] Managers and policy makers alike face questions about the most efficient mix of service strategies for the promotion of health in this more community-based and less institution-oriented system.

As the population of older adults (≥65 years) has increased, and as medical advances continue to convert once acute life-threatening diseases into chronic illnesses, there has been an associated increase in the prevalence of unremitting chronic conditions and frailty.[11–13] Over 80% of older people (≥65 years) have chronic medical conditions requiring daily self-care and management.[14] Chronic conditions, including cardiovascular diseases, diabetes, obesity, cancer, and respiratory diseases, account for 59% of the 56.5 million deaths annually and 45.9% of the global burden of disease worldwide.[15] Among those with chronic conditions, more than one half of older adults report having at least two of these diagnoses.[16] These unremitting chronic illnesses also have a significant economic impact. The total cost of ill health, disability, and death resulting from chronic diseases is about $80 billion annually for Canada.[17] Use of healthcare services is positively related to comorbidity—use increases as the number of chronic conditions goes up.[16] The gradient effect in health service use is most apparent for acute hospitalizations, general practitioner visits, and nursing consultations.[16] Left unchecked, these conditions have the potential to overwhelm the health care system and threaten its sustainability.[16] The long-term solution must involve health promotion to delay or better manage these conditions to contain costs and reduce demand for services.[18]

Approximately 15% of community-living seniors fall into the category of being "frail," defined as vulnerable to significant functional decline as a result of the accumulation of multiple, interacting illnesses, impairments, and disabilities.[13,19,20] Of those considered frail, 17% are at high risk for such decline that would jeopardize their ability to live independently at home in the community.[21] These people are typically 75 years of age or older and are living with multiple health conditions that are acute and chronic in nature as well as functional disabilities.[22] They may also have cognitive impairments or social support networks that are overextended or at risk of breaking down.[22,23] These characteristics put frail older adults at risk for increasing morbidity, disability, health service use, and death.[24]

However, chronic disease and frailty should not be considered an inevitable or irreversible consequence of aging.[25] Although it is true that as individuals age, they are at greater risk of developing chronic health problems, these conditions are not inherent in the aging process.[26] Older adults are quite heterogeneous, including those aging "successfully," "usually," and at "accelerated" rates.[27–29] A majority of the most costly health conditions are preventable, treatable, or manageable.[18] The World Health Organization[15,30] estimates that at least one third of the total economic and social burden of disease in developed countries is caused by a handful of largely avoidable risks: tobacco, alcohol, high blood pressure, high cholesterol, and obesity.[31]

For many of these risk factors for chronic disease, negative impacts can be reversed quickly, most benefits will accrue within a decade, and even modest changes in risk factor levels can bring about large improvements in people's health.[15,30] For example, with healthy eating, regular exercise, not smoking, and effective stress management, over 90% of cases of type 2 diabetes and 80% of cases of coronary heart disease could be avoided.[15,30] One review reported that even a 5% reduction in preventable illnesses could lead to substantial savings in medical costs, as well as cost savings beyond the health care sector.[18] Consequently, identifying modifiable factors that can reduce or delay health service use and increase quality of life in these populations is a priority.

A growing body of research in Canada suggests that older community-living adults can benefit significantly from proactive health promotion and preventive care interventions.[32–39] The ultimate goal of these programs is to proactively identify and address factors influencing health and to promote positive health behaviors and autonomy of older people living in the community, to prevent or delay institutionalization, reduce health care costs, and improve health-related quality of life and function.[40]

This chapter summarizes this research and identifies how health promotion and preventive care for community-living older adults can be improved. The specific objectives of this chapter are as follows: (1) to describe three separate groups of older adults and their need for health promotion and preventive care, (2) to describe a conceptual framework for health promotion and preventive care for frail older adults, (3) to describe a framework for economic evaluation of health care programs, (4) to argue in favor of the importance of screening to identify older adults who could benefit from health promotion and preventive care efforts, (5) to describe successful health promotion and prevention efforts among community-living older adults, and (6) to demonstrate the need for further policy and research on health promotion and preventive care for community-living older adults.

THE HETEROGENEITY OF OLDER ADULTS AND THE NEED FOR HEALTH PROMOTION

Older adults are a heterogeneous group, and aging occurs at different rates in different people. Chronologic age does not tell the full story of functional ability or quality of life, and most disabilities of old age are not inevitable, universal, or irreversible.[25] In the context of health, people who are aging successfully are those who continue to experience good health for an extended period of time. "This is the 65-year old who plans to take a cycling tour of France, the 75-year-old who plays tennis twice a week, or the 80-year-old who walks two miles each day."[29] Older adults who are *successfully aging* have minimal health problems, may visit their primary health care provider for preventive checks such as blood pressure, and may have a few risk factors (e.g., family history of heart disease), but they are quite healthy, with no modifiable risk factors. These older adults are likely to be on no medications or only prophylactic formulations. They watch what they eat and try to exercise. They typically develop signs of chronic disease late in life, such as starting medication for hypertension in their late 70s. Because of this delay in onset of chronic disease, successfully aging older adults spend less time dealing with its effects.[29]

Usually aging older adults have some signs that chronic disease has initiated. Typically, they take a few medications to manage conditions such as hypertension or dyslipidemia, they may be bothered by the occasional bout of arthritis pain, and their doctor sees them on a routine basis to monitor their conditions. These indicators or conditions do not drastically affect the quality of life of these older adults, as they still travel when they want and do most of the activities that they are interested in such as driving, babysitting their grandchildren, or taking cruises.[29] Approximately 80% of seniors are experiencing successful or usual aging,[41] although this proportion falls among the oldest old.[42]

The older adult experiencing *accelerated aging* appears frailer and more functionally dependent for his or her age. These people, who represent 15% to 20% of seniors, are typically over 75 years of age and have co-occurring physical health problems, both acute and chronic.[20,42] They are highly vulnerable, living in the community with supports that are prone to breakdown with any shift in their health and well-being.[21–23] Many live in isolation, cut off from community services because of a lack of information, transportation, or the will to initiate action on their own.[43] Another important consideration is that many seniors live in poverty or near-poverty conditions, as a growing number live alone without the benefit of two pensions for married older adults.[44] Additionally, the prevalence of depression among those experiencing accelerated aging is estimated at 26% to 44%, at least twice that among older people in general.[45] These characteristics lead to a greater risk for loss of functional independence, institutionalization, and death.[13] Long-term care facilities take care of approximately 5% of these seniors, and about 15% reside at home in the community.[20] These frail older adults pose a central challenge to current health systems, as they are frequently in contact with the health system including acute hospitalization and home care services.[23,29] A further consideration is that frail seniors living at home are particularly difficult to reach and are at high risk for loss of functional independence and for institutionalization.[13] These data underline the need for health promotion efforts in this group.

Before further discussing health promotion and preventive care in the frail older adult, it is important to clarify what is meant by frailty. Despite the dramatic increase in the use of the term *frailty* since the late 1980s, there is a lack of consensus in the literature regarding its meaning and use and no clear conceptual guidelines for establishing criteria to describe older adults as frail.[24] Is frailty a disease? Is it a part of aging? What does frailty look like? How is it defined, framed, and understood? Finally, exactly how frail is frail?[46,47] A first step in addressing the problem of frailty is to understand better how to identify those who are frail.[48] Despite calls for more research,[49,50] the components of frailty have not been sufficiently defined to identify populations at risk or in need of proactive interventions.[24]

One literature review of definitions and conceptual models of frailty in relation to older adults suggests that frailty is a multiple-determined state of vulnerability in which an individual is at risk of becoming more or less frail over time.[24] The implication of this is that the process of frailty can be modified or reversed.[24] This finding highlights the need for rational, theoretical interventions directed toward health promotion and preventive care for this population. This chapter gives guidelines for a taking a new theoretical approach to the concept of frailty in older adults, which is (1) multidimensional and considers the complex interplay among behavioral, biologic, social, and environmental determinants on health rather than a single influence[13,51,52]; (2) not age-related; (3) subjectively defined; and (4) considers both individual and environmental factors that influence health. (Table 98-1).[24]

Despite the differences in these three groups in terms of their needs, each one could benefit from health promotion and preventive care efforts targeted to its specific needs.[15,29] Programs and services that promote the health of older adults, focused on keeping them healthy rather than solely being reactive to symptoms, are underdeveloped in North

Table 98-1. Dimensions of Frailty

Dimension	Supporting Evidence
The concept must be multidimensional and consider the complex interplay among behavioral, biologic, social, and environmental determinants on health rather than a single influence.	This view is consistent with the observation that many social, socioeconomic, and lifestyle factors are associated with health and that determinants of health are often highly interrelated.[13,51,52] Theoretical models need to address the complexity of problems rather than focusing on a single problem, because older people typically have coexisting physical, emotional, and social problems that are interrelated with one another and with external factors.[24,170]
The concept must not be age related, suggesting a negative and stereotypical view of aging.	Theoretical models should reflect a positive view of aging that emphasizes the capacity for autonomy and independence and maximizes the person's strengths[171] as well as deficits.[24]
The concept must take into account an individual's context and incorporate subjective perceptions.	The trajectory of frailty is unique for each individual.[172] The emphasis is on the individual's perception of health rather than on the objective circumstances. Research supports the hypothesis that an individual's poor adjustment to chronic illness or affective state is not related to the specific physical disease or level of disability but rather to the negative meaning the individual attributes to it.[173] Theoretical models need to incorporate subjective measures and allow for individual variability.[24]
The concept must take into account the contribution of both individual and environmental factors that influence health.	Frailty can originate from within an individual or from conditions in the environment. Theoretical models need to address the constellation of individual and environmental factors that influence health.[24]

America.[28,53] Potentially, the lack of development of such programs is due to the narrow societal viewpoint that older adults cannot change behaviors such as smoking, eating, and exercising.[54] Chernoff[54] suggested that in some ways this belief is true, but there is also research that proves otherwise. Seniors are interested in changing and can change behaviors when given the support to do so. The goal of any health promotion program for older adults living in the community should be on optimizing their current health, even if minimal change in quantity of life is achieved.[1] Given the heterogeneity of older adults, it is essential to consider the differences in these three groups in terms of their health trajectories and quality of life when making decisions about the type and amount of health promotion activities required. As the population ages and the number of people aging in place increases, there is an urgent need to identify effective and efficient ways of promoting the health of community-living older adults.

CONCEPTUAL FRAMEWORK FOR HEALTH PROMOTION AND PREVENTIVE CARE FOR FRAIL OLDER ADULTS

Empirical evidence alone is insufficient to direct the design and evaluation of interventions. Theory is essential for program development, implementation, and evaluation, as it explains and can predict outcomes. Furthermore, theory enhances the generalizability of the results by providing the basis for informing the systematic development and implementation of intervention strategies that improve the health of older people as well as evaluation indicators.[55]

An adapted version of the model of vulnerability[56] incorporates the key concepts of frailty discussed earlier to guide the development, implementation, and evaluation of health promotion and preventive care interventions. Vulnerability is a net result of an interaction between the person's personal resources (cognitive, emotional, intellectual, behavioral) and environmental supports (social, material, cultural), both of which, along with biologic characteristics (age, gender, genetic endowment), are determinants of health. Within an individual, personal resources and environmental supports intersect, as shown in Figure 98-1, and can be synergistic and cumulative.[37] The base of the triangle represents the degree of vulnerability,[56] and thus also the individual's health

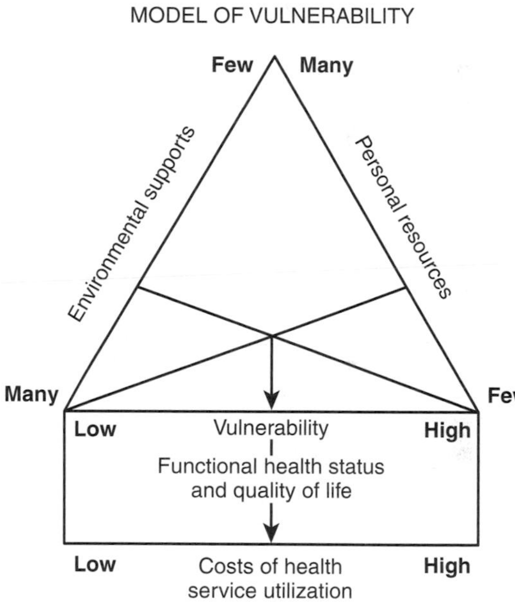

Figure 98-1. Model of vulnerability. *(Adapted from Rogers AC. Vulnerability, health and health care. J Adv Nurs 1997;26(1):65–72.)*

status and quality of life. Based on published evidence,[32] expenditure of use of health services increases proportionately with the level of vulnerability.

Even if personal resources hold constant, changes in an individual's environmental supports can greatly alter one's degree of vulnerability and thus his or her use of health and social services.[37] What is needed is "a 'fit' between the needs and resources of the person and the demands and resources of the environment (p. 68)."[56] This vulnerability model provides a schema of the basic components of a multidimensional health promotion and preventive care intervention for reducing functional decline, enhancing health, and promoting appropriate use of healthcare services. Proactive health promotion and preventive care interventions either targeted at the individual or the environment can identify and strengthen available resources, thereby reducing vulnerability and the on-demand use of expensive health services while enhancing quality of life. Hence, strategies for optimizing health in the model of vulnerability are multilevel.[56]

Table 98-2. Dimensions of Risk in Rogers' Model of Vulnerability

Risk Factors	Supporting Evidence
Personal Resources	
Inborn	Aday, 1993[174]; Rogers, 1997[56]
Age, gender, race, temperament, genetic predisposition to disease, susceptibility to illness, sensitivity to drugs and chemical imbalances	
Acquired	
Recently moved	Hebert, 1997[22]
Recently discharged from hospital	Hollander & Chappell, 2002[175]
Poor self-perceived health	Stuck et al, 1999[103]
Depression and anxiety	Schoevers et al, 2005[102]; Stuck et al, 1999[103]
Falling	Lin et al, 2007[176]; Markle-Reid et al, 2008[150]
Taking multiple medications	Hebert et al, 1997[22]; Hogan et al, 2003[51]
Cognitive impairment	Stuck et al, 1999[103]
Using assistance for activities of daily living	Challis & Hughes, 2002[131]; Markle-Reid et al, 2008[177]
Impaired vision or hearing	Stuck et al, 1999[103]
Social isolation	Stuck et al, 1999[103]
Comorbid health conditions	Stuck et al, 1999[103]; Wilkins, 2006[178]
Nutritional risk	Keller et al, 2004[146]
Low level of physical activity	Tinetti et al, 1999[153]
Excessive consumption of alcohol and smoking	Stuck et al, 1999[103]
Environmental Supports	
Societal attitudes and stereotypes of aging	Rogers, 1997[56]
Living alone, social isolation	Stuck et al, 1999[103]
Low income	Li et al, 2005[179]
Low levels of education	Aday, 1993[174]; Pressley, 1999[180]

Personal resources can be defined as either inborn or acquired characteristics, that interact with the environment to influence health.[56] Inborn characteristics that influence health include nonmodifiable factors such as the person's age, gender, race, temperament, genetic predisposition to disease, susceptibility to illness, sensitivity to drugs, and chemical imbalances. Acquired characteristics are modifiable factors known to increase risk for functional decline in older adults. *Environmental supports* can be defined as factors that interact with personal resources to influence health[56] (Table 98-2).

FRAMEWORK FOR ECONOMIC EVALUATION

Although the literature contains many evaluations of programs seeking to achieve improved outcomes for vulnerable populations, such as frail older community-dwelling adults, few of these outcome studies include measures of cost.[33] Economic analysis has now established itself as having an important role in the planning, management, and evaluation of healthcare. It consists of comparing both the effects and expense of alternative interventions for a single problem with the goal of maximizing improvements in health-related well-being using a fixed pool of available resources.[57] As depicted in Figure 98-2, the economic evaluation of healthcare programs[58] yields nine possible outcomes (the more favorable ones are highlighted by shading). In outcome 1, increased effects or health benefits are achieved with increased expenditure for additional resources consumed. This is called *cost-effective*, whereby more effect is achieved for more cost. Outcome 4 is also favorable, because increased effects are achieved with one approach over another at equivalent expenditures. Outcome 7 represents the win/win situation or unambiguous improvements in economic efficiency, whereby more effect is produced at lower expenditures. Outcome 8 represents the situation in which alternative health programs produce the same effect, but some approaches are associated with lower expenditure from a societal perspective. Options 7 and 8 are superior to the often implemented option 9, in which funding is cut, along with the potential for reduced effects, which releases resources for other purposes.[58]

This approach can be used to classify the main effects and expense of comparative community health interventions. In addition, this approach can be used to classify who (with what characteristics) benefits most and at what expense when various interventions are available. This is especially of concern in systems of national health insurance, in which people will use may use services (inappropriately).[59]

SCREENING AND ASSESSMENT: IDENTIFYING OLDER ADULTS WHO COULD BENEFIT FROM HEALTH PROMOTION AND PREVENTIVE CARE EFFORTS

There is a growing body of international evidence that suggests that early detection of older people at risk for functional decline or loss of autonomy is beneficial. Screening or other methods of early detection would identify older adults with risk factors that could lead to significant health problems and the use of costly health care resources. Several studies of screening and case finding among older adults have been conducted in an attempt to proactively identify and address problems to reduce the use of costly resources; these studies are reviewed later on.

Many older adults living the community have unrecognized risk factors. Health concerns or risk occur in almost all (92% to 99%) older adults in practice populations, with up to 83% having at least one unreported or unrecognized risk.[60–62] Many of these risk factors are social problems[62] that can affect a senior's support network and well-being and have the potential to increase health care expenditures if left undetected and, therefore, untreated. Unsolicited home

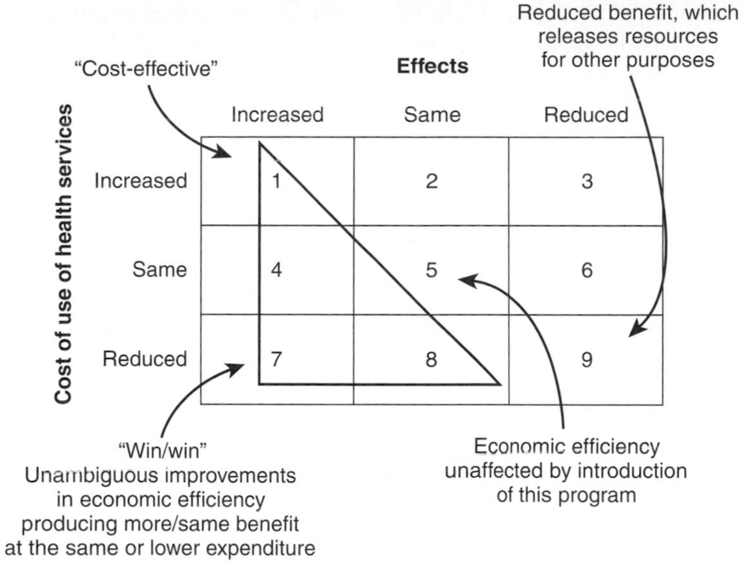

Figure 98-2. Framework for evaluating possible outcomes of economic evaluation of health care programs. *(From Birch S, Gafni A. Cost-effectiveness and cost utility analyses: methods for the non-economic evaluation of health care programs and how we can do better. In: Geisler E, Heller O, editors. Managing Technology in Healthcare. Norwell, MA: Kluwer Academic Publishers; 1996.)*

visits by a health visitor can be a means of recognizing these unmet needs. Harrison et al identified through this service that 35% of 110 patients over 70 years of age had previously unidentified risks that could benefit from preventive programs.[63] Similar results were reported by Brown et al, in an audit of 40 general practices in the United Kingdom of patients over 75 years of age.[64] In this study, 12% of the eligible practice population was seen over the study period; 44% were found to have at least one health problem that was previously undetected. Similarly, Ramsdell et al found that home-based assessment of older adults resulted in the detection of up to four new problems as compared to an office-based assessment.[65] Stuck et al identified several key advantages of in-home visits versus office-based visits.[66] A home-based assessment allows for an evaluation of the physical environment to identify risk factors and equipment needs, review of medications, observe contacts with family members, and provide better accessibility for clients with mobility problems. Further, an office-based visit often has a focus for the appointment and limited time affects solicitation of further risks.

Browne et al,[32] in a review of 12 randomized controlled trials evaluating a community-based approach to care in a Canadian setting, found that for clients with multiple problems (such as the frail older adult), it is more expensive in the same year to *not* provide these clients with proactive and comprehensive preventive care and health promotion. Similarly, Caulfield et al (p. 87),[60] in a review of the literature on geriatric screening programs, concluded that "home based, comprehensive screening of the older adult for undetected physical, mental and socio-economic problems by nursing or other trained personnel may be able to prolong survival, improve quality of life, and perhaps even postpone dependency or institutionalization." Screening eliminates a barrier between the need for help and gaining access to that help.

Discussed next are three areas—falls, nutrition, and depression—in which screening and assessment are advocated for older adults living in the community, as these conditions are readily preventable through health promotion efforts. The term *screening* refers to the process of detecting or identifying a health condition or risk factor among a specific population. The term *assessment* refers to the process that follows a positive screen and involves evaluating the problem and older adult in a more specific fashion in order to confirm the problem or establish the diagnosis and develop a treatment plan.[67]

Risk of Falls

Despite knowledge that most falls are both predictable and preventable, falls and fall-related injuries continue to negatively impact older adults' quality of life and health care resources (see also Chapter 106). Fall-related injuries are among the most common, serious, and expensive health conditions affecting community-living older adults.[68] Thirty percent of community-living adults over 65 years of age fall at least once a year, and the proportion increases to 50% by the age of 80 years.[69] In people aged 65 years and older, falls are the leading cause of injury-related admissions to acute care hospitals and in-hospital deaths[70] and explain 40% of nursing home admissions.[71] The costs of health care associated with fall-related injuries are staggering. The 1999/2000 costs of fall injuries to seniors in Canada were estimated to be $2.4 billion.[72] With an aging population and an associated increase in the number of falls and fall-related injuries, these cost estimates are projected to rise as high as $240 billion by 2040.[73]

The negative impact of a fall on health and related quality of life can be profound. Fall injuries often result in fear of falling,[74,75] leading to self-imposed restriction of activity and loss of confidence,[76] low self-esteem, depression,[75] chronic pain, and functional deterioration.[77] Falls and fall-related injuries and complications are the leading cause of death among seniors.[78] Frail seniors, exhibiting accelerated aging, are at increased risk for falls, with approximately 50% falling at least once per year (three times the risk of healthy seniors).[79] They are also more likely to sustain serious injury and take longer to recover after falling.[73] Falls are caused by multiple, interacting factors, some of which are modifiable. Factors such as postural hypotension, the use of multiple medications, and impairments in cognition, vision, balance, gait, and strength increase the risk of falling and fall injuries.[68] Although no single factor causes all falls, the risk of falling increases with the number of risk factors present.[80]

Evidence suggests that most falls are predictable and preventable. Previous intervention studies showed that approximately 30% to 40% of falls can be avoided.[81–83] A 10% reduction in the number of nonfatal falls would mean 7931 fewer falls and health care savings of $138.6 million.[18] Categorizing individuals into different levels of risk through screening is thus important from both clinical and economic perspectives; seniors with the highest risk of falling will benefit most from preventive efforts and from avoiding the negative consequences of falls.[82] The best approach to preventing falls in any group of older persons requires knowledge of where that group sits on the risk spectrum, because this will determine the type and amount of services required as well as the effectiveness of the program.[77] Essentially, fall risk screening is a means of targeting limited home and community care resources.

Home and community care providers are well positioned to play a major role in preventing falls in older people through screening and intervention. An understanding of the risk factors for falls (listed earlier) will increase the clinician's ability to effectively target the use of screening. Since the late 1990s, several fall risk screening instruments focused on community-living older adults have been developed due to the rising concern for fall-related injuries.[84] Considerable evidence now documents that the most effective fall reduction programs involve routine and systematic fall risk assessments or screens, followed by targeting of interventions to an individual's risk profile.[79,85] This research has been substantiated by meta-analyses of many randomized controlled trials[85,86] and by consensus panels of experts who have developed evidence-based practice guidelines for the detection and management of falls risk.[79,82,87,88] The importance of this direction cannot be overstated. Reducing just one fall risk factor can have great effect on the frequency and morbidity of falls.[83]

Risk of nutrition problems

As also discussed in Chapter 82, nutrition problems in older adults are common, because of the diverse individual and collective determinants of food intake in this age group.[27] Low intakes of various food groups, energy, protein, and micronutrients continue to be reported in those over the age 65 years.[29,89] Poor-quality food that is energy-dense and lack of exercise also are causes of obesity in this age group.[89] Obesity when coupled with poor function results in a precarious state for older adults. Those who are frail and exhibiting accelerated aging are also highly susceptible to malnutrition.[29,89,90]

Since the late 1990s, several nutrition screening indices have focused on community-living older adults,[91] because of the rising concern for the nutritional health of older adults and a desire to intervene as soon as possible.[29,54] Nutrition screening is viewed as a means of targeting limited nutrition resources, especially dietitian services.[92] Unfortunately, most of the research to date has focused on describing "at risk" populations or demonstrating the linkages between nutrition risk and negative health outcomes such as falls, other morbidity, institutionalization, and mortality, without demonstrating that nutrition screening can change practice and thus prevent these outcomes. Prevalence of risk varies depending on the index used and the subgroup of older adults screened; estimates range from 25% in "usually" aging seniors to 69% in those who are frail.[29,93–95] Risk factors associated with poor food intake or nutrition risk include poor self-rated health,[94,96] functional limitations,[27,96,97] low level of education, low income, lack of social support, poor dentition, smoking, vision problems,[96,97] stress,[93] lack of transportation, poor social networks, and living alone.[29] Food intake is complex due to its multifactorial determinants, and interventions to promote food intake need to be comprehensive and multisectoral.

In the United States, the Elderly Nutrition Program under the Older Americans Act has provided nutritious meals and other nutrition services to older adults that are especially vulnerable (e.g., those living in underserviced rural areas).[89] Although not mandatory, screening, assessment and interventions such as counseling and basic nutrition education can be provided within individual communities. Screening within the program is meant to target interventions,[89] but no research on the effectiveness of the screening process has been documented. Furthermore, only 20% of older adults who could benefit from this program are reached,[98] and targeting of services to those most in need is required.[99]

One article described a nutrition screening program with the NRS-2002 in 26 European hospital departments in 12 countries.[100] The average age of patients screened (n = 5051) was 60 years, and 33% were considered to be "at risk." These patients were more likely to have complications, fatal outcome, and a longer length of stay than those without risk. Unfortunately, the authors did not describe or evaluate the treatment options that may or may not have been provided to these patients, so the effectiveness of the screening is unknown. There is only one known evaluation of a nutrition screening program focused on older adults in the community, limited to describing and assessing the process of screening.[36]

The Bringing Nutrition Screening to Seniors in Canada project[36] involved developing, implementing, and evaluating screening programs in five diverse communities in Canada. Almost 1200 seniors were screened and, if found at risk, provided with referrals to community services. An ethical screening process that included follow-up postscreening helped to identify the impact of the program. Seniors indicated that screening helped them to recognize their problem areas and become aware of the various programs and services available in their community. Some individuals reported improving their food intake as a result of the screening, although objective data were not collected.[36] As with falls, now that nutrition screening tools are available, research needs to turn to determining the effectiveness of screening and early nutrition interventions in this population.

Risk of depression

Depression is among the most common, and potentially treatable, cause of death, morbidity, functional decline, and increased health care use and costs among community-living older adults.[101–103] Despite the high prevalence of depression in this population, the diagnosis of depression is often missed or suboptimally managed.[104] Depression affects between 5% and 10% of individuals in primary care but is only recognized in around one half of the cases.[105] In one study of older adults receiving home care services, only 12% of those with depression received adequate treatment.[104]

Both clinician and health care system factors impede the recognition and treatment of depression. First, older people at risk for or suffering or recovering from depression have limited access to community-based services directed toward promoting mental health. In many jurisdictions, eligibility for, and allocation of, home care services are directed toward addressing physical needs—mental health problems must be the secondary diagnosis in order to be eligible.[106] Second, there is limited collaboration and communication among home and community care providers, primary health care providers and others providing mental health services to community-living older adults, and a lack of continuity of care provider. Third, there is a lack of expertise among home and community care service providers in identifying and managing depression.[106,107] Older people generally have chronic medical conditions and disabilities that mask the presence of depression,[108] and attitudes and beliefs about mental illness discourage health care providers from asking patients about depression and patients from revealing depressive symptoms. Finally, there is a tendency to normalize symptoms of depression in this population.[109]

Unrecognized, untreated, and undertreated mood disorders generate enormous personal, economic, and societal costs.[104,108] Depression in older people often coexists with other chronic illnesses, and untreated depression is a significant risk factor for functional decline, diminished quality of life, death from comorbid medical conditions or suicide, dementia, social isolation, poor adherence to treatment, increased demands on unpaid caregivers and increased use of expensive health services.[110,111] In 1998, depression cost Canadians approximately $14.4 billion dollars per year.[112,113] These costs are compounded by indirect costs such as costs to unpaid caregivers. Unpaid caregivers of depressed seniors are more likely themselves to experience symptoms of depression.[114] Depression is also associated with unhealthy lifestyle factors such as smoking, alcohol use,[115] physical inactivity, and noncompliance with medical treatment.[116]

Those who are frail, exhibiting accelerated aging, are at increased risk for depression.[19,117] The prevalence of depression among older persons receiving home care services is estimated to be between 26% and 44%—at least twice that among older persons in general.[104,118,119] They also suffer from a fourfold increase in more severe forms of depression than the general population.[120] Clearly, recognition is key to referral and subsequent treatment for depression in this population.[109]

Multiple, interacting physical, psychological, and social factors increase the risk of depression in old age. These include factors such as having a comorbid health condition(s), functional limitations, taking medications (such as centrally acting antihypertensive drugs, analgesics, steroids, and antiparkinsonians), social factors (e.g., social disadvantage, low social support), or a previous history of depression.[121]

Routine depression screening and assessment have been shown to be effective in improving the recognition and management of depression in community-living older adults.[109,122–128] A variety of screening instruments have been developed for screening and assessing depression in older adults. These screening tools were developed to reflect the differences in presentation of depression in older adults and to address issues such as the presence of concurrent medical disorders (e.g., dementia).[129]

Community providers can play a pivotal role in screening for depression in community-living older adults. An understanding of the factors for depression (listed earlier) will increase the clinician's ability to effectively target the use of screening or inquire about symptoms that make up the diagnostic criteria for a depressive disorder, particularly when several risk factors are present.[67] The evidence suggests that screening is most effective when targeted to higher-risk groups.[67] Current Canadian recommendations suggest that screening for depression in primary care settings should be completed only if effective follow-up and treatment can be provided.[130] Although access to specialized geriatric mental health services remains limited in some settings, primary health care practitioners are able to provide appropriate follow-up and treatment.[67]

Importance and implementation of screening

Awareness of the importance of screening and assessment of risk is required at several levels: older adults, their families, their home care providers, and the community.[29] Although older adults appear to be interested in health promotion, they often do not think they are at risk for falls, poor nutrition, or depression. Screening may increase their attentiveness or self-awareness. More important, assessment of risk can be used to guide the allocation of limited home and community resources to those most likely to benefit from preventive efforts.

Overall, the data underscore the important role of home and community care providers in the early identification and management of risk factors for functional decline by performing a multifactorial assessment using validated screening instruments followed by targeting of interventions to an individual's risk profile.[85] In a review of the literature, Challis and Hughes[131] identified the need for greater standardization and multidisciplinarity of assessments as one of four factors that influenced the "margin" between institutional and community-based care for community-living seniors.

Screening in the community is a complex activity and providers need support to build capacity.[29] Furthermore, tools used for assessment of risk may not be standardized and often lack rigorous reliability and validity testing.[43,132] To be acceptable to practice and relevant for a diverse group of community-living older adults, risk screening instruments need to be reliable, valid, brief and easy to use and accurately discriminate between levels of risk. Different instruments may be required for different segments of the older adult population, as they are quite heterogeneous ranging from well and successfully aging to chronically ill.[133] They also need to be acceptable to the individual being assessed and the provider performing the assessment.[84]

In addition to an appropriate screening instrument, capacity for screening in the community is based on the development of an ethical screening process.[134,135] An ethical screening process includes referral to community resources or services and follow-up to ensure that identified needs are met.[135] Development of an ethical screening process is complex and time, resources, and effort are needed.[135] Research and best practice guidelines should be translated into practice so that risk assessment is implemented and appropriate interventions are tailored to individual needs.

PROMOTING HEALTH IN COMMUNITY-LIVING OLDER ADULTS: LESSONS FROM FIVE INTERVENTION STUDIES

Health promotion and disease prevention efforts are categorized as primary, secondary, or tertiary. Health promotion is the process of enabling people to take control over the determinants of health and thereby improve their health.[136] Health promotion strategies are based on a participatory model of health,[137] which seeks to expand an individual's positive potential for health. This is in contrast with preventive care, which is grounded in the traditional biomedical model of health[137] and seeks to avoid risks or decrease risks to health and well-being.[138]

A participatory approach to enhancing health involves activities that seek to empower individuals and promote positive attitudes, knowledge, and skills to maintain and enhance health.[139,140] Health promotion strategies involve goals such as autonomy, empowerment, and independent decision making.[37] Health promotion interventions are developed, implemented, and evaluated together with individuals, families, and stakeholders from different organizations.[141] Empowerment for health goes beyond illness and the management of a specific disease. Its success is seen in terms of enhanced health, well-being, quality of life, sense of self-esteem, and self-worth.[142]

According to the World Health Organization, health promotion strategies include developing personal health skills, creating supportive environments, strengthening community action, reorienting health services, and building healthy public policy.[142] Thus, health promotion strategies are multilevel, focusing not only on individuals but also on family, community, and societal health. Health promotion not only is concerned with enabling the development of life skills, self-concept, and social skills, but is also concerned with environmental intervention through a broad range of political, legislative, fiscal, and administrative means.[137]

Whereas health promotion is approach motivated, preventive care is avoidance motivated.[138] Preventive care, which is divided into primary, secondary, and tertiary levels, is aimed at reducing premature morbidity and mortality.[137,138,143] *Primary prevention* is focused on removal of risk factors for disease or functional decline from the individual or the environment. Activities of this type are implemented for successful or usual aging older adults who are asymptomatic and free of clinical evidence of the targeted disease or health condition. *Secondary prevention* activities focus on early identification and prompt treatment of risk factors before they lead to functional decline.[135] In essence, secondary prevention is the way to add "life to years."[1] Secondary prevention can avert successfully and usually aging older adults from progressing through the stages of functional decline, and they are thus more relevant. *Tertiary prevention* is typically provided to those with accelerated aging and includes activities or measures focused on those who currently exhibit some signs of functional decline. These interventions aim both to limit the progression of disease or functional decline or loss of independence[26] and to maximize function.

The current knowledge base concerning the potential role for health promotion and secondary prevention in older people remains relatively small.[26,29] Most community-based interventions for older adults occur at a tertiary prevention level, focusing on illness and the treatment of disease and largely ignoring health promotion, secondary prevention, and partnering approaches between and among all professionals and older people with chronic diseases.[37,144] In the United States, of the more than $1.7 trillion in health care spent nationally every year, less than 4 cents of every dollar is spent on prevention and public health.[18] This approach has come in for much criticism for its narrow focus on "downstream," diverting scarce resources away from primary and secondary prevention efforts that focus on early identification and prompt treatment of risk factors before they lead to functional decline. Functional disabilities and illnesses in older people often are managed as acute medical problems, not as ongoing life challenges that require continuous attention to health promotion and preventive care.[39] Older people need both health promotion and preventive care, so it is essential that health professionals become engaged in all areas of activity.[145]

This section describes five examples of health promotion and preventive care interventions designed for community-living older adults in which either falls, nutrition, or mental health (depression) were areas of focus:

I. Evergreen Action Nutrition: an example of a secondary prevention program[146–148]
II. Home support exercise intervention for frail older adults using home care services[149]
III. Nursing health promotion for frail older adults using home care services[38]
IV. Falls prevention for older home care clients at risk for falling[150]
V. Proactive screening, case finding, and treatment of older adults in primary care[151]

Studies I and II are prospective cohort studies of older adults living in the community with comparable types and severity of illnesses and disabilities who self-select to one community-based approach over another. Studies III to V are prospective randomized controlled trials (RCTs) that control for the methodological problems of self-selection that confound studies I and II. Measures of well-being and cost of use of health services provided to older adults randomly assigned to health-oriented, proactive care were compared with those of similar clients receiving reactive, unplanned, and disease-oriented approaches to care. The major findings from each study are described, and lessons as they relate to using results to informed practice, policy, and future research are described.

Study I. Evergreen Action Nutrition: an example of a secondary prevention program

Despite the importance of preventive nutrition interventions for older adults, secondary prevention programs are relatively absent or not documented.[29] Evergreen Action Nutrition is an education program provided since 1999 in a seniors recreation center in southern Ontario. Using a community-based approach, this program was developed, implemented, and evaluated by an advisory committee that included senior members of the center.[152] Nutrition screening was used throughout the program to identify needs, raise awareness, and evaluate activities. The program was voluntary, and seniors could participate solely through reading education materials or they could be involved in hands-on activities like cooking groups. Activities included resourcing the center library with quality nutrition books; a nutrition column in the monthly newsletter; monthly nutrition and nutrition displays; cooking groups for men; support groups for persons managing weight or diabetes; food demonstrations, which included hands-on activities and food consumption; celebrity chefs; and monthly deliveries of a fresh vegetable and fruit box. Process evaluation demonstrated that the program was effective.[148] The program had a large reach, with approximately two thirds of members (~2000 seniors) having participated in some way during a 3-year period. Respondents to a randomly mailed survey were significantly less likely to be at nutrition risk than those surveyed at baseline (38.9% vs. 56.7%, respectively). Participants, as compared with nonparticipants on the follow-up survey, had better fruit and vegetable intakes. Food demonstrations and cooking groups were effective at overcoming barriers to trying new foods and recipes.[146,147] Participants reported the intention to change cooking and eating behaviors based on these nutrition education formats. This program was conducted with funding from a research grant for the first 3 years of the program and has continued with minimal funding from the seniors association that runs the center and from monies collected for participation in activities. Lessons learned in this program are that diverse education activities are needed to reach a wide audience—no single intervention will appeal to all seniors. Seniors are interested and motivated to improve their nutrition knowledge and behaviors. A recreation center is an ideal setting for this activity, as it is a nonthreatening environment, and creating a program that has consistent educators and other staff is important for building trust and program continuity. Finally, a participatory approach that involved the target group was essential for developing and implementing meaningful education activities.

Study II. Home support exercise intervention for frail older adults using home care services

This prospective cohort study was designed to determine the effectiveness of a home support exercise program (HSEP) for frail older adults receiving home care services.[149] Home exercise is an effective means to prevent falls, to maintain functional independence, and to promote rehabilitation following injury or illness.[153] The study sample consisted of 98 frail older adults (≥65 years of age) using home support services in a home care program in southern Ontario, Canada. Sixty subjects were randomly selected to receive the HSEP, whereas 38 matched controls were allocated to receive standard home care without the HSEP. A total of 77 subjects completed the 4-month follow-up (40 HSEP, 37 controls). The HSEP is a 4-month in-home physical activity intervention provided by a trained home support worker. It consists of 10 simple, functional, and progressive exercises that are to be done on a daily basis. Once the exercises have been introduced, the home support worker continues to monitor the client's progress and to offer motivational support. Results showed that at 4 months, those who received the HSEP self-reported general improvement such as feeling better, being less stiff and stronger, and being able to walk more easily. Those in the control group reported that they felt worse than they did 4 months previously. Between groups, significant differences were observed for mobility and walking scores, with an average improvement of 14% to 34% in the HSEP group, compared with only minor improvement or functional decline in the control. Significant improvements for balance confidence were also observed, whereas the control group experienced little or no change in balance confidence. The findings support the effectiveness of the HSEP, as well as the importance of proactive and regular exercise interventions and support in this population.[149]

Study III. Nursing health promotion for frail older adults using home care services

This single-blind, randomized controlled trial, with a 6-month follow-up, conducted in a home care program in southern Ontario, Canada, was designed to determine the effects and expense of adding nursing health promotion and preventive care to usual home care services in a national system of health and social insurance.[38] The study sample consisted of 242 older adults (≥75 years of age) using home support services. Subjects were randomized to intervention (n = 144) or control groups (n = 144). A total of 242 (84%) subjects completed the 6-month follow-up. In addition to usual home care, the nursing group received a health assessment combined with regular home visits or telephone contacts, health education regarding management of illness, coordination of community services, and empowerment strategies to enhance independence. The primary outcome was functional health status and related quality of life. Secondary outcomes were depression, perceived social support, coping ability, and cost of use of health services from baseline to 6 months. Results showed that providing older adults with proactive nursing health promotion and preventive care compared with providing nursing services on a reactive and episodic basis results in better mental health functioning (P = .041) and a reduction in depression (P = .001) at no additional expense (e.g., both interventions cost the same). The overall conclusion of this study is that home-based nursing health promotion, proactively provided to frail older people with chronic health needs, enhances quality of life at no additional expense from a societal perspective. The results underscore the need to reinvest in nursing services for health promotion for older adults receiving home care services.[38]

Study IV. Falls prevention for older home care clients at risk for falling

This single-blind, randomized controlled trial, with a 6-month follow-up, conducted in a home care program in southern Ontario, Canada, was designed to determine the effects and costs of a multifactorial, interdisciplinary team approach to falls prevention compared to usual home care for older home care clients at risk of falling.[150] The study sample consisted of 109 older adults (≥75 years of age) using home support services who are at risk for falls. Subjects were randomized to intervention (n = 54) or control (n = 55) groups. A total of 92 subjects completed the 6-month follow-up. The intervention was a 6-month multifactorial and evidence-based prevention strategy involving an interdisciplinary team. The primary outcome was number of falls during the 6-month follow-up. Secondary outcomes were changes in fall risk factors and costs of use of health services from baseline to 6 months. Results showed that at 6 months, there was no difference in the mean number of falls between groups (−0.04 [95% CI:−1.27, 1.18]; $P = .702$). However, subgroup analyses showed that the intervention was effective in reducing falls in men ($P = .009$), 75 to 84 years of age ($P < .001$), with a fear of falling ($P < .001$) or a negative history of falls ($P < .041$). There was a greater reduction in number of slips and trips (−4.97 [95% CI:−10.7 to 0.84], $P = .03$) and a greater improvement in role functioning related to emotional health in the intervention group (−14.13 [95% CI: −0.28 to 28.54], $P = .054$). These improvements were achieved at no additional cost from a societal perspective (e.g., both interventions cost the same). The overall conclusion of this study is that a multifactorial, interdisciplinary team approach was more effective and no more expensive than usual home care in improving quality of life, reducing the incidence of slips and trips, and reducing falls among males (≥75 to 84 years) with a fear of falling or a negative history of falls.[150] This study is important because of the high prevalence of falls among older adults receiving home support services. The baseline fall rate of 72% in the present sample greatly exceeds the fall rates of 30% typically reported for representative samples of community-dwelling older adults.[79] Home care policy makers, agencies, and fund-raisers should work together to ensure that an interdisciplinary team approach is available to the subgroups of seniors who could benefit from it most to reduce future falls, enhance quality of life, and reduce on-demand use of health services.

Study V. Proactive screening, case finding, and treatment of older adults in primary care

This randomized controlled trial was designed to determine the effect and expense of proactive screening, case finding, and random treatment of ambulatory seniors having 1 of 28 unrecognized medical concerns, in a primary health care setting.[151] Seniors with unrecognized health concern were randomly allocated to treatment (n = 209) or nontreatment (n = 410) groups. Treatment consisted of one to two visits to an appropriate primary care professional (physician, nurse, or social worker) depending on the specific concerns. On the whole, there was no significant improvement in the overall functional capacity of seniors treated versus those not treated for their concerns. However, screening, case finding, and health-oriented, proactive primary care resulted in improved mental health and social functions (11% to 22%, respectively) for seniors who were 75 years of age and older and living alone. Similar seniors without treatment showed a deterioration of 2% in their scores over the 2-year period ($P = .04$). Seniors who were lonely and treated used $2610 per person per annum in services, compared with similar untreated seniors who used $10,971 per person per annum after 2 years. The overall conclusion of this study is that screening, case finding, and health-oriented, proactive primary care are more effective and less expensive for older adults with psychosocial risks.[151]

Lessons learned

Collectively, these studies of health promotion and preventive care interventions suggest that in a system of national health insurance, such as we have in Canada, proactive, comprehensive, and integrated interventions for older adults with varying characteristics can result in better heath outcomes for the same and sometimes lower cost compared with providing services on a limited, reactive, and piecemeal basis. The use of prospective studies allows for an estimation of change in client status over time. Studies I and II, which used a prospective cohort design, illustrate the benefit of health-oriented and proactive community services and support for older adults with comparable types and severity of illnesses and disabilities who self-select to one community-based approach over another. Studies III to V employed a randomized controlled trial design to compare the effects and costs of a health promotion and preventive care intervention with reactive, unplanned, and piecemeal approaches to care. Across these studies, subjects were assessed with different outcome measures appropriate to their circumstances, yet the same approach to the quantification of the cost of use of health services was employed.[154] Studies III and IV of frail, older, home care populations illustrate that health promotion and preventive care interventions compared with piecemeal and on-demand care result in improved outcomes at no more expense to society (rubric 4, Figure 98-3). In study V of ambulatory populations with chronic conditions who live alone, improved outcomes can be achieved at lower cost with health promotion and prevention care (rubric 7, Figure 98-3). Expenditure data in these four studies include the cost of the health promotion and prevention care interventions. The studies illustrate potential outcomes 4 and 7 in Figure 98-3 and collectively represent different kinds of economic efficiencies that are achieved with populations with more or less access to services to begin with.

As a whole, the results of these studies provide empirical support for the positive synergistic and cumulative effects of bolstering personal resources (e.g., physical, mental health, and social functioning) and environmental supports (e.g., community supports) on health status and related quality of life[56] to considerable economic effect (no additional or lower expense). Health care providers need to be able to assess older adults' areas of strength and vulnerability. Awareness of the sources of vulnerability and barriers to health care may assist health care providers to provide more holistic, comprehensive care to their clients.[56]

These five studies illustrate a number of features of successful community-based health promotion programs for community-living older adults. First, the results have shown that comprehensive and coordinated services aimed at all of the broad determinants of health are superior when compared to individual, fragmented, and disease-oriented approaches to care.[32] Because health is determined by many more things than physical needs, such approaches must extend beyond the care of medical problems to address other nonmedical determinants of health (e.g., social support, mental health, housing, income).[5] This approach represents a fundamental shift away from a *replacement function* focused solely on physical needs to an *empowerment function* to enhance seniors' independence, autonomy, and problem-solving skills.[155] The results of these studies suggest that, in a system of national health insurance, interventions that address single problems or single risk or protective factors are less effective in reducing health problems or enhancing competencies in people with synergistic risks than proactive, health-oriented, and comprehensive interventions.[33,37] Effective interventions include

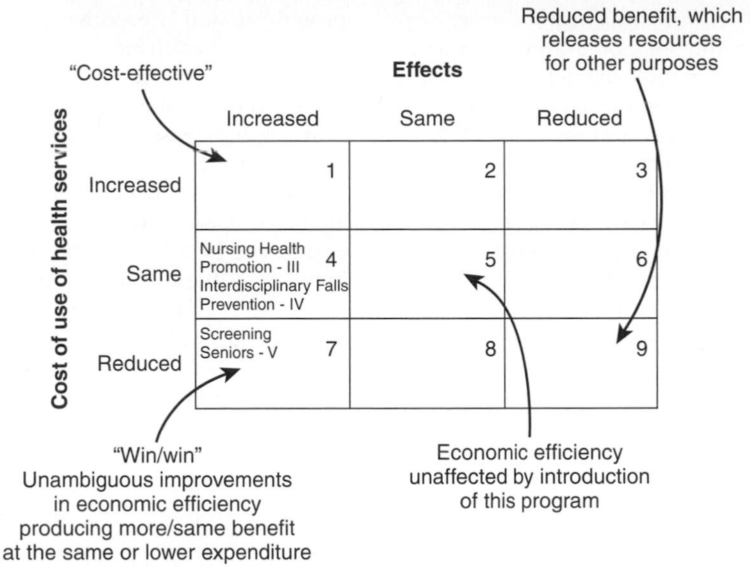

Figure 98-3. Framework for evaluating possible outcomes of economic evaluation of health care programs. *(From Birch S, Gafni A. Cost-effectiveness and cost utility analyses: methods for the non-economic evaluation of health care programs and how we can do better. In: Geisler E, Heller O, editors. Managing Technology in Healthcare. Norwell, MA: Kluwer Academic Publishers; 1996.)*

elements that ensure access to a comprehensive range of services provided in the right amount and delivered by the right care provider, in the right place and at the right time.[131]

Second, successful health promotion interventions need to be tailored to individual needs. The most expensive services are those that are not tailored to people's needs (or vulnerabilities).[33] No single intervention or mix of community services will meet the health promotion needs of all seniors. Hence, there is a need to classify who (with what characteristics) most benefits and at what expense, from various interventions, especially in systems of national health insurance where people will use, however, (in)appropriately, some service if another is made (un)available.[32] Screening plays a part in targeting those who are most likely to benefit. Seniors are interested and motivated to change their behavior to enhance health. Successful behavior change is associated with the empowerment of individuals through the provision of appropriate communication, information, and support. Interventions need to respond appropriately to an individual's readiness to change through various strategies tailored to an individual's needs. Models of care should be flexible and contextualized, taking into account individual needs and comorbidities and paying particular attention to vulnerable, at-risk populations. These data can be used to target scarce resources to those most likely to benefit from preventive efforts.

Third, to be successful, health promotion needs to occur across multiple sectors. In these studies, the interventions involved a wide range of actions operating at three levels: the individual clinician (e.g., promoting changes in practice behavior), the interdisciplinary team (e.g., fostering interprofessional collaboration), and the health care system (e.g., influencing the financing, management, and delivery of services). When health problems are chronic, care must be organized and coordinated over time, among providers, and across settings.[155] This multisector work requires good communication and a close affiliation so that individual home and community-based services do not operate in isolation but are part of a broader, more balanced, integrated approach to a comprehensive and coordinated system of services that address all of the factors that determine health.

Fourth, models of care need to be function based (from the client's perspective) rather than disease based. The emphasis is on the individual's perception of health, rather than on his or her objective circumstances, and in determining his or her decision to take action. The evidence is clear that increasing people's involvement in their health care management and decision making has been shown to improve health status and lower costs.[156]

Finally, it is important to take a comprehensive approach to examine expenditures associated with different approaches to home and community-based care.[32] In addition to savings within the health care sector, a program could expect to see a return on its investment in prevention in other sectors (e.g., education, social, and benefits other than reduction of disease).[18] Economists argue that the effect of a publicly funded home and community-based service on society as a whole should be considered when making decisions about the use of that service.[157] This comprehensive societal viewpoint is often ignored in the economic analysis of health care services.[32]

THE NEED FOR LEGISLATION AND POLICY

Despite the potentially important role of home and community-based services in health promotion and preventive care for older adults, several realities continue to impede this direction. Within the persistently biomedically and institutionally focused health care arena, in-home and community-based care still suffer from underfunding of services, underfunding of research to inform policy and practice, and limited consideration of the broader determinants of health in these sectors.[144] Since the late 1990s, health care systems have been challenged to provide more home and community care services to older, more vulnerable, and frail individuals while limiting the growth of health care expenditures.[158–160] Growing demand for home and community care is attributable to several factors—namely, technologic advancements, changing demographics, patient preference, and the presumed cost-effectiveness of home care.[158] With increasing life expectancy, substantial increases in home care expenditures are expected by 2026.[161] Often, the need goes unmet as resources are shifted from prevention and health promotion to meet the more pressing need for postacute care substitution.[162] This emphasis, coupled with the sustained biomedical orientation of services, can mean that the focus on prevention and health promotion for seniors with chronic needs is minimal at best.[144] The allocation of home and community services often is based on physical needs or medical services, suggesting that nonmedical services are unrelated to health outcomes, despite evidence to the contrary.[7]

A growing body of research, done mostly in a national system of health insurance, suggests that for older people with chronic health needs, these trends combine to create a fragmented system of health care delivery, characterized by providing health services on a reactive, episodic, and piecemeal basis rather than a comprehensive and proactive system of care.[23,33] Delays or errors in detecting and responding to chronically ill older people's changing health needs can contribute to more complications, cause functional decline and negative changes in quality of life,[163] and increase the demand for expensive institution-based care such as acute hospitalization.[33] Furthermore, this experience with the acute care system often undermines chronically ill seniors' self-confidence and their interest and ability to participate in their own care. The result is a vicious circle of reliance on institutionalized care.[140]

To address effectively the growing burden of chronic disease and frailty in older people living in the community, healthy home and community care policies are needed to provide vision, set priorities, and establish standards. Such policies and standards should support the development of basic competencies for health promotion and preventive care among providers, as well as systemic changes within home and community care organizations to allow the allocation of adequate resources for assessment of risk and delivery of health promotion and prevention strategies. There is a need to move away from a "find-it and fix-it" episodic orientation that does not match the ongoing care needs of older people with chronic condition, who need a "find-it, manage it, and prevent it" approach.[31]

Home and community-based programs need to provide a continuum of services including health promotion, prevention, and postacute care substitution services.[158] Enhanced funding and focused health promotion and preventive care activities should be applied to mitigate the risk factors for functional decline and loss of independence, so that living at home, even with significant challenges, can become a true reality for older populations. Without this legislation and resource provision, improvements in the health of older adults will continue to be an ad hoc affair with limited impact.[29]

THE NEED FOR MORE RESEARCH

With the increasing demand for home and community-based services for older people, there is increasing pressure for evidence to demonstrate that community-based health promotion and preventive care for older people is an efficient use of health care resources in developed countries.[164] A 2003 report by the World Health Organization for policy makers on the future direction of health-promotion evaluation emphasized the need for evidence about effective and efficient health-promotion and preventive care strategies.[15] This evidence is needed to ensure that the most appropriate services are available to those who most need them, to ensure the best health outcomes.[160] However, the current knowledge base concerning the potential role for health promotion and secondary prevention in older people remains relatively small.[26,29] Specifically, further investigation is needed regarding the most efficacious ways of providing health promotion and preventive care to the different groups of successfully, usually, and accelerated aging. These groups have different needs, risk factors, and comorbid conditions and experience different barriers and facilitators to health promotion,[165] and further research is needed to differentiate these influences.

Older adults with chronic conditions who are experiencing accelerated aging have been identified as at increased risk for functional decline, institutionalization, and death,[13] but these individuals are often excluded in community-based trials.[49,166] There is a need to establish a knowledge base about the needs of this vulnerable group. Understanding what factors in the individual and the environment are most predictive of morbidity and use of health services is needed to move forward with health promotion efforts in this group.

Large, randomized trials are required to test innovative approaches to health promotion and secondary prevention strategies for community-living older adults. Such studies should provide information on client-important outcomes, such as functional health status and related quality of life, mental health, and social support. These studies should also address more process-oriented outcomes associated with health promotion, such as autonomy, empowerment, and decision making.[137] Such studies should also compare outcomes achieved with different providers and different combinations of providers to inform how best to meet the needs of this client group. Future research also needs to incorporate a full economic evaluation and identify the specific subgroups of clients who will benefit most.

A major gap in the research on home-based health promotion is the lack of a theoretic framework.[37] As a result, it is difficult to assess the appropriateness of the intervention to the outcomes being measured or to formulate hypotheses regarding why or how a particular intervention should be expected to result in a particular outcome.[141,167] Future research is needed that uses a theoretical framework and provides descriptive and contextual details about the health promotion strategies and measures of process to enable their replication and provide information about why an intervention was or was not found to be effective.[168] Further testing of the vulnerability model is needed to provide a knowledge base for designing and evaluating health promotion strategies.

Finally, research is needed on older adults' awareness and perceived need for health promotion. Despite being identified as at risk and having an awareness of the benefits associated with certain health behaviors, not all older adults decide to make positive behavioral changes.[165] Furthermore, some people may be less likely to change health behaviors than others, such as the oldest cohorts and women,[169] and it may be necessary to target strategies to these groups. Qualitative studies would help to identify the processes involved in the decision to change behavior, including the factors that influence compliance with recommendations. This type of information can be used to identify the most effective ways of supporting health promotion behavioral change to ultimately improve older adults' quality of life. Overall, this research will assist with targeting limited home and community resources and improving the effectiveness of efforts.

ACKNOWLEDGMENTS

Dr. Maureen Markle-Reid holds a Career Scientist Award (2004–2009) from the Ontario Ministry of Health and Long-Term Care, Health Research Personnel Development Fund.

Dr. Heather Keller received a New Investigator Research Award (2000–2006) from CIHR, which allowed her to complete much of her work on the screening and community nutrition education interventions cited in this chapter.

Dr. Gina Browne is the founder and director of the System-Linked Research Unit, funded by the Ontario Ministry of Health and Long-Term Care, which supported many of the studies cited in this chapter.

For a complete list of references, please visit online only at www.expertconsult.com

CHAPTER 99

Preventive and Anticipatory Care

James T. Pacala

As illnesses and adverse conditions become more prevalent with advancing age, the opportunity for prevention becomes increasingly important for elderly people. Preventive activities can be divided into five broad categories: prevention of diseases, prevention of frailty, prevention of accidents, prevention of iatrogenic problems, and prevention of psychosocial illnesses. Disease-prevention practices are designed to do the following:

- Prevent illnesses from occurring in the first place (primary prevention)
- Detect and treat disease at an early stage, thereby minimizing the morbidity and mortality caused by that disease (secondary prevention)
- Optimize treatment of existing conditions, usually chronic illnesses, to prevent adverse sequelae from these diseases (tertiary prevention)

The accumulation of chronic diseases and adverse conditions with aging often leads to severely threatened or outright loss of function, widely known as "frailty"; efforts to prevent this often common end point are particularly pertinent in the older adult population. Elderly people are particularly prone to injuries from accidents, constituting another area of opportunity for preventive efforts. It is well established that medical care itself has a propensity to cause harm, which increases with aging, indicating a need for prevention of iatrogenic problems, particularly among those who are frail. Finally, psychosocial illnesses also commonly pose a threat to functioning in older adults, and prevention of these illnesses is gaining increasing attention.

Not all elderly people stand to benefit equally from each type of preventive activity. They exhibit great variability in health and functional status, ranging from highly functioning persons who are free of disease and injury to those who are frail and totally functionally dependent. Different types of preventive activities will have different yields, depending in part on the baseline health and functioning of the person. To maximize efficiency and patient benefit, individualizing prevention by devoting time and resources toward those activities that are most likely to prevent morbidity and mortality given the status of the older adult patient seems warranted.

This chapter describes modalities for each type of preventive activity. Then, strategies for prioritizing those activities by patient status are presented.

DISEASE PREVENTION

Primary and secondary disease prevention

Primary and secondary disease prevention encompasses several activities. Screening refers to activities that detect a previously unknown condition in asymptomatic individuals. Detected risk factors are then altered, and through lowering of risk, the target disease is primarily prevented. Diseases discovered in their early stages are treated, thereby secondarily preventing more severe manifestation of advanced disease. Immunoprophylaxis prevents significant illnesses through vaccination. Counseling promotes lowering of disease risk through behavioral change. Decreasing disease risk by administering medications is known as chemoprophylaxis.

The U.S. Preventive Services Task Force (USPSTF)[1] rigorously reviews a wide variety of primary and secondary prevention practices. Preventive services for elderly people that are recommended by the USPSTF and supplemented by immunization recommendations from the Centers for Disease Control and Prevention (CDC)[2] are shown in Table 99-1. Table 99-2 lists activities currently not recommended by either the USPSTF or the CDC but that have been endorsed by other specialty organizations. The preventive efficacy of the procedures in Table 99-2 is less well established; accordingly, they might be considered more selectively in elderly people.

Tertiary disease prevention

As some elderly people age, they accumulate chronic illnesses that pose a threat to their functioning and quality of life. Although chronic illnesses by definition cannot be cured, proper management of these diseases can prevent further disease-induced functional loss. Chronic diseases that commonly lead to morbidity and mortality in the older population include the following:

- *Arthritis.* Osteoarthritis and rheumatoid arthritis affect about one half of all people aged 65 and over and lead to mobility impairment, which in turn increases the risk for numerous other conditions—and a resultant decrease in disability-free life expectancy.[3] Therefore, aggressive management of arthritis through medication and exercise is indicated. (See Chapter 71 on arthritis.)
- *Diabetes.* Older adults exhibit significantly increased risk for retinopathy, nephropathy, and coronary disease when glycohemoglobin ($HgbA_{1c}$) fractions exceed 7.9%.[4] Clinicians should attempt to achieve $HgbA_{1c}$ concentrations at least below 8% in diabetic patients and less than 7% in those who are not frail. Aggressive prevention of foot ulcers should also be undertaken through patient education and foot exams at each visit. (See Chapter 96 on diabetes.)
- *Vascular disease.* Patients with prior history of coronary, cerebral, or peripheral arterial disease are at markedly increased risk for a disabling event. There is good evidence that treatment of vascular risk factors in older adults with prior myocardial infarction (MI), angina, prior stroke, or claudication significantly reduces the risk of a subsequent MI, stroke, or limb loss.[5,6] The risk factors include hypertension, smoking, diabetes, atrial fibrillation, and dyslipidemia. (See Chapters 34, 49, and 38 on coronary, cerebral, and peripheral vascular disease.)
- *Heart failure (HF).* HF accounts for a great deal of suffering in elderly people and carries a higher mortality rate than

Table 99-1. Recommended Disease-Prevention Activities*

Type of Activity	Disease to Be Prevented/Detected	Activity	Frequency
Screening	Hypertension	Blood pressure measurement	At least yearly
	Obesity, malnutrition	Height and weight measurement	At least yearly
	Breast cancer	Mammography	Every 1–2 years†
	Cervical, uterine cancer	Pap smear	At least every 3 years‡
	Colon cancer	Fecal occult blood testing (FOBT); sigmoidoscopy; colonoscopy	FOBT: yearly; sigmoidoscopy: every 3–5 years; colonoscopy: at least once
	Coronary artery disease	Serum lipid measurement	Every 5 years; more often in persons with prior myocardial infarction, angina, stroke, or who have peripheral arterial disease or diabetes mellitus
	Hearing deficit	Hearing test	Yearly
	Alcoholism	Alcoholism screening questionnaire	At initial visit and when problem drinking is suspected
	Abdominal aortic aneurysm	Ultrasonography	Once between ages 65–75 in men who have ever smoked
	Depression	Depression screening questionnaire	Yearly in clinical practices with systems to assure accurate diagnosis, effective treatment, and follow-up
	Osteoporosis	Bone mineral density measurement	At least once in women aged 65 and older
	Diabetes mellitus	Fasting plasma glucose, 2-hour postload glucose, and/or hemoglobin A_{1c}.	At least every 3 years in persons with BP >135/80 mm Hg
Immunoprophylaxis	Influenza	Flu shot	Yearly
	Pneumococcal disease	Pneumovax vaccination	Once at age 65§
	Tetanus	Tetanus booster	Every 10 years
	Herpes zoster	Herpes zoster immunization	Once in immunocompetent people without prior zoster
Counseling	Cardiopulmonary disease, several cancers	Smoking cessation	At every visit of patients who smoke
	Coronary artery disease; obesity	Behavioral dietary counseling	Yearly in those with risk factors for coronary artery disease or with BMI >30 kg/m²
Chemoprophylaxis	Coronary artery disease, stroke, colon cancer	Aspirin therapy 81–325 mg p.o.	Daily in persons at increased risk for coronary artery disease

*As endorsed by the U.S. Preventive Services Task Force or the Centers for Disease Control and Prevention.
†Should be continued past age 70 in women who have a reasonable life expectancy.
‡Stop at age 65 if regularly tested throughout adult life AND there were no positive results; if never tested, can stop after two normal pap smears 1 year apart. Women without a cervix should not receive a Pap smear.
§Consider repeating every 7 years.

many forms of cancer. Proper and aggressive treatment of HF, especially systolic dysfunction, has been shown to reduce hospitalization rates, functional decline, and even mortality.[7] (See Chapter 33 on HF.)

- *Osteoporosis.* With the availability of bone density measurement, osteoporosis can be detected before a disabling fracture. Treatment of osteoporosis, in patients both with and without prior fracture, has been shown to prevent new fractures. (See Chapter 70 on osteoporosis.)[8,9]

Tertiary prevention is accomplished through chronic disease management. The Wagner model of Chronic Disease Care is widely cited as definitive of state-of-the-art care for this category of older adults. The goal of the Wagner Chronic Care model is to establish a productive interaction between an informed activated patient and a prepared proactive practice team.[10] The model calls for four features that are essential in achieving this goal:

- Self-management support, featuring interventions for the patient to manage his or her own illness, with individual goal setting performed by the patient in conjunction with the health care team
- Delivery system design wherein all medical providers practice as a team with defined roles, featuring planned patient visits, use of evidence-based care, regular follow-up, and care coordination
- Decision support, wherein evidence-based guidelines are fully incorporated into daily practice
- Clinical information systems, including the establishment of a patient registry, a database of useful and timely information on all patients that assists providers in care planning and ongoing management

A disease-specific case management program can also be a powerful intervention for tertiary prevention, frequently employing a specially trained nurse to coordinate protocol-driven care, arrange support services, and provide patient education.[11] See Chapter 120 for more information regarding implementation of disease management programs in health systems.

PREVENTION OF FRAILTY

Aside from preventing individual diseases, the larger question remains of whether or not their frequent end point—frailty—can be prevented. Frailty refers to a condition in which loss of physiologic reserve makes the afflicted individual particularly susceptible to disability from minor stresses. Frail individuals commonly exhibit significant functional deficits, weakness, muscle wasting, deconditioning, slowed gait, and fatigue.[12]

Table 99-2. Additional Disease-Prevention Activities That May Be Applicable in All or Selected Elderly People

Type of Activity	Disease to Be Prevented/Detected	Activity	Frequency	Comment
Screening	Dementia, delirium	Mental status testing	Yearly	May grow in importance if early treatment of dementia is shown to change outcomes
	Falls	Inquiry about falls in the past year	Yearly	Inquiry should be extended to include balance and gait problems
	Prostate cancer	Digital rectal exam or prostate-specific antigen testing	Yearly	Effective for early detection; randomized trial data is inconsistent and shows a small mortality benefit, if at all
	Skin cancer	Skin exam	Yearly	Treatment of false positives has low morbidity
	Hypothyroidism	Thyrotropin measurement	Yearly	Some experts recommend screening women
	Glaucoma	Glaucoma screening	Yearly	
	Malnutrition, tooth decay, oral cancers	Dental visit	Yearly	
Chemoprophylaxis	Osteoporosis	Calcium 1200 mg/d and vitamin D 800 IU/d intake	Daily	
Counseling	Coronary artery disease; obesity; osteoporosis	Exercise counseling	Yearly	Should include aerobic conditioning (at least 30 minutes of moderate intensity five times per week) and muscle strengthening at least twice per week

Control of a chronic condition becomes labile, resulting in frequent functional decompensation and hospitalization.

Can frailty be prevented? Data from long-term cohort studies suggest that it can, primarily through exercise and proper nutrition. Healthy adults who exercise are at lower risk of becoming frail, and functionally impaired older adults who exercise are less likely to experience further functional loss. To be most effective, an exercise program should include the following components:[13]

- Aerobic conditioning—at least 30 minutes of moderate-intensity activity five or more times per week. Moderate-intensity activities are those that increase heart rate and would be rated at 5 to 6 on a 10-point intensity scale by the patient. Brisk walking is an activity that many older adults can perform for aerobic conditioning.
- Weight (resistance) training—8 to 10 exercises of major muscle groups, 10 to 15 repetitions per exercise, at least twice a week.
- Flexibility—at least 10 minutes of flexibility activities (e.g., static stretching, 10 to 30 seconds per stretch, three to four repetitions of major muscle/tendon groups) at least twice a week.
- Balance—balance exercises are recommended in persons with mobility problems or frequent falls.

Proper nutrition is important for prevention of many conditions contributing to frailty, including certain forms of cancer, osteoporosis, obesity, and malnutrition. Studies have consistently shown less morbidity and lower mortality rate in those who eat diets featuring the following:

- *Low fat.* Less than 30% of total calories, with no more than 10% coming from saturated fats.[14]
- *Low sodium.* A 2.4-gram sodium diet is recommended.[15]
- *High calcium.* Older adults need 1200 mg of calcium per day; most American diets contain only 600 to 700 mg per day. Calcium supplementation should be provided if the diet contains less than 1200 mg per day.[16]
- *Adequate vitamins and minerals.* These are ensured largely through eating fruits and vegetables. Some experts recommend supplementation with vitamin D (800–1000 IU/day) for bone health, folate (at least 200 mcg/d) to keep homocysteine levels low, and possibly the use of selenium (200 mcg/d) for its antioxidant effect.[16–18]
- *High fiber.* This is best obtained from eating fruits, vegetables, and grains.[14]
- *Moderate alcohol intake.* About 1 to 2 ounces of alcohol per day can actually promote health; more can be harmful.[19]

PREVENTION OF ACCIDENTS

Falls constitute a significant risk in older adults. Falls prevention programs (see Chapter 105 on falls) can be implemented for those who are at high risk for falls or who have already fallen.

Slowed reaction time, sensory deficits, dementia, and a host of other age-associated conditions place elderly people at higher risk of injuring themselves and others while driving. Correction of these conditions whenever possible and routine driving tests can minimize risks. All older adults should be reminded to use seat belts when traveling in an automobile. Cessation of driving poses a great threat to the autonomy of older persons, so addressing the driving ability of the geriatric patient should be undertaken with great care and sensitivity.

Household environments can also present a variety of accident hazards. For example, persons with peripheral neuropathy are at increased risk for burns from excessively hot water; setting the hot water temperature at less than 120° to 130°F can obviate this problem. Harm from fires can be reduced by the use of smoke detectors. Demented persons face many accident risks in the home, especially when operating electrical and gas appliances; the use of alarms and automatic shutoff features can be effective in these instances. A home safety checklist can be completed by patients or their caregivers to assess environmental hazards that could lead to an injurious fall. Many physical and occupational therapy (PT/OT) departments perform home visits for accident risk assessment. For elderly people who are particularly vulnerable to injury, PT/OT consultation can be extremely helpful in reducing their accident risk.

PREVENTION OF IATROGENIC PROBLEMS

Several age-associated factors place elderly people at increased risk of iatrogenic problems. As physiologic reserve progressively decreases, the margin for clinical error gets smaller, thereby increasing the risk of an adverse effect of a medical intervention. Older adults who accumulate chronic diseases also accumulate medical providers, often resulting in a lack of care coordination. Having multiple providers frequently leads to polypharmacy. Elderly people are hospitalized more frequently than younger persons; hospitalization presents a host of iatrogenic risks, such as nosocomial infection, adverse drug events, transfusion reactions, and so on.[20,21]

In addition to the preceding factors, the explosion of advances in medical technology has presented further opportunity for iatrogenic illness. Technologic interventions such as cardiopulmonary resuscitation (CPR), valve replacement surgery, carotid endarterectomy, combination intravenous antibiotic therapy, and use of artificial feeding tubes have dramatically increased the therapeutic options during life-threatening illnesses. Although their positive effects are often lifesaving, the potential adverse effects of these interventions are usually severe, such as brain damage from CPR, sudden death or MI from valve replacement surgery, stroke from carotid endarterectomy, fluid overload from combination intravenous antibiotics, and unwanted prolonged life from feeding tubes.

Compared with younger persons, older adults more often experience these untoward outcomes.[20] When elderly people confront critical illnesses, the decision of whether or not to undergo high-risk, potentially lifesaving interventions must be faced. Unfortunately, research has shown that physicians are frequently unaware of patients' preferences for aggressive care and often do not discuss these issues with patients.[22] The morbidity from a medical or surgical procedure that was not wanted in the first place is thus iatrogenic.

The first step in preventing iatrogenic problems is to recognize which patients are the most vulnerable to the adverse effects of medical care. Patients most susceptible to iatrogenic problems are those who have multiple chronic illnesses, see multiple physicians, and take multiple medications.[23,24] There is a direct correlation between the number of chronic illnesses and the chances that treatment of one illness will adversely affect the other.[25] Persons with multiple chronic illnesses frequently see multiple physicians. It is difficult for numerous providers to consult with each other every time they see a common patient. As a result, changes in a patient's therapeutic regimen are frequently made without the input of other providers, often increasing the risk of iatrogenic illness. Chronically ill and frail people also take numerous medications. The average elderly person takes two to three times the prescription and over-the-counter medicines taken by a younger person. Higher rates of drug use and chronic illness lead to a markedly increased risk of drug-drug or drug-disease adverse interactions. This risk of polypharmacy is particularly increased in patients who are malnourished or who have renal failure.

Another significant risk factor for iatrogenic problems is hospitalization. Acutely ill older adults are at increased risk for treatment-related delirium, adverse drug reactions, pressure sores, and nosocomial infections.[26,27] Patients with dementia or conditions causing immobility are at particular risk for hospital-induced iatrogenic problems, especially when undergoing surgery.[28,29]

Once high-risk patients are identified, several interventions can be implemented to prevent the following iatrogenic complications:

- *Case management.* The primary function of a case manager is care coordination. Case managers can be employed by physician groups, parent health plans, and community or governmental organizations. Research has shown that case management is most effective at achieving beneficial outcomes in elderly people who are frail.[30,31] Case managers facilitate communication between providers, ensure that needed services are provided, and avoid duplication of services.
- *Geriatric evaluation and management (GEM).* A GEM team can be called on to evaluate all of the patient's problems simultaneously and formulate a coordinated care plan. This intervention is resource intensive and should be applied to only patients with the most complex clinical problems.[32]
- *Pharmacist consultation.* A pharmacist's input can be particularly helpful to prevent complications from polypharmacy.[33]
- *Acute care for the elderly (ACE) units.* ACE units are specific wards of a hospital with dedicated staff, all designed to address the special needs of elderly inpatients. As such, these units are in tune with the iatrogenic risks of hospitalization and take specific measures to avoid these complications.[34]
- *Advance directives.* Advance directives, including designation of proxies for medical decision making, can be helpful in avoiding administration of undesired medical treatments during periods of critical illness when patients are unable to speak for themselves. Research on the effectiveness of advance directives has been somewhat disappointing, showing that they are rarely completed by patients, occasionally not obeyed by providers, and frequently changed when patients' conditions become dire; interventions designed to increase their effectiveness have been largely unsuccessful.[35] However, designation by the patient of a proxy for medical decision making can often circumvent many of these limitations.

PREVENTION OF PSYCHOSOCIAL ILLNESSES

Aging is frequently accompanied by loss and isolation. Spouses and close friends become disabled or die; children often move far away from home. Retirement brings not only stoppage of work but also distancing from one's peers. Immobility and other conditions make travel much more difficult. Increasing disability and functional dependence lead to loss of autonomy. Depression, loneliness, family discord, and other psychosocially derived illnesses and conditions can result from these challenges of aging.

Research has shown that older adults with psychosocial illness suffer higher rates of functional dependence and mortality.[36,37] Less well established is whether or not these illnesses can be prevented. The major challenge in psychosocial illness prevention is the fact that the usual major antecedents—death or relocation of loved ones—are essentially not modifiable. Despite this challenge, the preponderance of psychosocial illness and its strong association with morbidity and mortality in older adults warrant concerted preventive efforts.

Depression is common in elderly people. Although major depression leading to suicide attempts or hospitalization appears to be less common than in younger persons, depressive symptoms (sometimes called minor or situational depression) can be quite prevalent, with a frequency greater than 10%.[38] Unfortunately, depression is often unrecognized in primary care practice,[39] prompting the question of whether screening for depression in older adults is indicated. Screening would have a higher yield in patients with depressive risk factors: female, single, positive family history, financial problems, and lack of social supports. Several simple screening instruments have been developed that do not require a physician for administration. Coupling the ease of screening with the availability of effective and safe antidepressants, many clinicians have incorporated depression screening into their practices for older patients.[40]

It is well established that elders with increased social contact experience better health. Clinicians should take a social history from their patients, inquiring about situations of loneliness and isolation. In those who are isolated, efforts to increase social contact can theoretically prevent morbidity and mortality. Senior centers, social clubs, and increased family involvement are potentially effective interventions.

A sense of self-worth has also been linked to health in older adults.[41] Healthy seniors often speak of the importance of feeling needed by someone else. Remaining productive at work or leisure activities is also often cited as a correlate of successful aging. Again, though supporting research has not been performed, interventions such as obtaining a pet, performing volunteer work, contributing to household chores, or any other activities that confirm a sense of social connectedness are potentially effective in preventing psychosocial (and even physical) disability.

INDIVIDUALIZING PREVENTION

Because the elderly population exhibits marked heterogeneity of health status, tailoring preventive efforts to match the condition of the patient would seem indicated. Although a continuum in reality, the health and functional status of elderly people divides the population into three basic groups: healthy elderly (60% to 75%), chronically ill (25% to 35%), and frail (2% to 10%). Healthy older adults, constituting the majority of this population, have minimal or no chronic disease and are functionally independent. Those who are chronically ill have an accumulation of incurable conditions; these persons usually have no or mild functional impairment, frequently take several prescription medications, and occasionally are hospitalized from exacerbations of chronic illness. Frail older adults, the smallest group, typically have numerous and severe chronic illnesses, marked functional dependence, and loss of functional reserve. These persons are frequently hospitalized or institutionalized. Each of these three groups is presented with different threats to its health and functioning, calling for different preventive emphases.

Table 99-3 provides an overview of prevention in the elderly population, matching preventive priorities with patient condition. In healthy older adults who have yet to experience disease and functional decline, primary and secondary disease prevention as well as frailty prevention should be the focus of health maintenance efforts. In those who are chronically ill, it is most likely that complications from their long-standing illnesses will be the cause of future morbidity and functional decline. Thus, the highest preventive priority for these patients should center on tertiary prevention. This is not to say, however, that other preventive modalities should be completely ignored. For those patients who have become frail, there should be an increasing focus on accident prevention and iatrogenic illness prevention, as these events become much more common.

Another method of individualizing prevention is by factoring life expectancy, health status, and potential benefit of preventive activities together as the basis for decision making. The first step is to estimate an individual's life expectancy. This can be done through use of a mortality prognosticating instrument[42] or by adjusting life expectancy up or down based on the clinician's overall judgment of the patient's health status as being above, at, or below average for age-matched peers. Then the temporal payoff of the preventive activity is estimated and compared to the life expectancy of the patient. For example, the benefit of many cancer screening tests is not realized for approximately 5 years following detection of asymptomatic malignancies.[43] Thus, if a patient's life expectancy is 6 years based on age alone and that patient has poor overall health status compared with age-matched peers, the clinician would be disinclined to perform cancer screening in the patient, as the likelihood of benefit for the test is low. Guidelines on individualized decision making based on age and health status have been published for preventive activities in older adults.[44,45]

Two preventive activities are applicable to virtually all older adults regardless of condition. First, exercise can be effective for prevention of frailty, has a role in the primary prevention of diseases such as heart disease and cancer in both healthy and chronically ill older adults, and can help to preserve function and reduce accidents in patients who are frail. Second, immunization with influenza shots (yearly) and pneumococcal vaccine (once at age 65) is inexpensive, effective, and associated with minimal morbidity.

PREVENTIVE PRACTICE SYSTEMS

Provider knowledge of which preventive activities are indicated for the aging population is not sufficient for the appropriate delivery of preventive care. Implementation of an efficient disease-prevention and health-promotion system in a geriatric practice can be challenging, and delivery of routine preventive services in primary care settings is often shown to be deficient.[46] Older patients tend to have more acute care needs, manifested frequently as flare-ups of chronic conditions, the management of which occupies

Table 99-3. Prioritizing Preventive Activities by Health and Functional Status

	PATIENT HEALTH STATUS				DISEASE		
Type of Prevention	Primary	Secondary	Tertiary	Frailty	Accident	Iatrogenic Illness	Psychosocial Illness
Healthy	+++	+++	+	+++	+	0	+
Chronically Ill	+	+	+++	++	++	++	+++
Frail	0	0	++	0	+++	+++	+++

+++ = High priority; ++ = moderate priority; + = low priority; 0 = nonpriority.

a major portion of contact time with providers. Owing to the diverse nature of primary care practices, a "one size fits all" approach to implementing a disease-prevention and health-promotion program is not advisable. However, research has demonstrated that the following strategies result in greater degrees of successful preventive activities:

- *Use of nonphysician personnel.* Implementation of screening, immunoprophylactic, and counseling prevention activities are all essentially guideline driven and can be well managed by nurses or other personnel. Research has shown that nonphysicians do a better job of achieving greater compliance with cancer and other disease screening guidelines and that patients accept these activities being directed by a nonphysician.[47,48] Nonphysicians can be used for worthwhile but time-consuming counseling and behavioral change activities, such as those involved in smoking cessation and dietary weight reduction.[49]
- *Use of information systems.* Information technology has been shown to increase delivery of preventive services.[50] Computer reminders, guideline provision, and decision support, preferably at the point of care, all enhance preventive care.[50,51]
- *Patient and provider education.* Increasing the knowledge and awareness of patients and providers about preventive activities promotes such activities in clinical practice. Evidence-based guidelines aid medical personnel in the design of preventive systems.[51] Pamphlets, posters, and other education materials can increase the awareness of and demand for preventive activities among patients.[52]
- *Community-wide promotion.* Health care organizations, in partnership with community organizations, can promote preventive activities through mass mailings, public information, and advertisements such as through billboards and over the Internet to affect a more population-wide increase in prevention interest.[53]
- *Creation of incentives for prevention.* Reimbursement structures often favor acute care services over preventive services. Realignment of incentives to reward achievement of preventive guidelines can be a powerful intervention to increase disease-prevention activities.[54] Changing reimbursement to cover preventive services can also be a strong motivator of change.[54,55] Designing practice-based disease-prevention programs necessitates the direct involvement of the practitioners and staff. Working together, physicians and staff should review appropriate prevention literature, decide which disease-prevention activities will be emphasized, define barriers to practicing prevention, and design systems that will overcome those barriers.[47]

SUMMARY

Preventive medicine for older adults should address primary, secondary, and tertiary disease prevention as well as efforts for preventing frailty, injurious accidents, psychosocial illness, and iatrogenic conditions. Rigorous, evidence-based guidelines exist to aid clinicians in these activities, particularly for primary and secondary disease prevention. The relative emphasis of each type of preventive activity should be individualized according to the life expectancy and comorbid status of each patient. Prevention is most effective in practices that take a systems-based approach involving extensive use of nonphysician personnel, information technology linked to evidence-based guidelines, community involvement, and creation of appropriate incentives for preventive care.

KEY POINTS

Preventive and Anticipatory Care

- Five categories of conditions can be addressed for prevention: diseases (primary, secondary, and tertiary), frailty, psychosocial illness, injuries, and iatrogenic problems.
- Disease prevention and health promotion must be individually tailored to the elderly person's health status and functional level.
- Successful disease prevention and health promotion care systems usually feature use of nonphysician personnel, information technology support, educational interventions for both providers and patients, and alignment of incentives to promote preventive activities.

For a complete list of references, please visit online only at www.expertconsult.com

CHAPTER 100

Sexuality in Old Age

Robert N. Butler
Myrna I. Lewis

MISINFORMATION, MYTHS, AND PREJUDICES

Physicians frequently overlook the sexuality of older patients during the typical medical examination and evaluation. As a result, physicians may miss the opportunity to offer their older patients reassurance about the normal changes in sexuality that may be troubling them; they may not advise these patients about the side effects of medications that can adversely affect continuing sexual activity; and they may fail to diagnose sexual dysfunction and recommend treatment possibilities.[1]

Lack of public and professional medical education is partially to blame for this neglect of late-life sexuality in the medical encounter. Centuries of myths about aging, as well as prudery and ignorance, have helped close the minds of laypersons and professionals alike to the fact that many older people wish to, and do, continue expressing their sexuality until the end of their life. Because few studies have been conducted on sexuality in general, and on late-life sexuality in particular, data about the nature and frequency of sexual activity among older persons are limited. However, self-reports from surveys of older people have demonstrated that, for many, sexual desire and satisfaction remain important aspects of their lives. The main barriers to sexual expression in late life are medical and psychological problems and social obstacles. A problematic marital relationship or lack of a partner due to the death of a spouse or companion may also interfere.[1]

With the discovery of the therapeutic effect in men of sildenafil citrate in erectile dysfunction (ED) and its introduction in 1998, the attitudes of physicians and that of the public have moved to more positive approaches and acceptance of sexuality for older persons. This includes a growing awareness of the need for further understanding of female sexuality, including better diagnosis and treatment for older women that parallels current breakthroughs for older men.

NORMAL AGING AND CHANGES IN SEXUALITY

Sexuality may be defined as the quality or state that comprises sexual desire (libido), arousal, function, and activity; physical satisfaction; and emotional intimacy. Many older people maintain desire (libido) and sexual capacity and satisfaction as long as they have their health, a healthy partner, and a good relationship with that partner. They experience the same four stages of the sexual act as younger people: desire, arousal, climax, and recovery. Sexual expression remains a highly complex process in old age and may involve fantasy, the central nervous and peripheral nervous systems, the circulatory system, and all six senses. The capacity for fantasy may, however, decline for older men, according to the National Institute on Aging's Baltimore Longitudinal Study on Aging. We do not know if this is equally true for women because sexual fantasy in women was not documented in the study.

Normal change in sexual functioning is usually manifested as a gradual slowing—that is, more time is needed for arousal (erection in men; lubrication in women) and reaching a climax. Unlike women, healthy men can remain fertile until the end of life. There is no discrete climacteric for men, but rather a gradual decline of testosterone levels after age 30 that usually do not fall below normal. Testosterone levels in 70% of healthy older men are in the same range as those of younger men. With aging, the testes may become smaller and penile flaccidity greater. More direct stimulation of the penis may be necessary to reach engorgement and erection. For some older men, orgasm may last a shorter time than it did when they were younger. The force of ejaculation and the volume of ejaculate decrease. A great concern for older men (and for younger men as well) is their ability to maintain sexual potency. Impotence and ED are often automatically and inaccurately attributed to increasing age. They can, in fact, occur at any age for a variety of reasons and, once properly diagnosed, are often treatable[1] (see discussion of ED later in the chapter).

Because of cultural emphasis on a youthful female body image, older women tend to be more concerned than men about physical appearance and their sexual desirability. However, those women who are healthy can usually continue earlier patterns of sexual functioning, which includes maintaining orgasmic capacity. For some women, sexual interest may increase after menopause because they no longer experience concern about pregnancy. Nonetheless, reduced estrogen production resulting from menopause may present both physical and emotional problems for a number of older women. Physical problems include a change in vaginal shape, vaginal dryness, and thinning of the vaginal walls, which may lead to pain and bleeding during coitus and a less well-protected bladder and urethra, with recurrent cystitis as a result. Less acidic vaginal secretions may lead to greater incidence of vaginal infections. Emotional problems accompanying menopause include increased irritability and lability, often because of sleep deprivation, which is itself a menopausal symptom. Although estrogen replacement therapy (ERT) helps relieve some symptoms, extensive studies by the National Institutes of Health's Women's Health Initiative (WHI) have implicated ERT in the development of gallbladder disease and breast and uterine cancer. These studies also suggest that ERT may increase the risk of blood clots, which can result in strokes and heart attacks. However, since the results of the WHI were based on estrogen derived from the urine of pregnant mares (Premarin) that may be difficult to metabolize, further studies using other estrogen products are needed. In the meantime, diet, exercise, and drugs that lower cholesterol and blood pressure can lower risk of heart disease, and nonhormonal drugs such as bisphosphonates may be effective in cutting the risk of fractures in women with osteoporosis. Women can often find relief for vaginal dryness and irritation during intercourse with off-prescription water-based vaginal lubricants.[2–4]

Women who wish to remain sexually active in later life may face barriers that have nothing to do with physical symptoms. Because women typically live nearly 7 years longer than men and tend to marry men who are 3 or more years older, they have a much greater chance of surviving their male partners. About 60% of older women are without a spouse, as opposed to 20% of men, and many others may be living with a disabled spouse who cannot be a sexual partner. As they grow older, the ratio of women to men increases greatly, and the chances of finding another partner are greatly reduced. There are approximately 150 women to 100 men over the age of 65, and 250 women to 100 men over the age of 85.

It has been estimated that up to 10% of the general population is lesbian, gay, bisexual, or transgender (LGBT), although the exact number is unknown. As in the older heterosexual population, many LGBT individuals have long-term relationships and are emotionally stable, successful, and happy in their later years. When sexual difficulties occur for LGBT couples, they involve many of the same interpersonal, physical, social, and psychological problems faced by heterosexual couples. Physicians need to be sensitive to and accepting of alternative sexual expression.[2]

EXAMINATION AND EVALUATION OF THE PATIENT

The general medical evaluation of an older person should include a thorough sexual history, current sexual function, and a careful physical examination. The physician should initiate questions in these areas because older patients may not volunteer sexual information about themselves. Questions should be asked in an unintimidating and unembarrassing fashion. During the examination, the physician should pay special attention to the neurologic, circulatory, and endocrine systems. Because some medical conditions, surgical procedures, and medications can affect sexual functioning, the physician should be sure to include a discussion of sexuality when treating disease or prescribing medication to patients for whom continuing sexual activity is important.

The physician should be aware of the fact that sexually transmitted diseases (STDs) occur in old as well as young persons. People of all ages should practice "safe sex." Ten percent of all AIDS patients in the United States are over 55 years of age, and not all of them contracted HIV through blood transfusions. Hepatitis B is the only sexually transmitted virus preventable by vaccine.[2]

EFFECTS OF MEDICAL PROBLEMS, SURGERY, AND MEDICATIONS

Sexual interest and capacity wane in the presence of illness, and some diseases have a much more powerful effect on sexuality in the later years because of their frequency and character. Heart disease is three times more common in men than in women up to the age of 60, probably because of the protection afforded by estrogen, even postmenopausally. However, after menopause the incidence of heart disease in women begins to rise and eventually reaches that in men in their early 60s. Heart disease is a source of considerable concern to sexually active older people because sexual activity increases the heart rate. Many who have had angina or a heart attack become anxious about future sexual encounters. The fear of dying during intercourse may also compound depression that is already present in response to the heart disease itself. Physicians should point out to their concerned patients that, in fact, oxygen usage or "debt" in a sexual encounter is the rough equivalent of walking up one or two flights of stairs. Physicians should reassure their patients that anyone who can carry out usual daily activities is able to engage in sexual activity. A study published in 1996 of more than 800 men and women found that among individuals who had suffered a heart attack, the risk of a recurrent heart attack during sex was only 2 in 1 million.[5] An earlier large-scale study of more than 5500 coronary deaths found that less than 1% were related to sex, with a majority of these involving extramarital relations (suggesting that stressful aspects associated with such affairs—guilt, anxiety, the need to hurry—may play a role).[6] Thus, sexual activity poses extraordinarily little risk.

Patients are often uneasy about recommencing their sex lives following coronary bypass surgery. Some 4 weeks or more of abstinence is recommended before resuming sexual activity, to allow full healing to occur.

Other medical conditions that can impact significantly on sexuality are stroke, diabetes, osteoarthritis and rheumatoid arthritis, back pain, Parkinson's disease, chronic emphysema and bronchitis, chronic prostatitis in men, and stress incontinence in women. The effects on sexuality of these diseases and their treatment are summarized in Table 100-1.

Surgery can significantly impair sexual functioning as well. Common surgical procedures and their effects on sexuality are outlined in Table 100-2. Embarrassment or discomfiture from surgical procedures such as mastectomies or ostomies can inhibit sexual drive and performance. Prostate surgery is discussed in the section on ED.

Medications are among the most common causes of sexual dysfunction. Commonly prescribed medications that adversely affect sexuality are listed in Table 100-3. Physicians should familiarize themselves with medications that have fewer toxic effects on sexual function and prescribe them whenever possible. For example, angiotensin-converting enzyme (ACE) inhibitors taken for hypertension are less apt to cause sexual dysfunction than is methyldopa. Of the antidepressants, Wellbutrin is one of the least problematic. In addition, it is possible to reduce the dosage of some drugs to avoid adverse sexual and other effects without reducing the benefits of the drugs to the patient.[7] In certain cases, brief "drug holidays" may improve sexual function, but this requires discussion with a physician.

Abuse of substances such as alcohol and tobacco also impairs sexuality (see Table 100-3). Alcohol may increase desire but decrease performance. Tobacco use adversely affects male sexuality and causes wrinkles in both men and women.

ERECTILE DYSFUNCTION

Causes and diagnosis

Because even occasional ED can have significant emotional consequences for many men, which can, in turn, exacerbate physical problems, diagnosis should be made carefully. ED should be diagnosed only when failure in sexual encounters occurs in at least a quarter of all attempts.

It is estimated that 10 million to 20 million men in the United States experience some degree of ED. Although ED affects men of all ages, it tends to increase progressively with age because of the greater likelihood of accompanying medical conditions. The comprehensive Massachusetts Male Health Study found that 52% of men aged 40 to 70 experience some ED.[8]

It is estimated that 90% of ED cases are due to physical causes, including vascular disorders such as atherosclerosis

Table 100-1. Effects of Medical Conditions on Sexuality

Medical Condition	Effect on Sexuality	Treatment
Arthritis	Sexual desire is usually unaffected, but disability due to osteoarthritis and rheumatoid arthritis may interfere with performance	Trying sexual positions that do not aggravate joint pain; planning sexual activity for times of day when pain and stiffness are diminished
Chronic emphysema and bronchitis	Shortness of breath hinders physical activity, including sex	Rest; supplemental oxygen
Chronic prostatitis	Pain may diminish sexual desire	Antibiotics; warm sitz baths, prostatic massage; Kegel exercises
Chronic renal disease	Impotence, possibly with anxiety and depression	Dialysis; psychotherapy for underlying emotional problems; kidney transplantation may restore sexual capacity
Diabetes mellitus	Impotence is common	Very tight control of diabetes may restore potency
Heart and vascular disease		
Myocardial infarction	8- to 14-week recuperation period recommended before resuming sexual intercourse; depression and antidepressant drugs may reduce libido and capacity; fear of bringing on another heart attack if patient resumes sexual activity	Reassurance from the doctor about safety of sexual activity; exercise programs to improve cardiac function
Heart failure	Sexual dysfunction resulting from physical symptoms or medications; a 2- to 3-week week recovery period is advised before resuming sex in cases of pulmonary edema	Reassurance from the doctor about safety of sexual activity for patients with effectively managed heart failure; exercise programs to improve cardiac function
Coronary bypass surgery	4 weeks or more of abstinence is recommended before resuming sexual intercourse	Alternatives such as self-stimulation or masturbation can usually be started earlier in the recovery period; exercise programs to improve cardiac function
Pelvic steal syndrome	Example of vascular impotence—male loses erection as soon as he enters his partner and begins pelvic thrusting due to gravity's redirecting blood supply away from the pelvis	Changing position may help (man should lie on his back or side)
Hypertension	Incidence of impotence in untreated male hypertensive patients is about 15%; effects on women not established	Choose hypertensive drugs that do not impair sexual response
Parkinson's disease	Lack of sexual desire in both men and women; impotence in men	Levodopa can improve sex drive and performance in some men for a limited period
Peyronie's disease	Intercourse is painful for many men with the disease; penetration may be difficult or impossible when penis is angled too sharply	Psychotherapy to help patient adjust to changes in the penis; symptoms occasionally disappear spontaneously; surgery helps in some cases
Stress incontinence	Sexual dysfunction has been reported in up to 50% of women with this condition	Solving the underlying problem may help; Kegel exercises to strengthen muscles supporting bladder; estrogen taken orally or locally to firm up vaginal lining; biofeedback training
Stroke	Sexual desire may not be impaired, but sexual performance likely to be affected (e.g., male erectile dysfunction either because of physical or psychological reasons, anesthetic areas, or physical limitations due to paralysis)	Mechanical adjustments to assist positioning necessary for sexual activities; treatments for impotence

Data from Butler RN, Lewis MI. Sexuality. In: Merck Manual of Geriatrics, 3rd ed. Whitehouse Station, NJ: Merck Research Laboratories; 2000, pp. 1156–1164; and Butler RN, Lewis MI. The New Love and Sex after 60. New York: Ballantine Books; 2000.

Table 100-2. Effects of Surgery on Sexuality

Surgical Procedure	Effect on Sexuality
Hysterectomy	Need to refrain from sexual activity during healing (6 to 8 weeks after surgery); depression; possible reduction in sensation during orgasm
Mastectomy	Emotional reactions such as depression; loss of sexual desire because of emotional reactions of patient and partner
Prostatectomy	Need to refrain from sexual activity during healing (6 weeks); possible impotence because of surgery (nerve-sparing techniques help avoid this effect in some cases); possible psychogenic impotence
Orchiectomy	Impotence is common
Colostomy and ileostomy	Emotional reactions that can affect desire and potency (participation in ostomy clubs is recommended)
Rectal cancer surgery	Impotence is common

Data from Butler RN, Lewis MI. Sexuality. In: Merck Manual of Geriatrics, 3rd ed. Whitehouse Station, NJ: Merck Research Laboratories; 2000, pp. 1156–64; and Butler RN, Lewis MI. The New Love and Sex after 60. New York: Ballantine Books; 2000.

and pelvic steal syndrome (see Table 100-1); neurologic disorders such as trauma (e.g., sports injuries) and diabetic neuropathy; and endocrine disorders, such as thyroid disease, diabetes, and low testosterone levels, although low testosterone affects only about 4% of men. Testosterone is more likely to be associated with decreased libido than with ED. Radiation therapy and chemotherapy for cancer may destroy testicular function. In men with heart disease, fear that sex will cause a heart attack can cause sexual dysfunction.

ED may also be caused by structural abnormalities such as Peyronie's disease (see Table 100-1). Prostatectomies may create sexual problems. In some cases, a man who has had prostate surgery and has lost interest in sex may use the surgery as an excuse for avoiding sexual contact. ED may follow prostate surgery, but nerve-sparing surgical techniques, developed by Dr. Patrick Walsh of Johns Hopkins University, are available and can help avoid ED in many cases.[9]

As described earlier, certain drugs may also cause sexual dysfunction, including antihypertensives, antidepressants, antipsychotics, and others (see Table 100-3), as can overconsumption of alcohol.

Table 100-3. Selected Medications and Substances That May Adversely Affect Sexual Functioning

Psychotropics	β-Blockers
Tricyclic antidepressants	Propranolol
Clomipramine	Atenolol
Amitriptyline	Metoprolol
Doxepin	Bisoprolol
Imipramine	Timolol
Nortriptyline*	Betaxolol
Desipramine*	α1-Blockers
Monoamine oxidase	Prazosin*
inhibitors	Doxazosin*
Isocarboxazid	α2-Agonists
Phenelzine	Clonidine
Tranylcypromine*	Guanfacine
Serotonin reuptake inhibitors	ACE inhibitors‡
Fluoxetine	Captopril*
Paroxetine	Enalapril
Sertraline	Calcium-channel blockers
Fluvoxamine	Amlodipine
Venlafaxine	Verapamil
Mood stabilizers/	Diltiazem
anticonvulsants	Anticancer drugs
Lithium†	Vinblastine
Valproate*	5-Fluorouracil
Carbamazepine	Tamoxifen
Phenytoin	Cold/allergy medications
Phenobarbital	Chlorpheniramine
Antipsychotics/neuroleptics	Diphenhydramine
Phenothiazines	hydrochloride
Chlorpromazine	Pseudoephedrine
Fluphenazine*	Antiulcer medications
Perphenazine	Cimetidine
Thioridazine	Famotidine*
Other	Nizatidine*
Haloperidol	Ranitidine*
Thiothixene	Stimulants/anorectics
Risperidone	Phentermine
Antianxiety agents/	Fenfluramine
tranquilizers	Phenylpropanolamine
Benzodiazepines	Diethylpropion
Diuretics	Mazindol
Thiazide-type	Commonly abused substances
Chlorthalidone	Alcohol
Hydrochlorothiazide	Barbiturates
Indapamide*	Cannabis
Loop diuretics	Cocaine
Furosemide*	Opioids
Potassium-sparing	Methylphenidate
Spironolactone	Amphetamine
Antihypertensives	Nicotine
Reserpine	Hormones
Methyldopa	Progesterone
Guanethidine	Cortisol

Data from Crenshaw TL, Goldberg JP. Sexual pharmacology: drugs that affect sexual functioning. New York: WW Norton; 1996.

*Studies indicate that these drugs may have fewer sexual side effects than others in their class.

†Direct sexual side effects of lithium are confirmed only when it is taken in conjunction with benzodiazepines.

‡ACE inhibitors have fewer sexual side effects than other classes of antihypertensives.

Ten percent of cases of ED are due to psychological causes, including performance anxiety, stress, exhaustion, anger, bereavement, and depression. Sexual problems can be both the origin and a symptom of depression. Losing one's partner may be followed by grief, sometimes complicated by depression. It may lead to a kind of "enshrinement" of the lost partner. In such cases, "widower's guilt" may block the development of new relationships and cause ED when the man tries to engage in sexual activity with a new partner.[2]

Proper diagnosis of ED depends on taking a thorough history; asking questions about changes in libido, nocturnal erections, and problems with relationships; and reviewing diseases and medication and alcohol use. These steps should be followed by a physical examination and laboratory evaluation, including a testosterone level check. ED during sleep can be checked by rigiscan, a means of measuring nocturnal tumescence associated with rapid-eye movement sleep. It should be noted, however, that this is an imperfect method for diagnosing ED.

Treatment

In general, the old adage "use it or lose it" appears to be true. Erections bring oxygen-rich blood to the penis, which contributes to continuing healthful functioning. Good health habits promote sexual capability. In addition to helping people stay healthy, a balanced diet, no tobacco, moderate consumption of alcohol, and exercise programs all help prevent sexual dysfunction.

ED can often be treated successfully. For ED with a physical cause, the main treatment is of the underlying cause, such as diabetes or a reaction to medications. For psychogenic cases, psychotherapy, marital therapy, group therapy, and sex therapy—which is based on Masters and Johnson's use of "sensate focusing"—may be beneficial. These approaches are also useful when ED is physical in origin because there are often associated or concomitant emotional reactions to ED, and because such therapeutic approaches can reassure the patient and his partner.

However, it should be noted that ED may be an early sign of heart disease, hypertension, or diabetes. It is a sign, not a diagnosis. Therefore, ED should prompt careful evaluation.

PHARMACOTHERAPY

Sildenafil has become widely used. In dosages of 25, 50, or 100 mg (in most cases starting with 25 mg) and taken 1 hour prior to a sexual encounter, sildenafil will produce an erection, but only when the man is sexually stimulated. It is not an aphrodisiac but a "mechanical" means to facilitate intercourse. Nor does it substitute for intimacy; indeed, it may reveal strains in relationships. Sildenafil blocks the action of an enzyme, phosphodiesterase type 5, so that nitric oxide dilates the penile blood vessels. It also increases clitoral blood flow and some women report its usefulness; however, comprehensive studies have not verified this. Although there are currently no reliable measurements of female sexual response, efforts are under way to develop such instruments.

Sildenafil can cause hypotension when nitrates are used concurrently, so it is contraindicated in patients who take nitrates to relieve angina. A patient who has had an adverse heart event and has taken sildenafil that day should not be given a nitrate. Sildenafil can also cause headaches, upset stomach, bluish vision, and nasal congestion. Rarely, priaprism (4 hours of tumescence) occurs and must be treated to avoid damage to the penis.

Sildenafil has not been compared directly to other treatments for ED.[10] New oral drugs to treat ED are under study.

Other medications for ED include vasoactive compounds that are injected directly into the corpus cavernosum. Phentolamine, atropine, and prostaglandin E have been shown to be effective given individually or together. Prostaglandin E was the first prescription medication approved by the U.S. Food and Drug Administration (FDA) to treat ED. Erection should occur within 5 to 10 minutes after injection, and the erection can last

30 minutes or more. Injection with these substances should not be done more than once every 24 hours and not more than three times per week. Possible problems with this therapy include priapism (4%), which can be reversed with epinephrine or ephedrine; mild to moderate pain at the site of injection; and some scarring. Contraindications include sickle-cell anemia, multiple myeloma, leukemia, anatomic deformities, and implants (discussed later). Treatment of men with ED with transurethral alprostadil (a synthetic compound identical to prostaglandin E_1) is effective in nearly 70% of cases, regardless of age. A major advantage of this treatment is that the drug is delivered transurethrally via an applicator rather than through injection.[11]

Some studies of the substance yohimbine, which comes from the bark of an African tree, have shown that it has a positive effect on erection, probably because it acts on neurotransmitters such as acetylcholine and dopamine that are involved in the sexual response. However, undesirable side effects have been noted.

VACUUM THERAPY

This involves placing a cylinder over an unerect penis, sucking out air to produce an erection, and applying a wide rubber band at the base to maintain the erection. One third of individuals who try vacuum devices find them helpful. They should not be used by men taking anticoagulants or those who have low platelet counts.

IMPLANT

A permanent penile prosthesis may help a patient with an otherwise untreatable potency problem. Such a prosthesis is irreversible and therefore should be used only as a last resort. Penile implants can be noninflatable (positionable or semirigid rod prosthesis) and inflatable. Inflatable implants include an inflate/deflate pump with the cylinder in the penis or placed below the skin in the scrotum. There is a reservoir in the scrotum. Cylinders are placed behind the abdominal muscles. Contraindications to this treatment include psychiatric problems such as psychosis and untreated depression.[5] Complications include infection, mechanical failure, and penile fibrosis.

SURGERY

Revascularization surgery is still largely experimental.

THE "SECOND LANGUAGE OF SEX"

Some older people are not interested in sex because they were never interested in it, or their sexual desire has decreased, or their opportunities for sexual activity are significantly diminished, or other reasons. On the other hand, many older people are interested and want to continue to be sexually active. Whatever his or her point of view, each older person's wishes should be elicited and respected before treatment decisions are completed. There is a range of interest and degree of sexual activity among older people just as there is among other age groups, and treatment options can be as effective for them as for younger people.

The "first language" of sexuality, generally associated with youth, is biologic and intense. The "second language" of sexuality, broader than the first, is learned by experience over a lifetime. Of course, some younger people are naturally adept at expressing the second language of sexuality and, conversely, some older people never quite learn it. But for many people, the primary focus on genital contact gives way over time to a more encompassing definition of sexuality, which includes intimacy, mutuality, trust, love, romance, friendship, and caring.[2]

It is not known whether there is a clear association between sexual satisfaction and longevity, but there is evidence that love and sex enhance the quality of life. Some of the greatest obstacles to successful, intimate relationships in later life are the negative attitudes and practices toward older persons found among healthcare professionals and the public at large. Health professionals must recognize that their older patients have sexual interest, capacities, and pleasures and that—through education and other interventions—they have the means to repair many of the physical, emotional, and social impediments to continuing sexuality in late life.

SUMMARY

Physicians frequently fail to ask older patients about their sexual functioning during the typical medical examination and evaluation. Patients may be uncomfortable about revealing their sexual difficulties and may not be aware that sexual dysfunction in both sexes can often be treated. In addition, ED may be an early sign of diseases such as heart disease, hypertension, or diabetes.

Normal change in sexual functioning is usually manifested as a gradual slowing—that is, more time is needed for arousal (erection in men, lubrication in women) and reaching a climax. Healthy older women can usually continue earlier patterns of sexual functioning, but reduced estrogen production as a result of menopause may present physical and emotional problems. Ongoing studies at the National Institutes of Health are expected to help clarify indications, contraindications, and risks of hormone replacement therapy.

KEY POINTS
Sexuality in Old Age

- Some medical conditions, surgical procedures, and medications can affect sexual functioning. The physician should include a discussion of sexuality when treating disease in or prescribing medication to elderly patients for whom continuing sexual activity is important.
- It is estimated that 90% of cases of erectile dysfunction have a physical cause, whereas 10% are psychologically induced. Treatments for the latter include psychotherapy, marital therapy, group therapy, and sex therapy.
- Women who wish to remain sexually active in later life may face barriers that are unrelated to physical symptoms. For example, about 60% of elderly women are without a spouse, and many others live with a disabled spouse who cannot be a sexual partner.
- Medical conditions that can have a significant impact on sexuality are coronary bypass surgery, stroke, diabetes, osteoarthritis and rheumatoid arthritis, back pain, Parkinson's disease, chronic emphysema and bronchitis, chronic prostatitis in men, and stress incontinence in women.
- In men with heart disease, fear that sex will cause a heart attack can cause sexual dysfunction.
- With the discovery of the therapeutic effect in men of sildenafil citrate, the more positive attitudes of physicians and the public have moved to greater acceptance of the sexuality of older persons.

For a complete list of references, please visit online only at www.expertconsult.com

Exercise for Successful Aging

William J. Evans

INTRODUCTION

Both increased and decreased levels of physical activity are associated with meaningful outcomes in older people. Increased levels of physical activity have been linked to decreases in mortality, the risk of chronic diseases, nursing home admissions, development of cognitive disorders, and decreased functional capacity. Increased levels of physical activity have been associated with increased mortality, cognitive decline, obesity, and sarcopenia.

Exercise encompasses a broad range of activities. However, virtually every system in the human body is affected in some way by increasing levels of physical activity. *Exercise* can be defined as increased (above resting) muscular activity and may be categorized as anaerobic (sprinting), endurance (aerobic), or resistive (weight lifting). *Resistive* exercise defined as muscle contract a few times against a heavy load or with high tension. This type of exercise is also termed progressive resistance training (PRT) because the load or intensity is progressively increased as an individual becomes stronger. PRT is distinctly different *from aerobic or endurance exercise*, in which muscles contract against little, or no, resistance. *Anaerobic exercise* makes use *of the phosphocreatine* and/or *glycogenolysis for energy production*. Although this type of exercise is generally thought of as the sprinting type of exercise, an extremely deconditioned patient, such as an individual with chronic obstructive pulmonary disease or heart failure may perform anaerobic exercise simply by getting out of bed and walking across a room.

The adaptive response to regularly performed exercise has been repeatedly demonstrated to have remarkably beneficial effects. The list of these adaptive responses is extensive. The Centers for Disease Control and Prevention and the American College of Sports Medicine have suggested that everyone should accumulate at least 30 minutes of exercise on most (preferably all) days.[1] This recommendation is based on evidence of a substantial decrease in all-cause mortality, resulting from a moderate amount of increased physical activity.[2,3] The American Heart Association has stated that inactivity is a primary risk factor for cardiovascular disease.[4–6] Because far more Americans *are inactive than have elevated cholesterol or who smoke*, it is the predominant risk factor for heart disease in the United States. This chapter focuses on the acute and chronic adaptations to exercise with particular attention to substrate use and effects on risk factors for chronic disease and aging.

AEROBIC EXERCISE

Maximal aerobic exercise capacity is termed Vo_2max. Vo_2 (volume of oxygen consumed during maximal aerobic exercise) is defined by the Fick equation (Vo_2 = cardiac output × arteriovenous oxygen difference). Vo_2max is expressed as either mL of O_2 consumed × kg^{-1} body weight × min^{-1} or L of O_2 consumed × min^{-1}. Expressing it at mL × kg^{-1} × min^{-1} is most often used to define an individual's aerobic capacity as differences in body weight are controlled for. The Fick equation demonstrates that there are two important determiners of Vo_2max, central factors that control the delivery of oxygen to skeletal muscle and the capacity of skeletal muscle to extract and use oxygen for ATP during exercise. Regularly performed aerobic exercise increases Vo_2max through the following mechanisms: (1) increased cardiac output resulting from a plasma volume expansion (approximately 15%) and increased stroke volume as a result of cardiac hypertrophy and (2) improved capacity to extract and use oxygen by skeletal muscle. This enhanced oxidative capacity of muscle is due to increased capillarization, mitochondrial density, and myoglobin content. Under most conditions, the delivery of oxygen limits maximal aerobic performance. Increasing blood hemoglobin concentration (from anemic to normal or from normal to super normal) has been demonstrated to increase Vo_2max maximal and submaximal exercise performance.[7–10] Anemia due to malnutrition has been demonstrated to limit functional status and work capacity. On the other hand, aerobic exercise performance in athletes can be substantially improved by increasing hemoglobin levels above normal through the use of recombinant human erythropoietin.[11] Anemia is common in late life and may not always be associated with a clear cause.[12]

Maximal aerobic capacity (Vo_2max) declines with advancing age.[13] This age-associated decrease in Vo_2max has been shown to be approximately 1%/yr between the ages of 20 and 70 years. This decline is likely to be due to a number of factors, including decreased levels of physical activity, changing cardiac function (including decreased maximum cardiac output), and reduced muscle mass. Fleg and Lakatta[14] determined that skeletal muscle mass accounted for most of the variability in Vo_2max in men and women above the age of 60 years. Using data from the Baltimore Longitudinal Study on Aging, this group[15] also showed that the decline in maximal aerobic capacity with age accelerates after the age of 70 years. Because a decline in maximal heart rate is linear with advancing age, they ascribe this accelerated decline in late life to factors related to skeletal muscle, such as *capillary density and muscle oxidative capacity*. Short et al[16] showed that most of the age-related decline in maximal aerobic capacity can be explained by a decrease in muscle mass and muscle mitochondrial function (oxidative capacity). A number of studies have demonstrated that the age-related decline in Vo_2max is ameliorated by physical activity.[17–20] Bortz and Bortz[21] reviewed world records of master athletes up to age 85 for endurance events and noted that the decline in performance occurred at a rate of 0.5%/yr. They concluded that this decline of 0.5%/yr may represent the effects of age (or "biologic" aging) on Vo_2max and the remainder of the decline may be the result of an increasingly sedentary lifestyle. However, Rosen et al[22] examined predictors of this age-associated decline in Vo_2max and concluded that Vo_2max declines at the same rate in athletic and sedentary men and that 35% of this decline is due to *sarcopenia*.

Aerobic exercise has long been an important recommendation for the prevention and treatment of many of the chronic diseases typically associated with old age. These include type 2 diabetes mellitus (and impaired glucose tolerance), hypertension, heart disease, and osteoporosis. Regularly performed aerobic exercise increases insulin action. The responses of initially sedentary young (age 20 to 30) and older (age 60 to 70) men and women to 3 months of aerobic conditioning (70% of maximal heart rate, 45 min/day, 3 days/wk) were examined by Meredith et al.[23] They found that the absolute gains in aerobic capacity were similar between the two age groups. However, the mechanism for adaptation to regular submaximal exercise appears to be different between old and young people. Muscle biopsy specimens taken before and after training showed a more than twofold increase in oxidative capacity in older subjects, whereas those in the young subjects showed smaller improvements. In addition, skeletal muscle glycogen stores in the older subjects, significantly lower than those in the young men and women initially, increased greatly. The degree to which the elderly demonstrate increases in maximal cardiac output in response to endurance training is still largely unanswered. Seals et al[24] found no increases after 1 year of endurance training, while more recently, Spina et al[25] observed that older men increased maximal cardiac output, whereas healthy older women demonstrated no change in response to endurance exercise training. If these gender-related differences in cardiovascular response are real, this finding may explain the lack of response in maximal cardiac output when older men and women are included in the same study population.[24]

Aerobic exercise and carbohydrate metabolism

The 2-hour plasma glucose level during an oral glucose tolerance test increases by an average of 5.3 mg/dL per decade, and fasting plasma glucose increases by an average sp out of 1 mg/dL per decade.[26] The NHANES II study demonstrated a progressive increase of about 0.4 mM/decade of life in mean plasma glucose value 2 hours after a 75 g oral glucose tolerance test ([OGTT], which provides a specific amount of glucose drink in a solution and measures the changes in plasma glucose over a 2 to 3 hour period) (n = 1678 men and 1892 women).[27] Shimoka et al[28] examined glucose tolerance in community dwelling men and women ranging in age between 17 to 92. By assessing the level of obesity, pattern of body fat distribution, activity, and fitness levels they attempted to examine the independent effect of age on glucose tolerance. They found no significant differences between the young and middle-aged groups; however, the old groups had significantly higher glucose and insulin values (following a glucose challenge) than those in young or middle-aged groups. They concluded that "the major finding of this study is that the decline in glucose tolerance from the early-adult to the middle-age years is entirely explained by secondary influences (fatness and fitness), whereas the decline from midlife to old age still is also influenced by chronological age. This finding is unique. It is also unexplained." However, it must be pointed out that anthropometric determination of body fatness becomes increasingly less accurate with advancing age and does not reflect the intra-abdominal and intramuscular accumulation of fat that occurs with aging.[29] The results of this study may be due more to an underestimate of true body fat levels than age. Goodpaster et al have demonstrated that aging and obesity are associated with increased intramuscular lipid.[30,31] This increased intramyocellular lipid is associated with insulin resistance and muscle weakness.

The relationship among aging, body composition, activity, and glucose tolerance was also examined in 270 female and 462 male factory workers aged 22 to 73 years, none of whom were retired.[32] Plasma glucose levels, both fasting and after a glucose load, increased with age, but the correlation between age and total integrated glucose response following a glucose load was weak: in women only 3% of the variance could be attributed to age. When activity levels and drug use were factored in, age accounted for only 1% of the variance in women and 6.25% in men.

The fact that aerobic exercise has significant effects on skeletal muscle may help explain its importance in the treatment of glucose intolerance and type 2 diabetes. Seals et al[33] found that a high-intensity training program resulted in greater improvements in the insulin response to an oral glucose load compared with lower-intensity aerobic exercise. However, their subjects began the study with normal glucose tolerance. Kirwan et al[34] found that 9 months of endurance training at 80% of the maximal heart rate (4 days/wk) resulted in reduced glucose stimulated insulin levels; however, no comparison was made to a lower-intensity exercise group. Hughes et al[35] demonstrated that regularly performed aerobic exercise without weight loss resulted in improved glucose tolerance, rate of insulin stimulated glucose disposal, and increased skeletal muscle GLUT4 levels in older subjects with impaired glucose tolerance. GLUT4 is the glucose transporter protein found in skeletal muscle. More recently, Coker et al[36] examined the effects of intensity of exercise on insulin stimulated glucose uptake in older, overweight men and women. They examined the influence of moderate-intensity (50% Vo_2max) versus high-intensity (75% Vo_2max) aerobic exercise. Although intensity was different, energy expenditure during the exercise sessions was carefully controlled so that both groups used the same number of kilocalories. They demonstrated that after 4 months, only the high-intensity group demonstrated a significant improvement in insulin sensitivity. These data demonstrate that *higher-intensity exercise* (without weight loss) may be necessary to significantly reduce the risk of insulin resistance and type 2 diabetes.

Endurance training and dietary modifications are generally recommended as the primary treatment in the non–insulin-dependent diabetic. Cross-sectional analysis of dietary intake supports the hypothesis that a low carbohydrate/high fat diet is associated with the onset of type 2 diabetes.[37] This evidence, however, is not supported by prospective studies where dietary habits have not been related to the development of type 2 diabetes.[38,39] The effects of a high carbohydrate diet on glucose tolerance have been equivocal.[40,41] Hughes et al[42] compared the effects of a high carbohydrate (60% carbohydrate and 20% fat)/high fiber (25 g dietary fiber/1000 kcal) diet with and without 3 months of high-intensity (75% max heart rate reserve, 50 min/day, 4 days/wk) endurance exercise in older, glucose intolerant men and women. Subjects were fed all of their food on a metabolic ward during the 3-month study and were not allowed to lose weight. These investigators observed no improvement in glucose tolerance or insulin-stimulated glucose uptake in either the diet or the diet plus exercise group. The exercise plus high carbohydrate diet group demonstrated a significant and substantial increase in skeletal muscle glycogen content and at the end of the training, the muscle glycogen stores would be considered to be saturated. Since the primary site of glucose disposal is skeletal muscle glycogen, the extremely high muscle glycogen content associated with exercise and a high carbohydrate diet likely limited the rate of glucose disposal. Thus when combined with exercise and a weight maintenance diet, a high carbohydrate diet had a counter-regulatory effect. It is likely that the value of a high carbohydrate–high fiber diet in its effects on reducing excess body fat, which may be an important cause of the impaired glucose tolerance. Schaefer et al[43] demonstrated that an older subject consuming an ad libitum high carbohydrate diet lost weight. Hays et al[44,45] also demonstrated that an ad libitum *high carbohydrate diet resulted in weight loss in older men and women and a significant improvement in insulin sensitivity.* In this study, the weight loss was seen with no measurable decrease in energy intake during the 3-month duration of the study and compared with the control group consuming a higher fat diet.

There appears to be no attenuation of the response of elderly men and women to regularly performed aerobic exercise when compared with those seen in young subjects. Increased fitness levels are associated with reduced mortality and increased life expectancy. It has also been shown[46] to prevent the occurrence of type 2 diabetes in those that are at the greatest risk for developing this disease. Thus regularly performed aerobic exercise is an important way for older people to improve their glucose tolerance.

Aerobic exercise is generally prescribed as an important adjunct to a weight loss program. Aerobic exercise combined with weight loss has been demonstrated to increase insulin action to a greater extent than weight loss through diet restriction alone. In the study by Bogardus et al,[47] diet therapy alone improved glucose tolerance, mainly by reducing basal endogenous glucose production and improving hepatic sensitivity to insulin. Aerobic exercise training, on the other hand, increased carbohydrate storage rates, and therefore, "diet therapy plus physical training produced a more significant approach toward normal." However, aerobic exercise (as opposed to resistance training) combined with a hypocaloric diet has been demonstrated to result in a greater reduction in resting metabolic rate than diet alone.[48] Heymsfield et al[49] found aerobic exercise combined with caloric restriction did not preserve fat-free mass (FFM) and did not further accelerate weight loss when compared with diet alone. This lack of an effect of aerobic exercise may have been because of a greater decrease in resting metabolic rate (RMR) in the exercising group. In perhaps the most comprehensive study of its kind, Goran and Poehlman[50] examined components of energy metabolism in older men and women engaged in regular endurance training. They found that endurance training did not increase total daily energy expenditure because of a compensatory decline in physical activity during the remainder of the day. In other words, when elderly subjects participated in a regular walking program, they rested more, so that activities outside of walking decreased and thus 24-hour calorie expenditure was unchanged. However, older individuals who had been participating in endurance exercise for most of their lives have been shown to have a greater resting metabolic rate (RMR) and total daily energy expenditure than in age-matched sedentary controls.[51] Ballor et al[52] compared the effects of resistance training with those of diet restriction alone in obese women. They found that resistance exercise training results in increased strength and gains in muscle size and a preservation of FFM during weight loss. These data are similar to the results of Pavlou et al,[53] who used both aerobic and resistance training as an adjunct to a weight loss program in obese men and demonstrated a preservation in fat free mass.

STRENGTH TRAINING

Although endurance exercise has been the more traditional means of increasing cardiovascular fitness, the American College of Sports Medicine currently recommends strength or resistance training as an important component of an overall fitness program. This is particularly important in the elderly, in whom loss of muscle mass and weakness are prominent deficits.

Strength conditioning or progressive resistance training is generally defined as training in which the resistance against which a muscle generates force is progressively increased over time. Progressive resistance training involves few contractions against a heavy load. The metabolic and morphologic adaptations resulting from resistance and endurance exercise are quite different. Muscle strength has been shown to increase in response to training between 60% and 100% of the one-repetition maximum (1RM).[54] 1 RM is the maximum amount of weight that can be lifted with one contraction. Strength conditioning will result in an increase in muscle size and this increase in size is largely the result of increased contractile proteins. The mechanisms by which the mechanical events stimulate an increase in RNA synthesis and subsequent protein synthesis are not well understood. Lifting weight requires that a muscle shorten as it produces force. This is called a concentric contraction. Lowering the weight, on the other hand, forces the muscle to lengthen as it produces force. This is an eccentric muscle contraction. These lengthening muscle contractions have been shown to produce ultrastructural damage (microscopic tears in contractile protein muscle cells) that results in an acute phase response and an increase in muscle protein turnover.[55–59]

Effects of resistance exercise and insulin on protein metabolism

Studies of insulin secretion after resistance but not endurance exercise provides evidence for insulin's role in maintaining muscle mass. Arginine-stimulated insulin secretion is decreased with endurance training.[60,61] In contrast, acute resistance exercise in rats has been shown to increase insulin secretion.[62] As reviewed previously, regular aerobic exercise is known to increase insulin sensitivity and glucose tolerance. In addition to its effects on insulin action, aerobic exercise training results in decreased insulin secretion.[63] Regularly performed endurance exercise in young men is associated with an insulin pulse profile in the resting fasted state characterized by less insulin secreted per burst but a similar number of bursts over a 90-minute period. Thus training-induced elevations in target-tissue sensitivity to insulin may reduce the requirement for pulsatile insulin secretion. This coordinated response keeps glucose concentrations constant. Dela et al[60] demonstrated that aerobic exercise training decreases both arginine- and glucose-stimulated insulin secretion, indicating a profound β-cell adaptation.

A single bout of concentric exercise is a recognized enhancer of insulin action, whereas eccentric exercise transiently impairs whole body insulin action for at least 2 days after the bout.[64] Eccentric exercise also can result in a long-term delay in the rate of glycogen synthesis.[65] This decreased insulin action and delayed glycogen synthetic rate have been shown to result from decreased rate of glucose transport rather than decreased glycogen synthase activity.[66] This transient resistance to insulin and impaired resynthesis of glycogen can result in a systemic hyperinsulinemia that may result in an increase in the rate of muscle protein synthesis. One laboratory[67] has demonstrated age-related differences in the insulin response to hyperglycemia following a single bout of eccentric exercise. Two days following upper and lower body eccentric exercise, younger subjects demonstrated a pronounced pancreatic insulin response during a hyperglycemic clamp while this response was blunted in healthy elderly men.

The effects of resistance exercise on insulin availability appear to be opposite those of endurance exercise and thus stimulate net protein accretion. Insulin has been demonstrated to have profoundly anabolic effects on skeletal muscle. In the resting state, insulin has been demonstrated to decrease the rate of muscle protein degradation. Stable isotope amino acid studies in humans[68,69] clearly demonstrate that *insulin inhibits whole body protein breakdown* in vivo and stimulates muscle protein synthetic rate.[70]

Insulin has been demonstrated to increase the rate of muscle protein synthesis in insulin-deficient rats. However, in nondiabetic animals this effect was not seen. Fluckey et al have argued[62,71] that insulin is not likely to stimulate muscle protein synthesis in quiescent muscle. In my own experience, an insulin infusion does not increase the rate of protein synthesis in nonexercised muscle. However, using a resistance exercise model, investigators have demonstrated that resistance exercise did not stimulate an increase in the rate of protein synthesis. It was only with the addition of insulin that an exercise-induced increase in the rate of soleus and gastrocnemius protein synthesis was seen. This effect of insulin stimulation of the rate of protein synthesis was preserved with advancing age.

Protein requirements and exercise

High-intensity resistance training is clearly anabolic in both younger and older individuals. Data from our laboratory demonstrate a 10% to 15% decrease in nitrogen excretion at the initiation of training that persists for 12 weeks. That is, progressive resistance training improved nitrogen balance, thus older subjects performing resistance training have a lower mean protein requirement than do sedentary subjects.[72] This effect was seen at a protein intake of 0.8 g and 1.6 g, indicating that the effect of resistance training on protein retention may not be related to dietary protein intake. These results are somewhat at variance to our previous research,[73] demonstrating that regularly performed aerobic exercise causes an increase in the mean protein requirement of middle-aged and young endurance athletes. This difference likely results from increased oxidation of amino acids during aerobic exercise that may not be present during resistance training.

Strawford et al[74] also demonstrated similar effects of resistance exercise training on nitrogen balance in patients with HIV-related weight loss. The investigators examined the effects of an anabolic steroid (oxandrolone, 20 mg/day, and a placebo) and high-intensity resistance exercise training in 24 eugonadal men with HIV-associated weight loss (mean, 9% body weight loss). Both groups showed significant nitrogen retention and increases in lean body mass, weight, and strength. The mean gains were significantly greater in the oxandrolone group than in the placebo group in nitrogen balance, accrual of FFM, and strength. Results were similar whether or not patients were taking protease inhibitors. These results confirm the positive effects of resistance exercise on nitrogen retention and protein requirements.

These studies taken as a whole demonstrate the powerful effects of resistance exercise training on protein nutriture. The anabolic effects have important implications in the treatment of many wasting diseases and conditions such as cancer, HIV infection, aging, chronic renal failure, and undernutrition seen in many very old men and women. By effectively lowering dietary protein needs, resistance exercise can limit further losses of skeletal muscle mass while simultaneously increasing muscle strength and functional capacity.

Resistance exercise and aging

Our laboratory examined the effects of high-intensity resistance training of the knee extensors and flexors (80% of 1RM, 3 days/wk) in *older men (age 60 to 72 years)*. The *average increases in knee flexor and extensor strength were 227% and 107%*, respectively. Computed tomography (CT) scans and muscle biopsies were used to determine muscle size. Total muscle area by CT analysis increased by 11.4% while the muscle tissue showed an increase of 33.5% in type I fiber area and 27.5% increase in type II fiber area. In addition, lower body Vo_2max increased significantly, whereas upper body Vo_2max did not, indicating that increased muscle mass can increase maximal aerobic power. It appears that the age-related loss in muscle mass may be an important determinant in the reduced maximal aerobic capacity seen in elderly men and women.[14,15] Improving muscle strength can enhance the capacity of many older men and women to perform many activities, such as climbing stairs, carrying packages, and even walking.

This same training program was applied to a group of frail, institutionalized elderly men and women (mean age 90 + 3 years, range 87 to 96).[75] After 8 weeks of training, the 10 subjects in this study increased muscle strength by almost 180% and muscle size by 11%. More recently,[76] a similar intervention in frail nursing home residents demonstrated not only increases in muscle strength and size, but increased gait speed, stair climbing power, and balance. In addition, spontaneous activity levels increased significantly, whereas the activity of a nonexercised control group was unchanged. In this study the effects of a protein-calorie supplement combined with exercise was also examined. The supplement consisted of a 240-mL liquid supplying 360 kcal in the form of carbohydrates (60%), fat (23%), and soy-based protein (17%), and was designed to augment caloric intake by about 20%, and provide one third of the recommended daily allowance for vitamins and minerals. The men and women who consumed the supplement and exercised gained weight compared with the three other groups examined (exercise/control, nonexercise supplemented, and nonexercise control). The nonexercising subjects who received the supplement reduced their habitual dietary energy intake so that total energy intake was unchanged. In other words, the supplement did not add to total energy intake, but rather substituted one source of energy (the supplement) for another (their meals). In addition, investigators[77] demonstrated that the combined weight lifting and nutritional supplementation increased strength by 257 ± 62% (P = .0001) and type II fiber area by 10.1 ± 9.0% (P = .033), with a similar trend for type I fiber area (+12.8 ± 22.2%). Exercise was associated with a 2.5-fold increase in neonatal myosin (a form of myosin found in growing muscle) staining (P = .0009) and an increase of 491 ± 137% (P < .0001) in insulin-like growth factor-1 (IGF-1) staining. Ultrastructural damage increased by 141 ± 59% after exercise training (P = .034). Strength increases were largest in those with the greatest increases in myosin, IGF-1, damage, and caloric intake during the trial. Frail, very old elders respond robustly to resistance training with musculoskeletal remodeling, and significant increases in muscle area are possible with resistance training in combination with adequate energy intakes. It should be pointed out that this was a very old, very frail population with diagnoses of multiple chronic diseases. The increase in overall level of physical activity has been a common observation in our studies.[76–79] Since muscle weakness is a primary deficit in many older individuals, increased strength may stimulate more aerobic activities, such as walking and cycling. Indeed, Campbell et al[80] demonstrated that resistance training resulted in an approximately 15% increase in energy requirement in older men and women through an increase in resting metabolic rate and an increase in physical activity.

Strength training may increase balance through the improvement in strength of muscle involved in walking. Indeed, ankle weakness has been demonstrated to be associated with increased risk of falling in nursing home patients.[81] However, balance training, which may demonstrate very little improvement in muscle strength, size, or cardiovascular changes has also been demonstrated to decrease the risk of falls in older people.[82] *Tai chi,* a form of dynamic balance training that requires no new technology or equipment, has been demonstrated to reduce the risk of older people *falling by almost 50%.*[83] As a component of the National Institute on Aging FICSIT (Frailty and Injuries: Cooperative Studies of Intervention Techniques) trials, individuals aged 70 and older were randomized to tai chi (TC), individualized balance training (BT), and exercise control education (ED) groups for 15 weeks.[84] In a follow-up assessment 4 months after intervention, 130 subjects responded to exit interview questions asking about perceived benefits of participation. Both TC and BT subjects reported increased confidence in balance and movement, but only TC subjects reported that their daily activities and their overall life had been affected; many of these subjects had changed their normal physical activity to incorporate ongoing TC practice. The data suggest that when mental and physical control is perceived to be enhanced, with a generalized sense of improvement in overall well-being, older persons' motivation to continue exercising also increases. Province et al[85] examined the overall effect of many different exercise interventions in the FICSIT trials on reducing falls. Although each of these separate interventions were not powered to make conclusions about their effects on the incidence of falls in an elderly population, they did conclude that all training domains, taken together under the heading of "general exercise," showed an effect on falls. This probably demonstrates the "rising tide raises all boats" principle, in which training that targets one domain may improve performance somewhat in other domains as a consequence. If this is so, then the differences in fall risk correlated with the nature of the training may not be as critical compared with the differences in not training at all.

The use of a community-based exercise program for frail older people was examined[86] in a group of predominantly sedentary women over age 70 with multiple chronic conditions. The program was conducted with peer leaders to facilitate its continuation after the research demonstration phase. In addition to positive health outcomes related to functional mobility, blood pressure maintenance, and overall well-being, this intervention was successful in sustaining active participation in regular physical activity through the use of peer leaders selected by the program participants.

Although endurance training has been demonstrated to be an important adjunct to weight loss programs in young men and women by increasing their daily energy expenditure, its utility in treating obesity in the elderly may not be great. This is because many sedentary older men and women do not expend many calories when they perform endurance exercise because of their low fitness levels. Thirty to 40 minutes of exercise may increase energy expenditure by only 100 to 200 kcal with very little residual effect on calorie expenditure. Aerobic exercise training will not preserve lean body mass to any great extent during weight loss. Goran et al[50] showed that a vigorous walking program of up to 1 hr/day had no effect on total daily energy expenditure. They found that their older subjects compensated for their increased physical activity by becoming less active throughout the rest of the day. Because resistance training can preserve or even increase muscle mass during weight loss, this type of exercise for those older men and women who must lose weight may be of genuine benefit.

OTHER EFFECTS OF EXERCISE

Bone health

Nelson et al[87] examined the interaction of dietary calcium and exercise; the study included 41 postmenopausal women consuming either high calcium (1462 mg/day) or moderate calcium (761 mg) diets. Half of these women participated in a yearlong walking program (45 min/day, 4 days/wk, 75% of heart rate reserve). Independent effects of the exercise and dietary calcium were seen. Compared with the moderate calcium group, the women consuming a high-calcium diet displayed reduced bone loss from the femoral neck, independent of whether the women exercised. The walking prevented a loss of trabecular bone mineral density seen in the nonexercising women after 1 year. Thus it appears that calcium intake and aerobic exercise are both independently beneficial to bone mineral density at different sites.

The effects of 52 weeks of high-intensity resistance exercise training were examined in a group of 39 postmenopausal women.[79] Twenty were randomly assigned to the strength training group (2 days/wk, 80% of 1RM for upper and lower body muscle groups). At the end of the year significant differences were seen in lumbar spine and femoral bone density between the strength trained and sedentary women. However, unlike other pharmacologic and nutritional strategies for preventing bone loss and osteoporosis, resistance exercise affects more than just bone density. The women who strength trained improved their muscle mass, strength, balance, and overall levels of physical activity. Thus resistance training can be an important way to decrease the risk for an osteoporotic bone fracture in postmenopausal women.

Muscle power may be a more important determinant for functional capacity in older people than is strength. Bassey et al[88] demonstrated that power (force production × time) is more closely related to functional capacity than strength in frail nursing home residents. It is possible to design resistance exercise programs to increase both strength and power.[89] Increased muscle power should, perhaps, be the most important goal for a strength training regimen in older people.[90]

Memory disorders and exercise

Leisure activities (e.g., reading, playing board games, playing musical instruments, dancing) have been associated with a decreased risk of developing dementia in men and women over the age of 75.[91] A growing body of literature[92,93] suggests that regularly performed aerobic exercise will reduce the risk of dementia and Alzheimer's disease (AD). Resistance exercise has also been demonstrated to have a significant effect on memory in older people.[94] In animal studies[95–97] voluntary exercise results in direct effects on brain function through an increase in hippocampal brain-derived neurotrophic factor expression and a decrease in inflammation. A recent[98] randomized controlled trial of a 24-week physical activity intervention in 170 older subjects with memory problems but not diagnosed dementia, showed a persistent effect of the exercise memory over an 18-month period after the cessation of the exercise intervention. Walking at least three times per week has been demonstrated to reduce the risk of AD and dementia.

SUMMARY

Muscle strength training can be accomplished by virtually anyone. Many health care professionals have directed their patients away from strength training in the mistaken belief that it can cause undesirable elevations in blood pressure. With proper technique, the systolic pressure elevation during aerobic exercise is far greater than that seen during resistance training. Muscle strengthening exercises are rapidly becoming a critical component of cardiac rehabilitation programs as clinicians recognize the need for strength and endurance for many activities of daily living. There is no other group in our society that can benefit more from regularly performed exercise than the elderly. Although both aerobic exercise and strength conditioning are highly recommended, only strength training can stop or reverse sarcopenia. Increased muscle strength and mass in the elderly can be the first step toward a lifestyle of increased physical activity and a realistic strategy for maintaining functional status and independence.

In conclusion, exercise exerts a powerful acute and chronic effect on virtually every system in the human body. In assessing these effects and prescribing exercise, it is important to keep in mind the very different effects of aerobic versus resistance exercise. Both forms of exercise are recommended and should be a component of a comprehensive program of disease prevention and health promotion.

The effects of exercise in treating chronic debilitating disease are largely unexplored. For example, fatigue is the most common complaint of patients with cancer, yet the most common advice provided by oncologists is for increased rest. Just as cardiac rehabilitation has been demonstrated to provide an important mechanism for the post–myocardial infarction patient to improve fitness and reduce the risk of a second event, exercise can greatly improve fitness and reduce much of the fatigue associated with cancer and its treatment.[99] The proven effects of resistance training to enhance nitrogen retention and increase muscle size and strength can provide positive benefits for patients with wasting diseases (such as HIV infection) and cachexia. Resistance exercise may prove to have powerful effects on patients with chronic renal failure, who must consume low protein diets to slow the progression of their disease. Exercise therapy for those patients forced to undergo extended periods of inactivity during dialysis could also improve functional status and decrease the fatigue associated with disuse. The potential value of a reasonable and well-thought-out exercise program is great, and the exploration of this value should be a high priority for researchers. Indeed, a thoughtful and appropriate prescription of exercise for any geriatric patient should be the standard of care.[100]

KEY POINTS

Exercise for Successful Aging

- Maximal aerobic capacity (VO_2max) declines with advancing age.
- Aerobic exercise has long been an important recommendation for the prevention and treatment of many of the chronic diseases typically associated with old age.
- Strength or resistance training is an important component of an overall fitness program. This is particularly important in the elderly where loss of muscle mass and weakness are prominent deficits.
- A thoughtful and appropriate prescription of exercise for any geriatric patient should be the standard of care.

For a complete list of references, please visit online only at www.expertconsult.com

Injury in Older People

Mujtaba Hasan

An injury is defined as damage to tissues usually consequential to a disproportionate energy transfer.[1] The energy that produces an injury can be described as kinetic-causing fractures, contusions, and lacerations; thermal producing burns and scalds; chemical leading to poisoning; and electrical resulting in electrocution.[1] Injuries have been classified by type (a fracture, laceration, or burn), by intent (intentional or unintentional, also described as accidental or nonaccidental), and by cause (a road traffic accident, a fall, or a gunshot injury).[1]

Injury is one of the most underrecognized major health problems facing the world today.[1–3] Unintentional injuries pose a serious challenge for the health and well-being of older individuals. Although people aged 65 years and older make up less than 20% of the Western population, fatal injuries are much more common among older people, accounting for more than a third of all trauma-related deaths.[3–6] It is clear from studies that for the injuries of the same severity, older patients are more likely to be hospitalized and to have a longer hospital stays compared to younger adults.[2–10] However, little research has been carried out in older victims of trauma.

Falls are the leading cause of injuries and death in older people, accounting for 75% of all injuries, followed by road traffic accidents, which account for 13%.[7–16] In one study, almost half of all falls-related deaths occurred in older individuals despite forming only 14% of the entire falls-related trauma population.[17] It is estimated that approximately 30% of community-dwelling individuals aged 65 years and older suffer at least one fall each year.[3,7–8,18] Road traffic accidents account for the majority of multiple injuries.[13–16] Fatalities caused by fire and flames constitute the second most common cause of accidental death in older people.[19] Scalds are responsible for the majority of injuries resulting from burns, which are also associated with a high death rate.[3,4] Nonaccidental injury resulting from elder abuse is not a new phenomenon but is one that is being increasingly acknowledged as a growing problem.[20]

The consequences of injuries among older people include significant costs both in terms of human suffering and economic cost. The human costs among survivors of injuries are considerable, leading to disabilities, loss of independence, and institutionalization.[3–6] In addition, there can be profound psychosocial consequences including fear of further falls, loss of confidence, low self-esteem, isolation, and depression.[3,9,17,18] The economic costs are difficult to determine in view of the different type of injuries involved and the broad range of treatments used.[3]

In the United States it is estimated that older victims of trauma account for almost 38% of hospital bed days for all injury-related hospital admissions[11] and consume up to one third of trauma-related hospital expenditure, which was almost $100 billion in 1999.[21] The costs of treating hip fractures in the U.K. health service in a hospital setting is estimated to be approximately £160 million per year.[3] However, this does not include the costs associated with informal care and the direct costs of providing social services, domiciliary support, and institutional care.[3]

PHYSIOLOGIC CHANGES IN OLDER VICTIMS OF TRAUMA

The physiologic response that follows trauma in patients of any age is poorly understood. A number of physiologic responses have been identified that can be classified as (1) neuroendocrine responses and (2) metabolic responses.[22–24] Although the response in older individuals to injury is not dissimilar to that in younger adults and the aging is not associated with any impairment of these responses, the subject has not been adequately researched and the clinical importance of the physiologic response to injury that occurs in older patients remains unclear.

The neuroendocrine responses

The neuroendocrine response occurs immediately after an injury and leads to an increase in the activity of the sympathoadrenal system and the hypothalamic-pituitary-adrenal (HPA) axis.[22–24] The serum levels of growth hormone, prolactin, vasopressin, aldosterone, and glucagons also rise.[23–24] The degree and duration of such response is determined by the nature and severity of injury sustained by the individual patient and may be modulated by a number of factors such as volume depletion, hypotension, pain, hypoxia, and circulating cytokines.[22–24]

It has also been observed that the plasma cortisol concentration remains high in older individuals for a longer period after trauma compared to younger patients with injuries of similar severity.[25,26] Studies have shown that patients with hip fractures have increased rates of cortisol production and urinary-free cortisol excretion when compared with healthy controls at 2 weeks after the injury.[27] The reason for the continued cortisol production is unclear. It is also not known whether the posttraumatic persistent hypercortisolemia is an adaptive mechanism or has any benefit to the organism.[26–28]

It has been postulated that the persistently raised cortisol levels may indicate a reduced capability of older people to downregulate the response after resolution of the stimulus.[26–29] Similar observations have been made in old rats and is said to be due to a loss of corticosteroid receptors in the hippocampus resulting in a weakened feedback inhibition of the HPA axis as demonstrated by the dexamethasone suppression test.[28] The resistance to dexamethasone suppression has also been seen in patients with Alzheimer's disease and in elderly patients with depression and hip facture, possibly because of the loss of corticosteroid receptors in the hippocampus.[26,28,30] The clinical implications of such a sustained rise in the levels of cortisol in the context of trauma in older individuals remain unexplored.[30]

Metabolic changes

There has been little research carried out in this area, particularly in older victims of trauma. A study conducted in the 1930s in younger patients found that the two metabolic phases that occur in patients with injury are the *ebb phase* and the *flow phase* based on the degree of metabolic rate.[24] The ebb phase is associated with a decreased metabolic rate and an intensification of fuel generation.[24] The severity of injury determines the degree of rise in plasma glucose concentrations during the ebb phase both in the young as well as the old.[23,24] However, this is not associated with a corresponding rise in plasma insulin because of its suppression by circulating catecholamines.[23–24] Other changes that occur in both young and old people after injury include a rise in plasma glycerol, free fatty acids, and lactate concentrations.[24,31] On the other hand, it has been shown that older people have increased rates of lipolysis and reesterification of free fatty acids within adipose tissue for some unknown reasons.[24,31]

The increased metabolic rate that occurs in flow phase depends on the severity of injury and is associated with a concurrent rise in urinary nitrogen excretion resulting from the injury-related catabolic activities.[24] Studies have shown that the negative energy and nitrogen balance that occurs within a week after the trauma because of the catabolic activities in older hip fracture patients can be prevented in most patients by dietary supplementation of about 300 kcal/day energy and 20g/day protein.[32–34] The likelihood of survival in patients with more severe catabolic activity has been found to be significantly decreased.[33]

There is not only a transfer from carbohydrate to fat as the most desired fuel in the flow phase but also an age-related increase in the endogenous production of glucose after trauma.[31–35] In older individuals, glucose intolerance and insulin resistance that are observed after trauma are said to be notably greater in degree as well duration in comparison to the young for reasons that are not clear but may be due to the high cortisol concentrations following trauma.[31]

DOES RECOVERY OCCUR IN OLDER VICTIMS OF TRAUMA?

Although little work has been done in the elderly, recovery following injury probably takes place in the same manner in older patients as it does in younger adults. But the pace at which recovery takes place may be slower and depends on a number of factors including the nature and severity of injury, comorbidity, nutritional state, and premorbid functional status.[21–23] The key elements of recovery that have been identified include physiologic recovery and functional recovery.[21–23]

The physiologic recovery

This starts with the abatement of the catabolic flow phase and ends with the replenishment of the energy and protein deficits.[22,23,35] However, the subject of physiologic recovery has not been researched thoroughly, particularly in the older population. It is not clear, for example, what leads to the cessation of catabolic flow phase in order for the phase of anabolism to get established.[23,35] A study conducted in the 1950s on younger patients following major surgery concluded that the physiologic recovery could not proceed without patients being fed.[36]

The study also found that the pace of anabolic phase could not be hastened any further by interventions such as endocrine manipulations or tube feeding.[36] However, it is important that the dietary intake is increased in order for the patients to gain weight and for the recovery to continue unabated.[35,36] Another study that investigated glucose and protein kinetics in 8 patients aged 56 to 79 years following major surgery found that these patients could not oxidize glucose to carbon dioxide resulting in an increased production of lactate.[37] They also found that the glucose production was increased and the basal insulin concentrations were raised during the anabolic phase.

There appears to be a clear relationship between the nutritional status and the physiologic recovery in patients with trauma, particularly in terms of lean body mass, muscle strength and immune function.[38] These physiologic parameters have been reported to be adversely affected even in healthy older women if fed an energy rich but slightly protein deficient diet over 9 weeks.[39] Older patients with hip fracture if poorly nourished do badly, and there is evidence that the use nutritional supplements by overnight tube feeding can improve outcome.[40,41] Although the effectiveness of the oral multinutrient feeds has been confirmed by the Cockrane Review, it recommends that the tube feeding should only be used in situations where the patient is severely ill nourished.[42] Despite the high prevalence of malnutrition in older patients with hip fracture and other types of trauma, nutrition is not given the importance it deserves in the management of such patients in hospital settings.[43,44]

Functional recovery

The type of injury as well as its severity has an important bearing on how much recovery takes place in older individuals after trauma.[3,6,21–23] A study that explored the recovery of physical function after limb injuries in independent older people living at home demonstrated that not only hip fractures but also wrist fractures may reduce older people's chances of regaining independence.[45] The study also found that the prospects of any recovery 5 to 6 months after the injury are small.[45] The premorbid state is another important determinant of the extent to which functional recovery occurs in patients with trauma—only 40% of patients who were independently mobile before hip fracture have been shown to return to the same level of function.[46,47] The functional outcome is also dependent on the level of social support a patient has.[48]

Other factors that are known to be associated with an adverse outcome include delay in surgery, particularly in patients with hip fracture, and comorbid conditions such as stroke, dementia, arthritis, and malnutrition.[48–56] The impact of psychologic problems including depression on recovery from trauma is also being increasingly recognized, but the role of effective management of such problems on the hastening of the rate of recovery and in the improvement of the overall outcome remains unproven.[51,53] Studies in patients with hip fracture have demonstrated that the extensor muscle power in the fractured leg was the most important determinant of walking speed and stair climbing time.[57] The adequacy of the control of pain was an important factor in this study, which determined how much strength these muscles regained during recovery.[57]

The various measures that have been shown to improve functional recovery and outcome in patients with trauma include nutritional support, use of prophylactic antibiotics, and heparin prophylaxis.[35,55,56] Patients should also be encouraged to mobilize early to avoid complications such as muscle wasting, increased risk of venous thrombosis, and pressure ulcers.[58] However, some orthopedic surgeons do not recommend weight bearing early on after the insertion of a rigid fixation device to avoid the risk of failure of fixation, nonunion, osteonecrosis, or prosthetic dislocation.[52–54] But these problems were not reported to occur and benefits of early mobilization were shown to outweigh such risks in a study that allowed complete weight bearing soon after the surgical intervention.[52] Although different strategies have been adopted to help patients achieve functional recovery after hip fracture and other forms of trauma, one Cockrane review concluded that the most favorable approach to rehabilitate older patients with trauma has not yet been established.[59]

HOW TO ASSESS INJURY AND MEASURE OUTCOME?

A great majority of assessment scales and scoring systems that are in use for the victims of trauma have been developed from research carried out in young adults and have not been validated to be utilized in older individuals.[12,22,60,61] It is important to be aware of the limitations of the scoring systems when using in older population. Moreover, none of the commonly used scoring systems is completely suitable for every situation regardless of the age of the patient.[11,62] There are three different types of scorings systems for measuring injury in clinical practice: (1) the anatomic scales (based on the extent of the injury), (2) the physiologic scales (based on the physiologic responses of the recipient of the injury), and (3) a combination of these two (based on both the anatomic extent as well as the physiologic responses).[11,35,60–62]

Of the various anatomic scales—for example, the Abbreviated Injury Scale (AIS), Injury Severity Score (ISS) and the Anatomical Profile (AP)—the ISS is the one most commonly used in day-to-day practice.[63] It is valuable in service evaluation and in assessing outcome.[63] However, it has two major limitations. First, it has a limited role in acute settings as the data required may not be immediately available in the early stages of the assessment of a patient with trauma.[62,63] Second, it may overestimate the severity of injury in older patients as, for example, the force required to produce a fracture is likely to be less due to a reduction in the bone mass, and the associated soft tissue injury is also likely to be less severe.[23]

The Glasgow Coma Scale (GCS), the Revised Trauma Score (RTS), the Acute Physiology and Chronic Health Estimates (APACHE), and the Simplified Acute Physiology Score (SAPS) are some of the widely used scoring systems that are based on the changes in the physiologic parameters of a patient with trauma.[60,61] Their main roles are in determining when to manage patients in critical care facilities and to treat them more aggressively.[60,61] Their value in older victims of trauma, however, has been questioned in view of the impairment of the physiologic responses that occur with aging, which may result in an underestimation of the seriousness of the injury if these scales are used.[60,61] However, studies have shown that this is not of any clinical significance as older people usually develop more severe physiologic disturbances and once this and comorbid factors are taken into account, age alone does not appear to be a predictor of poor outcome or survival.[64–66]

The two widely used combined scoring systems, the Revised Trauma Score + Injury Severity Score (TRISS) and A Severity Characterization of Trauma (ASCOT), are said to be better predictors of survival.[35] A Geriatric Trauma Survival Score, based on the ISS plus cardiac and infective complications plus ventilator dependence, was developed in the 1970s to overcome some of the limitations of the commonly used measurement scales.[61] It has not been generally applied in clinical practice despite the claim that it was 92% accurate in predicting survival. Clearly, further studies are required to evaluate its role in the assessment of elderly injured patients.

INJURY PATTERNS IN OLDER PEOPLE

Although the patterns of injury in the elderly are not dissimilar to those in the young, fractures and serious injuries are more common in the older victims of trauma. The injured elderly patients also have certain differences in terms of injuries at specific sites and have special needs and considerations in view of the comorbidity and age-related decline in the functional reserve and ability to deal with stressors.[66]

Head injuries

There are a number of important differences between the old and the young victims of head trauma in terms of the epidemiology, types of injury, and outcome.[67] The incidence rates are slightly higher after 60 years of age, and more elderly men than women suffer a head injury.[67] But the predominance of women in older age groups may result in an underestimation of the true size of the problem in older individuals if the crude figures are not adjusted for sex.[67] The types of injury that are uncommon in older people include epidural hematomas because of the fact that dura becomes firmly attached to the skull in aging brain.[67] However, subdural hematomas are much more common because of a number of anatomic changes, including a relentless loss of brain volume, leading to an increase in the space around the brain and stretching of the bridging veins, and increased venous fragility.[67] The bleeding into the substance of the brain is also more common in older people.

There is also a clear disparity in outcome between the young and the old. Only a handful (about 10%) of older patients who sustain severe head trauma with a GCS score of 8 or less, survive the initial injury.[68] The survivors are reported to have a prolonged hospital stays and are usually left with a marked disability.[68] Moreover, older people sustaining trivial head trauma are said to have a high risk of significant intracranial injury and a worse prognosis in comparison to young adults despite no evidence of skull fracture, neurologic deficits, or altered level of consciousness.[69] A study in patients (both young and old) with acute subdural hematoma found that no functional recovery occurred in older patients when the GCS score was less than 13.[68] The reasons for such a universally poor outcome in older patients with head injury are not clearly understood, but factors that may be responsible include comorbidity, nihilistic attitudes among health professionals when managing older head trauma patients, a higher complication rate, and a reduced capacity of the aging brain to recover from injury.[64,68–70]

Thoracic trauma

Chest injuries carry a much higher risk of death and disability in older people compared to the young.[71–73] Studies report two to three times greater chance of death in older individuals with injuries limited to the chest in comparison to the young.[72,73] Even minor injuries to the chest wall can lead to a flail chest, pulmonary contusion, pneumothorax, or haemothorax.[74] As the chest wall loses its elasticity with aging, rib fractures occur more easily with even mild blunt trauma to the chest in older individuals.[75] Rib fractures are regarded as a marker of injury severity.[75] Their presence not only leads to the doubling of mortality in comparison to the younger patients but also the likelihood of the mortality rises significantly with increasing number of rib fractures.[74,75]

Complications occur more commonly in older patients with thoracic injury.[74] Older people can deteriorate rapidly even without fractures as the pain from chest trauma can lead to hypoventilation and failure to clear secretions, thereby causing pneumonia.[66,74,75] Regular assessment and closer monitoring of patients with thoracic injury are required in order to identify complications at an early stage.[74] Prompt mechanical ventilation may be needed in older patients if they develop features of respiratory distress.[35]

Abdominal trauma

Abdominal trauma frequently occurs in older people and has been observed in about 35% of patients with multiple injuries.[11,12,15] Abdominal injuries in older individuals differ from those in the young in several ways. First, the fatalities have been reported to increase fivefold in elderly patients with visceral injuries compared with younger patients, with the death rate reaching almost 80%.[6,11,12] Second, elderly patients with abdominal injuries require prompt attention and treatment as they are very intolerant of shock.[12–16,64] Abdominal examination alone is deemed less reliable in older patients and computed tomography (CT) examination of the abdomen should always be considered in all such patients.[66] It is particularly useful in patients with a history of significant abdominal surgery.

Third, as older individuals tolerate unnecessary laparotomy poorly, the possibility of complications following emergency surgery is greatly increased requiring a thorough perioperative evaluation before surgical interventions are contemplated.[35,76] However, delaying surgery has its downsides as older patients are intolerant of shock that may lead to multiple organ failure, which is invariably fatal.[76]

Fractures following falls

Fractures occur more commonly in the elderly population for two main reasons: their bones are weak and they are more prone to falls.[3] It has been observed that a reduction in bone mineral density by one standard deviation increases the risk of fracture two to threefold.[77,78] Injuries that may only result in soft tissue trauma or dislocation in the young produce fractures in the elderly. Several community studies have shown that elderly women are more likely than men to sustain fall-related fractures.[9] This is partly due to a higher prevalence of osteoporosis among older women.

Significant injuries have been reported among one tenth of fallers aged over 70 (10%).[79] It has been demonstrated that following a fall two fifths of women (40%) and a quarter of men (30%) aged 75 and over sustained fractures and that the proximal femoral fractures were responsible for the peak in trauma mortality in the old age.[80] Pelvic fractures also cause substantial mortality and morbidity, with fatalities approaching nearly 90% if the fracture is open.[11,12,15,21] A study of older patients has shown that the most common type of fracture after pelvic trauma was pubic rami fractures (56%), followed by acetabular fractures (19%), and ischium fractures (11%).[81] The study also found that over half of patients had multiple trauma and the mortality was four times greater than in a younger population.[81] The reasons why pelvic fractures carry such a high mortality and morbidity include an increased association with bleeding as well as visceral and multiple injuries.[82]

Falls are also responsible for most of the cervical injuries and fractures in the elderly.[83] Studies have shown that elderly trauma patients are twice more likely to reveal cervical fractures on X-ray examination compared to the young and are at an increased risk of fractures at multiple levels.[84,85] Upper limb fractures commonly occur in older people, with the preponderance of proximal humerus and distal radius fractures.[9,21,86] However, the incidence of tibial fracture declines with age in men but remains unaltered in women.[21,86] Moreover, the incidence of ankle fractures has been shown to be rising, particularly in older women.[21]

The type of the fractures observed depends on how falls occur.[35] Whereas falls on an outstretched arm that usually happen when a person is mobile lead to fractures of the wrist and proximal humerus, hip fractures are much more commonly associated with falls from a static position or when a person is moving slowly.[21,35,87] Long bone fractures without a clear history of injury or falls have been reported in frail older individuals. Although precise mechanisms as to how these fractures, also referred to as "minimal trauma fractures," develop are not clear, the factor that has been shown to be responsible includes mobility problems.[88]

To design strategies to prevent falls and fall-related fractures, it is important to develop a better understanding of why and how people fall and how this relates to the risk of fracture.[89,90] Some of the key reasons why people fall include environmental factors (poor lighting, loose carpets, etc.) and patient-related factors (arthritis, stroke, dementia, postural hypotension, etc.).[91] Although it is vital in falls prevention that these factors are managed effectively, it is also crucial that other factors that are responsible for a fracture are carefully taken into consideration.[92,93] These are the determinants of the strength of bone and the active and passive protective factors that determine how much kinetic energy of the fall is transmitted to the bone.[92–96]

A typical fall usually generates more than enough energy to break an old hip.[95] However, the risk of impact leading to fractures can be minimized by employing energy absorbing/dissipating mechanisms to reduce the force delivered to a bone: active mechanisms (e.g., muscular contractions and use of the outstretched hand) and passive energy absorption by soft tissue, clothing, floor coverings, and hip protectors.[94–97] As it has been found that fracture load is linearly related to bone mineral density, measures to increase bone mineral density of the proximal femur will have additional beneficial effect in order to reduce the risk of fracture.[98]

Multiple injuries

In general, patterns of injury are similar in young and old.[99] However, visceral injuries rarely occur in the elderly in the absence of major bony injuries.[6,15,99] The injuries that are associated with the majority of early fatalities are skull fractures leading to brain injuries and pelvic fractures that result from massive bleeding from lacerations to the pelvic venous plexus and visceral injury.[6,15,35,66]

Other common injuries that occur in patients with multiple trauma include long-bone fractures, especially of the tibia.[100] Such injuries call for an urgent assessment and treatment in order to control blood loss, reduce the risk of fat embolism, and enable early mobilization.[6,35,101,102] Older people are quite intolerant of delays in surgical intervention, as their condition can deteriorate rapidly even after isolated hip fractures.[103] Although a more recent study revealed that patients sustaining isolated hip fractures had similar injury severity scores, and a similar incidence of severe complications as the trauma population in general,[104] it is important to be aware of the negative impact of the age-associated decline in functional reserve and comorbidity on the outcome in older individuals.[22–23,66]

CONCLUSIONS

With the demographic changes predicting an increase in the population of older people worldwide over the next few decades, trauma in the old age will remain an important public health problem. Injuries are not only common in older individuals but are also a huge burden on the finance of a country's health service and pose considerable diagnostic as well as therapeutic challenges. Considerable progress has been made to develop a better understanding of the process of care of injured people, which has helped to reduce morbidity and improve survival.[66]

There is evidence that an early and appropriate use of investigations, invasive monitoring, and interventions including the support of a trauma center/team combined with an effective management of comorbid conditions and prevention of complications can influence outcome positively in older victims of trauma.[66,105–107] Although a great deal of work has been carried out to improve our knowledge and understanding of the impact of the age-associated physiologic changes, injury severity, comorbidity, and the patterns of injury in older trauma patients on the outcome, further research is clearly needed to identify the factors that adversely affect the functional recovery and outcome and to develop an evidence-based strategy to deal with them successfully.[108]

KEY POINTS

Injury in Older People

- Although injuries are more common in younger adults, older people are much more likely to die from their injuries (accounting for over a third of all trauma deaths).
- Fractures and serious injuries are more common in older victims of trauma, and there are certain important differences in terms of injuries at specific sites.
- Falls remain the leading cause of injuries and death in older people, accounting for 75% of all injuries.
- Older injured individuals consume a greater proportion of the health care budget in comparison to younger adults.
- A great majority of assessment scales and scoring systems that are in use for the victims of trauma have not been validated in older individuals, and it is important to be aware of the limitations of the scoring systems when applying them to the older population.
- The pace and extent of recovery that takes place in older victims of trauma depends on the nature and severity of injury, comorbidity, nutritional state, and premorbid functional status.
- There is evidence that an early and appropriate use of investigations, invasive monitoring, and interventions including the support of a trauma center/team combined with an effective management of comorbid conditions and prevention of complications can influence outcome positively in older victims of trauma.
- Further research is needed to identify the factors that affect the functional recovery and outcome adversely and to develop an evidence-based strategy to deal with them effectively.

For a complete list of references, please visit online only at www.expertconsult.com

CHAPTER 103

Rehabilitation: Therapy Techniques

Valerie M. Pomeroy
Marion F. Walker

Geriatric rehabilitation has a major impact on length of hospital stay and unnecessary admissions to institutionalized care, burden on caregivers, and numbers of crisis "social" admissions.[1] In recognition of the contribution of rehabilitation, the recent National Service Framework for Older People in the United Kingdom emphasizes the importance of promoting elderly people's health and independence.[2] Therapy is an important component of this service. Specific techniques are used to prevent the onset of disability and to restore, maintain, and control the deterioration of functional ability.

Loss of functional ability can take many different forms. These include the loss of the ability to communicate, remember, walk, perform personal care tasks, and/or perform social roles that are perceived as the norm. Indeed, loss of functional ability can itself lead to secondary difficulties such as depression, muscle wasting, and withdrawal from social interaction and activity.

Rehabilitation is therefore a multifaceted service with therapy provided by a multiprofessional team. For example, speech and language therapists provide interventions targeted at communication difficulties and swallowing problems; psychologists provide interventions targeted at emotional function and cognitive function (e.g., memory and perception); and nurses provide interventions targeted at personal care, mobility, and psychosocial interactions. Effective teamwork is central to the success of rehabilitation. Multiprofessional assessment is followed by treatment and goal-setting with individual patients who are also recognized as being members of the rehabilitation team. Most treatment packages are therefore complex and require continued teamwork to ensure integrated delivery and adjustment.

The complexity of the rehabilitation package is widely recognized and it is frequently perceived as a "black box," particularly by medical members of the team. The aim of this chapter is to describe for doctors some of the techniques that are used by therapists to help elderly people maintain or regain optimal independence. To make this task more manageable, the techniques described in this chapter are restricted to those provided by occupational therapists and physiotherapists. Of course, the therapy component of rehabilitation services for elderly people consists of much more than is outlined here, with many other professional groups making key contributions. The techniques outlined in this chapter are therefore presented as examples of therapy, illustrating how these are combined for specific patients and groups of patients. The findings of narrative and systematic reviews are used where these are available, but this chapter does not seek to provide a thorough review of the effectiveness of the interventions described.

Descriptions of therapy techniques would be meaningless without placing them in the context of professional expertise and clinical application. Therefore the next section outlines the core skills of occupational therapists and physiotherapists, the therapy research culture, and the process of therapy. Therapy techniques are then connected with the specific conditions of stroke, fractured neck of femur following a fall, Parkinson's disease, and frailty.

OCCUPATIONAL THERAPY AND PHYSIOTHERAPY

Occupational therapy

Occupational therapy has been defined as "the treatment of physical and psychiatric conditions through specific activities in order to help people reach their maximum level of function and independence in all aspects of daily life."[3] An earlier definition by Turner[4] captures the more holistic approach, still favored by many occupational therapists today: "Occupational therapy is the treatment of the whole person by their active participation in purposeful living."

The roots of occupational therapy were first established in the eighteenth century with the work of the French physician and psychiatrist Phillipe Pinel, and the Englishman William Tuke, who—in founding an asylum, "The Retreat at York"—made early attempts to rehabilitate the mentally ill.[5] By the twentieth century a group of professionals evolved the concept of occupation as a restorative agent and of the person as an active participant in promoting personal health.

George Burton coined the term "occupational therapy" in 1914 and the first school of occupational therapy in Great Britain was founded in Bristol in 1930.[6] The main impetus came to occupational therapy during World War II with the first curative workshop set up at Shepherd's Bush Military Hospital by Sir Robert Jones, an eminent British surgeon of the day. He enthused about the value of occupational therapy and urged the War Office to set up other centers. Unfortunately at this time treatment activities were limited to the field of crafts because the more realistic occupations were not possible because of trade prejudice.[6] This liaison with crafts is where the erroneous concept of the occupational therapist as "diversional therapist" originated.

Reed and Sanderson[7] list some basic concepts that do not belong to occupational therapy:

- Occupational therapy should not be used as a means of keeping a person busy.
- Occupational therapy does not provide employment.
- Occupational therapy should not be unplanned or a haphazard program of activities.

Since the early 1900s, occupational therapists have recognized the importance of having a strong theory of occupation to support their practice. Several authors have contributed to this theoretical base in the last 30 years, generating and expanding many models and approaches to be used in treatment.[5] The actual techniques used in day-to-day practice by occupational therapists are both numerous and diverse; and as clinicians primarily use a pragmatic eclectic approach to treat individual patients, it would be inappropriate simply to list them in a book of this nature. However, the main techniques used with elderly people are set out in this chapter.

The skills of the occupational therapist

Joice and Coia[8] describe the core skills of the occupational therapist as follows:

1. The use of selected activity which must be purposeful and meaningful to the individual. For example, in preparation for discharge from hospital to home, the occupational therapist would encourage the patient to practice making a hot snack. The task would be purposeful and meaningful either because the patient lives alone or the main caregiver is out at work all day.
2. Activity analysis to break activities down into physical, cognitive, interpersonal, social, behavioral, and emotional components. To use the example given above: Can the patient manage both the physical and the cognitive components of making a hot snack? Can the person stand for long periods at the sink and cook unaided, or does he or she require the use of a seat or perching stool? Can the person remember putting toast under the grill? Is the person aware of the sequencing of the tasks involved in making a hot drink? Does the person need to use any specialized equipment to achieve the task independently? If the individual's visual field has been affected by a stroke, can he or she see all the ingredients on the worktop and use them appropriately? Does the person have sufficient concentration and motivation to achieve the task?
3. Assessment and treatment of functional capabilities. The therapist must have the knowledge and ability competently to assess the functional, cognitive, and emotional capabilities of the individual and apply the appropriate treatment. A thorough knowledge of prehospital ability is essential for setting appropriate goals. "Competent assessment" in the current climate of evidence-based practice should, where possible, include the use of standardized, valid, and reliable measures. These will permit objective measurement of patients' progress.

The occupational therapist therefore strives to promote recovery through purposeful activity, and encourages the patient to retrain, to practice, and to become independent in some chosen activities of everyday life. These activities may incorporate personal care tasks such as washing, dressing, feeding, toileting, and bathing (known as activities of daily living [ADLs]) or more demanding tasks such as outdoor mobility, using public transport, household tasks, and leisure interests (known as extended activities of daily living [EADLs], or instrumental activities of daily living [IADLs]).

Occupational therapy training

In the United Kingdom, training in occupational therapy involves a 4-year course culminating in an honors degree. Topics covered during training include anatomy and physiology, behavioral science, psychology, clinical sciences medicine and psychiatry, research methods, management and social policy, profession-related practice, fieldwork education, theoretical frameworks, therapeutic activity, and core professional skills.

Occupational therapy settings

In the United Kingdom, occupational therapists work in a variety of settings: hospitals (ward-based), day-hospitals, day-centers, outpatient departments, social service departments, and health centers. In parts of the United Kingdom, and in response to government initiatives (see Chapter 103B online), new community occupational therapy posts are developing within primary care settings, such as in general practitioner surgeries or within health care centers. These posts mainly come under the jurisdiction of the primary care groups, or more recently, primary care trusts.

The social services occupational therapist (SSOT) can provide occupational therapy also in the patient's own home. Local health authorities currently fund these posts. This specialist group of occupational therapists is concerned mainly with clients who have permanent and substantial disability, with the aim of helping these people to live independently in the community. They can provide equipment to help a client function more independently or may supply equipment simply to ease the burden on the caregiver—such as by the provision of a hoist for bathing. Another remit of the SSOT is to give advice and facilitate structural changes within the disabled person's environment. This may range from outside ramps to enable wheelchair access to major adaptations such as building a ground-floor bathroom. Social services occupational therapists also provide advice on financial benefits when appropriate.

Surveys indicate that although social services occupational therapists are highly valued specialists, staffing levels and limited resources mean that their individual case contribution is often very limited.[9]

Physiotherapy

Since its inception in 1895, the profession of physiotherapy has been concerned with movement. Physiotherapists use many techniques to prevent the onset of movement problems to facilitate recovery in the acute phase following injury, and to rehabilitate people who have a longer-term movement problem. These therapies can be broadly classified as: exercise, manipulation and mobilization of joints and soft tissues, electrotherapy, acupuncture, and hydrotherapy. Physiotherapists also advise on the suitability of various types of devices (e.g., walking aids and orthoses) to assist movement and mobility. Problems with movement occur as the result of many processes, including fractures, arthritis, whiplash injuries, back pain, stress incontinence, repetitive strain injuries, cystic fibrosis, sports injuries, stroke, and stress disorders. Physiotherapists work in many health care, social care, and community settings.

The skills of the physiotherapist

Understanding how and why people move as they do underpins the core skill of physiotherapy. Physiotherapists have extensive knowledge and experience of "normal" movement throughout the life span and how this is altered by various pathologies and lifestyle processes. An initial assessment identifies what the person can do, what he or she cannot do, where movement becomes difficult, and why. From this a treatment plan is drawn up, in partnership with the patient if possible. Assessment and treatment are therefore based on theoretical knowledge and clinical experience of neural and musculoskeletal mechanisms involved in movement control and how these are affected by pathology, age, gender, lifestyle, and treatment modality.

Specialization is important to ensure that patients receive high-quality treatment. Physiotherapists specialize in a number of areas of health care, including orthopedics, intensive care, pediatrics, musculoskeletal injury, elderly care, sports injuries, psychiatry, neurology, and rheumatology. Consequently physiotherapists have additional core skills pertinent to their particular area of specialization. In addition to specialist knowledge and experience of particular conditions, specialist skills also include those relevant to the theory and practice of specific physical therapy techniques which are gained through postgraduate education and training. This chapter, which outlines only the physical therapy techniques used with elderly people, testifies to the range of skills deployed by physiotherapists.

Development of a research culture

In the United Kingdom, physiotherapy became an all-degree profession in 1992. Since then the number of physiotherapists with research skills has risen considerably. In the early 1980s only a few physiotherapists in the United Kingdom had been awarded a PhD. In 1997 there were 70 physiotherapists with doctorates and eight professors.[10] At the beginning of 2001 there were 100 physiotherapists with doctorates and 23 professors (nine without doctorates).[10] This is a dramatic increase, but still only a small proportion of the 35,000 physiotherapists in the United Kingdom.

Occupational therapy is also relatively new to the world of research, with many training schools introducing research modules into the curriculum only in the mid-1990s. The British College of Occupational Therapists has developed a research strategy to meet the research needs of occupational therapists.[11] Occupational therapists are required by the Code of Ethics and Professional Conduct to have: "A duty to ensure that wherever possible their professional practice is based upon established research findings."[12]

The increase in research-aware and research-active therapists is resulting in a more critical approach and a better evidence base for clinical practice. Despite these advances and the recommendations made in a position statement to the Department of Health in 1994,[13] standard career paths that include research activity have not yet been established. However, with the increase in the number of research-active therapists and the publication of high-quality research in peer-reviewed journals, this situation is likely to change.

THE THERAPY PROCESS

Rehabilitation is an active participatory process, so the first contact with the patient is crucial in establishing a good rapport and therapeutic relationship. Assessment, which is essential to determine subsequent interventions and should be an ongoing activity throughout the rehabilitation process, begins at the first meeting.[14] Assessment ascertains what the patient can do, what he or she cannot do, where activities become difficult, and importantly why difficulties are experienced.

For example, the Rivermead Perceptual Assessment Battery[15] can be used to assess individual components of perceptual competence. One subtest examines the ability of the individual to discern specific objects in the foreground of a complex picture (figure/ground). Any difficulty experienced with this subtest could explain why a patient cannot simply select trousers from a group of clothes lying on a bed. When a specific problem has been identified, the therapist can suggest the most appropriate therapy.

It is also important at this early stage to ascertain the prehospital history of functional ability. Was a patient who has suffered a stroke, for example, able to walk before the stroke, or is the deficit only part of a history of progressive disability? Specific information is needed about the type of activities the patient participated in before referral to therapy, such as how active the person was, what help is presently available at home, and what the person wishes to attain through the therapist's intervention. On interpreting a detailed assessment, movement, and functional diagnoses can be made and both are considered with the pathology and medical prognosis.

Goal-setting and treatment planning[16] are based on levels of existing functional and cognitive ability, discussion with the patient (and if appropriate the caregiver), and clinical judgment. Goals must always be realistic and attainable. As the patient progresses, they need to be reassessed and updated where necessary.

Therapists will also describe, to the patient and caregiver, their role within the multidisciplinary team and how they would hope to be able to contribute to the restoration of functional ability and social activity.

The framework for assessment, goal-setting, and intervention can be described by the bio-psycho-social approach of health care.[17] This holistic approach considers all elements of health: what is happening to parts of the body (pathology, impairment); what processes are happening at the level of the person's experience (disability); and what is happening in the person's wider social context (handicap). This framework is therefore complementary to the commonly used one proposed by the International Classification of Impairments, Disabilities and Handicaps (ICIDH),[18] which was recently updated with important terminological changes (see Chapter 103B online). As each framework is closely linked with the other, it is immaterial which is used by therapists.[19]

Once intervention has started, continued involvement and education of the main caregiver is essential if that person is to be able to use the techniques taught to best effect. This is particularly important when the patient is discharged from the hospital, at a time when therapeutic interventions are often minimal. Patients, caregivers, therapists, social services personnel, and homecare services are essential collaborators when planning a successful discharge back into the community.

It is also prudent for the therapist to listen to the patient and caregiver, as much can be learned from their experiences and suggestions for solutions to individual problems. Therapists also help and support caregivers throughout the rehabilitation process by providing an ear and an environment where they can express their feelings of frustration, anger, depression, and possibly guilt.[20]

SOME SPECIFIC THERAPY TECHNIQUES

The context for the description of therapy techniques is provided here by four of the most common conditions presenting to therapists: stroke; fractured neck of femur following a fall; Parkinson's disease; and frailty. However, it should be appreciated that a patient may have more than one problem. For example, an elderly person having recently sustained a cardiovascular insult may also demonstrate longer-term frailty with deconditioning and/or permanent impairment of the cardiovascular and musculoskeletal systems. In such circumstances, a therapist addressing each of a patient's difficulties may adopt a "mix and match" approach in devising a treatment program. Adaptability and flexibility are key therapy skills. This might explain why therapists report using a large number of different interventions for defined clinical presentations; for example, 31 interventions for gait apraxia[21] and 175 interventions for poststroke shoulder pain.[22] Such detailed description of techniques is important, especially if interventions are being tested in clinical trials; but as the aim of this chapter is to give an overview, techniques will be described here in rather less detail.

Although research into the effectiveness of specific therapy interventions for elderly people is limited at present, there are several therapy topics that are now the subject of Cochrane reviews. However, caution needs to be used when interpreting the results of these reviews. For example, it is difficult to collate the findings from different primary trials because of variation in aims, interventions, and outcomes,[23,24] and the identification of small numbers of compatible trials for meta-analysis.[25,26] Where adequate numbers of compatible trials are available, positive effects of some therapy interventions have been reported; for example, behavioral interventions and targeting environmental hazards to prevent elderly people sustaining a fall.[25] On the other hand, the optimum amount of therapy—its intensity, duration, and timing in the course of treatment[27]—is also uncertain. The descriptions that follow are therefore a snapshot of a changing science of therapy interventions for elderly people.

Stroke

Stroke is the commonest cause of permanent disability in elderly people and is an important area in rehabilitation as evidenced by its use as a "tracer" condition in the Audit Commission's report "The Way to Go Home: Rehabilitation and Remedial Services for Older People."[28] Therapy forms an important part of the multidisciplinary stroke care package which has been shown to prolong life and reduce disability,[29] an effect that is maintained 10 years after stroke.[30] The U.K. National Clinical Stroke Guidelines recommend that patients in the early phase should see a therapist each working day if possible and that they should be given as much therapy as they find tolerable.[31]

Before looking at some specific therapy techniques, it is important to touch on an issue of particular relevance to physical therapy—the use of "labels" to describe groups of techniques. Physical therapy given after stroke has historically been described by named approaches, and there have been a succession of these (Partridge[32] describes nine). Narrative reviews and trials, however, have not found any one "approach" to be better than any other at reducing disability.[33–35] Currently in the United Kingdom, the majority of physiotherapists and 50% of occupational therapists probably use the Bobath approach,[36–38] which emphasizes the facilitation of normal muscle tone and normal, good-quality movement[39] in preference to the direct training of movement tasks. Outside of the United Kingdom, the Bobath approach is not as predominant and other approaches are more favored—for example, the "movement science" approach, which emphasizes the importance of training everyday activities.[40] However, describing therapy by using these labels probably does not allow any inferences to be made about which specific techniques are used.[41] For example, a recent survey (already alluded to) of nurses, occupational therapists, and physiotherapists in England found that 175 different types of interventions were reported as used for poststroke shoulder pain, and suggested that there was intraprofessional variation.[22] These data support the clinical impression that the same label can be applied to different collections of therapy techniques, and so this chapter will not describe specific named approaches. Instead we want to give a flavor of the type of techniques that have been described in the stroke rehabilitation literature.

Initial steps

During the early period after stroke in patients with major motor impairment, positioning—the use of specific body postures—is advised in the U.K. National Clinical Stroke Guidelines.[31] A recent survey of physiotherapists found that the most common positions recommended during the first week after stroke were sitting in an armchair, side-lying on the hemiplegic side, and side-lying on the opposite side, with particular importance given to the position of the proximal joints of the limbs. For example, in side-lying on the hemiplegic side, the five most important components were found to be: head in neutral, scapular protraction, glenohumeral external rotation, hip extension, and knee flexion.[42]

During this early rehabilitation period, occupational therapists undertake a comprehensive ADL assessment and screen for perceptual and cognitive difficulties (e.g., the Rey figure screening tool[43]). Perceptual problems are common in both right and left hemiplegic stroke patients.[44] Perceptual screening involves asking the patient to copy a drawing of a complex figure made up of 18 components. This assessment is particularly important if the patient has the physical ability to complete a specified task but still remains dependent on assistance. If ADL difficulties are persistent and unexplained, the occupational therapist will then carry out a more detailed perceptual assessment, using perhaps the Rivermead Perceptual Assessment Battery.[15] This may clarify the type and nature of the perceptual problem and act as a pointer to the specific strategies to be used.

It is also important, early after stroke and throughout the rehabilitation process, to provide information to patients and caregivers on the nature of stroke, the difficulties they are experiencing, and the therapy interventions they are receiving. This will ensure that patients and caregivers are totally involved and knowledgeable about the therapeutic aims and objectives of the rehabilitation sessions. Compliance with the treatment regime will therefore be greater. Stroke Family Support Workers also provide much practical, psychological, and emotional support. This support is especially valuable when discharge from hospital is imminent.

Also from the very beginning of the rehabilitation process, therapists emphasize the importance of integration of interventions, and teach other members of the team (including informal caregivers) specific techniques for individual patients. For example, the occupational therapist may teach techniques to help with dressing, toileting, and/or feeding. These specifics may be directed at improving patients' ability to dress themselves. Some examples are:

- Cross the paretic leg over the nonparetic one to be able to reach the paretic foot.
- Use a footstool to reach the feet.
- Adopt clothes that are easier to put on and take off, such as elastic-waisted jogging trousers (this can be modified as function returns).
- Use visual cues—such as red thread around armholes, or red thread next to one button and one hole for correct alignment of buttons.
- Practice backwards chaining. Start with the last step in a functional task and then, when this is achieved, work backwards to the first step, so that eventually the person is able to complete the whole task.
- Encourage and exploit progression of ability by, for example, reducing the support provided by a firm chair with arms, to sitting on a bed while getting dressed.

The physiotherapist may place a description/diagram of recommended positions above the patient's bed and/or run study days on the principles of normal movement.[22]

Re-education of movement

Therapists are often concerned with the reeducation of movement, and many techniques have been used or are being developed.[41]

ACTIVE MOVEMENT

The patient can be asked to produce, or attempt to produce, a voluntary contraction of paretic muscle.[45,46]

BIOFEEDBACK

Biofeedback has been used to provide patients with information about muscle activity during movement.[47,48] The technique involves placing EMG electrodes over the belly of the target muscle and producing a visual display of the electrical activity during a movement or functional task.

CONSTRAINT-INDUCED THERAPY

This is based on experimental evidence of the benefits of "forced" use in monkeys (reviewed by Morris et al[49]). Essentially the technique involves using a sling or a bulky mitten to restrict the nonparetic upper limb. During the period of restriction, the patient is provided with an intensive functional exercise program and is encouraged to use the paretic upper limb during everyday activity.[50–56] This technique has not yet been the subject of evaluation in definitive clinical trials and is not in widespread clinical use. Research is ongoing.

ELECTROSTIMULATION

Electrodes are placed on motor points of wrist and finger extensor muscles to produce full wrist and finger extension with 10 seconds on and 10 seconds off, 1 hour a day for 15 sessions.[57,58] Francisco et al[59] placed electrodes on extensor carpi radialis and gradually increased the stimulus threshold with each session as voluntary recruitment increased. Functional electrical stimulation is also used particularly to improve ankle dorsiflexion during walking.[60] The technique involves stimulating the common peroneal nerve or tibialis anterior muscle, with the stimulation triggered during the swing phase of gait by a force-sensitive switch placed in the patient's shoe.

Facilitated muscle activity and movement An example is weight-bearing through the heel of the hand with an extended elbow.[45,46,61] A particular example relating to postural adjustment was described by Pomeroy et al.[22] The therapist sits behind the patient and the therapist's hands are placed each side of the patient's thorax while the therapist mobilizes the patient's trunk to produce lateral movement of the thorax on the pelvis.

Gross movement can also be facilitated. For example, stepping is effected by the therapist facilitating a patient to displace his or her weight diagonally forwards and outwards, so that balance reactions produce a forward stepping movement with the opposite lower limb. In effect the therapist is facilitating the accentuation of normal posture changes during movement. This technique can also be used to facilitate sit-to-stand. This activity requires an accentuation of the forward and downward movement of the head and shoulders, which occurs during normal standing from a chair.

These techniques require a detailed knowledge of the mechanisms of both normal and disrupted movement (see "Fractured Neck of Femur Following a Fall" section).

AEROBIC EXERCISE

An example is cardiorespiratory and musculoskeletal fitness training, typically over a period of about 10 weeks, using a cycle ergometer.[62] Over the first 4 weeks the initial workload of 30 to 50% of maximal effort is gradually increased to the highest level subjects could attain, and this level is then maintained for the last 6 weeks of the training period.

FUNCTIONAL ACTIVITIES

These include leg and arm training.[63] Training techniques for improving sitting balance include that described by Dean and Shepherd.[64] Patients are seated and undertake reaching tasks to retrieve different objects placed beyond arm's length. Distance and direction are varied, as are seat height, movement speed, object weight, and extent of thigh support on the seat. During reaching, patients are trained to give attention to placing weight through their paretic lower limb.[64]

Walking is a functional activity that is reeducated using numerous therapy techniques depending on the approach being used. A recent development has been to train walking as a whole activity using partial (<40%) body weight support while walking on a treadmill.[65–69] Essentially patients receive partial body weight support from a "parachute harness," which allows them to walk at a low velocity on a treadmill with or without manual guidance from a therapist to ensure that the gait pattern is as normal as possible.

MASSAGE AND SELF-STROKING

An example of this is tapping and rubbing the skin overlying the paretic muscle.[46]

ORTHOTIC ASSISTANCE

Orthoses might be provided to improve control of the ankle during walking. A variety of orthoses is available. Some, such as the air-stirrup brace, limit ankle eversion and inversion[70]; others "control" ankle dorsiflexion and plantarflexion.[70–73]

POSITIONAL FEEDBACK

Specific interventions include feeding information back to patients about weight distribution recorded by devices to measure force,[74–76] and about posture or joint angle recorded by devices to measure deviation from a set position.[77–80]

RESISTIVE EXERCISES

Resistive exercise training can be given for grasp, hand extension, and ballistic extension including flicking a table-tennis ball at a paper cup target.[81] Other techniques include training grip strength by squeezing two bars separated by springs, and performing wrist extension with weights attached to the dorsum of the hand.[82] Yet other interventions have involved the use of a dynamometer to produce the resistance.[83]

ROBOT-AIDED THERAPY

This is a novel therapy which is currently being developed and tested. The technique uses a robotic arm, which is programmed to guide the patient's hand to a target if the patient cannot produce the required movement unaided.[84]

Secondary complications

Prevention and management of secondary complications, such as pain and contractures, is important. Specific interventions include pain assessment and management, and passive movements and stretching.[45] Other specific techniques include providing information about the structure and function of the shoulder, giving frequent feedback to the patient about the position of the arm, and reminding the patient to support the arm all the time.[22]

Training of ADLs

Training of ADLs is another area for specific therapy interventions. For example, in teaching dressing techniques, the therapist can place the armhole of a garment between the patient's legs. The patient puts the paretic upper limb into the armhole with the paretic elbow resting on the paretic knee. The therapist then takes the sleeve over the patient's elbow and shoulder before the person puts his or her nonparetic upper limb into the garment.[22]

Attention is given to the supply of assistive equipment. Examples are a stocking aid, and special cutlery and kitchen equipment (such as belly clamp, one-handed tin-opener, Dycem matting, etc.).[85]

Prior to discharge

As hospital discharge approaches, therapists give particular attention to preparing patients for living with a disability outside the protected hospital environment. A predischarge home visit is essential to assess safety (see later in the "Fractured Neck of Femur Following a Fall" section) and to provide the opportunity for patients to test how they will manage essential personal care and move around their home after stroke. Important activities are practiced, such as getting out of bed, bathing, getting dressed, moving between rooms, and getting in and out of the house.

A home visit is an encounter with the real world and it is often the first time that patients and caregivers fully appreciate the impact of the stroke on their everyday life. The realization that "at a stroke" they have become disabled and that everything is not going to be fine when they go home can be devastating. Aspects of the home environment that were not even noticed before the stroke—such as a step down into the kitchen—are now seen to threaten a severe restriction on independence. For this reason the home visit and the days following it can be emotionally charged. Counseling is often required. Following these visits it may be necessary to refer the client on to a social services occupational therapist, particularly if larger pieces of equipment such as bath aids and ramps or structural changes to accommodation are required.

After discharge

After hospital discharge, therapy may continue and improvements continue to be made.[86–89] Specific interventions include problem-solving, repetitive practice of ADL activities, advice about self-management and re-education of abnormal components of gait by providing practice, and provision of appropriate walking aids.[86] Reintegration of social activity is promoted, and information is given on such facilities as Dial-a-Ride, shopmobility, and suitable swimming classes, where they are available. Leisure activities are promoted; and where previous leisure interests are no longer possible, alternative activities are explored. Where possible, every effort is made to regain the independence in every aspect of the patient's prestroke life. Unfortunately, rehabilitation in nursing or residential homes to date has been sparse, haphazard, and poorly defined[90]; this area is currently being researched.

Fractured neck of femur following a fall

During the acute postoperative period, therapists are most concerned with enabling patients to regain mobility and independence in personal self-care tasks. Of course all therapy interventions are influenced by the particular surgical procedure undertaken, so information given here can only be general in nature. Very early mobilization techniques frequently require patients to be assisted by one or two members of the therapy team so that they can practice fundamental skills such as moving around in bed and standing. Assistive devices such as tilt tables, wheelchairs,[91] raised toilet seats, and dressing aids (e.g., long-handled shoe-horn and stocking aids) might also be used. At this stage in rehabilitation it is also important to establish the patients' preinjury level of independence so that appropriate goals, both formal and informal, can be set with patients and caregivers. As patients become more independent in everyday tasks, more emphasis is given to the prevention of further falls.

Mobility training is often based on an understanding of "normal" biomechanical models of performing particular tasks. Deficient or missing biomechanical components are identified and individualized exercises are given to each patient to remedy the deficient component. Exercises to increase flexibility, strength, and movement control are given in the context of the task being trained. If patients are unable to complete the whole task, then components of the task are practiced in isolation before being incorporated into the desired activity.[92]

For example, sit to stand has two major phases of initial forward trunk lean (first 35% of rising) and upward movement.[93] This division of the task can be further divided into four phases[94]:

1. Flexion momentum is initiation of movement to just before buttocks "lift off." The trunk and pelvis rotate anteriorly while femurs, shanks, and feet remain stationary.
2. Momentum transfer is "lift off" to maximum ankle dorsiflexion. The center of mass moves anteriorly and upward.
3. Extension begins just after maximum ankle dorsiflexion and ends when the hips cease to extend.
4. Stabilization begins when the hips cease to extend and finishes when all motion associated with rising is complete—although the end point is not easy to define.

Some patients have difficulty with the momentum transfer phase because of lack of explosive power in the knee extensors. In this case, strength training of knee extensors combined with practicing "sit to stand" from an initial hip flexion angle of 120 degrees, and gradually reducing this to 90 degrees, is frequently used. Other aspects of functional mobility, such as transfers, gait and stair-climbing, are addressed through movement analysis.

In combination with specific techniques, opportunities are taken throughout the day to ensure that a conducive rehabilitation environment surrounds the patient. For example, the use of a perching stool (a high stool with slight downward slope to the seat) while shaving has the advantage over a standard chair of encouraging weight-bearing through the lower limbs.

A predischarge home visit identifies the potential risks that may cause the patient to fall. Such environmental hazards might include inappropriate heights of beds and chairs, loose or ill-fitting footwear, loose rugs, and slippery floor surfaces.[95] Of course it is not always possible to eliminate such hazards, so therapists need to respect the autonomy of patients and caregivers in making their own decisions—and remove, replace or modify any environmental hazards only with the person's consent.[96] At the very least, the therapist's role is to raise awareness of potential hazards and to teach patients and their caregivers the appropriate strategies to avoid them.

Other therapies designed to prevent further falls include[96–98]:

- Balance retraining (e.g., standing balance exercises in front of a mirror progressing through different feet positions, correction of a tendency to fall backwards (by applying pressure to the front of the body), and ADL practice
- Strengthening lower limb muscles
- Increasing flexibility of the trunk and lower limbs
- Providing mobility aids and appliances
- Raising awareness of unhelpful strategies adopted to avoid a fall (e.g., fixation on the target and therefore being unaware of environmental changes on the way, and tensing muscles to avoid falling (the "walking on ice" strategy), which does not allow for subtle postural adjustments.

Further falls do happen, nevertheless, so it is useful to teach methods of rising from the floor. The conventional method is to help the person on to the floor and then teach him or her how to get on to the knees, so that the person is in a position to rise by pulling on available furniture. An alternative method is to use backward chaining of the task (i.e., first teach the ability to achieve the last component of the task successfully, and then to work successively backwards through the preceding components so that eventually the person is able to stand up independently when placed on the floor.[99,100] It is also possible to teach methods of summoning help, moving about, and keeping warm while on the floor.

Fear of falling is a problem for elderly people—they perceive themselves to be at risk of falling, and then they anticipate adverse consequences of doing so.[101] Fear of falling may negate any gains made through rehabilitation[102] and therefore is a major focus of therapy intervention. This may be resolved by graded exposure to a hierarchy of anxiety-provoking situations agreed by the patient and therapist—starting with the situation least feared until fear is reduced and confidence increased, then moving on to the next situation in the hierarchy. Relaxation techniques may be used as an adjunct to therapy.[98]

Parkinson's disease

As Parkinson's disease is a progressive condition, it is clear that therapy techniques will alter as a patient's disability changes. For example, patients with mild disability might receive a preventative exercise program and counseling, while those with severe disability might receive respiratory exercises and assistive devices.[103] A range of specific techniques suitable for people with Parkinson's disease is described in this section, but it is important to appreciate that these will be modified for individual patients depending on factors such as cognitive impairment, medication, and secondary changes in musculoskeletal and cardiovascular systems.[104]

Early in the disease, interventions might be aimed at maximizing trunk and pelvic range of movement and strength. Interventions are focused on stretching and strengthening the trunk and pelvic muscles,[102,103,106] rhythmic walking, turning, and maintaining the length of flexor muscle groups. Particular techniques may include the therapist resisting the patient walking forward by placing hands on the patient's pelvis at the anterior superior iliac spines.[105] Group exercise to music is frequently encouraged with warm-up, aerobic conditioning, and cool-down sections to each session. One paper describing such exercise groups reported that participants exercised initially at 65% of their maximum heart rate and this was increased by 5% every 4 weeks over a 12-week exercise period. Participants were actively discouraged from exceeding 85% of their maximum heart rate.[107]

Functional mobility

As disability becomes more pronounced, other therapy techniques are incorporated into treatment. Techniques to improve functional mobility "are based on the assumption that normal movement can be obtained by teaching strategies to avoid the basal ganglia pathology."[103]

External cues can be visual, auditory, or sensory.[108] An example of the use of visual cues to aid mobility exercises would be placement of colored objects in boxes positioned at different levels on the side opposite to the active upper limb, to encourage trunk rotation.[109] Auditory cues include a metronome and music with a steady beat to increase temporal spatial parameters of gait, such as stride length and velocity.[108] Sensory cues might include repetitive movement alternatively to left and right, to initiate walking in those with gait initiation difficulty.[110]

Internally generated cues have also been given, such as training patients to concentrate on heel strike so that the foot is lifted from the ground and bigger steps are taken,[111,112] and counting while walking.[112] Interventions can increase awareness of abnormal posture and how to correct it by using a mirror and feedback from the therapist during gait training.[103]

Attentional strategies can be taught. For example, when turning consciously think of a clock and place feet at specific points on the clock face to ensure larger steps and turning circle. Other attentional strategies include asking the patient to focus on the point in the movement where difficulty begins and then beginning retraining activity. Specific retraining strategies are teaching people to walk with larger steps, encouraging them to lean forward when standing up, and promoting participation in everyday physical activity.

Cognitive strategies include mental rehearsal and visualization, and patients can be advised to concentrate on one task at a time so that available cognitive resources are used to "control" the required task, rather than relying on subcortical movement control mechanisms. Mental rehearsal involves patients thinking through the steps of a task before performing it. This may also include prior visualization, so that patients imagine themselves performing the activity before they physically attempt it.

One can change the form of the task. For example, patients can be taught to turn in a larger circle to avoid smaller and smaller steps and falls, and break down complex sequences of movement tasks into simpler components.

A recent therapy approach is based on the principle of improving functional mobility directly by repetitive practice. One example is treadmill training with partial body weight support[113] (as outlined above in the section on techniques used with people who have had a stroke). Another is practicing the components of walking on one spot.[103] It has been proposed that the current approach to therapy might change if further evidence emerges to support the finding that older people with Parkinson's disease (Hoehn and Yahr stages II and III) can improve the performance of movement following repetitive practice.[114]

In addition to the techniques used to improve the movement required for functional mobility, therapists also apply techniques to improve facial mobility. Techniques include brushing muscles, applying ice to muscles, and asking patients to blow through a straw.[115]

Therapists also use specific techniques aimed at limiting the effects of immobility, social isolation, and psychological withdrawal—so-called "secondary disability."[20] Depression is frequently encountered especially as mobility and communication skills decline. Group therapy provides a safe supportive environment in which to practice several types of skills.[20] For example, an integrated physical and occupational therapy rehabilitation program has been described that consists of 69 repetitive exercises to improve range of motion, endurance, balance and gait, and fine motor dexterity. These exercises were provided for 1 hour, three times a week, for 4 consecutive weeks.[116] Such a group activity has clear opportunities for communication practice and enables therapists to identify difficulties that might be alleviated by the provision of a word chart or communication device. A speech and language therapist should ideally be involved in such group activities.

Of course there are times when compensatory strategies are appropriate. Compensatory strategies to enable "sit to stand" include: training the patient to stand up by placing hands on the armrests of the chair and by edging to the front of the seat before beginning to rise; and raising the seat height of the chair. Changes to the environment might also be needed[104] similar to those outlined already. Assistive devices can be supplied, such as elastic shoelaces and the replacement of small fasteners with Velcro.

Environmental changes

Eating is often a particular problem and therapists advise the use of plate warmers to keep food hot. Other useful devices include enlarged handles on utensils (weighted to dampen tremor), and use of a Dycem mat under the plate to improve stability. Sometimes raising the table to a height at which the patient can use one elbow as a pivot can enhance control during eating.

Other simple changes can be made to the environment to ensure that the patient is able to continue with desired activities. For example, place all of the most frequently used kitchen ingredients on one shelf to avoid unnecessary stretching and bending, and/or use a kitchen trolley, which improves the walking patter increases stability, and reduces energy expenditure. There are a number of devices available to help, such as an electric tin-opener and teapot tipper.

Educating the caregivers

As in many other areas of geriatric rehabilitation, an important focus of therapy is educating the caregiver. Caregivers need to be advised that, although it may appear easier to carry out the task for the person, it is in fact kinder and indeed more therapeutic to let him or her struggle (within reason) with the task. This helps avoid inactivity and reduced self-esteem. Therapists work with caregivers and patients to set a hierarchy of tasks that should be done for the patient and those that the patients should do themselves. As the disease progresses, caregivers require training on positioning, moving, and handling. Specialist equipment might be needed such as a hospital bed, hoist, and/or wheelchair. Therapists work closely with patients and caregivers to ensure a best match of therapeutic interventions to abilities, needs, and the environment.

Frailty

In this chapter we shall use the definition of frailty proposed by Campbell and Buchner: "a condition or syndrome which results from a multi-system reduction in reserve capacity to the extent that a number of physiological systems are close to, or past, the threshold of symptomatic clinical failure."[117] The components of frailty appropriate for restorative therapy techniques are musculoskeletal function and aerobic capacity, which might interact with an adverse environment to result in difficulty with mobility, personal care, and social interaction.[118] Therapists are also involved in the prevention of decline in the mobility and daily activities of elderly people, and consider it important to maintain function at the highest level possible, especially during periods of acute inpatient hospital care.[119] The detrimental effects of immobility are well recognized and even a relatively brief period of nonuse of a limb or a limb segment can lead to muscle atrophy and shortening.[120]

People who are frail are clearly at risk from falls, immobility, and social isolation. The specific therapy techniques to address these problems have been outlined in previous sections. This present section will therefore concentrate on techniques to improve the mobility and daily activity of frail elderly people. Many of these techniques are contained within exercise programs to improve mobility of joints and body segments, stability in weight-bearing postures, and control of functional movement.[118,121–129]

Exercise programs

Knee contracture might be helped by therapist-provided low-load prolonged stretch to increase knee extension while the patient lies supine, and then maintaining the extended position using foam roll or wedges under the knee before strapping the knee into the position on the supporting surface.[129]

Exercises can be designed to move each joint passively through its full range of movement.[122] Progression is effected through a program of active exercises by patients to produce voluntary movement through a full range of joint movement,[122,124,125] and when appropriate resistance to movement is provided.[122,125] Resistance can come from the patient's own body weight,[127] arm pulleys,[130] external weights,[128,130] and Thera-band (a color-coded series of different resistive strength latex rubber, which can be cut to the required length for individual patients).[122,125,127,130] Resistive exercises are often provided for muscle groups, such as knee extensors, hip flexors, and deltoid and biceps brachii concentrically and eccentrically.[130,131] Some therapists also promote the use of resistance to movement, which is required for functional ability.[127,128] An isokinetic exercise system might be used to provide progressive resistance to the lower limb movement required during walking,[126] as might an exercise bike.[130]

An appropriate sized gymnastic ball[132–134] can be used by frail elderly people in sitting or standing, and the automatic responses stimulated by the ball's inherent stability can be used to improve dynamic balance. The attending therapist provides stability or instability as appropriate. To increase stability of the ball to enable elderly people to gain confidence in its use, it can be placed inside a cuff positioned on the floor to encircle the ball.[133]

There may be a need for functional training of tasks, such as transfers, walking, wheelchair propulsion, and personal care.[122] The biomechanical approach to analysis and remediation is usually followed as set out in the previous section on "Fractured Neck of Femur Following a Fall." The current trend seems to be toward use of assistive devices such as treadmill retraining of gait with partial body weight support.[135]

The techniques mentioned above are not applied in isolation and delivery is often in the form of group exercise to music. Schedules for these groups vary but include a selection of warm-up exercises, conditioning exercises (aerobic, balance, hand-eye coordination, hand-foot coordination, strengthening), a stretching period, functional exercises (walking, seated exercise to stretch trunk, chair rising, stair ascent and descent), and a relaxation/cool-down period.[136–138] Although exercise programs are frequently recommended, it is important to appreciate that frail elderly people may lack confidence in their ability to undertake exercise. Therapists therefore have to balance this lack of confidence with providing an exercise program that is sufficiently challenging to produce functional improvements quickly to motivate continuation.[139]

Exercise programs frequently provide a forum for the provision of information on exercise, safety in the home (set out in the earlier "Fractured Neck of Femur Following a Fall" section), and foot care. Footwear has been shown to affect performance of functional activities[140,141] and is addressed specifically in treatment programs.[124,142] Finlay[142] gives examples of dangerous footwear, including a shoe with excessive wear on the medial border thus "forcing" the foot into an everted position. Therapists provide information to patients and caregivers about the preferred shoe, avoiding in particular excessive heel height and using nonslip soles. It is sometimes necessary to refer to an orthotist for special footwear and/or to a podiatrist for special foot care; this is particularly important in diabetic patients. In addition the exercise classes, allow the therapist to assess the need for, and current condition of, assistive devices such as walking aids, wheelchairs, dressing aids, and hoists.[143] It is not uncommon for therapists to find patients using unsafe equipment or equipment in need of repair. Other areas of daily life may also benefit from a technology assessment and subsequent provision of appropriate assistive devices.

Cognitive impairment does not preclude the provision of therapy. However, the therapist must be adaptable and flexible.[144,145] Exercise programs involving treadmills, bicycles, and weight-lifting have all been used with frail elderly people with cognitive impairment.[146]

The environment

Good seating is important for elderly people. It helps to maintain mobility if it is easy to get in and out of the chair. It facilitates communication and social interaction if the chair is orientated in a room appropriately. A good chair can prevent or reduce postural pain and promote comfort and security—and thus reduce agitation. The chair can enable adequate nutrition and hydration, and maximize respiratory function through adequate postural support. Therapists consider the following important features of chairs.[147]

- The seat depth should be adequate to support the thighs while leaving about 5 cm behind the knees to avoid compression of the popliteal fossae, which would impair circulation and the nervous system.
- The seat should be wide enough to prevent compression of tissues but allow the sitter to use the armrests for support.
- The seat height should be at least equal to the floor-to-knee height of the user, to make it easier to stand up and sit down.
- The back rest should support the whole of the back, preferably with contoured spinal curve support.
- The seat-to-back angle should be 95 degrees ideally.
- The armrests should be level with the patient's elbow and as long as the seat depth.

Therapists can provide individualized cushioning to adapt chairs,[147,148] including pressure-relief cushions. It is very important for each patient to have more than one chair in which to sit because it is not normal to sit in one position or in one chair for long periods.

Also important for frail elderly people is the promotion of personal energy conservation. Organization of the environment can make best use of a person's abilities. For example, gather all garments before attempting to dress, dress all the lower half at once, reduce the difficulty of fastenings by applying Velcro, and reduce the burden of full weight-bearing by using a perching stool during kitchen activities.

FUTURE DIRECTIONS

The rapid expansion of rehabilitation doctorates, academic posts, and research output[10,149] is indicative of the increasing commitment of the therapy professions to base their practice on evidence. Therapists are now more critical of the methodology and rationale that governs their practice. As the research culture grows, therapists will test conventional techniques for their purported effects and implement those found to be most effective. Future innovations in therapy should therefore be based on research evidence in addition to clinical impressions.[150]

A recent U.K. Medical Research Council document[151] provides an excellent basis for a research strategy in geriatric rehabilitation, highlighting the need for systematic investigation of techniques, and combinations of techniques, in both exploratory and definitive clinical trials. However, in the present climate of a rapidly developing rehabilitation research base, it remains essential to remember that clinical evidence outside of formal research studies can also be an important source of information. Moreover, not all experimental evidence reaches peer-reviewed journals. Trials with positive results are still deemed to be more attractive by publishers and the inconclusive or negative trials are less likely to be published. Therefore the evidence base might actually be evidenced-biased.[152]

Expert opinion in the absence of scientific evidence has an important part to play in the rehabilitation process. Indeed, it is imperative that we do not throw away years of clinical judgment, especially in an area of rehabilitation as complex as elderly care. Specialist multidisciplinary groups such as SRR (Society for Research in Rehabilitation) and profession-specific bodies including OCTEP (Occupational Therapy for Elderly People) and AGILE (chartered physiotherapists working with older people) are essential networks from which future developments in elderly rehabilitation will flourish.

KEY POINTS

Rehabilitation Techniques

- Rehabilitation consists of a complex package of techniques delivered by a multiprofessional team and involving the active participation of patients and caregivers. It makes an important contribution to maintaining independence and quality of life of elderly people.
- To reduce the complexity of description, this chapter uses some of the techniques used by occupational therapists and physiotherapists as exemplars to illustrate the range of possibilities within the package.
- Although techniques are described here within sections of stroke, fractured neck of femur following a fall, Parkinson's disease, and frailty, these techniques are often used in different combinations to meet the complex needs of elderly people.
- The research culture in the therapy professions is growing fast as more therapists obtain doctorates and pursue research into the most effective techniques to maintain the independence of elderly people.

For a complete list of references, please visit online only at www.expertconsult.com

CHAPTER 104

Geriatric Pharmacotherapy and Polypharmacy

Joseph T. Hanlon
Steven M. Handler
Robert L. Maher
Kenneth E. Schmader

INTRODUCTION

Medications are the most frequently used and misused form of therapy for the medical problems of the aged. Geriatric health care professionals and their patients rely heavily on pharmacotherapy to palliate symptoms, improve functional status and quality of life, cure or manage diseases, and potentially prolong survival. There has been a major increase in our knowledge about the epidemiology and the clinical pharmacology of drugs in the elderly (see Chapter 23). This chapter examines efficacy and safety problems (including medication-related problems) of pharmacotherapy in aged populations, measures to reduce medication-related problems including polypharmacy in the elderly, and principles of optimal geriatric pharmacotherapy.

EFFICACY AND SAFETY OF PHARMACOTHERAPY FOR ELDERLY PATIENTS

The evidence for the efficacy of medication therapy in elderly patients has been bolstered by a number of seminal randomized controlled clinical trials for geriatric conditions (e.g., behavioral complications with dementia) and diseases (e.g., hypertension).[1,2] Moreover, a number of new and improved therapeutic medication entities have come to market and improved the ability of health care professionals to treat certain conditions (e.g., cholinesterase inhibitors for Alzheimer's disease, α-blockers for prostatic hyperplasia, and bisphosphonates for osteoporosis). In addition, the future seems bright for further medication discoveries that may benefit elderly people, as nearly 900 new medicines are currently in phase I to phase III testing.[3]

Despite these optimistic trends, there are still major limitations in our knowledge regarding the efficacy and safety of geriatric pharmacotherapy. Elderly patients are still underrepresented in premarketing clinical drug trials.[4] Although regulatory authorities have developed guidelines for pharmaceutical companies regarding new molecular entities that are likely to have significant use in elderly patients, the full impact of these guidelines has yet to be realized.[5] In addition, those trials that do include elders rarely include the "oldest-old" (i.e., 85+), those with multiple comorbidities, or those taking multiple medications.[4] These exclusions raise questions about the generalizability of the results to frail elderly people. Moreover, there is a paucity of postmarketing studies designed to compare the *effectiveness* of two drugs in the treatment of common conditions (e.g., duloxetine vs. gabapentin in management of postherpetic neuralgia). In addition, formal postmarketing surveillance of medications to determine adverse effects varies from country to country, but usually it consists of case reports of potential adverse effects—reports written by practitioners and published in medical journals or spontaneous reports written by practitioners, patients, or pharmaceutical companies and submitted to regulatory agencies.[6] These methods are limited by underreporting and the lack of denominator information about the population at risk. Thus, most safety information must come from formal postmarketing observational studies of specific therapeutic classes or conditions. This makes it difficult for prescribers to use evidence-based medicine to choose the "best" drug therapy for their frail elderly patients. Hopefully these deficiencies in pre- and postmarketing evaluation of efficacy and safety will be addressed in part by the Agency for Healthcare Research and Quality (funded by the University of Iowa), Older Adults Centers for Education and Research on Therapeutics in the United States (see www.iowacert.org for more details), and research utilizing national pharmacy dispensing data such as the Medicare Part D claims data in the United States (see http://www.cms.hhs.gov/PrescriptionDrugCovGenIn/08_PartDData.asp for more details).

MEDICATION-RELATED PROBLEMS IN ELDERLY PATIENTS

As mentioned previously, most information about medication-related problems must come from postmarketing observational studies of specific therapeutic classes or conditions. Problems commonly associated with medication use include medication errors and medication-related adverse events (Figure 104-1).[7] Medication errors can be defined as "a preventable event that may cause or lead to inappropriate medication use or patient harm while the medication is in the control of the health care professional, patient, or consumer."[7–9] These errors can occur at various stages of the medication use process—including the prescribing, order communication, dispensing, administering, and monitoring stages.

Medication errors may result in three different types of medication-related adverse patient events. The first type is an adverse drug reaction (ADR), which is defined as

> *"a response to a drug that is noxious and unintended and occurs at doses normally used for the prophylaxis, diagnosis, or therapy of disease, or for modification of physiologic function,"[10] pg. 289*

The second is an adverse drug withdrawal event (ADWE), defined as

> *"a clinical set of symptoms or signs that are related to the removal of a drug,"[6] pg. 30*

The third is a therapeutic failure (TF), defined as

> *"a failure to accomplish the goals of treatment resulting from inadequate drug therapy and not related to the natural progression of disease (e.g., omission of necessary medication therapy, inadequate medication dose or duration, and medication non-adherence),"[11] pg. 1092*

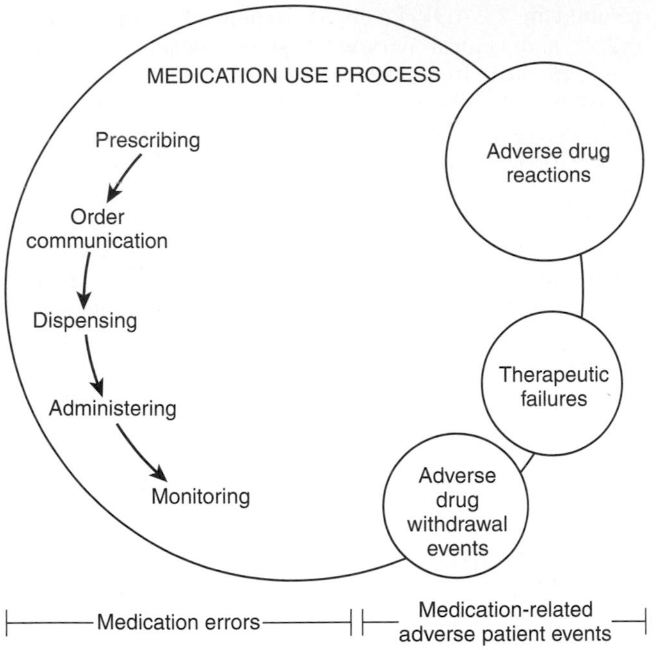

Figure 104-1. Conceptual model for medication-related problems in older adults. *(Adapted from Handler SM, Wright RM, Ruby CM, et al. Epidemiology of medication-related adverse events in nursing homes. Am J Geriatr Pharmacother 2006;4:264–72.)*

Medication-related patient adverse events were cited in an Institute of Medicine report as a major patient-safety concern in a variety of clinical settings including hospitals, ambulatory care, and nursing homes.[8] Two cost-of-illness analyses done in the United States suggest that morbidity and mortality associated with drug-related problems cost an estimated $177.4 billion per year in ambulatory patients and an estimated $4 billion per year in nursing home residents.[12,13] Next we describe the epidemiology of these three distinct medication-related adverse patient events.

EPIDEMIOLOGY OF ADVERSE DRUG REACTIONS

Several authors have reviewed the epidemiology of ADRs.[6,7,14] Here we summarize some studies published most recently. One of the worst adverse consequences of pharmacotherapy is emergency department evaluation and hospitalization. Budnitz et al evaluated the frequency and characteristics of ADRs that lead to emergency department visits in the United States over a 2-year period.[15] Using 21,298 ADR case reports, the authors concluded that 5.9% of all emergency department visits for adults over the age of 65 were for ADRs. Yee et al conducted a retrospective chart review of all older patients who visited the emergency department and found that 12.6% of all encounters were associated with an ADR.[16] Pirmohamed et al conducted a prospective evaluation of 18,820 patients who presented to large general hospitals in England.[17] The authors found that 6.5% (1225) of emergency department evaluations required hospital admission because of an ADR. The median age of a patient admitted for an ADR was 76 years, and the authors concluded that most ADRs were definitely or possibly avoidable.

Few investigators have studied ADRs in elderly outpatients or nursing home residents. In a large cohort study of older ambulatory adults, 5.5% (1523 of 27,617) experienced an ADR over a 12-month study period.[18] Of those that experienced an ADR, 27.6% (421) were considered preventable. In a group of 808 frail elderly outpatients, Hanlon et al documented that 33% experienced an adverse drug event over a 1-year follow-up period.[19] Of those that experienced an ADR, 37.6% (187/497) were considered preventable. Gurwitz et al studied the occurrence of ADRs in 18 Massachusetts nursing homes.[20] Over a 1-year period, they found that 2916 nursing home residents had 546 ADRs, an incidence rate of 1.89 ADRs per 100 resident-months. Overall, nearly 44% of the ADRs were fatal, life threatening or serious, and 51% were preventable. In a more recent study, Gurwitz et al examined the combined incidence of ADRs in two academic nursing homes.[21] In this 9-month prospective observational study, 815 ADRs were detected among 1247 nursing home residents, an incidence rate of 9.8 ADRs per 100 resident-months. As in their previous study, Gurwitz et al found that the majority (80%) of ADRs occurred at the monitoring stage of the medication-use process and a large proportion (42%) were considered preventable. Collectively, these studies from a variety of settings document that ADRs are a common phenomenon in elderly patients.

ADVERSE DRUG REACTION RISK FACTORS

Investigators have attempted to identify a uniform set of patient-level risk factors for the development of ADRs in order to direct prevention efforts at high-risk individuals.[15–21]

Only four risk factors were uniformly found to increase the likelihood of developing an ADR: presence of polypharmacy, use of central nervous system agents, anti-infectives, and anticoagulants. Multiple medication use or polypharmacy is an important factor because it is potentially modifiable. However, the reduction in number of medications in elderly patients with multiple diseases may be difficult because the diseases often require pharmacotherapy. It is also difficult to avoid the drug classes most associated with ADRs, because these drug classes are essential to the management of older persons.

Investigators have suspected that age-related alterations in pharmacokinetics and pharmacodynamics, fragmented medical care, suboptimal prescribing, suboptimal medication monitoring, and medication adherence influence the risk of ADRs.[22–30] The latter three items are clinically important and will be discussed further in this chapter.

There are two major categories of suboptimal prescribing that may contribute to ADRs: (1) overuse or polypharmacy and (2) inappropriate use.[26,27] Operational definitons of polypharmacy differ by clinical setting. One common definition (9+ drugs) in U.S. nursing homes is found in nearly 60% of patients.[31] There is limited information about polypharmacy defined as the administration of more medications than are clinically indicated.[26,27] Two studies showed that between 44% and 59% of outpatients were prescribed more than one unnecessary drug.[32,33]

Inappropriate prescribing can be defined as prescribing a medication whose risks outweigh the benefits.[26,27]

A common medical standard that has been applied and studied in a variety of care settings has been the Beers explicit criteria.[34–36] Results of recent epidemiologic studies suggest that the prevalence of prescribing a Beers criteria medication is 12% in the ambulatory care setting, 29% in the hospital setting, and 47% in the nursing home setting.[37–39]

Alternatively, inappropriate prescribing can be defined as prescribing that does not agree with accepted medical standards.[26,27] Hanlon et al found that 91.9% of 365 elderly ambulatory patients in the United States had one or more prescribing problems as evaluated by the Medication Appropriateness Index (MAI).[40] A study by Steinman et al found in a sample of 170 older patients very little concordance between those with polypharmacy (9+) drugs, or taking an inappropriate drug as per the Beers criteria, or taking an inappropriate drug as per the MAI.[41] Of note, the MAI was the most comprehensive approach, missing only 10% of patients identified as having either polypharmacy or taking a Beers criteria drug.[41]

Studies are starting to emerge describing problems associated with suboptimal medication monitoring and its relationship to ADRs in a variety of care settings. For example, two thirds of the ADRs experienced by older adults in the emergency department were due to toxicity from a relatively small set of drugs for which regular monitoring is commonly required to prevent acute toxicity.[15] In the ambulatory care setting, a substantial proportion of older adults do not receive appropriate laboratory monitoring while being prescribed chronic medications, which also leads to an increased risk of developing an ADR.[28,29,42] Finally, as many as 70% of the ADRs in nursing homes are related to a failure to appropriately monitor medications.[20,21]

Medication adherence may also be a risk factor for ADRs. However, the contribution of medication nonadherence to ADRs is likely to be minor as elderly patients may be adherent with up to 75% of their total number of medications overall.[30] Moreover, the most common type of medication adherence problems is underuse.[30]

EPIDEMIOLOGY OF ADVERSE DRUG WITHDRAWAL EVENTS

Adverse drug withdrawal events (ADWEs) are not formally examined in premarketing clinical trials so one must rely on clinical experience and published data in the postmarketing period to glean information about these problems. The clinical manifestation of ADWEs may appear either as a physiologic withdrawal reaction of the drug (e.g., β-blocker withdrawal syndrome) or as an exacerbation of the underlying disease itself.[43,44] There have been few studies of this phenomenon in elderly patients. Gerety et al investigated ADWEs in a single nursing home in Texas over an 18-month time period and found that 62 nursing home patients experienced a total of 94 ADWEs (mean 0.54 per patient), corresponding to an incidence of 0.32 reactions per patient-month.[45] Cardiovascular (37%), central nervous system (22%), and gastrointestinal drug classes were the most frequently associated with an ADWE. Over 27% of ADWEs were rated as severe. A study of ambulatory elderly patients by Graves et al in the United States investigated ADWEs in 124 patients and discovered that out of 238 drugs stopped, 62 (26%) resulted in 72 ADWEs in 38 patients.[46] Cardiovascular (42%) and central nervous system (18%) drug classes were the most frequently associated with an ADWE. In 26 of the ADWEs (36%), patients required hospitalization, emergency room admission, or urgent care clinic visits. Most of the ADWEs were exacerbations of an underlying disease, and some withdrawal events occurred up to 4 months after the medication was discontinued. Finally, in a study by Kennedy et al, ADWEs were investigated in the postoperative period in a single hospital.[47] Of 1025 patients studied, 50% were over the age of 60 years. Thirty-four patients suffered postsurgical complications resulting from drug therapy withdrawal. Specific drug classes involved in ADWEs included antihypertensives (especially angiotensin-converting-enzyme inhibitors), antiparkinson medications (especially levodopa/carbidopa), benzodiazepines, and antidepressants.

ADVERSE DRUG WITHDRAWAL RISK FACTORS

Little is known about the risk factors for ADWEs. In the study by Gerety et al, ADWEs were associated with multiple diagnoses, multiple medications, longer nursing home stays, and being hospitalized.[45] Graves et al found that the number of medications stopped was a significant predictor of ADWEs.[46] Analyses by Kennedy et al revealed that the risk of an ADWE increased as the length of time off the medication increased.[47]

EPIDEMIOLOGY OF THERAPEUTIC FAILURE

There have been few studies of this phenomenon in elderly patients. In a U.S. study of therapeutic failure leading to hospitalization, investigators used the reliable Therapeutic Failure Questionnarie (TFQ) to measure therapeutic failure in 106 frail older adults who were admitted to 11 Veterans Affairs hospitals.[48] Eleven percent of these individuals had probable therapeutic failure leading to hospitalization. The most common conditions associated with therapeutic failure involved congestive heart failure and chronic obstructive pulmonary disease. In the emergency department, Italian investigators found that 6.8% of patients had evidence of therapeutic failure with nearly two thirds occurring in patients over the age of 65 years old.[49] A U.S. investigation of drug-related emergency department visits in elderly patients found that 28% of drug-related visits were due to therapeutic failure.[16]

THERAPEUTIC FAILURE RISK FACTORS

Little is known about the risk factors for TFs. Reasons for therapeutic failure may include low prescribed dose, drug-drug interaction, drug resistance or nonresponse, inadequate therapeutic monitoring, nonadherence, or underprescrbing of necessary drug therapy. We discuss the latter two reasons next.

Nonadherence was the most common reason for therapeutic failure in the U.S. TFQ hospitalization study (58%) and in the U.S. emergency department visit study (66%).[16,48] Older patients may not fill the prescription, not take a filled prescription, skip doses, take the drug erratically, or reduce doses.

These behaviors may be intentional (e.g., adverse effects, health beliefs, concerns about taking too many drugs) or unintentional (e.g., cognitive impairment, poor vision or dexterity, lack of transportation).[50] Cost-related nonadherence is a particularly important and prevalent subtype of intentional nonadherence among older adults with limited means.[51,52]

Another major factor related to therapeutic failure is the underprescribing of medications, which can be defined as the omission of drug therapy that is indicated for the treatment or prevention of a disease or condition.[26,27] A study that applied the explict Assessing Care of Vulnerable Elders criteria found that 50% of 372 vulnerable adults were not prescribed an indicated medication.[42] The most common problems were no gastroprotective agent for high-risk nonsteroidal anti-inflammatory drug (NSAID) users, no angiotensin-converting enzyme inhibitor (ACE-I) in diabetics with proteinuria, and no calcium or vitamin D for those with osteoporosis.[42] A group of U.S. investigators using the Assessment of Underutilization of Medication (AOU) measure found evidence of underuse of medications in 62% of 384 frail elderly patients at hospital discharge.[53] The necessary medication classes most likely to be omitted were cardiovascular (e.g., antianginal), blood modifiers (e.g., antiplatelet), vitamins (e.g., multivitamin), and central nervous system (e.g., antidepressant) agents. Patients with limited ability to perform basic activities of daily living and greater comorbidity were at higher risk for undertreatment. Clinical researchers have consistently detected underuse of medications for specific diseases or conditions in older adults, including congestive heart failure, myocardial infarction, hypertension, hyperlipidemia, osteoporosis, depression, diabetes mellitus, and pain. For example, one study found that only half of a large cohort of 21,138 elderly patients with diabetes who also had hypertension or proteinuria received recommended therapy with an angiotensin-converting enzyme (ACE) inhibitor or angiotensin receptor blocker (ARB) to retard progression of chronic kidney disease.[54]

MEASURES TO REDUCE MEDICATION-RELATED PROBLEMS IN ELDERLY PATIENTS

Given that medication-related problems are common, costly, and clinically important, how can they be reduced? The specific answer to this question is surprisingly difficult because there are few health services intervention clinical trials in elderly patients that examine measures to reduce ADRs, ADWEs, or TFs. Therefore, health policy makers and clinicians must look to reasonable, empirical approaches that are based on existing epidemiologic and clinical information. These approaches, to be discussed here, include better health systems design, improved health services, and patient/caregiver education. Health professional education will be discussed in the last section on the principles of geriatric pharmacotherapy.

Health systems design

Medication-related problems can be reduced by designing health care systems that make it difficult for individuals to do the wrong thing and easy to do the right thing.[55] In the latest Institute of Medicine Report, *Reducing Medication Errors*, the authors provide a number of specific recommendations to improve medication safety.[8] One recommendation is that all health care organizations should immediately make complete patient-information and decision-support tools available to clinicians and patients. Another recommendation is that health care systems should capture information on medication safety and use this information to improve safety. Health care organizations should also implement the appropriate systems to enable providers to have (1) access to comprehensive reference information concerning medications and related health data, (2) assess the safety of medication use through active monitoring and use these monitoring data to inform the implementation of prevention strategies, (3) write prescriptions electronically, and (4) subject prescriptions to evidence-based, current clinical decision support. A recent systematic review assessed the effects that computerized physician order entry and clinical decision support systems have on the quality, efficiency and cost of health care for elders.[56,57] These studies suggest that although the amount of research available is limited, studies have been able to demonstrate improvements in the quality and efficiency of the medication use process. It is likely that the continued development and refinement of clinical decision support systems will lead to a reduction in medication errors and medication-related adverse events in a variety of care settings.

Health services approaches

Four reviews summarize clinical trials where two health services approaches, clinical pharmacist services and geriatric medicine services, have shown an improvment in suboptimal prescribing and medication adherence and reduced ADRs in older adults.[26,27,58,59] Clinical pharmacy is a health science discipline that is concerned with the science and practice of rational medication use. One study by Leape et al showed that clinical pharmacist activities reduced ADRs in intensive care unit patients.[60] Geriatric medicine services, also known as geriatric evaluation and management (GEM), utilizes a multidisciplinary team of specialists in geriatrics to manage patient care. The teams generally consist of a geriatrician, physician, nurse, social worker and pharmacist. An important component of GEM is the assessment and optimal management of medications. One study by Schmader et al showed that GEM care reduced the risk of serious ADRs in frail outpatients.[61] Additonal large, multicenter controlled trials are needed to determine the effectiveness of these and other approaches to optimizing medication use in older adults on medication-related adverse patient events.

Patient/caregiver education

Systematic education of patients and caregivers about ADRs may increase their ability to better report or avoid potential adverse drug events, thereby allowing clinicians to make medication changes before these adverse events become too serious. In addition, one study showed that when the pharmacist counsels patients about their medications upon hospital discharge, it can reduce the rate of adverse drug reactions.[62] One review summarized randomized controlled trials designed to enhance medication adherence and related outcomes in the elderly.[63] Patient education and compliance aids can improve medication adherence, which could potentially reduce therapeutic failure that may lead to hospitalization because of a patient or caregiver's decision to stop a beneficial medication.[63] Although not definitively shown, it is sensible that patient and caregiver education about ADWEs could prevent a patient or caregiver from stopping a medication abruptly that should be withdrawn slowly.

PRINCIPLES OF GERIATRIC PHARMACOTHERAPY

Clinicians who care for elderly patients need to know and apply principles of geriatric pharmacotherapy in order to maximize the benefits of medications in their elderly patients and minimize medication-related problems (Table 104-1). The first step in prescribing is to decide whether medication therapy is really necessary, as many medical problems in elderly patients do not require a pharmacologic solution. If the clinician decides that a medication is indicated and its benefits outweigh its risks, then the choice of the medication must factor in the medication's pharmacokinetics, the patient's renal and hepatic function, the medication's main potential adverse effects, and the patient's other medications and diseases. The starting dose for most medications in elderly patients must be lower, and the interval before modifying the dosage often must be extended. Cost and establishment of clear therapeutic end points are also important.

In the ongoing management of the patient and his or her medications, the clinician should monitor for potential ADRs via the history, physical examination, and, where appropriate, laboratory data.[6] The identification of ADRs can be a challenging task in elderly patients because their ADRs may present in a vague or atypical fashion and the causal link can be difficult to establish. The first step is to consider ADRs in the differential diagnosis of most geriatric syndromes. If the adverse event is a known side effect of one or more of the patient's medications, the clinician can further enhance his or her confidence in establishing ADR causality by considering the temporal relationship of onset of medication use to onset of event, competing causes, rechallenge, dechallenge, and other factors.[64] Nonetheless, in some cases, the clinician may find it difficult, and sometimes impossible, to establish the ADR causal link between medication effect and illness in elderly patients.

In patients who have recently stopped a medication, it is important to consider the possibility of an ADWE. ADWEs in elderly patients can be overlooked when the withdrawal event is mistaken for a patient's disease state. Common events that may happen in the everyday care of an elderly patient such as discontinuation of unwanted medications, intentional noncompliance, stopping medications before a surgical procedure, and managed care practices of medication substitution within classes of medications may lead to an ADWE. Table 104-2 lists medications commonly used by elderly patients that may be associated with withdrawal syndromes or exacerbation of the underlying disease.[43–46,65] To prevent ADWEs, the clinician should take into account the dose of the medication, the length of therapy of the medication, and the pharmacokinetics of the medication. Risk can be minimized or eliminated by a slow, careful tapering of the medication over a period of time. This approach is similar to the time taken in the initiation and titration of a new medication. Unfortunately, precise tapering schedules have not been established for most medications.

Table 104-1. Principles of Geriatric Pharmacotherapy

1. Consider whether medication therapy is necessary.
2. Know the pharmacology of the medication in relation to age.
3. Know the adverse effect profile of the medication in relation to the patient's other medication(s) and disease(s).
4. Choose initial dose, and adjust it carefully (doses will often need to be smaller in elderly people).
5. Select the least costly alternative.
6. Establish clear, feasible therapeutic end points.
7. Monitor for adverse drug reactions, an important cause of geriatric illness.
8. Slowly taper medications to prevent/minimize adverse drug withdrawal events (if possible).
9. Regularly review the need for chronic medications and discontinue unnecessary ones.
10. Assess whether there is omission of needed medication for the established diagnosis/condition.
11. Review adherence, simplify the medication regimen, if possible, and consider use of aids.

Table 104-2. Medications Associated With Adverse Drug Withdrawal Events in the Elderly

Medications	Type of Withdrawal*	Withdrawal Syndrome
Alpha-antagonist antihypertensives	P	Hypertension, palpitations, headache, agitation
Angiotensin-converting enzyme inhibitors	P, D	Hypertension, heart failure
Antianginal agents	D	Myocardial ischemia
Anticonvulsants	P, D	Seizures
Antidepressants	P, D	Akathisia, anxiety, irritability, gastrointestinal distress, malaise, myalgia, headache, coryza, chills, insomnia, recurrence of depression
Antiparkinson agents	P, D	Rigidity, tremor, pulmonary embolism, psychosis, hypotension
Antipsychotics	P	Nausea, restlessness, insomnia, dyskinesia
Baclofen	P	Hallucinations, paranoia, insomnia, nightmares, mania, depression, anxiety, agitation, confusion, seizures, hypertonia
Benzodiazepines	P	Agitation, confusion, delirium, seizures, insomnia
Beta-blockers	P	Angina, myocardial infarction, anxiety, tachycardia, hypertension
Corticosteroids	P	Weakness, anorexia, nausea, hypotension
Digoxin	D	Heart failure, palpitations
Diuretics	D	Hypertension, heart failure
Histamine-2 blockers	D	Recurrence of esophagitis and indigestion symptoms
Narcotic analgesics	P	Restlessness, anxiety, anger, insomnia, chills, abdominal cramping, diarrhea, diaphoresis
Nonsteroidal anti-inflammatory drugs	P	Recurrence of arthritis and gout inflammatory symptoms
Sedative/hypnotics (e.g., barbiturates)	P	Anxiety, muscle twitches, tremor, dizziness

*P, Physiologic withdrawal; D, exacerbation of underlying disease.

Table 104-3. Medication Appropriateness Index

Questions to Ask About Each Individual Medication

1. Is there an indication for the medication?
2. Is the medication effective for the condition?
3. Is the dosage correct?
4. Are the directions correct?
5. Are the directions practical?
6. Are there clinically significant drug-drug interactions?
7. Are there clinically significant drug-disease/condition interactions?
8. Is there unnecessary duplication with other medication(s)?
9. Is the duration of therapy acceptable?
10. Is this medication the least expensive alternative compared to others of equal utility?

At every visit, it is necessary to review and, if possible, simplify the patient's medication regimen. This may be achieved by altering the dosing schedule or discontinuing medicines that are no longer needed. To conduct the review when faced with an elderly patient taking multiple medications, the clinician can utilize any of the standardized approaches such as the Medication Appropriateness Index (MAI) (Table 104-3).[66] The clinician should also consider whether necessary medications have been omitted. A standardized tool such as the Assessment of Underutilization of Medication (AOU) can be used, which requires having a health professional match the complete list of chronic medical conditions to the prescribed medications after reviewing the medical record.[67] In this manner, one can determine whether there was an omission of a needed medication for an established disease or condition based on the scientific literature. For each condition, one of three ratings can be made: omission, marginal omission (e.g., have used appropriate nonpharmacologic approach), or no omission.

The clinician should also consider providing adherence aids for elderly patients. However, before providing the patient with methods to enhance adherence, it is important for the clinician to improve suboptimal prescribing and then to talk to the patient about how he or she takes the medications so that an individualized plan can be developed. It is also important to identify risk factors for poor adherence (e.g., impaired hearing, vision, and cognition).[30] Health care professionals should also follow up with compliance recommendations by monitoring their patients. Some general methods to enhance adherence in elderly patients include simplifying regimens, providing written instructions, and considering generic formulations to reduce costs. More specifically, pill boxes, increased font size on prescription labels, calendars, easy-to-swallow dosage forms, pill cutters, oral dosing syringes, insulin syringe magnification, tube spacer for inhalers, and easy-open caps may increase adherence in elderly patients. There are also some electronic devices available as compliance aids (e.g., alarm watches with messages, automated pill delivery systems, medication bottles with alarms) that may prove to be beneficial. Finally, active patient and family involvement should be encouraged.

SUMMARY

Geriatric pharmacotherapy may greatly enhance the quality of life of elderly patients by effectively palliating, preventing, or treating many diseases and conditions in late life. The evidence for the efficacy of medications in elderly patients has significantly increased over past decades thanks to some clinical trials, and many more potentially beneficial medications are in development. However, clinical trial data may be limited by the underrepresentation of older patients in many trials, the exclusion of frail elderly or oldest-old patients, and the lack of postmarketing studies designed to assess the effectiveness of competing medications. In addition, the benefits of medication therapy can be offset by ADRs, ADWEs, and therapeutic failure. Although variable in their estimates of the frequency of these medication-related problems, many epidemiologic studies agree that these are common, costly, and clinically important problems in elderly patients. Potential solutions to these problems include better health systems design, health services approaches, and patient and caregiver education. More research is needed to determine the feasibility and effectiveness of these approaches. Clinicians who care for elderly patients need to know and apply principles of geriatric pharmacotherapy in order to maximize the benefits of medications and minimize medication-related problems.

KEY POINTS
Geriatric Pharmacotherapy and Polypharmacy

- There are limitations in our knowledge about the efficacy and safety of medications in the elderly.
- Medication-related adverse patient events such as therapeutic failure, adverse drug withdrawal reactions, and adverse drug reactions are common and result in considerable morbidity in the elderly.
- Strategies to modify or reduce medication-related problems including polypharmacy will require that health systems design/institute new approaches to delivering care to elders.
- Clinicians should strive to conduct periodic systematic reviews of elderly patients' medication regimens as well as adhere to other principles to optimize geriatric pharmacotherapy.

For a complete list of references, please visit online only at www.expertconsult.com

CHAPTER 105

Impaired Mobility

Ruth E. Hubbard
Eamonn Eeles
Kenneth Rockwood

INTRODUCTION

In the popular imagination and in the scientific literature, impaired mobility and balance are each associated with aging. The association between aging and mobility impairment occurs because with age, there is an accumulation of deficits, including those that affect motor performance. This is not just a matter of diseases that give rise to disorders of mobility and balance. It is worth considering that even among elite athletes, performance is age-related. When assessing the metabolic power required to achieve running world records, sprint and endurance events show a relatively uniform decline with age across the different events.[1]

Chapter 106 considers the problem of falling. Here we focus on impaired mobility, although noting its relationship with balance; essential aspects of that will be covered here, too. To begin, we briefly review some essential features of how gait changes with age. Next we describe some common gait disorders and other common problems that can give rise to impaired mobility (e.g., joint and foot disorders), which can be assessed with reasonable efficiency. Moving from such specific problems, we consider how impaired mobility and balance affects older people in the hospital and in the community. Finally, we explore the relationship between impaired mobility and frailty, recognizing that the integrative aspects of reviewing high-order functions can be combined with a reductionist approach to particular disorders to make the care of frail older people better.

AGE-RELATED CHANGES IN MOBILITY

Changes in mobility and abnormalities of gait increase with increasing age; perhaps this is why the attribution of locomotion abnormalities to "old age" is a frequent occurrence among both older people and their physicians. The proportion of people with a normal gait falls from 85% of those aged 60 years to 18% aged 85 years.[2] Normal gait is dependent on the integrity and interaction of three components[3]:

- Locomotion, including initiation and maintenance of rhythmic stepping
- Balance, which engages *peripheral sensory receptors* for input, *central nervous system* structures for processing sensory input and planning motor output, and *effector organs* to carry out the movement plan (as reviewed in detail in Chapter 106).
- The ability to adapt to the environment

With aging, deficits accumulate across one or all of these systems, reducing the locomotor capability of most older adults. However, the extent to which this is due to "normal" aging is currently controversial.

The changing conceptualization of a phenomenon from normal-for-age to pathologic is exemplified by senile gait disorder. This slow, shuffling, cautious walking pattern is common in old age with no clear cause on clinical examination. And yet compared with age-matched individuals who walk normally, those with senile gait disorder have a significantly increased risk of developing dementia[4] and significantly reduced survival.[5] Similarly, gait or posture impairment, present in 25% to 30% of cognitively unimpaired older people, is associated with an increased risk of cognitive decline and dementia.[6] It is now thought that such gait abnormalities are a manifestation of subtle white-matter changes or vestibular, visual, or oculomotor dysfunction.[3] In consequence, it seems reasonable as a starting stance (pardon the pun) that little should be written off as "normal gait for age." Evaluation and treatment—stopping meds, starting exercise, etc.—should generally be considered. From an assessment standpoint, that might mean screening apparently high level people—if a geriatrician should care about them at all—with demanding tasks.[7]

Executive function

Walking was traditionally seen as an automatic task requiring little input from higher mental functions. However, an intricate interaction between gait and cognition is now recognized. The prediction of cognitive decline by senile gait disorder is matched by a converse relationship: those with established dementia are more likely to have gait abnormalities and have a significantly increased risk of falls.[8]

The link between cognition and walking may be mediated by executive function. In community-dwelling older adults after mild stroke, executive functioning is independently associated with performances of balance and mobility.[9] The prefrontal cortex, which plays a crucial role in executive functioning, seems to be particularly vulnerable to change with "normal aging.[10] Studies investigating dual tasks, which are dependent on intact executive function, provide further supportive evidence. Older people are less able to maintain normal ambulation while performing an additional task, particularly talking.[11,12] Even in physically fit older people, dual tasks influence balance during walking through a direct effect on body sway and stride variability and an indirect effect on gait velocity.[13] Task shifting when multitasking is also impaired with aging. Younger people prioritize walking safely when challenged with a secondary task, but this prudent strategy is diminished in older people.[12]

Walking speed

Most quantitative studies have found that "healthy" older people walk more slowly than young adults. Gait analyses suggest their 20% slower natural velocity is secondary to reduction in stride length and that cadence (steps per minute) is well maintained.[14] However, a slow gait should not be considered benign. In well-functioning community-dwelling older people, there is a continuous relationship between usual gait speed over a short course and subsequent risk of disability, hospitalization, and death.[15] Indeed, reduced gait speed has been advocated as a marker of frailty—either exclusively[15,16] or in combination with other markers of strength and vitality.[17] The dynamic nature of frailty has also been explored and underpinned by measurement of mobility changes.[18,19]

Gait initiation

Gait initiation requires the integrated control of limb movement and posture and is achieved with purposeful postural shifts (including relaxation of the triceps surae, synergistic contraction of the ventral muscles, swing hip abduction, and a few degrees of flexion in the support hip and knee). These culminate in a forward step, steady state velocity being achieved in less than two steps.[14] Gait initiation is well preserved in healthy older people.[20] Abnormalities of gait initiation are a sensitive but not specific sign of disease processes in older people, such as Parkinson's disease, multiple cerebral infarcts, normal-pressure hydrocephalus, progressive supranuclear palsy, and cervical myelopathy.

Rising from a chair

The ability to rise from a chair is a critical aspect of normal mobility. To carry out this so-called "chair stands" test, a straight-backed chair should be placed next to a wall so it cannot slip backwards. Participants should be asked to fold their arms across their chest and to stand up from the chair one time. A second assistant should be on hand if the participant seems at high risk of instability. If successful in standing once, participants can be asked to stand up and down five times as quickly as possible and timed from the initial sitting position to the final sanding position.[21]

Before standing, flexion of the knees brings the feet closer to the chair to reduce the distance that the center of mass must move anteriorly. This important preparatory movement is often omitted by patients with Parkinson's disease and other neurologic disturbances of gait.[14] Standing proceeds with bilateral hip flexion, ankle dorsiflexion, and anterior rotation of the trunk and pelvis, with reversal of these dynamic events when sitting. Reduced range of motion in the hips, pelvis, knees, and spine is common with aging and impedes the initial shift of the total body center of mass over the feet. Weakness of the hip girdle muscles is also a frequent finding in older people, a manifestation of general deconditioning, and those affected may need to use their arms to help themselves upwards. Chair stands are therefore sensitive to changes in postural control, strength, and coordination and have been included in physical performance measures to stratify highly functioning older adults. The Short Physical Performance Battery (SPPB), for example, includes walking, balance, and chair stands tests and independently predicts mobility disability and activities of daily living disability in community-dwelling older people.[21–23]

COMMON DISORDERS OF GAIT

Pragmatically, disorders of gait may be divided into those that are clinically obvious and others that are less so. The following gait patterns would be evident to experienced clinicians and are classified according to level of impairment/interaction with the nervous system[24]:

Middle level disorders

- The slow and shuffling gait of parkinsonism
- The stiff limb with clumsy circumduction and scuffing of footwear due to hemiparesis, most commonly observed in stroke
- Sensory and cerebellar ataxia and vestibular pathology share unsteadiness as a core feature but can be discriminated clinically by isolating and unmasking the affected organ
- Other middle level disorders include cervical spine disease and normal pressure hydrocephalus

Lowest level disorders

- The antalgic gait pattern in which a phase of the gait is shortened on the injured side to alleviate the pain experienced when bearing weight on that side, often secondary to disease in the ankle, hip, or knee.
- Arthritis or arthrodesis of the ankle may lead to a combination of lowest level disorders with altered load bearing and secondary stress in adjacent joints (antalgic gait), subsequent muscle weakness of the tibialis anterior (slap-foot or toe-drag gait), and compensatory gait patterns (steppage gait), and recruitment of long toe extensors with hammer toe deformity a consequence.[25]
- Other lower level disorders include peripheral neuropathy and myopathy.

Since these disorders are covered in other chapters, here we shall concentrate more on gait disorders that may present more of a diagnostic challenge.

The term gait apraxia has largely been superseded by higher-level gait disorder. This is based on "abnormalities of the highest sensorimotor systems" and assumes integrity in basic sensorimotor circuitry.[24] Gait pattern in higher level disorders is attributed to a motor programming failure comparable to the problems encountered in Parkinson's disease. These abnormalities can be classified according to their functional or neuroanatomic associations. Even so, the exact nature of these correlates is still debated; the present uncertainty is reflected by the many classification systems that have been proposed (Table 105-1).

It may be worthwhile reviewing just what higher level functioning achieves in relation to locomotion. Interrelated higher level structures (the cortico-basal ganglia-thalamocortical loop) meet the demands of personal desire to move and the maintenance of posture within the confines of environmental limitations.[26] Pathology in any of these regions or their connections therefore results in an array of gait disorders:

- Suppression of conversion of personal will into task execution manifesting as hesitation or freezing and problems initiating gait or making turns (particularly affected by abnormalities of the supplementary motor area and its connections).[26,27]
- Dysfunctional processing with gait adversely influenced by both emotional and environmental information
- Dysfunctional or absent postural righting reflexes resulting in injurious falls
- In contrast to hypokinesis implicit in basal ganglia underactivity, disturbance in basal ganglia function may also lead to excessive, involuntary and uncontrolled limb movements[28]

Classifications of gait have been criticized for their lack of consistency.[29] The Nutt classification, for instance,

Table 105-1. Classification of Higher-Level Gait Disorders

	LOCATION CLASSIFICATION*			
	Frontal Gait Disorder	**Frontal Dysequilibrium**	**Subcortical Dysequilibrium**	**Speculative**
Phenomenology classification*				Isolated gait ignition failure
Clinical findings	Extrapyramidal features, some postural imbalance	Bizarre ineffective gait	Loss of postural balance reflexes	Inability to initiate or continue movement
Liston classification†	Mixed gait apraxia	← Equilibrium apraxia → (spans Frontal Dysequilibrium and Subcortical Dysequilibrium)		Ignition apraxia
		← Mixed gait apraxia → (spans Frontal Dysequilibrium through Speculative)		
Elble classification‡	← Dysfunctional or absent postural righting → (spans Frontal Gait Disorder through Subcortical Dysequilibrium)			Gait ignition failure

Cautious gait, psychogenic gait, and extrapyramidal overactivity probably retain their separate identities and have been omitted from the table.
*Nutt JG, Marsden CD, Thompson PD. Human walking and higher-level gait disorders, particularly in the elderly. Neurology 1993;43:268–79.
†Liston R, Mickelborough J, Bene J et al. A new classification of higher level gait disorders in patients with cerebral multiinfarct states. Age Ageing 2003;32(3):252–8.
‡Elble RJ. Gait and dementia: moving beyond the notion of gait apraxia. J Neural Transm 2007;114(10):1253–8.

included frontal gait disorder, cautious gait, frontal dysequilibrium and cortical dysequilibrium as distinct entities.[24] The older person, with accumulation and overlap of pathology, may exhibit problems of higher gait, which are not reducible to such discrete categories. Distinct gait parameters were identified by Liston et al according to their own clinically proposed subtypes. This allowed for the theoretical inclusion of mixed pathology and gait subtypes.[29] The amalgamation of disordered balance in conjunction with ineffective gait by Elble[26] seems a sensible if not altogether precise way to overcome the lack of connection between the site of pathology and the physical characteristics of gait disturbance.

The phenomenological entanglement of **cautious gait** is worthy of consideration. This entity may be considered multifactorial and reflects the common pathway for expression of deficits anywhere within the locomotor system in an older person. Cautious gait may be entirely appropriate in the setting of a recent fall with loss of confidence or a perceived fear of falling.[30] Cross-sectional studies suggest that a cautious gait is common[31] and associated with poor standing balance, depression, anxiety, fear of falling, and reduced strength.[32] It is these properties that cite a cautious gait as a high risk group but one potentially amenable to targeted interventions. The distinction between dysfunctional/excessive compensatory mechanisms and a primary disturbance of gait is important.[32] Cautious gait should therefore not be labeled as a higher-level disturbance without first excluding and attempting to correct a primary disorder of locomotion.[31]

In direct contrast to cautious gait, those with careless gait[3] exhibit disinhibition of movement with an inability to match their judgment to their physical limitations or the hazards posed by the external environment. Though many studies report that older people with dementia walk slowly,[33] if their overall degree of physical impairment is taken into account (e.g., use of walking aids and functional impairment), they may actually walk too quickly.[34] Such recklessness implicates frontal lobe disturbance, as noted, and may account for the high level of injurious falls observed in dementia. Similarly, in hospitalized older people, those with delirium are at high risk of falls because of excessive ambulation and lack of insight into mobility problems.[35] Mismatch in confidence and ability, while difficult to measure, remain an important clinical indicator of gait stability.

Drugs can influence mobility and balance in as many ways as there are pathways involved.[36] The resulting gait disorder depends on the site of drug action and may be further complicated by polypharmacy, drug/drug interaction, and altered pharmacodynamics and kinetics associated with aging.[37] Since cognitive impairment is associated with disturbance in mobility and balance, it is not hard to conceptualize the careless gait of dementia or delirium becoming more precarious when disinhibiting sedatives or neuroleptics are prescribed.[38]

CLINICAL ASSESSMENT OF BALANCE AND MOBILITY

Mobility and balance provide an insight into the speed, stability, and adaptability of locomotion. Balance may be static (preserving upright posture while standing still) or dynamic (in response to an internal or external stressor). Contemporary studies have shown impairments in balance to be common and associated with adverse outcomes, particularly falls.[39] Performance measures have therefore been developed to quantify balance impairments, including:

- The Berg balance test.[40] This provides an ordinal measure of static and functional balance, has been validated in older patients in wide range of settings[41] and correlates with outcome and disability.[42] Although easy to use, it is limited by floor and ceiling effects.[43]
- The timed get-up-and-go is an integral measure of gait speed and balance in widespread clinical use.[44] It is reliable[45] and also correlates well with Barthel Index.[46] It seems to predict the patient's ability to go outside alone safely.[47]
- The Tinetti balance and mobility scale[48] tests for performance of balance and mobility across a wide range of tasks. The Tinetti scale is a valid predictor of future falls in older patients.[49] It is a reliable instrument across a range of rater experience.[50]

However, these tests lack well-described "norms" and it is not clear how much change to expect under different circumstances.[43] Performance-based measures also need to be sensitive to change to be informative. Yet if a patient is unable to complete the task asked of him or her by a performance-based measure then this results in missing data. For example, once a patient is unable to stand or walk then their abilities cannot be rated. This may exclude the very patients on whom more information would be helpful, the most frail.[51] Failure to complete performance-based measures is associated with poor health status and increased risk of death.[52]

Another method to assess mobility and balance involves observation of usual rather than extended performance. This may better represent the abilities of the frailest individuals. And being more inclusive of the functional abilities of a patient in the context of a geriatric service, the assessment of mobility incorporating a low functioning individual shines a light on overall state of health. The Hierarchical Assessment of Balance And Mobility[53–55] has been developed as a global means of tracking progression and recovery in frail older adults who become ill. By displaying changes in static and dynamic balance and in mobility graphically, it provides a standardized and transparent description of levels of mobility and balance in three areas: in bed mobility, transfers, and walking. In each area higher scores indicate greater mobility. Patients are observed and scored at their highest level of observed safe function using their usual aid. Despite a possible ceiling effect, which may be less relevant to the population group of interest, the HABAM (hierarchical assessment of balance and mobility) has demonstrated its validity, reliability, responsiveness, and sensibility as a measure of mobility and balance. The Elderly Mobility Scale[56] and the Physical Performance Mobility Examination[57] are other tools that are tailored to the assessment of older acutely unwell patients based on evaluation of the patients usual activity. Only the HABAM has been shown to represent a unidimensional measure of mobility and is validated as an interval measure. It has superiority in terms of ease and acceptability to users.[58]

The assessment of mobility in this way offers numerous clinical benefits:

- A risk stratification marker: using mobility and balance as a noninvasive tool to identify physiologic decline before conventional means of evaluation register such concern
- The opportunity to explore the relationship between specific diagnoses and/or geriatric syndromes with mobility and balance
- An objective threshold of improvement rather than gestalt can determine suitability and timing of more intensive rehabilitation techniques
- A visual prognostic tool with which to inform patients and caregivers, facilitate teaching and learning opportunities, and ease multidisciplinary working
- Assessment of mobility and balance provides a culture of clinically meaningful patient contact without redress to expensive technologies

Given the importance of mobility and balance as an overall correlate of an individual's state of health, the HABAM can be used to track daily changes in a patient's health. This has particular usefulness in elderly patients who are frail, in whom many of the traditional signs of illness often are not present. Consider, for example, a patient with pyelonephritis, whose presentation was one of being "off legs" or "taking to bed." In a younger patient it would be reasonable to track successful treatment of the infection by noting defervescence, the amelioration of the neutrophilic leukocytosis and settling of flank pain. If none of these was present at the start of the illness in a frail older adult, then their resolution can hardly be tracked as signs of recovery. Changes in mobility and balance, however, follow a reliable hierarchy, as illustrated in Figure 105-1. In the first patient (Panel A) mobility and balance had deteriorated considerably from baseline, so that one person could only move from side to side in bed, and required the assistance of two people to transfer and to walk even to the bathroom in one person hospital room. By the second hospital day, however, recovery had begun and accelerated after day 5. In another patient with a similar level of decline, however, continued worsening on the second and third hospital days signaled a rapidly fatal course that ended in death by day 6 (Panel B). In our experience, these observations can readily be taught to house staff and to other learners, who find it a useful way to quantify their nascent clinical judgment and so gain confidence in their ability to care for frail older adults who are acutely ill.

IMMOBILITY IN OLDER PEOPLE: IMPACT AND INTERVENTIONS

Older people in hospital

Prevention of age-associated decline in mobility is a major clinical and public health priority.[23] In the early 1940s, curative operations and antibiotics replaced bed rest as therapeutic strategies and pioneers of geriatric medicine were among the most vociferous advocates of early ambulation. Working in "chronic sick" wards where older people had spent years in the hospital because they had nowhere else to go, geriatricians found that rehabilitation and mobilization enabled many patients to be discharged home.[59] Asher famously expressed the disadvantages of bed rest in a 1947 BMJ paper: "Look at the patient lying in bed. What a pathetic picture he makes! The blood clotting in his veins, the lime draining from his bones, the scybala stacking up in his colon, the flesh rotting from his seat, the urine leaking from his distended bladder and the spirit evaporating from his soul".[60] The accuracy of Asher's observations has subsequently been confirmed. Prolonged bed rest in healthy young men has deleterious effects on nearly every organ system[61] and in older people in the hospital, bed rest contributes to deep vein thromboses, pressure sores, and incontinence.[62] Bed rest has such a major role in the pathogenesis of neuromuscular weakness in critically ill patients that a new approach for managing mechanically ventilated patients includes reducing deep sedation and early rehabilitation therapy and mobilization.[63] Finally, but by no means least importantly, Asher seems to have recognized the adverse psychological impact of immobilization,[64] though a minority argue that "the spirit evaporating from his soul" is more likely to result from enforced mobilization than judicious bed rest.[65]

Interventions to improve outcomes in hospitalized older people have centered on exercise. A recent Cochrane systematic review[66] determined the effect of exercise interventions for acutely hospitalized older medical patients on functional status, adverse events, and hospital outcomes. Of 3138 potentially relevant articles screened, 7 randomized controlled trials and 2 controlled clinical trials were

Hierarchical Assessment of Balance and Mobility

Completed By: ______________________ Date Completed: __________

Date Assessed	/	/	/	/	/	/	/	/	/	/	/	/	/	/	/	/	/	/
Instrument / **Day**	-14	01	02	03	05	06	07	08	09	10	11	12	13	14	15	16	17	18
BALANCE																		
21. stable ambulation	21								21	21	21	21						
14. stable dynamic standing								14										
10. stable static standing							10											
7. stable dynamic sitting						7												
5. stable static sitting		5	5	5	5													
0. impaired static sitting																		
TRANSFERS																		
18. Independent and vigorous	18									18	18	18						
16. Independent									16									
14 Independent but slow								14										
12. 1 person standby							12											
11. 1 person minimal assist						11												
7. 1 person assist			7	7	7													
3. 2 person assist		3																
0. total lift																		
MOBILITY																		
28. Unlimited, vigorous																		
26. Unlimited																		
25. Limited >50m, no aid																		
21. Unlimited, with aid																		
19. Unlimited with aid, slow																		
18. With aid >50m	18											18						
16. No aid, limited 8-50m										16	16							
15. With aid 8-50m									15									
14. With aid <8m+								14										
12. 1 person standby/+/- aid						12	12											
9. 1 person hands-on/+/-aid				9	9													
7. Lying-sitting independently		7	7															
4. positions self in bed																		
0. needs positioning in bed																		

Notes for scoring the HABAM.

- Baseline (-14) is taken as 2 weeks prior to the current assessment.
- Each domain (balance, transfers, mobility) is scored at the highest level attained.
- In Balance, "**dynamic**" refers to withstanding a force, either administered externally (e.g. a sternal nudge) or internally (e.g. reaching forward).
- In Transfers, **standby assist** refers to no hands-on assistance but presence of an aide for security; **minimal assist** refers to hands on with little force, chiefly for guidance.
- In Mobility, **<8m** corresponds to not being able to walk outside the room; **8-50m** mobility is being able to get to the nursing station and back; **>50m** is more than one trip around the ward.
- The HABAM should be scored using the patient's usual walking aid.

C. MacKnight, K Rockwood. *J Clin Epidemiol* 2000;53:1242-1247, K Rockwood et al. *J Am Geriatric Soc* 2008;56:1213-1217.

A

Figure 105-1. Hierarchical assessment of balance and mobility form. (A) A patient's mobility and balance had deteriorated considerably from baseline. The patient could only move from side to side in bed, and required the assistance of two people to transfer and to walk. By the second hospital day, however, recovery had begun and accelerated after day 5.

HIERARCHICAL ASSESSMENT OF BALANCE AND MOBILITY

Completed By: ______________________ Date Completed: ______________

Instrument / Day	-14	01	02	03	05	06	07	08	09	10	11	12	13	14	15	16	17	18
Date Assessed																		
BALANCE																		
21. stable ambulation	21																	
14. stable dynamic standing																		
10. stable static standing																		
7. stable dynamic sitting																		
5. stable static sitting		5																
0. impaired static sitting			0	0	0	0												
TRANSFERS																		
18. Independent and vigorous	18																	
16. Independent																		
14 Independent but slow																		
12. 1 person standby																		
11. 1 person minimal assist																		
7. 1 person assist																		
3. 2 person assist		3	3															
0. total lift				0	0	0												
MOBILITY																		
28. Unlimited, vigorous																		
26. Unlimited																		
25. Limited >50m, no aid																		
21. Unlimited, with aid																		
19. Unlimited with aid, slow																		
18. With aid >50m	18																	
16. No aid, limited 8-50m																		
15. With aid 8-50m																		
14. With aid <8m+																		
12. 1 person standby/+/- aid																		
9. 1 person hands-on/+/-aid																		
7. Lying-sitting independently		7																
4. positions self in bed			4															
0. needs positioning in bed				0	0	0												

Notes for scoring the HABAM.

- Baseline (-14) is taken as 2 weeks prior to the current assessment.
- Each domain (balance, transfers, mobility) is scored at the highest level attained.
- In Balance, "**dynamic**" refers to withstanding a force, either administered externally (e.g. a sternal nudge) or internally (e.g. reaching forward).
- In Transfers, **standby assist** refers to no hands-on assistance but presence of an aide for security; **minimal assist** refers to hands on with little force, chiefly for guidance.
- In Mobility, **<8m** corresponds to not being able to walk outside the room; **8-50m** mobility is being able to get to the nursing station and back; **>50m** is more than one trip around the ward.
- The HABAM should be scored using the patient's usual walking aid.

C. MacKnight, K Rockwood. *J Clin Epidemiol* 2000;53:1242-1247, K Rockwood et al. *J Am Geriatric Soc* 2008;56:1213-1217.

B

Figure 105-1—cont'd (B) Another patient with a similar level of decline continued worsening on the second and third hospital days, which signaled a rapidly fatal course that ended in death by day 6. *(Geriatric Medicine Research Unit, Dalhousie University, Halifax, Canada.)*

included. Although the effect of exercise on functional outcome measures was unclear, there was "silver" level evidence that multidisciplinary intervention that includes exercise may increase the proportion of patients discharged home and reduced length and cost of hospital stay for acutely hospitalized older medical patients.

Nutritional support also improves outcomes of hospitalized older people. Though mobility outcomes were not explicitly reported, dietetic assistance significantly reduced patients' risk of dying after hip fracture.[67] Randomized trials are underway to establish whether the combination of a 6-month, individualized exercise and nutrition program improves mobility and function after hip fracture.[68] Anabolic agents are theoretically attractive as therapeutic agents in hospitalized older people, reducing the negative nitrogen balance and improving body composition, but small randomized controlled trials have shown no effect on mobility or function and further studies with longer follow-up periods are needed.[69]

Community-dwelling older people

The impact of immobility for community-dwelling people has been investigated by Gill's group at Yale University. In a prospective study, illnesses and injuries leading to either hospitalization or restricted activity were strongly associated with the development of a disability, including the need for personal assistance walking inside the house or transferring from a chair.[70] The associations were present both in those who were and were not frail (with frailty defined on the basis of slow gait speed). In the same patient cohort, episodes of bed rest (staying in bed for at least one half a day due to illness, injury, or other problem) were associated with decline in function, including mobility impairment.[71] Additional research was called for to identify precipitants of bed rest and determine whether intervention or aggressive treatment would reduce functional decline.

Exercise programs of varying design have diverse positive effects in community-dwelling older people including improved muscle strength and gait speed,[72,73] reduction in falls,[74,75] and improved balance.[76,77] In longitudinal cohort studies, physical activity is protective of impaired physical function.[78–80] Participation in frequent and intense training can result in even greater improvements in reactive balance performance: older athletes undertaking long-term high intensity training demonstrate better and more rapid stabilization of posture following perturbation than healthy older adults under challenging conditions.[81]

Exercise programs for frail older people, however, have yielded conflicting results. A systematic review of physical training in institutionalized elderly patients indicated positive effects on muscle strength but effects on gait, disability, balance, and endurance were inconclusive.[82] In some studies, exercise programs in very frail older people result in no improvements in physical health or function[83] and increase musculoskeletal injury[84] and falls.[85] In contrast, other studies conclude that exercise improves physical performance scores[86] and reduces falls.[87] In an international observational study, physical activity in frail older people seemed to slow further functional decline.[88]

These conflicting results may be secondary to the use of different definitions of frailty and controversy about which outcomes have the best measurement characteristics.[23]

IMPAIRED MOBILITY AND FRAILTY

The most consistent independent predictors of future falls in older adults are gait or balance deficits.[89] This is consistent with the paradigm of frailty in older people as failure of a complex system. Walking on two legs is not exceptional to humans (birds and some lizards do it, too) but the complexity of this task, the kinematic features of our gait, and its dependence on central nervous system control makes human bipedalism unique and distinct from that found in animals.[90,91] Normal ambulation in people requires the coordination of many different muscles acting on multiple joints and is accomplished by the integration of activity in spinal neuronal circuitries with sensory feedback signals and with descending commands from the motor cortex.[90] The central nervous system coordinates this activity, adjusts it to fit environmental conditions, and refines it when required, all the while maintaining a remarkable degree of precision. For example, the position of the human foot during normal walking depends on the coordination of five joints and 15 muscles acting on the knee joint alone and yet with every step the foot is elevated by only 1 to 2 cm above the ground and its position varies by less than 4 mm.[92,93] The computational task solved by the human brain to accomplish this feat is extraordinary given the infinite number of combinations of joint and muscle positions that have to be attuned relative to each other to arrive at the desired outcome. Bipedalism is indeed a higher order function that requires a significant degree of connectivity and coordination between several interdependent components (muscular, skeletal, and nervous) of the complex system that is the human body. Consequently, it should not be surprising that frail individuals who have gait and balance deficits and who have lost the ability to integrate multiple inputs in the face of stress often experience impaired mobility and falls.[94]

There is a tension between this approach, and one that aims to tease out influence of the component parts. Several groups have emphasized the importance of sarcopenia (the reduction of muscle mass and function) in the pathogenesis of frailty.[95–97] Since immobility and lack of exercise are major factors responsible for sarcopenia, self-report and objective evaluation of physical performance are advocated as the best indicators of frailty in elderly subjects, a poor performance characterizing those who may benefit from intervention.[98]

Some components of frailty may be more predictive of adverse outcomes. Among very frail older people, those with mobility disability had a higher risk of mortality and nursing home placement than those without, and incidence of hip fracture and hospitalization was associated with severity of mobility limitations.[99] Similarly, mobility impairment is also of determining importance in high-functioning older women, with lower performances in mobility and balance tests (along with increasing age, poor perceived health, lower muscle strength, higher body mass index, lower educational level, and lower reported physical activity) being strong predictors of disability.[100] Furthermore, recent studies suggest the combination of certain frailty components may be critical. In participants of the MacArthur Study of Successful Aging, six frailty subdimensions were identified (different combinations of 4 or more of 10 criteria: weight loss, weak grip, exhaustion, slow gait, low physical activity, cognitive impairment, high interleukin-6, high C-reactive protein, subjective weakness, anorexia). Each had a different predictive validity for disability and mortality, suggesting "that pathways to frailty differ and that subdimension-adapted care might enhance care of frail seniors."[101]

Other groups have investigated component parts of frailty with even greater precision. For example, contributors to leg power (muscle strength and limb velocity) are each associated with different elements of balance performance in older people.[102]

So while some researchers in the aging field emphasize the conceptualization of frailty as a risk state and while others aim to clarify components of the risk state, the importance of mobility impairment is universally recognized. Both approaches to frailty are motivated by the need to increase our understanding of the pathways to poor health in old age and they are not irreconcilable. Inouye et al,[103] for example, identified impaired mobility as one of four shared risk factors (along with older age, baseline cognitive impairment, and baseline functional impairment) for five common geriatric syndromes (delirium, pressure ulcers, incontinence, falls, and functional decline) and for the "overarching geriatric syndrome of frailty." Pleiotropic interventions with effects on many different cells and tissues (such as antioxidants or exercise or improved nutrition) were advocated as the most promising preventive strategies. Thus it is feasible to unite the two different approaches to frailty, recognizing and investigating the importance of components of frailty yet managing it as a complex condition.

CONCLUSION

Mobility impairment is integral to frailty, however defined.[104–106] What is more, the clinical assessment of changes in mobility is an important aspect of evaluating change in physical frailty.[18,19] Since "you can't manage what you can't measure," the use of a standardized means of describing mobility can help improve the otherwise curiously moral language commonly employed at the bedside (e.g., mobility being "not too good"). Even though the dangers of going to bed have been known for generations,[60] it persists as the default method for providing care in many settings. Clearly, there is much that geriatricians need to do both to better understand mobility and balance and to better communicate why and how it should be assessed routinely in frail older adults, especially when they are ill.

KEY POINTS

Impaired Mobility

- Impaired mobility and balance are common in older adults who are frail.
- Impaired mobility and balance should be investigated as signs of illness, and not accepted as inevitable parts of aging.
- Exercise has a particular role in the treatment of impaired mobility and balance in elderly people.
- Though the dangers of going to bed have been known for generations, it persists as the default method for providing care in many settings.

For a complete list of references, please visit online only at www.expertconsult.com

CHAPTER 106

Falls

Stephanie A. Studenski

INTRODUCTION

Falls are a major focus of geriatric medicine because they are common among older adults and have complex interacting causes, serious consequences, and require multiple disciplines for effective management. The goals of this chapter are to present the scope and impact of the problem, explore various perspectives on causation, provide guidance about clinical evaluation and treatment, and examine opportunities to implement programs across health care settings and communities.

EPIDEMIOLOGY

Falls are common among older adults. Up to one third of community-dwelling persons over the age of 65 fall every year and about one fourth to one fifth of them will fall repeatedly.[1] Falling is more common among women than men and increases in prevalence with advancing age. In acute care settings, falls are the most commonly reported adverse incident with rates varying from 3 to 13 falls per 1000 bed days.[2] In chronic care settings, falls are so common that typically over half of residents are fallers and average rates can run from 1.5 falls per bed per year to two to six falls per resident per year.[3] The most obvious adverse consequence of falls are injuries, which develop in about 10% of community fallers and 30% of fallers in acute and chronic care.[1,2] Injuries are more likely in recurrent fallers.[1] Falls can be fatal; they are the fifth leading cause of death among older adults.[1] Falls are a major contributor to serious injuries, including not only hip fractures, but also other fractures, cervical spine injuries, and severe head trauma.[4,5] Falls are a common precipitator of hospitalization and contribute to the need for long-term institutionalization.[1,6] Falls in acute and chronic care institutions are also a source of complaints from families and even the source of litigation.[7] Although injuries and health care use are serious concerns, falling also creates other serious problems for the older adult, including functional limitations, fear of falling, restricted activity, and social isolation.[1,7] Falling can be a precipitator of a vicious cycle of failing health and function leading to death.

In the past, there has been no widely agreed-upon definition of falls. More recently, ProFaNE (Prevention of Falls Network Europe, www.profane.eu.org), a multinational work group dedicated to reducing falls and injuries through research and implementation of evidence-based interventions, has proposed the following as the most reliable and valid definition[8]:

"A fall is an unexpected event in which the participant comes to rest on the ground, floor or lower level."

Although this definition provides some consistency for reporting, there are still areas of confusion. It is not clear if it is appropriate to include in the definition of falls those events associated with loss of consciousness or overwhelming external forces such as being hit by a moving vehicle. Similarly, it may or may not be important to include events such as a "near" fall where the individual barely avoids a fall to the floor by suddenly grabbing for furniture or walls, or is caught by another person. Frequent near-falls, such as "stumbles" and "trips," are risk factors for future falls. There are also problems with fall reporting. Fall events may not be remembered retrospectively, especially if there were no injuries. Prospective monitoring improves accuracy but can be burdensome. Although falls in general are important, it is possible that the most clinically relevant concern is the recurrent faller or a fall injury. There are also serious health-related concerns for the population that does not actually fall because they have restricted their own activity. This group may also be at high risk for future falls, injuries, and social isolation.

CAUSATION

Falling is considered a classic geriatric syndrome because it is often due to multiple interacting conditions that create an organism with reduced tolerance to any type of external stress. The evidence base that has been used to define the causes of falls is highly dependent on the perspective and priorities of the researchers, the definitions of falling and fallers, the time frame and approach to monitoring for falls, the characteristics of the population under study, what factors were measured, and how interactions between factors were assessed in the analyses. Whatever the focus of the research, it is clear that many fallers demonstrate multiple abnormalities, and that the interactions among these abnormalities influence fall risk.

Epidemiologic perspective

Epidemiologic observational studies of older adults in community, acute, and chronic care institutions have identified risk factors for falls and all suggest that risk increases as the number of risk factors increases. Table 106-1 summarizes risk factor profiles by the setting in which older people were studied. Across settings, altered mobility and cognition are major risk factors for falls. Interestingly, it is possible to be too immobile to fall.[9] For example, in one chronic care setting, residents with fair standing balance had the highest fall rates, those with good standing balance had intermediate fall rates, and persons with poor standing balance had the lowest

Table 106-1. Predisposing Risk Factors for Falls in Older Persons in Three Types of Settings Based on Observational Studies

Community Dweller	Acute Care	Chronic Care
Fall history	Gait instability	Cognitive impairment
Weakness	Agitated confusion	Visual impairment
Balance problem	Urinary incontinence/frequency	Weakness
Gait problem	Fall history	Neurologic problems
Visual problem	High-risk medications	Gait/balance problems
Mobility limitation		Cardiovascular problem
Cognitive impairment		
Decreased functional status		
Postural hypotension		

fall rates.[10] Risk factor patterns and appropriate preventive interventions may differ substantially by overall mobility capacity; active older adults may experience falls and injuries for very different reasons than persons who stand and walk with difficulty, who in turn may fall for very different reasons than persons who cannot stand. Risk factors for injurious falls may differ from risk factors for all falls. In a recent study of older people in residential care facilities, fracture risk among fallers was higher in persons with better balance and no history of falls, perhaps suggesting that in some persons, activity increased the risk of producing sufficient force to fracture.[11] Risk factor profiles are also limited in that they generally only identify chronic and stable risk factors, sometimes called predisposing risk factors. Many falls might occur because an individual with predisposing risk confronts additional acute precipitating factors.[12] For example, an older adult with limited mobility and cognition might not become a faller until he or she develops diarrhea, becomes dehydrated and dizzy, and tries to rush to the bathroom. Because risk factor studies have rarely accounted for these more transient and dynamic precipitating contributors, much less is known about them.

Risk factors for falls overlap substantially with risk factors for other geriatric syndromes.[13] Older age and impairments in cognition, mobility, and function are risk factors for falls, incontinence, delirium, and frailty.[13] Thus there is a population of older adults with multiple impairments who are at risk for numerous geriatric syndromes, including falls and injuries. There may be other populations of older adults who are at risk for different types of falls; active older adults may fall and injure themselves during demanding activities, whereas very immobile older adults may fall out of bed and chairs or even be dropped by care providers. In the future, more distinct risk factor profiles might be defined based on overall mobility status.

Epidemiologic studies have also identified environmental risk factors for falls. Virtually all falls can be considered the result of interactions between a person and the environment. The individual has some level of ability to move and the environment has some level of challenge. The task of the moment is the context in which the person and the environment interact. The risk factors identified in Table 106-1 are sometimes called "intrinsic" factors because they relate to the individual. Risk factors associated with the environment are sometimes called "extrinsic" factors. The typical aged faller experiences a fall in an environment and while performing tasks that would not cause a healthy young person to fall. This phenomenon of falling under low challenge is the rationale for believing that many falls in older people are due largely to intrinsic factors. If an older adult has many intrinsic risk factors, it is possible that only modest problems with the environment or modest degrees of challenge in a task will precipitate a fall. Table 106-2 lists environmental risk factors for falls. Commonly reported indoor environmental factors are uneven walkways, loose rugs, absence of grab bars in the bathroom, and poor lighting.[14,15] Outdoor hazards are less frequently assessed but might be important, especially for more active older adults. Other extrinsic elements, such as the availability of human help, may be an important factor in falls among persons living in the community, and are even more likely to contribute to falls in the institutional setting.[10] Additional risk factors for falls include psychological and attitudinal characteristics such as risk preference.[9,16] Other risk factors for injury include osteoporosis, low body weight, and fall direction.[17]

Table 106-2. Environmental Risk Factors for Falls

Indoor Falls	Outdoor Falls
Poor lighting	Uneven and broken sidewalks
Loose or absent railings	Wet surfaces
Throw rugs	Poor lighting
Trailing cords and wires	Irregular steps
Uneven transitions such as level change between rooms	Unpredictable level changes
Lack of bars in the bathroom	
Slippery floors	
Cluttered walkways	

Physiologic perspective

Contributors to falls can be examined from the perspective of physiologic systems that contribute to balance. The rationale for using a framework of organ-based physiologic systems that affect balance is founded in models of disablement. These models draw links between pathologic processes and altered organ system performance (termed impairments), which combine to affect body movements (termed functional or performance limitations), then affect functional abilities and disability, and ultimately interfere with social roles, such as homemaker or volunteer (termed handicap). There are several disablement models. When assessing causation of problems of aging, these multisystem physiologic approaches are helpful for several reasons. First such approaches can address interactions between systems. Second, they can include mild or subclinical impairments that might affect function without being individually clinically obvious. Third, well-functioning systems might actually serve to compensate for problems with other systems. Thus both individual organ systems and even overall functions such as balance exist on a continuum; they might be obviously abnormal, subclinically abnormal under usual conditions, abnormal only under stressful conditions, normal, or even have "back up" or "reserve" excess capacity.

From a physiologic perspective, balance dysfunction results from impairment in one or more of the following systems: *peripheral sensory receptors* for input, *central nervous system* structures for processing sensory input and planning motor output, and *effector organs* to carry out the movement plan (Table 106-3). In many situations, it is the combination of deficits across these systems that produces instability and falls.

There are three main sensory systems used for balance: vision, somatosensation, and vestibular function. Visual functions such as acuity, depth perception, dark adaptation, contrast sensitivity, and peripheral vision help determine body position and trajectory in space and monitor the environment. Since bifocal glasses prioritize two focal lengths—one in the lower field at about 20 inches for reading and one in the upper visual field at about 20 feet for distance—bifocals can limit acuity in the critical zone in front of the feet while walking.[18] Diseases of the aging eye that affect multiple visual functions are common and include glaucoma, macular degeneration, and cataracts. Medications that cause miosis, or constriction of the pupil, can reduce dark adaptation.

Table 106-3. Components of Postural Control

Sensory Systems
Vision
Vestibular functions
Somatosensation
Central Nervous System
Perfusion
Speed/attention
Postural reflexes
Effector Systems
Strength
Flexibility
Endurance

Peripheral sensation is important for balance. These sensors provide information about the position of the body relative to the support surface and gravity, and reflect the relationship of one body part to another during rest and movement. Peripheral sensation is the most important system for monitoring the characteristics of the weight-bearing surface and the distribution of body weight onto the feet. Peripheral sensory loss is common in older adults because of diabetes and peripheral vascular disease. In the face of peripheral sensory loss, visual systems can compensate by supplementing information about body position. Thus a combination of vision loss and peripheral sensory loss can create serious problems with ability to monitor body position.

The vestibular system detects the position of the head with respect to gravity, monitors linear and angular acceleration of the head, and coordinates head and eye movements to maintain gaze and visual field stability while moving. Vestibular system impairments can occur with usual aging and are affected by ischemia or head trauma. Several widely recognized vestibular conditions, such as benign paroxysmal vertigo and perhaps Meniere disease, are common in older people. Others are also common but less well recognized, such as chronic bilateral vestibular hypofunction.

The central nervous system has numerous structures that contribute to balance. Structures in the brainstem and spinal cord are considered central pattern generators that produce stepping behaviors. Balance is further controlled by higher level brain structures including the frontal cortex, basal ganglia, cerebellum, motor cortex, and other areas. Degeneration of brain regions can affect balance, as in the basal ganglia in Parkinson disease and in cerebellar degeneration. All brain processes are dependent on adequate levels of brain perfusion, so any threats to perfusion affect central processes of gait and balance. Thus many of the conditions that produce syncope or presyncope can cause transient cerebral hypoperfusion and falls. Examples include orthostatic hypotension, tachy- and bradyarrhythmias, and critical aortic stenosis.[19] In recent years, there has been increased awareness of the role of more diffuse microvascular brain disease as a contributor to balance disorders and falls.[20] This mechanism is posited to involve ischemia in vulnerable brain areas, especially the frontal lobes and in important white matter tracts connecting the frontal lobes to critical subcortical areas. Radiologically this ischemia is manifested as leukoaraiosis or white matter disease on magnetic resonance imaging. White matter disease has been associated with specific patterns of cognitive dysfunction involving psychomotor slowing, and altered attention and executive functions such as sequencing and visual spatial organization.[20,21] These cognitive abnormalities have been associated with alterations in gait, especially excessively variable length and timing of stepping and with falls.[22,23] Thus there is an emerging concept of altered balance and gait due to abnormal nonamnestic cognitive functions and movement planning produced by regional microvascular brain disease. This condition may be manifest by irregular walking patterns and may be exacerbated by placing stress on cognition and movement. Tasks that simultaneously stress cognition and movement are part of an emerging conceptual approach to balance assessment called "dual tasking." Older persons whose performance worsens substantially when asked to walk and solve cognitive problems simultaneously may be at increased risk for falls.[24]

The central nervous system also operates a multisynaptic "righting reflex" that produces automatic correcting movements when balance is lost. Classically appearing as a stepping response that occurs much more quickly than can be done voluntarily, this righting reflex is lost in many central nervous system disorders including extrapyramidal diseases and other forms of multisystem atrophy. Sedation, either clinical or subclinical, may further reduce alertness and attention. Thus both sleepiness and sedative medications have been found to increase fall risk.[25,26] Less specific but potentially important are psychological factors such as fear of falling and risk preferences.[9,27]

Muscles and joints are effector organs that are critical for balance and mobility. Muscle weakness is widespread in older adults and can be due to primary muscle mass loss (sarcopenia), disorders of peripheral nerves or neuromuscular junctions, or to inactivity. Specific muscle diseases such as inflammatory myositis or steroid myopathy can produce proximal muscle and trunk weakness that occurs with falls. Lower motor neuron conditions, radicular nerve deficits due to spinal stenosis, or peripheral nerve damage can result in localizing strength deficits that affect specific muscle groups and more distinct functional movements. For example, a foot drop due to damage to the peroneal nerve prevents the forefoot from lifting to clear obstacles and can induce trips and stumbles. Recent evidence suggests that low vitamin D levels may contribute to muscle weakness and falls.[28] Low testosterone levels have been found to be associated with falls in men under age 80.[29] Other common conditions such as arthritis can reduce range of motion and produce pain that alters stepping and weight bearing.[30] Deformities distort the weight bearing surfaces of the foot and cause pain. Fatigue, either generalized or localized to muscle, can contribute to loss of balance. Thus acute conditions such as overworked muscles or chronic conditions associated with fatigue such as anemia[31] or congestive heart failure might increase risk for falls.

When fall onset is abrupt or there is a major change in balance, the likelihood is higher that there is a medical event that has affected the central nervous system. Any illness or episode that reduces cerebral perfusion through hypoxia, decreased oxygen carrying capacity, or hypotension could present as dizziness, lightheadedness, unsteadiness, and falls. Toxic or metabolic abnormalities due to medications, infection, or electrolyte disorders could present as unsteadiness and falls through effects on attention. New focal neurologic deficits due to stroke can also present as unsteadiness. Older

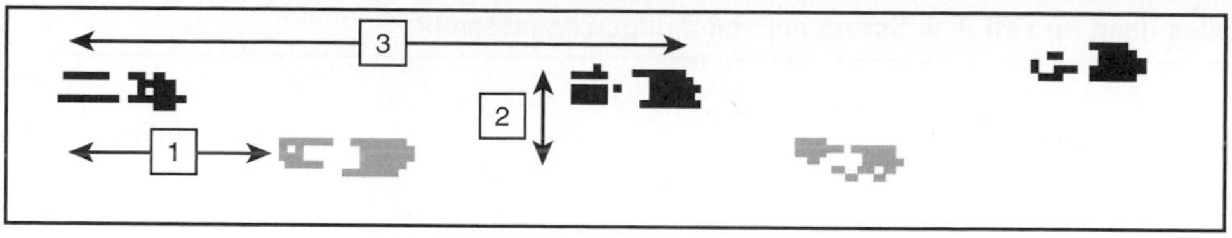

Figure 106-1. Terms used to describe normal walking (1: step length; 2: step width; 3: stride length).

adults with predisposing subclinical balance disorders could be more vulnerable to such precipitating factors. These types of physiologic acute and sometimes transient changes are harder to include in research studies because stable chronic effects are usually the focus of the investigation.

Biomechanical perspective

A biomechanical approach to fall risk is based on concepts of mass, force, momentum, and acceleration of the body as a whole and of body segments. The human body in standing is a long tall column that rests over a small base of support. The main task of movement is to displace and recover this column while the base of support changes. Thus the assessment of balance includes two main conditions, (1) static balance, defined as steadiness of the fixed column over a constant base of support and (2) dynamic balance, defined as control of the column and supporting structures during movement. The most essential and classic dynamic balance task is walking. Walking involves alternating use of one leg to support the body while the other swings from behind to in front of the body. There is an extensive knowledge base about normal and abnormal walking that is based on a set of biomechanical characteristics and uses a specialized terminology (Figure 106-1). Walking can be characterized by the pattern of steps using spatial factors such as step length, stride length (the distance between two heel contacts from the same foot), and step width. Walking can also be characterized by temporal factors such as double support time (the duration of the stride when both feet are on the ground at the same time) and cadence (step frequency). Walking has been described as "controlled falling" because the body column moves forward past the base of support and the feet must be timed to contact the support surface at the right location and time in anticipation of the moving location of the trunk.[32] When this timing is altered by disease, gait becomes irregular and trunk movement can be altered. Walking can also be characterized by changes in other body segments and joints. During normal walking, the foot begins a step with a push off from the toe, then lifting the foot to swing through and ending with a heel strike and forward rolling foot contact to initiate the next push off. The knee is in full extension at the time of toe push off, swings forward with slight flexion to aid foot clearance and then returns to full extension at the point of heel contact. The hip is in extension behind the trunk at push off and swings into flexion at heel contact. The arms swing alternately and in a sequence opposite to the step sequence of the legs. Biomechanical factors that have been found to be abnormal in fallers encompass both static and dynamic balance. Abnormal static balance associated with falling is manifested as increased sway during quiet standing. Some recent studies suggest that increased sway to the side, or medial-lateral plane, is especially associated with falls.[33] Alterations in dynamic balance among fallers are diverse depending on the underlying cause. Frequently observed abnormalities include prolonged double support time during walking, increased step width, increased trunk sway during movement, increased or decreased toe clearance, reduced hip extension, abnormal lateral stepping, and delayed correcting movements at the hip or ankle when the trunk is displaced.[34,35]

SCREENING

Screening for fall risk has two main goals: to identify persons at high risk and to identify remediable factors for intervention. Screening for risk alone can be more efficient than assessment for modifiable factors, so screening sequences that first identify risk and then assess remediable factors may make the best use of scarce resources. Since fall risk varies by population and type of fall, there is unlikely to be a single screening approach that works well in all settings. Certainly in diverse community populations, it makes sense to identify groups who are at low risk and who therefore can be spared more detailed, time-consuming assessments. Thus the American Geriatrics Society and the British Geriatrics Society have recommended falls screens that identify risk as (1) more than one fall in the last year, (2) one or more falls with injury, (3) self-report of unsteadiness, or (4) unsteadiness on performance testing.[36] Many older adults do not complain about falling to health care providers, so it is important to explicitly ask about falls. Some older adults fail to report falls because they forgot them. Some older adults may actively hide the fact that they are falling because they worry that family or providers will insist on relocation or activity restrictions. Screening in chronic care settings differs from screening in primary care. In chronic care settings, fall rates are often high and screening tools are more likely to have high false-negative rates. If prevalence is very high, it may be sensible to consider almost everyone as high risk and act accordingly. Fall risk screening in acute care is a high priority, but recently some have argued that no screening tool has high enough accuracy to justify the current investment in detailed admission fall screening since it consumes much nursing staff time with little real benefit.[37] In addition, general screens for functional problems in acutely ill hospitalized older adults may do as well at predicting falls as more specific falls screens and general screens can be used for multiple nursing issues.[38] There is some evidence that nursing global judgement is comparable in accuracy to formal screening tests in some chronic care settings.[39]

There are two main types of screening tools: those that are based on professional assessments of various historical and health factors and those that are based on observed performance of mobility and balance tasks. Some of the more common tools are described in Table 106-4. There are no clearly superior tools that have been shown to have high

Table 106-4. Scales Used for Fall Risk Screening and Balance Assessment

		SETTING		
Instrument	**Items**	**Community**	**Acute**	**Chronic**
Multifactorial Reports				
STRATIFY[55]	Five items: history of falls, agitation, visual impairment, frequent toileting, able to stand but needs assistance with moving		x	x
Morse falls scale[56]	Six items: history of falls, secondary diagnoses, parenteral therapy, use of ambulation aids, gait, mental status		x	x
FROP-Com [57]	13 risk factors in 26 items, fall and fall injury history, medications, medical conditions, sensory loss, feet, cognitive status, toileting, nutrition, environment, function, behavior, balance, gait (total score 0 to 60, fall risk high with score >24)	x		
Fall risk for residential care[58]	Among persons who can stand without assistance, poor balance, or (2 of 3 of fall history, nursing home residence, urinary incontinence) Among persons who cannot stand without assistance, any 1 of 3 (fall history, hostel residence, use of 9 or more medications)			x
Functional Mobility				
Berg balance test[40,59]	14 tasks scored 0 to 4; total range 0 to 56; fall risk increases as score decreases	x	x	x
Functional reach[60]	Distance reached in inches without moving the feet; fall risk <7 inches	x	x	x
Performance oriented mobility and balance[61]	Balance subscale score 0 to 16, gait subscale 0 to 12, summary score 0 to 28; summary score below 19 indicates high fall risk	x		x
Timed up-and-go[62]	Time in seconds to rise from a chair, walk 3 m, turn, walk back and sit down. <10 sec is normal. Fall risk increases with time >13.5 sec.	x		x
Dynamic gait index[41]	8 walking tasks scored 0 to 3, total score 0 to 24; <18 or 19 indicates fall risk	x		
Functional mobility tests[63]	Time to complete 8 step-ups (Alternate Step Test) >10 sec, timed sit to stand five times >12 sec, 6 m walk time >6 sec increased fall risk	x		
Physiologic profile assessment[64]	Performance in five domains: sway, reaction time, strength, proprioception, contrast sensitivity; total score 0 to >3. Fall risk increases with score of 2 or more.	x		

accuracy in multiple settings, so the optimal tool must be tailored to the population, the goals of screening, and the time and other resources available.

EVALUATION AND MANAGEMENT

Evaluation

When an individual has been identified as high risk for falls, then a more detailed evaluation is needed. The goals of evaluation are to (1) identify impairments that contribute to the problem, (2) gain an overall sense of mobility and balance capacity, and (3) consider special risk factors for injury. Since falling is multifactorial, multidisciplinary teams can provide a range of expertise. Disciplines that can make valuable contributions include physicians, nurses, physical therapists, occupational therapists, social workers, pharmacists, and others. Although the older adult should always be interviewed, other informants may be helpful. Table 106-5 illustrates elements of the history and physical examination that can be used to evaluate potential impairments. It is important to recall that older adults often have more than one impairment, so that finding one problem does not mean that there are not others as well. The history should include circumstances of one or more recent falls, history of injuries from falls, the course of the problem over time, associated symptoms and effect on overall mobility and activity. A fall description should include location, time of day, activity, symptoms, use of assistive devices, and ability to get up again. It is sometimes helpful to explore potential relationships to medication dosing schedules. Various patterns may suggest differing clusters of contributors. Recurrent backward falls tend to be associated with degenerative brain diseases. Acute onset is more likely to be due to a toxic or metabolic effect or perhaps an acute cerebrovascular or cardiac condition. Fear of falling can develop with or without a history of falling and can lead to severe activity restriction. Falls associated with dizziness may suggest some specific diagnoses (Table 106-6). Dizziness is common and nonspecific, so the interviewer must probe more deeply to distinguish potential contributors. True vertigo is defined as a hallucination of rotatory motion and is generally due to vestibular problems. Lightheadedness sometimes implies a sense of imminent loss of consciousness or presyncope. In this case, consider contributors to decreased cerebral perfusion. A third type of dizziness is perceived as "not in the head" and only occurs when upright. It may be an indicator of multisensory dysequilibrium, when more than one sensory impairment reduces the ability to monitor body position.

Medications are sometimes implicated in falls and can be among the most treatable contributors, so a thorough medication history is essential. Although there are long lists of medications with adverse effects on balance, there are just a handful of major mechanisms by which they cause falls. Common mechanisms include sedation, orthostatic hypotension, extrapyramidal effects, myopathy, and altered dark adaptation of vision. See Table 106-7 for examples of medications listed by potential mechanism. Persons who take multiple medications that alter balance are especially vulnerable.

Functional status should be assessed because mobility and balance are central to the ability to care for oneself and live independently. Many older adults use assistive devices for walking so it is important to explore when and how they were obtained, where they are used and not used,

Table 106-5. Clinical Assessment Based on Components of Postural Control

Organ System	Impairment	Clinical Evaluation	Potential Cause
Eye	Decreased acuity	Vision chart	Presbyopia, macular degeneration, cataracts
	Reduced visual fields	Confrontation, perimetry	Glaucoma, posterior circulation stroke
	Decreased depth perception	Stereo or depth testing	Monocular vision
	Decreased dark adaptation	Self-report, inability to dilate pupil in low light	Aging, miotic agents for glaucoma
Vestibular apparatus	Otoliths	Ability to detect true vertical, Hallpike maneuver	Benign positional vertigo
	Semicircular canals	Ability to detect position during rotation with eyes closed, nystagmus, visual acuity during head motion	Meniere's disease, vestibular hypofunction
Peripheral nerve	Peripheral neuropathy	Light touch, filaments, two point discrimination, vibratory sense	Diabetes, peripheral vascular disease, B_{12} deficiency
Circulation	Reduced cerebral perfusion	Low blood pressure, altered level of consciousness, lightheadedness	Medications, arrhythmias, postprandial hypotension
	Orthostatic hypotension	Positional change in blood pressure	Medications, autonomic dysfunction, dehydration
Brain	Reduced attention	Ability to perform dual tasks such as timed up-and-go with cup of water, executive function tasks	Mild cognitive impairment, dementia, medications
	Psychomotor slowing	Timed tapping, timed finger to nose test, trails A test (connect the dots)	Medications, degenerative and vascular brain diseases
	Altered postural reflexes	Absent or slowed righting reflexes	Parkinson's disease, other extrapyramidal and degenerative brain diseases
Muscle	Reduced strength	Manual muscle testing, strength-based functional performance (chair rise, squat)	Generalized: inactivity, sarcopenia, vitamin D deficiency, myopathies Focal deficits; spinal cord and peripheral motor nerve conditions
Musculoskeletal pain	Loss of flexibility	Contractures, decreased range of motion	Arthritis, inactivity
	Bone and joint deficits	Weight-bearing pain	Arthritis, fractures, periarticular conditions, foot problems
	Disturbance of spinal cord, roots, nerves	Leg and back pain with activity	Spinal stenosis, radiculopathies, peripheral neuropathies

Table 106-6. Differential Diagnosis and Management of Dizziness

Condition	Symptoms	Evaluation	Management
Orthostatic hypotension	Lightheadedness with change in position	Measure blood pressure in multiple positions, both immediately after change and then again after several minutes. Clinically important systolic drop is not well defined but is more likely to be significant if greater than 20 mm Hg or drops below 100	Taper or eliminate medications, fluorinated corticosteroids, salt loading, lower extremity muscle contractions before arising, compression hose
Arrhythmia, especially tachyarrhythmia or bradyarrhythmia	Lightheadedness or syncope not associated with position, occasionally with palpitations	Rhythm monitoring is important to capture symptomatic episode so monitoring may be prolonged.	Antiarrhythmic agents, medications for heart rate control, pacemakers
Benign paroxysmal positional vertigo (BPPV)	Short periods of true vertigo with head movement, even without upright body movement, such as rolling over in bed or looking up	Dix-Hallpike reproduces symptoms when in the head-down position and precipitates rotatory nystagmus in the direction of the involved ear.	Epley maneuver to reposition otolith debris; Brandt Daroff exercises
Meniere's disease	Severe episodes of vertigo with perceived ear pressure, decreased hearing, nausea, and vomiting	Usually diagnosed based on classic presentation, often incorrectly diagnosed when the true cause is not known	Diuretics, dietary modifications to reduce salt intake
Uncompensated vestibular hypofunction	Unsteadiness that worsens when vision is reduced; blurred vision with head motion	Rotational chair testing, caloric testing, dynamic visual acuity testing	Vestibular rehabilitation, optokinetic stimulation
Multisensory dysequilibrium	Sensation of lack of confidence in body position that only occurs when upright	Decreased sensory function in more than one sensory system (e.g., vision, vestibular, and peripheral sensation)	Treat sensory disorders, rehabilitation for use of sensory aids

and if there are areas of problem or concern. Since balance and mobility problems can limit function, it is important to determine if able and willing helpers are available. Older adults without access to helpers may be at special risk as they attempt to perform tasks that have become difficult.

Since the environment influences mobility and safety, a home assessment is an important element of falls evaluation. Although some aspects of the environment can be explored through an interview, a direct home assessment by professionals from a home visit agency can be invaluable. Key aspects of home assessment are described in Table 106-8.

Table 106-7. Medications That Affect Components of Postural Control

System Affected	Examples
CNS: attention and psychomotor speed	Benzodiazepines, sedating antihistamines, narcotic analgesics, tricyclic antidepressants, SSRIs, antipsychotics, anticonvulsants, ethanol
Basal ganglia and extrapyramidal system in general	Antipsychotics, metoclopramide, phenothiazines, SSRIs
Blood pressure regulation	Antihypertensives, antianginals, Parkinson drugs, tricyclic antidepressants, antipsychotics
Muscle: myopathy	Corticosteroids, colchicine, statins, ethanol, interferon
Pupil: miosis	Some glaucoma medications, especially pilocarpine

Table 106-8. Modifications for the Physical Environment

Area	Modifications
Lighting	• Nightlights in the bedroom, bathroom, and hallways leading to the bathroom • Keep a flashlight next to the bed • Timer or motion-activated lighting systems • Locate light switches near all doors and both ends of stairways
Flooring	• Nonglare, nonskid flooring • Avoid loose area rugs or used nonskid backing • Nonskid strips on steps • Bevel/ramp uneven transitions between rooms • Increase contrast at level changes
Stairwells	• Sturdy handrails, sometimes on both sides of steps • Chair lift (Stair Glide) • Rearrange rooms to achieve single-floor living
Bathroom	• Elevated toilet seat • Grab bars • Nonskid strips or mat on floor of shower or bathtub • Shower chairs • Tub bench
Kitchen	• Put common items at easily accessible height • Clear countertop clutter to maximize working space
Walkways	• Clear and straight as possible • Increase width by removing obstacles and furniture to accommodate walkers • Eliminate tripping hazards such as cords and tubing

The physical examination is useful to detect impairments that contribute to poor balance and to assess overall functional performance. Table 106-5 describes maneuvers that can be performed during the physical examination to detect impairments. Most of these assessments are familiar to health care providers, but a few are somewhat unique to balance assessment. Peripheral sensory testing is important since neuropathy is common among older adults. Although proprioception (joint position sense) is important for balance, testing is insensitive. Since proprioception and vibratory sensation use similar nerve fibers, testing vibratory sense may be more sensitive. A common strategy is to evaluate vibration detection using a 128 Hz tuning fork applied over a bony prominence such as the medial malleolus. The Romberg test, in which standing balance is compared with eyes open and closed, is a useful strategy for detecting visual dependence. An abnormal result suggests peripheral nerve or vestibular disorders. Abnormal muscle tone can indicate a variety of conditions. Increased tone implies upper motor neuron disease whereas decreased tone suggests lower motor neuron dysfunction. Increased tone can exist throughout the range of motion (lead pipe rigidity), or intermittently (cogwheeling rigidity). Coordination should be assessed in both the upper and lower extremities using tests of rapid alternating movements. Every balance assessment should include a test of righting reflexes. To perform the assessment, the examiner stands behind the patient, and asks the patient to prepare to respond to a push or pull with any reaction they prefer. The examiner pulls the patient's pelvis backwards sufficiently to displace the body outside the base of support. A normal response is a brisk step backwards. An abnormal response is a complete lack of stepping, called a "timber reaction." The patient can also be displaced to the side.

The evaluation is also used to determine functional mobility and balance capacity. Physical performance measures can serve as a guide, but it is important to target the performance assessment to the mobility capacity of the individual. Thus an older adult who is wheelchair-bound needs detailed assessment of bed mobility, transfers, and standing balance, whereas an active older adult may need more of a focus on high-level skills such as obstacle avoidance, dual tasks, and stair climbing. Table 106-4 includes commonly used functional performance assessment tools for mobility and balance. The Berg balance scale has been used to predict fall risk[40] but does not assess balance during walking. The dynamic gait index is especially helpful for detecting subtle higher level problems because it includes challenging conditions.[41] The performance-oriented mobility assessment (POMA) assesses static balance and gait and is widely used, but does not assess higher level functions.[42] Recently, balance assessments have added dual task tests that combine mobility assessment with distraction or a cognitive task. These divided attention tasks can sometimes uncover abnormal gait or balance not seen under usual simple conditions. Being unable to walk and talk at the same time is a risk factor for falls.[43] Reduced endurance during walking can create a sense of fatigue and leg weakness, so a long walk might be a useful element of the examination.

The third element of evaluation is to determine special risk factors for injury. Since fractures are a major cause of morbidity in fallers, every unsteady person should be assessed for osteoporosis. Another special concern is the risk of bleeding in persons who take anticoagulants. Loss of protective reflexes also increases the risk of injury. Since normal protective responses involve use of the upper extremity to moderate impact force and protect the head, injuries to the head, face, and orbit are especially worrisome. An absent righting reflex on physical examination is a significant indicator of increased risk of injury.

Management

The goals of management are to (1) treat impairments where possible, (2) build on systems that work well to compensate for deficits, and (3) provide physical and human resources to assist where necessary. Table 106-9 provides suggestions for management strategies based on the impairments

Table 106-9. Management of Impairments That Contribute to Instability and Falls

	Organ System	Impairment	Medical Management	Restorative Services	Environmental Modifications
	Eye	Decreased acuity	Corrective lenses	Low vision rehabilitation	Lighting
		Reduced visual fields	Prisms in spectacles	Low vision rehabilitation, teach to scan using head rotation	
		Loss of depth perception	Cataract removal if indicated	Teach to use shadows to detect depth	Lighting to accent shadows, contrast lighting
		Poor dark adaptation	Switch to glaucoma medications that do not cause miosis		
	Vestibular system	BPPV	Epley maneuver.	Vestibular rehabilitation	
		Meniere disease	Cautious use of meclizine, diuretics, rarely surgery	Vestibular rehabilitation	
	Peripheral nerve	Neuropathy	Footwear to protect foot and maximize sensation	Assistive devices for haptic enhancement	Handholds, railings
Central	Circulation	Reduced brain perfusion	Treatment varies by cause Arrhythmias: medications to control rate and rhythm, pacemakers Postprandial hypotension: frequent small meals		
		Orthostatic hypotension	Treatment varies by cause Adjust offending medications Autonomic neuropathy: salt loading, fluorinated corticosteroids Dehydration: hydration, reduce diuretic dose	Compression hose, calf muscle contractions	
	Brain	Reduced attention	Medication adjustment	Practice dual tasks	
		Psychomotor slowing	Medication adjustment	Practice movement speed	
		Abnormal righting reflexes	Antiparkinsonian medication helps bradykinesia more than balance	Assistive devices, practice getting up after a fall	Protective clothing
Effector	Muscle	Weakness	Reduced activity: treat contributing causes such as CHF, anemia, COPD, arthritis	Strength-training exercise	Raise chair height
			Focal motor deficit due to spinal stenosis: sometimes surgery	Orthotics, exercise, assistive devices	
			Myopathy: adjust offending medications, possibly steroids for myositis		
	Musculoskeletal	Decreased range of motion		Active and passive range-of-motion exercise, orthotics	
		Bone and joint pain	Analgesics, injections	Physical modalities such as heat, massage, assistive devices, orthoses, adaptive equipment	Place items within easy reach
		Spinal cord, roots, nerves	Injections, surgery, analgesics	Orthoses, assistive devices	Place items within easy reach

detected during the evaluation. As always, it is important to engage the older adult and family in the discussion of management options and to incorporate patient preferences into the plan.

Assistive devices can promote mobility in persons with balance problems through several mechanisms. In general, they all increase the base of support, thus increasing stability. Assistive devices can also provide sensory information about the walking surface directly to the upper extremity, and are especially helpful in this way to people with sensory loss in the feet. This ability to use sensory information from any part of the body to promote awareness of body position is called haptic sensation. Assistive devices should be professionally assessed and patients need training in proper use. Older adults notoriously acquire poorly fitting devices from family and friends. Canes increase the base of support and take up much less space than walkers. Walkers provide much more stability than canes but are more bulky and difficult to maneuver in tight spaces. Newer four-wheeled walkers are light weight and have hand-activated wheel locks, seats, and baskets that make them an attractive option for older adults. The larger wheels also make them more maneuverable on uneven sidewalks, grass, and gravel than the small wheels found on traditional walkers. Wheeled walkers also are easier to learn to use than traditional pick-up walkers.

Inappropriate footwear can be modified but there is no clear evidence to guide optimal characteristics of the shoe for falls reduction. Shoes with low wide heels promote stability. Shoes should fit comfortably but snugly so that the foot and the shoe move together. There is controversy about the optimal characteristics of the bottom of the shoe. Rubber soled shoes reduce pressure areas in persons with insensitive feet but also decrease sensory information about the walking surface. Hard leather soled shoes provide better sensory information and reduce tripping because they do not catch on surfaces, but increase the risk of slipping.

It is important to attend to the needs of the caregiver as well. Caregivers should receive training in body mechanics and transfer assists. They can also be educated about how to help get the older adult up after a fall.

Injury prevention is an important element of falls care. If a faller has had a fracture or is found to have osteoporosis, serious consideration should be given to prescribing appropriate medications. Hip protectors have been found to reduce injury in some studies but more recent data has shown less benefit.[44,45]

There is now a body of clinical trial evidence that supports the effectiveness of interventions to prevent falls.[46] Interventions that have been found to reduce falls include multiple risk factor reduction, professionally directed and individualized balance and strength rehabilitation, professionally led home hazard assessment and remediation, psychotropic medication withdrawal, Tai Chi group exercise, and cardiac pacemakers for fallers with cardioinhibitory carotid sinus hypersensitivity. Overall interventions yield about a 20% relative risk reduction and 10% absolute risk reduction, so there is certainly room for further improvement.

SYSTEMWIDE IMPLEMENTATION

There is now sufficient evidence from formal clinical trials to suggest that interventions to reduce falls may be effective in some settings.[7,47–49] Despite the evidence, these programs have not yet translated into systemwide changes in practice. Recent research suggests that translation to practice may be feasible and effective. A large nonrandomized study compared fall injury rates and medical service use between two comparable geographic regions before and after a systemwide intervention was implemented in one of the regions.[50] The intervention consisted of recommendations for medication reduction, management of postural hypotension, vision and foot problems, hazard reduction and training for balance, gait, and strength. Using multiple media, seminars, opinion leaders, and site visits, the intervention was targeted at primary care physicians, home health agencies, and emergency departments. Injury rates were lower in the intervention region and medical use increased less than in the usual care region. Other system interventions have been effective in emergency departments[51] but not nursing homes[52,53] or public health departments.[54] Keys to widespread implementation require that system barriers such as provider time limits, lack of knowledge, care fragmentation, and lack of reimbursement be addressed.[1]

SUMMARY

Falling is common and has serious consequences among older adults. Fallers often have multiple contributing impairments that interact to affect balance. Multidisciplinary interventions have been effective in some settings but evidence from research has not yet translated into usual clinical practice.

KEY POINTS

Falls

- Falling, especially recurrent falling, is a signal that health and function are failing in older adults.
- Most older adults who fall have multiple interacting impairments in the components of postural control.
- Systematic assessment and treatment planning is multidisciplinary and incorporates medical, rehabilitative, and psychosocial perspectives.
- The next major step in fall prevention is to disseminate evidence-based practices into health care systems.

For a complete list of references, please visit online only at www.expertconsult.com

Delirium

Eamonn Eeles
Ravi S. Bhat

INTRODUCTION

Delirium is typically an acute onset fluctuating disorder of consciousness. Profound alterations in the mental state of the affected person are manifest as impairments in arousal, attention, orientation, thinking, perception, and memory. Delirium often occurs in the setting of multiple physical illnesses and problems with a reciprocal impact on function. Not just a temporary suspension of cognitive abilities, delirium represents the susceptibility to adverse event through increasing functional dependence and aberrant behavior. Impaired mobility, falls, and fractures or pressure ulceration therefore add to the burden of illness.

Delirium is derived from the Latin *delirare,* meaning "to leave the furrow" and has long been recognized as a disturbance in the train of thinking.[1] The meaning of the term delirium has undergone many fluctuations over the last 200 years, but descriptions of delirium have maintained considerable stability over time with references to it in the writings of Hippocrates and,[2] in the Talmud,[3] and the Pancatantra.[4]

Delirium most commonly develops in frail elderly people. Thus rates of delirium are higher wherever there are greater numbers of frail elderly people, in other words, in hospitals and in long-term care settings such as nursing homes. However, despite equally greater density of health professionals in these settings delirium remains commonly underrecognized and thus poorly managed leading to a variety of adverse outcomes. By contrast, the prevalence of delirium in the community is low and may herald the presence of an underlying dementia.[5,6]

Evolution of the delirium concept and diagnostic criteria

Disturbance of consciousness is a characteristic feature of delirium that distinguishes it from the classical form of Alzheimer's disease and has also been the hardest to operationalize. It has been conceptualized in three different ways: as disruptions of the sleep-wake cycle; as part of continuum between alertness and coma; and as a disorder of attention.[7] Although sleep disturbances have long been recognized as a feature of delirium,[2] the evolution of consciousness and attention as features of delirium are relatively recent. Greiner's development of the concept "clouding of consciousness" in delirium[8] can be understood in the context of nineteenth century view that impairments in consciousness represented "organic" brain disease.[9] Clouding has come to refer to both a state of lowered arousal between alertness and coma[10] and a denseness of the medium in which psychic events occur,[11] leading to imprecision in its meaning. Geschwind's influential views,[12] based mainly on studies of delirium in younger adults,[13] paved the way for operationalization of delirium as an attentional disorder in modern classificatory systems.[14,15] However, disturbance of attention is not the sole cognitive disorder seen in, neither is it the sole preserve of delirium.[16] So it remains that disturbance of consciousness is the defining criterion for delirium.[17,18]

The international diagnostic criteria require different numbers and combinations of factors to diagnose delirium. For example the International Classification of Diseases-Tenth Edition (ICD-10)[18] requires five symptom characteristics to be present whereas the Diagnostic and Statistical Manual-Fourth Edition (DSM-IV)[17] requires only three and also specifies onset and causation more clearly. Unsurprisingly, DSM-IV is more inclusive and sensitive than ICD-10 in identifying delirium.[19–21] However, prognosis of delirium by different criteria sets of outcomes such as mortality and rates of institutionalization appear to be no different.[22]

Clinical features of delirium

Consciousness, or time-ordered serial awareness of self and the environment,[23] and its impairment may not be easily measured. Unable to gaze directly into the seat of consciousness, we can at least measure its component parts: arousal and attention. Alterations in arousal, or level of consciousness, may range from a hyperalert-hyperactive state—often accompanied by hallucinations, illusions, and delusions[24]—to a state of somnolence where the person is hypoalert and hypoactive.[25] Although the typical image of a delirious patient is one of a hyperactive and psychotic younger adult experiencing delirium tremens, older patients are more likely to be withdrawn and lying in bed or fluctuating between states of hyperalertness and somnolence.[26] This spectrum of psychomotor activity associated with delirium has been described since antiquity by terms such as *lethargus* and *phrenitis*.[2] The usefulness of the distinction has been called into question and is only of value if it relates to separate clinical outcomes.[7] In this regard, hypoactive delirium may represent a clinical casualty from the lack of an established definition; lack of archetypal "activated" features leaves it most vulnerable to misdiagnosis.[27,28] This poses a problem. The subtype of delirium that is most easily missed may also be associated with the worst outcome.[8,29] However, key components of established rating scales, namely delusions, variability, and mood lability have been shown to reproducibly discriminate between delirium subtypes.[30,31] The prospect of clinically systematizing psychomotor activity[32] may help to resolve some of the heterogeneity in delirium and improve the focus for future therapeutic interventions. Notwithstanding the abundant descriptive data concerning subtypes, the absence of standardized criteria represents a challenge and estimation of subtype frequency suffers.

As one of the core symptoms of delirium, the ability to focus, sustain and shift attention[12] forms a valuable, if incomplete, insight into the "sentry gate to consciousness."[33] Staff involved in daily care of older people often have difficulty in formally assessing inattention.[34] Accessibility to interview over a 2-minute period may be a simpler yet well validated measure to test attention.[35] Without formal assessment, cognitive decline may be unobserved and contributes to poor recognition of delirium in a variety of settings.[36–39]

Phenomenologic studies of delirium offer fresh insight into the development of psychopathology in delirium.[41] In their study Andersson et al[42] found that many patients simultaneously encountered past, present, and the realm of imagination as reality leading to apprehending these experiences both real and existing and unreal and nonexistent. Commonly patients think that they are being drugged, that there is a party going on or are in great danger. Patients may have visions of dead and yet not recognize family.[41] Within psychosis, hallucinations—visual or auditory—and delusions may be elicited and may be disturbing to patients and those around them.

Acuity of onset, usually over hours to days, is a core feature delirium of but is not peculiar to it?[17] Vascular dementia may share abrupt changes.[42,43] This may pose a diagnostic challenge as cerebrovascular insults are especially important in the occurrence of delirium in the elderly without significant predisposing factors.[44] Prevalence rates of these conditions may vary in acute settings[45] and may help in determining the likelihood of the diagnosis. Accurate history taking is helpful when patients come to the hospital as are serial cognitive assessments once patients are admitted.[46] Nursing staff may observe troublesome nocturnal behavior while their colleagues encounter with incredulity the same patient placid by day. Fluctuation of symptoms also is a characteristic of dementia with Lewy bodies (DLB)[47]; once again prevalence rates are helpful in determining the likelihood of the condition. Acuity of onset, fluctuating course, and classically but contentiously short lived and reversible, delirium is a consequence of underlying illness.[48] Early recognition then becomes important to addressing the cause and optimizing the outcome.

Differential diagnoses

Most patients with dementia that arrive acutely to the hospital will have, or will develop, a delirium (32% to 89%)[49] and represents a large, growing yet uncharted portion of hospital care.[49,50] As the clinical features may be similar, behavioral changes in an individual with dementia can be mistakenly normalized by the contribution of environmental change or perceived as a natural sequelae of dementia.[51] Greater than expected deterioration of cognition, along with new onset of hallucinations and delusions, is suggestive of a superimposed delirium.[52] Rating tools discriminate from dementia,[53] although they may not be entirely helpful in daily practice.[54]

Investigations, in particular the electroencephalogram (EEG), offer an adjunct to clinical assessment. Well described and replicated, the pattern of "diffuse slowing"[55] on EEG can help to distinguish a delirium from the following conditions: delirium superimposed on dementia,[56] temporal lobe epilepsy, and nonconvulsive status. Undoubtedly useful even in older patients,[57] an EEG requires a level of patient compliance and therefore becomes of questionable value where behavioral problems supervene. Further, it is supplementary to and not a replacement for the less invasive and more achievable focus of robust, bedside clinical and cognitive assessment.

Of all the dementias, DLB is perhaps the closest mimic of delirium with many features common to both the disorders. The sharply contrasting treatment strategies between both conditions make this a difficult but important distinction to make. The cause and natural history provides guidance to this predicament. DLB is a neurodegenerative disorder, and has an insidious onset in contrast to the acute onset with underlying systematic upset in delirium. Parkinsonian features should also alert the clinician to the possibility of underlying DLB. Delirium is an unwelcome but often frequented visitor among the dementias. DLB is no exception to the hazard of delirium, and dopaminergic therapies may potentiate this risk.[58] Careful follow-up and avoidance of precipitants for either condition is a pragmatic approach to management in the context of ongoing clinical uncertainty.

Depression and delirium may share "negative symptoms" and even a broad range of cognitive deficits.[59] The mood changes observed as part of the delirium syndrome, particularly hypoactive delirium, may account for the tendency to misdiagnose the two conditions. However, acute onset of mood change, particularly in a hospitalized older patient, represents a delirious event until proven otherwise. Failure to systematically exclude delirium may result in such patients receiving antidepressants mistakenly leading to a worsening of the condition both by the addition of a psychotropic[60] and the resultant inadequate treatment of delirium.

Prevalence

Delirium afflicts most acutely hospitalized, frail, older patients. The setting of the emergency department mixes increasing presentations of older patients with acute illness.[45] Such risk factors translate to a high prevalence of delirium within the emergency department of between 26% and 40% in older patients.[61] Clinicians who are more removed from the distal consequences of delirium often fail to undertake cognitive assessment.[61] Furthermore, even when cognitive assessment is performed, it does not always register with a diagnosis of delirium or affect management.[62] Pressures within an emergency department represent barriers to appropriate care for individuals at risk of delirium. These are not insurmountable; an education program and geriatrician support may help to realign the inequity of emergency health care provision to those most vulnerable.[61] In-hospital nonstandardized reported rates of delirium vary widely, typically 20% to 30%.[63] Delirium frequency is dependent on the hospital population under study with higher prevalence of 43% to 61% noted following hip fracture.[64] Prevalent delirium, encountered on admission and incident delirium, precipitated during the hospital stay, may represent different populations with the same syndrome. Both may occur with a similar frequency of around one third of acutely hospitalized patients.[63] The intensive care unit is a potent conflagration of illness severity and iatrogenic insult as to be inevitably bound with delirium[65] with a prevalence of around 70% in patients over 60 years of age.[66] Validated screening tools[67,68] have been developed for use even when individuals are unable to speak. As with all other clinical arenas that encounter delirium, mandatory screening has been recommended,[69] although the role of intervention strategies is as yet uncertain.

Delirium permeates beyond the acute sector. Prevalence of delirium in nursing homes varies from 32% to 62%.[70] Even with a conservative estimate, delirium and subsyndromal delirium[71] still represent a significant and largely unexplored health burden in postacute facilities. Chronicity of symptoms in these settings neither alleviates the consequences of delirium nor defines the best management for those in institutionalized care.[72] Many, if not most, individuals dying from chronic illness experience delirium.[73,74] The inextricable link between the two has called into question the poor outcome associated with delirium by not controlling for delirium experienced as part of the dying process.[75]

And yet the end stage of any chronic illness does not always have a predictable path nor does delirium impose an imminent sentence of death.[73] As yet, nothing within the delirium syndrome offers the ability to distinguish a temporarily recoverable process from a "terminal drop" but is worthy of future enquiry. In the meantime, an interdisciplinary focus with consensus driven management is advised.[76] A common pathway and range of causes is probable. General prevention and management strategies should be considered when an individual has not entered the terminal stage of illness or if they can be implemented without adding to the suffering of the dying process.

Causes and risk factors

Delirium is caused by multiple factors. Cause in medicine is often associated with the idea of a single cause that arose from the success of the germ theory in the nineteenth century.[77] There have been two major areas of focus on the pathophysiology of delirium: the cholinergic hypothesis[78,79] and more recently the role of proinflammatory cytokines.[80] The cholinergic hypothesis essentially attributes causation to reduced cholinergic input in the brain[79] and has lead to useful measures that offer the prospect of a role in delirium prevention.[81–83] However, this does not account for the other major player in delirium: infections, a problem addressed by proinflammatory cytokines. Recent studies have found an association generally between cytokines and delirium[84] and specifically with their rising levels and to onset of delirium.[85] The hypothesis is that with increased inflammatory activity in the dementing brain, peripheral cytokines lead to delirium.[80] In the end these remain unsatisfactory because they do not account for the multifactorial nature of delirium causation. Rationalizing the wealth of potential and multiple causes into commonly associated groups may assist in learning[86] and translate to better management. Despite its pragmatic appeal, this version lacks the ability to determine a hierarchy of cause and fails to offer a testable model of causation.

Given the conceptual limitations, development of a model of delirium has been refined to incorporate predisposing and precipitating factors.[87] Consistently identified, independently associated predisposing factors include older age, male gender, visual impairment, dementia and cognitive impairment, depression, functional dependence, immobility, fracture on admission, dehydration, alcoholism, increased comorbid conditions, previous stroke, and azotemia. Frailty is an underlying theme. Similarly, independently associated precipitating factors include medications, such as sedative hypnotics and narcotics; severe acute illness; infections, especially urinary tract infections; metabolic abnormalities especially hyponatremia; hypoxemia; shock; anemia; pain; physical restraint use; bladder catheter use; any iatrogenic event; intensive care unit treatment; surgeries; and high number of procedures in hospital.[88–91] From this list it is then possible to identify individuals who are predisposed to delirium upon whom preventative interventions have been successfully implemented.[92] However, this model while superficially similar to the vulnerability-stress models used in psychiatry,[93] has implicit assumptions which may not hold true in the context of delirium. Risk factors such as male gender are useful in predicting delirium but unlike vulnerabilities,[93] do not provide a template for causal mechanism. Moreover, the temporal separation between predisposing and precipitating factors may be relatively short, making separation of vulnerability and stress an arbitrary distinction. Finally, the model fails to provide an account for the multiple interactions between illnesses, physiologic states, and interventions that typically occur in the setting of delirium.

So how may we speculate on cause in delirium and under what conceptual framework? Illness can be considered as the somatic anomaly and its current or potential manifestations.[94] In older patients, each somatic anomaly individually is not sufficiently provocative enough to generate a delirium. Geriatric syndromes, such as delirium, are disorders of higher order function that are impaired because of complex interactions between multiple remote but interrelated components. This accounts for why tracking other higher state variables such as mobility and balance as markers of delirium progress makes sense. In the case of delirium, consciousness and its "clouding" is the victim of such physiologic disarray. The components of consciousness that are relevant in delirium are arousal, attention, and time perception.[95] In this untested model, delirium results when a critical number of mechanisms responsible for these functions in potentially different combinations fail.[95] This model accommodates the cholinergic and inflammatory cytokines because both these factors can significantly affect arousal mechanisms.[96–98]

Prevention of delirium

Is the occurrence of delirium in frail older individuals who are medically unwell an inevitability or can it be prevented? Landmark multicomponent intervention studies by Inouye et al[99,100] built on their predictive model have evolved to address multiple factors with favorable outcome unsurprisingly dependent upon adherence.[101]

The evidence for prevention of delirium is most compelling within a surgical setting.[102] A large study of proactive geriatric consultation versus usual care was undertaken in the setting of hip fracture.[103] The recommendations made, essentially basic aspects of good care, achieved a reduction of 33% in cases of delirium compared with usual care.[103] Delirium severity was also reduced with the greatest benefits extending to those without dementia and least functional limitations. Lundström et al[104] have since replicated these findings with reduced incidence, duration, and complication rate of multidisciplinary care in an orthopedic setting.

The benefits may extend to a reduced delirium rate in a cost-effective manner within a geriatric unit[105] associated with an improvement in outcome. What remains unanswered is the part of geriatricians' intervention that promotes success. The elixir may owe its healing properties to comprehensive geriatric assessment. If this is the case, then uptake relies on little more than initiative, support, and a basic skill set to be adopted by other disciplines.

The role of factors before engagement with acute care has up until recently received scant attention. The future is promising; exercise reduces the incidence of both dementia[106] and delirium[107] and promotes an active lifestyle for the maintenance of healthy cognition into midlife and beyond.

These studies endorse the function of geriatricians within a variety of settings and oppose the perception that delirium is inevitable, even in frail individuals who have experienced a grave insult such as a hip fracture. Clinicians, and in particular geriatricians, are in a position to direct education and implement multicomponent strategies with a deliverable reduction in delirium.

Delirium education can arguably play a role in delirium prevention. Nurses and personal care workers (nursing assistants or aides) are involved in the day-to-day care of many elderly, both in hospitals and residential care facilities, with doctors and specialists having intermittent contact. Training requirements, scope of practice, and philosophical orientation of these groups differ between themselves and from medical doctors and may contribute to different rates of delirium recognition. It has been suggested that philosophical orientation of nurses to health and aging may influence recognition.[108] Nurses using a healthful perspective, that is regarding "good health" in aging as normal, were most likely to differentiate between acute confusion and chronic confusion.[51]Delirium nonrecognition in this group may also be related to insufficient knowledge of cognitive deficits.[109] Studies of recognition of delirium by nurses have shown that nurses assessed disorientation the best or limit their assessment of cognition to disorientation[110–112] and failed to recognize behavioral aspects of delirium because of a tendency to normalize such behaviors.[110] Delirium education may thus have to address both teaching of clinical skills and enhancing the ability to question stereotypes.

Delirium evaluation

The identification and treatment of the underlying cause affords the only possibility of vanquishing delirium. Untreated delirium represents a high risk of adverse event through pressure ulcers, falls, and fractures[113] made worse by overbearing or constrictive medical endeavors to reduce behavioral problems. Great zeal may be given over to describing the array of possible causes.[114] However, ruthlessly pursuing pathology in an older patient with delirium, allowing for exceptions, may be inappropriate, threaten dignity,[115] and ultimately misses the point. In delirium, as with other geriatric syndromes, multiple common pathologies associated with aging and their treatments are most often responsible[116] and can be evaluated in the main without redress for invasive procedures. Firstly, recognizing that delirium is a sensitive marker of illness should trigger a sensible and proportionate screen for underlying causes. The presence of multiple co-morbidity and polypharmacy challenges standardized treatment regimes and an individualized approach to management of the cause in a frail, older patient should be considered. It should be recognized that delirium may persist even after discharge and highlights the need to track the course of delirium to resolution.

A few exceptions should be noted. Delirium in the older patient is sometimes a consequence of disease of the brain, such as stroke or infection, and should be considered, particularly when the clinical picture is associated with focal neurologic signs. In addition, drug withdrawal states, such as delirium tremens, usually comprise a different natural history and management strategy and are important to recognize and screen for. Regular cognitive assessment is important[46] to track the delirium, in addition to measurment of other higher state variables, such as mobility and balance that share sensitivity to disturbance of higher order failure.[54]

Rating scales in the evaluation of delirium have at least a couple of roles: identification of delirium and delineation of severity (see Table 107-1). The first allows for more systematic assessment of older people, such that delirium is clearly identified and the latter can help in evaluating change over time. In the absence of biologic markers, rating scales are dependent on operationalization of core features of a disorder. Delirium rating scales without some of the core features such as impaired attention have performed well in expert or trained hands in the identification of delirium. How can this be so? It may be that it is the systematic assessment of an older patient's mental state that is important because it allows for recognition of change in presentation based on clinical observation rather than reactions to patient behaviors. The research requirements of delirium rating scales are slightly but not vastly different to that in clinical practice. The issues of reliability and validity become more important. Many delirium rating scales have not been adequately tested for interrater reliability (IRR) and it has been suggested that IRR should be tested on all occasions when these scales are used in research.[117] The validity that is tested is often construct validity because delirium is a well-described but not well-validated entity.

Drug treatment

Not without promise, the role of cholinesterase inhibitors in delirium has been studied with the hope of correcting the central cholinergic deficit described as part of the syndrome.[78,79,118] Donepezil has failed to demonstrate a benefit[119] in terms of reduction in the incidence of delirium although larger studies are called for. Antipsychotic medications such as haloperidol have no preventative role in delirium.[120–121] However, low dose haloperidol (<3.0 mg/day) associated with decreased severity and duration but not incidence of delirium in postoperative patients compared with placebo controls in one study. Although haloperidol may be equally efficacious as risperidone or olanzapine,[121] it can pose a risk if DLB is mistaken for delirium. Atypical antipsychotics, by contrast, offer

Table 107-1. Clinical Tools and Their Role in Delirium Evaluation

Screening and Diagnosis	Screening, Diagnosis and Severity	Severity
Brief cognitive tests (Abbreviated Mental Test; Mini Mental State Examination)	Confusional State Evaluation (CSE)	Confusion Rating Scale (CRS)
Clinical Assessment of Confusion-A (CAC-A)	Delirium Assessment Scale (DAS)	Delirium Index (DI)
Cognitive Test for Delirium (CTD)	Delirium Rating Scale (DRS)	Delirium Severity Scale (DSS)
Confusion Assessment Method (CAM)	Delirium Rating Scale-Revised-98 (DRS-R-98)	
Confusion Assessment Method-ICU (CAM-ICU)	Delirium Symptom Interview (DSI)	
Delirium Observation Screening Scale (DOSS)		
NEECHAM Confusion Scale (NCS)		
Organic Brain Syndrome Scale (OBS)		
Saskatoon Delirium Checklist (SDC)		

less in the way of extrapyramidal side effects[122] but some may be associated with hyperglycemia[123] and increased risk of stroke.[124] Consideration should also be given to the inability to metabolize drugs in individuals who are frail[125,126] or delirious.[127] Drugs are not a replacement for good care and should be deliberated over only when adequate nonpharmacologic management strategies have been implemented. Neuroleptic agents may have a potentially justifiable role in the diminution of recall distress[128] but this is as yet without evidence.

Management of delirium

Recognition of delirium is half the battle yet one that is often poorly fought. Untreated delirium may have dire consequences. Educational strategies provide an improved knowledge base for clinicians[129] and better detection rates for delirium.[129,130] Unfortunately, consensus-based clinical guidelines fail to generate improvement in the management of delirium.[131] Interventions for other disorders that visibly impact on patient outcome have revolutionized how such conditions are perceived. Before thrombolysis, stroke received little interest compared to today, despite its ever present burden on disability and death. Delirium may lack a single dramatic intervention with which to inspire prescribers but this does not diminish its impact. Knowledge translation has the task of overcoming the obstacles to taking delirium seriously and challenge current attitudes and processes of care (see Table 107-2).

Multicomponent intervention has a sound basis on the grounds of the multifactorial nature of the condition (see Table 107-2). However, the evidence is far less clear than for preventative strategies.[132] Delirium, in a surgical setting, is amenable to reduction in duration and severity, but these benefits do not extend to the medical population.[133] Good geriatric care may hasten recovery from delirium with sustained cognitive outcomes at 1 year.[134] Any other health benefits observed have not extended to the longer term[100] and may only be cost-effective for targeted populations.[135] As yet, there is no robust evidence to direct management strategies for delirium superimposed on dementia.[136]

What is to be made of the limited body of evidence based recommendations in the management of delirium? It may simply reflect that such strategies do not work but does not excuse efforts to institute what makes sense and is good medicine.[137] The optimization of a patients environment has a sound basis and is worthy of consideration. Orientation represents assimilation of information acquired through sensory information from the outside world. Sensory deficits, accrued with advancing age, may be compensated for in a person's familiar environment to maintain orientation. Hospitals present a myriad of novel sensory stimulation. Inability to selectively process this external information as part of attention deficit within delirium may lead to misperception of sensory input, such as hallucinations or illusions, and worsen an already unravelled state of orientation. The interaction between the individual and his or her environment becomes readily appreciated as important for modulating the course of delirium. The role of optimization of sensory function is a standard of care in older hospitalized patients made more crucial by its speculated role in delirium.

Table 107-2. Strategies for Optimizing Care at an Institutional and Individual Patient Level in the Prevention and Management of Delirium

DELIRIUM PREVENTION AND MANAGEMENT			
SYSTEM APPROACH		INDIVIDUAL MANAGEMENT	
Challenge	**Management**	**Factor**	**Intervention**
Delirium knowledge gap	• Knowledge translation of established clinical guidelines to multidisciplinary team • Implementation of education strategies	Clinical uncertainty	• Intensity of management proportional to likely cause and commensurate with degree of frailty/expected outcome
Poor detection rate of delirium	• Mandatory screening in high risk and prevalence settings • Specialist delirium liaison services	Drugs	• Rationalize anticholinergic and other central nervous system acting medications
Postdelirium risk of dementia	• Development of memory clinics • Partnerships with other disciplines • Links with voluntary support groups • Raising the public awareness of delirium	Interventions	• Avoid if possible: integrate risk of delirium into judgment of best interests • Incorporate risk of delirium into informed consent/assent process
Inappropriate ward placement	• Prioritize timely transfer from acute to geriatric care • Reduce total ward transfers	Nutrition and hydration	• Assess and monitor • Consider guidance for feeding
Inappropriate ward environment	• Plan ward layout individual rooms and nursing input	Sensory abilities	• Screen visual and hearing abilities • Provide and optimize function of any aids used
Inadequate prior health care planning	• Encourage formal living will in frail/vulnerable individuals to assist future management and goals of care	Orientation	• Provide reorientation strategies: photographs, day-night lighting entrainment, encourage family involvement
Insufficient evidence to guide management	• Investigate the role of targeted intervention strategies • Flexibility to identify and pursue best location for management of the individual patient (e.g., palliative care, home, geriatrics)	Medical care	• Consider and correct multiple potential contributors • Track delirium with serial cognitive assessment, mobility, balance, and function • Early rehabilitation

The dearth of rigorous studies has prompted the evolution of largely consensus-based guidelines in the management of delirium.[138] Nevertheless, experts have a high level of agreement over recommendations[139] in the absence of supportive data that have a basis beyond just common sense.

Consideration of risk of delirium accompanying a procedure, while not always quantifiable,[140] should be integral to the informed consent process in an older patient.[141] The breakdown in cognitive abilities may affect the reliability of the history but also the competency of an individual with delirium to make decisions regarding their medical care and participation in research.[142–144] Proxy decision makers, because of the acute nature of onset, may not adjust easily to the gravitas of the decision-making process required by the condition. Nevertheless, collateral history is essential to ascertain the history, presence of prior cognitive impairment, and to clarify goals of treatment.[138] Comprehensive geriatric assessment provides an ideal framework with which to capture this information and affect outcomes.[145]

Prognosis

Delirium has profound and wide reaching consequences, including increased length of hospital stay,[146] higher rates of institutionalisation[147] and deaths,[20,72,148–150] cognitive impairment,[147,150] psychiatric morbidity,[151] patient distress,[128] functional decline,[152,153] and caregiver stress.[154,155]

As the demographic burden of delirium increases, so too will the number of survivors with impairment, the caregiver requirements, and economic cost of their care.[156] This may negate postdelirium interventions to affect outcome, which remains an unexplored area. Interdisciplinary services, despite the absence of evidence-based management strategies, should adapt to the perceived increase in need that follows in the wake of delirium.[138]

Conclusions and future directions

Delirium imposes a toll on the individual, caregiver, and society with personal, health care, and economic consequences. Delirium is well described and despite clinical tools, educational strategies, and clinical guidelines, its recognition is consistently poor and its burden continues to grow. It is no accident that delirium is most commonly seen within a hospital setting and illness severity offers some insight into this. Hospital process—fragmented care, multiple transfers, and iatrogenic events—provide the catalyst for much of delirium witnessed in this group of older, cognitively vulnerable individuals.[87] Yet delirium can be prevented by using a constellation of interventions that boils down to individualized but basic care without redress for additional high technology therapies. Prevention becomes all the more important when it is considered that management is based on unclear evidence. The lack of knowledge concerning management reinforces the need for regular screening for delirium because this affords the best prospect of diagnosing underlying illness that can be treated. Such insults should be sought and treated in the context of the patient and in the majority of cases will reflect commonly seen conditions.

Recognizing delirium is a challenge but by systematic application of validated tools in at risk older patients we can do better. Furthermore using the resources that are at hand, namely relatives and the multidisciplinary team, to gather a complete picture of an individual over time may enhance capture of this dynamic condition.

As frailty advances and death approaches, delirium becomes a common theme. Seen in nursing homes and the palliative care setting alike, interventions to prevent or dampen the course of delirium in the dying should be considered and implemented when not adding to the burden of suffering.

Understanding the interaction of pathophysiologic mechanisms in the determination of a deliriant threshold offers the prospect of using targeted strategies to prevent and manage delirium.

Geriatricians, psychiatrists, and the multidisciplinary teams are the groups with the greatest impact on outcomes in delirium. However, the growing burden of delirium is too overwhelming to deal with alone. Only by the dissemination of our skills beyond our conventional boundaries, including the community, can delirium be dealt a blow. Policy, inspiration, and knowledge translation have become the next frontier for geriatricians in the battle for minds in delirium.

KEY POINTS

Delirium

- Delirium is a common, underrecognized disorder among institutionalized and frail older patients.
- Education strategies improve knowledge and recognition of delirium and should be tailored to the health professional.
- Standardized assessment tools incorporating cognitive evaluation are an essential part of screening for delirium and monitoring its progress.
- Delirium is often multifactorial in etiology and the causes reflect common problems in older individuals.
- Delirium can be prevented by promoting good basic care in the form of multicomponent intervention strategies.
- Delirium is associated with a poor outcome and cognitive follow-up is recommended.

For a complete list of references, please visit online only at www.expertconsult.com

HAPTER 108

Constipation and Fecal Incontinence in Old Age

Danielle Harari

This chapter describes the epidemiology, risk factors, clinical presentation, assessment, and treatment of constipation and fecal incontinence (FI) in older adults. Data sources were a PUBMED/MEDLINE database was searched (1966 to 2008) for relevant abstracts and papers using the following keywords: constipation, impaction, anal, bowel, faecal, fecal, incontinence, urinary, laxatives, enemas, suppositories, and other relevant phrases such as "comprehensive geriatric assessment," "stroke," etc. Additional articles were identified by examining reference lists, Cochrane, and other recent systematic reviews. Levels of evidence are as used by the U.S. Preventive Task Force[1]:

- Good evidence: Level 1 - consistent results from well-designed, well-conducted studies
- Fair evidence: Level 2 - results show benefit, but strength limited by number, quality, or consistency of studies
- Poor evidence: Level 3 - insufficient because of limited number, power, or quality of studies

INTRODUCTION

Fecal incontinence (FI) in older people is a distressing and socially isolating symptom and increases the risk of morbidity,[2,3] mortality,[4,5] and dependency.[3,5] Many older individuals with FI will not volunteer the problem to their general practitioner or nurse. Regrettably, health care providers do not routinely inquire about the symptom, which is why it is a routine prompt in a standard comprehensive geriatric assessment. This "hidden problem" can lead to a downward spiral of psychological distress, dependency, and poor health. The condition can especially take its toll on informal caregivers of home-dwelling patients,[6] with FI being a leading reason for requesting nursing home placement.[7,8] Even when older people are noted by health care professionals to have FI, the condition is often managed passively (e.g., pads provision without assessment). Current surveys show limited awareness of appropriate assessment and treatment options among primary care physicians.[9] The importance of identifying treatable causes of FI in frail older people is strongly emphasized in national and international guidance,[8,10,11] but audit shows that adherence to such guidance is generally poor, with nonintegrated services, and suboptimal delivery by professionals of even basic assessment and care.[12,13]

Constipation is a common concern for adults as they age beyond 60, reflected by a notable increase in primary care consultations and burgeoning laxative use. Older people reporting constipation are more likely to have anxiety, depression, and poor health perception. Qualitative studies show they feel doctors can be dismissive about the problem, and that useful and empathic professional advice is hard to find,[14] and this is confirmed in primary care studies where GPs view constipation as less important than other conditions (such as diabetes).[15] Clinical constipation in frail individuals can lead to significant complications such as fecal impaction, FI, and urinary retention precipitating hospital admission. Constipation and FI are costly conditions, with high expenditure including laxative spending and nursing time.[6] For instance, it is estimated that 80% of community nurses working with older people in the United Kingdom are managing constipation (particularly fecal impaction) as part of their case-load.

DEFINITIONS

The WHO International Consultation on Incontinence defines FI as "involuntary loss of liquid or solid stool that is a social or hygienic problem.[11]" There is, however, a lack of standardization in defining FI in published prevalence studies hindering cross-study comparisons. Most community-based studies examine prevalence of FI occurring at least once over the previous year, which may overestimate prevalence, but does also provide the upper limit for FI occurrence. Nursing home studies mostly measure weekly or monthly occurrence. Systematic reviews examining FI prevalence have highlighted the need for consensus on definitions.[16,17]

Definitions of constipation in older people in medical and nursing literature have also been inconsistent. Studies of older people have defined constipation by subjective self-report, specific bowel-related symptoms, or by daily laxative use. Self-reported constipation (e.g., "Do you have recurrent constipation?") often means different things to different individuals.[15] It is now increasingly required in both clinical practice and research to use standardized definitions for constipation based on specific symptoms (Rome II and III criteria)[18–20] (Table 108-1). Important constipation subtypes affecting older people such as rectal outlet delay are easier to identify by using standard definitions.[18,20] Rome criteria are symptom-based: objective assessment relies on finding fecal loading in the rectum and/or colon. Such objective assessment is particularly important in frail older people in whom constipation can be underestimated (Table 108-2).

PREVALENCE OF CONSTIPATION AND CONSTIPATION-RELATED SYMPTOMS

Constipation is a hugely prevalent problem in older people. Approximately 63 million people in North America meet the Rome II criteria for constipation, with a disproportionate number being over 65 years old.[21] Age is strongly associated with nonspecific self-reporting of constipation.[22–24] It is therefore striking that the report of infrequent bowel movements (≤ 2 per week) is no more prevalent in older than younger people in community-based studies:

- Only 1% to 7% of both younger and older people report ≤ 2 bowel movements a week.[22,24,25]

- This consistent bowel pattern across age groups persists even after statistical adjustment for greater laxative use among older people.[22]
- Of older people complaining of constipation, less than 10% report ≤ 2 weekly bowel movements, and more than 50% move their bowels daily.[24,26]
- In contrast, two thirds have persistent straining and 39% report passage of hard stools.[26]

The symptoms predominantly underlying self-reported constipation in older people tend therefore to not be infrequent bowel movements, but straining and passing hard stools. Difficult rectal evacuation is a primary cause of constipation in older people. Twenty-one percent of community-dwelling people aged 65 and over have rectal outlet delay (Table 108-1),[27] and many describe the need to self-evacuate.[14,27] Two thirds of nursing home residents taking laxatives still report frequent straining.[28] Among these frailer individuals, difficult evacuation can lead to recurrent rectal impaction and overflow. Fecal impaction was a primary diagnosis in 27% of acutely hospitalized geriatric patients admitted over the course of 1 year in the United Kingdom,[29] and a survey of patients with FI found that fecal loading was present in 57% of older acute hospital inpatients and 70% of care home residents.[30] Frail older people do have a higher prevalence of ≤ 2 weekly bowel movements, affecting one third of care home residents reporting constipation.[31] Up to 80% of care home residents are constipated according to Rome III criteria,[32] a surprising figure considering that 50% to 74% of long-term care residents use daily laxatives.[31,32]

Table 108-1. Definitions of Constipation

Definition
Constipation (Rome III criteria)
Two or more of the following symptoms present on more than 25% of occasions for at least 12 weeks in the last 12 months:
2 or less bowel movements per week
Straining at stool
Hard stools
Feeling of incomplete evacuation
Rectal outlet delay (Rome II criteria)
Feeling of anal blockage at least a quarter of the time and
Prolonged defecation (>10 minutes to complete bowel movement); or
Need for self-digitation (pressing in or around the anus to aid evacuation) on any occasion
Clinical constipation
Large amount of feces (hard or soft) in rectum on digital examination and/or
Colonic fecal loading on abdominal radiograph

Table 108-2. Factors Potentially Leading to Underestimation of Constipation and FI in Frail Older People

Frail older people may:
• Be unable to report bowel-related symptoms due to communication or cognitive difficulties
• Have regular bowel movements despite having rectal or colonic fecal impaction
• Have impaired rectal sensation and inhibited urge to go and so be unaware of rectal stool impaction
• Have nonspecific symptoms associated with colonic fecal impaction (e.g., delirium, anorexia, functional decline)
• Be less likely to have symptoms of urgency associated with FI and more likely to have passive leakage

PREVALENCE OF FECAL INCONTINENCE IN OLDER PEOPLE

Table 108-3 summarizes data on prevalence and risk factors in FI. Meta-regression analysis of prevalence studies in community-dwelling people shows that age has a significant influence on rates of solid and liquid FI.[17] Prevalence is equal between genders in older people, except in the care home setting where it is greater in men.[33–36] One prospective study conducted in French nursing home residents[4] found a baseline FI prevalence of 54%, and a 10-month incidence in those continent at baseline of 20%. New-onset FI was transient (<5 days) in 62%, and long-standing in 38%. In the latter group, 1-year mortality was 26% compared with 7% in those who remained continent. The prevalence of FI varies according to the general health of the study population and therefore by proxy to the study setting:

- Community: 6% to 12% age over 65 and 18% to 29% age over 80[5,6,33,37–41]
- Acute hospital: 14% to 33% age over 65[42,43]
- Long-term care: 37% to 54%.[4,31,35,36,42]

Of note, United Kingdom care home studies have shown wide variations in prevalence between individual homes,[35,41] that may well be more reflective of different standards of care, rather than of different patient characteristics.

These prevalence data represent case-finding statistics within epidemiologic studies, but in real clinical settings FI is often overlooked. This is through both older people not help-seeking ("it is embarrassing" and "nothing that can be done"), and providers not case-finding and not following through when the problem is identified. Less than 50% of home-dwelling older people with FI (or their caregivers) have discussed the problem with a health care professional in British primary care surveys.[44] Younger women are more likely to seek help for less severe FI symptoms than older women,[45] yet even in younger cohorts in most cases of FI are still unrecognized by GPs.[46] Poor provider awareness of FI is just as prevalent in institutions despite greater opportunity for patient observation. In the acute hospital setting, only 1 in 6 of patients reporting FI have the symptom documented by ward nursing staff,[47] and care home nursing staff are aware of FI in only half of those residents self-reporting the condition.[31] Professional ignorance about how to treat FI may in part underlie this: a recent UK care home survey found that trained staff cited advanced age as the main cause of both urinary and fecal incontinence.[48] Auditing bowel care in care homes to improve quality of care may seem a solution but this proved challenging in a recent United Kingdom high profile nationwide audit of urinary and fecal incontinence care in older people.[13] Many care homes declined participation, and those who did partake generally reported hampered data collection due to limited access to clinical records and information technology, and staff shortages. The audit did however show that patients admitted to

Table 108-3. Epidemiology of FI in Older People and Recommendations for Identifying Cases

Epidemiologic Data Summary

- FI affects 1 in 5 older people (aged 65 and over) living in the community, and half of those resident in care homes.[1]
- Prevalence of FI increases with age alone, particularly in the eighth decade and beyond.[1]
- The prevalence of FI is higher in the acute hospital and nursing home setting than in the community,[1] thus the group most affected is frail older people.
- The prevalence of FI in frail older people is equal to or greater in men than women.[2] This predominance of older men over women with FI is most striking among nursing home residents.[2]
- The prevalence of FI varies dramatically between institutions in nursing home studies.[2]
- FI coexists with urinary incontinence in the majority of frail older people.[1]
- Aside from age, the following are primary risk factors for FI in older people[2]:
  - Loose stool
  - Impaired mobility
  - Dementia
  - Neurologic disease
  - Chronic medical conditions
  - Depression
- Fecal loading and constipation are clinically linked to FI, but there is little epidemiologic work assessing this association.
- Physicians and nurses in primary care, acute hospital, and long-term health care settings do not have a high awareness of FI in older people.[2]
- Within nursing homes, there is a low rate of referral by nursing staff of residents to primary care physicians or continence nurse specialists for further assessment of FI[2] and there is a tendency toward passive management (e.g., use of pads only without further evaluation).[2] Fecal loading is often present in older care home residents with FI.[2]
- Older people may be reluctant to volunteer the symptoms of FI to their health care provider[2] for social or cultural reasons, or due to a popular misperception that the condition is part of the aging process and therefore "nothing can be done about it."
- FI is associated with reduced quality of life and poor health perception.[2]

Recommendations: Identifying FI in Older People

- Bowel continence status should be established by direct questioning and/or direct observation in:
  - All nursing and residential home residents
  - Hospital inpatients aged 65 and over
  - People aged 80 and beyond living at home
  - Older adults with impaired mobility
  - Older adults with impaired cognition
  - Older adults with neurologic disease
  - Older adults with chronic disease
- Primary care staff, hospital ward staff, and long-term care staff should routinely inquire about fecal incontinence in frail older patients.
- Inquiry about FI should be systematic and include stool consistency, severity of FI, and impact on activities of daily living and quality of life.
- Health care providers should be sensitive to cultural and social barriers discouraging patients from talking about the condition.
- Frail older patients with restricted ability to access primary care, such as nursing home residents, and those with mobility, chronic illness, or cognitive impairments, should be screened for FI through systematic case-finding methods.
- Systematic outreach program that make it easier for frail older people and those who care for them to volunteer the problem to their primary care provider should be implemented.
- There are significant geographic variations in provision of specialist expertise in bowel care (both medical and nursing) nationally and globally, which may affect case-finding in older people.
- Further examination of underlying reasons for the variations in prevalence of FI between nursing homes (standards of care, patient case-mix, reporting) is needed.
- Urinary and fecal incontinence often coexist; continence care workers (e.g., nurse specialists) should be trained in identification and management of fecal and urinary incontinence in older people.
- Key requirements to improving detection in the practice setting should be implemented:
  - Education of health care workers to embed both a sense of value in identifying FI, plus confidence that the condition can be treated
  - Protocols should be in place clarifying all details of screening inquiry (who will ask, how to ask, when to ask, and who to ask)
  - Patients and caregivers should have access to educational materials at the point of inquiry

these care homes with preexisting FI tended to be placed on a containment management plan rather than being assessed for causes and possible treatment, and this was despite having good access to continence specialist care. On a similar theme, a recent U.S. National Institutes of Health State-of-the-Science Statement commented that health care provider education alone is not enough to improve the identification of adults with FI and recommended key requirements to improve detection in the practice setting (Table 108-3).[8]

RISK FACTORS FOR FI AND CONSTIPATION IN OLDER PEOPLE

Urinary incontinence is strongly linked to FI, with 50% to 70% coexistence in community-based studies.[2,34,39,49] Perhaps unsurprisingly, diarrhea or loose stool is a strong predictor for FI in all settings, but what is striking is the prevalence of chronic diarrhea in frail older people.[2,6,36,41] Medical comorbidity and physical disability are equivalent or greater than age in strength of assocation.[2,3,6,34,49] A cohort study of community-dwelling patients aged 65 and over found that severe FI (at least once weekly) was associated with increased mortality after 42 months, independent of age, gender, and poor general health.[5] Depression is repeatedly linked, though cause or effect is clearly impossible to discern from cross-sectional analyses.[2,49,34] Independent factors for FI in acutely hospitalized patients (in order of strength of association) are loose/liquid stool consistency, illness severity, and older age.[43] In elderly hospital inpatients, contributing factors are fecal loading (57%), functional disability (83%), loose stools (67%), and cognitive impairment (43%)[30]; those with loose stools and less comorbidity are more likely to have transient FI with resolution after 3 months.

Most risk factor studies for constipation are cross-sectional, but one prospective study examined baseline characteristics predictive of new-onset constipation (≤ 2 bowel movements per week or persistent straining) in elderly U.S. nursing home patients.[50] Seven percent (n = 1291) developed constipation over a 3-month period. Independent predictors were poor consumption of fluids, pneumonia, parkinson's disease, decreased bed mobility, greater than 5 medications, dementia, hypothyroidism, white race, allergies, arthritis, and hypertension (the latter 3 conditions were postulated to be associated primarily because of the constipating effect of drugs used to treat them). What is evident is that many of these factors are potentially modifiable. Table 108-4 summarizes practice guidance in constipation based on the epidemiologic data described below.

Reduced mobility

Greater physical activity (including regular walking) is associated with less constipation symptoms in older people living at home.[23,51] Reduced mobility is the strongest independent correlate (following adjustment for age and comorbidities) of heavy laxative use among nursing home residents,[52] and gut transit time in bedridden elderly subjects can be as long as 3 weeks.[53] Exercise increases colonic propulsive activity ("joggers diarrhea"), especially when measured postprandially.[54] In a survey of younger women (36 to 61 years), daily physical activity was associated with less constipation (≤ 2 bowel movements per week), and the association strengthened with increased frequency of physical activity.[55] This leads to speculation that increasing physical activity in adulthood may reduce the likelihood of constipation problems in older age. Epidemiologic studies in older people have repeatedly shown that poor mobility is also a strong risk factor for FI after adjustment for other variables.[3,4,6,34,36]

Polypharmacy/drug side effects

Polypharmacy itself increases the risk of constipation in older patients, particularly in nursing homes where each individual takes an average of six prescribed medications per day.[53] Certain drug classes are particularly implicated. Anticholinergic medications reduce contractility of the smooth muscle of the gut via an antimuscarinic effect at acetylcholine receptor sites, and in some cases (e.g., patients with schizophrenia taking neuroleptics), long-term use may result in chronic megacolon. Anticholinergic medications have been independently associated with daily laxative use in nursing home studies,[53] symptomatic constipation in community-dwelling older U.S. veterans,[56] and FI in elderly stroke survivors.[57] Although older people are certainly susceptible to the constipating effects of opiate analgesia, a study of nursing home residents with persistent nonmalignant pain showed equivalent constipation rates in chronic opiate users and nonusers over a 6 month period; those taking opiates showed improved function and social engagement.[58] Chronic pain is often undertreated in frailer older people, possibly through fear of adverse effects of analgesic drugs, so it is important to note that constipation in this context can be effectively managed by laxative and suppository coprescribing. Transdermal patches (e.g., fentanyl) are associated with lower constipation risk than sustained-release oral morphine.[59] All types of iron supplements (sulfate, fumarate,

Table 108-4. Practice Guidance for Constipation Based on Epidemiologic Evidence

Screening

- Constipation symptoms should be routinely asked about in patients aged 65 and over in view of the high prevalence of the condition in this population.
- Men and women in their eighth decade and beyond should be regularly screened for constipation symptoms, as prevalence increases with advancing age.
- Periodic objective assessment for constipation in elderly nursing home residents should be incorporated into routine nursing and medical care. Patients unable to report symptoms due to cognitive or communication difficulties should be especially targeted. Such an assessment should occur at minimum every 3 months (3 monthly incidence rate of new-onset constipation is 7% in nursing home residents), and optimally monthly.

Identifying Risk Factors

- The identification of risk factors for constipation in older people is critical to effectively managing the condition.
- The following are risk factors for constipation in older people:

Polypharmacy (5 medications)[2]
Anticholinergic drugs (tricyclics, antipsychotics, antihistamines, antiemetics, drugs for detrusor hyperactivity)[1]
Opiates[2]
Iron supplements[3]
Calcium channel antagonists (nifedipine and verapamil)[2]
Calcium supplements[2]
Nonsteroidal antiinflammatory drugs[2]
Impaired mobility[2]
Nursing home residency[2]
Dementia[2]
Parkinson's disease[1]
Diabetes mellitus[1]
Autonomic neuropathy[2]
Stroke[3]
Spinal cord injury or disease[1]
Depression[3]
Dehydration[2]
Low dietary fiber[3]
Hypothyroidism
Hypercalcemia
Hypokalemia
Uremia
Renal dialysis[3]
Mechanical obstruction (e.g., tumor, rectocele)
Lack of privacy or comfort
Poor toilet access[3]

- Systematic identification of multiple risk factors in vulnerable older people with constipation should be incorporated into good practice guidelines in all health care settings
- Patients at increased risk of constipation from recognized comorbidities (e.g., Parkinson's disease, diabetes) should be regularly assessed for the condition

Assessment

- Identifying specific bowel symptoms in older individuals reporting constipation is important to guide appropriate management of this common complaint.
- Reduced bowel movement frequency is not a sensitive symptom indicator for constipation in community-dwelling older people, though it is specific.
- Difficulty with evacuation and rectal outlet delay are primary symptoms in older individuals.
- An objective assessment should be undertaken in frail older people with constipation because these patients are at increased risk of developing complications.
- Increased wandering and agitation in patients unable to communicate due to dementia should prompt an assessment for constipation.
- Older patients being prescribed laxatives on a daily basis should be regularly reviewed for symptoms of constipation and rectal outlet delay, and treatment should be appropriately adjusted.

and gluconate) cause constipation in adults, the constipating factor being the amount of elemental iron absorbed.[60] Slow-release preparations have a lesser impact on the bowel because they carry the iron past the first part of the duodenum into an area of the gut where elemental iron absorption is poorer. Intravenous iron does not cause constipation and can be an alternative in patients with chronic anemia (e.g., chronic kidney disease) who become constipated on oral iron. Constipation was the main side effect in a 5-year study of calcium supplementation in older women (treatment 13.4% versus placebo 9.1%).[61] Calcium supplementation reduced bone turnover and fracture rates in women who took it, but long-term compliance was poor, and constipation may have contributed to this. Calcium channel antagonists impair lower gut motility, particularly in the rectosigmoid.[62] Severe constipation has been reported in older patients taking calcium channel antagonists, with nifedipine and verapamil being the most potent inhibitors of gut motility within this class. Nonsteroidal anti-inflammatory drugs (NSAIDs) increase the risk of constipation in older people, most likely through prostaglandin inhibition. In a large primary care study, constipation and straining were more prevalent reasons for stopping NSAIDs than dyspepsia.[63] NSAIDs have also been implicated in increasing the risk of stercoral perforation in patients with chronic constipation. Aluminium antacids have been associated with constipation in both nursing home[52] and community settings.[64]

Dietary factors

Low consumption of fiber in the form of wheat bran, vegetables, and fruit predisposes toward constipation, and in the United Kingdom, consumption of all of these decreases with advancing age. Community studies of older Europeans who eat a Mediterranean diet rich in fruit, vegetables, and olive oil show lower rates of constipation (4.4% in people aged 50 and over).[65] A study of nutritional factors within all the nursing homes in Helsinki found an association between malnutrition and constipation.[66] This may be two-way in that marked constipation can cause anorexia, whereas low calorie intake can promote constipation. Constipation is a recognized problem in patients receiving enteral nutrition. A prospective survey of older hospitalized patients receiving nasogastric tube feeding identified constipation as a complication of treatment in 30% of patients.[67] Enteric feeding products containing fiber are available, though there are no data on whether constipation is any less of a problem with their use.

Low fluid intake in older adults has been related to symptomatic and slow-transit constipation.[50,68] Withholding fluids over a 1-week period in young male volunteers significantly reduced stool output.[69] Elderly people are generally at risk of dehydration because of:

- Impaired thirst sensation
- Less effective hormonal responses to hypertonicity
- Limited access to drinks because of coexisting physical or cognitive impairments
- Voluntary fluid restriction in an attempt to control urinary incontinence

Population studies have suggested that alcohol consumption is a preventive factor for constipation symptoms in both men and women.[51,55]

Diabetes mellitus

Over half of diabetic outpatients report constipation symptoms, with neuropathy symptom scores correlating with laxative usage and straining.[70] Diabetic autonomic neuropathy can result in slow colonic transit and impairment of the gastrocolic reflex.[71] However, one third of diabetic patients with constipation do not have neuropathic symptoms,[70] so unrelated reversible factors (e.g., drugs, mobility, fluids) should be considered, particularly in older people. Colonic transit time in frail older people with diabetes and constipation is extremely prolonged at a mean of 200 hours.[72] Administering acarbose, an alpha-glucosidase inhibitor with a potential adverse effect of causing diarrhea significantly reduced transit in these patients.[72] Diabetes is a risk factor for the development of FI, especially in men.[73] FI may occur through mechanisms of[1] bacterial overgrowth resulting from prolonged gut transit causing characteristic nocturnal diarrhea and[2] multifactorial anorectal dysfunction (reduced basal and squeeze pressures, spontaneous relaxation of the internal anal sphincter, reduced rectal compliance, abnormal rectal sensation).[71,74] Acute hyperglycemia can further inhibit anorectal function and colonic peristalsis.

Neurologic diseases

Patients with Parkinson's disease (PD) suffer from multiple primary pathologies that lead to constipation:[1] dopaminergic neuron degeneration and increased presence of Lewy bodies in the myenteric plexus prolonging colonic transit (independent of age, physical activity, medications),[75,2] pelvic dyssynergia causing rectal outlet delay and prolonged straining,[75,3] and small increases in intraabdominal pressures on straining. Constipation can become prominent early in the course of the disease, even before motor symptoms developing. In a 24-year longitudinal study, less than one bowel movement a day was associated with a threefold risk of future PD in men.[76] Fifty-nine percent of PD patients report constipation according to Rome criteria, with 33% being very concerned by their bowel problem.[77] Antiparkinsonian drugs may further exacerbate constipation. Pelvic dyssynergia affects 60% of people with PD, and may be hard to treat. Botulinum toxin injected into the puborectalis muscle has been used to improve rectal emptying in PD patients with good effect, though repeat injections every 3 months are required to maintain clinical benefit.[78]

Dementia predisposes individuals to rectal dysmotility,[29] partly through ignoring the urge to defecate. Epidemiologic studies show a significant association between cognitive impairment and nurse-documented constipation in nursing home residents. Patients with non-Alzheimer's dementias (PD, Lewy body, vascular dementia) compared with those with Alzheimer's are more likely to suffer from constipation as part of autonomic symptoms.[79] Constipation in long-term care residents unable to communicate due to dementia has been linked to physically aggressive behavior[80] and development of wandering behavior[81] by independent association.

Depression, psychological distress, and anxiety are all associated with increased self-reporting of constipation and with FI in older persons. The symptom of constipation can also be somatic manifestation of psychiatric illness. A careful assessment is required to differentiate subjective complaints from clinical constipation in depressed or anxious patients.

Constipation affects 60% of those recovering from stroke on rehabilitation wards,[82] and a high number of these have combined rectal outlet delay and slow transit constipation.[83] Major FI is 4½ times more prevalent in stroke survivors than the nonstroke population.[84] FI may develop months after acute stroke and can be transient, consistent with constipation with overflow as one possible cause.[57] Epidemiologic data suggest that FI is associated more with disability-related factors (particularly functional difficulties in using the toilet, and anticholinergic medications) than stroke-related factors (e.g., severity and lesion location).[57,84,85] Weak abdominal and pelvic muscles following stroke also contribute to problems with evacuation.

Metabolic disorders

Hypokalemia and hypomagnesemia produce neuronal dysfunction that minimizes acetylcholine stimulation of gut smooth muscle, and so prolongs transit through the gut. This should especially be looked for and corrected in acute colonic pseudo-obstruction. Hypercalcemia causes conduction delay within the extrinsic and intrinsic gut innervation of the gut neuromuscular bowel dysfunction (which may be reversed following parathyroidectomy). Constipation is not an unusual presentation for clinical hypothyroidism, particularly in older women. Patients on long-term renal hemodialysis have prolonged age-adjusted transit time[86]; 63% complain of constipation, with important contributors being high (49%) use of resin to prevent hyperkalemia, suppression of the defecation urge while undergoing dialysis, and low fiber intake.[87] Resin administration can increase the risk of impaction in frail older patients also.

Colorectal cancer

Following adjustment for age and potential confounders, ≤ 2 reported bowel movements a week was associated with a greater than twofold risk of colon cancer in a U.S. study, with the association being stronger in women than men; no association was seen with laxatives.[88] Comparing underlying causes for FI in younger and older men shows colon and prostate cancer to be significantly more common in the older group,[89] so the index of suspicion for colorectal cancer should be higher in older adults with bowel symptoms.[90]

Diverticular disease

A case-control study of patients (mean age 68) with acute uncomplicated diverticulitis showed 74% to have prolonged transit.[91] Left-sided diverticulosis coli affects 30% to 60% of people over the age of 60 in developed countries. High intraluminal pressures while straining at stool in people who have a low fiber diet contributes to the cause of the condition.

PATHOPHYSIOLOGY OF CONSTIPATION AND FI IN OLDER PEOPLE

Physiologic studies suggest that changes in the lower bowel predisposing toward constipation in older people are not primarily age-related. This is compatible with the epidemiology showing that bowel movement frequency does alter with aging, and that constipation symptoms are more prevalent in older people with comorbidities. Extrinsic causes such as reduced mobility, fluid intake, dietary fiber, comorbidities, and medication all impact colonic motility and transit, and influence the pathophysiology of constipation. Studies of anorectal function do, however, show age-related changes predisposing to FI.

Colonic function

Colonic motility depends on the integrity of the central and autonomic nervous systems, gut wall innervation and receptors, circular smooth muscle, and gastrointestinal hormones. Propagating motor complexes in the colon are stimulated by increased intraluminal pressure generated by bulky fecal content. Studies of total gut transit time (passage of radiopaque markers from mouth to anus, normally 80% passed within 5 days), colonic motor activity, and postprandial gastrocolic reflex show no differences between healthy older and younger people.[92–94] Conversely, older people with chronic constipation do have prolonged transit of up to 9 days.[92,95] Markers pass especially slowly through the left colon with striking delay in the rectosigmoid, suggesting that total transit time is prolonged because of segmental dysmotility in the hindgut.[96] The prolongation is even greater in institutionalized or bedridden older patients with constipation, with transit time ranging from 6 to greater than 14 days.[53] Slow transit results in a cycle of worsening constipation by reducing stool water content (normally 75%) and shrinking fecal bulk, which then diminishes intraluminal pressures, and hence the generation of propagating motor complexes and propulsive activity. Aging is associated with some intrinsic physiologic mechanisms that may alter colonic function, predisposing older people to this "constipation cycle":

- Reduced number of neurons in the myenteric plexus and impaired response to direct stimulation,[96,97] leading to intrinsic myenteric dysfunction
- Increased collagen deposit in left colon leading to altered compliance and motility[97]
- Reduced amplitude of inhibitory junction potentials and hence inhibitory nerve input to circular colonic muscle causing segmental motor incoordination[98]
- Increased binding of plasma endorphins to gut receptors after age 60[99]

Anorectal function

In normal defecation, colonic activity propels stool into the rectal ampulla causing distention and reflexic intrinsically mediated relaxation of the smooth muscle of the internal anal sphincter (or anal canal). This is followed promptly by reflex contraction of the external anal sphincter and pelvic floor muscles, which are skeletal muscles innervated by the pudendal nerve. The brain registers a desire to defecate, the external sphincter is voluntarily relaxed, and the rectum evacuated with assistance from abdominal wall muscle contraction. There is a tendency toward an age-related decline in internal sphincter tone and thickness particularly beyond the eighth decade.[94,100–102] This reduction in internal anal sphincter pressure lowers the threshold for balloon (stimulated stool) expulsion, and is much more notable in frail older people with FI.[103,104] There is a clear age-related decline (greater in women than men) in external anal sphincter and pelvic muscle strength,[100,101] which may contribute to both incontinence and evacuation difficulties. Rectal motility appears to be unaffected by healthy aging,[94] but an age-related increase in anorectal sensitivity thresholds, and reduced rectal compliance has been observed, starting at an earlier age in women than men.[105] Patients with dementia and FI tend to exhibit multiple uninhibited rectal contractions in response to rectal distention.[103] Younger women with FI are more likely to have isolated anal sphincter defects (often child-bearing related),[106] whereas the anorectal pathology is more multifactorial in older women, including pudendal neuropathy, hemorrhoidectomy, diabetes, and rectal and vaginal prolapse.[45,107] Failure of the anorectal angle to open and excessive perineal descent in older women can also lead to constipation,[97] and consequent prolonged straining may compress the pudendal nerve further exacerbating any preexisting neuropathy. Table 108-5 describes the three main types of anorectal dysfunction that predispose older people to rectal outlet delay.

CLINICAL EVALUATION

The causes of FI and constipation in older people are usually multifactorial. Comprehensive geriatric assessment (evaluating medical, functional, and psychosocial factors in addition to the bowel) is key to identifying all contributing causes and developing a goal-focused management plan. There is much room for improving standards of bowel assessment in older people in current routine practice; surveys indicate a lack of thoroughness by doctors and nurses in all settings, with failure to obtain an accurate symptom history or to perform rectal examinations.[13,108] A recent U.K. audit in older patients with FI in primary care, acute hospital, and care home settings showed that only 50% of individuals within each setting had a history taken, only 22% to 33% had a basic examination documented (history and rectal), and cause(s) for FI was documented in only 27% to 49%, the 27% being in the acute hospital sector.[13]

Clinical history

It is helpful to have patients or caregivers keep a stool chart for 1 week to document bowel pattern and episodes of FI. Self-report of bowel symptoms are generally reliable and reproducible in older cohorts, including those in long-term care.[109–111] Proxy responses by informal caregivers for questions concerning FI have also been shown to concord well with index responses given by older patients.[112]

Documentation of stool consistency is diagnostically critical[8] for both FI and constipation, and the pictorial Bristol stool chart is commonly used to aid patients in describing their stool. Overflow fecal incontinence typically presents as frequent passive leakage of watery stool, sometimes confusing patients and caregivers (and occasionally health care providers) into thinking they have "diarrhea" rather than constipation. Patients with anal sphincter dysfunction tend to leak small amounts of stool, with urgency before leaking where external anal sphincter weakness predominates, and more passive (unconscious) leakage when internal sphincter dysfunction is the main cause.[113] Fecal urgency and/or loose stool should prompt investigation for diarrheal disease (see FI treatment). Patients with dementia-related incontinence tend to pass complete formed bowel movements, usually after meals. A recent history of altered bowel habit should prompt an exploration of precipitants (e.g., medications, stroke), and where unexplained, an evaluation for colorectal cancer. Abdominal pain, rectal bleeding, and certainly any systemic features such as weight loss and anemia should prompt further investigations for underlying neoplasm. IBS should be a diagnosis of exclusion in older people, and only made in those with a long history of IBS symptoms (Table 108-6). Abdominal pain is a warning symptom for constipation complications such as impaction with obstruction, stercoral perforation, sigmoid volvulus, or urinary retention. Rectal pain associated with defecation in older people may be due to rectal ischemia and other more common anorectal conditions. Urinary incontinence and lower urinary tract symptoms (frequency, urgency, straining and hesitancy, dysuria, nocturia) frequently coexist with FI and constipation[107,114] and should be characterized, and urinalysis and postvoid bladder residual volume measurement (preferably by hand-held scan) undertaken if present.

Fecal impaction

In frail patients, fecal impaction may present as a nonspecific clinical deterioration; more specific symptoms are anorexia, vomiting, and abdominal pain. Findings on physical

Table 108-5. Types of Anorectal Dysfunction Causing Rectal Outlet Delay in Older People

	Pathophysiology	Clinical Picture
Rectal dysmotility	Reduced rectal motility and contractions Increased rectal compliance Variable degree of rectal dilation Impaired rectal sensation with blunting of urge to pass stool Over time, increasing rectal distention required to reflexively trigger the defecation mechanism	Rectal hard or soft stool retention on digital examination of which patient may be unaware Chronic rectal distention leads to relaxation of the internal sphincter and fecal soiling One postulated cause is diminished parasympathetic outflow as a result of impaired sacral cord function (e.g., from ischemia or spinal stenosis). May also develop through persistent disregard or suppression of the urge to defecate as a result of dementia, depression, immobility, or painful anorectal conditions.
Pelvic floor dyssynergia	Paradoxical contraction or failure to relax the pelvic floor and external anal sphincter muscles during defecation Manometric studies show paradoxical increases in anal canal pressure on straining	Severe and longstanding symptoms of rectal outlet delay Parkinson's disease More common in younger women
Irritable bowel syndrome (IBS)	Increased rectal tone and reduced compliance Lower pain threshold on distending the rectum during anorectal function tests	Usually constipation-predominant in older people Rome criteria symptoms: abdominal distention or pain relieved by defecation, passage of mucus, and feeling of incomplete emptying

Table 108-6. Diagnosis of Constipation and FI in Older People

Bowel History
Number of bowel movements per week
Stool consistency
Straining/symptoms of rectal outlet delay
Fecal incontinence/soiling - frequency
Duration of constipation symptoms or FI
Irritable bowel syndrome symptoms (abdominal pain, bloating, passage of mucus)
Rectal pain or bleeding
Laxative use, prior and current
Psychological and quality of life impact of bowel problem
Urinary incontinence/lower urinary tract symptoms
Pad use and laundry changes
General History
Mood/cognition
Symptoms of systemic illness (weight loss, anemia)
Relevant comorbidities (e.g., diabetes, neurologic disease)
Mobility
Diet
Medications
Toilet access (location of bathroom, manual dexterity, vision)
Specific Physical Examination
Digital rectal examination including external and internal sphincter tone
Perianal sensation/cutaneous anal reflex
Rectal prolapse/hemorrhoids
Pelvic floor descent/rectocele
Abdominal palpation, auscultation
Postvoid residual volume
Neurologic, cognitive, and functional examination
Tests
Indications for plain abdominal radiograph
Empty rectum with clinical suspicion of fecal impaction
Persistent fecal incontinence despite clearing of any rectal impaction
Evaluation of abdominal distention, pain, or acute discomfort
Persisting complaints of constipation with increasing laxative usage
Indications for colonoscopy
Systemic illness (weight loss, anemia, etc.)
Bleeding per rectum
Recent change in bowel habit without obvious risk factors
Indications for anorectal function tests
Severe or persistent symptoms of rectal outlet delay, suggesting pelvic dyssynergia
Persistent FI with preserved anorectal sensation and clinically weak anal sphincter

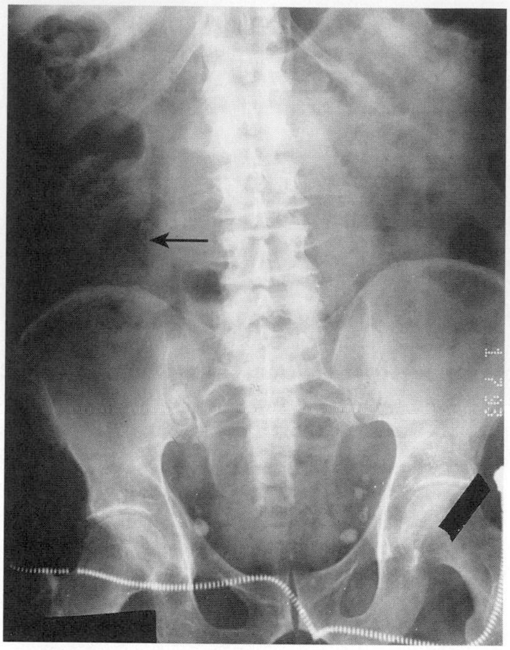

Figure 108-1. Abdominal radiograph of a 73-year-old man with chronic schizophrenia who has taken anticholinergic neuroleptics for many years. This was his third hospital admission for colonic impaction. The arrow points to the cecum, which is full of stool, indicative of slow transit. Fecaliths are visible in the pelvic region.

examination may include fever, delirium, abdominal distention, reduced bowel sounds, arrhythmias, and tachypnea secondary to splinting of the diaphragm. The mechanism for the fever and leucocytosis response is thought to be microscopic stercoral ulcerations of the colon. A plain abdominal radiograph will show colonic or rectal fecal retention associated with lower bowel dilation (Figure 108-2). Presence of fluid levels in the large or small bowel suggests advanced obstruction; the closer the fecal impaction is to the ileocecal valve, the greater the number of fluid levels seen in the small bowel.

Rectal and pelvic examination

Stool impaction on digital rectal examination does not have to be hard; soft stool retention is commonly seen in older people taking laxatives who have problems with rectal outlet delay. Absence of stool on rectal examination does not exclude the diagnosis of constipation.[23] A dilated rectum with diminished sensation and retained stool suggests rectal dysmotility. Digital assessment of squeeze and basal tone has been shown to be as sensitive and specific as manometry in discriminating sphincter function between continent and incontinent patients aged over 50.[115] Easy finger insertion with gaping of the anus on finger removal indicates poor internal sphincter tone, whereas reduced squeeze pressure around the finger when asking the patient to "squeeze and pull up" suggests external sphincter weakness. Preserved sensation (urge to stool, awareness of wind) improves likelihood of response to anal strengthening maneuvers. Absent cutaneous-anal reflex (gentle scratching of the anal margin should normally induce a visible contraction of the external sphincter) and, in particular, perianal anesthesia points to sacral cord dysfunction with possible related gut neuropathy. Proctoscopy is a simple, quick, and useful test for diagnosing internal hemorrhoids, and abnormalities of the rectal wall.

Perineal examination is relevant in view of the association between urogenital prolapse (particularly rectocele) and FI in older women.[107] An examination for posterior vaginal prolapse (bearing down in the gynecologic position) is appropriate in all women with constipation, especially those reporting incomplete rectal emptying. Excessive perineal descent is observed by asking the patient to bear down while lying in the lateral position. Normal perineal descent is less than 4 cm (can be eye-balled by drawing an imaginary line between that ischial prominences). Rectal prolapse may also be observed in this manner, though lesser degrees of prolapse may be only identified by having the patient strain while sitting on a toilet or commode. FI is a primary independent risk factor for pressure sores in older people,[6,116] so

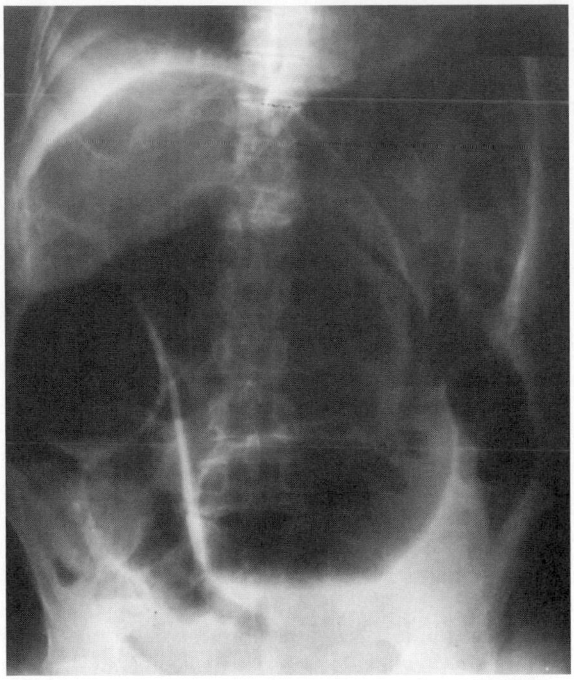

Figure 108-2. Abdominal radiograph of an 83-year-old man with Parkinson's disease and long-standing symptoms of continuous fecal leakage. As his caregiver at home, his wife was changing his clothing up to six times a day. The rectosigmoid colon is completely impacted, and the dilated bowel loop implies obstruction. He was briefly hospitalized for disimpaction with enemas and laxatives, resulting in complete resolution of incontinence. He and his wife were educated in regular use of laxatives and suppositories, and in lifestyle measures.

evaluation of skin integrity (with pressure ulcer risk assessment) is important.

Rectosigmoid fecal loading may impinge on the bladder neck causing a degree of urinary retention.[117,118] Constipation increased the risk of urinary retention fourfold (other predictors being urinary tract infection and previous urinary retention) in hospitalized women aged 65 and over.[118] Urinary symptoms of difficult voiding are unreliable in diagnosing retention in older people, so is good practice to do screening postvoid residual volumes in the setting of constipation and FI.

Plain abdominal x-ray

Incontinent patients without evidence of rectal stool impaction should ideally undergo a plain abdominal radiograph to establish or rule out the diagnosis of overflow. Abdominal x-ray is required in the presence of abdominal pain or dilation to identify impaction with obstruction and more severe complications, such as sigmoid volvulus, colonic pseudo-obstruction, and stercoral perforation.[95] Acute colonic pseudo-obstruction (Ogilvie's syndrome) is most likely to occur in hospitalized frail older people with a history of chronic constipation who are acutely medically ill or postoperative. It occurs with abdominal distention and colonic dilation on x-ray, with a cecal diameter of ≥ 10 cm. Marked fecal loading in the descending and sigmoid colon correlates well with prolonged transit time, as does the presence of feces rather than air in the cecum (Figure 108-2). Dilation of the colon (>6.5 cm maximum diameter) in the absence of acute obstruction points to a neurogenic component to bowel dysfunction, and thus identifies patients at risk of recurrent colonic impaction. Rectal dilation (>4 cm) implies dysmotility and evacuation problems.

Table 108-7. Bowel Preparation in Older People

- Older age, constipation, reported laxative use, tricyclic antidepressants, stroke, and dementia are associated with inadequate preparation and thus taking longer to instrument the cecum
- Even in those who take 75%–100% of their prescribed treatment, bowel preparation is satisfactory in only 50%

Guidance

- Give regular laxatives (e.g., Movicol 2 sachets daily) and enemas or suppositories for at least 1 week before the procedure, with a longer run up period in patients known to have constipation, or with comorbidities such as diabetes
- Individualize the cathartic regimen (e.g., 1–2 L of GoLYTELY daily over 2 to 3 days in those unable to drink 4 L, or use of alternative preparations such as sodium picosulfate)
- Identify potential nonadherence ("Can the patient drink 4 L of GoLYTELY in 24 hours?")
- Preempt unpleasant side effects ("Will the patient be able to reach the toilet in time to avoid fecal leakage?")
- Use oral phosphosoda with caution as administration in older people increases in serum phosphate, even in patients with normal creatinine clearance
- Consider preprocedure plain abdominal x-ray for evaluation of persisting fecal loading
- Where possible give clear fluid diet before administration of bowel preparation

Colonoscopy/bowel preparation

Chronic constipation alone is generally not considered an appropriate indication for colonoscopy; the range of neoplasia found is similar to that in asymptomatic patients undergoing primary colorectal cancer screening.[119] A review of 400 colonoscopies in people aged 80 and over showed a good safety profile but low cancer detection rate for symptoms (e.g., constipation, abdominal pain) other than bleeding (2% versus 12%).[120] Further investigation is of course warranted in the context of rectal bleeding, systemic illness, or laboratory abnormalities. Barium enema has now largely been superseded by colonoscopy in older patients. Colonoscopy causes significantly less discomfort than a barium enema and is diagnostically more sensitive. Inadequate colonoscopies are common in older people because of poor bowel preparation (Table 108-7).

Anorectal function tests

Anorectal physiology tests are not generally required in older people with constipation or FI because they do not tend to alter the clinical examination conclusions or the management plan.[121] They have a role in confirming pelvic dyssynergia in people with persistent rectal outlet delay, a condition amenable to biofeedback. Endoanal ultrasound or MRI measure the integrity of the anal sphincters and thus guide management of incontinence toward biofeedback therapy, or surgical intervention (sphincter reconstruction). This investigation is appropriate in those patients with clinically weak sphincters and preserved sensation whose FI persists after behavioral measures (pelvic floor exercises, loperamide).

Physical function and toilet access

Functional FI can occur in individuals who are unable to access the toilet in time due to impairments in mobility, dexterity, or vision, but who may even have normal lower gut function. Withholding evacuation because of access problems can lead to constipation. Evaluation of toilet access should ideally be multidisciplinary and include assessment of function (e.g., Barthel Index), mobility (e.g., "timed up-and-go"), visual acuity, upper limb dexterity (e.g., undoing buttons), and cognition. A practical assessment is to watch someone transfer and manage clothing on the toilet or commode. Toilet or commode design should be adapted to each individual (e.g., trunk support, adaptability, mobility, foot support).[122] For patients with functional difficulties, the physical layout of their home in relation to the bathroom should be assessed (location, distance from main living area, width of doorway for accommodating walking aids, presence of grab rails or raised toilet seat, lighting levels).

Psychological impact/quality of life

Constipation and FI affect quality of life, daily living, and morale in older people, even following adjustment for other chronic illnesses.[40,123] The Patient Assessment of Constipation Quality of Life questionnaire is a self-report tool that has been validated in elderly long-term care residents (QOL scores correlate with abdominal pain and constipation severity).[119] In routine practice, a person's attitude toward their bowel problem (positive, acceptance, denial, distress, apathy) and the impact on their quality of life (changes in usual family, social, physical, and work-related activities) should at least be included when taking a history.

TREATMENT OF CONSTIPATION IN OLDER PEOPLE

Nonpharmacologic treatment

The consultation between a general practitioner and an older person reporting constipation will more often than not result in a laxative being prescribed. Nursing home studies show high rates of self-reported constipation, despite very substantial levels of laxative prescribing. These observations suggest that nonpharmacologic treatments for constipation are underused. They should be first-line treatment in nonsevere constipation and combined with laxative treatment. A 1997 systematic review of nonpharmacologic treatment of chronic constipation in older people found no studies evaluating the effect of exercise therapy and only a few nonrandomized trials examining fiber and fluid supplementation,[124] and there has been little further robust research in this area since then. Available data, expert opinion, and practical recommendations are summarized below.

EDUCATION OF PATIENTS AND CAREGIVERS

Educating patients as to what constitutes normal bowel habit is helpful, and those with no or mild symptoms of constipation should be encouraged to discontinue laxative therapy. Patients who do require laxative treatment for constipation should be advised to aim for regular, comfortable evacuation rather than daily evacuation, which is often their preconceived norm.

Educational interventions promoting lifestyle changes should include written educational materials (ideally produced with input from users). A single nurse assessment and education session including provision of booklet in older stroke patients with constipation and FI showed that 1 year later they were still more likely to be altering their diet and fluid intake to control their bowel problem.[83] Table 108-8 illustrates some of the patient-centered instructions from this study booklet, which are relevant to all older people with constipation and FI.

Other RCTs have sought to influence fiber intake at a population level. Nutrition newsletters sent to older Americans in their homes significantly improved their dietary fiber intake. Another community intervention used media and social marketing in educational targeting of small retirement communities under the theme "Bread: It's a Great Way to Go," and reported a 49% decrease in laxative sales and 58% increase in sales of whole meal bread.

Educating home caregivers on maintaining fecal continence in patients with dementia (focusing on constipation and other contributors) increases knowledge levels,[125] though impact on FI is unknown. However, home caregiver involvement in bowel care plans is crucial in patients with FI, and should include awareness of caregiver needs.

DIET

Evidence for the effectiveness of fiber in treating constipation in elderly people is somewhat equivocal. In one community study, higher fiber intake was associated with lower laxative use among older women,[126] but in another study, higher intake of bran was associated with no reduction in constipation symptoms and greater fecal loading in the colon on abdominal radiography.[23] There have been several "before and after" studies in nursing home residents reporting that addition of dietary fiber (ranging from bran to processed pea hull) or fruit mixtures (apple puree to fruit porridge) to the daily diet improved bowel movement frequency and consistency, and reduced laxative intake and need for nursing intervention; despite the possibility of bias, these observational studies demonstrate the usefulness of increasing dietary fiber, fluid, and fruit in older people at high risk of constipation. In practical terms, at least 10 g of fiber with additional fluids should be recommended to patients. Although coarse bran rather than more refined fiber is more effective in increasing stool fluid weight, it is far less palatable, and is more likely to cause initial symptoms of increased bloating, flatulence, and irregular bowel movements. Fiber should therefore be recommended in the form of food, such as whole meal bread, porridge, fresh fruit (preferably unpeeled), seeded berries, kiwi,[127] raw or cooked vegetables, beans, and lentils.

FLUIDS

An RCT in adults with chronic constipation showed that the beneficial effect of increased dietary fiber was significantly enhanced by increasing fluid intake to 1.5 to 2 L daily.[128] Upping fluid intake by two 8-oz beverages a day for 5 weeks in dependent nursing home residents significantly increased bowel movement frequency and reduced laxative use.[129] This "hydration program" used a colorful beverage cart and four beverage choices to stimulate residents' interest in drinking. An RCT found that drinking carbonated versus tap

Table 108-8. Patient Education

Toilet Habits and Positioning
Do not delay having a bowel movement when you fell the urge.
Put aside a particular time each day (we would advise after breakfast) when you can sit on the toilet without being in a hurry.
A relaxed attitude to bowel evacuation will especially help if you have problems with straining or a feeling of anal blockage.
If straining is a problem, it is helpful to have a foot stool under your feet while sitting on the toilet because this increases the ability of your abdominal muscles to help evacuation of stool.
Abdominal Massage
Lie on the bed with pillows under your head and shoulders.
Your knees should be bent up with a pillow underneath them for support.
Cover your abdomen with a light sheet.
Massage your abdomen with firm but gentle circular movements starting at the right side and working across to the left side.
Continue the massage for about 10 minutes.
This massage should be a pleasant experience; if you feel any discomfort then stop.
Diet
To help prevent constipation, you should eat more of the food from List A and less of the food from List B. Food in list A tends to make the stool softer and easier to pass because they are high in fiber. Food in list B tend to make the stool harder because they bind together the contents of the bowel.
List A: Fresh fruit, prunes and other dried fruit, whole meal bread, bran cereals and porridge, salad, cooked vegetables (with skin where possible), beans, lentils
List B: Milk, hard cheese, yogurt, white bread or crackers, refined cereals, cakes, pancakes, noodles, white rice, chocolate, creamed soups
You should increase your fiber intake gradually because sudden change in fiber content may cause temporary bloating and irregularity. It is important to eat the food that contains fiber all through the day and not just at one meal such as breakfast
Increase the amount of fluid that you drink gradually up to 8–10 glasses a day. Try to drink more water, fruit juices, and fizzy drinks.
Sphincter Strengthening
Learning to do your exercises
Sit in a comfortable position with your knees slightly apart. Now imagine that you are trying to stop yourself passing wind from the bowel. To do this you must squeeze the muscle around the back passage. Try squeezing and lifting that muscle as tightly as you can. You should be able to feel the muscle move. Your buttocks, abdomen, and legs should not move at all. You should be aware of the skin around the back passage tightening and being pulled up and away from your chair. Really try to feel this. You are now exercising you anal sphincter muscles. (You do not need to hold your breath when you tighten the muscles!)
Practicing your exercises
Tighten and pull up the anal sphincter muscles as tightly as you can. Hold tightened for at least 5 seconds, then relax for at least 10 seconds.
Repeat this exercise at least 5 times. This will work on the strength of your muscles.
Next, pull the muscles to about half of their maximum squeeze. See how long you can hold this for. Then relax for at least 10 seconds.
Repeat at least 5 times. This will work on the endurance or staying power of your muscles.
Pull up the muscles as quickly and tightly as you can and then relax and then pull up again, and see how many times you can do this before you get tired. Try for at least 5 quick pull-ups. Try this quick pull-up exercise at least 10 times each day.
Do all these exercises as hard as you can and at least 5 times a day. As the muscles get stronger, you will find that you can do more pull-ups each time without the muscle getting tired.
It takes time for exercises to make muscle stronger. You may need to exercise regularly for several months before the muscles gain their full strength.
Instructions for Using Suppositories
These may be inserted into your rectum (back passage) by your nurse or caregiver or yourself if you are physically able to do it.
If necessary go to the toilet and empty your bowels if you can.
Wash your hands.
Remove any foil or wrapping from the suppository.
Either lie on your side with your lower leg straight and your upper leg bent toward your waist or squat.
Gently but firmly insert the suppository, narrow end first, into the rectum using a finger. Push far enough (about 1 inch) so that it does not come out again.
You may find you body wanting to push out the suppository. Close your legs and keep still for a few minutes.
Try not to empty your bowels for at least 10–20 minutes.

water significantly improved constipation scores, along with benefiting functional dyspepsia and gallbladder emptying.[130] Probiotic drinks have been shown to increase defecation frequency in older people.[131]

PHYSICAL ACTIVITY

An RCT in middle-aged inactive patients with chronic constipation showed that daily physical activity (30-minute brisk walk and 11-minute home exercises) decreased transit time and improved constipation, according to Rome II criteria.[132] Physical activity interventions in older adults are generally most effective if incorporated naturally into a person's day. Exercise interventions in older nursing home patients have shown disappointingly modest impact on constipation,[133,134] but existing evidence would support exercise programs (e.g., prompting to walk to toilet, bed exercises for chairbound[135] within context of addressing other risk factors also).

ABDOMINAL MASSAGE

There is some evidence to support abdominal massage in alleviating chronic constipation in spinal cord patients and older people.[135] A vibrating device that applied kneading force to the abdomen daily for 20 minutes in elderly constipated nursing home residents resulted in softening of stool, increased bowel movement frequency, and a 47% reduction in transit time after 3 months.[136] Patients can self-administer with training (Table 108-8).

TOILETING HABITS

Small nonrandomized studies show that regular scheduled toileting habits restore comfortable evacuation in stroke survivors[137] and in older postoperative inpatients. The preservation of the gastrocolic reflex with aging supports the rationale for postprandial toilet visits. Voluntary increase in intraabdominal pressure during defecation can compensate for rectal dysmotility to produce enough of an increase in rectal pressure for evacuation to occur, but older people are often limited by weakened abdominal musculature. Supporting the feet (on footstool or toilet block) can optimize the Valsalva manuever.[11]

TOILETING ACCESS—PRIVACY AND DIGNITY

A U.K. study asked frail older patients with FI about privacy during defecation.[138] Adequate privacy was reported by 23% of nursing home residents, and 50% of hospital inpatients. Lack of privacy, particularly in dependent older people in institutions, is a major care issue. Reluctance to use the toilet in institutional settings has been linked to residents developing severe fecal impaction in case reports. Table 108-9 summarizes basic but important recommendations relating to toileting and maintaining privacy and dignity.

PHARMACOLOGIC TREATMENT

Many reported trials of laxative treatment in older people are low quality, limited by unclear definitions for constipation, inconsistent outcome measurement, and underreporting of potential confounding factors during the trial period (e.g., fiber intake). The absence of good level evidence may in part underlie the somewhat empirical way in which laxatives are prescribed to older people. A 1997 systematic review of effective laxative treatment in elderly persons found that the few randomized controlled trials were potentially flawed,[124] and in the decade since there has been little new research in this area. The following evidence-based conclusions are drawn from recent meta-analytical reviews[124,139,140] of efficacy of laxatives in treating chronic constipation in adults:

- Availability of published evidence is poor for many commonly used agents including senna, magnesium hydroxide, bisacodyl, and stool softeners
- In trials conducted in older people, significant improvements in bowel movement frequency were observed with a stimulant laxative (cascara)[3] and lactulose,[2] while psyllium[2] and lactulose[2] were individually reported to improve stool consistency and related symptoms in placebo-controlled trials
- Level 1 evidence supports the use of PEG in adults
- Level 2 evidence supports the use of lactulose and psyllium in adults
- In trials conducted in older adults (>55 years), there is little evidence of differences in effectiveness between categories of laxatives
- A stepped approach to laxative treatment in older people is justified, starting with cheaper laxatives before proceeding to more expensive alternatives (Table 108-11)

Table 108-10 lists the indications, efficacy, and safety of laxatives, and Table 108-11 provides guidance to pharmacologic treatment of constipation in older people based on available evidence and best practice. Ineffective patterns of prescribing, such as giving docusate to care home residents,[141] may partly explain the reports of high constipation rates despite heavy laxative use. Another factor may be undertreatment of rectal outlet delay by enemas and suppositories.

Enemas have a role in both acute disimpaction and in preventing recurrent impactions in susceptible patients.[142,143] They induce evacuation as a response to colonic distention and by plain lavage; the commonest reason for a poor result from an enema is inadequate administration. Frail elderly patients with recurrent episodes of overflow FI despite regular laxative and suppository use can benefit from weekly enemas. In one study of nursing home residents with overflow incontinence associated with fecal impaction on rectal examination, daily phosphate enemas continued until no further result was effective in completely resolving incontinence in 94% of patients.[143] Regular use of phosphate enemas should be avoided in patients with renal impairment because dangerous hyperphosphatemia may occur.[144] Tap water enemas are the safest type for regular use, although they take more nursing administration time, and are not available in certain countries. Arachis oil retention enemas are particularly useful in loosening colonic impactions. In patients who have a firm and large rectal impaction, manual evacuation should be performed before inserting enemas or suppositories, using local anesthetic gel if needed to reduce discomfort.

The predominance of rectal outlet delay (including manual evacuation) in older people, many of whom take regular laxatives, is likely to be linked to underuse of *suppositories*. Although research data is lacking, in clinical practice suppositories are useful in symptoms of prolonged straining and incomplete rectal emptying. Regular suppository administration (usually three times a week, and ideally after breakfast) may be needed. With appropriate education, many older people can themselves use suppositories (see Table 108-8 for patient instructions). People with impaired dexterity can be

Table 108-9. Toilets and Toileting: Maintaining Privacy and Dignity

A multidisciplinary assessment should be made of older persons ability to access and use the toilet.[3]
Commodes/sani-chairs/shower chairs:
Should be available to residents in institutional settings.[3]
Should provide a safe seated position for prolonged use by older people with skin vulnerability and trunk support problems (e.g., padded seat, footstool if feet are unsupported, back and arm support, grab rails, etc.).[3]
Older people should be given the opportunity to use the toilet (either directly or by using a sani-chair or shower chair) rather than a bedside commode.[3]
Bedpans should be avoided for defecation purposes.
Transportation to the toilet and use of the toilet or commode should be carried out with due regard to privacy and dignity.
A direct method of calling for assistance should be provided when an older person is left on the toilet/commode.
When using a commode:
Methods to reduce noise and odor should be offered.
Methods to facilitate bottom wiping should be available.
If in living area and cannot be emptied immediately, a chemical toilet should be offered instead.[3]

Source: Adapted from Potter J, Norton C, Cottenden A. Bowel care in older people: research and practice. London: Royal college of physicians; 2002.

Table 108-10. Summary of Laxatives

Type and Agent	Indication, Action, Administration, Side Effects
Stimulant	Cheap, safe and effective for use in chronic constipation (ref)
Senna	Improves propulsive action (direct stimulation of myenteric plexus) and softens stool (Prostaglandin E-like effect)
(alternate is bisacodyl)	Onset 8–12 hr. Give at bedtime
	Long-term use associated with melanosis coli (mucosal pigmentation with no clinical significance) does not cause "cathartic colon"
Bulk	First-line laxative in ambulant older people with mild-moderate constipation, safe long-term, underprescribed in older people
Psyllium	First-line in diverticular disease (limits flare-ups of diverticulitis), facilitates painful defecation with hemorrhoids, reduces abdominal pain in IBS
Ispaghula husk	
Methyl cellulose	
Calcium polycarbophil	Reduces incontinent episodes in FI associated with loose stool
	Psyllium lowers cholesterol (binds bile acids in intestine)
	Hydrophilic fibers resistant to bacterial degradation, leads to bulkier and softer stool and peristaltic stimulation
	Onset 12–72 hr
	May initially cause bloating and unpredictable bowel habit, increased risk of impaction with poor fluid intake
Magnesium hydroxide (Milk of Magnesia)	Unsuitable for treatment of chronic constipation
	Rapid onset, so commonly prescribed to older hospital inpatients
	Stimulates release of cholecystokinin, increases secretion of electrolytes and water into gut lumen
	May cause watery stool, dehydration, FI, hypermagnesemia in renal insufficiency
Hyperosmolar	Second-line laxative for chronic constipation, relatively expensive
Lactulose	Nonabsorbable disaccharide degraded into low molecular weight acids, which osmotically draws water into the colon causing reflex prolonged tonic gut contractions. Shortens transit time, and softens stool
	Onset 24–48 hr
	May cause abdominal cramps and flatulence especially with fruit diet
Hyperosmolar	Useful for acute disimpaction (effective in care home residents and hospitalized patients)(refs) and rapid clear out for bowel preparation
Polyethylene glycol (PEG) "Movicol", GoLYTELY	Reduces recurrence of acute pseudo-obstruction if administered after initial resolution of colonic dilation
	Long-term use only in patients with neuropathic bowel or resistant constipation
	Potent hyperosmotic action, shortens transit time
	Onset 30–60 min, low starting dose and titrate against effect
	May cause nausea, abdominal cramps, FI and loose stool
Stool softener	Ineffective in treating constipation though commonly prescribed
Docusate	Reduces surface tension and promotes penetration of water into stool
	No effect on colonic motility or bowel movement frequency
	Increases risk of FI in care home residents
	Can cause perianal dermatitis in incontinent patients
Enterokinetic agents	No specific research in older people, so not recommended for routine use
5-HT4 agonists (e.g., Tegaserod)	Altered serotonin (5-HT) signaling may predispose to chronic constipation. 5-HT4 agonists (e.g., Tegaserod) stimulate gastrointestinal motility and increase stool water content.
	Efficacy and safety of Tegaserod in treating chronic constipation shown in RCT where 13% of participants were aged 65 and over, but no subgroup analysis. Tegaserod improves symptoms of constipation in IBS.
	Side effects includes headaches and diarrhea, postmarketing reports of ischemic colitis.

helped with suppository inserters designed for spinal cord injured patients. Glycerin, a hyperosmolar laxative used solely in suppository form, should be used first-line. If ineffective, bisacodyl suppositories in PEG base (effective in spinal cord injured patients)[145] should be substituted. Suppository onset of action varies by individual from 5 to 45 minutes (most likely influenced by the neurogenicity of the rectum), and so patients should be advised to set a quiet time aside for effective evacuation.

TREATMENT OF FECAL INCONTINENCE IN OLDER ADULTS

The algorithm summarizes the clinical evaluation and management of FI in this population emphasizing the structured comprehensive clinical approach, which can be undertaken by doctor or nurse specialist.[11] Table 108-12 provides a summary.

Multicomponent treatment of FI in frail older people

Although a multidimensional approach to FI treatment would clearly be indicated in view of the multifactorial causation in older people, there are few published studies of multicomponent interventions. An RCT in elderly stroke survivors with constipation and/or FI evaluated a one-off assessment according to the algorithm in Figure 108-3, leading to patient/caregiver education, and treatment recommendations to routine health care provider[83] showed benefit at 6 months in percent of "normal" defecations. A nursing home RCT found that a structured daily exercise program, combined with increased fluid intake and regular toileting opportunities, significantly improved FI and increased appropriate toilet use.[146] These types of evaluations do not identify any specific action to have a particular benefit, but do test a multicomponent approach that nonspecialist doctors and nurses could feasibly apply in various settings.

Lifestyle and diet

A U.S. study of self-care practices among home-dwelling older people with FI found that most commonly used strategies for managing FI were dietary change, wearing pads, and limiting activity.[147] Women, more so than men, altered their diet and missed meals to prevent FI. Reducing intake of fiber foods (whole grain bread, fruits, etc.) can limit FI in some people. Likewise, some individuals may benefit from limiting dairy products and sorbitol sweeteners. In the context of FI

Table 108-11. Pharmacologic Treatment of Constipation in Older People - Guidance

Chronic Constipation

In ambulant older people

Bulk laxative (psyllium) 1–3 times daily with fluids as required

If symptoms persist add senna 1–3 tablets at bedtime

In individuals with questionable fluid intake or those intolerant of bulk laxatives, start with senna 1–2 tablets at bedtime

If symptoms persist, add sorbitol or lactulose 15 mL daily as needed, titrating the dose to achieve regular (≥ 3 times a week) and comfortable evacuation

In high risk patients

- Bedridden individuals
- Patients with neurologic disease
- Patients with history of fecal impaction

Senna 2–3 tablets at bedtime and sorbitol or lactulose 30 mL daily, titrating upwards as needed

If symptoms persist, give PEG (½–2 sachets of Movicol daily)

Colonic Fecal Impaction

Clinical or radiologic obstruction

Daily retention enemas (e.g. arachis oil) until obstruction resolves, before starting oral laxatives

Colonic disimpaction

Daily enemas (preferably tap water) until no further washout result

PEG (½–2 L daily or 2–3 sachets of Movicol) with fluids

Ensure that patient has easy access to toilet to avoid fecal incontinence

When impaction resolves, give laxative regimen for chronic constipation in high-risk patients long-term to avoid recurrence

Rectal Outlet Delay

Rectal disimpaction

Manual disimpaction where necessary, followed by phosphate enema(s) for initial complete clearance of rectal impaction

Regular treatment

Glycerin suppositories at least once a week and as required to relieve symptoms

For persistent symptoms, use bisacodyl suppositories instead of glycerin suppositories

In patients at high risk of rectal impaction (rectal dysmotility, neurologic disease) give regular enemas (usually once weekly) and daily suppositories

If stool is hard or infrequent, add daily laxative as for chronic constipation

Table 108-12. Treatment of FI in Older People: Evidence-Based Summary and Recommendations

Overflow FI

- Stimulant laxatives, osmolar laxatives (PEG and lactulose), suppositories and enemas can be effective in treating fecal impaction in older people at risk of overflow[2]
- Complete rectal clearance is required to reduce overflow FI[2] but may be hard to achieve in frail older patients.[2] Weekly digital rectal examination and prolonged treatment is helpful in increasing effectiveness of a bowel clearance program.[2]

Frail Older People and Dementia-related FI

- Structured approaches to bowel care can reduce the frequency of FI in the nursing home setting.[2]
- Prompted toileting can be effective in reducing FI in patients with dementia within a structured bowel care plan.[2]
- Multicomponent structured nurse-led assessment and intervention can improve bowel symptoms and alter bowel-related habits in older stroke patients.[2]

FI Associated With Loose Stool

- Treatable causes of loose stool (e.g., infection) must first be identified.
- Dietary fiber supplementation can reduce episodes of FI associated with loose stool.[1]
- Caffeine reduction can reduce FI and urgency.[3]
- Some patients with FI benefit from limiting dietary dairy products, fiber (e.g., unpeeled fruit, vegetable, whole meal, etc.), sorbitol, and alcohol.
- Loperamide can reduce frequency of FI, particularly when associated with loose stool.[2]

FI Associated With Weak Anal Sphincters

- Older people with FI associated with weak sphincters and preserved sensation can benefit from sphincter strengthening exercises[3] and biofeedback.[2]

Lifestyle and Education

- Self-care practices are prevalent in older people with FI.[2] Women are more likely to alter their diet than men.
- Patient and caregiver education (using verbal and written materials) should be undertaken to promote self-efficacy and other coping mechanisms, and where appropriate self-management (e.g., reducing risk of constipation and impaction through dietary and lifestyle measures, advice on how to take loperamide). Advice on skin care, odor control, and continence aids is also important.

Privacy and Dignity

- Dependent older people with FI in care homes and hospitals often lack privacy during defecation.[3]
- Privacy and dignity of care during defecation should be afforded to all older people in institutionalized settings. Particular attention should be paid to this in patients with FI because privacy may be relatively overlooked in their care.

associated specifically with loose stool, an RCT of dietary fiber supplementation (psyllium or gum agar) significantly reduced incontinent episodes.[148] Caffeine reduction can also help—black coffee increased rectosigmoid motility within 4 minutes of ingestion in young healthy volunteers (a reaction not observed with ingestion of hot water), implying that caffeine triggers the gastrocolic reflex.[149] Caffeine has also been shown to stimulate defecation urgency in some patients with FI.[11]

TREATMENT OF OVERFLOW FI IN OLDER PEOPLE

An effective therapeutic program for overflow incontinence depends on:

- Regular toileting (ideally 2 hourly, which also promotes mobility)
- Monitoring of treatment effect by rectal examination and bowel chart
- Responsive stepwise drug and dosage changes
- Prolonged treatment (at least 2 weeks)
- Subsequent maintenance regimen to prevent recurrences

There are only two trials evaluating treatment of overflow FI, both involving frail elderly care home residents. One U.K. trial evaluated an intervention based on treatment recommendations to general practitioners.[143] Patients with rectal impaction and continuous fecal soiling were classed as having overflow and the recommended treatment was giving enemas until no further response, followed by lactulose. Complete resolution of incontinence was achieved in 94% of those who were fully treated, but GP and care home staff compliance with the recommended treatment was obtained in only 67% of patients. A French study found that treatment of constipation was only effective in improving overflow FI (incontinence at least once weekly associated with impaired rectal emptying) when long-lasting and complete rectal emptying (monitored by weekly rectal examinations) was achieved using daily lactulose plus daily suppositories, plus weekly tap water enemas.[142] The number of FI episodes was reduced by 35% and staff workload (based on soiled laundry

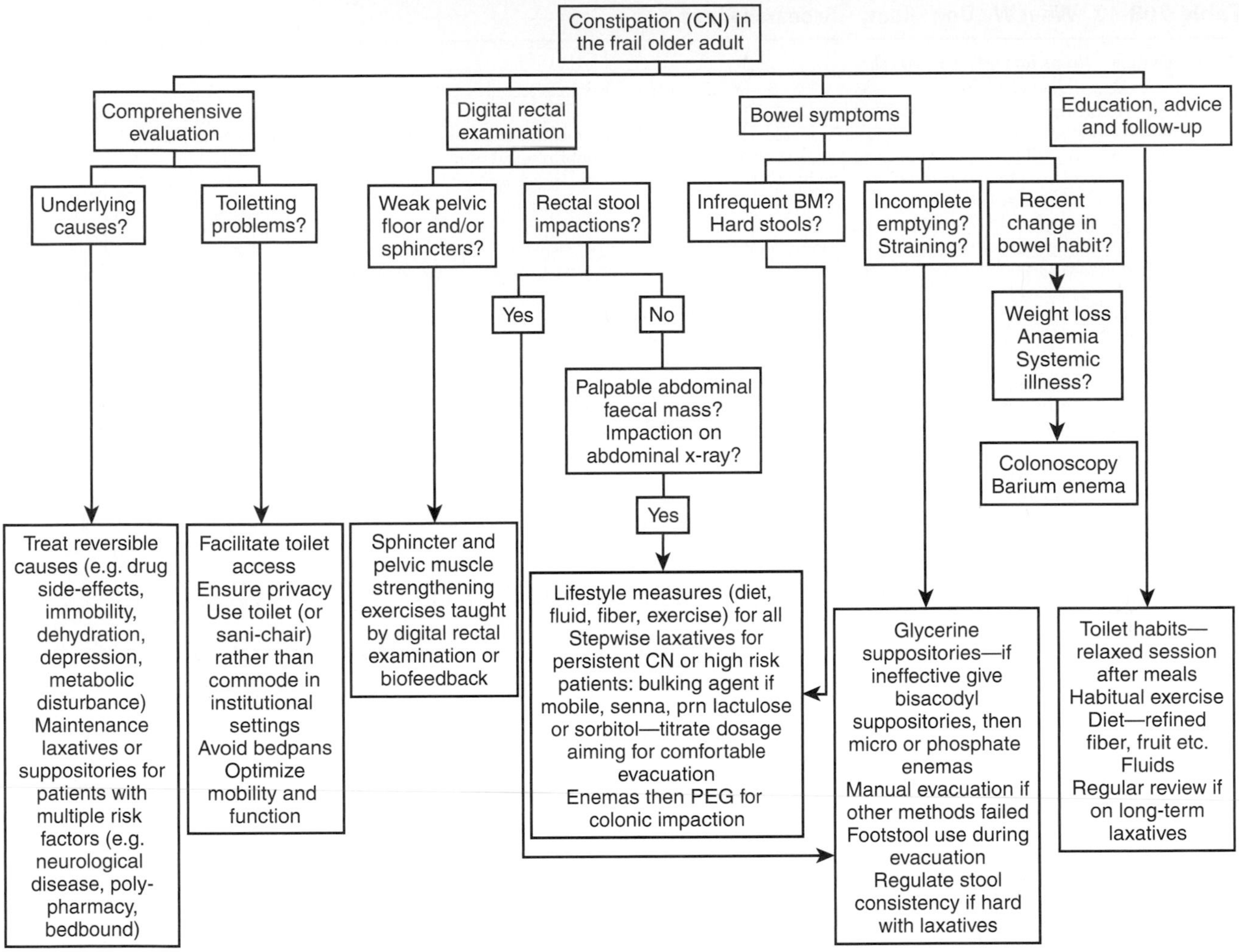

Figure 108-3. An algorithmic approach to assessment and treatment of constipation in older people.

counts) fell by 42% in those with complete rectal emptying; complete clearance was, however, only achieved in 40% of study subjects. These trials demonstrate the challenges of treating overflow FI in care homes where it is highly prevalent, both in terms of delivering the right care, and of needing to persevere with treatment to achieve good clear out and restoration of continence. They also emphasize the need for combined laxative and enema or suppositories, and for treatment persistence (lasting weeks rather than days) to achieve effective bowel clearance.

TREATMENT OF LOOSE STOOL

Treatable conditions affecting older people are:

- * Excessive laxative use - Stool softeners in particular have been linked to FI in frail older people.[35]
- * Drug side effects (e.g., proton-pump inhibitors [also increase risk of *Clostridium difficile*][150] selective serotonin reuptake inhibitors, magnesium-containing antacids, cholinesterase inhibitors
- * Lactose intolerance - Lactose malabsorption affects 50% of healthy women aged 60 and over compared with 15% in women aged 40 to 59 years.[151] Only certain individuals will develop a clinical intolerance to dairy products.
- * Antibiotic-related diarrhea - Among hospitalized patients, age, female gender, and nursing home residency significantly increases the risk for antibiotic-related *C. difficile* diarrhea.[152] The diarrhea also takes longer to resolve following treatment of *C. difficile* in more frail older patients.[152] Preliminary RCT data support the use of probiotic drinks in preventing *C. difficile* in older hospitalized patients on antibiotics.[153] Infective causes of loose stool should always be ruled out before settling on a chronic FI management plan (e.g., with loperamide or fiber).
- Diabetes - Treatment with erythromycin and metoclopramide is indicated where slow-transit with bacterial overgrowth is diagnosed. Acarbose may also be beneficial.[72]
- Crohn's disease - This condition has a second incidence peak in the sixth decade and beyond.

TREATMENT OF DEMENTIA-RELATED FECAL INCONTINENCE

It is important to look for all other causes of FI (e.g., constipation, drugs, reduced function) in patients with cognitive impairment because only those with severe cortical deficit will have FI-related primarily to dementia. Prompted

Table 108-13. What We Don't Know - Research Ideas

Constipation – Areas for Further Research

What are the different characteristics between constipation sufferers who seek help and those who do not? (Case-control study)
What drives constipation sufferers to seek help? (Qualitative research)
How can standardized "constipation protocols" for case-finding and risk assessment be implemented across community and institutional health care setting where frail older patients are cared for? (Action Research, Quality Improvement Study)
Why is the prevalence of constipation in nursing homes so high despite heavy laxative use? Is it:
- ineffective laxative prescribing?
- substandard assessment of patients?
- underuse of nonpharmacologic treatments? (Observational)

What is the impact of nonpharmacologic interventions targeting constipation risk factors on bowel and health-related outcomes in frail older people? (RCT)
What are the barriers to older people adopting bowel-related lifestyle measures? (Qualitative research)
What are the psychosocial and quality of life effects of chronic constipation on older individuals and caregivers? (Questionnaire population studies, qualitative research)
What is the effectiveness of enemas and suppositories in treating constipation and rectal outlet delay in older people? (RCT)
Is biofeedback an effective treatment for pelvic dyssynergia in older people with rectal outlet delay? (RCT)
How common is manual self-evacuation in older people, and does prolonged use affect anal sphincter function? (Questionnaire survey, anorectal function study)
What is the cost-effectiveness of a stepwise approach to laxative treatment in older people with constipation in different health care settings (community, hospital, long-term care) (RCT)
How effective and safe are new enterokinetic agents (serotonin agonists) in treatment of chronic constipation in older people, including frail individuals? (RCT)

FI – Areas for Further Research

- Trials of laxative and nonpharmacologic treatment and prevention of fecal impaction and overflow are needed to optimize standards of prescribing and care
- Multicomponent interventions to treat FI in frail older people should be evaluated as applied research to assess effective ways of delivering this type of intervention within routine health care settings
- There are challenges to undertaking RCT's in this area in frail older people. In particular, it is important to balance feasibility and practicality versus high strength intervention (i.e., a team of specialist continence nurses in nursing homes are likely to have an impact, but at what cost, and what carry-over will there be when they are gone). Methodologies other than RCTs (e.g., prepost with multivariate case-mix adjustment) should also be considered.
- Evaluation of case-finding methods for FI in different settings including the fundamentals of staff education, screening protocols, patient educational information
- Testing the feasibility of providing an integrative pathway approach to assessment of FI in the frail older person, including a range of health and social care providers and different health care settings (acute, intermediate, long-term care, community)
- Examination of the variability of FI rates between nursing homes within single nation states, (taking into consideration case-mix) to highlight problems areas both organizationally and clinically. Nursing home administrative factors such as resident:nurse staff ratios should be evaluated as a contributing factor to FI.
- Further epidemiologic studies are required to document causes of FI in frail older people in different health care settings. Such studies should include evaluation of the unmet need for patients and caregivers.
- Evaluation of etiologies, and in particular the pathophysiologic basis for high prevalence of FI in older men.
- Evaluation of potentially preventable causes of loose stools in institutionalized older people, and impact of their treatment on FI.
- Examine the research question, "Do educational interventions by health care providers to informal caregivers of home-dwelling older people with FI reduce caregiver burden and improve quality of life for patient and caregiver?"

toileting (by reminder or by accompaniment depending on cognition) is the mainstay approach in these patients and has been evaluated in two care home resident RCTs. One significantly increased the number of continent bowel movements but had no impact on FI frequency,[154] whereas the other significantly reduced the frequency of FI and increased the rate of appropriate toilet use, but interestingly did not impact the primary outcome measure of pressure ulcers.[146] Prompted toileting is also an appropriate intervention in hospital and at home, though it has not been evaluated in those settings. Pharmacologic control of disinhibited bowels in patients with dementia was demonstrated in a small care home study using daily codeine phosphate and twice weekly enemas; continence was achieved in 75% of those treated.[143] This approach can be effective in practice, but requires careful bowel planning and monitoring to prevent impaction.

TREATMENT OF ANORECTAL FI IN OLDER ADULTS

Older patients with a FI pattern suggestive of anorectal incontinence (small amounts of leakage, weak anal sphincters) should be taught sphincter strengthening exercises (Table 108-8). These are similar to pelvic floor exercises, a treatment shown to be effective in older women with urinary incontinence.[155] It is helpful to teach the exercises while placing the examining hand resting on the posterior vaginal wall, so that verbal feedback can be given as the patient contracts the pelvic floor; an RCT in older women with urge urinary incontinence showed that this teaching method was just as effective as formal biofeedback.[155] Similar verbal feedback can be given to men during digital examination of the anal sphincter. There is no evidence to suggest that frail older people without severe cognitive problems are any less able to adhere to such programs. Combined with the exercises should be advice to reduce caffeine intake and to increase fiber (psyllium can be prescribed). If FI persists after several months of this approach, biofeedback treatment should be considered. There is limited data on biofeedback in older people, but in one small study of older patients with no cognitive impairment, good motivation, and intact anorectal sensation, there was a 75% reduction in incontinent episodes short term.[156] There is no evidence to suggest that older patients selected by these criteria will not benefit.

KEY POINTS
Constipation and Fecal Incontinence in Old Age

- Constipation is a common problem as people age; the definition of constipation includes both quantitative (2 of fewer bowel movements per week; >10 minutes to complete bowel movements) and qualitative (straining, hard stools) components.
- Fecal incontinence is common among elderly people who are frail, but can be missed if not inquired about routinely. Such inquiry properly forms part of a comprehensive geriatric assessment.
- A wide range of problems can give rise to fecal incontinence in older adults, including problems in cognition, mobility, gastrointestinal motility, and anorectal dysfunction. A systematic approach is therefore essential.
- Common precipitants of constipation include low fluid volume intake, neurologic disorders, anticholinergic medications, iron supplementation, and dysautonomia.
- Fecal impaction can result in overflow diarrhea, so that the presenting complaint can be entirely at odds with the diagnosis. Note, too, that stool impaction on digital rectal examination does not have to be hard.
- In treating constipation, there is evidence for a variety of nonpharmacologic maneuvers, including increased fluid intake, dietary fiber, physical exercise, and abdominal massage although more research is needed, especially in relation to elderly people who are frail.
- A stepped approach to laxative treatment in older people is justified, starting with cheaper laxatives before proceeding to more expensive alternatives.
- Treatment of fecal incontinence starts with understanding the type (overflow, diarrheal, anorectal, functional, neurogenic)
- Many frail older adults will have more than one cause of fecal incontinence, and while a multidimensional approach would be indicated, there are few published studies of multicomponent interventions.

For a complete list of references, please visit online only at www.expertconsult.com

LOPERAMIDE

The most extensively tested drug treatment for FI associated with loose stools is loperamide. In one adult study loperamide significantly reduced FI, with no additional benefit when combined with fiber supplementation.[157] A small placebo-drug crossover trial in older adults showed that loperamide significantly reduced visual analogue scores for incontinence and urgency, prolonged colonic transit, and increased basal tone.[158] It is appropriate to start at low doses in older people (1 mg available in liquid form), with monitoring for impaction, and instruction on titration. Self-titration of loperamide can greatly restore confidence in older people whose social activites have been restricted because of FI.

FURTHER RESEARCH

Table 108-13 lists what we do not know about constipation and FI in older people, and ideas for further research. The overall aim in both clinical practice and research should be to develop common evidence-based policies, procedures, guidelines, and targets to promote integrated bowel care for older people within all health care settings.

CHAPTER 109

Urinary Incontinence

Adrian Wagg

Urinary incontinence is one of the giants of geriatric medicine. Despite this lofty status, however, it remains along with management of other associated lower urinary tract symptoms an entity largely neglected by geriatricians. Nevertheless, research-based evidence for the management of incontinence, even in the most frail elderly exists. Incontinence should not be a Cinderella subject, relegated to the realms of palliative nursing and should be approached seriously.

In the United Kingdom the prevalence of urinary incontinence increases in association with increasing age such that at age 60 moderate or more severe incontinence affects 22.3% of women and 10.2% of men and at age 80 and above, 33.4% of women and 23.5% of men are affected.[1] A recent survey has supported these observations and noted the increasing prevalence of lower urinary tract symptoms with advancing age.[2] The increased prevalence of incontinence in late life reflects a combination of physiologic change, an increased incidence of lower urinary tract disease, and the influence of associated morbidity in older people. It is both a marker of dependency of poorer health-related outcomes and also leads to an increased likelihood of institutionalization.[3] Incontinence also has a measureable negative impact on quality of life, although this appears not to be of the magnitude of that expressed by younger adults despite having a more severe extent of disease.[4] This may be because the coping mechanisms that people adopt become habituated, lessening the perceived impact. Older cohorts are generally more accepting of these or may expect conditions that they may associate with aging to afflict them and simply cope.

ANATOMY AND PHYSIOLOGY

The smooth muscle fibers of the detrusor muscle of the bladder appear to be randomly arranged over the dome of the bladder but funnel at the bladder neck to be continued into the urethra as longitudinal fibers forming a tube. In the male these fibers are inserted into the verumontanum, but in the female they terminate in the distal urethra. Contraction of the detrusor results in a rise in bladder pressure associated with shortening of the urethra. Contraction of the muscle of the trigone, the triangular baseplate with its apex at the bladder neck, and base running between both ureters results in funneling of the bladder neck. There are some fibers that are inserted into the external surface of the trigone distally. These pull the distal margins of the trigone apart, thus opening the bladder neck.

In normal circumstances the detrusor is highly compliant. This means that it is normal for a bladder to be filled to 500 mL and more, without an increase in intravesical pressure, other than the pressure head resulting from the volume of the fluid in the bladder, which would be approximately 8 cm H_2O at 500 mL. If the wall tension in the detrusor increases in association with filling, but then fails to relax (stress relaxation), the bladder is said to "lack compliance." "Low compliance" may result from fibrosis, detrusor hypertrophy, or an increased resting tone secondary to reduced neural inhibition.[5]

Control of the bladder and urethra depends upon a complex supraspinal neuronal network, which allows voluntary postponement of voiding and the ability to empty the bladder at a socially convenient time, even if there is little need to void. Animal studies and clinical observation have suggested that the main levels of control over the lower urinary tract are cortical (inhibitory), hypothalamic (excitatory), midbrain (inhibitory), and pontine (excitatory). With the advent of modern functional brain imaging, the sites of these control systems have been further identified. In adults, the normal mechanism for activating contraction of the detrusor is the release of acetylcholine from parasympathetic nerves, stimulated by a spino bulbospinal micturition reflex,[6] the main micturition reflex. Tension receptors in the detrusor activate afferents traveling in the pelvic nerves. These afferents pass through the lumbosacral dorsal roots to ascending tracts where they synapse in the midbrain periaqueductal gray (PAG). Their signaling intensity increases as the bladder fills and fibers from the PAG descend to the pontine micturition center (PMC), causing excitation. If left unmodulated, fibers from the PMC excitation causes activation of the descending motor efferents, which cause coordinated detrusor contraction and urethral relaxation.[7] However, afferent signals from the bladder do not automatically trigger the micturition reflex, but are relayed via the forebrain where a voluntary decision to empty the bladder can be made.[8]

Although much of the functional neuroanatomy of the lower urinary tract has been explored by animal experiments, the advent of functional imaging, (positron emission tomography, functional magnetic resonance imaging, single photon emission computed tomography) has allowed some impressive studies on humans, these methods map regional cerebral metabolism or blood flow and this is assumed to reflect neuronal activity. Many areas of the brain become active as the bladder is filled and studies have shown that humans and cats have remarkably similar arrangements. They show that micturition is associated with activity in the hypothalamus, periaqueductal gray matter, the right prefrontal cortex, anterior cingulate gyrus, and the dorsomedial pontine tegmentum.[9]

Since higher cerebral centers tend to inhibit the pontine micturition center, lesions above this area associated with detrusor overactivity of neurogenic origin. Frontal lobe lesions are associated with frequency, urgency, and urgency incontinence with a loss of warning of impending micturition. Strokes are often associated with detrusor overactivity, excepting those which primarily affect the occipital lobes. Any spinal cord injury that disrupts the normal connection between the sacral spinal cord and the supraspinal pathways controlling micturition will cause bladder dysfunction. Lesions of the spinal cord below the pons, but rostral to the sacral nuclei, result in bladder areflexia initially, lasting days to weeks before detrusor overactivity develops. However, if a spinal lesion involves complete destruction of the sacral nuclei, bladder areflexia will be permanent.[10,11]

The internal urethral sphincter is present only in the male, forming a circular collar continuous with the smooth muscle of the prostate. This sphincter is not part of the continence mechanism but contracts during ejaculation to prevent the retrograde flow of semen into the bladder. Failure of this sphincter leads to infertility, dry ejaculation, and seminuria. The internal sphincter is cut during transurethral resection of the prostate; however, continence is maintained.[12]

The external urethral sphincter is the principal mechanism for maintaining urethral continence in both sexes, although the smooth muscle and epithelium of the urethra is also important, particularly in women.[5] The urethra consists of an internal layer of longitudinal smooth muscle and an outer thinner layer of circular smooth muscle controlled by the action of adrenergic and cholinergic receptors and under modulation of NO and CO. Sympathetic control predominates, mediated by α_{1A} α-adrenoceptors.[13–16]

The striated muscles of the pelvic floor and the external sphincter are supplied by somatic efferents originating in the anterior horns of the sacral cord segments S2–S4. The motor neurons are grouped in a specific region called the Onuf's nucleus. This nucleus differs from other somatic motor nuclei, with histochemical appearances similar to sacral parasympathetic nuclei along with evidence of adrenergic innervation. The axons, originating from the Onuf's nucleus pass to the periphery through the pudendal nerve and the pelvic nerves. External sphincter activity is supported by the adrenergic smooth muscle of the urethra.

The sympathetic innervation for the lower urinary tract comes from postganglionic nerves traveling in the hypogastric plexus, the pelvic nerves, and the pudendal nerves. This sympathetic innervation inhibits the detrusor, providing an active component to relaxation and also stimulates the urethral smooth muscle and the sphincters.The inhibitory noradrenergic receptors on detrusor cells are β_3 subtype.[17–20] Motor activation of the detrusor in healthy humans is achieved by the stimulation of muscarinic receptors by acetylcholine; this activates second messengers causing release of Ca^{2+} ions from intracellular stores in the sarcoplasmic reticulum and an inward flow of Ca ions through L-type Ca^{2+} channels. The rise in intracellular Ca^{2+} ion concentration activates actin and myosin, thereby promoting contraction. The detrusor cell can depolarize with an inward current consisting of Ca^{2+} ions passing through L-type channels in sufficient magnitude to support depolarization, but the normal physiologic role of the L-type Ca^{2+} channel appears to be regulation of the filling of intracellular stores during the resting state. Cholinergic activation occurs independently of depolarization; its limited influence may explain the lack of efficacy of calcium channel blockers in the treatment of detrusor overactivity.[21–23] Ligand studies of the M_2 and M_3 muscarinic receptors in the bladder have shown that the greater proportion (85%) are M_2 receptors with only 15% being M_3. All of the contractile activity appears to be attributed to the M_3 receptor in healthy humans. However, the M_2 receptor is of increasing interest as its role in the appreciation and modulation of sensory inputs in both the detrusor and the urothelium have become apparent.[24,25]

It has been found that some muscarinic antagonists prove selective for the bladder, but this tissue specificity does not appear to be associated with either M_2 selectivity or lack of M_3 selectivity.[26–28]

It is now known that acetylcholine and noradrenaline are not the only significant neurotransmitters in the lower urinary tract. Nonadrenergic noncholinergic (NANC) neurotransmitters are neuropeptides that modulate the actions of the classical transmitters and may act as transmitters themselves. Neuropeptide-Y (NPY) and vasoactive intestinal polypeptides (VIP) are important neuromodulators, which are released at neuromuscular junctions so as to influence the release and uptake of acetylcholine and noradrenaline. Adenosine triphosphate (ATP) is thought to be an important neurotransmitter, coreleased with acetylcholine and it is known to cause depolarization of the detrusor. Although in the normal human bladder ATP is not important, there is evidence that in diseased states the activating mechanisms of the detrusor change and that NANC transmitters exert a much greater influence on the bladder, the ATP being broken down less effectively in the overactive detrusor.[29–31] More recently, an appreciation of the role of the sensory afferents in the detrusor and the role of the urothelium as an active, rather than a passive component of detrusor function has led to a greater understanding of the generation of detrusor overactivity, but not yet to therapeutic manipulation. Of resurgent interest is the concept of spontaneous detrusor activity and the role of the interstitial cell in the regulation of this.[32] These cells lie in the suburothelial space or within the detrusor and, indeed, throughout the lower urinary tract, and it has variously been postulated that these cells act as pacemaker cells, analogous to the interstitial cells of Cajal in the gastrointestinal tract.[33]

PRESENTATION

There is an outdated quote, often used, which states that the bladder is an unreliable witness and that the symptoms that a patient describes do not point to the true pathology.[34] This belief has arisen from the dubious assumption that patients can be fitted into clearly separate diagnostic categories where a set of unique symptoms leads to distinct diagnoses. Given that there is likely to be a spectrum of disease, reflecting the variability inherent in any biologic system, diagnostic categories most likely form intersecting continua that share some symptoms. Such faith in diagnostic absolutes is dangerous because it leads to dismissal of the significance of symptoms, which are the patients' experience of disease. The great majority of symptoms can be explained by the physiologic and mechanical principles that govern the lower urinary tract, and what the patients say usually makes sense. Experimental data have supported this thesis,[36] but there is a continual search for classification, discrimination, and scoring of disease variables that largely leads to no gain in terms of understanding of disease or advances in treatment.

Frequency, urgency, urgency incontinence, nocturia, and enuresis are symptoms associated with detrusor overactivity (DO) and have been observed to be associated with the involuntary detrusor contractions of DO,[37] and to reduce with documented resolution of the overactivity.[38,39]

Frequency and urgency may be more noticeable when out and about, when putting the key in the door on returning home, in cold weather, in anxiety-provoking situations, and to be subject to diurnal and seasonal variation. Intercurrent illness, particularly urinary infection, will exacerbate the symptoms. The subjective experience that is urinary urgency also varies between individuals, and probably, within the same individual. Some describe the idea of a growing potential for loss of bladder control, whereas others tell of a wholly physical sense of near incontinence. Clinically, the symptom complex is called the overactive bladder, or frequency-urgency syndrome, and it is defined as urinary urgency, with or without urgency incontinence, usually with frequency and nocturia in the absence of other lower urinary tract pathology that might lead to similar symptoms (such as bladder stones, tumor, or infection).[40]

Stress urinary incontinence is associated with coughing, sneezing, or other physical exertion. The term "genuine stress incontinence" is no longer used to describe stress incontinence caused by an incompetent urethral sphincter. The symptom of stress incontinence, which often coexists with varying degrees of overactivity, particularly in older people, is clearly associated with reduced sphincter function.[41,42] Where overactivity coexists, treatment of this may result in resolution of both urgency and stress-induced incontinence. This should be expected if the two pathologies work synergistically. Response to treatment of one pathology does not exclude the presence of the other.[43] On current evidence, if a woman describes stress incontinence, then there is a 78% probability that sphincter dysfunction exists. Although there is a reduction in the maximum closing pressure that can be generated in the urethra in association with increasing age, this closing pressure must exceed the pressure of urine at the bladder neck for continence to be maintained. As the bladder fills, a pressure will develop equal to the hydrostatic pressure of urine in the bladder plus the weight of any viscera pressing on it. If the maximum urethral closure pressure is reduced below this, then the woman will develop a sense of pending incontinence as the hydrostatic pressure rises; positional changes may exacerbate this. The woman will thus be forced to maintain a bladder capacity below the threshold. Frequency, urgency, and urge incontinence may all therefore be induced by an incompetent urethral sphincter. Additionally, rising during or at the end of the night with a full bladder, and suddenly applying an increased hydrostatic pressure to the faulty sphincter, will lead to very severe urgency and precipitancy.

Hesitancy, a reduced stream, intermittency of stream, straining to void, manual abdominal compression during voiding, terminal dribbling, postmicturition dribbling, and incomplete emptying are recognized symptoms of a voiding problem, be it obstructive or due to a failure of detrusor emptying function. Their presence correctly points to a requirement to check voiding efficiency. However, the physiology of micturition indicates that a high frequency will lead to similar symptoms. The bladder empties more efficiently from a higher capacity, but voiding efficiency is compromised by overdistention.[44,45] Elongation of the detrusor fibers in response to filling promotes optimum contact between the actin and myosin so that a better contraction can be obtained.[46] Flow rates are well known to be related to the voiding bladder volume. People with frequency and low-volume voids therefore commonly describe symptoms of poor voiding in the absence of either detrusor underactivity or obstruction.

Dysuria is the experience of pain in association with micturition. The classical symptom of a burning in the urethra during voiding, caused by infection, is well known. Less appreciated is the external dysuria experienced by women with vaginitis when urine passes over the labia.[47]

Table 109-1. Factors Associated with and Consequent upon Urinary Incontinence on Older People

Incontinence can be Associated with the Following:
Falls
Depression
Pressure ulcers
Bowel problems
Skin infection
Isolation
Impaired quality of life
Increased likelihood of institutional care
Incontinence is also a Consequence of the Following:
Lower urinary tract disease
Musculoskeletal disease
arthritis/contractures
Peripheral vascular disease
Stroke
Parkinson's disease
The dementias
Diabetes mellitus
Venous insufficiency
Chronic lung disease
Congestive heart failure
Neurologic disorders, for example: multiple sclerosis, spinal cord injury, and motor neuron disease

There are a number of conditions, labeled by the International Continence Society as painful bladder syndromes, which are beyond the scope of this chapter, that are poorly defined and require specialist management.

There are a variety of factors, unrelated to bladder physiology, relevant to older people that should be explored at the time of presentation. These commonly interact with a greater propensity for incontinence so as to cause it, such that correction will lead to continence. Conditions related to incontinence are listed in Table 109-1.

The importance of a medication review and alteration in the management of urinary incontinence in the elderly should not be underestimated. Table 109-2 lists the medications that may either precipitate or contribute to incontinence. Data from the National Audit of Continence Care for Older People suggest that, at best, this is only done for 33% of older people in primary care[48] but there is undoubted value in this.

MULTICHANNEL CYSTOMETRY

Multichannel cystometry "urodynamics" has been the principal method used to explore the physiologic changes in the lower urinary tract particularly seen in elderly people, but is also used, sometimes erroneously, as a diagnostic tool. A urodynamic study is not necessary for the initial conservative management of anyone presenting with urinary incontinence, be they young or old, and age should not influence the decision to use the investigation. However, an understanding of the test is certainly worthwhile.

The study describes a number of aspects of lower urinary tract function extremely accurately; for example, a urodynamic study measures urinary outflow obstruction precisely.[49]

However, the majority of urologists operate on the basis of symptoms rather than the physical demonstration of obstruction and do not routinely perform cystometry.[50] Because similar symptoms are found in roughly as many urodynamically obstructed and unobstructed men, it is inevitable that the

Table 109-2. Medications That May Either Precipitate or Contribute to Incontinence

Medications	Effects on Continence
α-adrenergic agonists	Increase smooth muscle tone in urethra and prostatic capsule and may precipitate obstruction, urinary retention, and related symptoms
α-adrenergic antagonists	Decrease smooth muscle tone in the urethra and may precipitate stress urinary incontinence in women
Angiotensin-converting enzyme (ACE) inhibitors	Cause cough that can exacerbate incontinence
Agents with antimuscarinic properties	May cause urinary retention and constipation that can contribute to incontinence; may cause cognitive impairment and reduce effective toileting ability
Calcium channel blockers	May cause urinary retention and constipation that can contribute to incontinence May cause dependent edema, which can contribute to nocturnal polyuria
Cholinesterase inhibitors (cognitive enhancers)	Increase bladder contractility and may precipitate urgency incontinence
Diuretics	Cause diuresis and precipitate incontinence
Lithium	Polyuria due to diabetes insipidus-like state
Opioid analgesics	May cause urinary retention, constipation, confusion, and immobility—all of which can contribute to incontinence
Psychotropic drugs	Mayc ause confusion and impaired mobility and precipitate incontinence
Sedatives	Some agents have anticholinergic effects
Hypnotics	
Antipsychotics	
Histamine$_1$ receptor antagonists	
Selective serotonin re-uptake inhibitors	Increase cholinergic transmission and may lead to urgency urinary incontinence
Other drugs	Can cause edema, which can lead to polyuria while supine and exacerbate nocturia and nighttime incontinence
Gabapentin	
Glitazones	
Nonsteroidal antiinflammatory agents	

clinical syndrome bearing the name "obstruction" is divorced from the urodynamic measure. Likewise, the requirement to demonstrate involuntary contractile behavior of the detrusor in association with symptoms to make the urodynamic diagnosis of detrusor overactivity also leads to up to 25% of subjects with urgency and urgency incontinence not having a diagnosis made. This is not a problem with the measure, but with the preoccupation that diagnoses should occupy specific "boxes" without overlap.[51]

On presentation, patients are asked to empty their bladders while urine flow rate is measured by means of a flow meter positioned in an adapted commode. A Jaques catheter (French gauge 10) and a nylon catheter (16 G) are placed in the bladder via the urethra, which is usually anesthetized with lidocaine gel. The postmicturition residual urine is drained off and measured. Another catheter (French gauge 10) tipped with a perforated latex sheath to prevent fecal plugging, is introduced into the rectum. The smaller bladder catheter and the rectal catheter are filled with normal saline and then connected to force displacement transducers mounted at the level of the superior ramus of the pubic bone. This reference point is used to establish atmospheric pressure. The detrusor pressure, generated by the walls of the bladder, is calculated by subtracting the intraabdominal pressure (measured via the rectal catheter) from the intravesical pressure (measured via the bladder catheter). The bladder is filled with a fluid at a rate of between 50 and 100 mL min^{-1}. The subject is asked to cough at intervals during the study to assess the quality of abdominal pressure subtraction and to report sensations of filling and urgency. The bladder is filled until either a maximum of 500 mL has been infused, or unstable detrusor activity prohibits further filling, or the patient is found to be unable to tolerate any further infusion. Unfortunately, filling rate, fluid temperature, and content are not standardized and vary with department preference. Videourodynamics uses radio-opaque contrast to fill the bladder. There has been an attempt to standardize the methods used for cystometry by both the international continence society and the British Society for Urogynaecology in the United Kingdom. Clearly some standardization is useful as this allows comparison of results and a quality assurance of the method by which these were obtained.

On completion of the filling study, the filling catheter is withdrawn from the bladder leaving the pressure measuring catheter in situ. The patient is then asked to void to completion. During voiding, the bladder and rectal pressure and the flow rate are recorded simultaneously.

During normal filling the detrusor pressure should only rise an amount consistent with the pressure head of the volume of fluid within it. If the detrusor contracts while the patient is attempting to inhibit micturition, then urodynamic detrusor overactivity is diagnosed. This should usually occur at the same time as the subjective sensation of urinary urgency, but the magnitude of the contraction may be small and not be associated with any sensation. In a subject with neurological disease, such as spinal cord injury or multiple sclerosis, this observation is termed detrusor overactivity of neurological origin.[40]

There is little evidence that the use of cystometry adds anything to history taking or makes a difference in outcome from treatment. When NICE made its recommendations on the rational, evidence-based use of cystometry, there was considerable adverse reaction from "clinical experts" often citing anecdotal evidence or conflating arguments about the utility of an additional investigation in the assessment of incontinent patients.[52]

AGE-RELATED PATHOPHYSIOLOGY

Early studies of age-related urodynamic findings were conducted on samples of elderly people without younger comparisons.[53–55]

In more recent studies, people with lower urinary tract symptoms have been compared across all age groups.[56–59]

Urgency incontinence is the commonest cause of urinary incontinence in elderly people, this being due chiefly to detrusor overactivity. This is particularly the case in elderly people living in institutions.[60,61] Among outpatients having lower urinary tract symptoms, between 75% and 85% of women aged 75 and over and 85% and 95% of similarly aged men will be found to have detrusor overactivity.[62] The observed changes associated with greater age in men and women with lower urinary tract symptoms undergoing cystometry are listed in Table 109-3 and illustrated in Figures 109-1 through 109-5.

It is interesting to note that men with lower urinary tract symptoms do not demonstrate all of the age-related changes associated with women. This probably relates to the higher urethral resistance caused by the prostate gland, causing detrusor muscle hypertrophy. The influence of this "obstructive" organ may dominate the evolution of bladder physiology.[63] In elderly people of both sexes, detrusor overactivity is associated with lower bladder capacities than in those with normal bladders. Contrary to expectations, lower bladder capacities, more aggressive detrusor overactivity, and older age do not appear to be associated with a poorer therapeutic prognosis. In fact, there do not appear to be any urodynamic variables indicative of a poorer outcome from treatment.[36]

Both sexes void less successfully in late life and voiding is associated with higher residual urine volumes and a higher proportion of patients with incomplete bladder emptying.

Table 109-3. Changes Associated With Greater Age in Men and Women With Lower Urinary Tract Symptoms Undergoing Cystometry

Decreased
Urinary flow rate
Speed of contraction of detrusor
Collagen:detrusor ratio (♀ only)
Maximum bladder capacity
Functional bladder capacity
Sensation of filling
Increased
Postvoid residual volume of urine
Urinary frequency
Outflow tract obstruction (♂ only)

The explanations for this are probably complex. Obstruction will play a part in men but it is by no means the only explanation. There is evidence for a reduced speed of detrusor shortening in late life and problems in sustaining adequate voiding contractions. The transmission of force from the detrusor in later life is damped by an accumulation of collagen and connective tissue, giving the impression of "impaired contractility" a common misnomer.

The combination of detrusor instability and incomplete bladder emptying in elderly people raises the controversy of "detrusor hyperactivity and impaired contractility" (DHIC). This was described by Resnick and Yalla when reporting on 32 elderly nursing home residents in 1987.[64] They identified a specific physiologic entity, being a subset of detrusor hyperreflexia in elderly people. The characteristics were involuntary detrusor contractions, a postmicturition residual urine volume, and a reduced speed and amplitude of isometric detrusor contractions. In studying a much larger sample of elderly people, such a distinct physiologic subgroup has not been identified. Voiding problems and detrusor overactivity, often coexist in elderly people but seem to be independent of each other.

Additionally, Elbadawi et al[65] have published data from electron microscopy studies of bladder biopsy specimens from elderly men (n = 11) and women (n = 24), which are in support of distinct pathophysiologic subgroups of detrusor function. They reported four structural patterns precisely matching four urodynamic groups with no overlap. Additionally two subsets, "normal contractility" (n = 11) and "impaired contractility" (n = 24) matched histologic subsets exactly. These findings have not been corroborated despite Carey et al[66] having reported finding some of the defining histologic characteristics described by Elbadawi et al[67] evenly distributed between normal women (n = 15) and women with detrusor overactivity (n = 22). In vitro studies of detrusor muscle contraction reveal a lower level of acetylcholine release in association with increasing age,[68] there are also data showing a reduction in the number of acetylcholinesterase containing nerves within the muscle.[69]

There are additionally changes in urethral function associated with aging in women. Figure 109-6 demonstrates a plot of the voiding detrusor pressure against flow rate recorded

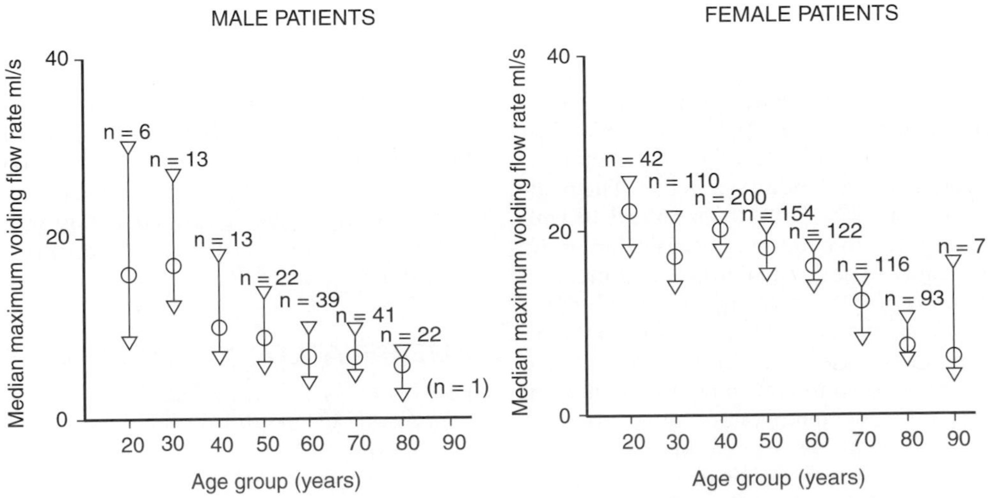

Figure 109-1. Urinary flow rate by decade of life in men and women with lower urinary tract symptoms.

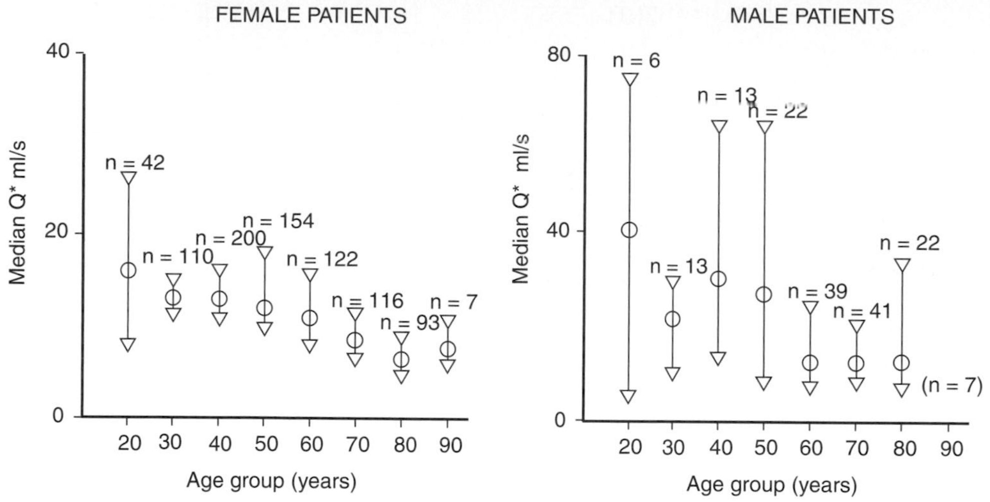

Figure 109-2. Speed of detrusor muscle shortening, calculated from the voiding pressure-flow plot in men and women with lower urinary tract symptoms in association with age.

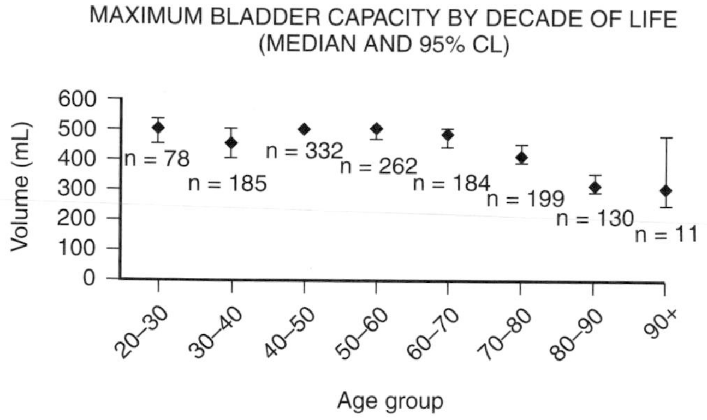

Figure 109-3. Maximum cystometric bladder capacity for women with lower urinary tract symptoms in association with age.

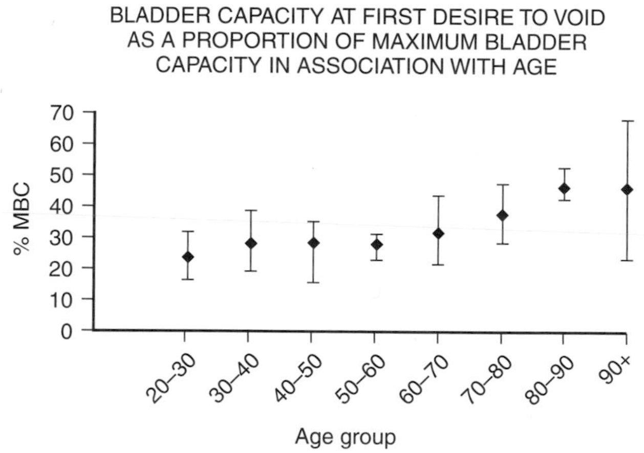

Figure 109-4. First desire to void, plotted as a proportion of maximum bladder capacity in women with lower urinary tract symptoms associated with age.

from a urodynamic study. The two pressure intercepts shown, $p_{det.clos}$ and $p_{det.open}$, are invariably elevated in the presence of detrusor overactivity and lower in the presence of stress urinary incontinence. Where both conditions exist, the values take the middle ground. Highest values are seen in neurologic diseases such as multiple sclerosis. Greater age in women is associated with lower values of both $p_{det.close}$ and $p_{det.open}$, even in the presence of detrusor overactivity (Figure 109-7). Data from studies measuring the maximum urethral closure pressure also show a similar decline in association with increasing age. Histologically, there is evidence of an age-related apoptosis of striated muscle cells of the urethral sphincter.[70,71]

ASSESMENT OF THE ELDERY INCONTINENT PATIENT

A screening question about bladder and bowel care as part of any interaction between an older person and a clinician is recommended. Many of the single assessment processes mandated by the National Service Framework for Older People contain a simple question such as "Do you have any problems with either your bladder or bowel?" A validated screening or case-finding questionnaire could be used in appropriate settings.[72]

Should the answer to that question be positive, then an assessment should be offered. However, this is not always the case. Essentially, problems can be divided into those relating to the storage of urine and those of emptying. Incontinence might be as a result of failure of either functions of the bladder. Useful questions are shown in Table 109-4.

Additional questions that should be asked relate to obstetric history (for example, the number of deliveries and if these were by forceps or were very prolonged), surgery, and bowel function, especially constipation and fecal incontinence because this can commonly coexist in frail, older people. Underlying causes of urinary incontinence may readily be identified. Characteristic features are shown in Table 109-5.

Assessing cognitive function

Older, cognitively impaired people are less able to cooperate in lifestyle interventions for their incontinence. They may also be at risk of developing further impaired cognition in response to drug therapy for their problem. Many older people are taking medication with antimuscarinic properties and

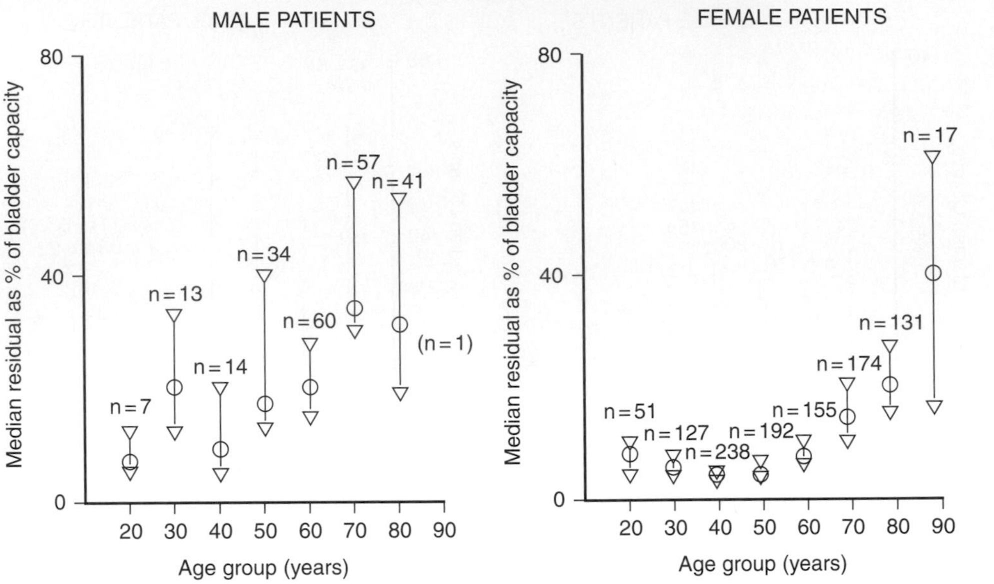

Figure 109-5. Postvoid residual volume of urine for men and women with lower urinary tract symptoms associated with age.

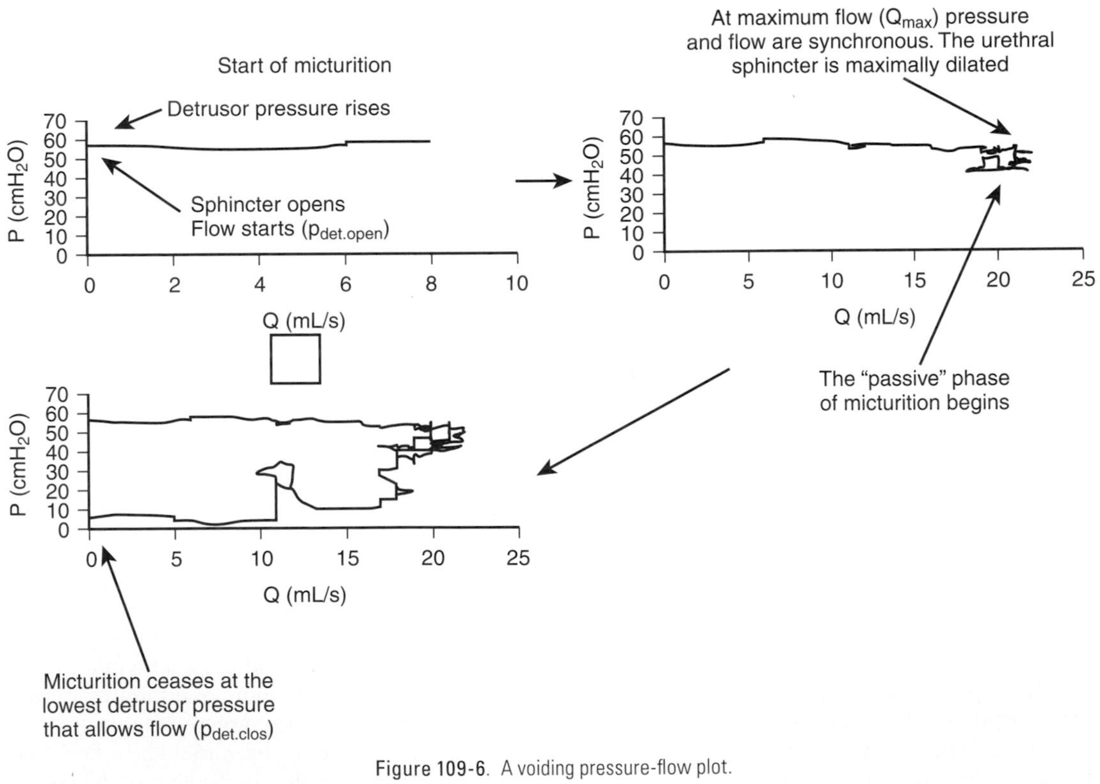

Figure 109-6. A voiding pressure-flow plot.

are at risk of subclinical cognitive impairment.[73] Oxybutynin, used for the treatment of overactive bladder, is associated with an impairment of cognition in normal older people.[74] There are also case reports of acute delirium in patients with preexisting cognitive impairment.[75,76] Therefore it is a good idea to assess this formally. Simple, robust, and reliable scoring such as the Folstein MMSE may be employed but, as yet, it is not known if this is sensitive enough to detect what might be subtle change. It can be performed in a short time and may serve as a baseline measure against which to judge the impact of treatment interventions or to assess what level of complexity of management the patient might tolerate.

Bladder diaries

Where possible, a bladder diary should be obtained to gain an understanding of the person's bladder habits and associated symptoms. A 3-day diary is usually sufficient. This can either be a tick chart of voiding frequency and incontinence episodes, or can include volume measurements at each void. This is most useful when polyuria or nocturnal polyuria is suspected (excessive nighttime voiding or enuresis). A bladder diary is difficult to obtain for the very old, frail, and cognitively impaired and obtaining a reliable recording requires considerable effort and observation, particularly if there are a considerable number of incontinent voids. The process will involve observation and regular "wet checks" to allow building up a pattern of voiding. Involvement of an informal caregiver, where one is available may be beneficial.

Examination

A physical examination should be performed for all people complaining of urinary incontinence. This at a minimum should consist of urinalysis to exclude infection and the presence of hematuria, and a rectal examination to exclude fecal loading as a precipitating factor for the incontinence. A digital rectal examination also allows the assessment of the prostate in men. Palpation of the abdomen will detect large volumes of urine in the bladder and can exclude large volume retention. For a more detailed examination and estimation of a postmicturition residual volume of urine, a portable ultrasound bladder scanner should be used.

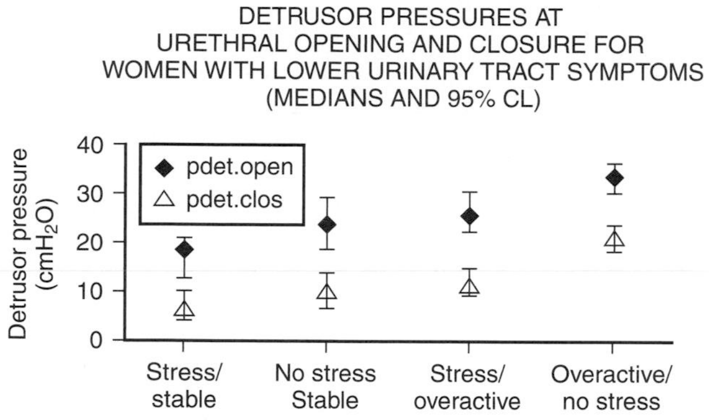

Figure 109-7. $p_{det.open}$ and $p_{det.close}$ associated with detrusor overactivity, normal cystometry, and urodynamic stress incontinence.

Vaginal examination

This is considered to be an important part of a continence assessment, however, this should only be undertaken by a professional with the necessary competence and probably as part of a specialist rather than generalist assessment. A visual examination though might reveal conditions such as urogenital atrophy or prolapse that can cause urinary symptoms. Typically, women complain of the presence of the "lump" in their vagina that may sometimes be visible, a dragging sensation or discomfort especially when sitting. The prolapse itself may cause voiding difficulty, leading to a postmicturition residual volume or occasionally may mask underlying stress urinary incontinence. What the generalist can do, though, is easily identify a significant urogenital prolapse — certainly those that protrude beyond the introitus should be referred for a specialist examination. Visual inspection of the skin will also help in the planning of treatment to maintain skin integrity where this is threatened.

Urinalysis

This should be done for all patients with urinary incontinence at first presentation, or if there is a change in symptoms suggesting infection of the urine. The presence of frank blood indicates the need for action to be taken. The best dipstick tests to use are those with leucocytes and nitrite test pads; if both tests are negative, the chance of there being an infection is low when compared with laboratory evidence of a UTI based upon microscopic pyuria and bacteruria.[77] Large amounts of glucose or ketones in the urine can make the nitrite test falsely negative and the utility of this test has recently been called into question.[78] If there are lower

Table 109-4. Questions About Urine Storage Symptoms

Symptom	Questions to Ask
Daytime frequency	How many times do you have to pass water in the day?
Nighttime frequency (nocturia)	How many times do you have to pass water at night?
Urgency	Do you get a desperate need to pass water that you find hard to hold?
Urgency incontinence	Do you wet yourself by accident because you do not reach the lavatory in time?
Stress urinary incontinence	Do you wet yourself if you cough, laugh, or exert yourself?
Aggravating factors	Do any of the following aggravate your symptoms: running water, cold weather, putting the key in the door and/or psychological stress.
The presence of the following symptoms should lead to specific action:	
Dysuria	Urinalysis and collect a urine sample for microscopy; treat according to findings
Hematuria	Assess for underlying pathology
Pain	
Questions About Voiding Symptoms	
Symptom	**Questions to Ask**
Continual (passive) urine loss	Does your urine leak continually by night and day? (Suggests either a fistula [women] or retention and overflow incontinence [men >> women])
Hesitancy or straining to void	Do you have to wait a long time in the lavatory before the urine flows? Do you have to push or strain to pass urine?
Poor or intermittent stream - indicating bladder outflow tract obstruction	Is the flow weak or does it stop and start as you empty you bladder?
Terminal dribbling - related to outflow tract obstruction	Do you continue to leak urine even after you have finished emptying your bladder?
Postmicturition dribbling - dribble from the penis due to urine staying in the urethra after bladder emptying	Do you leak urine a while after you have left the toilet? (men>>women)
Incomplete emptying	Do you feel that after you have emptied your bladder there is more to pass?
Prolapse	Do you feel a lump coming down your vagina when you pass water?

Table 109-5. Making a Distinction Between Stress and Urgency Incontinence

Factor	Stress	Urge/Urgency
Loss of urine with exertion (e.g., coughing, sneezing, lifting, or exercise	Typical	Uncommon
Nocturia	Uncommon	Typical
Frequency - voiding >8 times in a 24-hr period	Uncommon	Typical
Sudden uncontrollable urge to urinate	Uncommon	Typical
Volume of urine lost with each incontinence episode	Small	Moderate/large

Adapted from: Fantl JA, Newman DK, Colling J et al. Urinary incontinence in adults: acute and chronic management: clinical practice guideline, No. 2, 1996 Update. Rockville, Md: US Department of Health and Human Services, Public Health Service, Agency for Health Care Policy and Research; March 1996. AHCPR Publication No. 96-0682.

urinary tract symptoms or the patient has a delirium, then a midstream specimen of urine should be obtained if at all possible. For the very frail, there are pads that are similar to those used in pediatric practice that enable the collection if urine. For those doubly incontinent, an in and out catheter may be the only way of reliably obtaining a specimen.

Asymptomatic bacteriuria (the presence of bacteria in the urine that occurs without symptoms) is common in older women (in excess of 15%)[79] and treating this will have no effect on incontinence or on the general health of the individual. Antibiotic treatment will merely add to the likelihood of developing resistance to the antibiotic and expose the individual to antibiotic-related side effects. If the patient is already known to be chronically incontinent, then eradicating the bacteria will not help.[80] Women who do not have symptoms, and whose urine is negative for leukocyte esterase and nitrites, are most unlikely to have a UTI and do not require urine culture.

If dipstick-positive blood is found, it should be followed up by sending a sample for microscopy. If there is true microscopic hematuria, then a referral for investigation should be made because this can result from having urinary tract stones or a tumor. Clearly glycosuria, indicating either a low renal threshold for glucose or poorly controlled diabetes mellitus, requires further investigation and will cause polyuria.

Rectal examination

Whether or not a rectal examination should be routinely performed for all older people with urinary incontinence continues to promote discussion and opinion.

Although there is no published evidence that performing a rectal examination alters outcomes for the treatment of incontinence in women, expert opinion suggests that a loaded rectum may, because of its size, lead to voiding difficulty or the presence of a significant postvoid residual volume. Additionally, an assessment of prostate size and consistency in men will help to guide medical treatment. Occasionally, fecal impaction will lead to acute retention, resolution of which will lead to normal voiding.

THE TREATMENT OF URINARY INCONTINENCE

The overall aim in managing and treating incontinence is not cure; an absolute cure is seldom achieved and the best that any clinician might aim for is resolution of symptoms leading to a return to normal bladder habits and a normal lifestyle. Data from randomized, controlled studies of interventions for older people in this area are available but often exclude the frail elderly, thus extrapolations have to be made. In some instances, these may be perfectly valid but sometimes caution needs to be taken. This section will outline evidence based treatment interventions for the main incontinence syndromes in older people.

General measures

Fluid balance - Although many older people restrict the amount of fluid they drink, there are data to suggest that the achievement of a "normal" fluid balance (1 to 1.5 L/day in a temperate climate) and awareness of bladder habits can lead to an improvement in lower urinary tract symptoms.

Weight loss - In epidemiologic studies, more women with incontinence report themselves as being short for their weight or overweight. Evidence for the improvement of symptoms comes from two studies: one in which the intervention was a 3-month liquid only diet, achieving a median weight loss of 16 kg in the intervention group and resulting in a greater than 50% resolution of urinary tract symptoms, which was sustained for the 6 months of the study.[81] A more recent U.K. study[82] showed that 5% weight loss can improve incontinence severity and have a beneficial effect on quality of life in obese women with urinary incontinence.

Caffeine - There are conflicting epidemiologic data about the effect of caffeinated drinks on lower urinary tract symptoms but reduction is supported by one RCT.[83] There are no specific data for the elderly, but should a patient express the sentiment that tea or coffee appears to worsen their symptoms then it would seem sensible to attempt reduction.

Bladder retraining

The purpose of bladder retraining is to extend the intervoid interval, increase bladder capacity, and overcome urinary urgency. There are many methods espoused, and none are superior to others. Bladder diaries are often used as an adjunct to retraining, making people aware of their bladder habits and reinforcing change. The patient uses the chart to keep a record of episodes of micturition, while gradual efforts are made to delay micturition after the urge to void is experienced. The technique is effective.[84–86] However, it is not necessarily easy and clinical trial evidence illustrates the need for appropriate support in achieving a good outcome. Some patients with detrusor overactivity will experience pain while delaying micturition, and there is a real possibility of urge incontinence while working with the regime. Stretching the bladder can be augmented by encouraging higher fluid intake while at home, when an episode of incontinence can be dealt with in private. Increasing incontinence is more likely if the urethral sphincter is incompetent as the larger bladder volumes will increase pressure on the sphincter. As the bladder empties more efficiently from a capacity between 3 and 500 mL, it is logical to use a bladder retraining regime to treat voiding problems secondary to detrusor muscle lesions. Excessive delay, so that the bladder capacity rises substantially above 500 mL, should be avoided as such overdistention is associated with ineffective voiding. Should bladder retraining and lifestyle measures fail to achieve satisfactory symptom control, then pharmacologic options for treatment are available.

Up to 70% of people in their eighth decade of life report at least one life limiting coexistent medical condition, even those who report themselves as "fit." However, frailer and older men and women are often excluded from clinical studies in this field by virtue of these or the treatments for them.[87] Seldom do published papers report the number of people who were screened for inclusion in a study but were ineligible. Such studies that are published then include data on the physiologically, if not chronologically, younger group of older people. The results of these studies should thus be considered in this light.

The hypotheses underlying drug treatment for OAB have undergone a revolution over the last 8 years; it was widely held that the action of antimuscarinic agents was to suppress overactive contractions of the bladder acting via M_3 receptors, although data to support this were inconsistent.[88] It has become established that there is considerable sensory dysfunction associated with OAB and that M_2 receptors, found in the suburothelium, have a significant effect on the appreciation of urinary urgency. Newer drugs are now targeted to control urinary urgency, a central feature of the symptom complex that has a major impact on quality of life.[89,90] The role of antimuscarinics in patients with cognitive impairment is discussed later.

Oxybutynin is the most established antimuscarinic drug in use today. Trials comparing oxybutynin with placebo have consistently shown a reduction in symptoms with the active drug. Studies in older people, using lower doses of the drug than the usual licensed dose of 5 mg three times daily, have some efficacy with a concomitant reduction in the adverse effects and an enhanced level of tolerability of the drug, which at normal dosing resulted in up to 60% of subjects being unable to take it.[85,91,92] Oxybutynin is also effective when used in combination with prompted voiding schedules in the nursing-home environment. However, the drug had no effect on the requirement for nursing intervention in the management of incontinence, and the authors concluded that there was little justification for its use.[93] Extended-release oxybutynin was also reported to be an effective compound in the elderly, with 31% remaining free of urge incontinence in one 12-week study. However, 58.6% of subjects reported dry mouth, with 23.0% rating it moderate or severe; but despite this, only 1.6% of subjects withdrew.[94] There are two studies of extended release oxybutynin, one examining the effect of the drug on the management of cognitively impaired nursing home residents with urgency incontinence and the other covering women over the age of 65.[95,96]

Oxybutynin is also available in a transdermal preparation that is effective and avoids most antimuscarinic side effects associated with the oral preparation, and fewer systemic side effects than oral extended-release tolterodine. Side effects associated with transdermal delivery include local application-site irritation or erythema, generally managed by appropriate rotation of the application site, but described as severe in 2.5% of subjects.[97,98] Published analyses of the efficacy of transdermal oxybutynin included subjects of up to 100 years of age and those in institutional care settings.[99]

Solifenacin is a long-acting once-daily antimuscarinic agent that is effective in the treatment of OAB. A pooled analysis of results from older subjects taking solifenacin showed the drug to be effective in reducing urinary frequency, the number of urgency episodes, and sensation of urgency, with a restoration of continence in up to 49% of people.[100] In the pooled analysis, 13.5% of people on 5 mg reported dry mouth, which was mild to moderate. At the higher dose, a third of people complained of dry mouth, and in 1.9% this was reported as severe. In a randomized controlled trial versus tolterodine extended-release, solifenacin was shown to be equivalent in terms of reduction in micturition frequency and, in an analysis of secondary end points, better than tolterodine in several key indicators. There appeared to be no lessening of effect in those subjects aged over 65 years.[101]

Tolterodine is a nonselective antimuscarinic agent that appears to have some functional selectivity and greater affinity for bladder muscarinic receptors over those in the salivary glands. This appears to explain the lower incidence of dry mouth, 12.9% in one long-term study,[102] and the reduction in withdrawals from treatment seen with the use of the drug. The extended-release form of the drug gives greater tolerability and better efficacy than the immediate-release compound, which should be reserved for those older people with significant hepatic impairment. An effect of therapy can be seen within a week but the maximum effect is seen after 5 to 8 weeks of treatment.[103,104] There are published data specifically relating to the elderly that show efficacy, but there appears to be some diminution of effect in older people in some studies, although the clinical relevance of this is unclear.[105–107] Tolterodine does not appear to significantly worsen the postvoid residual urine volume and has been effective in treating men with both OAB and bladder outflow tract obstruction.[108,109] An evening dose of the drug is effective in reducing nocturnal voids and has been shown to be more tolerable.[110]

Imipramine appears to have a strong inhibitory effect on detrusor muscle. In the treatment of 10 elderly patients with detrusor instability, the use of imipramine was effective in achieving continence in six at doses of 25 to 150 mg. However, the existing evidence is of only moderate quality, and the incidence of side effects, particularly severe dry mouth, make it difficult to titrate to an effective dose.[111]

Propiverine hydrochloride has combined antimuscarinic and calcium channel blocking actions. Comparative trials against flavoxate and a placebo, and oxybutynin and a placebo, showed that propiverine has a similar efficacy to oxybutynin. Propiverine has a similar efficacy in treatment of symptoms to oxybutynin 5 mg twice daily, but with a statistically significantly milder and less common incidence of dry mouth. Although there are no specific data in older people, the elderly were not specifically excluded from studies. However, up to 20% of patients have adverse effects, which are mainly anticholinergic.[112,113]

Trospium chloride is a quaternary ammonium salt derived from atropine; it was effective in treating DO in several randomized controlled trials using urodynamic measures of diagnosis and extent of disease, and clinical and quality-of-life outcomes.[114–116] These studies included patients aged over 70 years, and there are no data to suggest that the elderly do less well. The drug was assessed in studies versus placebo and standard release oxybutynin, and was better in effect to placebo and equivalent in efficacy to oxybutynin, when treating DO at doses of 5 mg three times daily. Adverse effects occur less commonly with trospium than with oxybutynin. The drug has no significant drug-drug interactions and does not cross the blood-brain barrier, and thus it is unlikely to have an adverse effect on cognition. Except for one study on driving ability, changes in alpha wave activity on the electroencephalogram have been used as a surrogate end point.[117,118] Trospium might therefore be a useful drug where there is coexisting polypharmacy or concern about significant cognitive dysfunction.

Darifenacin is an antimuscarinic agent that has fiftyfold selectivity for M_3 over M_2 receptors, but only ninefold for M_3 over M_1. The drug has been specifically tested in older people in randomized controlled trials, and is effective in terms of objective and subjective variables and quality of life. Pooled data from the population aged over 65 years show a similar effect size to the younger groups.[119,120] In cognitively intact older people, darifenacin does not adversely affect cognition, probably due to its lack of M_1 receptor activity, and its CNS tolerability appears to be similar to a placebo.[121] The results of a study of darifenacin in the more elderly (over 75 years) failed to reach its primary end point, but more people on the drug than a placebo experienced a response to treatment.[122] The major side effects are constipation, affecting at most 23.6% of subjects at a dose of 15 mg, 10% of whom required treatment for this (although only 2.7% withdrew from treatment because of this) and dry mouth.

Fesoterodine, a prodrug that is converted into the active metabolite of tolterodine (5-hydroxymethyl tolterodine) has recently been launched in Europe and is due for launch in the United States in 2009. It is statistically significantly better than a placebo in all of the objective disease variables and has a favorable effect on quality of life.[123,124] For some outcome measures, the 8 mg dose appears to be more effective than the 4 mg dose. The side effect profile appears much the same as other available antimuscarinics with the exception of a lower incidence of reported constipation; whether this is borne out in current trials and clinical use remains to be seen.

OTHER PHARMACOLOGIC MEASURES

Although there is no evidence for estrogen therapy being of use in the treatment of incontinence in women, there are data to support the use of topical estrogens for treating OAB in postmenopausal women. One systematic review of studies involving 430 subjects found benefits in all of the relevant symptoms associated with the condition.[125] It may, however, have a role in the management of recurrent urinary infection. Estrogen withdrawal is associated with a fall in the levels of intravaginal glycogen on which lactobacilli depend. These bacteria cease to colonize the vagina, which is then occupied by colonic organisms that thrive in the higher pH associated with this change.[126] The atrophy of the urothelium encourages colonization by gram-negative fecal organisms and the bacteria adhere more easily. There is some evidence that estrogen replacement therapy may reverse this process and give protection to elderly women with recurrent urinary tract infection.[127–130]

Topical estrogen therapy appears to be associated with a negligible risk of endometrial hyperplasia and certainly, our oncologists are happy for its use even in those women with a previous breast cancer. A minimum of 3-months use is required as a trial of efficacy. Those women on systemic HRT are also just as likely to have urogenital atrophy as not; they should not be excluded from either an examination or treatment.

Desmopressin (synthetic antidiuretic hormone with no effect on blood pressure) can be useful in those individuals with nocturnal frequency or nocturnal polyuria. Its use might be hampered by drug-drug interactions, predisposing to hyponatremia or excessive drinking habits.[131] More recent data have been offered in support of careful, supervised use of desmopressin in older individuals.[132] In one meta-analysis of available trial data, dilutional hyponatremia occurred in 7% of patients, all within the initial phase of dose titration.[133] Given that this decrease in serum sodium may occur within 72 hours, it is worthwhile checking the levels before and 72 hours after initiation. Levels should be then checked again if there is any change to the disease state or treatment taken by the patient.

FLAVOXATE HYDROCHLORIDE (URISPAS)

At one time this drug was used extensively for treating the overactive bladder but its efficacy has not been shown in data from controlled clinical trials versus placebo. It is no longer considered to be an effective drug for the overactive bladder or detrusor overactivity.[134–136] There are no data from studies including the frailer elderly.

Surgery for detrusor overactivity

Surgical measures for the treatment of detrusor overactivity have developed over the years but there are, needless to say, few data on the elderly. There has been a rapid expansion in the intradetrusor usage of botulinum toxin, although an unlicensed indication, for both people with spinal cord injury and those with idiopathic detrusor overactivity, although evidence for the latter from randomized trials is lacking. The treatment appears to be efficacious, and the beneficial effect lasts up to 9 months per injection. The main adverse effect is voiding dysfunction, requiring the patient to revert to clean intermittent catheterization. In some studies of middle-aged women, the rate of this has reached 43%.[137] The elderly, with a higher prevalence of impaired voiding, may be at a higher risk of developing this complication. There are randomized, controlled trials underway.

For severe cases of urgency urinary incontinence not responding to conventional medical therapy, potential surgical approaches are sacral nerve modulation and the clam ileocystoplasty. Sacral neuromodulation appears effective for carefully selected individuals and some series have reported results in a few subjects over the age of 65. Approximately a third of subjects appear to require re-operation and reimplantation of the stimulator. Age over 55 years appears to be associated with a poorer outcome.[138,139] The precise mechanism by which neuromodulation has its effect still remains to be ascertained. Patients are committed to lifelong follow-up and many will require reoperation during the lifetime of the device.[140] Finally, the Clam ileocystoplasty is probably the only operation for detrusor overactivity for which there is evidence of efficacy. Some series have reported on patients in their eighth decade with good results.[141] However, since the procedure makes voluntary bladder emptying ineffective, patients require clean intermittent self-catheterization to empty.[142] Some elderly patients can cope with this, but the prevalence of multiple disabilities in late life demand careful selection and counseling.

Correcting sphincter incompetence

Pelvic floor muscle therapy remains the mainstay of conservative therapy for stress urinary incontinence. The evidence for their efficacy is limited in terms of quality but they are recommended by the Cochrane collaboration systematic reviews, and in England and Wales by NICE. Data are mostly from open studies or within group analyses of comparative trial data.[141] Data on pelvic floor exercises (PFE) in the elderly, however, are somewhat lacking, as might be expected but there are data from Japan, combining PFE with general physiotherapy for walking speed and muscle strength resulting in overall improvement in incontinence, although this may have been related to the loss of weight and greater ability to toilet effectively rather than any direct LVT effect.[142] The effect size for PFE in terms of incontinent episodes, leakage amount, and perceived severity for women older than 60 years of age was less than younger women but was still beneficial overall rather than but still is of statistically significant benefit.[143] Exercise programs need to be supervised and supported, and last for at least 3 months, with the minimal amount of effective exercises to achieve any benefit appearing to be 24 to 32 daily. PFE have not been found to be superior to surgery. Although they are advocated for the treatment of stress incontinence in older women, there is no specific evidence to support any specific efficacy in this group. It is regrettable that no large-scale studies of efficacy, which include age comparisons, have been conducted, so doubt hangs over their application. For men, PFE are used in the context of postprostatectomy incontinence where stress incontinence may affect up to 10% following a radical procedure. Evidence for their long-term efficacy is lacking and has been subjected to a Cochrane review.[144]

MEDICATION

Until recently there were no drug treatments with evidence of efficacy in the treatment of stress urinary incontinence. However, duloxetine, a combined serotonin and noradrenaline reuptake inhibitor was licensed in Europe in 2004. It is thought to act by increasing the tone of the urethral sphincter. There are data from randomized, controlled trials supporting its efficacy in women (it is not licensed for use in men) but there are no specific data in the elderly. The main side effect of the drug in clinical practice is nausea in 24% of women that caused 6.4% of all withdrawals within trials.[145] In clinical practice, even with slow titration of the dose, the withdrawal rate is higher.[146] The drug has not been considered by the FDA. In England and Wales, NICE does not recommend the drug for the treatment of stress urinary incontinence in women on pharmacoeconomic grounds.

SURGERY

Surgery for stress urinary incontinence has been revolutionized over the past 7 years by the wholesale adoption of the midurethral tapes, such as the tension-free vaginal tape (TVT). These have supplanted colposuspension as the primary procedure for urethral incompetence. There are now 10-year data showing efficacy and data also exist for older women[147] who, while not achieving the same extent of cure as younger women, did gain meaningful reductions in incontinence and were satisfied with their result. Other approaches to insertion of the tapes are possible; the transobturator route is often used in more obese women, with similar efficacy to the TVT, but a higher incidence of leg pain. The open Burch colposuspension remains the "gold standard" procedure for stress urinary incontinence with a sustained improvement up to 20 years postoperation.[148] For frailer, older women, the use of agents to bulk the urethral sphincter have been used with acceptable short- to medium-term results but these diminish with time and repeat injection may be required to achieve efficacy.[149]

THE AS ARTIFICIAL URINARY SPHINCTER

This is an option for the management of urethral sphincter failure in both sexes. It is best suited to people who do not have detrusor overactivity, but needless to say, there are no data in older people. The operation involves the insertion of a cuff around the urethra. This cuff is passively inflated from a reservoir of fluid placed in the pelvis. The cuff can be deflated, so as to allow voiding, by activating a pump placed in the scrotum or labia majora. After voiding, the cuff reinflates spontaneously. Complications include infection, displacement of the device, and mechanical failure. In one series with a 9 year follow-up, 35% of patients required a surgical revision.[150] In correctly selected patients, this prosthetic sphincter is highly effective.[151]

Treating voiding disorders

Intermittent self-catheterization is now the mainstay of management of voiding disorders associated with neurologic disease.[152,153]

Older people of both sexes have an increased tendency toward incomplete bladder emptying and this frequently coexists with detrusor overactivity. Voiding disorders may occur in the absence of symptoms but where there are symptoms, such as urinary frequency, recurrent urinary tract infection, or renal impairment, this can be managed by intermittent catheterization.[154]

There are no outcome data with regard to this technique in elderly people. It is clear, though, that asymptomatic individuals can probably be left alone. An assessment of the postmicturition residual urine volume is a routine part of our standard management protocol in men. There are data to suggest that women without voiding symptoms are unlikely to have a significant residual volume of urine. When we discover a significant problem, which we define as a residual of 200 mL or more, we institute a temporary, once daily intermittent catheterization program; this can be delivered by community nursing services if required. If this results in a rapid and significant improvement in symptoms, we then establish a more permanent regime, otherwise we take no further action.

The procedure may be difficult because of cognitive impairment and poor dexterity. It is more usual for us to enlist the services of a spouse or partner to administer the procedure, although a number of elderly people can self-catheterize. We have found that the fluid output in elderly people tends to be lower so that a less frequent regime of daily or twice daily catheterizations may prove adequate. Some older women, with delicate atrophic urethras, appear to be able to reduce urethral trauma by using estrogen replacement therapy.

Maintenance products

Pads continue to play an important role in the management of uncontrolled urinary or fecal incontinence. However, ambulant patients will need to use these devices while awaiting a surgical cure, or more likely as "an insurance policy" in case of incontinence. The design, technology, function, and performance of incontinence pads have been reviewed with meticulous detail elsewhere. Nowadays, there are some very effective products available, but care needs to be taken when choosing a suitable range.[155] There are now considerable data on which to base an informed judgment of the most suitable products and most guidelines suggest that patient preference should guide choice.[156] Too often decisions on the aids to provide for people are not given sufficient importance and tend to be based primarily on cost considerations.[157]

INDWELLING CATHETERS

These have a role in the management of some patients. They are best reserved for people with voiding problems, with or without controllable overactivity, who are unable to manage intermittent catheterization. They may also be employed for the frailest oldest group who are either not suitable for outflow tract surgery or for whom the frequent changing of pads may cause distress or considerable discomfort. A suprapubic catheter may be preferable because it is easier to maintain and does not traumatize the urethra.

Recurrent blocking and infections are complications of permanent catheterization; this tends to occur following the formation of a biofilm on the outside of the catheter, which is more likely to form in alkaline urine. Anecdotal reports favor the use of vitamin C, 1 g tds and cranberry juice to combat blockage and infection, but there are no clinical trial data to support this, although cranberry juice seems to have urinary antiseptic properties.[158] There are no data to support the use of silver-coated catheters in preventing urinary tract infection, only short-term bacteruria.[159] A successful indwelling catheter need be changed only once every 3 months. Asymptomatic bacteriuria should be left untreated.[160,161] The use of a flip-flow valve instead of an external drainage bag is often very acceptable to many, but requires cognitive and manual dexterity to operate. They are unsuitable for those with high pressure detrusor overactivity or those with upper renal tract damage.

EXTERNAL SHEATH DRAINAGE

Condom catheters, which are fixed to the penis using adhesives specifically developed for this purpose, may also be acceptable to men and are attractive as an alternative to pads. Urine drains from a tube connected at the apex of the sheath. The main problem is difficulty in attaching them because of penile retraction into the suprapubic fat pad. There are special attachments that can deal with this problem. Additionally, some patients have problems with displacement in response to the physical stresses of movement. A small randomized controlled trial versus indwelling catheters in men averaging 73 years of age resulted in a reduction in symptomatic UTI or bacteruria, increased level of comfort, and a reduction in the amount of associated pain.[162]

KEY POINTS

Urinary Incontinence

- Urinary incontinence is a highly prevalent condition in older people.
- Careful history, examination, and assessment is sufficient to make a diagnosis of the underlying cause of the urinary incontinence in the majority of cases.
- An assessment of coexisting medications and medical conditions is essential in the evaluation of an older person with urinary incontinence.
- Both asymptomatic bacteriuria and an asymptomatic postvoid residual volume of urine do not require treatment.
- The most common underlying cause of LUTS in the older person is the overactive bladder, regardless of the presence or absence of bladder outflow tract obstruction.
- There is evidence for the conservative management of UI in frail older people by the use of prompted voiding, individualized toileting, and scheduled voiding.

For a complete list of references, please visit online only at www.expertconsult.com

CHAPTER 110

Pressure Sores

Bryan D. Struck

Five centuries ago, French physician Ambroise Paré described one of the earliest pressure ulcers in the medical literature, noting that "the bedsore on the buttock has come from having been too long a time lying on it, without moving himself."[1] Today, pressure ulcers continue to be a significant problem, costing billions of dollars annually.[2,3] The United States, the United Kingdom, and the European medical community spent significant time and effort creating staging guidelines, identifying risk factors, and outlining prevention strategies.[4,5,6] Even with these guidelines, pressure ulcers continue to haunt medicine in the twenty-first century. The older adult population is especially at risk. Incidence rates of pressure ulcer in the United States approach 38% in acute care, 40% in critical care units, and 24% in long-term care facilities.[4] Prevalence rates in the United Kingdom range from 8% to 20% for hospitalized patients.[7,8] For fiscal year 2006, there were 322,426 pressure ulcers reported as a secondary diagnosis for hospitalized Medicare beneficiaries, at an average cost per stay of $40,381.[9] As a result, the Centers for Medicare and Medicaid will be making significant payment adjustments for this high cost and high volume hospital complication in October 2008.[9] This chapter will describe how normal aging affects the known risk factors for pressure ulcer development, review the pathophysiology of pressure ulcers, describe new staging classification, and discuss prevention and treatment options.

NORMAL AGING

With increasing age, several changes occur throughout the skin, resulting in increased risk of pressure ulcer development. Epidermal turnover rates decrease by 30% to 50% by the age of 70, resulting in rougher skin with decreased barrier function.[10] Theoretically, this change plays a role in decreased healing of epidermal wounds. The dermal-epidermal junction flattens resulting in decreased contact between the two layers. As a result the two layers may easily separate, making older skin more likely to tear and blister.

The dermis provides the basic structure of the skin between the epidermis and the deeper structures (muscle and bone). The dermis is a complex connective tissue matrix consisting of collagenous, elastic, and reticular fibers, which provide strength and elasticity. The blood vessels, lymphatics, nerves, and deeper portions of the hair follicles are located in the dermis. Normal aging changes the structure of and function of the dermis. Basal and peak levels of cutaneous blood flow are reduced by about 60%, resulting in compromised vascular responsiveness during injury or infection.[10] This change may be mediated by endothelial dysfunction.[11] With age, collagen synthesis decreases and degradation increases, resulting in a loss of the connective tissue matrix and impaired wound healing.[10] Elastic fibers decrease in number and size, resulting in decreased skin elasticity. Photo aging may worsen these normal changes.

Subcutaneous fat decreases with age, decreasing its ability to protect deeper structures from injury. Distribution of subcutaneous fat changes (decreasing in face and hands, increasing in thighs and abdomen), which decreases pressure diffusion over bony prominences.

PATHOPHYSIOLOGY OF PRESSURE ULCERS

Pressure that disrupts normal circulation to the skin and deep structures is the primary factor in the development of pressure ulcers. A complex vascular system, consisting of large vessels and a network of capillaries, courses through the dermis to supply the skin with oxygen, nutrition, and remove waste. Motor nerves monitor arterioles and excretion production.[12] Blood flow through the macrocirculatory system is controlled by the microcirculatory system. Small conductance vessels in between these two systems conduct blood and resist flow.[13,14] Dermis capillary blood flow pressures range from 11 mm Hg at the venule side to 32 mm Hg on the arterial side. If capillary pressures rises above 32 mm Hg, blood flow will be disrupted, causing ischemia within hours.[15,16] An elderly patient, supine on a bed, generates pressure between 50 to 90 mm Hg at the location of the heel and greater trochanter, well above the capillary filling pressure. Animal skin studies suggest damage can begin in 2 hours in the presence of only 100 mm Hg pressure.[17]

However pressure is not the only extrinsic factor that influences ulcer development. Friction and shear also are extrinsic factors. Friction causes epidermal injury, which can increase damage already present by pressure. This often occurs when objects such as bed linen or clothes are allowed to rub on the skin, removing the epidermis. The age associated decrease in epidermal turnover rate may delay repair. Moisturizer use can decrease effects of friction.

Shear is the internal force that is generated when a body shifts or moves in a direction parallel to the plane of contact.[18] As an elderly person slides down in the bed, the skin adheres to the bed surface but the underlying structures move with the body. This causes tearing of capillaries and disruption in blood flow. Now less pressure is needed to occlude blood flow. These phenomena may be worsened by the loss of subcutaneous fat seen with normal aging. Using a draw sheet and keeping a low head of bed elevation can minimize shear.

The final extrinsic factor is excessive moisture. Moisture from urinary or fecal incontinence or profuse sweating can lead to skin maceration and perhaps increased friction and sheer forces when left sticky and wet. Absorbent pads can improve moisture.

Aside from extrinsic forces, several intrinsic forces also impact the development of pressure ulcers. These factors include immobility, poor nutrition, decreased sensory perception, and low body mass.[16] Older adults are at increased risk for immobility because of increased rates of cerebral vascular disease, hip fracture, and increased recovery time from acute illness or surgery. If these comorbidities are present, physical therapy and occupational therapy consults may minimize the effects of immobility. Decreased sensory perception may be due to diabetic neuropathy or cerebral vascular disease, which may prevent an older adult from feeling the pain associated with damage from extrinsic forces. Inadequate nutrition increases risk for ulcer development and impairs healing.[19] Large wounds may require twice the normal protein intake to heal.[20] Tube feeding has not been associated with preventing or healing pressure ulcers in advanced dementia.[21]

Although the above extrinsic and intrinsic factors may initiate pressure ulcer formation, cell death results from ischemia-reperfusion (I/R) injury.[18] The initial ischemic injury occurs when blood flow ceases. Deeper structures such as skeletal muscle can tolerate only short periods of ischemia, compared to the epidermis, which can tolerate longer periods. Initially, the microcirculation dilates and releases histamine (blanchable erythema). Next the capillaries and venules engorge with red blood cells and then hemorrhage (nonblanchable erythema). Necrosis of all skin structures is seen by Stage III.[22] Reperfusion begins with removal of pressure. Damage seen with blanchable and nonblanchable erythema may be reversible. Nitrous oxide (NO) production decreases during ischemic periods, causing blood vessel constriction. During reperfusion, blood vessels dilate as NO production increases. If damage is extensive, the reperfusion spreads toxic metabolites and oxygen free radicals, destroying surrounding tissue.[18]

RISK ASSESSMENT

Prevention remains the mainstay of pressure ulcer treatment. The health care provider should carefully examine high-risk areas for pressure ulcer development, such as the occiput, spine, sacrum, ischium, heels, trochanter, knee, and ankle. Several scales exist to assess patients at risk for pressure ulcer development: the Norton, Braden, and Waterlow scales. The Norton scale assesses five areas on a four point scale: physical condition, mental condition, activity, mobility, and incontinence. A modified scale deducts one point for each of the following: comorbidities (diabetes, hypertension), low hemoglobin, low hematocrit, low albumin (<3.3 mg/dL), fever greater than 99.6° F, polypharmacy, and mental status changes/lethargy in the past 24 hours. A score of 10 is high risk.[23] The Braden scale is used both in research and clinic settings. This scale assesses risks in six categories: sensory perception, activity, mobility, nutrition, moisture level, and friction/shear (three point scale). The maximum score is 23. A score of 18 indicates increased risk for elderly patients.[24,25] The Waterlow scale is a modification of the Norton scale and assesses eight factors: build, sex and age, continence, mobility, appetite, medication, and special risk factors.[26] The higher the score on this complex scale indicates an increased risk. A 2007 review and study using the three scales in an inpatient geriatric setting showed that sensitivity and specificity of all scales depended on selected cutoff points sample changes.[27] The positive predictive value of the Braden and Norton scales is approximately 37%.[28] As a result it is recommended that the scales be used in conjugation with a good physical examination by a nurse or physician.[9,27] Recently, the Cochrane Database of Systemic Reviews attempted to determine whether using structured, systematic pressure ulcer risk assessment tools in any health care setting reduces the incidence of pressure ulcers. However, it found no randomized trials exist that compare assessment tools with clinical judgment or no risk assessment in terms of rates of pressure ulceration. Therefore, Cochrane could not conclude that assessment tools reduced the incidence of pressure ulcers.

PRESSURE ULCER CLASSIFICATION

The National Pressure Ulcer Advisory Panel (NPUAP) defines a pressure ulcer as localized injury to the skin and/or underlying tissue usually over a bony prominence as a result of pressure, or pressure in combination with shear and/or friction. Blanchable erythema or reactive hyperemia often precede pressure ulcer development and can resolve in 24 hours if treatment starts. However, once the skin changes go beyond the initial stage, pressure ulcer formation has started. The NPUAP uses a four-stage system of pressure ulcer classification.[29] In 2007, two new stages were added: suspected deep tissue injury and unstageable.[30]

Suspected deep tissue injury is a purple or maroon localized area of discolored intact skin or blood-filled blister because of damage of underlying soft tissue. The skin may be painful, different temperature compared to surrounding skin. Deep tissue injury may progress rapidly to a pressure ulcer, despite treatment. Stage I is intact skin with nonblanchable erythema of a localized area usually over a bony prominence. The skin may be painful, and a different temperature compared with surrounding skin. This indicates that there is inadequate perfusion to the cutaneous microcirculation. Stage II is a partial thickness loss of dermis presenting as a shallow open ulcer with a red-pink wound bed, without slough or bruising. An open or ruptured blister may also be present. At this stage, tissue anoxia has progressed to such an extent that the epidermis starts to necrose. Stage III is full thickness tissue loss associated with undermining and tunneling. Subcutaneous fat may be visible but bone, tendon, or muscle is not exposed. Ulcers on areas with no subcutaneous tissue (nose, ear, malleolus) may be very shallow compared with areas with significant subcutaneous tissue such as the sacrum. Stage IV is full thickness tissue loss with exposed bone, tendon, or muscle. It is often associated with slough or eschar, undermining and tunneling, and osteomyelitis. An unstageable ulcer is full thickness tissue loss in which the base of the ulcer is covered by slough (yellow, tan, gray, green, or brown) and/or eschar (tan, brown, or black) in the wound bed. The slough and/or eschar must be removed before the true stage can be determined. However, an eschar on the heels is considered stable if it is dry, adherent, and intact without erythema and should not be removed.

Once staging of the ulcer is completed, ulcer progression must be documented. One method of documenting a wound is as follows[31]: (1) stage the ulcer, time present, setting where occurred; (2) describe the location anatomically; (3) measure ulcer in centimeters (length × width × base); (4) describe percent of ulcer covered by granulation tissue versus yellow slough versus necrotic tissue/eschar; (5) note any odor; (6) describe the surrounding tissue; (7) document undermining or tunneling (use clock as reference point).

MANAGEMENT AND TREATMENT

As described earlier, pressure ulcer development occurs from a combination of extrinsic and intrinsic factors. Pressure ulcers are chronic wounds and amount of time to heal is very variable.[32] Management and treatment should focus on (1) pressure relief, (2) wound care, and (3) complications. In 2006, *Wound Repair and Regeneration* published *Guidelines for the treatment of pressure ulcers (GTPU)*, which were evidence and consensus based.[41] Evidence level (EL) were classified as I (multiple clinical trials supporting use), II (at least one trial), or III (suggestive but lacking sufficient data).

Pressure relief is the first line of treatment. According to the NPUAP, patients should be turned every 2 hours while in bed or 1 hour while seated. Patients should be positioned or padded as to minimize pressure on at-risk areas or minimize pressure on existing ulcers (GTPU EL II). Support surfaces can reduce pressure but not eliminate pressure, so repositioning is still important. Static support surfaces are usually foam, air, or water overlays and can reduce pressure, especially for stage I and stage II ulcers and if the patient can move.[33,34] (GTPU EL I). These surfaces lie over the existing mattress or replace the existing mattress and can be used in the home.

Dynamic support surfaces are low air loss beds, alternating pressure beds, and air fluidized beds. These devices are usually reserved for stage III and stage IV ulcers. (GTPU EL I) The low air loss beds and air fluidized beds reduce pressure by keeping the person floating on a bed of air or fluidized beads. By contrast, alternating pressure beds reduce pressure by reproducing the alternation of high and low pressure in the weight-bearing areas, which occurs in normal people as a result of postural changes in response to pressure pain. They consist of two alternating systems of air cells powered by a pump, which causes them to inflate and deflate reciprocally over a 5- to 10-minute cycle, thus continually changing the supporting areas of pressure on the body. These beds are expensive and large, so are difficult to use in the home setting and may increase immobility for older patients. One dynamic surface has not been shown to be superior to another one in treatment of pressure ulcers.[35]

Pressure ulcers require consistent wound care, which includes débridement, cleansing, and dressing. Necrotic tissue or slough may require débridement to promote healing (GTPU EL I). Sharp débridement uses a scalpel and scissors, removing only the dead tissue. Mechanical débridement uses wet to dry dressings, whirlpool, and irrigation. It is a nonselective method and may remove healthy tissue. Enzymatic débridement uses enzymes to slowly break down the fibrin and collagen in the necrotic tissue. The enzymatic ointments are expensive. Autolytic débridement uses the wounds own enzymes to slowly remove the necrotic tissue through use of an occlusive dressing.

Wound cleansing should be done with tap water or saline. Antiseptics should be avoided as their use will destroy healthy tissue (GTPU EL III).

The purpose of the dressing is to manage fluid balance in the ulcer by adding moisture or absorbing excess moisture (GTPU EL I). Films are semiocclusive or occlusive, usually transparent, promote autolytic débridement, and often used on stage II ulcers. Hydrogels provide moisture to the ulcer and are best used for ulcers that have adequate granulation tissue and minimal necrotic tissue. Hydrocolloid dressings are occlusive, adhere to the wound, and promote autolytic débridement. Alginate dressings are derived from seaweed and can absorb 20 times their weight in fluid, so are good for draining ulcers. Silver impregnated dressings are used to decrease microbial count and improve healing. Although they have been used in infection-prone wounds, such as burns and leg vein graft sites, their use in chronic wounds such as pressure ulcers is unclear, although data suggests that dressings may be changed less frequently saving clinician time, which offsets their expense. If stage III or IV pressure ulcers fail to progress from these therapies, consider using a negative pressure wound therapy such as a wound vac (GTPU EL I). However, hyperbaric oxygen therapy has not been shown to improve healing (GTPU EL I).

The primary complication of pressure ulcers is infection, resulting in poor healing, sepsis, or osteomyelitis. All ulcers are colonized and do not require antibiotics. However, if an ulcer does not progress in 14 days, infection should be considered (GTPU EL II). To prevent contamination with colonizing organisms, a culture should be obtained by deep aspiration or biopsy. Initiate treatment if greater than 10^5 colonies are present.[36]

QUALITY INIDICATOR AND LITIGATION

Google "pressure ulcer" and the search will return a list of law firm Web sites. Since pressure ulcers are considered preventable, their development is used as a quality indicator for long-term care facilities, hospitals, and effectiveness of a physician's care. It is argued that some pressure ulcers are unavoidable if the facility assessed the risk and implemented interventions or if the patient's medical condition (cachexia, metastatic cancer, severe peripheral vascular disease, or terminal illness) impedes healing or promotes development of ulcers.[37] Yet litigation over pressure ulcers in the United States continues to grow. A review of pressure ulcer cases against long-term care facilities showed that the number of cases increased 2.6 times from 1984 to 2002, with 87% of the plaintiffs receiving some type of recovery from the facility.[38] The mean recovery for the period 1984 to 1999 was $3,359,259 compared to a mean of $13,554,168 for the period 1999 to 2002.[38] In Great Britain, there is usually little to be gained in litigation as there would be little payable compensation. However, the National Health Service has a statutory procedure for handling pressure ulcer complaints in coordination with the Patient Advocacy and Liaison Service.[39]

Today when a family appears with a digital camera to photograph a pressure ulcer, one can conclude that the photo will be used in future litigation. When it appears that a family is contemplating legal action, the entire health care team should work with the patient and family. Table 110-1 summarizes risk management measures for pressure ulcers.[40] Pressure ulcer prevention programs also appear to limit litigation.[38]

CONCLUSION

The best plan for pressure ulcer prevention and treatment continues to be informed health care providers that are always vigilant in their examination of the elderly patient's skin and assessment of risk factors. Older adults have decreased epithelial cell turnover, decreased dermal blood flow, impaired collagen synthesis, and loss of subcutaneous fat. These changes make the skin more susceptible to pressure ulcers from extrinsic factors, such as pressure, friction, shear, and moisture. Since impaired mobility often accompanies illness in elderly people who are frail, the clinical index for suspicion for pressure ulcers must be high and require pressure reducing protocols immediately.

Table 110-1. Minimizing Litigation from Pressure Ulcers

Principle	Action
Avoid defensiveness, anger, and confrontation.	If family request help in documenting pressure ulcer, immediately ask administration for assistance.
Involve the entire team, even administration.	Maintain professionalism and avoid blame and finger pointing.
Attempt to reestablish trust with the family and patient.	Meet frequently with family, try new interventions.
Educate the family and provide realistic goals.	Notify family as soon as pressure ulcer noted, inform them end stage diseases will affect healing.
Review the history and reassess the patient.	Prepare a time line of events leading up to the pressure ulcer, discuss alternative pressure relief devices.
Reevaluate the care plan.	The best care plans are individualized, clearly state the role of each discipline in treatment.
Obtain proper studies and consultations.	Doppler for evaluation of peripheral vascular disease for leg ulcers, swallow study for patient with poor nutrition
Document problem behaviors and provide appropriate interventions.	Be specific in record with date, time. When describing behaviors, be objective, consistent with terms, and nonjudgmental (family interfered with care, patient had a leave of absence during care).
Establish a feedback loop for quality improvement.	When pressure ulcer occurs, review policy and procedures.

Adapted from Levine JM, Savino F, Peterson M, et al. Risk management for pressure ulcers: when a family shows up with a camera. J Am Med Dir Assoc 2008;9(5):360–363.

KEY POINTS

1. As skin ages, there is decreased epithelial cell turnover, decreased dermal blood flow, impaired collagen synthesis, and loss of subcutaneous fat. These changes make the skin more susceptible to pressure ulcers.
2. Extrinsic factors causing pressure ulcers are pressure, friction, shear, and moisture.
3. An elderly patient, supine on a bed, generates pressure between 50 to 90 mm Hg at the heel and greater trochanter, well above the 32 mm Hg arterial capillary filling pressure.
4. Intrinsic factors causing pressure ulcers are poor nutrition, decreased sensory perception, low body mass, and impaired mobility and endothelial dysfunction.
5. Impaired mobility often accompanies illness in elderly people who are frail; the clinical index for suspicion for pressure ulcers must be high.
6. Pressure ulcers can be reliably staged using the National Pressure Ulcer Advisory Panel classification (from nonblanchable erythema to full thickness tissue loss with exposed bone, tendon, or muscle).
7. Management relies on relieving pressure and a variety of treatments; no one treatment has yet been reliably shown to be superior.
8. Pressure ulcer development can be considered an indication of negligent care and lead to litigation.

For a complete list of references, please visit online only at www.expertconsult.com

CHAPTER 111

Sleep, Aging, and Late-Life Insomnia

Holly J. Ramsawh
Harrison G. Bloom
Sonia Ancoli-Israel

INSOMNIA

Epidemiology

In most,[1–6] but not all studies,[7–10] the prevalence of insomnia has been found to increase with age. It has typically been reported in one quarter to one third of people aged 65 and over (see Table 111-1). However, as more stringent definitions of insomnia are increasingly being used, lower prevalence rates have been estimated, particularly when daytime impairment has been used as a criterion.[3,4,6,11] Epidemiologic studies have also tended to show that insomnia is more common among older adult women than among older men[1,2,6,8,12] (Table 111-1), although a few surveys have found no gender differences,[7,10] or found differences for some but not all insomnia subtypes.[13] However, a recent meta-analysis of gender differences in insomnia found that women were indeed at greater risk for insomnia than men, and that this discrepancy in female insomnia risk relative to males increased after age 65. Findings also suggest that insomnia is higher among lower income and lower educational attainment groups.[1–4,8,9]

Insomnia appears to be widespread in medical settings, although it often goes unreported by patients and consequently underrecognized by providers.[14–18] Prevalence rates of insomnia symptoms in primary care settings have ranged from 30% to 69%.[14,15,17,18] In addition, one recent study found that 42% of new benzodiazepine prescriptions written for older adults in primary care settings were indicated for insomnia symptoms.[16] In addition, those reporting sleep problems tend to show significantly higher consumption of health care resources than those who do not.[19–21]

Information on the incidence of insomnia in older adults (i.e., the rate of onset of new cases of insomnia) is more limited. Using strict criteria for insomnia (see Table 111-1), the U.S. National Institute for Mental Health (NIMH) catchment study found a modest age-related increase in the 1-year incidence of insomnia, with incidence rising from 5.7% among those between ages 18 to 25, to 7.3% among those aged 65 and over.[11] In one large study of insomnia incidence in a sample of 6899 participants, Foley et al reported age-related rises in insomnia incidence for both men and women.[22] Within the age groups 65 to 74, 75 to 84, and 85 and over, this study found 3-year insomnia incidence rates of 12.4%, 15.1%, and 20.5% respectively, for men and 14.4%, 16.7%, and 13.7% for women.[22] The overall annual rate was 5%. In a more recent study examining the incidence of specific insomnia subtypes in older adults, the annualized incidence of trouble falling asleep was found to be 2.8% over a mean follow-up period of 3.5 years, and significantly higher in women than in men (3.4% versus 1.9% per year).[23] The annualized incidence of frequent awakenings was noticeably higher at 12.3%, with no significant effect of gender.[23]

Natural history of insomnia

The nature and duration of insomnia symptoms appear to change with advancing age. Table 111-2 shows the distribution of specific insomnia complaints among older adults (the categories are not mutually exclusive, as respondents may report more than one problem). Of the studies which report data for sleep onset, maintenance, and early morning awakenings (EMA), sleep maintenance problems are the most prevalent sleep complaint in the majority of these studies. Similar to other types of sleep complaints, rates of EMA show considerable variation across studies, ranging from 0.9% in China[6] to 45% in Japan.[7]

Several longitudinal studies suggest that insomnia symptoms persist over time. Foley et al reported that of nearly 2000 individuals reporting insomnia at baseline, more than half continued to report symptoms at 3-year follow-up.[22] One survey of general medical practice patients found that 69% of those with insomnia at baseline still had insomnia at 12-month follow-up.[24] Furthermore, persistence of insomnia symptoms was significantly associated with older age. Another study employing a sample of 1870 participants aged 45 to 65 years old from the general population found that at 12-year follow-up, 75% of those with insomnia at baseline still carried the diagnosis.[25]

Changes in sleep architecture

Numerous studies have reported age-related changes in sleep architecture. However, many of these studies have reported conflicting findings about a number of sleep indices. Importantly, a recent analysis of data from the Sleep Heart Health Study (SHHS) provides normative data on sleep architecture in almost 2700 adults, including a sizeable proportion of older adults.[26] The SHHS employed rigorous standards for scoring and analyzing of polysomnography data, and excluded individuals using psychotropics, those with restless leg syndrome, and individuals with systemic pain conditions. Whether participants had a history of each of several common medical conditions, including cardiovascular disease, diabetes mellitus, and chronic lung disease, was also recorded. The large sample size and exclusion of individuals with comorbid conditions known to impact sleep architecture suggest that the SHHS findings may be broadly representative of normative sleep architecture data in middle-aged and older adults. Thus the SHHS data figure heavily into the discussion of structural changes in the sleep of older adults.

CONTINUITY OF SLEEP

The sleep of older adults is more fragmented than that of their younger counterparts, being characterized by more frequent shifts between sleep stages and more periods of wakefulness during sleep (see Figure 111-1). Polysomnogram (PSG) evidence suggests increased awakenings at night

Table 111-1. Prevalence of Insomnia (Variously Defined) Among Older People Living in the Community Prevalence (%)

Location	Year	Age	No. of older respondents	Overall	Women	Men
National Sample, U.S.[1]	1985	65–79	798	25.0[a]	NR	NR
NIMH Catchment, U.S.[11]	1989	65+	1801	12.0[b]	NR	NR
East Boston, Mass.[2]	1995	65+	3537	33.7[c]	36.4	29.4
New Haven, Conn.[2]	1995	65+	2717	27.5[c]	31.1[l]	21.2[l]
Iowa[2]	1995	65+	3028	23.2[c]	25.4[l]	19.5[l]
4 states,* U.S.[12]	1997	65+	5201	NR	30.0[n]	14.0[n]
				NR	65.0[o]	65.0[o]
Japan[7]	2000	60+	766	29.5[d]	NR	NR
Norway[3]	2001	60+	NR	14.7[e]	NR	NR
Sourth Korea[4]	2002	65+	314	26.6[f]	NR	NR
				8.2[g]	NR	NR
Wisconsin[59]	2002	53–97	2800	49.0[h]	NR	NR
4 European countries†[5]	2003	65+	2759	24.1[i]	NR	NR
Taiwan[8]	2004	65+	2045	6.0[j]	8.0	4.5
Shandong, China[6]	2005	65+	1679	32.9[k]	36.4	28.7
				8.9[l]	10.1	7.5
National Sample, U.S.[9]	2006	65–74	3308	9.2[m]	NR	NR
National Sample, U.S.[9]	2006	75–84	2381	6.6[m]	NR	NR
National Sample, U.S.[9]	2006	85+	739	2.1[m]	NR	NR
Brazil[10]	2007	60+	6963	33.7[n]	NR	NR

NR = data not reported.

*North Carolina, California, Maryland, and Pennsylvania.

†Italy, Germany, Portugal, United Kingdom

[a]Insomnia defined as "had trouble and was bothered a lot" by "trouble falling asleep or staying asleep"

[b]"... had trouble falling asleep, staying asleep, or waking too early" for a period of 2 weeks or more, and consulted a professional about it, took medication for it, or stated that it interfered with life a lot, and "... if it was not always the result of physical illness"

[c]"trouble falling asleep and/or waking up too early and not being able to fall asleep again most of the time"

[d]"often" or "always" has trouble getting to sleep, staying asleep, or waking too early

[e]mean sleep latency >30 minutes, mean wake after sleep onset >30 minutes, or waking up at least 30 minutes earlier than preferred >10 days per month, and DSM-IV criteria met for insomnia disorder

[f]difficulty falling asleep, disrupted sleep, early morning awakenings, or nonrestorative sleep, at least one of which occurs 3+ days per week

[g]DSM-IV criteria met for insomnia disorder

[h]difficulty falling asleep, waking repeatedly, or "waking up and finding it difficult to fall back asleep," at least one of which occurring "often" (5–15 times per month) or "almost always" (16–30 times per month)

[i]difficulty falling asleep, staying asleep, or nonrestorative sleep *and* daytime impairment

[j]sleep latency >30 minutes or (wake after sleep onset > 3 times per night *or* early morning wakenings > 2 hours earlier than usual), either of which occurring 3+ times per week *and* accompanied by either poor subjective sleep quality or a moderate or greater degree of daytime dysfunction

[k]trouble sleeping due to sleep latency >30 minutes, "night awakenings," or early morning awakenings, at least one of which occurring 3+ times per week

[l]one or more insomnia symptoms *and* daytime consequences occurring one or more times per week

[m]regularly occurring insomnia or trouble sleeping in the past 12 months

[n]"fitful and disturbed sleep" in the past 30 days.

even among healthy older adults who do not complain about their sleep.[27] Nocturnal awakenings tend to be more common among men than women.[26] "Microarousals" (2 to 15 second bursts of alpha activity) have also been observed in the electroencephalograms (EEG) of sleeping older adults.[28] Microarousals, which are not accompanied by behavioral awakenings, are associated with daytime sleepiness.[28] In the SHHS, the arousal index (total number of EEG arousals from sleep divided by total sleep time) increased significantly with advancing age.[26]

DURATION OF SLEEP

Although sleep disruption becomes more pronounced with age, sleep duration appears to experience a decline. Van Cauter et al found that in a sample of men ages 16 to 83, total sleep time decreased on average by 27 minutes per decade from midlife until the eighth decade.[29] As a result, sleep efficiency (time spent asleep divided by time spent in bed) also tends to decrease.[26] A recent meta-analysis of 65 objective sleep studies representing 3577 participants ages 5 to 102 found that in adults, both total sleep time and sleep efficiency decreased with age.[30]

DEPTH OF SLEEP

With advancing age, there is a reduction in EEG slow waves (stages 3/4 or slow wave sleep; SWS; Figure 111-1).[30] In addition to a decrease in SWS, increases in stages 2 (light sleep) and 1 (drowsiness) have been reported.[30] SHHS data suggests that there are gender differences in sleep architecture in that men have lighter sleep as they age relative to women.[26] Specifically, the men had more Stage 1 and 2 sleep with increasing age, whereas there was no detectable effect of age on Stage 1 and 2 percentages in women. In addition, there were gender effects on SWS. Men had proportionally less SWS compared with women in each age group, and there was a steep and significant age-related decline in SWS in men, but no significant age-related changes in percentage of SWS in women. This putative gender effect on age-related SWS changes may explain why Ohayon et al found no significant change in SWS after age 60 in their meta-analysis of relevant studies.[30] Therefore, while there may be changes in depth of sleep with age, these changes may be confined to men, or at least more evident in males.

In addition, studies of auditory awakening thresholds (the minimum amount of noise required to wake a sleeping

Table 111-2. Distribution of Specific Complaints Among Older People With Insomnia Living in the Community Reported Problems (%) Among Older

		PEOPLE WITH INSOMNIA[†]		
Location	**Age**	**Onset**	**Maintenance**	**EMA**
4 states,[*] U.S. (men)[12]	65+	14.0	65.0	30.0
4 states,[*] U.S. (women)[12]	65+	30.0	65.0	34.0
National sample (Japan)[7]	60+	NR	77.0[‡]	45.1[‡]
National sample, Norway[3]	60+	18.1	26.7	27.9
National sample, S. Korea[4]	65+	7.5	21.0	5.3
Wisconsin[59]	53–97	21.2	36.2	24.1
National sample, Taiwan[8]	65+	6.7	4.7[§]	NR
Shandong, China[6]	65+	8.5	8.6	0.9

Onset, problems getting to sleep; *Maintenance*, problems staying asleep; *EMA*, early morning awakening; *NR*, data not reported.
*North Carolina, California, Maryland, and Pennsylvania.
†Categories not mutually exclusive.
‡Calculated from reported data.
§Data reported is combined prevalence of problems staying asleep and early morning wakenings.

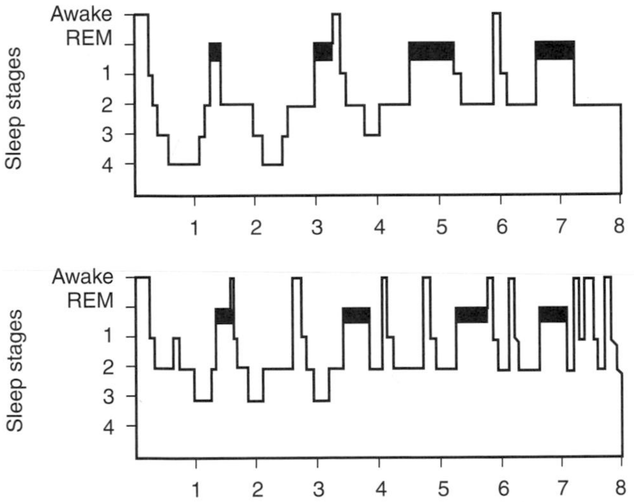

Figure 111-1. Sleep stage profiles for typical younger (above) and older (below) people. Note the decrease in stages 3 and 4, and the reciprocal increase in stages 1 and 2 with increasing age (for an 8-hour sleep).

person) show qualitative changes in the depth of individual sleep stages. It has been shown, for example, that during stages 2, 4, and REM, older people are more easily awakened by noise (i.e., have lower auditory awakening thresholds) than are younger people (this despite reductions in the hearing sensitivity of older subjects).[31] However, in a study of the effects of aircraft noise on the sleep of people living near a major airport, Horne et al[32] found that while awakenings in response to aircraft noise were most common in the oldest age group (ages 50 to 70), other factors, such as having children in the household, appeared to be more influential than aging in determining arousals.

REM SLEEP

The proportion of REM sleep has also been shown to decline with age.[33] Van Cauter et al found that REM sleep was reduced by as much as 50% in older adults compared with their younger counterparts.[29] However, Ohayon et al did not replicate this finding; they found that while REM sleep decreased between young and middle adulthood, percentage of REM sleep remained stable over time in adults older than 60.[30] A recent meta-analysis by Floyd et al, who used an analytic approach designed to detect nonlinearity in age-related REM change, found a small but significant decline in REM until the mid-70s, followed by a small increase in REM sleep percentage. Taken together, these studies suggest that REM is relatively well preserved in older adults, that if there is a decrease in REM sleep in older adults, it is modest, and that this small decline in REM sleep may begin to stabilize during the seventh decade of life.

The aging circadian rhythm

The circadian rhythm itself also shows evidence of age-related fragmentation, with sleep becoming more desynchronized and likely to impinge on daytime activities.[34,35] Recent research suggests that an age-related reduction in sleep promotion of the circadian pacemaker, along with decreased homeostatic pressure for sleep in older adults, may be involved in this desynchronization.[36]

Comorbidity

MEDICAL COMORBIDITY

There is a strong association between insomnia complaints and chronic medical conditions. Foley et al found that only 7% of new cases of insomnia in older adults occurred in the absence of health-related risk factors.[22] In community surveys of older adults, poor self-reported health, nocturnal micturition, and chronic pain are frequently associated with increased risk of insomnia.[3,6,8,10] In 2003, the National Sleep Foundation survey of adults aged 65 and older found a significant positive correlation between insomnia and current medical conditions, including cardiac and pulmonary disease.[37] In studies examining the prevalence of insomnia in specific medical conditions, it was found that 31% of arthritis and 66% of chronic pain patients report difficulty falling asleep; 33% of diabetes, 57% of end-stage renal disease, 81% of arthritis, and 85% of chronic pain patients report difficulty staying asleep; and 44% of cancer, 45% of gastroesophageal reflux disease, and 50% of patients with congestive heart failure report sleep initiation and maintenance difficulties.[38–44] In knee pain and osteoarthritis, predictors of greater insomnia complaints included a greater number of involved joints and knee pain severity.[43] In chronic obstructive pulmonary disease (COPD), insomnia also appears related to severity. A group of patients with moderate to severe COPD with demonstrated reduced oxygen saturation also reported poor sleep quality.[45]

PSYCHIATRIC COMORBIDITY

Psychiatric conditions are also highly associated with insomnia. Studies estimate that over 40% of individuals with persistent hypersomnia or insomnia have a psychiatric diagnosis.[11] Having insomnia has been associated with increased risk of onset of depression in the future, particularly for older women.[46,47] In one follow-up study on 1053 men who provided information on sleep habits in medical school and who had been followed since graduation, the authors found that those who went on to develop depression by 34-year follow-up were more likely to report experiencing insomnia during medical school.[48] Although the relationship between insomnia and depression has been more consistently studied, recent surveys also suggest that insomnia is also often associated with anxiety disorders in older adults.[24,49] Recent data from Ohayon et al,[5] which used a large community survey of individuals from four European countries, suggest that while insomnia typically precedes or cooccurs with the onset of depression, insomnia symptoms are more likely to develop at or after the onset of an anxiety disorder.

Treatment

Although pharmacologic treatments are available for insomnia, recent evidence suggests that behavioral approaches to insomnia treatment may be more effective than medications for older adults,[50,51] and thus may be considered either as a first-line treatment, or in combination with medication.[52] Combination treatment may allow patients to gain immediate relief from medication, whereas long-term relief of insomnia may be best achieved with behavioral treatment.

BEHAVIORAL TREATMENT

Behavioral treatment of insomnia, which involves a set of techniques collectively referred to as cognitive behavioral therapy (CBT), typically begins with psychoeducation about insomnia. During this phase, the behavioral model of insomnia is discussed, and factors that contribute to insomnia, such as heredity, medical and psychiatric comorbidity, and poor sleep hygiene, are introduced. Sleep hygiene involves promoting good sleep habits and avoiding sleep-incompatible behaviors in the bed/bedroom (e.g., establishing a set wake-up time, no napping during the day, keeping the bedroom at a cool temperature at night to promote sleep), which patients are instructed to adhere to in order to improve their sleep. Sleep hygiene instructions are tailored to each patient depending on his or her own sleep habits. The most frequently studied components of CBT for insomnia are sleep restriction and stimulus control. Although these components have sometimes been implemented as stand-alone treatments for insomnia, they are typically employed together in the context of the CBT approach to insomnia. Sleep restriction entails instructing patients to limit the time they spend in bed to the average number of hours slept per night plus 15 minutes (e.g., if a participant reports sleeping 6.5 hours per night on average over the past week, they will be instructed to spend 6.75 hours in bed per night). Time spent in bed is lengthened, typically in 15-minute increments, as sleep efficiency improves. Patients' time in bed is stabilized once their weekly sleep efficiency reaches 85% to 90% or higher, which is considered within the normal range. Stimulus control is used to decrease the alertness and arousal that many individuals with insomnia feel while in bed, and to increase the association of bed with sleepiness. It entails instructing the patient to sleep only in bed, to get out of bed whenever he or she feels alert and aroused or when awake more than 10 to 15 minutes, and to return to bed only when he or she begins to feel sleepy again. Although CBT for insomnia typically totals 6 to 8 sessions, abbreviated forms of CBT have been tested. One drawback of CBT is that clinical effects of treatment may take 2 to 4 weeks to emerge.[53]

PHARMACOLOGIC TREATMENT

Many classes of medication have been used to treat insomnia, including sedative-hypnotics, antidepressants, antipsychotics, antihistamines, and anticonvulsants, some of which are prescribed "off-label." However, a recent state-of-the-science report on insomnia from the National Institutes of Health concluded that there is no systematic empirical support for the effectiveness of antipsychotics, antihistamines, barbiturates, anticonvulsants, or antidepressants for treating insomnia.[52] In addition, the report expressed concern about the side effects of some of the off-label agents commonly used for insomnia, suggesting that the risks outweigh the benefits. Some of the risks associated with use of pharmacologic treatment of insomnia, such as increased risk of falls, may be particularly concerning for older adults. A newer class of medications known as type-1 γ-aminobutyric acid (GABA) benzodiazepine receptor agonists, which includes zaleplon, eszopiclone, zolpidem, and zolpidem MR, has been shown to be effective and safe in treatment of insomnia in older adults.[54–57] A melatonin agonist, ramelteon, has also been approved for insomnia associated with difficulty falling asleep, and has shown promise in older adults.[58]

Sleep-disordered breathing

Sleep-disordered breathing (SDB) refers to a range of periodic respiratory events that occur while asleep, from mild snoring to partial cessation of airflow (hypopnea) to complete airflow cessation (apnea).The severity of SDB is measured by the apnea hypopnea index (AHI). Data suggests that the prevalence of SDB increases with age.[59,60] Older individuals with dementia, and institutionalized elderly patients, have especially high rates of SDB, although reasons for these findings are not entirely clear.[61] One factor contributing to increased prevalence of sleep-disordered breathing in those with certain forms of dementia may be that areas of the brainstem involved in respiration and other autonomic functions are affected by the disease process in dementias.

Medical and behavioral risk factors for SDB include obesity, male gender, increasing age, family history, smoking, alcohol consumption, craniofacial features, and upper airway configuration.[62] In those with SDB, primary symptoms include snoring and excessive daytime sleepiness, which arise due to recurrent arousals from sleep and sleep fragmentation. About half of regular snorers have some degree of SDB, and snoring may also be a risk factor for SDB.[63] Other common presentations include daytime napping and falling asleep at inopportune times during the day. Functional impairment, particularly in social and occupational areas, is common in those with SDB. Cognitive deficits, such as short-term memory problems or difficulty concentrating, may also occur; in those with baseline cognitive impairment, these symptoms may be exacerbated.[64] SDB has been linked to cardiovascular disease, including coronary artery disease, heart failure, and stroke.[65–67]

Of the treatment options for SDB, continuous positive airway pressure (CPAP) is considered the gold standard. CPAP improves the symptoms of SDB, along with improving cognitive function in older adults.[68,69] However, adherence can sometimes be an issue because some patients find the mask inconvenient or uncomfortable; these patients should work with their provider to find a model that is tolerable for them. Alternatives to CPAP include dental devices and surgery; however, the outcomes for these methods are typically not as favorable as for CPAP, particularly in older adults. Patients should also be educated on the importance of healthy body weight, smoking cessation, and alcohol consumption because each contributes to favorable outcome of SDB. Medications such as long-acting benzodiazepines and narcotics should be avoided if possible because they have been shown to increase the frequency and duration of apneas.

Periodic limb movements in sleep/restless leg syndrome

Periodic limb movements in sleep (PLMS) are repetitive leg jerks or kicks that occur while asleep. These movements typically occur in clusters approximately 30 seconds apart, and can recur throughout the night, leading to brief arousals and fragmented sleep. Consequently, many of these patients may have complaints of insomnia, nonrestorative sleep, and excessive daytime sleepiness. Diagnosis is based on a periodic limb movement index (movements per hour during sleep) greater than 5. Restless leg syndrome (RLS) is commonly comorbid with PLMS, and is characterized by uncomfortable, "creepy crawly" sensations in the legs that typically occur during resting, wakeful states. Those afflicted find that moving the legs in response to these sensations temporarily relieves discomfort caused by these sensations. RLS also occurs while the patient is resting in bed, and may interfere with sleep initiation. Roughly 80% of adults with RLS also meet diagnostic criteria for PLMS.[70] The cause of both PLMS and RLS is not well understood, although RLS may be more likely to occur with iron deficiency (such as in pregnancy), radiculopathy, uremia, and peripheral neuropathy.

The prevalence of PLMS increases significantly with advancing age, with one study finding that 45% of older adults experiencing symptoms consistent with the diagnosis.[71] The presence of RLS also increases with age.[72] Although the gender distribution is roughly equal in PLMS, about twice as many older women experience RLS compared with men.[73]

Evidence-based treatment for PLMS/RLS includes agents that target leg movements or associated arousals. At present, dopamine agonists are recommended as a first-line treatment because they have been found to reduce the number of kicks and associated arousals.[74,75] Ropinirole and pramipexole are the only dopamine agonists currently approved by the U.S. Food and Drug Administration for the treatment of RLS.

Rapid eye movement (REM) sleep behavior disorder

Rapid eye movement sleep behavior disorder (RBD) occurs when the gross motor paralysis typically associated with REM sleep is intermittently absent. As a result, the sleeper may laugh, yell, kick, punch, or engage in other elaborate behaviors as they respond to dream content. RBD-related behavior typically occurs during the second half of the night, when REM periods are more frequent. These behaviors can often be violent or aggressive, and can result in injury to the patient or to bed partners. RBD occurs almost exclusively in older males,[76] and is highly prevalent in Parkinson's disease and related neurodegenerative conditions. In some cases, RBD may signal the onset of one of these neurologic conditions, and may occur years before diagnosis.[76,77] In cases of acute onset, RBD has been associated with posttraumatic stress disorder.[78] The overall estimated prevalence of RBD is 0.5% in the general population.[79]

Treatment of RBD is primarily pharmacologic, although strategies that decrease the likelihood of injury include placing pillows or cushions around the sleeper's bed, or having partners sleep in another room if behaviors are especially violent, can also be helpful. The pharmacologic treatment of choice is the clonazepam, a sedating benzodiazepine, which has been found to be beneficial for patients with RBD in up to 79% of cases.[80] In patients with RBD for whom clonazepam is contraindicated, melatonin has also shown promise in RBD treatment.[81]

Sleep in dementia

Demented patients have a high prevalence of disturbed sleep compared with healthy older adults, with 19% to 44% experiencing sleep disturbances. Sleep features in dementia can include abnormal nighttime behavior, wandering and confusion, agitation ("sundowning"), and daytime napping. These symptoms may be more prominent in institutionalized demented patients. One study showed that demented older adults living in institutions may not spend a single hour completely awake or asleep during a 24-hour period.[82] One contributing factor to this may be inadequate light exposure because previous studies have found that institutionalized patients with adequate light exposure had fewer sleep disruptions.[83] Many demented older adults have a comorbid sleep disorder such as SDB or a medical condition that contributes to the sleep disturbance such as chronic pain; the effects of medications to treat medical or psychiatric conditions may also interfere with sleep. However, sleep disturbance in demented patients may also occur in the absence of any contributing comorbid condition, and may be related to the dementing process itself. Supporting evidence includes findings that severity of sleep disturbance is positively correlated with dementia severity.[82]

After a thorough assessment of possible contributing factors to sleep disturbance, treatment should focus on the responsible sleep disorder, if one is detected. Nonpharmacologic interventions may include the introduction of increased activity via exercise or social activity, which may address the problem of unintended dozing during the day, particularly in institutionalized demented patients. Restriction of time in bed, increasing bright light exposure during the day, decreasing light at night, and making the environment more quiet at night have all been shown to improve sleep in this population will address poor sleep hygiene and inadequate light exposure. Nonpharmacologic approaches are preferable to medications for older individuals with dementia.

SUMMARY

Aging is associated with significant changes in sleep depth, duration, and architecture. Sleep disorders are often more common in older adults and thus may contribute to insomnia complaints in aging populations. However, sleep problems may also arise as a result of changes in the circadian rhythm, medical or psychiatric comorbidity, and the side effects of medications. Diagnosis of occult sleep disorders requires a thorough sleep and medical history, supplemented by overnight sleep recording when appropriate. Treatment may include somatic interventions, behavioral strategies, or combination treatment depending on the disorder. Successful treatment may significantly improve sleep and daytime functioning in older adults.

KEY POINTS

Sleep, Aging, and Late-Life Insomnia

- Sleep disorders are common in older adults.
- Sleep architecture changes with age, with sleep becoming lighter.
- Most sleep problems are a function of medical and psychiatric illness, medications, and primary sleep disorders, and are not a function of age per se.
- Diagnosis of sleep disorders requires a thorough sleep and medical history. For some primary sleep disorders, an overnight sleep recording should be considered.
- Treatment may include behavioral strategies, pharmacologic treatment, or combination of both.

For a complete list of references, please visit online only at www.expertconsult.com

Malnutrition in Older Adults

Larry E. Johnson
Dennis H. Sullivan

Malnutrition may refer to both deficiencies (such as protein, calorie, vitamin, mineral, etc.) and excesses (e.g., obesity and hypervitaminosis).[1] This chapter will focus on common nutritional concerns in older adults: protein-energy undernutrition (PEU), hydration, artificial feeding, and end-of-life nutrition. Vitamin health will be covered in Chapter 82 and obesity (i.e., overnutrition) in Chapter 83. As people age, the risks for undernutrition increase. Five to 10% of community-dwelling older adults are undernourished.[2] Undernutrition in hospitalized elderly persons is frequently unrecognized and untreated,[3] for example, hospitalized patients are often not fed for extended periods of time in preparation for various procedures. In one study of 700 older hospitalized men, 21% had a daily intake of less than 50% of maintenance requirements, and this low intake was associated with an eight times higher mortality risk.[4] Estimates for the prevalence for PEU in long-term and subacute care facilities vary from 12% to 85%.[5–8] As is true within hospitals, staff in these facilities also fail to recognize undernutrition.[9]

Weight loss is a cardinal sign for PEU and can develop in association with many disorders, including cancer, heart failure, pulmonary disease, diabetes mellitus, and thyroid disease. Detection of weight loss is important in the care of older adults. Older men who lose more than 3 kg/yr over 5 years have a 3.5 times greater mortality risk than those who have no weight change.[10] Losing 5% of weight in any one month is associated with a tenfold higher risk for death in long-term care residents compared with residents who gain weight.[11] Even much slower weight loss, such as 5% over 1 year[12] or 10% over several decades[13] is associated with an increased mortality risk.

Characterizing undernutrition using terms such as marasmus and kwashiorkor, clinical syndromes originally described in third-world children, has also been used with adult malnutrition. It is proposed that a distinction be made between persons who have "simple" starvation (which may be the same as what is referred to as marasmus) from those who have inadequate caloric intake in the presence of inflammatory states (which may be subclinical). This latter syndrome has variably been referred to as cachexia, kwashiorkor, hypoalbuminemic malnutrition, or wasting disease.[14,15] Although far more needs to be learned about the metabolic basis of PEU that develops in association with other disease states, there is growing evidence that disease-induced inflammation triggers a catabolic response that is relatively refractory to nutritional support alone. Even when protein and energy intakes are higher than estimated requirements, there is often continued catabolism of both fat and lean body mass, particularly skeletal muscle (see Chapter 73).[16] In addition, it is important to be wary of trying to distinguish voluntary from involuntary weight loss, particularly in the frail older adult[17]; any weight loss in this population, even in the obese, should be considered potentially serious. On the other hand, stable weight or weight gain in physically inactive older adults who are obese may mask muscle loss, leading to the condition of sarcopenic obesity.[18,19]

Failure to thrive and frailty

Weight loss and malnutrition are often associated with other physiologic and functional impairments and increased mortality. "Failure to thrive" is a poorly defined term that has been variously characterized as a syndrome in older adults accompanied by weight loss, anemia of chronic disease, reduced immune function, and low albumin and cholesterol, along with functional and cognitive decline.[20–22] This syndrome may be part of the spectrum of inflammation-induced catabolism described above with marked cachexia representing an advanced stage. Frailty is a related, but better defined, concept.[23] Indicators of frailty include unintended weight loss (defined as >5% weight loss over the previous 1 to 2 years), weakness/impaired walking, exhaustion, and poor physical activity.[23,24] Studies of both older males and females from the Cardiovascular Health Study and the Women's Health Initiative Observational Study have found that frailty is associated with increased risk of death, hip fracture, disability, and hospitalization.[23,24] The importance of a dysregulated inflammatory response as a contributor to frailty in older adults is being investigated. Weight loss may also precede the diagnosis of Alzheimer's disease.[25]

The anorexia of aging

With advancing age, appetite and food intake steadily decline, even in the absence of serious acute or chronic disease. Paralleling the change in appetite, there is usually an associated decline in energy expenditure (i.e., level of physical activity). Whether the declines in energy intake and expenditure are causally related is not known with certainty. However, both contribute to the progressive weight loss seen in many older adults after about age 60 to 70 years. The magnitude of this problem is indicated by population-based studies that reveal a progressive decline in the prevalence of overweight and obesity, and an increase in the prevalence of underweight (BMI < 18.5) with each decade of life after age 60.[26] With advancing age, the physiologic processes that regulate body weight and that link nutrient intake and energy expenditure apparently lose their compensatory responsiveness to changes in energy demands.[27] This was demonstrated in one study of young and old adults who were placed on energy restricted diets. Both groups lost weight. However, at the end of the fast, the older adults regained their lost weight more slowly and less completely than the younger subjects.[28] These findings suggest that a reduced ability to regulate appetite and food intake may contribute to the progressive loss of weight that many older individuals experience as they age.

A thorough assessment of any older adult who is losing weight is mandatory to determine if there are potentially reversible causes and to assess the severity of the anorexia.[29] Sometimes even an extensive evaluation fails to find any contributing causes for the weight loss. The term "Anorexia of Aging" has been coined to describe such older adults with isolated anorexia. It is hypothesized that this age-associated anorexia may result from any number of physiologic changes seen in older adults including impaired gastric motility, exaggerated adiposity signals from leptin and insulin, and/or postprandial anorexigenic signals from cholecystokinin (CCK) and peptide YY (PYY).[30] It may also entail a cytokine-dependent process as many older adults have elevated blood cytokine levels.[16,31]

Protein-energy undernutrition (PEU)

There is no "gold standard" laboratory test for PEU. Laboratory tests of so-called nutritional biochemical markers (e.g., serum albumin, transthyretin/prealbumin, α-acid-1 glycoprotein, or transferrin) have poor specificity. The synthesis and distribution of all of these serum proteins are probably more strongly affected by cytokine-associated inflammation (as "acute phase reactants") than nutrient intake. The sensitivity of these markers is also low. This is particularly true of serum albumin. The serum concentration of albumin may remain near normal during uncomplicated slow starvation. Thus it is possible to die of starvation with a normal serum albumin concentration. However, because of their responsiveness to physiologic stress, serum albumin and some of the other serum secretory proteins are important health status indicators; a low level is associated with increased morbidity and mortality, independent of nutritional status.[32] No biomarker is readily available to distinguish simple starvation from cachexia, and measuring nonspecific markers for inflammation, such as erythrocyte sedimentation rate or C-reactive protein, is not recommended.

Nutritional screening

There are a variety of screening tools to assess for nutritional risk. These instruments do not necessarily confirm that an individual has malnutrition, but they are useful for identifying those who need a more thorough nutritional evaluation. The Mini Nutritional Assessment (MNA) (Figure 112-1) has a six-question screening test.[33] If an older adult scores at nutritional risk, there are 12 more questions (including estimates of consumption, self-assessment, and anthropometric measures of midarm and calf circumference) to aid in assessing the probability of malnutrition. The Malnutrition Universal Screening Tool (MUST) (Figure 112-2) has also been validated for older adults and has alternative measurements for patients whose height cannot be measured or who cannot be weighed (for detailed information: www.BAPEN.org.uk).[34,35] In the United States, nursing home residents must have a minimum data set (MDS) completed within 14 days of admission, at any major change in condition, and at yearly intervals.[36] This document includes an assessment for nutritional risk, including chewing or swallowing problems, or mouth pain; complaints about the taste of food or complaints of hunger; IV fluids or hyperalimentation; feeding tube, mechanically altered or therapeutic diets, or oral syringe feeding; between meal supplements; adaptive feeding equipment; planned weight change programs; an estimate of percent calories consumed over the previous 7 days; height and weight over the previous 30 days; and weight loss or gain over the past 30 and 180 days. The MDS regulations for nursing home residents require a thorough evaluation for any resident who loses 5% of weight in 1 month or 10% in 6 months.[36]

Accurate estimates of a patient's height, weight, and weight loss are important. These measurements are sometimes difficult to obtain. Direct measurement of height may not be valid due to the presence of spine curvature. An older patient's memory of current or maximum adult height is frequently inaccurate; formulas to estimate height using demispan (half total arm span), ulna length, or knee height (using special calipers) are available. Identification of weight loss, using the MDS guidelines above, and an estimate of calorie intake, are important in identifying PEU. Weight measurement accuracy is highly dependent on the skill of the examiner; weights obtained by trained persons maintaining strict adherence to protocol are more reliable and can differ substantially from those obtained routinely by nursing staff. On the other hand, relying only on a patient's weight or body mass index (BMI) may not identify individuals who are malnourished but have fluid overload or sarcopenic obesity.

Chewing and swallowing

Healthy aging is generally associated with little clinical change in chewing and swallowing. Many medications (particularly anticholinergic and antimuscarinic drugs), Sjögren's syndrome, and radiation therapy for head and neck cancers decrease salivation, causing xerostomia and increasing the risk of dental caries and hampering chewing and swallowing.[37] Poor dental hygiene, missing teeth, poorly fitting or missing dentures are common, and cause reduced food intake, and require the evaluation of a dentist.[38] Proper routine dental care for the uncooperative patient requires training for the family, nursing staff, and the dentist. Finding a dentist especially trained in examining and treating resistive patients can be challenging if a gerodentist is not available.

The gastrointestinal tract generally shows little dramatic change with aging, though the accumulation of multiple small changes may contribute to the development of the anorexia of aging (see previous discussion).[39] Esophageal motility may be impaired ("presby-esophagus") with less efficient peristalsis. Medication transit and absorption may be affected by this change and pills may remain for a prolonged period in the esophagus of older persons who are supine. It is therefore recommended that older patients take more fluids with medications and then remain upright for at least 30 minutes rather than lying down immediately. This is a particularly important issue for older adults taking medications known to cause esophageal irritation. Gastroesophageal reflux and hiatal hernia increase with aging, with associated dyspepsia. In most cases, symptoms are managed with dietary avoidance of food that increase symptoms; universal avoidance of hot and spicy foods is not necessary. Widespread use of antacids for dyspepsia is extremely common; antacids reduce gastric symptoms but can increase the risk of pneumonia (stomach acid is valuable in killing bacteria that are swallowed) and may reduce absorption of some vitamins and minerals (e.g., B_{12} and iron) in very frail persons.[40,41] Further workup of uncomplicated dyspepsia is necessary only if alarm symptoms or signs appear such as weight loss, fall in hemoglobin, or gastrointestinal bleeding (see p. 623).

Dysphagia (or difficulty eating) can arise as a consequence of problems in any phase of eating including the anticipatory phase, preparatory phase, mastication (the oral phase), swallowing (pharyngeal phase), and/or passage of food or

Nestlé Nutrition INSTITUTE

Mini Nutritional Assessment MNA®

Last name: First name: Sex: Date:

Age: Weight, kg: Height, cm: I.D. Number:

Complete the screen by filling in the boxes with the appropriate numbers.
Add the numbers for the screen. If score is 11 or less, continue with the assessment to gain a Malnutrition Indicator Score.

Screening

A Has food intake declined over the past 3 months due to loss of appetite, digestive problems, chewing or swallowing difficulties?
0 = severe loss of appetite
1 = moderate loss of appetite
2 = no loss of appetite ☐

B Weight loss during the last 3 months
0 = weight loss greater than 3 kg (6.6 lbs)
1 = does not know
2 = weight loss between 1 and 3 kg (2.2 and 6.6 lbs)
3 = no weight loss ☐

C Mobility
0 = bed or chair bound
1 = able to get out of bed/chair but does not go out
2 = goes out ☐

D Has suffered psychological stress or acute disease in the past 3 months
0 = yes 2 = no ☐

E Neuropsychological problems
0 = severe dementia or depression
1 = mild dementia
2 = no psychological problems ☐

F Body Mass Index (BMI) (weight in kg)/(height in m^2)
0 = BMI less than 19
1 = BMI 19 to less than 21
2 = BMI 21 to less than 23
3 = BMI 23 or greater ☐

Screening score (subtotal max. 14 points) ☐☐
12 points or greater Normal – not at risk – no need to complete assessment
11 points or below Possible malnutrition – continue assessment

Assessment

G Lives independently (not in a nursing home or hospital)
0 = no 1 = yes ☐

H Takes more than 3 prescription drugs per day
0 = yes 1 = no ☐

I Pressure sores or skin ulcers
0 = yes 1 = no ☐

J How many full meals does the patient eat daily?
0 = 1 meal
1 = 2 meals
2 = 3 meals ☐

K Selected consumption markers for protein intake
• At least one serving of daily products (milk, cheese, yogurt) per day yes ☐ no ☐
• Two or more servings of legumes or eggs per week yes ☐ no ☐
• Meat, fish or poultry every day yes ☐ no ☐
0.0 = if 0 or 1 yes
0.5 = if 2 yes
1.0 = if 3 yes ☐.☐

L Consumes two or more servings of fruits or vegetables per day?
0 = no 1 = yes ☐

M How much fluid (water, juice, coffee, tea, milk...) is consumed per day?
0.0 = less than 3 cups
0.5 = 3 to 5 cups
1.0 = more than 5 cups ☐.☐

N Mode of feeding
0 = unable to eat without assistance
1 = self-fed with some difficulty
2 = self-fed without any problem ☐

O Self view of nutritional status
0 = views self as being malnourished
1 = is uncertain of nutritional state
2 = views self as having no nutritional problem ☐

P In comparison with other people of the same age, how does the patient consider his/her health status?
0.0 = not as good
0.5 = does not know
1.0 = as good
2.0 = better ☐.☐

Q Mid-arm circumference (MAC) in cm
0.0 = MAC less than 21
0.5 = MAC 21 to 22
1.0 = MAC 22 or greater ☐.☐

R Calf circumference (CC) in cm
0.0 = CC less than 31 1 = CC 31 or greater ☐

Assessment (max. 16 points) ☐☐.☐
Screening score ☐☐
Total Assessment (max. 30 points) ☐☐.☐

Malnutrition Indicator Score
17 to 23.5 points at risk of malnutrition ☐
Less than 17 points malnourished ☐

Ref. Vellas B, Villars H, Abellan G, et al. Overview of the MNA® - Its History and Challenges. J Nut Health Aging 2006;10:456–465.
Rubenstein LZ, Harker JO, Salva A, Guigoz Y, Vellas B. Screening for Undernutrition in Geriatric Practice: Developing the Short-Form Mini Nutritional Assessment (MNA-SF). J. Geront 2001;56A: M366–377.
Guigoz Y. The Mini-Nutritional Assessment (MNA®) Review of the Literature - What does it tell us? J Nutr Health Aging 2006; 10:466–487.

For more information: www.mna-elderly.com

Figure 112-1. The Mini Nutritional Assessment (MNA). The initial assessment is a six-question screening test. If an older adult scores at nutritional risk (11 points or less), there are 12 more questions to aid in assessing the probability of malnutrition. A score of 17 to 23.5 indicates a high risk for malnutrition and less than 17 indicates probable malnutrition.[33,130,131] *(Reprinted with permission from Societe des Produits Nestle S.A., Vevey, Switzerland.)*

BAPEN
Advancing Clinical Nutrition

'Malnutrition Universal Screening Tool' ('MUST')

MAG
Malnutrition Advisory Group
A Standing Committee of BAPEN

BAPEN is registered charity number 1023927 www.bapen.org.uk

'MUST'

'MUST' is a five-step screening tool to identify **adults**, who are malnourished, at risk of malnutrition (undernutrition), or obese. It also includes management guidelines which can be used to develop a care plan.

It is for use in hospitals, community and other care settings and can be used by all care workers.

This guide contains:
- A flow chart showing the 5 steps to use for screening and management
- BMI chart
- Weight loss tables
- Alternative measurements when BMI cannot be obtained by measuring weight and height.

The 5 'MUST' Steps

Step 1
Measure height and weight to get a BMI score using chart provided. *If unable to obtain height and weight, use the alternative procedures shown in this guide.*

Step 2
Note percentage unplanned weight loss and score using tables provided.

Step 3
Establish acute disease effect and score.

Step 4
Add scores from steps 1, 2 and 3 together to obtain overall risk of malnutrition.

Step 5
Use management guidelines and/or local policy to develop care plan.

Please refer to *The 'MUST' Explanatory Booklet* for more information when weight and height cannot be measured, and when screening patient groups in which extra care in interpretation is needed (e.g. those with fluid disturbances, plaster casts, amputations, critical illness and pregnant or lactating women). The booklet can also be used for training. See *The 'MUST' Report* for supporting evidence. Please note that 'MUST' has not been designed to detect deficiencies or excessive intakes of vitamins and minerals and is of **use only in adults**.

Step 1 BMI score + Step 2 Weight loss score + Step 3 Acute disease effect score

BMI kg/m^2	Score
>20 (>30 Obese)	= 0
18.5–20	= 1
<18.5	= 2

Unplanned weight loss in past 3–6 months

%	Score
<5	= 0
5–10	= 1
>10	= 2

If patient is acutely ill and there has been or is likely to be no nutritional intake for >5 days
Score 2

If unable to obtain height and weight, see reverse for alternative measurements and use of subjective criteria

Step 4
Overall risk of malnutrition

Add Scores together to calculate overall risk of malnutrition
Score 0 Low Risk Score 1 Medium Risk Score 2 or more High Risk

Step 5
Management guidelines

0
Low Risk
Routine clinical care
- Repeat screening
  Hospital – weekly
  Care Homes – monthly
  Community – annually
  for special groups e. g. those >75 yrs

1
Medium risk
Observe
- Document dietary intake for 3 days if subject in hospital or care home
- If improved or adequate intake – little clinical concern; if no improvement – clinical concern – follow local policy
- Repeat screening
  Hospital – weekly
  Care Home – at least monthly
  Community – at least every 2–3 months

2 or more high risk
Treat*
- Refer to dietitian, Nutritional Support Team or implement local policy
- Improve and increase overall nutritional intake
- Monitor and review care plan
  Hospital – weekly
  Care Home – monthly
  Community – monthly

*Unless detrimental or no benefit is expected from nutritional support e.g. imminent death.

All risk categories:
- Treat underlying condition and provide help and advice on food choices, eating and drinking when necessary.
- Record malnutrition risk category.
- Record need for special diets and follow local policy.

Obesity:
- Record presence of obesity. For those with underlying conditions, these are generally controlled before the treatment of obesity.

Re-assess subjects identified at risk as they move through care settings
See *The 'MUST' Explanatory Booklet* for further details and *The 'MUST' Report* for supporting evidence.

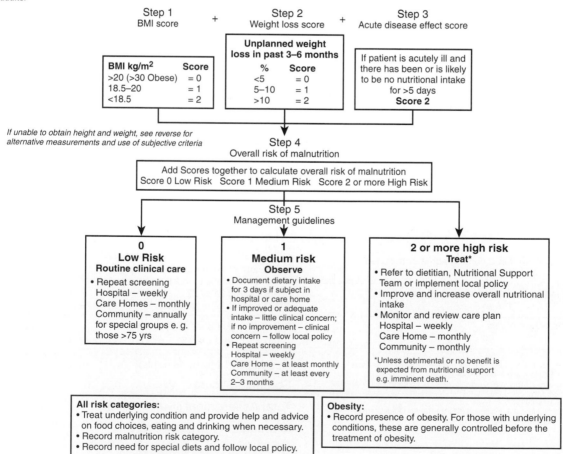

Figure 112-2. The Malnutrition Universal Screening Tool (MUST) has been validated for older adults, with low risk, medium risk, and high malnutrition risk.[34,35] *Reproduced with the kind permission of BAPEN (British Association for Parenteral and Enteral Nutrition). (For further information on this tool contact:* www.BAPEN.org.uk*)*

fluids down the esophagus (esophageal phase).[42] Details of the neurophysiology of swallowing can be found elsewhere.[43] Dysphagia may include signs and symptoms of difficulty chewing or swallowing, with the sensation of food getting stuck in the throat or chest and/or coughing or choking with swallowing. Patients with these symptoms require a thorough history and physical examination, especially of the head and neck regions to identify possible causes. The prevalence of dysphagia in community dwelling elderly varies from 7% to 28% (increasing with frailty)[44] but may also be relatively common even in younger adults.[45] Persons with degenerative neurologic disorders such as Alzheimer's disease and other dementias may have a tonic bite (refusing to open their mouths when fed) or hold food in the mouth for prolonged periods (swallowing apraxia). However, dysphagia may be present with less obvious symptoms, and should be considered whenever there is weight loss, decreased appetite, prolonged eating time, food falling from the mouth, food debris staying in the mouth, nasal or oral regurgitation, wet voice, or hoarseness after eating.[46] Any possible symptoms of oral or pharyngeal stage dysphagia that do not quickly resolve should be assessed by a speech-language pathologist (SLP) or an ENT (ears, nose, throat) specialist. Esophageal stage problems (e.g., esophageal cancer, candidiasis, reflux esophagitis, Zenker's diverticulum, hiatal hernia, varices, Barrett's esophagus, Schatzki's ring) will need assessment by a gastroenterologist, with esophagogastroduodenoscopy (EGD), string capsule endoscopy, or other specialized evaluations.[47] Dysphagia is an expected complication of head, neck, and esophageal cancers, and many of the therapies directed at these conditions; pretreatment swallowing exercises may benefit some of these patients.[48] There are a variety of survey instruments to screen for dysphagia; they are of limited usefulness for most clinicians but may be of benefit to SLPs.[49,50]

Oropharyngeal dysphagia occurs commonly after strokes and during the course of many neurodegenerative diseases, such as dementia and Parkinson's disease. Chronic swallowing disorders also appear to be common in independent-living elderly; 33% of older adults in one study reported a current problem.[51] Dysphagia following a stroke is associated with decreased survival in the 3 months after a stroke, and increased risk of nursing home placement.[52] SLP assessment can be very useful in assessing persons who are not chewing or swallowing normally, who cough with eating, or who are losing weight for unknown reasons. These experts can assess chewing and swallowing using many modalities, and often provide valuable treatment suggestions, although the evidence on the effectiveness of many of these strategies is limited. The most accurate diagnostic test for dysphagia is considered to be videofluoroscopy (or the modified barium swallow), but this requires radiation exposure. Fiberoptic endoscopic evaluation of swallowing (FEES) also appears to be quite accurate and can be performed at bedside, wherein air is blown through an endoscope in the nose down to the soft palate or pressure is applied to the pharyngeal muscles to trigger an observable swallow.[53,54] In the absence of SLP resources, several bedside tests may be useful, including the GUSS (Gugging swallow screen) (observing patients during a saliva swallow, then semisolid thickened liquids, thin liquids, and finally dry toast),[50] or the 3-oz (84 mL) water test, observing for coughing during, and for up to 1 minute following, drinking water.[55] A comprehensive nursing protocol to assess and manage swallowing problems in frail older adults is available.[56]

Table 112-1. Strategies to Reduce Dehydration in Older Adults

Prepare for dehydration in older adults in high risk situations (summer heat without air conditioning, acute illness, delirium, etc.)
Evaluate patient for possible benefit to drink using a straw
Offer a variety of fluids during recreational and social activities; "happy hours"; "tea times"
Consider offering options to water (juices, soups, water-rich fruits [watermelon, grapes, peaches] and vegetables [tomatoes, lettuce, squash])[132]
Discuss side effects/timing of diuretics to anticipate voluntary dehydration
Offer a choice of fluid options, rather than only one or two

A variety of treatment options are used by SLP experts to try to restore a normal swallow, including electrical stimulation, thermal stimulation, muscle exercises, and acupuncture.[57] More extreme interventions (cricopharyngeus muscle myotomy, botulinum toxin injections, etc.) have an uncertain role.[58] The use of modified diets can improve the safety of swallowing; SLPs and dietitians can provide guidance to patients, families, and staff on the use of such diets. For patients with difficulty swallowing thin liquids, adding thickening agents to provide nectar-like, honey-like, or spoon-thick, or fluids is an option.[59] However, thickened liquids are often less palatable and may increase the risk for dehydration.[60] Sitting patients upright when eating (and for some time afterwards), chin tucking when swallowing, eating more slowly, and use of various swallowing maneuvers are additional techniques (see Table 112-1). Methods that are more successful in persons with one cause for dysphagia may not work as well for another (see the "Aspiration and Aspiration Pneumonia" section).[61,62]

Constipation

The frail older adult is prone to constipation for many reasons (anticholinergic and opioid medications, poor fluid intake, poor fiber intake, little physical exercise, etc. [see Chapter 108]). Constipation is a common cause of poor food intake in the frail or bedbound older adult, and proper monitoring of bowel movements can be very useful in assessing reasons for reduced dietary intake of these patients.

Thirst and hydration

Adequate fluid intake may be associated with fewer falls, less constipation and laxative use, improved rehabilitation outcomes, less bladder cancer, and lower rates of postprandial orthostatic hypotension.[63,64] Risk for dehydration increases with advanced age, race (blacks have higher risk than whites), use of certain medications (diuretics, laxatives, psychotropics, and general polypharmacy), physical dependency, dementia, delirium, and chronic disease.[63,64] Healthy older adults have an age-associated decrease in thirst sensation (hypodipsia) and consume less fluid in response to the same degree of dehydration than younger adults.[65–67] Hypodipsia can be even more pronounced in older adults suffering from chronic disease; perhaps 30% of nursing home residents are dehydrated at any point in time.[68] Darker urine color in persons with adequate renal function, blood urea nitrogen:creatinine ratio (>25:1 mg/dL), serum osmolality (>300 mmol/kg), serum sodium (>150 mEq/L), urine specific gravity (>1.029), and urine output (<800 mL/day) may aid in the detection of dehydration.[69–71] Skin turgor is not an adequate tool to detect dehydration in older adults. Older adults at highest risk of dehydration include those who have a diminished thirst drive due to neurodegenerative conditions, those who cannot access or safely consume fluids due to physical or cognitive impairments or dysphagia, those who will not drink enough because of fears of urinary incontinence or have never consumed many fluids, and those at the end of life.[68] Distinguishing patients in this manner may aid in selecting the optimal prevention and treatment strategies.

Water requirements are not defined well for adults, let alone for older adults. In healthy adults, hydration status remains normal despite large individual differences in intake. Fluid goals should be tailored to each individual; for example, there may be competing goals with patients with fluid overload (as found with congestive heart failure) (Chapter 40), with hyponatremia with the syndrome of inappropriate secretion of antidiuretic hormone (SIADH) (Chapter 85), and with respect to activity level or environmental temperature. A daily water intake (including free water, water in other beverages, and water in food) of 3.7 L for men and 2.7 L for women meets the needs of most healthy persons, including advanced ages.[72] This should not be considered a minimum intake. A reasonable initial goal for sedentary older adults may begin with 30 mL/kg/day or 1500 to 2000 mL/day of fluids; this goal can then be adjusted based on blood urea nitrogen levels, urinary output, and clinical status. Possible intervention strategies are presented in Table 112-1. The poorer palatability of thickened liquids may reduce intake and not meet patients' fluid requirements.[60] In cases where oral fluid intake is temporarily decreased, for example, due to an acute infection, subcutaneous infusion of fluids (hypodermoclysis) for a day or two until adequate drinking resumes is easy to accomplish and may avoid intravenous access or hospitalization.[73]

Refeeding syndrome

Nutritional requirements are discussed in Chapter 82, and feeding someone can be based on those recommendations. There are several formulas that may be useful in initially calculating caloric needs; none are perfect but the Harris-Benedict equations (Table 112-2) serve as a starting point for average individuals.[74] However, in patients with significant chronic undernutrition (such as prolonged starvation), feeding too much and too rapidly can cause the refeeding syndrome, with rapid falls in blood phosphorus, potassium, and magnesium; sodium and water retention leading to fluid overload; and altered glucose homeostasis.[75,76] Electrolyte deficiencies, pulmonary edema, cardiac decompensation, and death become likely. High carbohydrate intake increases thiamine requirements and can precipitate acute Wernicke's encephalopathy in undernourished persons with unrecognized thiamine deficiency (e.g., alcoholics). It is critical to identify individuals at high risk for refeeding syndrome before beginning nutritional support, provide thiamine and other micronutrient

Table 112-2. Harris-Benedict Equations for Estimating Caloric Requirements

Men: 66.4 + [13.75 × weight (kg)] + [5.0 × height (cm)] − [6.8 × age]
Women: 655.1 + [9.6 × weight (kg)] + [1.85 × height (cm)] − [4.7 × age]

supplements immediately, and then begin feeding at about 25% of the estimated caloric goal (permissive underfeeding). As tolerated, intake can be increased slowly with the goal of reaching targeted daily intake after 3 to 5 days.[75,76] Electrolytes should be assessed before refeeding, and then monitored every 4 to 6 hours for the first day or two. Initial fluid intake should be restricted to less than 1000 mL per day in these individuals, and weights accurately measured daily. Weight gain more than 1 kg weekly is a warning for fluid overload.

Aspiration and aspiration pneumonia

Aspiration pneumonia is common in older frail adults, particularly those who are hospitalized or institutionalized, and those with acute or chronic neurologic disease. It may also make up 5% to 15% of all community-acquired pneumonias.[77] Highest predictors of aspiration pneumonia, which vary among differing patient populations, include the need for suctioning, COPD and CHF diagnoses, presence of feeding tube, feeding or oral care dependency, and being bedfast.[78,79] Patients on respirators are also at very high risk. Aspiration pneumonia in frail older adults frequently has few classic symptoms; delirium (confusion, agitation, lethargy), unexplained elevated white blood cell counts, or tachypnea may be the only early indicators. Aspiration itself may occur without any obvious clinical signs, or with only episodic fever or reduced oxygen saturation.[80–82] Approaches to reducing the risk of aspiration and aspiration pneumonia are outlined in Table 112-3.

In patients who have dysphagia, it is important to assess aspiration risk and whether this risk is influenced by the texture of the food consumed. In some of these patients, thin liquids present a particular problem. For these individuals, dietary modifications and adoption of specialized swallowing techniques may be important in reducing risk (see the "Chewing and Swallowing" section).[50] A recent study[83] did not find any clear difference in aspiration pneumonia risk between drinking thin liquids in a chin-down posture or thicker liquids in a normal posture in patients with dementia or Parkinson's disease (PD). Honey-like liquids appear to work better than nectar-like liquids or chin-down posture for many patients with dementia or PD.[61] However, half the patients receive no benefit from these maneuvers, particularly those with the most severe dementia. Many patients and their families refuse to accept thickened liquids and prefer to accept the aspiration risk of thin liquids; this decision process needs to be thoroughly documented. Videofluorographic swallow study (VFSS) currently appears to be the best test to assess aspiration risk, and is recommended before restricting intake of thin liquids.[53,54] Debilitated patients will continue to aspirate oral secretions and reflux, which are not prevented by SLP interventions or recommendations, and this is at least as important as prandial aspiration.[84]

Table 112-3. Reducing Risk of Aspiration and Aspiration Pneumonia in Older Adults*

All patients: Improve oral hygiene/frequent teeth brushing/properly fitting dentures
Hand feeding:
Provide a rest period (>30 minutes) before feeding time
Sit upright at 90 degrees, or highest position allowed by medical condition
Avoid rushed or forced feeding; feeding by syringe is risky
Alternate liquids with solids
Recognize the high risks of sedatives, hypnotics, and other psychotropic meds, and try to wean or reduce dosages
Speech-language-pathology referral: Evaluate patient for possible benefit of "chin down" position when swallowing or for possible benefit of adjusting liquid viscosity; thickened liquids of varying types may improve swallowing in some patients (ice cream and Jello are considered thin liquids)
Tube feeding (both nasogastric and gastrostomy tube feeding may *increase* aspiration risks):
Consider continuous feedings rather than intermittent (bolus) feedings
Keep backrest elevated at least 30 degrees during feedings, if possible
Consider pump-assisted feedings rather than gravity-controlled feedings
A gastric residual volume >200 mL during continuous feeding or before intermittent feedings may increase risk (but this remains controversial)[136]
Prokinetic agents such as metoclopramide or erythromycin may improve feeding tolerance, but are associated with their own serious potential side effects.
Placing the feeding tube tip beyond the pylorus (jejunostomy, gastrojejunostomy) may reduce aspiration in some patients
Using colored dye in tube feeding is contraindicated (it was originally felt that adding coloring to liquid tube feeding formulas would help to identify probable feeding aspiration if the coloring was found after throat and pulmonary suctioning)[137]

*(Note: most of these suggestions are consensus and expert opinions rather than evidence based [133–135].)

Several medications have been proposed to reduce the risk of aspiration pneumonia, most notably the angiotensin-converting enzyme (ACE) inhibitors, but the evidence to support this intervention remains inadequate.[77] Improved oral hygiene and regular tooth brushing may also reduce the risk of aspiration pneumonia.[85,86] Treatment of aspiration pneumonia will include coverage for both gram-positive and gram-negative organisms, including anaerobic mouth organisms.

Improving nutrition

Strategies to improve nutrition should be individualized, focusing on barriers specific to each person; strategies proven to be most successful entail multimodal interventions. Table 112-4 provides examples of such approaches. Appetite may improve when depression, pain, and constipation are treated, so these common disorders should be searched for whenever appetite is poor. For institutionalized older adults, appropriate social stimulation, one-on-one feeding support, increasing the variety of choices at and between meals, and a liberal food substitution policy are associated with increased calorie intake.[87] Nursing home residents who are physically unable to feed themselves are at particularly high risk for weight loss if adequate care is not provided. It is well established that this risk can be reduced by the provision of feeding assistance by appropriately trained staff. Less well recognized is that many nursing home residents assessed by the nursing staff to be physically independent are also at high risk for weight loss. Recent studies indicate that these individuals can also benefit from close supervision, verbal cuing, and other forms of staff support at mealtime.[88] Using non-nursing staff to transport patients to the dining room, deliver meals and provide substitute foods, document intake, and increase social stimulation may allow nursing staff to spend more time with mealtime feeding assistance.[88]

Weight loss in patients with dementia is often due to many interacting factors: self-feeding/chewing/swallowing difficulties; loss of hunger drive; and, occasionally, higher energy expenditure due to pacing coupled with failure of intrinsic regulatory systems for maintaining body weight.[89] Unless other diseases are present, there is no consistent evidence that patients with dementia have higher resting energy expenditure or other evidence of hypermetabolism. Obstinacy and feeding aversions (turning the head away when food is offered, keeping the mouth shut, pushing the spoon or hand away, and spitting out food) are common in dementia and often require individualized and creative and persistent approaches to maintain an adequate nutrient intake.[89–92]

Appetite stimulation

Medications designed to specifically improve appetite in older adults have not proven very effective, and many have considerable side effects or costs. Relatively few studies have targeted the frail older adult, and studies of cancer patients or persons with AIDS should not be presumed translatable to the aging patient. Corticosteroids, cyproheptadine, thalidomide, and human growth hormone lack proven effectiveness and are not recommended for appetite stimulation in older adults. Testosterone replacement or supplementation and other anabolic sex hormones (e.g., nandrolone) have important side effects and their use cannot be currently recommended in persons who are anorexic and losing weight without documented hypogonadism (see Chapter 58). Selective androgen receptor modulators (SARMS) have not yet been fully investigated but may play a future role.[93]

There is some evidence indicating that the cannabinoid, dronabinol, is effective in promoting weight gain in patients with Alzheimer's disease.[94,95] However, this medication is very expensive and many frail patients do not tolerate the dysphoria that is a common side effect. If careful monitoring can be provided, a trial of use in patients with anorexia can be considered. Megestrol acetate (MA) (a "progestagenic-corticoid-steroid") is another appetite stimulant that can be prescribed for frail older adults who are losing weight. Studies indicate that it is occasionally effective in increasing nutrient intake, inducing weight gain, and decreasing serum inflammation-associated cytokine levels.[14] However, the physiologic significance of this latter effect is not known, the weight gain is primarily fat, and MA often produces several potentially serious side effects. Many of its side effects are a consequence of its corticosteroid agonist and antagonist properties and include suppression of the pituitary-adrenal axis, muscle loss, insulin resistance, and salt and water retention. MA also suppresses testosterone levels to castrate levels and may increase the risk of venous thromboembolism and death.[96–98]

Table 112-4. Causes and Feeding Options in Patients Who Are Not Eating Enough[68,87,89]*

All Patients
Liberalize diet; offer variety of snacks between meals; offer food substitutions at meals
Reduce/eliminate "therapeutic" diets (e.g., low cholesterol, low fat, low salt)
Treat pain, constipation, depression
Dental evaluation
Give medications with high calorie liquid protein drinks
Reduce/eliminate sedating and other medications that often reduce appetite, if possible (e.g., anticholinergic, NSAIDs, some antidepressants and other psychotropic medications, dementia medications)
Train volunteers to feed patients/encourage family participation
Physically Capable
Independent: Educate, provide preferred/varied beverages, buffets, social stimulation, and encouragement
Assess for depression
Encourage exercise
Dementia: Offer food/variety of high-energy/high-protein snacks frequently between meals; integrate fluids into activities, happy hours; roving beverage and snack carts
Intensive dietitian involvement and staff education/awareness
Eat out of bed, in a chair at a table, if possible
Nonverbal and verbal cueing to encourage self-feeding, physical guidance; hand-over-hand technique to initiate and guide self-feeding; demonstrate eating movements for patient to imitate; show how to use utensils.
Reduce distraction, turn off television
Dentures in and eye glasses on
Simplify: one food/plate at a time
Observe for pocketing (cheeking) foods
Less emphasis on "healthy" eating and more on food preferences
Cannot Eat or Drink
Dysphagia:
SLP evaluation (see text)
Assess for mouth and throat infections
Physically dependent:
Adequate assistance, allow sufficient time to eat a meal
Will not eat or drink: (Patients who apathetic to eating or drinking may have frontal lobe dysfunction)
Sippers/eating disorders: Geropsychiatry evaluation
Fears incontinence: Adjust timing of diuretics/consider alternatives
End of Life
Review advance directives; discuss natural dying with patient and family, and the risks of artificial nutrition and hydration
Treat pain/constipation/depression; avoid medication side effects
Adequate hand feeding/assistance

*More suggestions are available at www.ConsultGeriRN.org. (Note: Persons with co-existing inflammation and cachexia may respond poorly to efforts at increasing nutritional intake.)

Appetite stimulation and weight gain are potential side effects of certain antipsychotics and antidepressants. This fact may have relevance in choosing therapies. Depression is common in older adults with anorexia, and should be actively and repeatedly screened for (see Chapter 57). Although antidepressants may either increase or decrease appetite in any individual patient, there is some evidence that mirtazapine can induce weight gain. Trials of antidepressant therapy, including mirtazapine up to its maximum dose, should be considered in any older adult who has unexplained anorexia and weight loss. Assessment by geropsychiatry is also recommended for patients who do not respond to initial therapy.

Current research on appetite stimulation is targeted on cytokines as these chemicals may play a significant role in cachexia[16,99,100]; this includes a potential role for antiinflammatory nutrients such as n-3 polyunsaturated fatty acids. Any role for ghrelin is unknown.

Enteral nutrition and tube feeding

When oral intake is inadequate and is likely to remain so for some time, artificial nutrition support should be considered. The nutritional assessment should consider several factors including the urgency of the need, the prognosis of the underlying condition, whether the individual has a functioning gastrointestinal (GI) tract, and the individual's personal preferences. If the GI tract is not functioning properly, peripheral or total parenteral nutrition support should be considered. If it is functioning and tube feeding is appropriate, it is then necessary to choose the type of tube and formula to be used, and the rate, schedule, and method of formula delivery.

The patient's overall prognosis is a critical consideration. If the underlying condition contributing to the older adult's loss of desire or ability to eat can be treated and the individual has a reasonable expectation of recovering independent function, it is often advisable to provide nutrition support during the recovery period.[101] This might be the case when the decline in nutrient intake occurs in association with major surgery, acute medical or psychiatric illness, or an acute and likely reversible exacerbation of a chronic medical condition. If the patient's BMI is greater than 18, the individual does not have a condition associated with exceptional metabolic demands, and volitional nutrient intake is expected to return to adequate levels within 5 days, nutrition support is probably not necessary.[101–103] In these cases, efforts should focus on identifying and eliminating any possible contributor to the patient's low intake. Older patients who have not had any appreciable nutrient intake for more than 5 days or who are unlikely to resume oral feedings within a comparable amount of time, nutrition support is warranted.[101–103] For patients with very little nutritional reserve (e.g., BMI <18), or high metabolic demands (e.g., extensive burns), initiate nutrition support if volitional intake cannot be restored within 2 or 3 days.[101–103]

If it is anticipated that tube feedings will be needed for less than 6 weeks, a soft (e.g., silicone or polyurethane), small-bore, nasoenteric feeding tube can be used. These tubes can be inserted at the bedside and their use avoids the need for an invasive procedure. The disadvantages of nasoenteric feeding tubes include increased risk of aspiration, sinusitis, and local nasal irritation; need for x-ray confirmation of correct placement before use; and the possibility of the tube being dislodged with coughing, vomiting, or poor patient tolerance. Tubes that are long enough to be passed into the duodenum or jejunum are useful when there is significant gastroparesis. Placement distal to the ligament of Treitz may also lower the risk of large volume aspiration, but it is often difficult to pass a tube beyond the stomach without endoscopic or fluoroscopic assistance.[104] Great care is required to prevent tube obstruction.

For patients requiring long-term enteral nutrition support (i.e., >6 weeks), a tube enterostomy is preferable. Tubes can be placed either endoscopically, radiologically, or surgically. Surgical placement is usually used only when there is a contraindication to less invasive procedures or the patient is going to surgery for another reason. Tubes placed radiologically or endoscopically can be used within hours and the procedure is often done as an outpatient. Special tubes that can be advanced into the jejunum can be used when there is pathology preventing gastric feedings, or when there is intractable intolerance to gastric feeding. Use of percutaneous jejunostomy tubes is usually limited to hospitalized patients with complex GI problems. Major complications of percutaneous endoscopic/radiologic gastrostomy occur in approximately 3% of patients and include hemorrhage, bowel perforation, fistula, aspiration, and erosion of the internal tube bumper into the abdominal wall.[101–103]

The type of formula to be used should be determined based on the needs of the patient. In most cases, a nutritionally complete, polymeric, lactose-free formula is the best option. The polymeric formulas differ in terms of the ratio of fat, protein, and carbohydrates, caloric density, and fiber content. Although some patients, such as those whose medical condition cannot tolerate high fluid intake, may benefit from high-calorie or high-nitrogen formulas, other patients do not tolerate the higher osmolality of such formulas, which may contribute to the development of diarrhea. With very narrow tubes, it is important to avoid use of formulas of high viscosity and not to insert crushed medications into the tube.

Partially digested and elemental (e.g., amino acid) formulas are available for patients who have difficulty digesting whole nutrients. However, these formulas are rarely required and are expensive. If the infusion rate of the formula is increased slowly or pancreatic enzymes are provided when needed, standard polymeric formulas can usually be used.

For patients who are severely undernourished, tube feedings should be started slowly to prevent metabolic complications (see the "Refeeding Syndrome" section).[75,76,105] Diarrhea, abdominal pain, and vomiting may occur when tube feedings are increased too rapidly. The use of tube feeding protocols to increase feeding rates to desired amounts, and closely monitoring laboratory values are recommended. Predictions of caloric intake are frequently inaccurate because tube feeding is frequently interrupted.

Some patients are eventually able to tolerate multiple, intragastric bolus feedings per day. This approach may be more physiologic and offers the advantage of allowing the patient to be intermittently disconnected from the feeding apparatus to enjoy more freedom of movement. This approach may also allow volitional oral feedings to be slowly introduced. Cyclic or nightly feedings may provide a similar advantage. For patients who do not tolerate bolus feedings or who need to be fed distal to the stomach, slow formula infusion by a pump is the preferred method. To minimize the risk of aspiration, the patient should be sitting upright at greater than 30 degrees during feedings, whether fed by bolus or slow infusion. Unless there is an absolute contraindication, patients receiving enteral nutrition support should always be allowed, and even encouraged, to resume volitional oral intake if tolerated. "Recreational" oral feeding, even if in small amounts, may be offered to patients with low aspiration risk to allow some of the hedonic sensations of eating.

Nutrition and hydration at the end of life (see also Chapter 116)

There are significant emotional, cultural, and religious aspects to providing nutrition and hydration to someone nearing the end of life and, in some cases, legal constraints as well.[106,107] It is often difficult to determine when aggressive nutritional support should be pursued and when someone should be allowed to die "naturally." Ideally, an ongoing dialogue among a patient, family members, and the health care team regarding advance directives should begin at adulthood when the patient is healthy and be based on the evidence of effectiveness before a health crisis.[108] Preferences regarding use of nutrition support at the end of life, how the individual defines quality of life, medical futility, dying naturally, unrealistic expectations, and medically prolonged death should be part of these discussions. As age advances and health changes, these directives should be reconsidered, again based on as much current evidence as is available. Encouraging the participation of nurses and nursing aides in the hospital or nursing home, and also providing them the latest clinical evidence,[109] may allow the health care team to present a unified, consistent, and supportive message, and maximize the chances for a peaceful death. Palliative care team referrals often benefit patients, families, and health care workers. Referral for hospice care is often delayed or avoided until shortly before death.[110]

The role of nutrition in end-of-life care is complex and controversial. Estimating life expectancy in patients with incurable disease is imperfect.[110,111] Average life expectancy after diagnosis differs significantly from one disease to another and there is considerable controversy as to how best to define the terminal stage of most conditions whether it be metastatic cancer, heart failure, or end-stage dementia. The issue is further complicated by the fact that the type of care provided may have a significant impact on the duration of life, but not necessarily the quality of life. This is particularly true of nutrition support. As discussed above, cancer-induced cachexia is generally resistant to increasing nutrient intake, and nutrition support is usually not effective in prolonging life. In contrast, some patients with Alzheimer's disease and other dementias can be kept alive for many years if provided adequate oral or enteral nutritional support (and excellent nursing care). However, there is no evidence that nutrition support slows the progression of the cognitive deficits or lowers the risk of aspiration, pressure sores, or infections, and it does not lead to improvement in physical function.[112–114] One observational study found no survival advantage for hospitalized patients with advanced dementia who receive a new feeding tube.[115] Whereas eating is associated with pleasure, enteral feedings are not felt to add to the quality of life. For these reasons, artificial nutrition and hydration are considered appropriate for reversible diseases, but decisions may become more complicated with irreversible illness and when the patient does not have advance directives and cannot make informed decisions (see Chapter 116). Complicating the issue further, clinicians' attitudes toward the role of nutrition support at the end of life differ significantly by specialty, region of the world, and personal beliefs.[116] Many health care providers, including oncologists and SLPs, encourage artificial nutrition and hydration and may cause confusion for patients and families (along with other staff) by using terms such as "life-sustaining" and "starvation.[84,117,118]" Dietitians and SLPs are more likely to recommend artificial nutrition and hydration than other health care professionals.[119,120] Diverse ethnic and religious backgrounds (of both patients and clinicians) may result in different goals and values, and different attitudes towards end of life care that are often poorly appreciated or anticipated.[121] Patient-family-health care provider discussions regarding prognosis, and education about the effectiveness or potential futility of various nutrition and hydration interventions are strongly recommended. If families need continuing support and education, and insist on artificial feeding and hydration, a therapeutic and finite trial of tube feeding can be instituted and can then be discontinued if the patient's condition has not improved or if the patient continues to be unable to consume enough food or fluids by mouth. This often allows family members to witness the futility of the purpose of the feeding and to come to terms with their depression and grief.

The dying process is often extremely stressful for families to observe. There are often many fears and unasked questions. Proactively discussing the natural dying process with patients and families can be very beneficial, including education regarding the dying patient's naturally slow cessation of food and fluid intake, and the evidence that there is no apparent suffering from this decline in intake.[122,123] Families need to be educated that intravenous (IV) hydration is unlikely to provide comfort, and may actually increase secretions and respiratory difficulty in the dying patient. Patients receiving IV hydration at the end of life often require diuretics for edema, ascites, and/or respiratory distress.[124] Families and patients need reassurance that pain management and treatment side effects (such as constipation, lethargy, confusion, etc.) will be anticipated and effectively treated.

Two clinical practice guidelines, from France and Canada,[125,126] address artificial nutrition in terminally ill cancer patients; parenteral nutrition is recommended only in selected persons with gastrointestinal obstruction due to cancer, a life expectancy of more than 6 to 12 weeks, and who have good functional status (Karnofsky score $>50\%$). These guidelines can improve decision making and reduce the inappropriate use of these interventions.[127] Educating patients, families, and staff that artificial feeding and nutrition in persons who are terminally ill may increase suffering and not improve outcome is recommended.[128,129]

For a complete list of references, please visit online only at www.expertconsult.com

CHAPTER 113

The Mistreatment and Neglect of Older People

Anthea Tinker
Simon G. Biggs
Jill Manthorpe*

Although medical practitioners are generally informed about child abuse, elder abuse, mistreatment, and neglect have only recently developed an evidence base of any significance. In this chapter, we first examine the development of concern, definitions, prevalence, and risk factors. We then discuss ways in which they may be identified and consider prevention and responses. We write from the perspective of developments in the United Kingdom, and from studies in a wider European and North American context. The publication of "Hidden Voices" by the World Health Organization (WHO) in 2001[1] revealed widespread recognition of this problem internationally. There is scope for continuing to draw lessons from cross-national perspectives, while recognizing differences in service and legal provisions along with cultural interpretations of abuse, between countries. Throughout we are concerned that, although there are lessons to be learned from child abuse, simplistic parallels should not be drawn. For example, there are dangers in interventions narrowly focused on the *protection* of older people, if they are ageist in philosophy, or undermine autonomy and rights in civil and criminal law. The European Convention on Human Rights, now incorporated into U.K. domestic law, offers an important counter to these dangers.

HISTORICAL DEVELOPMENT

Early concerns about mistreatment of older people were raised by doctors who saw a parallel with child abuse and placed the issue in the wider context of the care of older people both in their own homes and in institutions, emphasizing the importance of awareness and of good geriatric practice.[2,3] However, an evidence base was slow to develop with notable exceptions.[4,5] In its absence, abuse was linked to concerns about the stress placed on family caregivers by the care of older people, particularly those with dementia. Policy in many countries has drawn on developments from the United States. In England and Wales one policy response was the development of statutory guidance ("No Secrets[6]" and "In Safe Hands[7]") to establish multiagency (involving mainly health services, local government, and the police) systems through which concerns about the abuse of "vulnerable adults" might be addressed. The Mental Capacity Act 2005 created offenses relating to mistreatment or willful neglect of adults with mental incapacity. In the United Kingdom, policy developments have also responded to professional and pressure group concerns that elder abuse has been insufficiently resourced and prioritized (see Action on Elder Abuse[8] and Help the Aged[9]).

*With acknowledgments to Claudine McCreadie, who coauthored the original chapter with Anthea Tinker.

DEFINITIONS

Table 113-1 provides standard definitions and gives examples of both behavior and effect. Elder abuse, mistreatment, or neglect refer to the ill-treatment of an older person (usually defined as over age 65) by commission or omission. They may occur both in domestic settings (the older person's own home, a relative's home, or supported housing) and in institutions (care homes, nursing homes, and hospitals). Some kinds of behavior are criminal acts, such as assault and theft; others, such as verbal abuse, the restraint of someone who is aggressive, or overmedication, may be more contingent upon particular circumstances. Definitions are important because they determine "who will be counted as abused and who will not.[10] Abuse and neglect refer to behavior within a relationship connoting trust. This distinguishes actions by those closely linked to the older person, such as family members, or others in positions of responsibility (such as a member of staff) for their care, from actions by strangers.

Different types of abuse and neglect

There is now widespread agreement about five categories of abuse: physical violence; psychological abuse, often measured by persistent verbal aggression; financial abuse; sexual abuse; and neglect.[10,11] Although sexual abuse is sometimes subsumed under physical abuse, it has been increasingly recognized as a form of abuse in its own right. There is still very limited information on how much these types of abuse occur together and how much they are separate phenomena, but the research suggests that they both occur singly *and* in combination, and that the explanations for the abuse, and therefore the factors relevant to risk, may vary accordingly. The U.K. prevalence study[12] distinguished between forms of abuse that are interpersonal and of an intimate nature, financial forms, and neglect. Whether a common label and tendency to a common response are useful or not requires further research. The U.K. study gives a series of behavioral definitions of abuse that take frequency and severity into account that may be of greater use to professionals than ones intended for policy development.

Vulnerability of older people

In the context of elder abuse, vulnerability may be related to conditions of physical and mental frailty, and disability. Socioeconomic factors, such as low income, minority ethnic background, and bad housing, have been associated with enhanced risks.[13] The majority of prevalence studies has looked at older people living in community settings. Evidence for institutional forms of abuse tends to arise from public inquiries, inspection reports, and case studies. A study from the Czech Republic[14] suggests that 6% of care home residents suffer mistreatment either from staff or other residents. Residents of nursing homes, or of any institution providing social and health care, may be deemed vulnerable by virtue of their increased disability or their living situation. Professionals are likely to have contact with older people, who, because of their physical and/or mental impairments, are least able to protect themselves. However, while there are various discussions about individual risks, it may also be worth thinking about vulnerable situations. This means that we should be looking more at the context of the individual rather than about personal vulnerability. For example, not all people with dementia are at risk and those who are vulnerable are likely to be those who have few people to safeguard their best interests.

Table 113-1. Definitions of Types of Abuse, With Examples of Behavior and Effects[32]

Physical abuse: Nonaccidental infliction of physical force that results in bodily injury, pain, or impairment
- *Examples of behavior:* hitting, slapping, pushing, burning, physical restraint
- *Examples of effects:* bruises, fractures, burns, broken teeth, sprains, cuts, hair loss, bleeding from scalp, fear, anxiety, depression

Psychological abuse: The persistent use of threats, humiliation, bullying, swearing, and other verbal conduct, and/or of any other form of mental cruelty, that results in mental or physical distress
- *Examples of behavior:* treating an older person as a child, blaming, swearing, intimidating, name-calling, threatening violence, isolating older person
- *Examples of effects:* fear, depression, confusion, loss of sleep, loss of appetite

Financial abuse: Unauthorized and improper use of funds, property, or any resources of an older person
- *Examples of behavior:* misappropriating money, valuables, or property; forcing changes to will; denying access to personal funds
- *Examples of effects:* loss of money, etc., inability to pay bills, deterioration in health or standard of living, lack of amenities, unusual activity in bank accounts, signatures on documents uncertain, lack of solid arrangements for financial management, eviction or house sale notices

Sexual abuse: Direct or indirect involvement in sexual activity without consent
- *Examples of behavior*
- *Noncontact:* looking, photography, indecent exposure, harassment, serious teasing or innuendo, pornography
- *Contact:* touching breast, genitals, anus, mouth; masturbation of either or both persons; penetration or attempted penetration of vagina, anus, mouth, with or by penis, fingers, other objects
- *Examples of effects:* difficulty in walking or sitting, bruises, bleeding, venereal disease, psychological trauma

Neglect: Repeated deprivation of assistance needed by the older person for important activities of daily living
- *Examples of behavior:* failure to provide food, shelter, clothing, medical care, hygiene, personal care; inappropriate use of medication or overmedication
- *Examples of effects:* malnutrition, pressure ulcers, oversedation; untreated medical problems, depression, confusion

PREVALENCE AND INCIDENCE

Table 113-2 shows prevalence (in percentages) of elder mistreatment in North America, Canada, the United Kingdom, Amsterdam (in The Netherlands), and Spain. Studies have also taken place in Spain, the Czech Republic, Finland, Sweden, and Germany.[15] The Spanish study[16] is one of national community prevalence, indicating a figure of 0.8% reported by older people, but 4.5% by caregivers. The two major studies of community prevalence in North America[4,17] were based on telephone interviews. The U.K. survey was based on individual interviews with people aged 66 and over.[12] This found that overall 2.6% of people aged 66 and over living in private households reported that they had experienced mistreatment involving a family member, close friend, or care worker (i.e., those in a traditional expectation of trust or trust relationship) during the past year. When this 1-year prevalence of mistreatment is widened to include incidents involving neighbors and acquaintances, the overall prevalence increases to 4.0%.

One particular difficulty for studies using the general population is that people who are highly dependent on another person, and particularly people who have significant mental impairment, are unable to participate, except by proxy. In the United Kingdom and Spanish studies people with severe dementia or otherwise unable to take part were excluded from the research. In the Dutch study, nonresponse was relatively high for those with mental and physical incapacity.[18] Yet it is precisely these people whom practitioners would identify as most vulnerable. Clinical and forensic markers indicating abuse and neglect point to the importance of dementia, depression, psychosis, and alcohol abuse.[19] Declining health, loneliness, and depression have been associated with enhanced risk factors.[12] A key finding from the U.K. prevalence study was that types of mistreatment vary by gender and age, such that neglect increases with age for women, but other forms of mistreatment

Table 113-2. Prevalence of Elder Abuse in Boston, USA, 1986,[4] Canada, 1990,[17] United Kingdom,[12,33] Amsterdam (The Netherlands) 1994,[18] and Spain[16]

Type of abuse	Boston, USA 1986 (%)	Canada 1990 (%)	UK 2006 (%)	Amsterdam, The Netherlands 1994 (%)	Spain 2006 (%)
Physical	2	0.5	0.4	1.2	0.3
Psychological*	1.1	1.1	0.4	3.2	0.6
Financial	Not in study	2.5	0.7	1.4	0.9
Neglect	0.4	0.4	1.1	0.2	0.6
Sexual	Not in study	Not in study	0.2	Not in study	0.1
Multiple	Not in study	0.8	any 2.6	Not in study	0.8 any
Base:	2020	2008	2111	1797	

*Persistent verbal abuse.

decline. For men, however, abuse, especially financial abuse, increases with age.

RISK FACTORS

Physical abuse

The most thoroughly researched area of physical abuse is that taking place in domestic settings:

1. Risk is higher for older people who live with someone.[4,10,12,17] Older people may be abused by their partners, and by other relations including their adult children.
2. There is emerging research linking abuse with sociodemographic variables, such as marital status, occupation, and housing tenure.[12] Ethnic background has been the subject of more debate.[10,13] However, it is possible that these factors are overemphasized by both reporting bias and the confounding of race and poverty.
3. Some abuse is longstanding—Homer and Gilleard[20] refer to the "elderly graduates of domestic violence." The predominance of women as victims of domestic violence at younger age groups is not so marked in the case of elder abuse.[4,17] Lachs et al[21] conclude: "Clinicians should be particularly aware of high-risk situations in which functional and/or cognitive impairment are present, especially in circumstances where violent behavior has been known to exist previously."
4. Lachs et al[21] found that the number of activities of daily living (ADL) impairments approximately doubled the chance of reported abuse or neglect, and did not consider that reporting bias substantially influenced this finding.
5. There is little evidence that the stress of caring for an older person is on its own a cause of abuse. Large numbers of caregivers are under stress, but do not abuse their relative. How caregivers react to the stresses associated with caring may, however, be important.
6. Risk appears to depend more on problematic characteristics associated with the abuser—particularly their physical and mental health and notably, in many studies, their heavy consumption of alcohol or drug substances.[12,17,20,22] Research with general practitioners (GPs) (family physicians) linked identification of abuse with knowledge of these kinds of factor in patients' households. Those GPs who identified five or more of 15 risk situations were seven times more likely (all other variables held constant) to have identified a case of abuse.[23]
7. The role of dementia as a risk factor is controversial. Lachs et al[21] observed that cognitive impairment, particularly if it was new, was highly significant. Research specifically with people with dementia and their caregivers found that the factors distinguishing the abusive situations related to caregivers.[20] Behavioral and psychological problems among people with dementia, such as aggression, may be associated with aggression on the part of the person caring for them.[20]

Institutional settings

There is growing research about abuse in institutions.[24] Methods of caring assume significance, particularly as the prevalence of physical and mental disability is generally high among older people in institutions. Numerous inquiries in Britain into grave deficiencies in various areas of institutional care for all age groups have shown that abuse flourishes within a culture that allows it to be acceptable.[25] The leadership role of clinicians in such settings should include attention to complaints, staff turnover, risk management, and direct patient care. It is the worst of all possible worlds, as older people themselves are only too aware, to move an older person to an institution for safety's sake only for them to be abused there.

Sexual abuse

This type of abuse has been little researched. Those affected are overwhelmingly female and rely on others for their care but others may be at risk. Abusers may have problems themselves and need help. Attention should be paid to the potential for sexual abuse in residential and nursing home settings and to the risk of sexual abuse by other residents or visitors to the facility. Physical examinations should be alert to possible indicators of abuse, such as unexplained trauma in the genital area.

Financial abuse

Nearly all definitions of elder abuse include financial abuse. The U.K. prevalence study showed that this was the most common form of abuse (after neglect) with a rate of 0.7%.[12] It has been suggested that the boundaries are unclear between the financial mismanagement of people's affairs when they grow older and actual abuse. The financial affairs of older people with dementia appear often to be complex or confusing, thus increasing the risk of financial abuse. There is some evidence that financial abuse is more likely to be perpetrated by the extended family than by partners or paid care workers.[12,17,26] When allied with physical and psychological abuse, the perpetrator may be a close adult relation (usually an adult child) with problems of their own, particularly relating to alcohol misuse.[22] In England and Wales the Mental Capacity Act 2005 has strengthened the ability of people to make arrangements for their finances in the event of losing capacity to manage their money and set up a system of legal safeguards to reduce the likelihood of financial abuse. Other legal safeguards in England and Wales include systems to bar people from the paid and unpaid labor force if they are judged to have harmed or placed at risk of harm a vulnerable adult. This accepts a lower standard of proof than the criminal justice system. Financial abuse in the home has been discovered to be a major reason for banning staff working for older people.[27] The implications for medical professionals are that when an older person is in unexplained financial trouble, that where there seems to be a sudden drop in their living standards and if they seem unable to afford previously affordable items, then history taking may help to uncover matters of concern that should be reported to adult protective services.

Neglect

Neglect is generally interpreted as omission. However, opinion is divided about the appropriateness of classifying self-neglect as mistreatment in the context of adult protection

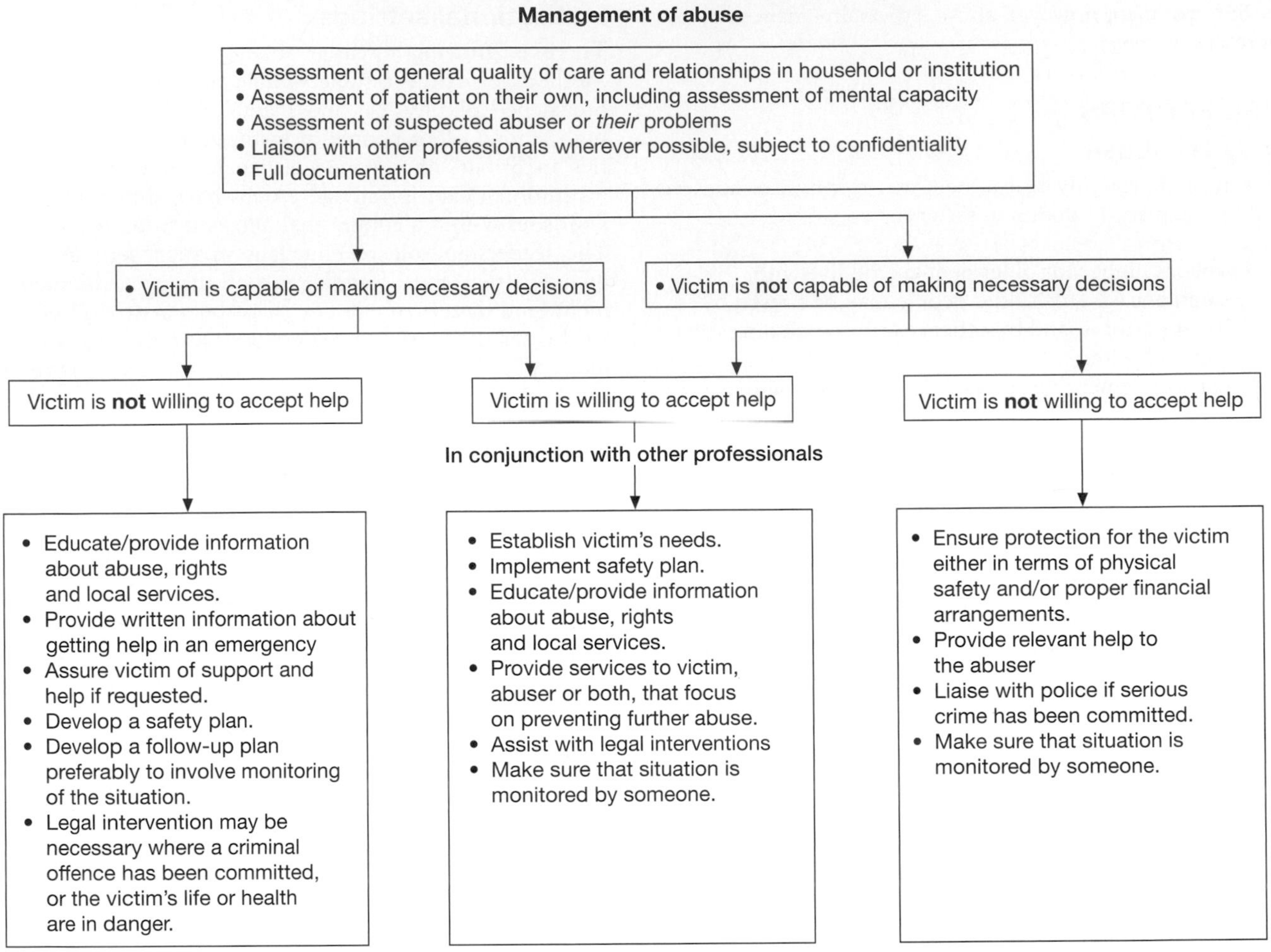

Figure 113-1. Management of abuse. *(Data from Fisk J. Abuse of the elderly. In Jacoby R, Oppenheimer C (eds): Psychiatry in the Elderly, ed 2. Oxford, 1997, Oxford University Press, pp. 736–48; Lachs MS, Pillemer KA. Abuse and neglect of elderly persons. N Engl J Med 1995;332:437–43; Kurrle S. Elder abuse: A hidden problem. Mod Med Aust 1993;9:58–72; and American Medical Association.)*

systems and local policies and procedures will assist in determining the clinical and care pathway. People whose needs are insufficiently met or ignored may be mentally frail, and unsurprisingly are in poor health.[17] The partner, closely followed by other members of the family, is the most likely to be unable to provide necessary care, which may lead to a situation of neglect among community-dwelling older people.[12]

IDENTIFICATION

Elder abuse is often hidden. The U.K. prevalence study,[12] for example, indicated that only approximately 3% of mistreated older people were in touch with adult protection services. It estimated that approximately 1 in 40 older people visiting their family physician would, statistically speaking, be suffering some form of mistreatment but that contact with adult protection services was far less than might be expected. The majority of cases, whether in domestic or institutional settings, are likely to arise in either primary or secondary care as part of some other presenting problem. People who are abused are unlikely to volunteer information and may either fear retribution, not trust formal authorities, or not wish to criminalize significant others. Identification often depends on a high index of suspicion. Two surveys in England showed that many family physicians might not recognize abuse and would welcome training in both identification and management.[23] Physical symptoms may be common to frail older people and be unreliable indicators alone.[20] As prevalence is relatively low, accurate diagnosis assumes great importance. Incorrect diagnosis followed by misplaced interventions may damage all those concerned. Apart from increased sensitivity and awareness of the possibility of abuse, the first general principle, common to all good practice in geriatric medicine and psychiatry, is that assessment must be holistic and interdisciplinary.[28] This may be time-consuming and some doctors may, under pressures of time and shortage of resources, be particularly unwilling to address issues of family violence. The logic of current research is that criminal justice and helping professionals should work together. Clinicians may be asked for opinions about possible abuse and their testimony may be vital in safeguarding an older person from further abuse but just as much in exonerating an innocent relative or care worker.

In the United States, where in some states the law requires mandatory reporting of alleged abuse cases, it is recommended that routine questioning should be built into daily practice and that in every clinical setting there should be a protocol for the detection and assessment of elder abuse. Knowing what to look for is key but so too is listening. There are benefits of a protocol or framework for questioning[11,29] and this can be useful in the context of possible financial abuse along with physical and psychological abuse.[26] Consultation with the older person on their own may be difficult but is advisable.[24]

Financial abuse is an issue that doctors may encounter in various ways.[11] They may be approached to advise on financial decision making and the capacity of people to make decisions when this is in doubt. For example, they may be asked whether a person has the mental capacity to make an advance decision or to dispose of assets. They need to know to whom to refer people for appropriate guidance, to know the professional and legal guidance in their national context, to be aware of protocols around data sharing and evidence collection, and to ensure that the person understands what they are agreeing to. They may come across possible abuse in the course of patient contact and it is then necessary to know about local safeguarding systems. A small study of the views of geriatricians working in the United States found that the average number of cases of elder abuse diagnosed per year was about eight per geriatrician.[30] Their diagnostic work rested on a combination of history taking and physical examination.

PREVENTION, TREATMENT, AND MANAGEMENT

The key objectives are the prevention of abuse and the promotion of the older person's human rights.[6,10] At the level of policy and guidance, it is essential that the medical profession is properly represented where any professional or local initiatives are taking place to develop a response to abuse. Experience from child protection suggests that this will not be easy to achieve. The issue of excessive or inappropriate medication being used as a form of abuse highlights the need for clinicians themselves to be careful of their own practices and those of their colleagues.

Two further general principles are meticulous documentation and liaison with other professionals, both within and outside medicine. The taking of photos or drawings, careful recording of suspected injuries, and conversations are important in collecting evidence. The difficulties of these and the time they take need to be taken into account when arranging consultations. The need to work interprofessionally raises difficult ethical questions in terms of confidentiality of the doctor-patient relationship, should the older person request the doctor to "do nothing." The older person's rights to autonomy have to be balanced with decisions that may need to be made in their best interests should they not have the capacity to consent or to refuse information sharing. The need for criminal justice intervention may arise if a crime is suspected to address possible dangers. The assessment of mental capacity, therefore, is of crucial importance and helps direct physicians to the options for intervention if the older person is unwilling to accept any help. Advocacy can be a particularly valuable service for the older person at the center of this concern, and in England and Wales this is now available for some people in situations of suspected abuse without mental capacity. Figure 113-1 should be interpreted in relation to the type of abuse and to the legal and service provision context in which medical practitioners are working. In most countries the number of laws that potentially bear on abuse are considerable, and advice may be needed from adult protection services. In the event of an emergency, the medical practitioner needs to make immediate contact with other responsible agencies and act to protect the older person from harm. Although safety of the alleged victim is the first priority, it is also essential to pay attention to the physical and psychological health of the other party, who themselves may be vulnerable.

SUMMARY AND CONCLUSION

Elder abuse can be divided into four distinct forms, including physical, psychological, sexual, and financial. Abuse is often associated with neglect, which together are often referred to as "elder mistreatment." The development of behavioral definitions, more precise targeting of risk factors, and the characteristics of the parties involved have led to a greater understanding of the risks associated with each form. Abuse and neglect can occur in community or institutional settings. In each case the principal aim should be to prevent abuse and neglect from occurring through building safe and responsive systems, regular monitoring, and interprofessional collaboration. Medical practitioners have key roles in ensuring that systems are safe and in responding to suspicions and allegations by providing expert medical intervention and testimony. Their responsibilities for the treatment of physical harm are evident but they also include offering support for

KEY POINTS

Elder Abuse

- Elder abuse refers to the mistreatment of an older person (usually defined as over age 65) by acts of commission or omission and key objectives are the prevention of abuse and the promotion of the older person's rights.
- It has been shown to affect between 2% and 6% of people aged over 65 depending upon definition and context and is generally understood to include physical, psychological, sexual, and financial forms.
- Risk of physical/verbal abuse appears to depend more on problematic characteristics associated with the abuser—particularly their physical and mental health and notably, alchohol and drug misuse. Those involved in suspected abuse may need support and may have health care needs of their own.
- Likelihood of having been mistreated may vary depending on gender, separation or divorce, socioeconomic position, declining health, and depression, and there is little evidence that the stress of caring for an older person is on its own a cause of such abuse.
- Identification may be enhanced by a high index of suspicion and is particularly important because of relatively low prevalence and physicians need to be aware of local protocols and their legal and professional responsibilities.
- Holistic assessment is necessary, through discussion with the older person and informants, physical examinations and history taking, including of mental capacity. The wider care team may be usefully involved.
- The severity of effect of the abuse, its frequency, how long it has been going on, and the intentions and capacity of those in the social network help practitioners judge the case for and type of intervention.

people in risky situations. That abuse takes place between adults, distinguishes it from child abuse. It has certain commonalities with domestic violence, but is wider in scope and form.

Abuse and neglect may best be currently understood within a human rights framework.

The primary aim should be to prevent abuse from occurring. There are at least four planks in prevention. The first is the provision of effective health and welfare services for older people, including income and medical provision.[31] The second is awareness among professionals, among which the medical profession is crucial, that abuse exists and requires a response, which may be most effective when it is multidisciplinary.[6,29] This may involve criminal justice interventions, skills development[11,24] and agreement to work within guidelines. It may also involve working with people who have mistreated older people or neglected them to prevent harm reoccurring. Third, in the context of a policy emphasis on care in people's own homes, is the need for recognition and action around caregivers, who may be both abuser and/or abused, older or younger themselves, and have physical and/or mental health problems. Finally, in the context of institutional care, monitoring or regulation of the quality of care is essential to respect the human rights of older people.

For a complete list of references, please visit online only at www.expertconsult.com

CHAPTER 114

Pain in the Older Adult

Patricia Bruckenthal

Despite its increased prevalence in older individuals, pain should not be considered a normal consequence of aging. Pain is always due to pathology, even if not easily identified or fully appreciated by the clinician. An understanding of the complex cellular, molecular, and genetic contributions to the experience of pain are beginning to emerge along with their relationship to physical, psychological, and environmental factors. Persistent pain interferes with enjoyment of life, and has deleterious effects on mood, social interaction, function, mobility, and independence. For many reasons, pain remains undertreated in this population. This chapter examines age-related changes in prevalence and perception of pain, and approaches to assessment and treatment. The focus is on pain and suffering, rather than the underlying causes of pain. The management of specific painful conditions is not discussed.

COMPONENTS OF PAIN

The pain experience is best understood by considering the influence of four determinants: nociception, pain perception, suffering, and pain behaviors.[1] *Nociception* is the detection of tissue damage by specialized transducers on primary afferent A delta and C nerve fibers in response to noxious stimuli. The subsequent *perception* of pain by the individual is affected by central processing of nociceptive input from the periphery, or from lesions in the peripheral and central nervous systems. Pain consequent upon nerve damage can occur with or without somatic nociceptive input. In the former case the perception of pain is altered from that which is usually reported following nociception. The intensity of pain under these circumstances bears little relationship to the extent and severity of observable pathology and tends to be less responsive to traditional analgesic medications. Adjuvant medications, or those formerly not used to treat pain, have demonstrated efficacy in treating pain that results from changes in the central and peripheral nervous system.

Suffering is a negative emotional response induced by pain, and also by fear, anxiety, loss, and other psychological states. Patients often use the language of pain to describe suffering, such as "heartache," although not all suffering is caused by pain. *Pain behaviors*, such as grimacing, lying down, limping, and avoidance of physical activity may result from pain perception and suffering. The clinician infers the existence of nociception, pain, and suffering from the patient's history, physical examination, and observation of pain behaviors.[1] Recognition of the multiple components of the pain experience will guide the clinician in assessing and planning age appropriate pain management.

TYPES OF PAIN

A simple classification differentiates pain as either acute or chronic. *Acute pain* can be of visceral or somatic origin. It usually has an identifiable temporal relationship with an injury or disease. Autonomic overactivity, such as diaphoresis and tachycardia, may be present. In this setting pain may be seen to serve a useful role in drawing attention to injured tissues, altering behavior, and hence preventing further tissue damage. Acute pain often leads the individual to seek medical attention. Pain often resolves before healing is complete. As people age there may be a blunting of protective warning signals. Age related dysfunction along pain pathways may account for age-related differences in pain perception.[2–4] Pain associated with visceral causes are prevalent and may present atypically in the older population. Visceral pain associated with cardiac, pulmonary, and abdominal disease is associated with morbidity and mortality, and can be difficult to diagnose in the elderly. Clinicians need to be especially vigilant in their pain assessment technique in this population.

Chronic pain persists beyond the normal duration of injury or tissue damage, or is associated with progressive disease. The time frame for the transition from acute to chronic pain is somewhat arbitrary, often determined by the underlying pathology, and not necessarily characterized by a change in quality or severity of symptoms. Chronic pain thus is often defined as pain persisting for longer than 3 to 6 months, or beyond the expected time of healing. There may be no identifiable pathology to account for the pain. Psychological and functional features are often associated with chronic pain and autonomic overactivity is not usually present. Chronic pain may be persistent (always present) or intermittent, such as migraine headache. Pain intensity may vary during the day or be related to activity level. Musculoskeletal disease, arthritis, orofacial, and neuropathic pain conditions are common in older persons. Once reversible factors have been excluded, the pain rather than the pathology is considered the major problem. At this stage, the goal of treatment shifts from a disease focus to reduction of pain, suffering, and disability.

Prevalence studies

Pain in older adults is common and has a tremendous impact on quality of life in this age group. There is great variability in the reported prevalence, likely due to differences in the reporting period for pain, the intensity of pain reported, and composition of the older population studies. Crook et al[5] reported age-specific rates 29% for those aged between 71 and 80 years when asked "how often are you troubled by pain during the past 2 weeks..." Brattburg et al[6] reported a 12-month prevalence of mild to severe pain in 75% in those over 75 years of age. Epidemiologic studies commonly show that pain affecting joints, feet, and legs is increased with age; that pain in the head, abdomen, and chest is reduced; but back pain frequency varies widely.[7,8,9] The high prevalence of degenerative joint disease overwhelms any contribution from other causes in all surveys. Studies in residential care settings for the elderly have shown prevalence rates of chronic pain between 49% and 85%,[10,11,12] with low back pain reported in 40%, arthritis of appendicular joints 24%, followed by old fracture site pain and painful neuropathies.[13] Moss et al[14] reported that during the last year of life 66% of individuals had frequent or continuous severe pain.

Among community-dwelling older adults, pain prevalence is reported between 25% to 83%;[15,16,17,18] women have a higher prevalence compared with men at any given age.[19–21] Lifestyle factors and preparedness to report pain may also be relevant.[22,23] Measurement of pain in the community is difficult and most likely underestimated. This is due to a combination of constitutional, lifestyle, and psychosocial factors.

Age-related changes in pain perception

Pain may not be the cardinal symptom of disease in older people. Silent myocardial infarction is more common with age.[24] Similarly, in a retrospective study of elderly patients with peritonitis, abdominal pain was absent in nearly half of the cases.[25] The physiologic basis of these observations is uncertain. Clinicians should not underestimate the potential seriousness of underlying pathology in an older person because of the absence of severe pain.

There are widespread morphologic, electrophysiologic, neurochemical, and functional changes within the nociceptive pathways, and psychological factors that may alter pain experience in elderly people.[26] Most studies of experimental pain support the view that pain thresholds to short-duration noxious stimuli are increased in older people.[27,28] Whether age also affects the level of discomfort and suffering associated with clinical pain is uncertain.[29] Controversy regarding the effect of age on pain thresholds exists, whereas pressure pain thresholds have been shown to both increase and decrease, with heat thresholds showing no changes with age.[2,3] A decrease in the function of the descending inhibitory pain control pathway as a person ages[30] suggests greater sensitivity to noxious experimental pain. In other studies, reticence, self-doubt, and reluctance to label a stimulus as painful underlie the perception that stoicism to pain increases with age. However, when pain is perceived, the experience is the same, or under some circumstances, enhanced or prolonged.[31,32] Tolerance to severe pain may even be reduced in older people.

Age-related loss of neurochemicals, such as serotonin,[33] glutamate, GABA,[34] and opioid receptors[35] implicated in pain modulation, may contribute to altered pain processing in older adults. Changes in the aging brain[36,37] have been associated with older persons processing and response to pain. Taken together these studies suggest that pain is dependent on a complex neuroprocessing system that is affected by aging and has implications for the pain experience in older adults.

PATHOPHYSIOLOGIC PERSPECTIVE

Inferences about the underlying pathophysiology of a painful condition assist the clinician in the selection of therapy and determining prognosis. Pain may be subdivided into three pathophysiologic subtypes: nociceptive, neuropathic, and psychogenic. Pain that arises from noxious stimulation of specific peripheral or visceral nociceptors is termed *nociceptive pain*. Examples include pain arising from osteoarthritis, soft tissue injuries, and visceral pathology. Pain arising from pathology of the peripheral nerves or within the central nervous system leading to aberrant somatosensory processing is termed *neuropathic pain*. This term encompasses a diverse range of conditions including painful peripheral neuropathies, phantom limb pains, postherpetic neuralgia, trigeminal neuralgia and central poststroke pain. Pain of neuropathic origin is often associated with abnormal and unpleasant sensations (dysesthesia) and may have a burning or shooting quality. Mild, normally nonnoxious stimuli in the affected region may cause pain (allodynia), and repetitive stimulation results in summation and pain persisting longer than the stimulus (hyperpathia). There may be a delay between the precipitating injury and the onset of pain. The onset of central poststroke pain syndrome occurs commonly between 1 and 3 months following the stroke, but may occur more than 1 year later.[38] Pain often persists in the absence of ongoing tissue damage.

The multidimensionality of chronic pain has long been recognized to include sensory-discriminative, affective-motivational, and cognitive-interpretative dimensions. These are influenced by biologic, psychological, and social factors. The ability of the individual to adapt to biopsychosocial changes in response to stress may be diminished with age. The term pain homeostenosis has been introduced to describe an organism's diminished ability to respond effectively to the stress of persistent pain.[37] Clinicians should be aware of factors that contribute to these phenomena, such as cognitive function, decreased density of opioid receptors, medical comorbidity, polypharmacy, and the effect of aging on pharmacokinetics and pharmacodynamics, social isolation, depression, and altered activities of daily living. There are specific assessment techniques and tolls to assist in assessing these factors.

Depression is common in people with chronic pain. Patients who are depressed may exhibit decreased energy, decreased engagement in treatment modalities or avoidance of pleasant diversional activities. Anxiety has also been closely associated with pain[39,40] and often coexists with depression in this population. Anxiety may play a part in fear-related behavior that might inhibit participation in physical rehabilitation efforts. Social networks and economic resources are important assessment parameters. Involvement with family and friends can provide pleasurable experiences and diversion away from a constant focus on pain. In addition to the availability of social support, the type of relationship should be assessed. Negative social reinforcement may present in the form of overly solicitous family members who encourage sedentary behavior. Other negative effects are likely if long-term caregivers become resentful of their support role. Economic resources have a great impact on access to potential treatment options and must to be identified.[41] Finally, beliefs and attitudes about pain can impact on the overall pain management plan. Pain can signify loss of independence, debilitating illness, or be regarded as a general consequence of the aging process and therefore underreported. If older patients have a good understanding of the underlying cause of pain, what it means in terms of functions, and possible treatment options, it is likely that they will participate in the plan of care and obtain more satisfactory outcomes.

EVALUATION

Pain is inherently subjective; the individual's self-report is the gold standard for assessment. The history should focus on the onset and temporal pattern of the symptoms, site, and quality of the pain, the severity, aggravating and relieving factors, and the impact that pain is having on the patient's lifestyle. The assessment of a patient with a complex pain problem may need to take place over several consultations. The reliability of the history can be affected by the chronicity of the pain, past interventions, and age-related conditions that affect cognition. A collaborative history from a family member is often helpful. Special emphasis should be placed on musculoskeletal and neurologic examinations because of their importance in the genesis of pain in elderly people. The assessment should include functional and psychological aspects and where possible the individual should be assessed within their own environment. The open-ended question, "What would you do if you no longer had pain?" often reveals valuable information regarding mood state, attitudes, and disability. Part of the assessment needs to focus on the patient's comorbidities, how these affect function, their contribution to altered mood state, and their propensity to affect management with medications, and physical or psychological interventions. One must be vigilant not to falsely attribute drug side effects to the underlying pathology.

Back pain is illustrative. An estimated two thirds of adults will experience back pain at some stage of their lives. Experimental studies reveal that pain may originate from any one of many structures. However, after clinical evaluation no precise pathoanatomic diagnosis can be established in 85% of cases.[42] Investigations are used to confirm a diagnosis and exclude more serious pathology. The diagnostic probabilities change with increasing age; cancers, compression fractures, and spinal stenosis becoming more common. Plain radiology is not highly sensitive but findings on computerized tomography (CT) and magnetic resonance imaging (MRI) are nonspecific and thus may be misleading. CT and MRI studies of asymptomatic individuals over 60 years of age reveal about 80% have abnormal findings, such as disk prolapse and spinal canal stenosis. Therefore the identification of pathology on diagnostic investigations does not necessarily indicate causality. Deyo and Weinstein[42] suggest that it is more helpful to address three questions during the assessment of a patient with low back pain: Is a systemic disease causing the pain? Secondly, is there social or psychological distress that may amplify or prolong pain? And thirdly, is there neurologic compromise that may require surgical evaluation? Under most circumstances, these questions can be answered from a careful history and physical examination without the need for further tests.

Several validated psychometric instruments can help to quantify and communicate the patient's pain experience. The widely used McGill Pain Questionnaire[43,44] consists of 78 adjectives describing emotional, sensory, and evaluative dimensions of the pain experience. Words such as throbbing, sharp, cramping, burning, and aching describe a sensory dimension, whereas tiring, exhausting, cruel, punishing, fearful, and sickening describe an affective component. Although older adults vary greatly in their use and understanding of self-report pain instruments, numeric rating scales and verbal descriptor are generally preferable.[45,46] Some visual analog scales have been found to be difficult to use among seniors.[47]

Psychological assessment

A comprehensive psychological assessment is not usually required in the setting of acute pain. However, chronic pain may have profound effects on mood, interpersonal relationships, and activity level, and it may be difficult to ascertain which is cause and which is effect. Psychological evaluation is indicated when medical evaluation fails to adequately explain the severity of pain behaviors. Psychological evaluation can also be valuable when the pain results in excessive health service use, or interference with normal activities or interpersonal relationships. Chronic pain patients are often resistant to psychological evaluation, considering this an inference that the pain is "in the head" rather than a physical problem. Patients often require careful explanation regarding the complex interaction between mind and body, which often influences pain, suffering, and disability.[48] Acknowledging that the pain is real preserves the patient's sense of legitimacy and allows for a more complete evaluation of the psychological factors contributing to the maintenance of pain.

It is important to evaluate how the patient and their relatives conceptualize the pain and goals of treatment. They may believe that the pain has persisted because the medical assessment has been inadequate or specific interventions denied. Each time a new intervention is tried and fails, the psychological distress is reinforced. Psychological strategies are not likely to be effective in teaching the patient how to manage with ongoing pain while the patient remains focused on seeking a cure. Pain behaviors such as limping, grimacing, inactivity, and verbalizing of pain complaints may be reinforced by social influences such as gaining attention, sympathy, or the ability to avoid unpleasant responsibilities. Fear of causing further pain or injury may lead to avoidance of activity. Attempts at management with medications and physical therapies, without addressing psychological factors, are often unsuccessful.

Assessment of pain in the presence of dementia

Dementia represents a major impediment to the evaluation and management of pain. Cognitive impairment may be aggravated by pain or medications used to treat the pain.[49] Bernabei et al reported that low cognitive performance and age greater than 85 years were independent risk factors for lack of appropriate treatment of pain in cancer patients.[50] The report of pain in demented individuals may be affected by memory impairment or limited communication skills. A corroborative history from relatives or previous therapists is often required. There is no convincing evidence of enhancement of pain by dementia. In fact, Parmelee et al[12] found a small negative relationship between pain intensity and cognitive impairment in a sample of 758 elderly institutionalized residents. Individuals with marked cognitive impairment were less likely to report pain in the back and joints. However, when pain was reported there was no difference in the presence or absence of a likely physical cause. Ferrell et al[51] reported that elderly nursing home residents with mild to moderate cognitive impairment required more time to assimilate and respond to questions regarding pain, but of the 62% reporting pain complaints, 83% could complete a unidimensional pain-intensity scale, with the Present Pain Intensity Scale of the McGill Pain Questionnaire having the highest completion rate of 65%. A pain report should therefore not be disregarded because the individual has cognitive impairment.

When assessing pain in severely cognitively impaired patients, the clinician must rely on behavioral indicators.

These include nonverbal cues such as restlessness and guarding, verbal cues such as crying, moaning, and groaning, and facial expressions such as grimacing.[52,53] Changes in usual activity may also indicate pain. There is tremendous variability in pain behavior and often certified nursing assistants will be the first to notice behavioral changes, including combativeness, resisting care, a decrease in social interactions, increased wandering, difficulty sleeping, and refusing to eat.[54,55] Behavioral indicators for pain in this population and pain assessment tools are developed for cognitively impaired long-term care residents. The assessment instruments vary greatly on their reliability, validity, and applicability for easy clinical use.[56,57] There are no shortage of geriatric assessment instruments available to clinicians. A recommendation from a comprehensive review of assessment of pain in older adults[58] suggests The Brief Pain Inventory[59] combined with the Short Form-McGill Pain Questionnaire[43] as an appropriate 10-minute battery for cognitively intact older adults.

Define the goals of therapy

Before embarking upon a treatment program, the patient and the clinician should agree on the goals of therapy, particularly when pain eradication is not feasible. Involvement of family members often assists with ensuring compliance and successful outcomes. A frank discussion about the prognosis and therapeutic options is often accepted with gratitude, particularly in individuals who have had unsatisfactory experiences in the past. Even if the sensory component of pain cannot be eliminated, improved outcomes can be achieved by addressing factors such as disability and mood disturbance. Management of severe pain often requires establishing a balance between the severity of sensory symptoms, the level of disability, and medication side effects. Disability may be more important to the patient than the pain. An improvement in the distance an individual is able to walk before being stopped by pain may be considered a positive outcome, although the intensity of maximum pain remains unaltered. Medication side effects may be more troublesome than the condition for which they were prescribed. Pain management programs combine cognitive and rehabilitative approaches to enhance coping strategies and minimize the impact that persistent pain has on the individual.

MANAGEMENT

Medications

Pharmacologic approaches with simple analgesics and nonsteroidal anti-inflammatory drugs (NSAIDs) are the mainstay, whether self-initiated or prescribed. This is often the most convenient and cost-effective approach. Selection of appropriate drug therapy for the older patient requires an understanding of age-related pharmacokinetic and pharmacodynamic changes, and needs to take into account any coexisting diseases and other medications, including those obtained without prescription. Selection of therapy needs to balance the potential efficacy with the potential for harm from the intervention. Timing is important. Analgesics may be prescribed on an "as required" basis for occasional pain or prophylactically for induced pain. However, for continuous pain, analgesics are best prescribed on a regular basis. Additional doses may be required before activities known to exacerbate pain or for breakthrough pain. Medications with long half-lives may be used to reduce the frequency of dosing. In general, medications should be commenced at low doses, titrating upwards and stopping at the lowest dose that achieves the desired outcome. Concern regarding potential adverse effects should not result in suboptimal treatment of pain. Although generally less effective when used for neuropathic pain, all analgesics can be reasonably trialed in that situation.

Simple analgesics

Summary of Management Algorithm

Paracetamol:
- First-line analgesic for older patients with chronic pain
- Often as effective as NSAIDs
- Best given regularly for persistent pain, rather than as required

NSAIDs:
- Increased risk of GI and renal complications in elderly
- Avoid if possible

Selective COX-2 inhibitors:
- Preferable to nonselective NSAIDs
- Similar nongastrointestinal side effects to nonselective NSAIDs

Adjuvant analgesic (e.g., antidepressants and anticonvulsants):
- Proven role in neuropathic pain states
- Total pain eradication is unlikely
- Selection of medication is based on side effect profile rather than comparative efficacy
- Start at low dose, increase slowly

Opioid analgesics:
- Have a role in chronic nonmalignant pain
- Treat constipation preemptively
- Drug dependence is uncommon in elderly people

Nonpharmacologic approaches (e.g., physical and psychological therapies):
- Will reduce reliance on medications
- Failure to employ these strategies often accounts for treatment failure

Acetaminophen is the preferred analgesic for older adults.[60] A trial of paracetamol is warranted as initial therapy on the basis of cost, efficacy, and toxicity profile. For many patients, paracetamol affords similar efficacy to that achieved with NSAIDs.[61] It is absorbed rapidly and metabolized by the liver. Because of the risk of hepatoxicity, acetaminophen should be used with caution in patients with liver disease, chronic alcoholism, malnutrition, and dehydration. Dosages should be limited to 4000 mg per 24 hours, with lower doses used for persons with diminished renal or hepatic function or for those requiring chronic use.

As a class, NSAIDs have been among the most frequently prescribed medications, particularly for pain associated with osteoarthritis and inflammatory arthropathies. Although effective in reducing signs and symptoms, they have no effect on the underlying musculoskeletal disease.[62] The side effect and drug interaction profile of NSAIDs is of particular concern. At least 10% to 20% of patients taking NSAIDs will experience dyspepsia. Complications of ulcer disease, such as hemorrhage and perforation, occur far more often in patients taking NSAIDs.[63] An estimated 16,500 deaths occurred from NSAID gastrointestinal toxic effects in the United States in 1997.[64] Renal toxicity is another concern. Risk factors for renal failure in patients with intrinsic renal disease treated with NSAIDs include age over 65 years, a history of hypertension, congestive cardiac failure, and concomitant use of diuretics or angiotensin-converting enzyme inhibitors. Most NSAIDs have a dose-response relationship with a ceiling effect. Increasing the dose above the recommended level or adding a second NSAID does not impart any greater analgesia, but increases the likelihood of drug toxicity.

The rate of NSAID-related serious gastrointestinal complications requiring hospitalization has decreased in recent years, in part due to extensive medical education campaigns and a move away from NSAIDs as first-line management of osteoarthritis.[64] Patients with inflammatory arthritides should preferentially be treated with disease modifying drugs. The options for management of patients with NSAIDs who are at high risk of serious upper gastrointestinal events are the use of a nonselective NSAID with gastroprotective therapy, or the use of a cyclooxygenase-2 (COX-2) specific inhibitor. Coadministration of misoprostol has been demonstrated to reduce the upper gastrointestinal complication rate of nonselective NSAIDs but is not well tolerated. Proton pump inhibitors are an acceptable alternative. H_2 receptor antagonists have been shown to prevent duodenal ulceration only, and cannot be recommended.[63] Celecoxib is the only COX-2 selective NSAID currently available in the United States.[4] The primary short-term advantage of this class of agents is the lack of effect on platelet function. As these drugs are frequently prescribed for pain control in rheumatoid arthritis and osteoarthritis, their usefulness for long-term therapy is limited. In addition, COX-2 inhibitors appear to affect renal function in a similar fashion to nonselective NSAIDs and particular care is required in patients with renal impairment, or those taking diuretics and angiotensin-converting enzyme inhibitors. COX-2 inhibitors may diminish the antihypertensive effects of ACE inhibitors and diuretic effects of frusemide and thiazides. Celecoxib inhibits CP450 (CYP2C9) enzyme and thus may cause elevation of plasma concentrations of drugs metabolized by this enzyme, such as some β-blockers, antidepressants, and antipsychotics.[65]

Topical NSAIDs are en effective and safe alternative for some patients, especially in the management of acute musculoskeletal and soft tissue inflammatory pain.[66,67] Diclofenac gel and patch formulations are currently available with several other NSAID formulations under development. Although GI side effects are less common than oral preparations, the risk exists especially in persons who have had previous side effects to NSAIDs.[68]

Opioid analgesics

In the past, opioid analgesics have been divided into weak and strong categories according to their potency. This distinction has now become less useful. All opioid analgesics have the potential to cause nausea, constipation, sedation, respiratory depression, and cognitive impairment. Increased cognitive impairment may itself lead to a diminished ability to cope with pain, thus leading to a paradoxical increase in pain with an increasing dose of opioid. Opioids are generally reserved for moderate or severe pain. Elderly patients tend to be more sensitive to equivalent doses and blood levels of opioids, receiving greater and more prolonged pain relief.[49] The analgesic effects of Codeine (methylmorphine) are mediated by its conversion to morphine via the cytochrome P450D6 (CYP2D6) system. About 8% of Caucasians and 2% of Asians are genetically deficient in CYP2D6 and obtain little pain relief with codeine. A number of medications frequently prescribed in elderly patients are capable of inhibiting CYP2D6, including cimetidine, quinidine, haloperidol, amitriptyline, and the selective serotonin reuptake inhibitors (SSRIs), including fluoxetine, paroxetine, and fluvoxamine. Side effects of codeine are common, particularly constipation, nausea, and confusion.

Other weak opioids include tramadol and propoxyphene. Tramadol is a centrally acting synthetic analgesic with opioid-like effects. Its mode of action is through binding to the μ-opioid receptor and inhibition of noradrenaline and serotonin reuptake. The efficacy of tramadol is comparable to ibuprofen in patients with hip and knee osteoarthritis. Dose reduction may be required in elderly patients. Propoxyphene should be used with caution or not at all in older adults because of the long half-life of its major metabolite and the potential for central nervous system side effects including hallucinations, seizures, and falls.[69,70] It has no clinical advantage over nonopioids such as acetaminophen. Combinations of nonopioids with weak opioids, such as aspirin or paracetamol with codeine offer enhanced analgesia.[71] The combined medications may result in a lower incidence of side effects as each analgesic can be used at a lower dose. The weak opioids have a ceiling effect for analgesia due to the combination and limits of acetaminophen. If adequate pain relief is not obtained at optimal doses, change to a strong opioid should be considered.

Morphine is the prototypic opioid. Its analgesic properties are not limited by a ceiling effect, but side effects are common. Tolerance to side effects develops more rapidly than tolerance to analgesic effects, although constipation tends to persist. Once the daily opioid requirements have been established through the administration of a short-acting opioid on a regular basis, then the use of delayed-release opioid agents should be considered. Delayed-release morphine and oxycodone preparations may be used in elderly patients but care must be taken to prevent drug accumulation. Other strong opioids include methadone, hydromorphone, (meperidine and fentanyl). Methadone must be used with caution because it has a long half-life of up to 2 or 3 days, resulting in accumulation in elderly patients.

Tolerance may develop with repeated administration of all opioids whereby higher doses are required to maintain equivalent analgesic effects. The rate of development of tolerance varies greatly, but is not as common as once believed. Before tolerance is suspected in a patient with a previously established opioid dose, evidence of advancing disease, new onset disease or injury, or psychosocial etiology should be investigated. If these are negative, the dose or frequency of dosing may be increased. Cross-tolerance with other opioids is not complete as they often act through different combinations of receptors. The problem may be overcome by changing to another oral opioid, commencing at one half of the equianalgesic dose. When a patient is unable to tolerate oral opioids, or has refractory pain, parenteral analgesia by the transdermal, subcutaneous, venous, epidural, or intrathecal route should be considered. A transdermal fentanyl patch offers the advantage of one application every 72 hours. It has a similar side effect profile to other opioids, although some subjects report less constipation than with other preparations. Fentanyl accumulates in skeletal muscle and fat and then is slowly released into the blood. Minimum effective concentrations are reached approximately 6 hours after application. Serum fentanyl concentrations fall by 50% approximately 17 hours after removing the patch. The clearance of fentanyl is delayed in elderly, cachectic, and debilitated patients. The 25 μg/hr transdermal fentanyl patch is equivalent to about 90 mg of morphine per day. It is not recommended for opioid-naive patients.

Adjuvant analgesics

Adjuvant analgesics are drugs that have a primary indication other than pain but are analgesic in neuropathic pain syndromes. They include medications from heterogeneous therapeutic classes, including tricyclic antidepressants, anticonvulsants, oral antiarrhythmics, and neuroleptics.

Antidepressants and anticonvulsants have a proven role in managing refractory neuropathic pain. Pain relief is usually only partial, with 30% reduction in pain scores usually being classified as success. For every three patients treated with either an antidepressant or anticonvulsant for postherpetic neuralgia or diabetic neuropathy, one patient experiences 50% pain relief that they would not have received with placebo.[72] Empirically, antidepressants have been used for neuropathic pain with a burning quality and anticonvulsants for shooting pain, despite lack of evidence linking efficacy to the characteristics of pain. Tricyclic antidepressants also have a role in managing tension and migraine headache, atypical facial pain, rheumatoid arthritis, chronic low back pain, fibromyalgia, and cancer pain.[73] Tricyclic antidepressants have been widely used in older individuals despite their propensity for side effects such as dry mouth, postural hypotension, falls, constipation, sedation, and urinary retention. The sedating side effect may be used to advantage for some individuals with pain-related insomnia. The analgesic effects of tricyclic antidepressants are independent of antidepressant effects, occurring more rapidly and at a lower dose than used for depression. The median effective analgesic dose of agents such as amitriptyline or nortriptyline is in the order of 50 to 70 mg daily.[74] A low starting dose of around 10 mg is recommended. Newer antidepressant medications, such as selective serotonin reuptake inhibitors (SSRIs), have fewer side effects but have not been demonstrated to be more effective than a placebo in achieving analgesia, although there are insufficient data to draw a final conclusion.[72,75] Newer selective SSRIs, venlafaxine[76] and duloxitine,[77] have been found effective for the treatment of peripheral diabetic neuropathy (PDN) and posthepatic neuralgia (PHN).

Anticonvulsants have been widely used for neuropathic pain despite surprisingly few trials of analgesic effectiveness.[78] Carbamazepine is the drug of choice for trigeminal neuralgia, with pain control achieved in about 75% of patients.[79] Anticonvulsants are considered second-line therapy following antidepressants for other neuropathic pain states.[78] Anticonvulsants shown to be of benefit for diabetic neuropathy and postherpetic neuralgia are carbamazepine, phenytoin, and gabapentin.[78] Gabapentin has a lower incidence of side effects than carbamazepine or phenytoin, but has not been proven to be more effective than the older anticonvulsants.[72,78] Other anticonvulsants that have been widely used to treat neuropathic pain without convincing evidence for benefit in clinical trials include valproate and lamotrigine.

The selection of an adjuvant analgesic agent for the management of neuropathic pain should be based on the side effect profile, and the potential for drug interaction, rather than relative efficacy of different agents. There is considerable individual variation in the response to these agents. Failure to respond to one agent is not predictive of the response to another agent within the same therapeutic class.

Topical lignocaine (lidocaine) patches have been licensed for use in postherpetic neuralgia in the United States. Extreme care must be used when using oral or parenteral local anesthetic agents, such as mexiletine and lignocaine to treat pain in older adults because of the potential for fatal arrhythmias. The use of neuroleptic medication for pain in older people is not indicated as side effects outweigh benefits. In addition herbal products and dietary supplements are used by many Americans. Marinac et al found that 21% of persons over 60 years old were using at least one herbal or dietary supplement with 19% at risk for a potential adverse drug reaction.[80]

Nonpharmacologic therapies

Nonpharmacologic approaches, either alone or in combination with pharmacologic approaches, should be an integral part of the care plan for older individuals with chronic pain.[60] Nonpharmacologic approaches encompass a broad range of physical and other treatment modalities. They are widely used by patients, often without the knowledge of their health care provider. Few of these therapies have undergone formal evaluation.

Physical therapies

Simple adjustments in posture and daily routines, such as preparing meals in a seated position, breaking up the housework, or the provision of a walking aid can reduce the impact of pain on daily life. The use of a walking frame, which causes a mild degree of lumbar flexion, will often ease the pain of lumbar canal stenosis.

Exercise is a major component of most pain management programs, either alone or in conjunction with pharmacologic and other nonpharmacologic approaches. Even frail and institutionalized elderly people may benefit. Exercise can lead to decrease in pain, improvements in function, and elevation of mood.[81] Hydrotherapy should be considered when weight-bearing exercises aggravate pain. The buoyancy effect of water reduces the weight of the body allowing joints to be moved with minimal friction through a full range of movements. The warmth of the water decreases pain and muscle spasm. Transcutaneous electrical nerve stimulation (TENS) is a popular method of symptom relief for a wide range of painful conditions in elderly people, such as low back pain, osteoarthritis, and postherpetic neuralgia. Other physical therapies used for a wide range of painful conditions include massage, cold and heat treatments, acupuncture, and electrotherapies such as ultrasound, infrared lamps, microwave, and shortwave diathermy.

Joint replacement surgery has had a major impact in alleviating the suffering of older people with degenerative joint disease who have experienced inadequate symptom control with conservative management.

Psychological approaches

Psychological factors may contribute to the maintenance of pain or be causally related to the pain. Regardless of the pathophysiologic basis of chronic pain, psychological strategies have a role in management. The essence of management is to establish appropriate pain coping strategies and discourage behaviors that may perpetuate the pain syndrome. Usually a combination of behavioral and cognitive strategies is employed. Cognitive strategies are aimed at modifying belief structures, attitudes, and thoughts to modify the experience of pain and suffering. This approach also includes distraction therapy, relaxation, biofeedback, and hypnosis. The patient is encouraged to take an active role and accept responsibility for pain management, rather than being a passive victim. These strategies have been demonstrated to be effective managing pain in older adults.[82,83]

Cognitive strategies are usually combined with a behavioral approach. Behavioral operant conditioning discourages pain behaviors, such as limping, grimacing, inactivity, and verbalizing of pain complaints. Usually, in conjunction with the patient's relatives, positive reinforcement is provided for behavior unrelated to pain and for successfully achieving preset goals. All other pain behaviors such as moaning are ignored. A number of studies have demonstrated increased activity, reduced analgesic consumption, and improved mood in middle-aged adults, with some reporting benefit for elderly patients with chronic pain.[84,85]

Other self-management strategies such as yoga, Tai Chi, and music therapy, show promise in reducing pain and increasing function in older adults.[86–88] The use on telephone and Internet delivered interventions may increase access to these therapies for older individuals.

Pain and cancer

Half of all cancers occur in the population over 65 years of age.[89] In the advanced stages of cancer, 70% experience pain, of which 80% is severe and persistent.[90] In up to 90% of cases, cancer pain can be managed by relatively simple means.[91] The World Health Organization (WHO) has developed the Cancer Pain Relief Program to offer adequate pain relief to all cancer patients in the world through the existing health system.[90]

The WHO method for relief of cancer pain is based on a three-step approach to the use of analgesia. The first step of the WHO analgesic ladder is the nonopioid analgesics, including paracetamol and NSAIDs. The second step is the weak opioids and the third step is the strong opioid group. Nonopioid analgesics are usually combined with an opioid in steps two and three to give additive analgesia. At each stage, adjuvant analgesic drugs, such as antidepressants and anticonvulsants, should be added when there is a specific indication. Zech et al[92] reported nearly 90% of 2118 palliative care patients were able to obtain satisfactory pain control on this regimen up to the time of death. Patients with residual pain were often content with the balance of analgesic efficacy and troublesome side effects. Emotional, spiritual, and functional aspects should not be neglected. Despite the widespread dissemination of the WHO ladder, most cancer pain patients around the world still appear to have inadequate analgesia.[93]

The use of opioids in chronic noncancer pain

There is clear consensus about the use of opioids in severe acute and malignant pain; however, the role of opioid therapy in the management of chronic pain of noncancer origin remains controversial. Clinical experience demonstrates that selected patients obtain considerable benefit.[94] Exaggerated fear of adverse effects should not prevent a trial of opioid therapy in appropriately selected individuals who have not responded to other therapies. Maintenance opioid therapy for chronic pain of noncancer origin should only be considered after the patient has been thoroughly evaluated and has not responded to other conventional pharmacologic and nonpharmacologic therapies. There is an increased onus on the clinician to ensure the patient understands the risks and benefits of this therapy. The more serious the risk, the more important it is for the physician to outline such risk, even if the probability of it eventuating is small. To overcome anxiety about this form of therapy, the clinician may need to explain to the patient the distinction between addiction, dependence, and tolerance. Physical dependence occurs with the prolonged use of all opioids. It is manifested by unpleasant symptoms following abrupt withdrawal, such as diaphoresis, abdominal cramps, malaise, and fear. Although the symptoms are similar to those experienced by opioid addicts, the normal person does not experience opioid craving. When there is a possibility of dependence, opioids should not be abruptly withdrawn. Addiction following the therapeutic administration of opioids is very rare, especially in older individuals. Opioid tolerance is manifested by reduced analgesic effect at the same dose. Its cause is unknown. Increased opioid dose requirements are more likely to be due to the progression of the underlying disease than the development of tolerance. With the relatively low doses of opioids used for the management of chronic noncancer pain in this population, the older individual is less likely to be troubled by these problems.[60]

The aims of treatment should be explicit, often aimed at easing the pain rather than total eradication. A technique such as Goal Attainment Scaling can be useful in this regard, indentifying ranges of desired outcomes, and allowing for side effects to be considered ahead of time.[95] Total eradication of pain may occur at the expense of intolerable side effects. Four factors should be regularly monitored; pain relief, side effects, overall functional status, and evidence of aberrant behavior. The dose may be increased to obtain better pain control or functional status. If, however, the opioid dose is escalating at a time when pain control or functional status is declining, management should be reviewed. The physician must be familiar with and observe statutory requirements regarding the supply of opioids. Both parties must agree to close supervision for the duration of therapy.

CONCLUDING REMARKS

Advancing age is associated with an increased incidence of painful pathology. Anyone who has persistent pain despite what appears to be conventional treatment should be carefully reassessed to determine why there has been a failure of response to therapy. One should never conclude that it is the patient who has failed to respond to treatment; it is the treatment that has failed to achieve the desired result. Severe unrelieved pain has a profound impact on the individual. Various factors may preclude the older patient from the benefit of definitive therapy to eradicate pain and under these circumstances, symptom management is indicated. This must take into consideration the effect of comorbidities on the expression, assessment, diagnosis, and treatment of the painful condition. Overemphasis on pharmacologic approaches ignores the potential benefits of physical and cognitive-behavioral strategies. The persistence of pain despite apparently appropriate therapy raises the possibility of unrecognized mood disturbance, pain of neurogenic origin, or advancing pathology. Under these circumstances a multidisciplinary pain management approach involving medical, physical, and psychological therapeutic modalities is often more effective than a single disciplinary approach.[96] Multidisciplinary pain management clinics have emerged over the past 30 years, but are limited geographically and by expertise in geriatric medicine. Age should not, however, be regarded as a barrier to successful outcomes from multidisciplinary management of pain problems. Even if pain cannot be eradicated, worthwhile improvements can often be achieved by addressing pain as a problem in a broader sense, not simply a sensory symptom.

KEY POINTS

Pain in the Older Adult

Assessments:

- Contribution of nociceptive and neuropathic factors
- Impact of pain on function and mood state
- Comorbidities affecting assessment, function, and treatment selection

Investigations:

- Presence of radiologic abnormalities does not prove causality
- Unexplained change in symptoms warrants reassessment to exclude serious pathology

For a complete list of references, please visit online only at www.expertconsult.com

Palliative Medicine for the Elderly Patient

Ilora Finlay
Margred Capel

This chapter will define palliative care and consider it in the context of the elderly patient. In addition it will consider briefly the impact age has on the illnesses encountered the social impact of this and the strategies available. The second part of this chapter will concentrate on symptom control.

INTRODUCTION

The hospice movement arose out of religious orders in the late nineteenth and early twentieth century, though arguably it has been practiced by medical practitioners in some form throughout history.[1,2] However, it was Cicely Saunders pioneering work that brought the advances in pain and symptom control, leading to the special skills known as modern palliative care.

Death is an inevitable consequence of life; increasing life expectancy and altered disease trajectories means that death from disease occurs more commonly in the elderly population. In developed countries, elderly people may be affected by multiple coexisting acute and chronic illnesses. In the twenty-first century palliative medicine aims to ensure the dying process itself does not have to be the excruciating struggle that many of the older generation recollect observing when their grandparents died.

Palliative medicine can have an important role when patients are entering their last days of life, but also can contribute to ameliorating the quality of life of patients suffering from chronic or intractable diseases.[1,2] Palliative care is defined by the World Health Organization (WHO) as "Palliative care is an approach that improves the quality of life of patients and their families facing the problems associated with life-threatening illness, through the prevention and relief of suffering by means of early identification and impeccable assessment and treatment of pain and other problems, physical, psychosocial, and spiritual."[3]

The aging process

Illnesses and coexisting morbidities encountered in the elderly population differ from those encountered in the young. The consequence of the aging process can mean patients have coexisting cardiac, metabolic, and rheumatologic disorders, such as ischemic heart disease, diabetes, and arthritis in addition to developing illnesses associated with age itself, such as neurodegenerative disorders (dementia, Parkinson disease), stroke, and cancer. The prevalence of failing organ function, such as heart failure and renal failure, can impose significant physical and psychological distress upon the individual, restricting activities and quality of life of the patient and the caregiver.

Providing palliative care to elderly patients with chronic illness may mean that at different stages of the illness the patient may require preventative or life-prolonging intervention, rehabilitation, or purely comfort measures depending on the needs of the individual that are identified and their place along the illness journey. Recognition and shifting emphasis of care may require sensitive communication with the patient and their care providers.

The aging process alters organ function, which impacts upon the pharmacokinetics of drug metabolism.[4] Pharmacodynamic processes are also affected by age with some receptors (including benzodiazepine and opiates) demonstrating greater sensitivity and others (including insulin) comparative insensitivity. The presence of coexisting disease risks compounding this through the consequences of polypharmacy.

Pressure ulcers

Immobility, incontinence, cachexia, malnutrition, and comorbidity contribute to the formation of decubitus pressure ulcers, which should be managed according to standard wound care guidelines.[5] The presence of a wound is an indicator of advanced disease and poor prognosis, but is not in itself an independent risk factor for death.[6,7]

Depending upon local access and availability, it may be appropriate to refer patients incapacitated from lymphedema to local lymphedema services to reduce size and restore function to limbs. General management of lymphedema includes careful skin hygiene and preventing acute inflammatory episodes.

Those at risk of pressure sores require an appropriate level of nursing intervention to turn and adjust the position of the patient regularly and systematically, when the patient is at home or in a long-stay accommodation family, and informal caregivers need instructions on how to protect vulnerable pressure points.

In the context of end of life care when a pressure sore is present it may be more appropriate to focus on comfort, including relief of pain and control of odor, bleeding, or discharge since healing may be an unrealistic goal. Pressure relieving equipment is still essential and dressings have a role in the relief of pain. Short-acting analgesia can be administered to the patient before painful dressing changes. There is some evidence that the application of topical analgesia in the form of diamorphine or morphine sulphate mixed in a medium such as Instillagel or lubricant jelly to painful wounds can cause local relief without the disadvantage of incurring systemic side effects.[8] Odor can be limited through use of adequate cleaning, frequent dressing changes, and use of topical metronidazole or silver sulfadiazine. Appropriate topical dressings such as charcoal dressings can contain odors. If the patient is not suffering from nausea, lemon or vanilla oils, or filtering/air purifiers can be used to mask smells in the immediate environment. A short prognosis should not preclude a patient from referral to local wound care services if their input could ameliorate suffering from a wound.

Care providers

Cultural and social differences exist within communities, affecting the availability of support and expectations of care for the patient. The burden of home care falls mainly on female members of the family with more women in developed countries now at home providing care for elderly people, rather than for children.[2,9] A minority of care of the elderly people is from paid caregivers. In addition to spouses providing care for their partners, in the absence of spouses or in the event of their ill health, children often provide care for their elderly parents. This role reversal impacts upon relationships, caregiver's physical and psychological health, and has economic consequences.[9,10] Care providers are at increased risk factor of death, major physical ill health, and depression.

Care providers of the elderly patient need increased support from the medical team during episodes of acute illness of the patient, and ongoing support during chronic stages, which may require them to provide care over many years. Caregivers need full explanations of the disease processes to help manage their expectations and help them cope with the uncertainty that disease brings.

The umbrella of palliative care may entitle patients and care provider's access to financial and social resources, to help alleviate the economic and social burdens of care provision. Access to a day center or sitting services may provide some respite to the care provider and respite care should be considered both if the caregiver has acute health needs and also at planned regular intervals to provide a break from the work of caring. Unrelieved stress and the burden of care can otherwise result in a breakdown in the relationship between the care provider and the patient, potentially spiraling down into situations of neglect, abuse, and worsening health in both parties.

Care providers frequently have concerns and feeling of guilt when the patient is being cared for in a nursing or residential home environment, so they need to be listened to and when necessary reassured of the reasons for the appropriateness of place of care. Often those who have cared for a long time want to continue to provide some care when the patient is transferred to a nursing home or hospice facilities; helping them do so can relieve the burden of guilt and worry they feel from relinquishing care in the home environment.

Following the death of the patient, the care provider may experience severe grief both for the profound loss they have experienced and for their loss of role in addition to readjusting to life, and organizing funeral arrangements and financial affairs. Such individuals are at risk of prolonged or complicated bereavement and referral to bereavement support groups and counselors may be beneficial.

Future planning

The importance of forward planning with elderly patients and their families or care providers cannot be underestimated. This can prevent considerable distress and disagreement, if family members and care providers have to make decisions concerning health and social care when the patient is unable to do so. The Mental Capacity Act 2005 directs medical teams to consider the information provided by those individuals who are familiar with the patient in the event that the patient is unable to communicate their wishes. The responsibility for medical decisions that have to be taken on behalf of a patient who has lost capacity still ultimately rests with the medical team and not the family. In the absence of family or friends, there is provision under the act for a court-appointed patient advocate who may input upon aspects of social and medical care.[11]

Use of advanced decisions, which are now legally binding, can enable the patient to consider the recognized complications of their illness or dying process, explore treatment options, and communicate their future preferred medical management in specific circumstances. An advanced decision can be useful as a preemptive tool when the patient has been diagnosed with neurodegenerative illnesses, such as dementia or motor neurone disease, so that the clinical team is fully aware of the patient's wishes. The advance decision to refuse treatment can set limits upon the interventions a patient would want to refuse in the future, for example, with respect to artificial feeding and nutrition, use of antibiotics, repeated venipuncture, resuscitation, and respiratory support. But an advance decision cannot direct the clinical team to undertake an intervention if it is not clinically indicated in the patient's best interest.

The four ethical principles of autonomy, beneficence, nonmaleficence, and justice create a framework within which all clinical decisions should be considered. Autonomy or self-governance requires respect for the individual's right to determine their own well-being; however, to do this patients require information in a comprehensible format to make informed choices concerning their future. Patient wishes for future care, values, and concerns can be recorded and some information can be used to form an advanced statement of wishes, bearing in mind that, anyway, the principle of nonmaleficence means patients should not be burdened with futile investigations, treatments, or useless information that does not enhance their life. Attempts at cardiopulmonary resuscitation may fall into this category in certain circumstances. Beneficence dictates that the anticipated benefits must outweigh the anticipated risks and burdens. Justice implies that all patients may have similar access to investigations and treatments without prejudice. It also implies that they may have the best possible care within the resources available but these have to be fairly allocated and divided among their community.

The use of ethical frameworks can be applied to decisions regarding withdrawal of active treatment to achieve the appropriate choice for the individual and prevent unethical blanket policies.

Oral intake

Dysphagia and disordered swallowing may occur as part of end-stage dementia, other neurodegenerative diseases, stroke, and some malignancies, predisposing the individual to malnutrition and to aspiration pneumonia. Changing the texture of food and fluid, use of thickeners, and careful positioning of the individual when eating, supports safe swallowing. Patients should be reassessed by speech and language therapists as their disease progresses and swallowing changes so that appropriate advice can guide care.

Eating is a social activity; altered diets or exclusion of the individual from family meals can lead to social isolation and diminish quality of life.[12] Providing food and drinks can be a source of stress between patients and their caregivers, with patients turning their heads away or clenching their teeth refusing to eat carefully prepared meals, so caregivers need support and explanation. Anorexia can be part of the natural dying process; in this situation artificial nutrition will not prolong life and indeed may be burdensome and distort the focus of care. But this matter must be communicated to and understood by any care providers via sensitive explanation to avoid the perception that the patient is being "starved to death" and food or fluid being forced into the mouth of an individual unable to swallow. Symptoms of thirst can be relieved with good oral hygiene, artificial saliva, and sips of water or ice cubes. These are practical interventions easily undertaken by the nurse or caregivers, if this does not appear adequate, subcutaneous fluids can be considered in the community or inpatient environment.

Artificial and supplemental feeding may need to be considered, depending upon the stage of the illness or acute intercurrent illness, with the patient's consent, particularly in the preterminal stages. However, subcutaneous fluid rehydration may provide comfort even in the last days of life to some patients. Nasogastric feeding should not be considered a long-term option as it is uncomfortable, may require frequent replacement with risk of pulmonary placement, nasal irritation, and aspiration pneumonia. For long-term nutrition gastrostomy and jejunostomy tubes should be considered. These confer their own risks related to the procedure and infection, and do not prevent the risk of aspiration if they are fed to the patient in a supine position; diarrhea is a potential complication. Parenteral feeding predisposes to infection and loss of integrity of the intestinal lumen. Patients should be considered as individuals and options tailored accordingly to the circumstance rather than adhering to a single policy.

Anosmia is a frequent concomitant of advancing years, particular in those who have smoked; lack of smell aggravates lack of appetite as taste is impaired. Good dentition is essential to eating, so oral hygiene is key. The loss of dentures should be considered an emergency because it immediately restricts the individual's diet, oral intake, communication, and socialization. Good dental care is increasingly important in those on bisphosphonates for osteoporosis because osteonecrosis of the jaw is a devastating potential complication.

Medication commonly causes dry mouth. In addition to discontinuing medication where possible, symptomatic relief can be achieved by sucking crushed ice, sips of fluid, artificial saliva, or sucking fresh or frozen pineapple pieces.[1,2] Oral candida infection is a relatively frequent finding, as the fungi adhere to denture plastic, but oral candida does not necessarily correlate with oral symptoms.[13] Dysphagia is an indication for systemic antifungals. However, radiologic imaging is indicated if the dysphagia does not resolve rapidly as other pathology may be concurrent. Oral ulcers can be systematically managed with a coating gel or mouthwash with topical lidocaine, topical steroid based cream, or topical coating agents, but the underlying cause, often ill-fitting dentures or poor nutrition must be sought.[1,2]

Place of care

Preferred place of care through life and when dying should be explored sensitively and honestly, making the elderly patient aware of the feasible options and their limitations. Inequalities of access to home care nursing exists throughout the United Kingdom and can preclude care at home. Primary care teams who keep palliative care registers can use the trigger for completing DS1500 and/or the question: "would you be surprised if the patient died within the next six months?" to identify patients for such a register. A register can be used to inform out of hours services of the patient's condition and tailor provision of health care to prevent unwanted or unnecessary admissions to the hospital via the emergency or out-of-hours services. Use of the Gold Standards Framework in Care Homes can reduce crisis hospital admissions and reduce the percentage of residents dying in the hospital and facilitate patient-centered care.[15]

Many hospices offer short-term admissions but cannot accommodate people for a prolonged period of terminal illness, which may mean the individual receives several admissions throughout the course of the terminal part of their illness. The introduction of the Integrated Care Pathway for the last days of life and application in the community and secondary care may improve the standard of care for patients in their terminal phase.[14] Approximately one fifth of the population die in care homes within the United Kingdom.

Patients can be considered terminally ill when they are likely to die within the foreseeable future from a specific progressing disease. Elderly patients often suffer from one or more chronic illnesses in addition to experiencing progressive or terminal diagnosis and can benefit from care with a palliative approach, quite apart from those who are actively dying and within their last days of life. Whenever symptoms occur, the potential cause of the symptom should be identified to guide treatment. Appropriate treatment of the cause may resolve the symptom and improve quality of life even in the face of concurrent terminal illness—such as treatment of hypothyroidism, Parkinson's disease, or intercurrent infection. Problem-orientated clinical notes prove particularly useful in patients with multiple comorbidities.

SYMPTOM CONTROL

Pain

Pain is what the patient says it is and the same principles apply to treating pain in elderly people as apply in younger patients. Each pain should be identified, characterized (including site, duration intensity) and separately recorded, and precipitating and relieving factors identified. Application of the simplistic pneumonic PQRST[16] may aid this process.

Eliciting the Cause of Each Pain Using "PQRST"

For each pain identify:

Precipitating or relieving factors

Quality of the pain (e.g., burning/in an area of altered sensation may point to neuropathic pain)

Radiation of the pain (e.g., radicular pain)

Severity (often rated using visual analogue or numeric on 0–10 scale)

Temporal factors (how long it has been present/how long it lasts if intermittent; whether worse at particular times of day)

Table 115-1. Causes of Pain Reported By 500 Patients on Admission to a Marie Curie Hospice Unit

Tumor bulk
Visceral, caused by compression of adjacent structures
Bone, metastases, and pathologic fractures
Intrinsic and extrinsic esophageal tumor mass
Organ capsule stretching, including liver capsule pain
Pleuritic pain from tumor nodules
Diaphragmatic pain, varying with respiration, from liver and diaphragmatic metastases
Nerve compression
Radicular pain from spinal cord compression
Headache from raised intercranial compression
Rectal tenesmus
Skin metastases
Pain not directly attributable to malignancy:
Concomitant infection: pleuritic chest pain, mouth discomfort, bladder spasm
Cystitis
Infected pressure sores
Herpes zoster (shingles)
Oral herpes simplex
Aches associated with debility, (but not attributable to malignancy)
Increased tone in paralyzed limb
Arthritis
Neuropathic pain
Skin burning following radiotherapy
Angina
Reflux esophagitis or dyspepsia
Peptic ulcer pain manifested as abdominal pain, referred pain to shoulder tip from perforation

The differential diagnosis of the pain should be recorded; this may determine pain treatments and possible disease modifying interventions. Meticulous physical examination is essential; for example, abdominal pain from urinary retention compared with pain from acute abdomen or tumor mass may give a similar history but have very different signs. The pain should be considered in holistic terms, including considering the impact this has upon the individual because effective control of the physical aspect of symptom control requires consideration and intervention to the social, emotional, and spiritual dimensions of the individual. Pain assessment should include mood, emotional functional, and cognitive assessment as these are recognized to impact upon pain perception and, unless addressed, may continue to be manifested as physical pain unresponsive to analgesia. Elderly patients in comparison to their younger counterparts are more likely to experience musculoskeletal, leg, and foot pain and less likely to experience headache and visceral pain (Table 115-1).[17]

After a baseline assessment of the pain, the situation should be evaluated every 24 hours until pain is controlled. A variety of tools can be used to assess pain including the Simple Descriptive Pain Intensity Scale, Numeric Pain Intensity Scale, and Visual Analogue Scale. The Functional Pain Scale has been validated for use in the elderly.[2] Altered behavior or agitation may be a manifestation of pain in patients with impaired communication.

Analgesia can be titrated in accordance with the WHO analgesic ladder, and depending upon the characteristics of the pain, appropriate adjuvants can be included in the regime. Consideration of tablet burden, medication compliance, and comorbidity may indicate the most simplistic regimen is appropriate, or alternatively a blister pack or dosset box may need to be considered for a patient at home with support from the appropriate community services.

Table 115-2. The Steps of the WHO Classification for Analgesic Use

Step 1	Step 2	Step 3
Nonopioid ± adjuvant	Weak opioids ± adjuvant ± nonopioid	Strong opioids ± adjuvant ± nonopioid
Paracetamol NSAIDS	Codeine Dihydrocodeine Tramadol [Buprenorphine is a mixed agonist/ antagonist]	Morphine Diamorphine Oxycodone Hydromorphone Fentanyl Alfentanil Methadone

Paracetamol is appropriate for osteoarthritis or musculoskeletal pains; the dose should be reduced in patients with liver impairment or probable malnutrition. Codeine is a prodrug of morphine. Co-codamol 30/500 is an effective analgesic administered 6 hourly; however, variations in metabolism through cytochrome P450 2D6 may significantly impair the analgesia available for use. Analgesia should be titrated upwards rather than adding additional drugs of the same class or step.

Morphine is a recommended first-line step 3 analgesic (Table 115-2); the dose can be titrated in increments of 30% to 50% until analgesia is achieved.[18] There is no ceiling dose for step 3 analgesics, rather these should be titrated stepwise if the pain responds (i.e., can be demonstrated on assessment to diminish or disappear with analgesia use). Presence of side effects or incomplete resolution of the pain despite opioid use should prompt addition of adjuvant, if not already commenced. In frail elderly people whose pain severity indicates they should go straight to step 3, oramorph 2.5 mg may be an appropriate starting dose of step 3 opioids given on a regular 4-hour basis reflecting the half-life of the drug.

Patients and care providers should be warned about potential side effects of medication used and where possible these should be minimized. For example a regular stimulant or mixed stimulant/softener laxative is almost always indicated when commencing step 3 strong opioids and about a third of patients will experience opioid induced nausea, so an antiemetic such as haloperidol may be indicated for the first 7 to 10 days on the drug. Reassurance and explanation is often needed for those patients and caregivers who feel the use of opioids risks could lead to the patient "becoming a drug addict" or becoming tolerant to the analgesic effect. Dosing interval or choice of opioids is influenced by coexisting organ failure. Persistence of side effects including drowsiness may be an indication for opioid rotation. Opioids that are extensively metabolized in the liver and do not accumulate in renal failure, such as fentanyl and alfentanil, would be of choice in patients with analgesic requirements and renal impairment. Fentanyl is poorly orally absorbed and subject to extensive first pass metabolism but is well absorbed from buccal, transdermal, and subcutaneous routes. However, the patch or transdermal route is a comparatively inflexible route of drug delivery and not suitable for a patient with unstable pain or rapidly escalating requirements; in such situations, subcutaneous administration may be needed.

The signs of fentanyl excess in the elderly can initially be more subtle than those classically associated with morphine excess. In fentanyl toxicity care providers may report that the patient is quieter and more sedentary than usual, where morphine toxicity usually causes drowsiness, confusion, hallucinations, grimacing, pinpoint pupils, slowed respiratory rate (respiratory depression), twitching, and myoclonus. Allodynia, hyperalgesia, are occasionally seen as a paradoxical hyperalgesia, but usually their presence indicates a neuropathic pain that is only partly opioid sensitive.

Tables exist comparing equivalent doses of step 2 and 3 opioids, and they should be applied when switching opioids.

The route of drug delivery depends on the patient's condition and ability to ingest, retain, and absorb oral medication. Potential routes of drug delivery in frail palliative care patients include oral, rectal, buccal, transdermal, and subcutaneous routes. Subcutaneous routes (including infusions and injections) are less painful than intramuscular injections and attenuate the rapid tolerance that may develop with repeated use of the intravenous route, making subcutaneous routes the parenteral route of choice. In cachectic patients several drugs can be combined with use of a syringe driver and compatibility tables exist demonstrating which medication and concentrations can be combined safely.[19]

Diamorphine is preferred in the United Kingdom for subcutaneous administration because it is highly soluble and so high concentrations can be given in small volumes. However, in many countries it is not available and morphine is the drug of choice. When analgesia is obtained that controls ongoing or background pain, provision must still be made for short-acting analgesia to be available to ameliorate any breakthrough pain.

Breakthrough pain is any pain which occurs over and above a background of well controlled pain. This is a different entity from patients who have increasing analgesic requirement which increases over time because of underlying disease progression rather than tolerance.[20] Oral transmucosal fentanyl citrate (OTFC) "lozenges" or dispersible tablets can be applied to the patients moist oral mucosa to provide rescue analgesia for breakthrough pain as the drug is absorbed transmucosally. Fentanyl or alfentanil preparations are also available by inhaler or nasal delivery systems, but specialist supervision is suggested for the initial test dose as drug delivery is rapid but comparatively short lived, making this of use for pain associated with movement or dressing changes. Theoretically any short lived opioids may be given in advance if the pain is predictable in nature. Pains which occur unpredictably require accurate diagnosis of the cause of the pain and interrupting the pathologic process where possible or if not possible, adding adjuvant medication or increasing the background dose of opioids.

BONE PAIN

Bone and joint pain may respond to adjuvant analgesia including nonsteroidal anti-inflammatory drugs which have a synergistic effect with paracetamol. NSAIDS should be prescribed with caution for patients already taking aspirin or steroids (increased risk of gastrointestinal bleeding), diuretics or ACE inhibitors amongst others as these increase the risk of renal failure due to altered renal blood flow and increased sodium reabsorption in the loop of Henle, aggravating any edema.

In malignant disease bone metastases can erode the bone cortex; this can be identified on plain radiographs. Prophylactic surgical intervention may prevent subsequent pathologic fracture. Radiotherapy provides analgesia in 80% of patients with pain from bone metastases and can be considered in frail individuals.[21] Patients with multiple bone metastases, in the absence of spinal cord compression and with a prognosis of greater than 6 weeks, may benefit from radioactive strontium injection. Bone pain, particularly from breast myeloma, or prostate primary may respond to infusions of intravenous bisphosphonates despite normal calcium, and there is some evidence that bisphosphonates protect against bone metastases in carcinoma of the breast.[22,23] Fractured bones should always be immobilized if possible. If immobilization is not possible, local injection into the fracture site with Depo-Medrone (methylprednisolone acetate) 80 mg and bupivacaine hydrochloride 0.5% may provide sufficient relief to allow the patient to be turned in the last days of life. An alternative would be an interventional anesthetic procedure and nerve block to the area.

MUSCULOSKELETAL PAIN

Topical capsaicin cream has been advocated for mild musculoskeletal and neuropathic pain. However repeated applications are required to prevent substance P reaccumulating and pain recurring. As the capsaicin is very irritant, it can cause a burning sensation on initial application and care must be taken to prevent any contamination of eyes and mucous membranes. Topical analgesic preparations or lignocaine patches may be useful alternatives in select circumstances.[24] Massage and heat therapy (if sensation is intact) may ameliorate musculoskeletal pain. Physiotherapy may prevent contractures developing in paralyzed limbs and the patient and care providers should also be taught maintenance therapy exercises. Skeletal muscle relaxants such as baclofen may relieve discomfort caused by stiffness under these circumstances, but the dose has to be titrated against the sedative side effects.[25]

NEUROPATHIC PAIN

Neuropathic pain is characterized by pain with a burning or electric shock quality or pain in an area of altered sensation and may occur as a result of nerve compression, destruction or infiltration. Patients may describe this pain in limbs affected by cerebrovascular events in particular if the thalamus is involved. The pain can be severe and associated with altered sensation including allodynia. Relief of nerve compression may be attempted through radiotherapy to diminish tumor size and high dose steroids (up to16mg dexamethasone in divided dose to be reduced over time) to reduce any peritumor edema. In certain circumstances surgical intervention may be appropriate.

Tricyclic antidepressants in low doses such as amitriptyline 10–25 mg at night, are useful adjuvant medication in neuropathic pain; the mode of action occurs through potentiation of opioids, serotonin reuptake inhibition and reduction in pain perception.[25] In the elderly use of tricyclic antidepressants, even in low dose, may be limited by anticholinergic side effects which include constipation, dry mouth, urinary retention, confusion, and tachycardia. The use of membrane-stabilizing anticonvulsants such as carbamazepine and valproate are also limited by side effects, the most significant of which in the elderly is drowsiness; their use in neuropathic pain has been largely overtaken by gabapentin. Gabapentin is licensed for use in neuropathic pain but the dose must be tapered against side effects of drowsiness and renal function; its precursor pregabalin is also marketed for neuropathic pain but its advantage seems relatively small and the cost is generally higher.

Ketamine, an anesthetic agent, has role in control of difficult neuropathic pain under specialist supervision in the inpatient environment. It is effective in low dose subcutaneous infusions 100–200mg/24 hours combined with low dose midazolam or antipsychotic medication to combat the side effects of dysphoria and hallucinations.[26] It is a cardiovascular stimulant so may be of use in combination with opioids as it counteracts their hypotensive effects and can be used in patients with renal failure.[27] Methadone can provide useful analgesia but its unpredictable half-life makes it difficult to use routinely because it tends to accumulate in the elderly and has been associated with prolonged QT interval on electrocardiograms (ECGs).

Nerve blocks

Nerve blocks have a role in the management of pain. Celiac plexus blocks in particular are useful for pain associated with pancreatic cancer, liver capsule stretch, and intraperitoneal and retroperitoneal structures. The block can be repeated after several months as required. Psoas compartment blocks can provide relief from hip pain. Epidural injections or indwelling catheters can provide relief from spinal nerve infiltration or compression. The medication used depends upon local policy and preference but tends to involve opioids and local anesthetic; steroids may also have a place. Complex pain with sympathetic involvement may also respond to sympathetic nerve blockade.

Nausea and vomiting

To treat nausea and vomiting effectively, it is essential to identify the underlying cause and then target the intervention accordingly; for example, vomiting can be an indication of hypercalcemia, renal failure, or bowel obstruction, which each require specific interventions in addition to tailored antiemetic therapy.

In the elderly patient causes related to comorbidity should always be considered such as benign positional vertigo, gastroparesis related to diabetes, and constipation. Nausea and vomiting can be an unwanted side effect of opioids and many other drugs, the opportunity to review an individual's medication with their general practitioner and discontinue any inappropriate medication to prevent polypharmacy should always be taken.

Vomiting is initiated by stimulus of different receptors on brain stem nuclei. Antiemetics can be selected to target different receptors depending upon the cause of the stimulus identified.[28] The specific neurotransmitters involved include dopamine, acetylcholine, histamine, and serotonin. Attention should be paid to comorbidities, such as Parkinson's disease, when selecting specific antiemetics to prevent exacerbating these conditions. Toxins, drugs, and metabolic abnormalities stimulate the chemoreceptor trigger zone lying next to the vomiting center on the floor of the fourth ventricle. Central dopamine antagonists including low dose haloperidol 1.5 mg to 5 mg or metoclopramide 10 to 80 mg orally or subcutaneously are effective.

Buccal or rectal prochlorperazine has limited use because it can cause confusion in the elderly as a side effect.

Cyclizine is an antihistamine anticholinergic drug, which may be used in combination with drugs acting at the central dopamine receptors to increase receptor blockade. It can be given orally; subcutaneous injections can be painful and associated with inflammation at sites. It may precipitate with certain drugs at high concentration in syringe drivers.

Prokinetics, such as metoclopramide or domperidone (available as suppositories or tablets), are of use if the individual has delayed gastric emptying as a consequence of extrinsic pressure from liver metastases, duodenal, mesenteric, or pancreatic tumor or ascites.

Patients with ascites caused by malignant pathology can receive symptomatic relief from nausea, vomiting, dyspnea, and discomfort from paracentesis. This can be performed in established inpatient centers as a day case. It is not always appropriate or necessary to perform paracentesis against intravenous administration of fluids.[29] Thought should be given to the pathologic and physiologic process contributing to the formation of ascites in the individual and to avoiding dehydrating the individual by removing excessive amounts of ascites while continuing diuretics or angiotensin-converting enzyme inhibitor medication. Patients on a therapeutic trial of diuretics aimed at reducing accumulation of ascites should be monitored for hypotension and the drugs discontinued if no discernable benefit is observed.

Nausea from liver metastases may respond to low-dose dexamethasone 2 to 4 mg daily. Serotonin receptor antagonists, such as ondansetron or granisetron, have a role in the short-term management of vomiting related to chemotherapy, radiotherapy, or nausea related to bleeding within the gastrointestinal tract. Constipation, headache, and expense limits prolonged use.

Hiccup can be distressing. Again, drug management must be tailored to the identified cause; for example, gastric distention through stasis may respond to prokinetic agents. Tumors involving the diaphragm or brain stem can respond to centrally acting drugs, including nifedipine,[28] baclofen,[29] and low-dose chlorpromazine.

Constipation

Constipation is a very common problem among the elderly community. Chronic conditions that predispose to constipation include Parkinson's disease, hypothyroidism, diabetes mellitus, depression, diverticular disease, and hemorrhoids.[2] Immobility and medication also significantly contribute to constipation. Constipation is a common side effect of opioids medication and all patients commenced upon opioids should be coprescribed laxatives. Nonopioid medications that predispose to constipation include iron and calcium supplements, calcium channel blockers, antihistamines, tricyclic antidepressants, and diuretics.

Assessment of constipation should include frequency, normal habit, consistency, pain, and diet. A rectal examination is useful to exclude impaction. High fiber preparations should be avoided because they may exacerbate constipation if used without adequate fluid intake. It may be prudent to avoid, or use with caution, stimulant medication in patients with known colonic lesions. Lactulose is an effective stool softener in large doses (60 to 90 mL daily) but can produce a lot of flatus.[32]

Unless contraindicated a stimulant (such as senna) and softener sodium docusate or magnesium hydroxide are appropriate combinations to use. Codanthramer has a mixed action and can be used if the patient dislikes liquid medication; it is licensed for use in terminally ill patients only, and can discolor urine and feces. It can cause severe skin irritation in patients with fecal incontinence. In severe constipation, high-dose polyethylene glycol 3350 (e.g., Movicol up to 8 sachets daily for 3 days) or sodium picosulfate (5 mg tds) may be needed. Fecal impaction can be treated with high-dose Movicol, enemas, or manual disimpaction with suitable analgesia cover. Arachis oil retention enemas (in patients who are not allergic to peanuts) followed by phosphate enemas the subsequent morning can be successful. Constipation should be actively prevented in breathless individuals because the effort of defecating can exacerbate dyspnea.

Bowel obstruction

Surgery is often not indicated in patients with bowel obstruction at multiple sites. This situation arises more commonly in ovarian and colon cancer. Patients who are identified to be at risk of this benefit from preventative management with stool softeners. Bowel obstruction is associated with vomiting, which can become feculent; additional late signs include pain and distention. The diagnosis can be made on clinical grounds; plain abdominal films may be surprisingly unremarkable early on.

Medical management of acute obstructive episodes requires antispasmodics such as hyoscine butylbromide for colic with an opioid to relieve abdominal pain. An antiemetic acting at the vomiting center, such as cyclizine, should be considered. In obstruction the oral route is unreliable, so medication is often best delivered in a syringe driver but cyclizine cannot be mixed in the same syringe with hyoscine butylbromide.

Corticosteroids sometimes are of benefit in obstruction, but unfortunately the characteristics that determine those patients who will benefit have not been elucidated.[33] It may be appropriate to try high-dose dexamethasone for a few days and discontinue this if there is no discernable improvement. Octreotide may reduce the volume of intestinal secretions, but should be used under specialist supervision.[34] There is no evidence to support drip and suck regimes in most patients with intestinal obstruction. Patients can usually take oral fluids and even light meals, but may have to contend with one or two vomits per day.

Diarrhea

Diarrhea can result in dehydration, electrolyte imbalance, exhaustion, and a loss of dignity. It can be exhausting and distressing for care providers who have to assist patients to the bathroom, or change pads, clothing, and bed clothes for the bed bound individuals.

Identifying the cause is essential. Radiotherapy, antibiotics, malabsorption, stress, and gastrointestinal bleeding are recognized precipitants. Rectal examination can exclude fecal impaction and overflow leakage, which are all too common; management of this is referred to under constipation. A stool specimen will exclude *Clostridium difficile* infection. Once reversible causes have been excluded, patients can be managed with rehydration, bulking agents, loperamide, or codeine-based products. Patients with fistulae, high output stomas, or secretory diarrhea as a consequence of underlying pathology can benefit from octreotide.[35]

Dyspnea

Shortness of breath is a subjective sensation, which can be experienced despite normal pulse oximetry and respiratory rate. It is a common symptom in both malignant and nonmalignant disease, which increases in prevalence in the last weeks of life.[2,36] Patients with nonmalignant disease but clear deteriorating health and recurrent hospital admissions should be encouraged to discuss their perceptions and fears and they may want to regain control of their condition through advanced care planning or an advance decision to refuse treatments should they suddenly deteriorate again.

Elucidating the cause of breathlessness requires a detailed history and examination; often modification of the disease process concurrently with palliation of the symptoms. Steroids, bronchodilators, diuretics, beta blockers, and angiotensin-converting enzyme inhibitors have a place in the management of chronic obstructive pulmonary disease (COPD) and cardiac failure, respectively. Acute cardiac failure may need intravenous frusemide, nitrates, and parenteral diamorphine. Uncontrolled arrhythmias should be identified and appropriately managed. Antibiotics have a place in symptom management even in the terminally ill to resolve pleuritic pain and the sensation of systemic ill health associated with pneumonia and infection. Draining of pleural effusions can provide prompt symptom relief. In selected individuals, endobronchial stents may relieve the dyspnea resulting from airways collapse and tumor occlusion.[1,2]

Patients with anemia rarely benefit from iron supplementation. Transfusion of packed cells may achieve the most rapid improvement, particularly when the hemoglobin is below 10 g/L.

Long-term oxygen therapy may improve exercise tolerance and longevity in patients with COPD but unless humidifiers are used can produce nasal irritation and dryness. The mask and tubing are cumbersome. Relief from dyspnea can often be achieved quite simply through use of a fan or open window to cool the face.[37]

Opioids reduce the symptoms of dyspnea.[37–39] Case reports and studies on small series of patients involving administration of various opioids via different routes exist, but the most robust evidence exists for the use of morphine. Research has demonstrated that in the doses used for symptom control there is no significant adverse effect on respiratory rate, oxygen, or carbon dioxide concentration.[39] In the opioid naïve patient 2.5 to 5 mg of oral morphine 4 hourly may suffice. In patients already receiving regular opioids, an increase in the background dose of 25% to 30% may give similar relief.[38] In patients unable to swallow, subcutaneous administration of diamorphine can be used to achieve the same effect. Patients in whom anxiety and fear are prominent may benefit from administration of benzodiazepine, either low-dose oral diazepam or subcutaneous midazolam.

Breathlessness clinics incorporating the principles of activity pacing, relaxation, breathing control, and efficient mobilization can improve symptoms[40] for those patients able to attend them.

Cough

Persistent cough can be an irritating and tiring symptom in both malignant and nonmalignant diseases. Common nonmalignant causes include esophageal reflux, postnasal drip, COPD, cardiac failure, pneumonia, and side effects of medication. The treatment should target the underlying pathology. Treatment of cough resulting from malignant pathology may include steroids and radiotherapy. Oxygen should be humidified if the cough results from dry airways or regular saline nebulizers can be used. Mucolytics, expectorants, bronchodilators, and chest physiotherapy may be useful in the management of productive coughs. Cough linctus containing preparations of codeine or regular low-dose opioids, including morphine, can have an antitussive effective.

Patients entering their last days of life with weak or absent cough reflex are unable to clear their airways and may develop "death rattle" the sound of air passing over fluid in the trachea. The sound can be distressing to families who need reassurance and explanation from staff. Anticholinergics, including hyoscine hydrobromide, hyoscine butylbromide, atropine, and glycopyrronium, can reduce secretions and can administered subcutaneously.[1,2,41] If it is important to prevent the sedative side effects and propensity to cause confusion or delirium then glycopyrronium or hyoscine butylbromide should be used because they do not cross the blood-brain barrier.

Dizziness

Dizziness is a commonly reported by older patients and is recognized as a syndrome in its own right. Unfortunately there is rarely a single etiologic cause for this distressing symptom, which may result in falls, syncope, functional disability, residential or nursing home placement, or death.[42] Cardiac arrhythmias, vascular disease, vestibular disorders, diabetic neuropathy, and altered proprioception may all contribute. In the absence of reversible causes, management involves educating the patient and care providers to prevent triggers and creating a safe home environment.

Fatigue

Fatigue is a common and distressing symptom experienced as a consequence of many diseases, including malignancy, and end-stage cardiac and respiratory failure. This symptom results in a loss of independence of the patient; the dependence on care providers can have a profound psychological impact on the patient who may perceive he or she is becoming a burden. Reversible causes are worth excluding and include anemia, depression, thyroid disease, hypokalemia, hypocalcaemia, and magnesium deficiency. Drugs which cause daytime somnolence such as anxiolytics, antipsychotics, and β-blockers should be rationalized. Antihypertensives should be reviewed with respect to the patient's current cardiovascular and fluid status.

Optimizing physical fitness, pacing activities, and sleeping routine, and working with the patient and care providers to set realistic and achievable goals, can help the patient to maximize his or her quality of life.

Anorexia-cachexia syndrome commonly occurs in patients with end-stage illness, often leading to protein undernutrition. The syndrome is caused by altered equilibrium and disrupted metabolism of inflammatory cytokines.[43] Communicating this information to the patient and care provider may help both understanding and acceptance of this. Treatment of nausea, altered taste, maximizing oral hygiene, and ensuring dentures fit adequately is essential. Various protein and calorie supplements exist but should not be forced on the patient if they are found to be unpalatable. Frequent small meals of favorite foods may be an acceptable alternative. Steroids are often used to augment appetite, but the effect is short lived; long-term steroid therapy may exacerbate myopathy and fatigue.[1,2]

Depression and adjustment disorder

Patients may undergo a bereavement process themselves as they become aware of their terminal illness, their loss of independence, and future. Patients may experience and express a range of emotions. The feelings experienced can be exacerbated by either unresolved bereavements or losses. Allowing time to explore the patients past may reveal these losses and provide support to enable patients to reconcile themselves to events.

Estimates vary about the number of terminally ill patients with depression (7% to 30%). Antidepressants may be appropriate for patients with early morning waking, anxiety states, lack of reactivity, feelings of pessimism toward others, anhedonia, or who are socially withdrawn. Symptoms including weakness, tiredness, loss of appetite, or pessimism concerning oneself are recognized manifestations of the terminal illness process and not necessarily pointers to depression.[44–46]

Confusion

Cognitive impairment unfortunately can accompany some chronic diseases and as eluded to earlier the patient should be encouraged to participate in advance preparation and sharing their wishes and preferences for future care. Elderly patients are particularly at risk of acute confusional states. The risk of delirium has been demonstrated to increase with age, cognitive impairment, infection, organ failure, and fracture.[47] Common causes of confusion are listed in Table 115-3.[1,2]

Management of acute confusion involves treating reversible causes and minimizing sensory impairment by restoring

Table 115-3. Common Causes of Confusion

Comorbidity	Cognitive impairment
	Neurodegenerative conditions
	Dementia
	Cerebrovascular disease
	Poor vision
	Hearing loss
Drugs	Anticholinergics
	Benzodiazepines
	Withdrawal from medication
	Opioids
Systemic	Infection
	Urinary retention
	Constipation
Metabolic	Hypoxia
	Uremia
	Organ failure
	Hypercalcemia
Malignancy related	Cerebral metastses
	Paraneoplastic syndromes

hearing aids and glasses. The individual should be cared for in a well lit room with minimal background noise and spoken to calmly and reassuringly. Low-dose antipsychotic medication may be helpful in treating the agitated confused individual expressing paranoid thoughts or experiencing hallucinations. Benzodiazepines can exacerbate the symptoms. Care providers require explanation and reassurance for a symptom that can be distressing to observe in a loved one.

The causes of confusion specifically related to malignancy include cerebral metastases and hypercalcemia. Paraneoplastic syndromes are uncommonly encountered and respond to modification of the disease process where this is possible.[46] Cerebral metastases may respond to high-dose dexamethasone (16 mg).[48] If there is no response after 5 days, the steroid can be stopped abruptly.

Hypercalcemia is a reversible cause of confusion. In the context of malignancy it usually confers a poor prognosis. It can occur in patients with bone metastases or those with tumors secreting a parathyroid-like hormone. Rehydration with intravenous fluid 0.9% sodium chloride should be commenced, followed by intravenous bisphosphonate. Pamidronate can be effective or zoledronic acid a more effective but expensive alternative may be considered.[1,2] Treatment for hypercalcemia may need to be repeated periodically, and the calcium monitored on discharge into the community.

Advanced illness can often be complicated by infection. Reduction of risk factors through maintenance of good skin care, individual nursing care to ensure appropriate toileting, repositioning of the immobile patient and careful feeding to minimize aspiration are necessary. Symptom relief measures including antipyretics and analgesics should be commenced if infection is identified. Antibiotics can be prescribed for symptom relief but may not be appropriate or confer any benefit in certain circumstances and advance planning with the patient and care providers is essential to identify the goals of care in the face of the changing needs of the patient. For example, antibiotics in advanced dementia do not improve survival benefit.[49,50] Disadvantages of antibiotic therapy include allergic reactions, developing resistant infections, *C. difficile* infection, diarrhea, bone marrow impairment, seizures, renal failure, and vomiting. Patients with severe cognitive impairment may not be able to rationalize the administration of intravenous antibiotics or accept painful intramuscular antibiotics.

Spiritual suffering

The religious or spiritual beliefs of elderly patients are important; or faced with debilitating illness with terminal illness patients may question self identity, the meaning and purpose of their life, and prior decisions or actions undertaken during their lives.[51] Faith leaders or religious customs may support both the individual patient and care providers, particularly during stressful periods and enable them to reconcile events.

Specific requests for euthanasia should be dealt with sympathetically and the request considered an opportunity to explore the deep distress the patient may be experiencing. The request may be associated with untreated physical or psychological symptoms; fear of the future, including fear of becoming a burden; anger and guilt concerning the effect the disease has had upon their life; and lack of an appropriate environment or dignity in their care delivery.[44,45,51,52]

Terminal stage

Accurately predicting an individual's prognosis is difficult, and fraught with misinterpretation by the patient and care providers.[1,2] Dying can be difficult to diagnose in patients who have been significantly unwell for a period of time through chronic ill health. The reflective question "Would you be surprised if your patient died within the next 6 months?"[15] is useful to trigger entering the patient on the palliative primary care palliative register and ensuring access to financial support, and guiding decision making and information giving.

In general the prognosis is likely to be measured in days when the patient's condition is deteriorating on a daily basis, if they are unable to take oral medication or tolerate more than sips of water, and are bedbound or semicomatose.[1,14] Sensitive communication of this information enables the patient and care providers to prepare for death but it can provoke various emotional responses in the face of a situation where care providers have looked after patients through various stages of health over a period of time.[52,53] This may be an opportunity for resolution of any outstanding family or interpersonal conflict, apologies, and reconciliations, or to express feelings and love. Poor communication surrounding dying underpins over half of the complaints received in the National Health Service.[54,55] Missed opportunities can result in bitterness, anger, and unresolved grief in care providers following the bereavement.

Realistic goals can then be set for care, which encompass the maintenance of dignity and comfort rather than prolonging the dying phase; this should be discussed with the care providers and where appropriate with the individual. Care providers may find that "death will be allowed to occur naturally" is far more acceptable than being told their loved one "will not be resuscitated." Explanation should include what to expect during the dying process (including the potential for "death rattle" and Cheyne-Stokes breathing pattern) and what to do after death occurs if the patient is dying at home.

Medication can be rationalized and many drugs omitted without detriment to the individual. Regular or routine monitoring of blood tests and many observations (for example blood pressure) can be discontinued although it can be useful sometimes to monitor respiratory rate to reassure relatives that the patient is not oversedated. Medications essential for symptom control can be given as subcutaneous injections or via infusion using a syringe driver.[2,14] If repeated subcutaneous injections are needed, a small subcutaneous butterfly cannula can be sited for administration. Fluid intake can be poor but careful oral care alluded to earlier may relieve the sensation of thirst. Occasionally patients will benefit from subcutaneous hydration to maintain comfort when dying and preventing dehydration; subcutaneous fluids can be given at home.

Preemptive planning allows medication to be prescribed and obtained in patients homes to be administered if needed to maintain a symptom control.[14] Medication should include opioids for administration for pain and dyspnea, antiemetic, anticholinergic for "death rattle," and sedative medication (such as midazolam) for use if the individual becomes agitated. Restlessness may have several potential causes, including urinary retention, constipation, metabolic abnormalities, pain, fear, and unresolved spiritual distress. Once reversible causes have been addressed the patient may benefit from sedative medication administered subcutaneously via a syringe driver.

Care providers should be encouraged to talk to the patient and each other. They should also be shown how to participate in care giving if they wish to, including mouth care and physical turning if the patient is dying at home in particular. Any religious ceremony or customs surrounding death should be undertaken. A care pathway outlining these measures for the last days of life has been developed to improve the standard of care for the dying.[14]

Many deaths in patients with chronic disease follow recognized patterns or illness trajectories.[56] Occasionally a sudden catastrophic event, such as a massive hemorrhage, stridor, or pulmonary embolism, occurs and death takes place within moments.[2,5] Staff are encouraged to maintain a calm and reassuring manner for the patient and any care providers present. If this situation has been foreseen and time permits the patients can be rendered unconscious and unaware through use of anxiolytic medication which has an amnesic effect. Care providers will require reassurance and explanation after the event to understand why the event occurred and that their loved one did not experience any distress.

Conclusion

Palliative care for elderly patients focuses on preserving function, dignity, and quality of life to enable the individuals to actively live their life. Attention should be paid to identifying and relieving caregiver stress. Preparation and open discussion around the future including end of life care and death enable the individual to regain control over their lives and relieve the stress caregivers experience from decision making.

KEY POINTS

Palliative Medicine for the Elderly Patient

- The definition of palliative medicine and its application along with the different stages of the illness journey of the elderly population
- Supporting decision making and future planning, a place for the Mental Capacity Act and ethical frameworks
- The origin of pain and the therapeutic management options
- Palliation of gastrointestinal and respiratory symptoms
- Confusion, depression, and spiritual suffering
- Identifying the terminal phase in patients with chronic illness and end of life care for common symptoms

For a complete list of references, please visit online only at www.expertconsult.com

CHAPTER 116

Ethical Issues in Geriatric Medicine

Søren Holm

In one sense there are no ethical issues or principles that are specific to geriatric medicine. Our moral status as persons do not change when we grow old and the old are due the same measure of respect and attention as the young.[1] The clinical situations in which ethical issues arise are also in most cases very similar to clinical situations that may arise in other areas of medical practice.

In another sense there are specific ethical issues in geriatric medicine caused by (1) a stereotypic social image in many Western societies of the elderly and old as less competent and less worthy of attention than the young, (2) the tendency in many health care systems to underfund geriatric medicine in comparison to other specialties, and (3) the complex interface between health care and social services for the old.

This chapter will briefly review some core general elements of medical ethics as they relate to geriatric medicine before considering some of the ethical problems that occur frequently in geriatric medicine, including decision making for incompetent patients, advanced decision making and the use of health care proxies, research involving the incompetent, and end of life issues. The final section will be concerned with resource allocation and the health care claims of the elderly and old.

Respect for autonomy

The cornerstone of clinical medical ethics is respect for autonomy or self-determination.[2] Competent patients who are informed about the available treatment options can decide which of the treatment options they prefer and can also decide not to have any treatment at all. It is generally accepted both in ethics and in law that competent patients can refuse treatment even if that treatment is simple and life saving.

The main reason that we ought to respect autonomy in health care is that the life the decisions are about is the life of the patient and he or she has a right to be able to shape that life according to his or her own values and ideas about the good life.

In most health care systems, respect for autonomy is institutionalized in clinical practice through a requirement for valid, informed consent for diagnostic and therapeutic procedures. And in research ethics, there is even stronger protection of autonomy through much more explicit informed consent requirements.

But respect for autonomy entails more than just respecting the decisions people make, it also entails respecting them as the primary decision makers in relation to their own life. This means first that patients have to be involved in decision-making processes at a point where there is real choice and before a default decision has been established by *fait à compli*; second that they should not be forced to make decisions before they are ready to make them; and third that patients have to be given the information that they require to make a decision, not only the information that I as a health care professional think is relevant.

Taking patients seriously as decision makers may therefore have implications for the way decision-making processes are designed and structured at the ward or department level to ensure that patients are involved at the right time and that there is time enough for them to be properly informed.

In a broader perspective, respect for self-determination also creates an obligation to promote people's abilities to make decisions by promoting their autonomy. If there is something we can do which will enable a person to make autonomous decisions we should do it. This may include clinically relatively trivial interventions (e.g., rehydrating a dehydrated and confused patient), but may also include patient education or the use of modern patient decision support programs.

Two common misunderstandings of what respect for self-determination means need to be mentioned. The first misunderstanding is that respect for autonomy entails that patients have to make all decisions themselves and that they cannot delegate decision making to other people. But delegating decision making is a perfectly autonomous thing to do! We all do it on a regular basis. And there is nothing ethically problematic in a patient asking a doctor to make the decision if that patient trusts that the doctor is able to make a better decision. Forcing patients to make decisions they do not want to make is not respecting the patient's self-determination.

The other common misconception is that you respect people's autonomy by giving them what they want and that this means that if you want something, for instance a specific treatment, I have a moral obligation to help you get it. But respect for autonomy only, strictly speaking, implies a negative duty of noninterference. Any positive duty to help cannot be derived from respect for self-determination, it has to be justified differently, for instance through some account of the professional obligations that flow from an established doctor-patient relationship.

Paternalism

Paternalism is the term used for actions we take or decisions we make for another person with the intention of benefiting that person. The word is derived from the Latin word for father and the idea is that a paternalist decision is like the decision a good father makes for his child. It is important to note that an action can only count as paternalist if it is done to benefit the other person. Actions chosen and performed to benefit the doctor, the health care system, or with mixed intentions are not paternalistic, but simply coercive.

Paternalistic decision making is not problematic if the person in question is incompetent (see latter discussion). This situation is sometimes referred to as genuine paternalism.

Paternalistic decision making is, however, problematic if the person is competent and wants to make his or her own decisions. In that case the paternalistic action overrides the autonomy of the person. Paternalistic decision making can be justified in emergency situations where there is no time to consult the patient and it can sometimes be justified in a public health context, but it is rarely, if ever justified in non-emergency interactions with individual patients.

An increasingly common form of paternalism is what can be called informational paternalism. Informational paternalism occurs when patient have clearly signaled that they do not want some piece of information about their condition (e.g., do not want to know the precise prognosis) but where they are given information nevertheless because the health care team thinks that it is... "best for them to know..." This is sometimes supported by the claim that health care professionals have a duty to tell the truth to their patients. But it does not follow from that duty, which is essentially a duty not to lie or to tell the truth if asked, that there is a duty to impress the truth on people who do not want to hear it. This is easily seen if we consider a parallel example: Every one of us have a duty to tell the truth to our friends but this does not generate an obligation to provide unsolicited evaluations of their dress sense or latest hair cut, even if those evaluations are the gospel truth!

Dignity

In the context of geriatric medicine, respecting and preserving the dignity of patients is the second ethical consideration that takes center stage. Respect for autonomy and for the decisions of a person can be seen as part of preserving and respecting the dignity of that person, but dignity is a complex concept that is not exhausted by respect for self-determination.[3]

To treat someone in a dignified manner is to treat them in a way that recognizes that they are a complete person with personal integrity and worth and a protected zone of privacy. Exactly what this means will vary from culture to culture and from time period to time period. But everyone within a culture will be able to identify a core set of behaviors that count as undignified and disrespectful behavior. This is also an area where research focusing on the experiences of patients can play a role in making it clearer when they experience care as impinging on their dignity. It should come as no surprise that many old people think it is undignified if they are shabbily dressed or if they are exposed naked or half naked to the gaze of others.[3]

In this context it is important to remember that some of the largest problems in relation to the protection of dignity are brought about by the numerous small routine violations of dignity that may erode both a person's sense of personal worth and the staff's sense of what is right and proper. Although the actions are done by individual health care professionals, the solution to this kind of problem is often organizational.

The incompetent patient

Not all patients are competent to make decisions about health care matters. Patients may become temporarily incompetent during an acute illness episode or they may become permanently incompetent (e.g., in the later stages of dementia). But health care and other decisions still have to be made even when the patient cannot make them himself.

The concept of incompetence initially seems to be straightforward. The normal adult is the paradigm case of an individual who is competent to make decisions, and that competence is lost if the person becomes unconscious, is very inebriated, or develops late stage Alzheimer's disease where almost all memory and most reasoning capacities are gone. Between the extremes of full competence and complete incompetence there is, however, a very wide range of situations where a person is either partially competent (i.e., competent to make certain decisions but not others), or where a person's competence is questionable. This grey area is created by two complicating factors (1) competence is always competence to make a specific decision and (2) we do not have a good account of exactly what it takes to be competent and how far you can deviate from the norm before you become incompetent.

That competence is always the competence to make a specific decision is very obvious in the case of children. It is not the case that one day they are completely incompetent to make decisions, and the next day they become fully competent. Even a 3-year-old is competent to decide which ice cream he or she wants when given the choice on a warm day at the beach. In the same way, someone with dementia may be incompetent to make decisions about his or her treatment, without being incompetent to make decisions about what to eat for dinner, or when to get up in the morning.

The second complicating factor in decisions about competence is that it is unclear how rational and how informed a decision has to be to count as competent. Most of the decisions the people make do not conform to strict rules of rationality and are performed in a situation of at least partial ignorance. Just think of the ways most of us decide on quite important things such as applying to medical school, buying a house, marrying, or starting to save for a pension. We do not seek all the information that we could have sought and we do not always think carefully through all the options. This means that unless we want to rule most decision making to be incompetent, and therefore possibly open to being overruled by others, we have to have a less stringent standard of competent decision making than full rationality and complete information.

We could try to say that what matters is not how the decision was made, but its content (i.e., what decision that was made). But this is a problematic argument since we generally allow people to make foolish choices, even about very important things. That a decision is not one that I would have made does not *eo ipse* make it an incompetent decision.

Here it is important to note that questions about incompetence are often only raised when our patients make decisions that we do not agree with. This is in itself problematic. There are probably as many patients who make decisions that we do agree with, but where we could have challenged their competence to make these decisions.

Decision making for the incompetent

In a situation where one person has to make important decisions for another, often called proxy decision making, there are in principle two different ways in which such a decision can be made. These are commonly referred to as the "substituted judgment standard" and the "best interest standard."[4]

According to the substituted judgment standard, the task of the decision maker is to try to make the decision the incompetent person would have made, if competent. This might involve empathic identification with the patient to discern what the patient would have decided. The problem with this standard for proxy decision making is that it is not obvious which of the incompetent person's characteristics that should play a role. Should I for instance make rash decisions for a patient who all his life was a rash decision maker or should I take account of a patient's needle phobia? Because of these problems the substituted judgment standard has fallen out of favor.

The best interest standard specifies the task of the proxy decision maker as making the decision that is in the patient's best interest (i.e., the decision that is most likely to benefit the patient). This is the standard that is accepted in most jurisdictions for legal decision making for the incompetent. The conception of best interest that is at play here is quite wide. A patient's best interest is not confined to his "medical best interest" (e.g., which treatment that is medically optimal), it also encompasses social issues, etc. It is furthermore generally accepted that what is in a patient's best interest is at least partly determined by the patient's prior values and life goals. If understood in this broad way and drawing on knowledge about the patient's values decision making guided by best interest will often come close to decision making guided by substituted judgment.

The term "best interest" seems to imply that there is one and only one decision and course of action that will promote the patient's best interest and that our task is to find that course of action. But this view rests on a mistake. There are many situations where we will be unable to decide which course of action will benefit the patient most because of uncertainties about the clinical situation and/or uncertainties about the patient's values.[5] We are often able to identify some decisions that are clearly not in the patient's best interest without being able to specify one of the remaining options as the one that clearly serves his or her interest the most.

Advanced decision making

Many jurisdictions now allow people to make legally valid advance decisions about health care that come into force if and when the person becomes incompetent. This can either be in the form of advance directives or in the form of the appointment of a designated proxy decision maker or a combination of the two.

Advance directives allow a person to specify what treatment he or she wants or does not want in specific future circumstances and are most useful for persons who suffer from a disease process with at least a somewhat predictable future course. In that situation it is also possible to help patients to clarify their wishes for future treatment by outlining the range of likely scenarios.

Advance directives formulated in more general terms such as "If I become unable to take care of myself, I do not want..." will always require a considerable amount of interpretation to decide whether they apply to the situation at hand and whether they should still be considered valid.

The problems in writing sufficiently specific advance directives have led to a move toward combining advance directives with the appointment of a designated proxy decision maker.

The task of the designated proxy is to make decisions on behalf of the patient when the patient is no longer competent to make those decisions. These decisions have to be made in the best interest of the patient (see previous discussion concerning "best interest"), just as decisions for patients who do not have a designated proxy. But the advantage of having a proxy is that patients can appoint someone who knows them and their values and preferences well and who is therefore more likely to evaluate best interest in the same way as the patient.

In jurisdictions where it is possible to designate a proxy it is usually the case that health care professionals can only override the proxy's decisions if they can show that they are clearly not in the patient's best interest.

The role of the family in decision making

In most Western countries family members have no formal role in decision making *qua* family members. There may be a requirement to consult them before decisions are made concerning an incompetent patient but there is usually no legal requirement to follow their advice unless they are the patient's legally designated proxy decision maker.

In reality families do justifiably play a larger role in decision making in many circumstances. Many competent patients want to involve their family members in the decisions and some may want to leave decisions to the family or some specific relative.

In relation to incompetent patient families often have a better understanding of the patient's value system than the health care team has and it is furthermore often the family that has to care for the patient outside of the health care context. This means that it will almost always be appropriate to consult the family before important decisions are made about incompetent patients. But it is also important to realize the interests of the patient and the family can be entangled in complicated ways that may make it difficult for family members to see clearly what is best for the patient. There may also be conflicting views among family members as to what should be done.

Research and incompetent persons

The traditional research ethics problem discussed in connection with dementia research is the problem of research involving persons who are incapable of giving valid informed consent. This problem has been extensively analyzed and at the regulatory level of research ethics a consensus has developed on the requirements that have to be fulfilled for such research to be deemed ethically acceptable. These requirements are: (1) consent must be sought from the person's representative (proxy); (2) if the person is able to assent or dissent, although unable to consent, the person's assent must be obtained; (3) the research must either be directly beneficial to the person, or it must be beneficial to the patient group to which the person belongs, and it must be impossible to perform the research in a group of patients who can consent; and (4) the risk to the person must be minimal in those circumstances where there is no direct benefit.

This consensus is, for instance expressed in paragraphs 27 to 29 of the most recent revision of the Helsinki Declaration from the World Medical Association.[6]

The restriction on types of research that an incompetent person can be included in can be justified in three different ways:

The first line of argument is based on the historical fact that vulnerable groups have often been used in ethically problematic research and that if the incompetent could be used as research participants in ordinary projects there is a risk that they would become an easy source of research material.

The second focuses on the intersection of interests between the person with a specific condition and the group of sufferers with that condition. The argument is that even if a person does not realize a personal benefit from the research, he is benefited indirectly through the benefits accruing to the group.

The third possible justification is the pragmatic one that unless we allow some kinds of research without consent into conditions where all sufferers are incompetent, very little progress will be made in the treatment of such conditions (the "golden ghetto" argument), but such research should be limited to those projects that cannot be performed in any other way to minimize the infringements caused by research without consent.

End of life issues

Three types of end of life issues are currently under discussion in medical ethics: (1) withdrawing and withholding treatment, (2) physician assisted suicide, and (3) active euthanasia.

There is no doubt that a doctor can withdraw or withhold any treatment if either (1) a competent patient refuses the treatment or (2) the treatment is futile (i.e., cannot benefit the patient). But there are still three open questions in relation to withdrawing and withholding:

- Is there a moral difference between withdrawing and withholding?
- What about treatments that are not completely futile, or not futile from all points of view?
- Is the provision of nutrition and hydration treatment?

Doctors often feel that there is a difference between withdrawing and withholding a given treatment. It feels more difficult to stop a treatment that is going on than it feels not to start a treatment. But it is very difficult to find any good justification for this feeling. The consequences of stopping and not starting are often the same (e.g., think of stopping and not starting respiratory support in a patient who needs it). And the reasons for the decision are almost always also very similar (e.g., it is not in the patient's best interest to continue/initiate this treatment). This has meant that there is a growing consensus that despite the phenomenological difference (i.e., the difference in how it feels), there is no real ethical difference between decisions to withdraw and decisions to withhold.

When thinking of withdrawing or withholding a treatment from a patient it is not difficult to reach a decision if the treatment in question is completely futile, if it has no chance of benefiting the patient in any way. But there are many situations where the treatment is not completely futile. It may have some small chance of being successful, or it may be likely to prolong the patient's life but raise the subsequent question of whether this longer life is worth having seen from the point of view of the patient. A typical situation where these issues arise is when contemplating cardiopulmonary resuscitation and the appropriateness of a do not resuscitate decision. If the patient is competent, all of this can be discussed with the patient and the patient can decide. But in the case of the noncompetent patient, others must decide what is in the best interest of the patient. It is not possible to give a percentage figure for when a treatment can be regarded as futile but it is generally agreed that a mere theoretical chance that something will work does not make it a worthwhile treatment.

The final controversial issue in relation to withdrawing and withholding is whether nutrition and hydration or "food and water" should be defined as treatment or as basic humane care that can never be withdrawn or withheld? Part of this controversy has been a discussion of whether withdrawal of nutrition and hydration leads to suffering and whether such suffering (e.g., thirst) can be relieved, but this discussion is in some sense a red herring. The real core issue in the controversy is not suffering but whether it can ever be justified not to provide this basic level of care. Legally the position is now settled in many jurisdictions by explicit legal judgments that it is acceptable to withdraw nutrition and hydration, but the ethical discussion is still not over, partly because it involves the thorny question of whether it is ever better for a person to be dead than alive. This links the withdrawing/withholding issue to the discussion of physician-assisted suicide and euthanasia.

Physician-assisted suicide and euthanasia

Physician-assisted suicide (PAS) is the situation where a doctor provides a patient with the means to commit suicide (e.g., by issuing a prescription for a lethal combination of drugs), but the patient performs the physical act of actually taking the drugs.

Active euthanasia is the situation where a doctor actively ends the life of a patient (e.g., by injecting a lethal combination of drugs). In relation to active euthanasia, it is possible to distinguish between voluntary euthanasia where the patient has requested euthanasia, nonvoluntary euthanasia where the patient is incompetent and nothing is known about his or her wishes, and involuntary euthanasia where a patient is killed against his or her will. Involuntary euthanasia is murder and nonvoluntary euthanasia raises a host of complex ethical and legal problems so the discussion about euthanasia is usually focused on whether or not voluntary active euthanasia should be legalized.

Physician-assisted suicide and/or voluntary active euthanasia has been legalized in a few countries. PAS is legal in Switzerland, the Netherlands. and the U.S. state of Oregon and active euthanasia is legal in the Netherlands and Belgium. In all cases, except in Switzerland, there are extensive procedural safeguards in place to try to ensure that the decision to ask for PAS or euthanasia is well considered and fully voluntary.

The ethical justification of PAS and/or euthanasia proceeds along two dimensions. The first line of justification relies on respect for autonomy. If people have a strong interest in leading their life according to their own values, then it is plausible that they also have a strong interest in how that life ends and that their choices should be respected. A hypothetical example which is often discussed in this line of argument is the successful academic with the first symptoms of Alzheimer disease who does not want his life to end in severe dementia and who claims that such an end would make a mockery of his life's achievements and would furthermore be undignified. Proponents of this line of argument often claim that it is the individual person who has to decide whether he would be better off dead and that only he can make that evaluation.

The second line of justification focuses on suffering and is based on the claim that if a person is in great pain, has breathing difficulties, or severe psychological suffering and there is no way to relieve the suffering then PAS or euthanasia may be justified to end the suffering.

The two lines of justification come together in the core cases of severe irremediable suffering in a person with terminal illness who wants the suffering to end.

The opposition towards legalizing PAS and/or euthanasia may either be opposition to the two practices as such, for instance based on the view that suicide or killing is never right, or it may be opposition to the legalization of the practices. It is quite common for people to agree that there are specific cases where active voluntary euthanasia is justified, but still argue that it should not be legalized.

The arguments against legalization are primarily of two kinds. One line of argument claims that it is important that the law symbolically upholds the view that taking the life of another human being is always wrong. The second line of argument is worried about slippery slopes and a gradual expansion from core cases to less core cases. Here the argument is that even if we write a law that only allows PAS or euthanasia for people with terminal illness and irremediable suffering who wish to die, then we will over time also allow euthanasia in cases where the voluntary element is less clear or in cases where the suffering is not present but merely predicted for the future. Some also worry that we will allow euthanasia in situations where the decision is formally voluntary but based on motivations that are perceived as problematic (e.g., if a patient wants euthanasia not to be a burden to family or an economic drain on the health care system). Would it not be better if these problems were solved in another way for instance by appropriate allocation of resources to health and social care for the elderly?

Priority setting and the elderly

Until this point the chapter has mainly been concerned with decision making in relation to specific identifiable patients but resource allocation decisions between groups of patients also raise ethical issues. No health care system has the resources to provide the medically optimal treatment to everyone who is ill. There is always a mismatch between the available resources and the claims on the health care system. This means that priority setting between patients and patient groups is a reality in all health care systems. Politicians may want to deny this, but it is nevertheless a fact.

This raises the question how the health care claims of the old should be prioritized? Should the claims of the old be given the same, greater, or lesser weight than the claims of the young? It is obvious that people's unreflective opinion on this issue vary according to how it is framed. We generally, and rightly agree that old people have the same worth and importance as young people and that, for instance there should be no difference in how we treat severe pain in the old and the young. But many people will express the opposite opinion if the issue is, for instance who should receive a kidney transplant and the hypothetical choice is between someone who is young and someone who is very old. People's views are often further complicated by considerations of merit and past contribution to the development of the welfare state. Those who are old now did not have access to the kind of health care we have today when they were young and may therefore have a stronger claim now.

It is difficult to devise a resource allocation system that takes into account of all these views concerning the relevance of age to priority setting and far beyond the scope of this chapter to try to settle which, if any is correct.

It is, however, important to note that some views on this issue raise considerable ethical worries. Some of the major tools of health economics directly institutionalize discrimination of the old. A range of these tools calculate the benefit of an intervention in terms of the increase in welfare/health or decrease in suffering/illness it produces and the time the patient experiences this benefit. But because the old have shorter life expectancy than the young, this has the consequence that a given curative treatment counts for less if given to an old person than to a young person, simply because the older person is likely to have less life left in which to benefit.[1] This is clearly unjust and against all principles of respecting every human being equally. The same is true of any kind of resource allocation that primarily bases itself on future contribution to society because that will also systematically discriminate against the elderly and old.

KEY POINTS

- The elderly and old have the same moral status and importance as anyone else.
- The health care claims of the elderly and old should be treated with the same attention as the health care claims of everyone else.
- Decision making for persons who are incompetent to make their own decisions have to be guided by what is in those persons' "best interest."
- The concept of "best interest" covers a wider range of considerations than merely "medical best interest."
- Advanced decision making is most useful for patients with a predictable clinical course.

For a complete list of references, please visit online only at www.expertconsult.com

CHAPTER 117

The Elderly in Society: An International Perspective

Robert N. Butler
Oleg Volkov

INTRODUCTION

The extraordinary growth in life expectancy at birth in nearly all countries of the world constitutes a revolution in longevity that is still going on. This revolution encompasses both survival of individuals to older ages and changing age profiles of entire populations.

The impact of the longevity revolution has been pervasive and profound, and perhaps will prove to be as important as the industrial revolution was in the 1800s. In the earlier years of the last century, public health programs, better nutrition, and improved living standards worked to increase life expectancy; in the later years of the century, achievements in medical science applied to personal medical care decreased dramatically the death rates from heart disease, stroke, and some types of cancer after 65 and significantly increased the number and proportion of persons aged 65+, 75+, and even 90+ years. In many countries men aged 65 can expect to live 13 to 16 more years, and women, 14 to 20 years. Today, however, demographic predictions are not secure because the spread of infectious diseases – notably AIDS – threatens the lives of younger populations in vulnerable countries: it can wipe out gains in longevity and hinder further advances.[1]

Women tend to live longer than men and several explanations have been offered aside from possible gender differences in biological endowment and development. Women's life style may be more healthful, with less smoking and alcohol use, and superior hygiene, while men, especially at younger ages, are more likely to pursue risky sports, to drive "under the influence," and to be in environments that promote violence. Women, as family health care representatives and users of reproductive health care, have tended to be more receptive to preventive services and more willing to accept help, which encourages early diagnosis. Yet in resource-scarce areas, tradition may favor allocation of household resources to the health of boys. Moreover, as women are more continuously exposed to workplace-related risks to health, the difference between the sexes may narrow. The strength of these diverse factors in different countries is likely to depend on cultural and economic patterns, including the degree of emancipation of women and the availability of modern health services.

Public concern with health and social services to maximize the personal and social benefits of increased longevity has spread. Furthermore, economic issues raised by such a rapid growth of older populations are now at the center of political debates in many developed and developing countries and on the agenda of international organizations. Much of the debate relates to the rising costs of pension and health programs.

Attention is also being directed to strengthening the quality of life of older persons, expanding their economic opportunities, and acknowledging their contributions to family and society. A major challenge has been meeting the needs of older men and women who can no longer manage daily functions because of physical or cognitive disabilities. Long-term care is beyond the financial and organizational capacities of most individual households, and countries with large older populations, such as Japan, Germany, and Sweden, have accepted public responsibility. This chapter reviews selected demographic aspects of the worldwide phenomenon of increased longevity and discusses the approaches used in different nations to provide economic security to their older residents.

Inequality of longevity: longevity in developed world and shortgevity in developing world

Not all nations are in a position to benefit from longevity, and in fact, a significant number suffer from its opposite—*shortgevity*. In the developed world average life expectancy is 75, while the developing world has an average life expectancy of 50. Thirty-two nations (31 countries in the African continent and Afghanistan) have a life expectancy of less than 50 years and a disability-free life expectancy of less than 40.

Shortgevity also occurs in countries that once achieved longevity but have subsequently lost years. This was dramatically illustrated when the Soviet Union was dissolved and the Russian Federation and separate states came into being. Female life expectancy in the Russian Federation is 58.5 years—the lowest in the developed world. Productive years of life were lost as a result of an increase in AIDS, and a spike in the incidence of alcoholism that occurred when people lost their sense of purpose and gave in to despair.

Most poor nations suffer from shortgevity, and indeed, poverty and shortgevity move in the same direction. It has been estimated that at the turn of the twenty-first century 200 million years of life were lost as a result of childhood and maternal malnutrition. Sierra Leone, for example, has an average life expectancy of 38 years and a disability-free life expectancy of only 26 years.

As long as there is shortgevity and nations have huge populations with 35% to 40% under 15 years of age, there will be too few healthy, productive citizens to buy, sell, and exchange the goods and services with the developed world.

Demographic trends

As early as 1960, at least 10% of the total population for each gender was aged 65+ in Europe, North America, and Oceania. By 2000, females aged 70+ had become a substantial proportion of all females in Europe and North America and the trend toward a high age profile will continue in these continents.

Table 117-1 shows changes in the size of the older population between 1960 and (projected) 2025, for individual countries, the world as a whole, and separately, for developed and developing countries. Worldwide, people aged 65 and older as a percent of the total population will have doubled, the same rate of change will apply to developing countries, and the increase will be even greater in developed

Table 117-1. Aging Countries: % of Men and Woman in Age Groups 65+, 65–79, and 80+, in 1960 and 2025

	65+ (% of Total)				65–79 (% of Total)				80+ (% of Total)			
Country	1960		2025 estimates		1960		2025 estimates		1960		2025 estimates	
	M	F	M	F	M	F	M	F	M	F	M	F
Japan	5.1	6.4	25.1	32.4	4.6	5.4	17.8	19.1	0.4	0.9	7.3	13.3
Switzerland	8.7	11.7	24.6	29.5	7.3	9.7	18.9	20.1	1.4	2.0	5.7	9.4
Italy	7.9	10.3	22.4	28.8	6.8	8.8	17.1	18.1	1.1	1.4	5.3	10.7
Finland	5.8	8.9	22.3	27.9	5.0	7.6	17.9	19.9	0.8	1.3	4.4	8.0
Sweden	11.0	12.9	23.0	27.7	9.3	10.9	17.2	18.6	1.7	2.1	5.8	9.1
Germany	9.9	12.9	21.6	27.6	8.6	11.2	16.3	18.1	1.4	1.7	5.3	9.5
Greece	7.2	9.0	21.7	26.8	6.0	7.6	16.2	18.4	1.2	1.4	5.5	8.4
Austria	10.0	13.9	21.6	26.8	8.6	11.8	16.5	18.1	1.3	2.1	5.1	8.7
Spain	7.0	9.4	20.6	26.4	6.1	7.9	15.9	18.1	0.9	1.5	4.7	8.3
Belgium	10.3	13.5	21.2	26.1	8.9	11.3	16.5	18.1	1.4	2.2	4.6	8.0
Hungary	7.8	10.0	16.7	25.5	6.8	8.8	14.1	18.9	0.9	1.2	2.6	6.6
Latvia	7.9	12.5	15.1	25.4	6.7	10.2	12.9	17.4	1.2	2.3	2.2	8.0
Ukraine	5.7	9.0	14.5	25.4	5.0	7.5	12.2	17.4	0.8	1.6	2.3	5.6
France	8.9	14.2	19.4	24.9	7.5	11.6	15.3	17.5	1.3	2.6	4.1	7.4
Denmark	9.8	11.3	20.3	24.6	8.4	9.6	15.9	17.3	1.4	1.7	4.4	7.3
U.K.	9.3	13.9	19.6	24.2	7.6	11.4	15.4	16.8	1.7	2.5	4.4	7.4
Bulgaria	6.6	8.4	16.9	24.2	5.9	7.3	14.4	18.9	0.7	1.1	2.5	5.3
Netherlands	8.1	9.2	19.6	24.1	7.2	8.1	15.9	17.6	0.9	1.1	3.7	6.5
Norway	10.1	12.2	19.6	24.0	8.4	9.9	15.6	17.0	1.7	2.3	4.0	7.0
Portugal	6.6	9.2	17.2	24.0	5.8	7.9	14.0	17.0	0.8	1.3	3.2	7.0
More developed	7.2	9.8	18.4	24.1	6.2	8.2	14.6	17.1	1.0	1.6	3.8	7.0
Poland	4.4	7.1	16.7	23.6	3.9	6.1	14.5	18.4	0.5	0.9	2.2	5.2
Lithuania	6.1	9.1	15.3	23.5	5.3	7.5	12.1	16.3	0.8	1.7	3.2	7.2
Singapore	1.6	2.6	19.8	23.1	1.4	2.2	16.8	18.6	0.2	0.4	3.0	4.5
Russian Fed.	4.1	8.1	14.2	22.8	3.6	6.7	12.5	18.3	0.5	1.4	1.7	4.5
Canada	7.2	7.8	18.7	22.6	6.1	6.5	15.1	16.8	1.1	1.3	3.6	5.8
Belarus	6.6	9.8	13.6	22.0	5.7	8.0	11.9	17.2	0.9	1.8	1.7	4.8
Hong Kong	1.6	4.1	19.1	21.1	1.5	3.6	15.8	16.7	0.1	0.5	3.3	4.3
USA	8.5	10.0	16.5	20.4	7.3	8.3	13.5	15.1	1.2	1.6	3.0	5.3
Australia	7.2	9.7	16.9	20.3	6.3	8.3	13.5	15.0	0.9	1.5	3.4	5.3
New Zealand	7.6	9.7	16.8	20.2	6.4	8.0	13.7	15.1	1.2	1.7	3.1	5.1
Romania	5.6	7.8	14.8	20.0	5.1	6.9	12.5	15.8	0.5	0.9	2.3	4.2
Barbados	4.9	8.5	15.3	19.5	4.3	6.9	13.5	15.5	0.6	1.6	1.8	4.0
Korea, Rep. of	3.1	4.4	14.4	19.3	2.6	3.6	12.3	14.7	0.5	0.8	2.1	4.6
Cuba	5.6	4.4	15.6	18.6	5.0	3.9	12.1	13.9	0.6	0.5	3.5	4.7
Armenia	5.7	6.9	13.1	18.5	4.8	5.6	11.6	15.4	0.9	1.3	1.5	3.1
Ireland	10.5	11.8	13.8	17.6	9.6	9.6	11.3	13.2	1.0	2.2	2.5	4.4
Israel	4.6	5.2	12.2	15.8	4.0	4.4	9.9	11.8	0.6	0.8	2.3	4.0
China	4.3	5.4	11.9	14.7	4.0	4.9	10.4	12.0	0.3	0.5	1.5	2.7
Argentina	5.4	5.9	10.3	14.3	4.8	5.1	8.4	10.7	0.6	0.8	1.9	3.6
Chile	4.3	5.3	11.2	14.2	3.8	4.6	9.3	11.0	0.5	0.7	1.9	3.2
Thailand	2.5	3.1	10.0	12.7	2.0	2.2	8.8	10.5	0.5	0.9	1.2	2.2
World	4.6	6.0	9.2	11.6	4.2	5.2	7.8	9.1	0.4	0.8	1.4	1.6
Brazil	2.8	2.9	8.8	11.6	2.3	2.3	7.6	9.6	0.5	0.6	1.2	2.0
Panama	3.6	3.7	9.6	11.4	3.4	2.8	8.1	9.3	0.2	0.9	1.5	2.1
U.A.Emirates	2.2	2.2	21.9	11.0	2.2	2.2	19.3	9.5	0.0	0.0	2.6	1.5
Jamaica	3.7	4.9	8.8	11.0	3.0	3.8	7.1	8.6	0.7	1.2	1.7	2.5
Turkey	2.7	4.3	8.6	10.4	2.3	3.6	7.5	8.6	0.4	0.8	1.1	1.8
Mexico	3.3	3.5	8.3	10.2	2.6	2.7	6.8	8.1	0.7	0.8	1.5	2.1
Colombia	2.6	3.6	7.8	10.2	2.4	3.2	6.8	8.5	0.2	0.4	1.0	1.7
Venezuela	2.4	2.7	8.1	9.9	2.2	2.4	6.9	8.1	0.2	0.2	1.2	1.8
Dominican Rep.	3.0	2.9	7.4	9.5	2.4	2.3	6.4	8.0	0.6	0.7	1.0	1.5
Less developed	3.6	4.2	7.6	9.3	3.3	3.8	6.6	7.7	0.3	0.4	1.0	1.6
Indonesia	3.2	3.5	7.6	9.2	2.9	3.2	6.7	7.8	0.3	0.3	0.9	1.4
India	3.3	3.5	7.6	9.0	3.1	3.3	6.6	7.5	0.2	0.3	1.0	1.5
Egypt	3.2	3.7	6.8	8.5	2.8	3.2	6.2	7.5	0.4	0.5	0.6	1.0
Philippines	2.7	2.8	6.1	7.6	2.2	2.4	5.4	6.5	0.5	0.3	0.7	1.1
Bangladesh	3.9	3.6	5.0	5.4	3.6	3.2	4.5	4.8	0.3	0.4	0.5	0.6
Nigeria	2.2	2.7	3.5	4.1	2.0	2.4	3.0	3.5	0.2	0.2	0.5	0.6

Sources: United Nations: World Population Ageing 1950–2050. Executive Summary. (Annex III. Profiles of Ageing). New York, 2001, World Population Prospects (2000). ST/ESA/SER.A/204. New York, 2001 ILC-USA: ESOP database.

countries. Both male and female populations will show these increases. The table presents countries in rank order by share of the female population in 2025; countries with less than 5.5 million persons aged 65 and older are shown in a lighter font. By 2025, females aged 80+ in developed countries will be 7% of the population in developed countries.

Countries with many older persons will need service development and implementation of social adjustments required to support health, living standards, and social integration. By 2010 there will be 21 countries having more than 3.5 million older men and women. These countries contain three quarters of the world population aged 65 and over.

Over the past century, very large gains in life expectancy both at birth and at age 65 have occurred and are evident in Table 117-2. This table contains statistics for 30 countries on six continents for which comparisons could be made. The greatest gain in life expectancy of males at birth was recorded for Spain—43.6 years; for females, Puerto Rico had the greatest gain—49.1 years.

Additional years of life gained during the past century did not result in larger labor force participation of older persons. Reports from the International Labour Office on about 200 countries for decades from 1950 to 2010 show that although the number of economically active older adults nearly doubled between 1960 and 2000 and will increase by about 15% in the next decade, their proportion of the labor force falls after 1960.

Overall, the number of males aged 60+ who are economically active grew from 65 million (1960) to 113.6 million (2000) and by 2010 will be 130.6. But their proportion of the total male labor force fell from 7.4% (1960) to 6.5% (2000) and will be about the same in 2010. Contrary to the general trend, Europe shows a decline in both numbers and proportions.

Overall, while the number of males aged 60 to 64 in the labor force almost doubled between 1960 and 2000 and is expected to reach 68.3 million in 2010, their share in the male labor force has stayed between 3% and 4%.

The trend for females aged 60 to 64 in the world labor force is similar to that of males. By 2010 one can expect 34.0 million such women. But their share in the total female labor force hovers at a little over 2%.

In Japan, where the standard retirement age was raised from 60 to 65 in 1996,[2] male workers aged 60+ more than doubled in number from 1960 to 2000 from 2.5 million (9.1% of all males in the labor force) to 5.6 million (14.1%), and an increase to 6.4 million (16.8%) is predicted by 2010 by the ILO experts. Their percentage of the entire male workforce is, and will continue to be the highest among all nations. In absolute numbers, however, the greatest growth took place in India, which added 12.3 million active males, 5.0 million

Table 117-2. Selected Countries: Gains in Life Expectancy at Birth and at 65+ years, 1900–2006

			Males		Females			Males		Females		Gain (at birth)	
NN	Country	Beginning Period	At birth	At 65+	At birth	At 65+	Closing Period	At birth	At 65+	At birth	At 65+	M	F
1	U.K.	1891–1900*	44.1	10.3	47.8	11.3	2006	77.0	16.9	81.3	19.7	32.9	33.5
2	Belgium	1891–1900	45.4	10.6	48.8	11.6	2006	76.6	16.9	82.2	20.6	31.2	33.4
3	India	1891–1901†	23.6	7.6	24.0	7.9	2006	61.8	12.3	63.8	13.1	38.2	39.8
4	Russian Fed.	1896–1897	29.4	...	31.7	...	2006	60.1	11.5	73.2	15.7	30.7	41.5
5	France	1898–1903	45.3	10.5	48.7	11.5	2006	77.2	18.1	84.2	22.4	31.9	35.5
6	Bulgaria	1899–1902	40.0	17.5	40.3	17.4	2006	69.1	13.1	76.2	16.1	29.1	35.9
7	Japan	1899–1903	44.0	10.1	44.9	11.4	2006	79.2	18.7	85.9	23.6	35.2	41.0
8	Spain	1900	33.9	9.0	35.7	9.2	2006	77.5	17.7	84.1	21.6	43.6	48.4
9	Hungary	1900–1901	37.1	...	37.9	...	2006	69.1	13.5	77.5	17.5	32.0	39.6
10	Ireland	1900–1902	49.3	...	49.6	...	2006	77.3	16.7	81.9	20.0	28.0	32.3
11	USA	1900–1902	47.9	11.5	50.7	12.2	2006	75.5	17.3	80.4	20.0	27.6	29.7
12	Trinidad & Tobago	1900–1903	36.7	8.5	38.8	9.8	2006	65.5	12.8	72.4	16.3	28.8	33.6
13	Netherlands	1900–1909	51.0	11.6	53.4	12.3	2006	77.7	16.8	82.0	20.2	26.7	28.6
14	New Zealand	1901–1905‡	58.1	12.2	60.6	13.3	2006	78.3	18.2	82.1	20.6	20.2	21.5
15	Denmark	1901–1905	52.9	11.9	56.2	13.0	2006	76.2	16.4	81.0	19.5	23.3	24.8
16	Austria	1901–1905	39.1	10.1	41.1	10.2	2006	77.2	17.3	82.7	20.6	38.1	41.6
17	Australia	1901–1910	55.2	11.3	58.8	12.9	2006	79.2	18.7	83.9	21.8	24.0	25.1
18	Norway	1901–1910	54.8	13.5	57.7	14.4	2006	78.1	17.5	82.7	20.7	23.3	25.0
19	Sweden	1901–1910	54.5	12.8	57.0	13.7	2006	78.7	17.7	83.0	20.8	24.2	26.0
20	Switzerland	1901–1910	49.3	10.1	52.2	10.7	2006	79.1	18.4	84.2	22.0	29.9	32.1
21	Iceland	1901–1910	48.3	11.7	53.1	13.4	2006	79.5	18.1	83.1	20.7	31.2	30.0
22	Finland	1901–1910	45.3	10.8	48.1	11.9	2006	75.8	16.8	82.8	20.9	30.5	34.7
23	Germany	1901–1910	44.8	10.4	48.3	11.1	2006	77.0	17.1	82.3	20.4	32.2	34.0
24	Italy	1901–1911	44.2	10.7	44.8	10.8	2006	78.4	17.7	84.0	21.5	34.2	39.2
25	Puerto Rico	1902–1903	29.8	10.3	31.0	12.2	2000–2005	71.2	16.0	80.1	19.7	41.4	49.1
26	Jamaica	1910–1912	39.0	10.8	41.4	12.6	2006	68.6	16.3	74.8	18.2	29.6	33.4
27	Guyana	1910–1912	29.9	7.8	32.4	9.6	2006	63.3	12.8	65.6	14.3	33.4	33.2
28	Argentina	1914	45.2	10.9	47.5	12.4	2006	71.5	14.6	78.3	18.5	26.3	30.8
29	Greece	1920	42.9	10.1	46.5	13.6	2006	77.4	17.6	82.5	22.0	34.5	36.0
30	Sri Lanka (Ceylon)	1920–1922	32.7	8.9	30.7	8.2	2006	68.7	14.5	76.3	16.8	36.0	45.6

Note: *Data relate to England and Wales only.
†Including Burma.
‡European population only.
Sources: UN Demographic Yearbooks; WHO Statistical Information System; ILC-USA ESOP database; Population of Russia 1897–1997.

of them 60 to 64 and 7.3 million 65+, over the course of 40 years, and in China, which added 10.6 million economically active males, 6.9 million aged 60 to 64 and 3.6 million 65+. However, these older males are not as large a proportion of the entire male labor force as in Jamaica and the Dominican Republic—9.4% and 8.6%, respectively.

In contrast, significant declines in the number of economically active older males were reported by Hungary and the United Kingdom. The rates of change in both numbers and older workers' share in the total working population of each sex vary from country to country. In 1960 males aged 60+ accounted for 10% or more of the male labor force in 11 countries. But in the 4 ensuing decades, these rates declined in 42 countries, while a drop in the numbers but not the rates occurred in 26 countries. Five countries, however, reported a substantial increase in the numbers of older males in the workforce, between 3.5 and 4.5 times their 1960 levels (China-Hong Kong, Nigeria, the Dominican Republic, Costa Rica, and Singapore).

There was a striking trend toward early retirement, shown by declines in the labor force participation rate of males aged 60 to 64 and 65+ in 52 countries with two other countries showing the decrease for 60 to 64+ only and one other for 65+ only.

Seven countries in Latin America and Asia reported steady growth in the numbers of older women in the labor force, and the proportion of older women in the total female labor force also grew. This trend is seen for 60+, 60 to 64, and 65+. In contrast, six European countries show a decrease in economically active older women. In Japan, where there will be 3.9 million women aged 60+ in the labor force in 2010, the proportion they represent of all women in the labor force is, and will continue to be the highest among all nations. The greatest growth in numbers has occurred in China (5.4 million added in 40 years; 2.0 million of them 65+) and India (4.2 million added; 2.0 million of them 65+).

Table 117-3 compares current (2010 projected) labor force involvement of males by age group with 1960 and shows significant declines at both 60 and 65. A major factor in this pattern of change has been the spread of pension systems enabling retirement (Africa being the continent least affected). Data for females (Table 117-4) show increased economic activity for all ages (chiefly due to growth in the age group 15–59) and relatively little activity after 60 in both 1960 and 2010. Change can be expected as costs of long retirement become personally and socially burdensome, and as productive capacity of older people is recognized as an asset.

With increased life expectancy at age 65 including more disability-free years ahead, the labor supply has the potential to increase. This will help keep the annual consumption expenditure (including health services) required to maintain daily living during the additional years of life in balance with annual incomes.

Paradoxically, recent history has shown a decline in the economic activity rate of men from age 60 onward in all continents, which is expected to continue in the years between 2000 to 2010. In 1960 work at older ages was relatively common in the world as a whole; of people aged 50 to 59, 92.8% were in the workforce, and the decline to 79.8% at ages 60 to 64 was relatively modest. Even at 65+, 48.3% of men were in the workforce. By 2000, there was a drop of about 7 percentage points at 50 to 59, but the economic activity rate for males aged 60 to 64 dropped by 12.9 percentage points, and at 65+, by 18.9 percentage points.

The economic activity rates are quite different for women. Globally, women's rate of economic activity for all ages has edged upward since 1960 to about half of the adult female population, but this has not yet made itself felt in older age groups, and for older women an increase in the next decade is not expected.

The interpretation of the rates of economic activity for women is complex. Their retirement age may be adapted to that of a spouse who is retiring early. Women's activity in the informal sector usually is not reflected in official data, in the same way that nonmarket work of males is poorly represented by official data, and household work and family caregiving generally are not part of labor force statistics. In fact, statistics on women are more likely to be substantially affected by these practices because they are more often working in the informal sector. Furthermore, cultural attitudes toward women working outside the home often limit their participation in the labor market of developing countries. Women's productive activities, whatever their form, generally support their consumption in old age. However, the scope of their activities is more limited and opportunities for mental stimulation would not be as extensive.

For men, the rate of labor force participation at age 60 and over declined between 1960 to 2000 in more than 40 of the 56 countries represented. Although low rates are more typical in industrialized countries that have well-established retirement systems and greater longevity, declines are also occurring in less developed countries as urbanization increases and job structures change. Some of the decline in economic activity of men after 65 is attributable to the emergence of disabling conditions with greater age, and to the higher age profile that appears within the 65+ population as longevity increases.

Gender differences in economic activity of older people are common. Labor force activity rates of women aged 60+ are above 20% in only 12 countries. After 65, only 7 countries reported labor force participation of more than 20%, and in 40 countries under 10% of women 65+ were economically active, including 10 countries where fewer than 2% were active.

In view of population aging, these statistics suggest major policy questions. Given the older populations' low labor force activity, how can individuals and societies finance additional anticipated years of life? Nations are in the early stages of gearing retirement programs, employment practices, workplace culture, and other institutional features to the new age profiles. How can older women, now the majority, be relieved of fear of poverty and isolation, provided with more avenues of activity, and be equipped financially to attain a good quality of life? Health care professions and industries are involved as well in maintaining work-readiness, reducing the burden of chronic illnesses, protecting populations against threats to longevity, and promoting attitudes that will assist in personal and social adjustment to the new opportunities and responsibilities.

Social protection for old age

NATIONAL RESOURCES

The standard of living of a country's older residents and the ability of the country to adjust smoothly to increased longevity are dependent on its overall resources and the

Table 117-3. Economically Active Males: Labor Force Structure and Labor Participation Rates

1960 and 2010 (percents)

Continent	Year	All Ages	Up to 14 yr	15–59 yr	50–59 yr	60+ yr	60–64 yr	65+ yr
A. Labor Force Structure By Selected Age Groups								
World	1960	100	5.1	87.4	12.2	7.4	3.6	3.9
	2010	100	1.3	92.1	14.2	6.5	3.4	3.1
Africa	1960	100	8.7	84.9	9.3	6.4	2.9	3.5
	2010	100	5.6	88.8	9.2	5.6	2.6	3.0
America, N.	1960	100	0.4	89.2	16.5	10.4	5.5	4.9
	2010	100	0.0	93.3	20.4	6.7	4.4	2.3
Latin Am. and	1960	100	5.1	87.3	10.6	7.5	3.3	4.2
Caribbean	2010	100	0.9	92.7	12.2	6.4	3.3	3.1
Asia	1960	100	6.7	86.3	10.9	7.0	3.1	3.9
	2010	100	0.8	92.2	14.1	7.0	3.6	3.4
Europe	1960	100	0.6	91.1	16.3	8.2	4.6	3.7
	2010	100	0.0	95.3	19.6	4.7	3.1	1.6
Oceania	1960	100	1.6	90.7	14.5	7.7	4.4	3.3
	2010	100	0.6	94.0	16.3	5.4	3.7	1.8
B. Labor Force Participation Rates By Selected Age Groups								
World	1960	57.9	28.3	91.9	82.8	59.6	79.8	48.4
	2010	58.4	9.0	86.0	86.6	38.3	57.8	28.1
Africa	1960	55.2	40.3	91.6	95.8	80.0	90.2	73.2
	2010	52.5	24.1	85.4	93.1	64.5	80.1	55.3
America, N.	1960	56.0	2.3	89.2	93.7	48.8	81.3	33.6
	2010	55.6	0.0	81.7	81.6	22.7	46.1	11.7
Latin Am. and	1960	53.9	24.0	92.0	92.0	69.5	82.0	62.0
Caribbean	2010	58.3	5.8	85.8	84.5	43.8	65.7	32.6
Asia	1960	58.4	36.1	92.8	93.8	67.6	82.6	58.9
	2010	60.5	5.8	87.0	88.7	44.5	63.1	34.2
Europe	1960	59.7	4.3	90.4	90.2	44.8	71.4	30.7
	2010	56.6	0.0	82.9	78.1	12.4	31.0	6.9
Oceania	1960	58.7	9.2	93.1	94.0	47.3	81.0	42.6
	2010	55.3	3.8	84.5	79.8	21.3	30.5	10.3

Source: Economically active population: 1950–2010. ed 4, International Labour Organization, Geneva, Switzerland, 1997.

Table 117-4. Economically Active Females: Labor Force Structure and Labor Participation Rates

1960 and 2010 (percents)

Continent	Year	All ages	Up to 14 yr	15–59 yr	50–59 yr	60+ yr	60–64 yr	65+ yr
A. Labor Force Structure By Selected Age Groups								
World	1960	100	6.4	88.7	10.5	5.0	2.6	2.4
	2010	100	1.6	93.6	12.4	4.5	2.4	2.0
Africa	1960	100	10.4	83.6	9.6	6.1	2.9	3.2
	2010	100	6.8	88.5	8.4	4.7	2.2	2.4
America, N.	1960	100	0.4	90.4	17.5	9.3	5.2	4.0
	2010	100	0.0	94.3	20.2	5.7	3.6	2.1
Latin Am. and	1960	100	7.1	87.0	8.5	5.9	2.6	3.3
Caribbean	2010	100	1.2	95.1	10.1	3.6	2.1	1.6
Asia	1960	100	8.2	87.7	8.8	4.1	2.1	2.0
	2010	100	1.0	94.3	11.8	4.6	2.5	2.1
Europe	1960	100	0.6	93.6	14.4	5.8	3.3	2.5
	2010	100	0.0	96.5	17.2	3.5	2.0	1.4
Oceania	1960	100	3.4	91.7	10.9	4.9	2.7	2.2
	2010	100	0.6	95.9	15.1	3.5	2.4	1.1
B. Labor Force Participation Rates By Selected Age Groups								
World	1960	33.2	21.1	53.6	42.8	18.3	28.8	13.1
	2010	41.5	8.0	63.5	52.7	15.4	28.1	10.0
Africa	1960	35.5	31.5	57.7	59.3	40.4	50.8	34.1
	2010	36.8	21.0	59.8	56.9	31.8	43.2	25.7
America, N.	1960	25.0	1.0	40.5	43.7	16.4	31.3	10.1
	2010	48.0	0.0	74.4	68.9	13.2	30.4	6.6
Latin Am. and	1960	14.2	8.9	24.0	19.1	12.6	15.7	10.9
Caribbean	2010	33.3	4.7	50.4	37.0	11.6	21.2	7.3
Asia	1960	36.2	28.2	54.2	45.4	21.1	30.8	15.9
	2010	43.0	5.3	64.1	52.1	18.1	30.8	12.2
Europe	1960	33.6	2.7	52.1	39.8	13.0	23.5	15.0
	2010	44.0	0.0	70.0	53.4	6.1	8.3	3.3
Oceania	1960	23.9	8.2	31.6	29.3	9.7	17.9	6.3
	2010	44.9	3.6	71.6	58.8	9.5	21.9	4.3

Source: Economically active population: 1950–2010. ed 4, International Labour Organization, Geneva, Switzerland, 1997.

commitment of the public sector to social expenditures. Important indicators of these factors include production per capita, government spending on consumption, and unemployment. In OECD countries, where population aging has been the most advanced, wide variation in these indicators can be observed.

Gross domestic product (GDP) per capita measures the annual total of national production available for all purposes, adjusted for population size. Government final consumption expenditure shows the extent to which household consumption of goods and services depends on public programs rather than private incomes. Sweden, with its tradition as a welfare state, leads with 26.2% of GDP. Social security and welfare programs account for as much as 6.7% of GDP in Denmark but less than 1% in several countries. These categories are important for older populations because they are likely to contain the programs intended to benefit older age groups.

The last of the selected indicators is unemployment. If the rate is high, the drain on unemployment insurance funds and social programs for supplementary income payments and job creation is likely to be substantial. Funds available for various services to older age groups will be more limited, and, furthermore, policymakers are less likely to be interested in expanding economic opportunities for older persons as an alternative to retirement.

Overview of pension systems

Income maintenance programs for old age were adopted throughout the world as market economies and industrialization spread along with institutions of political democracy. These programs varied widely in their coverage and specifications. The totality of the features vitally influences the standard of living of older populations, including ability to sustain healthful diets and living environments. Although the systems came earlier and were generally more extensive in the developed countries, even developing countries tended to cover public employees and special groups and branched out in time to broader coverage.

The income programs for old age have been referred to by several different names, each with its own shade of meaning. The term "social insurance" stresses the concept of pooling of risk through either a nationwide governmental fund, or funds under national supervision maintained by industry, occupation groups, or geographical divisions. "Insurance" implies adherence to actuarial requirements, that is, expected probabilities regarding length of life and other contingencies, although important modifications of actuarial control have been numerous (such as a floor under benefits for low-wage workers). "Social security" has a rather similar meaning since it embraces statutory programs that insure against loss of earning power "as a result of old age" (which is not actually a determinant of lost earning power but represents the risks of unemployment and disability, when applied to an older population). Both social security and social insurance have been associated with a goal of averting destitution and deprivation caused by various occurrences throughout the life course, such as death of a parent of minor children. This inclusive approach most likely helps adults to prepare financially for old age. Risk pooling and a benefit structure that allows for alleviation of poverty distinguish social security from individual investment programs.

The term "social protection" has come into use to express a broader ambition—the use of public, private, and combined initiatives to mitigate income problems, aid the vulnerable, and secure minimum standards of well-being for all. At the same time, social protection as an umbrella concept acknowledges that priorities will vary with each country's circumstances. It also features a proactive dimension-averting risk through the delivery of targeted or populationwide services and providing programs to help people move out of poverty.

Old age benefit programs in the developing world tend to have narrow coverage and modest benefits. Owing to difficulties in compliance with respect to mandated contributions and in asset management, the ability to deliver benefits has not always been maintained. These problems have also afflicted countries which, despite universal pension systems, are in transition from state to private enterprise. Additionally, at least one international agency (the World Bank) and others interested in developing capital markets have favored privatized programs as a stimulus and an infrastructure for economic growth.[3]

Social security systems use a variety of arrangements to deliver income in old age. Employment-related programs are mostly compulsory for defined categories of employees and employers, and sometimes permit self-employed persons to participate voluntarily. Length of employment and earning level determine benefit size. The government may contribute by subsidizing benefits for low-paid workers or meeting a fund deficit.

Universal or demogrant programs give a flat rate cash benefit upon retirement and are financed from general revenues. Some length of residency is required, and they are often combined with an earnings-related tier. Contributions by employers and employees may be used even though major support comes from income taxes.

The publicly operated provident funds that are sometimes used in developing countries (such as Singapore) are based on employer and employee contributions but the distribution at retirement is received as a lump sum (one time) rather than income over a period of years. Although the lump sum, which reflects the accumulated amounts credited to each worker's account plus accrued interest, may help a retiree to start a small business or to acquire additional training, in this method retirement assets may be depleted by emergency use or the risks endemic to small enterprises.

Supplementing or replacing these program types, mandatory private insurance requires that either the employee alone or the employee and employer contribute to an employee's individual retirement account. Survivor benefits are not included and must be acquired by private purchase. Other countries require employers to provide a lump sum refund of employer and employee contributions plus interest to an aged employee who leaves the firm. There is no pooling for risk across employers, although presumably in a large firm there is an implicit pool.

Complete or substantial retirement from the workforce is required for benefits in some countries (e.g., France, Finland, Egypt), but others start payments to all covered persons when they reach the specified retirement age. Some systems allow the individual to be credited for years out of the labor force for the purpose of child rearing. In some countries workers are allowed to accumulate wage credits after the normal retirement age, so as to entitle them to an adequate pension. Means-tested retirement pensions (as in Australia) may discourage labor force activity in the years preceding retirement by those who wish to reduce their earning record in order to qualify. This is a disincentive poorly adapted to the increased need for retirement savings created by greater life expectancy and a divergence from the objective of relieving poverty in old age.

The usual age of retirement ranges between 60 and 65 but sometimes it is length of service that establishes eligibility. Lowering of the qualifying age in response to public pressure was sometimes reversed to cut costs. Usually the age for women is 5 years less than for men but the trend is toward equalization.

Many pension laws include an early retirement option when special conditions are met, such as an unhealthy occupation, unemployment near the normal retirement age, and many years in covered employment. The wage base used in calculating benefits is critical in determining retirement income. Depending on individual work history, it makes a difference whether the last years of coverage or the highest-earning years are used. Indexing benefits for price changes protects against inflation and indexing for wage trends enables retirees to maintain the standard of living prevailing in the community. Such adjustments are subject to political trends and fiscal exigencies.[2]

Industrialized countries with extensive public pension systems have been facing fiscal and political problems as increasing longevity produces a growing number of pensioners. In some cases shifting older unemployed workers to pensioner status has alleviated general unemployment and drains on unemployment insurance funds. More generally, as macroeconomies grew workers became able to satisfy their desire to leave their long-term career jobs, especially physically demanding and psychologically stressful ones, for leisure or other uses of time, by early retirement.

This was made possible by provisions in social security laws that allowed benefits to start up to 5 years before the normal qualifying age when there were special circumstances, and also, without special circumstances but with actuarially reduced monthly pensions. The pronounced drop in labor force participation of older men that occurred after 1960 increased the annual obligations of public pension funds, while exits from the paid labor force reduced the productive resources of industrialized countries, in turn affecting (inter alia) the tax base supporting the pension system.

The trend of increased longevity and lower prevalence of disability in older age groups have led observers to question policies that tend to truncate the potentially active life years of aging persons. Specifically, provisions in pension laws that encourage early retirement are being scrutinized. If the normal retirement age is raised, economic support must be planned for those who can no longer work owing to impaired health; but disability insurance provides the community with the framework to handle this possibility.

A study of 11 industrialized countries measures the amount of wasted productive capacity implied by lowered economic activity rates. Although at age 50 about 90% of men are in the labor force, by age 69 this rate has dropped, but the decline varies among countries. In Belgium, virtually no male aged 69 works and in fact most have left by age 65; in Japan, almost 50% still work at age 69. In the examples given, unused capacity is 61% of potential capacity of older workers in Belgium but much less (22%) in Japan. These measures are crude in that hours of work may vary among those who remain in the paid labor force, and much of their work may be at less productive tasks, while for many of those who leave, nonmarket activities, including caregiving, may contribute to society.[4]

Privatization experiences of three countries

Individual retirement accounts with tax deferment privileges as a vehicle for household saving for old age have now appeared in countries on several continents, sparking extensive debate as to the relative merits, risks, and costs involved. Proponents have stressed the opportunity to accumulate returns from investment in financial markets that funnel capital to corporate economies and thus participate in the gains from growth, and the wider range of options at the disposal of each active employee (compared, for example, with national funds restricted to buying government bonds). At the same time, the need for regulation of the investment and management companies that handle the placement of retirement savings into investment outlets and the administration of benefits is acknowledged. Regulations plus fees charged by the companies plus costs of competing for enrollees narrow the difference in returns to retirees compared with conventional social security. Since a long horizon for saving is necessary for sufficient accruals to occur, averaging good and bad periods, privatization programs would be more appropriate for younger workers than those nearing retirement.

The circumstances that led to privatization varied by country. For example, in Chile, there was dissatisfaction with the public program owing to mismanagement and political corruption, failure to keep up with inflation, and uneven coverage across occupations. Policy makers supported the opportunity to promote investment in the economy.[5,6] In March of 2008, Chile reported adding public payouts for low-income elderly, granting public pensions to about a quarter of the nation's workforce by 2012. Nearly two thirds of elderly urban poor will benefit.

In China, pension cost allocation practices under the state system were obstructive to the transition to private enterprise, in which flexibility was important, and compliance with the state system was deficient. A potential problem is that low retirement ages were incorporated in the new legislation, limiting the amount that would be accrued in individual accounts, while the program was not fully geared to provide benefits for extended survival.[7]

The United Kingdom's privatized component was an outgrowth of an earnings-related tier that was added to the basic public pension system, and of allowing employers to offer their own plan as an alternative to the state system. Eventually, individuals were permitted to opt out of their employer's plan. When the economy declined, severe cuts in public pensions weakened support for the traditional system. The United Kingdom, like Chile, experienced problems under its new program, based on overselling, high charges, and limited utility of individual accounts to older workers that reduced overall net gains to participating workers.[8]

The privatization movement depends for success on a commitment of younger workers to save despite the stimulus of a consumerist economy, and has not had much to offer to those who could not afford to save much. Nor does "private security" provide accommodation, as can a state plan, for those whose work record is discontinuous because of child care, illness, or unemployment. Further experience will no doubt produce a more settled appraisal of the value of a substantial private investment component in the social planning for retirement security.[9]

Early retirement

Social security laws have the potential to influence both retirement before, and continued work after the statutory pensionable age. In OECD countries, provisions for receipt of pension benefits vary considerably from country to country. Twenty have early retirement options in their public pension programs, and among them 13 specify conditions under which early retirement is allowed. These provisions result in a difference between the standard retirement age stated in the law and the actual age at which pension benefits are awarded. The option allows older workers with sufficient credited years to change their time-use pattern. This could include self-employment and leisure pursuits and nonmarket services such as care of family members. Some countries, however, promoted early retirement as a response to high levels of unemployment, encouraging older workers receiving unemployment insurance benefits to leave the labor force. However, such a shift results in an increased social expenditure for pensions and loss of a productive resource to the labor market.

As pensions systems mature over time, more workers have sufficient earnings to become eligible for benefit payments before reaching the statutory qualifying age. Provisions for early retirement generally allow such workers to start drawing their pension. Pensionable age is also reduced for women with dependent children or children with disabilities and for men and women employed in difficult or unhealthy work.

Partial retirement, legally available in some countries, has become an attractive option for many persons, but its utility to older workers depends on whether part-time jobs are available.

Labor force participation in OECD countries declines as people approach pensionable age under prevailing programs, but the trend differs by gender. The rate for men aged 60+ is much greater than that for women, but the decreases in labor force participation among men age 65 and over is quite dramatic, dropping from 3 to 12 percentage points in several countries.

In contrast, economic activity rates among older women in these OECD countries vary enormously. Rates are high in developing countries, where pension and retirement support systems are relatively infrequent, and are very low in the developed countries.

CONCLUSION: THE GERIATRICIAN'S ROLE

The demographic trend of an increased life expectancy has already changed the age profile of many countries and is continuing to be felt throughout the world, resulting in significant changes, both in private lives and public discourse.

Older persons will be affected by national economic resources, systems that are set in place to protect them from destitution, and their involvement in the paid labor force. These in turn will have an impact on the agendas and goals of health care professionals. The long-term variations in economic growth rates, pension policies, anticipated shortage of workers that will necessitate that older persons remain in the labor force longer, among other considerations, constrain long-range predictions and create difficulties in planning for the well-being of the aging population. For example, since nations are likely to raise the normal age of retirement in response to longevity changes, the interests of older persons whose disabilities preclude full-time work will need to be safeguarded.

The ongoing demographic changes increase the numbers of individuals who will be strongly affected by the availability, perspective, and content of geriatric services. The health professions must be prepared for this growing number of older persons (projecting from numbers of persons already born) and for a variety of life alterations. The changing social and economic environment in which the health and

KEY POINTS
The Elderly in Society

- The extraordinary growth in life expectancy at birth in nearly all countries of the world has changed both survival rates of individuals and age profiles of whole populations. Since 1950, scientific achievements applied to personal medical care decreased death rates from heart disease, stroke, and some types of cancer after age 65.
- Women's survival advantage may be due to a healthier lifestyle, more risk avoidance, and receptivity to prevention and early care of illness. The gender difference in longevity may vary between countries, depending on whether tradition favors allocation of household resources to boys' health, whether women are increasingly exposed to workplace risks, and whether modern health services are available.
- Longevity creates economic problems because of the costs of retirement to individuals and society. Pension systems often contain counter-incentives to working, although use of the productive potential of older workers would help meet the costs of longevity to society and contribute to their morale and life quality.
- The labor force participation of older persons has not kept pace with the increase in their numbers and the control of late-life disability. Reports on about 200 countries show that although almost twice as many older adults were economically active in 2000 as in 1960, their proportion of the labor force had fallen.
- The spread of social security programs across the world means that both their built-in incentives to productive activity and their protective power against poverty are of wide interest at all levels of development. Indexing in benefit calculation, gender differences in the legal age of retirement, and incentives and disincentives relating to early retirement are among the features affecting whether the programs are compatible with the increased life expectancy and social goals of contemporary societies.
- Privatization of retirement programs has spread on several continents but is faced with many challenges. The problems include, among others, the level of fees charged by private companies administering the deposits, placement of investments, and payouts; the adequacy of retirement income afforded to older workers and low-wage workers, and the market risks encountered.

social care of older persons will be carried out will have an impact on important health service issues.

Geriatricians combine the application of medical science with a concern for the whole individual in responding to the challenge posed by demographic change. They must be prepared to make comprehensive assessments oriented (1) to preventive maintenance and restoration of function, and (2) not only to the seriously disabled but also to the mostly well. Doctors who care for older patients should be cognizant of their economic and social resources, and of the setting in which they live, not only their biologic parameters and organ integrity. The nature and stability of social support networks need to be understood, since changes in household composition, depletion of financial assets, and suitability of the housing environment can affect compliance with treatment, adherence to healthy regimens, and sources of morale and well-being. The death or disability of a spouse, migration of children, market fluctuations, and failures that affect the value of retirement savings are examples of risks embedded within the context of the individual's state of health. Thus, a patient's "fallback" options and the means of accessing them are important in effective care management.

Since most older persons are being treated for more than one ailment, the adoption of an integrated approach to care management can help doctors coordinate the stream of services that may be required. Geriatricians and other health care professionals, who have an understanding of the resilience and determination of many older persons, can be effective advocates and facilitators for preventive behaviors and the delay of functional loss. This advocacy should extend to the specifics of long-term care, including its coordination with acute-care services that chronically ill persons may require and the particular needs associated with hospice care.

It is anticipated that the activity level of the aging population will continue to increase, along with their access to information as the Internet becomes more accessible worldwide. As the strengths and options of older persons increase and more and more of them remain highly functional for long periods of time, the outlook of doctors who treat them will change.

For a complete list of references, please visit online only at www.expertconsult.com

CHAPTER 118

Geriatrics in Europe

Peter Crome

AGING IN EUROPE

In common with more developed countries throughout the world, the next 50 years will see a dramatic change in population demographics in Western Europe (Figure 118-1).

The EU-27 countries show a predicted increase for those aged 65 or more from 16.6 % of the total population in 2005 to 29.9 % by 2050,[1] although these increases are not uniform across the member countries. A greater, almost triple, increase for those aged 80 years or more is projected by 2050 to more than 50 million people.[1] These changes are due to reduced fertility and increasing life expectancy; however, there remain major differences in the latter between European countries. For example, for males in Estonia it is 67.3 and in Spain 77.0.[1] The differences for women are not as great but still substantial at 78.2 and 83.7, respectively.[1]

The rationale for public policies to adapt to meet this population change are similar in all European countries. The need for specialized services for older people has also been recognized. Geriatric medicine as a distinct specialty has developed at different rates in different countries despite the needs of older people being relatively similar. This chapter summarizes the state of geriatric medicine in Europe and the work of organizations whose work is focused on improving the health of frail older Europeans.

Health care in Europe

The requirement that in a civilized society all citizens should have access to good quality health care has been one of the principal features of European public policy. Different models have emerged based on state-funded systems, work-based or independent compulsory health insurance, or various combinations of the two. Some countries require co-payments, others do not. There has also been recognition that older people are disadvantaged in terms of their burden of illness, disability, and poverty in relation to the rest of community. Special arrangements have been introduced in most countries to try and reduce these disadvantages. For example, in England all those over 60 years do not pay for prescription medication. European Union citizens are also entitled to health care in every other EU country as if they were a citizen of that country. However, the specific way health care is funded and what services are provided and by whom is a matter for national and in some countries, regional determination.

THE DEVELOPMENT OF GERIATRIC MEDICINE

It is generally recognized that the identification of geriatric medicine as a distinct specialty resulted from the publications of Nascher in the United States.[2,3] However, the development of a national geriatric medicine service has been credited to the United Kingdom and the pioneering work of Marjorie Warren who implemented her service at the West Middlesex Hospital.[4,5] Fortuitously, this interest coincided with the introduction of a new universal National Health Service in 1948, which incorporated from its foundation a network of hospitals that provided care for the chronically disabled, most of whom were older people.

The history of the development of the specialty has been described in a previous edition of this textbook[6] and further information can be found in the excellent articles of Barton and Mulley[7] and of Morley.[8] Therefore only an abbreviated account will be given here. Until the reformation care for older disabled and sick people was provided under the auspices of the monasteries. These were closed during the reign of Henry VIII (1509–1547) and responsibility for this group of people passed to the civil authorities, who as time went on, built institutions for their incarceration in what were called workhouses. The basic principle was that of "less eligibility" with life being worse than that of the poorest laborer. The scandal of the workhouse, drawn to public attention through the work of Charles Dickens' Oliver Twist for example led toward the end of the nineteenth century into the establishment of Poor Law Infirmaries, which in turn were transferred to the management of county and city municipalities in the 1920s. These hospitals became the first geriatric medicine hospitals in 1948. The arrangements of the NHS allowed for services to develop in accordance with local needs and the existing hospital structures. Three different types of geriatric medicine services were developed. The integrated model had geriatricians working alongside general physicians, often sharing wards and support medical staff.[9] The age-related model saw medical emergency patients admitted to geriatric medicine or general medicine services according to age, most frequently 75.[10] The third model, the "needs-related" service, saw geriatric medicine services taking responsibility for older people with complex needs but often not until their acute needs had been treated first. In practice many services were not so rigidly demarcated.

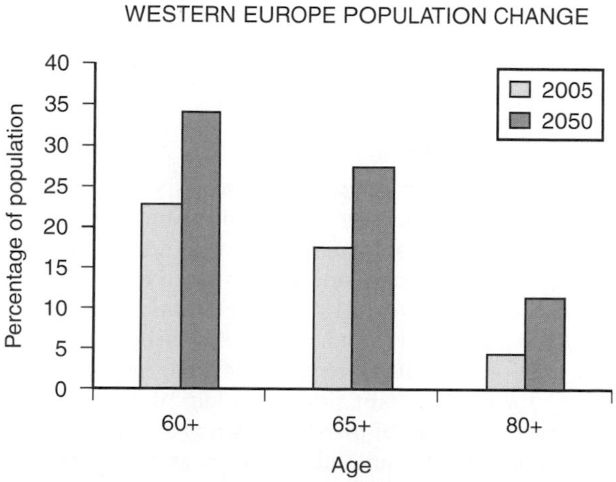

Figure 118-1. Western European countries population change. *(Data extracted from World Population Prospects: The 2006 Revision Population Database, http://esa.un.org/unpp)*

GERIATRIC MEDICINE IN SELECTED COUNTRIES TODAY

United Kingdom

The National Health Service came into being in July 1948 based on the principles of universality and provision on the basis of need rather than the ability to pay. Devolution of political power to the Nation's of the United Kingdom (England, Scotland, Wales, and Northern Ireland) has produced differences in organizational structures, financial arrangements for medical staff, and patient co-payments but the underlying premise of "free at the point of use" remains. Private sector medicine is essentially geared to provide services for simple one-off conditions, whereas the management of chronic disease remains within the National Health Service.

All people are eligible to register with a general practitioner who now usually works in small groups or practices although so called "single-handed" practitioners remain. There is a right to register with a general practitioner of one's choice but in practice this may be difficult for those in rural areas and those who live in underdoctored areas and with those doctors whose list might be "full." The range of services provided by the primary care team varies but might include therapy, minor surgery, and specialist outpatient clinics. In rural areas they might dispense drugs.

General practitioners presently undergo a 5-year training program, a 2-year foundation program common to all physicians, followed by 3 years as a general practitioner registrar, which comprises 2 years in a hospital post and 1 year in a general practice. There is no obligatory requirement to have a placement in geriatric medicine or old age psychiatry.

Most general practitioners are so-called "independent contractors" who are paid by a combination of basic allowances, capitation fees, meeting specific service targets (e.g., identifying patients with hypertension) and fees per item of service. Others are salaried employed by the practice partners or by the local health service. Medical consultations involve no direct payment by patients and medications for older people are free.

General practitioners may have their competence in geriatric medicine recognized by undertaking a diploma examination organized by the Royal College of Physicians of London and of Glasgow. A few general practitioners who undertake some degree of specialist work (e.g., falls investigation, care home medicine) may be employed as general practitioners with a special interest (GPwSI). They have to undergo specific training supervised by the local geriatrician.

SPECIALISTS

The training program for geriatricians lasts 9 years and has three components: the 2-year common foundation program, 2 years of core medical training followed by 5 years of training in geriatric medicine and general medicine. Entry into training is competitive and there are a range of assessment methods that are used to monitor and confirm progress. Successful completion of training renders a physician eligible to apply for a consultant post. In addition many hospitals will employ a number of physicians who have not completed the full training program and who work as assistants to consultants. Training takes place in the main teaching hospitals associated with medical schools, smaller district general hospitals, and in the community. Responsibility for the organization and delivery of postgraduate training rests with the National Health Service rather than the university, which is only responsible for the first year of the foundation program. Full details of training can be obtained from the Joint Royal Colleges Training Board Web site (www.jrcptb.org.uk) .The present training system is in a state of transition and is not yet fully implemented (for details see www.mmc.nhs.uk).

Table 118-1. Number of Consultants in the Larger Medical Specialties in the United Kingdom (2006)

Geriatric medicine	1092	Gastroenterology	886
Cardiology	827	Hematology	716
Respiratory medicine	707	Endocrinology and diabetes	635
Rheumatology	567	Neurology	520
Acute and general medicine	141		

Source: The Federation of the Royal Colleges of Physicians of the UK, 2007.

CONSULTANT NUMBERS

The Federation of the Royal Colleges of Physicians of the United Kingdom undertake an annual census of the numbers and work practices of consultants in the medical specialties in the United Kingdom.[11] Geriatric medicine is the largest of the medical specialties with 1092 consultants in post in 2006. The comparison with the other larger specialties is shown in Table 118-1. It should be noted that only a minority of physicians practice general or acute medicine as a standalone specialty, although it is expected that this will rise in the next few years. In contrast in 1993 there were only 658 consultant geriatricians and the growth has been steady over the last 15 years. Approximately 25% of the consultant workforce is female, but it is expected that this proportion will increase. Forty five percent of trainees in geriatric medicine are now women and women form the majority of new entrants into the profession.

THE WORK OF A GERIATRICIAN

The overwhelming number of geriatricians work as part of a multidisciplinary team based within an acute hospital. Geriatric medicine (often called care of the elderly or similar) is in turn usually placed within a medical division alongside specialties, such as diabetes and respiratory medicine. A few geriatricians work in smaller community hospitals as community geriatricians. Referral to geriatricians is via the patient's general practitioner, from other consultants or via emergency admissions. Typically there will be four or more consultant geriatricians in each acute hospital with support provided by doctors at different stages of training. The standard care pathway is for emergency admissions to be transferred either directly to the most appropriate inpatient service or to an acute all-specialty assessment unit. Patients no longer needing the services of an acute hospital may be transferred to a range of step-down (now often called intermediate care) facilities in community hospitals and care homes. A range of enhanced home care services are also usually available for the first month or so after discharge from the hospital. A list of U.K. government documents on health policy is contained in Table 118-2.

Most geriatricians have a subspecialty interest, such as orthogeriatrics, stroke, continence care, falls investigation,

Table 118-2. Recent United Kingdom Policy Documents Relevant to Geriatric Medicine

Document	URL
National Service Framework for Older People in Wales	http://www.wales.nhs.uk/sites3/documents/439/NSFforOlderPeopleInWalesEnglish.pdf
NSF Older People	http://www.dh.gov.uk/en/Publicationsandstatistics/Publications/PublicationsPolicyAndGuidance/DH_4003066
Better Health in Old Age Resource Document from Professor Ian Philp, National Director for Older People's Health	http://www.dh.gov.uk/en/Publicationsandstatistics/Publications/PublicationsPolicyAndGuidance/DH_4092957
A new ambition for old age: Next steps in implementing the National Service Framework for Older People	http://www.dh.gov.uk/en/Publicationsandstatistics/Publications/PublicationsPolicyAndGuidance/DH_4133941
National Dementia Strategy 2008	http://www.dh.gov.uk/en/SocialCare/Deliveringadultsocialcare/Olderpeople/NationalDementiaStrategy/index.htm
National Stroke Strategy 2008	http://www.dh.gov.uk/en/Publicationsandstatistics/Publications/PublicationsPolicyAndGuidance/DH_081062

and a few may practice exclusively or almost exclusively in this subspecialty. The training of geriatricians in acute care and in rehabilitation has made them ideally suited to lead the development of stroke care in separate acute stroke units and the majority of patients admitted to the hospital with stroke are now treated by geriatricians. Stroke has become a recognized subspecialty of geriatrics, neurology, general medicine, clinical pharmacology, and cardiovascular disease, although the number of physicians who have undergone the required extra training in stroke care is small.

Eighty per cent of geriatricians take part in unselected medical emergency work and geriatricians are the largest specialty providing this work (22.6%).[12]

GERIATRIC MEDICINE IN OTHER EUROPEAN COUNTRIES

There has not been a comprehensive review of the state of geriatric medicine in each of the countries of Europe. However, national societies have produced summaries of their own activities, key features of training, and the current state of development of the specialty for the Web sites of the EUGMS (www.eugms.org) and UEMS (http://www.uemsgeriatricmedicine.org). Principal features have been listed below.

Austria. The Austrian Society of Geriatrics and Gerontology is involved in research on the aging process and diseases in old age, the production of guidelines, and the organization of scientific meetings alone and in collaboration with other German speaking countries. Geriatric medicine is not recognized as a specialty, although attempts to create a subspecialty have been made. Similarly geriatric medicine is yet to establish itself in the undergraduate curriculum and in academia. The process of developing specialist services in acute hospitals is progressing slowly. The society publishes two journals: *geriatrie praxis Österreich* and *Journal für Geriatrir*. (www.geriatrie-online.at).

Belgium. The Belgian Society of Gerontology and Geriatrics organizes two conferences a year. Geriatric medicine has been recognized as a full specialty since 2006 and a geriatric medicine department (acute and rehabilitation is present in each of the over 100 general hospitals in the country).

Bulgaria. The Bulgarian Association on Aging was founded in 1997 although there had been other societies previously. The specialty is only starting its development and an optional training program for undergraduates has been instituted in the Sofia Medical School. The association holds regular meetings for its multidisciplinary membership.

Czech Republic. The Czech Society of Gerontology and Geriatrics engages in the development of clinical practice, education, research, and national and regional government policies. It organizes scientific conferences and publishes the Ceska geriatrická revue and together with the Slovak Society of Gerontology and Geriatrics Geriatria. Although comprehensive services for older people exist in many places they are not yet universal. Academic units have been established in three of the country's seven medical schools.

Denmark. In Denmark geriatric medicine developed as part of the assessment for care home admission. Today, however, geriatricians are involved in all aspects of the care of older people including the emergency department. Geriatric medicine is one of nine internal medicine specialties.

Estonia. The Estonian Association of Gerontology and Geriatrics was founded in 1997 and has a multidisciplinary membership. Its mission includes raising the profile of older people and training and organizing scientific conferences.

Finland. Finland has one of the oldest geriatrics societies (founded in 1948) and organizes an annual conference and other symposia. Geriatric medicine is a recognized independent specialty previously having been a subspecialty of internal medicine, neurology, and psychiatry. There are professors of geriatric medicine in all Finnish medical schools and geriatrics is a compulsory part of the undergraduate medical curriculum.

Germany. The first German Gerontology Society was founded in 1938, reconstituted after both World War II and the reunification of Germany. A separate medical geriatric society was founded in 1995. Geriatric medicine is recognized as a subspecialty of internal medicine, family medicine, and neurology and psychiatry although there are variations in each of the Länder. The German Geriatrics Society favors a training program that graduates joint internal medicine/geriatrics specialists. Although geriatric medicine is a compulsory part of the curriculum, academic departments have only been established in a minority of medical schools. The German Geriatrics Society organizes scientific meetings and publishes the European Journal of Geriatrics.

Hungary. The first Hungarian congress on gerontology as held in 1937 and the XV World Congress of Gerontology was held in Budapest in 1993. Recognition of the specialty occurred only in 2000.

Iceland. Geriatrics is recognized as a subspecialty of internal medicine and is being considered as a subspecialty of family medicine. Although it is possible to train in geriatric medicine entirely in Iceland, trainees are encouraged to train overseas. Geriatrics is taught in the medical school and the Icelandic Geriatrics Society was founded in 1989.

Ireland. Ireland has traditionally spent less on health than other Western European countries and this is reflected in generally lower numbers of specialists than in comparable countries. The development of geriatric medicine in Ireland has in many ways paralleled that in the United Kingdom, although the first geriatrician was not appointed until 1969. These similarities include: the presence of geriatricians in all general hospitals, the involvement of geriatricians in acute medicine on-call duties, and dual training in geriatric and general medicine. The review of O'Neil and O'Keeffe in 2003[13] reported that there were at that time 41 geriatricians in the country, the largest specialty with internal medicine. Two models of care existed; an age-related service in the major teaching hospitals and an integrated approach in smaller hospitals where there may be a solo geriatrician working alongside four or five other medical specialists. The pattern of postgraduate training is very similar to the United Kingdom and there is cross-representation on many postgraduate training bodies. The Membership of the Royal College of Physicians (MRCP) in Ireland examination is recognized as equivalent to that of the MRCP UK. Most Irish geriatricians will have undertaken part of their postgraduate training in the United Kingdom or other countries. The Irish Society of Physicians in Geriatric Medicine was founded in 1979 but geriatricians are also active in the Irish Gerontological Society whose membership extends into Northern Ireland, part of the United Kingdom.

Italy. The Italian Society of Gerontology and Geriatrics was founded in 1950 and has a biogerontology, nursing, and sociobehavioral sections in addition to its large clinical section. It has conducted large scale national studies and publishes a number of journals including *Ageing Clinical and Experiemental Research* and *Giornale di Gerontologia*. It organizes an annual scientific meeting and a summer school for fellows.

Luxembourg. Luxembourg Society of Gerontology and Geriatrics was founded in 1985. It holds an annual conference.

Malta. There are five geriatricians working in this small island country. They work mainly outside the country's main acute hospital.

Norway. In Norway geriatrics is a subspecialty of internal medicine. The Norwegian Geriatrics Society holds a scientific meeting every other year but also takes part in Nordic congresses. Geriatrics is part of the undergraduate curriculum and there are professors in Oslo, Bergen, Trondheim, and Tromsø.

Spain. The Spanish Society of Geriatrics and Gerontology was founded in 1948 and has clinical, biologic, and behavioral-social sections. There are 2500 members, the majority of whom are physicians. In addition to a national conference, the Society publishes Revista Española de Geriatría y Gerontolgía. A second society, the Spanish Society of Geriatrics and Gerontology, was founded in 2000 and holds biennial scientific meetings and has published a number of books. A survey conducted in 2003 revealed that there were no acute geriatric care units in seven of the country's regions amounting to two thirds of the country's acute hospitals.

Slovakia. Slovakia recognizes geriatric medicine as a specialty with training following European guidelines. The Slovakian Society of Geriatrics and Gerontology includes among its roles the dissemination of knowledge about older people to physicians and other health care workers, policy development, activities aimed at ending age discrimination, and organizing scientific meetings. Its journal *Geriatria* is published four times a year.

Sweden. Geriatrics is recognized as a full specialty. Most geriatricians work in specialist services for older people with a minority working in primary care or internal medicine. The Swedish Society for Geriatrics and Gerontology organizes a scientific conference each year.

Switzerland. Geriatric medicine was recognized as a specialty in 2000 and the Swiss Geriatrics Society was founded shortly after that in 2002. Before that geriatricians formed a section of the Swiss Gerontological Society. The two Societies share the same administrative office. Most geriatricians initially trained in internal medicine before undertaking geriatric medicine training but a small number first became family physicians. Specialist training comprises 2 years in geriatric medicine and 1 year in old age psychiatry after the 5 years in either internal medicine or family medicine. A recent review of the health care of older people in Switzerland, while recognizing that per capita spending on health was one of the highest in the world, highlighted a number of areas of concern.[14] There was a tenfold variation in the number of geriatricians between urban and rural areas. The Swiss National Science Foundation had no specific program on aging research. Only three of the five medical schools have academic departments and there were insufficient opportunities to train academic geriatricians.

The Swiss Geriatrics Society participates in meetings of the Swiss Internal medicine and Gerontology Societies and Congresses in French and German-speaking neighboring countries.

Turkey. The Geriatric Society-Turkey was founded in 2003 and publishes the *Turkish Journal of Geriatrics*. Its aims include the promotion of health of older people, teaching about their health care needs, public education, and organizing scientific meetings.

GERIATRIC MEDICINE ORGANIZATIONS IN EUROPE

There are three major European organizations whose principal *raison d'être* is the advancement of specialty of geriatric medicine and the improvement of health care for older people. These are:

- The International Association of Geriatrics and (IAGG) (www.iagg.com.br)
- The European Union Geriatric Medicine Society (EUGMS) (www.eugms.org)
- Union of Medical Specialists – Geriatric Medicine Section (EUMS-GM). (http://www.uemsgeriatricmedicine.org/)

Although three of these bodies are autonomous; they share common goals and cooperate in a number of ways by, for example, offering board membership to the other organizations and by organizing joint sessions at congresses. Their structure, functions, and successes are described below.

IAGG

The IAGG is a worldwide learned society for all those interested in the health and welfare of older people. Its member organizations come from more than 60 countries with a combined total membership of over 45,000. It has consultative status with the United Nations and its subsidiary bodies. Founded in 1950 it has held 18 World Congresses and plans to hold the nineteenth in Paris in 2009. Its official journal is *Gerontology – International Journal of Experimental, Clinical and Behavioral Gerontology*.

The IAGG is organized into five regions: Africa, Asia/Oceania, North America, Latin America and the Caribbean, and Europe (ER). The latter region, IAGG-ER, (http://www.iagg-er.org) is itself organized into three sections: clinical, biologic, and behavioral social science. Its affairs are coordinated by an executive board elected every 4 years by delegates from European societies affiliated with IAGG. Some countries have more than one member organization (Table 118-3). For example, the United Kingdom has three societies affiliated to IAGG: The British Geriatrics Society (clinical), the British Society of Gerontology (social science), and the British Society of Research on Ageing (biologic).

The principal activity of the IAGG-ER is to organize scientific conferences, which are presently held every 4 years. The next one will be held in Bologna in 2011. The conferences comprise plenary sessions, symposia, and free communications organized by the three sections together with some cross-sectional events. The clinical section has held eight separate congresses, the first being in Berlin in 1992 and latest in Ostend in 2006 in association with the annual meeting of the Belgian Society of Geriatrics and Gerontology. A joint symposium with the British Geriatrics Society will be held in April 2009. The clinical section has their own president and secretary-general but only the president is a member of the board of IAGG-ER. Membership of the IAGG-ER includes countries outside the European Union and some outside the traditional boundary between Europe and Asia (e.g., Georgia, Israel). Ribera Casado[15] has reviewed the history of the clinical section.

EUGMS

The EUGMS is a relatively new organization founded in 2000. It held its first congress in Paris in 2001. Individuals are members of the EUGMS on the basis that their national society is a member. As the European Union has enlarged to encompass countries from Middle and Eastern Europe, the number of affiliated societies and members has steadily increased. It is possible that all national geriatric medicine societies in Europe will eventually affiliate. Current affiliation is shown in Table 118-3. Its affairs are coordinated by a full board consisting of representatives of all member organizations and others. This meets once a year and elects an executive board. The secretariat is based in the British Geriatrics Society headquarters in London.

The goals of EUGMS include continuing professional development, representation of the specialty to the European Union, guideline development, and the promotion of research and education. However, its most obvious visible activity has been the organization of major international conferences every 2 years with smaller subject specific symposia in the intervening years. The next conferences are scheduled to take place in Copenhagen in 2008 and Dublin in 2010.

Other activities have included the publication of guidelines on type 2 diabetes mellitus (http://www.eugms.org/index.php?show=search&query=diabetes) and syncope (http://www.eugms.org/index.php?show=search&query=syncope). On the political front, EUGMS interacts with both the European Commission and the European Parliament. EUGMS also has an official scientific journal *The Journal of Nutrition Health and Aging*. A position paper setting out EUGMS' priorities is abridged in Table 118-4.

The desirability of having two separate clinical societies in Europe has been questioned,[15] particularly as many organizations are members of both and several geriatricians hold or have held office in both organizations.

EUMS - Geriatric Medicine Section

One of the basic tenets of the European Union is the free movement of workers between its countries with each nation's qualifications being recognized in all members of the European Union. As far as physicians are concerned, this means that undergraduate and postgraduate diplomas and certificates are acceptable in each country without the need for further examinations. The EUMS, now in its fiftieth year, is the body charged with coordinating specialist education within the European Union.

Responsibilities for specialist training are divided between national authorities and EUMS. National bodies are responsible for the duration and contents of training, quality control, determining entry procedures, assessment, and control of numbers. EUMS is allowed to set minimum standards, which have to be met in each country.

EUMS is organized into numerous specialist sections, including one for geriatric medicine—European Union of Medical Specialists (EUMS) – Geriatric Medicine (EUMS-GM). The activities of the section are coordinated through a board, the current president of which is Ian Hastie of the United Kingdom. Countries represented on the board are shown in Table 118-3. National representation is via the recognized national medical body in each country. In the case of the United Kingdom, this is the British Medical Association although this is then delegated to each specialty society.

Geriatric medicine is recognized as a specialty in Belgium, Denmark, Finland, France, Germany, Ireland, Italy, The Netherlands, Spain, Sweden, and the United Kingdom. However, it is not recognized in Austria, Greece, Luxembourg, and Portugal. The situation in the "new" European countries in central and eastern Europe is in transition, with the specialty being recognized in the Czech Republic, Hungary, and Slovakia although these countries are not yet integrated into EUMS-GM.

The goals of the section are to promote the recognition of geriatric medicine in all countries of the European Union, to standardize training standards and requirements, and as a consequence to ensure that all older people in Europe have access to adequately trained geriatric medicine specialists. It is tackling these issues through a wide range of activities (Table 118-5).

Training and the Curriculum

The EUMS-GM has produced a curriculum (http://www.uemsgeriatricmedicine.org/important_documents/geriatric_training_-_condensed_version.pdf), which should serve as a basis for those produced by national bodies. In summary, specialist training should take place over a 4-year period preceded by 2 years in general internal medicine. One of the 4 years may be in research. Training should

Table 118-3. Member Organizations of the IAGG, EUGMS, and EUMS-GM

Country	Society	Member IAGG	Member EUGMS	EUMS-GM*
Austria	Austrian Society of Geriatrics and Gerontology	✓	✓	✓
Belgium	Belgian Society for Gerontology and Geriatrics	✓	✓	✓
Bulgaria	Bulgarian Association on Aging	✓	O	
Czech Republic	Czech Society on Gerontology and Geriatrics	✓	✓	✓
Denmark	Danish Gerontology Society	✓	✓	✓
Estonia	Estonian Association of Gerontology and Geriatrics	✓	✓	O
Finland	Finnish Gerontology Society	✓	✓	✓
France	French Society of Geriatrics and Gerontology	✓	✓	O
Georgia	Georgian Geriatrics and Gerontology Society	✓		
Germany	German Society of Gerontology and Geriatrics	✓	✓	✓
Greece	Hellenic Association of Gerontology and Geriatrics	✓	✓	✓
Hungary	Hungarian Association on Gerontology and Geriatrics	✓	✓	✓
Iceland			✓	✓
Ireland	Irish Gerontological Society	✓	✓	✓
Israel	Israel Gerontological Society	✓	O	
Italy	Italian Society of Gerontology and Geriatrics	✓	✓	✓
Luxembourg			✓	
Macedonia			O	
Malta	Maltese Association of Gerontology and Geriatrics	✓	✓	✓
Netherlands	Netherlands Society for Gerontology	✓	✓	✓
Norway	Norwegian Gerontology Society	✓	✓	✓
Poland				✓
Portugal	Portuguese Society of Geriatrics and Gerontology	✓		✓
Romania	Romanian Society of Gerontology and Geriatrics	✓		
Russia	Gerontology Society of the Russian Academy of Sciences	✓		
Serbia	Gerontology Society of Serbia	✓		
Slovakia	Slovak Society of Gerontology and Geriatrics	✓	✓	✓
Slovenia			✓	
Spain	Spanish Society of Geriatric Medicine	✓		✓
	Spanish Society of Geriatrics and Gerontology	✓	✓	
Sweden	Swedish Gerontology Society	✓	✓	✓
Switzerland	Swiss Society of Gerontology	✓	✓	✓
Turkey	Geriatrics Society Turkey	✓	O	
	National Association of Social and Applied Gerontology – Turkey	✓		
Ukraine	The Ukrainian Gerontology and Geriatrics Society	✓		
UK	British Geriatrics Society	✓	✓	✓
	British Society for Research on Ageing	✓		
	British Society of Gerontology	✓		

*= Countries represented on EUGMS-GM Board
✓= Full member
O= Observer Member

take place predominately in hospitals. Training institutions should be capable of delivering training and have a broad range of high-quality services. Research ethics and therapeutics committees should be in place. The director of training should be a specialist of at least 5 years standing, although it is recognized that exceptions may be needed. Training should comply with all national and international requirements and each trainee should have a named educational supervisor. Trainees should keep a personal logbook or other record of training. Emphasis is stressed on following both national and EU regulations.

The duration of training varies slightly from country to country. In the United Kingdom those wishing to become a geriatrician undertake the 2 years foundation program that all doctors have to complete. This is followed by 2 years of core medical training and then 5 years further training in both geriatric medicine and acute medicine. This qualifies the doctor to work in both geriatric medicine and in acute medicine. This pattern is similar to other medical specialists (e.g., respiratory medicine, diabetes) who also undertake acute medicine. In other countries, different routes exist. For example, for those just wishing to practice as geriatricians in the Netherlands, there is a common trunk in general medicine of 2 years and 2 years in geriatrics and 1 year in old age psychiatry. Consultants in general medicine with a special interest in geriatric medicine have to undertake 4 years in general medicine and 2 years in geriatrics, of which 6 months has to be in old age psychiatry. In Belgium trainees have to complete 3 years in general medicine and 3 years in geriatric medicine.

Table 118-4. Key Points from a Position Paper on the State of Geriatric Medicine in Europe*

- Geriatric medicine is involved in the medical care of older people with acute, rehabilitation, and long-term health conditions in the community, care homes, and hospitals.
- There is a need to harmonize geriatric medicine throughout Europe.
- Geriatricians are able to undertake a comprehensive assessment of the patient with cognizance of atypical presentation, comorbidity, and functional state.
- Undergraduate medical students and postgraduate physicians need training in geriatric medicine from suitably qualified teachers.
- There is a need to develop an objective-based curriculum for specialists.
- There is a need to increase research capacity in aging research.
- Guidelines on ethical issues in old age should be developed.
- There is a need for geriatricians to collaborate with other medical specialties and with allied health professionals to improve the health of older people.

*Adapted from Duursma S, Castleden M, Cerubini A, et al. European Union Geriatric Medicine Society. Position statement on geriatric medicine and the provision of healthcare services to older people. J Nutr Health Aging 2004;8(3):190–5.

Table 118-5. Achievements and Activities of the EUMS - GM

- The production of standards and curricula for specialist training in geriatric medicine
- The production of guidelines for the training of medical undergraduates in geriatric medicine and gerontology
- The production of a system of inspection of training posts and their accreditation for equivalent training
- Contributing to the development of a Master's in Gerontology diploma
- Contributing to the EU Manual of Internal Medicine
- Developing a database of information about the training opportunities and organization in the individual member states
- Disseminating information about the organization and practice of geriatric medicine and other issues including revalidation and continuing professional development
- Establishing a Web site of the geriatric medicine section, with links to national associations of geriatrics and gerontology
- Encouraging participation by all members and their trainees in the International Meetings of the European Union Geriatric Medicine Society

Adapted from http://www.uemsgeriatricmedicine.org/

The EUMS-GM has also produced a summary curriculum that considers learning objectives under the following headings:

- Basis of care and provision of appropriate services
- Assessment and treatment
- Rehabilitation
- Discharge planning
- Assessment for long-term care
- Research
- Medical education
- Development of geriatric services
- Administration
- Contribution to the nation's health service
- Clinical audit
- Professional development

There are considerable differences in the state of development and the role of the specialty within the health service in each European country. However, EUMS-GM has been able to produce a consensus statement defining the purpose of the specialty (Table 118-6).

Table 118-6. Definition of the Specialty of Geriatric Medicine

- Geriatric medicine is a specialty of medicine concerned with physical, mental, functional, and social conditions occurring in acute care, chronic disease, rehabilitation, prevention, social, and end of life situations in older patients.
- This group of patients are considered to have a high degree of frailty and active multiple pathology, requiring a holistic approach. Diseases may present differently in old age, are often very difficult to diagnose; the response to treatment is often delayed and there is frequently a need for social support.
- Geriatric medicine therefore exceeds organ-orientated medicine offering additional therapy in a multidisciplinary team setting, the main aim of which is to optimize the functional status of the older person and improve the quality of life and autonomy.
- Geriatric medicine is not specifically age defined, but will deal with the typical morbidity found in older patients. Most patients will be over 65 years of age but the problems best dealt with by the specialty of geriatric medicine become much more common in the 80 and over age group.
- It is recognized that for historic and structural reasons the organization of geriatric medicine may vary between European Member Countries.

Adapted by EUMS-GM on May 3, 2008.

European Academy for Medicine for Ageing (EAMA)

The need for a concerted effort to increase academic capacity in geriatric medicine in Europe has long been recognized. The linking of the development of the specialty to the state of academic geriatrics was identified by the Group of European Professors in Medical Gerontology (GEPMG).[16] This group suggested a number of concerted activities, including training junior faculty, the development of a core curriculum at both the undergraduate and the postgraduate levels, and the establishment of a professorship in what they called medical gerontology in every medical school. One of the outputs from this report was the establishment of the European Academy for Medicine of Ageing, which graduated its first cohort of potential geriatric medicine leaders in 1996.[17] The format of teaching comprised four 1-week sessions held in Switzerland, which covered a broad range biologic and clinical topics. A subsequent evaluation reporting on the first 10 years of the program[18] identified a number of factors, which the authors thought were important. These included the involvement of international leaders, the intense interactive nature of the course, and the international nature of the student body, which now includes younger geriatricians from outside Europe. A large proportion of the students were able to advance their careers but whether they would have done so without their involvement in this course is not clear. Further information about EAMA is available from its Web site (http://www.healthandage.com/html/min/eama/).

The European Masters Program in Gerontology (EuMaG)

This program is coordinated by the Free University of Amsterdam and is designed for professionals from both health and social science backgrounds to study in an interdisciplinary-fashion. Modules are offered in different countries and students can study individual modules or undertake the whole course. At the present time modules are offered in the Netherlands (Introduction to Gerontology), Germany (Psychogerontology), United Kingdom (Social gerontology, and France (Health Gerontology and Summer School). Modules are often integrated with local teaching programs thus enhancing the mix of students. Further details are available on http://www.eumag.org/

COLLABORATIVE RESEARCH IN EUROPE

The European Union fosters collaborative international projects through its Framework programs, which have been in existence since 1984. The current program (framework 7) includes a number of projects relevant to the needs of older people. These include: PREDICT: Increasing the participation of the elderly in clinical trials; SMILING: Self mobility improvement in the elderly by counteracting falls; RESOLVE: Resolve chronic inflammation and achieve healthy aging by understanding non-regenerative repair; CAPSIL: International support of a common awareness and knowledge platform for studying and enabling independent living; and HERMES: Cognitive care and guidance for active aging. More information is available at http://cordis.europa.eu/en/home.html.

Links between nongovernmental organizations

Nongovernmental organizations have also formed European collaborations aimed at influencing European policy and for mutual support. The European Older People's Platform AGE has as its aim "to voice and promote the interests of older people in the European Union and to raise awareness of the issues that concern them most." (http://www.age-platform.org/EN/). The European Healthy Ageing Advocacy Forum has been set up with the main aim of sharing best practices among advocacy groups and charitable organizations. The forum is a network of independent organizations from eight countries.

CONCLUSIONS

As has been described, the development of the specialty of geriatric medicine has progressed at varying paces in different European countries despite the demographic needs being relatively similar. A number of organizations have been established whose aim has been to advance the health care of older people by professional development within the specialty of geriatric medicine and related disciplines. Several geriatricians hold office in more than one of these organizations and it is therefore not surprising that calls for closer working have been made.[15,19]

The demographic and technological changes that are taking place are having similar effects on the development of policy regarding health care of older people with the move to the provision of more care in the home and with ever shorter hospital stays. This will impact on the role of the geriatrician, which is likely to see a greater presence outside the hospital than is currently seen and a continued role in the general hospital. It is of interest that a majority of leading European geriatricians opted for a division of geriatrics into a community and a hospital branch.[20] However, there is consensus that older people, particularly those with physical and mental health comorbidity, in whatever setting they are, need to be treated by trained doctors and allied health care practitioners.

For a complete list of references, please visit online only at www.expertconsult.com

Geriatrics in North America

David B. Hogan

INTRODUCTION

In this chapter we will examine the history and current state of geriatrics in Canada (2008 estimated population 33.4 million; per capita gross domestic product $42,738) and the United States (2008 estimated population 304.9 million; per capita gross domestic product $43,594), two countries with strong historical and economic ties. Although geriatrics developed in response to similar demographic pressures in both countries, it has evolved in a different manner. In this chapter we will not be covering developments in the Caribbean or Latin America, where demographic aging is less advanced and the challenges differ from those encountered in more developed countries.[1] Nor will we be dealing with antiaging medicine and the effort to decelerate, if not fully arrest, aging.[2]

As with other parts of the more developed world, the absolute number and the relative proportion of older individuals (or seniors) in Canada and the United States are increasing. Defining what we mean by senior, though, is not straightforward. The use of the chronologic age of 65 to sharply demarcate the start of old age reflects an arbitrary choice made by our society. It is not driven by a strong biologic or clinical rationale. If the term senior is used in a relative sense to describe the oldest segment of the age pyramid in our countries, we should have continuously revised our age cutoff over the last half century. In 1971, 8% of the Canadian population was 65 years of age or older. Today, the 8% who make up the top of the age pyramid are 81 years of age or older.[3] In this chapter we will stick with the "usual" definition of a senior as an adult who is 65 years of age or older.

Both countries had large post-World War II baby booms from 1946 until 1964 in the United States and 1966 in Canada. Currently (2008) there are 37.3 million Americans 65 years of age or older (12% of the population).[4] Over the next 2 decades there will be on average 1.6 million seniors added to the United States population every year. It is expected that there will be more than 70 million seniors in America by 2030[5,6] and 86.7 million (21% of the population) in 2050.[4] Similar changes will be taking place in Canada. Between 2006 and 2026 the number of seniors is projected to grow from 4.3 to 8.0 million, with their share of the population increasing from 13.2% to 21.2%.[7] Both countries will have to meet the challenge of dealing with this unprecedented growth in the number of seniors.

There has been a degree of angst among at least some about the potential cost implications of these increases in the senior population.[8] As an extreme example of this, in 1984 the then Governor of Colorado, Richard D. Lamm, was inaccurately but widely reported as saying that older Americans "got a duty to die and get out of the way."[9] Although a Chicken Little, alarmist reaction is clearly inappropriate, there are legitimate concerns about issues such as how aging Americans and Canadians are planning (or more accurately not planning) for their later years. Rather than putting sufficient money aside to deal with retirements that might last for 30 years or longer, in the United States people are saving less for old age now than they have in any decade since the Great Depression.[10] The growth in the senior population will lead to increases in health care use and costs if their health status remains the same and we carry on with our current practices. Although the majority of American seniors are in good health, per capita health spending averages three to five times higher than for younger adults.[11] Seniors currently make up 12% of the American population, but they account for a quarter of physician office visits, a third of all hospitalizations, and a third of all prescriptions.[12] Those with complex, chronic health problems in particular use the health and social care system more. It is important, though, to take a balanced view on the impact of population aging on the health care system. Although it will add to costs in acute care, population aging does not rank with the pressures arising from other drivers such as increases in per capita use or the implementation of new technologies.[11] It is anticipated that the health care impact of population aging will be primarily on the home and residential care sector.[3]

Geriatrics is the branch of medicine that focuses on health promotion and the study, understanding, prevention, and treatment of disease and disability in later life. The rise in the number of older people during the twentieth and twenty-first century has led to an increase in interest about this field of practice. The history of geriatrics in North America goes further back than most realize. The word itself was coined nearly 100 years ago in 1909 by a New York physician, Ignatz Leo Nascher. He stated that old age was as "distinct [a] period of life... as... childhood" and deserved "a special branch of medicine."[13] He later authored the lengthy textbook *Geriatrics: The Diseases of Old Age and Their Treatment* that was published in 1914, but he failed in making it an inviting field of medical practice.[14]

During the first half of the twentieth century medical care in Canada and the United States was organized and financed in a similar manner. It was only in the 1950s that we began diverging in a significant manner. A number of Canadian physicians and researchers who emigrated to the United States, such as Sir William Osler, infamous for *The Fixed Period* controversy,[15] played important roles in shaping American attitudes and approaches toward the aged during the first half of the last century.[14] The birth of scientific gerontology can be said to have occurred in 1939 with the publication of *The Problems of Ageing*. This was edited by the noted anatomist Edmund Vincent Cowdry who was born and educated in Canada but spent most of his professional career in the United States, principally at Washington University in St. Louis.[14,16] The American Geriatrics Society was founded in 1942, before the Medical Society for the Care of the Elderly (in 1959 renamed the British Geriatrics Society) in the United Kingdom.[16] Five Canadians have served as its president. One of them, Willard O. Thompson, was the founding editor of the *Journal of the American Geriatrics Society*.[14,16]

Most North American physicians working in the field during the middle part of the last century had "day jobs" that consumed most of their time. With few exceptions they did not work full-time as geriatricians. Their clinical focus was on preventing problems. Healthy old age was felt to be dependent on the involvement of a physician in the care of the older person. Health maintenance activities were emphasized.[17] The development of geriatrics as a full-time specialty area lagged behind the United Kingdom. As noted by John Grimley Evans, while "Ignatz Nascher invented the word, Marjory Warren created the specialty."[18] Both formal recognition of the field and the creation of training programs in geriatrics were slow to occur. It was not until 1977 that the Council of the Royal College of Physicians and Surgeons of Canada (RCPSC) recognized of geriatric medicine as a subspecialty of internal medicine.[14] That year the Institute of Medicine of the National Academy of Sciences in the United States concluded that a formal practice specialty in geriatrics should not be established. It was only in 1988 that the first American certifying examination in geriatric medicine were held (the first Canadian examinations took place in 1981).[14,16] The first American fellowship in geriatric medicine was established in the late 1960s by Leslie Libow,[16] whereas Canadian residency training programs were in place by 1980.[14]

A particular strength of geriatrics in the United States has been the breadth and depth of its research enterprise, which has come to dwarf activities elsewhere in the world. More than half (53.9%) of the articles published in gerontology and/or geriatric journals during 2002 were authored or co-authored by Americans.[19] This compares with 9.7% for contributors from the United Kingdom and 6.7% for Canadians, who ranked second and third, respectively.[19] The establishment of the National Institute on Aging (http://www.nia.nih.gov/) in 1974 was an important milestone in the United States. It helped legitimize research into aging, while support from the institute was important in establishing geriatric programs within American medical schools.[16] In 2000 the Canadian Institutes of Health Research (CIHR) was established. One of the 13 Institutes making up the CIHR is an Institute on Aging (http://www.cihr-irsc.gc.ca/e/8671.html).

Care of older patients

There are important differences between older and younger adults that should affect the care provided. Seniors typically have diminished physiologic reserves. Chronic conditions such as cardiovascular disease, stroke, diabetes, cancer, chronic obstructive airway disease, musculoskeletal conditions, and dementia are more common and when present often more severe. Of even greater importance is the frequent presence within an aging patient of multiple morbidities occurring in many different combinations. The vast majority (82%) of seniors have at least one chronic condition with 24% having four or more.[6] Geriatric syndromes (e.g., delirium, falls, incontinence, frailty), malnutrition, sensory impairments, and disability including impaired mobility are also common among seniors. With both the physical and social environment of the patient, they are all important considerations in the provision of care. Polypharmacy (the consumption of many drugs together) to deal with the symptoms, diseases, and risk states (e.g., hypertension, hypercholesterolemia, osteoporosis) frequently encountered by older patients has become the rule rather than the exception. This in turn can lead to problems with adverse drug effects, prescribing cascades, disease-drug interactions, drug-drug interactions, inappropriate prescribing, and nonadherence. The inherent complexity of older patients unfortunately leads all too often to fragmented, uncoordinated care provided by an array of specialists and subspecialists.

Most older patients are (and will be) looked after by physicians without advanced training in geriatrics. These physicians will require sound knowledge about health and illness in older patients, and how to mobilize available resources to meet their needs.[20] "Gerontologize" is the awkward verb used to describe both the dissemination by education of the principles of effective care of older patients within the various fields of medical practice and the integration of these principles within clinical practice guidelines. Although progress has been made,[6,20,21] further work is required. As with other sociodemographic subgroups,[22] there is room for improvement in the quality of care provided to seniors. The Assessing Care of Vulnerable Elders (ACOVE) study found that the care provided to community-dwelling seniors fell short of acceptable levels for a wide variety of conditions. The care for geriatric conditions (e.g., falls, incontinence) was generally worse than that for general medical ones (e.g., diabetes, heart failure).[23] Within the acute care sector, the overall incidence of adverse events (unintended injuries or complications resulting in death, disability, or prolonged hospital stay that arise from health care management) during hospitalization of adult patients in Canada is in the order of 7.5 per 100 hospital admissions with increasing age a statistically significant risk factor for their occurrence.[23]

Dealing with the unique needs of seniors must be integrated within the broader context of health care planning, policy development, and service delivery for the entire population. An example of this would be in emergency care. Both the 2003 heat wave in France and Hurricane Katrina demonstrated how they are at particular risk during disasters. Emergency planning has to take this into account.[25,26] It is furthermore predicted that emergency departments will be strained by the pending influx of aged baby boomers.[27] How emergency care is provided, especially to frail seniors, will have to be modified to deal effectively with them.[28]

Although improving the care of *all* older patients must be a goal of our respective health care systems, how do geriatricians (i.e., those with advanced training in the care of older patients) fit within this overarching aspiration? In the next section I will address this question.

Specialty practice in geriatrics

In the United States geriatric medicine is recognized as a subspecialty of internal medicine by the American Board of Internal Medicine and a Certificate of Added Qualification by the American Board of Family Medicine. A certifying examination is jointly offered by the two boards on a yearly basis. After completion of a residency in either family medicine or internal medicine, trainees are required to take at least a year of additional training in geriatrics to be eligible for the certifying examination. Very few trainees take more than 1 year of training.[6] There are now 145 training programs in geriatric medicine with 514 residency positions, but only 62% were filled.[29] The decision to lower the duration of training from 2 to 1 year in 1998 was controversial.[6,16] It was recently suggested that training programs be strengthened so that geriatricians would be better able to fulfill leadership roles.[30] About half of all physicians certified in geriatric medicine before 1994 have pursued recertification.[6] This rate is substantially lower than that seen for other subspecialties of internal medicine, and raises concerns about retention. Currently (2008) there are approximately 7100 American physicians certified in geriatric medicine.[6]

There are two recognized training options available for Canadian physicians interested in geriatrics.[31] Physicians who have completed their training in family medicine can enroll in a 6- to 12-month residency in Care of the Elderly accredited by the College of Family Physicians of Canada. Graduates of these programs do not have to take a certifying examination. Their training is intended to equip them to provide primary medical care to older individuals, work within specialized geriatric programs, and/ or function as a medical resource in the care of older patients for their community. Since it was first offered in the early 1990s, there have been about 140 graduates of Care of the Elderly programs. The second option is for those trained in internal medicine. They can take a 2-year residency in geriatric medicine.[30] These programs are accredited by the RCPSC, which also administers a qualifying examination for those who have successfully completed their residency. Residents are trained to provide clinical consultations on older patients with complex health problems in a variety of settings, including hospitals. Currently (2008) there are about 220 Canadian specialists in geriatric medicine. Although both training streams are separate, graduates from either can be involved in medical education, program development, research, and medical leadership. To date internist geriatricians have been those principally engaged in these activities.

Geriatric psychiatry is the subspecialty of psychiatry that deals with the assessment and management of mental disorders in later life.[31] Notwithstanding its long history in Canada,[14] the RCPSC has just recognized it as a subspecialty of psychiatry. Currently there are about 200 geriatric psychiatrists in Canada.[31] The American Board of Psychiatry and Neurology recognized the subspecialty in 1989. The postgraduate training requirement is 1 year.[6] There are approximately 1600 certified geriatric psychiatrists in the United States.[6] In 2008–2009 there were 57 American trainees in geriatric psychiatry compared with 743 enrolled in a child and adolescent psychiatry training program.[29]

There is general agreement that American physicians with additional training in the care of older patients should have major roles in meeting academic requirements in education and research, and providing medical leadership. There is greater debate in the delineation of their clinical role. Indecision and inconsistency about what geriatricians should do has hampered the growth of the field.[32] In the United States it was initially thought that these physicians would be principally concerned with the medical care of the residents of long-term care facilities. Then it was thought that they would be consultants equipped to manage complex cases on referral. Next there was an effort to redefine geriatrics as a primary care field, but current and projected future numbers have made it clear that American geriatricians cannot have a major role in providing primary medical care to unselected older individuals. In the United States (and Canada) linkages frequently exist between geriatrics and palliative care. Although the two areas are complementary, they do have distinct roles.[33]

Compared to the American situation, geriatric medicine in Canada has been more consistently seen as a consulting field. A disconcerting finding of a recent survey of Care of the Elderly graduates was that less than half were restricting or focusing their practice to seniors.[34] The rest appeared to be working as a "typical" family physician, which raises questions about the utility (to themselves and society) of their additional training in geriatrics.

A critical issue on both sides of our border is recruiting sufficient numbers of physicians into the field. See Table 119-1 for an overview of the training situation in Canada. The 38 Care of the Elderly and geriatric medicine trainees in 2008–2009 represented less than 0.8% of all Canadian trainees in family medicine and internal medicine that year.[35] This compares to the 546 trainees in pediatrics excluding subspecialties. That year 10 Care of the Elderly and 6 geriatric medicine trainees, a total of 16, entered practice—well less than what is needed to correct the current physician resource deficit, deal with population growth, and replace retirees. Table 119-2 provides similar data for the United States. The 320 trainees in 2008–2009 represented about 0.3% of all residents in training.[29] That year there were 8089 trainees (7.5% of all residents) in pediatrics.[29] Assuming current rates of training and expected attrition rates, the Association of Directors of Geriatric Academic Programs has projected a daunting deficit of approximately 28,000 geriatricians in the United States by 2030.[6] In neither country is there evidence of significant increases in the number of trainees entering the field.

Table 119-1. Number of Trainees Enrolled in Postgraduate Training Programs in Care of the Elderly (6–12 Month Program) and Geriatric Medicine (2-Year Program) in Canada (1998–2008)–Data From Annual Reports of the Canadian Post-M.D. Education Registry

	Care of the Elderly	Geriatric Medicine	Total
1998–99	8	28	36
1999–00	14	29	43
2000–01	13	25	38
2001–02	14	23	37
2002–03	16	24	40
2003–04	13	15	28
2004–05	10	15	25
2005–06	12	15	27
2006–07	10	19	29
2007–08	14	24	38
2008–09	13	25	38

Table 119-2. Number of Trainees from Family Medicine and Internal Medicine Enrolled in Postgraduate Training (1 Year Program for Most) in Geriatrics in the United States (1998–2007)–Data from Annual JAMA Issue on Medical Education

	Family Medicine	Internal Medicine	Total
1998–99	37	298	335
1999–00	42	326	368
2000–01	28	293	321
2001–02	36	302	338
2002–03	41	327	368
2003–04	47	305	352
2004–05	46	288	334
2005–06	50	301	351
2006–07	44	243	287
2007–08	46	246	292
2008–09	64	256	320

Barriers to recruitment include the poor pay compared with other fields of medical practice and its perceived lack of glamour. In the United States the financial return on obtaining additional training in geriatrics is negative—internists who take this additional training end up making *less* money on average than those who do not.[36] As noted by Robert L. Kane the "prospect of working hard for less money is not a strong recruitment device."[32] An example of the perceived lack of "sparkle" compared with other fields is the exchange between two characters in the then hit television medical drama *Grey's Anatomy*:

George: "Maybe I should have gone into geriatrics. No one minds when you kill an old person."

Cristina: "Surgery's hot. It's the marines. It's macho. It's hostile. It's hardcore. Geriatrics is for freaks who live with their mothers and never have sex." (Episode - A Hard Day's Night; first aired March 27, 2005.)

Geriatrics has faced persistent opposition from within the medical profession. This might be due to factors such as the misconception that geriatrics just means taking care of an older patient, the perceived threat of the field to the identity and finances of existing practitioners and/or the subconscious fear of physicians to their own aging.[33] All of these misperceptions plus others were present within the RCPSC Specialty Committee for Internal Medicine in the late 1970s. It had not been consulted before the Council of the RCPSC recognized geriatric medicine as a specialty in 1977. Once informed they expressed strong disapproval and on two separate occasions (1978 and 1979) passed motions "deploring" the recognition. Comments from the minutes of their meetings included: "Geriatrics is the business of internists… [and] segregation [of older patients]… [is] not in their best interests"; British geriatricians were described as "curators of parking lots"; and, geriatrics in England was called "the refuge for failed internists, and the elderly receive very indifferent care in settings apart from other medical patients." Members of the committee declared that geriatrics had no specific knowledge base and that advances were not being made by geriatricians but by clinicians and scientists in other fields. One member stated that "geriatric practice can be very depressing, and that physicians are more likely to perform well with a broad spectrum of patients."[14] Their protests were to no avail as the decision by the Council of the RCPSC was not rescinded, but the inescapable conclusion is that within at least some corners of organized medicine, geriatrics "like its patients, is disrespected and marginalized[5]" with little recognition of our knowledge base and the clinical skills of geriatricians.[10]

Although recommendations have been made to improve recruitment, it is uncertain how effective they would be even if implemented.[6,30,31,34,37] Because of the shortage in the number of geriatricians there appears to be no option other than restricting practice to the subpopulation of seniors with the most complicated needs. This underscores as well the importance for geriatricians to focus on teaching the core principles of good elder care to medical students, postgraduate trainees in various fields, and practicing physicians. Another option would be to look outside the confines of medical practice and consider building up a cadre of nurses with additional training in the care of older patients who could assume a greater role in the primary care of seniors and/or the provision of health services within long-term care facilities.[10]

We are gradually acquiring the knowledge needed to improve the care we offer our older patients. Early North American contributions in the clinical care of older patients have included supporting the widespread use of standardized assessment instruments, emphasizing the importance of function in addition to traditional disease categories when assessing an older patient, and in developing the concept of comprehensive geriatric assessment.[16] Innovative models of care ranging from comprehensive community-based services (e.g., Program for the All-Inclusive Care of the Elderly, Système de services intégrés pour personnes âgées en perte d'automonie) to those based in hospitals (e.g., geriatric evaluation and management programs, Acute Care of the Elderly units, approaches to the prevention of delirium such as the Hospital Elder Life Program) have been developed in North America.[6,38–40] Particularly exciting research is taking place with regard to dementia and frailty.[40] Advances have also been made in other areas such as safe drug prescribing and advance directives/bioethics.[41,42] The conceptual work being done on geriatric syndromes such as delirium, falls, and incontinence is already influencing clinical practice and will pay further dividends in the future.[43] Exercise is showing promise as an intervention for challenges as diverse as preventing cognitive impairment/dementia,[44] improving outcomes in hospitalized older patients,[45] managing various chronic diseases,[46] and improving balance/preventing falls.[47,48] On the other hand, efforts to slow the aging process with hormone replacement therapy have yielded disappointing results.[49] Although much has been learned, even more remains to be discovered. Research on interventions and novel models of care must receive ongoing support.

Future directions

WHERE SHOULD WE GO FROM HERE? ADVICE IS NOT LACKING

Robert Kane offered a choice of six nonmutually exclusive alternatives for American geriatrics: carry on as a marginal activity primarily based in academic medical centers; become the dominant model for the primary medical care of complex older patients combined with a hospital practice to address their special needs; see geriatric primary care becoming the purview of geriatric nurse practitioners with geriatricians functioning as consultants for particularly complex cases; work primarily in long-term care facilities with geriatric nurse practitioners; palliative care; or, become role models for chronic disease care (his preferred option).[32] The responses to Kane's paper were generally negative. Some felt that no change was needed as our time would come,[50] while others expressed concern about prematurely restricting potential future roles for the specialty.[51] Leslie Libow called on American geriatricians to clarify their identity. Although he felt that there was a place for geriatrics in acute care, he feared the field would lose its way if it became too committed to that setting. Others disagree, feeling that hospital care should be emphasized.[52,53] He felt that American society should "nurture the growth of geriatrics... (as) to create and sustain a health care system for the elderly... we must first attend to the health of geriatrics."[33] The Canadian geriatrician Colin Powell advised us to work within multidisciplinary teams, focus our attention on frail older patients, develop alliances with older adults, and become accountable to them and society.[54] In response to a news item about the critical shortage of geriatricians in the United States, a *Lancet* editorial challenged geriatricians to take on "the opportunities of education, research, advocacy, and collaboration presented by an aging population" and called on all other health disciplines to cooperate with geriatricians in improving the care provided to seniors.[5] Some believe it is already too late to train an adequate number of geriatricians to deal with the clinical needs of the coming tsunami of the aged and that we should focus our limited resources on training both other physicians and nonmedical health care providers.[10]

According to the American Geriatrics Society future geriatricians will be engaged in the design and implementation of systems of care for older persons while maintaining key clinical (both primary medical care for some seniors and leading teams caring for frail seniors and those with complex medical conditions), teaching, research, administrative, and consultant roles. Frequently they will be leading these activities but often they will be partnering with other physicians and health care providers.[30]

At the 2007 Banff Conference on the future of geriatrics in Canada there was discussion among attendees about what should be the principal responsibilities of geriatricians.[34] Advocacy for older persons and their care was considered important. The primary clinical role identified was to provide consultations on older patients with complex health needs (e.g., multiple chronic medical conditions, those requiring interdisciplinary/multidisciplinary care, frailty). A majority, albeit slim (57%), of attendees did not believe that geriatricians should provide primary medical care to even this subgroup of seniors. From an academic standpoint, it was felt that teaching should be primarily directed to those in medicine and other health care providers while clinical and health service research relevant to aging were highlighted as investigative areas requiring emphasis. It was felt that those trained in geriatrics had much to offer in policy and system development and program leadership/administration.

The challenges facing geriatrics in North America include more clearly defining the field of practice and marketing it to various stakeholders, in particular physicians in training. The path we should take is not clear and the direction followed might well differ in our two countries. The only given is that we must not fail in crafting the future of geriatrics to best meet the needs of our grandparents now, our parents shortly, and ourselves before long.

KEY POINTS

Geriatrics in North America

- Physicians without advanced training in geriatrics will provide most of the medical care received by seniors. Geriatricians have an important role to play in ensuring that these physicians receive appropriate training in the principles of effective care of older patients.
- In both Canada and the United States, the recruitment and retention of geriatricians has been poor. With the anticipated growth in the number of seniors, the short-fall in physician resources will reach a crisis level.
- In each country, steps must be taken now to clarify the desired roles and responsibilities of geriatricians within the health care system, the number required to fulfill these obligations, and to put into place a comprehensive strategy for the recruitment and retention of these physicians.

For a complete list of references, please visit online only at www.expertconsult.com

CHAPTER 120

Geriatrics in the Rest of the World

Jean Woo

There is variable information on elderly populations in countries other than Europe and North America. In general, characteristics of elderly populations in economically developed countries are similar to Europe and North America. This chapter describes the impact of demographic and economic changes on life expectancy, morbidity, and disability and responses of health and social systems to these changes, using countries representing different stages of economic development in the Western Pacific and Southeast Asian regions.

Life Expectancy, Morbidity, and Disability

In 2007 the percentage of population aged 65 years and above ranged from 3% to 4% in Laos and Cambodia, to 12% to 13% in New Zealand, Hong Kong, and Australia, to 21% in Japan (Figure 120-1). In general, with economic development, life expectancy increases and morbidity changes from higher prevalence of communicable to noncommunicable diseases. The causes of death from chronic noncommunicable diseases ranged from approximately 90% in New Zealand and Australia, 80% in Singapore, South Korea, Japan, and China, 50% in India and Myanmar, to 35% in Cambodia and Laos.[1] Life expectancy at birth is highest in Japan and the Hong Kong Special Administrative Region (SAR) of China (80%), and lowest in Laos (56%) (Figure 120-2). Ideally increasing life expectancy should be accompanied by compression of morbidity and disability. There is little available data to determine whether there is compression of morbidity and disability in Asia, nor what chronic diseases make the largest contribution to disability. In Hong Kong SAR, China, active life expectancy at age 70 years is approximately 10 years for both men and women; however, total life expectancy and the life expectancy lived with disability (DLE) are longer in women compared with men, DLE being 4.4 years in women and 2.2 years in men. Diseases making the largest contribution to disability are stroke, dementia, fractures, Parkinson's disease, and diabetes mellitus.

Chronic diseases of major impact in the elderly population

The prevalence of cognitive impairment among elderly Hong Kong Chinese aged 70 years and over is approximately 15% in two community surveys carried out in 1990–91 and 2001–02. Age, female gender, history of Parkinson's disease and stroke, functional disability, low education level and low social class and income, were predisposing factors. A review of epidemiologic studies on dementia in China showed rates at the lower end of the rates in Caucasians, with regional variation in the ratio of vascular dementia to Alzheimer's diseases.[2] The prevalence of dementia ranged from 0.46% to 7.0%, whereas the annual incidence ranged from 0.81% to 2.02%, being slightly higher in women and those with lower education. Alzheimer's disease was the predominant type of dementia, followed by vascular dementia. In contrast to western studies, the prevalence of Lewy body dementia was lower in Hong Kong Chinese, with a prevalence rate of 2.9% over a 2-year period.[3] Similar to Caucasian populations, presence of the apolipoprotein epsilon-4 allele is associated with more rapid deterioration in cognitive function,[4] and an association has also been observed between promoter polymorphism of the interlenkin-10 gene and Alzheimer's disease.[5]

Osteoporotic fracture is another common problem with major impact in terms of disability and mortality. It has been projected that 50% of all hip fractures in the world will occur in Asia by 2050. Increasing incidences have been documented for many regions, in Hong Kong, Japan, and Singapore, the rates being higher in urban compared with rural areas.[6,7] Risk factors were similar to those in Caucasian populations: lack of load bearing activity, smoking, alcohol consumption, past-history of stroke, fractures, greater height, use of sedatives and thyroid drugs, and low calcium intake.[8]

Chronic respiratory disease also causes considerable disability and mortality, being among the top causes of hospital admission and mortality for the elderly. Unfortunately the trend in respiratory symptoms appear to be increasing among the elderly, likely a result of environmental factors such as increasing air pollution, since smoking prevalence decreased at the same time.[9] Unfortunately governments in Asia tend to lag behind the West in acknowledging the health impacts of air pollution, and to take definitive action.

Frailty

The transition state from a fully functional state, with gradual decline and development of dependence toward death, may be viewed as a state of frailty. Geriatric medicine is largely care for frail elderly persons. The concept of frailty as an accumulation of deficits covering physical, functional, psychological, nutritional, and social domains, with the balance tipped toward deficits rather than assets, had been developed initially in a Canadian elderly population, and an index consisting of summation of deficits in many domains used as a quantitative indicator of frailty,[10] and shown to predict mortality, and may be used as a measure of biologic age. This concept of a frailty index had been tested in a Hong Kong Chinese elderly population aged 70 years and over, and shown to be equally applicable in a different ethnic and cultural setting irrespective of which particular variables were measured.[11] It was able to predict mortality, functional, and cognitive decline,[12] and was influenced by social and environmental factors in keeping with the concept of frailty being multidimensional.[13]

A characteristic feature of frailty is sarcopenia, which describes the age-associated loss of skeletal muscle mass and loss of strength even in the absence of disease. The underlying cause is thought to be a consequence of a decrease in androgens, growth hormone, and IGF-1 that occurs with aging, accompanied by an increase in inflammatory cytokines. This is an important concept in geriatric medicine

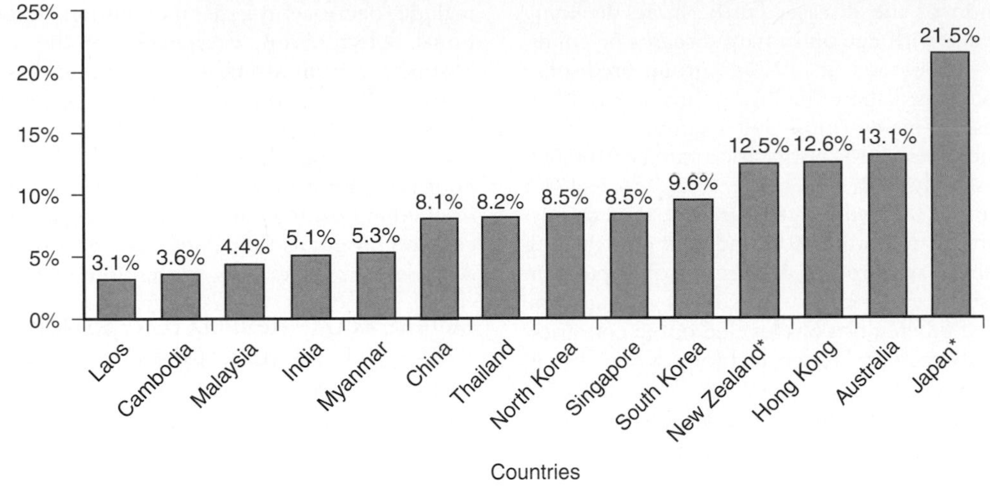

Figure 120-1. Percentage of population aged 65 and above, 2007. *(Sources: Sources: CIA World Factbook; Department of Statistics of Malaysia; China Population Information & Research Centre; Department of Statistics of Singapore; Statistics New Zealand; Census and Statistics Department of Hong Kong; Australian Bureau of Statistics; and Statistics Bureau & Statistical Research and Training Institute of Japan.)*

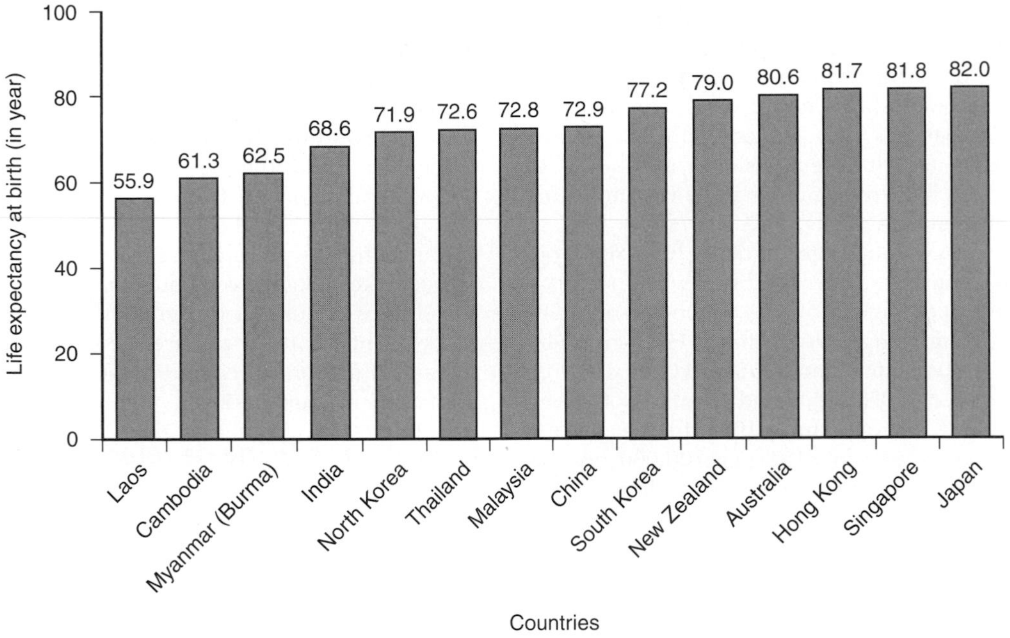

Figure 120-2. Life expectancy at birth (both sexes), 2007. *(Source: CIA World Factbook.)*

because it affects function and hence independence, and predisposes to falls. It was initially defined as a mean value of appendicular skeletal muscle mass divided by [height]^2 less than 2SD below mean values for young adults, analogous to the definition of osteoporosis. Using this definition, sarcopenia exists in elderly Hong Kong Chinese aged 70 years and over, but apparently at a lower prevalence (12.3% in men and 7.6% in women) compared with Caucasians (between 16% and 57.6% in men and 11% and 60% in women).[14] However, the Asian young adult mean value was about 15% lower compared with published Caucasian figures, so that the actual prevalence may be similar between Chinese and Caucasians. Older age, cigarette smoking, chronic lung disease, atherosclerosis, underweight and physical inactivity were associated risk factors, while the consequences include poorer physical well-being, slower walking speed and chair stand, and reduced grip strength.

Communicable diseases

Elderly people are particularly susceptible to pneumonia, with common infection agents being tuberculosis, *Streptococcus pneumoniae, Haemophilus influenzae,* and a virus affecting the respiratory tract.

TUBERCULOSIS

Many of the current generation of people aged 70 years and above would have been exposed to *Mycobacterium tuberculosis* before chemotherapy and vaccination became available, particularly during periods of deprivation such as during the World Wars. Therefore tuberculosis in the elderly is largely due to reactivation of the disease. Furthermore declining immunocompetence with age and many diseases or conditions commonly encountered in this age group predispose to tuberculosis, such as diabetes mellitus, chronic renal failure, malignancies, or malnutrition. For example, in Hong Kong in 2007, the tuberculosis notification rate per 100,000 population rose steeply with age, being 55.2, 156.5, 464.5 in the 20 to 24, 65 to 69, and 85+ age groups, respectively. Similarly the mortality rate was 0, 9.4, and 63.9 per 100,000, respectively, in these age groups. As a result of population aging and increased prevalence of tuberculosis with age, the falling incidence of tuberculosis has leveled out in countries, with significant tuberculosis burden in Hong Kong, Japan, Singapore, and Malaysia.

Certain clinical features of tuberculosis are distinctive for elderly patients. Diagnosis is often delayed in the elderly.[15] A study of patients with tuberculosis in Hong Kong showed that elderly patients had more frequent nonspecific complaints and less frequent hemoptysis, more extensive lung infiltration on chest x-ray, and lower serum albumin concentrations.[16] Mortality from tuberculosis is higher in the elderly, likely due to delayed diagnosis, more extensive disease, and presence of multiple morbidity. The elderly are also more susceptible to adverse effects from antituberculous drugs as a result of pharmacokinetic changes with age,[17] hepatic involvement in military tuberculosis, and undernutrition, as in some parts of India. Reduced protein binding of antituberculous drugs with age and slower metabolism of toxic metabolites such as hydrazine, may contribute to the increased incidence of side effects.

Residents of old age homes are particularly at risk from tuberculosis, as a result of factors predisposing to reactivation of latent tuberculosis and also cross infection. For example, a survey in Hong Kong SAR China in 1993 showed a rate of between 1200/100,000 and 2600/100,000 compared with a rate of between 100/100,000 and 400/100,000 in the general population.[18] A larger study 10 years later gave a prevalence of between 530 to 1101 per 100,000 population,[19] indicating perhaps improvement in the old age home environments. In an environment where TB prevalence is high in the general population, the Mantoux test is not a useful method for screening or surveillance, and chest x-ray and sputum examination would be more useful. For the same reason, isoniazid prophylaxis for those who have a positive Mantoux test is not adopted, more attention being paid toward infection control, such as optimal nutrition, adequate ventilation, and avoidance of overcrowding.

INFLUENZA-LIKE ILLNESS (ILI)

ILI is of particular concern among elderly people living in old age homes, as a potential cause of epidemic outbreaks, and a common cause for hospitalization. A prospective clinical and microbiologic survey of ILI in a cohort of people living in old age homes in Hong Kong SAR China over a 1-year period recorded 259 episodes in 194 out of a total of 771 subjects, with mild peaks in winter and summer, over a sustained level throughout the year.[20] An infection agent was identified in 61.4% of episodes, 58.3% of which were bacterial and 46.7% were viral. Organisms encountered in order of frequency were *S. pneumoniae*, respiratory syncytial virus, *Pseudomonas aeruginosa*, metapneumovirus, and parainfluenza viruses types 1 and 3. Presenting clinical features commonly include "decrease in general condition," cognitive and functional deterioration, irrespective of the underlying cause. Distinction from aspiration pneumonia was difficult and an unknown proportion could have this as the underlying cause. Mortality was high, being 10% for the episode, predisposing factors being MRSA infection, low body mass index, and poor premorbid function. Eighty-seven percent of episodes resulted in hospital admissions. There may be a role for vaccination programs to include organisms other then influenza A alone, as is the current prevention policy.

SEVERE ACUTE RESPIRATORY SYNDROME (SARS)

The occurrence of the SARS outbreak in Hong Kong in 2003 was a very good example of failure to recognize atypical presentation of disease in the elderly resulting in outbreaks in old age homes caused by elderly people contracting the disease from hospital admissions during the epidemic and then spreading to other residents on discharge, as the diagnosis was missed. In an effort to curb the spread in old age homes, the Hong Kong Geriatric Society issued a position statement pointing out the limitations of the World Health Organization criteria for SARS, stating some elderly people may have geriatric syndromes only, such as falls, confusion, incontinence, and poor feeding.[21,22] Furthermore, diarrhea may be mistaken for fecal incontinence. Multiple morbidity such as aspiration pneumonia further confuse the picture. Therefore a contact history was a key factor in consideration of the diagnosis. Other points to note are a lengthened incubation period from 14 to 21 days, higher incidence of side effects to ribavirin and corticosteroids, and a higher mortality rate. The latter could be a result of delayed diagnosis or reduced likelihood of ventilator support for those with multimorbidity. Failure to recognize the diagnosis constituted a risk of infection for all caregivers, and this pathway was repeatedly demonstrated during the months of the epidemic from March to June in 2003.

Geriatric medicine development

Apart from Australia and New Zealand, where geriatric medicine is well developed, care of elderly people tends to follow an organ-based approach, with the focus on individual diseases rather than on geriatric syndromes and frailty. The spectrum of geriatric medicine from the biomedical model to functional capacity, the immediate surroundings of an elderly person, ethical issues, and quality of life requiring interdisciplinary continuity of care, is not widely recognized. Countries that have been under British rule or influence, and that are economically developed, tend to adopt a perspective following that in the United Kingdom and North America. To address this issue, ideally undergraduate curricula should contain mandatory geriatric medicine teaching, with structured postgraduate training. Provision of undergraduate and postgraduate training is highly variable, being well-developed in some countries such as Australia, New Zealand, and Hong Kong. In mainland China, although large cities have developed geriatric clinical services and research centers, most of the physicians are from system-based specialties, so that training in geriatric syndromes and a holistic approach is lacking. However, there are developments in this area in collaboration with countries where geriatric medicine training is well developed. For example, the China Medical Board of New York funded a 4-year project between John Hopkins

University School of Medicine and Peking Union Medical College Hospital in Beijing, where Chinese staff were initially trained in the United States and then established demonstration services in Beijing using the train the trainer concept.[23] The geriatric units in Hong Kong have also participated in training staff from the mainland.

Comprehensive geriatric assessment

A key feature of geriatric medicine is comprehensive assessment. Some of the tools used in comprehensive geriatric assessment developed in Western populations may not be applied to other populations with different ethnicity, language, and culture. Translation and validation are required before tools can be incorporated into part of the assessment procedure. This process has been carried out among Chinese for the Mini Mental State Examination,[24] where a cover cut-off point of 18 was used as a large majority of the current elderly population received no or little education; the Geriatric Depression Scale (cut-off point of 8)[25]; the London Handicap Scale (LHS)[26]; and the Philadelphia Geriatric Morale Scale (PGMS).[27] The LHS appears to be applicable across cultures, with subjects from mainland China, Hong Kong, and the United Kingdom sharing similar perceptions on selected handicap scenarios.[26] The factor structure of the PGMS has also been confirmed in Hong Kong Chinese.[27]

Scales are particularly useful in assessment of dementia. The Alzheimer's disease assessment scale cognitive subscale (ADAS-log) has been validated in elderly Chinese in Hong Kong, and discriminant function analysis between demented and nondemented subjects yielded a canonical discriminant function with three question items, word recall test, orientation, and comprehension of speech.[28] The short version had a sensitivity of 90%, specificity of 94.6%, and overall accuracy of 92.5%. The clock drawing test as a quick screening assessment of dementia has also been validated, a cut-off score of 3/4 having a positive predictive value of 98%.[29] Likewise, the Chinese version of the Community Screening Instrument for Dementia (CSI-D) has been validated as an educationally independent instrument sensitive enough to detect early stages of the disease.[30] A short memory questionnaire has also been developed for screening of mild cognitive impairment, which also correlated with subjective memory complaints.[31]

Another important domain for assessment, particularly among elderly living in institutional settings, is the detection of undernutrition or malnutrition. The latter is a recognized risk factor for adverse health outcomes and mortality. One of the widely used nutrition screening tools is the Mini Nutritional Assessment (MNA) originally developed in Europe. It consists of questions regarding intake of particular food items and anthropometric measures, with classification into three categories of nutritional status. However, it may not be easily translated into populations with different body size and dietary habits. Furthermore, in some settings it may not be possible to measure body weight due to absence of suitable scales for dependent subjects and lack of manpower, as in many old age homes in China and Hong Kong. A screening tool that does not depend on weighing is all the more important in such settings. The MNA was adapted for use in the Chinese population in such settings and validated in institutional settings in Hong Kong and Shanghai (The Chinese Nutrition Screen: CNS).[32] A cut-off value of ≥ 21 was found to be useful in screening out those at risk or had malnutrition, correctly identifying 90% of those with normal nutritional status.

Health and social services

To complement the development of comprehensive geriatric assessment, appropriate health and social services meeting the needs of the elderly in the acute, convalescent, rehabilitative settings, along with long-term care in the community or residential care setting are required.

PRIMARY AND SECONDARY HEALTH CARE

Accessibility to good primary health care partly depends on provision of health care professionals and the health care financing system. A wide spectrum of health care systems exists in Asia, Australia, and New Zealand. At one extreme there is the predominantly government subsidized low cost system in Hong Kong SAR, China, to the other extreme of largely user pays private system dictated by market forces in mainland China. In between are systems sustained by insurance, government contributors, and part self-payment, as in Singapore, Japan, Australia, and New Zealand. The system of one primary care doctor as the first contact point, as in the British National Health Service, is particularly suited for care of the elderly. The development of health care centers, with the primary care doctor coordinating all health social needs using the case management model, would have provided a more flexible response to the needs of people with increasing frailty. Variations of such systems exist in Australia and New Zealand, but are poorly developed particularly where primary care largely relies on a user-pays system.

For example, the change from a government-funded to a market-orientated health care system in mainland China in the 1980s has resulted in the system serving a small proportion of the population who can afford to buy insurance, mainly in urban areas, where employers may make a contribution to a medical savings account. However, in rural areas, health care expenditure is largely out of pocket.[33,34] In one recent survey, 87% of rural and 37% of urban residents were uninsured, and seniors, ethnic minorities, and residents in less-developed regions (where there are few doctors and geographic barriers exist) visited physicians less than those who were insured. Urban residents also used hospitals more compared with rural residents. Therefore it is likely that both financial barriers and adequacy of provision of health care will affect health of the elderly in mainland China.

In contrast, the health and social care system in Hong Kong SAR China represents the other extreme, where the government largely subsidizes the health care system, with the user paying a small fee. For those who cannot afford the fee, after means testing, the same level of care is provided entirely free. Although more than 85% of primary care is provided by private doctors, those who cannot afford it are cared for by government outpatient clinics, or users may make use of 24-hour access of the accident and emergency departments. The standards of care supplied by government hospitals are as high, if not higher than private hospitals, patients having access to the latest drugs and technology. The comprehensive range of medical and social services have developed over the years based on the U.K. model. There are well-developed acute and nonacute geriatric and psychogeriatric services that extend to the community and old age homes, palliative care for both cancer and noncancer patients, day hospitals, various types of social welfare allowances and community support home care services. Currently models for chronic disease management and transitional care in the community are being developed.[35] However, the current health care financing system is considered unsustainable and insurance and user pays models are being developed.

There is little data reporting on the health profile of elderly people cared for under different health and social care systems. The question of whether there is one particular model that would result in better health outcomes, while of key importance, is difficult to address as a result of many confounding factors. A comparison of health profile of three elderly Chinese cohorts carried out at approximately the same (1990–1991) under opposite extremes of the spectrum of health care systems (predominantly government subsidized or predominantly self-paying), showed that the Beijing rural cohort had the best health profile while the Hong Kong cohort had the worst profile, despite better lifestyle practices and higher socioeconomic status in the Hong Kong and Beijing urban cohort. However, the Beijing rural cohort also had the highest prevalence of functional limitations.[36] The findings suggest that while the relationship between health care systems and life expectancy may be more direct, the influence on health profile elderly people may be more complex, as lifestyle, socioeconomic, and psychosocial factors are likely to play important roles.

LONG-TERM CARE

The number of frail elderly people with multiple morbidities, functional, and psychological impairments requiring care by others, will increase with aging populations. Although development in community support services is important in enabling elderly people to remain at home, development in the residential care sector both in terms of number of places and quality of care will be equally important. The anticipated shift from community to residential care is partly the result of changing social patterns from large extended families living together, to smaller units or to living alone. For example although the percentage of elderly people in Japan living with adult children is higher then Western populations, it fell from 50% in 2000 to 45.5% in 2004.[37] This is in contrast to 30% of men and 38% women aged 80 years and older living alone in Australia. In both Japan and Australia, the number of residential care places is increasing rapidly, while at the same time the provision of community care services also increased, although the provision ratio per 1000 persons aged 70 years and over is actually decreasing in Australia. In Hong Kong, the percentage of elderly people living in residential care institutions has also risen rapidly from about 5% to 9% over a 12-year period. Therefore it would be unrealistic to expect that improvement and increased provision of community service alone would be sufficient to meet the needs of increasingly frail aging populations.

An essential feature of community care is a seamless interface between health and social services, and between care by different disciplines of health care professionals and volunteers. Coordination is required to provide care plans specific to individual needs. The actual models vary depending on health care financing systems. For example in Hong Kong, various types of community care centers run by nongovernment organizations have evolved, covering a wide spectrum of support from social centers; day care centers, which provide personal and rehabilitative care during daytime; and enhanced home care (visits by allied health staff, nurses, or doctors).

There is a role for information technology support for those living in the community. In Hong Kong, for those living alone, they can subscribe to an alarm system where an alarm bell can be worn as a necklace and connected via the telephone system to community centers. In an emergency such as a fall, the center can arrange ambulance transport to the nearest hospital. Home rehabilitation via teleconferencing with a rehabilitation center has also been pioneered; a group therapy in community centers conducted by staff from a partner hospital via teleconference has also been developed and evaluated for older persons with memory problems,[38] knee pain,[39] diabetes,[40] urinary incontinence,[41] and stroke.[42] Evaluation showed that this mode of service delivery is feasible and resulted in beneficial objective outcomes.

As in many parts of the world, the quality of care in residential care homes is variable and there is much room for improvement. The change in philosophy in residential care from an institutional environment to a home environment with dedicated trained care workers pioneered by the Green House Project homes in the United States, while producing impressive results,[43] have yet to be replicated in Asia. In this region, quality of care is largely governed by fiscal concerns and the rising demand despite questionable quality. Regulating standards of care effectively determines the number and the care staff needed, with resulting increases in fees that adversely influence affordability. In many regions, a pragmatic balance exists between total lack of care, and residential care of variable quality that is affordable to individuals and governments. Poor quality has repeatedly been documented in the past 20 years among residential care homes in Hong Kong, for example in the area of undernutrition[44] and restraint use.[45] Twenty-five percent of residents have a body mass index of less than 18.5 kg/m^2, while use of restraints is among the highest in the world. Nevertheless efforts have been made in providing health care support by geriatric and psychogeriatric outreach teams supplemented with teleconference consultation.

The future of long-term care of acceptable quality likely depends on a health care financing system consisting of a mixture of government subsidy, insurance, and self-payment. Geriatricians will have a vital role in developing systems appropriate to the culture and region, with a key element of comprehensive assessment to tailor made services in response to individual needs.

END OF LIFE CARE

There is a general consensus that end of life care could be improved, and palliative services should also cover those who are dying of chronic diseases such as heart failure, chronic lung disease, or end-stage neurodegenerative diseases, in addition to those dying of cancer, even though the trajectories toward death may be different. The core components of symptom control and attention to psychospiritual needs remain the same. However, there may be cultural differences in management of patients and their families in these settings. For example, many elderly people defer to their families, who sometimes adopt an approach that is futile against the recommendation of the physician, out of a wish of "doing their best" for their relative. Improved public education would be desirable to discuss these issues. In Western cultures, spending the last few days in privacy with relatives in a side room in the hospital may be considered desirable, but among Chinese people in Hong Kong, it may be reviewed as neglect by staff and relatives have sometimes complained about such management that was assumed by health care workers as desirable.

Prevention of chronic diseases and functional decline

Health promotion efforts have been made by many countries in an attempt to lessen the morbidity and disability burden of aging populations by advocating healthy lifestyles. A key to effectiveness of dietary and physical activity counseling is the strategy for achieving behavioral change, since simple impartment of knowledge is unlikely to be effective. An interesting cultural addition to these efforts is the role of traditional Chinese Medicine (TCM) in healthy aging.[46] The philosophy of TCM is to treat diseases before they appear, thus fulfilling the role of prevention very well. Theoretically and at cellular level or in animal studies, TCMs have been shown to inhibit uptake of neurotransmitters, to have anabolic effects, immunoenhancing effects, and antiproliferative effects on tumor cells, antioxidant properties, stimulate nitric oxide production in endothelial cells and erectile tissues, inhibit platelet aggregation, improve glucose tolerance, and have estrogen-like properties. However, few have been subjected to randomized controlled trials to document benefits in humans. Nevertheless, TCM is widely used in prevention of various conditions associated with aging, which may or may not be effective. However, adverse side effects have also been documented.

CONCLUSION

The importance of geriatric medicine appears to be proportional to demographic changes with increasing life expectancy and the shift from communicable to noncommunicable disease, and it is in variable stages of development in parts of the world other than Europe and North America. Training systems and models of care in the latter would be relevant, with adaptation to local needs. The principles of care of the elderly remain unchanged, and could form the basis of training irrespective of geographic or political regions. Development in previous British colonies or commonwealth countries show how this diffusion of knowledge has occurred and is ongoing, through formation of the Asian Pacific Geriatrics Network. The latter has annual meetings where geriatric problems from different countries in the region are discussed and provides a forum for continual sharing of knowledge.

KEY POINTS

Geriatrics in the Rest of the World

- Life expectancy and the proportion of population aged 65 years and over increase in parallel with economic development of countries
- Patterns of diseases change from dominantly communicable to noncommunicable, in parallel with this transition
- Chronic diseases of major impact include dementia and other neurodegenerative diseases. Communicable diseases of impact are tuberculosis, and bacterial and viral causes of pneumonia
- Frailty is a key component in geriatric medicine, and measurements are applicable across ethnic and cultural groups
- Scales used for comprehensive geriatric assessment may need to be adapted and validated for local use
- Health and social care systems vary across countries, and the impact on health of the elderly is uncertain
- Geriatric training and service development follow the principles developed in Europe and North America, with adaptation to local systems and needs

For a complete list of references, please visit online only at www.expertconsult.com

CHAPTER 121

Geriatrics in Latin America

Jorge H. Lopez
Renato Maia Guimarães

INTRODUCTION

From Mexico in the north to Chile and Argentina in the south, there are 20 countries in Latin America (LA) and some other greater economies in the Caribbean. Notwithstanding the cultural interface, countries are not uniform in showing great diversity in demography, economy, and political organization. From the 561 million people living in this region, about 5.7% are 65 years and over.[1] From the middle twentieth century to the present, the region has shown an accelerated aging of its population. The rate of this demographic change has been so fast that the state, society, and families have been unable to develop adequate mechanisms to confront the health, cultural, and economic demands of the aged.[2,3,4,5] In the region, the process of population aging is very different from that experienced by the developed countries; in the latter, the process took place at a rather slow pace (over a period of 2 or more centuries) and was preceded by improvements in social and sanitary conditions. The dependency ratio (people 65 and over / people 15 to 64 years old) reflects the economic impact of aging. It will increase from 9% in 2000 to 13.4% by the year 2020 (Table 121-1).This makes clear the economy in the region will have to grow vigorously to be able to support pension schemes and other social needs of old people.

Life expectancy at birth for the quinquennium 2005 to 2010 in LA is expect to reach 73.3 years for both sexes; 70.1 years for men and 76.6 for women, lower than in the United States where it is expect to be 79.4 years (75.5 for men and 83.3 years for women). Table 121-2 shows life expectancy at birth in selected countries. It is noteworthy that countries such as Costa Rica and Chile have reached life expectancy near to that of United States, with differences smaller than a year for both men and women. However, life expectancy at birth in less developed countries may be misleading because it includes deaths at early ages and does not reflect that millions are living longer. Life expectancy at age 65 shows little difference in relation to the United States where it is 18.4 years compared with 17.5 years in LA.[6] Thus Latin Americans who achieve the age of 65 may remain alive for as many years as old people living in more developed countries.

The socioeconomic situation in LA is far from ideal.[7,8] The unemployment rate in the region is 8%, reaching 15% in the Dominican Republic, in Haiti more than two thirds of the labor force does not have a formal job. The illiteracy rate among people 15 years and older is 9.5% for LA as a whole, with Uruguay having the lowest rate (2%), and Haiti the highest (45%). Furthermore, poverty indices are very high; it is estimated that about 31% of the total population is poor and 8.6% are indigent. In countries such as Bolivia and Honduras more than half of the population live under the poverty line.[1] Some examples are shown in Table 121-3.

Demographic transition

The demographic transition model of a population begins with a sustained decline in mortality, followed by a decline in fertility. The early stage of this model is characterized by high rates of fertility and mortality contrasting with the very advanced stage, which has low mortality and fertility, added to population growth near zero or even negative.[5]

In the middle of the twentieth century. the majority of countries in LA were in the early stage of demographic transition with Uruguay being the only country in the full stage, with low mortality, stable fertility, and limited population growth. At present no country is in the early stage, even in Guatemala and Haiti mortality is decreasing. Most countries are in the full demographic transition stage. Argentina, Brazil, Costa Rica, and Chile are in the advanced stage, with a population annual growth rate that fluctuates between 1% and 1.4%, whereas Uruguay and Cuba are in the very advanced stage, with annual population growth rates of 0.6% and 0.3%, respectively.[3] By 2030, Brazil will rank sixth in the world in absolute number of old people with 30 million being 60 years and over.[9] It is of concern that the majority of the older population, a group that poses great demands on health care, will live in less developed countries, where little resources are available to attend to those demands.[10] At the beginning of the demographic transition, the rate of dependency is high as a result of high fertility, followed by certain relief as fertility declines. In LA this situation is only temporal, as the rapid aging population will increase the demographic dependence, something expected to occur around 2020.[3] Inequality in LA is very wide and grows deeper with advanced age.[11] Aging and its health and social consequences may act like an amplifier of inequality. It is difficult to be young and poor; however, it is worse to incorporate the burden of some condition that may be present in old age to an already poor person.

Epidemiologic transition

In 1971, Omran[12] formulated his epidemiologic transition theory, proposing that mortality is a fundamental factor in population dynamics; that a long-term shift in mortality and disease patterns occur during the transition; that the deepest changes in the models of health and disease appear in children and women in fertile age, and changes in health and disease are associated to the demographic and socioeconomic transition. A model characteristic of less developed countries proposed by Omran describes the changes over time in three major stages: (1) pestilence and famine, (2) receding pandemic, and (3) the triple health burden. Most of the countries of LA are in the third stage of the epidemiologic change.[13,14,15] The triple burden of health refers, in the first place, to the persistence of some old diseases, especially infections. In LA for example, many countries still have higher rates of infection such as tuberculosis, malaria, or dengue, among others.[16] A second aspect of the triple load refers to the increase in the rate of prevalent pathologies, especially chronic diseases such as obesity, blood hypertension, and diabetes mellitus.[17] An ill-prepared health care system characterizes the third stage, emphasizing that a particular country is not in a good position to cope with the new challenges.[9,10,18]

In Peru, for example, the mortality rate declined from 21 per 1000 in 1950 to 6 per 1000 in 1995, period infant

Table 121-1. Ratio of the Population Aged 65 and Over to the Population Aged 15–64 (percent)

Country	2000 %	2020 %
Argentina	15.7	18.0
Cuba	15.1	21.1
Mexico	8.4	13.0
Brazil	8.3	13.2
Colombia	7.5	12.0
Venezuela	7.3	11.8
Latin America	9	13.4

Source: Cepal. 2007.[1]

Table 121-2. Life Expectancy (Years) at Birth for the Quinquennium 2005 to 2010 in Some Selected Latin American Countries and United States

Country	Total	Men	Women
Bolivia	65.5	63.4	67.7
Brazil	72.4	68.9	76.1
Colombia	72.8	69.2	76.6
Venezuela	73.8	70.9	76.8
Argentina	75.2	71.6	79.1
Mexico	76.1	73.7	78.6
Uruguay	76.2	72.8	79.9
Cuba	78.3	76.8	80.4
Chile	78.5	75.5	81.5
Costa Rica	78.8	76.5	81.2
Latin America	73.3	70.1	76.6
United States	79.4	75.5	83.3

Source: Cepal. 2007.[1]

Table 121-3. People Living in Poverty and Indigence in Latin America (% of the total population)

Country	Poverty*	Indigence†
Chile	13.9	3.2
Argentina	21.0	7.2
Mexico	26.8	4.4
Brazil	29.9	6.7
Peru	31.2	4.9
Colombia	45.4	18.2
Bolivia	53.8	20.2
Honduras	59.4	30.0
Latin America	31.1	8.6

Source: Cepal.[1]

**Percentage of population having incomes amounting to less than twice the cost of a basic food basket. Includes indigent population.*

†Percentage of population having incomes amounting to less than the cost of a basic food basket.

Table 121-4. Percentage of People 65 Years and Over With Pension in Some Latin American Countries

Country	People Older Than 65 Years With Pension (%)
Brazil	81.5
Argentina	66.2
Chile	45.5
Venezuela	39.0
Peru	37.0
Costa Rica	36.0
Bolivia	11.9

Source: Suarez, Pesceto.[5]

mortality declined from 159 per 1000 to 42 per 1000. The reduction in the mortality rate in LA has been very fast when compared with the developed Western countries, where the rate of mortality dropped from 25 per 1000 inhabitants in 1860 to near 10 per 1000 in 1930; it means this phenomenon lasted almost the double when compared to what happened in several LA countries.[16] Nevertheless, the epidemiologic transition process in some countries of the region did not follow the same course of the developed ones because there is an overlap in stages. There is an increase in the prevalence of chronic noncommunicable diseases coexisting with a resurgence of certain infectious diseases, such as malaria and leishmaniosis, a phenomenon that has received the name countertransition.[19] Cardiac diseases in countries such as Cuba, Costa Rica, and Chile represent approximately 30% of the deaths, whereas in El Salvador, Guatemala, and Ecuador they represent less than 5%.[20] For instance, about 1955 in Mexico transmissible diseases accounted for 70% of all deaths, but now are 12%; on the other hand, in the same time period the ratio of deaths due to noncommunicable diseases increased from 23% to 75% of all deaths.[21]

It is then evident that the LA epidemiologic transition model varies between certain countries, and there are even variations within different regions of a same country, given the great social and economic gaps existing among them.[16,20,22] Three major groups of epidemiologic transition can be distinguished in the region: (1) countries that are in the advanced stage, (2) countries that are in the initial stage, and (3) an intermediate group of countries in an epidemiologic transition known as a prolonged polarized model, with superposition of stages; prolonged transition; countertransition, and epidemiologic polarization.[20]

The answer of Latin America to the new demands

RETIREMENT POLICIES

In the countries of the world with highest incomes per capita, people retire younger, so that the participation of elders in the workforce is lower, and only 13% of men older than 65 years are economically active. In contrast, in the less favored countries, 39% of men older than 65 years are still economically active,[6] with percentages in LA ranging between 18% in Uruguay and up to 47% in Bolivia.[3] This is due to a limited coverage by the pension programs and to pensions being insufficient to cover the basic needs. In most of the social security systems of the region, pensions values are defined in accordance with the person's income at the age of retirement, and by the time the employee contributed to social security. In many countries the social security system coexists with social care systems based on pensions, subsidies, or bonuses to poor elderly and handicapped people who did not have any formal work and were unable to make contributions to social security.[5,23] Half of the people 65 years and over in LA do not have any pension system or savings that allows them to cover their needs, and they depend to a great extent on the support of their families or charitable organizations. The proportion of old people that receive some type of pension or retirement varies between the countries, Nicaragua being lowest with a coverage of only 6.3% and Brazil the highest with 81.5%.[5] Table 121-4 shows the percentage of people older than 65 years with pension in some LA countries.

As a consequence of the demographic changes there have been substantial reforms in the social security pension systems in the majority of the LA countries in recent years. These reforms are of such magnitude that experts consider this to be the biggest change in just so short a time ever to happen in the history of social security so far.[24] Chile has made a deeper reform and th World Bank considers it an example for the world. The type of reform preferred by the governors of the region was one directed toward the privatization of the pension system, moving from a collective system to an individual one. The argument, not yet validated, was that this system would grant the financial viability of pensions, making them more efficient, by increased savings and investment.[25] Another challenge identified with pension reform is the accentuation of gender inequality. In several countries of the region, it has become evident that women are less covered by social insurance than men, and that the amount of their pensions is inferior.[25] The average amount of annual pension received by the beneficiaries varies from approximately $960 per year in Peru and Venezuela, up to $6000 a year in Chile and Costa Rica.[5]

HEALTH

The theory of compression of morbidity proposes that health prevention and assistance could delay the expression of morbidity allowing people to age with less morbidity and disability.[26] Nevertheless an analysis of old people health in developing countries suggests expansion more than compression of morbidity.[27,28] This can be explained by the concept of health capital and aging proposed by Guimarães.[29] It posits that health status in old age reflects life time events, including genetics, social economic factors, formal education, and health support. Thus the health condition of elderly people who survive in adverse conditions in many Latin American underdeveloped countries reveals a low health capital, with a low functional reserve and high prevalence of disability, as consequence of a lifetime of deprivation.

In Latin American countries the share of the gross domestic product (GDP) destined to health fluctuates between 1.6% (Venezuela) to 6.9% (Cuba), with the vast majority being below the 5%.[3] At times of economic crises the mortality among the elderly can increase. This was the case in Cuba at the time of embargo, when an increase of 15% in the mortality of people 65 years and older was observed. A similar increase was observed in Mexico in 1995 due to the economic crisis.[30] Notwithstanding, health goes beyond the viability of doctors. It can appreciated how some countries such as Nicaragua have a limited health human resource with a doctor for every 2568 inhabitants, whereas in Uruguay there is a doctor for every 248 persons. (Table 121-5).[3]

Like in most of the world, women in LA live longer, but they also live more years with disability.[31] A study in Brazil found that although men at the age of 60 years have a life expectancy of 17.6 years, from which 14.6 (83%) are free from functional disability. At the same age women can hope to live 22.2 years, 16.4 years (74%) without disability.[32] Studies on the health of the elderly in Mexico have found that approximately 40% of those over 80 years old, and 66% of those over 90 years old are unable to perform lighter domestic tasks and, likewise, this functional limitation is greater among women.[30] The major study on health of the old people in LA is the SABE study (Salud, Bienestar y Envejecimiento: Health, Well-being, and Aging), a multicentric project conducted by the Pan-American Health Organization (PAHO). It included 10,891 people 60 years and older, living in seven big cities of the region (Bridgetown; Buenos Aires; Havana; Mexico City; Montevideo, Uruguay; Santiago, Chile; and Sao Paulo). Data from that study show that a high percentage of old people have a poor self-perception of their health. For example, 49.1% in Bridgetown, 53.4% in Sao Paulo, 62.6% in Havana, 63.2% in Santiago, and 69.4% in Mexico DF, perceived their health as being either fair or poor. This study also documented that the prevalence of basic daily life activities fluctuated between 13.8% in Bridgetown to 23.7% in Sao Paulo, where 40.3% also referred to difficulties with instrumental activities.[33] The SABE study also focused on basic problems, such as falls and dementia. The prevalence of falls varied from 21.6% in Bridgetown to 34,0% in Santiago.[34] The prevalence of cognitive decline evaluated by the Mini Mental State Examination (MMSE) was 1.1% in Montevideo and 12% in Sao Paulo.[33] The wide difference may reflect problems in methodology because it also contrasts with the result of a survey that of 2,000 old people living in the community in Brazil using the DSM IV criteria (Diagnostic and Statistical Manual of Mental Disorders), where a 2% prevalence of dementia was found.[35]

Table 121-5. Some Health Indicators in Latin America - 2005

Country	Inhabitants/ Physician	Hospital Beds/ 1000 People
Uruguay	248	1.8
Argentina	319	—
Brazil	356	2.4
Costa Rica	558	1.3
Ecuador	696	1.6
Chile	776	2.3
Mexico	738	0.7
Nicaragua	2568	0.8

Source: Cepal. 2007.[3]

There is a cultural tradition in Latin America of families given support for their older relatives. The Latin caregiver (usually a daughter) tends to spend more time with their old or ill relative,[36] a fact that can cross the borders. A study done in San Francisco, for example, found that female Latin caregivers delayed the institutionalization of their old relatives with dementia when compared with female caregivers with Caucasian origin. In addition, when comparing both groups using Kaplan-Meier curves, a higher life expectancy was found among the Latin elderly with dementia compared with Caucasians.[37]

HEALTH OF THE ELDERLY IN RURAL AREAS

Twenty three percent of the total population in Latin America lives in rural areas.[3] In contrast to what happens in developed countries,[38] these areas usually have precarious sanitary and health services, which render the old particularly vulnerable and prone to suffer serious health situations. It has been seen that, even when sick, elders living in rural areas look less for health services than those living in urban areas.[22] In Costa Rica, a country with a high percentage of rural population (37%),[3] it has been demonstrated that old people living in the countryside are at a high risk of not being seen by specialists or not being hospitalized when they merit it because of their health conditions.[39]

Several studies have analyzed other health topics of the elderly in LA rural areas. In Mexico, for instance, it was found that the chronic diseases most frequently reported by old people in rural areas were blood hypertension, diabetes mellitus, and cardiopathies,[40] that is to say, pathologies similar to those found in urban zones. In the countryside of the Colombian coffee region, 1668 people with an age average of 71 years were studied; 83% of them reported a fear of falling, and half of them restricted their activities as a result of this fear.[41] Nevertheless a study in Brazil found that women who live in the countryside have a significantly smaller risk of having walking limitations than the women from urban areas.[42]

Development of geriatric medicine in Latin America

In LA the increase of the old population has not been matched by a parallel increase of professionals and services in gerontology and geriatrics. Doctors specialized in geriatrics are few, a characteristic also shared by developed countries. In the United States, there are about 7000 geriatricians to take care of 38 million old people, which is equivalent to one geriatrician for each 5500 people 65 years and older,[43] a number similar to that in Uruguay with 5000, and Costa Rica with 5300 (see Table 121-6). The development of geriatrics in Latin America is quite heterogeneous, with countries that have already gone a long way on the matter such as Brazil, Mexico, and Argentina, passing by other countries where the specialty is relatively young, such as Colombia and Peru. In many countries such as Paraguay, Panama, and Bolivia, geriatrics do not exist or is rather scarce. Apart from a few exceptions, geriatric medicine is not integrated into hospitals and it is practiced more as an outpatient service. A progressive inclusion of geriatric medicine in the national health system can be observed in Chile and Brazil.

The Argentinean Society of Gerontology and Geriatrics (Sociedad Argentina de Gerontología y Geriatría) was created in 1951 and the specialty approved in 1977.[44] Brazil was also one of the first LA countries in developing a Society of Geriatrics, which is already older than 45 years, and has training programs in geriatrics for doctors since the late 70s. However, there is only one specialized doctor in geriatrics for every 37,000 old people.[45] Table 121-6 shows the number of people 65 and over per geriatrician in some LA countries.

Table 121-6. People 65 Years and Over Per Geriatrician in Some Latin American Countries

Country	65 Years and Over Per Specialized Doctor in Geriatrics
Uruguay	5.000
Costa Rica	5.300
Argentina	7.200
Mexico	18.000
Peru	19.000
Brazil	37.000
Ecuador	41.000
Chile	48.000
Colombia	100.000

Source: Values obtained from geriatricians of every country, and references 1, 44, and 45.

Geriatrics and geriatric research in Latin America

One of the main recommendations expressed in the Madrid International Plan of Action on Aging is to stimulate research on aging, mainly in less developed countries.[46] This makes sense considering the enormous demographic, social, economic, and health burden that these countries will face in coming years, added to the little amount of research originated in these countries. An investigation done in 2002 to analyze the origin (by countries) of the investigation in gerontology and geriatrics supports this appreciation: 95% of the research in aging came from the wealthiest countries. More than half (54%) of the research was done in the United States, followed by the United Kingdom (10%), and Canada (7%). Only 1.4% of the published works come from Latin America, with 85% of the scientific publications in this region coming from only three countries: Argentina (37%), Brazil (31%), and Mexico (17%).[47] Only 122 scientific articles on geriatrics and gerontology were found in LA between 1980 and 2000, most of them indexed in the LILACS database (Literatura Latinoamericana y del Caribe en Ciencias de la Salud or Latin American and Caribbean Health Sciences Literature), 32 of them published between 1980 and 1989, and 90 published between 1990 and 2000. This demonstrates an increasing interest on the subject, although research clearly continues to be scarce. However, it should be noted that the best researchers tend to publish their papers in international journals. The majority of papers published in Latin America were qualitative (approximately 60%), whereas the rest (approximately 40%) were quantitative. In 54% of them the main subject was geriatrics, whereas in the remaining 46% the main subject was gerontology.[48] Added to the fact that research on the subject is scarce, it is also noteworthy to point out that, in some cases, the publication of scientific research is very little, as it was demonstrated by an investigation in Peru, where it was found that only 19% of the research work was published, with 86% of it being a descriptive investigation.[49]

The scarcity of research in LA is also demonstrated when the clinical trials database from the United States National Institutes of Health is reviewed: from approximately 60,000 trials registered, little more than 3000, or only about 5%, are being carried out in the region. Table 121-7 shows some examples in LA and Table 121-8 shows them broken down by regions.[50]

Perspectives of geriatric medicine in Latin America

As in the rest of the world, the fast population aging in LA contrasts with the slow development of economic, social, and health policies necessary to deal with the huge challenges that this great and unprecedented change demands. It is widely documented that there are not enough highly qualified human resources necessary to take care of the older population. This situation is evident not only in health sciences but also, and perhaps in a more marked way, in other areas of knowledge on aging, and, in the short term, there seems not to be strategies designed to attend to this need.

Table 121-7. Top 10 Latin America and Caribbean Countries, According to Number of Trials Registered in the US NIH Clinical Trial Database

Country	Number of Clinical Trials
Brazil	897
Puerto Rico	800
Mexico	742
Argentina	657
Chile	335
Peru	293
Colombia	201
Costa Rica	83
Guatemala	77
Panama	57

Source: www.clinicaltrials.gov.[50]

Table 121-8. Number of Clinical Trials Studies Registered in the US NIH Clinical Trial Database By Regions

Region	Number of Clinical Trials
North America	36.843
Europe	12,415
Asia	8324
Latin America and the Caribbean	3221
Oceania	1815
Africa	1309

Source: www.clinicaltrials.gov.[50]

Although the great majority of countries in LA signed the Madrid International Plan of Action on Ageing, 2002,[46] very few governments can show concrete results after 6 years. In most medical schools students are trained in the care of children, pregnant women, and adults, but training in care for the elderly is little, especially from a bio-psycho-social perspective. Teaching geriatrics is in its first steps. It is also necessary to qualify nonmedical health personnel such as nurses, physical therapists, dentists, psychologists, and social workers with the purpose of integrating interdisciplinary teams able to attend the old.[51]

At the postgraduate level in medicine, besides to prepare geriatricians, it is also important to train specialists from other clinical and surgical areas in the care of the old. It is widely known that, among others, urologists, ophthalmologists, orthopedists, and anesthesiologist, attend to a high volume of geriatric patients, although they have received very little or no formal training at all in how to attend to the elderly.[52,53]

ACKNOWLEDGMENTS

Thanks to Dr. Diana Palacios for revising and correcting part of the manuscript, and to Dr. Carlos Gonzalez' helpful aid in translating part of the paper. The following doctors also gave invaluable help to the authors: Luis M. Gutierrez-Robledo (Mexico), Laura Bazaldua (Mexico), Jose Gonzalez (U.S.), Daniel Valerio (Costa Rica) Patricio Buendía (Ecuador), Pedro P. Marin (Chile), Luis Varela (Peru), Ricardo Jaúregui (Argentina), Clever Nieto (Uruguay), and Fernando Gómez (Colombia).

KEY POINTS

Geriatrics in Latin America

- From the 561 million people living in Latin America, about 5.7% are 65 years and over and life expectancy at birth for the quinquennium 2005 to 2010 is expected to reach 73.3 years for both sexes.
- In this region, it is estimated that about 31% of the total population is poor and 8.6% are indigent.
- In the countries of the world with the highest incomes per capita, only 13% of men older than 65 years are economically active; in contrast, in the less favored countries, 39% of men older than 65 years are still economically active.
- Half of the people 65 years and over in Latin America do not have any pension system. They depend to a great extent on the support of their families or charitable organizations.
- The major study on the health of old people in Latin America is the SABE study (Salud, Bienestar y Envejecimiento: Health, Well-being, and Aging); data from that study show that more than half of old people perceived their health as being either fair or poor.
- Twenty three percent of the total population in Latin America live in rural areas, which usually have precarious sanitary and health services and render the old particularly vulnerable and prone to suffer serious health situations.
- As in the rest of the world, the fast population aging in Latin America contrasts with the slow development of economic, social, and health policies necessary to deal with the huge challenges that this change demands.

For a complete list of references, please visit online only at www.expertconsult.com

CHAPTER 122

Long-Term Care in the United Kingdom

Clive Bowman

LONG-TERM CARE IN THE UNITED KINGDOM

The history of long-term care in the United Kingdom is curious mix of benevolence, denial, and pragmatism driven more by social conscience and political pressure than intelligent epidemiologic understanding of needs and planned services. The key issue of quality of life rather than its length being a guiding principle is widely accepted, in stating "I would want to live as long as my quality of life is good and I can look forward to each new day."[1] Kirkwood succinctly represents a widely held view. It is a curious phenomenon that while strenuous medical endeavors to prolong life continue, the nature of life in long-term care remains inadequately described and understood.[2]

Poor law policies of the nineteenth century sought to provide refuge for the destitute, the unemployed, the sick, the blind, people with epilepsy and the elderly. The principle was to offer a standard of life below the lowest achievable by anyone in employment with the intention of deterring idleness. The advent of the National Health Service (NHS) in 1948 incorporated beds providing long-term care for elderly and disabled people into the service. The NHS inherited a motley collection of chronic sick wards in municipal hospitals, workhouse infirmaries, former infectious diseases hospitals, and sanatoria. From this unpromising estate geriatric medicine (GM) emerged. The main purpose of GM was the supervision of patients in these beds (and the many hundreds on lists waiting to occupy them). The reports by Warren and other pioneers highlighting the potential for rehabilitation and restoration to independence through accurate diagnosis, effective treatment, and the provision of rehabilitation[3] kick-started more positive attitudes. Through the 1950s and 1960s the management of long-term care remained the core of geriatric practice, but this concerned primarily the activity of managing a scarce resource, avoiding long-term care through comprehensive clinical and social assessment, treatment and rehabilitation together with increasing support at home. Although there were individual initiatives and innovation, the profile and the clinical and social aspects of the care of people in long-term care did not receive such attention or investment.

In 1962 Townsend published "The Last Refuge," a study of residential institutions and homes for the aged in England.[4] The study concluded that communal homes were "not adequately meeting the physical, psychological, and social needs of the elderly people living in them, and that alternative services and living arrangements should quickly take their place." The number of geriatric beds in the NHS remained virtually unchanged from 1959 to 1985, with improved and new treatments, rehabilitation, and community care counterbalancing increasing numbers of older people. From 1986 to 1994, the number of these beds declined with beds in private and voluntary nursing homes increasing dramatically (see Table 122-1). Similar trends were apparent in the local authority residential home sector with an increase of 136% in private and voluntary homes. Hospitals for patients with mental illness also provided a good deal of long-term care for elderly people but the psychogeriatric beds were separately counted and distinguished in official statistics from 1988.[5]

Cochrane's monograph of 1971,[6] "Effectiveness and Efficiency," predicted the inflation of acute health care and a widening gap in the standards between curative endeavor and caring. Isaacs et al[7] described in 1972, "The Hard Core" of patients that a geriatric service traditionally looked after and emphasized that only well coordinated health and care services could respond effectively to the needs of this group. In the early 1970s, these people were still largely the result of neglect, poverty, and despondency of the frail, isolated, sick, and dispossessed old. Improvements in both living standards and aspects of health and care have considerably addressed the issues of, "filth, hunger, cold, and danger" confronting the frailest. However, Cochrane's prescient concerns regarding the organization of care have largely been unheeded.

In the early 1980s, a crisis in housing and health care resources led to social security payments being made available on demand, without assessment of needs, for residential and nursing home care. This resulted in a rapid development of an independent sector eager to satisfy a seemingly unending demand. The total scale of this expenditure escalated from $14.5 million (£10 million) in England and Wales in 1979 to $275.5 million (£190 million) in 1983, $636.5 million (£439 million) in 1986, and $3.62 billion (£2.5 billion) in 1992.[8] The rapid, uncontrolled expenditure favored institutional care and prompted a review from which the report "Caring for People" in 1989[9] emerged. This resulted in renewed promotion of domiciliary services to enable people to live in their own homes whenever feasible and sensible, with an emphasis on proper assessment of need and case management, in essence these introduced needed hurdles to access care. The role of the independent sector was affirmed along with good quality public services. Social service departments became responsible for the assessment of need, offering various choices, including wherever possible, domiciliary support as an alternative to residential care. These recommendations were enshrined in the National Health Service Community Care Act, 1990.[10] Means testing, a longstanding feature of social services support, was effectively extended to frail older people who previously could have anticipated free NHS care, albeit typically in outdated Victorian wards. The architects of the welfare state did not include a commitment to fully state-funded care and support for older people. With greater personal wealth, care has increasingly become dependent on "self-funding" until personal resources are diminished to a proscribed level. Concurrently an increasing reliance on top up payments has emerged to be paid from remaining savings, family, friends, or charity to supplement fees from local authorities. Although testing has hallmarked social care there remains a provision for fully NHS funded or "free" care either in hospitals or more recently in

Table 122-1. Provision of Residential Care Places, United Kingdom 1980–1994/5

	1980	1985	1991–92	1994–95
LA residential homes	134,500	137,100	117,400	86,400
Independent residential homes	80,000	130,400	203,100	218,200
Independent nursing homes	26,900	38,000	147,300	194,800
NHS geriatric/ long stay	46,100	46,300	44,300	34,700

Source: Department of Health, UK.

the community at large and in care homes for people with a poorly defined level of complexity and frequency of care.

The anomaly of access to free NHS care for some and means tested care for others based perhaps as much by chance as assessed need has proved particularly unpopular especially among middle-class families, many of whom saw their inheritance threatened, often successfully challenging flawed decision making. Difficulties in eligibility assessment have continued with complaints for fully funded care dwarfing all others to the health service ombudsman and repeated revisions to policy reflecting more a need to control resource allocation than understand the health care needs of the aging population. Present policies for funding care are widely considered to be unfit for the purpose and at the time of writing (June 2008) there is intense consultation and a hope that a green paper will pave the way to a sustainable political solution to the issue of overall care funding and its financing for the individual.

The cost of long-term care has dominated debate and with some 80% of government funding committed to care home fees together and the desire to maintain people in their own homes unsurprisingly has meant continued pressure to keep people out of care homes. On occasion extraordinary packages of domiciliary care have been provided to maintain people often socially isolated in their own home, while the limited supply of community workers has meant that people with lower levels of support have found access to care much more difficult. At the same time pressure on funding in social care has led to people being placed in residential care rather than professionally led care in nursing homes. Financial settlements of local authorities have competing statutory demands such as child protection services placing further pressure on funding. One of the many frustrations is that policies that attempt to modernize or change the place of care tend to be substitutional rather than encouraging a spectrum of solutions to provide for a range of needs.

Rigorous eligibility assessment, and improved availability of housing options led to a reduction in the number of care home beds, in 2000, 9700 beds were reported to have closed, 7267 from the private and voluntary sector, and 2481 places from local authority homes.[11] The number of care home places have fallen steadily for more than a decade, from 511,000 at a peak in 1993 to 420,000 in 2007.[12] More recently a point of inflection has been reached with the reduction of beds seems to have slowing.

The dissolution of medical leadership in long-term care

The medical supervision, leadership, and multidisciplinary care that had been a feature of traditional geriatric care in the United Kingdom since the inception of the NHS has not followed patients to community care whether it be in the individual's own home or in care homes, and the established professional time and clinical teams have been redirected largely to support acute hospital medicine. Increasingly, general practitioners have had the responsibilities thrust upon them, generally without contractual incentives or training to develop appropriate patterns of care often in the absence of input from specialists.[13] Discontinuities and inconsistencies in health care rapidly have become evident.[14] Two surveys of consultant involvement in long-term care,[15,16] produced similar findings with between 60% and 66% carrying out ward rounds once weekly or more often, although 15% visited the wards only monthly or less frequently. The day-to-day care of patients was generally by doctors in training or contracted general practitioners, these arrangements provided a continuity of the skills and craft of the medicine of long-term care and a defined responsibility to a consultant.

The demands on general practitioners to support patients housed in care homes have generally have been incorporated into existing work routines rather than attributed defined time. As there are some three care home beds for every NHS hospital bed, it is unsurprising that care has been reactive rather than planned, proactive, or anticipatory. The consequence has been that an inadequate model of care[17] has evolved. The tradition of geriatric care has been compromised[18] with both primary and secondary health care now offering little more than a fire-fighting service to the most vulnerable. Local innovation and adaptations have occurred but their effectiveness is largely unknown; moreover, the clinical oversight of long-term care has become largely unregulated and beyond scrutiny.

Despite emphasizing on the need for preadmission assessment to avert inappropriate institutionalization, evidence continues to indicate shortcomings. A multicenter audit in the late 1990s of nursing home admissions revealed that only 40% of admissions had undergone specialist geriatric or psychogeriatric preadmission assessment.[19] A small single center prospective study accepted older people referred by their general practitioners for long-term care for whom the responsible social workers had misgivings of the need, remarkably 8 out of 33 were admitted to Nursing Home Care with 13 being able to return home.[20] Attempts in the National Service Framework[21] of 2001 to embed a single assessment process, failed through a combination of a lack of proportionality in assessment tools and commitment. Although it remains difficult to determine the reason for people to be in long-term care, a census in 2003 of more than 15,000 care home residents described the drivers for care home admission and the dependencies of residents (Tables 122-2 and 122-3). Although this data was limited to a national provider (Bupa)[22] of care, the findings were validated in a larger survey of homes in 2006.[23]

Within the case mix and dependencies recorded, there is a further complication in that the discharge and transfer rate

Table 122-2. Reasons for Admission to Care Homes

	Nursing	Residential	All residents
Dementia	38% (4272)	31% (1164)	36% (5456)
Frality	22% (2499)	34% (1282)	25% (3799)
Stroke	25% (2877)	12% (453)	22% (3287)
Slight Impairments	12% (1349)	16% (600)	13% (1958)
Arthritis	12% (1392)	15% (560)	13% (1957)
Family/Social Reasons	9% (968)	20% (773)	12% (1748)
Heart	10% (1160)	10% (382)	10% (1547)
Diabetes	9% (993)	7% (284)	8% (1280)
Hearing Impairments	6% (695)	9% (328)	7% (1025)
Depression	6% (673)	8% (319)	7% (998)
Other	7% (766)	6% (222)	7% (992)
Fractures	7% (777)	4% (167)	6% (951)
Parkinsonism	5% (613)	5% (187)	5% (807)
Lung of Chest Disease	5% (519)	4% (144)	4% (664)
Cancer	5% (508)	4% (139)	4% (651)
Osteoporosis	4% (459)	4% (142)	4% (604)
Epilepsy	4% (400)	2% (81)	3% (481)
Unknown	2% (177)	6% (214)	3% (392)
Neurological Trauma	2% (201)	1% (26)	2% (229)
MS	2% (207)	1% (19)	1% (226)
Learning Difficulties	1% (167)	1% (54)	1% (221)
Housing	1% (130)	2% (90)	1% (220)
Schizophrenia	1% (167)	1% (40)	1% (208)
Missing Limp	1% (165)	1% (43)	1% (208)
Manic Depression	1% (81)	1% (38)	1% (119)
Motor Neurone	0% (50)	0% (3)	0% (53)
Huntingdon's	0% (45)	0% (7)	0% (52)
Cerebral palsy	0% (38)	0% (9)	0% (47)

from care homes means that much temporary care is being provided and so actually understanding the actual numbers of long-term care residents remains difficult.

Extrapolation using population projections and present patterns of care home use suggests that between 2003 and 2051[24] that the number of care home places will need to rise by 150% in the United Kingdom. This projection is reflected in a review by the King's Fund's Wanless,[25] which estimated that the costs of social care could increase in England from \$17.4 billion (£12 billion) in 2002 to \$43.5 billion (£30 billion) in 2026. The single greatest driver for care home admission is and increasingly will be dementia.

DEVELOPING QUALITY IN CARE

For a long time, no statutory mechanism for the routine inspection of the long-term care within the NHS existed. A government agency—The Hospital Advisory Service, later renamed The Health Advisory Service (HAS)—was established in 1969 in response to a series of reports of patients mistreated in psychiatric hospitals. The HAS was charged with visiting geriatric and psychiatric departments of hospitals in rotation, the intention being to advise and encourage good practice rather than to admonish. A visiting team consisting of a consultant geriatrician, manager, nurse, and therapist would spend 1 to 2 weeks in a hospital and present a detailed report and recommendations to the Health Authority and would follow with the director reporting to Parliament annually. The final report of the outgoing director of the HAS in 1987 stated, "The quality of long-term care offered to elderly people in hospital is still generally very poor. There is a growing contrast with the individual personal care offered in many local authority homes to elderly people with degrees of disability not significantly different from those seen in hospital.[21]" The scope of the HAS inspections did not fully extend to the care in the community provided by independent nursing and residential care homes. Care homes have been subject to regulation primarily by a variety of bodies using largely social and personal care derived standards, most recently administered by the Commission for Social Care Inspection, generally separate from the regulation of health care.

Table 122-3. Patterns of Mobility, Mental State and Continence in Care Homes

	Residential	Nursing	Overall
1. Mobility	n=3894	n=11,335	n=15,287
Ambulant	40% (1566)	18% (2059)	24% (3642)
Ambulant with assistance	43% (1687)	28% (3228)	32% (4933)
Entirely dependent	16% (641)	53% (6048)	44% (6712)
2. Mental State	n=3849	n=11,104	n=15,015
Normal	31% (1175)	19% (2110)	22% (3295)
Confused or forgetful	60% (2319)	65% (7231)	64% (9591)
Challenging behavior	11% (423)	23% (2549)	20% (2989)
Depressed or agitated	12% (479)	21% (2352)	19% (2840)
3. Continence	n=3832	n=11,278	n=15,166
Continent	53% (2044)	20% (2253)	28% (4311)
Urinary incontinence only	24% (930)	19% (2151)	20% (3089)
Fecal incontinence only	1% (45)	1% (95)	1% (141)
Urinary and fecal incontinence	21% (813)	60% (6779)	50% (7625)

Table 122-4. Basic Principles That Underlie the Rights Accorded to All Who Find Themselves in the Care of Others

1. Respect for privacy and dignity
2. Maintenance of self-esteem
3. Fostering of Independence
4. Choice and control
5. Recognition of diversity and individuality
6. Expression of beliefs
7. Safety
8. Citizens' rights
9. Sustaining relationships with relatives and friends
10. Opportunities for leisure activities

Source: A Better Home Life Center for Policy on Aging, London, UK, 1996.

The personalization and empowerment of care home residents has been encouraged through many reports, notably "Home Life" and its successor "A Better Home Life," which provided a code of good practice for residential and nursing home care.[22] This latter report espoused principles to guide daily life in a continuing care setting (see Table 122-4).

Currently a project promoting personalization through "My Home Life"[28] aims to improve the quality of life of those who are living, dying, visiting, and working in care homes for older people has championed good practice and engagement in quality of care.

Although the enthusiasm to support improving the experiences of people in care remains important, it contrasts with the wider understanding of the needs of people in care, their clinical dependencies, and reliance on structured health care support. In 1998 The Royal College of Physicians, British Geriatrics Society, and Royal Surgical Aid Society drew up clinical guidelines to enhance the health of older people in long-term care.[29] This report gave guidance on the management of dementia, depression, disability, autonomy, continence, medication, falls, and pressure care. The media and public more generally have a poor regard for care and although awareness of dignity issues is a theme, the greatest sense of outrage surrounds clinical issues, in particular the management of medication and specifically the use of neuroleptic drugs. Medication, particularly sedation, has and remains poorly managed despite many reports that have criticized care homes in their use of drugs. Slowly, but inevitably, understanding that there is a medical responsibility in prescribing drugs is gaining understanding[30] and at some point it will become apparent that inadequate commissioning of services with limited staff resources can only be squared through poor practices.

The present and future of long-term care in the United Kingdom

As levels of clinical complexity and dependency in long-term care has evolved, patients have become paradoxically redesignated "residents and clients" with greater emphasis on the social aspects of care. Often the potential for fulfilling personal autonomy and ability to choose are undermined by great physical and mental impairment. In reality the outcome of care is dependent, as never before, on clinical care and well-being. As hospitals become more focused on procedural investigation and treatment with increasingly short lengths of stay and rapid discharge, the level of advocacy, navigation, and support for older people can confidently be predicted to increasingly be found in postacute care settings, particularly care home facilities. Not only will care homes have more complex long-stay care case mix, but also patients without clear anticipated outcomes. For instance, consider a patient with a devastating stroke for whom enteral feeding is necessary to maintain hydration and nutrition. Such patients have traditionally remained in the hospital with continuity of specialist care being a positive contribution to difficult decision making. Now an increasingly initial investigation, assessment, and insertion of feeding tube will signal the end of the hospital episode with discharge before an agreed long-term care plan and realistic set of objectives can be established, placing a significant responsibility on a system of care not equipped to provide such decision making. The implication is that geriatric medicine will have to rapidly develop or be reinvented!

The political problem of long-term care prompted the establishment of a Royal Commission on long-term care.[31] The commission examined various funding options for the future provision of housing and personal care. In an authoritative review, the commission described the epidemiologic uncertainties regarding future needs as a "funnel of doubt"; however, the failure by the commissioners to agree a single solution dissipated their impact. The government's response to the Royal Commission on long-term care was to determine that from October 2001 the separation of personal care and health care be clarified through an eligibility assessment with the funding of the professional nursing component of care being provided by the state and the remaining costs of care being met through a means-tested process. Real difficulties pervade the definition of "nursing care" as opposed to "personal care." Subsequently, the subject has continued to be contentious with a number of "sticking plaster" solutions to what are increasingly viewed as system failures.

Most recently the increasing volume of critical reports from a wide range of respected foundations and think tanks has led to a renewed commitment to change. A continuing difficult problem with long-term care has been its resources, especially beds to be used to meet a range of needs just as many of the original geriatric NHS beds were used for "slow stream" rehabilitation, "respite care" or "end of life care" so it is been with care homes and community care more widely. Inevitably, this lack of precision in definition of long term care adds difficulties to the understanding of funding requirements with means-tested social care, free at the point of delivery health care, and determining budgetary allocations.

Table 122-5. Recommendations for a Comprehensive Interdisciplinary Approach to the Health and Care of Older People in Care Homes

1. An agreed comprehensive assessment tool should be adopted that records diagnoses along with disabilities to enable commissioning, inform care planning, and governance.
2. Individual care planning should address clearly assessed needs and wishes of the individual. It should also identify expectations, responsibilities, and limitations of health and care. The care plan provides an individual benchmark from which an individual's care may be monitored.
3. A population-based approach should be used for the planning and provision of services to residents in care homes. Integrating all the professions into an organization sized to address the care home population needs is most likely to produce effective and efficient care.
4. A specialist gerontological nurse should be the lead clinical practitioner for the identification and integration of health care support to the home in the care of its residents. Recognition, definition, development, and training within interdisciplinary care are required.
5. General practitioners need their roles and responsibilities to be defined and supported in care homes. New ways of working should greatly improve patterns of care; training and qualifications should be encouraged and recognized.
6. There is an urgent need to reengage specialist geriatric medicine and old age psychiatry in a structured manner to the care home population.
7. The management of medication and the role of the pharmacist may be enhanced through an institutional approach.
8. The organization, application, and governance of all the professions allied to medicine may be enhanced through integration with other professionals and through core institutional-based care rather than individual contracting.
9. A major investment in training, learning, and development is required for medical, nursing, social work, and paramedical professions. The concept of a "teaching nursing home" as a learning organization should be developed.
10. Research is needed to inform further developments that aim to improve health and care outcomes through evidenced-based practice for care home residents through evidence-based practice.

If the purpose of care is poorly understood, there has been no shortage of commitment to regulation of care. The Care Standards Act[32] presented national standards for residential and nursing homes for older people from April 2002. These were initially administered by The National Care Standards Commission (NCSC), supplanted after several years by the Commission for Social Care Inspection (CSCI), and in the near future to be replaced by a new commission that will integrate health care regulation with social care regulation.

It should be clear that what is missing in the United Kingdom is a comprehensive strategy of need, funding financing, and perhaps most relevant to readers, the organization of health care. A proposal formulated by a working party of the Royal College of Physicians in partnership with the Royal College of Nursing and the British Geriatrics Society in 2000[33] features 10 recommendations that could collectively provide a comprehensive interdisciplinary approach to care (Table 122-5), this report, like so many others remains a testament to the authors commitment rather than a landmark of progress!

Finally, the availability and organization of the staffing of care remains fragile. Low fee levels have meant poor levels of remuneration, dissuading some potential care staff and undermining staff retention particularly in the prevailing economic climate of near full employment. Care workers from around the globe have sustained the United Kingdom care needs, whether changing economics will make this sustainable remains uncertain.

KEY POINTS

Long-Term Care in the United Kingdom

- Long-term care remains underdeveloped in the United Kingdom, with attention principally being focused on avoiding care rather than on the care itself.
- Inadequate epidemiologic information regarding the population in long-term care has seriously undermined policy planning.
- Diminishing use of care as a substitue for inadequate housing provision for older people has been "offset" by the epidemiologic impact of dementia and other neurodegenerative diseases.
- Policy concerns have addressed the cost of care rather than determining the funding necessary to deliver care of an acceptable standard and then determining financing mechanisms for individuals confronting the need for care.
- A whole system formulation for long-term remains elusive and is required to determine the needs to be met and the means by which they are provided.

For a complete list of references, please visit online only at www.expertconsult.com

CHAPTER 123

Institutional Long-Term Care in the United States

Luis F. Samos
Enrique Aguilar
Joseph G. Ouslander

HISTORY OF INSTITUTIONAL LONG-TERM CARE

This chapter will provide an overview of institutional long-term care (LTC) in the United States. Long-term care is the broad range of medical and nonmedical services that are designed to meet the needs of people with chronic illnesses and variable degrees of disability. These services may be needed on a temporary basis going from weeks to months or may be needed permanently. The need for long-term care may also be due to terminal illness. There are two basic types of LTC institutions in the United States: nursing homes (NH) and assisted living facilities (ALFs).

In the early 1900s, there was no federal program to support health care for the elderly, so that impoverished seniors were sent to "poor farms" or almshouses. In the 1920s, a U.S. Department of Labor report increased the awareness of the problem and the public began demanding reform. In 1935 the Social Security Act was signed by President Franklin D. Roosevelt, which created the "Old Age Assistance Program." This provided financial support for older people, but discouraged almshouse living, paving the way for the creation of private old-age homes.[1,2]

In 1954 a change in federal law provided grants for the construction of nursing homes, which were modeled after hospitals. In 1965 President Lyndon Johnson declared: "thirty years ago, the American people made a basic decision that the later years of life should not be the years of despondency and drift."[2] Soon after Medicare and Medicaid were passed into law and these programs provided additional support for LTC. There was an enthusiastic response to Medicare but also overwhelming costs, so that in 1969 the government restricted much of the coverage for NH care. In the 1970s a new policy authorized Medicaid to pay for NH care on a reasonable cost and needs related basis.

In the 1970s and 80s significant concern about the quality of care in NHs began to be voiced.[1,2,3] In 1986 a study conducted by the Institute of Medicine at the request of Congress found that many residents of NHs were receiving substandard care. This led to the passage of the Nursing Home Reform act as a part of the Omnibus Budget Reconciliation Act (OBRA) in 1987. The purpose of this legislation was to ensure that residents in NHs would receive quality physical and mental care. This act included guidelines for the use of antipsychotics and physical restraints, and created the NH Resident Bill of Rights (Table 123-1).[2,4]

OBRA 1987 also mandated the creation of a resident assessment system, which led to the development of the minimum data set (MDS). The MDS is a structured tool designed to comprehensively assess NH residents from a general clinical and functional point of view. Screening with the MDS may trigger the use of one or more resident assessment protocols (RAPs), which address 18 common conditions. The RAPs in turn are used for care planning for individual residents. In addition, data from the MDS is submitted to state governments electronically and used to calculate reimbursement for Medicare-reimbursed skilled nursing stays, and to examine quality of care (see later discussion).[1,2]

DEMOGRAPHICS AND ECONOMIC CONSIDERATIONS

Demographics

With current trends towards a rapidly aging population in the United States, the health care system and its LTC services will face many challenges. According to the U.S. Census Bureau, 37 million people age 65 and over lived in the United States in 2006, accounting for more than 12% of the population. Over the twentieth century this population grew from 3 million and is projected to be 86.7 million in 2050, comprising 21% of the population. The estimated percentage increase of this age group between 2000 to 2050 is projected to be 147%.[5,6] By comparison, the population as a whole will have increased only 49% over the same period. The older (65 and over) population is expected to more than double between 2000 and 2030 going from 35 million to 71.5 million,[7] but this growth rate will slow after 2030, when the "Baby Boomers" enter the group of the oldest-old population (those 85 and older). The oldest-old population is projected to grow rapidly after 2030. For example, the population 85 and over grew from just over 100,000 in 1900 to 5.3 million in 2006.[8,9]

Life expectancies at both age 65 and age 85 have increased. Current mortality trends suggest that people who survive to age 65 can expect to live an average of 18.7 more years, almost 7 years longer than people age 65 in 1900. The life expectancy of people who survive to age 85 today is 7.2 years for women and 6.1 years for men.[9]

From the above numbers, the growing importance of LTC services is not surprising. Estimates indicate that approximately 35% of Americans age 65 will receive some NH care in their lifetime, 18% will live in a NH at least a year, and 5% for at least 5 years.

Approximately 2% of Americans age 65 to 84 and 14% age 85 and older live in NHs. There are currently close to 1.8 million residents in NHs in the United States, which represents an increase from 1.6 in 2004, although the percentage of elderly living in NHs has declined in recent years from 8.1% of those 75 and older in 2000, to 7.4% in 2006. This is likely due in part to improved short-term rehabilitation and an increasing number of residents returning home, along with the increasing number of ALFs.

Almost half of all individuals living in NHs are 85 years or older and about 70% are women. Residents with dementia account for more than half of the population, more than half are confined to a bed or wheelchair, and 80% need help with four or five activities of daily living. NH residents can be divided into two basic groups: one that stays a short period of time because they are undergoing rehabilitation or because they are medically ill and are hospitalized or die; and a second group of long-stayers (Figure 123-1).[10,11,12]

Economics

Economic considerations in LTC are of paramount importance in an era of ever increasing health care costs. The average cost of residing in a NH in 2008 is $187 per day for a semiprivate room and $209 per day for a private room. An ALF costs about $3,000 per month for a one-bedroom unit, and the cost for a home health aide is $29 per hour. The federal government does not provide for ALF care; some states provide limited support through Medicaid or other programs.

The total amount spent on LTC in the United States in 2005 was $207 billion, excluding informal care (provided by family or friends). There are only two basic ways to pay for NH care in the United States—out-of-pocket from savings (or private LTC insurance which generally has limited coverage), or Medicaid, which essentially requires impoverishment to qualify. About half of NH and other LTC services are in fact covered by Medicaid, which is a federal and state program for low income individuals (not just the elderly). Medicaid expenditures on NH and other LTC services now amount to more than $100 billion.[13,14]

Medicare, which is federal health insurance for the elderly and disabled, has two parts: Medicare Part A, which pays for hospital and related care, and Medicare Part B which pays for outpatient services including physician fees. Medicare Part A will only pay for a skilled nursing facility stay after a 3-day qualifying stay in an acute hospital. Thus, in the United States, Medicare does not pay for direct admission to a NH or for long-stay NH care. This is because Medicare was originally designed to protect older people from the costs of catastrophic acute illnesses—thus Medicare Part A benefits are linked to the care of acute conditions. Medicare will pay for short-term NH care if the resident needs frequent medical and/or nursing services, or rehabilitation with goal of returning home. Although Medicare will theoretically pay for 100 days, most stays are in the 30 to 40 day range, after which long-stay NH care is paid for privately or by Medicaid (see later discussion).[16]

For skilled NH care (short-stay), Medicare uses a Prospective Payment System (PPS) that makes payments based on predetermined amounts. As opposed to the diagnosis-related groups (DRGs) used in inpatient hospital settings, a system that is based on the expected amount of resources needed according to the resident's physical functioning, diagnoses, health conditions, and treatments as documented in the MDS. This system is called the Resource Utilization Groups (RUG), and currently includes 53 groups. RUG payments cover all services except physician fees (which are paid for by Medicare Part B). Since the RUG system was implemented, it has changed the relationship between physicians and NH administrators because the costs of services ordered by the physician are now bundled into the RUG payment. Previously, Medicare paid for medications, diagnostic tests, and rehabilitation therapy separately, so the NH administrators were not as concerned about what physicians ordered.[17]

A relatively small proportion of older people are in Medicare managed (or capitated) care plans (the proportion varies considerably across the United States). In these programs, the 3-day acute hospital requirement can be waived for skilled care. Thus the Medicare managed care plan enables these individuals to be directly admitted to a NH for short-term care for conditions such as deep vein thrombosis, pneumonia, congestive heart failure, pelvic fracture, etc.[16,17]

Table 123-1. The Nursing Home Residents' Bill of Rights

The Nursing Home Reform Act of 1987 established the following rights for nursing home residents:
- Freedom from abuse, mistreatment, and neglect
- Freedom from physical restraints
- Privacy
- Accommodation of medical, physical, psychological, and social needs
- Participation in resident and family groups
- Treatment with dignity
- Exercise of self-determination
- Free communication
- Participation in the review of one's care plan, and to be fully informed in advance about any changes in care, treatment, or change of status in the facility
- The right to voice grievances without discrimination or reprisal

Types of services

Most NH residents require mainly nonskilled or maintenance care such as help with activities of daily living like bathing, dressing, eating, getting in or out of a bed or chair,

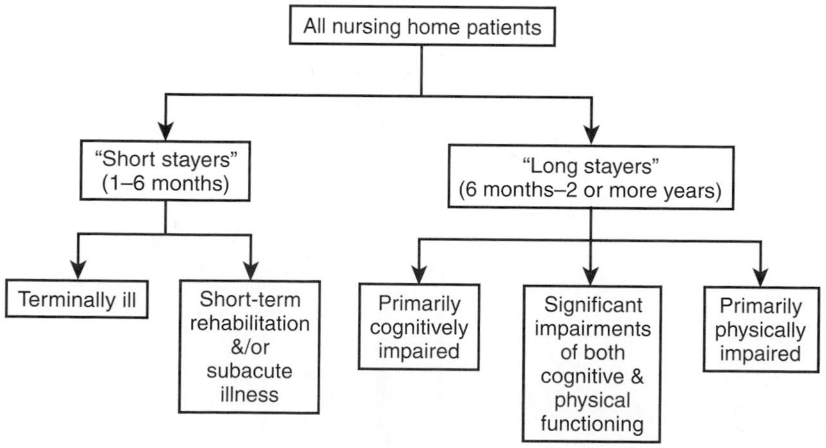

Figure 123-1. Types of patients in U.S. long-term care facilities. *From Kane RA, Ouslander JG, Abrass IB. Essentials of clinical geriatrics. ed 4, New York, 1999, McGraw-Hill.*

and using the bathroom. These individuals have generally already maximized their rehabilitation potential. This care does not require skilled health care personnel and Medicare does not pay for this level of care, but Medicaid does if the individual qualifies financially. Skilled care requires the intervention of medical, nursing, and rehabilitation personnel. Examples of skilled NH care include intravenous injections, wound care, and physical, occupational, and speech therapy (including cardiac, neurologic, pulmonary, or orthopedic rehabilitation).

Hospice care is also provided in both NHs and ALFs. Hospice programs provide medical, psychological, and spiritual support to terminally ill patients and their loved ones. The emphasis of hospice is quality of life, comfort, and dignity. A major point of hospice is to control pain and other symptoms so the patient can remain as alert and comfortable as possible. Hospice services are available through Medicare to persons who can no longer benefit from curative treatment and are estimated to have a limited life expectancy. Enrollment in a Medicare hospice program enables additional support to be brought into the NH or ALF through private hospice providers.

Settings

In the United States, institutional long-term care takes place either in NHs or ALFs. ALFs offer a housing alternative for older adults who are relatively independent. The services generally provided or arranged for in ALFs are listed in Table 123-2. ALF residents generally do not require the intensive medical and nursing care provided in NHs, and usually perform their basic activities of daily living themselves or with little help. The philosophy of ALF care is to allow older people to enjoy freedom and independence.

According to the National Center for Assisted Living, there are more than 36,000 ALFs in the United States, housing more than 1 million people. Since there is no strict definition of what constitutes an ALF, it is difficult to indicate the exact number of facilities. The average age of ALF residents is 83. About 74% of the residents are women and about half need assistance with dressing or bathing. According to NCAL, the average size of an assisted living residence is 43 units and ranges from 3 to 200 units. The average number of residents in a facility is 40, with a range up to 175. Residents are assessed on admission and periodically thereafter, and monthly fees are often based on the number of services provided.[19–22]

ALFs encourage their residents to "age in place." This has resulted in a substantial number of ALF residents being functionally disabled, and a blurring in the distinction between ALFs and long-stay NHs. Moreover, with relatively few exceptions, physicians and nurse practitioners do not visit ALFs, and many geriatric conditions, such as dementia, fall risk, incontinence, and others are inadequately recognized and managed in the ALF setting.

NHs provide assistance with activities of daily living but also offer an array of medical and nursing care within a 24-hour per day supervised environment. There are approximately 17,000 NHs in the United States. Most of them are free-standing facilities, but some are a part of a retirement community that usually includes independent living, an ALF, and other elderly services (Continuing Care Retirement Communities). Approximately half of U.S. NHs are owned by multifacility chains. Table 123-3 shows selected characteristics of NHs in the United States.[11–13,23]

Individuals admitted to a NH are usually more dependent than ALF residents on admission, especially those admitted for long stay, which can extend to years of institutional living. About half of residents spend at least a year in the NH and 21% of them live there for almost 5 years. Among residents admitted for short stay, which could last from days up to 3 months, many are admitted for rehabilitation, usually after a qualifying stay in the hospital (as described previously). Other individuals admitted for short stay are admitted for respite care. Respite programs involve a temporary admission, so that the family member or caregiver can take some time off. Respite care is not supported by Medicare, but may be by Medicaid in some states. The Veterans Health Administration, which has over 100 NH care units and state Veteran's Homes, offers respite free of charge for up to 30 days a year to qualifying veterans.

Table 123-2. Services Generally Provided in an Assisted Living Facility*

- 24-hour supervision
- Three meals a day in a group dining room
- A range of services that promote the quality of life and independence of the individual, such as:
  - Personal care services (help with bathing, dressing, toileting, etc.)
  - Assistance with medication management, or with self-administration of medicine
  - Social services
  - Supervision and assistance for persons with Alzheimer's or other dementias and disabilities
  - Recreational and spiritual activities
  - Exercise and wellness programs
  - Laundry and linen service
  - Housekeeping and maintenance
  - Arrangements for transportation

*Residents are assessed on admission and periodically, and monthly fees are often based on the number of services provided.

Table 123-3. Selected Characteristics of U.S. Nursing Homes*

Number of Facilities
17,000 total nursing homes
1.8 million beds with 80%-85% occupancy rates
Average size of 107 beds
13% of facilities are based in an acute care hospital

Ownership
66% for profit
27% not-for-profit
7% government

Direct Care Staff (Average numbers)
53 total direct care staff
35 certified nurse assistants
11 licensed practical nurses
6 registered nurses

Reimbursement
67% Medicaid
23% private pay
10% Medicare

*Figures shown are based on older data; current data may differ slightly.

Provision of care

Key leadership in a U.S. NH includes the administrator (who may or may not have had training as a nurse or other direct care health professional), the director of nursing, and the medical director. All licensed NHs are required to have a physician medical director. The medical director performs several functions and must integrate clinical best practices with regulatory issues. The medical director can be extremely important in establishing a professional and caring culture in the organization. In most facilities the medical director also has direct patient care responsibility; in some cases they care for the majority of residents. The medical director is also instrumental in ensuring that the NH meets state and federal regulations. He or she must ensure medical coverage and quality care, participate in policy and procedure development and implementation, infection control, and other quality improvement initiatives. The American Medical Directors Association (AMDA) has professionalized the role of the U.S. NH medical director over the last several years, and offers advanced training and certification for this role.[11,24]

In the majority of U.S. NHs, there is infrequent presence of physicians, nurse practitioners, or physician assistants; though some NHs, especially the larger ones, have on-site medial staff most days of the week. Nurses, both registered nurses (RNs) and licensed practical nurses (LPNs) are the key members of the clinical staff in NHs. Certified nurse assistants (CNAs) provide 90% of the hands on care, and support the services of RNs and LPNs. NHs also have either on a part of full-time basis physical, occupational, and speech therapists, social workers, psychologists, dietitians, pharmacists, and one or more chaplains. All of these professionals form part of the interdisciplinary team.[11,25,26]

Optimally care is delivered to NH residents by an interdisciplinary team that specializes in geriatric care. Interdisciplinary team care can be complex and time-consuming, but it is essential for the delivery of high quality care in the NH setting.

The basic paradigm for clinical care in the NH is theoretically guided by the resident assessment instrument, which is composed of the MDS and 18 RAPs (Table 123-4). Completion of the MDS is mandated within 14 days of admission and whenever there is a major change in status (such as a hospitalization), and specific sections are updated quarterly. When a condition is identified, the interdisciplinary team must document whether further assessment is indicated, and use one or more of the RAPs as appropriate to the clinical situation to generate an individualized care plan. MDS data must be entered into a computer data base, which is downloaded to the state government. These data are then used to calculate RUG rates (for residents on the Medicare Part A benefit) and to generate a series of quality indicators (see later discussion). In actual practice in the majority of U.S. NHs, an MDS coordinator (usually a nurse) completes the MDS with variable input from team members, and medical evaluations are done separately with little coordination with the MDS and care planning process.[27,28,29]

Quality of care

Quality of care in U.S. NHs is highly variable. Some facilities provide outstanding care. However, despite intensive efforts by federal and state governments and professional and advocacy organizations, the quality of care in many NHs remains suboptimal.

TABLE 123-4. Conditions Addressed by Resident Assessment Protocols

- Delirium
- Cognitive loss
- Visual function
- Communication
- ADL/functional/rehab potential
- Urinary incontinence/indwelling catheter
- Psychosocial well-being
- Mood state
- Behavioral symptoms
- Activities
- Falls
- Nutritional status
- Feeding tubes
- Dehydration/fluid maintenance
- Dental care
- Pressure ulcers
- Psychotropic drug use
- Physical restraints

NH care delivery in the United States is highly regulated. NHs are subject to regular (at least annual) surveys by state and/or federal surveyors, and can be fined, lose the ability to admit new residents, or closed depending on the scope and severity of violations of regulations cited by the surveyors. Extensive reforms and regulatory changes were enacted as part of Omnibus Reconciliation Act in 1987 and they have continued to evolve. These regulations establish quality standards and related guidance to surveyors, minimum staffing and training requirements, reinforce residents' rights and quality of life, and limit restraints and the use of psychoactive medications as a mean to control resident behavior.

The major focus of quality improvement efforts in NHs is based on a series of quality indicators (QIs) that are derived from the MDS. QIs now address both short-stay and long-stay residents, and are publicly reported on the "Nursing Home Compare" section of the Medicare Web site (www.Medicare.gov/nhcompare) so that consumers can view QIs of NHs they are considering. Table 123-5 lists the quality measures monitored by the federal and state governments. At the level of the individual NH, these measures can be benchmarked against other NHs in the same multifacility chain, in the state, or nationally. These analyses can be used to target specific quality improvement initiatives. State and federal surveyors also use the QIs to target areas of concern for their surveys.

The Center for Medicare and Medicaid Services supports Quality Improvement Organizations (QIOs) in each state in the United States that are contracted to assist NHs (as well as other health care providers) with quality improvement efforts. The effects of the QIO programs are difficult to prove, but there is evidence that NH care quality has improved in association with QIO efforts. The focus of the QIO NH initiatives over the last several years have been on reduction of the use of physical restraints, pressure ulcers, pain, and depression, and on culture change in NHs (see later discussion) with a specific focus on resident and staff satisfaction, "person-centered care," and staff turnover (which averages 50% to 100% among certified nursing assistants in many U.S. NHs).[30,31,32] A wide variety of quality

Table 123-5. Quality Measures for Nursing Home Care in the United States

Quality Measures	MDS Observation Time Frame
Long Term Measures	
Percent of long-stay residents given influenza vaccination during the flu season	October 1 thru March 31
Percent of long-stay residents who were assessed and given pneumococcal vaccination	Looks back 5 years
Percent of residents whose need for help with daily activities has increased	Looks back 7 days
Percent of residents who have moderate to severe pain	Looks back 7 days
Percent of high-risk residents who have pressure sores	Looks back 7 days
Percent of low-risk residents who have pressure sores	Looks back 7 days
Percent of residents who were physically restrained	Looks back 7 days
Percent of residents who are more depressed or anxious	Looks back 30 days
Percent of low-risk residents who lose control of their bowels or bladder	Looks back 14 days
Percent of residents who have/had a catheter inserted and left in their bladder	Looks back 14 days
Percent of residents who spent most of their time in bed or in a chair	Looks back 7 days
Percent of residents whose ability to move about in and around their room got worse	Looks back 7 days
Percent of residents with a urinary tract infection	Looks back 30 days
Percent of residents who lose too much weight	Looks back 30 days
Short-Stay Measures	
Percent of short-stay residents given influenza vaccination during the flu season	October 1 thru March 31
Percent of short-stay residents who were assessed and given pneumococcal vaccination	Looks back 5 years
Percent of short-stay residents with delirium	Looks back 7 days
Percent of short-stay residents who had moderate to severe pain	Looks back 7 days
Percent of short-stay residents with pressure sores	Looks back 7 days

Source: http://www.cms.hhs.gov/NursingHomeQualityInits/10_NHQIQualityMeasures.asp (accessed September 18, 2008).

improvement resources and tools are available from the QIO program at: http://www.qualitynet.org/dcs/ContentServer?pagename=Medqic/MQPage/Homepage.

CULTURE CHANGE IN U.S. NURSING HOMES

"Culture change" is a current buzzword in the U.S. NH industry. Numerous professional and advocacy organizations are focused on changing the culture of NHs to one that focuses on quality first. A multiorganization initiative, "Advancing Excellence in America's Nursing Homes" (http://www.nhqualitycampaign.org/) is focused on culture change and other aspects of quality improvement in U.S. NHs. The culture-change movement grew slowly at first and since 2005 has now begun to spread rapidly. It focuses on empowering staff to deliver person-centered care and improve quality of life for residents, and advocates changing the environment from an institutional or hospital model to a more homelike or social model, considering the facility as the residents own home. Table 123-6 illustrates some of the differences between these two models. Table 123-7 lists some of the other key components of culture change.[33]

FUTURE PERSPECTIVES

Many challenges lie ahead for institutional LTC in the United States. Growing need and complexity of chronic illnesses and their treatment will stress the system. ALFs will continue to care for an increasingly complex population, with little medical and nursing input. This will place them at risk for poor quality of care, regulatory sanctions, and legal liability, unless good geriatric care is incorporated into this setting. NHs will continue to serve an increasingly frail resident population with high medical and nursing needs, especially as the reimbursement system begins to provide financial disincentives to hospitalize NH residents. These changes will come at a time when there is a crisis in terms of shortage of trained nurses, nurse practitioners, and physicians who specialize in geriatrics and long-term care. Blending the medical needs with the person-centered culture described above will be extremely challenging. Fiscal constraints in the Medicare and Medicaid programs will serve to exacerbate these challenges.

At the same time, there are opportunities. Opportunities to build upon the early successes of the culture change movement and quality improvement initiatives that have begun to permeate some U.S. NHs.[34] There are strategies that can be employed to improve care quality and reduce avoidable expenditures. Examples include preventing complications of chronic illnesses and avoiding iatrogenic problems, reducing polypharmacy, using care protocols and improved communication tools to reduce avoidable hospitalizations, and

Table 123-6. Institutional vs. Homelike Model of Nursing Home Care

Institutional (Hospital) Model	Homelike (Social) Model
Residents follow facility routine	Facility follows residents' routine
Staff float	Permanent assignments
Staff make decision for patients	Residents make their own decisions
Facility belongs to staff	Facility is residents' home
Staff know residents' diagnosis	Staff knows residents as individuals
	Nurture the human spirit in addition to providing treatments

Table 123-7. Key Components of Nursing Home Culture Change

Gathering together for socialization and activities	Natural sights
Natural light	Natural sounds
Line of sight	Contact with nature
Control of equipment	Group bonding
Natural smells	Celebrations
New technologies	Contact with other generations
Home like artificial lighting	Home like meals

more proactive use of advance directives to avoid unnecessary and expensive care at the end of life. Some of the cost savings might be reinvested in pay-for-performance initiatives that incentivize quality and culture change. NHs and ALFs also have the opportunity to partner with hospitals and home health care programs to improve transitions in care, a major quality and patient safety issue in the United States. This is a major focus of the current Medicare QIO program. Finally, and very importantly, there are opportunities to use health information technology—electronic medical records, remote monitoring devices, and others—to improve care quality, make care more efficient, and focus efforts on person-centered care that improves the quality of life of elderly people in need of institutional LTC.

For a complete list of references, please visit online only at www.expertconsult.com

CHAPTER 124

Education in Geriatric Medicine

Ruth E. Hubbard

INTRODUCTION

Education in geriatric medicine is currently failing to meet its objectives. Although geriatricians report the highest satisfaction with their specialty,[1] few medical students opt to join our ranks, particularly in the USA[2] and Canada.[3] Worldwide, populations are aging with the oldest old the most rapidly growing segment of society.[4] Yet many physicians and family doctors remain unfamiliar with key principles and practices of geriatric medicine.[5]

In this chapter, motivators for improvements in geriatric medicine education are contrasted with barriers to change. Newer educational theories have generally placed greater emphasis on processes of learning and the personal development of students. A working summary of these learning theories is provided, with examples of innovative educational programs linked to each approach. This education evidence base is intended to inform clinical geriatricians, optimizing the effectiveness of both their teaching and their own learning.

Motivators for change

Several factors are motivating improvements to the education of geriatric medicine (Table 124-1). Improving the care of older people has been prioritized at a governmental level, particularly in Australia[6] and the United Kingdom[7] and the teaching of geriatric medicine in the undergraduate curriculum is advocated by the World Health Organization,[8] General Medical Council[9] and the Association of American Medical Colleges.[10]

In the United States, philanthropic institutions are driving improvements in health care for older people. Between 1997 and 2008, the Hartford Foundation (www.jhartfound.org) and the Reynolds Foundation (www.dwreynolds.org) committed $118 million to U.S. medical schools to fund comprehensive programs to strengthen the geriatrics training of medical students, residents, and/or practicing physicians. The Reynolds Foundation has also provided support to the Association of Directors of Geriatric Academic Programs (ADGAP) to facilitate information exchange. This has included the development of an online system to share geriatric educational materials (www.pogoe.org).

Perhaps the most powerful motivator for change is the yawning gap that currently exists between service provision and care need. Two thirds of hospital inpatients in the United Kingdom are now aged over 65 years.[11] Older, dependent patients with rehabilitation need are not confined to Care of the Elderly units but are scattered throughout intensive care, medical, and surgical wards.[12] All doctors looking after adult patients therefore need the skills to work with older people. Yet the list of knowledge deficits in geriatric medicine identified by physicians[13,14] encompasses many essential domains:

- Medication prescribing
- Neurologic and behavioral problems
- Urinary incontinence and falls
- Health screening
- Ethical issues such as capacity to make treatment decisions
- Multidisciplinary working
- Navigating transitions to or from the acute hospital

Knowledge deficits result in greater medical uncertainty and feelings of inadequacy and frustration for the physician.[14] This frustration may manifest as negative stereotyping and suboptimal care. Ageist practices and undignified care of older people are all too apparent to geriatricians in our day to day practice[15] and continue to make the headlines in the medical[16] and lay press.[17]

Barriers to change

The barriers to improvements in geriatric medicine education include logistical and philosophical factors (Table 124-2). The medical school curriculum is already overcrowded, there may be difficulties coordinating teaching across nontraditional sites, such as nursing homes, and qualified teachers are a scarce resource.[18,19] In the United Kingdom, for example, the infrastructure for teaching and promoting geriatric medicine is being eroded. Between 1986 and 2006 numbers of both medical schools and medical students increased but the number of academic departments of geriatric medicine declined.[20] Moreover, teaching is the dual casualty of the escalating pressures of clinicians' service commitments and academics' research output accountability.

Some physicians openly question the need for geriatric medicine. Increasing numbers of older complex inpatients and the positive results achieved by nongeriatricians supervising multidisciplinary teams have both been used as arguments to abolish the specialty.[21] It is hard to imagine similar debates about the existence of cardiology ("we all manage patients with ischemic heart disease") or endocrinology ("we too use oral hypoglycemics to lower blood sugar") being countenanced by leading medical journals. These negative attitudes act as impediments to geriatric medicine education. Before attitudes can be changed, the reasons for them must be explored.[22]

Medical attitudes

Most medical students do not consider pursuing a career in geriatric medicine.[23–25] Students not interested in geriatrics rate performing procedures, technical skills, and not managing chronically ill patients as important practice characteristics.[23] Some students feel older people are "to blame" for their illnesses through life-style choices.[26] A more positive attitude to older people increases the likelihood of choosing a career in geriatric medicine.[24] Early exposure to geriatric medicine has been advocated[25] as students with more experience of older people, both positive and negative, are less likely to resort to stereotype and show more interest in geriatric medicine as a career.[26]

The presentation of geriatric medicine as a specialty founded on utilitarian values ("our interventions work") may have compromised its appeal. Modern concepts of frailty have the potential to provide a scientific framework, helping

Table 124-1. Motivators for Improving Education in Geriatric Medicine

Motivators for Change
Increasing numbers of older people
Current lack of knowledge → frustration for the physician and suboptimal care for the older patient
Improving the care of older people prioritized at governmental level
Funding initiatives in United States
Wide support (e.g., WHO, GMC) for increased teaching of geriatric medicine in the undergraduate curriculum

Table 124-2. Barriers to Improving Education in Medical Education

Barriers to Change
Shortage of time in the curriculum
Lack of funding
Few qualified teaching staff
Negative attitudes of students
Problems integrating teaching in nontraditional sites such as nursing homes

us understand and explain why these interventions work, and for whom.[27] Fifty years ago, "senile dementia" was viewed as an inevitable consequence of aging but "Alzheimerization" has changed public perceptions and motivated enhanced research endowments.[28,29] A clear description of clinical features, insights into pathogenesis, and development of modifying interventions have been essential components in this transformation. The "frailterization" of decrepitude and decline through comparable investigative steps is a tantalizing prospect.

Perceptions of prestige also contribute to negative attitudes. In one survey,[30] medical students, and junior and senior doctors consistently ranked neurosurgery and thoracic surgery as the highest prestige specialties. Only dermatovenerology rivaled geriatric medicine for the lowest prestige rating. Highest prestige conditions, such as myocardial infarction, leukemia, and brain tumor, seem to share an acute onset, definitive diagnostic strategies, high-tech interventions, and the possibility of complete cure. They reinforce the doctor's role as healer (anticipated by medical students as "Your job is to make the person better and help them live"[26]). Low prestige conditions, such as fibromyalgia and anxiety neurosis, often require a shift in philosophy from cure to care and demand communication skills rather than procedural finesse. Indeed, the knowledge and skills required to manage such conditions are the very ones that physicians report most difficulty in mastering.[13,14]

Societal attitudes

Medical student beliefs are shaped not just by their own experiences but by the attitudes of wider society.[31] The following opening gambits may stimulate discussion and act as a means to explore societal attitudes:

- In 2005, a U.K. survey of 2000 adults aged over 16 years reported that one third of people thought that the demographic shift toward an older society would make life worse in terms of standards of living, security, health, jobs, and education and one in three respondents viewed the over 70s as incompetent and incapable.[32]
- Charities that work with older people in the United Kingdom report difficulties generating financial support, with a quarter of the total income of charities that work with children and adolescents and half that of animal charities.[33]
- Simone de Beauvoir described two stereotypes of older people[34]: "The purified image of themselves that society offers the aged is that of the white haired and venerable sage, rich in experience, planing high above the common state of mankind; if they vary from this then they fall below it; the counterpart of the first image is that of the old fool in his dotage, a laughing stock for his children. In any case either by their virtue or by their degradation, they stand outside humanity."
- Older people have not always been undervalued. Before advancement of the written word, "elders" acted as collective memories during long evenings and at legal proceedings.[35]
- Societies that value physical beauty tend to depreciate old age whereas those that aim at a spiritual ideal entertain a more abstract aesthetic ideal.[36]

Educational theory

BACKGROUND

Teaching methods within the medical profession have traditionally been hierarchical, both at undergraduate and postgraduate level.[37] Medical knowledge is seen as the possession of experts, Socratic figures who transmit this knowledge to passive learners,[38] conforming to objectivist philosophy that knowledge is an entity that "exists in the world" outside the minds of individuals.[39]

Any teaching session may be seen by the well-intentioned traditional medical educator as an opportunity to "pass on" as much of this knowledge as possible, perhaps by recalling numerous "facts" for the students to transcribe. The learners are expected to commit the information to memory, becoming "little living libraries" capable of regurgitating the same information at a later date.[40] But increasing the density of information given to students has detrimental effects on the amount of information actually retained.[41] The objectivist, pedagogic teaching model is being supplanted by teaching methods based on alternative educational theories.

Those theories stem from five main sources[42]: behaviorism, adult learning (andragogy), constructivism, cognitivism, and social learning. Concern has been raised that these theories lack a solid evidence base and are founded on metaphor rather than science.[43] However, a familiarity with educational epistemology [coupled with an awareness that epistemology means "theory of knowledge"] can improve the effectiveness of teaching practice by providing a basis for the selection of instructional and evaluation strategies to match intended goals of learning.

Behaviorism

LEARNING THEORY

The behaviorist model involves a teacher-centered approach and has traditionally been used for the development of competencies and for demonstrating psychomotor skills. The focus of learning (as espoused by Skinner) is on observable behavior: environment shapes behavior and reinforcement is central to the learning process.[44] A behavioral objective should include the performance (what behavior will be performed), conditions (under which the behavior must be performed), and criteria (the measure of acceptable performance).[45] Behaviorists deny the importance of consciousness and cognitive processes and define mental state solely in terms of environmental input and behavioral output.[46] Behaviorist-medical methodology is said to conform to a Western "dominator" paradigm reinforcing "masculine" values and traits.[47] Though educational programs are now more often based on andragogy and constructivism, behaviorism still has an important role in developing competency based curricula.[42]

APPLICATION IN GERIATRIC MEDICINE EDUCATION

As already discussed, students not interested in geriatrics rate performing procedures and technical skills.[23] Geriatric medicine has been dismissed as "an approach centered on gentle symptom management."[21] Behaviorist teaching may therefore be particularly useful to counteract the perception that geriatricians use no special skills. Behaviorist objectives (performance, conditions, criteria) improved the functional assessment of an older person at the University of Michigan Medical School.[48] Performance included history taking (e.g., asking about falls and memory impairment) noting visual and hearing impairments and gait assessment. This was evaluated at a Standardized Patient Instructor station of an Objective Structured Clinical Examination (OSCE). The measure of acceptable performance was a score of 50% on a 17-item check list. Student performance was initially poor (with a mean score of 43%) but improved significantly after the introduction of an integrated geriatric curriculum. The curriculum included more geriatric content in preclinical courses, experience in an outpatient clinic, and clearly stated learning objectives related to clinical skills in functional assessment.

Adult learning theory

LEARNING THEORY

The objective of education in adult learning (andragogy) is for the learner to become autonomous and self-directed.[49] The role of the teacher is to facilitate the growth and development of the overall person. Maslow's contention that self-actualization could only occur once when threats were minimized[50] challenged the teaching methods of Lancelot Spratt characters, whose gentle humiliation of students for comedic effect engendered fear as well as the desired respect. Key characteristics of adult learning described by Carl Rogers[51] include personal involvement of the student such that learning is self-initiated and self-evaluated. Significant andragogical learning only occurs when the subject matter is perceived to be relevant.

APPLICATION IN GERIATRIC MEDICINE EDUCATION

The andragogical principle of self-directed learning was the driving force behind the General Medical Council guidance in the United Kingdom that student-selected components should comprise a quarter to a third of medical school curricula.[9] Geriatric medicine may not benefit from such initiatives since students are unlikely to choose self-selected modules to address knowledge deficits. Self-ratings correlate poorly with externally generated measures of ability[52] and adult learners tend to gravitate to studying things they enjoy and are already good at.[53]

Another tenet of andragogy is that significant learning is acquired through doing.[45] Experiential learning improves knowledge of and attitudes to the subject taught.[54] A randomized controlled trial of an experiential educational intervention in geriatric medicine was undertaken at the University of Western Ontario.[55] The experiential session included:

- A game-show style quiz on demographics
- Use of specialized goggles and footwear to simulate visual and physical impairments often felt by older people
- Group interview of an older lady in a wheelchair and hospital gown. She suddenly disrobed to reveal her exercise wear and led the class through the fitness exercises she taught at the local community center.

Assessment 1-year later showed no greater knowledge in the intervention group but student behavior and feedback suggested improved attitudes to older people and more chose geriatric medicine as a clinical elective.

Constructivism

LEARNING THEORY

Constructivists believe that learners build knowledge from their own perceptions and experiences. Learning is an active process, occurring within the minds of each individual.[40] The role of the constructivist teacher is therefore to support the learners' own construction of knowledge.[38] This differs fundamentally from the traditional role as conveyor of information. Learners are thought to possess a current field of knowledge, described by Vygotsky as the "zone of proximal development."[56] The role of subject experts as preferred teachers for medical students is questioned (since their knowledge may be beyond the zone of proximal development of the students) and peer teaching promoted. Constructivism has gained popularity as a framework for medical education. The emphasis on processes of learning and personal development of students is considered to be particularly effective in fostering professional attitudes and beliefs.[57]

APPLICATION IN GERIATRIC MEDICINE EDUCATION

The principle of building on knowledge through the curriculum has been employed in the geriatric medicine program at the Southern Illinois School of Medicine.[58] Students encounter a simulated older couple through standardized couple patient experiences, small group sessions, and paper-based learning modules. The couple ages 10 years between each annual, 4-hour session. The woman represents healthy aging whereas her husband becomes frail, with multiple comorbidities, polypharmacy, and functional decline. Thus the students gain insights into health promotion/illness prevention and caregiver burden along with medical complexity and the impact of frailty. Discussions are guided by the SEMPACE model, which aims to address all areas affecting older people's health: Social, Environmental, Medical, Psychological, Activities of Daily Living, Caregiver, and Economic domains. Although Aging Couple Across the

Curriculum is currently in the development phase, and may require a more appealing acronym to have a truly pervasive impact, early student evaluations have been positive and an increased interest in geriatric medicine is suggested by more students choosing geriatric electives.

Cognitivism

LEARNING THEORY

The emergence of cognitive science precipitated a significant change, some would even say a Kuhnian revolution[59] in education and teaching methods. Although radical behaviorists minimize the importance of consciousness and mental processes, cognitive scientists focus on the learner's thought processes.[42] The teacher's role is to develop the learner's capacity for effective self-directed learning.

Reflective practice, integral to cognitivism to develop critical thinking, is an increasingly advocated concept in the fields of medical and nursing education. Reflective practice was first described by Schon in the early 1980s[60]: reflection *in* action occurs during the experience whereas reflection *on* action occurs, perhaps axiomatically, after the event. Reflection is more than simply replaying or thinking about practice.[61] It is "not complete without action[62]" and should lead to the development of new perspectives, behaviors, and practices.[63] Some argue that reflection may lead to anxiety[64] and psychological harm[65] and that discussion of case histories may compromise patient confidentiality.[66] Reflection has even been compared with Orwellian thought control since participants are encouraged to express their own feelings and amend them to harmonize with the majority view.[67] Despite these criticisms, reflection has been widely extolled as the pathway to medical professionalism.[68]

APPLICATION IN GERIATRIC MEDICINE EDUCATION

A mandatory 4 week clerkship in geriatric medicine introduced at McGill University, Montreal involved elements of independent and self-directed study, learning in and on practice, and web-based teaching to reinforce learning.[69] An electronic evaluation portfolio seemed to motivate students' self-reflection[70] and induce a positive change in attitudes.[71]

Concept maps are a cognitivist technique in which students create a 2-dimensional diagram exploring their understanding of important topics.[72] Concept maps reflect expected differences due to experience and training and can be scored reliably.[73] However, the absence of correlation between concept map assessment scores and conventional measures of learning such as final course grades suggests different knowledge characteristics are being tapped.[74] Geriatric medicine, replete with complexity, may be particularly suitable for concept mapping. Student understanding of the geriatric giants, for instance, could be explored. Examples of how a concept map may evolve as knowledge increases and complexity is appreciated are shown in Figures 124-1 and 124-2.

Social learning

LEARNING THEORY

Social learning is the result of a continuous interplay between three factors: the person, the learning environment, and the desired behavior.[74] Role modeling, bedside teaching, and applications of social learning have long been the mainstay of teaching to students and junior doctors.[42] The teacher is responsible for creating the desired model (e.g., history taking, cognitive assessment) and should then observe and correct the student's performance.

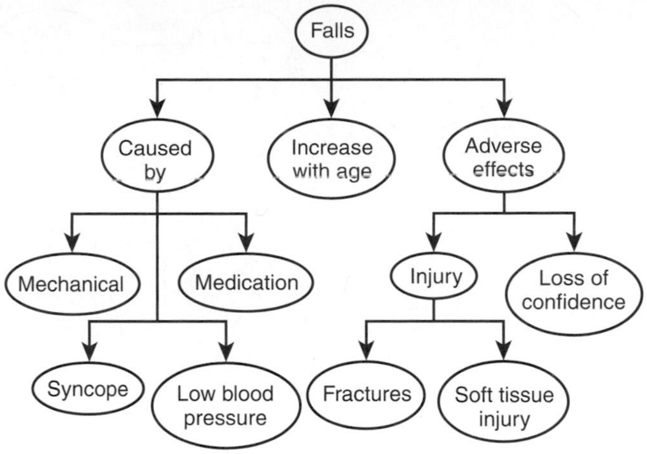

Figure 124-1. Concept map of *falls*. The absence of cross-links and the consistent use of 2 to 3 levels of hierarchy would result in a low score.

APPLICATION IN GERIATRIC MEDICINE EDUCATION

Clinical geriatricians may be unaware of the extent to which we impact students attending ward rounds or outpatient clinics. As role models, knowledge is essential but we also need to understand and articulate the reasons for actions.[75] The factors militating against referral for major surgery, for example, may be carefully weighed by an experienced geriatrician but without exploration and explanation, the observing student may interpret that the decision was based on chronologic age alone.

Hafferty and Franks' seminal work[76] on the learning of ethics proposed that the "broader cultural milieu" or "hidden curriculum" of medical schools had a greater influence than the formal curriculum on physicians' personality and conduct. This hidden curriculum may be particularly disadvantageous to geriatric medicine. Positive forces such as governmental edicts to abolish ageist practices[7] are undermined by what medical students hear and see on the wards.[15] Qualitative studies of trainees have confirmed that "clinician-teachers sometimes make disparaging remarks about particular medical specialties which may act as a barrier to recruitment."[75] At a time when even the British Geriatrics Society debates changing its name since "geriatrics" has "acquired negative connotations,"[77] we should be careful about the message this sends to others about the patients we care for. Through explicit consideration of the hidden curriculum, students may learn to challenge rather than accept ageist practices and behaviors.

SUMMARY

Educational theories emerging since the 1960s have shifted the emphasis of teaching from transmission of medical knowledge to support of learners as they develop. There is considerable overlap between different constructs; reflective practice and self-directed learning, for example, are commonly occurring themes. This should not compromise

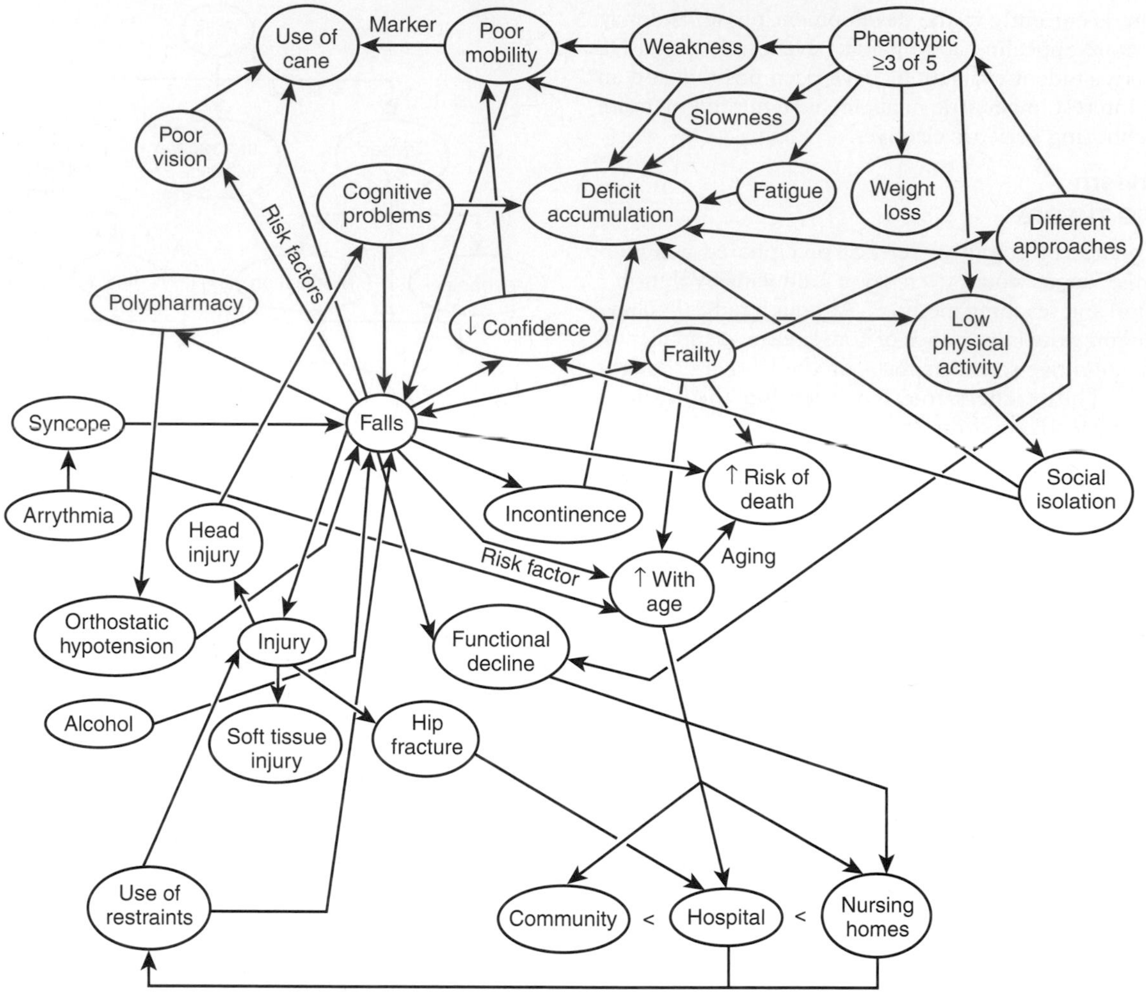

Figure 124-2. Higher scoring concept map of *falls* with frequent cross-links and consistent use of 5 or more levels of hierarchy.

curriculum design, the purpose of which is to optimize learning rather than exclusively apply a single educational theory.

The focus on learning processes and personal development of students is particularly relevant for the education of geriatricians. Younger patients having a single pathology such as chest pain, benefit from a rich evidence base and decision making can chiefly follow algorithm. Decision making for older, complex patients, on the other hand, is often guided by wisdom and prudence, described by Thomas Aquinas as "a keen understanding of the present that is informed by a memory of the past and modulated by current counsel."[78] Geriatricians therefore need to be able to integrate knowledge gained though management of each patient ("memory of the past") and keeping up to date with a rapidly evolving evidence base ("current counsel"). Newer learning strategies—reflection on experience, social collaboration, identification of own learning needs—may foster these skills.

CONCLUSION

Geriatricians understand that caring for older people is a dynamic, complex, and richly gratifying specialty but this has not always been appreciated by others. We need charismatic and motivational teachers to raise the profile of geriatric medicine at medical schools and attract a higher number of trainees. To become an excellent clinical teacher, knowledge of our specialty is necessary but

KEY POINTS
Education in Geriatric Medicine

- Currently, few students consider becoming geriatricians and physicians and family doctors remain unfamiliar with key principles and practices of geriatric medicine.
- Barriers to change in medical schools include negative attitudes of students, an overcrowded curriculum and lack of motivated teachers.
- Educational theories emerging since the 1960s have shifted the emphasis of teaching from transmission of medical knowledge to support of learners as they develop.
- Geriatricians should be familiar with techniques to optimize the effectiveness of both their teaching and their own learning.
- Charismatic educators with geriatric knowledge and teaching skills have the potential to increase recruitment of geriatricians and improve standards of care by our colleagues in other specialties.

not sufficient. Enthusiasm, communication skills, and the ability to create a supportive learning environment are noncognitive attributes that may need to be cultivated.[79,80]

Ultimately, though, education in geriatric medicine should not just be targeted at recruiting and training a workforce of talented geriatricians. Old, dependent patients with rehabilitation need comprise the majority of the inpatient population.[12] We cannot directly provide care for all these older patients but have a responsibility to ensure that effective practices and essential skills are shared. In so doing, our colleagues in other specialties would find geriatric medicine less frustrating and more rewarding and, most importantly of all, the quality of care for all older people would be improved.

ACKNOWLEDGMENTS

Dr. Hubbard has received research funding from the Peel Medical Research Trust, London and the Fountain Innovation Fund of the Queen Elizabeth II Health Sciences Centre, Halifax, Canada.

For a complete list of references, please visit online only at www.expertconsult.com

CHAPTER 125

Improving Quality of Care in the United Kingdom

David A. Black

Improving quality of care is difficult and controversial. Over the last 20 years in the United Kingdom there have been growing pressures from an increasing number of stakeholders to demonstrate and deliver quality improvement. From the inception of the National Health Service (NHS), politicians have been seen to be held responsible for a state-funded health service; patients are becoming increasingly knowledgeable and empowered to act and insist on improvements; health care purchasers have a particular interest in risk management processes owing to the influence of litigation; and finally the professions themselves have a growing interest in evidence-based medicine and delivering the best possible care. Yet the problems of improving care have recently been summarized by Brook, who in a review states "in the last 30 years research has demonstrated that quality of care can be measured, the quality varies enormously, that where you go for care affects its quality far more than who you are, improving quality of care, while possible, is difficult, and in general has yet to be successfully accomplished."[1] Although this seems a pessimistic view, the gain from improving quality of care, when successful, can be spectacular. During the Crimea War, by enforcing improved standards of care and hygiene, Florence Nightingale reduced the mortality rates at the Scutari Military Hospital from 42.2% to 2% within 6 months.

Some may view the quality improvement movement as a management fashion. Yet the very success of geriatric medicine in the United Kingdom is a result of continuous improvements in the care of older people, starting in 1946 when Dr. Marjory Warren identified the large numbers of older people confined in atrocious workhouse settings who were denied effective health care. From those beginnings at the very onset of the NHS have evolved the comprehensive systems of assessment and care that are so different from the world of 1946. The development of geriatric medicine has been largely based on a persistent striving at the local level for more and better services in the face of policy weakness, professional neglect, and resource starvation, coupled with poor training and a neglected research base. The health care of older people remains one of the major challenges for quality improvement within the health service, particularly in the face of continual pressures to manage the growing number of the very old in the population.

The purpose of this chapter is to provide a theoretical understanding of the background to quality improvement by describing quality initiatives in the wider world of business and relating these to current health service policy with practical examples in geriatric medicine. A major problem for practitioners is the confusion of terminology and definitions. The experience of other areas, such as industry, has not been properly understood and the health service has been showered with initiatives, activities, jargon, and buzz words. The problems for clinicians have included failure to provide adequate commitment of time, significant problems with the information gathered, and difficulties implementing change when the needs have been identified. This chapter attempts to explain how the history of quality initiatives in business and the health service have led to the current government's approach, in particular the concept of clinical governance.

WHAT IS QUALITY?

At its very simplest, a basic working definition of highest quality care is "doing the right things well." In business, quality can be seen to have a number of dimensions[2]:

1. *Performance* - the primary operating characteristics or the product of services.
2. *Features* - add-ons or supplements.
3. *Reliability*.
4. *Conformance* - the degree to which a product's design and operating characteristics meet established standards.
5. *Durability* - measures of a product's life.
6. *Serviceability* - the speed and ease of repair.
7. *Esthetic* - the product's look, feel, and taste.
8. *Perceived quality* - as viewed by a customer or client.

These dimensions do not map immediately to health care, and experts have struggled to find generally applicable definitions of the quality of health care.

The situation is especially complex as a service may have multiple customers, including the patient, the general practitioner (GP), and the local health authority. The World Health Organization divided quality into four aspects[3]:

- Professional performance (technical quality)
- Resource usage (efficiency)
- Risk management (the risk of injury or illness associated with the services provided)
- Patient satisfaction with the services provided

Whatever definition is used, it must capture the complexity and variability of health care. One of the most widely used definitions was published by the Institute of Medicine in 1990 and states that quality consists of: the degree to which health services for individual and populations increase the likelihood of desired health outcomes and are consistent with current professional knowledge.[4]

Blumenthal has noted that health care professionals tend to define quality in terms of the attributes and results of care provided by practitioners.[5] This technical quality of care has two dimensions: the appropriateness of the services provided; and the skill with which appropriate care is performed. The biggest change for health care professionals has been to understand that care has also to be responsive to the preferences and values of consumers, particularly the individual patient.

A further view of quality, particularly in the United Kingdom, has been espoused by Maxwell.[6] This takes into account not just the individual patient but a wider population approach. Maxwell's six dimensions of quality are:

1. *Access* (issues such as physical accessibility and waiting times).
2. *Relevance to need* (appropriate to the assessed needs of the whole community).
3. *Effectiveness* (ability of the treatment or service to produce the desired result).
4. *Equity* (fair distribution of resources within the publicly funded system).
5. *Social acceptability* (including issues such as the environment and privacy).
6. *Efficiency and economy* (the best possible for the best possible price).

This model has been widely used for the purchasing or commissioning of services over the last decade in the United Kingdom.

MEASURING QUALITY OF CARE

Once the dimensions of quality have been identified, it should be possible to set standards and indicators of good practice (see later discussion). However, we cannot start to improve the quality of care unless we are able to measure it. The real challenge is to find measures that are effective, that can be obtained inexpensively, and ideally that are part of the care process itself.

Quality of care may be assessed using measures of structure, process, or outcome. These three attributes were originally described by Donabedian.[7]

1. *Structure* - includes the building blocks and characteristics of health care, including buildings, equipment, and staff.
2. *Processes* - refers to all the activities forming the encounter between the health care professional and the patient, including diagnosis, tests, treatments, and record-keeping.
3. *Outcomes* - refers to the patient's subsequent health status and other effects of care, including knowledge and satisfaction.

These three attributes are interlinked, with both structure and process contributing to the outcome of care. There are implications:

- If quality-of-care criteria based on structural and process data are to be believed, it must be possible to show that variation in either process or structure leads to a difference in outcome.
- If outcome criteria are to be believable, it must be shown that differences in outcome will result if the processes under the control of the health professionals are altered.

Brook et al[8] argue that, in health care, process measures are the most valid. Outcome measures, which may seem at first to be the most obvious measure, have also been widely used to assess quality but there are problems. Outcomes may be due, at least in part, to factors not related to the quality of care (e.g., a patient's physiologic reserve or age). Also, some outcomes of care may become obvious only many years later; this will seriously limit their use as a tool for quality improvement. An example is the long-term outcome of good diabetic care in preventing vascular disease.

Measures of process are currently thought to be the tool of choice. An example is the management of stroke disease. The Cochrane Collaboration review of stroke units demonstrated that bringing together multidisciplinary teams and changing the process of care brought major benefits: patients managed within specialist stroke units are much more likely to be alive and at home a year after stroke than those managed on general medical wards.[9] Local measures of outcome would not have shown this as *individual* stroke units do not have enough patients to demonstrate improved survival. Process measures, however, are useful in enabling comparisons to be made with those processes shown in the Cochrane Collaboration.

Although there are exceptions to this rule (an example might be of the outcomes of carotid artery surgery in carotid artery stenosis), process measures then are most commonly used to assess quality. Several issues arise:

1. Which data should be used?
2. Are the data reliable? The problems of completeness and accuracy of data in the National Health Service are well described.
3. Are the data valid? Are we choosing the right measures to reflect changes in quality care?
4. Are the data sensitive enough?
5. Is the evidence generalizable? For example, are data about the management of incontinence applicable to both an acute hospital and a nursing home?
6. Does the importance of the quality data justify the cost of collecting them?
7. Are the measures understandable to all users, both professionals and patients? For example, are the patient surveys that are currently used as a measure of quality helpful and understandable by all parties?

RECENT QUALITY IMPROVEMENT INITIATIVES IN THE UNITED KINGDOM

Clinical audit

Audit was formally introduced into the NHS in 1989 and was the main quality improvement technique used by clinicians in the 1990s. Clinical audit can be described as "systematically looking at processes used for diagnosis, care and treatment, examining how associated resources are used, and investigating the effect that care has on the outcome of quality of life for the patient."[10]

Clinical audit is usually described in the form of a cycle in which teams are encouraged to move through a process of setting standards, collecting and analyzing data, comparing the data with the standards set in a peer-review environment, and finally planning changes to improve the quality of care to meet the original standards set. The cycle is then repeated. In an environment of elderly care, it is essential that audit is undertaken by multiprofessional teams and is focused on the needs of patients.

Clinical audit is not clinical research although, like research, it requires systematic collection of standardized data. Clinical audit is not simply counting but it is not necessarily complicated. It can be done just as effectively with a pencil and paper as with a computerized system. Clinical audit produced a great deal of activity among health care professionals, and by 1996 it was estimated that 20,000 projects had taken place with the majority of consultants (83%) and general practitioners (86%) participating. Projects in geriatric medicine included the Royal College of Physicians' CARE scheme[11] and regional audits of hip fractures, for example in East Anglia.[12]

The criticism and challenges of clinical audit include:

- Failure to use nationally set standards, and the use of resources on many small local projects with ill-defined standards and aims
- Failure to complete the audit cycle—projects demonstrate problems but changes are not made and no further re-audits are carried out to demonstrate improvement (or otherwise) in quality
- A lack of patient-focused audits
- A lack of links between audit and management, and between audit and education
- Far too few audits being multidisciplinary or multisectoral
- Constraints of time, staff shortages, and limitations of information technology and the failure of some staff to participate at all

Recently the General Medical Council (GMC) has made it a requirement that all doctors in the United Kingdom take part in clinical audit, and it will be a requirement for revalidation.

The problems of single department or hospital audits being able to provide meaningful changes in quality have led to newer initiatives across networks of hospitals or even on a national basis. Examples include work of the clinical effectiveness and evaluation unit of the Royal College of Physicians (rounds 1-3), voluntary audit of stroke care involving more than 80% of hospitals nationally, allowing all hospitals to measure their own performance against the national picture.[13] Current work includes Falls and Bone Health in Older People, and Continence Services as part of the assessment of progress with the National Service Framework.[13]

Standards, guidelines, and protocols

To support clinical audit it is necessary to be clear about the standards that are being measured. During the 1990s many national and local organizations started to produce standard guidelines and protocols to inform the audit process, and to encourage a "clinical effectiveness" approach. Clinical effectiveness is seen as the extent to which the health status of patients can be expected to be enhanced by clinical interventions. Specific examples include the British Geriatrics Society's compendium of guidelines,[14] and the work of the Royal College of Physicians' Clinical Effectiveness and Evaluation Unit.

Another major stimulus for assembling the evidence of effectiveness of interventions has been the Cochrane Collaboration launched in 1993. Cochrane reviews are systematic reviews of randomized control trials of health care carried out in a very precise way using the techniques of meta-analysis to pool the results of trials.[9] The six principles of the Cochrane Collaboration are: collaboration, building on people's enthusiasm and interest, minimizing duplication of effort, avoidance of bias, keeping up to date, and ensuring access.

NHS guideline production is now principally in the hands of the National Institute for Clinical Excellence ([NICE] see later discussion) and they have set out 10 key principles for NHS guideline production (Table 125-1). The Clinical Resource and Audit Group[15] defined standards, guidelines, and protocols as follows:

- *Standards* - specific statements relevant to particular criteria of care against which practice can be assessed.
- *Guidelines* - a systematically developed set of statements that assist in decision making about appropriate health care for specific clinical conditions.
- *Protocols* - a fixed set of instructions to follow in the management of conditions, designed to reduce treatment variation and improve outcomes.

In practice, guidelines are seen as advisory and protocols as mandatory. The challenge for clinicians is to integrate guidelines or protocols into everyday care, usually in the form of integrated care pathways, which aim to both ensure best care and allow easy audit to determine variation from the best pathway of care. This seems to be effective for single diseases, but becomes much more complex in the elderly-care environment, even when there is a single primary defined problem such as stroke.[16]

THE AUDIT COMMISSION

The Audit Commission is an independent organization reporting to Parliament. It has a statutory role to report on value for money in both health services and local authorities. The auditors have a duty to examine the economy, efficiency, and effectiveness of use of public resources. Each year a small number of topics are chosen for detailed investigation, resulting in a report describing the issues and currently

Table 125-1. Principles for NHS Guideline Production

1. The objective of NHS clinical guidelines is to improve the quality of clinical care by making available to health professionals and patients well-founded advice on best practice.
2. Quality care is based on clinical effectiveness—the extent to which health status of patients can be expected to be enhanced by clinical interventions.
3. Quality of care in the NHS necessarily includes giving due attention to the cost-effectiveness of health care interventions.
4. NHS clinical guidelines are relevant to the care provided by the NHS throughout England and Wales.
5. NHS clinical guidelines are advisory.
6. NHS clinical guidelines are based on best possible research evidence, expert opinion, and professional consensus.
7. NHS clinical guidelines are developed using methods that command the respect of patients, the NHS, and NHS stakeholders.
8. Although NHS clinical guidelines are focused around clinical care provided by clinicians, patients are treated as full and equal partners along with relevant professional groups involved in a clinical guideline development.
9. All those who might be affected by NHS clinical guidelines deserve consideration within the clinical guideline development (usually including patients and their caregivers, service managers, the wider public, government, and health care industries).
10. NHS clinical guidelines should be both ambitious and realistic in nature. They should set out clinical care that might reasonably be expected throughout the NHS.

identified best practice. The following year all organizations in the NHS offering these features are reviewed by the commission. Those for whom indicators suggest problems have an in-depth review and detailed recommendations are produced for the board of the organization. Follow-up to review progress against the objectives set usually occurs a year later.

Reports relating to older people include[17]: *United They Stand* (update 1999)—reviewing the coordinated care of elderly people with hip fractures; *Fully Equipped* (2000)—the provision of equipment to older or disabled people by the NHS and social services in England and Wales; *The Way To Go Home* (2000)—rehabilitation and remedial services for older people; and *Forget Me Not: developing mental health services for older people* (2000).

ACCREDITATION

In the United Kingdom and elsewhere there are external inspection systems, which may lead to accreditation. For example, within industry, the British Standards Institution has accreditation standards BS5750 and ISO9000. These are voluntary schemes that identify organizations that have reached basic standard procedures to ensure that customer requirements are met. Accreditation depends upon documentation of procedures and policies, and assessment by an accrediting team visit. In the health services this has been used mostly in facilities departments, but clinical departments, including mental health services, have on occasion achieved these standards.

Currently accreditation is out of favor as a quality management tool in the National Health Service. The Healthcare Commission (see later discussion) do yearly assessment of performance of every NHS Trust in England, the "annual health check." The National Service Litigation Authority will charge differential fees to trusts based on an assessment of their risk management service, while postgraduate deaneries will approve the delivery of standards of training for junior doctors. Although these bodies have some inspecting function and in some cases can remove or close down services, they do not formally accredit services.

Complaints procedures

Complaints form another mechanism for monitoring the quality of health care delivery. In the United Kingdom, any complaint to a hospital must be acknowledged by the chief executive within 48 hours, and there is a national standard of the complainant receiving a reply following a completed investigation within 20 working days. It is expected local resolution should resolve the vast majority of complaints in the NHS organizations, and NHS organizations all have a Patient Advice and Liaison Service (PALS), which will support complainants.

However if complainants are not satisfied, they may ask the Health Care Commission for an independent review of their case. The Healthcare Commission will appoint a care manager, who can decide how far to investigate the case; to refer the case back for local resolution; or to provide a final report and recommendations for the NHS Trust. If a complainant is still dissatisfied, the complainant has a right to refer the matter to the National Health Service ombudsman, who may decide to investigate the complaint further. The ombudsman provides an annual report to Parliament, which may "name and shame" publicly.

Since most complaints against doctors relate to poor communication, there may be particular challenges in elderly medicine both in avoiding complaints and in learning from them.[18] There are distinctive features that affect communication between older patients and physicians. For example, ageism can occur in medical encounters, with physicians trivializing older people's problems. Physicians may spend less time with older people and may consider older patients to be more difficult to deal with than younger patients. Clinical discussion with older people is sometimes unusual in that a third person is often present, which complicates the communication process. These problems are additional to the generic problems of communication between doctor and patient.

The rise in the number of complaints about hospital-based elderly care was one of the main drivers that led to the setting up of the National Service Framework for Older People, an initiative from the Department of Health.

LESSONS FROM INDUSTRY ON QUALITY MANAGEMENT

The main advances in the business world in the field of quality improvement came during the 1970s and early 1980s with the understanding that quality could not be improved simply by inspection, and problems corrected by removing those defective goods or poorly performing individuals found by the inspection. In health care this is called by Berwick "the bad-apple theory."[19] The bad-apple theory of improving health care suggests that, as there are increasingly sensitive and specific tools for identifying poor outlier performance (for example this might be the bottom performing 5% in a population of doctors, services, or hospitals), then by removing these outliers it is possible to improve quality. This is still the theory behind accreditation, revalidation, and purchasing to set standards.

The radical conceptual change to this was introduced by the management theorists William Deming and Joseph Duran who brought back from Japan to America the theory of continuous improvement. They found that problems in business were usually implicit in the complex production processes, and that problems with quality could only rarely be attributed to the lack of ability, will, or intention of the people involved with the processes. Thus removing the "bad apples" rarely worked. The problems were not of motivation or effort but of poor job design, failure of leadership, or unclear purpose. From this basic concept a number of models of quality improvement evolved in the business world, which have subsequently been applied patchily to the health care environment. These include total quality management (TQM), re-engineering, and benchmarking. Continuous quality improvement in its widest sense remains the major influence on U.K. health care quality improvement.

Total quality management (TQM)

The most widely used quality intervention, certainly in business, is TQM. This has been defined as[20]:

The management of activities involved in improving the quality of the organization's product or service. TQM is a philosophy and a set of guiding principles for continuous improvement. It applies human resources and analytical tools focused on meeting the customer's current and future needs and tries to integrate these into management's efforts.

There are several widely recognized key characteristics of TQM systems that must always involve the whole organization and focus on the customer.[20]

- TQM has to take into account all parts of the organization.
- The chief executive and all top managers must visibly support it.
- TQM is ingrained as a value in the organization and the culture. It is not an add-on, TQM is "how we do things around here."
- Partnerships with customers and suppliers are encouraged, and the aim is to exceed the customer's expectations.
- Everyone in an organization should be trying to exceed the expectations not just of external customers but of everyone with whom they interact within the organization who may equally be a customer.

  - Cycle times can be reduced by focusing on doing the job faster.
  - Statistical quality control and the use of self-managed work teams can improve processes.
  - Do it right first time. Do not rely on inspection to identify defects, but correct the process to ensure that defects do not occur.
  - There should be corporate citizenship. The organization values everyone, both those within it and those it serves—these are often called "stakeholders."
  - No single formula works for everyone. Each organization is unique and must find its own way rather than taking an "off the shelf" approach.

Business process reengineering (BPR)

Reengineering, such as TQM, is a systemwide change approach focusing on changing the basic processes of the organization.[21] BPR can be defined as the fundamental rethinking and radical redesign of business processes to achieve dramatic improvements in performance. Reengineering seeks to make all processes more efficient by combining, eliminating, or restructuring tasks, and the idea is to achieve large improvements in performance. Claims from the original studies suggested 100% improvement or more. Whereas TQM often looks at small continuous changes or improvements, reengineering tries to take a radical approach to large-scale changes. Certainly in the business world, reengineering can be seen as a high-risk strategy. Its success rate is under 50% and perhaps much less.

Benchmarking

Benchmarking, developed in the early 1990s, is the detailed study of productivity, quality, and value in different departments and activities in relation to performance elsewhere. The idea is basically simple. Find an organization that is good (ideally the best) at the particular process that you also carry out. Study carefully how it does well what it does, and then incorporate its technique into your own organization. This might involve looking at an organization in a completely different sector of the economy. An example in health care might be a hospital that looked at how a hotel managed its room booking processes to maximize the use of elective beds.

Outcomes in the health service

These three techniques for quality improvement and organizational development have been applied, sometimes indiscriminately, in the health care environment. Pollitt noted how difficult it has been to implement them within the health service.[22]

Seventeen pilot total TQM projects were set up by the Department of Health in 1989, and the term "total quality management" has also been applied to other projects in the health service. A number of trusts also received considerable investment for pilot schemes of reengineering. Leicester Royal Infirmary made a considerable name for itself for its one-stop neurology clinic, but demonstrable quality gains across a whole organization have not been found, at least in the NHS projects. Benchmarking as a specific project does not appear to have had an independent systematic evaluation in the health service.

Pollitt points out that these quality initiatives were difficult to implement within the health service.[22] In particular, they fail to take account of the professions and the complexity of standards and guidelines emanating from professional bodies. They all require considerable time and resources and yet specialist quality training is a resource that few health care organizations have been able to deliver. Moreover, a hospital environment is far more complex than the single-process environment of a manufacturing business. Hospitals fail to match many of the key elements that would be required to translate these business approaches into the NHS. Existing quality improvement activities reflect fragmented occupational structures and relationships within the organizations. In the NHS quality still remains, in large part, as a "bolt-on" extra.

Continuous improvement

Despite the problems set out above, it is widely accepted that a continuous improvement model is most likely to succeed in achieving quality improvement in health care. It is clear that quality improvement is a painstaking and time-consuming business and that team working, team building, and leadership skills are all required for quality improvement.

One goal that has been suggested for health care is that the medical profession should move to so-called "six sigma quality."[23] The sixth-sigma goal aims for a rate of errors that lies six standard deviations outside of the normal distribution (i.e., fewer than 3.4 errors per 1 million events). Currently in anesthesia, using many techniques of quality improvement, deaths have been reduced to 5.4 per million, very close to the sixth-sigma goal. Yet 79% of eligible survivors after myocardial infarction do not receive β-blockers, a rate equal to about one sigma.[23]

Berwick uses the term "continuous improvement" to mean "continuously improving systems."[24] He suggests a very simple model of system improvement, described by Langley et al.[25] This comprises three basic questions and a cycle for testing innovations (Figure 125-1). The Plan-Do-Study-Act cycle describes the growth of knowledge through making changes and reflecting on the consequences. A simple model with clear leadership is often the best place to start quality improvement processes.

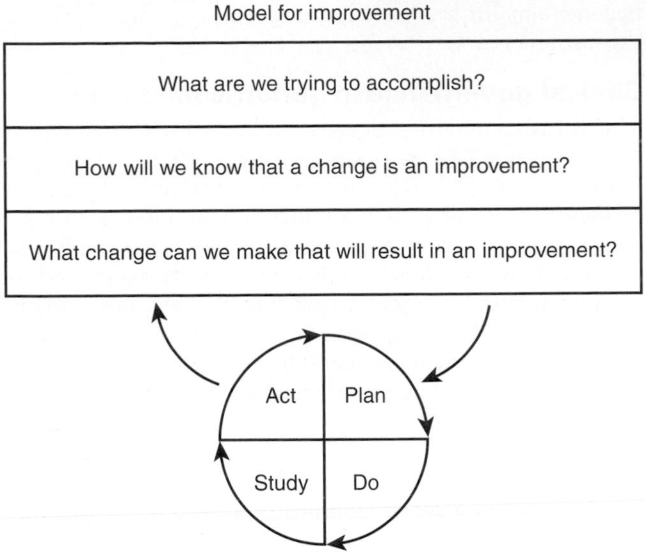

Figure 125-1. A model of improvement adapted by Berwick from Langley et al.[25] *Reproduced from Berwick DM: A primer on leading the improvement of systems. BMJ 1996;312:619–22.*

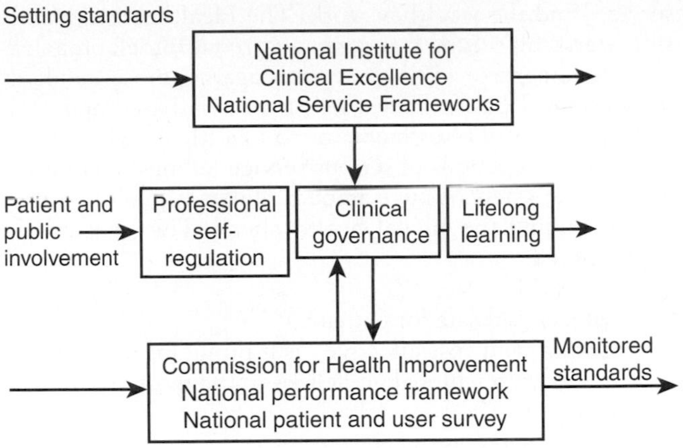

Figure 125-2. A model for quality improvement in the NHS.

THE CURRENT NHS APPROACH

Service standards, delivery, and monitoring

Based on the 1997 NHS white paper[26] and the subsequent white paper, *A First Class Service*,[27] the government set out a new model for quality improvement within the health service. This has three main parts: clear standards of service; dependable local delivery; and monitored standards (Figure 125-2).

Clear standards of service and the national institute of clinical excellence (NICE)

Clear standards of service are being increasingly defined through two approaches. The first is the National Institute for Clinical Excellence (NICE). NICE is an independent organization responsible for providing national guidance on promoting good health and preventing and treating ill health.[28] It promotes clinical and cost effectiveness through guidance and audit. It advises on best practice in existing treatment options, appraises new health interventions, and advises the health service on how they can be implemented. Examples of importance for older people include: clinical guidelines on Parkinson's disease, technology appraisals of drugs in the treatment of Alzheimer's disease, guidelines on supporting people with dementia and their caregivers in Health and Social Care, and guidelines on the assessment and prevention of falls in older people. However, a major challenge for all organizations is the effective implementation and follow through of NICE guidance.

The second approach to setting standards is through the National Service Frameworks (NSFs). These set national standards and define care models for specific services or care groups, put in place programs to support implementation, and establish performance measures against which the progress and timetable can be measured. A National Service Framework should bring together the best evidence of clinical and cost effectiveness with the views of the service users to determine the best ways of providing particular services. The National Service Framework in Elderly Care was published in May 2001.[29] It contained guidelines on the management of specific conditions such as stroke and falls, on the organization of services with an emphasis on patient-centered care, and on the use of intermediate-care facilities. It has policy statements about rooting out ageism whereby older people are denied some treatments simply on account of their age. The National Service Framework has proved to be a focus for quality improvement, although the impact in geriatric medicine may not have been as dramatic as the National Service Frameworks in other areas, such as cancer and heart disease.[30]

Dependable local delivery

The second strand of *A First Class Service* is ensuring that arrangements are in place to support dependable local delivery of good care. Professional self-regulation includes the introduction of appraisal for all doctors and revalidation through the General Medical Council. It encourages programs of lifelong learning based on effective appraisal, and the introduction of personal development plans for all staff.

For over 10 years the GMC and the government discussed concept and framework for licensing and revalidation of doctors. This will finally be introduced in 2009 in two parts. The first is relicensing for all doctors as demonstration of their fitness to practice and to continue with a license in medicine. The second aspect is recertification in the specialty that they are currently documented in the Medical Register. This recertification in specialty will occur on a 5-year rolling basis, but the detail of the standards—how they will be assessed for all clinicians—remains to be agreed on between the GMC and Royal Colleges.

It also involved the quality improvement tool of "clinical governance" (see later discussion).

Monitoring and publicizing standards

Thirdly, the government put in place systems to monitor and publicize standards. The Healthcare Commission is the independent inspection body for both the NHS and independent health care.[31] It is responsible for assessing and reporting on the performance of health care organizations to ensure they are meeting expected standards of care while encouraging them to continually improve their services and the way they work. The Healthcare Commission works by setting standards and requiring all organizations to undertake a self-assessment against those standards on an annual basis. They then use a risk-based approach to validate those assessments or to investigate where there have been allegations of serious service failings or concerns for patients' safety. A huge amount of data is published each year including the annual health check. The standards of care covered:

- Safety - is it safe for patients?
- Clinical and cost-effective - is it providing treatment in line with national guidelines in the most effective way.
- Governance - is it well run?
- Patient focused - does it organize it services around the needs and preferences of patients?
- Accessible and responsive care - is it easy to get the care you need without unreasonable delays?
- Environment and amenities - is the place where you are treated well designed and maintained?
- Public health - does it improve, promote, and protect the health of local people?

The Healthcare Commission reports annually to Parliament. If the Healthcare Commission has concerns that an organization is unsafe, it does have statutory powers of enforcement.

Clinical governance

Within the process of inspection, standard-setting, and attempts to measure quality, the main driver for clinical quality improvement at the local level is the concept of "clinical governance.[32]" Clinical governance is defined as: "a system through which NHS organizations are accountable for continuously improving the quality of their services and safeguarding high standards of care by creating an environment in which excellence in clinical care will flourish."

Clinical governance is seen as a process of continuous quality improvement in health care along the lines described by Berwick.[24] This aims to put quality at the heart of what health care organizations do in the United Kingdom as opposed to merely bolting it on or "inspecting it in." For the first time, the chief executives of trusts became personally responsible for the quality of health care provided in their organizations.

The seven pillars underpinning clinical governance include: clinical effectiveness, risk management effectiveness, patient experiences, communication effectiveness, resource effectiveness, strategic effectiveness, and learning effectiveness. At a local level this involves integrating a focus on safety and risk management with continuous professional development and lifelong learning. Also understanding an individual practitioner's performance with both patients and their colleagues while setting this in the wider context of organizational delivery and the expectations of the Healthcare Commission. Tools at a local level include patient surveys, appraisal systems including 360 degree feedback, audit data about comparative individual and team performance and outcomes, and a rigorous approach to clinical incidents and risk management. Patient safety issues, for example, reducing health care related infections, have become a major focus of clinical governance activities over the last few years.

Clinical governance in geriatric medicine

The British Geriatrics Society and the Royal College of Physicians published a position paper in 1999 on interpreting clinical governance and its implications for geriatric medicine.[33] Along with recommending an integrated common scheme for clinical governance, the paper made specific recommendations for individual practitioners, and for services within an organization and the services crossing organizations. An integrated common scheme was based on the clinical governance cycle (Figure 125-3). This requires practitioners or services to consider each aspect of the cycle.

- *Standards* include those set by NICE and the National Service Framework, along with professional standards from the GMC and legal standards.
- *Professional qualities* are based around the individual or the service needs for differing knowledge and skills. These may vary over time and are not exclusively clinical.
- *Service delivery and organization* includes the use of guidelines and protocols, and analysis of whether the structures available within the organization can deliver the care that is required.
- *Monitoring* includes systematic evaluation of clinical audit, both local and national; complaints; risk assessment; national performance indicators; critical incident reviews; national patient surveys; and external body reviews such as the Healthcare Commission.
- *Change management* includes all those processes that can be used to improve the quality of care, such as the quality improvement tools discussed within this chapter.

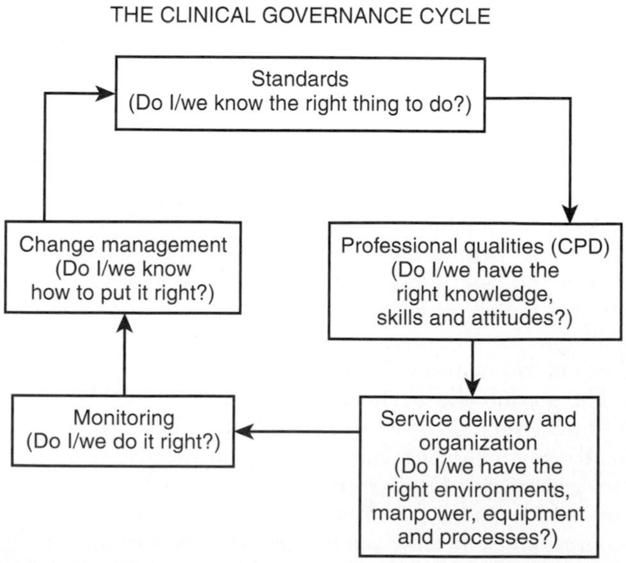

Figure 125-3. The clinical governance cycle. *Reproduced from British Geriatrics Society and Royal College of Physicians of London: Clinical Governance: A Position Paper. London, 1999.*

The British Geriatrics Society has further considered guidelines for implementing clinical governance at the departmental level.[34] Key areas of implementation are:

1. Each department of geriatric medicine should have a nominated lead consultant in organizational service quality.
2. The appropriate participation of consultants in geriatric medicine in processes covering each element of the clinical governance cycle should be clearly demonstrable.

If clinical governance is to be successful, it must have the same strengths as corporate governance: it must be rigorous in its application, have an organizationwide emphasis, and be accountable in its delivery, developmental in its thrust, and positive in its connotations. The drive to clinical governance is by far the most ambitious quality initiative that has ever been implemented in the NHS. It is too early to say whether clinical governance will bring about the revolution in quality improvement that was promised at its launch; however, it can be seen how the various quality initiatives of the previous 20 years have been drawn together into an integrated common scheme, which is more closely in touch with the reality of the National Health Service rather than the business world.

Long-term care

Geriatric medicine in the United Kingdom grew out of long-term care with attempts to improve the quality of care of older people in that environment.

Changes in social security funding led to massive expansion of private sector provision, in particular nursing-home care in the 1980s and 1990s. The vast majority of long-term nursing-home and residential-home care is now in the private and "not-for-profit" sector. The main driver for standards remains inspection. The Commission for Social Care Inspection is now the regulatory and inspecting body for all social care services in the private, public, and voluntary sectors including all care homes. Inspection processes in the past have been very much based on structure rather than process of outcome. There is an increasing move to try and produce more data regarding overall quality with a new star rating system being introduced in 2008.

In 1992, the Royal College of Physicians and the British Geriatrics Society produced the first document on guidelines and audit measures in long-term care followed by a clinical audit scheme called the CARE (Continuous Assessment Review and Evaluation) scheme.[11] This allowed users to audit seven main domains (Table 125-2) and encouraged a process of continuous review and reassessment. Although not widely used, where it has been used there is some evidence of improvement.[35] Yet the problems of improving quality in long-term care, particularly the medical aspects, remain.[36] Among the recommendations are reengagement of physicians in geriatric medicine in long-term care within the community, a whole-system approach to planning care, and the development of a new nursing role for the gerontological specialist. The current drive in the NHS to move specialty care out into the community to support community activity is an opportunity to revitalize and improve medical care for older people in the community particularly in long-term care.

Table 125-2. Key Audit Indicators for Long-Term Care

Preserving autonomy
Promoting urinary continence
Promoting fecal continence
Optimizing drug usage
Managing falls and accidents
Preventing pressure sores
Environment and equipment
Aids and adaptations
The medical role in long-term care

KEY POINTS
Improving Quality of Care in the United Kingdom

- Quality in health care has a number of dimensions, which makes definitions, standard setting, and measurement complex.
- Until recently the main approaches to improving quality involved inspection of services and encouragement for clinical audit.
- During the 1990s, new approaches from business introduced the ideas of continuous quality improvement, although implementation, in large part, has been haphazard and inadequately understood and resourced.
- The U.K. government has introduced the concept of "clinical governance," which now places a responsibility on all professionals to be accountable for not only maintaining but also improving standards of care within the health service.
- There is still huge room for improvement in our approaches to improving the quality of care of older people in the United Kingdom.

For a complete list of references, please visit online only at www.expertconsult.com

CHAPTER 126

Preserving Medicare Through a "Quality" Focus

Richard G. Stefanacci

MEDICARE'S NEW FOCUS ON QUALITY

Guardians of Medicare believe that the answer to preserving Medicare is to focus on quality improvement. The Institute of Medicine (IOM) describes quality health care as care that is, "safe, effective, patient-centered, timely, efficient, and equitable." These six determinates were part of their watershed document, Crossing the Quality Chasm: A New Health System for the 21st Century.[1] The Agency for Healthcare Research and Quality (AHRQ), an arm of the federal government, defines health care quality as, "doing the right thing for the right patient, at the right time, in the right way to achieve the best possible results."[2]

Both definitions provide a clear picture of quality health care based on scientific evidence. It is also clear that by focusing on quality, not only will Medicare beneficiaries benefit, but Medicare as a whole will through reduction in expenditures. These reductions in expenditures are the result of decreased waste and preventive measures resulting in a decrease in our current and future health expenditures. This is a shift from health care reform that has traditionally started with the presumption that the major problem is high costs.

In 1965 when Medicare was born the expenses were limited both because of the limited availability of services and the demand. The total number of Medicare beneficiaries was around 10 million while the average life expectancy for a Medicare senior at that time was about 4 years. Today with almost an unlimited availability of innovative expensive services in the face of exploding demand, Medicare is facing resource management challenges. This demand for services is driven by baby boomers now numbering over 40 million with life expectancy when they reach Medicare of an additional 20 years. Rather than restrict benefits, Medicare instead is looking toward quality improvement as a means to operate more efficiently and effectively.

The evidence of quality shortcomings is substantial and growing. The following are a few examples:

Researchers from the RAND Corp. have found that, on average, Americans receive the care indicated by medical evidence as necessary only 55% of the time. Most of these results reflect underuse of necessary care that can lead to needless complications, adding to health care costs and reducing productivity. Some results reflect overuse of unnecessary care that increases costs directly, and if complications occur, can further increase costs and threaten the health of patients.

A 1999 Institute of Medicine (IOM) report estimated that as many as 98,000 Americans die each year as a result of avoidable patient safety errors, while the Centers for Disease Control and Prevention has estimated that 90,000 Americans die each year due to hospital-based infections. These reflect misuse, another quality problem that leads to preventable deaths and injuries.

There also are examples of enormous variations in delivery of care nationally, regionally, and locally. A report to Congress by the Agency for Healthcare Research and Quality (AHRQ) found that the proportion of elderly patients with pneumonia who received recommended pneumococcal screenings or vaccinations in the highest-performing state was 7.5 times higher than in the lowest-performing state. Researchers at Dartmouth University have shown that Medicare expenditures in Los Angeles were twice as high compared with Sacramento for care given to persons in the last 2 years of their lives. These results indicate that care for these Medicare beneficiaries was not based on standardized or evidence-based guidelines. Similarly, a recent analysis of data from the Hospital Quality Alliance (HQA), the first initiative to report routinely on hospital performance, showed that the quality of hospital care varies widely, not only by geographic region and hospital type, but also across conditions within individual hospitals.

This focus on quality has been demonstrated both behind and in front of the scenes. Perhaps the most expressive of which was the name change from the Health Care Finance Administration to the Centers for Medicare and Medicaid (CMS). As CMS, Medicare is now exerting a greater influence on quality rather then simply on finance, although Medicare's focus on quality improvement is hoped to have a substantial effect on extending Medicare's resources. They are dearly needed as the number of Medicare beneficiaries doubles over the next 2 decades.

Historically, Medicare reimbursement has been based on volume of acute care services provided. However, the current belief is that if we just keep paying the bills the same old way, we will not get higher quality, more efficient care. Medicare has long provided critical support for hospital and doctor care when beneficiaries have complications from their diseases. But Medicare's benefits have not kept up with the shift toward preventing diseases and their complications that has been such an integral part of the progress in medical care in the past 35 years. Medicare has not paid for many preventive tests to detect diseases early or prevent them in the first place, or for programs that help our beneficiaries with chronic illnesses to take proven steps to prevent their complications, or for the prescription drugs that can head off the costly and often deadly consequences of chronic illnesses. Consequently, Medicare has seen rapid spending growth on the complications of diabetes, heart disease and failure, lung disease, advanced cancers, and many other illnesses. By closing the gap in prevention-oriented coverage, Medicare believes it can foster the health care system to deliver higher-quality care.

It is often stated that the three most important measures for a health care system are access, cost, and quality. Although much of the focus has been on the components of cost (price times use), perhaps the most difficult to define and measure is quality. In addition to being the most difficult to assess, quality is not necessarily directly effected by the cost of health care, making it even more difficult to improve since simply adding more dollars does not always improve quality. In fact several studies demonstrated that regions of high Medicare spending did not enjoy better quality.[3] Fisher found that higher spending was the result of a greater use of inpatient-based and specialist-oriented patterns of practice. So to achieve better health outcomes, it takes more than just added dollars but an approach focused on quality.

Of course the focus on quality is not entirely new. Since its beginning, Medicare has been keenly interested in ensuring quality care for its beneficiaries. This push for quality health care has evolved slowly over time; first, focusing primarily on a regulatory approach while at the same time building some assistive programs for providers to achieve quality care delivery standards. Most recently Medicare has moved to effecting the demand and supply for quality Medicare services by using market forces. Medicare has undertaken a strategy of measuring, reporting, and rewarding performance in health care through both the demand and supply side. On the demand side this is accomplished through the use of public reporting of quality data. The thought is that consumers will be driven toward higher quality providers and away from lower quality providers. On the supply side, the focus is pay-for-performance measures and a reimbursement system that rewards high-quality providers financially, providing them the resources to expand their services.

Starting with a regulatory approach

In the early days of Medicare the focus for achieving quality outcomes was strictly regulatory. This regulatory approach to assuring quality has existed since the beginning of the Medicare program. The focus here has primarily been on fraud and abuse prevention. Regulation against fraud and abuse is thought in many circles to be the best defense against this problem, which is currently estimated to cost Medicare and Medicaid about $33 billion each year. Medicare fraud is defined as purposely billing Medicare for services that were never provided or received. This is of course not to say that CMS regulations all fall in the area of fraud and abuse. In the area of nursing home care, for example, state surveyors are armed with volumes of regulations to enforce such things as food temperature and the storage of medications.

In the move toward quality many have outlined plans for achieving better quality results that go beyond regulations; Steinberg published his four actions needed to produce the greatest effect.[4] His actions included the following:

- Quality of care should be measured and reported routinely at both the national and provider-specific levels.
- We must make greater use of information technology.
- We should draw on the power of patients to improve the quality of care they receive and their health outcomes.
- Current financial incentives need to be redesigned so as to not discourage quality improvements.

Movement away from a pure regulatory focus is in part due to the fact that quality problems persist despite a decline in deficiencies. Also there is concern that over time effectiveness of regulations decline.[5]

Reporting quality to push demand

For Medicare's first 3 decades very little public reporting of data was available. Even the commercial world data was limited to information available in HEDIS (Health Plan Employer Data and Information Set.) CMS began its move in the collection and use of data on a grassroots level through peer review organizations (PROs), now referred to as Quality Improvement Organizations. PROs systematically promoted improvements in quality measures tracked using voluntary, collaborative, and educational approaches.

Initial reporting of quality measures was viewed as a way to promote self-improvement as providers compared themselves to their competitors. This role of reported quality data has evolved. The first change was to use the data to promote movement of patients to higher quality providers.

This worked especially well as payers shifted more of the cost of insurance to patients and their families and asked them to take a greater role in decisions about their care. This model of "consumer-directed health care" aims to give patients incentives to make informed decisions and choose necessary, cost-effective care. However, this model assumes that patients will have sufficient information about the quality, performance, and costs of hospitals, doctors, health plans, and others that deliver care. Consumers report that they do not generally have this kind of information available to them.

To help patients gain access to this information companies such as HealthGrades have developed. HealthGrades is the leading health care ratings organization, providing ratings and profiles of hospitals, nursing homes, and physicians to consumers, corporations, health plans, and hospitals. Millions of consumers and hundreds of the nation's largest employers, health plans, and hospitals rely on HealthGrades' independent ratings to make health care decisions based on the quality of care. Visitors to HealthGrades.com find quality ratings of the nation's 5000 hospitals and 16,000 nursing homes along with in-depth profiles of the nation's 650,000 physicians. As a leader in the consumer revolution in health care, HealthGrades receives more than 2.5 million unique visitors to its consumer Web site each month. It is thought that this type of information is what is needed to move toward consumer driven health care. This is moving the medical market on the demand side through the use of public reporting of quality data. Again, the thought is that consumers will be driven toward higher quality providers and away from lower quality providers.

Quality measurement and reporting in health care are crucial for identifying areas in need of improvement, monitoring progress, and providing consumers and purchasers with comparative information about health system performance. Although several measurement systems are used routinely to assess ambulatory, hospital, and long-term care, a systematic assessment of quality across spectrums of care is lacking. Spurred by rising costs and lagging quality improvement, large purchasers, health plans, and others have developed and implemented a variety of approaches that seek to reward high performance and create incentives for quality improvement. Efforts to improve and increase care measurement and align the incentives of providers through pay-for-performance programs are important building blocks in developing a health care system that performs more effectively and efficiently. Federal leadership is important to provide consistency to measurement and incentive systems so that the nation can gain the full value of these tools.

The measuring and reporting of quality measures is a very active process as there continues to be many barriers.

Barriers that include: limited availability of data, the burden associated with collecting or obtaining data, and the generally poor quality of data, including insufficient level of detail and lack of timeliness.

Even with following guidelines consensus regarding appropriate quality measures is not always agreed upon. Many feel that quality cannot be reflected in a single, meaningful criterion because it involves many criteria emerging from preferences of multiple constituencies— policymakers, health care professionals, administrators, owners, investors, third-party insurers, and consumers. Such values and preferences may overlap, but they may conflict as well.[6]

In evaluating measures that are important to measure, the following criteria have been recommended to follow:

- The disease is prevalent and a major source of morbidity or mortality in the Medicare population
- There is strong scientific evidence and practitioner consensus that there are processes of care that can substantially improve outcomes
- Reliably measuring the delivery of these processes is feasible
- There is a substantial "performance gap" between current
- performance and desirable performance
- There is at least anecdotal evidence that QIOs can intervene effectively to improve these performance measures.

As a result the first series of measures focused on acute myocardial infarction, heart failure, stroke, treatment and prevention of pneumonia, breast cancer, and diabetes.

A change in direction: pay-for-performance (P4P)

In 2001, the Institute of Medicine (IOM) identified the flat-rate fee schedule as a barrier to quality improvement and recommended that CMS adopt reimbursement policies linked to quality improvement such as through a pay-for-performance system.[7]

Thus data can be used to drive demand for services but on the other side CMS is also using data to drive supply by increasing the resources given to high-quality providers through pay-for-performance initiatives. Here the focus is pay-for-performance measures and reimbursement systems that reward high-quality providers financially, providing them the resources to expand their services. Medicare is testing two quality-based bonus reimbursement models for hospitals and large physician groups. On the hospital side, Medicare is awarding bonus Medicare payments to hospitals based on their performance on evidence-based quality measures for inpatients with heart attack, heart failure, pneumonia, coronary artery bypass graft, and hip and knee replacements. Within these five clinical areas, CMS will evaluate hospital performance on 34 measures. The Physician Group Practice Demonstration tests a hybrid payment method for paying physicians by combining Medicare fee-for-service payments with a bonus pool derived from savings achieved through improved management of patient care and services.

The pay-for-quality concept is not new, as insurers such as Independence Blue Cross (IBC) and Highmark Blue Cross Blue Shield have for years offered reimbursement bonus in addition to their capitation payments to primary care physicians who follow clinical guidelines such as Health Plan Employer Data and Information Set (HEDIS).

There is a growing belief that current payment systems not only fail to reward or encourage quality and quality improvement but sometimes actually penalize them. Many payment systems pay for each service rendered on a fee-for-service basis. As a result, if a hospital, physician, or other provider performs fewer or less intensive services by following evidence-based guidelines, the organization or provider receives less money. As the IOM stated in its Quality Chasm report, policymakers must align payment incentives with the drive to improve quality.

Today, the Medicare payment policy is structured so as to align payments with provider performance. The Medicare Payment Advisory Commission (MedPAC) is required to consider a variety of measures because the direct relevance, availability, and quality of information in each potential indicator varies among providers.[8] In the development of measurements the focus has started in the areas of structural capacity and process standards before moving to outcome measures. The reason for these starting points before moving to outcome measures is the following:

- There is more consensus on appropriate processes.
- Measuring processes of care are generally easier, requiring no need for risk adjustment.
- It is easier for practitioners to identify and fix the reasons why critical processes of care are not being met.
- Many outcome measures take years to calculate their effect.[9]

The AMA House of Delegates amended and approved the AMA Principles and Guidelines for the formation and implementation of pay-for-performance programs.

As the pay-for-performance concept becomes more commonplace, the physician community will work to ensure pay-for-performance programs are positively structured and appropriately applied. The AMA believes pay-for-performance programs must be aligned with the following five principles:

- Ensure quality of care
- Foster the relationship between patient and physician
- Offer voluntary physician participation
- Use accurate data and fair reporting
- Provide fair and equitable program incentives

In the end CMS's movement toward quality measures as a means to push the demand and supply of provider systems will have profound effects on how physicians practice

MEASURING QUALITY

Physician

Medicare payments for physician services are made on the basis of a fee schedule, which has been in place since 1992. The Medicare fee schedule is intended to relate payments to the actual resources used in providing the health care services. The fee schedule assigns relative values to services that reflect physician work (i.e., time, skill, and intensity it takes to provide the service), practice expenses, and malpractice costs. These relative values are adjusted for geographic variations in costs.

In addition to responding to external pressures to measure quality performance, some payers have taken the initiative to measure the quality performance of individual physicians or physician groups.[6,7] Typically, physician or physician group performance is compared with peers, adjusting for differences in case mix. This profiling of physician performance relative to peers often includes comparisons on health care use and cost along with measures of quality. The objective of the payer is to compensate physicians on the basis of quality and use management.

In practice, producing credible physician profiles of quality are difficult for individual HMOs to do. The physician's contribution to health care usage and costs is known to the health plan from administrative records (claims paid for services provided under fee-for-service, and capitation payments made for services provided under capitation). The physician's quality performance is more difficult to measure with the claims data typically used by health plans for this purpose. In particular, primary care physicians under capitation will generate limited claims for services assessed in process measures of quality. An exception is the fee-for-service reimbursement of immunizations to remove any disincentive to provide the preventive measure and to provide data to the health plan. Furthermore, some services of quality performance such as whether a diabetic in the health plan received a hemoglobin A_{1c} are not available on many payers databases.

The 2006 Tax Relief and Health Care Act (TRHCA) (P.L. 109–432) required the establishment of a physician quality reporting system, including an incentive payment for eligible professionals who satisfactorily report data on quality measures for covered services furnished to Medicare beneficiaries during the second half of 2007. CMS named this program the Physician Quality Reporting Initiative (PQRI).

The Medicare, Medicaid, and SCHIP Extension Act of 2007 (MMSEA) was enacted on December 29, 2007 (Pub. Law 110–173). MMSEA authorizes CMS to make PQRI incentive payments for satisfactorily reporting quality measures data. Eligible professionals who meet the criteria for satisfactory submission of quality measures data for services furnished will earn an incentive payment of 2% of their total allowed charges for Physician Fee Schedule (PFS) covered professional services furnished during that same period. This incentive payment has been increased since the introduction of the program in 2007.

The 2008 PQRI consists of 119 quality measures, including two structural measures. One structural measure conveys whether a professional has and uses electronic health records (EHR) and the other electronic prescribing. Besides providing PQRI information during a patient encounter in the form of a completed billing/HCFA 1500 form, CMS has also opened up submission through registries. In an era of EHR this is especially efficient. Providers can manage and submit data on the PQRIs of their choosing from their EHR database.

To test the effectiveness of the pay-for-performance system, CMS implemented a demonstration program. The Physician Group Practice demonstration provided rewards to large, multi-specialty group practices for improving the quality of care and reducing the cost increases for their patients. Unfortunately in this first application of the pay-for-performance initiatives, the "Physician Group Practice Demonstration" found that a number of groups did not earn performance payments because they did not generate savings to the Medicare program despite incurring upfront costs to improve care management systems that totaled millions of dollars in some cases.[10]

Besides the effectiveness in providing a return back to physicians who participated in this pay-for-performance program, another barrier to their impact on quality is the fact that since many physicians contract with several payers in their market area, only a portion of the physician's patients will be a member of a given payer. A profile produced by any given payer may be based on a small sample of the physician's patients. Furthermore, performance measures may differ on the profiles produced by the different payers for which the physician contracts. Because physicians are more likely to dismiss as flawed the results of profiles produced under these circumstances, their effectiveness in improving performance may be limited. Furthermore, some performance measures monitored by the payer are population-based; however, a fraction of payer members do not see their physicians regularly. Physicians have no opportunity or infrequent opportunities to demonstrate that they have provided quality care for this fraction of the payer's members for which they are responsible. Again, physicians will not view such measures as credible gauges of performance. However, with Medicare as the major driving force in the development and implementation of physician quality measures, the thought is that other payers will follow making these quality measures universally accepted.

Hospital

CMS hospital quality measures come from information collected by hospitals that volunteer to provide data for public reporting. The information is intended to illustrate how quality of care can vary between hospitals. Currently, the quality information relates to the care given for patients with three serious medical conditions that are common in people with Medicare:

- Myocardial infarction (i.e., heart attacks)
- Congestive heart failure
- Pneumonia

CMS first attempted to collect this information on a purely voluntary basis, but could not garner sufficient interest from hospitals. When voluntary participation failed, CMS tied submission of quality data to payments for services administered to Medicare patients. Today, hospitals that fail to submit data are not eligible for the payment increase applied to the payment, which can translate to as much as a 0.4% reduction in revenue for some facilities. This increased financial support resulted in almost 99% of U.S. hospitals (over 4200 hospitals) providing data for comparative quality measures. It is now been proposed that the measures will be expanded to include outcomes such as patient satisfaction and surgical complications. Measures of hospital efficiency are also under consideration.

Measures of hospital quality have been developed through the Hospital Quality Alliance (HQA). The HQA consists of more than a dozen organizations including AARP, AFL-CIO,

AHRQ, AHA, AHIP, AMA, ANA, and JCAHO to facilitate nationwide public reporting of useful quality measures by hospitals. All of this activity was done in a transparent, collaborative fashion with the goal of providing more information to consumers and practitioners to lead to better performance.

The hospital data is reported online through Medicare's Hospital Compare site. In this tool information on how well hospitals care for patients with certain medical conditions or surgical procedures, and results from a survey of patients about the quality of care they received during a recent hospital stay is reported. This information is provided to help patients compare the quality of care hospitals provide, again as a means to drive demand to the higher quality providers.

Expansion of this program is being tested through CMS demonstration programs. One such program has CMS collaborating with Premier, Inc., a group of nonprofit hospitals, to operate a demonstration to improve their quality of care. This demonstration tracks and reports quality data for 34 measures at each of about 270 participating hospitals. Under the demonstration, top-performing hospitals will receive incentive payments for the care of inpatients with any of five conditions: acute myocardial infarction, heart failure, community acquired pneumonia, coronary artery bypass graft, and hip and knee replacement. Participating hospitals will get composite scores for each of the five clinical conditions, and the hospitals will be ranked in order of their scores. Hospitals with scores in the top 10% will get a 2% bonus of their payments for Medicare fee for service patients, whereas hospitals with scores in the second 10% will get a 1% bonus. Early results are promising, showing improvement in quality scores for the participating hospitals. It is expected that lessons learned from the Premier demonstration will shape our future hospital pay-for-performance initiatives.

Nursing home

With 3 million of the frailest Americans relying on services provided by a nursing home at some point during the year and of them 1.5 million staying long enough to consider the nursing home their main residences,[11] it should come as no surprise that nursing homes are heavily governed to assure appropriate care. But even with heavy oversight one in five nursing homes nationwide were cited for serious deficiencies, deficiencies that caused actual harm or placed residents in immediate jeopardy.[12]

Some major areas of focus identified by nursing home medical directors include the following[13]: telephone conversations, transitional care, falls and hip fracture, Coumadin use, pressure ulcers, inappropriate medications, pain control, urinary incontinence, weight loss, and exercise.

Under the Omnibus Budget Reconciliation Act (OBRA) of 1987, nursing homes participating in the Medicare and Medicaid programs are required to monitor nursing-home residents using the Resident Assessment Instrument (RAI). The RAI consists of the Minimum Data Set for nursing home resident assessment and care screening (MDS), which assesses functioning on activities of daily living (ADLs), cognition, continence, mood, behaviors, nutritional status, vision and communication, activities, and psychosocial well-being. Problems or risks for decline identified through the MDS assessment will trigger further assessment on one or more of the RAI's 18 resident assessment protocols, which are used to identify treatable causes of problems common to nursing home residents.[10] The OBRA 1987 requirements, which became federal law in 1990, were the result of widespread evidence of poor quality of care in nursing homes. Prior studies found prevalent use of physical restraints, inappropriate use of psychotropic medications, overuse of urinary catheters, and inadequate treatment of incontinence, pressure ulcers, nutritional problems, and behavioral problems.

Several studies compared process quality and patient outcomes before implementation of the RAI with the postimplementation period and found evidence of improvements. More specifically, in a study of 254 nursing homes in 10 states, accuracy of information in medical records, comprehensiveness of care plans, presence of advanced directives, participation in activities, and use of toileting programs for those with bowel incontinence improved after implementation of the RAI. Use of physical restraints declined by 25% and use of indwelling catheters declined by 29%. Another study of 267 nursing homes showed that the rate of decline in ADLs, social engagement, and cognitive function was reduced after the introduction of the RAI.

Nursing Home Compare includes information only on nursing homes that are Medicare or Medicaid certified. The data on this Web site refers to the regulatory requirements that the nursing home failed to meet but does not reflect the entire inspection report (which, in some cases, may be well over 100 pages in length). The detailed inspection report (the form HCFA-2567) contains the specific findings that support the state's determination that the requirement was not met. A complete inspection report and the nursing home's corresponding plan of correction to address the deficiencies found during the inspection are available from the state survey agency or from the nursing home itself.

The Department of Health and Human Services (DHHS) has a national Nursing Home Quality Initiative to improve the quality of nursing home (NH) care. A critical part of this initiative is CMS's posting of quality indicators for every NH on 10 quality indicators.[14] These "report cards" are intended to be used by consumers to make informed decisions and motivate providers to improve their care. The CMS quality initiative is a major redirection to focus on clinical care needs of the frail elder instead of historically focusing on the process of care. This is the result of a shift toward the resident and away from the institution. Although fairly well received, these nursing home report cards have been said to have limited value because of their failure to adjust for differences in risk in different long-term care facilities.[15]

Measures of nursing home quality as part of the Nursing Home Quality Initiative, has already achieved important improvements in aspects of nursing home care such as use of restraints and controlling pain. This alliance recently expanded and refined its measures and is taking further steps to improve additional important outcomes and efficiency, such as to reduce pressure ulcers and avoid hospital admissions with preventable complications.

CMS under its 2007 Action Plan[16] addresses nursing home quality through:

- Web-based report card "Nursing Home Compare"
- Expanding the certification and survey process
- Adding a pilot test pay-for-performance under the heading of "value-based purchasing"

In the Nursing Home Value-Based Purchasing Demonstration, the hypothetical savings for the incentive payments would come from reductions in hospitalizations and subsequent skilled nursing facility stays. The problem is that if no savings are generated, no performance payments will be made, regardless of the nursing homes' performance.[17]

Managed care plans

Medicare beneficiaries began enrolling in Medicare MCOs in 1985 under provisions of the Tax Equity and Fiscal Responsibility Act (TEFRA). However, it would be more than a decade later that the Medicare program would begin ongoing review of health care quality in Medicare MCOs. This was because PROs had access to Medicare fee-for-service claims for random case selection, but did not have access to Medicare MCO claims for the same purpose. In the interim, comprehensive evaluations of quality performance were conducted under contract with CMS by Mathematica Policy Research for both the Medicare HMO demonstrations and the Medicare MCOs contracting in the first 5 years of the TEFRA risk-contracting program.[18] The evaluations, which compared measures of process and outcomes for beneficiaries receiving care in Medicare MCOs to Medicare fee-for-service, reported that quality performance under MCOs and fee-for-service were quite similar. Although comprehensive, these evaluations did not have the surveillance effect of the ongoing review of cases by the PROs. In addition, standards for quality performance and quality improvement measurement in commercial MCOs (i.e., MCOs other than Medicare and Medicaid), such as HEDIS and NCQA accreditation, were in notable contrast to the lack of comparable quality performance standards for Medicare HMOs.

The lack of ongoing quality performance measurement in Medicare managed care ended in 1998, when CMS first required HEDIS reporting by Medicare MCOs. In addition, CMS required Medicare MCOs to submit for audit the beneficiary-level data used in the computation of the HEDIS measures. As part of the current HEDIS reporting set, CMS requires Medicare MCOs to conduct a longitudinal survey of health status for a random sample of the MCO's Medicare beneficiaries. Using the SF-36, the Health Outcomes Study compares the health status of beneficiaries surveyed in a baseline year with their health status measured 2 years later.

Under the 1997 Balanced Budget Act, the Quality Improvement System for Managed Care (QISMC) was established and became operational in 1999. QISMC applied many of the same principles of CQI adopted by the PROs in the Health Care Quality Improvement Program. More specifically, Medicare MCOs were required to measure clinical performance in the prevention or treatment of acute and chronic conditions, high-volume services, high-risk services, and continuity and coordination of care. Similarly, QISMC requires measurement of performance in nonclinical areas such as availability of and accessibility to care, quality of provider encounters, and resolution of appeals, grievances, and other complaints. For clinical and nonclinical areas selected by HCFA and the MCO, QISMC requires Medicare MCOs to develop and implement interventions for improving performance, and remeasure performance over time to demonstrate quality improvements. QISMC also imposes standards on methods of performance measurement; for example, they must be unambiguous, based on current clinical knowledge or health services research, and measure outcomes such as health status, functional status, beneficiary satisfaction, or valid proxies of the measures (ref. 4 QISMC standards). Performance must be measured over all relevant providers and beneficiaries at risk, and valid sampling methods must be used if performance is not measured for all beneficiaries at risk. A quality-improvement project under QISMC standards requires a minimum of 3 years: measurement of baseline performance in the first year, remeasurement of performance in the subsequent year when significant performance improvement is demonstrated, and continued measurement for a year beyond achieving significant improvement to demonstrate that a higher performance has been sustained over time.[4]

CMS is also paying organizations in Medicare to help chronically ill beneficiaries get better continuity, support, and treatment for their care. This includes Medicare Advantage health plans, including HMOs, PPOs, and fee for service plans that offer additional benefits. Medicare is moving to full "risk adjustment" of payments to these plans, so that to do well in Medicare, a health plan must pay particular attention to providing benefits that are attractive to beneficiaries who are chronically ill, frail, or dually eligible. This year, Medicare Advantage plans are more widely available than ever before in the history of the program, with well more than 90% of beneficiaries having access. And beneficiaries can save about $100 a month on average compared with the traditional plan with or without a Medigap plan they purchase on their own, with beneficiaries in fair or poor health able to save even more. In fact, this year, there are over 50 plans specializing in coordinated care for dual-eligible and chronically ill beneficiaries around the country, and many more such plans are expected to be available next year although Medicare Advantage plans may be subject to substantial reductions in their revenue from CMS as a result of a political switch toward traditional Medicare.

Working beyond Medicare Advantage plans, CMS is also working to bring better continuity of care and support for chronically ill beneficiaries in the traditional Medicare plan, by creating financial incentives through our Medicare Chronic Care Improvement Program (CCIP). Medicare CCIP is designed to help beneficiaries who account for a majority of Medicare costs today - those with diseases including congestive heart failure, complex diabetes, and chronic lung diseases. The evidence shows that it is possible to improve outcomes and lower costs by avoiding disease complications, by helping beneficiaries understand their disease, their physician's treatment plan, how they can improve their outcomes through medication compliance and certain lifestyle steps, and what to do with early signs of poor disease control. Now, organizations participating in Medicare CCIP initiative will get paid by Medicare when they get improvements in valid clinical quality measures, patient and physician satisfaction measures, and total Medicare costs. Their payments will come from some of the savings they create, and successful programs will have an opportunity to expand.

Prescription drug plans

Quality measures and reporting is involving all areas of Medicare including its newest benefit, Medicare Part D, the prescription drug benefit. Medicare Part D plans since their beginning in 2006 have been responsible for providing medication therapy management (MTM). MTM is viewed by

CMS as an opportunity for prescription drug plans (PDPs) to improve the health outcomes of their patients. Although the structure of MTM has to date been left in the hands of the specific plans, CMS is establishing standards and will expect plans to adhere to them. Organizations such as the Pharmacy Quality Alliance are developing the frame work of measurable standards for MTM programs.

COST EFFECTIVE QUALITY

Although the historic focus of CMS has been on coverage for acute services, there is a growing realization that to preserve Medicare a focus on quality is required. This is based on the findings that a small portion of seniors with chronic comorbid conditions use a disproportionately large amount of resources. Focus on preventive care using primary care providers in community-based settings of care can improve quality and at a reduced cost (Table 126-1).

Primary care expansion

Our current reimbursement structure rewards procedures and the use of technology but not time spent with patients or coordinating care. There is little incentive for primary care although there are plans to revise this trend by providing loan repayment, training grants, and improved provider reimbursement as a means to increase the availability of primary care services.

When comparing the United States to other countries that enjoy better health at lower costs, one major contributing factor is their focus on convenient primary care services. The United States has slowly moved in that direction through the increased use of nurse practitioners (NPS), convenient care clinic, and the demonstration project operating under the heading of the medical home.

It should come as no surprise that NPs are increasingly providing primary care to our seniors. NPs are advanced practice nurses whose field was born in 1965 at the University of Colorado. Today there are over 115,000 NPs practicing with additional 6000 added annually as a result of programs at over 300 academic centers. NPs are able to reach patients in a unique manner by blending nursing and medical care.

This unique manner combined with the increased availability of NPs has not been lost on the Governor of Pennsylvania Ed Rendell who believes strongly in the value of NPs. The governor stated that "We should employ nurse practitioners in the delivery of health care services far more than we do." A major reason for this support is an estimate by academics that a nurse practitioner can perform about 70% of the things that a primary care physician can do, often at 50% or less of the costs. The Pennsylvania plan calls for expanding the scope of nurse practitioners through unlocking of regulations that restrict their scope of practice.

Federal legislators are also attempting to expand the scope of NPs with an aim for long-term care involvement as current law requires that all care in a skilled nursing facility be provided under the direct supervision of a physician. The Long-term Care Quality and Modernization Act of 2006 would amend this to include that "at the option of a state, under the supervision of a nurse practitioner, clinical nurse specialist, or physician assistant who is working in collaboration with a physician." This would expand the role and responsibilities of NPs in skilled nursing facilities. In addition this legislation would amend current law that does not permit nonphysician practitioners to be employed by the skilled nursing facility. By removing this language, NPs could be employed by the facility and supervise resident care.

Besides a focus on primary care, a back to basics approach also calls for encouraging coordination of care. Under our current system care is often fragmented into silos. Medicare is engaging in reimbursement systems that promote greater coordination of care. One example is Medicare demonstration in bundling Medicare Part A and B payments.

Providers such as skilled nursing facilities and hospitals will have Medicare Part B payments included in their Medicare Part A reimbursement. Instead of physicians billing Medicare directly under Medicare Part B, they will instead be engaged by these Part A providers (hospitals and subacute nursing centers) who will be responsible for paying for their services. As such it is likely that these Part A providers will employ physicians directly, thus resulting in greater coordination of care.

Yet another example of the promotion of coordination of care is the Medical Home Demonstration. This demonstration mandates a trial in up to eight states to provide targeted, accessible, continuous, and coordinated family-centered care to Medicare beneficiaries who are deemed to be high need (that is, with multiple chronic or prolonged illnesses that require regular medical monitoring, advising, or treatment.) The objective is to bring greater coordination of care to the Medicare fee for services system.

Coordinated care models

Medicare has for some time been expanding programs that care for LTC residents in and outside of the traditional nursing home. In 1987, United Healthcare launched a program known as Evercare. Evercare uses NPs within nursing homes to increase onsite the primary care thereby reducing the need for emergency room evaluations and increasing preventive care and timely acute care assessment and treatment, all of which help reduce avoidable admissions. In addition the Evercare program is able to provide a skilled level of services without Medicare's requirement for a hospitalization of 3 days.

More recently the Medicare Modernization Act allowed for the development of these types of programs and a broader range of options under Medicare Advantage (MA) and specifically their Special Needs Plans (SNP). SNPs are permitted to focus solely on one of three distinct groups: residents of nursing homes, dual eligible seniors (those who are entitled to Medicare Part A and/or Part B and are eligible for some form of Medicaid benefit), or those suffering from multiple chronic illnesses. These are managed care programs

Table 126-1. Focus of Medicare

	Original Medicare	Future Medicare
Level of Care	Acute	Preventive
Providers	Specialist	Primary Care (PCP, NP, PA)
Facility	Hospital	Community
Integration	Silos	Coordinated Care
Technology	na	eRx, EHR, monitoring devices

to specific populations that have the same incentives as any Medicare managed care plan. The incentive is to provide care to improve health outcomes, thereby avoiding preventable hospitalizations.

A predecessor to the SNPs is PACE—the Program for All-inclusive Care for the Elderly. The PACE model began to evolve in the early 1970s in an effort to help the Asian American and other non-English speaking communities of San Francisco care for elders in their own homes. For these ethnicities, placing frail, elderly family members in a nursing home was not a culturally acceptable solution; therefore On Lok Senior Health Services created an innovative way to offer a comprehensive array of medical supervision, physical and occupational therapies, nutrition, transportation, respite care, socialization, and other needed services.

The benefits for these seniors living outside of the nursing home have been demonstrated in several studies. For instance, a 1996 study of Washington, Oregon, and Colorado seniors that were eligible for a nursing home concluded that the expansion of home and community-based services were a cost-effective alternative to institutional care in these states.[19] In addition to the cost-effectiveness of home-based services being offered in the community, medical directors should realize the advantage of developing a referral source to the nursing home for those that truly require that level of care. Also by expanding the reach of the clinical team it can afford significantly more depth, including not only the ability to be dedicated full time to this endeavor, but to enable other disciplines that require a larger base population than a traditional nursing facility can afford.

Technology

Often talked about as the cornerstone for improvement in technology in the form of electronic prescribing, health records and monitoring devices – these opportunities have yet to reach their full potential.

To motivate providers to use electronic prescribing[20] CMS has included a financial bonus through the Physician Quality Reporting Initiatives. The Medicare Improvement for Patients and Provider Act of 2008 (MIPPA) authorizes a new incentive program for eligible professionals who are successful electronic prescribers (E-Prescribers) as defined by MIPPA. This new incentive program is in addition to the quality reporting incentive program authorized by Division B of the Tax Relief and Health Care Act of 2006 - Medicare Improvements and Extension Act of 2006 (MIEA-TRHCA) and known as the Physician Quality Reporting Initiative (PQRI). The e-prescribing incentive is similar to the PQRI incentive in that reporting periods are 1 year in length and the incentive is based on the covered professional services furnished by the eligible professional during the reporting year. In addition, MIPPA requires that quality measures that can be reported for purposes of qualifying for the PQRI incentive payment not include e-prescribing measures. Reporting periods are for a calendar year, beginning with calendar year 2009 through 2013.

The e-prescribing incentive amount is based on the secretary's estimate (based on claims submitted not later than 2 months after the end of the reporting period) of the allowed charges for all such Physician Fee Schedule (PFS) covered professional services furnished by the eligible professional during the reporting period. The e-prescribing incentive percent amount for reporting years 2009 to 2010 is 2.0%; for reporting years 2011 to 2012 is 1.0%; and for reporting year 2013, it is 0.5%.

CMS is also making sure that providers have the support they need to take advantage of health information technology (IT) to lower costs and improve quality. First, CMS is working with the Veterans Administration to adapt their VISTA system for electronic records to the public domain. Second, CMS is providing technical support through our state-based Quality Improvement Organizations (QIOs). In their new 3-year quality improvement strategy, the QIOs will assist providers in using evidence-based approaches to achieve measurable quality improvements and get the most benefit from quality-based payment systems. One important method for doing so is to help them choose and implement health IT systems using advice and support that has worked well for similar providers and that is well-coordinated with other administration efforts to support effective, interoperable IT systems. These IT systems will help physician offices and other providers measure quality of care and improve it. The emphasis for technical assistance is on small offices, rural areas, and underserved areas.

Combined with increasing financial support for higher quality and lower overall costs, these steps to make it easier to adopt and use effective health IT. A study supported by the Office of the National Coordinator for Health Information Technology published in the *New England Journal of Medicine* found optimism for expanded use of EHRs; 17% of doctors used some kind of EHR system, 16% had acquired a system but hadn't booted it up yet, and 26% volunteered that they planned to buy one inside of 2 years. A less optimistic view was noted in a survey of about 3,000 doctors by a research team at the Institute for Health Policy at Massachusetts General Hospital.[21] This study found that only 4% of physicians had a fully functional system that could satisfy some of the basic standards set by the Certification Commission for Healthcare Information Technology. With a price tag of between $35,000 and $50,000 per doctor over 3 years implementation of an EHR can be costly (Table 126-2).

Table 126-2. Development of Clinical Records for Quality Data Assessment*

Essential Features of Clinical Records for Quality Data Assessment
Specifies Data Elements
Establishes linkage capability among data elements and records
Standardizes the element definitions
Is automated to the greatest possible extent
Specifies procedures for continually assessing data quality
Maintains strict controls for protecting security and confidentiality of the data
Specifies protocols for sharing data across institutions under appropriate and well-defined circumstances
Preparing for Quality Data Reporting
Expanding and improving the capture and use of currently available data
Creating an environment that rewards the automation of data
Improving the quality of currently automated data
Implementing national standards
Improving clinical data management practices
Establishing a clear commitment to protecting the confidentiality of enrollee information
Careful capital planning

*Schneide EC, Riehl V, Courte-Wienecke S, et al. Enhancing performance measurement: NCQA's road map for a health information framework. JAMA 1999;282(12):1184–90.

RESOURCES: "QUALITY" ORGANIZATIONS

Several government and nongovernmental organizations are dedicated to quality. These organizations work to ensure quality through identification/analysis of quality issues, resources to address these quality issues, including providing accreditation to notate quality organizations.

There are a few key organizations dedicated to identification/analysis of quality issues, the most influential at least to the public is the Institute of Medicine (IOM); the most influential to Congress is MedPAC, which is tasked with providing Congress advice on issues involving Medicare including quality. CMS has tasked the Quality Improvement Organizations (QIO) with the job of helping health care providers, whereas other organizations work with the federal government to place a stamp of quality on organizations and products (Table 126-3).

Identification/analysis: institute of medicine (IOM)

With a focus on quality, the Institute of Medicine (IOM) in 1996 launched a concerted, ongoing effort focused on assessing and improving the nation's quality of care, which is now in its third phase. The first phase of this quality initiative documented the serious and pervasive nature of the nation's overall quality problem, concluding that "the burden of harm conveyed by the collective impact of all of our health care quality problems is staggering."[22]

The initial phase built on an intensive review of the literature conducted by Dr. Mark A. Schuster at RAND to understand the scope of this issue and a framework was established that defined the nature of the problem as one of overuse, misuse, and underuse of health care services. During the second phase, spanning 1999 to 2001, the Committee on Quality of Health Care in America, laid out a vision for how the health care system and related policy environment must be radically transformed to close the chasm between what we know to be good quality care and what actually exists in practice. Phase three of the IOM's Quality Initiative focuses on operationalizing the vision of a future health system described in the Quality Chasm report.

The IOM report Leadership by Example: Coordinating Government Roles in Improving Health Care Quality (2002) encourages the federal government to take full advantage of its influential position as purchaser, regulator, and provider of health care services to determine quality for the health care sector. The vision for each of these distinct federal roles is very much in concert with ideas laid out in the Quality Chasm report. Other efforts in this area include Envisioning the National Healthcare Quality Report (2001) and Guidance for the National Healthcare Disparities Report.

Resources: quality improving organizations

Since the inception of the Medicare program, the quality of care received by beneficiaries has been monitored. The earliest organizations responsible for quality performance measurement were the professional services review organizations (PSROs), local review boards who reviewed care received by a limited number of beneficiaries during an inpatient hospital stay. The jurisdiction of PSROs was typically for one or several counties within a state, and had a primary focus on whether the health care received was medically necessary.

Table 126-3. "Quality" Organizations

Agency Within the Department of Health and Human Services (HHS) – Identification/Analysis	
Agency for Healthcare Research and Quality (AHRQ)	Supports health services research initiatives that seek to improve the quality of health care in America. AHRQ's mission is to improve the quality, safety, efficiency, effectiveness, and cost-effectiveness of health care for all Americans.
Independent Congressional Agency – Identification/Analysis	
Medicare Payment Advisory Commission (MedPAC)	Established to advise the U.S. Congress on issues affecting the Medicare program such as payments to private health plans participating in Medicare and providers in Medicare's traditional fee-for-service program, and analyzing access to care, quality of care, and other issues affecting Medicare.
Private, 501(c)(3) Not-For-Profit Organization – Accreditation	
National Committee for Quality Assurance (NCQA)	Dedicated to improving health care quality. The NCQA seal is a widely recognized symbol of quality. Organizations incorporating the seal into advertising and marketing materials must first pass a rigorous, comprehensive review and must annually report on their performance. For consumers and employers, the seal is a reliable indicator that an organization is well-managed and delivers high-quality care and service.
Utilization Review Accreditation Commission (URAC)	A leader in promoting health care quality through its accreditation and certification programs. URAC offers a wide range of quality benchmarking programs and services that keep pace with the rapid changes in the health care system, and provide a symbol of excellence for organizations to validate their commitment to quality and accountability. Through its broad-based governance structure and an inclusive standards development process, URAC ensures that all stakeholders are represented in establishing meaningful quality measures for the entire health care industry.
Joint Committee for the Accreditation of Healthcare Organization (JCAHO)	To continuously improve the safety and quality of care provided to the public through the provision of health care accreditation and related services that support performance improvemen The Joint Commission accredits and certifies more than 15,000 health care organizations and programs in the United States. Joint Commission accreditation and certification is recognized nationwide as a symbol of quality that reflects an organization's commitment to meeting certain performance standards.
A Private, 501(c)(3) Not-For-Profit Organization – Resources	
Institute of Healthcare Improvement (IHI)	Works to accelerate improvement by building the will for change, cultivating promising concepts for improving patient care, and helping health care systems put those ideas into action.
Quality Improvement Organizations (QIO)	Improving quality of care for beneficiaries and protecting the integrity of the Medicare Trust Fund by ensuring that Medicare pays only for services and goods that are reasonable and necessary and that are provided in the most appropriate setting, and protecting beneficiaries by expeditiously addressing individual complaints.

In 1984, the PSROs were replaced by the peer review organizations (PROs) with jurisdiction for an entire state (and for several of the 43 PROs, jurisdiction for more than one state). Initially PROs monitored inpatient care by selecting random samples of inpatient admissions from computerized Medicare hospital claims records. Initial review of medical necessity and quality of care for the sampled admissions were performed by nurse reviewers. Admissions identified with problems were then reviewed by physician reviewers, who requested medical records for review if they concurred with the initial case review. Admissions judged to have problems after the review of medical records resulted in denial of payment for the admission.

By the end of the 1980s, the PROs extended their review beyond inpatient care to include skilled nursing facilities, outpatient hospital departments, ambulatory surgery centers, and home health agencies. In addition, the reviews by the PROs increasingly focused on quality performance measures. By the early 1990s, the effectiveness of the PROs in successfully monitoring quality performance and improving quality was questioned. The reliability of physician reviews done by the PROs was questioned in some influential studies. In particular, one study showed that the agreement between reviews of PRO reviewers compared with reviewers at Johns Hopkins were no better than what would be expected by chance. The effectiveness of retrospective review in identifying the source of quality problems and preventing them was also questioned, given the elapse in time since specific cases were reviewed. Also, in contrast to provider profiling in which quality performance is based on some or all of the provider's patients, a PRO's retrospective review of a random sample of cases will identify at most very few cases per provider subject to review and no cases for many providers. Under the PRO's system of review, this paucity of cases for any given provider invites attribution of quality problems for a specific case to random variation in outcomes rather than systemic problems with a physician or health care facility.[23]

In light of this criticism of PROs, their activities were redefined under the Health Care Quality Improvement Program in 1993. Under this initiative, retrospective case review was replaced by collaborative initiatives with hospitals and physicians to improve quality that was closer to the model of CQI. Although the aggregate impact of this new initiative is difficult to assess, case studies suggest success in specific settings. For example, results from one quality-improvement initiative for patients with congestive heart failure (CHF) showed that evaluation of left ventricular function improved from 53% to 65% and that appropriate use of ACE inhibitors improved from 54% to 74%.[24]

The mission of these organizations is to improve the effectiveness, efficiency, economy, and quality of services delivered to Medicare beneficiaries. Based on this statutory charge, and CMS' program experience, CMS identifies the core functions of the QIO program as:

- Improving quality of care for beneficiaries
- Protecting the integrity of the Medicare Trust Fund by ensuring that Medicare pays only for services and goods that are reasonable and necessary and that are provided in the most appropriate setting; and
- Protecting beneficiaries by expeditiously addressing individual complaints, such as beneficiary complaints; provider-based notice appeals; violations of the Emergency Medical Treatment and Labor Act (EMTALA); and other related responsibilities as articulated in QIO-related law

CMS relies on QIOs to improve the quality of health care for all Medicare beneficiaries. Furthermore, QIOs are required under Sections 1152–1154 of the Social Security Act. CMS views the QIO program as an important resource in its effort to improve quality and efficiency of care for Medicare beneficiaries. Throughout its history, the program has been instrumental in advancing national efforts to motivate providers in improving quality, and in measuring and improving outcomes of quality.

The Medicare Quality Improvement Organization (QIO) Program (formerly referred to as the Medicare Utilization and Quality Control Peer Review Program) was created by statute in 1982 to improve quality and efficiency of services delivered to Medicare beneficiaries. In its first phase, which concluded in the early 1990s, the program sought to accomplish its mission through peer review of cases to identify instances in which professional standards were not met for purposes of initiating corrective actions. In the second phase, quality measurement and improvement became the predominant mode of program operation. As a result of significant changes that have occurred in our understanding of how to improve quality, and changes in the environment to promote public reporting of provider performance and the development of performance-based payment programs, the QIO is now positioned as an agent of change.

CMS views the QIO program as a cornerstone in its efforts to improve quality and efficiency of care for Medicare beneficiaries. The program has been instrumental in advancing national efforts to measure and improve quality, and it presents unique opportunities to support improvements in care in the future. Consequently, CMS is undertaking these activities to ensure that the program is focused, structured, and managed so as to maximize its ability for creating value. These improvements support broader initiatives to provide transparency for beneficiaries and create performance-based payment programs for providers. Most health care providers deliver care to Medicare beneficiaries and patients insured by commercial insurers. Recent efforts to improve quality reflect the idea that shared quality improvement goals and consistent quality measures for all patients will result in fewer burdens to providers and an opportunity to identify and achieve meaningful performance improvements. Thus, to achieve demonstrable and significant improvement in care for Medicare beneficiaries, the program is supporting partnerships that engage a broad group of stakeholders for the purpose of improving quality of care for all patients based on common goals and measures. This approach facilitates leveraging private sector resources and expertise at the local and national level, with a potentially more significant impact on the quality and efficiency of the health care system.

Currently on their ninth scope of work (SOW), the QIOs are focused on the following:

- Beneficiary protection - reviewing the quality of care provided to beneficiaries and implementing quality improvement activities as a result of case review activities.
- Patient safety - working with hospitals and nursing homes to improve performance on a set of important processes and results that will reduce patient risk factors.

- Prevention - improving immunization rates for influenza and pneumonia along with key cancer screening. Some QIOs will also work to improve care for chronic kidney disease patients and/or work to reduce health disparities for specific underserved populations.
- Care transitions - selected QIOs will work on encouraging the coordination of care across the spectrum of health care; promoting seamless transitions from the hospital to home, skilled nursing care, or home health care; and promoting efforts to reduce unnecessary rehospitalizations in specified regions of several states.

In addition, through their work in that above themes, the QIOs help CMS promote and achieve three overarching goals for American health care:

- Adoption of value-driven health care
- Supporting the adoption and use of health information
- Technology
- Reducing health care disparities

THE FUTURE OF "QUALITY"

The foundation for CMS quality improvement is focused on the vision of "the right care for every person every time." This is based on CMS seeking to make care safe, effective, efficient, patient-centered, timely, and equitable (Table 126-4).

To achieve this CMS has strengthened its quality council, which now is chaired by the administrator and meets every 2 weeks, and has created workgroups in the areas of health information technology, performance measurement and pay-for-performance, technology and innovation, prevention, Medicaid and State Children's Health Insurance Program (SCHIP), long-term care, cancer care, and methods for breakthrough improvement.

These groups, with membership drawn from across CMS, report to the quality council, which reviews, approves, and tracks their work plans. The quality coordination team supports the quality council by managing this tracking and planning process and providing a variety of technical support to the workgroups. Accountability for individual tasks remains with the CMS unit that carries them out, but accountability for overall integration, and for adjusting the plan in response to events, remains with the workgroup and the quality council to which it reports.

The cross-cutting nature of the quality council workgroups has already been mentioned, but the same principles can produce clinical breakthroughs. For example, promoting influenza immunization in nursing homes might involve a partnership with stakeholders (by the CMS Long-term Care Task Force), addressing the payment for administering vaccine (Center for Medicare Management), requiring that vaccine be offered to every patient (Office of Clinical Standards and Quality), enforcing that requirement (Center for Medicaid and State Operations), including immunization status in information that nursing homes report to CMS (Office of Clinical Standards and Quality), publishing each home's immunization rate (Center for Beneficiary Choices), and providing technical assistance and promoting staff immunization (Office of Clinical Standards and Quality). These actions rarely require new organizational units because existing units of CMS already have responsibility for most of the needed activities, but strong planning and coordination are necessary to make activities of so many CMS components come together to change care.

These are strategies, not goals; highways, not destinations. The destination is safe, efficient, effective, patient-centered, timely, and equitable care. But the five strategies are critical to getting us there and will be carried out through systematic efforts that span all parts of CMS, because all parts of our agency can and must support quality improvement.

It is hoped that through this five-part roadmap, CMS and providers can work together to establish a health care system for seniors that is safe, effective, efficient, patient-centered, timely, and equitable. As we strive to make these improvements to the health care system our collective ideas, thoughtful consideration and broad participation are needed. CMS will work to do its part, by strengthening our partnerships and using them to strengthen ability to identify, support, and improve high-quality, personalized care. This is absolutely essential for the sustainability of Medicare, Medicaid, and our health care system: increasingly, high-quality care is the only kind of care we can afford.

Table 126-4. Highways on the CMS Quality Roadmap*

The CMS quality roadmap features five main strategies to achieve the goal of high-quality care:

1. Work through partnerships—within CMS, with Federal and State agencies, and especially with nongovernmental partners—to achieve specific quality goals.
2. Develop and provide quality measures and information as a basis for supporting more effective quality improvement efforts.
3. Pay in a way that reinforces our commitment to quality, and that helps providers and patients take steps to improve health and avoid unnecessary costs.
4. Promote effective electronic health systems to support quality improvement.
5. Bring effective new treatments to patients more rapidly and help develop better evidence so that doctors and patients can use medical technologies more effectively.

*http://www.cms.hhs.gov/CouncilonTechInnov/downloads/qualityroadmap.pdf

KEY POINTS

Preserving Medicare Through a "Quality" Focus

- The change from the Health Care Finance Administration (HCFA) to the Centers for Medicare and Medicaid Services (CMS) signaled more then a name change; rather it marked a movement beyond simply paying claims to one of value-based purchasing. As a value-based purchaser CMS now plays a critical role in promoting quality outcomes.
- There is now a shift to more comprehensive models of care rather then continued support of a fragmented siloed payment system. In addition there is also a shift toward focusing on quality of life rather then simply extending years lived.
- Use of technology to improve quality through electronic prescribing and health records is being viewed as a major opportunity to reduce waste through improvements in quality.
- By reporting quality outcome data on providers CMS expects seniors to be driven to "quality" providers thus resulting in improvements in outcomes and cost savings.
- Support is available through CMS for improving quality through Quality Improvement Organizations (QIO) and other organizations.

For a complete list of references, please visit online only at www.expertconsult.com

Managed Care for Older Americans

Richard G. Stefanacci

The current care delivery system for older Americans requires significant reform to improve the care of this population.[1] One of the growing delivery systems that is well positioned to improve the care for older adults is provided through managed care. This is in part due to the fact that managed care shares some common goals and processes with geriatric medicine.[2,3]

In its broadest sense, managed care refers to a system where a payment is made to a provider or health plan that is then responsible for a group of services. A more traditional and focused view of managed care refers just to health plans that are responsible for providing all of the services available under the entire Medicare program with the exception of hospice services. These services can be provided either directly through a closed system of providers or through an open system using contracted community providers. The closed system uses a full complement of employed providers. Medicare Advantage (MA), under The Centers for Medicare and Medicaid Services (CMS), administered this program as provided under the Medicare Part C program. Previous to the Medicare Modernization Act of 2003 these plans were referred to as Medicare+Choice or simply a health maintenance organization.

Medicare managed care plans have several potential advantages over the traditional Medicare fee-for-service program. These advantages include having lower deductibles and copayments, and offering benefits that are not part of the Medicare fee-for-service coverage, such as payments for preventive care including reimbursement for eyeglasses and hearing aids; health education, and health promotion programs such as case management and disease management. Managed care plans can also provide discounts on or improved access to transportation, day care, respite care, or assisted living. Plans are also not restricted by Medicare fee-for-service rules such as the requirement for 3 hospital days plus a discharge day to qualify for subacute services; instead Medicare managed care plans can admit members directly to skilled nursing facilities, thus avoiding a hospitalization and related costs, both financial and health. This subacute level of care is for services requiring skilled nursing care, such as intravenous therapy or rehabilitation.

Although coverage for pharmaceutical costs had historically been a major reason why older adults enrolled in Medicare managed care, the introduction of free-standing prescription drug plans under Medicare Part D, which started Jan 1, 2006, removed this differential from fee-for-service in traditional Medicare. As a result of Medicare Part D both FFS Medicare and Medicare managed care plans both provide the opportunity for coverage of prescription medications.

Thus principles of managed care are moving beyond MA plans into portions of Medicare fee-for-service. Through such programs as pay-for-performance and some unique demonstration programs, Medicare is applying the principles of managed care so older adults in traditional Medicare can also benefit.

MANAGED CARE TIMELINE

The modern era of managed care was heralded by a new law enacted by the U.S. Congress in 1974. This law permitted the establishment of health maintenance organizations (HMOs) whose purpose was to encourage the development of prepaid health plans. From their start in the mid-1970s until the late 1990s, managed care saw a slow and consistent growth. Participation in Medicare managed care increased steadily in the 1990s, reaching a peak of 6.3 million beneficiaries (16%) in 2000.

In 1997 revisions enacted by Congress that increased administrative burden and reduced payments to the health plans resulted in many plans exiting the market or limiting their enrollment.[4] Enrollment declined between 2000 and 2003 because of plan withdrawals from some areas, reduced benefits, and higher premiums.

A rebirth of managed care for Medicare beneficiaries occurred as a result of the Medicare Modernization Act (MMA). MMA (passed in 2003) changed managed care for older adults in several ways. First, it changed the name from Medicare+Choice (M+C) to Medicare Advantage, and added different managed care options such as demonstration programs and special needs plans (SNP). MA plans also received increased payments, which were used to raise payments to providers, lower enrollee premiums, enhance existing benefits, and increase stabilization funds. As a result of these changes, enrollment in MA plans rose slightly from 2003 to 2004 and continues to rise each year (Figure 127-1).

MEDICARE MANAGED CARE IN FEE-FOR-SERVICE

Under the Medicare Part A benefit, also referred to as hospital insurance, providers are paid a defined amount for providing a bundle of services. Medicare Part A providers include acute care hospitals, skilled nursing facility subacute care, and hospice. It is important to note that while Medicare Part C (Medicare Advantage) includes Medicare Part A, B, and in most cases Part D, hospice is still provided as a separate benefit. Since Medicare Part A providers are paid a capitated payment, they are encouraged to use managed care principles to control cost and improve outcomes.

Medicare Part B, also referred to as medical insurance, covers physician provider services. Although historically these services were paid simply on the basis of the number and type of services provided, (CMS) is applying managed care principles to this program as well. The 2006 Tax Relief and Health Care Act required the establishment of a physician quality reporting system, including an incentive payment for eligible professionals who satisfactorily report data on quality measures for covered services furnished to Medicare beneficiaries. CMS named this program the Physician Quality Reporting Initiative (PQRI). In 2008 PQRI consisted of

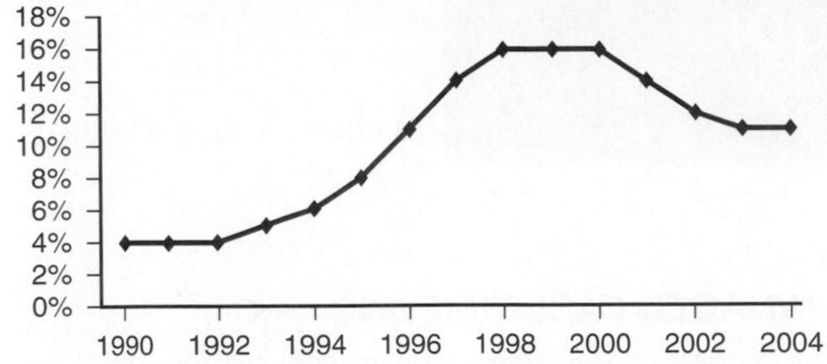

Figure 127-1. Percentage of beneficiaries enrolled in Medicare managed care. *(Source: Kaiser Family Foundation calculations using data from the Centers for Medicare and Medicaid Services, Medicare Managed Care Contract Plans Monthly Summary Reports for December 1 of each year, at* http://www.cms.hhs.gov/healthplans/statistics/mmcc;/ *(Medicare managed care enrollment), and total Medicare enrollment data from the Centers for Medicare and Medicaid Services, Office of the Actuary, personal communication.* http://www.kff.org/insurance/7031/ti2004-2-17.cfm*)*

119 quality measures, including two structural measures. One structural measure conveys whether a professional has and uses electronic health records and the other electronic prescribing.[5] These measures are a movement to encourage the use of managed care principles in the Medicare FFS program.

Prescription drug plans as previously mentioned are authorized under the Medicare Part D program. In addition to general managed care principles to assure appropriate medication use, prescription plans are required by CMS to provide medication therapy management programs (MTMP).[6] CMS's objective with regard to MTMP is to control costs and improve quality. Plans provide MTMP through implementation of managed care principles.

Care for beneficiaries with chronic illnesses, such as heart disease and diabetes, is a major expense to the Medicare program, and a major detriment to beneficiaries' quality of life. For example, just under one half of all beneficiaries in 1997 were treated for one or more of eight categories of chronic illnesses, and they accounted for three fourths of all Medicare spending in 1998 (Brown et al, 2004). Furthermore, beneficiaries often have multiple chronic illnesses, which compounds the cost and complexity of their care. The 12% with three or more of the eight chronic health problems accounted for one third of all Medicare spending. Coordinating the care of these patients is difficult because patients with chronic illnesses see an average of 11 different physicians per year.[7]

The CMS conducts and sponsors a number of innovative demonstration projects to test and measure the effect of potential program changes. CMS's demonstrations study the likely impact of new methods of service delivery, coverage of new types of service, and new payment approaches on beneficiaries, providers, health plans, states, and the Medicare Trust Funds. Evaluation projects validate CMS research and demonstration findings and help CMS monitor the effectiveness of Medicare, Medicaid, and the State Children's Health Insurance Program (SCHIP).

Many of the demonstration projects are focused on managing care for those Medicare beneficiaries suffering from chronic illnesses. The following are examples of some of the many demonstration projects that CMS has funded in the past and continues to fund.

Coordinated care demonstration[8]

The Medicare Coordinated Care Demonstration (MCCD) tests whether case management and disease management programs can lower costs and improve patient outcomes and well-being in the Medicare fee-for-service population. The evaluation of this demonstration project by Mathematica Policy Research, Inc. showed no clear benefit of this program. Based on the patterns of differences in hospitalizations, Medicare Part A and B expenditures, and total Medicare expenditures including the care coordination fees, six of the programs are not cost neutral, four probably are not, and five may be cost neutral, over their first 25 months of operations. Given the results, the continuation of this demonstration is in doubt.

Senior risk reduction program[9]

The Senior Risk Reduction Demonstration was established to test whether health promotion and health management programs that have been developed and tested in the private sector can also be tailored to and work well with Medicare beneficiaries to improve their health and reduce avoidable health care use.

Care management for high-cost beneficiaries demonstration[10]

This demonstration was established to evaluate various care management models for high-cost beneficiaries in the traditional Medicare fee-for-service program.

ESRD disease management demonstration[11]

The End-Stage Renal Disease (ESRD) Disease Management Demonstration was established to increase the opportunity for Medicare beneficiaries with ESRD to join integrated care management systems. The demonstration is designed to test the effectiveness of disease management models to increase quality of care for ESRD patients while ensuring that this care is provided more effectively and efficiently.

Program for all-Inclusive care for the elderly (PACE)[12]

Some demonstration programs that have proven their value have gone on to become permanent programs. The Program of All-Inclusive Care for the Elderly (PACE) is such a program. The PACE model is centered on the belief that it is better for the well-being of seniors with chronic care needs and their families to be served in the community whenever possible.

PACE serves individuals who are age 55 or older, certified by their state to need nursing home care, are able to live safely in the community at the time of enrollment, and live in a PACE service area. Although all PACE participants must be certified to need nursing home care to enroll in PACE, only about 7% of PACE participants nationally reside in a nursing home. If a PACE enrollee does need nursing home care, the PACE program pays for it and continues to coordinate the enrollee's care.

A study[13] of the PACE model by Dr. Catherine Eng and her team found positive outcomes. Specifically the results demonstrated good consumer satisfaction, reduction in use of institutional care, controlled use of medical services, and cost savings to public and private payers of care, including

Medicare and Medicaid. The study concluded by stating that the PACE model's comprehensiveness of health and social services, its cost-effective coordinated system of care delivery, and its method of integrated financing have wide applicability and appeal.

Social/health maintenance organization (S/HMO)[14]

Another similar program to PACE that did not achieve permanent status but instead was terminated because of the lack of demonstrated effectiveness was the social/health maintenance organization (S/HMO). S/HMOs were a four-site national demonstration located in: Portland, Ore.; Long Beach, Calif.; Brooklyn, N.Y.; and Las Vegas. This program combined Medicare Part A and B coverage, with various extended and chronic care benefits into an integrated health plan.

A social HMO is an organization that provides the full range of Medicare benefits offered by standard HMOs, plus additional services that include care coordination, prescription drug benefits, chronic care benefits covering short-term nursing home care, a full range of home and community-based services such as homemaker, personal care services, adult day care, respite care, and medical transportation. Other services that may be provided include eyeglasses, hearing aids, and dental benefits.

These plans offered the full range of medical benefits that are offered by standard HMOs plus chronic care/extended care services. Membership offers other health benefits that are not provided through Medicare alone or most other senior health plans.

MANAGED CARE PRINCIPLES

Managed Care Principles

- **Screening** enrolled population to identify individuals with special needs.
- **Coordinating** the actions of all providers across the continuum of enrolled beneficiaries' care.
- Offering effective **health promotion,** disease prevention, and self-management programs.
- Making available the services of **interdisciplinary** health care professionals, including physicians, nurses, social workers, pharmacists, and rehabilitation therapists.
- Using **geriatric expertise** available for designing and administering geriatric programs and for consultation with primary care physicians, case managers, and other providers.

Managed care can be an efficient approach for Medicare to finance high-quality, cost-effective geriatrics. The American Geriatrics Society (AGS) wrote in their position statement[15] on Managed Care that to realize the potential flexibility and creativity inherent in capitated financing, MCOs should develop special processes for providing high-quality health care to enrollees who need complex health services.

The starting point is identifying those members most at need for special attention by screening the enrolled population to identify individuals with special needs. Plans should use valid and reliable instruments to screen their enrollees regularly. They should assess the clinical needs of high-risk enrollees for both functional status and quality of life. The rationale for this approach is that about 10% to 15% of beneficiaries, most of who have several chronic conditions, account for 70% to 80% of Medicare's annual payments for health care. Early identification of those who are at highest risk for requiring expensive care—and assessing their clinical needs—would facilitate coordination of care and timely preventive interventions designed to improve the clinical and financial outcomes of care.[16]

Assessment for risk is typically accomplished through a health risk assessment (HRA). One of the tools used for identifying members is the Pra and PraPlus.[17] Many organizations use the Pra or the PraPlus to screen older populations to identify individuals who are at risk for using health services heavily in the future. MCOs can then offer special forms of health care, such as case management, comprehensive geriatric assessment (CGA), or geriatric evaluation and management (GEM) to these at-risk individuals.

Coordinating the actions of all providers across the continuum of enrolled beneficiaries' care is important for quality care. The rationale here is that coordination improves the quality and the outcomes of health care, including safety, cost, and satisfaction with care. The coordination of care can be made more efficient and effective by using integrated medical records and improved communication tools.[18,19] Offering effective health promotion, disease prevention, and self-management programs can prevent or delay the progression of disease, resulting in better patient outcomes and lower costs of health care. In addition programs that provide education of patients and their caregivers with regard to their conditions and self-management initiatives empower them to be proactive and choose wise alternatives.[20–22] Making available the services of health care professionals from several disciplines, including physicians, nurses, social workers, pharmacists, and rehabilitation therapists is needed. These professionals should function as interdisciplinary teams in managing not only the medical conditions but also social factors that affect high-risk beneficiaries' well-being. The interdisciplinary team approach allows for comprehensive, coordinated assessment and management of beneficiaries' medical, psychological, social, and functional needs—and those of their unpaid caregivers.[23–26] Geriatric expertise should be available for designing and administering geriatric programs and for consultation with primary care physicians, case managers, and other providers. MCOs would be well served by using a geriatrician in a medical director role to help guide the development and management of programs necessary for success in caring for seniors. Geriatricians have the background necessary in efficiently and effectively managing patients in teams, and managing the care of complex patients with multiple problems across the continuum of care.[27,28] The quality of the health care provided to beneficiaries by MCOs should be measured consistently and reported regularly to the plans' executives and providers, to CMS, and to the public. New instruments designed to measure the quality of outpatient care and coordination of care must be developed and tested for reliability and validity. Credible, understandable information about the quality of health care is essential to organizations' processes for improving quality and to consumers' efforts to make informed choices from among the available health plans and providers.[29]

PLAN REIMBURSEMENT

For payment purposes, there are two different categories of MA plans: local plans and regional plans. Local plans may be any of the available plan types and may serve one or more counties. Medicare pays them based on their enrollees' counties of residence. Regional plans, however, must be PPOs and must serve all of one of the 26 regions established by the CMS. Each region comprises one or more entire states.

Under the MA program, Medicare buys insurance coverage for its beneficiaries from private plans with payments made monthly. The coverage must include all Medicare Part A and Part B benefits except hospice. These payments are based on a number of factors including age and geographic variations in health care costs.

Recommendations to Medicare on payments, including changes to the MA program are made by the Medicare Payment Advisory Commission (MedPAC), the official, independent federal advisory body to Congress on Medicare payment policy. There is pressure to decrease reimbursement to Medicare managed care because of a belief that private plans, which were initially brought into the Medicare program to reduce costs, have actually increased costs. Both MedPAC and the Congressional Budget Office have found that private plans are paid 12% more, on average, than it would cost traditional Medicare to cover the same beneficiaries. According to an analysis by The Commonwealth Fund, these overpayments are estimated to average about $1000 for each beneficiary enrolled in a private plan. CBO estimates that these overpayments will equal at least $54 billion over the next 5 years and $149 billion over 10 years.[30,31]

In a June 2005 report, MedPAC recommended various changes in how Medicare pays managed care plans under MA to reduce inefficient and wasteful Medicare payments.[32] The Congressional Budget Office has estimated that the MedPAC proposals would save $20 billion to $30 billion over 5 years.[33] Based on the MedPAC recommendations to decrease payments to MA plans, Congress passed the Medicare Improvements for Patients and Providers Act of 2008, which includes many reductions in MA reimbursement which is likely to force a reduction in benefits and thus a reduction in enrollment.

In the case of prescription drug plans (PDPs), which operate under the Medicare Part D program, payment is made for providing prescription drug coverage for those Medicare beneficiaries that enroll in that specific plan. Overall, for prescription drug plan payments Medicare subsidizes premiums by about 75% and provides additional subsidies for beneficiaries who have low levels of income and assets. Medicare's payments to prescription drug plans are determined through a competitive bidding process, and enrollee premiums are also tied to plan bids. Payments from Medicare to these prescription drug plans is risk-adjusted based on the likely drug spending for that specific enrollee. On average these payments from Medicare equal $104 per month, which when combined with the average monthly premium equal about $124 per month. The prescription plan is responsible for paying the costs of medications (excluding the member's responsibility) and administrative overhead, which include medication therapy management services.

Those health systems that are more integrated, such as the MA plans, typically offer greater pharmaceutical benefits because they benefit from pharmaceutical use that reduces hospitalization and medical services. Evaluations of these plans has shown that MA plans offer greater pharmaceutical benefits; 73% versus 17% of MA plans offered enhanced prescription coverage versus prescription drug plans (PDP). In addition the same evaluation noted that 28% of MA plans versus 6% of PDPs provided coverage in the coverage gap.[34] MA plans offering enhanced drug benefits and therefore spending more on medications can reduce other Medicare expenditures.

CAPITATION AND PAY-FOR-PERFORMANCE

Capitation rates in all regions of the country should be sufficient for providing high-quality health care for all Medicare beneficiaries, regardless of the intensity of their clinical needs. Specifically, the CMS should provide capitation that reflects the probable cost of caring for each enrolled beneficiary. This should be accomplished by risk-adjusting capitation payments according to individual beneficiaries' diagnosis, functional status, and use. Capitation payments that acknowledge that beneficiaries with chronic conditions require more health care than those who are healthy would encourage MCOs to enroll beneficiaries who have chronic conditions and to provide them with special services designed to address their needs for complex care. In contrast, inadequate risk-adjustment of capitation payments is a disincentive for plans to enroll frail or medically complex beneficiaries or to offer special services that might encourage such beneficiaries to enroll.[35–37]

Beyond capitation is a movement to base payment on outcomes. Termed pay-for-performance (P4P), it has the potential to improve care to this population. Current payment systems do not consider quality in determining reimbursement. The incentives of the current reimbursement systems sometimes promote poor quality care. The present fee-for-service payment systems pay providers based on the number and complexity of services provided to patients without regard to quality, efficiency, or impact on health outcomes. Pay-for-performance has been proposed as one strategy designed to correct this deficiency.

A value-based purchasing system for the Medicare system must address the care of the large portion of Medicare beneficiaries who have multiple chronic conditions, are frail, of advanced age, or require palliative care and not focus only on the care provided to the typical beneficiary.[38] For these beneficiaries, measures should account for comorbidities and assess aspects of health that are common to multiple conditions (e.g., cognitive status, functional status, and pain.) Measures should be constructed so that providers are not penalized when they honor patients' preferences for care or their cultural or religious beliefs.

The older adult population served by Medicare is extremely heterogeneous. Many people are healthy and functional, but up to one third of the Medicare population are vulnerable, with multiple comorbidities and geriatric conditions (functional and cognitive impairment, falls, and frailty). In addition, some older adults will place different values on participation in self-management and adherence to medical recommendations, especially in the setting of multiple comorbidities and health status vulnerability. Some older adults may put more emphasis on improved functioning and quality of life rather than traditional indicators of clinical care quality.

It is essential that a pay-for-performance program not unwittingly lead to a decrease in quality for vulnerable elders or those who may have different clinical care goals. Assessing and rewarding performance using indicators that have been developed for and commercially (non-Medicare) insured population and may not be relevant to vulnerable older adults has the potential to detract attention away from essential care and services. A pay-for-performance system needs to produce quality results that are meaningful and appropriate to the overall goals of clinical care for the patient population as a whole and for particularly vulnerable populations including the frail elderly. Failing to take this important policy concern into account could adversely affect access to primary and specialty care among those Medicare beneficiaries who might benefit the most from high-quality care.[39–42]

It has been proposed that payment reform is needed to drive practice change. Effective pay-for-performance systems support and stimulate the structural capabilities necessary for the provision, documentation, measurement, and continuous improvement of high-quality care. The need for different provider settings to care for unique patient populations must also be considered when designing and implementing payment based upon performance. For example, larger practices may have more resources to implement quality care processes. Such resources include providing patient education materials for patients and their caregivers, language translation services, and other outreach activities to facilitate good patient care. A smaller practice may have fewer resources to measure and report quality, yet be an essential care provider, such as a rural care provider or home-bound elderly care team. Certain practices may be focused on a population subset for which there are no performance measures at this time. Payment reform should lead to improved practice design without eliminating essential care providers.

MEASURING QUALITY OF CARE

Providers who use innovative approaches that improve quality of care find that most current payment systems do not provide them with the resources needed to sustain these activities. Today's fee-for-service payment system does not provide payment for services such as health education or development of the infrastructure to measure and report quality. The result is that providers are unable to invest in activities that have great potential to improve quality and avoid unnecessary medical costs. An example of such activities is health information technology (HIT), including electronic health records and ePrescribing. Providers typically cite the cost of these HIT systems and lack of a clear return on investment as barriers to their implementation. In addition to the incentive of higher reimbursement for provision of better quality care, funds should be made available through direct grants and low interest loans for the infrastructure responsible for implementation of a HIT system within a practice. HIT systems are not only used for the management of clinical records, but are critical elements in data collection, clinician feedback, quality improvement, and population tracking. Each of these is essential to practice improvement as the final desired outcome of pay-for-performance programs.[43–45]

Structure, process, and clinical outcomes measures used must be valid and relevant for the unique care needs of frail or vulnerable older adults. These measures should be evidence-based, clinically relevant, have clear association with improved outcomes of care, and be applicable to all patients whose care they assess.

Technical specifications for numerators and denominators of measures should be constructed so that measures are not applied to special populations where evidence of linkage to performance of care processes to improved outcomes is lacking. These populations include persons of very advanced age, those with multiple comorbidities, limited life expectancy, or moderate to severe dementia.

More importantly, specific measures are needed to assess the quality of care of persons over age 75, those who are vulnerable and/or frail and who are receiving palliative care near the end of life. Clinical performance measures relevant to the Medicare population are of three types:

1. Structure measures - used to recognize systems of care associated with improved health outcomes. Multidisciplinary teams for care, capacity for patient education in self-care management, disease registries, electronic health records, and systems to support the use of intervisit interval patient contacts, and monitoring are important aspects of the chronic care model. Important processes of care are difficult to deliver absent such structure(s). Initial reward systems should recognize investment in such delivery structure.
2. Process measures - used to determine whether care that is known to be effective is provided. The AGS believes that specific measures are needed to assess the quality of care of persons over age 75, those who are frail or vulnerable, and those who are receiving palliative care near the end of life. The Assessing the Care of the Vulnerable Elders (ACOVE)[46] measures were developed by the RAND Corporation in response to the needs of persons at risk for frailty or persons aged 75 and older. They have been tested in cohorts of community-dwelling vulnerable older adults. Adoption of some or all of these indicators in addition to disease- and prevention-based measures appropriate for the younger population will greatly enhance attaining the goal that quality of care can be measured for all Medicare beneficiaries and that the providers who care for these patients have measures of accountability.
3. Clinical outcome measures - must be appropriate to the usual health care needs and goals of the patient population in which they are used. Many of these measures are disease-specific, originally developed in commercially insured populations, and do not account for other comorbidities. If not previously

tested in the heterogeneous Medicare population, such measures may be particularly problematic. In frail or vulnerable older persons, the goals of treatment for chronic disease are more variable than in younger adults, and the linkage between process of care delivered and clinical measures is often imperfect.

High-quality geriatric care requires providing services to a heterogeneous population with varied health care service needs and goals of care, including many with multiple chronic illnesses and geriatric conditions. Fundamental to the definition of quality is that the standard of care being measured is applicable to the individual to whom it is applied. Many available clinical performance measures have been developed in the middle-aged commercial population. Some of these measures have been tested in older adult populations, but some have not, so the applicability of untested measures to older adult, heterogeneous populations is not known. The complexity of delivering high-quality care to this population can only be guided by rigorous scientific testing of performance indicator measures. Such testing can allow us to adapt measures to the specific needs of vulnerable patient populations. These measures need to be developed and validated by individuals with expertise in the care of frail elders. Measurement development and testing is a dynamic process so even in the setting of value-based purchasing there should be an established process for continual evolution of performance indicator measures. Key stakeholders should remain involved.[47–50]

A pay-for-performance system must provide positive reinforcement for quality performance and improvement and not promote the avoidance of patients for whom providing high-quality care will be more challenging. When applied to individual providers, these measures should be constructed so that both achievement of target thresholds (excellence) and progress toward achievement of targets (improvement) can be positively reinforced. In addition, the collection of data that are used to evaluate performance should not be burdensome to providers and should accurately reflect the performance of care processes on an individual patient basis. Failure to consider these factors may unduly penalize providers who practice in small groups or care for special populations.

Linking a portion of payments to valid measures of quality and effective use of resources will result in providers having direct incentives and financial support to implement the innovative approaches that result in improved outcomes. All monies that are set aside for pay-for-performance should be distributed to providers achieving the quality criteria. Savings from improved care are likely to accrue to Medicare funds that are not part of the physician resource pool. Performance-based funds should not be used in a withhold approach or a Medicare Part B budget neutral manner. To the fullest extent possible, norms should be established for like populations and risk adjustment should occur. Although it is recognized that value-based purchasing should not be delayed while such adjustments are refined, such an approach will minimize the risk of providers avoiding patients (e.g., the frail and medically complex) who present the greatest challenge in meeting quality indicators used for pay-for-performance (Figure 127-2).[51,52]

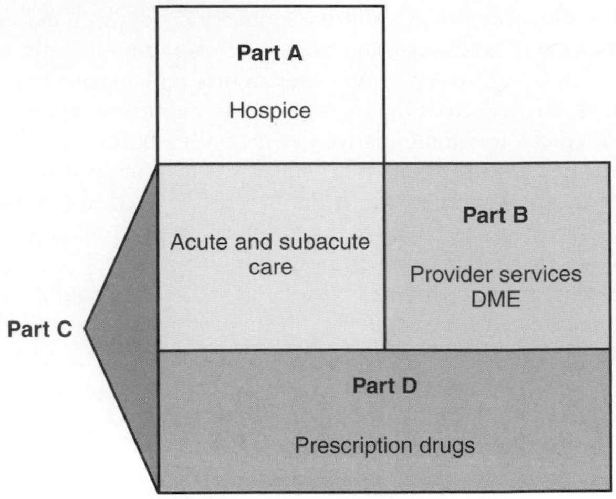

Figure 127-2. Medicare programs.

A VISION FOR CARE IN THE FUTURE

As managed care for older adults evolves a direction likely to follow has been laid out by the Institute of Medicine. The IOM identified three key principles that need to form the basis of an improved system of care delivery for older Americans. These principles are in alignment with the six aims of quality defined in Crossing the Quality Chasm.[53]

First and foremost, the health needs of the older population need to be comprehensively addressed, and care needs to be patient-centered. For most older adults, care needs to include preventive services (including lifestyle modification) and coordinated treatment of chronic and acute health conditions. For frail older adults, social services may also be needed to maintain or improve health. These social services need to be integrated with health care services in their delivery and financing. Furthermore, efforts need to be made to reduce the wide variation in practice protocols among providers, which should further enhance the quality of care for older adults.

The principle of comprehensive care also includes taking into account the increasing sociodemographic diversity of older adults. The number and percent of ethnic minorities in the older population is increasing dramatically, and even within ethnic groups there is tremendous cultural diversity. Health care providers need to be sensitive to the wide variety of languages, cultures, and health beliefs among older adults. Other segments of the older population face additional challenges. For example, older adults in rural areas often face isolation and barriers to access for some services.

The second principle underlying the vision of care in the future is that services need to be provided efficiently. Providers will need to be trained to work in interdisciplinary teams and financing and delivery systems need to support this interdisciplinary approach. Care needs to be seamless across various care delivery sites, and all clinicians need to have access to patients' health information and population data, when needed. Health information technology, such as interoperable electronic health records and remote monitoring, needs to be used to support the health care workforce by improving communication among providers and their patients, building a record of population data, promoting interdisciplinary patient care and care coordination, facilitating patient transitions, and improving quality and safety overall. Giving providers immediate access to patient information, especially for patients who are cognitively impaired and unable to provide their own clinical history, may reduce the likelihood of errors, lower costs, and increase efficiency in care delivery.

This vision for the future is being tested through the Medicare Medical Home Demonstration. Section 204 of the Tax Relief and Health Care Act of 2006 (TRHCA)[54] mandates a demonstration in up to eight states to provide targeted, accessible, continuous, and coordinated family-centered care to Medicare beneficiaries who are deemed to be high need (i.e., with multiple chronic or prolonged illnesses that require regular medical monitoring, advising, or treatment.) The objective is to bring managed care principles to the Medicare fee-for-services system.

Efficiency can be further improved by ensuring that health care personnel are used in a way that makes the most of their capabilities. Expanding the scope of practice or responsibility for providers has the potential to increase the overall productivity of the workforce and at the same time promote retention by providing greater opportunities for specialization (e.g., through career lattices) and professional advancement. Specifically, this would involve a cascading of responsibilities, giving additional duties to personnel with more limited training to increase the amount of time that more highly trained personnel have to carry out the work that they alone are able to perform. Although the necessary regulatory changes would likely be controversial in some cases, the projected shortfall in workforce supply requires an urgent response. This response will most likely have to involve expansions in the scope of practice at all levels, while at the same time ensuring that these changes are consistent with high-quality care.

In the end, the U.S. system of care for older adults will rely on improving the effectiveness and efficiency of our current system. Many of the systems for efficient and effective care are already being provided through today's managed care program. The key will be further improvements in the current managed care system along with allowing these principles to work in the larger fee-for-service Medicare program.

KEY POINTS
Managed Care for Older Americans

- Managed care shares some common goals and processes with geriatric medicine.
- Increasingly managed care principles are being applied outside of traditional managed care organizations in Medicare fee-for-service programs.
- Despite the benefits of managed care there continues to be pressure to decrease reimbursement to these plans.
- Managed care principles include a focus on screening, coordination, health promotion, and interdisciplinary health care professionals with geriatric expertise.
- Future successes of the American system for caring for older adults is reliant on the application of managed care principles for efficiency and effectiveness beyond managed care organizations.

For a complete list of references, please visit online only at www.expertconsult.com

CHAPTER 128

Telemedicine Applications in Geriatrics

Stuti Dang
Adam G. Golden
Herman S. Cheung
Bernard A. Roos

BACKGROUND

Health care systems are struggling with the issue of how to provide high-quality services to the increasing number of older adults in an era of limited financial and workforce resources. Many people recognize that the current system for health care delivery is unsustainable because of increasing costs and a shortage of nurses and other staff to provide care. More effective and efficient models of care based on preventive and person-centered health systems are urgently needed.

The current fee-for-service system of provider payment in the United States is often viewed as a barrier to achieving effective, coordinated, and efficient care.[1,2] By emphasizing acute episodic care, the current system often rewards the overuse of costly specialized services and involvement of multiple physicians in the treatment of individual patients. There is an emerging consensus and legislative initiatives to "reward" the sharing and exchange of information, provide coordination and continuity of care, and effectively control chronic conditions to prevent hospitalization.[3]

Care coordination programs blended with technology could prevent or limit hospitalizations and emergency room visits of frail elderly patients with chronic disease. Monitoring and information technology could transform the health care system, lowering costs and increasing benefits. Such approaches and applications would substantially improve the quality of care and reduce the overall economic burden of these chronic diseases.

CARE COORDINATION IN CHRONIC DISEASE MANAGEMENT

The chronic disease model advocates that care should be continuous, coordinated between the patient and the care team, and provide self-management support to patients.[4] Although distinctions have often been drawn, the terms "care coordination," "case management," "care management," and "disease management" are often used interchangeably. All four terms focus on the chronic disease model and implementation of care standards.

The most promising results in terms of effectiveness and efficiency involving care coordination have been in the management of patients with congestive heart failure (CHF) and diabetes mellitus. Heart failure disease management programs that monitor a patient's self-reported changes in weight and symptoms have been shown to reduce hospital readmissions.[5] Systematic reviews suggest that nurse case management leads to improvements in patient outcomes and processes of care for diabetes patients.[6,7]

Using well-established guidelines and carefully scripted protocols, care coordinators are able to provide disease-related education, bolster family support, and identify barriers to medical compliance. Some care coordination programs rely primarily on home-based visits, whereas others employ telephone-based interventions, either by themselves or in combination with home visits. Establishing such a care coordination program with home-based visits and/or telephone surveillance is normally labor intensive and expensive. Operationally, even telephone surveillance requires a chart review, telephone contact by health care personnel, and often multiple calls to pharmacists or physicians. In many cases, the surveillance protocol is informal; typically the patient is instructed to call the practice if a change in health status is perceived. Reporting may occur at variable intervals.

CARE COORDINATION IN THE MANAGEMENT OF THE FRAIL OLDER ADULT

Although care coordination has had much success when targeted to high users with congestive heart failure and diabetes, models that can improve the quality of care for frail older adults "at risk" have also been developed. The goals of these models may include decreased health care use and decreased institutional placement along with decreased morbidity and mortality. A review of care coordination studies showed decreased readmission rates, emergency department visits, and health care expenditures in some, but not all studies.[8,9] These studies differed with regard to their success in increasing efficiency and decreasing cost, the population served, the interventional model, and the outcome measures used. Part of the problem is that the care coordinators in these types of programs must address many issues in patients who suffer from multiple chronic illnesses and geriatric syndromes. Another major limitation to these models is the high cost of employing and training staff who can care for the complex frail older adult.

Despite the limitations found in these research studies, many states have taken the initiative to develop care management-based programs for older Medicaid recipients. Florida's Nursing Home Diversion Program, for example, has used care coordination for about 14,000 indigent homebound elders who meet both medical and financial criteria for nursing home placement under Florida Medicaid. The cost to the state per client is less than half of what it would be if the person was living in a nursing home.[10]

BASIC PRINCIPLES OF TELEMEDICINE/ TELEHEALTH

The Institute of Medicine defines *telemedicine* as "...the use of electronic information and communications technologies to provide and support health care when distance separates the participants."[11] Telemedicine employs telecommunications and computer technology as a substitute for face-to-face contact between provider and client.[12] *Telehealth* and *telecare* are used by some health care professionals to encompass potential preventive and educational applications of telemedicine, such as remote monitoring, patient education, and data collection.[13] In reality, the words telemedicine, telehealth, and telecare are often used interchangeably.

Interest in telehealth as a way of providing care is being spurred by the rising cost of medical treatment and by the difficulties patients face accessing care and navigating the complex health care system. Rapid advances in technology and broadband transmission capability and the wider availability of low-cost, patient-friendly equipment are responsible for much of this interest. Some of the perceived benefits of telehealth are listed in Table 128-1.

There are two different categories of clinical telemedicine applications: (1) *Asynchronous* (store-and-forward) applications acquire and store clinical information (e.g., radiographic images, photographs of dermatologic lesions, and pathologic histology) that is then forwarded to (or retrieved by) another practitioner at a later time for the purposes of providing a consultation. (2) *Synchronous* (real-time) applications involve a two-way interactive exchange between the patient and provider(s), which allows physicians to assess patients who are at a distance. Examples of synchronous applications include telemental health, telerehabilitation, telecardiology, and teleneurology.

Telehealth can facilitate chronic management of patients in the home/community environment through video-conferencing and messaging reminders. Electronic sensors can also be used to monitor vital signs, weight, glucose, and movement throughout the home. Ideally, the properly identified technology may make the task of the care coordinator more efficient and effective. For the health care professional, the right technology can improve medication management, identify early signs of worsening illness, and guide follow-up care after a discharge from the hospital or skilled nursing facility. With all the information that is collected on patients, there is also an opportunity for artificial intelligence and computer analysis for decision support for health care professionals. Telehealth offers other benefits to managed care organizations, providers, patients, and caregivers (Table 128-1).

Table 128-1. Potential Advantages of Home Telehealth Systems

For the Managed-Care Organization
- Cost-effective approaches in managing geographically dispersed, multilingual populations
- Reliable outcomes assessment
- Centralized data management
- Patient follow-up and case management by exception
- Automated message reminders (e.g., medications, appointments)

For the Patient
- Improved patient adherence
- Increased patient access to care
- Enhanced patient satisfaction
- Opportunity for early intervention
- Reduced hospital/emergency room visits
- Enhanced provider access to patient
- Empowered patient participation in care
- Improved communication between patient and provider
- Access to health care information, resources, and databases
- Decreased need for patient to travel
- Treatment changes without office visit through feedback to providers

For the Provider
- Increased patient access to care
- Enhanced clinician access to patients
- Enhanced ability to monitor patients
- Efficient use of clinician time

For the Caregiver
- Support
- Access to health care information, resources, and databases
- Sense of comfort that their loved one is being watched

By providing interactions that are ongoing, disease-specific, and individualized, an in-home messaging device can empower patients and their caregivers to become involved in managing their chronic illness. This sense of empowerment may increase patient adherence and foster self-monitoring. The in-home messaging technology may create a sense of partnership with the health care system as the patients believe that the system is watching over them. This device also provides opportunities for improved communication between clinicians and patients. Telehealth allows for "just-in-time" education in a private learning environment.[14]

APPLICATIONS OF HOME TELEMEDICINE/ TELEHEALTH IN THE ELDERLY

Chronic disease management

Telehealth can assist care coordination programs to monitor for potential critical, disease-specific parameters (e.g., blood sugar in diabetes and weight change in CHF). The daily measures allow for the "real time" reassessment and readjustment of the care plan. Telehealth technology may improve monitoring—for example, by the daily prompting of the patient for his or her weight, information that could be used to facilitate behavior modification. Selective daily monitoring via telehealth technology of specific critical parameters leads to focused communications between the patient and care manager. Most systems also offer information and support to improve patient self-control and management. In this patient-centered model, the patient is empowered both in disease self-management and communication with health care providers. Putatively, such a competent patient could take on more of the responsibility and burden of disease management, ultimately leading to earlier and preventive intervention and a decrease in major encounters and health care cost.[15] In all chronic diseases models that have been studied, the frequent assessment and contact through home telehealth appear to increase patient and caregiver confidence and sense of security.[16] In the United States, the Veterans Health Administration and Department of Defense have taken the lead in implementing telehealth technology to about 30,000 patients in their care coordination programs nationally.

Congestive heart failure (CHF)

The Weight Monitoring in Heart Failure (WHARF) trial used twice-daily automated monitoring of signs or symptoms with a system consisting of an electronic weight scale and a monitor for patients to answer questions about symptoms. No differences in terms of health services use were observed. However, there was a 46% reduction in the mortality rate among the monitored group.[17] Another study compared Internet-based monitoring of weight, blood pressure, heart rate, and oxygen saturation, relayed to the patient's cardiologist, versus nurse home visits. A 40% reduction in heart failure admissions and health care costs was observed among the telemonitored group compared with the nurse home-visit group.[18]

"Telephone-based" monitoring and education by nurses combined with decision support systems to determine call frequency and prioritize education topics have produced a reduction (20% to 47%) in hospitalizations, death, or emergency room visits in CHF patients.[19,20] In two studies comparing "telephone-based" systems for CHF to "more complex" telemonitoring, the telephone-based monitoring demonstrated equal effectiveness and was less expensive.[21,22]

A meta-analysis analyzed data from 14 randomized controlled trials (4,264 patients) of remote monitoring in CHF.[23] Four of these studies had employed telemonitoring, nine had structured telephone support as interventions, and one had evaluated both telemonitoring and structured telephone support. This meta-analysis concluded that remote monitoring programs reduced the rates of hospital admission for CHF by 21% and all-cause mortality by 20%. Four of the nine studies using structured telephone support examined health care costs. Of these, three reduced cost and one had no effect. Other reviews of telehealth interventions in CHF have been equivocal about the benefits of telemonitoring.[24,25] Although the data have been mixed regarding cost reduction by reducing hospitalizations, overall the results are promising.

Diabetes mellitus

In the Informatics for Diabetes Education and Telemedicine (IDEATel) project, one of the largest randomized controlled trials in diabetics in the United States, telemedicine case management resulted in improved glycemic control, blood pressure levels, and total and LDL cholesterol levels at 1 year of follow-up.[26] The elderly patients demonstrated significantly improved diabetes self-efficacy, but depression and diabetes distress did not improve.[27] Close monitoring of diabetic patients via technology showed a reduction in Hb A_{1c}, good receptiveness by patients, and patient empowerment and education.[28,29] In other studies, patients required fewer clinic visits when they were monitored daily via home telehealth.[30] Another intervention, which included both a Web-based medical record and longitudinal health care professional support, accomplished significant benefits in Hb A_{1c} levels and compliance with diabetic guidelines.[31]

Hypertension

A recent study randomized patients to usual care, home BP monitoring and secure patient Web site training only, or home BP monitoring and secure patient Web site training plus pharmacist care management delivered through Web communications. In this Web-based intervention, blood pressure control was significantly improved only in the group that had telehealth contact with the pharmacist.[32]

Chronic wounds

Telemedicine using video technology has been used to monitor the progress of chronic wounds (e.g., pressure, foot, or venous stasis ulcers among homebound patients who were not receiving routine monitoring by specialized nurses or doctors).[33]

Supporting caregivers

DEMENTIA

Several studies have focused on the use of technology to support dementia caregivers.[34,35] A review of this literature shows that intervention usage varied between studies and was generally low.[36] The outcomes were inconsistent, with only moderate effects on improving caregiver stress and depression. Treatment effects were found to vary by ethnic groups, formal support, and baseline burden. However, these findings should be treated cautiously, since they often come from multiple subgroup analyses.

PALLIATIVE CARE

The use of telemedicine is also being explored in providing support at the end of life, mostly using videophone technology. Telehealth can provide psychological support and symptom monitoring and management, while reducing the need for visits for the nurse.[37]

Safety and security monitoring

Telemedicine allows care coordinators to closely monitor seniors with limited caregiver support. Care coordinators can use the technology to provide social support and health care reminders. Technology applications have also been examined in the areas of home alert systems and fall-detection devices for seniors at risk for falls. Although it is proposed that home alert systems may reduce hospital admissions and improve discharge rates, leading to cost savings, few good quality studies have been published. One case control study in the United Kingdom found that a home alert system for persons with dementia may help such patients stay in their homes and improve functional status.[38] The use of technologies for locating elderly persons with dementia who wander also appears promising.[39] Automatic fall detectors have been developed to prevent, detect, and predict falls. A recent small study of older people living in sheltered housing in the United Kingdom examined the results of an intervention consisting of automatic fall detectors. After a 12-month monitoring period, there was no noticeable change in the fear of falling. However, significant improvement was found in the social functioning domain ($P = 0.049$), with scores 8% higher in the intervention group, suggesting a beneficial effect of telecare. Positive trends were also evident in the length of time spent out of the home and in improved feelings of safety during the day and night.[40]

e-Health

e-Health is an emerging field in the intersection of medical informatics, public health, and business, which refers to health services and information delivered or enhanced through the Internet and related technologies. In a broader sense, the term characterizes not only a technical development, but also a way of thinking, and a commitment for networked, global thinking to improve health care locally, regionally, and worldwide by using information and communication technology.[41] e-Health is a broader term than either telemedicine or telehealth, including telehealth, telecare, electronic medical records, and use of the Internet, among many other applications.

The search for health care information and resources is one of the most common uses of the Internet by the elderly. Potential uses of the Internet by seniors are listed in Table 128-2. Unfortunately, many health care Web sites are designed in ways that make them difficult for the elderly to use. Research suggests three main categories of Web design problems, all arising from "ability" changes with aging: (1) visual,

Table 128-2. Potential Roles of the Internet in the Care of the Aged Patient

- Resource for medical information
- Medium for enhanced communication between patients/caregivers and providers/care managers
- Access portal to billing information
- Resource for information about health care facilities and long-term care institutions
- Means for diagnosis and treatment of patients at distant locations
- Monitor of patients with chronic illness/disease
- Delivery of automated message reminders (e.g., medications, appointments)
- Online support groups

(2) motor, and (3) cognitive. For example, visual problems occur for the elderly when type faces are too small or in unusual fonts, and motor problems occur when navigation elements are too small or too closely spaced. Even in the use of the computer mouse there are age-related changes, especially in more complex tasks such as clicking and double clicking, which require longer movement times and more submovements. Errors in such tasks are related to manual dexterity, and not to age, per se, and not to prior mouse experience.[42] Alternative site designs and navigation elements such as larger keyboard buttons could make these sites more usable for the elderly. Cognitive problems exist when site navigation imposes excessive demands on elders who have reduced working memory capacity. Web sites that will be used by the elderly present specific challenges for designers, who need to pay attention to usability research.[43]

USABILITY ISSUES IN THE ELDERLY

Although results have been promising in studies with telephone use, many older adults have difficulty learning to use and operate other technologies, such as computers, the Internet, videocassette recorders, automatic teller machines, and telephone menu systems.[44,45] Yet, many studies have reported the satisfaction and comfort of older patients with carefully selected telehealth technology. In one study older patients with obstructive lung disease or CHF felt comfortable with the videoconference and other peripheral devices used in the study.[46] In another study, American veterans who were suffering from noncognitive diseases reported that the home messaging technology was easy to use and helpful in managing their chronic conditions.[47]

On the other hand, home telecare is not always user-friendly for people who have Alzheimer's disease; they have difficulties in learning a new task and hence in the use of a telemedicine device. In one study, dementia patients failed to respond to the establishment of a videoconference session after it was initiated from the center.[48,49] In another study they were unable to transmit their data successfully.[50]

The technology must be simple and user-friendly and operate reliably without interruptions if it is going to be used by a population with a high incidence of cognitive and sensory impairment. In such cases complicated technology will serve only to increase program costs and decrease patient adherence. A selection bias could emerge whereby only the patients who are well-educated and highly motivated will remain. Therefore, technology interfaces should place minimal cognitive demands and provide environmental supports, such as cues and reminders or navigational aids. Seniors should be adequately trained in a self-paced, comfortable, and nonthreatening environment, where they receive positive feedback.[51] It is also important for care coordinators to properly screen older adults for their ability to use the technology.[52]

Overall, adoption of technology in the elderly is a complex issue, influenced by a variety of factors, including sociodemographic elements, attitudinal variables, and cognitive abilities.[53] Widespread dissemination of telemedicine will be facilitated if the technology is "accepted" and "usable" by the patients and caregivers. The easiest technology to use is whatever elders are already used to. In some cases, a selected device must be adapted to the needs of the patient. We believe that the telehealth field will eventually move to commonly used devices, such as the cell phone, the home phone with a caller-ID box, or the television. For some people, cell phones and other handheld devices are more practical, while for those with poor vision and dexterity, larger devices (larger special cell phones or television) may be more applicable.

BARRIERS TO WIDESPREAD USE OF TELEMEDICNE

In addition to usability factors, several other barriers have limited the widespread use and implementation of telemedicine. These impediments include: (1) clinician attitudes, (2) factors related to the technology, (3) economic elements, (4) policy, and most overwhelmingly, (5) lack of evidence. Each of these areas are briefly described below (Table 128-3).

Clinician attitudes

Many health care professionals express concern that telemedicine applications will not benefit them in their day-to-day practice. Others describe practical difficulties incorporating

Table 128-3. Issues to Be Considered before Instituting a Home-Telehealth Program

- Identify patient most likely to benefit from such an intervention
  - o At risk for institutionalization
  - o With multiple impairments/chronic conditions
  - o Needing multiple services
  - o Without available social supports
  - o Where preventive services may avoid/delay institutional care
  - o Ability to participate
    - Appropriate medical condition
    - Manual dexterity
    - Vision
    - Commitment to program
  - o Appropriate technology
- Staffing issues
  - o Background and training
  - o Workload/census issues
  - o Level of decision making/management ability
- Limitations of technology:
  - o Connections
  - o Picture quality
  - o Cost
  - o Maintenance
  - o Usability
- Policy factors
- Privacy factors
- Reimbursement/workload issues

telemedicine into their existing space, schedule, practice, and clinical workflow.

Technology factors

There are few hardware and software standards; the systems are proprietary, vendor-specific, and often do not interoperate. Rapid advancement and changes in technology also make both hardware and software options confusing and vulnerable to obsolescence. Breakdowns and equipment failures must be expected. Care coordinators need to have procedures in place for expected malfunctions and equipment repair downtime.

Most users are patients and families, often with little or no training in using complex electronic devices. Telehealth technology must therefore design fail safe systems and operating procedures. Set-up and use should not require instruction manuals.

Economic elements

Lack of reimbursement by agencies, including Medicare, is probably the biggest disincentive in telehealth. To overcome the other barriers, providers must have incentives to use telehealth technology, either financial or as a model advocated by the health care umbrella under which they practice. Quickly changing hardware and software options are confusing and also result in an expensive capital investment that is vulnerable to being outdated. Capital investment costs include the units given to the patient, the equipment used by the care coordinators, and the coordinating/decision support software. The overall cost per patient will decrease as the program increases the number of subjects enrolled. Once a system is in place, it cannot be immediately replaced because of the cost. The use of telemedicine must also budget for equipment maintenance and replacement.

Policy factors

Policy affects how telehealth is implemented and regarded. There are a number of legal issues, such as cross-state licensure and potential physician malpractice risk. Security and privacy issues will be decisive to the success of future telemedicine services. Robust ethical guidelines must be debated and developed so as to best preserve the appropriate control, privacy, and dignity of all users under all circumstances.

Lack of evidence

Many telemedicine programs have not been subject to rigorous comparative studies to assess their effects on quality, accessibility, cost, or acceptability.[54,55] Some limited studies have shown the benefits of home-based telemedicine interventions in chronic diseases. However, the potential benefits described above of telehealth interventions are difficult to generalize since the studies have had significant variation in patient characteristics (e.g., demographics, ability for self-management, medical condition), sample selection, care coordination design, and technology modalities and devices. The interventions assessed are very heterogeneous, with regard to outcome measures and length of follow-up. The exact contribution of telehealth technology to the effectiveness and efficiency of care provision for chronic diseases cannot now be determined, given the broad range of interventions and absence of standard practices. Other shortfalls include difficulty discerning how much of the observed benefit is actually because of commitment of the research staff.

Telehealth care coordination programs have met with variable degrees of success, and the basis for success in these programs is not fully understood. Good results may depend on the ability of the care coordinator to influence physician and patient behavior. Care coordination programs vary as to the participation/involvement of the treating physician. In most cases, the care coordinators alert the physician about issues involving the patient. Programs where the coordinator can make management decisions about a patient's treatment and implement decisions independently may be more efficient than care coordination models where the information is simply passed on to the physician. The effects and relative importance of other staffing and operational issues to the success of a telehealth care coordination program remain to be identified and understood: qualifications and training of the care coordinator, frequency of monitoring, the ideal technology, the ideal duration of an intervention, the ideal morbidity, and patient characteristics.

Good evaluation is also restricted by limited resources for conducting studies. Choices among measurement options are often shaped by practical considerations, such as cost, human resources, timetable, and organizational relationships. Once an investment is made, it may discourage rigorous research designs, including experimental clinical trials and quasi-experimental clinical studies.

FUTURE DIRECTIONS

Despite the concern expressed about the progressive dehumanization of interpersonal relationships encouraged by widespread telemedicine use, technology's rapid evolution appears to be moving toward more sophisticated and invasive forms of interventions. Telehealth technology will address three main functions: information gathering, information exchange, and intelligence processing. Electronic health records (EHR) and information technology connectivity will lead to an information explosion and lend the capability of making the electronic communication seamless. Artificial intelligence and advanced computational capabilities could generate very sophisticated decision-support programs that would themselves generate decisions, occasionally with human help. Novel methods for the delivery of quality health care could increase the effectiveness of management while containing costs and using scarce human resources to maximum effect. Increasing access to the millions who do not have health care is also envisioned as one of the possibilities of telemedicine.

In a perfect world, every elder would be monitored 24/7, looking for any change in status, and intervening. But because resources are always finite in an era of infinite wants, it will be crucial to tailor the intervention, targeting it to patients and conditions with the highest probability of benefiting from the introduction of telemedicine, patients who will provide the best "bang for the buck," so to speak. Different times in the history of the world bring different prime movers. Although outcomes and quality are important, the main driver of the telemedicine innovation will be the extreme and ever increasing cost of health care for the elderly. Although telemedicine is not the solution in and of itself, the current view is that telemedicine holds promise to make health care cheaper, safer, and better quality and therefore deserves further exploration.

The ultimate goal is that the increase in benefit should exceed the cost. Therefore, telemedicine programs will have to be rigorously evaluated for cost-effectiveness, efficiency, scalability, safety, and acceptability to patients.[56] Greater attention must be given to issues associated with scientific rigor such as sample size, statistical power, and research design.

The use and the speed of dissemination of telemedicine in any health care environment depend on the value being added to that system of care. The value added will depend on the careful selection of technology that meets the specific needs of the administrators, health care professionals, and patients. In the managed care sector, technology will be implemented only if it shows immediate profitability in a financial cycle from the administrators' viewpoint. From the point of view of health care professionals, telemedicine must improve quality of care while improving productivity. It must also not result in an increase in costs or workload. Consideration also must be given to how best to integrate technologies with more traditional intervention approaches.

The patient's perspective is also essential in the development of these models; it will be important to use technology suited to patient needs. Users will need training in the use of specific technology, taking into account level of expertise (if any) and comorbidities. The training of patients and caregivers must be culturally and ethnically sensitive. Telemedicine can enable care coordination organizations to deploy limited multilingual staff to provide support to minority patients and caregivers over a large geographic area.[57]

Other metrics must also be taken into account, such as compliance issues and process efficiency. By providing the evidence base for all these metrics, the concerns of the payers and the policymakers will be addressed and the full potential of the telemedicine dream can be approached.

KEY POINTS

Telemedicine Applications in Geriatrics

- Health care as it is structured now is fragmented and inefficient, with a lot of duplication and inefficiency in the system, leading to rising health care cost.
- Coordination of care is a key focus of the Institute of Medicine and of the chronic disease model, both of which advocate that care should be accessible, centered around patients and families, comprehensive, continuous, and coordinated.
- The coordination of care can be greatly facilitated through proper use of telemedicine technologies, in combination with appropriate organizational changes and skills.
- Telemedicine is viewed as a promising tool for improved management for chronic diseases, improved efficiencies of care provision, enhanced self-management, timely medical decision making, improved outcomes, enhanced access to health care services, and as a tool to potentially decrease the economic burden of chronic diseases in the elderly.
- The effectiveness and efficacy of telemedicine needs to be rigorously evaluated for impact on quality, accessibility, cost, or acceptability of health care, to impact policy and payment.

For a complete list of references, please visit online only at www.expertconsult.com

Index

Page numbers followed by f indicate figures; t, tables; b, boxes.

A

A Severity Characterization of Trauma (ASCOT), 867
Abbreviated Injury Scale (AIS), 867
Abciximab, 291
Abdominal aortic aneurysm, 352–355, 353f–354f
  aneurysm repair in elderly, 355
  complications of aneurysm surgery, 354–355
  diagnosis of, 353, 353f–354f
  natural history of, 353
  presentation of, 353
  prevalence of, 352–353
Abdominal computed tomography, 649–650, 661–662
Abdominal massage, for constipation, 919, 919t
Abdominal pain, 108
Abdominal trauma, 868
Abdominal ultrasound, 637
Abdominal x-rays, for constipation and FI, 917, 917f
Abnormal movements, of old age, 103
ABPM. *See* Ambulatory blood pressure monitoring
Abscess
  in brain, 549
  of liver, 644
Absorption
  of drugs, aging effects on, 139
  by small bowel, 652. *See also* Malabsorption
Abuse. *See* Alcohol abuse
Acarbose, 510, 768b, 769
ACC/AHA guidelines. *See* American College of Cardiology/American Heart Association guidelines
Accelerated aging. *See* Premature aging
Accelerated atrioventricular rhythm, 336
Access, of quality of care, 1039
Accident prevention, 850–851
Accreditation, for quality of care improvement in United Kingdom, 1041
ACE inhibitors. *See* Angiotensin-converting enzyme inhibitors
ACE units. *See* Acute care for the elderly units
Acetabular fractures, 584–585, 585f
Acetaminophen. *See* Paracetamol
Acetazolamide, 141t, 462, 820
Acetylcholinesterase inhibitors (AChEI)
  for dementia, 400–401, 432
  for myasthenia gravis, 530–531
  for Parkinson's disease, 517
Acetylcysteine, 373
Acetylsalicylic acid, 296–297
Achalasia, 611, 613, 613f
AChEI. *See* Acetylcholinesterase inhibitors
Acid phosphatase, as prostate disease marker, 704
Acid-base homeostasis, aging effects on, 56
Acid-reducing drugs, bacterial overgrowth syndrome and, 654–655
Acne, in Down syndrome, 448–449
ACOVE. *See* Assessing Care of Vulnerable Elders
Acquired immunodeficiency, in old age, secondary causes of, 88–90
ACTH. *See* Adrenocorticotropic hormone
Actinic keratosis (AK), 805
Active movement, stroke and, 874
Active surveillance, for prostate cancer, 712
Activities of daily living (ADLs)
  dementia effects on, 393–394, 393t, 409–410
  disability assessment and, 10
  obesity and impairment of, 686
  in social functioning, 224
  therapy for, 871, 875
Activity analysis, in occupational therapy, 871
Acute arterial mesenteric ischemia, 657–658
Acute care for the elderly (ACE) units, for iatrogenic problems prevention, 851
Acute cholecystitis, 647–648
Acute coronary syndromes, 290–291
Acute hyperthyroidism, 743
Acute limb ischemia
  management of acute thrombosis, 349, 350f
  management of femoral embolism, 349
  outcome of limb salvage for, 349, 350f
Acute liver failure (ALF), 638, 638t, 643
Acute mitral regurgitation, 324
Acute myelogenous leukemia (AML), 787–788, 788t
Acute nerve root entrapment, in degenerative disease of lumbar spine, 544
Acute pain, 965
Acute pancreatitis, 631–633, 631f, 632t
Acute Physiology and Chronic Health Estimates (APACHE), 867
Acute renal failure (ARF), 691, 692t
Acyclovir, 472, 550–551, 550b, 692, 803–804
AD. *See* Alzheimer's disease
Adalimumab, 570t, 656–657, 669t
ADAM questionnaire. *See* Androgen Deficiency in the Aging Male questionnaire
Adaptive capacity, successful aging due to, 184–186
Adaptive program theory, 18–19
Addison's disease, 732–733, 808
Adenocarcinoma
  of gallbladder, 648
  gastric, 624
  of pancreas, 627–631, 628f
    blood tests for, 628
    chemoradiotherapy for, 631
    diagnosis of, 628
    epidemiology and age incidence of, 627, 628f
    imaging of, 628–629
    management of, 629–631
    presentation of, 627
  of small bowel, 659
Adenomatous polyps, of large bowel, 673
Adenosine, for SVT, 336
Adenosine diphosphate inhibitors, 495
Adenosine echocardiography, for CAD, 287
ADGAP. *See* Association of Directors of Geriatric Academic Programs
Adjustment disorder, palliative care for, 980
Adjuvant analgesics, for pain, 970
ADLs. *See* Activities of daily living
ADR. *See* Adverse drug reaction
Adrenal androgens, physiologic responses to, 730
Adrenal cortex disorders, 730–733
  adrenocortical function in normal aging, 731–732
  biochemical actions of steroid hormones, 730–731
  clinical patterns of, 733–735, 734f
Adrenal cortex disorders (*Continued*)
    adrenal carcinomas, 733–734, 734f
    adrenal insufficiency, 732–733
    Cushing syndrome, 732–734, 734f, 808
    glucocorticoid excess, 732–734
    incidentaloma, 734–735
  cutaneous complications of, 808
  physiologic responses to adrenocortical steroids, 730
  regulation of adrenal function, 731
  tests of adrenal function, 732–733
Adrenal insufficiency, 732–733
α-Adrenergic blockers, 339t
β-Adrenergic drugs, 519
β-Adrenergic stimulation, response of aging heart to, 95–96
Adrenocortical steroids, 730–731
Adrenocorticotropic hormone (ACTH)
  aging effects on, 125–126
  isolated deficiency of, 736
  for ulcerative colitis, 667–668
Adriamycin, 753
ADT. *See* Androgen deprivation therapy
Adult learning theory, in geriatric medicine education, 1034
Advance directives
  for iatrogenic problems prevention, 851
  for incompetent patients, 985
  palliative medicine and, 974
Advanced glycation end products (AGEs), 35
Adverse drug reaction (ADR), 880–882, 881f
Adverse drug withdrawal event (ADWE), 880, 881f, 882, 884, 884t
ADWE. *See* Adverse drug withdrawal event
AEDs. *See* Antiepileptic drugs
Aerobic conditioning, for frailty prevention, 850
Aerobic exercise
  aging effects on capacity for, 56
  carbohydrate metabolism and, 860–861
  for stroke therapy, 874
  for successful aging, 859–860
AF. *See* Atrial fibrillation
Agarotoban, 789
Age groups, epidemiology of aging and definitions of, 6, 6t, 7f
Age-associated disease, physiologic damage resulting from, 52–53
Ageism, in the workplace, 195–196
Agency for Healthcare Research and Quality (AHRQ), quality health care, 1046
Age-related model, of geriatric medicine, 997
AGEs. *See* Advanced glycation end products
Aging. *See also* Cognitive aging; Old age
  allostasis and allostatic overload in, 158
    consequences of being "stressed out" and sleep deprivation, 159–160
    definition of stress, allostasis, and allostatic load, 158, 159f
    effects of stress on human brain, 160–161
    measurement of allostatic load, 158–159, 160t
    protection and damage as response to stressors, 158, 160f
    role of adverse early life experience in, 161
    role of brain in response to stress, 160, 161f
    role of positive affect, self-esteem, and social support, 161

Aging (*Continued*)
of auditory system, 822–824
autonomic cardiovascular control and, 501–503, 502f
autonomic response to stress and, 503–504
biology of, 30
cell death, cell replacement, and stem cells, 33
cell proliferation, telomerase, and telomere function, 32–33
insulin-signaling pathway and longevity regulation, 30–32, 31f
longevity dividend concept and reasons for investing in aging research, 35–38
progeroid syndromes and normal aging, 33–34
protein damage and sarcopenia, 34–35
biomedical inputs to, 13–15
of blood, 127
B cells, 132–133
circulating blood cells, 130
eosinophils, basophils, and mast cells, 130
epigenetics, 128–129
granulocytes, 130
hematopoiesis, 127
hematopoietic stem cells, 127–128
lymphoid development, 131
monocytes and macrophages, 130
progenitor compartment, 129–130
red cells, 130–131
sites of blood cell development, bone marrow, and stroma, 127–128
T cells, 131–132
telomeres and senescence, 128
of bones and joints, 117, 118f
articular cartilage, 117–119, 118f–119f
consequences of, 122
future of, 122–123
skeleton, 119–121, 119f–120f
soft tissues, 121–122
cancer and, 791–792
of cardiovascular system, 54, 91
aging-associated changes in vascular structure, 91, 92f
arterial stiffness in aging arteries, 92–93, 93f, 93t
endothelial function in aging, 91–92
heart structure changes with age, 93–94, 96t
myocardial function in aging heart at rest, 94–95, 96t
response of aging heart to exercise, 95–96, 96t
cellular mechanisms of, 42
cell senescence, 45–48
destructive agents in cellular aging, 42–45
in extracellular matrix, 49
in protein synthesis and degradation, 48–49
in signaling pathways, 49
changes in quality of life and disability associated with, 5
of connective tissues, 73
aging and properties of connective tissues, 77–80
properties of connective tissues, 73–74
definition of, 30
as dementia risk factor, 385–386
Down syndrome and, 448–449
of endocrine system, 123
andropause, 124–125
dehydroepiandrosterone, 125
growth hormone/insulin-like growth factor-I axis, 123–124
hypothalamic-pituitary-adrenal axis, 125–126

Aging (*Continued*)
hypothalamic-pituitary-thyroid axis, 126
menopause, 124
epidemiology of, 3
quality of life and disability, 4–9, 4f, 6t, 7f–9f, 9t
in Europe, 997, 997f
evolutionary theory and mechanisms of, 18
evolution of aging, 18–19, 19f
genetics of life span, 19–21, 20f
tests of, 21–22
frailty index relationship to, 64, 64f
future of, 15–18
gastroenterology and, 106
altered manifestation of adult gastrointestinal diseases, 107–109
gastrointestinal problems unique to elderly, 109–110
normal physiology of aging, 106–107
genetic mechanisms of, 38
chromosomal gene mutations, 39–41
epigenetics, 41
integrative approach to, 41
mitochondrial genetics, oxidative stress, and aging, 38–39
telomeres, 40–41
of genital tract, 716
of GI tract, 106–107
glucose tolerance impairment and, 761, 761f, 762t
heart disease treatment decisions and, 295–298, 296t–297t
of immune system, 82–85, 85t, 86f
B-cell function changes, 84–85
cell lysis changes, 83
clinical consequences of immune senescence, 85–88
cytokine dysregulation, 85, 85t, 86f
immune enhancement, 89
immune function assessment, 89
nonspecific host defense changes, 82
phagocytosis changes, 82–83
secondary causes of acquired immunodeficiency in old age, 88–90
specific host defense changes, 83
T-cell function changes, 83–84
immunologic markers of, 85t
inevitability of, 8
introduction to frailty, geriatric medicine, and, 1
of liver, 107, 635
mathematical models of, 59
development of frailty index based on comprehensive geriatric assessment, 62–65, 63f–65f, 65t
phenotypic definition of frailty, 60–62, 61f
metabolic-insulin signaling in control of, 154–157, 155f–156f
mitochondrial genetics, oxidative stress, and, 38–39
neurobiology of, 150
generation of reactive oxygen/nitrogen species, 151–152
metabolic-insulin signaling in control of aging and neurodegeneration, 154–157, 155f–156f
nitrosative and oxidative stress in, 150, 151f–152f
protein misfolding in neurodegenerative disease, 150–151
protein S-nitrosylation and neuronal cell death, 152–154, 153t
neuroendocrinology of, 163
brain metabolism and neurodegenerative disease in, 167–169

Aging (*Continued*)
reproductive aging in men, 166–167
reproductive aging in women, 163–169
normal. *See* Normal aging
orthostatic hypotension and, 342
pain in, 965
palliative medicine and, 973
of pancreas, 107, 626
of parathyroid glands and calcium homeostasis, 755–756, 756t
of people with intellectual disability, 447
of personality, 178
personality stages and ego development, 178–181, 179t
social-cognitive approaches to personality, 181–182
synthesis and future directions, 182–183
pharmacology of, 138
altered pharmacodynamics, 141, 141t
altered pharmacokinetics, 139–140, 139t–141t
drug interactions, 141–143, 141t–143t
epidemiology of drug use, 138
physiology of, 51
age changes in organismic function, 55–57, 57f
interspecies and intraspecies variation in physiologic deterioration, 53
physiologic deterioration and the aging phenotype, 51–53, 52f
in specific organs and organ systems, 53–55, 54f
of populations, causes and results of, 3
premature, 20–21, 836
processes behind, 3–4
productive. *See* Productive aging
progerin in, 68–71, 69f
research on, reasons for investing in, 35–38
of respiratory system, 97
functional changes, 98–99
pulmonary host defense and immune response changes, 99–101
respiratory function tests, 97
structural changes, 98
of skin, 133
extrinsic aging, 133–135
hair, 136
immune function, 136
intrinsic aging, 133
mechanism of, 78, 136
nails, 136
nerves and sensation, 136
subcutaneous tissue, 136
sweat glands, 135–137
treatment and prevention of, 136–137
in women, 136
successful. *See* Successful aging
telomerase and, 32
of thyroid, 126, 738
of urinary tract, 111
lower urinary tract: bladder and outlet, 112–116, 113t
upper urinary tract: kidneys and ureters, 111–112
Aging index, 8
α-Agonists, 143t, 345
β-Agonists
for asthma, 364–365, 367, 367t–368t
for COPD, 373
sensitivity to, 99, 141, 141t
tremor caused by, 519
AHI. *See* Apnea hypopnea index
AHRQ. *See* Agency for Healthcare Research and Quality

AICD. *See* Automatic implantable cardioverter-defibrillator
AIH. *See* Autoimmune hepatitis
Airflow obstruction
  in asthma, 364
    reversibility of, 364–365, 365f
  diseases of, 362, 363t
Airways, of smokers, 370
AIS. *See* Abbreviated Injury Scale
AK. *See* Actinic keratosis
Akinesia, 512
Akinetic-rigid syndromes, 511, 511t
Albumin, 641–642
Albuterol, 373
Alcohol
  altered mental status due to, 205
  cardiovascular risk and, 303
  in chronic cardiac failure, 283
  chronic pancreatitis and, 633
  cluster headache due to, 470
  constipation and, 913
  delirium due to, 241
  dementia associated with, 386–387
  ED and, 856, 857t
  frailty prevention and, 850
  gastropathy due to, 619
  heart failure precipitated by, 274–275, 274t
  herbal-drug interactions of, 142t
  in hypertension management, 308
  liver metabolism of, 635–636
  myalgia and myopathy induced by, 529
  orthostatic hypotension and, 508b
  sexuality in old age and, 855, 857t
  sleep-disordered breathing and, 946–947
  syncope caused by, 339t
Alcohol abuse, 441–442
Alcoholic liver disease (ALD), 639
ALD. *See* Alcoholic liver disease
Aldosterone, regulation of production of, 731
Aldosterone antagonists, 292, 641
Alemtuzumab, 787
Alendronate, 556, 556t, 558, 586, 616
ALF. *See* Acute liver failure
Alfacalcidol, 557, 561, 759b
ALFs. *See* Assisted living facilities
Alfuzosin, 709t
Alkylating agents
  for intracranial tumors, 537–538
  leukemia after, 788t
  myelodysplasia after, 777–778
  for ovarian cancer, 724
Allergic asthma. *See* Atopic asthma
Allopurinol, 381, 574, 692
Allostasis and allostatic load, in aging, 158
  consequences of being "stressed out" and sleep deprivation, 159–160
  definition of stress, allostasis, and allostatic load, 158, 159f
  effects of stress on human brain, 160–161
  measurement of allostatic load, 158–159, 160t
  protection and damage as response to stressors, 158, 160f
  role of adverse early life experience, 161
  role of brain in response to stress, 160, 161f
  role of positive affect, self-esteem, and social support, 161
Alprazolam, 140t, 142t
Alprostadil, 725, 857–858
Altered mental status (AMS), as nonspecific clinical presentation of disease in elderly, 205–206
Aluminium antacids, 912–913
Aluminum hydroxide, 622
Alzheimer's disease (AD), 411
  aerobic exercise and, 864
  aging of connective tissues in patients with, 80
  behavioral symptoms in, 417
  biologic markers of diagnosis and disease progression, 417–419, 418f
  clinical diagnostic criteria for, 414–415, 414t
  clinical evaluation for, 415
  constipation and, 913
  delirium v., 903
  epidemiology and genetics of, 412–414
  insulin/insulin-like growth factor-I signaling effects on, 123
  laboratory studies of, 416–417, 416t
  neuroendocrinology of aging in, 167–169
  neurologic examination for, 415–416
  neuropsychology in diagnosis and treatment of, 404–405, 409t
  pathology and mechanisms of, 411–412, 412f
  previously accepted but ineffective therapies for, 420
  risk factors for, 385
  S-nitrosylation of PDI in protein misfolding and neurotoxicity in cell models of, 153–154
  treatment of, 419–420, 419t
Amantadine (Symmetrel)
  delirium and, 513
  elimination of, 141t
  for influenza, 376
  for levodopa-induced dyskinesia, 516
  for parkinsonism, 515t, 517–518
Ambulatory blood pressure monitoring (ABPM), 304
Ambulatory electrocardiography, 287
American College of Cardiology/American Heart Association (ACC/AHA) guidelines, for perioperative cardiovascular evaluation before noncardiac surgery, 236–237, 236t
American College of Sports medicine, exercise recommendations by, 859, 861
Amiloride, 641, 698
Amino acid derivatives, for glucose control, 769
Aminocaproic acid, 528
Aminoglycosides
  for cholecystitis and cholangitis, 648
  elimination of, 140, 141t
  ototoxicity of, 824
  renal failure due to, 691–692
5-Aminosalicylate therapy
  for Crohn's disease, 670
  for diverticular disease, 664
  for lymphocytic and collagenous colitis, 671
  for ulcerative colitis, 667–668, 667t
Amiodarone
  for AF, 333
  anticoagulation therapy and, 358
  for atrial flutter, 335
  for chronic cardiac failure, 278b, 282
  cytochrome P450 reaction with, 141t
  drug interactions of, 143, 281
  herbal-drug interactions of, 142t
  hyperthyroidism due to, 740–741
  hypothyroidism due to, 745
  interstitial lung disease induced by, 381
  for maintaining sinus rhythm, 333
  myalgia and myopathy induced by, 528–529
  after myocardial infarction, 293, 293t
  nonalcoholic fatty liver disease risk and, 639–640
  parkinsonism induced by, 518
  syncope caused by, 339t
  thyroid hormone secretion and metabolism in response to, 738
  tremor caused by, 519
Amiodarone (*Continued*)
  for ventricular arrhythmias, 328–329, 329t–330t
  for ventricular rate control in patients with AF, 332
Amitriptyline
  codeine and, 969
  for headache, 469–470, 476
  herbal-drug interactions of, 142t
  liver metabolism of, 635–636
  for migraine, 468
  for postherpetic neuralgia, 472, 477b
  for vulval discomfort, 719–720
AML. *See* Acute myelogenous leukemia
Amlodipine, 140t, 278b, 281–282, 290–291
Ammonium lactate, 802
Amnesia
  psychogenic, 459
  transient epileptic, 458
  transient global, 458–459
Amoxicillin, 620, 663t, 664
Amphetamine, 519
Amphotericin B, 550
Ampicillin, 548, 548t, 648, 664–665
Ampullary tumors, 649
Amputation
  of lower limb, for diabetes mellitus, 763–765, 764t–765t, 765b
  for traumatic fracture, 584, 584f
AMS. *See* Altered mental status
Amylin analogues, 774
Amyloid plaques, of Alzheimer's disease, 411–412, 412f
β-Amyloid proteins, of Alzheimer's disease, 411–413, 420
Amyloidosis
  connective tissue disorders associated with, 581–582
  upper gastrointestinal tract in patients with, 625–626
Anabolic steroids, herbal-drug interactions of, 142t
Anagrelide, 780
Anal endosonography, 662
Analgesics, 797
  for apatite deposition disease, 576
  for calcium pyrophosphate crystal deposition, 575
  for chronic pancreatitis, 634
  constipation and, 912–913
  dementia due to, 417
  depression and, 841
  for diverticular disease, 663t
  for eye pain, 476
  for headache, 469, 472–474
  headache due to overuse of, 469–470, 475, 477b
  for migraine, 467–468, 468t, 477b
  for neurologic complications of degenerative disease of lumbar spine, 545
  for pain, 968–969
  for palliative care, 973, 976–977, 976t
  for pancreas adenocarcinoma, 630
  renal failure and, 693–694
  as secondary cause of acquired immunodeficiency in old age, 89
Anatomical Profile (AP), 867
Androgen, adrenal, 730
Androgen Deficiency in the Aging Male (ADAM) questionnaire, 147, 147t
Androgen deprivation therapy (ADT), for prostate cancer, 713–714
Androgen therapy
  for breast cancer, 728, 728t
  for reproductive aging in men, 167
  sexual motivation and, 724–725

Andropause, 124–125, 166–167
Anemia, 775–777, 775t–777t
  autoimmune hemolytic, 786–787
  autonomic failure and, 508
  of inflammation, 776
  pathogenesis of, 776–777, 776t–777t
  prevalence of, 775–776, 775t
Anesthesia
  cognitive functioning after, 242
  delirium due to, 241
  in old age, 230–232
    age, surgery, and outcome, 230–231
    anesthetic drugs, 231
    anesthetic factors, 231–232
    cardiac problems in elderly surgical patient, 235–237, 236t
    CNS problems, 241–242
    fluid and electrolyte imbalance, 239–241
    future trends, 244–245
    long-term medications, 232
    morbidity and mortality following, 231
    obesity, 239
    online computerized risk assessment and guidance, 243
    preoperative assessment, 232–234, 232t–233t
    prophylactic preoperative β-blockade, 232
    for prostate surgery, 709–710
    respiratory problems in older surgical patient, 234–235, 235t
    surgical and anesthetic audits, 243–244
    trends in, 230
    undernutrition and, 237–239, 239t
  for orthopedic geriatrics, 584–586
Anesthetic audits, 243–244
Anesthetics
  acute liver failure induced by, 643
  for epilepsy, 459
  in old age, 231
  for pruritus, 803
  for vulval discomfort, 719–720
Aneurysm
  abdominal aortic, 352–355, 353f–354f
    aneurysm repair in elderly, 355
    complications of aneurysm surgery, 354–355
    diagnosis of, 353, 353f–354f
    natural history of, 353
    presentation of, 353
    prevalence of, 352–353
  small, management of, 355
Angelman syndrome, 445, 446t–447t
Angina pectoris
  of CAD, 286
  stable, 290
  unstable, 290–291
Angiodysplasia, in large bowel, 675
Angioplasty, for carotid disease, 352
Angiosarcoma, of skin, 807
Angiotensin antagonists, for chronic cardiac failure, 277, 281
Angiotensin II blockers, 112
Angiotensin receptor agonists, 93
Angiotensin receptor blockers (ARBs)
  acute renal failure due to, 691
  for chronic cardiac failure, 279
  for chronic kidney disease, 695
  hyperkalemia due to, 698, 698t
  for hypertension, 309
  after myocardial infarction, 292
  for nonalcoholic fatty liver disease, 639–640
  for stroke prevention, 495–496
  for vascular cognitive impairment, 426–427
  for ventricular arrhythmia, 330
Angiotensin-converting enzyme (ACE) inhibitors, 15–16
  for acute coronary syndromes, 291
  acute renal failure due to, 691
  for aortic regurgitation, 319
  for blood pressure control in diabetes mellitus patients, 772
  for bone pain, 977
  for CAD, 288–289
  for chronic cardiac failure, 277–285, 278b, 285b
  for chronic mitral regurgitation, 325
  for CKD, 695
  for diabetic retinopathy, 763
  dry mouth and, 605
  in elderly patients undergoing surgery, 232
  elimination of, 141t
  in frail elderly, 295–297
  hyperkalemia due to, 698, 698t
  for hypertension, 305t, 308–310
  interstitial lung disease induced by, 381
  longevity due to, 14
  after myocardial infarction, 292, 292t–293t
  for nonalcoholic fatty liver disease, 639–640
  orthostatic hypotension and, 503
  in preventing age-related decline in renal function, 112
  renal artery stenosis and, 305
  for sarcopenia, 592–593
  sexuality in old age and, 855, 857t
  for STEMI, 291
  for stroke prevention, 495–496
  syncope caused by, 339t
  for ventricular arrhythmias, 327, 329–330
Angle-closure glaucoma, 814
Animal-assisted therapy, for dementia management, 400
Anorectal aging, 107
Anorectal fecal incontinence, treatment of, 922t, 924
Anorectal function, constipation and FI and, 914–915, 915t, 917
Anorexia, 949–950, 974–975
Anosmia, 975
Antacids
  constipation and, 912–913
  drug interactions of, 141
  for heartburn, 612–613
  for peptic ulcer disease, 622
  respiratory infection associated with, 99–100
  for stomatitis, 609
Antalgic gain, 887
Anthracyclines, 14, 788
Antiaging medicine, 145
  antioxidants as, 148, 148t
  caloric restriction as, 146
  exercise as, 146
  history of, 145–146
  hormonal fountain of youth, 147–148, 147t
  for photoaging, 148, 148t
Antianxiety drugs, dementia due to, 417
Antiarrhythmic drugs
  for AF, 333–334
  hypothyroidism due to, 745
  for maintaining sinus rhythm in patients with AF, 333–334
  after myocardial infarction, 292–293, 293t
  for ventricular arrhythmias, 327, 330t
    class I drugs, 327–328, 328t
    class III drugs, 329, 329t
Antiarthritic drugs, as secondary cause of acquired immunodeficiency in old age, 89
Antibiotics, 797
  acute liver failure induced by, 643
  acute pancreatitis and, 631–633
  anticoagulation therapy and, 358
  for aortic regurgitation, 319
  for aortic stenosis, 316
  for bacterial overgrowth syndrome, 655
  for bronchiectasis, 379
  C. difficile infection and, 664
  candidiasis associated with, 608, 617
  for cholecystitis and cholangitis, 648
  for chronic mitral regurgitation, 325
  for CNS infection, 547–549, 548t
  coagulation defects due to, 789–790
  for colonic ischemia, 672
  for confusion, 981
  for COPD, 373
  for Crohn's disease, 656–657, 669
  for diabetic foot ulcers, 598b
  for diverticulitis, 663, 663t
  enteral nutrition and, 683, 683t
  esophageal injury due to, 616
  functional recovery and, 866–867
  for *H. pylori*, 15–16, 620–621
  for hepatic encephalopathy, 642
  for herpes zoster, 803–804
  for hyperthyroidism, 743
  for infectious colitis, 664–665
  loose stool and, 923
  for MALT lymphoma, 785
  for mitral stenosis, 324
  for multiple myeloma, 783
  myalgia and myopathy induced by, 529
  for osteomalacia, 561
  Parkinson's disease and, 517
  for patients with mitral annular calcium, 322
  for peptic ulcer disease, 622
  for pneumonia, 377
  for pressure ulcers, 941
  for prostatitis, 705
  for pyogenic liver abscess, 644
  renal failure and, 691–694
  as secondary cause of acquired immunodeficiency in old age, 89
  for spontaneous bacterial peritonitis, 641–642
  for stasis dermatitis, 803
  for stomatitis, 609
  systemic complications of, 820
  for thyroid nodule management, 753
  for uterovaginal prolapse surgery, 720
  for UTIs, 690–691
  weight gain due to, 689
Anti-CCP. *See* Anticyclic citrullinated peptide antibodies
Anticholinergic antihistamines, 143t
Anticholinergic tricyclic antidepressants, 143t
Anticholinergics
  adverse effects of, 110
  altered mental status due to, 205–206
  in Alzheimer's disease, 417
  for asthma, 365
  constipation and, 912–913
  for COPD, 373
  for cough, 980
  delirium and, 241, 513
  dementia associated with, 387, 395, 417
  drug interactions of, 143
  for dysphagia and chest pain, 614
  for dystonia, 519
  falls due to, 208
  fatigue due to, 206–207
  for overactive bladder, 721
  for parkinsonism, 515t, 517–518
  systemic complications of, 820
  weight loss due to, 206

Anticholinesterase inhibitors, 605, 820
Anticholinesterase miotics, 813
Anticipatory care
accident prevention, 850–851
disease prevention, 848–849
frailty prevention, 849–850
iatrogenic problem prevention, 851
individualizing, 852, 853t
preventive practice systems, 852–853
psychosocial illness prevention, 851–852
Anticoagulation therapy
for acute arterial mesenteric ischemia, 657–658
for AF, 333–334
for aortic valve replacement, 316, 316t
for atrial flutter, 335–336
for carotid and vertebral artery dissection, 474
for chronic cardiac failure, 282
chronic subdural hemorrhage and, 474
coagulation defects due to, 790
for diabetes mellitus patients, 774b
drug-disease interactions of, 143t
in elderly, 358–359, 358f
for femoral embolism, 349
hemorrhage associated with, 388
for Hutchinson-Gilford progeria syndrome, 71
with inferior vena caval filters, 359
management of bleeding due to, 359
after myocardial infarction, 291–292
outcomes measurement of use of, 248t–265t
in patients with hyperthyroidism, 743, 754b
sensitivity to, 141
for stroke, 334–335, 482, 490–491
for venous thromboembolism, 357–360, 358t, 360b
Anticonvulsants. *See also* Antiepileptic drugs
for chronic daily headache, 469–470
for epilepsy, 459
for essential tremor, 519
for frontotemporal dementia, 432
for insomnia, 946
isoniazid use with, 378
low thyroxine due to, 738
for mania, 440
for migraine, 468
osteoporosis due to, 585
for pain, 970
as secondary cause of acquired immunodeficiency in old age, 89
weight gain due to, 689
Anticyclic citrullinated peptide antibodies (Anti-CCP), 567
Antidepressants, 161–162
antiepileptic drugs and, 463
for anxiety disorders, 440–441
Cox 2 inhibitors and, 969
dementia and, 401, 417
for depression, 435–436, 443b, 980
drug interactions of, 143
ED and, 856, 857t
for headache, 469, 475
for insomnia, 946
for late life delusional disorders, 438–439
for migraine, 468, 468t
orthostatic hypotension and, 503, 508b
for pain, 970
as secondary cause of acquired immunodeficiency in old age, 89
for smoking cessation, 372–373
for somatization, 110b
for stroke, 495
weight gain due to, 689
Antidiabetic drugs, 142t
Antidiarrheal agents, 665, 671
Antiemetics, 468, 468t, 477b, 797
Antiepileptic drugs (AEDs), 459, 462–464, 463t, 465b
adverse effects of, 462–463, 463t
dementia associated with, 387
drug-drug interactions of, 463, 463t
initiation of, 465–466
osteomalacia and, 559
osteoporosis due to, 554–555
role of newer generation drugs, 465
therapeutic plasma monitoring of, 463
withdrawal from, 464
Antifibrotic agents, for primary sclerosing cholangitis, 646
Antifungals
hypothyroidism due to, 745
for onychomycosis, 805
for seborrheic dermatitis, 802
Antiglutamate agents, 530
Antihistamines
drug-disease interactions of, 143t
dry mouth and, 605
fatigue due to, 206–207
for insomnia, 946
for pruritus, 803
for scabies, 804
sensitivity to, 141t
Antihypertensives, 308–309
aging effects on, 141
for CAD, 288–289
dementia and, 400, 417
depression and, 841
drug interactions of, 143
dry mouth and, 605
ED and, 856, 857t
ED due to, 724
fatigue due to, 206–207
in frail elderly patient, 298
for Hutchinson-Gilford progeria syndrome, 71
for hypertension, 305t, 310–311, 310b
orthostatic hypotension and, 342, 503, 508–510, 508b
in preventing age-related decline in renal function, 112
as secondary cause of acquired immunodeficiency in old age, 89
for stroke, 481–482, 492, 496–497
syncope caused by, 339t, 346
Anti-inflammatories. *See also* Nonsteroidal antiinflammatory drugs
for apatite deposition disease, 576
for arthritis, 568–569, 568t
for asthma, 364–365, 367, 367t
for dementia, 400
for neurologic complications of degenerative disease of lumbar spine, 545
for sarcopenia, 593
Antimalarial agents, 528–529
Antimuscarinic drugs, 721
Antioxidants
as antiaging medicine, 148, 148t
for dementia, 400
for macular degeneration, 813b, 818
for nonalcoholic fatty liver disease, 639–640
reactive oxygen species reaction with, 44
Antiparkinson drugs, 506–507
delirium and, 513
depression and, 435, 841
hallucinations and, 513
Antiphospholipid antibody syndrome, 492
Antiplatelet agents
for aortic regurgitation, 319
for carotid and vertebral artery dissection, 474
chronic subdural hemorrhage and, 474
for diabetes mellitus patients, 774b
in frail elderly patient, 295
Antiplatelet agents (*Continued*)
for intermittent claudication, 355b
for mitral annular calcium, 323
for stable angina, 290
for stroke, 482, 490–493, 495
for thrombotic thrombocytopenic purpura, 789
Antipsychotics, 161–162
Cox 2 inhibitors and, 969
for delirium, 906–907
dementia due to, 417
dry mouth and, 605
ED and, 856, 857t
for frontotemporal dementia, 432
for graduates, 439
for insomnia, 946
for late life delusional disorders, 438–439
for late-onset schizophrenia, 438
for mania, 440
as secondary cause of acquired immunodeficiency in old age, 89
weight gain due to, 689
Antipyretics, 743
Antirheumatic drugs, 571
Antiseptics, 745
Antispasmodics, 143t, 663t
Antithrombotic therapy
for aortic valve replacement, 316, 316t
in elderly patients undergoing surgery, 232
for mitral annular calcium, 323
for thromboembolic stroke in patients with cardiac arrhythmias, 334–335
for venous thromboembolism, 361
Antithyroid antibodies, 739–740
Antithyroid drugs
for hyperthyroidism, 742–743, 754b
as secondary cause of acquired immunodeficiency in old age, 89
Anti-TNFα agents, 593, 667
Antituberculous drugs, acute liver failure induced by, 643
Anti-VEGF agents, 813b, 816–819, 817f
Antivirals, for herpes zoster, 472, 803–804
Anxiety
chronic pain and, 966
constipation and, 913
Anxiety disorders, 440–441
epidemiology of, 440
generalized anxiety disorder, 440
obsessive-compulsive disorder, 441
panic disorder, 440
phobic disorders, 440
posttraumatic stress disorder and bereavement, 440–441
Anxiolytics, 158, 161–162, 440
Aortic aneurysm, abdominal, 352–355, 353f–354f
aneurysm repair in elderly, 355
complications of aneurysm surgery, 354–355
diagnosis of, 353, 353f–354f
natural history of, 353
presentation of, 353
prevalence of, 352–353
Aortic regurgitation (AR), 317–320
echocardiography and Doppler echocardiography for, 318–319
electrocardiography and chest roentgenography for, 318
etiology and prevalence of, 317
medical and surgical management of, 319–320, 319t
natural history of, 319
pathophysiology of, 318
signs of, 318
symptoms of, 318

Aortic stenosis (AS), 312–317
  aortic valve replacement for, 315–317, 316t
  balloon aortic valvuloplasty for, 317
  echocardiography and Doppler echocardiography for, 314
  electrocardiography and chest roentgenography for, 314
  etiology and prevalence of, 312
  medical management of, 316
  natural history of, 314–316, 315t
  pathophysiology of, 312–313
  percutaneous transcatheter implantation of aortic valve prostheses for, 317
  signs of, 313–314, 313t
  symptoms of, 313
Aortic valve prostheses, 317
Aortic valve replacement (AVR)
  for aortic regurgitation, 319–320, 319t
  for aortic stenosis, 315–317, 316t
AOU. *See* Assessment of Underutilization of Medication
AP. *See* Anatomical Profile
APACHE. *See* Acute Physiology and Chronic Health Estimates
Apatite deposition disease, 575–577
APCs. *See* Atrial premature complexes
Aphasias, primary progressive, 407–410, 409t
Apnea hypopnea index (AHI), 946
Apocrine sweat glands, 135
APOE gene, mutations in, 413
Apomorphine (Britaject), 515t, 516–517
Apoptosis. *See* Cell death
APP gene, mutations in, 412–413
Appendicitis, 208–209, 209t, 664
Appetite stimulation, 955–956
Aprindine, 328, 333–334
AR. *See* Aortic regurgitation; Audiologic rehabilitation
Arachis oil retention enemas, 920, 979
ARBs. *See* Angiotensin receptor blockers
Archaic reflexes. *See* Primitive reflexes
ARF. *See* Acute renal failure
Aripiprazole, 401
Aromatase inhibitors, for breast cancer, 727–729, 728t, 799
Aromatherapy, for dementia management, 400
Arousal, delirium and, 903
Arrhythmia. *See* Cardiac arrhythmias
Arsenic trioxide, for leukemia, 788
Arterial aging
  in aging of connective tissues, 80
  arterial stiffness in, 92–93, 93f, 93t
  via arterial remodeling, 91, 92f
Arterial disease of the limb, 348–349, 350f
  acute limb ischemia, 349, 350f
  chronic peripheral vascular disease, 348–349
Arterial emboli, in acute limb ischemia, 349
Arteriosclerosis, in aging and Hutchinson-Gilford progeria syndrome, 70–71
Arthritis, 566, 566t
  aging of connective tissues in patients with, 79
  in apatite deposition disease, 575–577
  in calcium pyrophosphate crystal deposition, 574–575
  comorbidity of, 848
  disease mechanisms of, 566–570, 567t
  in Down syndrome, 448
  drug therapy in, 568–569, 568t–570t
    anti-inflammatories, 568–569, 568t
    biologics, 569–570, 570t, 576b
    DMARDs and immunosuppression, 569, 569t, 576b
    steroids, 570
Arthritis *(Continued)*
  gait and, 887
  in gout, 573–574
  insomnia and, 945–946
  investigations of, 566–568, 567t
  osteoarthritis. *See* Osteoarthritis
  in polymyalgia rheumatica and giant cell arteritis, 573
  rheumatoid. *See* Rheumatoid arthritis
  seronegative spondylarthritis, 571–572
  supportive nondrug therapy for, 570
  symptoms and signs of, 566
Arthrodesis, gait and, 887
Articular cartilage, aging of, 117–119, 118f–119f
Arzoxifene, 164–165
AS. *See* Aortic stenosis
Asbestosis, 382
Ascites, 641
ASCOT. *See* A Severity Characterization of Trauma
Asia
  demographics in, 991
  geriatric medicine in, 1010
    chronic disease and functional decline prevention, 1015
    chronic diseases of major impact, 1010
    communicable diseases, 1011–1012
    comprehensive geriatric assessment, 1013
    development of, 1012–1013
    frailty, 1010–1011
    health and social services, 1013–1015
    life expectancy, morbidity, and disability, 1010–1015
Aspiration pneumonia, 602–603, 954–955, 955t
Aspirin
  for acute coronary syndromes, 290–291
  for antiphospholipid antibody syndrome, 492
  for aortic valve replacement, 316, 316t
  asthma provoked by, 366
  for chronic cardiac failure, 282
  for CKD, 695
  colon cancer risk and, 673
  for dementia, 400
  drug-disease interactions of, 143t
  gastropathy, peptic ulcer disease, and, 620
  for giant cell arteritis, 473–474
  herbal-drug interactions of, 142t
  for Hutchinson-Gilford progeria syndrome, 71
  for hypertension, 306–307, 311
  for intermittent claudication, 355b
  longevity due to, 14
  for migraine, 467–468, 468t, 477b
  for myeloproliferative disorders, 780
  after myocardial infarction, 291–292, 293t
  for prostate cancer, 713–714
  for stable angina, 290
  for STEMI, 291
  for stroke, 334–335, 482, 492–493, 495–497
  for vascular prophylaxis in diabetes mellitus, 773
  for ventricular arrhythmia, 327
Assessing Care of Vulnerable Elders (ACOVE), 883, 1006, 1061
Assessment. *See also* Multidimensional geriatric assessment; Preoperative assessment; Social assessment
  in community-living older adult
    depression, 840–841
    fall risk, 839–840
    for health promotion and preventive care, 838–842
    nutrition, 840
  description of, 839
  of disability, 10–11
  home-based v. office-based, 838–839
Assessment *(Continued)*
  of mobility, 9–10, 888–889
    life spaces, 10
    timed walking test, 9
  of rehabilitation potential, 7–9, 8t
    mobility, 9–10
    standardized v. professional, 8–9, 8t
  in therapy, 871–872
Assessment of Underutilization of Medication (AOU), 883
Assisted living facilities (ALFs), 1026, 1028, 1028t
Assistive devices, for falls, 901
Association of Directors of Geriatric Academic Programs (ADGAP), 1032
Asteatotic eczema, 801–802
Astemizole, 140t
Asthma, 362
  airflow obstruction in, 364
    reversibility of, 364–365, 365f
  atopic, 366
  bronchial hyperresponsiveness in, 365–366
  clinical features of, 366
  differential diagnosis of COPD and, 374–376, 375t
  as disease of airflow obstruction, 362, 363t
  epidemiology of, 362–363
  histopathologic findings of, 364
  management of, 367–368, 367t–368t
  outcomes of, 368–369
  pathogenesis of, 364
Asymptomatic cerebrovascular disease, 303
Asynchronous telemedicine, 1065
Atenolol, 332, 468, 742
Atherosclerosis
  ED and, 855–856, 856t
  longevity and, 13
  in stroke pathology, 482
Atomoxetine, 508b, 510
Atopic asthma, 366
Atorvastatin, 496
Atracurium, 231
Atrial fibrillation (AF), 330–334, 331t
  antiarrhythmic drugs for maintaining sinus rhythm in patients with, 333–334
  associated risks with, 330–331
  cardiovascular risk and, 302
  clinical symptoms of, 331
  control of fast ventricular rate with, 332
  control of very fast rapid ventricular rate with, 332
  diagnostic tests for, 331
  elective cardioversion for, 333
  general treatment measures for, 331–332
  hyperthyroidism in patients with, 743
  nondrug therapies for, 332
  in patients with mitral annular calcium, 321
  predisposing factors for, 330, 331t
  slow ventricular rate with, 332–333
  in tachycardia-bradycardia syndrome, 332
  ventricular rate control in patients with, 334
  in Wolff-Parkinson-White syndrome, 332
Atrial flutter, 335–336
Atrial premature complexes (APCs), 336
Atrophy, noninfarct, 423
Atropine, 605, 671, 857–858, 980
Attention
  aging effects on, 171–172
  delirium and, 903
  therapy techniques for, 877
Attentional strategies, for Parkinson's disease therapy, 877
Atypical antipsychotics, 438, 440
Atypical facial pain, 472
Atypical neuroleptics, 417, 517

Audiologic rehabilitation (AR), 826, 829–830, 829t–830t
Audit Commission, for quality of care improvement in United Kingdom, 1040–1041
Auditory awakening thresholds, with advancing age, 944–945
Auditory system, aging of, 822–824
Audits, surgical and anesthetic, 243–244
Aura, with migraine, 466–467
Auranofin, 569t
Austria, geriatric medicine in, 999
Autism, 445
Autoimmune autonomic ganglionopathy, 507–508
Autoimmune hemolytic anemia, 786–787
Autoimmune hepatitis (AIH), 640, 643
Autoimmune thrombocytopenic purpura. *See* Idiopathic thrombocytopenic purpura
Autoimmunity
  dementia associated with, 387
  immune senescence and, 85–86
Automatic implantable cardioverter-defibrillator (AICD)
  after myocardial infarction, 293
  for ventricular arrhythmias, 329–330, 330t
Autonomic dysfunction
  aging effects on autonomic cardiovascular control, 501–503, 502f
    baroreflex function, 501
    cardiac parasympathetic function, 501
    end-organ responsiveness, 502
    neuroendocrine changes, 503
    systemic sympathetic function, 502, 502f
    vascular changes, 503
  aging effects on autonomic response to stress, 503–504
    orthostatic hypotension, 503
    postprandial and heat-induced hypotension, 503–504
  with dementia, 389–390
  in elderly, 504–506
    baroreflex failure, 504–505
    chronic autonomic failure, 505
    neurally mediated syncope, 504
    primary autonomic failure, 505–507, 506f
    secondary autonomic failure, 507–508
  orthostatic hypotension and, 342, 508–510, 508b
Autonomic nervous system disorders, 498
  assessment of baroreflex function, 501
    biochemical assessment of sympathetic function, 501
    estimation of norepinephrine spillover, 501
    muscle sympathetic nerve activity, 501
  basic concepts of autonomic physiology, 498–501, 499f–500f
    autonomic pathways, 498, 499f
    methods for testing autonomic function, 498–501, 499f–500f
    spectral analysis of heart rate and blood pressure, 500–501
Autonomic testing, for primary autonomic failure, 506–508, 506f
Autonomy, respect for, 983
AVR. *See* Aortic valve replacement
5-Aza-2'deoxycytidine (decitabine, DAC), 129, 778–779
Azacytidine, 129, 778–779
Azathioprine
  for arthritis, 569t
  for autoimmune hepatitis, 640
  for bullous pemphigoid, 807
  for Crohn's disease, 656–657, 669t, 670
  for idiopathic pulmonary fibrosis, 381
  for inclusion body myositis, 528
  for lymphocytic and collagenous colitis, 671
Azathioprine (*Continued*)
  for myasthenia gravis, 531
  for polymyositis or dermatomyositis, 527
  for steroid-induced myopathy, 529
  for ulcerative colitis, 667t, 668
Azilect. *See* Rasagiline
Azithromycin, 379, 666

B

B cells, aging of, 84–85, 132
Bacitracin, 803
Back pain, 967
Baclofen, 471–472, 477b, 977
Bacterial endocarditis, 322
Bacterial meningitis, 546–549, 548f, 548t, 550b
Bacterial overgrowth syndrome, of small bowel, 654–655
BAHA. *See* Bone-anchored hearing aid
Balance
  clinical assessment of, 888–889, 898t
  evaluation for, 898t, 900
  sensory systems for, 895–896
Balance exercises
  for fractured neck, 876
  for frailty prevention, 850
  strength training and, 863
Balloon aortic valvuloplasty, for aortic stenosis, 317
Balsalazide, 667t
Barbiturates
  chronic daily headache due to, 469–470
  drug-disease interactions of, 143t
  for epilepsy, 464
  herbal-drug interactions of, 142t
  for insomnia, 946
  liver metabolism of, 636t
  nephrotoxicity of, 693–694
  syncope caused by, 339t
Bariatric surgery, 689
Barium contrast studies, of large bowel, 661
Baroreflex, 498, 499f, 500–501
  assessment of, 501
  effects of aging on, 501
  failure of, 504–505
Barrett metaplasia, 615, 615f
Barthel index, disability assessment and, 10
Basal cell carcinoma (BCC), 806
Basophils, effects of aging on, 130
Bazedoxifene, 164–165, 557–558
BCC. *See* Basal cell carcinoma
Beers explicit criteria, pharmacotherapy and, 881–882
Behavioral and psychological symptoms (BPSDs), of dementia, 393t, 394
Behavioral implications, of hearing loss, 824–825, 825t
Behavioral mechanisms, of social factors influencing health, 203
Behavioral symptoms, in Alzheimer's disease, 417
Behavioral treatment, for insomnia, 946
Behavioral variant frontotemporal dementia. *See* Frontal variant frontotemporal dementia
Behaviorism, in geriatric medicine education, 1033–1034
Belgium, geriatric medicine in, 999
Benchmarking, for quality management, 1042
Benign prostatic hyperplasia (BPH), 706–708, 706f–707f
  detrusor dysfunction associated with, 706
  investigation of, 708
  management of, 708–709, 709t
  new modalities for treatment of, 709
  symptom complexes and terminology of, 706, 706f
Benign tumors
  gastric, 624
  of liver, 644
  of small bowel, 658
Benzathine penicillin, for CNS infection, 551
Benzbromarone, 574
Benzocaine, 803
Benzodiazepines
  for alcohol withdrawal, 639
  altered mental status due to, 205
  for anxiety disorders, 440
  dementia associated with, 387
  for detoxification, 442
  drug interactions of, 143
  drug-disease interactions of, 143t
  for epilepsy, 459
  herbal-drug interactions of, 142t
  isoniazid use with, 378
  liver metabolism of, 635–636
  for lower esophageal ring, 616
  sensitivity to, 141, 141t, 144, 144b
Bereavement, 440–441
Berg balance test, 888, 900
Betadine, 745
Betaxolol, 820
Bevacizumab, 728t, 816–817
BHR. *See* Bronchial hyperresponsiveness
Bicalutamide, 713–715
Bile ducts, obstruction of, 646–649
  gallstones, 646–648
  malignant obstruction, 648–649
Biliary stents, 630
Biliary tract diseases, 645
  bile duct obstruction, 646–649
  investigations of, 649–651
    abdominal CT, 649–650
    ERCP, 650
    EUS, 650
    liver ultrasound, 649
    MRI, 650
    PTC, 651–651
  isolated disorders of bilirubin metabolism, 645
  liver disease, 645–646
Bilirubin, 645
Biochemical assessment, of sympathetic function, 501
Biofeedback, for stroke therapy, 874
Biologic variation, in geriatric reference intervals, 219
Biologics, for arthritis, 569–570, 570t, 576b
Biology, of aging, 30
  cell death, cell replacement, and stem cells, 33
  cell proliferation, telomerase, and telomere function, 32–33
  insulin-signaling pathway and longevity regulation, 30–32, 31f
  longevity dividend concept and reasons for investing in aging research, 35–38
  progeroid syndromes and normal aging, 33–34
  protein damage and sarcopenia, 34–35
Biomarkers
  of Alzheimer's disease, 417–419, 418f
  of frontotemporal dementia, 431–432
  of vascular cognitive impairment, 426
Biomechanical disorders, of foot, 594–595, 595f–596f
Biomechanics, of fall causation, 897, 897f
Biomedical inputs, to aging, 13–15
Biopsy
  for intracranial tumor diagnosis, 535–536
  of large bowel, 662
  of liver, 637–638
  of muscle, 523

Biosynthesis, of collagen of connective tissue, 74
Bisacodyl suppositories, 920–921
Bismuth preparations, for *H. pylori* infection, 620
Bismuth subsalicylate, 671
Bisoprolol, 278b, 280
Bisphosphonates
for bone loss, 109, 124, 164
for bony metastases, 728t, 729
for Hutchinson-Gilford progeria syndrome, 68
hyperparathyroidism and, 757, 757b–758b
for multiple myeloma, 783
for osteoporosis, 527, 531, 556–558, 586
for Paget disease of bone, 563–564, 564b, 578
Black cohosh, for menopause, 718
Bladder
aging of, 112–116, 113t
bladder function and structure, 114–115
outlet function and structure, 115–116
physiologic assessment, 113–114
system-based perspective of, 116–117
benign prostatic hyperplasia effect on, 706–708, 707f–708f
control of, 926
dysfunction and retention of, 708
function and structure of, 114–115, 926–927
Bladder diary, for urinary incontinence assessment, 932–933
Bladder overactivity, 115, 706–707, 707f, 709, 721
Bladder retraining, for urinary incontinence, 934–936
Bleeding
in GI tract, 623, 659–660, 674–677, 675t, 676f
in large bowel, 659–660, 664
with overanticoagulation, 359
Bleomycin, 786
Blindness. *See* Visual loss
Blinking reflex. *See* Glabellar tap reflex
α-Blockers, 138
drug-disease interactions of, 143t
for hypertension, 305t, 309
for voiding problems due to benign prostatic hyperplasia, 708–709, 709t
β-Blockers, 15, 161–162
for accelerated atrioventricular rhythm, 336
for acute coronary syndromes, 291
for AF, 334
for alcohol withdrawal, 639
for aneurysm surgery, 354
for aortic stenosis, 315
for APCs, 336
asthma provoked by, 366
for atrial flutter, 335
for atypical facial pain, 472
for blood pressure control in diabetes mellitus patients, 772
for CAD, 288–289
carotid sinus reflex sensitivity and, 344
for chronic cardiac failure, 277, 278b, 279–285, 285b
for cirrhosis complications, 641
Cox 2 inhibitors and, 969
depression associated with, 435
diabetes secondary to, 760
distribution of, 139
drug interactions of, 143
dry mouth and, 605
in elderly patients undergoing surgery, 232
fatigue due to, 206–207
in frail elderly patient, 295–297
for glaucoma, 813
for hypertension, 305, 305t, 308–310
for hyperthyroidism, 742–743, 754b
β-Blockers (*Continued*)
hypoaldosteronism and, 733
for hypothyroidism, 748
for migraine, 468, 468t, 477b
for mitral stenosis, 324
after myocardial infarction, 292–293, 292t–293t
orthostatic hypotension and, 503, 510
for Parkinson's disease, 517
preoperative, 232
sensitivity to, 141, 141t
for stable angina, 290
for STEMI, 291
for SVT, 336
systemic complications of, 820
for ventricular arrhythmia, 327–330, 328t
for ventricular rate control in patients with AF, 332
Blood
aging of, 127
B cells, 132–133
circulating blood cells, 130
eosinophils, basophils, and mast cells, 130
epigenetics, 128–129
granulocytes, 130
hematopoiesis, 127
hematopoietic stem cells, 127–128
lymphoid development, 131
monocytes and macrophages, 130
progenitor compartment, 129–130
red cells, 130–131
sites of blood cell development, bone marrow, and stroma, 127–128
T cells, 131–132
telomeres and senescence, 128
production of, 127
Blood disorders, 775
acute myelogenous leukemia, 787–788, 788t
anemia, 775–777, 775t–777t
chronic lymphocytic leukemia, 786–788
hemostasis disorders, 789–790
lymphoma, 783–786
multiple myeloma, 781–783, 782t
myelodysplasia, 777–779, 778t–779t
myeloproliferative disorders, 779–781
Blood flow, pressure ulcers and, 939–940
Blood monitoring
of antiepileptic drugs, 463
of glucose, 771
Blood pressure. *See also* Hypertension
ambulatory monitoring of, 304
arterial stiffness effects on, 93, 93f
asymptomatic cerebrovascular disease and, 303
autonomic regulation of, 498, 499f
autonomic testing using, 498–501
cardiovascular risk and, 300–301
in diabetes mellitus patients, 772
diurnal variation of, 510
measurement of, 304
prevention of secondary stroke and, 495–496
target levels of, 306–307
Blood tests
for diagnosing stroke risk factors, 492
for pancreas adenocarcinoma, 628
Blood vessels, pressure ulcers and, 940
BMI. *See* Body mass index
Bobath approach, 873
Body composition, 687
Body mass index (BMI), 302, 685, 686t
Body temperature, aging effects on, 57
Bone
in aging male, 166–167
aging of, 117, 118f
articular cartilage, 117–119, 118f–119f
consequences of, 122
future of, 122–123
Bone (*Continued*)
skeleton, 119–121, 119f–120f
soft tissues, 121–122
health of, exercise and, 863–864
involutional loss of, 554
menopause and postmenopause effects on, 124, 164
metabolic disease of. *See* Metabolic bone disease
nonmetabolic disease of, 577–578, 578f
pain in, 714, 977
remodeling of, 119–120, 120f, 553
Bone marrow, aging effects on, 127–128
Bone mineral density
aging effects on, 56
peak, 554
weight loss and, 687
Bone-anchored hearing aid (BAHA), 830–832
Bortezomib, 783
Botulinum toxin, 148t, 495, 519, 611
Botulism, 507
Bowel. *See* Large bowel; Small bowel
Bowel obstruction, palliative care for, 979
Bowel preparation, for constipation and FI, 917, 917t
BPH. *See* Benign prostatic hyperplasia
BPR. *See* Business process reengineering
BPSDs. *See* Behavioral and psychological symptoms
Brachytherapy, for prostate cancer, 712
Braden scale, 940
Bradyarrhythmias, 336–337
Brain
abscess in, 549
imaging of
for intracranial tumor diagnosis, 535
for late-onset schizophrenia, 437–438
for primary autonomic failure, 506–507, 506f
for stroke, 489–490, 491f
infarct of. *See* Stroke
metabolism of, neuroendocrinology of aging in, 167–169
stress and, 160–161, 161f
tumors of. *See* Intracranial tumors
Breast cancer, 726, 792, 797
diagnosis of, 726
management of, 727–729, 728t, 798–799
pathology and molecular markers of, 726–727, 727t
presentation of, 726
screening for, 793–794
staging of, 726
Bright light therapy, for dementia management, 400
Bringing Nutrition Screening to Seniors, 840
Britaject. *See* Apomorphine
British Geriatrics Society, 1024, 1024t, 1045
Bromocriptine (Parlodel), 515t, 516–517, 536
Bronchial hyperresponsiveness (BHR), 365–366
Bronchiectasis, 378–379, 379t
Bronchitis, 362, 363t
Bronchodilators
before aneurysm surgery for abdominal aortic aneurysm, 354
for asthma, 364–365, 367t
for bronchiectasis, 379
for cough, 980
Budd-Chiari syndrome, 641
Budesonide
for Crohn's disease, 656, 669t, 670
for lymphocytic and collagenous colitis, 671
for ulcerative colitis, 668
Bulgaria, geriatric medicine in, 999
Bulking agents, for diarrhea, 979

Bullous pemphigoid, 807
Bumetanide, 278, 278b
Bupropion, 143t, 283, 372–373, 435
Burden, of stroke, 478, 478t, 480–481
Business process reengineering (BPR), 1042
Buspirone, 517

C

CAA. *See* Cerebral amyloid angiopathy
Cabasar. *See* Cabergoline
Cabergoline (Cabasar), 515t, 516–517
CAD. *See* Coronary artery disease
CADASIL. *See* Cerebral autosomal dominant arteriopathy with subcortical infarcts and leukoencephalopathy
Caffeine
chronic daily headache due to, 469–470
herbal-drug interactions of, 142t
for hypertension management, 308
for hypnic headache syndrome, 476
metabolism of, 140t
for orthostatic hypotension, 343t, 508–509
for postprandial hypotension, 347, 510
for urinary incontinence, 934
Calciferol, 758b
Calcific periarthritis, 575–576
Calcilytics, 558
Calcimimetic medications, 758
Calcineurin inhibitors, 803
Calcitonin, 164, 557, 563–564, 578, 586
Calcitriol, 557, 561
Calcium
for acute renal failure, 693
assay of, 756t
bone loss and, 164, 448, 554
in cellular aging, 44–45
for chronic kidney disease, 695–696
constipation and, 912–913
for dementia associated with hypoparathyroidism, 387
drug interactions of, 141
hypercalcemia and, 757t
hyperparathyroidism and, 756–757, 759, 757b–758b
for hypertension management, 308
for hypoparathyroidism, 759
nutritional requirements for, 681–682, 687–688
for osteomalacia, 561
for osteoporosis, 527, 531, 556t, 557–558, 583, 585–586
Calcium antagonists
for chronic cardiac failure, 281–282
for hypertension, 305t
orthostatic hypotension and, 503
sensitivity to, 141t
Calcium channel blockers
for acute coronary syndromes, 291
for blood pressure control in diabetes mellitus patients, 772
constipation and, 912–913
drug-disease interactions of, 143t
for dysphagia and chest pain, 614
in frail elderly patient, 297–298
headache due to, 475t
for hypertension, 306–310, 310b
for hypothyroidism, 748
for migraine, 468, 468t
after myocardial infarction, 292, 293t
parkinsonism induced by, 511t, 518
sensitivity to, 141
for stable angina, 290
for STEMI, 291
syncope caused by, 339t
for ventricular arrhythmias, 328
Calcium consumption
exercise and, 863–864
frailty prevention and, 850
Calcium homeostasis, 698–700, 755–756, 756t
Calcium ion influx
generation of ROS/RNS and, 152
NMDA receptor-mediated glutamatergic signaling pathways inducing, 151–152
Calcium pyrophosphate crystal deposition (CPCD), 574–575
connective tissue disorders associated with, 581
Caloric restriction
aging response to, 51–52, 52f
as antiaging medicine, 146
lifespan prolongation by, 41
longevity and neurodegeneration response to, 155–157, 156f
role of mitochondria in response to, 39
Campbell de Morgan spots, 803
Campylobacter species, colitis caused by, 666
Canada
demographics in, 1005
geriatric medicine in, 1005–1009, 1007t
Canadian Institutes of Health Research (CIHR), 1006
Cancer, 791. *See also* Neoplasms; Tumors
adrenal, 733–734, 734f
aging and, 791–792
altered phenotype due to replicative senescence and, 10006#u0060, 40
of breast. *See* Breast cancer
chemotherapy for. *See* Chemotherapy
colon. *See* Colon cancer
colorectal, 674, 914
diagnosis of, 795
drug therapy for, 797–798
gynecologic, 721–724, 723t
of cervix, 722, 794–795
of corpus uteri, 722–723
of ovary, 723–724, 723t
of vagina, 722
of vulva, 722
hormonal manipulations for. *See* Hormonal manipulation
immune senescence and, 86–87
incidence of, 795
insomnia and, 945–946
of lung. *See* Lung cancer
nursing care for, 799–800
pain and, 971
prevention of, 792–795
of prostate. *See* Prostate cancer
radiotherapy for. *See* Radiotherapy
rehabilitation after treatment for, 800
screening for, 792–795
skin, 805–807, 805b
staging of, 795–796
surgery for, 797
survival of, 800–801
telomerase activity and, 32, 40
of thyroid, 750–754, 751t
treatment of, 796–797
Candesartan, 281, 426–427
Candidiasis
esophageal, 617
of oral cavity, 608–609
Capecitabine, 728–729
Capitation, in managed care in United States, 1060–1061
Capsaicin (Zostrix), 472, 594, 597, 977
Captopril, 278b, 279, 281, 292t
Captopril renography, 305
Carbachol, 820
Carbamazepine
for alcohol withdrawal, 639
cytochrome P450 reaction with, 141t
for dementia, 401
for epilepsy, 462–463, 463t
for glossopharyngeal neuralgia, 472
low thyroxine due to, 738
for mania, 440
for pain, 970
for postherpetic neuralgia, 472, 477b
for trigeminal neuralgia, 471, 477b
Carbohydrate consumption, diabetes and, 860–861
Carbohydrate metabolism, aerobic exercise and, 860–861
Carbonic anhydrase inhibitors, 813, 819–820
Carboplatin, 383, 724
Carcinoid tumor, of small bowel, 659
Carcinoma. *See also* Adenocarcinoma
adrenal, 733–734, 734f
gastric, 624
hepatocellular, 638–639, 642
of oral cavity, 610
pancreatic, 648
of skin, 805–806
Carcinoma in situ, of breast, 727
Cardiac arrhythmias, 327
accelerated atrioventricular rhythm, 336
AF, 330–334, 331t
APCs, 336
atrial flutter, 335–336
bradyarrhythmias, 336–337
multifocal atrial tachycardia, 336
paroxysmal atrial tachycardia with atrioventricular block, 336
in patients with heart failure, 282
SVT, 336
thromboembolic stroke in patients with, 334–335, 334t
ventricular arrhythmias, 327–330, 328t–330t
Cardiac assessment, of noncardiac surgical patient, 235–236
Cardiac complications, of aneurysm surgery for abdominal aortic aneurysm, 354
Cardiac disease. *See* Heart disease
Cardiac events
hypertension management and, 306
in patients with mitral annular calcium, 322, 322t
Cardiac failure. *See* Chronic cardiac failure
Cardiac management
for acute pancreatitis, 632
for Hutchinson-Gilford progeria syndrome, 71
Cardiac pacing. *See* Pacing
Cardiac parasympathetic function, effects of aging on, 501
Cardiac problems, in elderly surgical patient, 235–237, 236t
ACC/AHA guidelines for perioperative cardiovascular evaluation before noncardiac surgery, 236–237, 236t
cardiac assessment of noncardiac surgical patient, 235–236
cardiac surgery, 237
incidence of postoperative cardiac complications, 235
Cardiac resynchronization therapy (CRT), 284
Cardiac surgery, in elderly surgical patient, 237
Cardiorespiratory reserve, preoperative estimation of, 233, 233t
Cardiovascular control, autonomic, effects of aging on, 501–503, 502f
Cardiovascular disease
as dementia risk factor, 386
in Down syndrome, 448
menopause and, 717
oral health and, 603

Cardiovascular risk
blood pressure and, 300–301
factors to be considered along with hypertension, 302–303
AF and left ventricular hypertrophy, 302
alcohol and diet, 303
body mass index, 302
diabetes mellitus, 302
hormone replacement, 303
lipid abnormalities, 302
physical exercise, 303
smoking, 302
pulse pressure and, 301, 301f
systolic blood pressure, diastolic blood pressure, and, 301
Cardiovascular system, aging of, 54, 91
aging-associated changes in vascular structure, 91, 92f
arterial stiffness in aging arteries, 92–93, 93f, 93t
endothelial function in aging, 91–92
heart structure changes with age, 93–94, 96t
myocardial function in aging heart at rest, 94–95, 96t
response of aging heart to exercise, 95–96, 96t
Cardioversion, for AF, 333
Cardioverter-defibrillator. *See* Automatic implantable cardioverter-defibrillator
CARE. *See* Continuous Assessment Review and Evaluation
Care coordination
in chronic disease management, 1064
in frail older adults, 1064
Care management for high-cost beneficiaries demonstration, 1058
Care providers, for palliative medicine, 974
Care Standards Act, 1025
Caregiver
burden of, 226–227
education of
for constipation, 918
for delirium, 906–907
falls and, 901–902
for Parkinson's disease, 877
to reduce medication problems, 883
telemedicine for support for, 1066
Caries, 604
Carmustine, 537
β-Carotene, 44, 148, 818
Carotid artery
asymptomatic stenosis of, 352
dissection of, 474
Carotid disease, 349–352, 351f–352f
carotid surgery for, 351–352
angioplasty and stenting, 352
benefits of, 351–352
mortality from, 352
timing of, 352
diagnosis of, 349
investigations of, 349–351, 351f–352f
Carotid endarterectomy, for prevention of secondary stroke, 496
Carotid sinus hypersensitivity, 343–345, 344f
epidemiology of, 344
evaluation of, 344–345, 344f
management of, 345
pathophysiology of, 343–344
presentation of, 344
Carotid sinus massage, 344–345, 344f
Carotid sinus syndrome, 343–345, 344f
epidemiology of, 344
evaluation of, 344–345, 344f
management of, 345
pathophysiology of, 343–344
presentation of, 344
Cartilage. *See* Articular cartilage
Cartilage disorders, 578
Carvedilol, 278b, 280, 292t
Case control studies, for researching aging and related conditions, 24
Case management, for iatrogenic problems prevention, 851
Cataracts, 813b, 814–815, 814f
Cathepsin K inhibitors, 557–558
Cavities. *See* Caries
CBT. *See* Cognitive behavioral therapy
CCIP. *See* Chronic Care Improvement Program
CDC. *See* Centers for Disease Control and Prevention
CDH. *See* Chronic daily headache
Cefotaxime, 548, 548t, 641–642
Ceftazidime, 548
Ceftriaxone, 548t, 551–552, 552b
Celance. *See* Pergolide
Celecoxib, 143t, 568, 568t, 621
Celiac disease, 653–654
Celiac plexus block, 630, 634
Celiac sprue, age-related changes in manifestation of, 108
Cell aging, destructive agents in, 42–45
environmental agents, 42
intracellular calcium homeostasis and, 44–45
reactive oxygen species, 42–44
Cell attachment proteins, 77
Cell biology, of Hutchinson-Gilford progeria syndrome, 66–68, 68f
Cell death
in articular cartilage, 119
protein S-nitrosylation and, 152–154, 153t
role of stem cells in, 33
sarcopenia and, 589–590, 593
Cell lysis, age-related changes in, 83
Cell proliferation, 32–33
Cell replacement, role of stem cells in, 33
Cell senescence, 45–48
in aging of connective tissues, 77
of blood cells and hematopoietic stem cells, 128
genomic instability in, 46–48
telomeres and telomerase in, 46
Cellular mechanisms, of aging, 42
cell senescence, 45–48
destructive agents in cellular aging, 42–45
in extracellular matrix, 49
in protein synthesis and degradation, 48–49
in signaling pathways, 49
Centenarians, 184
definitions of healthy aging in, 184
demography of, 184
distinguishing between compression of morbidity and compression of disability and the role of resilience, 184–186
gender disparity in, 185, 185f
heritability and familiality in, 185–186
supercentenarians, 186
Centers for Disease Control and Prevention (CDC)
disease prevention activities and, 848, 849t
exercise recommendations by, 859
Centers for Medicare and Medicaid Services (CMS)
demonstration projects of, 1058
care management for high-cost beneficiaries demonstration, 1058
ESRD Disease Management Demonstration, 1058
Medicare Coordinated Care Demonstration, 1058
Program for All-inclusive Care for the Elderly, 1058–1059
Centers for Medicare and Medicaid Services (CMS) *(Continued)*
Senior Risk Reduction Demonstration, 1058
social/health maintenance organization, 1059
Medicare Advantage and, 1057
Central nervous system (CNS)
balance and, 896
falls and, 895, 896t
infections of, 546
focal lesions, encephalitis, and chronic meningitis, 549–553, 550b
meningitis, 546–549, 548f, 548t
and problems in elderly surgical patient, 241–242
postoperative delirium, 241–242
postoperative dementia, 242
postoperative stroke, 241
Cephalosporins
for bacterial overgrowth syndrome, 655
C. difficile infection and, 664
for CNS infection, 547–548, 548t, 550b, 552b
drug interactions of, 143
for pyogenic liver abscess, 644
Cerebellar signs, of dementia, 390
Cerebral amyloid angiopathy (CAA), 423–424
Cerebral autosomal dominant arteriopathy with subcortical infarcts and leukoencephalopathy (CADASIL), 423, 427
Cerebral infarct. *See* Stroke
Cerebral tumors, epilepsy and, 460
Cerebral vessel occlusion, 482
Cerebral vessel rupture, 482–483
Cerebral white matter lesions, 485, 489
Cerebrospinal fluid (CSF), examination of, 535, 547
Cerebrovascular disease
epilepsy and, 460
headache with, 474
as hypertension complication, 303
Cerebrovascular events, in patients with mitral annular calcium, 322–323, 323t
Certified nurse assistants (CNAs), in nursing homes, 1029
Certolizumab, 656–657
Cervical myelopathy and radiculopathy, 539–541, 540f
Cervical spondylosis, 472, 539–541, 540f
Cervix
aging of, 716
cancer of, 722, 794–795
CGA. *See* Comprehensive geriatric assessment
Challenge. *See* Stressors
Chamber size, of patients with mitral annular calcium, 321
Chamomile, 142t
Chemoradiotherapy
for pancreas adenocarcinoma, 631
for uterine cancer, 723
Chemotherapy, 797
for breast cancer, 727–729, 727t–728t, 729b
candidiasis associated with, 608
for cervical cancer, 722
for colorectal cancer, 674
dementia associated with, 389
dental implant failure with, 605
dry mouth and, 605
elderly preference for and compliance with, 796–797
elimination of, 140
for esophageal neoplasms, 618
fatigue due to, 206–207
for gastric tumors, 624–625
gout associated with, 574

Chemotherapy (*Continued*)
for intracranial tumors, 536–538, 538b
for Kaposi sarcoma, 807
for leukemia, 788
for lymphoma, 784–786
for malignant mesothelioma, 384
for metastasis to eye, 819
myelodysplasia after, 777–778
for non-small cell lung cancer, 383
for ovarian cancer, 723–724
for pancreas adenocarcinoma, 631
for pancreatic neuroendocrine tumors, 631
for prostate cancer, 713–715
side effects and toxicity of, 796–798
for small bowel tumors, 659
for small cell lung cancer, 383–384
stomatitis associated with, 609
thrombocytopenia associated with, 789
for thyroid nodule management, 753
Cherry angiomas, 803
Cherry hemangiomas, 803
Chest pain, noncardiac, 614
Chest roentgenography
for aortic regurgitation, 318
for aortic stenosis, 314
Chest x-ray, of chronic cardiac failure, 275–276
Chewing, malnutrition and, 950–953
CHF. *See* Congestive heart failure
Chile, pension system privatization in, 994
China, pension system privatization in, 994
Chlorambucil, 519, 724, 785, 787, 807
Chloramphenicol, 547, 549, 645, 820
Chlordiazepoxide, 139–140, 140t, 639
Chlorhexidine gluconate, 609
Chloromycetin, 655
Chloroquine, 528–529, 819–820
Chlorothiazide, 789
Chlorpromazine, 143t, 819–820
Chlorpropamide, 141t–142t, 768, 771
Chlorthalidone, 298, 309
CHMP$_2$*B* mutations, 428–429, 429t, 431
Cholangiocarcinoma, 648–649
Cholangitis, 641, 645, 647–648
Cholecalciferol, 695–696
Cholecystitis, 209, 209t, 647–648
Cholesterol
age-related changes in, 221, 221f, 221t
as CAD risk factor, 289
cardiovascular risk and, 302
as stroke risk factor, 492
Cholestyramine, 640, 664–665, 803
Cholinergic failure, 507
Cholinergic hypothesis, for delirium, 905
Cholinergic supplementation, for dementia, 400
Cholinesterase inhibitors
for Alzheimer's disease, 419–420, 420b
for CADASIL, 423
chronic cardiac failure and, 284
for delirium, 906–907
for dementia, 398f, 432
for vascular cognitive impairment, 426b, 427
Chondrocalcinosis, 574–575
Chorea, 519
Chromosomal gene mutations, in aging, 39–41
Chronic autonomic failure, 505
Chronic bronchitis, 362, 363t
Chronic cardiac failure, 272
chest x-ray of, 275–276
device therapy for, 284
diagnosis of, 274–275, 274t–275t
disease course and prognosis of, 273, 273t
drug burden in, 284
ECG of, 276
echocardiography of, 276–277, 276f
epidemiology of, 272–273
Chronic cardiac failure (*Continued*)
etiology of, 274, 274t
natriuretic peptides in, 277
palliative care for, 284
pathophysiology of, 273–274
problematic disease interactions, 283–284
cognitive impairment, 284
COPD, 283
depression, 284
urinary incontinence, 283
treatment of, 277–283, 278b
ACE inhibitors, 277–285, 278b, 285b
alcohol consumption, 283
angiotensin antagonists, 277, 281
β-blockers, 277, 278b, 279–285, 285b
diet, 283
digoxin, 277, 278b, 280–282, 285, 285b
diuretics, 277–281, 278b, 283–285, 285b
exercise, 282–283
general issues, 277
multidisciplinary team interventions, 282
other pharmacologic agents, 281–282
role of heart failure nurse, 282
smoking cessation, 283
spironolactone, 278, 278b, 280, 285, 285b
Chronic Care Improvement Program (CCIP), 1051
Chronic daily headache (CDH), 469–470, 470t
Chronic disease management
care coordination in, 1064
telemedicine for, 1065
Chronic idiopathic myelofibrosis (CIF), 779–781
Chronic kidney disease (CKD), 694–696, 695t
anemia and, 777
cutaneous complications of, 808
Chronic liver disease, 638–639, 638t
Chronic lymphocytic leukemia (CLL), 786–788
Chronic medical conditions
insomnia and, 945–946
of major impact, 943
prevalence of, 835
prevention of, 946
Chronic meningitis, 549–552
Chronic mesenteric ischemia, 658
Chronic mitral regurgitation, 324–325, 325t
Chronic myelogenous leukemia (CML), 779–781
Chronic myelomonocytic leukemia (CMML), 777, 778t
Chronic nerve root entrapment, in degenerative disease of lumbar spine, 544, 544f
Chronic obstructive pulmonary disease (COPD), 369–375
changes in airways of smokers, 370
chronic cardiac failure in patients with, 283
clinical features of, 372, 372t
COPD exacerbation, 372
physical exam and laboratory tests, 372
symptoms, 372
systemic inflammation and COPD, 372, 372t
differential diagnosis of asthma and, 374–375, 375t
as disease of airflow obstruction, 362, 363t
epidemiology of, 369
insomnia and, 945–946
management of, 372–374
pharmacologic therapy, 373
pulmonary rehabilitation, 373–374
smoking cessation, 372–373
natural history of, 370–372, 371f
pathogenesis of, 370, 370f
prognosis of, 374
progression to, 370
pulmonary function testing in, 365f, 370, 371f
surgery for, 374
weight loss and malnutrition in, 374
Chronic pain, 965
multidimensionality of, 966
opioids for, 971
Chronic pancreatitis (CP), 633–634
Chronic subdural hemorrhage, headache with, 474
Ciclopirox (Loprox, Penlac), 595–596
Ciclosporin, 140t, 569t
CIF. *See* Chronic idiopathic myelofibrosis
Cigarette smoking. *See* Smoking
CIHR. *See* Canadian Institutes of Health Research
Cimetidine
codeine and, 969
cytochrome P450 reaction with, 141t
depression associated with, 435
drug interactions of, 141–143
elimination of, 141t
headache due to, 475t
for peptic ulcer disease, 622
thrombocytopenia associated with, 789
Cinnarizine, 511t, 518
Ciprofloxacin
for Crohn's disease, 669t, 670
cytochrome P450 reaction with, 141t
for diverticular disease, 663t
drug interactions of, 141–143
for infectious colitis, 665
renal failure due to, 692
for spontaneous bacterial peritonitis, 641–642
for UTIs, 691
Circadian rhythm, with advancing age, 945
Circulating blood cells, aging of, 130
Cirrhosis, 638–642, 638t
Cisplatin, 14–15, 383–384, 724
Citalopram, 401, 463, 517, 635–636
CKD. *See* Chronic kidney disease
Clarithromycin, 141–143, 620, 666
Class I antiarrhythmic drugs, 292–293, 293t, 327–328, 328t
Class III antiarrhythmic drugs, 329, 329t, 333
Claudication, 348–349
neurogenic, 525–526, 545
Clavulanate, 663t
Clear standards of service, with NHS, 1043
Clindamycin, 609, 655, 663t, 664, 672
Clinical audit, for quality of care improvement in United Kingdom, 1039–1040
Clinical care, for Hutchinson-Gilford progeria syndrome, 71–72
Clinical governance
with geriatric medicine, 1044–1045, 1044f
with NHS, 1044
Clinical history
of chronic cardiac failure, 275
for constipation and FI, 915, 916t
Clinical immunology. *See* Immunology
Clinical information systems, for tertiary disease prevention, 849
Clinical state variable, frailty index as, 64–65, 65f, 65t
Clinical trials, for researching aging and related conditions, 25–26
Clinician attitudes, towards telemedicine, 1067–1068
CLL. *See* Chronic lymphocytic leukemia
Clobazam, 462, 463t
Clofibrate, 528, 608
Clomipramine, 441, 476
Clonazepam, 462, 463t, 471, 477b, 517, 519
Clonidine
for alcohol withdrawal, 639
depression associated with, 435
for menopause, 718

Clonidine (*Continued*)
for orthostatic hypotension, 510
in patients with primary autonomic failure, 506–508
syncope caused by, 339t
Clopidogrel
for acute coronary syndromes, 290–291
drug-disease interactions of, 143t
in frail elderly patient, 297
herbal-drug interactions of, 142t
after myocardial infarction, 291–292, 293t
for stable angina, 290
for STEMI, 291
for stroke prevention, 482, 495–497
for thromboembolic stroke in patients with cardiac arrhythmias, 335
for vascular prophylaxis in diabetes mellitus, 773
Clostridium difficile
diarrhea and, 979
large bowel infection with, 664–665, 665t
Clotrimazole (Lotrimin, Mycelex), 595
"Clouding of consciousness," 903
Clozapine, 140t, 143t, 517
Cluster headache, 470
CML. *See* Chronic myelogenous leukemia
CMML. *See* Chronic myelomonocytic leukemia
CMS. *See* Centers for Medicare and Medicaid Services
CMV. *See* Cytomegalovirus
CNAs. *See* Certified nurse assistants
CNS. *See* Central nervous system
CNS depressants, 142t, 143
CNS lymphoma. *See* Primary CNS lymphoma
CNS stimulants, 143t
Coagulation defects, in elderly, 789–790
Coal workers pneumoconiosis, 382
Co-amoxiclav, 636t, 655
Co-beneldopa (Madopar), 515–516, 515t–516t
Co-careldopa (Sinemet), 515–516, 515t–516t
Coccidiomycosis, 550
Cochlear implants, 830–832
Codanthramer, 979
Codeine
for diarrhea, 979
headache caused by, 469–470, 475
metabolism of, 140t
for neurogenic claudication and spinal stenosis, 526
for pain, 969
for restless legs syndrome, 519
Cognitive aging, 101
normal, 170
attention and processing speed, 171–172
executive functions, 174–175
intelligence and aging, 170–171
lifestyle factors associated with cognitive functioning, 175–176
memory, 172–173
verbal abilities, 173–174
Cognitive assessment, for vascular cognitive impairment, 424–425
Cognitive behavioral therapy (CBT), for insomnia, 946
Cognitive decline
with delirium, 908
social factors associated with, 202
Cognitive deficits, sleep-disordered breathing and, 946–947
Cognitive function
hypertension and, 310
as outcomes measurement for multidimensional interventions, 245
in urinary incontinence, 931–932
Cognitive impairment. *See also* Mild cognitive impairment; Vascular cognitive impairment
chronic cardiac failure in patients with, 284
as complication of hypertension, 303–304
depression and, 435–436
in frail elderly with heart disease, 298–299
postoperative, 242
Cognitive reserve, 171
Cognitive stimulation therapy (CST), for dementia management, 399
Cognitive symptoms, of dementia, 393, 393t
Cognitive testing, for dementia diagnosis, 395, 403–404
Cognitive training, for dementia management, 399
Cognitivism, in geriatric medicine education, f0010, 1035, 1036f
Cohesion. *See* Social cohesion
Cohort effects, 54
Cohort studies, for researching aging and related conditions, 24–25
Colchicine
for apatite deposition disease, 576
for calcium pyrophosphate crystal deposition, 575
for gout, 574
for primary sclerosing cholangitis, 646
Colitis. *See also* Inflammatory bowel disease
in Crohn's disease, 670
infectious, 664–666, 665t
lymphocytic and collagenous, 670–671
ulcerative, 666–667, 667t
Collaborative research, in Europe, 1004
Collagen
in articular cartilage, aging effects on, 118–119
of connective tissues, 73–74
cross-linking of, 79
in dermis, aging effects on, 134–135
Collagenous colitis, 670–671
Colon. *See* Large bowel
Colon cancer, 673–674, 797
screening for, 673–674, 794
ulcerative colitis and risk for, 668–669
Colonic function, constipation and FI and, 914
Colonic ischemia, 671–672
Colonic pseudo-obstruction, 672
Colonoscopy, 662, 917, 917t
Colorectal cancer, 674, 914
Commission for Social Care Inspection (CSCI), 1025
Common duct stones, 647–648
Communicable diseases, in regions of world, 1011–1012
influenza-like illness, 1012
severe acute respiratory syndrome, 1012
tuberculosis, 1011–1012
Communication
with older adults with intellectual disability, 451
with patients with hearing loss, 825t
Community
epidemiology of drug use in, 138
oral health of elderly residents in, 603–604
Community Care Act, 1990, 1021–1022
Community Care Act, National Health Service and, 3
Community-living older adult
falls prevention for, 843–844
health promotion for, 835
benefits of, 835
economic evaluation framework, 838, 839f
for frail older adults, 837–838
Community-living older adult (*Continued*)
intervention study lessons, 842–845
legislation and policy needs, 845–846
lessons learned, 844–845, 845f
need for, 836–837
research needs, 845–846
screening and assessment for, 838–842
immobility and, 892
screening and assessment for
depression, 840–841
fall risk, 839–840
nutrition, 840
Community-wide promotion, for preventive practice systems, 853
Comorbidity
health service use v., 835
with obesity, 686
in people with intellectual disability, 448
in personality disorders, 443
as secondary cause of acquired immunodeficiency in old age, 89
Compensatory strategies, for Parkinson's disease therapy, 877
Complaints procedure, for quality of care improvement in United Kingdom, 1041
Complexity, of geriatric medicine, 1, 59–60, 61f, 245
Comprehensive assessment protocols, for social assessment of geriatric patients, 224
Comprehensive geriatric assessment (CGA), 7, 8t, 215
frailty index based on, 62–65, 63f–65f, 65t
preoperative, 232
social assessment as part of, 223
Compression
of disability, 184–186
of morbidity, 184–186, 188–189
of spinal cord, 539–541, 540f
in degenerative disease of lumbar spine, 544–545, 544f
from intradural tumors, 542
in Paget's disease, 543–544
in rheumatoid arthritis, 541, 542f
thoracic disk protrusion and, 541–542
Compression stockings, for venous thromboembolism, 360
Computed tomography (CT)
abdominal, 649–650, 661–662
for CAD, 287–288
for epilepsy, 461–462
of liver, 637
for pain, 967
for pancreas adenocarcinoma, 628–629
for prostate assessment, 703
of stroke, 489–490, 491f
Computed tomography angiography, of stroke, 490
Computerized risk assessment, for surgery and anesthesia in old age, 243
COMT inhibitors, for parkinsonism, 515t
Comtess. *See* Entacapone
Concept maps, in cognitivism, f0010, 1035, 1036f
Conduction defects, in patients with mitral annular calcium, 321
Confusion
causes of, 980–981, 980t
palliative care for, 980–981
Congenital heart disease, in Down syndrome, 448
Congestive heart failure (CHF), 945–946, 1065–1066
Congregate group settings, social assessment within, 228
Conjunctiva, disorders of, 811, 811f

Connective tissue
  aging and, 73–74, 77–80
  diseases of, 577
    cartilage disorders, 578
    fibrous tissue, ligament, and tendon disorders, 578–579
    immune-mediated, 580, 581f
    of lung, 381
    metabolic disorders, 580–582
    neoplasms, 579–580, 579f–580f
    nonmetabolic diseases of bone, 577–578, 578f
  properties of, 73–74
    aging and, 77–80
    collagens, 73–74
    elastin, 74
    proteoglycans, 75, 75t
    structural glycoproteins, 75–77
Connectivity graph, of health in old age, 59–60, 60f
Constipation, 909
  age-related changes in manifestation of, 108
  assessment of, 923f
  clinical evaluation of, 915–918
  definitions of, 909, 910t
  in Down syndrome, 448
  further research for, 924t, 925
  malnutrition and, 953
  palliative care for, 978–979
  pathophysiology of, 914–915
  prevalence of, 909–910
  risk factors of, 912, 912t
  treatment for, 918–921, 923f
Constraint-induced therapy, for stroke, 874
Constructivism, in geriatric medicine education, 1034–1035
Continuous Assessment Review and Evaluation (CARE), 1045
Continuous positive airway pressure (CPAP), 947
Contrast studies, of large bowel, 661
Convulsive status epilepticus (CSE), 459
Coordinated care models, for cost effective quality of care, 1052–1053
COPD. *See* Chronic obstructive pulmonary disease
Co-proxamol, for migraine, 467–468
Cornea, disorders of, 811–812, 812f
Coronary artery disease (CAD), diagnosis and management of, 286
  acute coronary syndromes, 290–291
  clinical manifestations, 286
  coronary revascularization, 293t, 294
  coronary risk factors, 288–290
  diagnostic techniques, 286–288
  hormone replacement therapy, 293–294, 293t
  recognized and unrecognized myocardial infarction, 286, 286t
  stable angina, 290
  STEMI therapy, 291
  therapy after myocardial infarction, 291–293, 292t
Coronary revascularization, 293t, 294
Coronary risk factors, 288–290
  cigarette smoking, 288
  diabetes mellitus, 289
  dyslipidemia, 289
  hypertension, 288–289
  left ventricular hypertrophy, 289
  obesity, 289–290
Coronary syndromes, acute, 290–291
Corpus uteri, cancer of, 722–723
Corticosteroid receptors, in older victims of trauma, 865
Corticosteroids
  adverse effects of, 110b
  for appetite stimulation, 955
  asteatotic eczema and, 802
  for asthma, 362, 365, 367–369, 367t
  for autoimmune hepatitis, 643
  for bowel obstruction, 979
  for bronchiectasis, 379
  for bullous pemphigoid, 807
  cataracts and, 815
  for celiac disease, 654
  for chronic meningitis, 550
  for CNS infection, 548
  for colonic ischemia, 672
  for COPD, 373
  for Crohn's disease, 656–657, 669t, 670
  dementia and, 387, 400
  drug interactions of, 143
  for giant cell arteritis, 473–474, 818
  for gout, 574
  headache due to, 475t
  hip fractures and, 565
  for hypersensitivity pneumonitis, 382
  for hyperthyroidism, 743
  for idiopathic pulmonary fibrosis, 381
  for idiopathic thrombocytopenic purpura, 789
  for intracranial tumors, 536–537
  for lymphocytic and collagenous colitis, 671
  for macular degeneration, 817–818
  for myasthenia gravis, 531
  for necrobiosis lipoidica, 808
  for neurogenic claudication and spinal stenosis, 526
  for ocular inflammation, 819
  ophthalmic complications of, 820
  for optic nerve disorders, 819
  in patients with diabetes, 221
  for primary sclerosing cholangitis, 645–646
  for pulmonary vasculitis, 381
  renal failure due to, 692
  respiratory system aging and, 98
  for sarcoidosis, 381
  for stasis dermatitis, 803
  for thyroid ophthalmopathy, 819
  for ulcerative colitis, 667–668
  for uveitis, 812
  for vulval discomfort, 719–720
Corticotropin, 667t
Cortisol, 125–126, 865
Costs, of stroke, 479
Cotrimoxazole, for UTIs, 691
Cough, palliative care for, 980
Council of the Royal College of Physicians and Surgeons of Canada (RCPSC), 1005–1006
Cox 2 inhibitors, 161–162
  for arthritis, 568–569, 568t
  gastropathy, peptic ulcer disease, and, 621
  for gout, 574
  for pain, 968b, 969
CP. *See* Chronic pancreatitis
CPAP. *See* Continuous positive airway pressure
CPCD. *See* Calcium pyrophosphate crystal deposition
Cranial nerve function, in old age, 101–102
  hearing and vestibular function, 102
  smell and taste, 101–102
  vision, 102
Craniofacial features, sleep-disordered breathing and, 946–947
Creative activities, for dementia management, 400
Cricopharyngeal achalasia, 611
Crohn's disease, 655–657, 666, 669, 669t
  age-related changes in manifestation of, 109
  clinical picture and investigations of, 656
  ileocolitis and colitis of, 670
  loose stool and, 923
  management of, 656–657
Cross-sectional data, longitudinal data v., 5–6
Cross-sectional studies, for researching aging and related conditions, 24
Crotamiton, 804
CRT. *See* Cardiac resynchronization therapy
Cryptococcal meningitis, 550
Cryptogenic epilepsy, 456–457
Crystal deposition disease. *See* Apatite deposition disease; Calcium pyrophosphate crystal deposition; Gout
Crystalline lens, disorders of, 814–815, 814f
Crystallized intelligence, aging and, 170
CSCI. *See* Commission for Social Care Inspection
CSE. *See* Convulsive status epilepticus
CSF. *See* Cerebrospinal fluid
CST. *See* Cognitive stimulation therapy
CT. *See* Computed tomography
Cushing syndrome, 733–734, 734f, 808
Cutaneous aging, mechanisms of, 78
Cutaneous cancer, 805–807, 805b
Cyclizine, 978
Cyclopentolate, 820
Cyclophosphamide, 797–798
  for arthritis, 569t
  for bullous pemphigoid, 807
  for chronic lymphocytic leukemia, 787
  for idiopathic pulmonary fibrosis, 381
  for inclusion body myositis, 528
  for lymphoma, 784–786
  for myasthenia gravis, 531
  for ovarian cancer, 724
  for polymyositis or dermatomyositis, 527
  for pulmonary vasculitis, 381
Cycloplegics, systemic complications of, 820
Cyclosporin, 15, 585, 667–668, 698, 698t, 807
Cyclosporin A, 645, 810–811
Cyclosporine gravis, 531
Cyproheptadine, 659, 955
Cysteinyl leukotriene antagonists, 367t
Cystic islet cell tumors, of pancreas, 627
Cystic tumors, of pancreas, 627
Cytarabine, 784
Cytochrome P450 monooxygenase enzymes
  drug metabolism by, 139–140, 140t
  inducers and inhibitors of, 141–143, 141t
Cytokine dysregulation, with aging, 85, 85t, 86f
Cytokine inhibitors, 593
Cytokines. *See* Proinflammatory cytokines
Cytomegalovirus (CMV), colitis caused by, 666
Cytosine arabinoside, 788
Cytotoxic drugs, 574, 617
Cytoxan, 753
Czech Republic, geriatric medicine in, 999

D

Dabigatran etexilate, 360
DAC. *See* 5-Aza-2'deoxycytidine
Dacarbazine, 786
Daily living aids, for rehabilitation, 14–15
Danazol, 780–781, 789
Dandelion, herbal-drug interactions of, 142t
Danshen, herbal-drug interactions of, 142t
Dapsone, 807
Darifenacin, 721, 936
Dasatinib, 781
Daunorubicin, 788
Daytime napping, sleep-disordered breathing and, 946–947

DCIS. *See* Ductal carcinoma in situ
DDAVP. *See* Desmopressin
Decision making, for incompetent patient, 984–985
  advanced, 985
  family role in, 985
Decision support, for tertiary disease prevention, 849
Decitabine. *See* 5-Aza-2'deoxycytidine
Decongestants, 142t, 473
Deep tendon reflexes, age-related changes in, 103–104
Deep vein thrombosis (DVT), 356–357
Defibrillator. *See* Automatic implantable cardioverter-defibrillator
Deficit accumulation, frailty in relation to, 60–62, 61f
Degeneration, of intervertebral disk, 578
Degenerative disease, of lumbar spine, 544–545, 544f
Degradation, of protein, aging effects on, 48–49
Dehydration, 681, 681t
  malnutrition and, 953–954, 953t
  surgery and anesthesia in old age and, 240
Dehydroepiandrosterone (DHEA), 125, 148
Dehydroepiandrosterone replacement therapy, 125, 730
Delayed-type skin hypersensitivity (DTH), 84
Delirium, 385–386, 903
  causes and risk factors of, 905
  clinical features of, 903–904
  concept and diagnostic criteria evolution, 903
  differential diagnoses of, 904
  drug treatment for, 906–907
  drug-induced, 513
  evaluation of, 906, 906t
  management of, 907–908, 907t
  as nonspecific clinical presentation of disease in elderly, 205–206
  in older adults with intellectual disability, 451
  postoperative, 241–242
  prevalence of, 904–905
  prevention of, 905–906
  prognosis for, 908
Delivery system design, for tertiary disease prevention, 849
Delusional disorders. *See* Late life delusional disorders
Dementia. *See also specific diseases of dementia, e.g.,* Alzheimer's disease
  aerobic exercise and, 864
  constipation and, 913
  definitions of, 385, 392
  depression and, 435–436
  with diabetes mellitus, 765–766
  diagnosis of, 385
    autonomic dysfunction, 389–390
    cerebellar signs, 390
    clinical examination features in differential diagnosis, 389
    gait impairment, 390
    laboratory investigations in, 390–391
    limitations of current classification, 385
    neuropathy and other motor neuron findings, 390
    ocular and visual findings, 390
    other disorders associated with, 386–389
    Parkinsonian disorders, 390
    pyramidal disorders, 390
    risk factors, 385–386
    seizure and myoclonus, 390
  differential diagnosis of, 394–397, 396f
    reaching a diagnosis, 395–397, 396f
    telling a diagnosis, 397–398, 397t
Dementia (*Continued*)
  disclosure of diagnosis of, 397–398, 397t
  in Down syndrome, 448
  hypertension and, 310
  management of, 398–402, 398f
    drug management, 400–401
    memory aids and cognitive training, 399
    nonpharmacologic therapies, 399–400
    safety and risk, 398–399
  neuropsychology in diagnosis and treatment of, 402
    challenges to, 402–404
    neuropsychological tests, 404–407, 404t, 409t
    reasons for neuropsychological assessment, 402
  in older adults with intellectual disability, 451
  pain assessment with, 967–968
  postoperative, 242
  poststroke, 422, 426
  presentation of, 392–394, 393t
    behavioral and psychological symptoms, 393t, 394
    clinical presentation, 392–394, 393t
    diagnostic criteria, 392
  rehabilitation detection of, 9
  sleep in, 947–948
  social factors associated with, 202
  social functioning and, 227–228
  telemedicine support for, 1066
Dementia with Lewy bodies (DLB), 407–408, 409t, 904
Dementia-related fecal incontinence, 922t, 923–924
Denmark, geriatric medicine in, 999
Denosumab, 557–558
Dental devices, for sleep-disordered breathing, 947
Dental disease, headache and facial pain due to, 473
Dentistry, geriatric, 599
  changing need for dental care in elderly, 601–602, 601f–602f
  for community dwelling v. long-term care facility residents, 603–604
  oral health
    definition of, 599
    measures of, 599–601, 599f–601f
    systemic health response to, 602–603
  recognition and management of common oral conditions in elderly, 604–607, 605f–606f
Dentition
  in Down syndrome, 448
  menopause and, 717
Dentures, 604–605, 605f
Dependable local delivery, with NHS, 1043
Dependency
  indices of, 8
  social factors associated with, 202
  structured, 188
Dependency ratio, 8
Depo-Medrone. *See* Methylprednisolone acetate
Deposition disease. *See* Apatite deposition disease; Calcium pyrophosphate crystal deposition; Gout
Depression
  chronic cardiac failure in patients with, 284
  chronic pain and, 966
  constipation and, 913
  delirium and, 904
  dementia v., 394–395, 408–409, 409t
  insomnia and, 946
Depression (*Continued*)
  in old age, 433–436
    clinical features of, 434–435
    dementia and, 435–436
    epidemiology of, 433
    etiology of, 433
    gender and, 433
    genetic susceptibility to, 433
    management of, 435–436
    neurobiologic risk factors, 433–434
    personality and social factors, 434
    physical health and, 434
    prognosis of, 436
    suicide and, 436
  palliative care for, 980
  prevalence of, 840–841
  rehabilitation detection of, 9
  screening and assessment for, 840–841, 852
  vascular, 435
  with vascular cognitive impairment, 425
Deprivation. *See* Sleep deprivation
Dermatitis
  seborrheic, 802
  stasis, 803
  of vulva, 718
Dermatologic disorders
  of foot, 595–596, 596f
  of vulva, 718–719
Dermatology, in Down syndrome, 448–449
Dermatomyositis (DM), 526–528
Dermis, aging of, 134–135, 939
Dermovate, 719
DES. *See* Diethylstilboestrol
Desflurane, 231
Desipramine, 140t, 472, 789
Desmopressin (DDAVP), 343, 343t, 508b, 509, 936
Destructive agents, in cellular aging, 42–45
  environmental agents, 42
  intracellular calcium homeostasis and, 44–45
  reactive oxygen species, 42–44
Detrusor
  aging effects on, 114–115
  benign prostatic hyperplasia and dysfunction of, 706, 709
  in bladder function, 926–927
  voiding pressure v. flow rate, 930–931, 933f
Detrusor hyperactivity and impaired contractility (DHIC), 930
Detrusor hyperreflexia with impaired contractility (DHIC), 115
Detrusor overactivity (DO), 115, 721
Developed nations, longevity in, 988
Developing nations
  longevity in, 988
  productive aging in, 196–197
Developmental reflexes. *See* Primitive reflexes
Devil's claw, herbal-drug interactions of, 142t
Dexamethasone
  for CNS infection, 548, 550b
  for intracranial tumors, 537
  for lymphoma, 784
  for metastatic spinal tumors, 542–543
  for multiple myeloma, 783
  for nausea and vomiting, 978
  for neuropathic pain, 977
  in older individuals, 125
Dexamethasone suppression test, 732–733
Dextromethorphan, 140t
Dextropropoxyphene, 435
DHEA. *See* Dehydroepiandrosterone
DHIC. *See* Detrusor hyperactivity and impaired contractility; Detrusor hyperreflexia with impaired contractility

Diabetes mellitus, 760, 760t
aerobic exercise and, 860–861
aging of connective tissues in patients with, 78–79
blood pressure control in, 772
cardiovascular risk and, 302
care issues and future initiatives for, 773–775, 774b
comorbidity of, 848
connective tissue disorders associated with, 581–582
constipation and FI and, 913
cutaneous complications of, 807–808
definition, classification, and diagnosis of, 760–761, 760t–761t
in elderly population, 762–766, 763f, 764t–765t, 765f, 765b
dementia, 765–766
foot disease, 597–598, 598b, 763–765, 764t–765t, 765b
mortality of, 765, 765f
residential care and housebound patients, 766–767, 767t, 767b
visual loss, 763, 764t
epidemiology of, 761–762, 762t
foot problems in, 597–598, 598b
glucose control in, 767–768, 768t–770t, 768b
choice of treatment for glucose control, 770
monitoring of, 771
pathologic basis for treatment of type 2 diabetes, 767–768
treatments for glucose control, 768–770, 769t–770t
home monitoring for control of, 771
hyperglycemic coma in patients with, 771–772, 771b
hypertension and, 310
and hypoglycemia in elderly patient, 767, 768t, 771
impairment of glucose tolerance with aging, 761, 761f, 762t
insomnia and, 945–946
lipid control in, 772–773
loose stool and, 923
as risk factor for CAD, 289
telemedicine for, 1066
upper gastrointestinal tract in patients with, 625
vascular prophylaxis in, 773
Diabetes specialist nurses, for elderly, 774, 774b
Diabetic ketoacidosis (DKA), 771–772
Diabetic neuropathy, 524–525, 524t
Diabetic retinopathy, 763, 764t, 813b, 815–816, 816f
Diagnosis-related groups (DRGs), in Medicare, 1027
Diagnostic and Statistical Manual-Fourth Edition (DSM-IV), delirium and, 903
Dialysis, 694
Diamorphine, 976t, 977
Diarrhea, 923, 979
Diastolic blood pressure, cardiovascular risk and, 301
Diastolic function, in aging heart at rest, 94–95
Diastolic heart failure. *See* Heart failure with preserved systolic function
Diazepam, 139–141, 140t, 639
Diazoxide, 771
Dibucaine, 803
DIC. *See* Disseminated intravascular coagulation
Diclofenac, 140t, 467–468, 568, 568t, 574, 805
Dicyclomine, 663t
Diet
cardiovascular risk and, 303
in chronic cardiac failure, 283
constipation and, 913, 918, 919t
fecal incontinence and, 921–925
for glucose control, 768
malnutrition and, 953
for weight loss, 687–688, 688t
Dietary restriction. *See* Caloric restriction
Diethylstilboestrol (DES), 713–714
Dieulafoy lesions, in large bowel, 675–676
Differentiated type vulvar intraepithelial neoplasia, 719
Diffuse esophageal spasm, 613–614
Diffuse large B-cell lymphoma (DLBCL), 784–786
Diffuse Lewy body disease (DLBD), 505–506
Diffuse parenchymal lung disease (DPLD), 380, 380f
Digitalis
for acute arterial mesenteric ischemia, 657–658
for aortic stenosis, 316
colonic ischemia and, 671
hyperkalemia due to, 698t
ophthalmic complications of, 820
toxicity due to, 327, 333, 336
Digitalis glycosides, for ventricular rate control in patients with AF, 332
Digitoxin, 789
Dignity, 984
Digoxin
antacids and, 622
for aortic regurgitation, 319
for atrial flutter, 335
carotid sinus reflex sensitivity and, 344
for chronic cardiac failure, 277, 278b, 280–282, 285
drug interactions of, 143
elimination of, 140, 141t
in frail elderly patient, 298
herbal-drug interactions of, 142t
for mitral stenosis, 324
for paroxysmal atrial tachycardia with atrioventricular block, 336
potassium balance and, 698
for SVT, 336
syncope caused by, 339t
toxicity of, 281, 344–345
for ventricular rate control in patients with AF, 332
for Wolff-Parkinson-White syndrome, 332
Dihydroergotamine, 345
Dihydropyridines, 305t, 306–309, 310b, 772
1,25-Dihydroxycolecalciferol, 756
Diltiazem
for acute coronary syndromes, 291
for atrial flutter, 335
drug interactions of, 143
for mitral stenosis, 324
for stable angina, 290
for STEMI, 291
for SVT, 336
for ventricular rate control in patients with AF, 332
for Wolff-Parkinson-White syndrome, 332
Dimethicone, 804
Diogenes syndrome. *See* Senile self-neglect
DIP. *See* Drug-induced parkinsonism
Dipeptidyl peptidase-IV inhibitors, 774
Diphenhydramine, 205–206, 609
Diphenoxylate, 671
Diphosphate therapy, 699t
Diphosphonate, 714
Dipyridamole, 142t–143t, 475t, 482, 495
Dipyridamole-thallium imaging, for CAD, 287
Direct thrombin inhibitors, 360–361, 360b
Disability
assessment of, 10–11
compression of, 184–186
in epidemiology of aging, 4–9, 4f, 6t, 7f–9f, 9t
age group definitions in, 6, 6t, 7f
changes over time in, 5
cross-sectional v. longitudinal data in study of aging, 5–6
ethnicity, emigration, and immigration effects on, 9, 9t
features of younger v. older people, 8, 8f
indices of dependency in, 8
inequalities among older individuals, 9
inevitability of aging, 8
living alone and, 9, 9f
marital status in, 7–8, 7f
measuring differences in, 5–8, 6t, 7f–8f
predicting future of, 5
sex in, 6–7, 7f
illness v. role, 6
prevention of, 2–3
process leading to, 5–6
revised ICIDH model of, 6–7, 7f
after stroke, 494
WHO classification of, 6
world statistics on, 1010–1015
Disclosure, of dementia diagnosis, 397–398, 397t
Disease based models of care, function based v., 845
Disease prevention, 848–849
other activities for, 848, 850t
primary, 848, 849t–850t
secondary, 848, 849t–850t
tertiary, 848–849
USPSTF and CDC recommended activities for, 848, 849t
Disease-modifying antirheumatic drugs (DMARDs), 569, 569t, 576b
Disengagement theory, 188
Disopyramide
for AF, 333
drug-disease interactions of, 143t
for maintaining sinus rhythm, 333–334
for SVT, 336
syncope caused by, 339t
for ventricular arrhythmia, 327–328
for Wolff-Parkinson-White syndrome, 332
Disposable soma theory, 19–22, 19f–20f
Disseminated intravascular coagulation (DIC), 790
Distribution, of drugs, aging effects on, 139
Disulfiram, 442
Diuretics
for acute renal failure, 693
for aneurysm surgery for abdominal aortic aneurysm, 355
for aortic regurgitation, 319
for aortic stenosis, 316
for ascites, 641
for blood pressure control in diabetes mellitus patients, 772
for CAD prevention, 288–289
for chronic cardiac failure, 277–281, 278b, 283–285, 285b
dementia due to, 416–417
diabetes secondary to, 760
diabetic ketoacidosis and, 771
in diagnosis of heart failure, 275
in frail elderly patient, 298
gout associated with, 573–574, 581
hepatic encephalopathy induced by, 642
for HONK coma, 771

Diuretics (*Continued*)
hypercalcemia and, 757t
hyperkalemia due to, 698, 698t
for hypertension, 305, 305t, 308–311, 310b
hypoaldosteronism and, 733
for hypoparathyroidism, 759
for mitral stenosis, 324
myalgia and myopathy induced by, 528–529
orthostatic hypotension and, 343t, 503, 508–509, 508b
for paroxysmal atrial tachycardia with atrioventricular block, 336
renal failure due to, 692
as secondary cause of acquired immunodeficiency in old age, 89
for stroke prevention, 495–496
syncope caused by, 339t
urinary incontinence and, 721
Diurnal blood pressure variation, 510
Diversity
personality stage theories and, 179
personality trait theories and, 180
social-cognitive theories to personality and, 181–182
Diverticula
epiphrenic, 616
esophageal, 616
midesophageal, 616
pharyngeal, 611–612, 611f
Diverticular disease, 663, 663t, 914
Diverticulitis, 663–664, 663t
Diverticulosis, 662–664, 663t
Dizziness
differential diagnosis and management of, 898, 899t
as nonspecific clinical presentation of disease in elderly, 207
palliative care for, 980
DKA. *See* Diabetic ketoacidosis
DL threo-dihydroxyphenylserine (DL-threo-dops, DOPS), 510
DLB. *See* Dementia with Lewy bodies
DLBCL. *See* Diffuse large B-cell lymphoma
DLBD. *See* Diffuse Lewy body disease
DM. *See* Dermatomyositis
DMARDs. *See* Disease-modifying antirheumatic drugs
DNA damage, in cell senescence, 47–48
DNA methyltransferase inhibitors, for myelodysplasia, 778–779
DNA mutations, in cell senescence, 46
DO. *See* Detrusor overactivity
Dobutamine echocardiography, for CAD, 287
Docetaxel, 383, 714
Docusate, 920
Dofetilide, 333, 335
Domperidone, 468, 468t, 515, 516t, 517, 978
Donepezil, 419, 419t
for delirium, 906–907
for dementia, 400, 432
dry mouth and, 605
for Parkinson's disease, 517
Dong quai, 142t, 164
Dopa decarboxylase inhibitors, 515
Dopamine agonists
delirium and, 513
orthostatic hypotension and, 508–509
for parkinsonism, 515t, 516–517
for restless legs syndrome, 519
sensitivity to, 141
Dopamine antagonists, 144, 144b, 978
Dopaminergic agents, 141t, 536
Doppler echocardiography
for aortic regurgitation, 318–319
of aortic stenosis, 314
DOPS. *See* DL threo-dihydroxyphenylserine
Dosing regimens, aging effects on, 140
Down syndrome, 445–449, 446t–447t
Doxazosin, for hypertension, 309
Doxorubicin
for breast cancer, 728–729
for Kaposi sarcoma, 807
longevity due to, 14
for lymphoma, 784–786
for multiple myeloma, 783
for skin angiosarcoma, 807
for thyroid nodule management, 753
Doxycycline, 552
DPLD. *See* Diffuse parenchymal lung disease
DRGs. *See* Diagnosis-related groups
Driving, accident prevention and, 850
Dronabinol, 955
Drug burden, in chronic cardiac failure patients, 284
Drug delivery route, for palliative care, 977
Drug interactions, 141–143, 141t–143t
of antiepileptic drugs, 463, 463t
drug-disease interactions, 143, 143t
with herbs, 142t
pharmacodynamic interactions, 143
pharmacokinetic interactions, 141–143, 141t–142t
as secondary cause of acquired immunodeficiency in old age, 89
Drug therapy. *See also* Pharmacotherapy, geriatric; Polypharmacy
absorption of, aging effects on, 139
access to, 138
associated with ADWE, 884, 884t
dementia associated with, 386–387
distribution of, aging effects on, 139
in elderly patients undergoing surgery
anesthetics, 231
long-term medications, 232
elimination of, aging effects on, 140, 141t
epidemiology of use of, 138
access to medications, 138
in community, 138
in hospitals, 138
in LTCFs, 138
falls and, 898, 902
liver metabolism of, 140, 140t, 635–636
loose stool and, 923
management of, for dementia treatment, 400–402
metabolism of, aging effects on, 139–140, 140t
ophthalmic complications of, 819–820
orthostatic hypotension caused by, 339t, 342
for pain, 968
for palliative care, 976–977, 976t
physiologic and homeostatic mechanisms and response to, aging effects on, 141
postural control and, 898, 900t
problems with, 880–881, 881f
seizures due to, 460
sensitivity to, aging effects on, 141, 141t
sexuality in old age and, 855, 857t
syncope caused by, 339t
underutilization of, 883
urinary incontinence and, 928, 929t, 931–932, 937
Drug-induced acute liver failure, 643
Drug-induced headache, 475, 475t
Drug-induced hyperkinetic movement disorders, 519–520
Drug-induced interstitial lung disease, 381
Drug-induced myalgia and myopathy, 528–529
Drug-induced parkinsonism (DIP), 518
Dry mouth. *See* Xerostomia
DSM-IV. *See* Diagnostic and Statistical Manual-Fourth Edition
DTH. *See* Delayed-type skin hypersensitivity
Ductal carcinoma in situ (DCIS), 726–727
Duloxetine, 435, 463
Duodenal mucosa, injury of, 618–619
Duodenal ulcers, 622, 622f
Dupuytren disease, 10071#t0015, 578–579
Dutasteride, 709, 709t
DVT. *See* Deep vein thrombosis
Dynamic support surfaces, for pressure ulcers, 941
Dysequilibrium, 207
Dyskinesia. *See* Levodopa-induced dyskinesia
Dyslipidemia
as CAD risk factor, 289
cardiovascular risk and, 302
in Down syndrome, 448
Dyspepsia, nonulcer, 622–623
Dysphagia, 612–613, 950–953
in elderly, 109
oropharyngeal, 610–611, 611t, 953
palliative medicine and, 974–975
postintubation, 611
Dysphagia aortica, 616
Dyspnea, 979
Dystonia, 519
Dysuria, 928

E

EADLs. *See* Extended activities of daily living
EAMA. *See* European Academy for Medicine for Ageing
Early life experience, aging response to, 161
Early retirement options, 994–995
Easycare assessment, 11
Eating, palliative medicine and, 974–975
Ebb phase, of metabolism in victims of trauma, 865–866
Eccrine sweat glands, aging of, 135
ECG. *See* Electrocardiography
Echinacea, herbal-drug interactions of, 142t
Echocardiography
of aortic regurgitation, 318–319
of aortic stenosis, 314
of CAD, 287
of chronic cardiac failure, 276–277, 276f
of stroke, 490–491
Echothiophate, 820
ECM. *See* Extracellular matrix
Ecologic studies, for researching aging and related conditions, 24
Economic evaluation, framework for, 838, 839f
Economics
of long-term care in United States, 1027
telemedicine and, 1068
Economy, of quality of care, 1039
Ectropion, 810, 811f
Eczema, 448–449, 718
Eczema craquelé, 801–802
Eczematous disorders, 801–802
ED. *See* Erectile dysfunction
Edentulism, 604–605, 605f
Education. *See also* Patient education
in geriatric medicine, 1032
adult learning theory, 1034
barriers to change in, 1032, 1033t
behaviorism, 1033–1034
cognitivism, f0010, 1035, 1036f
constructivism, 1034–1035
medical attitudes towards, 1032–1033
motivators for change in, 1032, 1033t
social learning, 1035
societal attitudes towards, 1033
theory for, 1033

EEG. *See* Electroencephalogram; Electroencephalography
Effector organs, falls and, 895, 896t
Efficacy
of geriatric pharmacotherapy, 880
of quality of care, 1039
Efficiency
of managed care in United States, 1063
of quality of care, 1039
Effusion. *See* Pleural effusion
Ego, development of, 178–181, 179t
e-Health, 1066–1067, 1067t
Elastin
of connective tissues, 74
in dermis, aging effects on, 135
Elastofibroma, 579–580, 580f
Eldepryl. *See* Selegiline
Elderly. *See also* Old age
care of, 1006
mistreatment and neglect of, 959
definitions of, 959–960, 960t
historical development of, 959
identification of, 962–963
prevalence and incidence of, 960–961, 960t
prevention, treatment, and management of, 962f, 963
risk factors for, 961–962
younger people v., 8, 8f
Elderly in society, international perspective on, 988
demographic trends, 988–991, 989t–990t, 992t
early retirement, 995
inequality of longevity, 988
pension systems, 993–994
privatization experiences, 994–995
social protection for old age, 991–993
Elderly Nutrition Program, 840
Elective cardioversion, for AF, 333
Electrocardiography (ECG)
for aortic regurgitation, 318
for aortic stenosis, 314
for CAD, 286–287
for chronic cardiac failure, 276
for epilepsy, 460
Electroencephalogram (EEG), for delirium, 904
Electroencephalography (EEG), of epilepsy, 460–461, 461f
Electrolyte balance and imbalance, 697–698, 698t
surgery and anesthesia in old age and, 239–241
assessment of fluid and electrolyte status, 240
dehydration, 240
fluid and electrolyte therapy, 240–241
fluid regimen over perioperative period, 241
salt and saline depletion, 240
water depletion, 240
Electromyography (EMG), for neuromuscular disorder diagnosis, 523
Electronic health records (EHR)
for cost effective quality, 1053, 1053t
physician and, 1049
Electrophysiology, for neuromuscular disorder diagnosis, 523
Electrostimulation, for stroke therapy, 874
Elimination, of drugs, aging effects on, 140, 141t
Eltrombopag, 789
Emboli. *See also* Pulmonary embolism; Venous thromboembolism
arterial, in acute limb ischemia, 349
femoral, in acute limb ischemia, 349
EMG. *See* Electromyography
Emigration, in epidemiology of aging, 9, 9t
Emphysema, 98, 362, 363t, 374
Empowerment function, replacement function v., 844–845
Empyema, subdural, 549
EN. *See* Enteral nutrition
Enalapril, 140t, 278b, 279
Encainide
for AF, 333
for maintaining sinus rhythm, 333–334
metabolism of, 140t
after myocardial infarction, 292–293
syncope caused by, 339t
for ventricular arrhythmia, 327–328, 328t
Encephalitis, 549–552
herpes simplex, 550–551, 550b
Encephalopathy, hepatic, 642
End of life issues, 957–958, 986, 1014–1015
Endarterectomy, for prevention of secondary stroke, 496
Endocarditis, 322
Endocrine disorders
dementia associated with, 387–388
in Down syndrome, 448
sarcopenia and, 588–589
Endocrine function, of pancreas, 626
Endocrine myopathies, 529
Endocrine system. *See also* Neuroendocrinology
aging of, 123
andropause, 124–125
dehydroepiandrosterone, 125
growth hormone/insulin-like growth factor-I axis, 123–124
hypothalamic-pituitary-adrenal axis, 125–126
hypothalamic-pituitary-thyroid axis, 126
menopause. *See* Menopause
Endometrial cancer, 722–723
End-organ responsiveness, effects of aging on, 502
Endoscopic retrograde cholangiopancreatography (ERCP), 629, 650
Endoscopic ultrasound (EUS)
of biliary tract, 650
for pancreas adenocarcinoma, 629
Endoscopy, of small bowel, 653
Endosonography, anal and rectal, 662
Endothelial function, in aging, 91–92
Endovascular aneurysm repair (EVAR), 355
Endovascular techniques, 355
Endovascular therapy, for prevention of secondary stroke, 496
End-stage renal disease, insomnia and, 945–946
End-Stage Renal Disease Management Demonstration, 1058
Endurance training, in old age, 863
Enemas, 920
Energy requirements, aging effects on, 680, 680t
Enflurane, 231
Engagement. *See* Social engagement
Enoxaparin, 360
Entacapone (Comtess), 515t, 516
Entactin/nidogen, 76
Entamoeba histolytica, colitis caused by, 666
Enteral nutrition (EN), 682–683
for malnutrition, 956–957
for surgery, 239t
Enthesopathy, 579
Entropion, 810, 811f
Environmental agents, in cellular aging, 42
Environmental changes
for frailty therapy, 878–879
for Parkinson's disease therapy, 877
Environmental supports
description of, 838
personal resources v., 837, 837f, 838t
Eosinophils, effects of aging on, 130
Ephedrine, 343, 345
Epidermis, aging of, 134
Epidermoid carcinoma, of oral cavity, 610
Epigenetics, of aging, 41, 128–129
Epilepsy, 453
antiepileptic drugs for. *See* Antiepileptic drugs
classification of, 153–155
convulsive status epilepticus, 459
definition of, 453
diagnosis of, 457
differential diagnosis of, 457–459, 458t, 459f
in Down syndrome, 448
epidemiology of, 453, 454f
epileptic seizures in, 453, 455–456, 455t
etiology of, 460, 461f
future research in, 464–465
impact of, 464, 464t
investigation of, 460–462, 461f
nonconvulsive status epilepticus, 459
services for patients with, 464–465
sudden unexplained death in, 460
syndromes, 456–457
Epiphrenic diverticula, 616
Episodic memory, aging effects on, 173
Eplerenone, 292, 641
e-Prescribing incentive, 1053
Eptifibatide, 291
EQ-5D, for quality of life measurement, 4, 4f
Equity, of quality of care, 1039
ER stress, in protein misfolding and neurotoxicity in cell models of Parkinson's disease and Alzheimer's disease, 153–154
ERCP. *See* Endoscopic retrograde cholangiopancreatography
Erectile dysfunction (ED)
age and, 854
causes and diagnosis of, 855–857, 856t
sildenafil for, 854
treatment for, 857–858
Ergocalciferol, 695–696, 756b, 758b
Ergot compounds, 470
Ergotamine, 468, 468t, 475, 510
Erlotinib, 383
ERT. *See* Estrogen replacement therapy
Erythrocytes, aging effects on, 130–131
Erythromycin
C. difficile infection and, 664
cytochrome P450 reaction with, 141t
drug interactions of, 141–143
for gastric outlet obstruction, 631
for infectious colitis, 666
liver metabolism of, 636t
metabolism of, 140t
Erythropoietic stimulating agents, for multiple myeloma, 783
Erythropoietin
for chronic cardiac failure, 278b, 282
for myelodysplasia, 778–779
for myeloproliferative disorders, 780–781
for orthostatic hypotension, 343, 343t, 509–510
Escherichia coli, colitis caused by, 665–666
Escitalopram, 463
Esophagus, 612–618
aging effects on, 106
disorders of
achalasia, 613, 613f
Barrett metaplasia, 615, 615f
candidiasis, 617
diffuse esophageal spasm, 613–614
dysphagia and heartburn, 612–613
dysphagia aortica, 616
epiphrenic diverticula, 616
esophageal diverticula, 616

Esophagus (*Continued*)
hiatus hernia, 614, 614f
intramural pseudodiverticulosis, 616–617, 617f
lower esophageal ring, 615–616, 615f
medication-induced, 616, 617f–618f
midesophageal diverticula, 616
motility disorders, 613
neoplasms, 617–618, 618f
"nutcracker" esophagus and noncardiac chest pain, 614
reflux esophagitis, 614–615
secondary motility disorders, 613
Essential thrombocythemia (ET), 779–781
Essential tremor (ET), 518–519
Established renal failure, 696
Estonia, geriatric medicine in, 999
17β-Estradiol, for preserving brain metabolism, 168
Estradiol therapy, for bone loss, 56
Estren-β. *See* 19-Nor-4-androstene-3β,17β-diol
Estrogen
age-related decline in, 124
chorea caused by, 519
in Down syndrome, 448
high thyroxine due to, 739
menopause and, 854
sarcopenia and, 589, 592
sexual motivation and, 724–725
Estrogen antagonists, for breast cancer, 727–728, 728t, 792
Estrogen replacement therapy (ERT)
for Alzheimer's disease, 413, 420
as antiaging medicine, 147
bladder overactivity and incontinence response to, 113
for bone loss, 56, 164
for breast cancer, 728, 728t, 798
for dementia, 400
depression associated with, 435
disease development and, 854
for lichen sclerosis of vulva, 719
longevity due to, 14
for males, 166–167
in menopause, 124, 717–718, 808–809, 854
oral estrogen, 717
subcutaneous estrogen implants, 718
topical estrogen, 717–718
transdermal estrogen, 717
for osteoporosis, 586
for overactive bladder, 721
for preserving brain metabolism, 168
for prostate cancer, 714
for reproductive aging in women, 164–167
skin aging response to, 136
for ulceration, 720
urinary incontinence and, 936
uterine cancer and, 722
Eszopiclone, 946
ET. *See* Essential thrombocythemia; Essential tremor
Etanercept, 570t
Ethacrynic acid, 824
Ethambutol, 378, 820
Ethical issues, 983
dignity, 984
end of life issues, 986
incompetent patient, 984
decision making for, 984–985
research and, 985–986
of nutrition in aging, 684
paternalism, 983–984
physician-assisted suicide and euthanasia, 986–987
priority setting and the elderly, 987
respect for autonomy, 983
Ethnicity, in epidemiology of aging, 9, 9t
Ethosuximide, 462
Etidronate, 556, 563, 759b
Etoposide, 383, 807
Etoricoxib, 568t, 574
EUGMS. *See* European Union Geriatric Medicine Society
EuMaG. *See* European Masters Program in Gerontology
EUMS-GM. *See* European Union of Medical Specialists - Geriatric Medicine Section
Europe
aging in, 997, 997f
collaborative research in, 1004
geriatric medicine in, 997–1004
organizations, 1000–1004
other countries, 999–1000
United Kingdom, 998–999
health care in, 997
nongovernmental organization links, 1004
European Academy for Medicine for Ageing (EAMA), 1003
European Masters Program in Gerontology (EuMaG), 1003–1004
European Union Geriatric Medicine Society (EUGMS), 1001, 1002t–1003t
European Union of Medical Specialists - Geriatric Medicine Section (EUMS-GM), 1001–1003, 1002t–1003t
Euthanasia, 986–987
EVAR. *See* Endovascular aneurysm repair
Evening primrose oil, 164
Evercare, 1052
Evergreen Action Nutrition, 842–843
Evista, 164–165
Evolution, of aging, 18–19, 19f
comparison of theories on, 19
disposable soma theory, 19–22, 19f–20f
genetics of life span, 19–21, 20f
natural selection and age, 18–19
programmed or "adaptive" aging, 18
tests of, 21–22
Exacerbation, of COPD, 372
Exclusion of elderly
due to frailty, 204
from research, 26
Executive functions
aging effects on, 174–175
mobility and, 886
Exercise. *See also* Aerobic exercise
as antiaging medicine, 146
CAD risk and, 290
cardiovascular risk and, 303
constipation and, 912
definition of, 859
for frailty, 849–850, 878
in heart failure, 282–283
immobility and, 889–892
for pain, 970–971
response of aging heart to, 95–96, 96t
sarcopenia and, 588, 591
for stroke therapy, 874–875
for successful aging, 859
aerobic exercise, 859–861
aerobic exercise and carbohydrate metabolism, 860–861
bone health, 863–864
memory disorders and, 864
protein requirements for, 862
resistance exercise and, 862–863
resistance exercise and insulin and protein metabolism, 861–862
strength training, 861
for weight loss, 688
Exercise capacity, aging effects on, 56
Exercise stress testing, for CAD, 287
Exocrine function, of pancreas, 626
Expectorants, 373, 980
Explicit memory, aging effects on, 172–173
Exploding head syndrome, 476
Extended activities of daily living (EADLs)
disability assessment and, 10
occupational therapy for, 871
External hip protectors, 558
External sheath drainage, for urinary incontinence, 938
Extracellular matrix (ECM)
aging effects on, 49, 77–80
components of, 73–74
collagens, 73–74
elastin, 74
proteoglycans, 75, 75t
structural glycoproteins, 75–77
Extracranial artery ultrasound, of stroke, 490
Extramedullary Paget's disease, of vulva, 719
Extrinsic aging
in physiologic deterioration, 51–52, 52f
of skin, 133–135
Eye. *See also* Vision
disorders of, 810
conjunctiva disorders, 811, 811f
cornea disorders, 811–812, 812f
crystalline lens disorders, 814–815, 814f
eyelid disorders, 810, 810f–811f
glaucoma, 813–814, 813f, 813b
lacrimal apparatus disorders, 810–811
low-vision rehabilitation for, 820–821
neuro-ophthalmology disorders, 819
ophthalmic complications of systemic diseases, 819
ophthalmic complications of systemic medications, 819–820
optic nerve disorders, 819
orbit disorders, 819
retina and vitreous disorders, 815–819, 816f–817f
systemic complications of ophthalmic medications, 820
uveal tract disorders, 812–813
headache and, 475–476
Eyelids, disorders of, 810, 810f–811f

F

Facial neuralgias, 470–472
glossopharyngeal neuralgia, 471–472
postherpetic neuralgia, 472
trigeminal neuralgia, 470–471
Facial pain
atypical, 472
from sinus disease and dental disease, 473
Factor Xa inhibitors, for venous thromboembolism, 360–361, 360b
Failure to thrive, frailty and, 949
Falls, 894
assessment of, 558
causation of, 894–897
biomechanical perspective on, 897, 897f
epidemiologic perspective on, 894–895, 894t
physiologic perspective on, 895–897, 896t
description of, 894
epidemiology of, 894
evaluation for, 898–902, 899t–900t
fractures following, 868
as injury cause, 865
management of, 900–902, 901t
as nonspecific clinical presentation of disease in elderly, 207–208

Falls *(Continued)*
prevention of, 843–844, 850, 868
risk of
fractured neck and, 876
screening and assessment for, 839–840, 897–898, 898t
Famciclovir, 472, 803–804
Familiality, in successful aging, 185–186
Family burden, 226–227
Family history
as dementia risk factor, 386
sleep-disordered breathing and, 946–947
Famotidine, 621–622
Farnesylation, of progerin, in Hutchinson-Gilford progeria syndrome, 68
Farnesyltransferase inhibitors, 68
Fat consumption
diabetes and, 860–861
frailty prevention and, 850
Fat mass, aging effects on, 56
Fat-free mass (FFM)
aerobic exercises and, 861
aging effects on, 56
Fatigue
as nonspecific clinical presentation of disease in elderly, 206–207
palliative care for, 980
Fatty liver, 109
Fecal impaction, with constipation and FI, 915–916, 916f
Fecal incontinence (FI), 909
clinical evaluation of, 915–918
definition of, 909
epidemiology of, 910, 911t
further research for, 924t, 925
pathophysiology of, 914–915
prevalence of, 910–911, 911t
risk factors of, 910–912, 911t
treatment of, 921–925, 922t
Fecal occult blood tests (FOBTs), 662
Federation of the Royal Colleges of Physicians of the United Kingdom, 998
Feeding, palliative medicine and, 975
FEES. *See* Fiberoptic endoscopic evaluation of swallowing
Felbamate, for epilepsy, 462
Felodipine, 290–291, 306–307
Femoral emboli, in acute limb ischemia, 349
Fentanyl, 139, 912–913, 969–970, 976–977, 976t
Fenugreek, 142t
Ferrous sulphate, 278b, 282, 616
Fesoterodine, 936
Fever, as nonspecific clinical presentation of disease in elderly, 208
Feverfew, 142t, 469
FFM. *See* Fat-free mass
FI. *See* Fecal incontinence
Fiber consumption
constipation and, 913, 918, 919t
diabetes and, 860–861
frailty prevention and, 850
laxatives and, 918
Fiberoptic endoscopic evaluation of swallowing (FEES), 953
Fibrate, 289, 291, 528
Fibronectin (FN), 75–76
Fibrous tissue, disorders of, 578–579
Filling phase, of bladder, 706–707, 707f
Financial abuse, risk factors for, 961
Finasteride, 709, 709t
Finland, geriatric medicine in, 999
"First language of sex,", 858
Flavoxate hydrochloride, 936–938
Flecainide
for AF, 333
for maintaining sinus rhythm, 333–334
after myocardial infarction, 292–293
for SVT, 336
syncope caused by, 339t
for ventricular arrhythmia, 327–328, 328t
Flexibility activities
for fractured neck, 876
for frailty prevention, 850
Florinef. *See* Fludrocortisone
Flosequinan, 282
Flow phase, of metabolism in victims of trauma, 865–866
Flow volume loops, of airway obstruction, 365, 365f
Fluconazole
for candidiasis, 609, 617
cytochrome P450 reaction with, 141t
for meningitis, 550
for onychomycosis, 805
Flucytosine, 550
Fludarabine, 784–785, 787
Fludrocortisone (Florinef)
for carotid sinus syndrome, 345
for orthostatic hypotension, 343, 343t, 508b, 509–510
for Parkinson's disease, 517
for postprandial hypotension, 347
for vasovagal syncope, 346
Fluid collection management, for acute pancreatitis, 633
Fluid imbalance, surgery and anesthesia in old age and, 239–241
assessment of fluid and electrolyte status, 240
dehydration, 240
fluid and electrolyte therapy, 240–241
fluid regimen over perioperative period, 241
salt and saline depletion, 240
water depletion, 240
Fluid intake, constipation and, 913, 918–919
Fluid intelligence, aging and, 170
Flunarizine, 476
Fluoroquinolone
C. difficile infection and, 664, 666
for CNS infection, 548
for infectious colitis, 665–666
for pneumonia, 377
Fluorouracil, 148t, 674
5-Fluorouracil (5-FU)
for actinic keratosis, 805
for cholangiocarcinoma, 649
for pancreas adenocarcinoma, 631
for skin carcinoma, 805–806
Fluoxetine
codeine and, 969
cytochrome P450 reaction with, 141t
for frontotemporal dementia, 432
for migraine, 468
parkinsonism induced by, 518
for tension headache, 469
for vasovagal syncope, 346
Flutamide, 713
Fluvastatin, 141t
Fluvoxamine, 141t, 432, 969
FN. *See* Fibronectin
FOBTs. *See* Fecal occult blood tests
Focal lesions
of CNS, 549–552
of liver, 644
Focal seizures, 455–456, 455t
Folate, 682, 776–777
Folic acid, 13, 176
Follicular lymphoma, 784–785
Fondaparinux, 360
Food hygiene, longevity due to, 13
Foot disease, 594
dermatologic disorders, 595–596, 596f
with diabetes mellitus, 597–598, 598b, 763–765, 764t–765t, 765b
nail disorders, 596–597
orthopedic/biomechanical disorders, 594–595, 595f
for patients with diabetes, 597–598, 598b
ulcers of legs, feet, and toes, 596–597, 598b, 764, 765t
Footwear, falls and, 901
Forearm fractures, in elderly, 564
Formoterol, 373
Foscarnet, 666
Fosinopril, 140t
Fractures, 577
aging effects on rate of, 118f, 122
in elderly, 564–565
following falls, 868
of neck, therapy techniques for, 875–876
orthopedic geriatrics for, 583–584, 584f
periarticular fractures, 584–585, 585f
periprosthetic fractures, 585, 585f
traumatic fractures, 583–584, 584f
osteoporotic, 554, 583, 585–586
prevention of, 585–586
Fragile X syndrome, 445, 446t–447t
Fragility fractures, 554, 583, 585–586
Frailty, 59, 835, 849–850
care coordination and, 1064
constipation and, 909, 910t
deficit accumulation in relation to, 60–62, 61f
delirium and, 903, 905
dimensions of, 836, 837t
exclusion and "silence by proxy" due to, 204
failure to thrive and, 949
falls prevention for, 843–844
FI and, 909, 910t, 921, 923f
health promotion for, 837–838
heart disease and, 295
age and treatment decisions, 295–298, 296t–297t
manifestations of heart disease in older adults, 298
outcomes of heart disease treatment in older persons, 297, 297t
polypharmacy and cognitive impairment in heart disease, 298–299
home support exercise program for, 843
impaired mobility and, 892–893
introduction to aging, geriatric medicine, and, 1
nursing health promotion for, 843
phenotypic definition of, 60–62, 61f
preventive care for, 837–838, 849–850
in regions of world, 1010–1011
rehabilitation and, 1
resistance exercise and, 862–863
social factors associated with, 203
therapy techniques for, 877–878
environment, 878–879
exercise programs, 878
Frailty index
as clinical state variable, 64–65, 65f, 65t
comprehensive geriatric assessment for use in, 62–65, 63f–65f, 65t
validation of, 62–64, 64f
Free radical stress. *See also* Reactive nitrogen species; Reactive oxygen species
in neurobiology of aging, 150
generation of reactive oxygen/nitrogen species, 151–152

Free radical stress (*Continued*)
metabolic-insulin signaling in control of aging and neurodegeneration, 154–157, 155f–156f
nitrosative and oxidative stress in, 150, 151f–152f
protein misfolding in neurodegenerative disease, 150–151
protein S-nitrosylation and neuronal cell death, 152–154, 153t
in protein damage and sarcopenia of aging, 34–35
Freudian theory, on personality stages and ego development, 178
Friction, pressure ulcers and, 939
Frontal lobe seizures, 456
Frontal variant frontotemporal dementia, 429
Frontotemporal dementia (FTD), 428
biomarkers of, 431–432
clinical presentation of, 429
diagnosis of, 430–431
epidemiology of, 429–430
etiology of, 428–429, 429t
neuropsychology in diagnosis and treatment of, 407, 409t
risk factors for, 385–386
treatment of, 432
Frontotemporal lobar degeneration (FTLD), 428
biomarkers of, 431–432
clinical presentation of, 429
diagnosis of, 430–431
epidemiology of, 429–430
etiology of, 428–429, 429t
treatment of, 432
Frusemide, 278, 278b, 281, 285, 285b, 771
FTD. *See* Frontotemporal dementia
FTLD. *See* Frontotemporal lobar degeneration
5-FU. *See* 5-Fluorouracil
Function based models of care, disease based v., 845
Functional abilities
assessment of, 211–215, 213f, 214t, 898–899
falls and, 898–899
of geriatric patients, social assessment of, 224
obesity and impairment of, 686
Parkinson's disease and, 876–877
stroke and, 874
Functional decline
with delirium, 908
forms of, 870
prevention of, 946
social factors associated with, 202
Functional psychiatric illness, in old age, 433
depression, 433–436
late life psychosis, 436–439
Functional recovery, in older victims of trauma, 866–867
Functional reserve
preoperative estimation of, 233, 233t
successful aging due to, 184–186
Functionalism theory, in social gerontology, 188
Fungal infection, of skin, 804–805
Furosemide
acute pancreatitis due to, 631–632
for ascites, 641
elimination of, 141t
in frail elderly patient, 298
low thyroxine due to, 738
sensitivity to, 141, 141t
Future of old age, 11
current and future biomedical inputs to aging, 13–15
future of aging, 15–17
historical determinants of future health of elderly, 12–13
Future planning, for palliative medicine, 974
Future predictions, in quality of life among older individuals, 5

G

Gabapentin
for chronic daily headache, 469–470
for epilepsy, 462–463, 463t
for neuropathic pain, 977–978
for postherpetic neuralgia, 472, 477b
for trigeminal neuralgia, 477b
for vulval discomfort, 719–720
GAGs. *See* Glycosaminoglycans
Gait
age-related changes in, 103
disorders of, 887–888
with dementia, 390
higher level, 887, 888t
lowest level, 887–888
middle level, 887
initiation of, 887
Galantamine, 400, 419, 419t, 432
Gallbladder
adenocarcinoma of, 648
aging effects on, 107
Gallstones, 646–647
age-related changes in manifestation of, 109
complications of, 647–648
Gamma interferon tests, for tuberculosis, 378
Ganciclovir, 666
Ganglionopathy, autoimmune autonomic, 507–508
GAPs. *See* Geriatric assessment programs
Garlic, herbal-drug interactions of, 142t
GAS. *See* Goal Attainment Scaling
Gastric adenocarcinoma, 624
Gastric lymphoma, 624–625, 625f
Gastric mucosa, injury of, 618–619
Gastric outlet obstruction (GOO), 630–631
Gastric tumors, 624–625, 625f
Gastric ulcers, 622
Gastritis, 619–620, 619f
Gastroduodenal ulcer disease, atypical presentation of, 108
Gastroenterology, aging effects on, 106
altered manifestation of adult gastrointestinal diseases, 107–109
gastrointestinal problems unique to elderly, 109–110
normal physiology of aging, 106–107
Gastroesophageal reflux disease (GERD)
atypical presentation of, 108, 208, 209t
in Down syndrome, 448
insomnia and, 945–946
Gastrointestinal stromal tumors (GISTs), 659
Gastrointestinal (GI) tract. *See also* Upper gastrointestinal tract
bleeding in, 659–660, 674–677, 675t, 676f
diseases of
age-related changes in manifestation of, 107–109
in Down syndrome, 448
of old age, 109–110
normal aging of, 106–107
Gastropathy, NSAIDs and, 619–622, 625b
GCS. *See* Glasgow Coma Scale; Graduated compression stockings
GDP. *See* Gross domestic product
Gefitinib, 383
Gegenhalten. *See* Paratonia
GEM. *See* Geriatric evaluation and management
Gemcitabine, 383, 631, 728–729
Gemtuzumab, 788
Gender
depression in old age and, 433
disparity in successful aging and, 185, 185f
epidemiology of aging and, 6–7, 7f
sleep-disordered breathing and, 946–947
Gene mutations, chromosomal, in aging, 39–41
Gene overexpression, in cell senescence, 47
Gene repression, in cell senescence, 46–47
General anesthetic, delirium and, 233t, 241
Generalized anxiety disorder, 440
Generalized seizures, 455, 455t
Genetic counseling, for Hutchinson-Gilford progeria syndrome, 71
Genetic testing, for frontotemporal dementia, 431
Genetics
aging mechanisms involving, 38
chromosomal gene mutations, 39–41
epigenetics, 41
integrative approach to, 41
mitochondrial genetics, oxidative stress, and aging, 38–39
telomeres, 40–41
of Alzheimer's disease, 412–414
as dementia risk factor, 386
depression in old age and, 433
of frontotemporal dementia, 428–431, 429t
of Hutchinson-Gilford progeria syndrome, 66–68, 68f
of life span, 19–21, 20f
human progeroid syndromes, 20–21
species differences in longevity, 19
variation within species, 20, 20f
sarcopenia and, 590, 593
Genital tract, aging of, 716
Genomic instability, in cell senescence, 46–48
Gentamicin, 663t, 672
GEPMG. *See* Group of European Professors in Medical Gerontology
GERD. *See* Gastroesophageal reflux disease
Geriatric assessment. *See also* Multidimensional geriatric assessment
as outcomes measurement for multidimensional interventions, 246
Geriatric assessment programs (GAPs), 215–217
Geriatric day hospital, 16–17
Geriatric dentistry. *See* Dentistry, geriatric
Geriatric evaluation and management (GEM), for iatrogenic problems prevention, 851
Geriatric individuality, in laboratory medicine, 218–219, 219f
Geriatric interventions. *See* Multidimensional geriatric intervention
Geriatric medicine. *See also* Old age
care of older patients, 1006
clinical governance with, 1044–1045, 1044f
development of, 997, 1005–1010
education in. *See* Education
in Europe, 1000
collaborative research, 1004
organizations, 1000–1001
other countries, 999–1000
United Kingdom, 998–999
introduction to aging, frailty, and, 1
laboratory medicine in. *See* Laboratory medicine
in Latin America, 1016
demographic transition, 1016
development of, 1019, 1019t
epidemiologic transition, 1016–1017
health in, 1018, 1018t
perspectives of, 1019–1020
research, 1019, 1020t
retirement policies, 1017–1018, 1017t
rural health in, 1018–1019

Geriatric medicine (*Continued*)
monitoring in, 220–221
in North America, 1005
future direction, 1008–1010
specialty practice in, 1006–1008, 1007t
social assessment in. *See* Social assessment, of geriatric patients
in world, 1010
chronic disease and functional decline prevention, 1015
chronic diseases of major impact, 1010
communicable diseases, 1011–1012
comprehensive geriatric assessment, 1013
development of, 1012–1013
frailty, 1010–1011
health and social services, 1013–1015
life expectancy, morbidity, and disability, 1010
Geriatric minimum data set (GMDS), 28t
Geriatric oncology. *See* Cancer
Geriatric orthopedics. *See* Orthopedic geriatrics
Geriatric pharmacotherapy. *See* Pharmacotherapy, geriatric
Geriatric psychiatry, 1007
Geriatric Trauma Survival Score, 867
Geriatric ulcers, 621–622, 621f
Geriatrician, work of, in United Kingdom, 998–999, 999t
Germany, geriatric medicine in, 999
Gerontology. *See also* Social gerontology
definition of, 1
GFR. *See* Glomerular filtration rate
GH. *See* Growth hormone
Ghrelin agonists, 147
GI tract. *See* Gastrointestinal tract
Giant cell arteritis, 580, 581f, 818
arthritis in, 573
headache due to, 473–474
Giant duodenal ulcers, 622, 622f
Giant gastric ulcers, 622
Ginger, 142t
Gingko, 142t, 400
Ginseng, 142t, 164
GISTs. *See* Gastrointestinal stromal tumors
Glabellar tap reflex, aging effects on, 105
Glasgow Coma Scale (GCS), 867
Glasgow Scoring System, for acute pancreatitis, 632, 632t
Glaucoma, 813–814, 813f, 813b
Glibenclamide, 142t, 768, 771
Gliclazide, 768
Gliomas, 537–538
Glitazones, 413–414
Glomerular filtration rate (GFR), 111, 690, 691t
Glomerulonephritis, 692, 693t
Glossopharyngeal neuralgia, 471–472
Glucagon, 616, 771
Glucagon stimulation test, 732
Glucocorticoid therapy
for Addison's disease, 732–733
for arthritis, 570
diabetes secondary to, 760
for hypothyroidism, 748, 754b
for intracranial tumors, 536–537, 538b
osteoporosis due to, 555, 585–586
for stomatitis, 609
Glucocorticoids
excess of, 732–734
physiologic responses to, 730
regulation of production of, 731
Glucosamine, 15, 142t
Glucose control, in diabetes mellitus, 767–768, 768t–770t, 768b
choice of treatment for glucose control, 770
monitoring of, 771
pathologic basis for treatment of type 2 diabetes, 767–768
treatments for glucose control, 768–770, 769t–770t
Glucose homeostasis, aging effects on, 57, 57f
Glucose intolerance, in older victims of trauma, 866
Glucose regulators, for glucose control, 769
Glucose testing, for diagnosing stroke risk factors, 492
Glucose tolerance
impairment of, with aging, 761, 761f, 762t
successful aging and, 860–861
α-Glucosidase inhibitors, 768b
Glutamate, age-related perception of pain and, 966
Glutamatergic signaling pathways, NMDA receptors mediation of, 151–152
Glycerin, 820, 920–921
Glycerol injection, 471
Glycoproteins, of connective tissues, 75–77
entactin/nidogen, 76
fibronectin, 75–76
integrins and cell attachment proteins, 77
laminin, 76
thrombospondin, 76–77
Glycopyrronium, 980
Glycosaminoglycans (GAGs)
of connective tissues, 75, 75t
in dermis, aging effects on, 135
Glycosylation, in aging of connective tissues, 79
GMDS. *See* Geriatric minimum data set
GnRH agonists, 167
GnRH antagonists, 167
Goal Attainment Scaling (GAS)
for measuring outcomes of multidimensional interventions, 247–249, 247t–248t
for pain, 971
Goal-setting
for rehabilitation, 13
for therapy, 872
Gold, for arthritis, 569t
Gold salts, taste perception and, 608
Gold Standards Framework in Care Homes, 975
Golden age, 188–189
GOO. *See* Gastric outlet obstruction
Gossypol, 142t
Gout, 209t, 210, 573–574, 581
Graduated compression stockings (GCS), for venous thromboembolism, 360
Graduates, late life psychosis in, 439
Grand mal seizure, 455
Granulocytes, aging of, 130
Granulocyte-stimulating factor, 778–779, 788
Grasp reflex, age-related changes in, 104–105
Griseofulvin, 805
Gross domestic product (GDP), 993
Group of European Professors in Medical Gerontology (GEPMG), 1003
Group settings, social assessment within, 228
Growth factors, in aging of connective tissues, 77–78
Growth hormone (GH)
age effects on, 123–124
deficiency of, 735–736
sarcopenia and, 589
Growth hormone therapy, 735–736
as antiaging medicine, 147
for appetite stimulation, 955
for bone loss prevention, 121
risks and benefits of, 123–124
for sarcopenia, 589, 591–592
Growth hormone/insulin-like growth factor-I axis, aging of, 123–124
Guaifenesin, 373
Guanethidine, 339t
Guar gum, 142t
Gugging swallow screen (GUSS), 953
GUSS. *See* Gugging swallow screen
Gustatory sensation, aging effects on, 106
Gut management, for acute pancreatitis, 632
Gynecologic disorders, 716
age-associated changes in genital tract, 716
anatomic changes, 716
hormone changes, 716
cancer, 721–724, 723t
of cervix, 722, 794–795
of corpus uteri, 722–723
of ovary, 723–724, 723t
of vagina, 722
of vulva, 722
menopause. *See* Menopause
sexuality and aging, 724–725
management of couples with sexual problems, 725
sexual behavior and age, 724–725
sexual response and age, 725
urinary incontinence, 721
uterovaginal prolapse, 720
vulval disorders, 718–720, 719t
dermatologic conditions, 718–719
premalignant disorders, 719, 719t
symptoms of, 718
vulval discomfort, 719–720

H

H_1-antihistamines, 141t
H_2 blockers, 99–100
HABAM. *See* Hierarchical assessment of balance and mobility
Hair, aging of, 136
"Hairy tongue," 609
Haloperidol, 140t, 639, 906–907, 969, 978
Halothane, 231, 643
Handicap
assessment of, 10–11
mobility, 10
after stroke, 494
Hartford Foundation, geriatric medicine education and, 1032
HAS. *See* Health Advisory Service
HATS. *See* Hearing assistive technologies
HAV. *See* Hepatitis A
Hawthorne, 142t
HBV infection. *See* Hepatitis B
HCC. *See* Hepatocellular carcinoma
HCV. *See* Hepatitis C
HE. *See* Hepatic encephalopathy
Head injuries, in older people, 867
Head trauma, dementia and, 386, 388
Headache, 466
diagnostic approach to, 476–477
drug-induced, 475, 475t
eye and, 475–476
intracranial tumors and, 474–475
low-pressure headache syndrome, 475
miscellaneous causes, 476
from neck, 472–473
primary headache disorders, 466–467
chronic daily headache, 469–470, 470t
cluster headache, 470
migraine, 466, 468t
tension headache, 469
from sinus disease and dental disease, 473
with trauma, 474

Headache (*Continued*)
vascular disorders and, 473–474
carotid and vertebral artery dissection, 474
cerebrovascular disease and hypertension, 474
chronic subdural hemorrhage, 474
giant cell arteritis, 473–474
subarachnoid hemorrhage, 474
Health Advisory Service (HAS), 1023
Health care
in Europe, 997
use of, as outcomes measurement for multidimensional interventions, 245, 248–265, 266–267
Health in old age
cognitive functioning in response to, 176
depression and, 434
oral health effects on, 602–603
personality stage theories and, 179
personality trait theories and, 180
self-rated, as outcomes measurement for multidimensional interventions, 245, 248–265, 266–267
social associations with, 201–204
social capital and, 199
social cohesion and, 199
social engagement and, 199
social isolation and, 199
social networks and, 199
social support and, 198
social vulnerability and, 199
social-cognitive theories to personality and, 182
socioeconomic status and, 198
study of social influences on, 199–201, 200t
Health maintenance organizations (HMOs), 1057
Health Plan Employer Data and Information Set (HEDIS), 1047
Health promotion, 842
for community-living older adult, 835
benefits of, 835
economic evaluation framework, 838, 839f
intervention study lessons, 842–845
legislation and policy needs, 845–846
lessons learned, 844–845
need for, 836–837
research needs, 845–846
screening and assessment for, 838–842
for frail older adults, 837–838
for older adults with intellectual disability, 451–452
participatory approach to, 842
preventive care v., 842
Health risk assessment (HRA), 1059
Health screening tools, for older adults with intellectual disability, 449
Health service use, comorbidity v., 835
Health services, in regions of world, 1013–1015
end of life care, 1014–1015
long-term care, 1014
secondary health care, 1013–1014
Health services approach, to reduce medication problems, 883
Health status
individualizing prevention and, 852
in Latin America, 1018, 1018t
rural, 1018–1019
Health systems design, to reduce medication problems, 883
Healthcare Commission, 1043–1044
HealthGrades, 1047
Hearing
aging effects on, 102
in Down syndrome, 448
loss of, 822
Hearing (*Continued*)
age-related changes within auditory system, 822–824
behavioral implications of anatomic and physiologic changes, 824–825, 825t
demographics of aging and hearing loss, 822
psychosocial consequences of decrements in pure-tone sensitivity and speech understanding, 825–826
referral to specialists for, 833–834
screening for, 832–833, 833f, 833t
technologies for, 826–832, 827t, 828f, 829t–830t, 831f
Hearing aids, 826–832, 827t, 828f, 829t–830t
bone-anchored, 830–832
Hearing assistive technologies (HATS), 830–832, 831f
Hearing Handicap Inventory for the Elderly (HHIE-S), 832–833, 833f, 833t
Heart, aging of
myocardial function in, 94–95, 96t
response to exercise and, 95–96, 96t
structural changes in, 93–94, 96t
Heart disease. *See also* Valvular heart disease
clinical manifestations of, in older adults, 298
as complication of hypertension, 304
in Down syndrome, 448
in frail elderly patient, 295
age and treatment decisions, 295–298, 296t–297t
manifestations of heart disease in older adults, 298
outcomes of heart disease treatment in older persons, 297, 297t
polypharmacy and cognitive impairment in heart disease, 298–299
insomnia and, 945–946
ventricular arrhythmia prognosis and, 327
Heart failure (HF), 848–849. *See also* Chronic cardiac failure
Heart failure nurse, role of, 282
Heart failure with preserved systolic function (HFPSF), 273–274
Heart murmur
of acute mitral regurgitation, 324
of aortic regurgitation, 318
of aortic stenosis, 313–314, 313t
of chronic mitral regurgitation, 324
of mitral regurgitation in patients with mitral annular calcium, 321–322, 321t–322t
of mitral stenosis, 323–324
of mitral stenosis in patients with mitral annular calcium, 321t–322t, 322
Heart rate, autonomic testing using, 498–501
Heartburn, 612–613
Heat-induced hypotension, 503–504
HEDIS. *See* Health Plan Employer Data and Information Set
Hematology. *See* Blood disorders
Hematopoiesis, 127–128
Hematopoietic stem cells (HSCs)
aging effects on, 127–128
epigenetics of, 129
progenitor cells derived from, 129–130
Hemiballismus, 519
Hemiparesis, gait and, 887
Hemochromatosis, 640–641
Hemodialysis, 694
Hemodynamic instability, with pulmonary embolism, 359
Hemorrhage
subarachnoid, headache with, 474
subconjunctival, 811, 811f
subdural, headache with, 474
upper gastrointestinal, 623
Hemorrhagic stroke, 485, 485f
acute treatment of, 493
diagnosis of, 489, 491f
intracerebral, 479
pathologic mechanisms underlying, 482–483
subarachnoid, 479
Hemostasis, disorders of, 789–791
Heparin. *See also* Low molecular weight heparin; Unfractionated heparin
for acute arterial mesenteric ischemia, 657–658
for acute coronary syndromes, 291
for acute thrombosis, 349
for disseminated intravascular coagulation, 790
for femoral embolism, 349
functional recovery and, 866–867
herbal-drug interactions of, 142t
for hyperglycemic coma, 772
hyperkalemia due to, 698
laboratory results affected by, 221t
for lower GI bleeding diagnosis, 677
osteoporosis due to, 585
for STEMI, 291
for stroke, 492–493
thrombocytopenia associated with, 789
for uterovaginal prolapse surgery, 720
for venous thromboembolism, 357, 360, 360b
Hepatic encephalopathy (HE), 642
Hepatic metabolism, of drugs, 140, 140t, 635–636
Hepatitis
age-related changes in manifestation of, 109
autoimmune, 640, 643
ischemic, 643
Hepatitis A (HAV), acute infection with, 643
Hepatitis B (HBV), 638, 643
Hepatitis C (HCV), 638–639, 643
Hepatitis E (HEV), 643
Hepatocellular carcinoma (HCC), 638–639, 642
Hepatorenal syndrome (HRS), 642
Herbal-drug interactions, 142t, 143
Herceptin, 16
Heritability, in successful aging, 185–186
Hernia
hiatal, 614, 614f
paraesophageal, 614, 614f
Herpes simplex encephalitis, 550–551, 550b
Herpes zoster, 88, 803–804
HEV. *See* Hepatitis E
Hexamethonium, 339t
Hexobarbital, 139–140
HF. *See* Heart failure
HFPSF. *See* Heart failure with preserved systolic function
HGPS. *See* Hutchinson-Gilford progeria syndrome
HHIE-S. *See* Hearing Handicap Inventory for the Elderly
Hiatus hernia, 614, 614f
HiCy. *See* High-dose cyclophosphamide
Hierarchical assessment of balance and mobility (HABAM), 889, 890f
High pressure/low flow voiding, 708–709, 709t
High-dose cyclophosphamide (HiCy), 132
Higher level gait disorders, 887, 888t
High-risk approach, to stroke prevention, 481–482
Hip fractures, in elderly, 565–566
Hip protectors, 558, 902
Hirudin, 789
Histamine antagonists, 622–623
Histamine blockers, 15–16, 89
Histology, of pancreas, 626

Histopathology
of asthma, 364
of Crohn's disease, 669
of large bowel, 662
Historical determinants, of future health of elderly, 12–13
History. *See also* Clinical history, Family history, Natural history
of antiaging medicine, 145–146
of geriatric assessment, 211
of vascular cognitive impairment, 421
History taking
for dementia diagnosis, 395
for neuromuscular disorders, 520–521, 524t
HIV, as secondary cause of acquired immunodeficiency in old age, 89
HL. *See* Hodgkin lymphoma
HMOs. *See* Health maintenance organizations
Hodgkin lymphoma (HL), 783, 786
Home support exercise program (HSEP), 843
Home visit, stroke therapy and, 875
Home-based assessment
of disability and rehabilitation, 11
office-based assessment v., 838–839
Home-based rehabilitation, 15–16
Homeostasis, calcium, in cellular aging, 44–45
Homeostatic mechanisms, aging effects on, altered pharmacodynamics and, 141
Homocysteine, 13
HONK coma. *See* Hyperglycemic hyperosmolar nonketotic coma
Hormonal manipulation, 798–799
for breast cancer, 727–729, 727t–728t, 798–799
for prostate cancer, 713–715
Hormone replacement therapy (HRT)
as antiaging medicine, 147–148, 147t
for bone loss, 56
for CAD, 293–294, 293t
cardiovascular risk and, 303
dental implant failure with, 605
for immune function improvement in old age, 83
longevity due to, 14
in menopause, 124, 716–718
migraine and, 467
OA response to, 119
for osteoporosis, 556, 558, 586
for reproductive aging in men, 167
for reproductive aging in women, 164–167
sarcopenia and, 589
sexual motivation and, 724–725
skin aging response to, 136
stroke risk and, 480, 480t
uterine cancer and, 722–723
Hormones, age-associated changes in, 716
Horseradish, 142t
Hospice care, in United States, 1028
Hospital
epidemiology of drug use in, 138
iatrogenic problems and, 851
quality measurement of, 1049–1050
Hospital Quality Alliance (HQA), 1046, 1049–1050
Host defense, pulmonary, age-related changes in, 99–101
Hot flashes, 163–165
Housebound elderly, diabetes mellitus in, 766–767, 767t, 767b
Household environments, accident prevention and, 850–851
HPA axis. *See* Hypothalamic-pituitary-adrenal axis
HQA. *See* Hospital Quality Alliance
HRA. *See* Health risk assessment
HRS. *See* Hepatorenal syndrome
HRT. *See* Hormone replacement therapy
HSCs. *See* Hematopoietic stem cells
HSEP. *See* Home support exercise program
Human growth hormone. *See* Growth hormone
Hungary
demographics in, 991
geriatric medicine in, 999
Hutchinson-Gilford progeria syndrome (HGPS), 21
arteriosclerosis in, 70–71
clinical care for, 71–72
farnesylation of progerin in, 68
insights into normal aging from, 66
description of HGPS, 66, 67f
molecular genetics and cell biology, 66–68, 68f
similarities and differences between aging and HGPS, 68–71, 69f
normal aging and, 33–34
Hydralazine
for aortic regurgitation, 319
for chronic cardiac failure, 281–282
in frail elderly patient, 298
glomerulonephritis due to, 693t
headache due to, 475t
for hypertension, 309
syncope caused by, 339t
Hydration
at end of life, 957–958
malnutrition and, 953–954, 953t
Hydrochlorothiazide, 296, 298
Hydrocolloid dressings, for pressure ulcers, 941
Hydrocortisone, 609, 667–668, 667t, 735–736, 802
Hydrogels, 941
Hydromorphone, 969
α-Hydroxy acids, 802
Hydroxychloroquine, 569t, 819–820
1α-Hydroxycolecalciferol, 756
α-Hydroxyl acids, 148t
β-Hydroxyl acids, 148t
Hydroxyurea, 780
Hyoscine butylbromide, 980
Hyoscine hydrobromide, 980
Hyoscyamine, 663t
Hyperbaric oxygen therapy, for pressure ulcers, 941
Hypercalcemia
confusion and, 981
constipation and, 914
with primary hyperparathyroidism, 756–758, 757f–758f, 757t, 757b
Hyperfiltration theory, 112
Hyperglycemic coma, 771–772, 771b
Hyperglycemic hyperosmolar nonketotic (HONK) coma, 771–772
Hyperkalemia, 698, 698t
Hyperkinetic movement disorders, 518–519
chorea, 519
drug-induced disorders, 519
dystonia, 519
essential tremor, 518–519
restless legs syndrome, 519
Hypernatremia, 697–698
Hyperparathyroidism
lithium-induced, 758, 758b
primary, 756–758, 757f–758f, 757t, 757b
secondary, 756, 756b
tertiary, 758–759, 759f, 759b
Hyperphosphatemia, 699–700, 699t
Hypersensitivity. *See* Carotid sinus hypersensitivity
Hypersensitivity pneumonitis, 382
Hypertension, 300
arterial stiffness effects on, 93, 93f
as CAD risk factor, 288–289
complications of, 303–304
asymptomatic cerebrovascular disease, 303
cognitive impairment, 303–304
heart disease, 304
stroke, 303
in diabetes mellitus patients, 772
diagnosis and evaluation of, 304–305
ambulatory blood pressure monitoring, 304
clinical assessment and investigations, 304–305
general issues, 304
measuring blood pressure, 304
epidemiology of, 300–301, 301f
blood pressure and cardiovascular risk, 300–301
prevalence and incidence, 300
pulse pressure and risk, 301, 301f
systolic blood pressure, diastolic blood pressure, and risk, 301
headache with, 474
management of, 305–309, 305t, 306f
drug treatments, 308–309
nonpharmacologic methods, 307–308
prophylaxis, 307
published trials, 305–306, 305t, 306f
statin use, 307
orthostatic hypotension and, 342
other cardiovascular risk factors and, 302–303
AF and left ventricular hypertrophy, 302
alcohol and diet, 303
body mass index, 302
diabetes mellitus, 302
hormone replacement, 303
lipid abnormalities, 302
physical exercise, 303
smoking, 302
pathogenesis of, 301–302
portal, 641
in special cases, 309–311
80 and over group, 309–310
cognitive function, dementia, and quality of life, 310
stroke, 310–311
type 2 diabetes, 310
stroke and, 303, 310–311, 480–481, 496
supine, 510
telemedicine for, 1066
Hyperthyroidism, 740–743, 741t–742t, 808
acute, 743
AF and, 743
clinical presentation of, 741–742, 742t
demography of, 740
diagnosis of, 742
etiology of, 740–741
management of, 742–743, 754b
subclinical, 743–745, 744t, 754b
T_3 toxicosis, 741
Hypnic headache syndrome, 476
Hypnotics
dementia due to, 417
falls due to, 208
fatigue due to, 206–207
as secondary cause of acquired immunodeficiency in old age, 89
Hypoaldosteronism, 733
Hypoglycemia, 767, 768t, 771

Hypoglycemic drugs
for diabetes mellitus, 767–768, 768t–770t, 768b
choice of treatment for glucose control, 770
pathologic basis for treatment of type 2 diabetes, 767–768
treatments for glucose control, 768–770, 769t–770t
orthostatic hypotension and, 503
as secondary cause of acquired immunodeficiency in old age, 89
Hypokalemia, 914
Hypomagnesemia, 914
Hypoparathyroidism, 759–760
Hypophosphatemia, 699–700, 699t
Hypopituitarism, 735–737
Hypotension. *See also* Orthostatic hypotension
postprandial, 346–347, 503–504, 510
Hypothalamic-pituitary-adrenal (HPA) axis
aging of, 125–126
in older victims of trauma, 865
Hypothalamic-pituitary-thyroid axis, aging of, 126
Hypothalamic-pituitary-thyroid regulation, 737
Hypothyroidism, 741t, 745–748, 808
clinical presentation of, 746–747
demography of, 745
in Down syndrome, 448
etiology of, 745–746
laboratory diagnosis of, 747
myxedema coma, 747–748
subclinical, 748–750, 749t, 754b
therapy for, 747–748, 754b
Hypoxemia, postoperative, 234–235

I

IADLs. *See* Instrumental activities of daily living
IAGG. *See* International Association of Gerontology and Geriatrics
Iatrogenic glucocorticoid excess, 734
Iatrogenic problem prevention, 851
Ibandronate, 556, 556t, 586
IBD. *See* Inflammatory bowel disease
IBM. *See* Inclusion body myositis
Ibuprofen, 467–468, 510, 568, 568t, 635–636
Ibutilide, 333, 335
ICD-10. *See* International Classification of Diseases-Tenth Edition
ICDs. *See* Implantable cardioverter-defibrillators
Iceland, geriatric medicine in, 999
ICIDH. *See* International Classification of Impairments, Diseases and Handicap
ICIDH-2. *See* International Classification of Impairments, Diseases and Handicap, revised
ICP. *See* Integrated care pathway
IDEATel project. *See* Informatics for Diabetes Education and Telemedicine project
Identity, self and, 181
Idiopathic focal epilepsy, 456
Idiopathic generalized epilepsy (IGE), 456
Idiopathic parkinsonism. *See* Parkinson's disease
Idiopathic pulmonary fibrosis (IPF), 380–381, 380f
Idiopathic thrombocytopenic purpura (ITP), 789
IGE. *See* Idiopathic generalized epilepsy
IGF-I. *See* Insulin-like growth factor-I
IIS. *See* Insulin/insulin-like growth factor-I signaling
IL-2. *See* Interleukin-2
IL-6. *See* Interleukin-6
IL-10. *See* Interleukin-10
Ileocolitis, in Crohn's disease, 670
ILI. *See* Influenza-like illness
Imaging. *See also* Neuroimaging
for adrenal disease, 733
in arthritis, 567–568, 567t
of brain
for intracranial tumor diagnosis, 535
of late-onset schizophrenia, 437–438
for primary autonomic failure, 506–507, 506f
for stroke, 489–490, 491f
of large bowel, 661–662
of pancreas adenocarcinoma, 628–629
of thyroid, 739
Imatinib, 659, 781
Imipramine
liver metabolism of, 635–636
for maintaining sinus rhythm, 333–334
metabolism of, 140t
for overactive bladder, 721
for urinary incontinence, 935
for ventricular arrhythmia, 328
Imiquimod, 805–807
Immigration, in epidemiology of aging, 9, 9t
Immobility
community-living older adult and, 892
in older people, 889–892
Immune function
assessment of, 89
of skin, aging effects on, 136
Immune response, of respiratory system, age-related changes in, 99–100
Immune-mediated connective tissue disease, 580, 581f
Immunization. *See* Vaccination
Immunodeficiency. *See* Acquired immunodeficiency
Immunoglobulins, thyroid-stimulating, 740
Immunologic markers, of aging, 85t
Immunologic tests, for arthritis, 566–567
Immunology, 82
changes in human immune system with aging, 82–85, 85t, 86f
B-cell function changes, 84–85
cell lysis changes, 83
cytokine dysregulation, 85, 85t, 86f
nonspecific host defense changes, 82
phagocytosis changes, 82–83
specific host defense changes, 83
T-cell function changes, 83–84
clinical consequences of immune senescence, 85–88
autoimmunity, 85–86
cancer, 86–87
infection, 87
influenza, 87–88
pneumococcal disease, 88
varicella zoster virus, 88
immune enhancement, 89
immune function assessment, 89
secondary causes of acquired immunodeficiency in old age, 88–90
comorbidity, 89
HIV and other infections, 89
malnutrition, 88
polypharmacy, 89
stress, 89
Immunosuppressants
for arthritis, 569, 569t
candidiasis associated with, 617
for celiac disease, 654
for Crohn's disease, 656–657
for dementia, 400
glucuronidation of, 645
for myasthenia gravis, 530–532
for polymyositis or dermatomyositis, 527
Immunosuppressants (*Continued*)
for primary biliary cirrhosis, 640
for rheumatoid arthritis, 541
for uveitis, 812
Impaired glucose tolerance, with aging, 761, 761f, 762t
Impaired mobility, 886
age-related changes, 886–887
executive function, 886
gait initiation, 887
rising from chair, 887
walking speed, 886
balance and mobility assessment, 888–889
frailty and, 892–893
gait disorders, 887–888
immobility, 889–892
Implant
for ED, 858
oral, 604–605, 605f
Implantable cardioverter-defibrillators (ICDs), 284
Implantable hearing devices, 830–832, 831f
Implicit memory, aging effects on, 172–173
Impotence, age and, 854
In situ carcinoma, of breast, 727
In vitro diagnosis, objectivity as basic principle of, 218
Incentive creation, for preventive practice systems, 853
Incidentaloma, 734–735
Inclusion body myositis (IBM), 528
Incompetent patient
decision making for, 984–985
ethical issues involving, 984
research and, 985–986
Incontinence. *See* Fecal incontinence; Urinary incontinence
Indapamide
for blood pressure control in diabetes mellitus patients, 772
for CAD prevention, 288
in frail elderly patient, 295
for stroke, 310–311, 495–496
for vascular cognitive impairment, 426–427
Indices of dependency, 8
Individuality. *See* Geriatric individuality
Individualized assessment, for measuring outcomes of multidimensional interventions, 247–249, 247t–248t
Indomethacin
drug interactions of, 143
for headache, 470, 476
headache due to, 475t
for orthostatic hypotension, 510
for postprandial hypotension, 347
Indoramin, 709t
Indwelling catheters, for urinary incontinence, 938
Inequalities
in later life, 190–191
among older people, 9
Infection
of bone, 577
of CNS, 546
focal lesions, encephalitis, and chronic meningitis, 549–552, 550b
meningitis, 546–549, 548f, 548t
dementia associated with, 388
immune senescence and, 87
of large bowel, 664–666, 665t
of prostate, 705
respiratory, 99–100, 376
as secondary cause of acquired immunodeficiency in old age, 89
of skin, 803–805
of urinary tract, 209t, 210, 690–691

Inferior vena caval filters, 359
Inflammation
in aging of connective tissues, 77–78
anemia of, 776
with COPD, 372, 372t
dementia associated with, 387
Inflammatory bowel disease (IBD), 666–667, 667t
age-related changes in manifestation of, 109
Crohn's disease, 655–657, 666, 669, 669t
age-related changes in manifestation of, 109
clinical picture and investigations of, 656
management of, 656–657
ulcerative colitis, 666–667, 667t
Inflammatory markers, for stroke, 492
Inflammatory myopathy, 526–528
Infliximab
for arthritis, 570t
for Crohn's disease, 656–657, 669t, 670
for ulcerative colitis, 667t, 668
Influenza, 87–88, 376
Influenza-like illness (ILI), in regions of world, 1012
Informatics for Diabetes Education and Telemedicine (IDEATel) project, 1066
Information systems, for preventive practice systems, 853
Informed consent, for conducting research involving older individuals, 26–27
Injury
definition of, 865
in old age, 865
injury assessment and outcome measurement, 867
patterns of, 867–869
physiological changes in, 865–866
recovery in, 866–867
of spinal cord, 543
Injury Severity Score (ISS), 867
Innate immunity. *See* Primary immunity
Inotropes, 282
Insomnia, 943
architecture changes in sleep, 943–945
comorbidity with, 945–946
epidemiology of, 943, 944t
natural history of, 943, 945t
periodic limb movements in sleep, 947
rapid eye movement sleep behavior disorder, 947
restless leg syndrome, 947
sleep-disordered breathing, 946–947
treatment for, 946
Institute of Medicine (IOM)
Pay-for-performance and, 1048
quality health care, 1046
quality of care and, 1054
safety errors, 1046
Institutional abuse, risk factors for, 961
Institutionalization
for delirium, 908
rates of, 835
social factors associated with, 202–203
Instrumental activities of daily living (IADLs)
dementia effects on, 409–410
occupational therapy for, 871
in social functioning, 224
Insulin
for acute renal failure, 693
for glucose control, 767, 768t, 768b, 769–771, 770t, 774b
for hyperglycemic coma, 771b, 772
after myocardial infarction, 773
orthostatic hypotension and, 508b
protein metabolism and, 861–862
Insulin (*Continued*)
sarcopenia and, 588–589
thrombocytopenia associated with, 789
Insulin resistance, in older victims of trauma, 866
Insulin signaling, in control of aging and neurodegeneration, 154–157, 155f–156f
Insulin/insulin-like growth factor-I signaling (IIS)
aging effects on, 49
lifespan-affecting modulations of, 10020#s0065
longevity regulation and, 30–32, 31f
mechanisms by which lifespan and neurodegenerative disease are affected by, 10020#s0070
mutations affecting, 39
organismal aging and, 10020#s0060, 155f
Insulin-like growth factor-I (IGF-I), 123–124, 589
Integrated Care Pathway (ICP), 12–13, 975
Integrated model, of geriatric medicine, 997
Integrins, 77
Intellectual disability, 445
communication with older adults with, 451
definitions and etiology of, 445, 446t
epidemiology of, 445–447, 446t
health assessment in older adults with, 449–451, 450f, 451t
health promotion for older adults with, 451–452
syndromic and nonsyndromic age-related disease in, 447–449
syndromic and nonsyndromic biologic aging in, 447
Intelligence, aging and, 170–171
cognitive reserve, 171
premorbid ability, 170
Interconnectedness, of health in old age, 59–60, 60f
Interdisciplinary team care, for rehabilitation, 12
Interferon, 659, 807
Interferon α, 631, 638–639
Interindividual variation, in geriatric reference intervals, 219
Interleukin-2 (IL-2), 85
Interleukin-6 (IL-6), 85
Interleukin-10 (IL-10), 15
Intermediate care services, 4–5, 4t, 5b
Intermittent claudication. *See* Claudication
International Association of Gerontology and Geriatrics (IAGG), 1000–1001, 1002t
International Classification of Diseases-Tenth Edition (ICD-10), delirium and, 903
International Classification of Impairments, Diseases and Handicap, revised (ICIDH-2), 6–7, 7f
International Classification of Impairments, Diseases and Handicap (ICIDH), 6
International Continence Society, 928
International perspective on elderly in society, 988
demographic trends, 988–991, 989t–990t, 992t
early retirement, 995
inequality of longevity, 988
pension systems, 993–994
privatization experiences, 994–995
social protection for old age, 991–993
Internet, elderly care and, 1066–1067, 1067t
Interspecies variation, in physiologic deterioration, 53
Interstitial lung disease, drug-induced, 381
Intervertebral discs, 121, 578
Intracellular calcium, in cellular aging, 44–45
Intracerebral hemorrhage, 479, 485, 493
Intracranial tumors, 533
classification of, 533
clinical presentation of, 534–535
epidemiology of, 533–534
headache due to, 474–475
investigations and diagnosis of, 535–536
management algorithm for, 536b
treatment of, 536–538
Intraductal papillary mucinous neoplasm (IPMN), of pancreas, 627
Intradural tumors, spinal cord compression from, 542
Intramural pseudodiverticulosis, 616–617, 617f
Intraspecies variation, in physiologic deterioration, 53
Intravascular volume, reduced, 508
Intravenous immunoglobulin (IVIG)
for autoimmune autonomic ganglionopathy, 507–508
for idiopathic thrombocytopenic purpura, 789
for inclusion body myositis, 528
for myasthenia gravis, 532
for polymyositis or dermatomyositis, 527
Intravenous urogram, for prostate assessment, 702–703, 703f
Intrinsic aging, of skin, 133
Intrinsic living processes, damage resulting from, 51
Intrinsic renal failure, 691–692, 693t
Intubation, for Hutchinson-Gilford progeria syndrome, 71
Invasive intervention, for ventricular arrhythmias, 329
Involutional bone loss, 554
Iodide, 740–741, 743, 745, 754b
Iodine, 740–742, 741t, 745. *See also* Radioactive iodine
Iodine uptake, measures of, 739
Iodoquinol, 666
IOM. *See* Institute of Medicine
IPF. *See* Idiopathic pulmonary fibrosis
IPMN. *See* Intraductal papillary mucinous neoplasm
Ipratropium, 373
Ireland, geriatric medicine in, 1000
Irinotecan SN-38, 645
Iron
constipation and, 912–913
drug interactions of, 141
fecal occult blood tests and, 662
herbal-drug interactions of, 142t
for lower gastrointestinal bleeding, 675
Iron chelating therapy, for myelodysplasia, 778–779
Iron deficiency anemia, 776
Ischemia
colonic, 671–672
of limbs
management of acute thrombosis, 349, 350f
management of femoral embolism, 349
outcome of limb salvage for, 349, 350f
mesenteric, 657–658
myocardial, of CAD, 286–287
noninfarct, vascular cognitive impairment associated with, 423
small bowel, 657
Ischemic hepatitis, 643
Ischemic stroke, 479
acute treatment of, 492
CT of, 489
echocardiography of, 490–491
pathologic mechanisms underlying, 482
subtypes of, 485–486, 486t
thrombolysis for, 493

Islet cell tumors, of pancreas, 627
Isoflurane, 231
Isolation. *See* Social isolation
Isoniazid, 110b, 378, 550
Isophane, 770
Isoprenaline, 346
Isosorbide dinitrate, 281–282, 298
ISS. *See* Injury Severity Score
Italy, geriatric medicine in, 1000
ITP. *See* Idiopathic thrombocytopenic purpura
Itraconazole (Sporanox), 596, 805
Ivermectin, 804
IVIG. *See* Intravenous immunoglobulin

J

Japan
  demographics in, 990–991
  productive aging in, 196
Jaundice, 628, 630. *See also* Biliary tract diseases
JIPs. *See* Joint Investment Plans
Joint arthroplasty, 584
Joint Investment Plans (JIPs), 4–5
Joint replacement surgery, for pain, 971
Joint Royal Colleges Training Board, 998
Joints
  aging of, 117, 118f
    articular cartilage, 117–119, 118f–119f
    consequences of, 122
    future of, 122–123
    skeleton, 119–121, 119f–120f
    soft tissues, 121–122
  in foot, orthopedic/biomechanical disorders of, 594

K

KA. *See* Keratoacanthoma
Kaolin-pectin, 609
Kaposi sarcoma (KS), 807
Kava, 142t, 164
Kelp, 142t
Keratinocytes, aging effects on, 134
Keratoacanthoma (KA), 806
Ketamine, 978
Ketoacidosis. *See* Diabetic ketoacidosis
Ketoconazole, 141t–142t, 698, 802
Kidney, aging of, 54–55, 54f, 111–112
  glomerular filtration rate, 111
  mechanistic considerations, 112
  renal blood flow, 111
  structural changes, 112
  system-based perspective of, 112
  tubular function, 111–112
Kidney disease, 690
  acute renal failure, 691, 692t
    immediate management of, 693
    intrinsic, 691–692, 693t
    postrenal, 692–693
    prerenal, 691
    subsequent management of, 693–694, 694t
  chronic, 694–696, 695t
    anemia and, 777
    cutaneous complications of, 808
  cutaneous complications of, 808
  diagnostic problems in older adults, 690, 691t–693t
    atypical disease presentation, 690
    renal function measurement, 690, 691t
    urine specimen collection and interpretation, 690
    UTIs, 690–691
  established renal failure, 696
  renal replacement therapy for, 694
Klinefelter syndrome, 445, 446t
KS. *See* Kaposi sarcoma

L

Labetalol, 339t
Laboratory medicine
  for Alzheimer's disease diagnosis, 416–417, 416t
  for COPD, 372
  for dementia diagnosis, 390–391, 396
  in geriatrics, 218
    geriatric individuality, 218–219, 219f
    medical significance of laboratory results in elderly, 221–222, 221f, 221t
    monitoring in geriatrics, 220–221
    objectivity as basic principle of in vitro diagnosis, 218
    screening and monitoring in, 219–220, 219f, 220t
Lacrimal apparatus, disorders of, 810–811
β-Lactams, 377, 549, 552b, 620
Lactinex, 664–665
Lactose intolerance, loose stool and, 923
Lactulose, 642, 978
Lambert-Eaton myasthenic syndrome (LEMS), 507, 530–531
Lamin A, in Hutchinson-Gilford progeria syndrome, 66, 68f
Laminin (LM), 76
Lamisil. *See* Terbinafine
Lamivudine, 638
Lamotrigine, 462, 463t, 477b
Lanreotide, 659
Lapatinib, 727–728, 727t–728t
Large bowel, 661
  aging effects on, 107
  anatomy of, 661
  appendicitis in, 664
  bleeding in, 659–660, 664
  cancer of. *See* Colon cancer
  colonic diverticulosis in, 662–664, 663t
  diagnostic testing of, 661
  fecal occult blood tests for, 662
  functions and symptoms of, 661
  histopathology of, 662
  imaging of, 661–662
  infectious diseases of, 664–666, 665t
  inflammatory bowel disease in, 666, 667t
  ischemia of, 671–672
  lower gastrointestinal bleeding in, 659–660, 674–677, 675t, 676f
  lymphocytic and collagenous colitis (microscopic colitis) of, 670–671
  neoplasms of, 673–674
  polyps of, in elderly, 109
  pseudo-obstruction of, 672
  volvulus of, 672–673
Large vessel disease, vascular cognitive impairment associated with, 422
L-arginine, for cancer, 792
Late life delusional disorders, 436, 438–439
  graduates, 439
  management and outcome of, 438–439
  pathogenesis and etiology of, 438
Late life psychosis, 436–439
  alcohol abuse, 441–442
  anxiety disorders, 440–441
  late life delusional disorders, 436, 438–439
  late-onset schizophrenia, 436–438
  mania, 439–440
  personality disorders, 442–444
  somatoform disorders, 441
Late paraphrenia, 436
Late postoperative hypoxemia, 234–235
Late-acting deleterious mutations theory, 18–20
Latent tuberculosis, 378
Late-onset schizophrenia, 436–438
  assessment, treatment, and course of, 438
  brain imaging of, 437–438
  epidemiology of, 436–437
  etiology of, 437
  neuropsychological testing for, 437–438
  presentation and clinical features of, 437
Lateral pharyngeal diverticula, 612
Latin America
  demographics in, 991
  geriatric medicine in, 1016
    demographic transition, 1016
    development of, 1019, 1019t
    epidemiologic transition, 1016–1017
    health in, 1018, 1018t
    perspectives of, 1019–1020
    research, 1019, 1020t
    retirement policies, 1017–1018, 1017t
    rural health in, 1018–1019
Laxatives
  biopsy of large bowel and, 662
  for constipation, 920, 921t
  for diverticular disease, 663t
  fiber consumption and, 918
  loose stool and, 923
  myalgia and myopathy induced by, 528–529
LCIS. *See* Lobular carcinoma in situ
L-dopa, taste perception and, 608
Learning disability. *See* Intellectual disability
Lecithin, 400
Leflunomide, 569, 569t
Left ventricular filling, in aging heart at rest, 94–95
Left ventricular hypertrophy, 289, 302
Legs, ulcers of, 596–597, 598b, 764, 765t
Leisure activities, cognitive functioning in response to, 175
LEMS. *See* Lambert-Eaton myasthenic syndrome
Lenalidomide, 778–779, 783
Lens, disorders of, 814–815, 814f
Lesbian, gay, bisexual, or transgender (LGBT), sexual difficulties and, 855
Leucovorin, 674
Leukemia
  acute myelogenous, 787–788, 788t
  chronic lymphocytic, 786–788
  chronic myelogenous, 779–781
  chronic myelomonocytic, 777, 778t
Leukoplakia, in oral cavity, 609–610
Levamisole, 674
Levetiracetam, 462–463, 463t
Levodopa
  chorea due to, 519
  for drug-induced parkinsonism, 518
  herbal-drug interactions of, 142t
  metabolism of, 140t, 516
  for multiple system atrophy, 518
  orthostatic hypotension and, 508–509
  for parkinsonism, 513, 515–517, 515t–516t, 519b
  for restless legs syndrome, 519
  sensitivity to, 141
Levodopa plus entacapone (Stalevo), 515t, 516
Levodopa responsive parkinsonism, 511
Levodopa-induced dyskinesia, 514–517
Levofloxacin, 377, 663t
Levonorgestrel, 717
Levothyroxine, 400
Lewy bodies, 512
Lewy body disease, 407–408, 409t, 505–506, 904
LFTs. *See* Liver function tests
LGBT. *See* Lesbian, gay, bisexual, or transgender

LHRH therapy, for prostate cancer, 713
Lice, 804
Lichen planus, of vulva, 718
Lichen sclerosis, of vulva, 719
Lichen simplex, of vulva, 718
Lidocaine
for candidiasis, 617
cimetidine and, 622
distribution of, 139
for maintaining sinus rhythm, 333–334
metabolism of, 140, 140t
for stomatitis, 609
for ventricular arrhythmia, 327–328
for vulval discomfort, 719–720
Life expectancy
epidemiology of, 3, 4f
golden age and, 188–189
individualizing prevention and, 852
pension system and, 988–991, 995–997
world statistics on, 1010–1015, 1011f
Life review, 179
Lifespan
caloric restriction and prolongation of, 41
genetics of, 19–21, 20f
human progeroid syndromes, 20–21
species differences in longevity, 19
variation within species, 20, 20f
mechanisms of insulin/insulin-like growth factor-I signaling effects on, 123
modulations of insulin/insulin-like growth factor-I signaling affecting, 123–124
Lifestyle
cognitive functioning in response to, 175–176
depression and, 841
fecal incontinence and, 921–925
Lifestyle intervention, for weight loss, 687–689
Ligaments, disorders of, 10071#t0015, 578–579
Lignocaine, 970, 977
Limb, arterial disease of, 348–349, 350f
acute limb ischemia, 349, 350f
chronic peripheral vascular disease, 348–349
Limb salvage, for acute limb ischemia, 349, 350f
Lindane, 804
Lipid abnormalities
as CAD risk factor, 289
cardiovascular risk and, 302
Lipid control, in diabetes mellitus, 772–773
Lipid-lowering agents
for chronic kidney disease, 695
in frail elderly patient, 295
for lipid control in diabetes mellitus, 772–773, 774b
myalgia and myopathy induced by, 528
for nonalcoholic fatty liver disease, 639–640
for prevention of secondary stroke, 496
α-Lipoic acid, 44, 148
5-Lipoxygenase inhibitors, 367t
Lisinopril, 278b, 279
Lithium
for depression in old age, 435
elimination of, 141t
for headache, 470, 476
headache due to, 475t
herbal-drug interactions of, 142t
hypercalcemia and, 757t
hypothyroidism due to, 745
for mania, 440
mania and, 439
nephrotoxicity of, 693–694
parkinsonism induced by, 518
restless legs syndrome due to, 519
taste perception and, 608
tremor caused by, 519
Lithium-induced hyperparathyroidism, 758, 758b
Litigation, pressure ulcers and, 941, 942t
Liver, 635
acute failure of, 638, 638t, 643
aging of, 107, 635
biopsy of, 637–638
cirrhosis complications, 641–642
disease of, 638–641, 638t, 645–646
age-related changes in manifestation of, 109
drug and alcohol metabolism by, 635–636
focal lesions of, 644–645
function of, 635
investigations of, 636–637, 636t–637t
radiology of, 637
structure of, 635
transplantation of, 643–644
ultrasound of, 649
Liver function tests (LFTs), 636–637, 636t–637t
Liver metastases, 644
Living alone, in epidemiology of aging, 9, 9f
LM. *See* Laminin
LMNA gene, 66, 68f
LMWH. *See* Low molecular weight heparin
Lobular carcinoma in situ (LCIS), 726–727
Localization related seizures. *See* Focal seizures
Lomustine, 537
Longevity
in developed and developing world, 988
epidemiology of, 3, 4f
gender disparity in, 185, 185f
heritability and familiarity of, 185–186
insulin-signaling pathway in regulation of, 30–32, 31f
metabolic pathways affecting, 155–157, 156f. *See also* Insulin/insulin-like growth factor-I signaling
species differences in, 19
within species differences in, 20, 20f
Longevity dividend, 35–38
Longitudinal data, on aging, cross-sectional data v., 5–6
Longitudinal studies, for researching aging and related conditions, 24–25
Long-term care (LTC)
current approach to improvement of, 1045, 1045t
in regions of world, 1014
in United Kingdom, 1021
developing quality in care, 1023–1024, 1023t
dissolution of medical leadership in, 1022–1024, 1023t
history of, 1021–1022, 1022t
present and future of, 1024–1026, 1024t
in United States, 1026
demographics, 1026, 1027f
economics, 1027
future perspectives of, 1030–1031
history of, 1026
nursing home culture changes, 1030, 1030t
provision of care, 1029, 1029t
quality of care, 1029–1030, 1030t
settings, 1028, 1028t
types of service, 1027–1028
Long-term care facilities (LTCFs)
epidemiology of drug use in, 138
oral health of residents in, 603–604
Long-term memory, aging effects on, 172–173
Loop diuretics, 277–280, 278b, 641
Loose stool, 922t, 923
Loperamide, 671, 925, 979
Loprazolam, 141
Loprox. *See* Ciclopirox
Lorcainide, 327
Losartan, 281
Lotrimin. *See* Clotrimazole
Low molecular weight heparin (LMWH)
for stroke, 492–493
for venous thromboembolism, 357, 360, 360b
Lower esophageal ring, 615–616, 615f
Lower gastrointestinal bleeding, 659–660, 674–677, 675t, 676f
Lower limb amputation, with diabetes mellitus, 763–765, 764t–765t, 765b
Lower urinary tract (LUT), aging of, 112–116, 113t
bladder function and structure, 114–115
outlet function and structure, 115–116
physiologic assessment, 113–114
system-based perspective of, 116
Lowest level gait disorders, 887–888
Low-pressure headache syndrome, 475
Low vision rehabilitation, 820–822
LTC. *See* Long-term care
LTCFs. *See* Long-term care facilities
L-thyroxine
hyperthyroidism due to, 741
for hypothyroidism, 747–748, 750, 754b
as test of thyroid nodule malignancy, 752
for thyroid nodule management, 753
Lumbar puncture, for CNS infection, 547
Lumbar spine, degenerative disease of, neurologic complications of, 544–545, 544f
Lung
aging of, 97
functional changes, 98–99
pulmonary host defense and immune response changes, 99–101
respiratory function tests, 97
structural changes, 98
nonobstructive disease of, 376
bronchiectasis, 378–379, 379t
connective tissue disease, 381
diffuse parenchymal lung disease, 380, 380f
drug-induced interstitial lung disease, 381
hypersensitivity pneumonitis, 382
idiopathic pulmonary fibrosis, 380–381, 380f
influenza, 376
nontuberculous mycobacterial infection, 378
occupational lung disease, 382
pleural effusion, 379, 379t
pneumonia, 376–377, 377t
pneumothorax, 379–380
pulmonary vasculitis, 381
respiratory infections, 376
sarcoidosis, 381
tuberculosis, 377–378
obstructive disease of. *See* Asthma; Chronic obstructive pulmonary disease
thoracic tumors involving. *See* Lung cancer
Lung cancer, 382–383, 382t
malignant mesothelioma, 384
management of, 382–383, 382t
non-small cell, 383
presentation and investigation of, 382
screening for, 794
small cell, 383–384
Lung volume reduction surgery (LVRS), 374
LUT. *See* Lower urinary tract
Lutein, 818
Luxembourg, geriatric medicine in, 1000
LVRS. *See* Lung volume reduction surgery
Lyme disease, in CNS, 552–553
Lymphocytic colitis, 670–671
Lymphoepithelial cyst, of pancreas, 627
Lymphoid development, aging effects on, 131

Lymphoma, 783–786
celiac disease and, 654
clinical features, prognosis, and management of, 784
diagnosis and workup of, 783–784
epidemiology of, 783
etiology of, 783
gastric, 624–625, 625f
Hodgkin, 783, 786
primary CNS, 533, 536–538
of small bowel, 659
T-cell, 785–786

M

MA. *See* Megestrol acetate
Ma huang, 142t
MAC. *See* Mitral annular calcium
Macrolide antibiotics, 141–143, 358, 377, 620, 666
Macrophages, aging effects on, 130
Macular degeneration, 813b, 816–818, 816f–817f
MADIT. *See* Multicenter Automatic Defibrillator Implantation Trial
Madopar. *See* Co-beneldopa
Magnesium, 308, 561
Magnesium hydroxide, 979
Magnetic resonance angiography, of stroke, 490
Magnetic resonance imaging (MRI)
of biliary tract, 650
for CAD, 287–288
of cervical radiculopathy and myelopathy, 540–541, 540f
for epilepsy, 461–462
of liver, 637
for pain, 967
for pancreas adenocarcinoma, 629
for primary autonomic failure, 506–507, 506f
for prostate assessment, 703–704, 704f
of stroke, 489–490
stroke patterns, 490
MAI. *See* Medication Appropriateness Index
Malabsorption, 652
Malathion, 804
Malignancy, pancreaticobiliary, 649
Malignant gliomas, 537–538
Malignant mesothelioma, 384–385
Malignant obstruction, of bile duct, 648–649
Malignant tumors
gastric, 624–625, 625f
of small bowel, 658–659
Malnutrition, 949
anorexia of aging, 949–950
appetite stimulation for, 955–956
aspiration and aspiration pneumonia, 954–955, 955t
characterization of, 949
chewing and swallowing, 950–953
constipation and, 953
in COPD, 374
dementia associated with, 388–389
at end of life, 957–958
enteral nutrition and tube feeding for, 956–957
failure to thrive and frailty, 949
improvements for, 955, 956t
nutritional screening, 950
protein-energy undernutrition, 950
refeeding syndrome, 954, 954t
as secondary cause of acquired immunodeficiency in old age, 88
thirst and hydration and, 953–954, 953t
Malnutrition Universal Screening Tool (MUST), 950, 952f
MALT lymphoma. *See* Mucosa-associated lymphoid tissue lymphoma
Malta, geriatric medicine in, 1000
Managed care, for older Americans, 1057
capitation and pay-for-performance, 1060–1061
in fee-for-service, 1057–1059
future of, 1062–1064
measuring quality of care, 1061–1062, 1062f
plan reimbursement in, 1060
principles for, 1059–1060, 1059b
timeline of, 1057
Managed care plans, quality measurement of, 1051
Mangle cell lymphoma, 784
Mania, 439–440
Mannitol, 355, 820
MAOIs. *See* Monoamine oxidase inhibitors
MAPT mutations, 428–431, 429t
Marginal cell lymphoma, 785
Marital status, epidemiology of aging and, 7–8, 7f
Mass approach, to stroke prevention, 481
Massage
abdominal, for constipation, 919, 919t
carotid sinus, 344–345, 344f
for stroke therapy, 874
Mast cells, effects of aging on, 130
MAT. *See* Multifocal atrial tachycardia
Material mechanisms, of social factors influencing health, 203
Mathematical models, of aging, 59
development of frailty index based on comprehensive geriatric assessment, 62–65, 63f–65f, 65t
phenotypic definition of frailty, 60–62, 61f
Maximal aerobic capacity, 859
MCCD. *See* Medicare Coordinated Care Demonstration
McGill Pain Questionnaire, 967
MCI. *See* Mild cognitive impairment
MDS. *See* Myelodysplasia
Mecamylamine, 339t
Mechanisms of aging. *See also* Cellular mechanisms
evolutionary theory on, 18
evolution of aging, 18–19, 19f
genetics of life span, 19–21, 20f
tests of, 21–22
Medicaid, creation of, 1026
Medical conditions
chronic, prevalence of, 835
insomnia and, 945–946
sexuality in old age and, 855, 856t
Medicare
cost effective quality, 1052–1053, 1052t
coordinated care models, 1052–1053
primary care expansion, 1052
technology for, 1053, 1053t
creation of, 1026
economics of, 1026
future of quality for, 1056–1057, 1056t
organizations for quality improvement in, 1054–1056, 1054t
identification and analysis, 1054
resources for, 1054–1056
parts of, 1057–1059
preservation through quality focus, 1046
pay-for-performance, 1048
regulatory approach to, 1047
reporting of quality data, 1047–1048
quality measurement of, 1026
hospital, 1049–1050
managed care plans, 1051
nursing home, 1050–1051
physician, 1026
prescription drug plans, 1051–1052
Medicare, Medicaid, and SCHIP Extension Act of 2007 (MMSEA), 1049
Medicare Advantage plans, 1051, 1057–1059
Medicare Coordinated Care Demonstration (MCCD), 1058
Medicare Improvement for Patients and Provider Act of 2008 (MIPPA), 1053
Medicare Modernization Act (MMA), 1052–1053, 1057
Medicare Payment Advisory Commission (MedPAC), 1060
Medication Appropriateness Index (MAI), pharmacotherapy and, 882, 885, 885t
Medication therapy management (MTM), 1051–1052
Medication therapy management programs (MTMP), 1058
Medication-induced esophageal injury, 616–618, 617f–618f
Medication-misuse headache, 475
Medications. *See* Drug therapy
Mediterranean diet, constipation and, 913
MedPAC. *See* Medicare Payment Advisory Commission
Megasigmoid syndrome, 672
Megestrol acetate (MA), 955
Meglitinides, 769
Melanocytes, aging effects on, 134
Melanoma, 806–807
Melatonin, as antiaging medicine, 148
Melphalan, 783
Memantine
for Alzheimer's disease, 419–420, 419t, 420b
for dementia, 400–401, 432
for vascular cognitive impairment, 427
Memory
aging effects on, 172–173
long-term memory, 172–173
overall changes, 173
working (short-term) memory, 172
in Alzheimer's disease, 404–405
Memory aids, for dementia management, 399
Memory disorders, exercise and, 864
Men, reproductive aging in
andropause, 166–167
therapeutic horizons, 167
unresolved issues, 167
Meningitis
bacterial, 546–549, 548f, 548t, 550b
chronic, 549–553
cryptococcal, 550
tuberculosis, 549–550
Menopause, 163–164, 716–718
cardiovascular disease and, 717
cutaneous complications and, 808–809
endocrine system changes in, 124
estrogen implants in, 718
estrogen replacement during, 147, 808–809
hormone replacement therapy in, 124, 716–718
oral estrogen for, 717
osteoporosis and, 716–717
sexual interest and, 854
skin and dentition and, 717
topical estrogen in, 717–718
transdermal estrogen in, 717
MENT. *See* 7a-Metnyl-19-nortestosterone
Mental Capacity Act 2005, 974
Mental health, social factors associated with, 203
Mental health assessment, for older adults with intellectual disability, 451
Mental rehearsal, for Parkinson's disease therapy, 877
Mental retardation. *See* Intellectual disability

Mental state assessment, for dementia diagnosis, 395
Mental status
altered, as nonspecific clinical presentation of disease in elderly, 205–206
in old age, 101
Meperidine, 139, 663t, 969
Mephobarbital, 139–140
6-Mercaptopurine, 656–657, 667t, 668, 669t, 670
Mesalamine, 656, 667t, 668, 669t
Mesenteric ischemia, 657–658
Mesothelioma, malignant, 384
Mestinon. *See* Pyridostigmine
Metabolic bone disease, 553
in Down syndrome, 448
fractures in elderly, 564–566
osteomalacia, 558–564, 559t, 560f, 561t
osteoporosis. *See* Osteoporosis
Paget's disease of bone, 561, 562f
Metabolic changes, in older victims of trauma, 865–866
Metabolic disorders
connective tissue affected by, 580–582
constipation and, 914
dementia associated with, 388–389
Metabolic myopathies, 529
Metabolic pathways, in neurobiology of aging, 150
generation of reactive oxygen/nitrogen species, 151–152
metabolic-insulin signaling in control of aging and neurodegeneration, 154–157, 155f–156f
nitrosative and oxidative stress in, 150, 151f–152f
protein misfolding in neurodegenerative disease, 150–151
protein S-nitrosylation and neuronal cell death, 152–154, 153t
Metabolic syndrome, testosterone association with, 168–169
Metabolism
of drugs, aging effects on, 139–140, 140t
skeletal, aging effects on, 121
Metastases
of breast cancer, 728
intracranial, 533
to liver, 644
primary, 533
of prostate cancer, 713–714
spinal, 542–543
Metformin
elimination of, 141t
for glucose control, 768–770, 768b, 769t
herbal-drug interactions of, 142t
for nonalcoholic fatty liver disease, 639–640
Methacholine inhalation challenge, 365
Methadone, 969, 978
Methazolamide, 820
Methicillin, 548, 548t
Methimazole, 742–743
Methodological problems, of research in older people, 23
exclusion of older people from research, 26
obtaining informed consent, 26–27
outcomes measurement, 28–30, 28t
qualitative methodologies, 23–26
recruitment and retention, 27, 27t
study designs, 23
Methotrexate, 797–798
for arthritis, 569–570, 569t–570t
for bullous pemphigoid, 807
for Crohn's disease, 656–657, 669–670, 669t
drug interactions of, 143
Methotrexate (*Continued*)
herbal-drug interactions of, 142t
for idiopathic pulmonary fibrosis, 381
for inclusion body myositis, 528
interstitial lung disease induced by, 381
for intracranial tumors, 538
for lymphocytic and collagenous colitis, 671
for lymphoma, 784
osteoporosis due to, 585
for polymyositis or dermatomyositis, 527
for primary sclerosing cholangitis, 646
Methylcellulose, 671
Methyldopa, 309, 855, 857t
α-Methyldopa, 339t, 344, 605
Methylphenidate, 143t
Methylprednisolone acetate (Depo-Medrone), 574, 977
Methysergide, 468–469, 468t
7a-Metnyl-19-nortestosterone (MENT), 167
Metoclopramide
drug-disease interactions of, 143t
enteral nutrition and, 683
for gastric outlet obstruction, 631
for gastroparesis, 625
for migraine, 468
for nausea and vomiting, 978
for orthostatic hypotension, 510
parkinsonism induced by, 518
sensitivity to, 141, 141t
Metolazone, 278
Metopirone test. *See* Metyrapone
Metoprolol
for acute coronary syndromes, 291
for AF, 334
for chronic cardiac failure, 278b, 280
for hyperthyroidism, 742
metabolism of, 140t
for migraine, 468
after myocardial infarction, 292t
for ventricular arrhythmia, 330, 330t
Metoprolol succinate, 232
Metronidazole
for bacterial overgrowth syndrome, 655
for brain abscess, 549, 552b
for Crohn's disease, 669t, 670
for diverticular disease, 663t
for *H. pylori* infection, 620
for infectious colitis, 664, 666
for pyogenic liver abscess, 644
taste perception and, 608
Metyrapone, 698, 733–734
Metyrapone (Metopirone) test, 732
Mexiletine, 327–328, 328t, 333–334
Mezlocillin, 648
MG. *See* Myasthenia gravis
MGUS. *See* Monoclonal gammopathy of undetermined significance
"Microarousals," 943–944
Microscopic colitis, 670–671
MID. *See* Multiinfarct dementia
Midazolam, 139, 140t, 141, 637–638
Middle level gait disorders, 887
Midesophageal diverticula, 616
Mid-gastrointestinal bleeding, 659–660
Midodrine (ProAmatine)
for carotid sinus syndrome, 345
for orthostatic hypotension, 343, 343t, 508b, 509
for vasovagal syncope, 346
Migraine, 466–470, 468t
Mild cognitive impairment (MCI), 405–406, 409t
Mineral intake, frailty prevention and, 850
Mineral ion balance, 697–700, 699t
Mineral oil, adverse effects of, 110b
Mineralocorticoids, 345, 730, 733
Mini Nutritional Assessment (MNA), 950, 951f
Mini-Mental Status Examination (MMSE), 403, 415–416, 416t, 430, 1018
Miotic eyedrops, for glaucoma, 814
MIPPA. *See* Medicare Improvement for Patients and Provider Act of 2008
Mirapexin. *See* Pramipexole
Mirtazapine, 401, 463
Misfolding. *See* Protein, misfolding
Misoprostol, 568–569, 621
Mistreatment, of older people, 959
definitions of, 959–960, 960t
historical development of, 959
identification of, 962–963
prevalence and incidence of, 960–961, 960t
prevention, treatment, and management of, 962f, 963
risk factors for, 961–962
Mitochondrial dysfunction, sarcopenia and, 589
Mitochondrial genetics
damage of, in cell senescence, 48
oxidative stress and aging in, 38–39
Mitoxantrone, 784
Mitral annular calcium (MAC), 320–323
AF in patients with, 321
bacterial endocarditis in patients with, 322
cardiac events in patients with, 322, 322t
cerebrovascular events in patients with, 322–323, 323t
chamber size of patients with, 321
conduction defects in patients with, 321
diagnosis of, 321
mitral regurgitation in patients with, 321–322, 321t–322t
mitral stenosis in patients with, 321t–322t, 322
mitral valve replacement in patients with, 322
predisposing factors for, 320–321
prevalence of, 320
Mitral regurgitation
acute, 324
in patients with mitral annular calcium, 321–322, 321t–322t
Mitral stenosis (MS), 323–324
diagnostic tests for, 324
management of, 324
pathophysiology of, 323
in patients with mitral annular calcium, 321t–322t, 322
prevalence and etiology of, 323
symptoms and signs of, 323–324
Mitral valve replacement, 322
MM. *See* Multiple myeloma
MMA. *See* Medicare Modernization Act
MMSE. *See* Mini-Mental Status Examination
MMSEA. *See* Medicare, Medicaid, and SCHIP Extension Act of 2007
MNA. *See* Mini Nutritional Assessment
MND. *See* Motor neuron disease
Mobility
age-related changes in, 886–887
executive function, 886
gait initiation, 887
rising from chair, 887
walking speed, 886
assessment of, 9–10, 888–889
life spaces, 10
timed walking test, 9
constipation and, 912
evaluation for, 898t, 900
immobility, 889–892
impaired, 886
frailty and, 892–893
gait disorders, 887–888
social factors associated with, 202
walking aid for, 9–10

Mobility training, for fractured neck, 875–876
Modafinil, 517
Model of vulnerability, 837, 837f, 838t
Moisture, pressure ulcers and, 939
Molecular genetics, of Hutchinson-Gilford progeria syndrome, 66–68, 68f
Molecular markers, of breast cancer, 726–727, 727t
Monitoring. *See also* Blood monitoring
  in geriatrics, 220–221
  with laboratory medicine for geriatric population, 219–220, 219f, 220t
Monitoring standards, by NHS, 1043–1044
Monoamine oxidase inhibitors (MAOIs)
  drug-disease interactions of, 143t
  headache due to, 475t
  herbal-drug interactions of, 142t
  syncope caused by, 339t
  for tension headache, 469
  toxic serotonin syndrome and, 519
Monoamine oxidase-B inhibitors, 515t, 516
Monoclonal antibodies, to β-amyloid proteins, 413, 420
Monoclonal gammopathies, of old age, 86–87
Monoclonal gammopathy of undetermined significance (MGUS), 781–782, 782t
Monocytes, aging effects on, 130
Montelukast, for asthma, 367t
Morbidity
  of asthma, 363
  compression of, 184–186, 188–189
  following anesthesia in old age, 231
  of obesity, 686–687
  in people with intellectual disability, 448
  world statistics on, 1010
Moricizine, 292–293, 327–328, 328t, 333–334
Morphine
  absorption of, 139
  constipation and, 912–913
  for diverticular disease, 663t
  glucuronidation of, 645
  liver metabolism of, 635–636
  metabolism of, 140t
  for pain, 969
  for palliative care, 976
  for STEMI, 291
Morphine sulfate, 290
Mortality
  from abdominal aortic aneurysm rupture, 354
  from aneurysm surgery for abdominal aortic aneurysm, 354–355
  of aortic regurgitation, 319
  of aortic stenosis, 314–316, 315t
  of asthma, 363
  from carotid surgery, 352
  of diabetes mellitus, 765, 765f
  following anesthesia in old age, 231
  hypertension management and, 305–306
  of intellectual disability in old age, 446–447
  of obesity, 685–687
  as outcomes measurement for multidimensional interventions, 248t–265t, 266t–267t
  of stroke, 478–479, 478t
  weight loss and, 687
Motesanib diphosphate, 753
Motility disorders, esophageal, 613
Motivation, in rehabilitation, 13–14
Motor features, of Parkinson's disease, 512
Motor neuron disease (MND), 529–532
Motor neuron findings, of dementia, 390
Motor signs, of old age, 102–103
  paratonia, 103
  tremor and abnormal movements, 103
Mouth, nutrition and, 608
Movement, abnormal, of old age, 103
Movement disorders, 511
  akinetic-rigid syndromes, 511, 511t
  hyperkinetic disorders, 518–519
  Parkinson's disease. *See* Parkinson's disease
  parkinsonism not due to Parkinson's disease, 518
    drug-induced parkinsonism, 518
    parkinsonism-plus, 518
    vascular parkinsonism, 518
MPDs. *See* Myeloproliferative disorders
MRI. *See* Magnetic resonance imaging
MS. *See* Mitral stenosis
MSA. *See* Multiple system atrophy
MSCTA. *See* Multislice computed tomography angiography
MTM. *See* Medication therapy management
MTMP. *See* Medication therapy management programs
Mucinous cystic neoplasm, of pancreas, 627
Mucolytics, 373, 379, 980
Mucosa
  duodenal, injury of, 618–619
  gastric, injury of, 618–619
  oral, 608
Mucosa-associated lymphoid tissue (MALT) lymphoma, 785
Multicenter Automatic Defibrillator Implantation Trial (MADIT), 293
Multichannel cystometry, for urinary incontinence, 928–929
Multidimensional geriatric assessment, 211, 212f
  effectiveness of geriatric assessment programs, 215–217
  history of geriatric assessment, 211
  social assessment as part of, 223
  structure and process of, 211–215, 213f, 214t
    assessment in office practice setting, 214–215
    comprehensive geriatric assessment, 215
Multidimensional geriatric intervention, measuring outcomes of, 245
  geriatric assessment outcomes and quality of life measures, 246–249
  individualized outcome assessment, 247–249, 247t–248t
  randomized controlled trials of geriatric interventions and associated outcome measures, 248t–265t
  standardized assessment systems, 246–247
  summary of outcome measures used in randomized controlled trials of geriatric interventions, 266t–267t
Multidisciplinary assessment, in older adults with intellectual disability, 449
Multidisciplinary team care, for rehabilitation, 11–12
Multifocal atrial tachycardia (MAT), 336
Multiinfarct dementia (MID), 421
Multiple myeloma (MM), 781–783, 782t
Multiple system atrophy (MSA), 505–507, 506f
  levodopa for, 518
  orthostatic hypotension associated with, 342
Multislice computed tomography angiography (MSCTA), for CAD, 287–288
Murmur. *See* Heart murmur
Muscle biopsy, for neuromuscular disorder diagnosis, 523
Muscle relaxants, for prostatitis, 705
Muscle sympathetic nerve activity, 501–502, 502f
Musculoskeletal system
  aging of, 117, 118f
    articular cartilage, 117–119, 118f–119f
    consequences of, 122
Musculoskeletal system (*Continued*)
    future of, 122–123
    skeleton, 119–121, 119f–120f
    soft tissues, 121–122
  disorders of, 566t
  in Down syndrome, 448
  pain in, palliative care for, 977
Music therapy, 400, 971
MUST. *See* Malnutrition Universal Screening Tool
Mutations
  of Alzheimer's disease, 412–413
  chromosomal, in aging, 39–41
  DNA, in cell senescence, 46
  in frontotemporal dementia, 428–431, 429t
  in *LMNA* gene, in Hutchinson-Gilford progeria syndrome, 66, 68f
Myalgia, 521, 528–529
Myasthenia gravis (MG), 530
Mycelex. *See* Clotrimazole
Mycobacterial infection, 378. *See also* Tuberculosis
Mycophenolate mofetil, 381, 531, 807
Mydriatic, 820
Myelodysplasia (MDS), 777–779, 778t–779t
Myelopathy, cervical, 539–541, 540f
Myeloproliferative disorders (MPDs), 779–781
Myerson sign. *See* Glabellar tap reflex
Myocardial function, in aging heart at rest, 94–95, 96t
Myocardial infarction
  atypical presentation of, 209, 209t
  coronary revascularization after, 293t, 294
  postoperative, 235
  recognized and unrecognized, 286, 286t
  therapy after, 291–293, 292t
Myocardial ischemia, of CAD, 286–287
Myoclonic jerk, 455
Myoclonus, with dementia, 390
Myopathy
  drug-induced, 528–529
  endocrine and metabolic, 529
  inflammatory, 526–528
  steroid-induced, 529
Myositis, 526–528
Myostatin, 592
Myxedema coma, 747–748

N

N-acetyl-cysteine (NAC), 381, 643
N-acetylprocainamide, 141t
Nafcillin, 548, 548t
NAFLD. *See* Nonalcoholic fatty liver disease
Nails
  aging of, 136
  of foot, 596–597
Naloxone, 803
Naltrexone, 640
Naproxen, 139, 467–468, 568, 568t, 574
Narcotics
  for diverticular disease, 663t
  hypothyroidism due to, 746–747
  for neurogenic claudication and spinal stenosis, 526
  for orthopedic geriatrics, 584
  orthostatic hypotension and, 503
  weight loss due to, 206
Nascher, Ignatz, 1
Nasogastric feeding, palliative medicine and, 975
Nateglinide, 769
National Beds Enquiry, 4
National Care Standards Commission (NCSC), 1025

National Health Service (NHS)
Community Care Act and, 3
current approach to quality of care improvement, 1043–1045, 1043f
clear standards of service, 1043
clinical governance, 1044, 1044f
dependable local delivery, 1043
long-term care, 1045–1045, 1045t
monitoring and publicizing standards, 1043–1044
primary care-led, 4
of United Kingdom, 997
National Institute for Clinical Excellence (NICE), 1043
National Institute on Aging, 1006
National Pressure Ulcer Advisory Panel (NPUAP), 940
National Service Frameworks (NSFs), 1043
Natriuretic peptides, in chronic cardiac failure, 277
Natural history
of aortic regurgitation, 319
of aortic stenosis, 314–316, 315t
of COPD, 370–372, 371f
Natural selection, age effects on, 18–19
Nausea, palliative care for, 978
NCSC. *See* National Care Standards Commission
NCSE. *See* Nonconvulsive status epilepticus
Nebivolol, 280
Neck, headache arising from, 472–473
Necrobiosis lipoidica, 808
Necrosis, pancreatic, 633
Needs-related model, of geriatric medicine, 997
Nefazodone, 141t–142t
Neglect, of older people, 959–960, 960t
historical development of, 959
identification of, 962–963
prevalence and incidence of, 960–961, 960t
prevention, treatment, and management of, 962f, 963
risk factors for, 961–962
Neomycin, 609, 642, 803
Neoplasms
celiac disease and, 654
of connective tissue, 579–580, 579f–580f
esophageal, 617–618, 618f
of large bowel, 673–674
of small bowel, 658–659
of thyroid, 750–754, 751t
Neoplastic disorders, dementia associated with, 389
Neo-Synephrine, 820
Nerve blocks, for palliative care, 978
Nerve root disorders. *See* Spinal cord disorders
Nerve root entrapment, in degenerative disease of lumbar spine, 544, 544f
Nerves, of skin, aging effects on, 136
Network theory of aging, 41
Networks. *See* Social networks
Neural pain modulators, for stroke, 495
Neuraminidase inhibitors, 376
Neuroanatomy, of social factors influencing health, 204
Neurobiologic risk factors, for depression in old age, 433–434
Neurobiology, of aging, 150
generation of reactive oxygen/nitrogen species, 151–152
metabolic-insulin signaling in control of aging and neurodegeneration, 154–157, 155f–156f
nitrosative and oxidative stress in, 150, 151f–152f
Neurobiology, of aging *(Continued)*
protein misfolding in neurodegenerative disease, 150–151
protein S-nitrosylation and neuronal cell death, 152–154, 153t
Neurodegeneration
epilepsy and, 460
mechanisms of insulin/insulin-like growth factor-I signaling effects on, 123–124
metabolic-insulin signaling in control of, 154–157, 155f–156f
neuroendocrinology of aging in, 167–169
nitrosative and oxidative stress in, 150, 151f–152f
other metabolic pathways affecting, 155–157, 156f
protein misfolding in, 150–151
Neuroendocrine changes, autonomic system aging and, 503
Neuroendocrine responses, in older victims of trauma, 865
Neuroendocrine testing, for primary autonomic failure, 506–508, 506f
Neuroendocrine tumors, of pancreas, 631
Neuroendocrinology, of aging, 163
brain metabolism and neurodegenerative disease in, 167–169
reproductive aging in men, 166–167
reproductive aging in women, 163–169
Neurofibrillary tangles (NFTs), of Alzheimer's disease, 411–412, 412f
Neurogenic claudication, 525–526, 545
Neuroimaging
for dementia diagnosis, 396–397
for epilepsy, 461–462
of frontotemporal dementia, 430
of vascular cognitive impairment, 425–426, 425f
Neuroleptic malignant syndrome, 519
Neuroleptics. *See also* Atypical neuroleptics
aging effects on, 141
for Alzheimer's disease, 417
chorea due to, 519
for delirium, 906–907
for dementia, 401, 432
drug interactions of, 143, 143t
for hemiballismus, 519
involuntary movement induced by, 519
for late life delusional disorders, 438–439
for mania, 440
parkinsonism induced by, 511t, 513t, 518
sensitivity to, 141, 141t
for vulval discomfort, 719–720
Neurologic complications, of degenerative disease of lumbar spine, 544–545, 544f
Neurologic disease
constipation and, 913–914
in Down syndrome, 448
Neurologic examination, for Alzheimer's disease, 415–416
Neurologic signs, 101, 102t
cranial nerve function, 101–102
deep tendon reflexes, 103–104
gait and station changes, 103
glabellar tap reflex, 105
mental status, 101
motor signs, 102–103
primitive reflexes, 104–105
sensory signs, 104
Neuromuscular blocking agents, in elderly patients, 231
Neuromuscular disorders, 520
approach to patient with, 520–523, 520t
examination, 522
history taking, 520–521, 524t
investigations, 522–523
Neuromuscular disorders *(Continued)*
drug-induced myalgia and myopathy, 528–529
endocrine and metabolic myopathies, 529
inclusion body myositis, 528
inflammatory myopathy, 526–528
motor neuron disease, 529–532
myasthenia gravis, 530–532
neurogenic claudication and spinal stenosis, 525–526
peripheral neuropathies, 523–525, 524t
diabetic neuropathy, 524–525, 524t
Neuromuscular function, sarcopenia and, 588
Neuromuscular transmission, pathophysiology of myasthenia gravis and, 531
Neuronal cell death, protein S-nitrosylation and, 152–154, 153t
Neuro-ophthalmology disorders, 819
Neuropathic pain, 966, 977–978
Neuropathology
of Parkinson's disease, 512–513
of vascular cognitive impairment, 425
Neuropathy. *See* Peripheral neuropathies
Neurophysiology, of social factors influencing health, 204
Neuroprotective agents, for stroke, 492–493
Neuropsychiatric profiles, of vascular cognitive impairment, 425
Neuropsychology
in dementia diagnosis and treatment, 402
challenges to, 402–404
neuropsychological tests, 404–407, 404t, 409t
reasons for neuropsychological assessment, 402
in frontotemporal dementia diagnosis, 430
in late-onset schizophrenia diagnosis, 437–438
NeuroSERMs, for reproductive aging in women, 164–166
Neurosyphilis, 551
Neurotoxicity, in cell models of Parkinson's disease and Alzheimer's disease, S-nitrosylation of PDI in, 153–154
Neutrophils, aging of, 130
NFTs. *See* Neurofibrillary tangles
NH. *See* Nursing homes
NHS. *See* National Health Service
Niacinamide, 807
NICE. *See* National Institute for Clinical Excellence
Nicotine replacement, 283, 372–373
Nicotinic acid, 289, 291
Nifedipine
for aortic regurgitation, 319
cimetidine and, 622
in frail elderly patient, 298
herbal-drug interactions of, 142t
metabolism of, 140t
Nilotinib, 781
Nitrates
for acute coronary syndromes, 291
for acute renal failure, 693
for aortic regurgitation, 319
for aortic stenosis, 316
for chronic cardiac failure, 278, 278b, 281–282, 284–285, 285b
cluster headache due to, 470
for dysphagia and chest pain, 614
in frail elderly patient, 297
headache due to, 475t
after myocardial infarction, 292, 293t
orthostatic hypotension and, 503
sildenafil and, 857
for stable angina, 290
for STEMI, 291
syncope caused by, 339t

Nitrazepam, 141
Nitric oxide, aging effects on release of, 92
Nitrofurantoin, 381
Nitroglycerin
for acute coronary syndromes, 290–291
for stable angina, 290
for STEMI, 291
for vasovagal syncope evaluation, 346
Nitroprusside, 501
Nitrosative stress, in neurobiology of aging, 150, 151f–152f
Nitrous oxide (NO), pressure ulcers and, 940
NMDA antagonists, 426b, 427
NMDA receptors
in mediating glutamatergic signaling pathways and inducing calcium ion influx, 151–152
in neurobiology of aging, 150, 151f
N-methyl-D-aspartate receptor antagonists, 400
NO. *See* Nitrous oxide
Nociception, 965
Nociceptive pain, 966
Nocturnal micturition, insomnia and, 945–946
Nodal zone lymphoma (NZL), 785
Nodular thyroid disease, 750–755, 751t
Nonalcoholic fatty liver disease (NAFLD), 109, 639–640
Noncardiac chest pain, 614
Nonconvulsive status epilepticus (NCSE), 459
Nonenzymatic glycosylation, in aging of connective tissues, 79
Nonepileptic seizure. *See* Psychogenic attack
Non-Hodgkin lymphoma, 783–786
Noninvasive autonomic tests, 498–500, 499f–500f
Nonobstructive lung disease. *See* Lung, nonobstructive disease of
Nonparoxysmal AV junctional tachycardia. *See* Accelerated atrioventricular rhythm
Nonphysician personnel, for preventive practice systems, 853
Non-small cell lung cancer, 383
Nonspecific host defense, aging-related changes in, 82
Nonsteroidal antiandrogens, 713, 733
Nonsteroidal antiinflammatory drugs (NSAIDs)
acute liver failure induced by, 643
acute pancreatitis due to, 631–632
acute renal failure due to, 691
for Alzheimer's disease, 413, 420
for apatite deposition disease, 576
for arthritis, 568–569, 568t
asthma provoked by, 366
for bone pain, 977
for calcium pyrophosphate crystal deposition, 575
for cervical radiculopathy and myelopathy, 541
colon cancer risk and, 673
constipation and, 912–913
Crohn's disease and, 656
for diabetic neuropathy, 597
drug interactions of, 143, 143t
in elderly patients, 231, 571
esophageal injury due to, 616
gastrointestinal damage caused by, 106, 108, 110, 110b
gastropathy, peptic ulcer disease, and, 619–622, 625b
for giant cell arteritis, 473–474
for gout, 574
for headache, 469, 472
heart failure precipitated by, 274t, 275
herbal-drug interactions of, 142t
hyperkalemia due to, 698, 698t
Nonsteroidal antiinflammatory drugs *(Continued)*
liver metabolism of, 636t
longevity due to, 14
lymphocytic and collagenous colitis and, 671
meningoencephalitis associated with, 387
for migraine, 467–468, 468t, 477b
for neurogenic claudication and spinal stenosis, 526
for orthopedic/biomechanical disorders of foot, 594
for orthostatic hypotension, 343
for pain, 968–969, 968b
for pancreas adenocarcinoma, 630
renal impairment and, 309, 692
as secondary cause of acquired immunodeficiency in old age, 89
ulcerative colitis and, 668
for upper gastrointestinal bleeding, 623
Nontuberculous mycobacterial infection, 378
19-Nor-4-androstene-3β,17β-diol (Estren-β), 167
Norepinephrine, 501, 657–658
Norfloxacin, 641–642, 655
Normal aging, 52–53
adrenocortical function in, 731–732
Hutchinson-Gilford progeria syndrome and insights into, 66
description of HGPS, 66, 67f
molecular genetics and cell biology, 66–68, 68f
similarities and differences between aging and HGPS, 68–71, 69f
pressure ulcers and, 939
progeroid syndromes and, 33–34
sexuality and, 854–855
Normal pressure hydrocephalus (NPH), dementia associated with, 389
Normal-tension glaucoma, 814
North America, geriatric medicine in, 1005
future direction, 1008–1009
specialty practice in, 1006–1008, 1007t
Norton scale, for pressure ulcers, 940
Nortriptyline, 140t, 435, 472
Norway, geriatric medicine in, 1000
Nosocomial pneumonia, 377
Nosotropics, for dementia, 400
"Not because they are old," 4
NPH. *See* Normal pressure hydrocephalus
NPs. *See* Nurse practitioners
NPUAP. *See* National Pressure Ulcer Advisory Panel
NSAIDs. *See* Nonsteroidal antiinflammatory drugs
NSFs. *See* National Service Frameworks
NSTEMI, 290–291
Nurse practitioners (NPs), for cost effective quality of care, 1052
Nursing care
for cancer, 799–800
in rehabilitation, 12
Nursing health promotion, 843
Nursing home. *See* Long-term care facilities; Residential care
Nursing Home Compare, 1050
Nursing Home Quality Initiative, 1050
Nursing Home Reform Act, 1026
Nursing Home Residents' Bill of Rights, 1026, 1027t
Nursing homes (NH)
bill of rights for, 1026, 1027t
culture changes in United States, 1030, 1030t
for long-term care, 1026, 1028, 1028t
quality measurement of, 1050–1051
"Nutcracker" esophagus, 614
Nutrition, 678, 679f
common problems and deficiencies, 681–682
in COPD, 374
cutaneous complications and, 808
dementia associated with deficiencies of, 388–389
at end of life, 957–958
ethical considerations, 684–685
for frailty prevention, 850
functional recovery and, 866–867
immobility and, 892
improvements of, 955, 956t
longevity due to, 12–13
mouth and, 608
nutritional requirements, 680–681, 680t–681t
physiologic recovery and, 866
programs and services, 683–684
sarcopenia and, 590–592
screening and assessment for, 678–680, 840, 950
strategies for nutrition optimization, 682–683, 683t
surgery and anesthesia in old age and, 237–239, 239t
for weight loss, 687–688, 688t
Nystatin, 609
NZL. *See* Nodal zone lymphoma

O

OA. *See* Osteoarthritis
Obesity, 682, 685
adverse effects of, 685–686, 686t
benefits of, 686
as CAD risk factor, 289–290
causes of, 685
increased mortality and morbidity of, 686–687
measurement of, 685, 686t
prevalence of, 685
sleep-disordered breathing and, 946–947
surgery and anesthesia in old age and, 239
treatment of, 687–689, 688t, 688b
weight loss effects in older adults, 687
Objectivity, as basic principle of in vitro diagnosis, 218
Obscure gastrointestinal bleeding, 659–660
Obsessive-compulsive disorder (OCD), 441
Obstruction
of bile ducts, 646–649
of bowel, 979
Obstructive lung disease. *See* Asthma; Chronic obstructive pulmonary disease
Occipital seizures, 456
Occlusion, of cerebral vessels, 482
Occupational lung disease, 382
asbestosis, 382
coal workers pneumoconiosis, 382
pneumoconiosis, 382
Occupational therapy, 870–871
historical overview of, 870–871
for Hutchinson-Gilford progeria syndrome, 71–72
research culture for, 872
settings for, 871
skills for, 871
training for, 871
OCD. *See* Obsessive-compulsive disorder
OCSP Classification. *See* Oxfordshire Community Stroke Project Classification
Octreotide
for bacterial overgrowth syndrome, 655
for bowel obstruction, 979
for orthostatic hypotension, 343, 510
for pancreatic neuroendocrine tumors, 631
for postprandial hypotension, 347, 510
for small bowel tumors, 659

Ocular findings, in dementia, 390
Office practice setting, multidimensional geriatric assessment in, 214–215
Office-based assessment, home-based assessment v., 838–839
Ogilvie syndrome, 672, 917, 917f
OGTT. *See* Oral glucose tolerance test
Olanzapine, 140t, 143t, 438, 443b
Old age
  future of, 11
    current and future biomedical inputs to aging, 13–15
    future of aging, 15–18
    historical determinants of future health of elderly, 12–13
  health in. *See* Health in old age
  inequalities in, 9, 190–191
  methodological problems of research in, 23
    exclusion of older people from research, 26
    obtaining informed consent, 26–27
    outcomes measurement, 28–30, 28t
    qualitative methodologies, 23–26
    recruitment and retention, 27, 27t
    study designs, 23
  presentation of disease in, 205
    atypical presentation of common diseases, 208–210, 209t, 690
    kidney disease, 690
    nonspecific clinical presentations, 205–208, 206t
  "problem" of, 187–188
  social vulnerability in, 198
    associations with health, 201–203
    background and definitions, 198–199, 198f
    frailty, exclusion, and "silence by proxy,", 204
    policy ramifications and potential for interventions, 204
    study of social influences on health, 199–201, 200
    successful aging, 201
Omalizumab, 367t
Omega-3 fatty acids, 818
Omeprazole, 140t–141t, 568–569, 621
Oncology, geriatric. *See* Cancer
Ondansetron, 659
Online computerized risk assessment, for surgery and anesthesia in old age, 243
Onychomycosis, 804–805
Open reduction internal fixation (ORIF), 584–585
Open-angle glaucoma, 813
Operative mortality, of aneurysm surgery for abdominal aortic aneurysm, 354–355
Opiates
  for acute renal failure, 693
  adverse effects of, 110b
  for cholecystitis and cholangitis, 648
  for chronic cardiac failure, 284
  in elderly patients, 231
  for eye pain, 475
  hyperparathyroidism and, 756b
  hypoxemia after, 234
  for medication-misuse headache, 475
  for postherpetic neuralgia, 472
  for prolonged rest ischemia, 350f
Opioid receptors, age-related perception of pain and, 966
Opioids
  for cancer, 800
  for cervical radiculopathy and myelopathy, 541
  chronic daily headache due to, 470
  for chronic pain, 971
  for dyspnea, 979
Opioids (*Continued*)
  herbal-drug interactions of, 142t
  metabolism of, 140
  for pain, 968b, 969–970
  for palliative care, 976–977, 976t
  for pancreas adenocarcinoma, 630
  sensitivity to, 141, 141t, 144, 144b
Opportunity age, 189–190
Optic nerve disorders, 819
Optiset pen, for glucose control, 770
Oral candida infection, palliative medicine and, 975
Oral cavity, 608
  disorders of
    candidiasis, 608–609
    epidermoid carcinoma, 610
    "hairy tongue,", 609
    leukoplakia, 609–610
    stomatitis, 609
    vascular lesions, 608, 609f
  mouth and nutrition, 608
  oral mucosa, 608
Oral contraceptives, stroke risk and, 480, 480t
Oral glucose tolerance test (OGTT), 860
Oral health, 599. *See also* Dentistry, geriatric
  measures of, 599–601, 599f–601f
  systemic health response to, 602–603
Oral intake, palliative medicine and, 974–975
Oral lesions, 600f–601f, 606–607, 606f
Oral transmucosal fentanyl citrate (OTFC), 976t, 977
Orbicularis oculi sign. *See* Glabellar tap reflex
Orbit disorders, 819
Organismic function, age-related changes in, 55–57, 57f
Organs, age-related changes in physiology of, 53–55, 54f
ORIF. *See* Open reduction internal fixation
Oropharyngeal dysphagia, 953
Oropharynx, 610–612
  disorders of
    cricopharyngeal achalasia, 611
    oropharyngeal dysphagia, 610–611, 611t
    pharyngeal diverticula, 611–612, 611f
    postintubation dysphagia, 611
Orthopedic disorders, of foot, 594–595, 595f, 596f
Orthopedic geriatrics, 583
  anesthetic considerations, 584–586
  follow-up, 586
  geriatric-orthopedic co-care, 586
  for osteoporosis, 583
  for periarticular fractures, 584–585, 585f
  for periprosthetic fractures, 585, 585f
  prevention of fractures, 585–586
  for trauma, 583–584, 584f
Orthostatic headache, 475
Orthostatic hypotension, 341–343, 343t, 503
  aging effects on, 342
  evaluation of, 343
  hypertension effects on, 342
  management of, 343, 343t, 508–510, 508b
    nonpharmacologic treatment, 508–509
    pathophysiology-guided therapy, 508
    pharmacologic treatment, 509
    treatment of related conditions, 510
  medication effects on, 339t, 342
  other conditions affecting, 342
  pathophysiology of, 341–342
  presentation of, 342–343
  primary autonomic failure syndromes associated with, 342
  secondary autonomic dysfunction associated with, 342
Orthostatic test. *See* Posture test
Orthotic assistance, for stroke therapy, 875
Oseltamivir, 376
Osmotic agents, for glaucoma, 814
Osteoarthritis (OA), 117–119, 119f, 572–573, 572t
  aging of connective tissues in patients with, 79
  clinical features of, 572–573, 572t
  clinical subgroups of, 573
  comorbidity of, 848
  epidemiology of, 572
  pathogenesis of, 119
  soft tissue aging and, 121
Osteomalacia, 558–561, 559t, 560f, 561t
  biochemical findings in, 560–561, 561t
  clinical features of, 559–560
  diagnosis of, 561
  in elderly, 559
  radiology in, 560, 560f
  treatment of, 561
Osteomyelitis, 577
Osteoporosis, 120–121, 120f, 553–558, 555t–556t, 559f
  aging of connective tissues in patients with, 79–80
  antiepileptic drugs and, 462–463
  clinical features of, 554
  comorbidity of, 849
  diagnosis of, 554–555
  investigation of, 555, 555t
  management of, 555–558, 556t
    choice of treatment, 558, 559f
    future treatments, 557–558
  menopause and, 716–717
  orthopedic geriatrics for, 583
  pathogenesis of, 554
  prevalence of, 553–554
  prevention of, 585–586
  treatment of, 164–165
OTFC. *See* Oral transmucosal fentanyl citrate
Outcomes
  age, surgery, and, 230–231
  of asthma management, 368–369
  of heart disease treatment in older persons, 297, 297t
  of quality of care, 1039
Outcomes measurement
  of multidimensional geriatric interventions, 245
    geriatric assessment outcomes and quality of life measures, 246
    individualized outcome assessment, 247–249, 247t–248t
    randomized controlled trials of geriatric interventions and associated outcome measures, 248t–265t
    standardized assessment systems, 246–247
    summary of outcome measures used in randomized controlled trials of geriatric interventions, 266t–267t
  in old age, 867
  in research involving older individuals, 28–30, 28t
  in United States managed care, 1061–1062
Outlet, aging of, 112–117, 113t
  bladder function and structure, 114–115
  outlet function and structure, 115–116
  physiologic assessment, 113–114
  system-based perspective of, 116–117
Ovarian cancer, 723–724, 723t
Ovary, aging of, 716
Overactive bladder, 115, 706–707, 707f, 709, 721
Overexpression, in cell senescence, 47
Overflow fecal incontinence, treatment of, 922–923
Oxacillin, 548
Oxcarbazepine, 462, 463t, 471

Oxfordshire Community Stroke Project (OCSP) Classification, 486, 486t
Oxidative stress
in aging
in neurobiology, 150, 151f–152f
in protein damage and sarcopenia, 34–35
in cellular aging, 42–44
mitochondrial genetics, aging, and, 38–39
respiratory system aging and, 97–98
Oxybutynin, 605, 721, 931–932, 935
Oxygen therapy, for dyspnea, 979

P

PACE. *See* Program for All-inclusive Care for the Elderly
Pacing. *See also* Cardiac resynchronization therapy
for carotid sinus syndrome, 345
indications for, 337t
Paclitaxel, 383, 724, 807
PAF. *See* Pure autonomic failure
Paget's disease
of bone, 561, 562f, 577–578, 578f
spinal cord compression in, 543–544
of vulva, 719
Paid employment, productive aging with, 194–195
Pain, 965
age-related perception of, 966
in aging, 965
cancer and, 971
components of, 965
differential diagnosis for, 976, 976t
evaluation of, 966–968
with dementia, 967–968
psychological, 967
management of, 968–971
adjuvant analgesics, 970
chronic pain, 971
medications for, 968
nonpharmacologic therapies for, 970
opioid analgesics, 969–970
physical therapies, 970–971
psychological approaches, 971
simple analgesics, 968–969, 968b
palliative care for, 975–978, 975b
of pancreas adenocarcinoma, 628, 630
pathophysiologic perspective on, 966
prevalence studies of, 965–966
therapy goals for, 968
types of, 965–966
Pain behaviors, 965
Pain radiology, 967
Painful diverticular disease, in large bowel, 663, 663t
Palliative care, 973
aging process, 973
care providers for, 974
for chronic cardiac failure, 284
future planning for, 974
oral intake and, 974–975
for Parkinson's disease, 517
place of care for, 975
for pressure ulcers, 973
for small cell lung cancer, 384
symptom control, 975–982
bone pain, 977
bowel obstruction, 979
confusion, 980–981, 980t
constipation, 978–979
cough, 980
depression and adjustment disorder, 980
diarrhea, 979
dizziness, 980
dyspnea, 979
Palliative care (*Continued*)
fatigue, 980
musculoskeletal pain, 977
nausea and vomiting, 978
nerve blocks, 978
neuropathic pain, 977–978
pain, 975–978, 975b
spiritual suffering, 981
terminal stage, 981–982
telemedicine support for, 1066
Palliative chemotherapy, for non-small cell lung cancer, 383
Palliative radiotherapy, for non-small cell lung cancer, 383
Palmomental reflex, age-related changes in, 104
PALS. *See* Patient Advice and Liaison Service
Pamidronate, 563, 981
Pancreas, 626
acute pancreatitis, 631–633, 631f, 632t
aging effects on, 107, 626
anatomic relationships of, 626
background, 626, 627f
chronic pancreatitis, 633–635
development of, 626, 627f
endocrine function of, 626
exocrine function of, 626
histology of, 626
tumors of, 626, 628f
cystic tumors, 627
solid tumors, 627–631, 628f
Pancreatic carcinoma, 648
Pancreatic necrosis, 633
Pancreatic neuroendocrine tumors (pNET), 631
Pancreaticobiliary malignancy, 649
Pancreatitis
acute, 631–633, 631f, 632t
chronic, 633–634
Pandysautonomia, 507
Panic disorder, 440
Pantoprazole, 108
Papain solution, 616
Papaverine, 657–658
Papaya, 142t
Papilledema, 819
Paracentesis, for nausea and vomiting, 978
Paracetamol
acute liver failure induced by, 643
for bisphosphonate administration, 556
glucuronidation of, 645
for migraine, 467–468, 468t, 477b
for pain, 968, 968b
for palliative care, 976
for tension headache, 469
Paraesophageal hernia, 614, 614f
Paraneoplastic disorders, dementia associated with, 389
Paranoid disorders. *See* Late life delusional disorders
Paraphrenia, 436
Parasomnias, epilepsy v., 459
Parasympathetic function, cardiac, effects of aging on, 501
Parasympathomimetic miotics, 813, 820
Parathyroid gland disorders, 755
calcium homeostasis and changes with age, 755–756, 756t
hypoparathyroidism, 759
lithium-induced hyperparathyroidism, 758, 758b
physiology of parathyroid hormone, 755
primary hyperparathyroidism, 756–758, 757f–758f, 757t, 757b
secondary hyperparathyroidism, 756, 756b
tertiary hyperparathyroidism, 758–759, 759f, 759b
Parathyroid hormone therapy (PHT)
assay of, 756t
for bone loss and osteoporosis, 164, 557
physiology of, 755
sarcopenia and, 589
Paratonia, of old age, 103
Parenteral feeding, palliative medicine and, 975
Parenteral nutrition (PN), 683, 683t
Parietal seizures, 456
Parkin, S-nitrosylation and, 153
Parkinson's disease (PD), 511–518, 513t–516t
clinical diagnosis of, 513–514, 513t
clinical features of, 511
clinical subtypes of, 514, 514t
constipation and, 913
delirium and, 904
epidemiology of, 514
etiology of, 514–515
gait and, 887
headache due to, 476
motor features of, 512
neuropathology of, 512
nonmotor features of, 512–513
orthostatic hypotension associated with, 342
primary autonomic failure with, 505–508
prognosis of, 518
S-nitrosylation and, 153
S-nitrosylation of PDI in protein misfolding and neurotoxicity in cell models of, 153–154
therapy techniques for, 876
caregiver education, 877
environmental changes, 877
functional mobility, 876–877
treatment of, 515, 515t–516t
drug strategies in advanced disease and palliative care, 517
drug treatment of motor features, 515–518, 515t–516t
drug treatment of nonmotor features, 517
surgical treatment, 517–518
Parkinson's disease dementia (PDD), 407–408, 409t
Parkinsonian disorders, with dementia, 390
Parkinsonism not due to Parkinson's disease, 518
drug-induced parkinsonism, 518
parkinsonism-plus, 518
vascular parkinsonism, 518
Parkinsonism-plus, 518
Parlodel. *See* Bromocriptine
Paromomycin, 666
Paroxetine
codeine and, 969
cytochrome P450 reaction with, 141t
for frontotemporal dementia, 432
herbal-drug interactions of, 142t
metabolism of, 140t
for migraine, 468
parkinsonism induced by, 518
for tension headache, 469
Paroxysmal atrial tachycardia (PAT), with atrioventricular block, 336
Part A, of Medicare, 1027
Part B, of Medicare, 1027
Partial edentulism, 604–605, 605f
Partial seizures. *See* Focal seizures
Participatory approach, to health promotion, 842
PAS. *See* Physician-assisted suicide
PAT. *See* Paroxysmal atrial tachycardia
Paternalism, 983–984
Patient Advice and Liaison Service (PALS), 1041
Patient education
for constipation, 918
for preventive practice systems, 853
to reduce medication problems, 883
for rehabilitation, 14

Pay-for-performance (P4P)
in managed care in United States, 1060–1061
Medicare preservation through, 1048
PBC. *See* Primary biliary cirrhosis
PCG/T. *See* Primary Care Group/Trust
PD. *See* Parkinson's disease
PDD. *See* Parkinson's disease dementia
PE. *See* Pulmonary embolism
Peak bone mass, 554
Pediculosis, 804
Pegaptanib sodium, 816–817
Pelvic examination, for constipation and FI, 916–917
Pelvic floor, 716, 927
Pelvic steal syndrome, ED and, 855–856, 856t
Pemetrexed, 384
Penicillamine, 646
D-Penicillamine, 526, 529
Penicillins
for aortic regurgitation, 319
C. difficile infection and, 664
for CNS infection, 548, 548t, 550b, 551
for dementia, 400
drug interactions of, 143
glomerulonephritis due to, 693t
thrombocytopenia associated with, 789
Penlac. *See* Ciclopirox
Pension systems, 993–994
early retirement, 995
Pentostatin, 787
Pentoxifylline, 639
Peptic ulcer disease
atypical presentation of, 208, 209t
in elderly, 621–622, 621f–622f
H. pylori and, 619–620, 619f
NSAIDs and, 619–622, 625b
Perception, of pain, 965–966
Percutaneous cholangiography (PTC), of biliary tract, 651–652
Percutaneous transcatheter implantation, of aortic valve prostheses for aortic stenosis, 317
Performance oriented mobility assessment (POMA), 900
Pergolide (Celance), 515t, 516–517
Perhexiline, 528–529
Perianal disease, in Crohn's disease, 670
Periarticular fractures, orthopedic geriatrics for, 584–585, 585f
Perimenopause, 163–164
Perindopril
for CAD prevention, 288
for chronic cardiac failure, 278b, 279
in frail elderly patient, 295, 297
after myocardial infarction, 292t
for stroke, 310–311, 495–496
for vascular cognitive impairment, 426–427
Perineal examination, for constipation and FI, 916–917
Periodic limb movements in sleep (PLMS), 947
Periodontal disease, 603–604
Perioperative period, fluid regimen over, 241
Peripheral neuropathies, 523–525, 524t
diabetic neuropathy, 524–525, 524t
Peripheral sensory receptors
balance and, 896
falls and, 895, 896t
testing of, 899t, 900
Peripheral vascular disease, 348–349
with diabetes mellitus, 764
Periprosthetic fractures, orthopedic geriatrics for, 585, 585f
Peritonitis, spontaneous bacterial, 641–642
Permethrin, 804
Peroxisome proliferator-activated receptor γ agonists, for glucose control, 768b
Peroxynitrite, 150, 152f
Personal autonomy, as aspect of social functioning, 227
Personal preferences, as aspect of social functioning, 227
Personal resources, 838
environmental supports v., 837, 837f, 838t
Personal values, as aspect of social functioning, 227
Personality
aging of, 178
personality stages and ego development, 178–181, 179t
social-cognitive approaches to personality, 181–182
synthesis and future directions, 182–183
depression in old age and, 434
measurement of, 179–182
social-cognitive approaches to, 181–182
stages of, 178–181, 179t
diversity and, 179
health and, 179
Personality disorders, 442–444
Personality traits, 179–180, 179t
diversity and, 180
health and, 180
Petit mal seizure, 455
PEU. *See* Protein-energy undernutrition
Peyronie disease, ED and, 856, 856t
PGRN mutations, 428–431, 429t
Phagocytosis, aging-related changes in, 82–83
Pharmacist consultation, for iatrogenic problems prevention, 851
Pharmacodynamic interactions, 143
Pharmacodynamics, aging effects on, 141, 141t
alterations in physiologic and homeostatic mechanisms, 141
altered sensitivity, 141, 141t
Pharmacokinetic interactions, 141–143, 141t–142t
Pharmacokinetics, aging effects on, 139–140, 139t–141t
absorption, 139
distribution, 139
elimination, 140, 141t
metabolism, 139–140, 140t
Pharmacologic stress testing, for CAD, 287
Pharmacology
of aging, 138
altered pharmacodynamics, 141, 141t
altered pharmacokinetics, 139–140, 139t–141t
drug interactions, 141–143, 141t–143t
epidemiology of drug use, 138
for insomnia, 946
Pharmacotherapy, geriatric, 880
adverse drug reactions, 881–882
adverse drug withdrawal events, 882
efficacy and safety of, 880
measures to reduce problems with, 883–884
health services approach to, 883
health systems design, 883
patient/caregiver education, 883–884
principles of, 884–885, 884t–885t
problems with, 880–881, 881f
therapeutic failure in, 882–883
Pharyngeal diverticula, 611–612, 611f
Phenobarbital, 462, 463t, 464, 803
Phenothiazines, 104, 339t, 503
Phenotypic definition, of frailty, 60–62, 61f
Phenoxybenzamine, 339t, 709t
Phentolamine, 857–858
Phenylephrine, 143t, 501
Phenytoin
cimetidine and, 622
cytochrome P450 reaction with, 141t
distribution of, 139
drug interactions of, 141
for epilepsy, 459, 462–463, 465b
herbal-drug interactions of, 142t
liver metabolism of, 635–636, 636t
low thyroxine due to, 738
for maintaining sinus rhythm, 333–334
metabolism of, 140t
for trigeminal neuralgia, 471, 477b
for ventricular arrhythmia, 327–328
Phobic disorders, 440
Phosphatase, as prostate disease marker, 704
Phosphate binders, 759b
Phosphate enemas, 920
Phosphate homeostasis, 698–700, 699t
Phosphodiesterase-5 inhibitors, 143, 282
Photoaging, 78
antiaging medicine for, 148, 148t
of skin, 133
PHT. *See* Parathyroid hormone therapy
Physical abuse, risk factors for, 961
Physical activity. *See also* Exercise
cardiovascular risk and, 303
cognitive functioning in response to, 175
constipation and, 912, 919
for dementia management, 400
sarcopenia and, 588, 591
for weight loss, 688
Physical environment, falls and modification of, 899, 900t
Physical examination
for COPD, 372
for dementia diagnosis, 395
for falls and balance, 899t, 900
for urinary incontinence assessment, 933
Physical function
as outcomes measurement for multidimensional interventions, 245, 248t–267t
weight loss and, 687
Physical health. *See* Health
Physical inactivity, as risk factor for CAD, 290
Physical performance, sarcopenia and, 590–591, 591f
Physical therapy
for Hutchinson-Gilford progeria syndrome, 71–72
for pain, 970–971
Physician
preoperative role of, 232, 232t
quality measurement of, 1026
Physician Quality Reporting Initiative (PQRI), 1053, 1057–1058
Physician-assisted suicide (PAS), 986–987
Physiologic assessment, of lower urinary tract, 113–114
Physiologic deterioration, 51–53, 52f
causes of deterioration, 51–53, 52f
interspecies and intraspecies variation in, 53
Physiologic recovery, in older victims of trauma, 866
Physiological changes, in older victims of trauma, 865–866
metabolic changes, 865–866
neuroendocrine responses, 865
Physiological mechanisms
aging effects on, altered pharmacodynamics and, 141
of social factors influencing health, 203

Physiology
of aging, 51
age changes in organismic function, 55–57, 57f
interspecies and intraspecies variation in physiologic deterioration, 53
physiologic deterioration and the aging phenotype, 51–53, 52f
in specific organs and organ systems, 53–55, 54f
autonomic, 498–501, 499f–500f
of falls causation, 895–897, 896t
of urinary incontinence, 926–927
Physiotherapy, 871
for cough, 980
for musculoskeletal pain, 977
research culture for, 872
skills for, 871–872
PhytoSERMs, for reproductive aging in women, 164–166
PICH. *See* Primary intracerebral hemorrhage
Pick bodies, in frontotemporal dementia, 428
Pilocarpine, 820
Pimecrolimus, 802–803
Pindolol, 510
Pioglitazone, 768–769
Pipeline, 462
Piperacillin, 648, 663t
Piroxicam, 139–140, 140t
Pituitary disorders, 735–737
Pizotifen, 468–469, 468t, 477b
Plasma monitoring, of antiepileptic drugs, 463
Platelet defects, purpura resulting from, 789
Platinum-based chemotherapy
for lung cancer, 383–384
for ovarian cancer, 724
Pleiotropic genes theory, 18–19, 21
Pleural effusion, 379, 379t
PLMS. *See* Periodic limb movements in sleep
PM. *See* Polymyositis
PN. *See* Parenteral nutrition
pNET. *See* Pancreatic neuroendocrine tumors
Pneumococcal disease, immune senescence and, 88
Pneumococcal meningitis. *See* Bacterial meningitis
Pneumococcal vaccine, for meningitis prevention, 549
Pneumoconiosis, 382
Pneumonia, 376–377, 377t
aspiration, 602–603, 954–955, 955t
atypical presentation of, 209–210, 209t
management of, 377
nosocomial, 377
vaccination for, 377
Pneumothorax, 379–380
PNFA. *See* Progressive nonfluent aphasia
POCD. *See* Postoperative cognitive dysfunction
Podiatry. *See* Foot disease
Podophyllin, 609
Policy ramifications
social vulnerability in old age, 204
telemedicine and, 1068
Polycythemia vera (PV), 779–781
Polyethylene glycol, 979
Polymyalgia rheumatica, 573, 580, 581f
Polymyositis (PM), 526–528
Polymyxin B, 803
Polypharmacy, 880
adverse drug reaction, 881–882
adverse drug withdrawal event, 882
constipation and, 912–913
dementia due to, 417
in frail elderly with heart disease, 298–299
measures to reduce problems with, 883–884
Polypharmacy (*Continued*)
health services approach to, 883
health systems design, 883
patient/caregiver education, 883–884
as secondary cause of acquired immunodeficiency in old age, 89
therapeutic failure, 882–883
Polyps, of large bowel, 109, 673–674
POMA. *See* Performance oriented mobility assessment
Poor Law Infirmaries, 997
Population
aging of, causes and results of, 3
younger v. older people in, 8, 8f
Population approach, to stroke prevention, 481
Portal hypertension, 641
Positional feedback, stroke and, 875
Positive affect, in allostasis and allostatic overload, 161
Positron emission tomography, for pancreas adenocarcinoma, 629
Possible selves model, 181
Post-Freudian theory, on personality stages and ego development, 178–179
Postherpetic neuralgia, 472, 803–804
Postintubation dysphagia, 611
Postmenopause, 164
Postmortem diagnosis, of frontotemporal dementia, 430–431
Postoperative cardiac complications, in elderly surgical patient, incidence of, 235
Postoperative cognitive dysfunction (POCD), 242
Postoperative delirium, 241–242
Postoperative dementia, 242
Postoperative hypoxemia, 234–235
Postoperative myocardial infarction, 235
Postoperative outcomes, age, surgery, and, 230–231
Postoperative respiratory complications, in elderly, incidence of, 234
Postoperative stroke, 241
Postprandial hypotension, 346–347, 503–504, 510
Postrenal acute renal failure, 692–693
Poststroke dementia (PSD), 422, 426
Posttraumatic stress disorder (PTSD), 440–441
Postural changes, of old age, 103
Postural control, 895, 896t
clinical assessment based on, 898, 899t
drugs and, 898, 900t
Postural hypotension. *See* Orthostatic hypotension
Posture test, 498
Potassium, for accelerated atrioventricular rhythm, 336
Potassium balance, 698, 698t
Potassium channel blockers. *See* Class III antiarrhythmic drugs
Potassium chloride, 336, 616
Potassium intake, 303, 307–308
Potassium iodide, 745
Potassium-sparing diuretics
for chronic cardiac failure, 278
hyperkalemia due to, 698t
for hypertension, 309
hypoaldosteronism and, 733
Pout reflex. *See* Snout reflex
PPS. *See* Prospective Payment System
PQRI. *See* Physician Quality Reporting Initiative
PQRST, for pain, 975, 975b
Practice setting, multidimensional geriatric assessment in, 214–215
Pramipexole (Mirapexin), 515t, 516–517
Pramlintide, 774
Prandial glucose regulators, 769
Pravastatin, 496, 773
Prazosin, 281–282, 339t, 709t
Prednisolone
for arthritis, 570
for autoimmune hepatitis, 640
for cluster headache, 470
for Crohn's disease, 656
Cushing syndrome due to, 734
for giant cell arteritis, 473–474
for idiopathic pulmonary fibrosis, 381
for polymyositis or dermatomyositis, 527
for ulcerative colitis, 667t
Prednisone
for asthma, 367t
for bullous pemphigoid, 807
for chronic lymphocytic leukemia, 787
for chronic meningitis, 550
for Crohn's disease, 669t, 670
for idiopathic thrombocytopenic purpura, 789
for lymphocytic and collagenous colitis, 671
for lymphoma, 784–786
for multiple myeloma, 783
for myasthenia gravis, 531
for thyroid nodule management, 753
for ulcerative colitis, 667t
Pregabalin, 462–463, 463t, 472, 477b
Pregnenolone, 148
Premalignant disorders, of vulva, 719, 719t
Premature aging, 20–21, 836. *See also* Hutchinson-Gilford progeria; Werner syndrome
Preoperative assessment, of elderly patients, 232–234, 232t–233t
functional reserve estimation, 233, 233t
general strategy of, 232–233, 233t
preoperative role of physician, 232, 232t
"routine" preoperative testing, 233–234
Preoperative β-blockade, in old age, 232
Prerenal acute renal failure, 691
Presbycusis, 823–824
Prescription drug plans, 1058
plan reimbursement for, 1060
quality measurement of, 1051–1052
Presenilin-1, mutations in, 413
Pressor agents, for orthostatic hypotension, 509–510
Pressure sores. *See* Pressure ulcers
Pressure ulcers, 939
classification of, 940
management and treatment of, 940–941
normal aging and, 939
palliative care for, 973
pathophysiology of, 939–940
quality indicator and litigation with, 941, 942t
risk assessment of, 940
Presyncope, 207
Preventive care
accident prevention, 850–851
of cancer, 792–795
for community-living older adult, 835–836
benefits of, 835
economic evaluation framework, 838, 839f
for frail older adults, 837–838
intervention study lessons, 842–845
legislation and policy needs, 845–846
lessons learned, 844–845, 845f
need for, 836–837
research needs, 845–846
screening and assessment for, 838–842
of delirium, 905–906, 907t
disease prevention, 848–849
Evergreen Action Nutrition, 842–843
of fractures, 585–586
frailty prevention, 849–850

Preventive care (*Continued*)
health promotion v., 842
iatrogenic problem prevention, 851
individualizing, 852, 853t
levels of, 842
preventive practice systems, 852–853
psychosocial illness prevention, 851–852
of respiratory problems in older surgical patient, 234, 235t
of secondary stroke, 495–496
of skin aging, 136–137
of stroke, 481, 481t
high-risk approach, 481–482
mass approach, 481
of vascular cognitive impairment, 426–428
of venous thromboembolism, 359–360
Preventive practice systems, 852–853
Primary aging, 51
Primary autonomic failure, 342, 505–508, 506f
Primary biliary cirrhosis (PBC), 640
Primary care expansion, for cost effective quality of care, 1052
Primary Care Group/Trust (PCG/T), 4
Primary care setting, occupational therapy in, 871
Primary CNS lymphoma, 533, 536–538
Primary disease prevention, 848, 849t–850t
Primary headache disorders, 466–467
chronic daily headache, 469–470, 470t
cluster headache, 470
migraine, 466, 468t
tension headache, 469
Primary health care, in regions of world, 1013–1014
Primary hyperparathyroidism, 756–758, 757f–758f, 757t, 757b
Primary immunity, aging-related changes in, 82
Primary intracerebral hemorrhage (PICH), 485
Primary progressive aphasias, 407–410, 409t
Primary sclerosing cholangitis (PSC), 641, 645
Primidone, 462, 463t, 464, 519
Priming, aging effects on, 173
Primitive reflexes, age-related changes in, 104–105
Prion disease, 388
Privatization experiences, of pension systems, 994–995
ProAmatine. *See* Midodrine
Probably symptomatic epilepsy, 456–457
Probenecid, 143
Procainamide
for AF, 333
drug interactions of, 143
elimination of, 141t
for maintaining sinus rhythm, 333–334
after myocardial infarction, 292–293
for SVT, 336
syncope caused by, 339t
for ventricular arrhythmia, 327–328, 328t
for Wolff-Parkinson-White syndrome, 332
Procedural memory. *See* Implicit memory
Process measurement, in United States managed care, 1061
Processing speed, aging effects on, 171–172
Prochlorperazine, 518, 978
Proctoscopy, for constipation and FI, 916
Productive aging, 189–190, 193
ageism in the workplace, 195–196
demography, 193
in developing nations, 196–197
in Japan, 196
with paid employment, 194–195
in retirement, 193–194
with unpaid work, 196
Professional services review organizations (PSROs), quality improvement and, 1054–1055
Progenitor compartment, of blood, aging of, 129–130
Progerin
in aging process, 68–71, 69f
in arteriosclerosis of aging and Hutchinson-Gilford progeria syndrome, 70–71
farnesylation of, in Hutchinson-Gilford progeria syndrome, 68
in Hutchinson-Gilford progeria syndrome, 66, 68f
Progeroid syndromes, 20–21. *See also* Hutchinson-Gilford progeria; Werner syndrome
normal aging and, 33–34
Progesterone therapy
depression associated with, 435
for menopause, 717–718
for vaginal cancer, 722
Progestin therapy, 124, 728, 728t
Program for All-inclusive Care for the Elderly (PACE), 1053, 1058–1059
Programmed aging, 18
Progressive nonfluent aphasia (PNFA), 407, 409t, 428–430
Progressive resistance training (PRT), 859
Proinflammatory cytokines, 589, 905
Prokinetics, for nausea and vomiting, 978
Proliferative lymphocyte disorders, of old age, 86–87
Propafenone
for AF, 333
for maintaining sinus rhythm, 333
for orthostatic hypotension, 510
for SVT, 336
for ventricular arrhythmia, 327, 330t
Propantheline, 663t
Propiverine, 721, 935
Propoxyphene, 969
Propranolol
absorption of, 139
for AF, 334
cimetidine and, 622
for cirrhosis complications, 641
depression associated with, 435
drug-disease interactions of, 143t
for essential tremor, 519
for hyperthyroidism, 742–743
metabolism of, 139–140, 140t, 635–636
for migraine, 468, 468t
after myocardial infarction, 292t
for orthostatic hypotension, 510
for paroxysmal atrial tachycardia with atrioventricular block, 336
for SVT, 336
thyroid hormone secretion and metabolism in response to, 738
for ventricular arrhythmia, 328t
for Wolff-Parkinson-White syndrome, 332
Propylthiouracil, 742–743
Prospective memory, aging effects on, 172–173
Prospective Payment System (PPS), in Medicare, 1027
Prostaglandin analogues, 568–569, 813
Prostaglandin inhibitors, 495, 510
Prostaglandin therapy, 725, 857–858
Prostate, 701
assessment of, 702–704, 703f–704f
clinical aspects of disease of, 705–714, 706f–708f, 709t, 710f, 711t, 715f
benign prostatic hyperplasia, 706–708, 706f–707f
prostatitis, 705
development of, 701–702, 701f–702f
morphology of, 701–702, 702f
serum markers of disease of, 704–705, 705f
surgery involving, 709–710
Prostate cancer, 710–711, 710f, 711t
localized cancer, 711–712, 711t
local-regional disease, 712–713
metastatic disease, 713–714
screening for, 794
synopsis of elderly patient with, 714–715, 715f
Prostate-specific antigen (PSA), 704–705, 705f, 711–712
Prostatitis, 705
Prostrate surgery, ED and, 856, 856t
Protection, as response to stressors, 158, 160f
Protein
accumulation, connective tissue disorders associated with, 581–582
aging effects on synthesis and degradation of, 34–35, 48–49
intake, sarcopenia and, 590–592
metabolism, resistance exercise and insulin, 861–862
misfolding
in cell models of Parkinson's disease and Alzheimer's disease, S-nitrosylation of PDI in, 153–154
in neurodegenerative disease, 150–151
of parkin, 153
requirements
aging effects on, 680–682
for exercise for successful aging, 862
Protein-energy undernutrition (PEU), 949–950
Proteoglycans, of connective tissues, 75, 75t
Prothrombinex, 495
Proton pump inhibitors
for dexamethasone, 537
for GERD, 108
for *H. pylori* infection, 620
for nonulcer dyspepsia, 623
for NSAID use, 568–569, 574
for peptic ulcer disease, 622
for protection, 473–474
renal failure due to, 692
Provider education, for preventive practice systems, 853
Provoked seizures, 460
PRT. *See* Progressive resistance training
Pruritus, 802–803, 802t
PSA. *See* Prostate-specific antigen
PSC. *See* Primary sclerosing cholangitis
PSD. *See* Poststroke dementia
Pseudodementia, 394–395, 408, 435
Pseudodiverticulosis, intramural, 616–617, 617f
Pseudoephedrine, 143t
Pseudogout, 574–575, 581
Pseudo-obstruction, of large bowel, 672
Psoriatic arthritis, 571–572
PSROs. *See* Professional services review organizations
Psychiatric disorders, 386, 946. *See also* Functional psychiatric illness
Psychiatric medications, dementia associated with, 387
Psychoactive drugs, 241, 339t
Psychogenic amnesia, epilepsy v., 459
Psychogenic attack, epilepsy v., 457–458, 458t
Psychological approaches, to pain, 971
Psychological distress, constipation and, 913
Psychological impact, of constipation and FI, 918
Psychological mechanisms
ED and, 857
of pain, 967
of social factors influencing health, 203
Psychological symptoms, of dementia, 393t, 394
Psychosis. *See* Late life psychosis
Psychosocial consequences, of hearing loss, 825–826

Psychosocial function, as outcomes measurement for multidimensional interventions, 245
Psychosocial illness prevention, 851–852
Psychotropics, 138, 474
Psyllium, 142t, 671
PTC. *See* Percutaneous cholangiography
PTH. *See* Parathyroid hormone
Ptosis, senile, 810, 811f
PTSD. *See* Posttraumatic stress disorder
Pulmonary disease, insomnia and, 945–946
Pulmonary embolism (PE), 356–361, 379t
Pulmonary function testing, in COPD, 365f, 370, 371f
Pulmonary host defense, age-related changes in, 99–100
Pulmonary rehabilitation, for COPD, 373–374
Pulmonary vasculitis, 381
Pulmonic regurgitation, 326
Pulse pressure, cardiovascular risk and, 301, 301f
Pulsion diverticula. *See* Epiphrenic diverticula
Pure autonomic failure (PAF), 342, 505–506
Pure-tone sensitivity
  behavioral implications of loss of, 824–825, 825t
  psychosocial consequences of loss of, 825–826
Purpura
  from platelet defects, 789
  senile, 789
PV. *See* Polycythemia vera
Pyogenic liver abscess, 644
Pyramidal disorders, in dementia, 390
Pyrazinamide, 378, 550
Pyrethrin, for pediculosis, 804
Pyridostigmine (Mestinon), 508b, 510, 531
Pyridoxine, 378
Pyrosis. *See* Heartburn

Q

QALYs. *See* Quality-adjusted life years
QIOs. *See* Quality Improvement Organizations
QIs. *See* Quality indicators
QISMC. *See* Quality Improvement System for Managed Care
Qualitative methodologies, for research in older people, 23–26
Quality Improvement Organizations (QIOs), 1029–1030
  quality improvement and, 1055–1056
  technical support through, 1053
Quality Improvement System for Managed Care (QISMC), 1051
Quality indicators (QIs)
  for nursing homes, 1029
  pressure ulcers as, 941, 942t
Quality of care
  accreditation for, 1041
  Audit Commission for, 1040–1041
  clinical audit for, 1039–1040
  complaints procedure for, 1041
  cost effective, 1052–1053, 1052t
    coordinated care models, 1052–1053
    primary care expansion, 1052
    technology for, 1053, 1053t
  description of, 1038–1039
  future of, 1043, 1056t
  improvement of
    benchmarking, 1042
    business process reengineering, 1042
    continuous, 1042, 1043f
    current NHS approach, 1043–1045, 1043f
    outcomes of, 1042
    total quality management, 1041–1042
    in United Kingdom, 1038
Quality of care *(Continued)*
  management of, 1041–1042
  measurement of, 1039, 1048–1052
    hospital, 1049–1050
    managed care plans, 1051
    nursing home, 1050–1051
    physician, 1048–1049
    prescription drug plans, 1051–1052
    in United States managed care, 1061–1062, 1062f
  Medicare preservation through, 1046
    pay-for-performance, 1048
    regulatory approach to, 1047
    reporting of quality data, 1047–1048
  organizations promoting, 1054–1056, 1054t
    identification and analysis, 1054
    resources for, 1054–1056
  standards, guidelines, and protocols for, 1040–1041, 1040t
Quality of life
  constipation and FI and, 918
  in epidemiology of aging, 4–9, 4f, 6t, 7f–9f, 9t
    age group definitions in, 6, 6t, 7f
    changes over time in, 5
    cross-sectional v. longitudinal data in study of aging, 5–6
    ethnicity, emigration, and immigration effects on, 9, 9t
    features of younger v. older people, 8, 8f
    indices of dependency in, 8
    inequalities among older individuals, 9
    inevitability of aging, 8
    living alone and, 9, 9f
    marital status in, 7–8, 7f
    measuring differences in, 5–8, 6t, 7f–8f
    predicting future of, 5
    sex in, 6–7, 7f
  fall and, 839–840
  hypertension and, 310
  love and sex for, 858
  obesity effects on, 686
  as outcomes measurement for multidimensional interventions, 246
  weight loss and, 687
Quality-adjusted life years (QALYs), for quality of life measurement, 4–5
Quantification, of sarcopenia, 587–588
Quetiapine, 140t, 517
Quinapril, 279
Quinidine
  for AF, 333
  antacids and, 622
  for atrial flutter, 335
  cimetidine and, 622
  codeine and, 969
  cytochrome P450 reaction with, 141t
  distribution of, 139
  drug interactions of, 141–143, 281
  esophageal injury due to, 616
  for maintaining sinus rhythm, 333–334
  metabolism of, 139–140, 140t
  after myocardial infarction, 292–293
  for SVT, 336
  syncope caused by, 339t
  for ventricular arrhythmia, 327–328, 328t
  for Wolff-Parkinson-White syndrome, 332
Quinolone, 141, 620, 648, 691

R

Radiculopathy, cervical, 539–541, 540f
Radioactive iodine
  for hyperthyroidism, 742–744, 754b
  hypothyroidism due to, 745
  for thyroid nodule management, 753
Radiographs, of cervical radiculopathy and myelopathy, 540–541, 540f
Radiology
  of large bowel, 661
  for liver, 637
  in osteomalacia, 560, 560f
  of small bowel, 653
Radiotherapy, 799
  for bone pain, 977
  dementia associated with, 389
  for intracranial tumors, 537
  for neuropathic pain, 977
  for non-small cell lung cancer, 383
  for pancreas adenocarcinoma, 631
  for prostate cancer, 712
RAI. *See* Resident Assessment Instrument
Raloxifene, 164–165, 556, 556t, 558, 586
Ramelteon, for insomnia, 946
Ramipril, 278b, 279, 292t, 495–496
Randomized controlled trial (RCT)
  barriers to participation in, 27, 27t
  of geriatric interventions and associated outcome measures, 248t–265t, 266t–267t
  for researching aging and related conditions, 25–26
Ranibizumab, 816–817, 817f
Ranitidine
  drug interactions of, 143
  elimination of, 141t
  headache due to, 475t
  for peptic ulcer disease, 622
  for ulcer prevention, 621
Ranolazine, 290
Rapid eye movement (REM) sleep, with advancing age, 945
Rapid eye movement sleep behavior disorder (RBD), 947
Rasagiline (Azilect), 515t, 516
RBD. *See* Rapid eye movement sleep behavior disorder
RCPSC. *See* Council of the Royal College of Physicians and Surgeons of Canada
RCT. *See* Randomized controlled trial
RE. *See* Refractory anemia
Reactive nitrogen species (RNS), 151–152
Reactive oxygen species (ROS)
  calcium ion influx in generation of, 152
  in cellular aging, 42–44
  generation of, 151–152
  intracellular calcium in generation of, 44–45
  mitochondrial genetics, aging, and, 38–39
  in neurobiology of aging, 150, 151f–152f
  skin aging due to, 136
Reality orientation, for dementia management, 399
Recognized myocardial infarction, 286, 286t
Recombinant erythropoietin. *See* Erythropoietin
Recombinant factor VII, for stroke, 493
Recombinant tissue plasminogen activator (rt-PTA), for pulmonary embolism, 359
Recruitment, for conducting research involving older individuals, 27, 27t
Rectal endosonography, 662
Rectal examination
  for constipation and FI, 916–917
  of prostate, 702
  for urinary incontinence assessment, 934
Rectal outlet delay, 910t
  anorectal dysfunction and, 914–915, 915t
  suppositories and, 920–921
Red cells, aging effects on, 130–131
Red clover, 164, 718
5α-Reductase inhibitors, 138
α-Reductase inhibitors, 708–709, 709t
Refeeding syndrome, 954, 954t

Reference intervals
geriatric, 219–220, 219f, 220t
geriatric individuality and, 218–219, 219f
for laboratory diagnosis, 218
Reflexes
deep tendon, age-related changes in, 103–104
glabellar tap, aging effects on, 105
primitive, age-related changes in, 104–105
Reflux esophagitis, 614–615
Refractory anemia (RE), 777, 778t
Registered nurses (RNs), in nursing homes, 1029
Regulation, of longevity, 30–32, 31f
Regulatory approach, to Medicare preservation, 1047
Rehabilitation
assessment and potential for, 7–9, 8t
audiologic, 826, 829–830, 829t–830t
after cancer treatment, 800
content of, 13–15, 13f
definitions of, 1–2
disability
assessment of, 10–11
illness v. role, 6
prevention of, 2–3
process of, 5–6
revised ICIDH model, 6–7, 7f
WHO classification of, 6
general principles of, 1
historical overview of, 1
older age and need for, 2, 2t
policy framework in United Kingdom, 3–5
pulmonary, 373–374
services for, 15–17
geriatric day hospital, 16–17
home-based, 15–16
location of, 15
teamwork in, 11–13
therapy techniques, 870
for fractured neck, 875–876
for frailty, 877–879
future directions for, 879–880
groups of, 873
occupational therapy, 870–871
for Parkinson's disease, 876–877
physiotherapy, 871–872
process for, 872
for stroke, 873–875
for visual loss, 820–822
Rehydration
for confusion, 981
for diarrhea, 979
Reimbursement, by Medicare, 1046
Relaxation therapy, for dementia management, 400
Relevance to need, of quality of care, 1039
REM sleep. *See* Rapid eye movement
Reminiscence, for dementia management, 399
Remodeling. *See* Bone, remodeling of
Remote symptomatic, 456
Renal blood flow, aging effects on, 111
Renal complications, of aneurysm surgery for abdominal aortic aneurysm, 354
Renal disease. *See* Kidney disease
Renal failure
acute, 691, 692t
established, 696
intrinsic, 691–692, 693t
tertiary hyperparathyroidism due to, 758–759, 759f, 759b
Renal function, measurement of, 690, 691t
Renal insufficiency, anemia and, 777
Renal management, for acute pancreatitis, 632
Renal replacement therapy (RRT), 694, 696
Repaglinide, 769–770
Replacement function, empowerment function v., 844–845
Replicative senescence, 45–48
of blood cells and hematopoietic stem cells, 128
genomic instability in, 46–48
phenotypical changes due to,
telomere structure and, 32, 40
telomeres and telomerase in, 46
Repression, gene, in cell senescence, 46–47
Reproductive aging
in men
andropause, 166–167
therapeutic horizons, 167
unresolved issues, 167
in women, 163–164
perimenopause to menopause, 163–164
postmenopause, 164
therapeutic horizons, 164–165
unresolved issues, 165–167
Requip. *See* Ropinirole
Research
on aging
in Latin America, 1019, 1020t
in North America, 30
reasons for investing in, 35–36
collaborative, in Europe, 1004
for constipation and fecal incontinence, 924t, 925
incompetent patient and, 985–986
in occupational therapy and physiotherapy, 872
in older people, 23
exclusion of older people from research, 26
obtaining informed consent, 26–27
outcomes measurement, 28, 28t
qualitative methodologies, 23–26
recruitment and retention, 27, 27t
study designs, 23
Resection, for pancreas adenocarcinoma, 629–630
Resident Assessment Instrument (RAI), 1050
Residential care. *See also* Assisted living facilities; Long-term care facilities
diabetes mellitus in patients receiving, 766–767, 767t, 767b
Resilience, successful aging due to, 184–186
Resistance exercise, 859
memory disorders and, 864
protein metabolism and, 861–862
for stroke therapy, 875
successful aging and, 862–863
Resource Utilization Groups (RUG), in Medicare, 1027
Respiratory complications, of aneurysm surgery for abdominal aortic aneurysm, 354
Respiratory disorders, dementia associated with, 389
Respiratory function tests, 97
Respiratory infection, 99–100, 376
Respiratory management, for acute pancreatitis, 632
Respiratory problems, in older surgical patient, 234–235, 235t
estimation of respiratory risk and possible preventive strategies, 234, 235t
incidence of postoperative respiratory complications, 234
late postoperative hypoxemia, 234–235
pathophysiology of respiratory problems in elderly surgical patients, 234
Respiratory risk, in older surgical patient, 234, 235t
Respiratory system, aging of, 97
functional changes, 98–99
pulmonary host defense and immune response changes, 99–100
respiratory function tests, 97
structural changes, 98
Resting electrocardiography, for CAD, 286–287
Resting metabolic rate (RMR), aerobic exercises and, 861
Restless leg syndrome (RLS), 519, 947
Retention
for conducting research involving older individuals, 27, 27t
of urine, 708
Retina disorders, 815–819, 816f–817f
Retinoic acid, 14–15, 788
Retinoids, 137, 148t
Retinopathy, diabetic, 763, 764t, 813b, 815–816, 816f
Retinovascular occlusive disease, 818–819
Retirement
age of, 994
early options, 994–995
productive aging in, 193–194
social role during, 187
golden age of increasing life expectancy and compression of morbidity, 188–189
inequalities in later life—continuities and impact, 190–191
opportunity age—successful aging and the third age, 189–190
"problem" of old age, 187–188
theoretical approaches: from functionalism to structured dependency, 188
Retirement policies, in Latin America, 1017–1018, 1017t
Revascularization, coronary, 293t, 294
Reversibility, of airflow obstruction in asthma, 364–365, 365f
Revised Trauma Score (RTS), 867
Revised Trauma Score + Injury Severity Score (TRISS), 867
Reynolds Foundation, geriatric medicine education and, 1032
Rheumatoid arthritis, 570–571, 571t
aging of connective tissues in patients with, 79
atypical presentation of, 209t, 210
clinical assessment of, 570–571, 571t
clinical features of, 570, 571t
clinical outcomes of, 571
comorbidity of, 848
in elderly, 571
epidemiology of, 570
spinal cord compression in, 541, 542f
Rheumatoid factors, 566
Ribavirin, 638–639
Rifamixin, 655
Rifampicin, 378, 640
Rifampin, 141t, 548, 550, 803
Rigidity, 512
Riluzole, 530
Rimantadine, 376
Ring, esophageal. *See* Lower esophageal ring
Risedronate, 556, 556t, 563, 586
Risk
of adverse drug reactions, 881–882
of adverse drug withdrawal event, 882
of AF, 330–331
of delirium, 905
dementia and, 385–386, 398–399
for depression in old age, 433–434
of falls, 894–895, 894t
environmental, 895, 895t
injuries and, 900

Risk (*Continued*)
of FI, 910–912, 911t
online computerized, for surgery and anesthesia in old age, 243
of pressure ulcers, 940
for stroke, 479–480, 480t
blood tests for diagnosis of, 492
modifiable factors, 480, 480t
nonmodifiable factors, 480, 480t
of therapeutic failure, 882–883
of thromboembolic stroke in patients with cardiac arrhythmias, 334–335, 334t
for venous thromboembolism, 356, 356t
Risperidone, 140t, 401, 438, 443b
Ritonavir, 141t
Rituximab
for arthritis, 569–570
for chronic lymphocytic leukemia, 787
for idiopathic thrombocytopenic purpura, 789
for lymphoma, 784–785
for myasthenia gravis, 531
Rivaroxaban, 360
Rivastigmine, 400, 419, 419t, 432, 517
Rivermead Perceptual Assessment Battery, 872
RLS. *See* Restless leg syndrome
RMR. *See* Resting metabolic rate
RNS. *See* Reactive nitrogen species
RNs. *See* Registered nurses
Robot-aided therapy, for stroke therapy, 875
Roentgenography. *See* Chest roentgenography
Ropinirole (Requip), 515t, 516–517, 635–636
ROS. *See* Reactive oxygen species
Rosiglitazone, 768–769
Rosuvastatin, 312
Rotigotine, 516–517
"Routine" preoperative testing, 233–234
Royal Colleges of Physicians of the United Kingdom, 998, 1024, 1024t
Royal Surgical Aid Society, long-term care and, 1024, 1024t
RRT. *See* Renal replacement therapy
rt-PTA. *See* Recombinant tissue plasminogen activator
RTS. *See* Revised Trauma Score
Rufinamide, 462
RUG. *See* Resource Utilization Groups
Rupture
of abdominal aortic aneurysm, mortality from, 354
of cerebral vessels, 482–483

S

SAECG. *See* Signal-averaged electrocardiography
Safety
in dementia management, 398–399
of geriatric pharmacotherapy, 880
telemedicine for monitoring, 1066
SAH. *See* Subarachnoid hemorrhage
Salbutamol, 693
Salicylates, 141, 143, 693–694, 738, 824
Salicylic acid, 802
Saline depletion, surgery and anesthesia in old age and, 240
Saliva, 605–606
Salivary glands, 605–606
Salivation, aging effects on, 106
Salmeterol, for COPD, 373
Salt depletion, surgery and anesthesia in old age and, 240
Salt restriction
for hypertension management, 307
for stroke prevention, 496
stroke risk and, 481
SAP. *See* Severe acute pancreatitis
SAPS. *See* Simplified Acute Physiology Score
Sarcoidosis, of lung, 381
Sarcoma, of small bowel, 659
Sarcopenia, 587
in aging, 34–35, 102, 121–122
consequences of, 590–593, 590f–591f
definition of, 587–588
epidemiology of, 587
etiology of, 588–590
frailty and, 1010–1011
treatment and future perspectives of, 591
Sarcopenic obesity, 587–589
SARMs. *See* Selective androgen receptor modulators
SARS. *See* Severe acute respiratory syndrome
Satisfaction, as aspect of social functioning, 227
SBP. *See* Spontaneous bacterial peritonitis
Scabies, 804
Scalp disease, in Down syndrome, 448–449
SCC. *See* Squamous cell carcinoma
Schatzki ring. *See* Lower esophageal ring
Schizophrenia, 439. *See also* Late-onset schizophrenia
SCI. *See* Spinal cord injury
Screening, 839
for cancer, 673–674, 792–795
cognitive, 403–404
in community-living older adult
depression, 840–841
fall risk, 839–840
for health promotion and preventive care, 838–842
nutrition, 840
for delirium, 906, 906t
for disease prevention, 848
for fall risk, 897–898, 898t
for hearing loss, 832–833, 833f, 833t
with laboratory medicine for geriatric population, 219–220, 219f, 220t
nutritional, 678–680
for small bowel disorders, 652
for thyroid dysfunction, 740
SDB. *See* Sleep-disordered breathing
Sebaceous glands, aging of, 135–136
Seborrheic dermatitis, 802
"Second language of sex,", 858
Secondary aging, 51
Secondary autonomic dysfunction, orthostatic hypotension associated with, 342
Secondary autonomic failure, in elderly, 507–508
Secondary disability, therapy for, 877
Secondary disease prevention, 848, 849t–850t
Secondary health care, in regions of world, 1013–1014
Secondary hyperparathyroidism, 756, 756b
Secondary osteoporosis, 554
Secondary stroke, prevention of, 495–496
Secondary thrombocytopenia, 789
Secretase inhibitor drugs, 401
β-Secretase inhibitors, 420
γ-Secretase inhibitors, 420
Sedation
in delirium or confusion, 233t
dementia associated with, 395
Sedative hypnotics, 143, 946
Sedatives
for dysphagia and chest pain, 614
falls due to, 208
fatigue due to, 206–207
for hyperthyroidism, 743
hypothyroidism due to, 746–747
orthostatic hypotension and, 503
as secondary cause of acquired immunodeficiency in old age, 89
Seizure
with dementia, 390
epileptic, 453, 455–456, 455t
provoked, 460
Selection. *See* Natural selection
Selective androgen receptor modulators (SARMs), 167, 558
Selective estrogen receptor modulators (SERMS), 163–166, 556–558
Selective serotonin reuptake inhibitors (SSRIs)
for anxiety disorders, 440–441
chronic cardiac failure and, 284
codeine and, 969
for dementia, 401
for depression in old age, 435
dry mouth and, 605
for frontotemporal dementia, 432
for obsessive-compulsive disorder, 441
for pain, 970
for Parkinson's disease, 517
toxic serotonin syndrome and, 519
Selegiline (Eldepryl, Zelapar), 513, 515t, 516–517
Selenium sulfide, 802
Self
aging of, 178
personality stages and ego development, 178–181, 179t
social-cognitive approaches to personality, 181–182
synthesis and future directions, 182–183
identity and, 181
Self-assessed health, social factors associated with, 203
Self-esteem, in allostasis and allostatic overload, 161
Self-management support, for tertiary disease prevention, 849
Self-neglect, senile, 443
Self-rated health, as outcomes measurement for multidimensional interventions, 245
Self-stroking, for stroke therapy, 874
Self-worth, psychosocial illness prevention and, 852
Semantic dementia, 407, 409t, 428–430
Semantic memory, aging effects on, 173
Senescence. *See also* Aging; Replicative senescence
definition of, 51
immune, clinical consequences of, 85–88
Senile emphysema, 98
Senile ptosis, 810, 811f
Senile purpura, 789
Senile self-neglect, 443
Senior Risk Reduction Demonstration, 1058
Sensation, of skin, aging effects on, 136
Sensitivity, to drugs, aging effects on, 141, 141t
Sensory signs, of old age, 104
Sensory systems, for balance, 895–896
Sentinel lymph node, 727
SERMS. *See* Selective estrogen receptor modulators
Seronegative spondylarthritis, 571–572
Serotonin, age-related perception of pain and, 966
Serotonin antagonists, 346, 468–469, 477b
Serotonin-norepinephrine reuptake inhibitors (SNRIs), 435
Serous cystadenoma, of pancreas, 627
Sertraline
for anxiety disorders, 440
for dementia, 401, 432
for depression in old age, 435
herbal-drug interactions of, 142t
for Parkinson's disease, 517
for primary biliary cirrhosis, 640
for vasovagal syncope, 346

Serum antigens, for pancreas adenocarcinoma, 628
Serum cholesterol testing, for diagnosing stroke risk factors, 492
Serum glucose testing, for diagnosing stroke risk factors, 492
Serum markers, of prostate disease, 704–705, 705f
Serum thyroglobulin, 740
Service provision, for geriatric patients, social assessment for determination of, 224
SES. *See* Socioeconomic status
Severe acute pancreatitis (SAP), 632
Severe acute respiratory syndrome (SARS), in regions of world, 1012
Sevoflurane, 231
Sexual abuse, risk factors for, 961
Sexuality
- definition of, 854
- epidemiology of aging and, 6–7, 7f
- in old age, 724–725, 854
  - ED, 855–858
  - examination and evaluation of patient, 855
  - lesbian, gay, bisexual, or transgender, 855
  - management of couples with sexual problems, 725
  - medical problems, surgery, and medications, 855, 856t–857t
  - normal aging and, 854–855
  - "second language of sex,", 858
  - sexual behavior and age, 724–725
  - sexual response and age, 725

Sexually transmitted diseases (STDs), in old age, 855
Shankhapushpi, 142t
SHHS. *See* Sleep Heart Health Study
Shiga toxin producing *E. coli* 0157:H7, 665–666
Shigella, large bowel infection with, 665
Shingles. *See* Herpes zoster
S/HMO. *See* Social/health maintenance organization
Short-term memory, aging effects on, 172
Shy-Drager syndrome. *See* Multiple system atrophy
Sick sinus syndrome. *See* Tachycardia-bradycardia syndrome
Sigmoidoscopy, 662
Signal-averaged electrocardiography (SAECG), for CAD, 287
Signaling pathways, aging effects on, 49
Sildenafil
- drug interactions of, 143
- for ED, 725, 854, 857
- ophthalmic complications of, 820

"Silence by proxy," due to frailty, 204
Silent brain infarcts, 485, 488–489
Silver, for pressure ulcers, 941
Simplified Acute Physiology Score (SAPS), 867
Simvastatin, 142t, 289, 496, 772–773
Sinemet. *See* Co-careldopa
Sinus disease, headache and facial pain due to, 473
Sinus rhythm, antiarrhythmic drugs for maintenance of, 333–334
Sirolimus, 807
Sitagliptin, 774
SIVD. *See* Subcortical ischemic vascular disease
Skeletal muscle
- aerobic exercise and, 860
- pressure ulcers and, 940

Skeletal muscle mass index (SMI), 587–588
Skeletal muscle relaxants, 143t
Skeleton, aging of, 119–121, 119f–120f
- skeletal metabolism changes, 121
- structural changes, 120–121, 120f

Skin
- aging of, 55, 133
  - extrinsic aging, 133–135
  - hair, 136
  - immune function, 136
  - intrinsic aging, 133
  - mechanism of, 78, 136
  - nails, 136
  - nerves and sensation, 136
  - normal, 939
  - subcutaneous tissue, 136
  - sweat glands, 135–137
  - treatment and prevention of, 136–137
  - in women, 136
- disease of, 801–809, 801b, 802t, 805b
  - approach to patient with, 801
  - cutaneous cancer, 805–807, 805b
  - eczematous disorders, 801–802
  - epidemiology of, 801
  - infectious diseases, 803–805
  - pruritus, 802–803, 802t
  - systemic disease with cutaneous complications, 807–809
  - vascular-related disease, 803
- menopause and, 717
- types of, aging and, 133–134

Skin test, for tuberculosis, 378
Slap-foot gait, 887
Sleep, 943
- architecture changes in, 943–945
- circadian rhythm, 945
- continuity of, 943–944, 945f
- in dementia, 947–948
- depth of, 944–945
- duration of, 944
- insomnia, 943
  - comorbidity with, 945–946
  - epidemiology of, 943, 944t
  - natural history of, 943, 945t
  - periodic limb movements in sleep, 947
  - rapid eye movement sleep behavior disorder, 947
  - restless leg syndrome, 947
  - sleep-disordered breathing, 946–947
  - treatment for, 946
- REM, 945

Sleep deprivation, aging consequences of, 159–160
Sleep disorders, dementia associated with, 389
Sleep Heart Health Study (SHHS), sleep architecture changes and, 943
Sleep hygiene, for insomnia, 946
Sleep restriction, for insomnia, 946
Sleep-disordered breathing (SDB), 99, 946–947
Slovakia, geriatric medicine in, 1000
Slow wave sleep (SWS), with advancing age, 944, 945f
Small bowel, 652
- aging effects on, 107
- diseases of, 653–660
  - acute arterial mesenteric ischemia, 657–658
  - bacterial overgrowth syndrome, 654–655
  - celiac disease, 653–654
  - chronic mesenteric ischemia, 658
  - Crohn's disease, 655–657
  - neoplasms, 658–659
  - obscure gastrointestinal bleeding, 659–660
  - small bowel ischemia, 657
- investigation of, 652–653
  - absorption tests, 652
  - radiology and endoscopy, 653
  - screening tests, 652

Small cell lung cancer, 383–384
Small vessel disease, vascular cognitive impairment associated with, 422–423
Smell, aging effects on, 101–102, 106
S-mephenytoin, metabolism of, 140t
SMI. *See* Skeletal muscle mass index
Smoking
- airways changes induced by, 370
- cardiovascular risk and, 302
- in chronic cardiac failure, 283
- COPD due to, 369–373, 371f
- cutaneous complications of, 809
- respiratory system aging and, 97
- as risk factor for CAD, 288
- skin aging due to, 133
- sleep-disordered breathing and, 946–947
- stroke risk and, 480

S-nitrosylation
- chemical biology of, 152–153, 153t
- in neurobiology of aging, 150, 152f
- neuronal cell death and, 152–154, 153t
- parkin and, 153
- of PDI, in protein misfolding and neurotoxicity in cell models of Parkinson's disease and Alzheimer's disease, 153–154

Snoezelen light therapy, for dementia management, 400
Snoring, sleep-disordered breathing and, 946
Snout reflex, age-related changes in, 104
SNPs. *See* Special Needs Plans
SNRIs. *See* Serotonin-norepinephrine reuptake inhibitors
Social activities
- assessment of, 225
- cognitive functioning in response to, 176

Social assessment, of geriatric patients, 223
- aspects of social functioning, 224–228
- assembling the assessment protocol, 229
- assessment within congregate group settings, 228
- descriptive overview of social assessment batteries, 223–224
- emerging areas of assessment, 228–229
- social assessment as part of comprehensive assessment, 223

Social capital, health in old age and, 199
Social cohesion, health in old age and, 199
Social contact, psychosocial illness prevention and, 852
Social engagement, health in old age and, 199
Social factors, depression in old age and, 434
Social functioning, aspects of, 224–228
- caregiver burden, 226–227
- dementia patients, 227–228
- personal autonomy, preferences and values, 227
- problems in assessment of, 225
- satisfaction, 227
- social relationships, activities, and resources, 225
- social support, 226
- subjective well-being, 226

Social gerontology, 187
- golden age of increasing life expectancy and compression of morbidity, 188–189
- inequalities in later life—continuities and impact, 190–191
- opportunity age—successful aging and the third age, 189–190
- "problem" of old age, 187–188
- theoretical approaches: from functionalism to structured dependency, 188

Social influences, on health in old age, 199–201, 200t
Social insurance, 993
Social isolation, health in old age and, 199
Social learning, in geriatric medicine education, 1035

Social networks, 199, 225
Social protection, 991–993
Social relationships, 225
Social security, 993
Social Security Act, 1026
Social services, in regions of world, 1013–1015
  end of life care, 1014–1015
  long-term care, 1014
  secondary health care, 1013–1014
Social services occupational therapy (SSOT), 871
Social support
  in allostasis and allostatic overload, 161
  assessment of, 226
  health in old age and, 198
Social vulnerability. *See also* Model of vulnerability
  health in old age and, 199
  in old age, 198
    associations with health, 201–203
    background and definitions, 198–199, 198f
    frailty, exclusion, and "silence by proxy," 204
    policy ramifications and potential for interventions, 204
    study of social influences on health, 199–201, 200t
    successful aging, 201
Social vulnerability index, 200
Social-cognitive theories, to personality, 181–182
Social/health maintenance organization (S/HMO), 1059
Socioeconomic status (SES)
  cognitive decline and, 202
  health in old age and, 198
Socioemotional selectivity theory (SST), 181
Sodium balance, 697–698
Sodium channel blockers. *See* Class I antiarrhythmic drugs
Sodium docusate, 979
Sodium intake, 508b
  cardiovascular risk and, 303
  frailty prevention and, 850
  for hypertension management, 307
  stroke risk and, 481
Sodium picosulfate, 979
Sodium valproate, 401, 440, 462, 471, 477b, 519
Soft tissues, of bones and joints, aging of, 121–122
Solar elastosis, 78, 135
Solar keratosis. *See* Actinic keratosis
Solid tumors, of pancreas, 627–631, 628f
Solid-pseudopapillary neoplasm, of pancreas, 627
Solifenacin, 709, 721, 935
Somatoform disorders, 441
Somatopause, 123
Sorbitol, 683
Sotalol, 333, 339t
d,l-Sotalol, 293, 293t, 329–330, 329t
d-Sotalol, 293, 329t
Spain, geriatric medicine in, 1000
Spasm, esophageal, 613–614
Special Needs Plans (SNPs), 1052–1053
Species
  differences in longevity in, 19
  variation in longevity within, 20, 20f
  variation in physiologic deterioration between and within, 53
Specific host defense, aging-related changes in, 83
Spectral analysis, of heart rate and blood pressure, 500–501
Speech understanding
  behavioral implications of loss of, 824–825, 825t
  psychosocial consequences of loss of, 825–826
Spinal cord compression, 539–541, 540f
  in degenerative disease of lumbar spine, 544–545, 544f
  from intradural tumors, 542
  in Paget's disease, 543–544
  in rheumatoid arthritis, 541, 542f
  thoracic disk protrusion and, 541–542
Spinal cord disorders, 539
  cervical myelopathy, 539–541, 540f
  cervical radiculopathy, 539–541, 540f
  cord compression from intradural tumors, 542
  cord compression in rheumatoid arthritis, 541, 542f
  cord injury, 543
  metastatic spinal tumors, 542–543
  neurologic complications of degenerative disease of lumbar spine, 544–545, 544f
  Paget's disease, 543–544
  spinal cord compression and thoracic disk protrusion, 541–542
  vascular disorders, 543
Spinal cord injury (SCI), 543
Spinal stenosis, 525–526
Spinal tumors, 542–543
Spiritual suffering, palliative care for, 981
Spirochetal infections, of CNS, 551
Spironolactone
  for ascites, 641
  for chronic cardiac failure, 278, 278b, 280, 285, 285b
  in frail elderly patient, 298
  hyperkalemia due to, 698
  for ovarian cancer, 724
Splenic marginal zone lymphoma (SZL), 785
Spondylarthritis. *See* Seronegative spondylarthritis
Spondylosis
  cervical, 472, 539–541, 540f
  lumbar spine, 544
Spontaneous bacterial peritonitis (SBP), 641–642
Sporanox. *See* Itraconazole
Squamous cell carcinoma (SCC), of skin, 805–806
SSOT. *See* Social services occupational therapy
SSRIs. *See* Selective serotonin reuptake inhibitors
SST. *See* Socioemotional selectivity theory
St. John's wort, 141t–142t
Stable angina, therapy of, 290
Staging
  of breast cancer, 726
  of cancer, 795–796
  of prostate cancer, 711t
Stalevo. *See* Levodopa plus entacapone
Standardized assessment systems, for measuring outcomes of multidimensional interventions, 246–247
Standards, for quality of care improvement in United Kingdom, 1040–1041, 1040t
Stasis dermatitis, 803
Statins
  for acute coronary syndromes, 291
  for Alzheimer's disease prevention, 413–414
  for aortic stenosis, 312, 315
  for CAD prevention, 289
  for chronic cardiac failure, 282
  for dementia, 400
  in elderly patients undergoing surgery, 232
  in frail elderly patient, 296–297, 296t
  for Hutchinson-Gilford progeria syndrome, 68
Statins (*Continued*)
  hyperparathyroidism and, 756b
  for hypertension management, 307, 311
  for lipid control in diabetes mellitus, 772–773
  myalgia and myopathy induced by, 528
  for STEMI, 291
  for stroke, 492, 496
  for vascular cognitive impairment, 427
  for ventricular arrhythmia, 327, 330
Station changes, of old age, 103
STDs. *See* Sexually transmitted diseases
Stem cells, in cell death and cell replacement, 33
STEMI, therapy for, 291
Stenosis
  aortic. *See* Aortic stenosis
  of carotid artery, 352
  mitral. *See* Mitral stenosis
  spinal, 525–526
  tricuspid, 325–326
Stent-grafts, endovascular, 355
Stenting, for carotid disease, 352
Steppage gait, 887
Steroid-induced myopathy, 529
Steroids. *See also* Adrenocortical steroids; Corticosteroids; Glucocorticoids; Mineralocorticoids
  acute pancreatitis due to, 631–632
  for alcoholic liver disease, 639
  for apatite deposition disease, 576
  for arthritis, 569–570
  asteatotic eczema and, 802
  for autoimmune hemolytic anemia, 786–787
  for bullous pemphigoid, 807
  for calcium pyrophosphate crystal deposition, 575
  for cluster headache, 470
  cognitive dysfunction associated with, 387
  for COPD, 373
  for Crohn's disease, 109, 656–657, 669t, 670
  Cushing syndrome due to, 734
  dementia due to, 416–417
  depression and, 841
  diabetes secondary to, 760, 760t, 770
  diabetic ketoacidosis and, 771
  for eye pain, 475–476
  for giant cell arteritis, 473–474, 477b
  for gout, 574
  herpes zoster flare and, 803
  for hypopituitarism, 735
  for hypothyroidism, 748
  for inclusion body myositis, 528
  for intracranial tumors, 536–537
  for lichen sclerosis of vulva, 719
  for lymphocytic and collagenous colitis, 671
  for medication-misuse headache, 475
  for metastatic spinal tumors, 542–543
  myalgia and myopathy induced by, 529
  osteoporosis due to, 554–555
  for polymyalgia rheumatica, 580
  for polymyositis or dermatomyositis, 527–528
  for postherpetic neuralgia, 472
  for primary biliary cirrhosis, 640
  for rheumatoid arthritis, 541
  and risk of NSAID-related complications, 621
  for scabies, 804
  for seborrheic dermatitis, 802
  as secondary cause of acquired immunodeficiency in old age, 89
  for thrombotic thrombocytopenic purpura, 789
  for vulval eczema/dermatitis, 718
  weight gain due to, 689
  for xerosis, 802
Stilbestrol, 714–715
Stimulants, 142t

Stomach, 618–625, 619f, 621f–622f, 624f–625f
aging effects on, 106
disorders of
benign tumors, 624
gastric and duodenal mucosal injury, 618–619
H. pylori, gastritis, and peptic ulcer disease, 619–620, 619f
malignant tumors, 624–625, 625f
nonulcer dyspepsia, 622–623
NSAIDs, gastropathy, and peptic ulcer disease, 619–622, 625b
peptic ulcer disease in elderly, 621–622, 621f–622f
upper gastrointestinal bleeding, 623
volvulus, 623–624, 624f
Stomatitis, 609
Strength training
balance and, 863
falls and, 902
for fractured neck, 876
for successful aging, 861
Stress. *See also* Oxidative stress
in aging, 158
consequences of being "stressed out" and sleep deprivation, 159–160
definition of stress, allostasis, and allostatic load, 158, 159f
effects of stress on human brain, 160–161
measurement of allostatic load, 158–159, 160t
protection and damage as response to stressors, 158, 160f
role of adverse early life experience in, 161
role of brain in response to stress, 160, 161f
role of positive affect, self-esteem, and social support, 161
autonomic response to, aging effects on, 503–504
role of brain in response to, 160, 161f
as secondary cause of acquired immunodeficiency in old age, 89
Stress testing, for CAD, 287
Stress urinary incontinence, 721, 928
artificial urinary sphincter for, 937
medication for, 937
surgery for, 937
treatment for, 937
urgency urinary incontinence v., 934
"Stressed out," aging consequences of, 159–160
Stressors
organismic ability to cope with, aging effects on, 55
protection and damage as response to, 158, 160f
Stroke, 484
with carotid disease, 349–352, 351f–352f
clinical presentation of, 487–489
constipation and, 914
definitions of, 484–485
delirium and, 906
epidemiology of, 478–482
burden of stroke, 478, 478t, 480–481
costs of stroke, 479
heterogeneity of stroke, 479
incidence of stroke, 478t, 479
mortality of stroke, 478–479, 478t
prevalence of stroke, 478t, 479
prevention of stroke, 481, 481t
risk factors for stroke, 479–480, 480t
hypertension and, 303, 310–311, 480–481
investigations of, 489–493, 491f
blood tests for diagnosing stroke risk factors, 492
brain imaging, 489–490, 491f
diagnosis of stroke mechanism, 490–491
Stroke (*Continued*)
management of, 492–493
acute treatment of intracranial hemorrhage, 493
acute treatment of ischemic stroke, 492
antiplatelet therapy, 493
emerging treatments, 493
organized stroke unit care, 492–493
thrombolysis for acute ischemic stroke, 493
oral health and, 603
organization of services for, 497
pathologic mechanisms underlying, 482–483
hemorrhagic stroke, 482–483
ischemic stroke, 482
postoperative, 241
prevention of primary stroke, 496–497
prevention of secondary stroke, 495–496
antiplatelet therapy, 495
blood pressure reduction, 495–496
carotid endarterectomy, 496
endovascular therapy, 496
lipid lowering agents, 496
TIA clinics, 496
warfarin, 495
recovery from, 493–494
rehabilitation of, 494–495
risk factors for, 479–480, 480t
modifiable factors, 480, 480t
nonmodifiable factors, 480, 480t
therapy techniques for, 873
ADL training, 875
after discharge, 875
initial steps, 873–874
prior to discharge, 875
re-education of movement, 874–875
secondary complications, 875
timing of carotid surgery after, 352
types of, 485–486, 485f, 486t
ischemic stroke subtypes, 485–486, 486t
Stroke units, 492–493, 497
Stroma, of bone marrow, aging effects on, 127–128
Strontium ranelate, 164, 556–558, 556t
Strontium^{89}, 714
Structural glycoproteins, of connective tissues, 75–77
entactin/nidogen, 76
fibronectin, 75–76
integrins and cell attachment proteins, 77
laminin, 76
thrombospondin, 76–77
Structural lesions, dementia associated with, 389
Structure, of quality of care, 1039
Structure measurement, in United States managed care, 1061
Structured dependency, 188
Study designs, for research in older people, 23
Subarachnoid hemorrhage (SAH), 474, 479, 485
Subclinical hyperthyroidism, 743–745, 744t, 754b
Subclinical hypothyroidism, 748–750, 749t, 754b
Subconjunctival hemorrhage, 811, 811f
Subcortical ischemic vascular disease (SIVD), 423
Subcortical syndrome, 424–425
Subcutaneous estrogen implants, 718
Subcutaneous tissue, aging effects on, 136
Subdural empyema, 549
Subdural hemorrhage, headache with, 474
Subjective well-being, assessment of, 226
Successful aging, 184, 189–190, 201, 836
definitions of, 53, 184
demography of centenarians, 184
distinguishing between compression of morbidity and compression of disability and the role of resilience, 184–186
exercise for, 859
aerobic exercise, 859–861
aerobic exercise and carbohydrate metabolism, 860–861
bone health, 863–864
memory disorders and, 864
protein requirements for, 862
resistance exercise and, 862–863
resistance exercise and insulin and protein metabolism, 861–862
strength training, 861
gender disparity in, 185, 185f
heritability and familiality in, 185–186
supercentenarians, 186
Suck reflex, age-related changes in, 104
Sucralfate, 141, 609, 622
Sudden unexplained death in epilepsy (SUDEP), 460
SUDEP. *See* Sudden unexplained death in epilepsy
Suffering, with pain, 965
Suicide, depression in old age and, 436
Sulfasalazine
for arthritis, 569, 569t
for Crohn's disease, 656, 669t
taste perception and, 608
for ulcerative colitis, 667–668, 667t
Sulfonamides, 665, 789
Sulfonylureas
for glucose control, 767–771, 768t, 768b
in patient with CAD, 289
Sulfur, for scabies, 804
Sumatriptan, 468, 468t, 470, 472
Supine hypertension, 510
Support. *See* Social support
Support surfaces, for pressure ulcers, 941
Suppositories
bisacodyl, for constipation, 920–921
rectal outlet delay and, 920–921
Supraventricular tachycardia (SVT), 336
Surgery. *See also* Vascular surgery
in old age, 230
age, surgery, and outcome, 230–231
anesthetic factors, 231–232
cardiac problems in elderly surgical patient, 235–237, 236t
central nervous system problems, 241–242
fluid and electrolyte imbalance, 239–241
future trends, 244
obesity, 239
online computerized risk assessment and guidance, 243
preoperative assessment, 232–234, 232t–233t
respiratory problems in older surgical patient, 234–235, 235t
surgical and anesthetic audits, 243–244
trends in, 230
undernutrition and, 237–239, 239t
Surgical audits, 243–244
Surveillance, for prostate cancer, 712
Survival
of cancer, 800
geriatric assessment programs effect on, 215–216
social factors associated with, 201–202
SVT. *See* Supraventricular tachycardia
Swallowing, malnutrition and, 950–953
S-warfarin, metabolism of, 140t

Sweat glands, aging of, 135–137
Sweden, geriatric medicine in, 1000
Switzerland, geriatric medicine in, 1000
SWS. *See* Slow wave sleep
Symmetrel. *See* Amantadine
Sympathetic function
  biochemical assessment of, 501
  effects of aging on, 502, 502f
Sympathetic nerve activity, of muscle, 501
Sympathoadrenal system, in older victims of trauma, 865
Sympatholytics, 504–505
Sympathomimetics, 331–332, 366, 475t, 813
Symptomatic epilepsy, 456
Synchronous telemedicine, 1065
Syncope, 338
  carotid sinus syndrome and carotid sinus hypersensitivity causing, 343–345, 344f
  definition of, 338
  epidemiology of, 338, 339f
  epilepsy v., 457, 458t
  evaluation of, 340–341, 341f
  neurally mediated, 504
  orthostatic hypotension causing, 341–343, 343t
  pathophysiology of, 338, 339t–340t
    individual causes, 338, 339t–340t
    multifactorial causes, 338, 339t
  postprandial hypotension causing, 346–347
  presentation of, 340
  vasovagal, 345–346
Synovial joint, aging of, 117–118, 118f–119f
Synthesis, of protein, aging effects on, 48–49
α-Synucleinopathies, 505–506
Syphilis. *See* Neurosyphilis
Systemic inflammation, with COPD, 372, 372t
Systolic blood pressure, cardiovascular risk and, 301
Systolic hypertension, 93, 93f, 306
SZL. *See* Splenic marginal zone lymphoma

T

T cells, aging effects on, 131–132
T_3. *See* Triiodothyronine
T_4. *See* Thyroxine
Tabes dorsalis, 551
Tachycardia-bradycardia syndrome, 332
Tacrine, 143t, 419
Tacrolimus, 531, 645, 698, 802–803
Tadalafil, 725
Tai Chi
  falls and, 902
  for pain, 971
Tamarind, 142t
Tamoxifen, 14–16, 727
  for breast cancer, 729, 798–799
  depression associated with, 435
  high thyroxine due to, 739
  for reproductive aging in women, 164–165
  uterine cancer and, 722
Tamsulosin, 709t
Tap water enemas, for constipation, 920
Tar, for seborrheic dermatitis, 802
Target of rapamycin (TOR), 49, 156
Tasmar. *See* Tolcapone
Taste, aging effects on, 101–102
Tau, in frontotemporal dementia, 428, 430–431
2006 Tax Relief and Health Care Act (TRHCA), 1049
Tax Relief and Health Care Act of 2006 (TRHCA), 1063
Taxanes, 724
Tazarotene, 148t
Tazobactam, 663t
T-cell function, aging-related changes in, 83–84
T-cell lymphomas, 785–786
TDDs. *See* Telecommunication systems for the deaf
TDP-43 proteinopathy, 431
TEA. *See* Transient epileptic amnesia
Teamwork, in rehabilitation, e11–e13
  integrated care pathway, e12–e13
  interdisciplinary team care, e12
  multidisciplinary team care, e11–e12
  nurse in, e12
  promotion of, e12–e13
Technology
  for cost effective quality of care, 1053, 1053t
  telemedicine and, 1068
Telecommunication systems for the deaf (TDDs), 831–832
Telemedicine, 1064
  applications of, 1065–1067
    chronic disease management, 1065
    chronic wounds, 1066
    congestive heart failure, 1065–1066
    diabetes mellitus, 1066
    e-Health, 1066–1067, 1067t
    hypertension, 1066
    safety and security monitoring, 1066
    supporting caregivers, 1066
  background on, 1064
  barriers to widespread use of, 1067–1068, 1067t
    clinician attitudes, 1067–1068
    economic elements, 1068
    lack of evidence, 1068
    policy factors, 1068
    technology factors, 1068
  basic principles of, 1064–1065, 1065t
  elderly usability issues of, 1067
  future directions of, 1068–1069
Telmisartan, 495–496
Telomerase, 14, 32–33, 128
  aging and, 32
  cancer and, 32, 40
  in cell senescence, 46
Telomeres
  aging and, 4, 14, 40–41
  as biomarker of physiologic age, 33
  of blood cells and hematopoietic stem cells, 128
  in cell senescence, 46
  functioning of, 32–33
  in people with intellectual disability, 447
  replicative senescence and, 32
Temazepam, 141
Temozolome, 538
Temozolomide, 537–538
Temporal arteritis. *See* Giant cell arteritis
Temporal lobe seizures, 455–456
Tendons, disorders of, 578–579
TENS. *See* Transcutaneous electrical nerve stimulation
Tension headache, 469
Terazosin, 709t
Terbinafine (Lamisil), 596, 805
Terfenadine, 140t
Teriparatide, 556t, 557, 586
Terlipressin, 641–642
Terminal stage, palliative care for, 981–982
Tertiary disease prevention, 848–849
Tertiary hyperparathyroidism, 758–759, 759f, 759b
Testosterone
  age-related decline in, 124–125, 166–167
  in Down syndrome, 448
  levels of, 854
  metabolic syndrome association with, 168–169
  sarcopenia and, 589, 592
  sexual motivation and, 724–725
Testosterone therapy, 125
  as antiaging medicine, 147, 147t
  in Down syndrome, 448
  growth hormone therapy with, 123
  longevity due to, 14
  for reproductive aging in men, 167
Tetrabenazine, 518–519
Tetracosactin, for ACTH-stimulation test, 732–733
Tetracycline
  antacids and, 622
  for bacterial overgrowth syndrome, 655
  for bullous pemphigoid, 807
  drug interactions of, 141
  esophageal injury due to, 616
  for *H. pylori* infection, 620
  for infectious colitis, 665
  for stomatitis, 609
  thrombocytopenia associated with, 789
TGA. *See* Transient global amnesia
Thalidomide, 593, 783, 955
"The coming of age," e3–e4
Theophylline
  for asthma, 366, 367t
  cimetidine and, 622
  for COPD, 373
  drug-disease interactions of, 143t
  headache due to, 475t
  herbal-drug interactions of, 142t
  metabolism of, 139–140, 140t
Therapeutic failure, 882–883
Therapeutic Failure Questionnaire (TFQ), 882
Therapy techniques, 870
  for fractured neck, 875–876
  for frailty, 877–878
    environment, 878–879
    exercise programs, 878
  future directions for, 879
  groups of, 873
  occupational therapy, 870–871
    research culture for, 872
    settings for, 871
    skills for, 871
    training for, 871
  for Parkinson's disease, 876
    caregiver education, 877
    environmental changes, 877
    functional mobility, 876–877
  physiotherapy, 871
    research culture for, 872
    skills for, 871–872
  process for, 872
  for stroke, 873
    ADL training, 875
    after discharge, 875
    initial steps, 873–874
    prior to discharge, 875
    re-education of movement, 874–875
    secondary complications, 875
Thermoregulatory system, aging effects on, 57
Thiamine, 400, 442
Thiazide diuretics
  for blood pressure control in diabetes mellitus patients, 772
  for CAD prevention, 288–289
  for chronic cardiac failure, 278, 278b
  diabetes secondary to, 760
  diabetic ketoacidosis and, 771

Thiazide diuretics (*Continued*)
drug interactions of, 143
drug-disease interactions of, 143t
gout associated with, 574
herbal-drug interactions of, 142t
hypercalcemia and, 757t
for hypertension, 305, 305t, 308–311, 310b
for hypoparathyroidism, 759
Thiazolidinediones (TZDs), 639–640, 769–770, 774
Thioridazine, 140t, 143t
Thiothixene, 143t
Third age, 189–190
Thirst, malnutrition and, 953–954, 953t
Thoracic disk protrusion, 541–542
Thoracic injuries, in older people, 867–868
Thoracic tumors
lung cancer, 382–383, 382t
management of, 382–383, 382t
non-small cell, 383
presentation and investigation of, 382
small cell, 383–384
malignant mesothelioma, 384
Thrombocytopenia, 789
Thromboembolic stroke
in patients with cardiac arrhythmias, 334–335, 334t
in patients with mitral annular calcium, 322–323, 323t
Thromboembolism. *See* Venous thromboembolism
Thrombolysis, for acute ischemic stroke, 493
Thrombolytic agents
for acute thrombosis, 349
for lower gastrointestinal bleeding diagnosis, 677
for pulmonary embolism, 359
for STEMI, 291
for venous thromboembolism, 357
Thromboprophylaxis, 359–360
Thrombosis. *See also* Deep vein thrombosis
in acute limb ischemia, 349, 350f
Thrombospondin (TSP), 76–77
Thrombotic risk factors, stroke risk and, 492
Thrombotic thrombocytopenic purpura (TTP), 789
Thymic hormone replacement, 83
Thyroglobulin, 740
Thyroid
aging of, 126, 738
assessment of function of, 738–740
imaging of, 739
morphology of, 737–738
Thyroid disorders, 737
acute hyperthyroidism, 743
cutaneous complications of, 808
dementia associated with, 387–388
eye disorders, 819
hyperthyroidism, 740–743, 741t–742t, 754b, 808
subclinical, 743–745, 744t, 754b
hypothyroidism, 741t, 745–748, 754b, 808
subclinical, 748–750, 749t, 754b
myopathy due to, 529
nodular thyroid disease and neoplasia, 750–754, 751t, 754b
screening for, 740
Thyroid hormone
action of, 738
circulating levels of, 738
secretion and metabolism of, 737–738
Thyroid hormone therapy, 743
hyperthyroidism due to, 741, 741t, 743–744
for hypothyroidism, 746–748, 750
as test of thyroid nodule malignancy, 752
for thyroid nodule management, 752–753
Thyroid storm. *See* Acute hyperthyroidism
Thyroid-stimulating immunoglobulins, 740
Thyrotoxicosis. *See* Hyperthyroidism
Thyrotropin-releasing hormone test, 739
Thyroxine (T_4), 737
action of, 738
aging and, 738
circulating levels of, 738
herbal-drug interactions of, 142t
high states of, 739
for hypopituitarism, 735
low states of, 738–739
for myopathy, 529
secretion and metabolism of, 737–738
Tiagabine, 462, 463t
TIAs. *See* Transient ischemic attacks
Tibolone, 592, 717, 724–725
Ticlopidine, 142t–143t, 482, 495
Tiludronate, 563
Timed get-up-and-go, 888
Timed walking test, for mobility assessment, e9
Timolol, 292t, 820
Tinetti balance and mobility scale, 888
Tiotropium, 373
Tirofiban, 291
Tissue plasminogen activator (tPA), for stroke, 491f, 492–493
TNF inhibitors. *See* Tumor necrosis factor inhibitors
Tobacco. *See also* Smoking
cutaneous complications of, 809
sexuality in old age and, 855, 857t
Tobramycin, 663t
Tocainide, 327–328, 333–334
Toe drag gait, 887
Toes, ulcers of, 596–597, 598b, 764, 765t
Toilet access, constipation and FI and, 918
privacy and dignity for, 920, 920t
Toileting habits, constipation and, 920
Tolbutamide, 139, 140t, 768, 770
Tolcapone (Tasmar), 515t, 516
Tolterodine, 143t, 605, 709, 721, 935
Tongue, "hairy tongue,", 609
Topical estrogen, in menopause, 717–718
Topiramate, 462, 463t, 468–470, 468t, 476, 477b
Topoisomerase inhibitors, 777–778, 788t
TOR. *See* Target of rapamycin
Torsemide, 283
Total quality management (TQM), 1041–1042
Toxic serotonin syndrome, 519
Toxins, dementia associated with, 386–387
tPA. *See* Tissue plasminogen activator
TQM. *See* Total quality management
Traction diverticula. *See* Midesophageal diverticula
Traits. *See* Personality traits
Tramadol, 969
Trandolapril, 292t
Tranquilizers
chronic daily headache due to, 469–470
delirium due to, 241
hypothyroidism due to, 747
ophthalmic complications of, 819–820
for somatization, 110b
Transabdominal ultrasound, for pancreas adenocarcinoma, 628
Transcutaneous electrical nerve stimulation (TENS), for pain, 970–971
Transdermal estrogen, in menopause, 717
Transdermal patches, constipation and, 912–913
Transient epileptic amnesia (TEA), epilepsy v., 458
Transient global amnesia (TGA), epilepsy v., 458–459
Transient ischemic attacks (TIAs)
clinical presentation of, 487
clinics for, 496
definition of, 484–485
epilepsy v., 459, 459f
migraine and, 467
Transplantation, of liver, 643–644
Transrectal ultrasound, for prostate assessment, 703, 703f
Trastuzumab, 727–728, 728t
Trauma
head, dementia and, 386, 388
headache due to, 474
orthopedic geriatrics for, 583–584, 584f
Traumatic enthesopathy, 579
Trazodone, 142t, 401
Tremor, 103, 512
Tretinoin, 137, 148t
TRHCA. *See* 2006 Tax Relief and Health Care Act; Tax Relief and Health Care Act of 2006
Triamterene, 698
Triazolam, 140t
Tricuspid regurgitation, 325
Tricuspid stenosis, 325–326
Tricyclic antidepressants
aging effects on, 141
for anxiety disorders, 440
for atypical facial pain, 472
chronic cardiac failure and, 284
for depression in old age, 435
for diabetic neuropathy, 597
distribution of, 139
drug-disease interactions of, 143t
dry mouth and, 605
herbal-drug interactions of, 142t
metabolism of, 140
for migraine, 468, 468t, 477b
for neuropathic pain, 977–978
ophthalmic complications of, 819–820
orthostatic hypotension and, 508b
for overactive bladder, 721
restless legs syndrome due to, 519
syncope caused by, 339t
taste perception and, 608
for tension headache, 469, 477b
tremor caused by, 519
for vulval discomfort, 719–720
Trigeminal neuralgia, 470–471
Triiodothyronine (T_3), 737
action of, 738
aging and, 738
circulating levels of, 738
low states of, 739
secretion and metabolism of, 737–738
toxicosis of, 741
Trimethaphan, 506
Trimethoprim, 143, 690–691, 698
Trimethoprim-sulfamethoxazole, 665, 691, 698
Triptans, 470, 477b
TRISS. *See* Revised Trauma Score + Injury Severity Score
Trospium, 721, 935–936
TSP. *See* Thrombospondin
TTP. *See* Thrombotic thrombocytopenic purpura
Tube feeding, for malnutrition, 956–957
Tuberculin skin test for, 378
Tuberculosis, 377–378
gamma interferon tests for, 378
investigation of, 377–378
latent, 378
management of, 378
presentation of, 377
prognosis of, 378
in regions of world, 1011–1012
tuberculin skin test for, 378

Tuberculosis meningitis, 549–550
Tubular function, aging effects on, 111–112
Tumor necrosis factor (TNF) inhibitors, 569–570, 570t
Tumors. *See also* Neoplasms
ampullary, 649
cerebral, epilepsy and, 460
gastric, 624–625, 625f
intracranial. *See* Intracranial tumors
intradural, spinal cord compression from, 542
of pancreas, 626, 628f
pituitary, 735
of small bowel, 658–659
spinal, 542–543
Turkey, geriatric medicine in, 1000
Turner syndrome, 445, 446t
Type 2 diabetes, treatment of, 767–768
Type 5 phosphodiesterase inhibitors, 725
Tyrosine kinase inhibitor, 781
TZDs. *See* Thiazolidinediones

U

UAO. *See* Upper airway obstruction
UDCA. *See* Ursodeoxycholic acid
UFH. *See* Unfractionated heparin
UIP. *See* Usual interstitial pneumonia
Ulcerative colitis, 666–667, 667t
age-related changes in manifestation of, 109
colon cancer risk and, 668–669
Ulcers. *See also* Peptic ulcer disease
gastroduodenal ulcer, atypical presentation of, 108
of legs, feet, and toes, 596–597, 598b, 764, 765t
Ultrasound. *See also* Endoscopic ultrasound
abdominal, 637
of liver, 649
of stroke, 490
transabdominal, for pancreas adenocarcinoma, 628
transrectal, for prostate assessment, 703, 703f
Underactive detrusor, management of patients with, 709
Undernutrition, surgery and anesthesia in old age and, 237–239, 239t
Unemployment, 993
Unexplained anemia, 777, 777t
Unfractionated heparin (UFH), 357, 360, 492–493
United Kingdom
demographics in, 991
geriatric medicine in, 998–999
consultant numbers, 998, 998t
geriatrician work, 998–999, 999t
specialists in, 998
long-term care in, 1021
developing quality in care, 1023–1024, 1023t
dissolution of medical leadership in, 1022–1024, 1023t
history of, 1021–1022, 1022t
present and future of, 1024–1025, 1024t
National Health Service of, 997
pension system privatization in, 994
quality of care improvement in, 1038
continuous, 1042, 1043f
current NHS approach, 1043–1045, 1043f
description of, 1038–1039
lessons from industry on, 1041–1042
measurement of, 1039
outcomes of, 1042
recent initiatives, 1039–1041
United Kingdom *(Continued)*
recent policy documents, 990t, 998
rehabilitation policy framework in, e3–e5
intermediate care services, e4–e5, e4t, e5b
National Beds Enquiry, e4
NHS and Community Care Act, e3
"Not because they are old,", e4
primary-care led NHS, e4
"The coming of age,", e3–e4
United States
demographics in, 1005
geriatric medicine in, 1005
future direction, 1008–1009
specialty practice in, 1006–1008, 1007t
long-term care in, 1026
demographics, 1026, 1027f
economics, 1027
future perspectives of, 1030–1031
history of, 1026
nursing home culture changes, 1030, 1030t
provision of care, 1029, 1029t
quality of care, 1029–1030, 1030t
settings, 1028, 1028t
types of service, 1027–1028
managed care in, 1057
capitation and pay-for-performance, 1060–1061
in fee-for-service, 1057–1059
future of, 1062–1063
measuring quality of care, 1061–1062, 1062f
plan reimbursement in, 1060
principles for, 1059–1060, 1059b
timeline of, 1057
Unpaid work, productive aging with, 196
Unrecognized myocardial infarction, 286, 286t
Unstable angina pectoris, 290–291
therapy for, 290–291
Upper airway configuration, sleep-disordered breathing and, 946–947
Upper airway obstruction (UAO), 374–375, 375t
Upper gastrointestinal bleeding, 623, 659–660
Upper gastrointestinal tract, 608
esophagus, 612–618, 613f–615f, 617f–618f
oral cavity, 608, 609f
oropharynx, 610–612, 611f, 611t
stomach, 618–625, 619f, 621f–622f, 624f–625f
systemic disease and, 625
amyloidosis, 625
diabetes mellitus, 625
Upper urinary tract, aging of, 111–112
glomerular filtration rate, 111
mechanistic considerations, 112
renal blood flow, 111
structural changes, 112
system-based perspective of, 112
tubular function, 111–112
Ureidopenicillin, 648
Ureters, aging of, 111–112
Urethra, control of, 926
Urethral sphincter
external, 927
incompetence of
artificial replacement, 937
treatment for, 937
internal, 926–927
Urgency incontinence, 927, 929–930, 934t
Uricosuric, 574
Urinalysis, for urinary incontinence assessment, 933–934
Urinary incontinence, 721, 926
age-related pathophysiology of, 929–931, 930f–932f, 930t
anatomy and physiology of, 926–927
assessment of, 931–934, 933t
bladder diaries for, 932–933
cognitive function, 931–932
physical examination, 933
rectal examination, 934
urinalysis, 933–934
vaginal examination, 933
chronic cardiac failure in patients with, 283
external sheath drainage for, 938
indwelling catheters for, 938
maintenance products for, 938
management of patients with benign prostatic hyperplasia and, 708
multichannel cystometry for, 928–929
presentation of, 927–928, 928t
treatment of, 934–936
bladder retraining, 934–936
general measures, 934
medication, 937
sphincter incompetence correction, 937
surgery, 936–937
for voiding disorders, 937
Urinary sphincter, function and structure of, aging effects on, 115–116
Urinary symptoms, constipation and FI and, 917
Urinary tract, aging of, 111
lower urinary tract: bladder and outlet, 112–116, 113t
upper urinary tract: kidneys and ureters, 111–112
Urinary tract infection, 209t, 210, 690–691
Urine specimens, 690
Urosepsis, atypical presentation of, 210
Ursodeoxycholic acid (UDCA), 640, 646, 803
U.S. Preventive Services Task Force (USPSTF), disease prevention activities and, 848, 849t
User-led physical health assessment, for older adults with intellectual disability, 449, 450f, 451t
USPSTF. *See* U.S. Preventive Services Task Force
Usual interstitial pneumonia (UIP), 380–381, 380f
Uterovaginal prolapse, 720
Uterus
aging of, 716
cancer of, 722–723
UV radiation (UVR)
cellular aging due to, 42
skin aging due to, 133
Uva-ursi, herbal-drug interactions of, 142t
Uveal tract, disorders of, 812–813
UVR. *See* UV radiation

V

Vaccination
for Alzheimer's disease, 401, 413, 420
for herpes zoster, 803–804
for influenza, 87–88, 376
pneumococcal, for meningitis prevention, 549
for pneumonia, 88, 377
for preventing age-related changes in immune system, 89–90
sensitivity to, 141t
for varicella zoster virus, 88
Vacuum therapy, for ED, 858
VaD. *See* Vascular dementia
Vagifem, 717–718

Vagina
aging of, 716
cancer of, 722
Vaginal examination, for urinary incontinence assessment, 933
Valacyclovir, 472, 803–804
Valerian, 142t
Valganciclovir, 666
Validation therapy, for dementia management, 399–400
Valproate
for dementia, 401
for headache, 469–470
herbal-drug interactions of, 142t
for migraine, 468, 468t, 477b
for trigeminal neuralgia, 471, 477b
Valproic acid, 141, 462, 463t
Valsartan, 281
Values. *See* Personal values
Valvular heart disease, 312
acute mitral regurgitation, 324
aortic regurgitation, 317–320
echocardiography and Doppler echocardiography for, 318–319
electrocardiography and chest roentgenography for, 318
etiology and prevalence of, 317
medical and surgical management of, 319–320, 319t
natural history of, 319
pathophysiology of, 318
signs of, 318
symptoms of, 318
aortic stenosis, 312–317
aortic valve replacement for, 315–317, 316t
balloon aortic valvuloplasty for, 317
echocardiography and Doppler echocardiography, 314
electrocardiography and chest roentgenography for, 314
etiology and prevalence of, 312
medical management of, 316
natural history of, 314–316, 315t
pathophysiology of, 312–313
percutaneous transcatheter implantation of aortic valve prostheses for, 317
signs of, 313–314, 313t
symptoms of, 313
chronic mitral regurgitation, 324–325, 325t
mitral annular calcium, 320–323
AF in patients with, 321
bacterial endocarditis in patients with, 322
cardiac events in patients with, 322, 322t
cerebrovascular events in patients with, 322–323, 323t
chamber size of patients with, 321
conduction defects in patients with, 321
diagnosis of, 321
mitral regurgitation in patients with, 321–322, 321t–322t
mitral stenosis in patients with, 321t–322t, 322
mitral valve replacement in patients with, 322
predisposing factors for, 320–321
prevalence of, 320
mitral stenosis, 323–324
diagnostic tests for, 324
management of, 324
pathophysiology of, 323
prevalence and etiology of, 323
symptoms and signs of, 323–324
pulmonic regurgitation, 326
tricuspid regurgitation, 325
tricuspid stenosis, 325–326
Vancomycin
for CNS infection, 548, 548t, 550b, 552b
elimination of, 141t
for infectious colitis, 664–665
for stomatitis, 609
Varenicline, 372–373
Varicella zoster virus (VZV), immune senescence and, 88
Varices, 641
Vascular changes, autonomic system aging and, 503
Vascular cognitive impairment (VCI), 421
biomarkers of, 426
diagnosis of, 424–426, 424t, 425f
clinical evaluation, 424
cognitive assessment, 424–425
neuropsychiatric profiles, 425
disease progression of, 426
epidemiology of, 421
etiology and pathophysiology of, 422–424
historical overview of, 421
neuroimaging of, 425–426, 425f
neuropathology of, 425
prevention and treatment of, 426–427
subtypes of, 421–422
Vascular cognitive impairment that does not meet dementia criteria (VCI-ND), 421–422, 426
diagnosis of, 424
Vascular dementia (VaD), 421–427
delirium and, 904
diagnosis of, 424
neuropsychology in diagnosis and treatment of, 406–407, 409t
treatment of, 427
Vascular depression, 435
Vascular disease, comorbidity of, 848
Vascular disorders
headache and, 473–474
carotid and vertebral artery dissection, 474
cerebrovascular disease and hypertension, 474
chronic subdural hemorrhage, 474
giant cell arteritis, 473–474
subarachnoid hemorrhage, 474
of spinal cord, 543
Vascular lesions, of oral cavity, 608, 609f
Vascular parkinsonism, 518
Vascular prophylaxis, in diabetes mellitus, 773
Vascular structure, aging-associated changes in, 91, 92f
Vascular surgery, 348
for abdominal aortic aneurysm, 352–355, 353f–354f
for arterial disease of the limb, 348–349, 350f
for carotid disease, 349–352, 351f–352f
endovascular techniques, 355
management of small aneurysms, 355
Vascular-related skin disease, 803
Vasculature, of dermis, aging effects on, 135
Vasculitis
in large bowel, 675
pulmonary, 381
Vasoactive drugs
carotid sinus reflex sensitivity and, 344
orthostatic hypotension due to, 342–343
Vasoconstriction, deficient, 508
Vasoconstrictors, 642, 657–658
Vasodilators
for acute arterial mesenteric ischemia, 657–658
for aortic regurgitation, 319
for aortic stenosis, 316
for chronic cardiac failure, 278
for chronic mitral regurgitation, 325
Vasodilators *(Continued)*
cluster headache due to, 470
for dementia, 400
for hypothyroidism, 748
for lower gastrointestinal bleeding diagnosis, 677
for mitral stenosis, 324
syncope caused by, 339t
vasovagal syncope due to, 345–346
Vasopressin, for lower gastrointestinal bleeding, 677
Vasovagal syncope, 345–346
VCI. *See* Vascular cognitive impairment
VCI-ND. *See* Vascular cognitive impairment that does not meet dementia criteria
VCP mutations, 428, 429t, 431
Venlafaxine, 435, 463, 718
Venodilators, 508b
Venous lakes, 803
Venous thromboembolism (VTE), 356
clinical presentation and diagnosis of, 356–357
deep vein thrombosis, 356–357
pulmonary embolism, 357
graduated compression stockings for, 360
inferior vena caval filters, 359
management of overanticoagulation and bleeding, 359
monitoring warfarin therapy, 359
practical aspects of oral anticoagulant therapy in elderly, 358–359, 358f
prevention of, 359–360
prognosis of, 360–361
risk factors for, 356, 356t
treatment of, 357–358, 358t
treatment of pulmonary embolism with hemodynamic instability, 359
Ventricular arrhythmias, 327–330
ACE inhibitors for, 327, 329
AICD for, 329–330, 330t
β-blockers for, 327–330, 328t
calcium channel blockers for, 328
class I antiarrhythmic drugs for, 327–328, 328t
class III antiarrhythmic drugs for, 329, 329t
general therapy for, 327
invasive intervention for, 329
prognosis of, 327
in patients with heart disease, 327
in patients with no heart disease, 327
Ventricular premature complexes (VPCs), 327–330
Ventricular rate control
for fast ventricular rate with AF, 332
in patients with AF, 334
for slow ventricular rate with AF, 332–333
for very fast rapid ventricular rate with AF, 332
Ventricular tachycardia (VT), 327–330
Verapamil
absorption of, 139
for acute coronary syndromes, 291
for atrial flutter, 335
for cluster headache, 470
drug interactions of, 143
herbal-drug interactions of, 142t
liver metabolism of, 635–636
metabolism of, 140t
for mitral stenosis, 324
for multifocal atrial tachycardia, 336
for stable angina, 290
for STEMI, 291
for SVT, 336
for ventricular rate control in patients with AF, 332
for Wolff-Parkinson-White syndrome, 332

Verbal abilities, aging effects on, 173–174
Vertebral artery dissection, headache due to, 474
Vertebral fractures, in elderly, 564–565
Vertigo, 207
Vestibular function, aging effects on, 102
Vestibular system, balance and, 896
Videofluoroscopy, 953
Vigabatrin, 462
Vildagliptin, 774
VIN. *See* Vulvar intraepithelial neoplasia
Vinblastine, 786
Vincristine
  for Kaposi sarcoma, 807
  for lymphoma, 784–786
  for multiple myeloma, 783
  myalgia and myopathy induced by, 528–529
  for thyroid nodule management, 753
Vinorelbine, 383
Vision
  aging effects on, 102
  in dementia, 390
  in Down syndrome, 448
Visual loss. *See also* Eye, disorders of
  with diabetes mellitus, 763, 764t
  rehabilitation for, 820–821
  treatments for major causes of, 813b
Visualization, for Parkinson's disease therapy, 877
Vitamin A, 13, 15, 682, 757t
Vitamin B, 13, 282
Vitamin B_6, 13, 681–682
Vitamin B_{12}, 13
  anemia and, 776–777
  deficiency of, cognitive functioning and, 176
  for dementia, 400
  nutritional requirements for, 681–682
Vitamin C, 13, 15
  as antiaging medicine, 148
  as antioxidant, 44
  for hypertension management, 308
  for macular degeneration, 818
  for preventing age-related changes in immune system, 89
Vitamin D, 13–15
  as antiaging medicine, 147, 149b
  assay of, 756t
  bone loss and, 121, 164, 448, 554–555
  for dementia associated with hypoparathyroidism, 387
  hypercalcemia and, 757t
  hyperparathyroidism and, 756–757, 756b–757b
  hypoparathyroidism and, 759
  nutritional requirements for, 681–682, 687–688
  for osteoporosis, 527, 531, 556t, 557–558, 583, 585–586
  sarcopenia and, 589, 592
  toxicity of, 699–700, 699t
Vitamin D deficiency osteomalacia, 558–561, 559t
Vitamin D metabolites
  for osteomalacia, 561
  for osteoporosis, 557
Vitamin D_3 analogs, 14–15
Vitamin E, 13, 15
  for Alzheimer's disease, 420
  as antiaging medicine, 148
  as antioxidant, 44
  for dementia, 400
  for macular degeneration, 818
  for reproductive aging in women, 164
Vitamin intake, frailty prevention and, 850
Vitamin K
  for overanticoagulation and bleeding, 359
  for warfarin reversal, 495
Vitreous disorders, 815–819, 816f–817f
Voiding disorders, 928, 937
Voiding phase
  of bladder, 707–708, 708f
  management of patients with benign prostatic hyperplasia and problems with, 708–709, 709t
Volvulus
  of large bowel, 672–673
  of stomach, 623–624, 624f
Vomiting, palliative care for, 978
Von Hippel Lindau syndrome, of pancreas, 627
VPCs. *See* Ventricular premature complexes
VT. *See* Ventricular tachycardia
VTE. *See* Venous thromboembolism
Vulnerability. *See* Social vulnerability
Vulva
  aging of, 716
  cancer of, 722
  care of, 718
Vulval disorders, 718–720, 719t
  dermatologic conditions, 718–719
  premalignant disorders, 719, 719t
  symptoms of, 718
  vulval discomfort, 719–720
Vulvar intraepithelial neoplasia (VIN), 719, 719t
Vulvodynia, 719
VZV. *See* Varicella zoster virus

W

Wagner model of Chronic Disease Care, 849
Waist circumference, 685, 686t
Waldenström macroglobulinemia (WM), 785
Walking
  biomechanics of, 897
  speed of, 886
  stroke and, 874
  terms for, 897, 897f
Walking aid, selection of, e9–e10
Warfarin
  for AF, 333–334
  antiepileptic drugs and, 463
  for antiphospholipid antibody syndrome, 492
  for aortic valve replacement, 316t
  for atrial flutter, 335–336
  for chronic cardiac failure, 278b, 282
  for chronic mitral regurgitation, 325
  cimetidine and, 622
  coagulation defects due to, 790
  in elderly patients undergoing surgery, 232, 232t
  in frail elderly patient, 298
  herbal-drug interactions of, 142t
  liver metabolism of, 635–636, 636t
  metabolism of, 139–140
  for mitral annular calcium, 323
  for mitral stenosis, 324
  monitoring of, 359
  after myocardial infarction, 291–292
  outcomes measurement of use of, 248t–265t
  in patients with hyperthyroidism, 743
  for prevention of secondary stroke, 495
  sensitivity to, 141t, 144, 144b
  stroke and, 490–491, 495–497
  thrombocytopenia associated with, 789
Warfarin (*Continued*)
  for thromboembolic stroke in patients with cardiac arrhythmias, 334–335
  for venous thromboembolism, 357–361, 358t, 360b
Watchful waiting, for prostate cancer, 712
Water, required amount of, 681, 681t
Water balance, 697
Water content, of dermis, aging effects on, 135
Water depletion, surgery and anesthesia in old age and, 240
Waterlow scale, for pressure ulcers, 940
Weakness, 521
Weight bearing, functional recovery and, 866–867
Weight loss
  aerobic exercises and, 861
  anorexia of aging, 949–950
  in COPD, 374
  in elderly, effects of, 687
  failure to thrive and frailty, 949
  for hypertension management, 307
  interventions for, 687–689, 688t, 688b
  malnutrition and, 949
  as nonspecific clinical presentation of disease in elderly, 206
  with pancreas adenocarcinoma, 628
  for urinary incontinence, 934
Weight Monitoring in Heart Failure (WHARF), 1065–1066
Weight training, for frailty prevention, 850
Well-being. *See* Subjective well-being
Wellbutrin, sexuality in old age and, 855, 857t
Werner syndrome, 20–21, 33–34, 80
WHARF. *See* Weight Monitoring in Heart Failure
White matter lesions. *See* Cerebral white matter lesions
WHO analgesic ladder, 976, 976t
WHO classification, of disability, 6
Williams syndrome, 445, 446t–447t
Withdrawing treatment, ethical issues of, 986
Withholding treatment, ethical issues of, 986
WM. *See* Waldenström macroglobulinemia
Wolff-Parkinson-White syndrome, 332
Women
  reproductive aging in, 163–164
    perimenopause to menopause, 163–164
    postmenopause, 164
    therapeutic horizons, 164–165
    unresolved issues, 165–167
  skin aging in, 136
Working memory, aging effects on, 172
Workplace, ageism in, 195–196
World, geriatric medicine in, 1010
  chronic disease and functional decline prevention, 1015
  chronic diseases of major impact, 1010
  communicable diseases, 1011–1012
  comprehensive geriatric assessment, 1013
  development of, 1012–1013
  frailty, 1010–1011
  health and social services, 1013–1015
  life expectancy, morbidity, and disability, 1010
Wound care
  for palliative care, 973
  for pressure ulcers, 941
  telemedicine for, 1066

X

Xanthine oxidase inhibitors, 574
Xerosis, 801–802
Xerostomia, 605–606, 975

X-ray
  of chronic cardiac failure, 275–276
  of prostate, 702

Y

Yoga, for pain, 971
Yohimbine, 142t, 508b, 510, 606, 858
Younger people, older people v., 8, 8f

Z

Zafirlukast, 367t
Zaleplon, 946
Zanamivir, 376
Zeaxanthin, 818
Zelapar. *See* Selegiline
Zenker diverticulum, 611–612, 611f
Zileuton, 367t
Zinc, 89, 813b, 818
Zinc pyrithione, 802
Zofenopril, 292t
Zoledronate, 556, 556t, 563
Zolpidem, 946
Zonisamide, 462, 463t
Zostavax, 803–804
Zostrix. *See* Capsaicin